COMPREHENSIVE
ADOLESCENT HEALTH CARE
SECOND EDITION

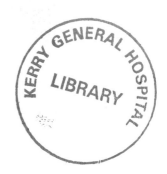

SECOND EDITION

COMPREHENSIVE ADOLESCENT HEALTH CARE

Stanford B. Friedman, M.D.
Professor of Pediatrics
Albert Einstein College of Medicine
Bronx, New York
Division of Adolescent Medicine
Montefiore Medical Center
Bronx, New York

Martin Fisher, M.D.
Associate Professor of Clinical Pediatrics
Cornell University Medical College
New York, New York
Chief
Division of Adolescent Medicine and Behavioral Pediatrics
North Shore University Hospital-Cornell University Medical College
Manhasset, New York

S. Kenneth Schonberg, M.D.
Professor of Pediatrics
Albert Einstein College of Medicine
Bronx, New York
Director
Division of Adolescent Medicine
Montefiore Medical Center
Bronx, New York

Elizabeth M. Alderman, M.D.
Assistant Professor of Pediatrics
Albert Einstein College of Medicine
Bronx, New York
Attending Physician
Division of Adolescent Medicine
Montefiore Medical Center
Bronx, New York

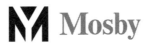

St. Louis Baltimore Boston Carlsbad Chicago Naples New York Philadelphia Portland
London Madrid Mexico City Singapore Sydney Tokyo Toronto Wiesbaden

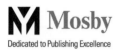

Mosby
Dedicated to Publishing Excellence

A Times Mirror
Company

Vice President and Publisher: Anne S. Patterson
Editor: Laura DeYoung
Developmental Editor: Laura Berendson
Project Manager: Linda Clarke
Senior Production Editor: Veda King
Designer: Carolyn O'Brien
Manufacturing Manager: William A. Winneberger, Jr.

SECOND EDITION
Copyright © 1998 by Mosby–Year Book, Inc.

Previous edition copyrighted 1992 by Quality Medical Publishing, Inc.

Printed in the United States of America
Composition by Graphic World, Inc.
Printing/binding by Maple-Vail Book Manufacturing Group

Mosby–Year Book, Inc.
11830 Westline Industrial Drive
St. Louis, Missouri 63146

Library of Congress Cataloging in Publication Data

Comprehensive adolescent health care   /   [edited by] Stanford B.
    Friedman   . . .   [et al.].—2nd ed.
        p.   cm.
    Includes bibliographical references and index.
    ISBN 0-8151-3386-3
    1. Adolescent medicine.   I. Friedman, Stanford B. (Stanford
Barton), 1931-
    [DNLM: 1. Adolescent Medicine.   2. Adolescent Health Services.
WS   460   C7375   1998]
RJ550.C67   1998
616'.00835—dc21
DNLM/DLC
for Library of Congress   96-51485
                                                              CIP

98   99   00   01   02   /   9   8   7   6   5   4   3   2

CONTRIBUTORS

Elizabeth A. Abel, MD
Clinical Associate Professor of Dermatology
Department of Dermatology
Stanford University School of Medicine
Stanford, California

Steven Ablon, MD
Associate Clinical Professor of Psychiatry
Harvard University Medical School at
Massachusetts General Hospital
Training and Supervising Adult and Child Analyst
Boston Psychoanalytic Society and Institute

Gerald R. Adams, BS, MA, PhD
Department of Family Studies
College of Family Studies
University of Guelph
Guelph, Ontario, Canada

Harvey W. Aiges, MD
Professor of Clinical Pediatrics
New York University School of Medicine
Associate Chairman, Pediatrics
North Shore University Hospital
Manhasset, New York

Elizabeth M. Alderman, MD
Division of Adolescent Medicine
Department of Pediatrics
Albert Einstein College of Medicine
Montefiore Medical Center
Bronx, New York

Ramin Alemzadeh, MD
Assistant Professor
Department of Pediatrics
University of Tennessee Medical Center
Knoxville, Tennessee

Paula Thomas Ardron, MD
Fellow in Pediatric Asthma and Immunology
Children's Hospital at Strong
University of Rochester Medical Center
Rochester, New York

Carolyn Ashworth, PhD
Department of Pediatrics
University of Alabama at Birmingham
Division of General Pediatrics & Adolescent Medicine
Birmingham, Alabama

H. Verdain Barnes, MD, FACP, FSAM
Professor of Internal Medicine
Family Medicine and Pediatrics
Eastern Virginia Medical School
Chair, Department of Medicine
Director, Center for Generalist Medicine
Norfolk, Virginia

Ronald G. Barr, MA, MDCM, FRCP(C)
Professor of Pediatrics and Psychiatry
McGill University
Head, Child Development Programme
Montreal Children's Hospital
Montreal, Quebec
Canada

Roberta K. Beach, MD
Associate Professor of Pediatrics and Adolescent
  Medicine
University of Colorado School of Medicine
Assistant Director of Community Health Services
Denver Department of Health
Denver, Colorado

Jeffrey L. Berman, MD
Maine Eye Center
University of Vermont School of Medicine
Portland, Maine

Robert James Bidwell, MD
Associate Professor of Pediatrics
Department of Pediatrics
John A. Burns School of Medicine
University of Hawaii
Honolulu, Hawaii

Frank M. Biro, MD
Associate Professor, Clinical Pediatrics
University of Cincinnati
Cincinnati, Ohio

Jeffrey L. Black, MD
Luke Waites Child Development Center
Texas Scottish Rite Hospital for Children
Clinical Assistant Professor
University of Texas Southwestern Medical Center
Dallas, Texas

v

Robert Wm. Blum, MD, MPH, PhD
Professor & Director
Division of General Pediatrics & Adolescent Health
Director
WHO Collaborating Centre on Adolescent Health
Department of Pediatrics
University of Pediatrics
Minneapolis, Minnesota

Marjorie A. Boeck, MD, PhD
Medical Director, The Davisson Clinic
Dallas, Texas

Lynn J. Bonitz, RN, MS
Long Island Medical Center
Schneider Children's Hospital
New Hyde Park, New York

Lynn Borgatta, MD
Medical Director
Planned Parenthood of Westchester/Rockland, Inc.
Clinical Associate Professor
New York Medical College
Department of Obstetrics and Gynecology
New York, New York

Roberta H. Friedman, MLS
Retired

Norman M. Brier, PhD
Clinical Professor of Pediatrics & Psychiatry
Albert Einstein College of Medicine
Bronx, New York

Claire D. Brindis, DrPH
Director, Center for Reproductive Health Policy
   Studies
Department of Pediatrics
University of California, San Francisco

Richard R. Brookman, MD
Professor of Pediatrics
Chairman, Division of Adolescent Medicine
Medical College of Virginia
Virginia Commonwealth University
Richmond, Virginia

Nathaniel A. Brown, MD
Senior Clinical Program Head, Hepatitis
Glaxo Wellcome
Research Triangle Park, North Carolina
Research Associate Professor, Pediatrics
University of North Carolina School of Medicine
Chapel Hill, North Carolina

Philip A. Brunell, MD
Cedars-Sinai Medical Center
UCLA School of Medicine
Los Angeles, California

Brian N. Campolattaro, MD
Clinical Assistant Professor of Ophthalmology
New York Medical College
Valhalla, New York

Mary A. Carskadon, MD
University of California, Los Angeles
Department of Pediatrics
Cedars-Sinai Medical Center
Los Angeles, California

Cecilia D. Cervantes, MD
Department of Pediatrics
Division of Endocrinology and Metabolism
North Shore University Hospital
Manhasset, New York,

France Chaput, MD
Division of Child Psychiatry
New York State Psychiatric Institute
New York, New York

Naula M. Chaudry, PhD
Strong Center for Developmental Disabilities
University of Rochester Medical Center
Rochester, New York

Anupama Chawla, MD
Department of Pediatrics
North Shore University Hospital
NYU School of Medicine
Manhasset, New York

Andrew Clark, MD
Child Psychiatry Service
Massachusetts General Hospital
Boston, Massachusetts

Maria R. Coccia, MD, PhD
Ohio State University
Division of Infectious Diseases
Columbus, Ohio

Alwyn T. Cohall, MD
Chief, Division of Adolescent and Young Adult
   Medicine
St. Luke's Roosevelt Hospital Center
New York, New York

Renee Mayer Cohall, ACSW
Senior Social Worker
Division of Adolescent and Young Adult Medicine
St. Luke's Roosevelt Hospital Center
New York, New York

Michael W. Cohen, MD
Clinical Professor
Department of Pediatrics
University of Arizona
College of Medicine
Director
Attention Disorder Center of Tucson
Tucson, Arizona

Stephen Commins
Chief, Division of Behavioral Pediatrics
Neumours Children's Clinic
Assistant Professor of Pediatrics
Mayo Medical School
Rochester, Minnesota

Edward E. Conway, Jr., MD, MS, FAAP, FCCM
Associate Chairman
Director, Pediatric Critical Care Medicine
Beth Israel Medical Center
New York, New York

Lynda B. Cooper, ACSW, BCD
Department of Social Work
North Shore University Hospital
Manhasset, New York

Rubin S. Cooper, MD, FAAP, FACC
Professor of Clinical Pediatrics
Cornell University Medical College
North Shore University Hospital
Manhasset, New York

Jean Corrigan, RN
Division of Pediatric Endocrinology and Metabolism
North Shore University Hospital
Manhasset, New York

Susan M. Coupey, MD
Professor of Pediatrics
Albert Einstein College of Medicine
Associate Director, Division of Adolescent Medicine
Montefiore Medical Center
Bronx, New York

Barbara A. Cromer, MD
Columbus Children's Hospital
Columbus, Ohio

Mihaly Csikszentmihalyi, PhD
Professor of Human Development
Department of Psychology
The University of Chicago
Chicago, Illinois

Angela Damiano
New York University Medical Center
Department of Otolaryngology
New York, New York

Fredric Daum, MD
New York University School of Medicine
North Shore University Hospital
Manhasset, New York

Margot Davey, MBBS, FRACP
Royal Children's Hospital
Melbourne, Australia
Monash Medical Center
Melbourne, Australia

Nelson W. Davidson, MD
Clinical Assistant Professor
Division of Adolescent Medicine
Department of Pediatrics
University of Maryland at Baltimore
Private Practice, Baltimore, Maryland
Staff Physician, Johns Hopkins University
Student Health and Wellness Center
Baltimore, Maryland
Staff Physician, St. Joseph's Medical Center
Towson, Maryland
Physician Contractor, Baltimore City Health
    Department,
Division of School Based Clinics
Baltimore, Maryland

Philip W. Davidson, PhD
Professor of Pediatrics and Director
Strong Center for Developmental Disabilities
University of Rochester School of Medicine and
    Dentistry
Rochester, New York

Robert W. Deisher, MD
Professor Emeritus
University of Washington
School of Medicine
Department of Pediatrics
Seattle, Washington

Everett P. Dulit, MD, PhD
Associate Clinical Professor
Department of Psychiatry
Albert Einstein College of Medicine
New York, New York

David Elkind, PhD
Department of Child Study
Tufts University
Medford, Massachusetts

Elliot F. Ellis, MD
Professor of Pediatrics Emeritus
State University of New York at Buffalo
Medical Director
Muro Pharmaceutical, Inc.
Tewksbury, Massachusetts

Robert E. Emery, PhD
Department of Psychology
University of Virginia
Charlottesville, Virginia

Abigail English, JD
National Center for Youth Law
Chapel Hill, North Carolina

Candace J. Erickson, MD, MPH
Assistant Professor of Clinical Pediatrics
Department of Pediatrics
Columbia University College of Physicians and
    Surgeons
New York, New York

Theresa M. Exner, PhD
Associate Professor of Medical Psychology
Department of Psychiatry
Columbia University College of Physicians and
    Surgeons
New York, New York

Jordan W. Finkelstein, MD, MSC
Department of Biobehavioral Health
Pennsylvania State University
College of Health and Human Development
University Park, Pennsylvania

Martin Fisher, MD
North Shore University Hospital
New York University School of Medicine
Manhasset, New York

Donald J. Forrester, DDS, MSD
Pediatric Dental Consultant
Germantown, Maryland

Pavel Fort, MD
Department of Pediatrics
Division of Endocrinology and Metabolism
North Shore University Hospital
Manhasset, New York

Ilona J. Frieden, MD
Associate Clinical Professor
Dermatology and Pediatrics
University of California
San Francisco, California

Stanford B. Friedman, MD
Department of Pediatrics
Division of Adolescent Medicine
Montefiore Medical Center
Albert Einstein School of Medicine
Bronx, New York

Donna Futterman, MD
Associate Professor of Pediatrics
Director, Adolescent AIDS Program
Montefiore Medical Center
Albert Einstein College of Medicine
Bronx, New York

Jack Gladstein, MD
Associate Professor of Pediatrics
Associate Dean for Student Affairs
University of Maryland School of Medicine
Baltimore, Maryland

Melanie A. Gold, DO
Assistant Professor of Pediatrics
General Academic Pediatrics/Adolescent Medicine
Children's Hospital of Pittsburgh
University of Pittsburgh School of Medicine
Pittsburgh, Pennsylvania

Mark N. Goldstein, MD
New York Eye and Ear Infirmary
Clinical Assistant Professor of Otolaryngology
Department of Otolaryngology
New York Medical College
New York, New York

Elizabeth Goodman, MD
Division of Adolescent/Young Adult Medicine
Children's Hospital
Boston, Massachusetts

James Tait Goodrich, MD, MPhil, PhD
Division of Pediatric Neurosurgery
Leo Davidoff Department of Neurosurgery
Albert Einstein College of Medicine
Montefiore Medical Center
Bronx, New York

Siobhan Gormally, MD
Child Development Program
Montreal Children's Hospital
Montreal, Quebec, Canada

Jack D. Gorvoy, MD
Director, Division of Pediatric Cystic Fibrosis
Schneider Children's Hospital
Associate Clinical Professor of Pediatrics
Albert Einstein College of Medicine
New Hyde Park, New York

Morris Green, MD
Perry W. Lesh Professor of Pediatrics
Indiana University School of Medicine
James Whitcomb Riley Hospital for Children
Indianapolis, Indiana

Bruce Greenstein, MD
Albert Einstein College of Medicine of Yeshiva
   University
Bronx, New York

Mary Beth Gregor, RPA-C
Department of Pediatric Surgery
Montefiore Medical Center
Albert Einstein College of Medicine
Bronx, New York

Patricia L. Haber, MD
Montefiore Medical Center
Albert Einstein College of Medicine
Bronx, New York

Craig D. Hall, MD
Associate Professor
University of Medicine and Dentistry of New Jersey
Newark, New Jersey
St. Joseph's Hospital and Medical Center
Department of Craniofacial Surgery
Hackensack University Hospital and Medical Center
Department of Plastic Surgery
St. Barnabus Hospital and Medical Center
Department of Craniofacial Surgery
Hackensack, New Jersey

Beatrix A. Hamburg, MD
Professor of Psychiatry and Pediatrics
Department of Psychiatry
Mount Sinai School of Medicine
New York, New York

Karen Hein, MD
Executive Officer
Institute of Medicine
National Academy of Sciences
Washington, D.C.

Scott W. Henggeler, PhD
Family Services Research Center
Department of Psychiatry and Behavioral Sciences
Medical University of South Carolina
Department of Psychiatry and Behavioral Sciences
Charleston, South Carolina

James V. Hennessey, MD
Assistant Professor of Medicine
Brown University School of Medicine
Department of Medicine
Division of Endocrinology
Providence, Rhode Island

S. Paige Hertweck, MD
Co-Director
Pediatric Adolescent Gynecology Fellowship
Assistant Professor
Department of Obstetrics and Gynecology
University of Louisville School of Medicine
Louisville, Kentucky

Neal Hoffman, MD
Montefiore Medical Center
Adolescent AIDS Program
Assistant Professor of Pediatrics
Albert Einstein College of Medicine
Bronx, New York

Kent P. Hymel, MD
Lt. Col.
U.S. Air Force Medical Corp.
Chief Military Consultant for Child Abuse

Charles E. Irwin, Jr., MD
Professor, Department of Pediatrics
Director, Division of Adolescent Medicine
University of California, San Francisco

Victor Israele, MD
Associate Professor of Pediatrics
UCLA School of Medicine
Co-Director Pediatric Infectious Diseases
Ahmanson Pediatric Center
Cedars-Sinai Medical Center
Los Angeles, California

Marc S. Jacobson, MD
Professor of Pediatrics
Albert Einstein College of Medicine
Director, Center for Atherosclerosis Prevention
Schneider Children's Hospital of Long Island Jewish
    Medical Center
New York, New York

Michael Jellinek, MD
Department of Psychiatry
Massachusetts General Hospital
Boston, Massachusetts

Gloria Johnson-Powell, MD
Professor of Child Psychiatry
Harvard Medical School
Director, Partnerships in Prevention
Judge Baker Children's Center
Boston, Massachusetts

Linda W. Juszczak, MS, MPH, CPNP, RN
Deputy Director
School Health Policy Initiative
Department of Pediatrics
Division of Adolescent Medicine
Montefiore Medical Center
Bronx, New York

Ronald Nathaniel Kaleya, MD
Department of Surgery
Montefiore Medical Center
Albert Einstein College of Medicine
Bronx, New York

Murray M. Kappelman, MD
University of Maryland, School of Medicine
Baltimore, Maryland

Theodore Kastner, MD
Director
Center for Human Development
Morristown Memorial Hospital
Morristown, New Jersey
Associate Professor of Pediatrics
New Jersey Medical School
University of Medicine and Dentistry of New Jersey
Associate Professor of Clinical Pediatrics
Columbia University
College of Physicians and Surgeons
New York, New York

Diana King, MD
Assistant Professor of Pediatrics
Albert Einstein College of Medicine
Montefiore Medical Center
Bronx, New York

Michele D. Kipke, MD
Division of Adolescent Medicine
Children's Hospital of Los Angeles
Department of Pediatrics
USC School of Medicine
Los Angeles, California

Sylvain Kleinhaus, MD
Professor of Surgery and Pediatrics
Albert Einstein College of Medicine
Director, Pediatric Surgery
Montefiore Medical Center
Bronx, New York

Lorraine V. Klerman, DrPH
Professor and Chairperson
Department of Maternal and Child Health
School of Public Health
University of Alabama at Birmingham
Birmingham, Alabama

Leonard R. Krilov, MD
Chief, Pediatric Infectious Disease
North Shore University Hospital
New York, New York
University Medical School
Associate Professor of Pediatrics
New York University School of Medicine
New York, New York

Richard D. Krugman, MD
Professor of Pediatrics and Dean
University of Colorado School of Medicine
Denver, Colorado

Michael A. LaCorte, MD
Chairman, Department of Pediatrics
The Brooklyn Hospital Center
Professor of Clinical Pediatrics
New York University School of Medicine
Brooklyn, New York

Gary W. Ladd, EdD
Department of Educational Psychology
University of Illinois at Urbana-Champaign
Champaign, Illinois

Cristina Lammers, MD
Assistant Professor
Obstetrics and Gynecology
Hospital de Clinicas
Universidad de la Republica Oriental del Uruguay
Montevideo

Julia Graham Lear, PhD
Director
Making the Grade
The George Washington University
Washington, D.C.

Melvin D. Levine, MD
The Clinical Center for the Study of Development
   and Learning
University of North Carolina
Chapel Hill, North Carolina

Fima Lifshitz, MD
Chairman of Pediatrics
Maimonides Medical Center
Brooklyn, New York

Nathan Litman, MD
Associate Director
Department of Pediatrics
Montefiore Medical Center
North Central Bronx Hospital
Professor of Pediatrics
Albert Einstein College of Medicine
Bronx, New York

Deborah Lopez, MD
Albert Einstein College of Medicine
Pediatric Critical Care Medicine
Montefiore Medical Center
Bronx, New York

Richard G. MacKenzie, FSAM, MD
Director
Division of Adolescent Medicine
Children's Hospital, Los Angeles
Associate Professor of Pediatrics
School of Medicine
University of Southern California
Los Angeles, California

Neil J. Macy, MD
Assistant Professor
Departments of Orthopaedics and Pediatrics
Albert Einstein College of Medicine
Bronx, New York

Robert W. Marion, MD
Professor of Pediatrics
Albert Einstein College of Medicine
Director
Center for Congenital Disorders
Montefiore Medical Center
Bronx, New York

James F. Markowitz, MD
Division of Pediatric Gastroenterology
Department of Pediatrics
North Shore University Hospital
NYU School of Medicine
Manhasset, New York

Andrea Marks, MD
Associate Clinical Professor of Pediatrics
Mt. Sinai School of Medicine
New York, New York

Marguerite M. Mayers, MD
Associate Professor of Pediatrics
Department of Pediatrics and Ambulatory Medicine
Albert Einstein College of Medicine
Montefiore-North Central Bronx Hospital
New York, New York

Lezley P. McIlveen, BDS, MS
Private Practice
Pediatric Dentistry
Herndon, VA
Former Clinical Director
Department of Pediatric Dentistry
Children's National Medical Center
Washington, D.C.

Donna Moreau, MD
Associate Clinical Professor of Child Psychiatry
Department of Psychiatry
Columbia University College of Physicians and
    Surgeons
Director, Child and Anxiety Clinic
Presbyterian Hospital
Research Scientist
New York State Psychiatric Institute
New York, New York

Danielle Morris, PsyD
Senior Instructor
Department of Pediatrics
Strong Center for Developmental Disabilities
University of Rochester
Rochester, New York

Marva M. Moxey-Mims, MD
Children's National Medical Center
Department of Nephrology
The George Washington University School of
    Medicine
Department of Pediatrics
Washington, D.C.

Laura Mufson, PhD
Assistant Professor
Clinical Psychology in Psychiatry
Columbia University College of Physicians
    and Surgeons
Research Scientist
New York State Psychiatric Institute
Assistant Director
Children's Anxiety and Depression Clinic
New York, New York

Michael A. Nelson, MD
Clinical Associate Professor of Pediatrics
Department of Pediatrics
University of New Mexico
Albuquerque, New Mexico

Lawrence C. Newman, MD
Director of the Montefiore Headache Unit
Assistant Professor of Neurology
Albert Einstein College of Medicine
Bronx, New York

Amy S. Paller, MD
Professor
Pediatrics and Dermatology
Northwestern University Medical School
Head
Division of Dermatology
The Children's Memorial Hospital of Chicago
Chicago, Illinois

Anthony L. Palomba, MD
Department of Pediatrics—Critical Care
Bronx-Lebanon Hospital
Bronx, New York

Jennifer T. Parkhurst, PhD
Department of Educational Psychology
University of Illinois
Champaign, Illinois

Doris R. Pastore, MD
Adolescent Health Center
Mt. Sinai Medical Center
New York, New York

Cynthia R. Pegler, MD
Clinical Instructor of Pediatrics
New York Hospital
Cornell University Medical College
Lenox Hill Hospital
New York, New York

Ellen C. Perrin, MD
Professor of Pediatrics
Division of Developmental and Behavioral Pediatrics
University of Massachusetts Medical Center
Worcester, Massachusetts

Sheridan Phillips, PhD
Director
Clinical Psychology Internship Program
Division of Child and Adolescent Psychiatry
Department of Psychiatry
University of Maryland School of Medicine
Baltimore, Maryland

Gregory E. Prazar, MD
Pediatrician
Exeter Pediatric Associates
Exeter, New Hampshire

Michael Pugliese, MD
Assistant Professor of Pediatrics
State University of New York
School of Medicine at Stonybrook
Stonybrook, New York

Leonard A. Rappaport, MD
Assistant Professor of Pediatrics
Harvard Medical School
Associate Chief
Division of General Pediatrics
Children's Hospital
Boston, Massachusetts

Milton J. Reitman, MD
Director of Pediatrics
Pediatric Cardiology
St. Francis Hospital
The Heart Center
Roslyn, New York

William Risser, MD, PhD
Professor of Pediatrics
Director, Division of Adolescent Medicine
University of Texas—Houston Medical School
Houston, Texas

Arthur L. Robin, PhD
Department of Psychiatry and Behavioral
  Neurosciences
Wayne State University
Detroit, Michigan

Joseph Lee Rodgers, PhD
Professor
Department of Psychology
University of Oklahoma
Norman, Oklahoma

Audrey Rogers, PhD, MPH
Pediatric, Adolescent, and Maternal
ALDS Branch
National Institute of Child Health and Human
  Development
Bethesda, Maryland

William M. Rogers, II, MD, MPH
San Francisco Department of Public Health and
  Student Health Service
San Francisco State University
San Francisco, California

Reuben D. Rohn, MD
Professor of Pediatrics
Eastern Virginia Medical School
Director
Adolescent Medicine and Endocrinology
Children's Hospital, Kings Daughters
Norfolk, Virginia

Elizabeth Rose, MD
Staff Attending Adolescent Medicine
Morristown Memorial Hospital
Morristown, New Jersey
Assistant Clinical Professor of Pediatrics
College of Physicians and Surgeons
Columbia University
Morristown, New Jersey

Richard G. Rosen, MD
Associate Professor of Surgery
Montefiore Medical Center
Albert Einstein College of Medicine
Bronx, New York

Walter D. Rosenfeld, MD
Director
Adolescent/Young Adult Center for Health
Morristown Memorial Hospital
Morristown, New Jersey
Associate Professor of Clinical Pediatrics
College of Physicians and Surgeons
Columbia University
Morristown, New Jersey

John S. Rubin, MD
Honorary Senior Lecturer
United Medical and Dental School of Guy's and
  St. Thomas's Hospital
University of London
Consultant Ear Surgeon, Clinical Tutor
Lewisham NHS Trust
Visiting Associate Professor
Department of Otolaryngology
Albert Einstein College of Medicine
Bronx, New York

Edward J. Ruley, MD
Medical Director
Pediatric Kidney Center
INOVA Hospital for Children
Falls Church, Virginia
Clinical Professor of Pediatrics
Uniformed Services University of the Health Sciences
Bethesda, Maryland

Desmond K. Runyan, MD, DrPH
Department of Social Medicine
The University of North Carolina at Chapel Hill
Chapel Hill, North Carolina

Sheryl A. Ryan, MD
University of Rochester School of Medicine and
    Dentistry
Division of Adolescent Medicine
Department of Pediatrics
Rochester General Hospital
Rochester, New York

Robert Sammartano, RPA-C
Attending Physician Assistant
Division of Pediatric Surgery
Department of Surgery
Albert Einstein College of Medicine
Montefiore Medical Center
Bronx, New York

Adrian D. Sandler, MD
Medical Director
Olson Huff Center for Child Development
Thomas Research Rehabilitation
Asheville, North Carolina

Joseph S. Sanfilippo, MD
University of Louisville
School of Medicine
Louisville, Kentucky

Richard M. Sarles, MD
Professor and Director
Division of Child and Adolescent Psychiatry
University of Maryland, School of Medicine
Baltimore, Maryland

Janet Schebendach, MA, RD
Schneider Children's Hospital of Long Island Jewish
    Medical Center
Division of Adolescent Medicine
Albert Einstein College of Medicine
New Hyde Park, New York

Russell J. Schiff, FAAP, FACC, MD
Department of Pediatrics
Division of Pediatric Cardiology
North Shore University Hospital
Manhasset, New York

Alice Schlegel, PhD
Department of Anthropology
University of Arizona
Tucson, Arizona

Marcie B. Schneider, MD
Assistant Professor of Pediatrics
North Shore University Hospital
New York University School of Medicine
Manhasset, New York

Edward L. Schor, MD
Medical Director,
Division of Family and Community Health
Iowa Department of Public Health
Des Moines, Iowa

S. Kenneth Schonberg, MD
Professor of Pediatrics
Albert Einstein College of Medicine
Bronx, New York

Robert H. Schwartz, MD
Clinical Professor of Pediatrics
Director, Clinical Pediatric Allergy
Children's Hospital at Strong
University of Rochester Medical Center
Rochester, New York
Medical Director
Allergy and Asthma
Rochester Resource Center (AARRC)
Fairport, New York

Stephen R. Setterberg, MD
Assistant Professor
Department of Neuroscience
Psychiatry Division
University of North Dakota School of Medicine
Psychiatric Medicine Associates
Fargo, North Dakota

I. Ronald Shenker, MD
Chief, Adolescent Medicine
Schneider Children's Hospital
Professor of Pediatrics
Albert Einstein College of Medicine
New Hyde Park, New York

William A. Shine, AB, EdD, EdM, MA
Superintendent of Schools
Great Neck Union Free School District
Great Neck, New York

Shlomo Shinnar, MD, PhD
Professor of Neurology and Pediatrics
Director, Comprehensive Epilepsy Management Center
Montefiore Medical Center
Albert Einstein College of Medicine
Bronx, New York

Daniel Silbert, MD
Assistant Professor
Department of Pediatrics
State University of New York
Stony Brook, New York
Nassau County Medical Center
East Meadow, New York

Mervin Silverberg, MD
Chairman, Department of Pediatrics
North Shore University Hospital
Manhasset, New York

Lewis P. Singer, MD
Pediatric Critical Care
Montefiore Medical Center
Bronx, New York

Margaret Thaler Singer, PhD
Emeritus Adjunct Professor
University of California, Berkeley
Private Practice
Berkeley, California

Saranjeet Singh, MD
Director of Critical Care
Department of Pediatrics
Jamaica Hospital
Jamaica, New York

Carol A. Smith, MD
New York Medical Group
Yonkers, New York

Alfred J. Spiro, MD
Professor of Neurology and Pediatrics
Director, MDA Muscle Disease Clinic
Albert Einstein College of Medicine of Yeshiva
    University
Bronx, New York

Suzanne P. Starling, MD
Vanderbilt University Medical Center
Nashville, Tennessee

Mitchell Steinschneider, MD, PhD
Department of Neurology
Albert Einstein College of Medicine
Bronx, New York

Victor C. Strasburger, MD
Department of Pediatrics
UNM School of Medicine
Albuquerque, New Mexico

Berish Strauch, MD
Department of Plastic Surgery
Montefiore Medical Center
Albert Einstein College of Medicine
Bronx, New York

Murray Straus, MD
Family Research Laboratory
University of New Hampshire
Durham, New Hampshire

David E. Suttle, MD
US Army-ROTC
Cadet Command
ATCC-S
Fort Monroe, Virginia

Virginia Bishop Townsend, MD
University of Illinois
Department of Pediatrics
Chicago, Illinois

Guochuan E. Tsai, MD
Instructor
Laboratory of Molecular and Developmental
    Neuroscience
Department of Psychiatry
Massachusetts General Hospital and Harvard Medical
    School
Boston, Massachusetts

Mary Ellen Turner, MD
Nephrology Department
Children's National Medical Center
Washington, D.C.

David R. Updegraff, BA, MSW, PhD
President
St. Mary's School for the Deaf
Buffalo, New York

Claudio Violato, BSc, MA, PhD
Professor
Department of Educational Psychology
University of Calgary
Calgary, Alberta, Canada

Frederick M. Wang, MD
Clinical Professor of Ophthalmology and Visual
    Science
Albert Einstein College of Medicine
Bronx, New York

Gerard Weinberg, MD
Associate Professor of Pediatrics and Surgery
Albert Einstein College of Medicine
Montefiore Medical Center
Bronx, New York

Mark E. Weinblatt, MD
Associate Chief
Division of Pediatric Hematology
North Shore University Hospital
Associate Professor of Clinical Pediatrics
New York University School of Medicine
Manhasset, New York

Irving B. Weiner, PhD
Department of Psychiatry and Behavioral Medicine
University of South Florida
Tampa, Florida

Esther H. Wender, MD
Director
Child Health Services
Westchester County Department of Health
Hawthorne, New York
Clinical Professor of Pediatrics
Albert Einstein College of Medicine
Bronx, New York

Morris A. Wessel, MD
Clinical Professor of Pediatrics
Yale University School of Medicine
Consulting Pediatrician
Clifford Beers Guidance Clinic
New Haven, Connecticut

Bryan J. Williams, DDS, MSD
Director, Department of Dental Medicine
Children's Hospital and Medical Center
Seattle, Washington

Murray Wittner, MD, PhD
Department of Pathology
Albert Einstein College of Medicine
Bronx, New York

The editors and authors of this textbook have combined their experience and expertise to develop a truly wonderful resource for healthcare providers. The book contains essential information that will enable providers to recognize and manage the medical, surgical, psychosocial, and gynecologic sexuality-related conditions commonly encountered in adolescents. It should be a required component of the library of all adolescent medicine specialists as well as any other provider of primary health care to this age group.

Adolescents have traditionally been considered a healthy lot. If one judges health status based on mortality rates, adolescents are indeed among the healthiest of U.S. citizens. However, analysis of existing data by the United States Congress Office of Technology Assessment (OTA) has resulted in the conclusion that "the conventional wisdom that American adolescents as a group are so healthy that they do not require health and related services *is not justified*." The data suggest that as many as 1 in 5 adolescents has at least one serious health problem. Furthermore, it has been estimated that between 5% and 10% of adolescents have a serious *chronic* physical condition significant enough to limit their daily activities in 50% of the affected individuals.

Clearly there is a need to provide health resources to this vulnerable population. Medical interventions must include both preventive care and treatment of acute and chronic conditions. Although prevention is the traditional cornerstone of pediatric and adolescent medicine, it has been proven to be a formidable task to convince not only the potential recipients but also the third party payors of the value of such services. Therefore, a disproportionate share of current healthcare expenditures is directed toward treatment services.

It is well documented that adolescents access the healthcare system less frequently than any other age group. They have fewer physician visits and the lowest hospitalization rate of any age group. Whereas nearly 75% of adolescents have annual contact with a physician, nearly 15% report not having seen a physician in over 2 years. Why, if a need for health services is so compelling, do adolescents have such low utilization rates? The answer is simple: there are formidable barriers to basic healthcare for adolescents. These barriers can be categorized into two general groups, financial and nonfinancial.

Approximately 85% of U.S. adolescents, aged 10 to 18 years, are covered by some form of health insurance: 72% have private insurance, 10% are insured through Medicaid, and 3% are covered by other plans. This means that approximately 15% of the adolescent population, or 4.5 million, are uninsured. Interestingly, the majority of adolescents who lack any form of insurance coverage are most likely to come from two-parent, white families in which at least one parent is employed and earns an income greater than the federal poverty line. A unique problem faces older adolescents in that when they reach age 18 they often are no longer covered under their family's insurance plan. Therefore, nearly a quarter of the 19- to 24-year-olds have no health insurance. Even with insurance coverage, many plans do not cover services that adolescents need most. Preventive services are lacking in most plans, and those that cover mental health and treatment for substance abuse contain stringent limitations. Low reimbursement rates, particularly for the Medicaid eligible, results in low provider participation.

There are a number of nonfinancial barriers to health care that either limit access or include resources where less than optimal care is available. A major barrier is the lack of physicians and other healthcare providers that are trained and skilled to deliver comprehensive and coordinated medical care to this age group. Less than 0.2% of all physicians in the American Medical Association masterfile listed adolescent medicine as their primary or secondary specialty. Given the current situation regarding funding of graduate medical education, it is obvious that there will never be a sufficient number of adolescent medicine specialists to meet the healthcare needs of this population. It would appear that adolescent medicine specialists will be of greatest service if they are concentrated in the faculties of academic institutions—to teach students and housestaff how to successfully incorporate adolescents into their practice, to serve as referral resources for the more complex clinical cases, and to provide the research necessary to perpetuate the discipline.

Other than the workforce issues, the main nonfinancial barriers tend to center around issues related to comprehensiveness of care and maintenance of confidentiality. There are but a few comprehensive health centers for adolescents in the United States. The majority of these are either hospital-based programs in teaching institutions or they are one of a variety of community-based models. An innovative approach to healthcare delivery, which began in the 1970s, is the school-linked health centers. These clinics are able to provide a wide variety of services in an obviously convenient setting within or near the school. The major drawback to this model has been community acceptance, particularly of those that offer reproductive services.

Confidentiality is a prerequisite to the establishment of an effective healthcare relationship with an adolescent.

The mature minor doctrine enables cognitively mature adolescents to give informal consent for medical treatment, and specific legal statutes allow confidential treatment for conditions such as substance abuse, sexually transmitted diseases, and pregnancy. Thus, a contract of confidentiality between the adolescent and the provider has become the standard of practice in adolescent medicine. A barrier to care is created because parents are generally held responsible for payment for services rendered. This could potentially result in an unintentional breach of the confidentiality contract. Fear of disclosure through the billing process is known to prevent or delay the young person from seeking medical care.

The current mechanisms in vogue in the United States for financing health care do not bode particularly well for the adolescent or the specialist provider. Managed care tends to focus on treatment rather than preventive services. Confidential care delivered in a comprehensive manner is difficult in this model, which is motivated by profit. Likewise, adolescent clinics and school-linked clinics are probably not viable options in this financial environment. Efforts underway to restructure the Medicaid system ultimately could result in reduced funding for this program, which provides a safety net for a large number of poor children and adolescents. Thus, in addition to providing direct health services to this age group we have another professional obligation, and that is to serve them in an advocacy role. We must be steadfast in our resolve that adolescents need and deserve their fair share of the healthcare resources that this country has to offer, and our appeals must constantly resound at all local, state, and federal levels.

Joe M. Sanders, Jr., MD
Executive Director
American Academy of Pediatrics

There have been major developments in the field of Adolescent Medicine since the 1992 publication of the first edition of *Comprehensive Adolescent Health Care*. Residency training in both internal medicine and pediatrics requires experience in adolescent medicine, and many medical students now are exposed to adolescents during their pediatric rotations. Quality research in the field continues to increase as reflected in recent decisions by the *Journal of Adolescent Health* to expand from eight to twelve issues per year and the *American Journal of Diseases of Children* to include "Adolescents" in its new title *(Archives of Children and Adolescents)*. Within the field itself, membership in the Society for Adolescent Medicine has grown steadily (currently there are more than 1,300 members) and a most significant development has been the establishment of adolescent medicine as a subspecialty, with an examination leading to Board certification.

Despite the changes that have taken place within the field, the primary health services of adolescents will not be the exclusive domain of subspecialists in adolescent medicine. The vast majority of adolescents will continue to seek attention from general pediatricians, family medicine physicians, internists, gynecologists, and other providers of primary care. In addition, mental health professionals in many disciplines provide critical services to adolescents. It is our hope that this text will be helpful to all professionals devoted to the care of adolescents and their families, although we must acknowledge that our contributors often refer to "pediatricians" in their text, reflecting the background of most medical professionals in the field of adolescent medicine.

For purposes of this book, adolescence is considered to extend from approximately 12 to 21 years of age, although this range is arbitrary. Furthermore, some individuals enter puberty and adolescence early, and others remain adolescents (from a psychosocial and/or physiologic point of view) beyond 21 years of age. Please also note that some of our contributors have used the terms "teenager" and "adolescent" interchangeably.

This second edition has 20 new chapters. In addition, many previous chapters have undergone major revisions, all chapters have been updated, cross-referencing among chapters has been expanded, and special attention has been given to issues outlined by the American Board of Pediatrics for inclusion in the Adolescent Medicine Subspecialty Certifying Examination. Major additions include a section on medical emergencies (e.g., Overdose, Toxic Shock Syndrome) and an expanded section on psychiatric disorders (e.g., Posttraumatic Stress Disorder, Obsessive-Compulsive Disorder). Other new chapters include *Financing Adolescent Health Services, Psychoeducational Tests for Adolescents, Attention Deficit-Hyperactivity Disorder,* and *Sexual Assault*.

The editors are deeply indebted to Mary Sharkey, who coordinated all of our efforts. We appreciate the efforts of the staff at Mosby, especially Laura DeYoung, Laura Berendson, and Anne Patterson. Christine Schmidt at North Shore University Hospital was very helpful in the preparation of this textbook. And, most of all, our thanks go to the contributors, who collectively spent numerous hours in sharing their expertise and experiences.

Stanford B. Friedman, MD
Martin Fisher, MD
S. Kenneth Schonberg, MD
Elizabeth M. Alderman, MD

CONTENTS

PART ONE

Principles of Adolescent Medicine

CHAPTER 1

History of Adolescence

•

Claudio Violato

Adolescence is as much a social phenomenon as a psychological one. As societies change over time, so does the conceptualization of adolescence. The modern scientific concept of adolescence began with the now famous two-volume work of G. Stanley Hall, *Adolescence,* first published in 1904. Hall (1844-1924) has since been accorded the status of the father of the psychology of adolescence. The concept of adolescence—although the term *adolescence* did not appear until the fifteenth century—has its roots in antiquity, especially in the works of the early Greeks. Both Plato and Aristotle attached special significance to the transitional period between childhood and adulthood. Like many modern-day psychologists, these early thinkers regarded adolescence as a time of turbulence and passion when young people begin to face the responsibilities of adulthood. This view has remained remarkably stable over time. In this chapter we trace the history of adolescence from its ancient roots to medieval views, through the Renaissance, to modern conceptions in the eighteenth and nineteenth centuries, and finally to the present-day view in the twentieth century.

ANCIENT VIEWS

While Plato (427-347 BC) did not specifically develop a theory of development or adolescence, accounts of youth appear in various of his works, particularly in his dialogues, *Laws* and *The Republic.* He did, however, develop a rather extensive theory of human nature with a dualist assumption as the cornerstone of the theory. His famous dictum *soma sema* (the body is the seat of the soul) sums up the division of body and soul. Only the soul can develop to the highest rational level, but it is fettered by the body. For Plato, rational and critical thought is absent in children and appears mainly in adolescence, as it is at this time that the soul is beginning to achieve its highest plane. Moreover, innate ideas—another of Plato's pivotal concepts—are brought out fully in adolescence when reason develops. Passion and excitability were central themes in the affective aspect of adolescence for Plato, as they have been since throughout the millennia. Finally, in the third part of Plato's tripartite system of human nature (reason, appetite, and spirit), young people developed such headstrong will (spirit) that they argue merely for argument's sake. Indeed, adolescents are so excitable, according to Plato, that they should not be allowed to drink wine before 18 years of age because "fire must not be poured upon fire."

Aristotle (384-322 BC), one of Plato's most successful students, diverged from his teacher on the point of dualism or mind-body separation. Rather, he began with a doctrine of the unity of the physical and mental worlds. Like modern materialist psychologists such as Freud, Aristotle saw the soul as the function of the body that provides the structure. The soul, then, cannot exist without the body just as the mind cannot exist without the brain.

Like Plato, Aristotle accepted the view that human development is a process whereby the soul evolves to progressively higher states, culminating in young manhood (14 to 21 years of age), in which the highest plane is achieved. Aristotle's description appears in *Rhetorica* and foreshadows G. Stanley Hall's descriptions of adolescence as a time of *Sturm und Drang* (storm and stress). The adolescent, in Aristotle's description, shows strong passions, especially sexual, that are indiscriminately gratified if possible. These impulses are intense and can be violent, but are of short duration and are extinguished quickly. These youths can be gullible, optimistic, and future oriented, but at the same time they can be obstinate and complain constantly of not being understood and of unfair treatment at home and by society generally.

MEDIEVAL VIEWS

During the medieval period, or Dark Ages as it is also referred to, a moratorium existed on independent thinking and the discovery of new knowledge. Remarkably, for nearly 1000 years from the total collapse of the Roman Empire in the fifth century to the fifteenth century and the Renaissance, the view of the world was based strictly on Christian theology and religious dogma.

During this period, children and adolescents were not accorded separate status but were regarded as miniature adults. Moreover, humanity was considered to be essentially depraved, each person entering the world tainted with original sin. Indeed, it was the original transgressions of Adam and Eve that caused the downfall of humanity into sin and introduced death: "Sin came into the world through one man and death through sin" (Genesis 3: 6-7). Plato's dualism was thus revived, as the soul had a separate existence from the body. While corporeal death was inevitable, the soul would live on for eternity either happily (in heaven) or in perpetual misery and torture (in hell) if redemption had not been achieved.

This doctrine of depravity underscores innate tendencies toward badness and ungodliness. During these Dark Ages, development was seen as a process whereby the person became progressively worse and removed from God. The path to redemption lay in stern discipline of the child and repression of childish (sinful) impulses. The child had to be civilized. These were particularly strong views in Catholic theology before the Reformation, and were subsequently revived in Calvinism in Europe and Puritanism in the United States.

RENAISSANCE VIEWS

The Renaissance, or rebirth, after the Middle Ages marked a sharp break with medieval ideals and practices, particularly in the arts, literature, and science and in the concept of human nature. These changes began in Italy primarily during the fifteenth and sixteenth centuries and later spread throughout the world. The most pertinent views on human nature and human development are those of three philosophers: Comenius, Locke, and Rousseau.

The major break of Renaissance thought with medieval doctrine was over the doctrine of preformationism. Both John Comenius (1592-1670) and John Locke (1632-1704) rejected the concept of innate ideas and evil in humans and focused instead on experience and individual development. Locke, in his 1753 work *An Essay Concerning Human Understanding,* developed the theme that all knowledge is obtained directly through the senses, because the mind of the neonate was a *tabula rasa* (blank slate). For Locke, development was a gradual process from initial mental passivity to increased cognition during adolescence and not the emergence of innate depravity. Locke's view clearly foreshadowed the work of the behavioral psychologist J.B. Watson, who extended this idea of the *tabula rasa* in his 1924 book *Behaviorism* when he declared: "Give me a dozen healthy infants, well-formed, and my own specific world to bring them up in and I'll guarantee to take any one at random and train him to become any kind of specialist I might select."[1] For both Comenius and Locke, adolescence was the final stage of human development in which the individual acquires abstract thought and rationality, becomes self-directed, and achieves an identity. These are themes of development that are also central to the twentieth-century theories of Jean Piaget and Erik Erikson.

Probably the most influential thinker of the Renaissance vis-à-vis human development was Jean Jacques Rousseau (1712-1778). In contrast to Comenius and Locke, Rousseau focused on affect rather than cognition. Like many of his contemporaries, Rousseau adhered to the dominant themes of his day of romanticism and primitivism as the Romantic Era prevailed in a spirit of revolt against the dogma of "reason" inherent in medieval scholasticism. Ultimately the static mechanistic universe of the Dark Ages was discarded for a dynamic evolutionary one.

Primitivism encompassed the belief that the natural or earliest conditions of humanity are glorious and ideal and are reflected in children and childhood. It was in this context that Rousseau wrote his famous book *Émile* (1780) about the development of a fictitious boy, wherein he expounded his view of children, adolescents, and development. The child was close to nature, primitive and thus intrinsically good. As a noble savage, the child was naturally endowed with a sense of right and wrong. Four stages of development were proposed by Rousseau that culminated during the period of adolescence (15 to 20 years of age) when the person shifts from selfish motivations to social concerns and develops an identity. Conscience is acquired so that morality and virtuous behavior become possible; this leads into maturity, which is dominated by spiritualism. Rousseau considered adolescence to be a "second birth," an idea that has been elaborated by contemporary psychoanalytic psychologists such as Peter Blos, who sees adolescence as the "second individuation" (the first is completed by the end of the third year of life with the child's ability to distinguish between self and mother). As the Romantic Era gave way to the Modern Period, the revolutionary ideas embodied in the work of Charles Darwin, Rousseau, and other Renaissance thinkers had firmly established the concept of childhood and adolescence.

MODERN VIEWS

Eighteenth and Nineteenth Centuries

In both Europe and the United States, industrialization radically transformed life during the eighteenth and nineteenth centuries. As society shifted from an agrarian mode of production to an industrial one, people moved to cities, with the resultant urbanization of society. Work now occurred outside the home (in the factories), but women and children remained at home doing "homework" while men did "real work." Thus, home became separated from work and children became feminized as much as women became childish. This period was also characterized by the introduction of mass education, child labor laws, and mass communications, first through print and finally through electronic media.

Such was the setting, then, when Charles Darwin (1809-1882) published his book *The Origin of Species* in 1859. A number of revolutionary ideas are contained in that work, but two of the most pertinent for current purposes are that (1) species change (evolve) over time from simple to complex forms and (2) humans are part of the natural order, with direct ancestry from infrahumans. As a result, the idea was finally accepted (grudgingly by many) that humans are part of the natural organic world rather than apart from nature and above it, as had been held by Aristotle and many others since. Darwin's ideas influenced many twentieth-century psychologists, including Sigmund Freud, Jean Piaget, and Arnold Gessel, but probably had the most direct impact on the work of G. Stanley Hall.

Hall expanded Darwin's concept of biologic evolution into a psychologic theory of recapitulation. He adhered to the dictum that ontogeny recapitulates phylogeny, that the development of the individual (ontogeny) replays the entire biologic history of humanity (phylogeny). Accordingly, each individual must pass through the entire development of humanity as a whole, from animal-like primitivism (infancy) to savagery (childhood), into early social forms (late childhood), and finally into more recent civilized ways of life that characterize modern times (adolescence and beyond). For Hall, "bad" behavior (during infancy and childhood) was natural, normal, and inevitable, but one could take consolation in the fact that it would disappear as development progressed. This concept has been borrowed and expanded in modern popular culture when adults reassure each other that badly behaved children and adolescents are "just going through a phase."

The most lasting contribution that Hall has made to the study of adolescence is the idea that it is a time of *Sturm und Drang,* as mentioned earlier. Hall borrowed this theme from eighteenth- and nineteenth-century German literature, especially the works of Goethe and Schiller, who depicted youth as full of idealism, with commitments to goals, and riddled with passion and suffering. In this genre, adolescents were depicted as moody, given to outbursts of deep personal feelings, and revolting against the established and old. This theme of storm and stress was not original with Hall, can be traced at least as far back as the works of Plato and Aristotle, and has been a common theme throughout the millennia, but Hall formalized this idea and legitimized it as "scientific." It has been a dominant theme governing adolescent research and therapy throughout the twentieth century, even though the bulk of empirical evidence now indicates that adolescence is a relatively tranquil period of smooth transition: most adolescents do not experience undue trauma and turbulence.[2,3]

Twentieth Century

In addition to the main theme of *Sturm und Drang* and youth as a time of renewal and struggle against injustice, a number of dominant images and stereotypes of adolescence have dominated the twentieth century. These stereotypes of youth coincide roughly with each decade of this century beginning in the 1920s.

Modern depictions of 1920s youth characterize those adolescents as fun loving, carefree, and self-indulgent. The depictions of youthful gaiety in the 1920s reflect the magnanimous mood of the period buttressed by economic expansion.

Conditions changed drastically in the 1930s. Life under conditions of the "dirty thirties" was bleak. Young people are depicted during this period not as fun loving and carefree, but rather as having a social conscience and heightened awareness of others. Nevertheless, the young of the 1930s did not actively protest or rebel against the social system; that would be left to a later generation.

The end of the 1930s was marked by the cataclysm of World War II. The previously dislocated youth now had a clear goal: young men went to war and young women assisted the war effort at home. Adolescents during the 1940s were depicted as serious, committed to a purpose, patriotic, and heroic.

The United States emerged from World War II triumphant. It was the most powerful nation on Earth with a vibrant economy and a hopeful outlook to the future. In the expansive mood of the times, the image of youth paralleled that of the 1920s: adolescents were seen as silly, flighty, fun loving, and foolish. By the end of the 1950s, the images began to change. The adolescent as portrayed by James Dean in *Rebel Without A Cause* began to dominate. As the title of the film indicates, the young were becoming rebellious without understanding the underlying reason. The storm and stress theme was emphasized; adolescents were portrayed as emotionally turbulent and ready to strike out, frequently for no apparent reason.

By the 1960s the dominant image of youth characterized young people as visionaries. Visionaries were distinguished by a purity of moral vision, saintlike creatures battling heroically against the immense forces of evil surrounding them as embodied in "The Establishment." Popular theories of adolescence such as those of Erik Erikson, as well as influential books such as *The Vanishing Adolescent* (1959) by Edgar Z. Friedenberg and *The Making of a Counterculture* (1960) by Theodore Roszak, together with films, television depictions, adolescent psychology textbooks, and novel and magazine descriptions, helped to create, legitimize, and sustain the stereotype of the young as engaged in a gallant, if hopeless struggle against the corruption of the adult world.

Protest, dissent, and rebellion began to wane by the early 1970s and a new stereotype of youth arose: the "me" generation. In marked contrast to the visionary victim, the youth of the "me" generation did not care about social causes, their fellow humans, or justice. Moreover, they endorsed "The Establishment" and certainly did not want to overthrow it. The main goal was to fully exploit its potential and to get for oneself as much out of it as possible.

The 1980s again produced a new stereotype of adolescence. This image of young people as "serious but troubled" shows adolescents as committed to school and work but troubled by economic uncertainty, the possibility of nuclear war, world famine, and the break-up of the family. Unlike the visionary, however, the serious but troubled young are not willing to protest or rebel, as they see these problems fatalistically and hopelessly. Many of the elements of this stereotype appeared in an article entitled "Growing Pains" in a popular magazine: "If a generalization had to be made, I would say most of us are scared . . . our attitudes are colored by hints of pessimism that arise from other issues that confront us . . . Part of that pessimism may reflect the fact that we do not seem to be as idealistic as past generations," wrote a 17-year-old high school graduate.[4] These serious but troubled youth are realistic rather than idealistic.

A new stereotype of adolescence has emerged for the 1990s. This image of young people as "young fogies" shows adolescents as world-weary and living with broken families, AIDS, a drug abuse epidemic, environmental degradation, economic uncertainty, a collapsing world order, and a bleak future generally. In this stereotype, these weighty problems of adult society are cast upon young people before they are prepared to deal with them. The image of the world-weary "young fogy" is depicted in television shows such as "Blossom," "Fresh Prince of Belair," and "Beverly Hills 90210." This image also abounds in the print media and was captured aptly in a cover story in *MacLean's* (February 22, 1993).[5] Robertson Davies' statement that "One of the really notable achievements of the twentieth century has been to make the young old before their time" is cited favorably in this cover story as capturing the essence of today's youth. So, like the "serious but troubled" youth of the 1980s, this new image of young people characterizes them as troubled and pessimistic. Beyond that, they are also depicted as jaded, world-weary, and hopeless, forced into the concerns and problems of middle age before their time.

FUTURE OF ADOLESCENCE

These are the social, cultural, and historical milieux in which we currently study adolescence. It is now a specialty unto its own in medicine, psychology, and education. There are several learned and scientific journals such as *Adolescence, Journal of Youth and Adolescence,* and *Journal of Adolescence* that publish research findings in the area. Two handbooks of adolescence have been published in the last decade, *Handbook of Adolescent Psychology* (1987) edited by Vincent Van Hasslet and Michel Hersen, and another with the same title edited by Joseph Adelson (1980). Adolescence as a scientific, medical, and educational specialty is here to stay.

As we approach the end of the twentieth century, two main and contradictory themes govern theory and research in adolescence.[6] The first is the classic or storm and stress view; the second is the empirical view, which holds that adolescence is relatively peaceful and harmonious. Psychiatrists, clinical psychologists, and social workers who study abnormal adolescents tend to adhere to the classic view while those who study normal adolescents espouse the latter view. The main task for researchers and theoreticians in the next several decades is to integrate and synthesize these apparently contradictory points of view into a more satisfactory explanation and understanding of adolescence.[7]

References

1. Watson JB: *Behaviorism,* New York, 1924, Norton.
2. Offer D, Ostrov E, Howard KI, Atkinson R: *The teenage world,* New York, 1988, Plenum Press.
3. Violato C, Holden W: A confirmatory factor analysis of a four-factor model of adolescent concerns, *J Youth Adolesc* 17:101-113, 1988.
4. *MacLean's* (September 7) 1987; p. 45.
5. *MacLean's* (February 22) 1993.
6. Coleman JC: Current contradictions in adolescent theory, *J Youth Adolesc* 7:1-11, 1978.

7. Violato C, Travis LD: *Advances in adolescent psychology,* Calgary, Alberta, 1995, Detselig.

Suggested Readings

Aries P: *Centuries of childhood,* New York, 1962, Random House.
> *An authoritative account of the concept of childhood and depiction of children. The analysis of childhood through the art of various historical epochs is particularly good.*

Kett JF: *Rites of passage,* New York, 1977, Basic Books.
> *A detailed description of adolescent experiences in the United States during three major historical phases from 1790 to the present.*

Violato C, Travis LD: *Advances in adolescent psychology,* Calgary, Alberta, 1995, Detselig.
> *A detailed and in-depth analysis of central issues in adolescent psychology. While research and theoretical problems are addressed, there is also an attempt to deal with more conventional and socially relevant topics in adolescence.*

Violato C, Wiley AJ: Images of adolescence in English literature: the Middle Ages to the modern period, *Adolescence* 25:253-264, 1990.
> *An analysis of the imagery of youth and adolescence in the works of major authors, including Chaucer, More, Locke, Shakespeare, Bayly, Milton, Prior, Wordsworth, Coleridge, Hazlitt, and Dickens.*

CHAPTER 2

Evolution of Adolescent Behavior

•

Mihaly Csikszentmihalyi

Several adolescent disorders, especially those of a psychosocial nature, have their origin in a mismatch between genotypic instructions on the one hand and environmental conditions affecting the phenotype on the other. Over millions of years of evolution, the human organism has become programmed to act in certain predictable ways from puberty into young adulthood. For instance, males have been selected for aggressiveness, adventurousness, and independence. Traits that were relatively more important for young females include sociability, affiliation, and nurturance.[1,2] However, rapidly changing cultural conditions in the last few thousand, and especially the last few hundred, years no longer allow the expression of these ingrained traits for either gender, thereby causing a great deal of inner stress in adolescence, which in turn is responsible for many of the notorious pathologies of this stage of life. The bad news is that this conflict will not go away by itself, and it may become increasingly pathogenic if nothing is done about it. The good news is that we are beginning to better understand the conditions responsible for the conflict, thereby enabling us to initiate constructive action to solve the conflict.

In terms of biologic development, the teenage years should be the best part of one's life. Most physical and psychological functions are especially efficient in adolescence; speed, strength, reaction time, and memory reach their peak. This is the time when one enjoys most the movements of one's body, when food tastes best, when sleep is sweetest, and when music is most seductive. In adolescence, new ideas, beliefs, and works of art have the greatest impact on the imagination.

Unfortunately, all of this potential for positive experience runs afoul of the limitations inherent in complex social systems, with the result that the teenage years are often the most stressful rather than the most fulfilling period of one's life. For many young people, the habits they develop in adolescence to reduce conflicts result in pathologic adaptations that impair physical and mental health for the rest of life. By obtaining a better idea of the parameters of the conflict, it is possible to eliminate some of its causes, thus restoring the potential for optimal experience and preventing the emergence of both acute and chronic pathologies.

TURMOIL

Reality of Turmoil

The argument whether the Sturm und Drang (storm and stress) of the teenage years is a natural and even a desirable stage in the life cycle has been intensely debated. Some authors see considerable conflict, and a few believe that normal psychological development requires teenagers to be rebellious and defiant. Others deny that stress at this stage is inevitable and point out that most teenagers do not show evidence of unusual conflict or stress.[3,4]

On the whole, however, it seems that in diverse cultures in China, Africa, and South America and in all historical periods stretching back to written records, adolescence has been considered a "time of troubles."[5] It is unlikely that this historical, cross-cultural consensus is based on a misapprehension. It is more likely that the passage through physical puberty does indeed precipitate a variety of conflicts, making this a particularly problematic age. Health statistics in our society indicate that individuals in the second decade of life are particularly vulnerable to vehicular accidents, substance abuse, and several other kinds of reckless deviance.[6,7] Of course, this does not mean that every teenager will be a delinquent or display rebelliousness. However, it does suggest that the probability of such behaviors is highest during this period of the life cycle.

Sources of Turmoil

The causes of this widespread conflict cannot be understood by considering only the individual teenagers involved or by examining only external environmental influences. To explain the conditions involved, one must take a very long view of the *interaction* between human physiology and its environment. It is not difficult to realize that the stresses result from a lack of fit between human organisms shaped by evolutionary forces that act very slowly and are difficult to change and opportunities for action determined by social conditions that change relatively quickly.

Our species would have become extinct long ago if individual humans had not been at their most active mentally, physically, and sexually as soon as their bodies were most vigorous and mature. Natural selection, evolving presumably for millions of years, perfected a particular type of mammalian adaptation based on a relatively short period of development in utero and a relatively long and protected childhood. This combination made possible the unprecedented opportunity for prolonged learning of cultural instructions that have given such a great advantage to our species. At the same time, no species could postpone too long the adult productive and reproductive tasks of its members with impunity. Given the narrow edge of survival that competition for scarce resources typically allows, it has been essential that as soon as individuals were ready, they would begin to provide for the necessities of life, including the next generation.

Thus, our genetic program is likely to contain strong instructions for engaging in behavior that leads to predation on the one hand and to cooperative reproduction on the other, behavior activated by the hormonal changes following puberty. If teenagers had not been programmed to be boisterous, aggressive, and sexy, we would not be here now. Currently, however, we are living in an environment that forces adolescents to ignore many of the instructions contained in their genes, and we brand as deviant their efforts to follow the call of nature.

The development of what we call "civilization," or a form of life increasingly dependent on culturally transmitted behavioral instructions as opposed to genetically transmitted instructions, has produced this friction in the timing of such behaviors. As soon as farming became the main form of human adaptation around the world, by approximately 8000 BC, a new set of behavioral requirements came into effect that conflicted with the simpler requirements of hunting, gathering, and herding. Successful farmers must have extensive agricultural knowledge, patience, and a willingness to do repetitive work that brings slow results; they must also be willing to be tied down to a particular place. In many respects these traits conflicted with the characteristics that had made hunters successful. While hunting was, relatively speaking, a young man's game, farming relied on qualities possessed by more mature men and women.

Ever since the "agricultural revolution," cultural evolution has tended to reduce the opportunities for action available to adolescents in favor of greater opportunities for more mature individuals. These changes have become especially obvious in the last few centuries. For instance, in the thirteenth century 7-year-old students in the Paris schools were routinely armed with daggers to defend their lives in the turbulent and lawless urban environment.[8] In almost all parts of the world, girls were expected to marry promptly after their first menses. A few generations ago, boys as young as 5 or 6 years old were expected to work in factories for 70 or more hours a week.

Fortunately, these conditions no longer exist. However, it could be argued that the realistic involvement of teenagers in adult behaviors is more congruent with their genetic programming, whereas the current isolation of teens from "real" life, useful as it is for their adaptation to future niches in our society, creates a great deal of frustration. Ironically, these frustrations often cause *maladaptive* behaviors in later life.

The claim that the constraints of civilized life cause undesirable repressions is very old. It was vigorously expressed by Freud in his *Civilisation and Its Discontents* (1929). The present argument, however, differs from his on at least two important points. First, a perspective informed by evolutionary theory suggests that the genetic programming that constitutes "human nature," although difficult to modify over short periods, is nevertheless more open and flexible than it had been previously thought to be. Second, while sexual "drives" are of central importance for the survival of humankind, they do not have the privileged status that they acquired in Freudian theory. To survive, humans have been programmed for taking chances, helping each other, competing with each other, using their bodies and their minds to their fullest potential, and enjoying sexual stimulation. These other sources of pleasure are presumably as primary as the sexual ones, and it does not make much sense to consider them sublimated transformations of sexuality. On the other hand, this view suggests that there are several reasons why a person might feel conflict and be unfulfilled. Individuals prevented from following their genetic instructions regarding physical or mental activity, nurturance, and risk taking may be just as frustrated as those who are sexually repressed.

In summary, adolescent psychosocial disorders are to a large extent caused by teenagers being genetically primed for behaviors that are no longer necessary or desirable at the present stage of sociocultural evolution. The two obvious solutions—to change the genetic programming or to return to a social system that would give full scope to adolescents' needs—are not feasible at the moment, but a third possibility exists that might reduce some of the conflict. It may be helpful to discover what adolescents enjoy doing that is consistent with their genetic programming *and* with social requirements as well as making opportunities available for such activities, while reducing or modifying those that satisfy only one or neither of these requirements.

ACTIVITIES: WHAT DO TEENAGERS ENJOY DOING?

A homeostatic model of human motivation would suggest that adolescents will seek a state of relaxation as soon as their basic needs are satisfied. In reality, several studies have shown that teenagers the world over value activities that present them with incremental challenges and that make it possible for them to improve their skills. Teenagers are most happy and satisfied when they are involved in sports and hobbies, music or art, and intimate friendships.[9-11] These activities allow them to expand their skills, to grow in competence, and consequently to feel good about themselves. When these outlets are not available, teenagers often turn to deviance because it presents an alternative set of challenges.

Vandalism, juvenile delinquency, and indiscriminate use of mind-altering substances are often seen primarily as pathologies of deprived, socially marginal adolescent males. This is true to a large extent, but surprisingly, such forms of deviance have been increasing with extraordinary rapidity among the affluent and the privileged. These behaviors are driven by the need to relieve a boring, unchallenging environment. When young people are deprived of meaningful opportunities for action, stealing a car, breaking a school window, or ingesting forbidden substances becomes the challenge. "If you could show me something that is as much fun as stealing jewelry from a house without waking the owners up, I would do it," says a middle-class adolescent caught in a burglary. Like other teenagers, by "fun" he means something exciting and slightly dangerous, something one can be proud of having done.

Similarly, promiscuous sexuality, which results in unwanted pregnancies and various kinds of venereal diseases, for most teenagers is a way of testing skills in a challenging context rather than a way of reducing homeostatic needs. We often ask incredulously why intelligent, well-to-do adolescent girls become pregnant. Do they not know any better? Adults who ask this question do not understand that "safe sex" is generally not a priority for teenage girls. They want to prove their ability to attract young males, they want to feel desirable, they want to act as adults, they want to attract attention and control power, and on some level they very much want to prove their ability to nurture and to be responsible for another life. All this has been programmed in their genes. For some girls the only way to comply with these instructions is to become pregnant in defiance of adult wishes.

The empirical evidence concerning teenagers confirms what one would deduce from evolutionary theory, namely, that they enjoy and seek out situations that make them feel competent and fully functioning. When such opportunities are lacking, they are driven to invent them. Because these opportunities created by teenagers are, by definition, outside the existing social norms, they are generally seen by adults as "deviant." Occasionally, however, youths' attempts to overcome stifling limitations result in new forms of art, music, ideology, and life style, which become acceptable to the culture at large. According to Thomas Kuhn, even scientific revolutions occur because young scientists eventually get bored with the theoretical paradigms invented by their elders.

OBSTACLES TO ENJOYMENT

We have seen that in a very general sense the structural sources of conflict in adolescence consist of a mismatch between genetically programmed desires and culturally programmed opportunities. How specifically does this mismatch manifest itself? Reviewed here are five main areas in which teenagers are typically prevented from expressing their potential in contemporary society.

Restrictions on Physical Movement and Freedom

The most basic possession of an individual is his or her body. Especially in adolescence, some of the most satisfying experiences involve physical sensations that result from movement in hard work, sports, and dancing. In contemporary life, opportunities for physical activities have become increasingly reduced, and when they are present, they are often isolated from the rest of life and therefore relatively trivialized. Playing football or biking is fun, but it has little to do with one's family or occupation.

Another crucial issue concerns control over one's location. Freedom to move and to choose situations is a fundamental need, especially for young people. Since the introduction of compulsory education, this need has been severely compromised. Spending a good part of the day in the confines of a school is ipso facto repressive. For this reason, even academically talented teenagers wish they were doing something different when at school, even when they are involved in a favorite subject in a favorite class.[6]

Another obstacle to physical mobility is the layout of our living arrangements. Compared with previous communities, the typical suburb is extremely homogeneous, dispersed, and impervious to adolescent interaction. In many ways teenagers are confined until they obtain their own driver's license, which is the major rite of passage in contemporary adolescence. However, even when there is access to a car, most communities offer only the most stereotyped and superficial opportunities for action to young people.

Absence of Responsibility

Erikson[12] first described adolescence in modern Western societies as a "moratorium," a period of freedom from responsibilities that allows thinking of alternatives and experimenting with options before committing oneself to a lifelong career. It is true that such a moratorium may be necessary in a culture with numerous and quickly changing occupational roles and life styles. However, excluding young people from responsibilities for too long has its own dangers, because they may never learn how to run their own lives or how to care for those who depend on them.

The worst consequence of not having clear and real expectations is that adolescents feel that what they do does not matter and that therefore they do not matter. Depression and suicidal behavior often result when they feel that no one really cares. It is true that when parents have excessively high expectations of their children, stress and anxiety may result. However, the opposite is more often true: no expectations communicate an indifference that can be very traumatic to teenagers.

In any case, the range of responsibilities open to adolescents is very limited. For many, the only expectation is to be a good student. Not all youngsters can be good students, and even if they were, being a good student hardly exhausts the potential of a young person. In past historical periods, the difference between adult performances and responsibilities and those of teenagers was mainly a matter of degree. Today it is definitely a difference in kind: many adolescents have no idea what their parents actually do or feel.

Problems of Sexuality and Intimacy

In every society the advent of sexual maturity presents particular problems and requires the application of social controls. As we have belatedly learned in the last decades, promiscuity, or "sexual liberation" as its idealistic advocates preferred to call it, is still not a viable option in terms of either health, personal growth, or social well-being.

During the sexual revolution of a generation ago, it was believed that adolescents would be happier and freer than any other cohort because—thanks to the car, the pill, and new enlightened views—they would no longer be sexually repressed. This assumption has now revealed itself to be rather crude and simplistic. Sex without intimacy, commitment, and responsibility is neither satisfying nor liberating. Although our culture provides adequate opportunities for adolescent physical sexuality, it provides few clues about how to express commitment or intimacy.

Isolation from Adult Role Models

One of the peculiarities of our present social environment is age segregation. In previous historical periods, young men and women apprenticed with their elders so that they acquired the cultural instructions necessary for later functioning. At present, adolescents spend most of their time in a peer culture that bears little relation to adulthood. Typical American adolescents spend only 3 minutes a day alone with their fathers, and half of that time is spent watching television.[6] How many values, skills, and beliefs can be passed on in a minute and a half a day? The only adults many teenagers encounter on a sustained basis are schoolteachers. This relationship is not very satisfactory because first, being an obligatory relationship, it is believed to be constraining; second, it is usually limited to the transmission of limited, abstract information; and third, students rarely interact with teachers on a one-on-one basis—the classroom is actually not an adult-centered context but part of the peer culture.

Although teenagers prefer spending time with peers to being with adults, the opportunities for action in peer groups are often much more limiting and often only afford opportunities for deviant behavior. The lack of meaningful and enjoyable cross-generational activities clearly contributes to the pathologies of adolescence.

Absence of Control and Power

The obstacles previously listed imply that adolescents have little control over their lives. Their freedom is curtailed, their opportunities are few, and they have few meaningful roles and responsibilities. These limitations are in turn dependent on increasingly age-based asymmetries of power.

One of the effects of cultural evolution has been to allow the concentration of resources, property, and power. Hunter/gatherers were forced to be egalitarian and democratic. With the advent of agriculture, it became possible to store resources, which in turn made economic inequality possible. Gerontocracies, or societies ruled by elders, were one of the outcomes. In technologic societies, control of resources is increasingly abstract and knowledge based, thus favoring relatively older individuals. It is true that a few young athletes and entertainers command sizable incomes, and that affluent teenagers are usually well provided for materially. However, it is common for adolescents to feel that they are "second-class citizens," estranged from the sources of decision making and societal power.

MEANS OF FULFILLMENT

The list of obstacles to adolescent fulfillment suggests what needs to be done to alleviate the pathologies endemic to adolescence. Much can be done, either on a societal scale or at the level of each parent, to improve the fit between what teenagers need and what is available to them. Unfortunately, adults assume that growing up is a "natural" process and that teenagers will sooner or later turn into well-adjusted adults on their own. This, however, is not the case. Growing up is no longer "natural." Sociocultural conditions have made it difficult for young people to acquire those experiences their natures require. Hence, remedial actions are necessary to make teenagers' lives enjoyable and worth living.

When a teenager has symptoms of depression, excessive rebelliousness, or any of the other host of diseases typical of this stage of life, questions to ask include the following: Is this young person stifled physically or sexually? Does he or she have appropriate responsibilities? Is he or she integrated at all in the adult world? How much control over life does he or she have? It is likely that many behavioral and physical symptoms would improve if adjustments were made in the more troublesome areas.

It would be even better if community leaders and parents were able to anticipate adolescent needs and if they took these into account when deciding on educational curricula, work legislation, urban planning, and other issues involving the quality of life. However, while we are waiting for societal solutions, parents and other concerned adults can do a great deal more than is now done to help young people get involved with life. Doubling the time fathers spend with their teenagers to 6 minutes a day would probably help, but it would still be only less than one twentieth of the time spent watching television.

What do these facts suggest to the practicing pediatrician? Given that the strongest causes of adolescent mortality are linked to accidents, suicides, drugs, and violence, a physician must be on the alert for symptoms suggesting excessive boredom and frustration, which are often their causes. A teenager who is generally bored or anxious, who is either always lonely or always in the company of peers, and who lacks intense interests and seems to have few sources of joy is vulnerable to the typical adolescent psychic pathologies.

The specific prescription must vary from person to person, but depending on the personal strengths and on the opportunities in the environment, the general principle is the same: Healthy growth requires that the individual be fully functioning and involved with meaningful challenges. If these requirements are obtained, teenagers will not need to seek refuge in self-destructive alternatives. Whatever the physician can do to awaken the natural curiosity and set off the teen's involvement with meaningful challenges is bound to be helpful. This can be done either directly or through parents, therapists, school counselors, youth workers, religious personnel, or the natural friendship of peers. In any case, prevention of problems can be accomplished if the physician takes into account the importance of optimal functioning for the health of patients, especially in the teenage years.

References

1. Savin-Williams RC: *Adolescence: an ethological perspective,* New York, 1987, Springer-Verlag.
2. Weisfeld G: Aggression and dominance in the social world of boys. In Archer J (ed): *Male violence,* London, 1994, Routledge, pp 42-69.
3. Offer D: *The psychological world of the teenager,* New York, 1969, Basic Books.
4. Offer D, Ostrov E, Howard K: *The adolescent: a psychological self-portrait,* New York, 1981, Basic Books.
5. Kiell N: *The universal experience of adolescence,* London, 1969, University of London Press.
6. Csikszentmihalyi M, Larson R: *Being adolescent,* New York, 1986, Basic Books.
7. U.S. Department of Commerce: *Statistical abstracts of the United States, 1986,* Washington, DC, 1986, Bureau of the Census.
8. Aries P: *Centuries of childhood,* New York, 1962, Vintage.

9. Csikszentmihalyi M: *Flow: the psychology of optimal experience,* New York, 1990, Harper & Row.
10. Csikszentmihalyi M, Wong M: The situational and personal correlates of happiness: a cross-national comparison. In Strack F, Argyle M, Schwartz N, eds: *The social psychology of subjective well-being,* London, 1991, Pergamon Press.
11. Csikszentmihalyi M, Rathunde K, Whalen S: *Talented teenagers: the roots of success and failure,* New York, 1993, Cambridge University Press.
12. Erikson E: *Childhood and society,* New York, 1962, WW Norton.

CHAPTER 3

Epidemiology of Mortalities and Morbidities in Adolescents

•

Melanie A. Gold and Jack Gladstein

Epidemiology is the study of patterns of health and illness in human populations, and the factors that influence these patterns. The epidemiology of disease can be used to understand or investigate the causes of disease, determine public health policy, and plan treatment. Epidemiologists study the prevalence of disease and its variation by season, geographic location, age, and development. They also assess the influence of risk factors such as socioeconomic status, educational level, or sexual activity as determinants of susceptibility or resilience to disease. Epidemiologic data can assist society in making informed decisions regarding the allocation of health resources. Vital statistics also describe the health status of populations. In adolescent medicine, epidemiologic studies may help to determine the allocation of personnel resources as well as educational and research funding.

Terminology

Mortality rates provide a standard way to compare the numbers of deaths occurring in different populations. An age-specific mortality rate is the mortality rate in a specific age group, and the cause-specific mortality rate is the mortality rate in a population from a specific disease or cause. The case-fatality rate is the number of deaths from a specific disease occurring in a given time divided by the number of individuals with the specific disease during the same period.[1] Morbidity rates are similar to mortality rates, but many epidemiologists believe they are a more direct measure of the health status of a population. The numerator is the number of individuals with the

disease and the denominator is the number of people in a population at risk. Prevalence is the number of individuals with a given disease at a given point in time divided by the population at risk at that point in time. Incidence is the number of new cases that have occurred during a given interval of time divided by the population at risk at the beginning of the time interval. Incidence should always be expressed in terms of units of time.[1,2]

Data Sources

To study the mortality and morbidity statistics of adolescent health, it is important to identify the sources of the data. Statistics are only as good as their sources and the method of data collection. Information on morbidity and mortality statistics may come from a variety of government and locally funded collection sources, including the records of individual physicians, diseases reportable to state or local health departments, hospitalization rates, death rates, motor vehicle collision rates, youth risk behavior surveys, census reports, police reports, and school and social service agency reports. Several problems exist in assessing epidemiology in adolescents. Agencies use different age categories in aggregating data. Thus, some of the data may include children who are too young, or adults who are too old. Morbidity and mortality rates vary between jurisdictions because of differences in mandated reporting. Measures used to collect health data on adolescents are often unreliable. These instruments have rarely been pilot tested for validity and reliability among the populations in which they are used, and there are currently no established standard measuring instruments for measuring health-compromising behavior such as substance use, sexual activity, or violence, or for measuring the developmental process of mental illnesses that do not meet full diagnostic criteria.[3,4] Crime and victimization statistics depend on the reporting procedures of police departments and miss those crimes that are not reported. These data measure only adolescents who have been apprehended, and sometimes include only those youths who have been convicted.

Many data sources sample select populations of adolescents (high school surveys). Thus, data may not be generalizable to adolescents not in school (e.g., incarcerated youths, youths in special education, high school dropouts, youths who are absent on the day of the survey). For example, Youth Risk Behavior Surveillance—United States, 1995,[5] a nationwide survey that monitored six categories of priority health risk behaviors in youths and young adults (unintentional and intentional injury, tobacco use, alcohol and other drug use, sexual behaviors, dietary behaviors, and physical activity), may not reflect all adolescents. It is a national, school-based survey conducted by the Centers for Disease Control and Prevention and state and local education agencies. Although a rich source of direct information on adolescents, the survey is limited to collecting data solely from youths "in school." The survey depends on self-report, and students may fear lack of confidentiality, despite assurances of anonymity. Data were collected from only 25 states, omitting more than half the states in the country. In addition, much of the data on adolescents are reported secondhand, for example, by parents or physicians, who may not know the true prevalence of a high-risk activity. Adolescents may seek health services confidentially and without parental knowledge for issues such as family planning or sexually transmitted disease.

ADOLESCENT POPULATION AND MORTALITY STATISTICS

Despite the limitations of data collection, much is known about adolescents in the United States.

General Population Trends

According to the U.S. Bureau of Census, in 1990 there were over 63 million children in the United States under the age of 18 years, of whom 20 million were between the ages of 12 and 17 years. Although the percentage change in population of children under 6 years of age has increased by 12.5% in the past decades, the increase in the size of the population of children aged 6 to 11 years was only 3.4%, and in contrast the change in the population of adolescents (ages 12 to 17 years) decreased by 14.1%.[6]

Mortalities

In 1990, the top four causes of death in the United States for people of all ages were, in descending order of frequency, heart disease, malignant neoplasms, cerebrovascular disease, and unintentional injuries.[7] In 1990, for children aged 5 to 14 years, the leading cause of death was accidents, followed by malignant neoplasms, homicide, congenital anomalies, heart disease, and (lastly) pneumonia and influenza.[8] Among children aged 10 to 14 years in 1988, the leading cause of death was motor vehicle injury, as either a passenger or a pedestrian. The second and third causes of death were homicide and suicide, respectively. From 1985 to 1991, the rate of total homicides and firearm-related homicides increased significantly for persons aged 15 to 24 years, whereas from 1992 to 1994 the rates of total and firearm-related homicides for this age group were stable.[9] Intentional injuries accounted for almost 20% of the total injury deaths in this age group.[10] In 1990, the ranking order of disease or conditions causing death in Americans aged 15 to 24 were, in descending order, accidents, homicide, suicide, cancer, heart disease, HIV/AIDS, birth defects, stroke, pneumonia/influenza, and lung disease.[11]

Mortality Trends

Death rates of young people aged 15 to 24 years between 1980 and 1990 decreased overall for males, from 172 per 100,000 in 1980 to 147 per 100,000 in 1990. However, these trends, when evaluated by race only, show a true decline in mortality for white males, whereas for African-American males the mortality rate has actually increased from 209 per 100,000 in 1980 to 252 per 100,000 in 1990. A similar, though less pronounced change can be seen for females aged 15 to 24 years, with an overall drop in mortality from 1980 to 1990 of 58 to 49 per 100,000. However by race, African-American females showed virtually no change in mortality (71 per 100,000 in 1980 to 69 per 100,000 in 1991) (Table 3-1).[12]

ACCIDENTS. In 1991, 25.6% of total traffic fatalities were among adolescents aged 10 to 14 years, 42.5% among those aged 15 to 19 years, and 34.2% among those aged 20 to 24 years.[13] Bicyclist fatalities for 1991 in 10- to 15-year age groups were 189 per million population, and in 16- to 20-year age groups 62 per million population. Males were four to seven times more likely than females in these age groups to be bicyclist fatalities.[14] Likewise, in 1991, pedestrian fatality rates by age and gender were 295 per 100,000 in adolescents aged 10 to 15 years and 366 per 100,000 in those aged 16 to 20 years, with males in both age groups two to three times more likely to suffer a fatal injury than females (Table 3-2).[15]

	1980	1990
Gender		
Male	172	147
Female	58	49
Race and Gender		
White male	167	131
Black male	209	252
White female	56	46
Black female	71	69

Adapted from the 1993 Statistical Abstracts of the United States on CD-ROM: CD-ABSTR-93, Washington, DC, 1993, US Department of Commerce, Economics and Statistics Administration, Bureau of the Census, Data User Services Division.

TABLE 3-2.
Bicyclist and Pedestrian Fatalities by Age and Gender: 1991 (Rate per million population)

	Bicyclist Deaths	Pedestrian Deaths
Total		
10-15 yr	189	295
16-20 yr	62	366
Males		
10-15 yr	153	191
16-20 yr	55	251
Females		
10-15 yr	36	104
16-20 yr	7	115

Adapted from U.S. Department of Transportation: National Highway Traffic Safety Administration. National Center for Statistics and Analysis. 1991 Pedacyclist Fatal Crash Facts and Traffic Fatality Facts, Washington, DC, c. 1991, National Center for Statistics and Analysis, Research and Development, pp 3-4.

The 1993 Youth Risk Behavior Survey addressed the following behaviors associated with injury among high school students.[5]

SEAT BELT USE. 21.7% of students never or rarely used safety belts when riding in a car or truck driven by someone else. Fewer white males than white females used safety belts. There was a large variation of seat belt usage from state to state.

HELMET USE. Nationwide, 25.1% of students had ridden a motorcycle. Of these students, 43.8% never or rarely used a helmet. In comparison, nationwide, 76.2% of high school students rode a bicycle in the year before the survey. Of these students, 92.8% never or rarely wore a bicycle helmet.

RIDING WITH A DRIVER WHO DRANK ALCOHOL. During the month before the survey, 38.8% of students had ridden in a vehicle with a driver who had been drinking alcohol. Prevalence increased with increasing grade (ninth to twelfth).

WEAPON CARRYING. 20.0% of high school students nationwide carried a weapon (gun, knife, or club) in the month before the survey. Male students were significantly more likely than females to carry a weapon. A total of 7.6% of students nationwide carried a gun in the month before the survey, males more than females.

ENGAGING IN A PHYSICAL FIGHT. A total of 38.7% had been in a physical fight in the year before the survey and 4.2% had been treated by a doctor or nurse for injuries sustained in a physical fight. Boys were more likely than girls to be involved in a fight.

SCHOOL-RELATED VIOLENCE. A total of 4.5% had missed at least 1 day of school during the preceding month because they thought it was unsafe at school or felt unsafe traveling to or from school; 9.8% carried a weapon on school property in the month before the survey; 8.4% were threatened or injured with a weapon at school in the past year; 15.5% had been in a physical fight on school property during the year before the survey. In all racial groups, males were more likely than females to be involved in a fight. Students in earlier grades were more likely to be involved in fights than students in higher grades (see Chapter 112, Violence).

SUICIDAL IDEATION AND ATTEMPTS. A total of 24.1% of students had seriously considered attempting suicide in the year preceding the survey. Across ethnic/racial groups, females were more likely than males to consider attempting suicide. Hispanic females (34.1%) were more likely than black (22.2%) and white (31.6%) females to consider suicide. Nationwide, 8.7% of adolescents had actually attempted suicide during the year preceding the survey; 2.8% reported an attempt that resulted in an injury that had to be treated by a doctor or a nurse. Across all grades and racial/ethnic groups, females were more likely than males to have attempted suicide (see Chapter 123, Suicidal Behavior and Suicide).

MORBIDITIES

Substance Use (See Chapter 108, Substance Use and Abuse)

ALCOHOL. In 1991, 46.4% of adolescents aged 12 to 17 years and 90.2% of those aged 17 to 25 years had had some lifetime experience with alcohol (Table 3-3). In the older group (18 to 25 years), over 80% had used alcohol

TABLE 3-3.
Percentage Substance Use by Type, Frequency, and Age

	Ever	Past Year	Past Month
Alcohol			
12-17 yr	46.4	40.3	20.3
18-25 yr	90.2	82.8	63.6
Illicit drugs*			
12-17 yr	20.1	14.8	6.8
18-25 yr	54.7	29.2	15.4
Marijuana			
12-17 yr	13.0	10.1	4.3
18-25 yr	50.5	24.6	13.0
Cocaine			
12-17 yr	2.4	1.5	0.4
18-25 yr	17.9	7.7	2.0
Hallucinogens			
12-17 yr	3.4	2.1	0.8
18-25 yr	13.2	4.8	1.2
Inhalants			
12-17 yr	7.0	4.1	1.8
18-25 yr	10.9	3.5	1.5

*Includes marijuana, inhalants, cocaine, hallucinogens, heroin, and nonmedicinal use of psychotherapeutics.
Adapted from U.S. Department of Health and Human Services, Public Health Service: Alcohol, Drug Abuse, and Mental Health Administration, National Household Survey on Drug Abuse; Population Estimates, 1991, Rockville, Md.: U.S. Department of Health and Human Services, Public Health Service: Alcohol, Drug Abuse, and Mental Health Administration, n.d.; pp. 19-21, 31-33, 37-39, 49-51, 91-93, 109-111, 121-123.

during the past year, with more than 60% reporting use in the previous month. In all three use categories (ever, past year, and past month), whites reported higher percentages of use than blacks and Hispanics.[16] According to the Youth Risk Behavior Survey—United States, 1993,[5] 80.4% of all high school students had at least one drink of alcohol in their lifetime. Eleventh and twelfth graders were significantly more likely than ninth and tenth graders to have drunk alcohol. More than half of all students (51.6%) had had at least one drink of alcohol in the month preceding the survey. Nationwide, 32.6% of students had had five or more drinks of alcohol in the month preceding the survey. Across ethnic/racial and upper grade subgroups, male students were significantly more likely than females to report episodic heavy drinking.

ILLICIT DRUGS. Approximately one in five 12- to 17-year-olds, and over half of those aged 18 to 25, reported having used an illicit drug (Table 3-3). Within the older age group, use during the previous month approximated 15%.[16]

Marijuana use. Over half of adolescents and young adults (aged 18 to 25 years) had had some lifetime experience with marijuana, with 13% of this age group reporting use during the previous month (Table 3-3). In the 1995 Youth Risk Behavior Survey, nearly one third (42.4%) of high school students nationwide had used marijuana in their lifetimes, and 17.7% had used marijuana at least once in the month preceding the survey.[5]

Cocaine use. In 1991, 2.4% of 12- to 17-year-olds had tried cocaine at least once in their lifetime, and 17.9% of youths 18 to 25 years old had ever used cocaine. In 1991, reported crack use was lower than that of cocaine, with 0.9% of 12 to 17-year-olds and 3.7% of 18- to 25-year-olds having ever used crack, 0.4% of 12- to 17-year-olds and 1% of 18- to 25-year-olds having used crack in the previous year, and 0.1% of 12- to 17 year-olds and 0.4% of 18- to 25-year-olds having used crack in the previous month.[16] In the 1995 Youth Risk Behavior Survey, nationwide, 7.0% of high school students had used cocaine during their lifetime, and 3.1% had used cocaine in the month preceding the survey. Hispanic students, irrespective of gender, were more likely to report lifetime and current cocaine use than black or white students. Nationwide, 4.5% of high school students used crack or free-based forms of cocaine during their lifetime.[5]

Hallucinogens. Lifetime use of hallucinogens reported by 12- to 17-year-olds was 3.4% and by 18- to 25-year-olds 13.2%. A total of 2.1% of 12- to 17-year-olds had used them in the past year, while 0.8% had used them in the past month. In comparison, 4.8% of older teens 18 to 25 years old had used hallucinogens in the past year and 1.2% had used them in the past month.[16]

Inhalants. A total of 7% of 12- to 17-year-olds and 10.9% of 18- to 25-year-olds had ever used inhalants, but 4.1% of younger adolescents used inhalants in the previous year, compared with only 3.5% of 18- to 25-year-olds. Also, 1.8% of younger teens used inhalants over the previous month compared with 1.5% of young adults aged 18 to 25 years.[16]

Injected drugs. According to the 1995 Youth Risk Behavior Survey, nationwide, 2.0% of high school students had injected illegal drugs during their lifetime. Males were more likely to report use than females.[5]

Trends of drug use. An overall comparison of drug use patterns in high school seniors between the class of 1980 and that of 1990 show that the percentage of drugs used in the previous 30 days had declined for alcohol, as well as for illicit drugs.[17] Compared with a decade before, previous month alcohol use among youth aged 12 to 17 years had dropped from 27% in 1982 to 20% in 1991.[18]

CIGARETTE USE. According to the 1995 Youth Risk Behavior Survey, nationwide, 71.3% of students had ever tried cigarettes. Older grade students were more likely to have smoked than students in ninth or tenth grade. More than one third of students (34.8%) smoked more than one cigarette in the month preceding the survey; 16.1% had smoked for more than 20 of the 30 days preceding the survey; and nearly one third had smoked at least one cigarette a day for 30 days. White students were more likely than black or Hispanic students to smoke regularly.[5] Over one third (37.9%) of 12- to 17-year-olds and almost three quarters (71.2%) of 18- to 25-year-olds had used cigarettes at least once during their lifetime, and 10.8% of 12- to 17-year-olds had smoked tobacco in the previous month, while 32.2% of 18- to 25-year-olds had smoked in the past month.[16] Compared with a decade earlier, past month cigarette use among youths aged 12 to 17 years had dropped from 15% in 1982 to 11% in 1991.[18]

SMOKELESS TOBACCO. Nationwide, 11.4%, or more than one in ten students, had used smokeless tobacco in the month preceding the 1995 Youth Risk Behavior Survey.[5] Males were more likely than females to chew. White males were significantly more likely than black or Hispanic males to chew. Smokeless tobacco use was seen predominantly in white males, with 11.8% of 12- to 17-year-olds and 21.8% of 18- to 25-year-olds ever having engaged in this behavior.[18]

ANABOLIC STEROIDS. Although anabolic steroids were not always considered a drug of abuse, their use, particularly by athletes, has been the subject of study. According to the 1995 Youth Risk Behavior Survey, 3.7% of high school students had at one time or another used steroids without a doctor's prescription. Not surprisingly, males were far more likely than females to report use.[5]

Sexual Activity

Sexual behaviors among adolescents contribute to sexually transmitted disease and unintended pregnancy. According to the 1995 Youth Risk Behavior Survey,[5] more than half (50.3%) of all high school students had sexual intercourse during their lifetimes. Black students were significantly more likely to be nonvirginal than white students. Among female and male students, prevalence rates increased significantly from ninth to twelfth grade. Nationwide, 17.8% of students had sexual intercourse with four or more partners. More than 37.9% had had sexual intercourse within the three months before the survey, an indicator of current sexual activity. The prevalence of current sexual activity increased with grade. Both black and Hispanic males were more likely than females to be currently sexually active, whereas white females were more likely than white males to be currently sexually active. In that same survey,[5] 54.4% of sexually active high school teens nationwide reported condom usage during their last sexual intercourse. Males were more likely than females to report that a condom was used, whereas 17.4% of sexually active high school students nationwide reported that they or their partners were using birth control pills during the last sexual intercourse (see Chapter 141, Contraceptive Technology).

SEXUALLY TRANSMITTED DISEASES. Three million adolescents acquire sexually transmitted diseases (STDs) annually. In 1992, of the estimated 12 million new cases of STD, one quarter were among adolescents 19 years old and younger, while 41% were among young adults aged 20 to 24 years.[19] The most commonly contracted infections were from *Chlamydia,* gonorrhea, *Trichomonas,* human papillomavirus (HPV), genital herpes, hepatitis B, syphilis, and human immunodeficiency virus (HIV). Between 10% and 29% of sexually experienced adolescent females tested for STDs have been diagnosed with *Chlamydia* infection.[20] Although 1995 was the first year genital infections with *Chlamydia* were nationally notifiable, this condition was the most commonly reported disease for 1995, however age data remain unavailable.[21] Sexually experienced adolescents between the ages of 15 and 19 years have higher rates of gonorrhea than any other 5-year age group between 20 and 44 years.[20] In 1995, gonorrhea remained the most frequently reported infectious disease (645 per 100,000) among persons 15 to 24 years.[23] In 1995, the adolescent syphilis rate was 13.7 per 100,000, which has more than doubled since the 1980s.[19,23] Up to 1% of sexually experienced female adolescents are infected with HPV, of which some strains have been associated with cervical dysplasia.[24] (see Chapter 140, Sexually Transmitted Disease).

PREGNANCY TRENDS. In addition to the high prevalence of STDs, female adolescents experience high rates of unintended pregnancy. Twelve percent of all adolescents aged 15 to 19 years and 21% of those who are sexually experienced become pregnant each year, resulting in over 1 million adolescent pregnancies annually. At least 85% of the pregnancies are unintended. Half of these pregnancies are carried to term, while a third end in elective abortion.[22] (see Chapter 142, Adolescent Pregnancy, Chapter 143, Adolescent Parenting, and Chapter 144, Abortion).

ABORTION TRENDS. In 1992 the national abortion-to-birth ratio was the lowest recorded since 1977. From 1973, when abortion was legalized, to the mid-1980s the abortion ratio increased and peaked in 1984 at 364 per 1,000 live births. The abortion ratio has since declined steadily to 335 per 1,000 in 1992. The national abortion rate (the number of abortions per females of reproductive age) increased from 17 per 1,000 women aged 15 to 44 years in 1974 to 25 per 1,000 in 1980 and has since remained unchanged at a rate of 23 to 24 per 1,000.[26] In 1992 adolescents 19 years of age or younger obtained 165,675 abortions. Abortion ratios were highest for those adolescents who were under 15 years of age (790 per 1,000 live births) as compared with those who were 15 to 19 years of age (440 per 1,000 live births). In contrast, abortion rates were highest for women aged 20 to 24 years (42 per 1,000 women) and for those 15 to 19 years (26 per 1,000) while they were lowest for adolescents under 15 years of age (3 per 1,000 women). For most age groups, the abortion ratio rose from 1974 to the mid-1980s and then declined until 1992.[26] The abortion ratio for adolescents under the age of 15 years remains the highest ratio among all the age groups, however, the abortion ratio for adolescents 15 to 19 years has decreased for 5 consecutive years with the lowest ratio for that age group reported in 1992. The majority of women (87%) nationwide obtained abortions during the first 12 weeks of pregnancy, however, women 19 years or younger were more likely than older women to obtain abortions later in pregnancy. Increases in the number of adolescents giving birth, rather than decreases in pregnancy rates, may account for the decline in the abortion ratio. These trends may reflect changes in adolescents' attitudes toward carrying unplanned pregnancies to term, as well as changes in access to abortion services and changes in abortion laws such as parental consent or notification laws and mandatory waiting periods, which may disproportionately affect adolescents' abortion decisions.

SUMMARY

Morbidity and mortality rates in adolescents reflect the broader society. The increasing rates of violence and crime, drug use, and pregnancy warrant closer evaluation to develop solutions. The evolution of antibiotics and medical technology has minimized the impact of infectious illnesses. Formerly fatal diseases now render adolescents survivors with a chronic illness. The impact of these chronic illnesses on other risk factors and behavior is an area of study in its earliest phases.[27] Morbidity and mortality secondary to adolescent behavior have emerged as the major health issues of this era. In this chapter we have outlined some basic concepts of epidemiology, cited some of the problems in this area, and shared some statistics with regard to the most vexing problems facing adolescents today. It is our hope that, over time, mortality and morbidity rates will decline, so that adolescents can live healthier and more fulfilling lives.

References

1. Elston RC, Johnson WD: *Essentials of biostatistics,* ed 2, Philadelphia, 1994, FA Davis, pp 3-9.
2. Dawson-Saunders B, Trapp TG: *Basic and clinical biostatistics,* Norwalk, CT, 1990, Appleton & Lange, pp 1-6.
3. American Psychiatric Association: *Diagnostic and statistical manual of mental disorders (DSM-IV),* ed 4, Washington DC, 1994, American Psychiatric Association.
4. American Academy of Pediatrics: *Diagnostic and statistical manual for primary care: child and adolescent version (DSM-PC: child and adolescent version),* Elk Grove Village, IL, 1996, American Academy of Pediatrics.
5. Youth Risk Behavior Surveillance—United States, 1993: *MMWR* 44:1-56, 1995. US Department of Health and Human Services, Public Health Service, Centers for Disease Control and Prevention, Atlanta, GA.
6. US Bureau of the Census: 1990 Census of Population and Housing, 1990 CPH-1 and summary tape file 1C.
7. US Department of Health and Human Services: Public Health Services. Centers for Disease Control and Prevention. National Center for Health Statistics. *Health, United States,* Hyattsville, MD, 1993, Public Health Service, pp 49-51.
8. 1993 Statistical Abstracts of the United States on CD-ROM: CD-ABSTR-93, Washington, DC, 1993, US Department of Commerce, Economics and Statistics Administration, Bureau of the Census, Data User Services Division.
9. Trends in rates of homicide—United States, 1994-1995, *MMWR* 45:460-464, 1996.
10. Children's Safety Network, 1991: *A data book of child and adolescent injury,* Washington, DC, 1991, National Center for Education in Maternal and Child Health, p 10.
11. Anon: Top ten killers of teens, *Curr Health* 2:8, 1993.
12. 1993 Statistical Abstracts of the United States on CD-ROM: CD-ABSTR-93, Washington, DC, 1993, US Department of Commerce, Economics and Statistics Administration, Bureau of the Census, Data User Services Division.
13. US Department of Transportation. National Highway Traffic Safety Administration. National Center for Statistics and Analysis. 1991 Fatality Facts. Washington, DC, c. 1991, National Center for Statistics and Analysis, Research and Development, p 1.
14. US Department of Transportation. National Highway Traffic Safety Administration. National Center for Statistics and Analysis. 1991 Pedacyclist Fatal Crash Facts. Washington, DC, c. 1991, National Center for Statistics and Analysis, Research and Development, p 3.
15. US Department of Transportation. National Highway Traffic Safety Administration. National Center for Statistics and Analysis. 1991 Traffic Fatality Facts. Washington, DC, c. 1991, National Center for Statistics and Analysis, Research and Development, p 4.
16. US Department of Health and Human Services. Public Health Service. Alcohol, Drug Abuse, and Mental Health Administration, National Household Survey on Drug Abuse: Population Estimates, 1991. Rockville, MD, US Department of Health and Human Services, Public Health Service. Alcohol, Drug Abuse, and Mental Health Administration, pp 19-21, 31-33, 37-39, 49-51, 91-93, 109-111, 121-123.

17. US Department of Education. Office of Educational Research and Improvement. National Center for Education Statistics. Digest of Education Statistics, 1992. Washington, DC, 1992, US Government Printing Office, p 139.

18. Use of selected substances in the past month by youths 12-17 years of age and young adults 18-25 years of age, according to age, sex, race, and hispanic origin: United States, selected years 1974-91, Health United States 1992 and Health People 2000 Review, 1993, US Department of Health and Human Services, Table 66, pp 97-99, 104-105.

19. Centers for Disease Control and Prevention: Division of STD/HIV Prevention, 1992 Annual Report, Atlanta, GA, 1993.

20. Schacter J: Why we need a program for the control of *Chlamydia trachomatis, N Engl J Med* 320:802-804, 1989.

21. Ten leading nationally notifiable infectious diseases—United States, 1995, *MMWR* 45:883-884, 1996.

22. Centers for Disease Control and Prevention: Division of STD/HIV Prevention, 1991 Annual Report, Atlanta, GA, 1992.

23. Centers for Disease Control and Prevention Summary of Notifiable Diseases, United States—1995, *MMWR* (suppl) 44:1-86, 1996.

24. Moscicki A, et al: Human papillomavirus infection in sexually active adolescent females: prevalence and risk factors, *Pediatr Res* 28:507-513, 1990.

25. Spitz AM, Ventura SJ, Koonin LM, et al: Surveillance for pregnancy and birth rates among teenagers by state—United States, 1980 and 1990. CDC Surveillance Summaries, *MMWR* 42:1-27, 1993.

26. Koonin LM, Smith JC, Ramick M, Green CA: Abortion surveillance—United States, 1992, *MMWR* 45:1-36, 1996.

27. Gold MA, Gladstein J: Substance use among diabetic adolescents: preliminary findings, *J Adolesc Health,* 14:80-84, 1993.

CHAPTER 4

International Health

•

Cristina Lammers and Robert Wm. Blum

Adolescence is often viewed as the healthiest life stage in which, compared with other age groups, mortality rates are comparatively low. However, mortality is but one measure of health status, and in this chapter we explore not only the major causes of death for adolescents around the world but also the major causes of morbidity.

It has always been assumed that mortality in poorer countries is due to infectious diseases such as tuberculosis. However, recent data show that causes of morbidity and mortality in developing countries are to a great extent the same as in nonindustrialized countries.

MORTALITY

One trend of the 1980s is that, for many countries where data are available, mortality rates in the second decade of life have declined. In France, for example, there was a downward trend in juvenile fatalities from 6545 deaths in 1990 to 6085 deaths 2 years later. In Latin America, adolescents represented 7.4% of all deaths in 1986, which was a 3.5% decline from 7 years earlier. Looking regionally, we see substantial variations among countries. In Costa Rica, juveniles represent 4.4% of deaths; in the Southern Cone (Chile, Argentina, Paraguay, and Uruguay), it is 7.4%; and in the Andean Region of Latin America (Bolivia, Colombia, Ecuador, Peru, and Venezuela), it is 12.7%. In comparison, juvenile deaths account for 5.5% of all mortality in the United States.

A closer look at mortality figures for almost every country where data are available indicates that juvenile males are at least at twice the risk of dying as their female counterparts. In Switzerland, for example, excess mortality among male adolescents is four times that of females. In Latin America, overall male mortality is twice that of adolescent females. These trends reflect the externalizing and violent risk taking of males, while it appears that females throughout the world are more internalizing.

Another trend observed around the world is the jump in mortality rates between the ages of 15 and 19 years. Data from Australia, Switzerland, Israel, and the United States all indicate that mortality risk declines steadily from 1 to 14 years of age, and then increases thereafter. Similar trends are seen in Latin America. Improved immunization coupled with control of infectious diseases has resulted in unprecedented child survival in much of the developing world; however, behavioral etiologies appear to account for the rise in juvenile mortality worldwide during middle and late adolescence.

When causes of death are explored, the trends become more understandable, for there is a striking similarity of etiologies for juvenile mortality in both industrialized and developing nations around the world: unintentional injuries, suicide, homicide, maternal mortality (in developing nations) and, increasingly, AIDS. There are some notable differences, however, especially in Asia. In Hong Kong, the leading causes of death in young people 10 to 14 years of age are unintentional injuries, malignancies, and infections. For older adolescents, unintentional injuries and suicide are the leading causes, with malignancies third. Similar variations are seen among the top five causes of juvenile mortality, reflecting cultural norms such as attitudes toward suicide or the extent of interpersonal violence. However, in most countries, external causes of death predominate during the second decade.

Unintentional Injury

Fatal vehicular injuries range from 6.8% in Chile to 24.1% in Venezuela for young people aged 10 to 19 years. Likewise, as automobiles become more available in developing countries, so too do the rates of juvenile vehicle-related deaths. Thus, for example, there was a 600% increase in juvenile fatalities related to automobiles in Mexico in the years 1965 to 1985 and a 250% increase in Venezuela. Conversely, in industrialized countries where availability of automobiles has been widespread for a longer period, most of the reduction in juvenile mortality overall is related to reduction in vehicular deaths. Factors that have had greatest impact on reducing vehicular deaths include reduction of highway speeds, improved automotive safety technology (e.g., air bags), and an increased legal age for the purchase of alcohol from 18 to 21 years. Similar trends have been seen in most industrialized countries, with significant reductions in automotive fatalities in the 1980s.

Suicide

Deliberate self-harm is the second leading cause of death in many countries. In many Latin American countries such as Costa Rica, Chile, Uruguay, and Ecuador, suicide accounts for 5% of all deaths among adolescents. However, even these data are incomplete, for where there is a religious or cultural taboo, suicide is underreported. Despite that fact, global trends suggest that suicide rates are on the increase. In Israel, suicide rates have shown a notable rise, especially among non-Jewish males 15 to 19 years of age. These data are very similar to those in Australia, where suicide is the second most common cause of death for youths 15 to 24 years of age, accounting for 22.6% of male mortality and 12.4% of female mortality in those age groups. New Zealand data are comparable, as are those of much of

Europe. In Portugal and Switzerland, suicide is second to unintentional injuries as the leading cause of death in the second decade. In Switzerland, suicide accounts for 20.1% of all adolescent male deaths and 4.0% of adolescent female deaths. For juvenile males in Norway and Holland, suicide represents 15.6% of all causes of death.

Not every country has shown an increase in suicide rates. Mediterranean countries have shown less of an increase than Northern Europe. Why this is the case is uncertain, but the extent of social flux within a country may be highly predictive of juvenile suicide rates. Perhaps social role changes (e.g., dual parent employment, secularization, women's roles) in Northern Europe are significantly greater than those in Mediterranean countries, explaining at least in part the differences seen. Hong Kong, with relatively low rates, has seen little change since the mid-1970s. What has paralleled the West, however, in Hong Kong are the increases with age: 0.55% for those aged 10 to 14, 3.6% for those aged 15 to 19, and 9.8% for 20- to 24-year-olds. Despite the increased prevalence of suicide attempts with age, there has also been a dramatic increase in suicides among the youngest adolescents. In Hong Kong and elsewhere in Asia (e.g., Singapore and Taiwan), there is a more narrow gender differential: male-to-female ratio of 1.3:1 rather than between 1.8:1 and 3.0:1 as is seen in many Western countries.

Where survey data are available, it appears that significant numbers of young people are at risk for both injury and death as a consequence of deliberate self-harm. Data from France for 1994 indicate that 15.4% of all adolescents attempt suicide at least once—rates very similar to those reported in the United States.

One significant factor associated with increased mortality from homicide and suicide is the increased lethality of the methods used. In the United States, 81% of the increase in suicide among youths 15 to 19 years of age since the mid-1980s was related to the use of guns. As has been historically true, males are significantly more likely than females to use firearms in suicide attempts. In Asia, jumping from high buildings predominates as the method of choice for suicide in young people.

Homicide

While less common than death from injury or suicide in many countries, homicide is increasingly being acknowledged as a major cause of death among young people. Homicide is responsible for 16.9% of all juvenile deaths in Puerto Rico, 12.4% in Mexico, and 8.3% in Brazil. In many countries in Europe, although homicide rates remain low among young people, there are clear and worrisome upward trends.

Maternal Mortality

Maternal mortality remains one of the leading causes of death for young people in developing countries where labor complications and septic abortions are not uncommon. Clearly, in many countries, young women are at significantly higher risk than older women for perinatal death. Such risks include toxemia, cephalopelvic disproportion, and placenta previa for the mother; and low birthweight, trauma, postpartum infections, and prematurity for the infant. Among teens 15 to 19 years of age, pregnancy complications account for 19.4% of all deaths in the second decade in Paraguay, 13.0% in Ecuador, 8.2% in the Dominican Republic, and 7.2% in El Salvador. In Chile, pregnancy complications are the leading cause of hospitalizations, other than for obstetric services, among women 15 to 24 years of age.

The perinatal period is not the only risk for the pregnant adolescent. Abortion is illegal in all of sub-Saharan Africa and Latin America (except Cuba). The World Health Organization (WHO) estimates that approximately half of all maternal mortality stems from septic abortions almost exclusively in countries where abortion is outlawed. In Nigeria, the International Planned Parenthood Federation found that abortion accounted for 72% of all mortality among women 19 years of age and younger. In countries where abortion is legal and performed under medical supervision, mortality among young women is less than two per 100,000. Where it is illegal, the risk increases nearly 100 times with the major causes of death secondary to uterine perforation, sepsis, and hemorrhage. In Kenya, for example, where sterile abortions are uncommon, 50% of all gynecologic admissions of young females to Kenyatta Hospital in Nairobi are for abortion complications. These data become even more tragic when it is realized that, in some developing countries, individuals most likely to resort to abortion are those who are young, urban, and on an education and career track that would be ended by an out-of-wedlock pregnancy.

HIV and AIDS

Increasingly, AIDS is becoming a major cause of death among young people. In Africa, AIDS accounts for 52% of the mortality among young adults and 28% overall. In Uganda, 30% of adults in the reproductive age range (15 to 44 years) are estimated to be HIV positive. In high prevalence areas, certain special populations such as prostitutes have HIV prevalence rates of over 75%.

In summary, there appears to be a convergence of causes of mortality among young people in both industrialized and developing countries such that external causes of death (injuries, homicide, and suicide) account for the majority of deaths in most countries. In developing countries, maternal mortality is an additionally important cause of death. Death from vehicular injuries appears to be declining in many countries, but deaths from suicide and interpersonal violence appear to be in the ascendant. This trend is especially true for males and older adolescents. Death from AIDS is likewise increasing among young people in many countries.

INFECTIOUS DISEASES IN THE DEVELOPING WORLD

Helminths

The WHO estimates that approximately 400 million school-age young people are infected with intestinal helminths affecting growth, nutritional status, physical fitness, and school performance. The quartet of common helminthic infections includes ascariasis, trichuriasis, strongyloidiasis, and hookworm. Hookworms have a peak prevalence during late adolescence and early adulthood. Adolescent females and young adult women appear to be more heavily infected than males. High "worm burden" is associated with iron deficiency anemia, since worms use iron as their source of nutrition. In sub-Saharan Africa in 1991 the estimated prevalence rate for hookworm for women of childbearing age was 32%, with between 7.5 and 7.8 million women both pregnant and infected—a combination highly associated with morbidity.

Schistosomiasis

Schistosomiasis is the second most common parasitic infection after malaria that is endemic in much of Africa, the Eastern Mediterranean, South America, and the Caribbean. Associated symptoms include dysuria and/or hematuria. Contact with contaminated fresh water is the major source of infection, with the snail serving as the host. Males tend to be more commonly infected than females. Peak prevalence is in the second decade of life. Specifically, at puberty there is a marked increase in prevalence, intensity of infection, and manifestations of morbidity. Not uncommonly the genital lesions associated with this condition are confused with sexually transmitted diseases (STDs), thereby causing social stigma. In endemic countries, hematuria is considered *the* pubertal rite of passage.

Tuberculosis

The WHO estimates that 1.3 billion people worldwide have tuberculosis, of whom 3 million die annually. Although it is well known to be associated with the immunocompromised host, tuberculosis appears to be more aggressive around the time of puberty. Thus, adolescents who acquire the disease are more likely than younger children to develop cavitary lesions. Such virulence has been attributed to hormonal changes and to altered protein and calcium metabolism associated with adolescent growth. Clearly, the problem is compounded by poverty, crowding, and insanitary living conditions. Gender distribution appears to be approximately equal until 15 years of age, after which time the risk is higher for males. Bacille Calmette-Guérin (BCG) vaccine is commonly given at birth in many developing countries, but its effectiveness in preventing adult disease remains controversial. For children under 14 years, effectiveness estimates are in the range of 40% to 70%.

MORBIDITY: A FOCUS ON RISK FACTORS

As the major causes of death among the world's adolescents are external in etiology, so too are the major morbidities predominantly behavioral rather than infectious in etiology. A range of social factors influence the nature of the problems: poverty and extreme poverty, rural to urban migration, international migration, increasing education of both females and males, the changing roles of women, the decline of the agrarian society, urban overcrowding, and the changing nature of marriage and the family. This section focuses on two major domains of adolescent risk behaviors that result in morbidity: sexual behaviors and substance abuse.

Sexual Behaviors and Sexually Transmitted Diseases

The age at marriage increases around the world, and so do the number of years between puberty and marriage, increasing the risk of out-of-wedlock childbearing. With the increase in education of young women in many countries, early pregnancy frequently has more dire consequences today than in previous generations. Further complicating this picture is the trend in many countries to earlier ages of sexual debut. One out of six adolescents in Mexico City, 30% of young people in Guatemala, and 40% of teenagers in El Salvador and Brazil have initiated intercourse before the age of 15 years. Likewise, 45.5% of males in Spain report having had intercourse on or before their fifteenth birthday. These figures are consistent with European countries where data are available as well as in North America. While cultural and socioeconomic factors influence variance among countries, the differences are not as dramatic as they once were.

There are no vast differences in trends in sexual activity, nations responding to those trends differ dra-

matically. These responses, in turn, greatly influence morbidity data. For example, in Sweden, family planning, STD treatment and prevention services have been widely available for adolescents since 1975. As a consequence, adolescent birth rates are low, with youths aged 10 to 19 years accounting for only 3.3% of all births in 1990. Similar data are found in Norway, where adolescents account for 2.9% of births, Holland (2.2%), and Switzerland (1.7%), compared with 12.8% of all births in the United States in 1989. In Latin America, El Salvador, Guatemala, and Honduras have continued to have the highest adolescent birth rates in Latin America at more than 150 per 1000. In Mozambique, Africa, the rate is nearly double that of El Salvador.

Because of inconsistent use of contraception, myths about and aversion to barrier methods, and more frequent changing of partners than their adult counterparts, young people are at high risk for acquiring a sexually transmitted infection. Even in countries where sex education is emphasized and family planning services are available, young people all too often remain poor users of contraception. Notable exceptions include Switzerland, where 90% of young people report using contraception at first intercourse, and Scandinavia. In the United States, as in Europe, condom use declines with advancing age as young people switch to oral and injectable forms of contraceptives. The decline with age in the use of barrier contraception clearly predisposes the older adolescent to STDs and AIDS. In many countries of Latin America, Asia, and Africa, policies restricting adolescent access to contraception combine with the lack of availability, keeping pregnancy and STD rates high.

Data from Australia indicate that *Chlamydia trachomatis* is the most common cause of STD, representing 17% of genital infections among 13- to 19-year-old females. Swiss data indicate that 9% of sexually active female adolescents and 14% of their male counterparts have received antibiotic treatment for an STD.

According to the Pan American Health Organization, by 1995, 153,087 cases of AIDS had been reported in the Americas, with the highest prevalence in the United States, followed by Brazil, Mexico, the Dominican Republic, Honduras, and Haiti in descending order. In the Americas, youth from the United States represent 9.8% of all cases of HIV infection. In comparison, 8.3% of HIV-positive individuals and, for the Americas in general, 4% of all AIDS cases occur in adolescence. Even more significant than HIV prevalence in adolescence is the reality in many countries that AIDS incidence is strikingly higher among young adults aged 20 to 29, most of whom were probably infected as adolescents. According to the WHO, half of all HIV-infected people are under 25 years of age. Additionally, ethnic minorities and economically disadvantaged populations are overrepresented among the HIV-infected population.

It does appear that concern over AIDS, coupled with sex education, has an impact on adolescent contraceptive behaviors. Specifically, studies in the United States, Italy, Germany, and Sweden have shown that knowledge about AIDS and condom use have increased among adolescents. However, the age of first intercourse continues to decline in many countries, and little change has been observed in patterns of sexual behavior.

Substance Abuse

Besides illicit substances, the WHO classifies alcohol and tobacco as drugs. In many countries, it appears that drug use and abuse continues to rise among young people and is often a contributing factor to juvenile mortality. In Chile, 65% of all young people who committed suicide, and 71% of those who were involved in fatal vehicular injuries, were intoxicated. Drug use is also associated with fighting, poor academic performance, and the carrying of weapons. Among those 15 to 19 years of age, alcohol use increased 400% between 1958 and 1981 in Latin America. In Australia, weekly use of alcohol was reported by 11% of seventh graders, rising to 47% of those in the eleventh grade. In Switzerland, 3% of adolescent males and 1% of adolescent females are daily drinkers. In France, 12% of youths report regular drinking. Not only does there appear to be an increase in the prevalence of adolescent drinking in many countries, but European studies suggest that the amounts consumed have also increased, creating a very dangerous situation.

In many countries of Europe and North America, there was a decline in the percentage of juvenile cigarette smokers during the latter half of the 1980s. In Austria, 20% of youths are current smokers, a decline from 1987; in Chile, it is 28%. In France, smoking rises dramatically through adolescence to reach 43% of 18-year-old males. Large-scale surveys throughout Europe show little change in juvenile smoking prevalence during the 1990s. In Latin America and Africa, where data on tobacco use are less available, it appears that smoking use has increased among juveniles, perhaps coinciding with a major shift of focus of multinational tobacco companies from the northern to the southern hemisphere. China remains the largest tobacco producer in the world.

Marijuana appears to be the most widely used illicit substance in the world. Fifteen percent of young people in Mexico and Chile and 40% of youths in Brazil report regular use. Among Australian youths, marijuana use was reported by 28% of adolescents 16 years of age and older.

While cocaine and its derivatives are an increasing problem in many countries in Latin America and Europe, their use remains significantly less than that of the "big three" drugs of abuse: alcohol, tobacco, and marijuana. They also tend to be drugs used more by young adults than by adolescents. Younger teens are more likely to abuse inhalants in many countries where drug use patterns have been studied.

In summary, the use of all drugs (except inhalants) appears to increase throughout the teenage years. In many countries of the developing world, tobacco use among young people is increasing, and in some industrialized countries such as France, there appears to be a new trend toward increased usage. In the case of most drugs of abuse, males use more than females. Cigarettes are a notable exception to this trend: in most countries, female adolescents appear more likely to smoke than male adolescents. While illicit drug use appears to be a more urban than rural phenomenon, many countries report at least as high or higher use of alcohol and tobacco in the rural areas. Clearly, alcohol and illicit drugs are not only associated with long-term morbidity but also highly correlated with juvenile mortality.

YOUTHS' VIEWS OF THEIR OWN HEALTH

Despite the causes of morbidity and mortality in young people around the world, it is evident that they utilize health services less than do their adult counterparts. One reason may lie in their perception of their own health status. Most youths report their health as *good* to *excellent;* however, when specific questions are asked, concerns emerge.

In Switzerland, youths aged 15 to 20 years described their main health concerns as stress, depression, school problems, nutrition, sports-related injuries, and conflicts with parents and peers. Far down the list of concerns was substance abuse. Similar issues have been identified in Australia, Canada, and Israel.

Adolescents acknowledge major health concerns but are reluctant to seek health care services, frequently reserving a medical visit for a time when they are very ill. Barriers to health care are similar to those in the United States and include embarrassment, time and financial costs, taboos, confidentiality, and a perception that health care professionals are often unwilling to provide the time required to meet the needs of youth. As a consequence, delay in seeking help is common.

In truth, where it has been studied, it appears that health care professionals throughout the world are often ill-prepared to address the social and behavioral etiologies that underlie many adolescent morbidities. If we are to be effective in meeting the needs of youth, we must understand their health concerns not only in relation to morbidity and mortality trends but also from the perspectives of young people themselves.

Acknowledgment

Supported, in part, by the American Association of University Women, International Fellowship Award. Additional support from the Maternal and Child Health Bureau, MCJ #00095.

References

1. Choquet M, Ledoux S: *Adolescents—enquette nationale analyses et prospective,* Paris, 1994, Inserm.
2. Boss P, Edwards S, Pitman S, eds: *Profile of young Australians—facts, figures and issues,* 1995, Cambera.
3. Maddaleno M, Silber TJ: An epidemiological view of adolescent health in Latin America, *J Adolesc Health* 14:595-604, 1993.
4. DiClemente R: Epidemiology of AIDS, HIV prevalence and HIV incidence among adolescents, *J School Health,* 62:325-330, 1992.
5. Males M: Teen suicide and changing cause of death certification, 1953-1987, *Suicide Life Threat Behav* 21 (3):245-259, 1991.
6. Maddaleno M, Munist M, Serrano C, Silber T, Suares Ojeda E, Yunes J, eds: *La salud del adolescente y del joven,* Washington, DC, 1995, Organizacion Panamericana de la Salud.
7. The National Council for the Child: *The state of the child in Israel,* statistical abstract, Tel Aviv, 1995, Minister of Health.
8. Narring F, Tschumper A, Michaud PA, et al: La santé des adolecents en Suisse. Rapport d'une enquete nationale sur la santé et les styles de vie des 15-20 ans, Lausanne, 1994, Institut Universitaire de Medecine Sociale et Preventive.
9. Mortality trends and leading causes of death among adolescents and young adults—United States, 1979-1988, *MMWR* 42:459-462, 1993.
10. Bacci A, Manhica GM, Machungo F, Bugalho A, Cuttini M: Outcome of teenage pregnancy in Maputo, Mozambique, *Int J Gynaecol Obstet* 49:19-23, 1993.

CHAPTER 5

Endocrine Physiology at Puberty

•

Jordan W. Finkelstein

Puberty is the process that transforms the child into a sexually mature person capable of reproduction. This process involves changes in the secretion of numerous hormones, enzymes, and other physiologically active substances and is accompanied by marked changes in physical growth and maturation and in many behaviors. This chapter describes the most important changes in the secretion of hormones that accompany the pubertal process. An understanding of the physiologic and hormonal changes that take place during puberty provides a basis for comprehending both the physical and the behavioral changes that occur during this phase of the life cycle.

CONCEPTS OF HORMONAL REGULATION

Most studies elucidating changes in hormone secretion during puberty have been cross-sectional in design. The research has consisted of two basic types. First, groups of children and adolescents of varying chronologic or developmental ages have been examined. Such studies are useful for understanding hormonal change over long periods (months to years). Second, smaller groups of youths have had the concentrations of hormones measured at frequent intervals (minutes to hours) over a short period (usually a maximum of 24 hours). Both types of studies are necessary to a full understanding of the dynamics of change in adolescents.

The major hormonal changes involve alterations in the functioning of the hypothalamic-pituitary-target endocrine organ axis. In general, stimuli impinge on neurosecretory neurons in the hypothalamus, which results in the production and secretion of releasing hormones in the hypothalamus. The releasing hormones are transported by the pituitary portal plexus to the pituitary gland, which then releases a trophic hormone. This trophic hormone is transported in the bloodstream to the target gland, where it binds to receptors and stimulates hormone synthesis. For example, in one of the most important systems in puberty, the hypothalamic-pituitary-gonadal axis, the hypothalamus contains neurosecretory neurons located mainly in the medial basal hypothalamus and the arcuate nucleus. The axons terminate in the central portion of the basal hypothalamus, the median eminence. At this site, gonadotropin-releasing hormone (GnRH—a decapeptide) is synthesized and released into the portal plexus, which carries it to the pituitary. In the pituitary the releasing hormone causes the synthesis and secretion of the gonadotropins follicle-stimulating hormone (FSH) and luteinizing hormone (LH) into the circulation, which stimulates the gonadal cells to produce germ cells (sperm or ova) and sex steroids (estrogens and androgens).

The hypothalamic-pituitary-gonadal system has three modes of interaction with the gonads: tonic, cyclic, and episodic (or pulsatile). In most other systems, only the tonic and pulsatile systems of interaction apply. *Tonic* secretion is regulated by the classic negative feedback system. When the concentration of sex steroids is low, the hypothalamus secretes more releasing hormone, which then stimulates the pituitary to release more gonadotropins, and this in turn stimulates the gonads to release more sex steroids. When the concentration of sex steroids is high enough, releasing hormone and gonadotropin release are inhibited. *Cyclic* secretion occurs only in females and relates to the menstrual cycle. In this instance, just before ovulation a positive or stimulatory feedback system is in operation. A high concentration of estrogen causes the release (rather than inhibition) of large amounts of gonadotropins, which in turn stimulate ovulation. *Episodic* secretion occurs when the hypothalamic pulse generator (a signal-producing mechanism acting independently of either of the two feedback systems previously mentioned) causes the secretion of a releasing hormone in a periodic manner. All the major pituitary hormones are secreted episodically, with pulses occurring in adults about every 90 minutes. It is important to recognize that this phenomenon occurs because the concentration of any hormone that is secreted episodically may change significantly from one minute to the next. Laboratory results obtained from single samples of blood for clinical purposes may not yield sufficient information; therefore, samples obtained over the course of an hour or several hours may be required for diagnostic purposes.

In addition to releasing hormones, inhibiting hormones may play a role in regulation of the pituitary hormones and therefore in target gland secretion. Somatostatin inhibits the release of growth hormone, thyrotropin, glucagon, and insulin. Some hormones also act to regulate the cells that secrete them (autocrine actions) or to regulate the cells that lie adjacent to them (paracrine actions). Thus, local regulation of secretion also occurs. In some instances, pituitary hormones act on organs not traditionally thought to be endocrine glands. This occurs with growth hormone, which acts on the liver to produce insulin-like growth factor 1 (IGF-1). Other organs, such as the gastrointestinal tract, secrete molecules that some researchers now consider to be hormones. The list of putative hormones is therefore steadily increasing. The role of the classic neurotransmitters in the stimulation and inhibition of hormones must be acknowledged. Details of these hormones and their actions are beyond the scope of this discussion, and little is known about changes in their secretion during adolescence. (See Suggested Readings.)

ONSET OF PUBERTY

Throughout the period from the end of the first year of life until 6 to 8 years of age, the concentration of most hormones involved in pubertal development changes very little from day to day. The negative feedback system seems to be functional and pulsatile secretion occurs for most of the hormones, but the positive feedback system is not operative. At approximately 6 to 8 years of age, secretion of androgenic hormones from the adrenal gland increases. This is referred to as *adrenarche*. At this time, dehydroepiandrosterone and other related weakly androgenic compounds are secreted by the adrenal glands independently of trophic hormone control (no increase occurs in either adrenocorticotropic hormone [ACTH], or the gonadotropins [FSH or LH]). During adrenarche the concentration of androgens is significantly higher than that seen in younger children. This change occurs several years before the appearance of any clinical effects, such as the development of sexual hair, but in some children increases in sebaceous and apocrine gland activity may occur, causing oily skin and adult body odor. Some endocrinologists consider adrenarche to be the initiating factor controlling the onset of puberty.

Others, however, have documented another mechanism responsible for the changes in hormone secretion at puberty. This mechanism involves a change in the sensitivity of the negative feedback system. A part of this system, which is presumed to be located in the brain and has been termed the *gonadostat*, seems to be very sensitive to low concentrations of sex steroids during the prepubertal period. At puberty, but before clinical puberty is evident, the sensitivity of the gonadostat decreases so that higher concentrations of sex steroids are required to induce negative feedback. Because of this change, greater amounts of gonadotropins are secreted, which results in greater production of sex steroids by the gonads. A new set point for the gonadostat is then established. Thus, in late prepuberty and at the onset of puberty, adrenarche occurs, and there is decreasing sensitivity of the gonadostat to sex steroids, resulting in increased concentrations of FSH, LH, androgens, and estrogens. All of these hormones are secreted episodically, and studies that used the frequent sampling technique report that the average concentration of gonadotropins is minimally higher during sleep than during wakeful states, when the concentration is clearly in the prepubertal range. At this early stage in puberty, positive feedback is not yet established.

CHANGES IN THE HYPOTHALAMIC-PITUITARY-GONADAL AXIS

As puberty progresses, significant changes in concentrations or patterns of secretion occur in two important hormonal systems. Changes in the hypothalamic-pituitary-gonadal system are described in this section; changes in the growth hormone–IGF-1 system are discussed in the section on growth hormone. The change in the hypothalamic-pituitary-gonadal axis is called *gonadarche*. A significant increase in the mean concentration of FSH and LH occurs during the sleep period, but there is no increase in the mean concentration during wakefulness. Pulsatile secretion of gonadotropins occurs. Several investigators have demonstrated this change in normal children, and it may be used to define the onset of puberty. Because this change occurs before any obvious increase in the size of the gonads takes place, it can be termed *hormonal puberty*. Although this has not been demonstrated, it is assumed that during the very earliest part of this phase, increased release of GnRH occurs, with little or no increase in the secretion of sex steroids. It is not known how long this sleep-associated augmentation phenomenon for gonadotropins must occur before a corresponding increase in the secretion of sex steroids from the gonads or the appearance of secondary sexual characteristics takes place. During wakefulness the mean concentration of FSH, LH, and sex steroids is the same as that found in prepubertal children. This accounts for the sometimes puzzling clinical finding in which an early adolescent has some secondary sexual development despite gonadotropin concentrations in the prepubertal range. Over time gonadotropin stimulation of the gonads continues, with a significant increase in the concentration of testosterone in males during the sleep phase, coincident with release of FSH and LH, and the earliest signs of male puberty appear. This increased secretion of gonadotropins and testosterone is linked to sleep and not to the time of day. In females the increase in estradiol caused by increased FSH and LH secretion does not occur during the sleep phase but takes place at about 3:00 to 5:00 PM. The reason for this delay in the secretion of estradiol is not known. The earliest signs of puberty occur in females at this time. This phase is usually called early puberty (see Table 5-1 for a description of the physical changes).

Changes in Hypothalamic-Pituitary Secretory Patterns

As puberty progresses, the concentration of gonadotropins and sex steroids continues to rise in both sexes. By midpuberty, concentration of these hormones increases during wakefulness as well as during sleep, but the concentration of FSH, LH, and testosterone during sleep remains significantly higher than during wakefulness (Fig. 5-1). During the late afternoon the concentration of estradiol remains significantly higher than it is during sleep. It has been suggested that gonadotropin secretion pulses occur at a lower frequency in the prepubertal child and increase to approximately every 90 minutes as puberty progresses. In addition, the amplitude of these pulses increases significantly compared with early puberty.

During late puberty the amplitude of pulses increases further so that peak concentrations of FSH and LH during sleep may exceed those seen at any time in adults. The mean concentration of testosterone and estradiol also increases at the same times, as previously described; they do not exceed the concentrations seen in adults. Peak height velocity is reached in most individuals some time during midpuberty to late puberty. There is good correspondence between the maximal concentration of estradiol and peak height velocity in females, but at the time of peak height velocity in males the concentration of testosterone is only about 45% of the maximal level. This suggests that estrogen may play an important role in the regulation of growth in both sexes. At the end of puberty, the concentration of gonadotropins and sex steroids is the

TABLE 5-1
Physical (Tanner) Stages of Puberty

Male Genital Staging

Stage	Testicular Length	Volume	Average Age (95% Range) of Attainment* Chronologic Age	Bone Age
I	Prepubertal	<4 mL		
II	>2.0 cm	4-6 mL	11.2 (9.2-14.2)	11.5 (9.0-13.5)
III	>3.0 cm	>6-<10 mL	12.9 (10.5-15.4)	13.2 (10.5-15.0)
IV	>4.0 cm	10-15 mL	13.8 (11.6-16.0)	14.5 (12.5-16.0)
V	>5.0 cm	>15 mL	14.7 (12.5-16.9)	
Peak height velocity			13.9 (12.3-15.5)	14.5 (12.0-16.0)
Spermarche			13.4 (11.7-15.3)	

Female Breast Staging

Stage	Description	Average Age (95% Range) of Attainment* Chronologic Age	Bone Age
I	None		
II	Bud < diameter of areola	10.9 (8.5-13.3)	10.5 (8.5-13.2)
III	Breast > areolar diameter	12.2 (9.8-14.6)	12.0 (10.2-14.0)
IV	Areola mounded above plane of breast	13.2 (11.4-15.0)	13.5 (11.5-15.0)
V	Adult	14.0 (11.6-16.4)	15.0 (12.5-16.0)
Peak height velocity		12.2 (10.2-14.2)	12.5 (10.0-14.5)
Menarche		12.7 (10.5-15.5)	

(Tanner breast staging does not quantitate breast volume.)

Continued.

same during sleep and wakefulness. The disappearance of the sleep-augmentation phenomenon thus can be used as one method of defining the end of the pubertal process. Sexual maturation has been completed at this time.

Gonadal Changes

Most of the sex steroids in blood are bound to a specific carrier protein called sex hormone–binding globulin. It is thought that only the proportion of sex

TABLE 5-1
Physical (Tanner) Stages of Puberty—cont'd

Pubic Hair Staging

Stage	Description	Male Chro-nologic Age*	Male Bone Age*	Female Chro-nologic Age*	Female Bone Age*
I	None				
II	Sexual hair barely visi-ble at base of phallus or on scro-tum (M); on mons or labia (F)	12.2 (9.2-15.2)	13.5 (11.5-14.5)	10.4 (8.0-12.8)	11.5 (8.5-13.0)
III	Easily visible sexual hair at base of phallus or on mons	13.5 (11.1-15.9)	14.2 (11.5-15.5)	12.2 (9.8-14.6)	12.2 (10.0-14.5)
IV	Sexual hair confined to the su-prapubic region	14.2 (12.0-16.4)	14.2 (12.5-16.5)	13.0 (10.0-15.2)	13.2 (11.0-15.0)
V	Adult—sex-ual hair on medial thighs	14.9 (12.9-16.9)		14.0 (11.6-16.0)	
VI	Sexual hair up linea alba				

*Years.
Adapted from Sizonenko PC: Normal sexual maturation, *Pediatrician* 14;191-201, 1987.

steroid that is free (not bound to sex hormone–binding globulin) is physiologically active. The concentration of sex hormone–binding globulin decreases during puberty and the amount of free sex steroid increases. This may play a role in the rate of progression of puberty.

In males the production of mature sperm occurs sometime during midpuberty. During the course of pubertal development, positive feedback becomes established in females. This system is not completely established in many females until several years after the occurrence of menarche, which accounts for the irregular menstrual pattern seen in many young women (in whom anovulatory cycles occur). During ovulatory cycles, the concentration of FSH gradually increases throughout the early follicular phase; this is responsible for the growth and development of a group of follicles. During the latter half of the follicular phase, the concentration of FSH decreases. The concentration of LH also increases during the follicular phase. The concentration of estradiol increases slowly during the first half of this phase and

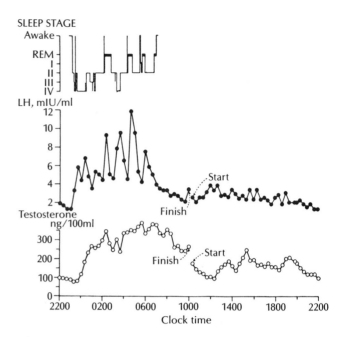

Fig. 5-1. Plasma luteinizing hormone (LH) and testosterone in midpuberty. (From Boyar RM, et al: Human puberty: simultaneous augmented secretion of luteinizing hormone and testosterone during sleep, *J Clin Invest* 54:609, 1974.)

then more rapidly until the positive feedback surge of estradiol occurs at midcycle, when its concentration increases rapidly by severalfold. About 24 hours after this surge of estradiol, the concentration of LH markedly increases and is accompanied by a somewhat less striking increase in FSH that lasts 1 to 3 days. Ovulation occurs during this time.

After ovulation, the concentrations of FSH, LH, and estradiol fall sharply; FSH and LH continue to fall during the luteal phase and increase slightly just before menses. Estradiol levels rise slightly to a secondary peak about 6 to 8 days after the LH surge and then fall to a low concentration just before menses. The corpus luteum is formed after ovulation. The corpus luteum secretes progesterone, the concentration of which peaks about 6 to 8 days after the LH surge. As the corpus luteum degenerates, the concentration of progesterone falls to a nadir just before menses. Androstenedione and testosterone also increase at the time of the midcycle LH surge, probably as a result of LH stimulation of the ovarian cells responsible for production of androgen.

In summary, the earliest change in the hypothalamic-pituitary-gonadal axis is increased FSH and LH secretion during sleep; this sleep augmentation continues throughout puberty. Pulse frequency is established at about one pulse every 90 minutes, and the amplitude of pulses increases to a maximum during late puberty. The pattern of testosterone secretion is similar to that of the gonadotropins, but the maximal concentration is not reached until early in adult life. The pattern of estradiol secretion differs only in that the highest peaks occur during the late afternoon rather than during sleep. In the young adult the sleep-augmentation phenomenon no longer occurs, and the concentration of gonadotropins and sex steroids is the same during sleep and wakefulness.

CHANGES IN GROWTH HORMONE

During childhood, secretion of growth hormone occurs mainly during the sleep phase. Growth hormone is secreted in a pulsatile manner, and the pulses seem to be associated with slow-wave sleep. This phase of sleep usually takes place within the first few minutes after onset of sleep and at the beginning of each sleep cycle. Growth hormone may be released during wakefulness, but pulses are of low magnitude and frequency.

In early puberty, little change in growth hormone secretion takes place, although some increase takes place in the amplitude of pulses during wakeful hours. However, by midpuberty secretory episodes occur during both wakefulness and sleep. Both the amplitude and the duration of pulses increase significantly, but pulse frequency remains unchanged and is still associated with slow-wave sleep, occurring at about one pulse every 90 minutes. The mean concentration of growth hormone during sleep is significantly higher than during wakefulness and in comparison with the pulses in the prepubertal period. During late puberty, frequent pulses during wakefulness are of greater amplitude than those that occurred during midpuberty. The sleep-associated pulses also have significantly greater magnitude but the same frequency as those that occurred during earlier stages. In adults, growth hormone secretory patterns are not significantly different from those seen during childhood (i.e., few wakeful pulses, and secretion is mainly related to sleep).

Growth hormone seems to promote growth through its action on the liver, which produces IGF-1. This protein hormone acts on the diaphyseal and epiphyseal cartilaginous growth plates to stimulate growth in length. The concentration of IGF-1 rises significantly during puberty and reaches maximal concentrations coincident with peak height velocity in both males and females.

Both androgens and estrogens are necessary for optimal growth effects. Estrogen seems to play a very important role in termination of linear growth, through its role in increasing epiphyseal maturation and fusion.

In summary, growth hormone is secreted episodically, mainly during sleep in the prepubertal child. During adolescence, increased secretion of growth hormone takes place during sleep, with the greatest amounts secreted during the first sleep cycle in association with slow-wave sleep and lesser amounts secreted during later sleep cycles. As puberty progresses, increased

amounts are secreted during wakefulness, but most growth hormone secretion still occurs during sleep. In the adult, growth hormone secretion resembles that of the prepubertal child. Growth hormone acts through the production of IGF-1, which is produced in the liver, rising in concentration during adolescence and reaching maximal concentration during peak height velocity.

OTHER HORMONAL CHANGES

Secretion of ACTH and cortisol also shows a distinct diurnal variation. The majority of ACTH and cortisol secretion (and presumably corticotropin-releasing factor) occurs between 4:00 and 8:00 AM. Several peaks, often overlapping, take place during this time. Several small peaks commonly occur during waking hours. At approximately midnight, the concentration of cortisol falls to almost undetectable levels and may remain low for several hours. It would seem that the negative feedback system is inoperative at those times. Significant episodes of secretion follow. No significant changes occur in this pattern during puberty. The secretion of cortisol seems to be linked to clock time rather than sleep.

Prolactin is also secreted episodically during childhood. The pattern of secretion resembles that of growth hormone, with most secretion occurring during sleep. This pattern is reached by ages 3 to 6 years and does not seem to change during puberty. Basal (random) concentrations of prolactin are higher in females than in males.

The secretion of thyroid-stimulating hormone (TSH) is similar to that of prolactin, with most of the secretion taking place during sleep and a lesser amount during wakeful hours. No change in TSH secretion is noted during puberty. However, slight decreases occur in the concentration of total thyroxine, triiodothyronine, and thyroxine-binding globulin, which correlate with advancing pubertal development. No significant change takes place in the concentration of free thyroxine during puberty.

No changes have been demonstrated in the secretion of either insulin or glucagon during puberty. However, a decrease in sensitivity to insulin, as measured during intravenous administration of glucose, does seem to occur in normal pubertal adolescents as compared with children or postpubertal adolescents. This is also true for adolescents with diabetes—a fact to keep in mind when managing adolescents with diabetes, who commonly have problems achieving control of blood glucose. Lack of good control is commonly attributed to noncompliance or to stress. Although this may be true in some instances, the change in insulin sensitivity may be a contributing factor.

Melatonin appears to have no role in mediating pubertal development in humans.

Suggested Readings

Bertrand J, Rappaport R, Sizonenko PC: *Pediatric endocrinology: physiology, pathophysiology and clinical aspects,* ed 2, Baltimore, 1993, Williams & Wilkins.
> Along with Kappy (see below), this is the most up-to-date source on hormonal biosynthesis and secretion, feedback control, endocrine rhythms, and neurotransmission concerning children. Also excellent clinical material.

Boyar RM, Wu RHK, Roffwarg HP, Kapen S, Weitzman ED, Hellman L, Finkelstein JW: Human puberty: twenty-four hour estradiol patterns in pubertal girls, *J Clin Endocrinol Metab* 43:1418, 1976.
> Discusses changes in luteinizing hormone and estradiol secretion during puberty in girls.

Cora JF, Rosenfield RL, Furlanetto RW: A longitudinal study of the relationship of plasma somatomedin-C concentration to the pubertal growth spurt, *Am J Dis Child* 141:562, 1987.
> Focuses on change in insulin-like growth factor 1 during puberty.

Delemarre-van de Waal HA, Plant JM, van Rees GP, Schoemaker J: *Control of the onset of puberty,* vol III, Amsterdam, 1989, Elsevier.
> Third in a series of the same name describing the latest research in pubertal development in animals and humans. Best single sources for detailed research in puberty. (Vol II was published after Vol III.)

Grumbach MM, Sizonenko PC, Aubert ML: *Control of the onset of puberty,* vol II, Baltimore, 1990, Williams & Wilkins.
> Second in a series of the same name describing the latest research in pubertal development in animals and humans. Best single source for detailed research in puberty.

Kappy MS, Blizzard RM, Migeon CJ: *The diagnosis and treatment of endocrine disorders of childhood and adolescence,* ed 4, Springfield, IL 1994, Charles C Thomas.
> Along with Bertrand (see above), this is the most up-to-date source on hormonal biosynthesis and secretion, feedback control, endocrine rhythms, and neurotransmission concerning children. Also excellent clinical material.

Martha PM, Rogol AD, Mauras N, Kerrigan JR, Blizzard RM: Growth hormone secretion in puberty. In *Control of the onset of puberty,* vol II. eds Delemarre-van de Waal HA, Plant JM, van Rees GP, Schoemaker J, editors: *Control of the onset of puberty,* vol III, Amsterdam, 1989, Elsevier.
> Offers a description of change in growth hormone secretion during puberty.

Parker LN: The adrenarche, *Endocrinologist* 3:385, 1993.
> Describes hormonal changes during adrenarche.

Rebor RW, Kenegsberg D, Hodgen GD: The normal menstrual cycle and the control of ovulation. In Becker KL, Bilezikian JP, Bremner WJ, Hung W, Kahn RC, Loriaux DL, Rebor RW, Robertson GL, Wantofsky L, editors: *Principles and practice of endocrinology and metabolism,* Philadelphia, 1990, JB Lippincott, p 97.
> Offers a good description of the menstrual cycle.

Rose SR, Nisula BC: Circadian variation of thyrotropin in childhood, *J Clin Endocrinol Metab* 68:1086, 1989.
> Discusses changes in thyroid-stimulating hormone and thyroid hormones during puberty.

Sizonenko PC, Aubert ML: Pituitary gonadotropins prolactin and sex steroids: secretion in prepuberty and puberty. In Grumbach MM, Sizonenko PC, Aubert ML, editors: *Control of the onset of puberty,* vol II, Baltimore, 1990, Williams & Wilkins.
> Describes changes in gonadotropin, sex steroid, and prolactin secretion during puberty.

Veldhuis JD, Urban RJ, Sollenberger MJ, Evans WS, Rogol AD, Johnson ML: Neuroendocrine regulation of the human gonadotropin releasing hormone pulse generator. In Amura H, Shizume K, Yoshida S, editors: *Progress in endocrinology,* New York, 1988, Elsevier, p 433.
> Focuses on the pulse generator controlling gonadotropin-releasing hormone.

CHAPTER 6

Physical Growth and Development

•

Frank M. Biro

PUBERTAL MATURATION

At any given chronologic age, adolescents are in various stages of maturity. These stages may be defined along several lines: cognitive, psychosocial, and biologic. This chapter concentrates on the biologic changes that occur during the adolescent years and discusses the impact of these changes on cognitive and psychosocial factors. In comparison with changes that occur before or after pubertal maturation, the status of psychological and social factors, as well as that of several organ systems, are more closely correlated to pubertal status than to chronologic age.[1]

The most visible and prominent changes are skeletal

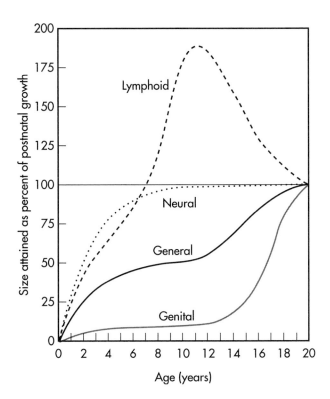

Fig. 6-1. Growth curves in humans.

growth and secondary sexual changes; no less profound are changes in the neuroendocrine axis, alterations in body composition, and the achievement of fertility. The various organ systems mature at different rates, as noted by Scammon and others (Fig. 6-1).[2] This helps to account for certain clinical observations, such as the lower frequency of tonsillectomy during the middle to late teen years. Pubertal maturation affects other systems as well. For example, there are normal cardiovascular changes during puberty, including those noted on electrocardiograms[3]; changes in blood pressure[4]; and changes in cardiac output and heart rate.[5] Teens acquire greater aerobic power reserves as a consequence of the greater stroke volume, decreased heart rate at rest, decreased maximal heart rate, increased cardiac reserve, increased hemoglobin concentration (especially in males), and greater systolic pressure with exercise.[6]

Nearly 25% of adult height occurs during pubertal maturation. Linear growth takes place in two parts: limbs and trunk. The limbs accelerate before the trunk, with the distal portions growing before the proximal portions; literally, in early puberty, the adolescent is "all hands and feet." The timing of the growth spurt (peak height velocity) varies by gender; in girls, there is a consistent temporal relationship to menarche. The disparity in mean height between genders is a result of the timing and peak of the growth spurt. When girls start their spurt, boys are, on the average, 2 cm taller. At that time, because boys continue to grow 3 to 4 cm per year for an additional 1 to 2 years, the delay in

the boys' spurt accounts for 7 cm more. The peak in boys' spurt is greater, accounting for an additional 4 cm. The peak height velocity is 10.3 cm/year in males, and 9.0 cm/year in females; however, when calculated over a 12-month span, these values fall to 9.5 cm/year in males and 8.4 cm in females.

Several important observations are associated with the height spurt. There is an increase in alkaline phosphatase associated with peak height velocity.[7] Whereas testosterone stimulates cartilage growth in early puberty, it leads to a rapid advance in epiphyseal fusion in later puberty. Insulin-like growth factor I (IGF-I) levels peak later than the mean age of peak height velocity. In a 1994 study, the effects of age were significantly different between pubertal stages, consistent with the observation that those who experience early-onset puberty have a more pronounced growth spurt than those who undergo late-onset puberty.[8]

It is important to look at whole year changes in height because of the seasonal variability in growth. On average, greater growth occurs in March, April, and May, although the time of the year varies in which a given individual has a seasonal peak.[9] Growth charts are generated by either longitudinal or cross-sectional data. Cross-sectional charts do not follow the growth of any given individual. Longitudinal charts can determine individual patterns and allow the distinction to be made between early, average, and late maturers.[9] Although late-maturing boys may be incredulous, the timing of the height spurt in normal children does not affect their final height attainment.

Weight changes occur in the context of gender, height, pubertal maturation, and chronologic age. Standards have been constructed for weight curves, such as those by Tanner and Davies.[9] Weight changes, particularly during pubertal maturation, reflect gender-specific changes in body composition, especially in lean body mass and proportion of body fat. Adolescent girls have a greater proportion of body fat, with adipose tissue distributed along the upper arms, thighs, and upper back.

There are several methods the clinician can use to define obesity, such as a preestablished body mass index (BMI) percentile (such as 85th percentile), weight for height, weight percentile by age, percentage body fat, or skinfold percentile (see Chapter 33, "Obesity"). Prospective studies have established that obesity tracks from adolescence to adulthood.[10] The weight pattern and timing of onset of adiposity are associated with adult cardiovascular risk factors; an increase in the ratio of abdominal to lower body fat demonstrates an independent association with hypertension, elevated glucose, and hypertensive heart disease.[11] However, weight gain in early adult life, rather than during childhood or adolescence, may be a more sensitive indicator of later cardiovascular morbidity and mortality.[12]

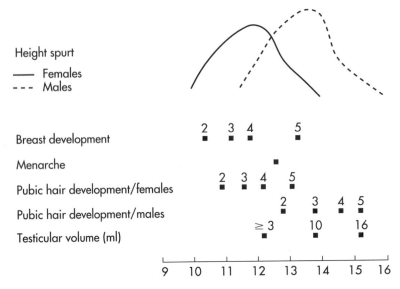

Fig. 6-2. Sequence of pubertal events in North American adolescents based on evaluations of 515 boys, ages 10 to 15 years at intake, seen every 6 months over 3 years, and 864 girls, ages 9 and 10 at intake, seen every 12 months over 6 years.

Changes in muscle mass and bone mineral density occur during puberty. There is an increase in muscle mass 3 months after the height spurt, with a strength spurt after the increase in muscle mass.[5] In women, 50% of total body calcium is laid down during puberty,[13] and in males, 67%; by the end of puberty, males have nearly 50% more total body calcium than females.[14] Nearly all (99%) body calcium resides in bone. Among females, the increase in bone density that occurs during puberty is greater in African-American than in Caucasian adolescents.[15]

Secondary Sexual Development

Over the past three decades, clinicians and researchers have used the pubertal staging systems published by Marshall and Tanner.[5,16,17] This system is based on evaluation of consecutive examinations and photographs (see Chapter 13, "Physical Examination"). Briefly, both pubic hair and breast staging are based on five categories, with stage 1 representing prepubertal development, and stage 5 adult development. Pubic hair stage 2 is the appearance of fine, straight hair along the lateral borders of the genitals. In stage 3, the hair is more coarse and curly, as well as darker, and extends over the pubic bone. In stage 4, the hair continues to become darker and curlier but does not yet extend to the thighs. Tanner breast stage 2 is the breast bud stage. In stage 3, there is further enlargement of the breasts and areola, but not until stage 4 do the areola and papilla form a secondary mound (separation of contour). There is some variability in a given individual's timing, sequence, or tempo, but most

adolescents follow a predictable path through pubertal maturation, as shown in Figure 6-2.

Physiology of Male and Female Maturation

The earliest secondary sexual characteristic to appear in most girls is breast/areolar development,[1,16] although a substantial minority have pubic hair as the initial manifestation. The specific initial manifestation may have an association with body morphology and composition both at the onset and throughout pubertal maturation.[18] As noted in Figure 6-2, peak height velocity occurs soon after entry into puberty.

The earliest stage of male maturation is an increase in testicular volume. In a longitudinal study, 95% of boys were noted to have an increase in testicular volume (≥3 ml) before the appearance of pubic hair; this stage (designated as pubertal stage 2A by the authors[19]) had a mean duration of 0.61 years. It was significantly different from Tanner pubic hair stage 1 without testicular development, as well as pubic hair stage 2, in the anthropometric variables studied, such as height, weight, and BMI, as well as hormonal measures (testosterone, free testosterone, and dehydroepiandrosterone sulfate [DHEAS]). Of note, if one considers only pubic hair in the assessment of early male puberty, it may lead to unnecessary tests in clinical situations and misclassification in research studies.[19] Although graphs have been published regarding the relationship of testicular volume and/or pubic hair with chronologic age, clinical

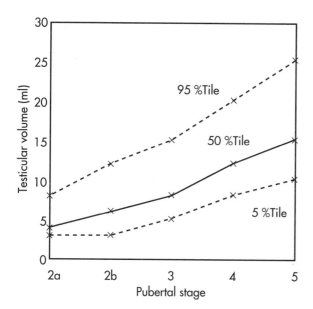

Fig. 6-3. Testicular volume in adolescents as a function of pubertal stage based on evaluations of 539 boys, ages 10 to 15 years, seen every 6 months over 3 years. (From Biro FM, Lucky AW, Huster GA, Morrison JA: Pubertal staging in boys, *J Pediatr* 127:100-102, 1995.)

problems may arise regarding whether testicular volume is appropriate for a given pubic hair stage (e.g., when one is concerned about endogenous or exogenous androgens). Figure 6-3, based on the above study, allows the clinician to evaluate the relationship between testicular volume and pubic hair.

Researchers have also proposed an alternative to Tanner's breast staging system. Four areolar stages were constructed by Garn and Falkner[20] on the basis of areolar diameter, pigmentation, and contour. Areolar stage 1 is prepubertal; stage 2 has palpable subareolar tissue, an increase in size and pigmentation of the areola, and little development of papilla; stage 3 has further increase in size and pigment of the areola, with separation of areola and papilla from the contour of the breast; and stage 4 has elevation of the papilla and regression of the areola, with mature size and color of the areola. There is a high correlation (Spearman correlation coefficient 0.94), when comparing the Garn and Falkner areolar staging system with Tanner's breast staging system.[20]

Although menarche will be covered more extensively in the sections on adolescent gynecology, there are some interesting issues regarding menarche from the perspective of pubertal maturation and research on puberty. There have been secular changes in menarche; menarche has decreased 3 to 4 months per decade, although this has stabilized since the mid-1970s. The correlation between actual and recalled age of menarche is 0.81.[21] When menarche occurs under the age of 12 years, it is associated with increased weight and BMI[22]; additionally, early

maturers are at an increased risk for obesity compared with late maturers.[23]

PERILS OF PUBERTY

The healthcare provider of adolescents may be asked to evaluate aspects of pubertal maturation that may be viewed by the patient, family, or provider as abnormal but are part of normal pubertal development. Included among these "perils of puberty" are acne, psychological correlates of puberty, gynecomastia, scoliosis, myopia, anemia, types of sports-related injuries, dysfunctional uterine bleeding, and subfertility among adolescent females and males. For example, there is an accelerated progression of the degree of scoliosis during puberty as a result of the growth in the axial skeleton. The greatest incidence of myopia (i.e., new cases) occurs during puberty, as a result of the growth in the axial diameter of the eye.[5] Hemoglobin levels change as a function of gender and pubertal stage.[24] Iron requirements may not be met by diet during the growth spurt or with onset of menses.[25]

The overall prevalence of pubertal (as distinguished from adult) gynecomastia is 49%. The onset is generally during early or middle puberty, may be unilateral or bilateral, and persists for 6 to 18 months.[26] There is little to distinguish boys with or without gynecomastia. Those with gynecomastia demonstrated a more rapid tempo through puberty, were lighter and leaner, and had lower free testosterone. Those with persistent gynecomastia (i.e., 2 years or more) had a diameter of palpable tissue greater than or equal to 2 cm during the first year (odds ratio 8.7).[27] Although the underlying diagnosis is "idiopathic pubertal gynecomastia" in the majority,[28] other etiologies include drugs, hypogonadism, testicular tumors, and hyperthyroidism. In a study investigating the etiology in 27 young adult males hospitalized with a diagnosis of gynecomastia, 24 were otherwise healthy, but two had testicular cancer, one of whom presented with new-onset gynecomastia.[27]

Acne, similar to gynecomastia, is extremely common during the adolescent years (see Chapter 72, "Dermatologic Problems"). It is a disorder of the pilosebaceous unit, characterized by follicular occlusion and inflammation, caused by androgenic stimulation of the unit. When the follicular opening becomes plugged, a comedo is formed. If the opening is widely dilated, there is oxidation of keratinous material and formation of a blackhead; open comedones rarely lead to inflammatory acne. With a small opening, there is the formation of a closed comedo (whitehead) that may lead to inflammatory acne if the contents of the comedo rupture into the dermis. There is an increase in the number of acne lesions with advancing maturation in both boys and girls, with a greater number of comedones than inflammatory lesions at all stages.[29]

Acne begins on the central face, and may predate development of secondary sexual characteristics in some girls.[30] In girls, the severity of acne is associated with greater serum levels of DHEAS, as well as a greater number of acne lesions, in early puberty.[31] Despite its high prevalence during puberty, the presence of acne, particularly moderate or severe acne in early puberty, should alert the clinician to the possibility of an endocrinologic disorder (e.g., congenital adrenal hyperplasia).

Pubertal status may help predict the specific type of musculoskeletal injuries that adolescents may encounter during participation in sports.[32] For example, the greatest risk of damage to epiphyseal growth plates occurs during the period of peak height velocity. The asynchronous growth of body parts may result in limited range of motion of some joints; together with the increase in muscle mass that occurs shortly after peak height velocity, the limited range of motion and increased muscle mass may lead to sprains or strains. A common overuse injury in teens is Osgood-Schlatter disease, an inflammation of the tibial tubercle apophysis (see Chapter 151, "Orthopedics").

There exist biologic correlates of adolescence as well as psychological manifestations of puberty. There is no relationship between pubertal maturation and cognitive development,[33] although the timing of pubertal maturation does appear to affect psychosocial functioning. The younger age at the onset of puberty in girls leads to younger age at growth spurt; consequently, there is a gender reversal in height from ages 10.5 to 13 years. Whereas boys develop a more positive self-image and mood as they progress through puberty, girls feel a decreased sense of attractiveness.[34] There are conflicting findings regarding associations between sex hormones and emotional dispositions or aggressive attributes[35] and between sex hormones and body image[36]; among girls in early adolescence, there appears to be a curvilinear effect of estradiol levels with depressed affect (increased then decreased), impulse control (decreased then increased), and psychopathology (increased then decreased).[37]

Pubertal development may have an especially negative impact when there is desynchrony between timing of pubertal development and chronologic age, such as seen in the early maturing girl, or when pubertal changes are not viewed as desirable.[38] There is an association between problem behavior and early pubertal development[39]; the early-maturing girl is more likely to have older friends,[40] and this has been associated with earlier onset of sexual intercourse, smoking, and drinking.[41]

Dysfunctional uterine bleeding is excessive, prolonged, and/or irregular endometrial bleeding unrelated to anatomic uterine lesions; anovulation/disruption of ovarian function accounts for eight of ten cases. There is unopposed estrogen on endometrium, leading to a sustained proliferative, rather than maturation to a secretory, endometrium. Estrogen levels ultimately are unable to sustain hyperplastic endometrial lining, leading to a breakdown with irregular, sometimes heavy bleeding.

Progression from anovulatory to ovulatory cycles is shorter with an earlier age of menarche. When menarche occurs under the age of 12, 50% will become ovulatory within the year; when menarche occurs between 12 and 13 years, 50% will ovulate within 3 years. When menarche occurs over the age of 13, 50% will ovulate within 4.5 years.[42]

There also appears to be a physiologic subfertility among adolescent males. Among mothers 15 years of age or younger, one would expect most male partners to be under 16 years of age, but few of the fathers to these mother's children were under 16.[43]

Sexually active adolescents are at the highest risk for nearly all sexually transmitted diseases (see Chapter 140, "Sexually Transmitted Diseases").[44] The etiologic factors are both behavioral and biologic. Behavioral issues that increase the risk for sexually transmitted diseases include younger age at the onset of intercourse and number of partners. Biologic factors include age of menarche (which influences behavioral factors) and specific biologic maturation. In the first few years after menarche, there is persistence of a transformation zone of columnar to squamous epithelial cells on the exocervix. Columnar cells are the site of infection by *Chlamydia*[45]; the transformation zone is the area of greatest activity with human papillomavirus urogenital infection.

References

1. Taranger J, Engstrom I, Lichtenstein H, Svennberg-Redegren I: Somatic pubertal development, *Acta Paediatr Scand* 258S:121-135, 1976.
2. Harris JA, Jackson CM, Patterson DG, Scammon RE, editors: *Measurement in man,* Minneapolis, 1930, University of Minnesota Press.
3. Stafford EM, Weir MR, Pearl W, et al: Sexual maturity rating: a marker for effects of pubertal maturation on the adolescent electrocardiogram, *Pediatrics* 83:565-569, 1989.
4. Rosner B, Prineas RJ, Loggie JMH, Daniels SR: Blood pressure nomograms for children and adolescents by height, sex and age in the United States, *J Pediatr* 123:871-886, 1993.
5. Tanner JM: *Growth at adolescence,* ed 2, Oxford, England, 1962, Blackwell Scientific Publications.
6. Bailey DA, Malina RM, Mirwald RL: Physical activity and growth of the child. In Falkner F, Tanner JA, editors: *Human growth,* New York, 1986, Plenum Press, pp 147-170.
7. Round JM, Butcher S, Steele R: Changes in plasma inorganic phosphorus and alkaline phosphatase activity during the adolescent growth spurt, *Ann Hum Biol* 6:129-136, 1979.
8. Juul A, Bang P, Hertel NT, et al: Serum insulin-like growth factor-I in 1030 healthy children, adolescents, and adults: relation to age, sex, stage of puberty, testicular size, and body mass index, *J Clin Endocrinol Metab* 78:744-752, 1994.

9. Tanner JM, Davies PS: Clinical longitudinal standards for height and height velocity for North American children, *J Pediatr* 107:317-329, 1985.
10. Cronk CE, Roche AF: Longitudinal trends in subcutaneous fat thickness during adolescence, *Am J Phys Anthropol* 61:197-204, 1983.
11. Gillum RF: The association of body fat distribution with hypertension, hypertensive heart disease, coronary heart disease, diabetes, and cardiovascular risk factors in men and women aged 18-79 years, *J Chronic Dis* 40:421-428, 1987.
12. Manson JE, Willett WC, Stampfer ML, et al: Body weight and mortality among women, *N Engl J Med* 333:677-685, 1995.
13. Lloyd T, Rollings N, Andon MB, et al: Determinants of bone density in young women. I. Relationships among pubertal development, total body bone mass, and total body bone density in premenarchal females, *J Clin Endocrinol Metab* 75:383-387, 1992.
14. Forbes GB: Body composition in adolescent children. In Falkner F, Tanner JA, editors: *Human growth,* vol 2, New York, 1986, Plenum Press; pp 119-145.
15. Gilsanz V, Roe TF, Mora S, et al: Changes in vertebral bone density in black girls and white girls during childhood and puberty, *N Engl J Med* 325:1597-1600, 1991.
16. Marshall WA, Tanner JM: Variations in the pattern of pubertal changes in girls, *Arch Dis Child* 44:291-303, 1969.
17. Marshall WA, Tanner JM: Variations in the pattern of pubertal changes in boys, *Arch Dis Child* 45:13-23, 1970.
18. Biro FM, Lucky AW, Simbartl LA, Morrison JA: Pathways through puberty: a longitudinal study of pubertal maturation in girls, *Pediatr Res* 33:3A, 1993.
19. Biro FM, Lucky AW, Huster GA, Morrison JA: Pubertal staging in boys, *J Pediatr* 127:100-102, 1995.
20. Biro FM, Falkner F, Khoury P, et al: Areolar and breast staging in adolescent girls, *Adolesc Pediatr Gynecol* 5:271-272, 1992.
21. Bergsten-Brucefors A: A note on the accuracy of recalled age at menarche, *Ann Hum Biol* 3:71-73, 1976.
22. Wellens R, Malina RM, Roche AF, et al: Body size and fatness in young adults in relation to age at menarche, *Am J Hum Biol* 4:783-787, 1992.
23. Garn SM, LaVelle M, Rosenberg KR, Hawthorne YM: Maturational timing as a factor in female fatness and obesity, *Am J Clin Nutr* 43:879-883, 1986.
24. Daniel WA: Hematocrit: maturity relationship in adolescence, *Pediatrics* 52:388-394, 1973.
25. Nutrition monitoring in the United States: a progress report from the Joint Nutrition Monitoring Evaluation Committee, 1986. DHHS Pub No (PHS) 86-1255. Baltimore, 1986, U.S. Department of Health and Human Services, U.S. Department of Agriculture.
26. Biro FM, Lucky AW, Huster GA, Morrison JA: Hormonal studies and physical maturation in adolescent gynecomastia, *J Pediatr* 116:450-455, 1990.
27. Biro FM, Lucky AW, Huster GA, Morrison JA: Difficulties in differentiating transient from persistent gynecomastia in adolescents, *Pediatr Res* 27:3A, 1990.
28. Braunstein GD: Gynecomastia, *N Engl J Med* 328:490-495, 1993.
29. Lucky AW, Biro FM, Huster GA, et al: Acne vulgaris in early adolescent boys, *Arch Dermatol* 127:210-216, 1991.
30. Lucky AW, Biro FM, Huster GA, et al: Acne vulgaris in premenarchal girls: an early sign of puberty associated with rising levels of dehydroepiandrosterone, *Arch Dermatol* 130:308-314, 1994.
31. Lucky AW, Biro FM, Simbartl L, et al: Predictors of severity of acne vulgaris in young adolescent girls: results of a five-year longitudinal study, *J Pediatr* 130:30-39, 1997.
32. Backous DD, Farrow JA, Friedl KE: Assessment of pubertal maturity in boys, using height and grip strength, *J Adolesc Health Care* 11:497-500, 1990.
33. Orr DP, Brack CJ, Ingersoll G: Pubertal maturation and cognitive maturity in adolescents, *J Adolesc Health Care* 9:273-279, 1988.
34. Crockett JL, Petersen AC: Pubertal status and psychosocial development: findings from the Early Adolescence Study. In Lerner RM, Foch TT, editors: *Biological-psychosocial interactions in early adolescence: a life-span perspective,* Hillsdale, NJ, 1987, Erlbaum, pp 173-188.
35. Susman EJ, Inoff-Germain G, Nottelmann ED, et al: Hormones, emotional dispositions, and aggressive attributes in young adolescents, *Child Dev* 58:1114-1134, 1987.
36. Slap G, Khalid N, Paikoff R, et al: Evolving self-image in young adolescents: relationships with pubertal manifestations and hormones, *J Adolesc Health* 13:42, 1992.
37. Warren MP, Brooks-Gunn J: Mood and behavior at adolescence: evidence for hormonal factors, *J Clin Endocrinol Metab* 69:77-83, 1989.
38. Simmons RG, Blyth DA, McKinney KL: The social and psychological effects of puberty on white females. In Brooks-Gunn J, Petersen AC, editors: *Girls at puberty: biological and psychosocial perspectives,* New York, 1983, Plenum Press, pp 229-272.
39. Silbereisen RK, Petersen AC, Albrecht HT, Kracke B: Maturational timing and the development of problem behavior: longitudinal studies in adolescence, *J Early Adolesc* 9:247-268, 1989.
40. Magnusson D, Stattin H, Allen VL: Differential maturation among girls and its relation to social adjustment: a longitudinal perspective. In Featerman DL, Lerner RM, editors: *Life-span development and behavior,* New York, 1986, Academic Press, pp 135-172.
41. Brooks-Gunn, J: Antecedents to and consequences of variations in girls' maturational timing, *J Adolesc Health Care* 9:365-373, 1988.
42. Apter D, Vihko R: Early menarche, a risk factor for breast cancer, indicates early onset of ovulatory cycles, *J Clin Endocrinol Metab* 57:82-86, 1983.
43. Hardy JB, Duggan AK, Masnyk K, Pearson C: Fathers of children born to young urban mothers, *Fam Plann Perspect* 21:159-163, 187, 1989.
44. Biro FM: *Adolescents and sexually transmitted diseases.* Maternal and Child Health Technical Information Bulletin. Washington DC, 1992, National Center for Education in Maternal and Child Health in cooperation with the Maternal and Child Health Bureau, Health Resources and Services Administration, Public Health Service, U.S. Department of Health and Human Services.
45. Harrison HR, Phil D, Costin M, et al: Cervical *Chlamydia trachomatis* infection in university women: relationship to history, contraception, ectopy, and cervicitis, *Am J Obstet Gynecol* 153:244-251, 1985.

CHAPTER 7

Cognitive Development

•

David Elkind

Since the time of Descartes, the process of knowing, or cognition, has been wedded to the notion of identity or being. At no point in development is this connection between knowing and being more evident than during adolescence. For the first time, thanks to new mental abilities that emerge coincidentally with puberty, young people are able to "think about thinking" and to appreciate the privacy of their own thoughts. At this age, young people are reluctant to share their newly discovered private thoughts, and the characteristic response of young adolescents to parental questions such as "Where did you go?," "Out," "What did you do?," "Nothing" reflects the young person's newly discovered private world of ideas.

It is within this private arena of their own thoughts that adolescents are also struggling to construct a sense of "personal identity." This construction will eventually enable them to integrate the disparate parts of their self-experiences—as brother or sister, son or daughter, athlete and/or scholar, and so on—to provide both continuity with the past and guidance and direction for the future. It is because adolescents use their newfound powers of cognition to construct a sense of personal identity that Descartes' classic phrase "I think, therefore I am" seems most descriptive of the adolescent.

While the new cognitive abilities of adolescents are closely tied to the construction of a sense of identity, they are also connected to some of the more deviant aspects of adolescent thought and behavior. Because of newfound abilities attained in adolescence, teenagers often engage in characteristic exaggerations and distortions that will eventually decrease once they have become more accustomed to and proficient with these new intellectual powers. It is the cognitive vulnerability of young adolescents, coupled with inappropriate demands for decision making, that contributes to much dysfunctional adolescent behavior.

COGNITIVE DEVELOPMENT AND IDENTITY FORMATION

One of Inhelder's and Piaget's major contributions to our knowledge regarding the development of intelligence, adaptive thought, and action was their discovery of a "second age of reason" that makes its appearance at the time of puberty.[1] Since ancient times, the age of 6 or 7 had been regarded as the age of reason, the point at which a child can be held responsible for knowing the difference between right and wrong. The reasoning abilities children acquire at that age is, however, the syllogistic reasoning described by Aristotle:

All men are mortal (major premise)

Socrates is a man (minor premise)

Socrates is mortal (conclusion)

What Piaget and Inhelder discovered was that adolescents acquire a higher order form of logic that was first described by logicians in the nineteenth century, namely, propositional logic. Propositional logic is to syllogistic logic as algebra is to arithmetic. In arithmetic numbers stand for quantities of things, but in algebra letters represent numbers and not things. Algebra is thus much more general and much more powerful than arithmetic; it is a higher order of arithmetic. Algebra allows us to solve mathematical problems that we could not solve with arithmetic operations alone.

In the same way, propositional logic operates on syllogistic reasoning and allows us to deal with concepts such as *formal truth* that cannot be dealt with at the level of syllogistic reasoning. A proposition such as "snow is black" may be formally true (if the question is "In a world where coal was white, what color would snow be?") while factually false. The propositions of syllogistic logic refer to persons, things, or properties (snow, whiteness), but those of propositional logic refer to other propositions (the proposition that snow is black is true). Propositional logic, then, deals with the logical truth or falsehood of propositions, not with their empirical truth. The proposition that "snow is black" is true if, and only if, the proposition that "coal is white" is also true.

Inhelder and Piaget termed the new mental abilities that enable adolescents to deal with symbolic logic *formal operations.* These operations, propositional logic, enable young people to reason about contrary-to-fact ideas (such as the idea that coal might be white), to construct ideals, and to muster many different kinds of evidence to support a particular argument. In many ways the attainment of formal operations brings about a sort of Copernican revolution in the adolescent's thinking that helps account for many of the well-known behavioral phenomena of early adolescence.

For example, consider the common experience of many parents who have a well-mannered, respectful 10-year-old who loves to be with the family, go on family outings, and so on. To such a youngster the parents can do no wrong. Within 2 years this well-mannered, respectful youngster no longer wants to participate in family affairs, challenges parental authority, and often seems to believe that parents can do nothing right. What has happened? The parents have not changed that much during the 2 years that marked the transition from child to preteen.

What has happened is the attainment of formal operations. For the first time the pre- or early teen can construct ideal parents and then contrast these ideal parents (often modeled on the parents of friends) to his or her own parents and finds them wanting. This negative appraisal of parents is reinforced by another set of circumstances also occasioned by formal operations. The young person can now construct gender ideals and may form "crushes" on members of the opposite sex. This may make the youth feel guilty about withdrawing love from parents. To assuage his or her guilt, a teenager may often look for negative things about the parents to justify the withdrawal of love.

The attainment of formal operations in adolescence also makes possible what Erikson has called the sense of "personal identity."[2] Erikson believed that the sense of personal identity is a construction that pulls together all of the young person's diverse, and often conflicting, social roles (e.g., son, daughter, brother, sister, nephew, niece, athlete, scholar, friend), talents (e.g., musical, artistic, culinary), values, and attitudes into some meaningful and workable whole—a personality. This sense of personal identity, or personality, provides a basis for continuity with the past and guidance for the future. The construction of a sense of personal identity takes time and effort. In addition, it presupposes the formal operations of

intelligence, since these permit the coordination and integration of the many different, sometimes opposing, strands of the individual's selfhood. For various reasons, not all teenagers are able to arrive at this sense of personal identity. Instead, they may be left with a sense of "role diffusion" in which they have no clear-cut sense of themselves and often speak and act inappropriately. Some construct what may be called a kind of "patchwork self" of disparate attitudes and values that do not fit with one another and give the young person the appearance of arbitrariness and lack of conviction.[3]

Although Erikson assumed that the process of identity formation was roughly the same for young men and women, a number of researchers have challenged this position. Gilligan and colleagues have made a number of studies of young adolescent girls and find that their process of identity formation is somewhat different from that of young men.[4] First of all, Erikson argued that a sense of personal identity preceded a sense of intimacy (he argued that to really give yourself in a true intimacy relationship, you had to have a strong enough sense of self not to fear losing it as a result of the closeness of intimacy). However, for women the relations between intimacy and identity are more closely entwined than is true for men. In part this may be because early in development boys must break their identification with the mother in order to identify with the father, which girls do not have to do. Early on, boys must give up intimacy for identity, so later they must reestablish intimacy. For girls no such break occurs, and thus there is less need to separate intimacy from development.

Gilligan and colleagues found another difference between young men and young women with respect to identity formation.[4] Whereas teenage boys usually find themselves by opposing themselves to authority, girls often need to find themselves by submitting to authority. This is clearly social and cultural, and the process is unwittingly contributed to by both mothers and female teachers. Although this is changing as the opportunities for women are enlarged, the pattern of demanding that young women conform while young men rebel in their identity formation process has long-term personality implications for both genders.

Our understanding of identity formation has been broadened in other ways as well. Marcia[5] has developed scales to measure four statuses in the process of identity formation as described by Erikson. Performance on these scales has been linked to different personality profiles. Those who have an *achieved* identity status have successfully experimented with different roles, challenged values, and come up with a consistent and workable sense of self and identity. Such individuals tend to set realistic goals, to perform well under stress, and to choose friends and romantic partners who will further their growth and independence.

Individuals who, according to the Marcia scales, are in a *moratorium status,* are generally undergoing a delayed or drawn-out struggle for identity. They tend to be anxious, unsure of what they want to do and where they want to go in life. Such young people may be perennial students yet rebellious of authority and also guilty about not achieving in the manner their parents might have liked them to achieve.

A third group of young people fall into a group that Erikson described as *identity foreclosure.* Young men and women who from an early age know what they are going to do in life, either because of a family history or because of being in a particular profession such as law or medicine, or who are expected to take over the family farm or business, may never grow through the struggles to find out who and what they are because they can assume a preformed identity. Although many who have attained this status are successful, they are more anxious and less satisfied and happy with their lives than those who have come by their identity in other ways. These students are respectful of authority and choose friends and romantic partners who reinforce their dependency orientation.

The last identity status assessed by the Marcia scales is that of *identity confusion.* The young people who fall within this category have been found to have high levels of anxiety, to be somewhat rigid, and to exhibit strong feelings of inadequacy. They often continue to put off making serious life choices and get caught up in an active, if immature social life, often with younger people and involving a lot of parties, sex, and drugs. Other young people who fall into this category may become loners or drifters. Still others may join cults or other groups that offer them an intense group identity.

Although most young people move through these identity status positions and eventually arrive at an achieved status, some people get stuck at one or another of these positions, with the personality results described above.

In addition to its role in identity formation, the system of formal operations makes possible a whole new level of intellectual functioning and academic achievement. The elementary school curriculum, for example, might be characterized as "making the unfamiliar familiar." Children learn about new countries, new plants and animals, new substances, new measures, and so on. At the secondary level, however, the curriculum centers on "making the familiar unfamiliar." The teenager discovers that water on which some objects float and into which other objects sink is really not a liquid but two gases. In algebra they find that a letter, such as "a," which as children they had learned to identify with sounds now represents not sounds but numbers. They now discover that books such as *Alice in Wonderland* and *Gulliver's Travels,* which they once read as interesting stories, are

"allegories" with a whole new set of different metaphoric meanings.

In short, the new mental abilities that appear at adolescence bring the young person into the adult estate. They enable the adolescent to construct a sense of personal identity and to begin to think in the complex and multileveled thought patterns so characteristic of adult thought and so foreign to the cognition of children. At the same time, these abilities also contribute to the diversity of personality and to the differences associated with gender and identity status.

COGNITIVE DEVELOPMENT AND DEVIANT BEHAVIOR

Adolescence is generally regarded as a period of social experimentation, limit testing, and risk taking. This is particularly true today, now that premarital sexual activity has become socially acceptable and that mind-altering drugs are readily available to young people at ever younger ages. Yet even during those periods in history when social behavior was more rigidly controlled than it is today, adolescents took risks. How can we understand this risk-taking propensity of adolescents? Although numerous factors contribute to adolescent risk taking, some mental constructions that appear once young people attain formal operations probably play a part. This is true because the attainment of new mental abilities does not carry with it immediate proficiency in the use of those abilities, no less than the attainment of new height and weight gives the adolescent instantaneous skilled coordination in the use of his or her new body configuration. Some new mental constructions are products of the teenager's inexperience in using formal operations.

As previously mentioned, formal operations make it possible for adolescents to think about thinking. Children think, of course, but they do not reflect on their own thinking. Adolescents can think about their own thinking and about the thinking of other people. Nonetheless, they tend to make a characteristic error when they engage in this kind of thinking. Because they are going through such a radical transformation in height, weight, physical appearance, emotional expansion, and intellectual transformation, they tend to be self-centered. Accordingly, when they think about other people's thinking, they automatically assume that others are thinking about what they are thinking about, namely, themselves.

As a result, young teenagers construct what I have called an "imaginary audience," a belief that everyone in their immediate vicinity is watching them, thinking about them, and interested in their every thought and action.[6] This imaginary audience gives rise to a heightened sense of self-consciousness unique to early adolescence when the audience is most powerful.[7] This new self-consciousness can be seen in the young adolescent's enormous concern with physical appearance, and with the sometimes elaborate efforts young people will engage in to alter their appearance through diet or exercise.

Another mental construction complements that of the imaginary audience. The teenager reasons, "If everyone is watching me and concerned about and interested in me, I must be somebody special, somebody truly original." This way of thinking contributes to the construction of what has been called the "personal fable," the belief that the teenager is special and unique.[6] "Other people will grow old and die," the teenager thinks, "but not me." "Other people won't realize their life's ambitions, but I will." The personal fable also gives rise to a sense of invulnerability. "Bad things will happen to other people but not to me." Sometimes the fable can take a negative form: "Nobody in the whole world could have done or said something so stupid, so embarrassing, so hurtful." Like the imaginary audience, the personal fable is most prominent in early adolescence.

These powerful constructions of early adolescence—the imaginary audience and personal fable—help us to understand why young teenagers are greater risk takers than they will be later, when these constructions have been tempered and modified by disconfirming experiences. To illustrate, in early adolescence some teenagers will experiment with drugs to please the audience, to show them that the adolescent is "cool" and "with it." Likewise, many young people take risks because their personal fable leads them to believe that nothing will happen to them as a result: "Other people get hooked on drugs, not me!" "Other girls will get pregnant, but not me." It is this strong belief in their invulnerability to harm that encourages many young teenagers to take risks.

Education alone will not counter the young teenager's sense of audience and fable. Probably every adult who smokes knows the dangers of smoking. Education is not the issue for these individuals; the issue is *why* they continue to smoke, knowing the health hazards of the practice. Adults take risks for the same reasons adolescents do: because of the belief in their own invulnerability. If we wish to address risk taking in a preventive way, we need to look for ways of attacking the teenager's or, for that matter, the adult's sense of invulnerability.

One of the most powerful and effective techniques in this regard is to arrange for teenagers who have been addicted to drugs, have become pregnant, or have contracted a venereal disease to talk to groups of young teenagers. When young people listen to peers who have taken risks and paid the price, this challenges them to examine their own sense of speciality and invulnerability. Education is important, but it needs to be coupled with some form of experience that will help counter the young teenager's imaginary audience sensitivity to peer group pressure and personal fable-induced sense of invulnerability.

CONCLUSION

Adolescence is often portrayed as a period of Sturm und Drang, or storm and stress. However, this image of the young may be more of an adult projection than a reality. To be sure, young people are testing limits and taking risks, but most do so in socially acceptable ways. If young people today are suffering more from stress-related death and disease than was true in earlier generations, this is not due to decadence on the part of youth. Rather, it reflects the new social pressures to make decisions regarding peer conformity, drug use, and sexual activity at an age when the imaginary audience and the personal fable are most powerful and teenagers are most vulnerable to their influence. To improve the mental health of youth, we need not only to offer them effective education but also to provide the kinds of input from peers that will help them attain more realistic appreciation of the audience and of their own speciality and vulnerability.

References

1. Piaget J, Inhelder B: *The growth of logical thinking from childhood to adolescence,* New York, 1958, Basic Books.
2. Erikson E: *Childhood and society,* ed 2, New York, 1963, WW Norton.
3. Elkind D: Egocentrism in children and adolescents, *Child Dev* 38:1025-1034, 1967.
4. Gilligan C, Lyons NP, Hammer TJ, editors: *Making connections. The relational worlds of adolescent girls at the Emma Willard School,* Cambridge, 1990, Harvard University Press.
5. Marcia JE: Identity and self development. In Lerner RM, Peterson AC, Brooks Gunn J, editors: *Encyclopedia of adolescence,* vol 1, New York, 1991, Garland.
6. Elkind D: *All grown up and no place to go,* Reading, MA, 1984, Addison-Wesley.
7. Elkind D, Bowen R: Imaginary audience behavior in children and adolescents, *Dev Psychol* 15:38-44, 1979.

CHAPTER 8

Psychosocial Development

●

Beatrix A. Hamburg

Over the course of recorded human history and across a broad range of societies, adolescence has been considered a highly significant period of life transition. Its importance has been recognized almost universally through ceremonial practices that represent "rites of passage." However, the nature and duration of adolescent experience have shown substantial variation.

In earlier times (and currently in less developed, simpler societies), adolescence constituted a very brief transition in the life span. As soon as children completed the biologic changes of puberty and attained adult physique and physiology, adolescence would end. Often this ending was acknowledged in puberty rites signaling induction into adult roles and responsibilities.

In modern industrialized societies, the transition from adolescence to adulthood has become increasingly prolonged and complex. At present, it spans about one decade, starting at approximately 11 years of age. Adolescence has been lengthened at both ends. Although entry into adolescence is still linked to pubertal changes, these changes now occur at much younger ages than previously. With age of menarche used as a marker, there has been a secular trend over the past century in which puberty has demonstrated an age decline of about 4 months per decade. This remained consistent until about 1960, when biologic limits may have been reached in affluent societies.[1]

In the United States the average age of menarche currently is approximately 12.5 years, which can be compared with approximately 16.0 years in 1860. This change has been attributed largely to improved health and nutrition. Although pubertal changes are a prominent feature of early adolescence, pubertal status by itself does not signal entry into adolescence. In the United States this milestone is almost universally marked by graduation from elementary school (grade 6) and entry into junior high school or middle school.

The upper end of adolescence has been marked by an increasingly older age of entry into adult work and family roles. Compulsory schooling in the United States has been extended into high school, and almost one half of those in the 18- to 22-year-old population attend college. Since about 1950, educational requirements for good jobs in most industrial countries have included both high school graduation and some college or specialty training.

In addition to being a later event, the transition to adulthood is characterized by ambiguity about how and when adult status is attained. There are differing ages for obtaining a driver's license; acquiring the right to vote, to marry, to negotiate legal contracts, and to legally purchase alcohol and cigarettes; and being inducted into the armed services. For several years individuals of adult physique and physiology are held in a limbo between childhood roles and adult status and expectations.

There have been important and enduring social changes in the latter half of this century that have profoundly affected the social environment in which adolescents are growing up. One important example is a major shift in the labor market away from low-skill but high-pay factory jobs to high-skill technologic and service jobs. Another example is the evolution of family forms and functions as demonstrated by new roles for women, including greatly increased participation in the labor force; associated changes are a rise in the divorce rate, the development of birth control technology, and the legalization of abortion. There has also been a trend toward increasing permissiveness in regard to sexuality, which is demonstrated by provocative media images and an emphasis on sexuality in entertainment and advertising. In addition, the media have reflected and amplified society's endorsement of violence and the use of firearms. Finally, there has been a widespread increase in the "recreational" use of mind-altering substances such as marijuana and cocaine.

Because the lengthening of the adolescent period is a rather recent development, well-developed social institutions for the socialization and support of adolescents in this new social climate are lacking. This is particularly true for urban disadvantaged youths. The widespread sharp rise in problem behaviors among adolescents since the 1960s can be viewed as evidence that certain developmental needs of adolescents are not being met by contemporary society. There are deep concerns about the high rates of school dropout, pregnancy, suicide, violence, and substance abuse among adolescents. Although a great many young people are not involved in these problem behaviors, there are major psychosocial challenges for all youths in negotiating the crucial and prolonged transition from adolescence to adulthood in the current social climate.

Coming of age in America now includes three distinct developmental stages: early adolescence, middle adolescence, and late adolescence. Yet there is a persisting tendency to consider all adolescents together and to think simply in terms of an "adolescent" or a "teenager" regardless of whether the individual is in junior high school, high school, or college. The failure to appreciate the distinct stages of adolescent development has imposed particular burdens on very young adolescents. Members of this age group have been poorly understood, and their needs have been largely unmet because popular adolescent stereotypes actually derive from late adolescence. However, early adolescents have very little in common with late adolescents. Each stage of adolescence has its own characteristic developmental tasks, biologic and psychological resources, and coping possibilities. Late adolescents are at the threshold of the adult world, trying to establish themselves as independent persons. Middle adolescents have reached a period of consolidation after the major biologic and psychosocial changes of early adolescence. However, early adolescents are still moving erratically in and out of the world of childhood. They are groping for guidelines and looking for support as they attempt to define their new status.

Throughout adolescence, certain themes recur: identity, autonomy, achievement, and intimacy (including sexuality). As young people move through the stages of adolescence, they meet successive challenges in these areas. With ever-increasing physical and intellectual maturity, they can build on the learning experience of prior periods. Ultimate success in negotiating these life challenges and setting patterns for adult functioning is crucially linked to how the individual coped with the earliest stage of adolescent development. Failure to cope with the stresses of early adolescence has both immediate and long-term consequences.

Adolescent behaviors have always been a matter of great popular interest and have provoked strong reactions, both positive and negative, ranging from bafflement and outrage to admiration of youthful idealism and commitment. Until recently, however, there has been relatively little systematic research on this subject. As a result, there is still considerable ignorance, confusion, and myth about adolescence among the general public.

One of the strongest myths is that adolescence is inevitably a time of storm and stress linked to the biology of puberty. This view was originally set forth in 1904 by G. Stanley Hall[2] in a major volume on adolescence. Hall's treatise was not based on research, and some of his distinguished colleagues dissented from his view. However, Hall's ideas have prevailed and are still influential today. One reason is that certain psychoanalytic theorists have held views that tended to support the concept of storm and stress. Among psychoanalysts, adolescence was seen as the "genital" stage of development in which the "latency period" of the school-age child is terminated by the hormonal and bodily changes of puberty that powerfully reactivate the earlier conflicts of infantile and early childhood sexuality. Influential psychoanalysts such as Anna Freud,[3] Pauline Kestenberg,[4] and Peter Blos[5] have all associated the resolution of these conflicts in adolescence with the experience of intrapsychic turmoil. Such turmoil was thought to be a necessary ingredient of normal adolescent development and a requirement for reworking the old conflicts and achieving independence from parents in order to attain personal autonomy. These classic psychoanalytic views tended to reinforce the view that troubled, turbulent adolescence is a normal and transient phase.

Erik Erikson[6] modified the classic psychoanalytic approach to adolescence by shifting the emphasis toward the psychosocial tasks of adolescence and away from an exclusive focus on powerful biologic influences in adolescence. He introduced a life-span model of development with eight stages specified: infancy, early childhood, preschool, school age, adolescence, young adulthood, adulthood, and senescence. The psychosocial developmental tasks and negotiation strategies for each stage were outlined. Erikson emphasized the interdependent and incremental aspects of his theory of stages. In his view the legacy of success or failure in prior stages determines the likely outcome of each succeeding stage. However, Erikson did emphasize the possibility of modifying or buffering earlier adverse outcomes by successes at a later period in development.

Erikson focused his attention on the adolescent stage, in particular the transition from late adolescence into adulthood. He outlined a detailed and influential description of the psychosocial tasks and challenges in consolidating identity, achieving adult autonomy, committing to an enduring partner relationship, and establishing a work or career path. These concepts form the basis of most of the current thinking about adolescents and have guided the attitudes and behaviors of many parents, teachers, and youth-service personnel. Although the Erikson model is most applicable to the late adolescence of mainstream white males, more recent adolescent research has given new insights into the differing psychosocial tasks of early adolescents, women, and minority youth.

ADOLESCENT TURMOIL

The belief that adolescent turmoil is normal may lead to the assumption that emotional difficulties in adolescence will be outgrown and therefore do not need to be assessed or treated. However, such a serious clinical decision should be based on data rather than on conventional beliefs and assumptions. In recent adolescent research, systematic studies have examined the extent to which turbulence is a widespread part of normal development and whether or not it truly represents disturbances that will be transient and possibly growth promoting.

Large-scale surveys of public high school students, involving extensive interviews and questionnaires, were carried out in the 1960s and were based on a representative sample of a nonclinical population.[7] The investigators found only minor evidence of turmoil among the adolescents. Typical findings demonstrated a high degree of agreement between parents and their adolescents regarding basic values. This was the first significant challenge to the established beliefs of inevitable rebellion and turmoil. Other subsequent surveys have confirmed these findings.

Another landmark study was Offer's longitudinal Normal Adolescent Project, in which a panel of boys entering high school as freshmen were followed up over the 4-year period until graduation by means of in-depth interviews, self-reports, and psychological testing.[8] A smaller subset of this group was also studied through annual follow-ups during the 4 years after graduation. Offer and colleagues confirmed that most adolescents do not experience turmoil. They made a further contribution by identifying three major developmental routes of adolescence: continuous growth, surgent growth, and tumultuous growth. They found that 25% of the group experienced continuous growth, a pathway characterized by smooth, well-adjusted functioning throughout adolescence, even in the face of stressful circumstances or adverse life events. Surgent growth was identified in 34% of the population. In this route, well-adjusted adolescents showed good adaptation to the minor vicissitudes of ordinary life, but with unanticipated stressful events they experienced noticeable difficulty and distress for a short time. In general, adolescents in both these groups were well adjusted and successful. Only 21% of the adolescents in Offer's study showed a pattern of tumultuous growth, which is the only category that could be considered as representing adolescent turmoil. Adolescents in this group had mood swings and troublesome feelings of anxiety, depression, and guilt or shame. The researchers noted that this group was characterized by economic disadvantage, family and marital conflicts, and a high rate of family mental illness.

Rutter et al[9] shed further light on the prevalence of adolescent turmoil through an epidemiologic study of the mental health status of British adolescents aged 14 to 15 years who were living on the Isle of Wight. In response to a self-report questionnaire, 50% of the adolescents noted sadness or "misery." However, only 12.5% of boys and 14.8% of girls were found to be actually depressed when assessed in an in-depth interview. Therefore, some of the self-reported feelings of "misery" on the questionnaire were unrelated to impairment of functioning or true mood disturbance. Diagnosable psychiatric disorder was noted in 16.3% of the subjects. Rutter estimated that about 10% of the community (i.e., nonclinical) population of adolescents actually suffer from diagnosable low-level depression and/or anxiety. This group seems most comparable with the tumultuous-growth group described by Offer.[8]

Taken together, the studies by Offer[8] and Rutter[9] affirm that adolescent turmoil is not a frequent or normative finding. These data indicate that there is, however, a small segment of the adolescent population who experience a fairly high level of serious distress or turmoil.

Current evidence shows that when true turmoil exists, it usually represents psychopathology and will not be simply "outgrown." Careful assessment and treatment are required. Two longitudinal studies have shown that for a majority of severely disturbed adolescents severe adolescent disturbance continues into adult life.[10,11] These studies also demonstrated that a significant percentage of disturbed adolescents had previously shown psychiatric disturbance throughout childhood. On the basis of the above studies, it can be concluded that there has been excessive reliance on the assumption that severe adolescent disturbance is normative or situational. When such turbulence is found, it should be given serious clinical attention.

A consensus exists that, in general, adolescents give self-reports of more mood swings and depressive feelings than do either children or adults. Yet researchers such as Rutter et al[9] have found that on direct interview the self-reports of dysphoria by adolescents are not always confirmed by mental status evaluation or demonstrated by impairment of functioning. Offer[8] suggested that this phenomenon may represent greater introspection on the part of adolescents and more willingness to be open about negative feelings. Others have pointed to the egocentrism of adolescence and the related self-consciousness, hypersensitivity, irritability, and overreaction to perceived criticism. In addition, adolescence is a time of exploratory activity. New behaviors are used to directly challenge family values or community norms. Although these "transgressions" may lead to disturbing guilt and remorse, such responses are generally only temporary.

In summary, normative fluctuations of mood are linked to adolescent developmental processes and are characterized by their transient nature, commonly measured in hours or days. These fluctuations can and should be distinguished from the unremitting, long-standing mood and behavior changes of serious depressive disorders.

DEVELOPMENTAL PERIODS OF ADOLESCENCE

Developmental processes are dynamic throughout the life span and reflect the interactions between the developing person and the changing context. In the first part of this century, some theorists believed that early experiences, occurring primarily before 5 years of age, had a determining influence and charted the course for future development of the individual. Subsequent research has shown that the impact of preceding life experiences is continually being reshaped by later experiences.

The major psychosocial influences on development can be characterized as normative or nonnormative. Normative refers to the experiences and expectations that occur in a regular and predictable way in society, such as entry into school or the workplace. Nonnormative relates to events that occur on a chance basis, for example, accidents, illness, divorce, and personal defeats or triumphs.

In general, normative influences are graded according to age. There are normative social ages for most life transitions, such as entering elementary school, junior high school, high school, or college; getting married; entering the world of work; and retiring. In addition, there are informal norms, such as the age to begin dating and the age for having one's first child. These social norms are used to judge whether the individual is "on time," too young, or too old to engage in a given behavior. Normative expectations reflect the social climate of the times. For example, the permissiveness of the current social climate has led to a younger age norm for dating and a later age for marriage. Such variations often show differential impact for individuals at specific developmental stages. In general, adolescents are very sensitive to changes in social climate and are highly influenced by them. Descriptions of normal psychosocial development rely most heavily on normative influences.

Early Adolescence

Early adolescence marks the transition from childhood to adolescence and spans ages 11 to 15 years. Until recently there has been little understanding of the fact that early adolescence represents a specific developmental stage with its own tasks and challenges. This lack of understanding has imposed a burden on early adolescents because their role expectations have been derived from the concepts and stereotypes related to late adolescence, in which the major task is transition to adulthood. As a result, the psychosocial context for early adolescents has been based on the importance of encouraging independence. This emphasis on independence has been linked to a withdrawal of parental presence and supervision in a social climate of pressures for "grown-up" behaviors such as smoking, drinking, drugs, and sexuality. However, unlike late adolescents, who are much more mature and knowledgeable, early adolescents need more, not less, guidance. Therefore, independence is not a valid issue for early adolescents. Because they will be living at home for up to 8 years longer, they are not yet facing the real prospect of being on their own as adults.

In early adolescence, ages 11 to 15 years, the almost total discontinuity from the world of childhood makes the coping skills and strategies of that period virtually useless. New preemptive demands emerge in all the major spheres of functioning in early adolescence. The pervasive nature of the crucial changes occurring defines this as a critical life transition.[12] First are the challenges posed by the biologic changes of puberty. The years from ages 11 to 15 represent a period of drastic and rapid bodily change that is equaled only in gestation and infancy. Unlike infants, in whom self-awareness and resulting psychological impact are lacking, adolescents are exquisitely sensitive to the timing, rate, and duration of their pubertal changes as well as to the nature of their "luck" in terms of bodily changes: for example, whether or not they have severe acne. Developing adolescents may also perceive that their bodily changes are occurring too early or too late or that their emerging physique, with its transitional awkwardness or perceived imperfections, will characterize their adult status. As a group, early adolescents have deep concerns about their body and physical attractiveness. Girls often want to lose weight and become thinner. Many boys wish to be taller, heavier, and more muscular.

In the midst of their concerns about pubertal change, most early adolescents have little information about the wide range of normalcy in the timetables of physical development or the patterns of physical change. Boys may be confused by evidence of sexual stirrings such as nocturnal emissions. Despite the prevalence of provocative sexual imagery and the explicitness of television and movies, many early adolescents are both ignorant of and have considerable misinformation about sexuality, sexually transmitted diseases (STDs), and AIDS. They are unprepared for peer pressures regarding sex. In general, they do not understand the biologic fundamentals of puberty or the related health and behavioral issues.

Classic studies that have systematically compared the behavior and personality of early- and late-maturing adolescents have found that the timing of puberty has a significant psychological impact on adolescents. Overall, early maturation into adult physique carries distinct advantages for males. Research has shown that boys with adult-like physique were given more leadership roles, were more proficient in sports, were perceived as more attractive and smarter than their peers, and were more popular than others in their age group. In general, they also demonstrated high self-esteem in early adolescence. Late-maturing boys who were short and childlike in appearance until age 15 or older tended to show more personal and social maladjustment over the entire course of adolescence. They tended to be insecure, suggestible, and vulnerable to peer pressure. Members of this group were seen as weak, immature, and often less competent than average. This was particularly true among working class and minority groups, which placed heavy emphasis on virility, strength, and "macho" attributes.[13]

With girls a more complex pattern emerged. Those who were "on time" in their pubertal development perceived themselves as more attractive and felt more positively about their bodies than girls who were either early or late in their timing.[14] Early-maturing girls, who are actually the most "off time" with both their male and female peers, had more problems in adaptation than girls who were late maturing. The discomfort of early-maturing girls is notably accentuated when they are in a junior high school setting rather than the extended elementary school context (kindergarten through grade 8). In junior high these well-developed, mature-looking young girls are objects of sexual attention by older males (grade 9) and tend to be drawn into cliques or crowds of much older peers. One of the striking aspects of junior high school is the wide variation in pubertal development of the students. There are sometimes startling differences in the height, size, and shape of students in grades 7 through 9 as well as in their social maturity and range of exploratory behaviors.

As noted earlier, graduation from elementary school and entry into junior high or intermediate school has become the informal societal marker for the end of childhood and entry into adolescence in the United States. However, junior high school has not proved to be a good context for early adolescent development. Only recently has there been increasing recognition of the importance of the school experience in adolescent development. The junior high school structure represents a sharp break from that of elementary school. In elementary school there was one classroom with a single teacher and a stable group of classmates throughout the day. Elementary schools are generally small in size and designed to be a supportive environment for children. In contrast, junior high schools are generally many times larger than elementary schools, sometimes having well over 1000 students. When they enter grade 7, youngsters are often overwhelmed by the size and complexity of the school. The security of a single classroom with one teacher is replaced by rotating classes with a different teacher and different set of classmates each hour. The size difference may accentuate the other stresses felt by the early adolescent. In fact, research has shown that very large secondary schools—whether they are intermediate, junior high, or high school—foster a sense of alienation for students at all grade levels.

In junior high school the adolescent's peer group is greatly expanded. There are more choices of friends and also more chances for rejection. Conformity to the peer group, which is partly related to developmental processes, peaks in early adolescence. It seems to reflect the insecurity of early adolescents about meeting their new role requirements and expectations and their heightened need for affirmation. Slavish adherence to peer norms is greatest among those young adolescents with minimal parental and other adult support.

Typically, there is a drop in academic performance in junior high school that is related to motivation rather than to ability. Studies of adolescent cognition suggest that modes of school instruction for this age group should be modified to include more practical experiences and meaningful contexts for presenting school material. Also, early adolescents seem to benefit from regular discussions and guided verbal interactions to sharpen their reasoning skills. However, much current teaching instead depends on rote learning.

Some urban junior high schools pose risks of intimidation and physical harm from other students or young adult "visitors" to the school grounds. Many schools attended by urban disadvantaged youths have a prison-like environment rather than one that is conducive to learning. This type of environment has very negative consequences for learning and motivation to attend school. It is in junior high school that youngsters are making decisions about the value of schooling and whether to work toward high school graduation or to drop out. For many, particularly urban disadvantaged youngsters, the experience of junior high school is especially alienating and therefore dropping out becomes the likely choice.

The decision-making processes of early adolescents are not understood in detail. This is a serious lack because early adolescents are making important decisions about the value of schooling and crucial decisions about sexuality, substance use, health behaviors, societal attitudes, future life options, and their own self-worth. The few existing studies show that, unlike middle or late adolescents, early adolescents are still in the concrete and operational stages of thinking. They are just beginning to be capable of abstract thinking in limited areas. Cognitive skills are noticeably lacking in their psychosocial and interpersonal transactions. In future studies of cognitive styles and information processing of early adolescents, links to newer studies of brain maturation during puberty need to be explored. There is evidence of a brain maturation spurt in early adolescence, as shown by neuronal changes and patterns of decreased oxygen and glucose consumption of the brain.[15,16]

Developmental studies of cognition have established that adolescent thinking differs from that of either children or adults in several important aspects of processing. Over the course of adolescence, there are progressive gains in speed, efficiency, and potential for abstract thought, and by late adolescence these reach levels comparable with those of adults. However, adolescents' motivations are specific to their developmental stage, and their knowledge and life experiences are shallow and do not form a substantial basis for efficient decision making. Young adolescents have been shown to have many strong beliefs that are based on misinformation, particularly in social and health matters. These misconceptions are often firmly held, and any challenge to them through education or persuasion may be met with strong resistance. Therefore, adolescent thinking styles must be taken into account when attempts are made to offer health education.

The thinking skills of early adolescents have been studied in relation to the ability to generate options, to understand that situations may be viewed from several perspectives at the same time, to foresee long-term consequences, and to evaluate the reliability and value of information as well as the relation to the tendency to overgeneralize from personal experience without also weighing other evidence. All these aspects show a developmental progression from childhood through adolescence to adulthood. In early adolescence, transition points have been noted at ages 11 to 12 years and at 15 to 16 years. By middle adolescence, decision making has become very much like that of adults. However, across the entire span of adolescence there seems to be a greater variability than among adults in higher order thinking skills and use of these advanced cognitive skills beyond school, in real-world situations. In social situations adolescents are often highly emotionally involved. Their social cognitive skills are far less mature and less effective than their cognitive skills in academic, nonemotional, and supportive situations. Unfortunately, many crucial decisions—about drinking, drugs, sex, and delinquent behavior—are made under highly emotional circumstances and with competing motivations. More needs to be learned about how to help adolescents use higher-order thinking skills in difficult social decisions. Group discussion, modeling by peers, and role playing are some of the techniques being investigated for preventive intervention programs on topics such as substance abuse and sexuality to help adolescents use their full potential for social cognitions and effective decision making.

Middle Adolescence

Middle adolescence is a distinctive developmental period that corresponds to the high school years, generally from ages 15 through 17 years. For the most part, middle adolescence is a period of relative quiescence characterized by consolidation of the multiple changes and transitions of the early adolescent pubertal period and preparation for the major transition to late adolescence, when autonomy becomes the central issue.

Middle adolescence is less demanding and less stressful than early adolescence because it involves no new biologic or hormonal changes. Also, both school structure and social and academic demands are familiar and continuous with prior experience. Middle adolescents have a clearer concept of self as an adolescent, and this role clarity is shared by the adults around them. They almost never revert to the childhood behaviors that occasionally appeared in early adolescence.

Although they still live at home, middle adolescents are significantly less involved with their parents. There is a sharp drop in earlier bickering and conflict over rules and responsibilities. More autonomy is granted not only by parents but by society. Two major examples are the ability to obtain a driver's license and to procure a work permit. Both greatly enhance the status and independence of middle adolescents.

Middle adolescents spend much less time with their families than do early adolescents. They are either with their peers or, when at home, often alone in their rooms. Although their relationships with peers are more extensive, they show more discrimination than in early adolescence. There is less dependence on the peer group and little of the earlier slavish adherence to peer norms or demands. Instead, friendships become differentiated both among males and among females.

Peer Relations

Peer influence does not replace parental influence in determining the basic values of adolescents. In childhood most activities are home and neighborhood based and are characterized by the presence and involvement of adults. However, as the individual moves out of childhood and through adolescence, peer influence gains greater importance and the amount of time spent with peers increases. By the end of junior high school and beyond, more than twice as much of the adolescent's time is spent with peers as with adults.

The earlier view of a monolithic, strongly pressuring peer group is now yielding to a more complex picture of overlapping peer influences. To meet their developmental needs, adolescents use peers as models, mentors, foils, competitors, confidants, and supporters. These needs are met through a few close friendships; membership in a clique defined by special interests or attributes (e.g., jocks, populars, nerds, punkers, druggies); and participation in a larger crowd defined by race, ethnicity, neighborhood, or school for its identity. Certain casual relationships with classmates may also be useful to development in specific ways. Although a great many of these peer associations are selected by the individual adolescent, some important ones are not. Unselected peer relations commonly include racial, ethnic, social class, and neighborhood peer groups. In other instances the adolescent is not admitted to the clique or group that he or she wants to join. Rather than becoming a loner, some adolescents settle for joining whatever group will have them. These less selective peer groups may be marginal or deviant groups.

Adolescents vary substantially in their susceptibility to peer-group pressures. Vulnerability to such pressure has many determinants and can be associated with factors such as the desire to emulate the behavior of group members, immaturity and insecurity about social skills, and personal or behavioral problems. Thus, adolescents use peer influences to construct their own environments as they explore possibilities and seek to meet their needs. The groups that they choose may have a positive or negative impact on their development. Adolescents may reinforce or reject their preexisting tendencies based on the influence of peer groups.

Efforts are now being made to use peer influence in systematic ways to educate and influence adolescents in interventions to prevent problem behaviors such as drug use, sexual activity leading to pregnancy, and delinquency. There have been promising results with peer counseling and peer leaders in adult-sponsored groups.

Sexuality

The most significant issue for middle adolescents in the United States today is initiation into sexuality. Making the transition from virginity to sexual activity has become a central marker for adolescents. Without question, the adolescents of today are much more sexually tolerant than their predecessors. They are more sexually active than their parents were at the same age, and recent findings indicate that they are also more sexually active than adolescents of any earlier time, including their older siblings.

Many parents tacitly permit their adolescents considerable sexual freedom. This permission is often accompanied by another tacit understanding: that sex will not be discussed with the parents and that they will not be directly confronted with the sexual behaviors of the adolescent. Because most parents continue to be uneasy about discussing sexual matters, sex remains a taboo subject. As a result, much of an adolescent's learning about sex comes from peers and from the media.

It has always been difficult to obtain data on the sexual activity of adolescents and adults in the United States, but the available statistics clearly show certain trends. In 1953, Kinsey et al[17] reported that, on the basis of data from 1938 to 1950, 7% of white females had intercourse by age 16 and 20% by age 20. From these baseline rates, female sexual activity began to rise dramatically starting in 1968. (See Chapter 3, "Epidemiology of Mortalities and Morbidities".)

Contemporary adolescents in the United States live in a world where adults are much more sexually active and permissive than in previous times. They are exposed to sexual explicitness in popular music, movies, television, and magazines. In addition, various types of advertising are often highly sexually provocative. However, only very recently has there been a growing concern that adolescents receive effective sexual education and display safe and responsible sexual behavior. For at least a decade, the United States has had the highest rates of teenage pregnancy and childbearing of any comparable industrialized nation. Since adolescents in those nations have similar ages of sexual initiation and levels of sexual activity and lower rates of abortion, the difference in rates of childbearing is due to lack of responsible and competent contraception.

The evidence of high and rising rates of adolescent infection with STDs and the specter of AIDS have heightened the urgency for ensuring that today's adolescents receive full, frank, and effective sex education. In many school districts where sex education was avoided a few years ago, it is now mandatory; this education includes information on AIDS and the use of condoms. The current emphasis on male responsibility through the use of condoms is a dramatic change from the earlier focus on use of the pill and other female methods of contraception.

Although masturbation is probably the most common sexual activity in adolescence, particularly among males, it receives little formal attention in research, sex education courses, or discussions with health personnel. Yet there does appear to be a general acceptance of the practice without the harsh messages about potential harm that were formerly used to restrict and frighten adolescents.

In this era of AIDS, homosexuality among adolescents is beginning to be studied more intensively. On the basis of existing data, the rates of increase in homosexual activity among adolescents do not appear to be as high as the reported heterosexual trends.[18] A current rate of 2% to 3% of homosexuality among adolescents, mainly males, is reported.

It is in middle adolescence that gender identity becomes consolidated. Intensification of gender role behaviors had their beginning in early adolescence.[19] At that time the peer group was most rigidly defined. Early adolescent males displayed conspicuously "masculine" interests and behaviors, and girls were highly "feminine." The masculine stereotype included assertiveness, independence, competence, mastery, expectation to act as the aggressor in sexual encounters, and containment of emotions. The feminine stereotype involved emotionality, dependence, emphasis on interpersonal relationships rather than achievement, and well-developed social skills. In middle adolescence the rigid adherence to these social norms yields to the understanding that gender roles are not rooted in biology, and that they are arbitrary and can vary independently of an individual's sex. Increasingly, emphasis is placed on the individual's freedom to act in accordance with personal preference. However, most young persons still tend to feel more comfortable in traditional gender roles.

This sophistication in dealing with gender roles reflects the fact that middle adolescents have a greater range of cognitive skills, including the capacity for more abstract reasoning, as well as more life experiences on which to base their thinking. There is also a broadening of perspective. Showing increasing attention to neighborhood concerns and certain societal issues, such as war or peace and the environment, some middle adolescents are readily recruited for community activities.

Although planning ahead on a short-term basis begins to become apparent in some areas, one important area where this does *not* occur is sexuality. Contraception is rarely used for first intercourse. Since sexual activity is often sporadic and unplanned, contraception may be used infrequently even by more sexually experienced middle adolescents. Therefore, the likelihood of unplanned pregnancy is high. For girls, becoming a teenage mother can signal an abrupt end to middle adolescence. For others, both girls and boys, dropping out of school may bring an end to middle adolescence.

Late Adolescence

Just as leaving elementary school and entering junior high school or middle school has become a convenient marker for entry into early adolescence, the senior year of high school is a key marker for imminent transition to the adult world, late adolescence. Although the end point of this transition is less easily defined than the beginning, it generally refers to adoption of adult work roles, formation of a family, and demonstration of responsible citizenship. Achievement of autonomy and further consolidation of identity are viewed as major tasks of this period.

Erikson[21] presented a concept of identity that gives a primary but not exclusive emphasis on identity consolidation as a task of late adolescence. He sees identity formation as a process that is continuous from late infancy through old age. This is a compelling formulation that has had ample validation from other sources.

Nonetheless, Erikson's emphasis on late adolescence is still appropriate. The structuring of a definitive, coherent sense of identity and individuality is a central and notable achievement that becomes possible only in late adolescence. Until then the necessary ingredients for synthesis of self-image have not been accumulated. The earlier self-perceptions of attractiveness, talent, mastery, and value to others are now reexamined, to be either confirmed or rejected.

Body image is a critical aspect of identity that cannot be fully developed until after the physical changes of puberty are completed. Relationships with parents and family are gradually renegotiated to a more adult-adult basis. By the end of late adolescence this status, optimally, has progressed to autonomy for the adolescent in the context of continuing strong affectional ties to the family.

Late adolescents have attained an adult level of reasoning skills. They have the capacity for formal thought, abstraction, and metacognitions. The level of cognitive development for a given adolescent depends, in part, on training and practice. The highest order of thinking skills and manipulation of symbols do not tend to be used in daily life. However, most late adolescents possess and use adult thinking skills in introspections about themselves and significant others. They can make very complex and sophisticated judgments about human relationships. They no longer base their judgments about people on overt behaviors but have good understanding of inner motivations, including multiple determinants of an action. Late adolescents have a well-developed sense of the future and possess the ability to plan ahead effectively. They can critically examine the logic and the consistency of statements made by adults, not only in personal discussions but also in political statements. They see fallacies in arguments and reasoning and are often quite skeptical. In late adolescence, enduring personal and societal attitudes and values are entrenched.

Over time, the adolescent's exploratory behaviors and interactions with peers have helped to define preferences, values, talents, sensuality, coping styles, ways of regulating emotions, and methods of handling conflicts. These experiences are also important in shaping the adolescent's sense of self-worth and feeling of belonging to a valued group. In addition, a personal identity is built through a mosaic of identifications with teachers, parents, peers, or media figures. This composite of identifications will determine the individual's future aspirations, career choices, stance toward society in terms of deviance or conventionality, adoption of health-promoting or health-damaging behaviors, and sexual preference. Throughout late adolescence, crucial decisions are made and shaped into the patterns and behaviors that will characterize the adult. A substantial number of late adolescents have established their sexuality and entered into an intimate, committed partner relationship.

Much of this final shaping of identity centers on the adolescent's perceptions of his or her future options as an adult. Among contemporary late adolescents, roughly one half attend college and the other half enter the world of work. The immediate pathway is clearer for those adolescents who go to college, since academic goals are sharply focused for them in high school. The immediate and attainable goal is getting into college, and this route holds much promise for future career success. In some significant ways the years in college offer a "moratorium," a time to engage in further consolidation of identity. There are new arenas for exploration, new role models and mentors, and new peers against whom to test oneself. College life offers both maximal autonomy and a structured, supportive environment in which to complete developmental tasks in a prolonged adolescence.

Adolescents who do not take the college route have quite different tasks and experiences.[21] They are likely to consolidate their identity earlier, since they do not have the added time and supportive structures of the college experience to delay facing the issues of earning a living, forming a family, and accepting other adult responsibilities. The pathways for young people who do not go to college are diverse. Many follow a traditional path of finding a job with good long-term prospects, getting married, having children, and building a self-sufficient life. Others become single parents. Many young persons return to live with their parents. A significant percentage may have legal problems and become incarcerated.

At present, the rates of youth unemployment and underemployment are high. Many young people, particularly school dropouts, will settle for low-paying, dead-end jobs, such as in fast-food restaurants, banks, or grocery stores. Some enter the underground economy of "off-the-books" jobs or illegal activities. Such choices do not enrich skills, give a basis for optimism about future career prospects, or enhance the likelihood that the adolescent will be successful in adult society.

Among late adolescents there is a high prevalence of living together without marriage. When children are conceived by or born to cohabiting couples, many of these couples decide to marry. However, many times the child is born out of wedlock and raised in a household headed by an adolescent single mother. Such households are often at the poverty level and supported by welfare.

When adaptations to the challenges of achieving autonomy and consolidating identity are problematic, options for future growth and development may be foreclosed and a troubled adulthood may lie ahead. Adolescents in this population, often heavily composed of minorities and the disadvantaged, also tend to have notably higher than normal physical and mental health problems. For them, the consequences of early and continuing adverse experiences are difficult to overcome. Earlier influences determined the opportunities that were encountered and shaped the choices that were made.

There are common factors associated with young persons, whether affluent or disadvantaged, who complete their adolescent development with a coherent sense of identity, confident autonomy, capacity for loving relationships, and competence and capacity to be successful in adult roles. These factors can be summarized as follows:

1. Involvement with caring adults and prosocial peers
2. Consistent messages about adult role expectations and positive, respected role models
3. Group solidarity in support of conventional values and goals (family, peers, school, community)
4. Opportunities to succeed in a context of clear and demanding but attainable expectations and standards of performance
5. Meaningful rewards and reinforcement for positive achievements
6. Work opportunities that promote self-respect and self-sufficiency

CHRONIC ILLNESS OR DISABILITY

It is a paradox of modern medicine that therapeutic triumphs and advances in biotechnology have resulted in a growing population of children and youth who no longer die of diseases and disorders but who survive and are treatable, but cannot be cured. Today substantial numbers of persons live out a full lifetime with chronic disease or disability. Among these individuals there are disorders of varying degrees of severity, with medical regimens that may or may not be burdensome. The disorders may be visible, disfiguring, or disabling to different degrees. Some, such as diabetes, may have no apparent signs at all to the casual observer. However, for all affected individuals there are additional developmental tasks and challenges in adolescence.

Certain fundamental similarities exist for all youngsters as they negotiate the transitions of adolescence, regardless of health status, ethnicity, or socioeconomic level. These are the universal themes of identity, autonomy, achievement, and intimacy (sexuality). However, just as ethnic and socioeconomic disadvantages often pose special problems for the young, adolescents who are disabled or chronically ill face significant additional and unique challenges. In many ways chronic illness poses dilemmas in which the normative tasks of adolescence often come into sharp and direct conflict with adaptation to the disorder or disability. Youngsters in this population often lack the ability, experience, or opportunity to fulfill normative personal and societal expectations for their adolescent developmental processes. Across the entire range of disorders and disabilities, a set of comparable and systematic obstacles complicate the tasks of these adolescents and may impair their ability to resolve successfully the challenges that confront all adolescents.

Identity

Since one important aspect of identity is body image, the biologic changes of puberty are enormously significant. The timing, rate, and outcome of these changes have separate influences on the developing adolescent. Many chronically ill youngsters experience delayed puberty because of the retarding effects of the illness itself. For all males, significantly delayed puberty is problematic. For the chronically ill, such a delay compounds many problems. These youngsters, as they enter adolescence, have begun to reappraise the significance of their disability and have concerns about their bodily integrity. When on-time pubertal development fails to occur, special anxieties arise. Will they ever develop in an acceptable way? How can they face their peers, who are mostly very mature and well developed? These doubts and uncertainties have profound effects on an adolescent's feelings of self-worth.[22] Typical pubertal adolescents have been shown to have normative concerns about their own body image and to be intolerant of imperfections in others. Therefore, at the height of adolescent self-consciousness, chronically ill adolescents experience greater peer intolerance of their condition and often encounter rejection. The immature appearance of late-developing, chronically ill adolescents may lead their parents to persist in treating them as children and cause resistance to their age-appropriate moves toward more independence.

Pubertal changes are not always synchronous. For example, although an adolescent may be physically immature, that individual may show significant advances in cognitive maturity. The young person may have new introspective abilities—to reflect on the meaning of having a particular health condition and to appraise his or her prospects for the future in terms of health, personal relationships, and career options. Depending on the individual, this type of thinking may lead to realistic planning and behavior or to harmful denial and lack of compliance with the medical regimen. In some instances it may lead to self-pity or sadness and a tendency to withdraw. For most chronically ill or disabled adolescents, there is some degree of lowering of self-esteem as the adolescent comes to terms with an identity that involves compromised bodily integrity and lifelong disorder.

Family Interactions

The most constructive developmental outcomes for these adolescents occur when there is a consistent, supportive family environment. It is important to note that "supportive" does not mean indulgent and overprotective. Parents must be willing to loosen ties and permit incremental and responsible autonomy. The adolescent must eventually take responsibility for self-care and management of the disorder. The family should encourage open discussion of the illness, and offer realistic expectations for the adolescent and practical suggestions of how to maximize the individual's potential. Parents must help the youngster to avoid using the illness as an excuse for avoiding challenges or unpleasant responsibilities or a means of engendering guilt and securing special favors.

Parents who convey the message that they feel sorry for their youngster often reinforce negative feelings in the child, for example, a sense of being "damaged goods" that others will never value. When parents rigidly maintain the same degree of protection and control that they exerted in their offspring's childhood, they may precipitate rebellious, risk-taking behaviors on the part of the adolescent. When parents deny the illness and insist that the youngster needs no special consideration and "must live in the real world just like everyone else," extreme insecurity, anxiety, and depression may ensue. This may lead to fearfulness, inactivity, and isolation from peers and outside interests or to hostile and resentful attitudes toward others.

Achievement

When chronically ill or disabled adolescents develop a negative self-concept, a significant adverse impact on motivation may occur. Since many of these youngsters expect to do poorly or fail, their achievement level is low. In addition, lack of understanding on the part of teachers often leads to unrealistic expectations for these youngsters. Some expectations may be too high for those who have a substantial physical disability. Although such youngsters may be intelligent and motivated, they may have missed a significant number of school days because of illness; when in school, they may have had times when they were inattentive for health reasons. Inadvertently, teachers may set up these adolescents for failure. Other times, expectations are set too low. For example, the teacher may expect too little and therefore only a low level of performance is elicited.[23] Parents and physicians need to help the youngster, teachers, and other significant persons to understand what expectations are realistic and to aid the youngsters in achieving their highest potentials. Ensuring positive achievement motivation in this adolescent transition is crucial because attitudes about adult self-efficacy and motivational patterns are being adopted at this time.

Peer Relations

Beginning in early adolescence, youngsters rely heavily on their peers to reflect information on their acceptability, attractiveness, and performance. This feedback helps them define who they are in terms of how they are perceived. Peer attentiveness and concern with peer evaluation peaks in early adolescence. Affiliation with the peer group peaks in middle adolescence. For all adolescents, positive peer interaction is a determining factor in the development of positive self-esteem and sense of self-worth. The quality of peer relations not only has a significant impact on social development but also affects academic success. Chronically ill and disabled adolescents frequently have difficulty with peer relationships, but this is only partly their fault. Studies have confirmed that healthy students are not accepting of youngsters who have disabilities. This intolerance is at its highest among early adolescents.[24] It has been shown that in classrooms students without disabilities tend to exclude those with disorders and sometimes may be unpleasant to them and even taunt them. This intolerance has been attributed to the fact that early adolescents are concerned about their own bodily integrity and sensitive to the unpredictable bodily changes of puberty that they are undergoing. They seem to be made anxious when confronted with disfigurement, disorder, or disability in others and therefore they actively reject such persons.

This rejection process is made more likely because chronically ill or disabled youngsters often have less social competence and fewer skills than their healthy peers. They have often missed some of the earlier social learning experiences involving the give-and-take of peer interaction. They may be more self-absorbed because of their disorder and less efficient in reading social cues in others. As a result, they are deficient in the perspective taking that would give them empathy with their peers and offer clues for relating and communicating with them more effectively. However, these are social skills that can be taught.

Sexual Identity

This is a particularly problematic area for chronically ill or disabled adolescents. When there is social distance or poor peer relations, these adolescents lack the usual opportunities to compare ideas, to gain information, and to explore sexual feelings. They also lack models of chronically ill or disabled adults who are portrayed or seen as competent social and sexual persons. The sense of isolation and ignorance is coupled with these adolescents' own negative body image and perceptions that they are unappealing and unlovable. Furthermore, social myths reinforce the image of chronically ill or disabled persons as being asexual even though there is no evidence to support such beliefs. Youngsters in this situation need special understanding and support in the area of sexuality. Their parents and the medical personnel involved with them should examine their own attitudes to be sure that they personally do not accept these myths or have doubts or negative beliefs that will be conveyed to the adolescent. To promote a positive sexual identity, they must be able to provide accurate information to these youngsters about their sexual capabilities and guide them toward realistic expectations for sexual functioning. This can be done in conjunction with helping them to learn social skills and achieve age-appropriate social competence.

In evaluating their future lives and considering options for adult roles, chronically ill or disabled adolescents will have more doubts and uncertainties about their chances for finding fulfilling careers and achieving secure intimate relationships than will their healthy peers. These issues need to be dealt with realistically but with emphasis on the many positive options that do exist.

The needs of chronically ill or disabled adolescents are the same as for all adolescents. Despite their illness or disability, these youngsters need to feel that they are worthwhile, competent persons who are respected. They need to be accepted by others as valued members of family and peer groups. They need a sense of a positive future. With adequate understanding given to their special needs, realization of the goals of adolescent development is possible for substantial numbers of adolescents despite illness or disability.

References

1. Harrison GA, Tanner JM, Pilbeam DR, Baker PT: *Human biology,* ed 3, Oxford, 1988, Oxford University Press, p 382.
2. Hall GS: *Adolescence: its psychology and its relations to physiology, anthropology, sociology, sex, crime, religion and education,* Englewood Cliffs, NJ, 1904, Prentice-Hall.
3. Freud A: *Normality and pathology in childhood: assessment of development,* ed 6, New York, 1977, International Universities Press.
4. Kestenberg P: Phases of adolescence with suggesstions for a correlation of psychic and hormonal organizations. III. Puberty growth, differentiation and consolidation, *J Am Acad Child Psychiatry* 6:426, 1967.
5. Blos P: *The young adolescent,* New York, 1970, Free Press.
6. Erikson EH: *Childhood and society,* New York, 1950, WW Norton.
7. Douvan E, Adelson J: *The adolescent experience,* New York, 1966, John Wiley.
8. Offer D: *The psychological world of the teenager,* New York, 1969, Basic Books.
9. Rutter M, Graham P, Chadwick OFD: Adolescent turmoil: fact or fiction, *J Child Psychol Psychiatry* 17:35, 1976.
10. Masterson JF. The symptomatic adolescent five years later: he didn't grow out of it, *Am J Psychiatry* 123:1338, 1967.

11. Weiner IB: Psychopathology in adolescence, *Arch Gen Psychiatry* 33:193, 1976.
12. Hamburg BA: Early adolescence: a specific and stressful stage of the life cycle. In Coelho G, Hamburg D, Adams J, editors: *Coping and adaptation,* New York, 1974, Basic Books, pp 101-124.
13. Clausen J: The social meaning of differential physical and sexual maturation. In Dragastin SE, Elder GH Jr, editors: *Adolescence in the life cycle: psychological change and social context,* New York, 1975, John Wiley.
14. Brooks-Gunn J, Petersen A, editors: *Girls at puberty: biological and psychosocial perspectives,* New York, 1983, Plenum Press.
15. Kety SS: Circulation and metabolism of the human brain in health and disease, *Am J Med* 8:205, 1950.
16. Huttenlocher P: Synaptic density in human frontal cortex: developmental changes and the effects of aging, *Brain Res* 163:195, 1979.
17. Kinsey AC, Pomeroy WB, Gebhard PH: *Sexual behavior in the human female,* Philadelphia, 1953, WB Saunders.
18. Dreyer PH: Sexuality during adolescence. In Wolman BB, editor: *Handbook of developmental psychology,* Englewood Cliffs, NJ, 1982, Prentice-Hall.
19. Galambos N, Olmeida D, Petersen A: Masculinity, femininity and sex role attitudes in early adolescence: exploring gender intensification, *Child Dev* 61:1905-1914, 1990.
20. Erikson EH: *Identity and the life cycle,* New York, 1980, WW Norton.
21. William T. Grant Foundation Commission on Work, Family and Citizenship: *Youth and America's future. The forgotten half: non-college youth in America,* New York, 1988, The Foundation.
22. Lerner RM, Bracking BE: The importance of inner and outer body parts in the self-concept of late adolescence, *Sex Roles* 4:225, 1978.
23. Felson RB: Physical attractiveness, grades and teachers and attributions of ability, *Rep Res Soc Psychol* 11:64, 1980.
24. Kleck R, DeJong W: Physical disability, physical attractiveness and social outcomes in children's small groups, *Rehab Psychol* 28:79, 1983.

CHAPTER 9

Development of Sexual Behavior

•

Joseph Lee Rodgers

In the popular press the American adolescent is often portrayed as a package of "raging hormones" constantly in search of sexual gratification. At the other extreme, a minority of adults and policymakers who oppose sex education in school and community programs would deny even the existence of libido—much less actual sexual behavior—among adolescents: "What we don't talk about can't be happening." The truth about adolescent sexuality is certainly somewhere between these two extremes. Although the biologic and psychologic responses to puberty are real and potent, most adolescents are not as sexually active as those depicted in many best-selling novels and movies. On the other hand, increasing levels of adolescent pregnancy provide overt evidence that sexual activity is indeed occurring among adolescents in the United States.

How sexually active are U.S. adolescents? How has adolescent sexual behavior changed over time? What does it mean for an adolescent to be "sexually active?" What behavioral transitions exist through which adolescents pass during the development of their sexuality? What are the characteristics of adolescents who are becoming sexually active—or considering it? How carefully do they use contraceptives? Who are their partners? Where do they have sex? When? Why? This chapter provides an objective picture of sexual activity among heterosexual adolescents in the United States. Very little empirical information is currently available regarding the development of homosexual behavior. The disciplinary approach is psychosocial, and demographic treatment concerns the "typical adolescent." The portrayal will rely on research data collected by psychologists, sociologists, economists, and demographers, noting important differences in sex and race.

ADOLESCENT COITAL ACTIVITY: TRENDS AND LEVELS

Adolescents in the United States have become increasingly sexually active over time. Information collected before the 1970s was obtained from predominantly white respondents, from local and state data, which were not national estimates. In the data of Kinsey et al,[1,2] collected during the 1940s, 3% of white females and 39% of white males reported being nonvirgins by age 15. The data collected in Michigan in 1972 by Vener and Stewart[3] showed that 24% of white females and 38% of white males had had sexual intercourse by this same age. Inner-city data from Baltimore in 1981 and 1982 showed the percentage of nonvirgins to be 35% for white females and 66% for white males at age 15.[4]

National estimates (i.e., ones that can be generalized to the United States as a whole) are available only from about 1970 onward. Zelnik and Kantner's National Survey of Young Women (NSYW)[5] was based on longitudinal data from females living in metropolitan areas from 1971 to 1982. In 1971, approximately 28% of females aged 15 to 19 were nonvirgins (including 23% of whites and 52% of blacks); 8 years later, this figure peaked at 46% and then dropped slightly to around 42% (40% of whites and 53% of blacks) by 1982.

A number of important and high-quality datasets collected around 1980 provided an excellent "data snapshot" of the climate of adolescent sexuality in the United States in the early 1980s. The National Longitudinal Survey of Youth (NLSY) is a nationally representative dataset used to define precise estimates of national levels of sexuality. Analysis of this dataset provided the following percentages of nonvirgin adolescent 15-year-olds in the United States in 1983 by race-sex subgroup: white males, 12%; white females, 4.7%; black males, 42%; black females, 10%; Hispanic males, 19%; Hispanic females, 4.3%. Another survey, the National Survey of Family Growth (NSFG), showed somewhat higher figures in 1982 estimates.[6] Nonvirginity reported among 15.5-year-old females was 18% in whites and 28% in blacks. These figures reflect considerable sexual activity among our youth at an aggregate national level.

Results from the most comprehensive survey of sexual behavior that has ever been conducted were published in 1994.[7] The National Health and Social Life Survey (NHSLS) obtained responses from a random sample of U.S. adults in 1991, but asked a number of questions that indicated patterns of adolescent sexual behavior. When these respondents were divided into birth cohorts from 1933 to 1942, 1943 to 1952, 1953 to 1962, and 1963 to 1967, age at first intercourse showed a "small but discernible" decline in all gender and race categories. The results from this survey were compared with those from other national surveys (in particular, the National Survey of Family Growth), and results were almost identical (supporting the validity of findings in both this and previous data sources).

Of particular note for defining a picture of the typical adolescent is that by far the majority of American adolescents are *not* sexually active by age 15. The mean age at first intercourse in the 1983 NLSY data was 17.5 years for white males, 15.5 years for black males, 17.0 years for Hispanic males, 18.5 years for white females, 17.5 years for black females, and 18.5 years for Hispanic females (all rounded to the nearest half-year). By age 19, approximately 55% of all whites and 75% of all blacks reported being nonvirgins.

Race-sex differences reflected in these figures are consistent across all national datasets. At any particular age, the average black adolescent is more sexually precocious than the white and Hispanic adolescent, and the average male adolescent is more sexually precocious than the average female adolescent. Theorists have been especially interested in these group differences.

Several explanations have been offered to account for the sex differences. Because females reach puberty earlier than males, why their first intercourse is later than that for males is an interesting question. One cause may be rooted in the differential costs of pregnancy for males and females. Other psychosocial explanations rely on different social norms for males and females, a still extant double standard of sexual ethics. Recent work has shown a relationship between androgens and sexuality (attitudes and behaviors) for both males and females: males have considerably more androgens than females, which can help explain sex differences. In the ADSEX survey,[8] more than a trivial number of males, especially black males, reported prepubertal coital behavior; around 35% of black males and 10% of white males reported first coitus at age 9 or younger; virtually no females reported first intercourse before age 10. Thus, puberty may not be as important a marker for male coital activity as for females. These figures probably reflect some male bravado in responding to survey questions about sexual activity. Prepubertal males' descriptions of their first sexual partner were often inconsistent in several ways with the characteristics of the females with whom they would have had contact. Ages they gave for their first partner were often much younger than the earliest ages reported by the females. Another explanation that can plausibly explain this apparent inconsistency is that males and females may account differentially for prepubertal sex play. Little research has been done on prepubertal sexual activity.

Race difference has also received some attention; cultural, social, and biologic theories have been proposed. One physical theory[9] is particularly interesting. Both male and female blacks reach puberty before whites. Early studies discounted this effect because the differences are fairly small (less than a year, on the average). However, once nonlinear effects of sexually precocious adolescents looking for partners over several years are accounted for, even a few months of difference in physical maturation can have long-term effects (especially at young ages where only a few new nonvirgins represent a large percentage increase). Social and cultural explanations have had only limited success in explaining this race difference.

Demographic researchers have focused on aggregate figures like those reported above; the percentage of nonvirgins and the age at first intercourse are standard ways to measure levels of sexual activity in an adolescent population. However, these two measures are fairly superficial reflections of much more complex behavioral processes. Sophisticated models portray the development of sexuality as more than simply a question of whether sexual intercourse has occurred or not.

NONCOITAL SEXUAL ACTIVITY

Hand holding, kissing, going on dates, light petting, heavy petting, and oral sex are all noncoital partner-oriented behaviors indicating levels of sexuality; fantasizing and masturbation are personal behaviors in which a majority of adolescents engage. If we posit a latent developmental continuum reflecting general sexuality, then each of these behaviors is simply an indicator, which in combination with other behaviors can help to identify the adolescent's current position on the continuum. We must distinguish explicit sexual behavior from sexual attitudes or biologic disposition, because both opportunity and social or religious sanctions can affect behavioral responses. An adolescent may be highly sexually motivated in a physical sense but refrain from some or all sexual behavior for other reasons. The process can also work in the opposite direction. An adolescent with little biologic motivation may respond to social pressure to become sexually active. Recent theorists have treated biologic, psychologic, and social influences on sexuality as separate but interacting processes. Therefore, different, although clearly correlated, latent continua explain sexual drive, attitudes, and behavior. In the following discussion the focus is on sexual behaviors themselves, rather than their underlying causes. The Suggested Readings contain causal explanations and formal models.

The ADSEX survey provided information about noncoital sexual behavior.[10] This survey was administered in schools in two metropolitan communities in the southeastern United States between 1978 and 1982. First-round data were obtained from junior high students (grades 7 to 9, mean age of 14.1, age range 12 to 15); the second-round data were collected 2 years later (when students were in grades 9 to 11). This survey contained information linking adolescents to their friends and siblings with a broader range of information about noncoital sexual behaviors than the national surveys.

An interesting question is whether adolescents make a smooth transition during their sexual development. That is, do most adolescents hold hands before they kiss, kiss before they pet, and pet before they have intercourse? Research on this question suggests that among whites, the answer is usually "yes." The longitudinal structure of the ADSEX data showed a systematic progression through

"necking," "feel breast clothed," "feel breast directly," "feel female sex organs directly," "feel penis directly," and "intercourse." However, blacks moved in a different sequence across these "sexual stepping stones" and in a somewhat less consistent manner than whites. For blacks, coital activity moved up in the order as being more common than any of the three unclothed petting behaviors. In other words, typically, blacks reported sexual intercourse as occurring before many of the apparently less intimate behaviors. Further, black females were relatively inconsistent in their progression through these sexual behaviors. This difference has practical implications for healthcare professionals. If white adolescents report that they have not engaged in petting, further information about more intimate behaviors is usually carried along with that response; such inferences for black adolescents would be more tenuous.

During the 2-year period in which these junior high students in grades 7 to 9 advanced to grades 9 to 11, the median "advance" through these behaviors for whites was slightly more than two behaviors. For example, a white male or female who said "yes" to the question on "necking" in the eighth grade was likely to respond "yes" to the questions on "necking," "feel breast clothed," and "feel breast directly" by the time he or she was in grade 10. Black adolescents had a less predictable progression through these behaviors.

A fairly large proportion of the adolescents in this survey reported no sexual experience of any kind. In the first-round ADSEX data for junior high school students (mean age of 14.1, with a range of 12 to 15), one fourth had not engaged in any of the behaviors listed above. Race-sex data showed that 21% of white males, 34% of white females, 6% of black males, and 25% of black females responded "no" to all of the social-sexual activities.

Apparently, white adolescents have a more extended "preparation" for sexual intercourse than do black adolescents. This finding, and the earlier pubertal maturation of blacks, can help explain the higher levels of both sexuality and premarital pregnancy among blacks than among whites. To some degree, white females are protected from pregnancy longer than black females by the progression through which they pass before engaging in coitus.

Rates of oral sex among the 1980 ADSEX respondents were considerably higher than those found by Kinsey's surveys in the 1940s. In the ADSEX survey, slightly more total teenagers reported oral sex than reported sexual intercourse; more females reported oral sex than reported intercourse, and slightly more males reported intercourse than reported oral sex. An interesting hypothesis is that adolescents often have oral sex as a substitute for genital sex to reduce pregnancy risk; of the virgins, 24% of males and 16% of females reported oral sex, providing support for this hypothesis. Among both sexes, fellatio was less common than either intercourse or cunnilingus.

FIRST INTERCOURSE EXPERIENCE

Although sexual behavior is far more complex than indicated by responses to a question about virginity status, this response (or age at onset) is the most important indicator of sexuality. First, coital behavior is (virtually) a prerequisite for pregnancy. One of the aggregate predictors of fertility rates is the amount of time that women are "at risk" of pregnancy; obviously, the sooner intercourse begins, the longer is the at-risk period. Second, a number of health risks are linked to onset and amount of coital activity, in particular the risk of sexually transmitted disease. Finally, evidence collected during the 1980s and 1990s suggests that many nonsexual adolescent behaviors—including schoolwork; friendship interactions; and use of drugs, alcohol, and cigarettes—may have subtle but important relationships to coital behavior (which in turn is obviously linked to noncoital sexual behavior). The information that follows comes from the ADSEX study, unless otherwise indicated.

Both males and females typically had a first partner older than themselves (in the NLSY data, an average of 1 year older for males and 3 years older for females). Among the NHSLS respondents (adults retrospectively reporting on their first intercourse experience), 10% of males and 22% of females had their first intercourse with their spouse. In all, 78% of the males and 93% of the females had first intercourse with someone they knew well (a spouse, someone with whom they were in love, or a close friend). Five percent of the males and 1% of the females had their first intercourse with someone they had just met. In the ADSEX data, approximately two thirds lost their virginity with someone they knew well, either a fiancé, a steady, or a close friend. About one fifth of the respondents lost their virginity with someone they had just met; males were more likely to give this response than females. These ADSEX frequencies are shown in Figure 9-1. Approximately 40% of the respondents were sure or believed that their first partner was also a virgin; about 35% were sure or thought their partner was not a virgin. There was a large sex difference; many more females than males thought their partner was not a virgin, and many more males than females thought their partner was a virgin.

Reasons cited for first intercourse typically involved the partner, and almost half of both males and females responded "so that my partner would love me more." Approximately 20% of males and females said the reason was either "to please the partner" or "so not to hurt the partner." About 15% of the males indicated

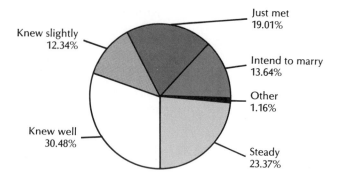

Fig. 9-1. Relationship of first sexual partner.

that "I forced my partner" the first time they had intercourse (compared with approximately 2% of the females). About 15% of the females indicated that "my partner forced me," compared with around 7% of the males. The national data in the recently collected NHSLS also contained information about the reason for first intercourse. Eight percent of the males and 25% of the females reported that they did not wish to engage in their first intercourse experience but "went along with it" anyway. Conversely, 91% of the males and 71% of the females reported that they wanted their first intercourse to occur when it did. Of those who wanted it to happen, over half of the males gave as a reason "curiosity about sex" and one fourth said it was because of affection for their partner. Among females, almost half gave affection as the reason, while just under one fourth gave curiosity as the main reason. Three percent of females and 12% of males reported that physical pleasure was the main motivation.

Characteristics of friends, siblings, and parents are also a consideration. The sexual behavior of black respondents, especially black males, has been difficult to predict from that of their friends or siblings. White adolescents have more than a chance similarity in their intercourse status to their friends and siblings, females particularly so. White males appear to *select* friends who are similar, while white females *influence* their friends to become similar. These same patterns also occur in relation to siblings. Whites, and especially white females, are even more similar to their siblings than to their friends, controlling for age differences. Research on mothers and daughters (both blacks and whites) also shows that a daughter's sexual experience is related to the mother's sexual experience when she was an adolescent. Furthermore, both males and females are more likely to be sexually active if they have lived in a single-parent household. Note that these relationships are not necessarily causal in nature. Parents who divorce are undoubtedly different from nondivorced parents in many ways; some of these differences may be the cause of increased sexual activity among their children, rather than divorce per se.

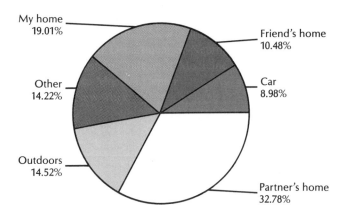

Fig. 9-2. Location of first intercourse.

The environmental location of first intercourse is shown in Figure 9-2. Almost one third of the adolescent respondents reported loss of virginity in their partner's home; one third, in either their own home or a friend's home; and one third in a car, outdoors, at school, or in a hotel. Almost half of adolescents lost their virginity during the months of June, July, or August. In the NLSY data, the summer sexuality peak was reduced substantially after high school, suggesting that the free time and activities of summer may promote sexual behavior. Evidence shows that general levels of coital behavior in humans increase during the heat of summer, perhaps because of hormonal shifts; however, pure biologic models do not explain the change in loss of virginity patterns after high school.

In the NSYW data, almost one half of adolescent females used contraception at first intercourse in 1982 (up from 40% in 1976). The likelihood of using contraception increased with age. Whites were more likely than blacks to use contraception at first intercourse, but blacks were more likely to use a prescription method of contraception (the pill, an intrauterine device, or a diaphragm); white females were more likely to rely on condom use by their partner. Those who planned their first intercourse were more likely to use contraception than those who did not. In the recently collected NHSLS data, approximately one fourth of the earlier birth cohorts reported using contraception at first intercourse. This proportion increased to 50% for the youngest cohort, matching the NSYW findings.

CONTINUING ADOLESCENT INTERCOURSE

In American society and in many other societies, the first intercourse experience is considered a marker of adulthood. However, continuing sexuality is in many ways more important because it is ongoing sexual behavior that increases the risk of pregnancy and sexually transmitted diseases. In the NSYW study, 14% of white female nonvirgins had had intercourse only once; 13% of black female nonvirgins had had a single experience.

In the ADSEX data, respondents indicated continuing intercourse with their first partner. Approximately 35% of the nonvirgins indicated only one intercourse experience with their first partner (by far the model response), and males were more likely to give this response than females. (In the recent NHSLS data, 28% of males and 14% of females reported having sex with their first partner only once.) Another 30% of the ADSEX respondents had sex two to five times with their first partner. About 35% indicated only one sex partner, again by far the model response; another 40% reported two to five partners; 3% reported 20 or more partners, almost all of those males. During the previous month, 35% of the nonvirgins reported no partners; another 35% reported one partner, 10% reported two partners, and 5% reported three partners. The same 35% reported zero coital acts during the past month, 20% reported one coital act, 10% reported two, and 10% reported three. Approximately three fourths of the nonvirgin adolescents in this survey had sex less often than once a week.

Temporally, continuing sexual intercourse is more evenly distributed across the year than first intercourse (which peaks in June and July). There is a slight increase in overall intercourse rates during the late summer. However, the peak is much lower than for first intercourse.

The NSYW study showed that about one half of all first premarital pregnancies occurred within 6 months of loss of virginity (which is not surprising, because approximately one half of first coitus experiences in females are unprotected). In 1983 almost three fourths of teenage females aged 15 to 19 reported using contraception at last intercourse; this figure increased from slightly under one half in 1971. Older and more sexually precocious adolescents are generally more careful in contraceptive use. Even though the efficacy of contraception increased between the early 1970s and the 1980s, overall intercourse rates increased substantially, leading to increased pregnancy rates even as contraceptive use increased.

CONCLUSION

The picture of the typical American adolescent suggests that (1) typicality depends on the race and/or sex subgroup; (2) sexual behavior, both coital and noncoital, is clearly occurring among our youth and at salient levels; and (3) the figures cited belie the popular media view that adolescents actively participate in a "bubbling caldron of sexuality." Even among the minority of 15-year-olds who have had sexual intercourse, most do not have intercourse on a regular basis. Those who have considerable sexual experience have sex only occasionally. A small minority have sex often and with many partners, but this small minority is probably overrepresented in television, movies, and books.

Perhaps the major challenge to parents and policymakers concerned about adolescent pregnancy relates to the relatively *infrequent* coital behavior of most sexually active adolescents. Such infrequency is linked to lack of planning. Coital activity among young teenagers is *not* behavior that is carefully discussed and for which its participants prepare. Conversations of adolescents with researchers and policymakers repeatedly support the fact that sexual encounters often "just happen" rather than being planned. High levels of denial and repression occur among many adolescents. However, both coital and noncoital sexuality is highly reinforcing behavior, contributing to an adolescent's desire for peer support, expression of maturity, and physical stimulation. Given these levels of reinforcement and the adolescent's short-term view of the future, it is easy to explain why many teenagers do experiment sexually and then quickly enter at least occasional sexual encounters into their behavioral repertoire, despite the obvious health and pregnancy risks associated with such behavior.

References

1. Kinsey A, Pomeroy W, Martin C: *Sexual behavior in the human male,* Philadelphia, 1948, WB Saunders.
2. Kinsey A, Pomeroy W, Martin C: *Sexual behavior in the human female,* Philadelphia, 1953, WB Saunders.
3. Vener AM, Stewart CS: Adolescent sexual behavior in middle America revisited, *J Marriage Fam* 36:728, 1972.
4. Zabin LS, Hirsch MB, Smith EQ, Hardy JB: Adolescent sexual attitudes and behavior: are they inconsistent? *Fam Plann Perspect* 16:181, 1984.
5. Zelnick M, Kantner JF: Sexual activity, contraceptive use and pregnancy among metropolitan-area teenagers: 1971-1979, *Fam Plann Perspect* 12:230-231, 1980.
6. Kahn JR, Kalsbeek WD, Hofferth SL: National estimates of teenage sexual activity: evaluating the comparability of three national surveys, *Demography* 25:189-204, 1988.
7. Laumann EO, Gagnon JH, Michael RT, Michaels S: *The social organization of sexuality: sexual practices in the United States,* Chicago, 1994, University of Chicago Press.
8. Rodgers JL, Billy JOG, Udry JR: The rescission of behaviors: inconsistent responses in adolescent sexuality data, *Soc Sci Res* 11:280-296, 1982.
9. Rowe DC, Rodgers JL: A social contagion model of adolescent sexual behavior: explaining race differences, *Soc Biol* 41:1-18, 1994.
10. Rodgers JL, Rowe DC: Social contagion and adolescent sexual behavior: a developmental EMOSA model, *Psych Rev* 100:479-510, 1993.

Suggested Readings

Hayes CD, editor: *Risking the future: adolescent sexuality, pregnancy, and childbearing,* vol I, Washington, DC, 1987, National Academy Press.
   This book, along with the working papers, statistical appendix, and annotated bibliography in volume II (Hofferth SL, Hayes CD, editors), provides by far the most comprehensive treatment of this topic that exists. Chapters written by a dozen or so experts in the field provide reviews of the literature on almost every aspect of adolescent pregnancy, sexuality, and childbearing.

Kahn JR, Kalsbeek WD, Hofferth SL: National estimates of teenage sexual activity: evaluating the comparability of three national surveys, *Demography* 25:189-204, 1988.
   This article combines information from three high-quality national surveys. Excellent developmental curves showing age at first intercourse among U.S. adolescents in the early 1980s are presented.

Laumann EO, Gagnon JH, Michael RT, Michaels S: *The social organization of sexuality: sexual practices in the United States,* Chicago, 1994, University of Chicago Press.
   This book reports results from the most comprehensive sexuality survey ever conducted in the United States to date. Most reported findings concern adult sexual practices. One chapter (Chapter 9) is concerned with first intercourse, which for many of the respondents occurred during adolescence.

Miller BC, Card JJ, Paikoff RL, Peterson J: *Preventing adolescent pregnancy,* Newbury Park, N.J., 1992, Sage.
   This book reviews many different U.S. pregnancy prevention programs and reports on evaluations of these programs.

Miller BC, Fox GL: Theories of adolescent heterosexual behavior, *J Adoles Res* 2:269-282, 1987.
   This article reviews a broad array of different theoretical perspectives that have been used by researchers to organize and understand adolescent sexual behavior.

Rodgers JL, Billy JOG, Udry JR: The rescission of behaviors: inconsistent responses in adolescent sexuality data, *Soc Sci Res* 11:280-296, 1982.
   This article highlights some of the reliability and validity issues involved in collecting both coital and noncoital adolescent sexuality data.

Rowe DC, Rodgers JL, Meseck-Bushey S: An "epidemic" model of sexual intercourse prevalences for black and white adolescents, *Soc Biol* 36:127-145, 1989.
   This article proposes that sexuality spreads through an adolescent network primarily through a contagion process whereby nonvirgins "transmit" coital behavior to virgins. Race differences are shown to be highly related to differences in maturational rates between whites and blacks.

Rodgers JL, Rowe DC: Social contagion and adolescent sexual behavior: a developmental EMOSA model, *Psych Rev* 100: 479-510, 1993.
   This article proposes a theory of social contagion that accounts for transitions through five levels of sexual intimacy. Each stage (naivety, kissing, light petting, heavy petting, and sexual intercourse) is "spread" either through contagious contact (an experienced opposite-sex adolescent transmitting the behavior to a virgin) or through noncontagious contact (two virgin adolescents engaging in the behavior). Transition parameters are estimated that account for each type of transition, separately for race and sex subgroups.

CHAPTER 10

Practice Settings

•

Martin Fisher

Adolescents receive health care from many different professionals in a wide variety of settings. In the private practice domain, physicians in all specialties (pediatrics, family practice, internal medicine, obstetrics and gynecology, psychiatry, and the surgical subspecialties), nurse practitioners, social workers, and psychologists are involved in adolescent care. Increasing numbers of adolescents are obtaining care through prepaid group practices such as health maintenance organizations, and many continue to require hospital-based care. Special services are available in high schools, colleges, the military, and correctional facilities. The provision of first-rate comprehensive adolescent health care in any available setting is a laudatory goal. In fact, the scope and quality of care differs for each style of practice, and several articles have described the issues involved in delivery of adolescent health care in each of the different settings. To aid the clinician caring for adolescent patients, this chapter reviews the strengths and limitations inherent in the different medical environments.

OFFICE-BASED PRACTICE

In 1991 the U.S. Department of Health and Human Services, reporting data from a 1985 survey, indicated that adolescents 11 to 20 years of age made approximately 59 million visits per year to office-based physicians (Table 10-1).[1] These visits represented 9% of all patient visits and were similar in demographic profile (i.e., primarily female, white, and non-Hispanic) to all other age groups. A breakdown of all adolescent office visits shows that 35% are to general and/or family practitioners, 18% to pediatricians, 8% to obstetrician/gynecologists, 7% to dermatologists, 5% to internists, 5% to ophthalmologists, 2% to psychiatrists, and 20% to all other

(primarily surgical) specialties. Distribution of these visits by age groupings (11 to 14 years versus 15 to 20 years) are as expected; younger adolescents make more visits to pediatricians and older adolescents make more visits to other specialties, especially obstetrician/gynecologists. Each of these specialties faces specific issues in attracting adolescent patients and in managing their health needs in an appropriate and efficient manner.

Pediatrics

During the past several decades, attempts have focused on incorporating adolescent health care into general pediatric practice. Both economic incentives and the growth of adolescent medicine as a subspecialty primarily within pediatric departments have supported this movement. Currently, 33% of all visits by those aged 11 to 14 years, but only 10% of those aged 15 to 20, are to pediatricians.[1] This situation exists despite the official pronouncements of the American Academy of Pediatrics that pediatricians should continue to supervise the health care needs until the patient is 21 years of age.[2]

Several factors are responsible for this discrepancy. Since pediatricians have been traditionally known as "baby doctors," it requires a shift in thinking by all concerned (parents, patients, and physicians) for adolescents, especially older adolescents, to become incorporated into the practice style of pediatrics.[3,4] Surveys show that many pediatricians still maintain age "cut-off" policies in early or middle adolescence for the acceptance of new patients or the continuation of old patients in their practices. Many also express concern over their ability to manage such psychosocial issues as sexuality-related concerns, substance abuse problems, and eating disorders.[5-9] Lack of knowledge, time constraints, difficulty with balancing the confidentiality of the adolescent with

TABLE 10-1
Number of Office Visits Made by Persons of All Ages and by Adolescents 11-20 Years of Age, and Percentage Distribution by Sex, Race, Ethnicity, and Physician Specialty: United States, 1985

Number of Visits in Thousands	All Ages 683,386	11-20 (yr) 58,996	11-14 (yr) 19,360	15-20 (yr) 39,637
	Distribution (%)			
Sex				
Female	60.9	57.4	50.1	61.0
Male	39.1	42.6	49.9	39.0
Race				
White	90.0	89.3	90.8	88.6
Black	8.2	8.8	7.5	9.4
Other races	1.8	1.9	1.7	2.0
Ethnicity				
Hispanic	6.4	7.5	6.2	8.2
Non-Hispanic	93.6	92.5	93.8	91.8
Physician specialty				
General and/or family practice	30.5	35.4	30.8	37.7
Internal medicine	11.6	5.1	4.0	5.7
Pediatrics	11.4	17.6	33.3	9.9
Obstetrics and gynecology	8.9	8.1	1.3	11.4
Ophthalmology	6.3	4.6	4.9	4.5
Orthopedic surgery	4.9	7.3	8.0	7.0
General surgery	4.7	3.7	2.1	4.5
Dermatology	3.8	6.5	3.7	7.8
Psychiatry	2.8	2.0	1.9	2.1
Otorhinolaryngology	2.5	2.6	2.9	2.4
Urologic surgery	1.9	0.6	0.5	0.7
Cardiovascular disease	1.7	0.1	0.0	0.2
Neurology	0.8	0.6	0.7	0.6
All other specialties	8.2	5.8	6.0	5.7

From Nelson C: *Office visits by adolescents,* DHHS Pub No (PHS) 91-1250, Washington, DC, 1991, U.S. Department of Health and Human Services.

the needs of the parents, and inability to establish appropriate fees are factors cited to explain the problems in managing adolescent issues in pediatric practice.[10] Younger pediatricians, especially those exposed to adolescent medicine training during their residencies, are expressing more confidence in managing these problems, and many established pediatricians whose patient population is aging with them are becoming more aware of adolescent issues. It is hoped that these trends, along with the availability of increasing numbers of articles on management of adolescent issues in pediatric practice,[11-14] will lead to an increase in the care of adolescents by pediatricians in office-based practice during the years ahead.

Many adolescents with a chronic illness identify their pediatric specialist as their only physician. Specialists often administer immunizations (e.g., influenza vaccine for the adolescent with asthma) and perform sports preparticipation examinations. It is important for pediatric specialists to ensure that their adolescent patients receive primary care, including appropriate anticipatory guidance related to sexuality and substance use.

General and Family Practice

Slightly more than one third (35%) of all office-based visits by adolescents, 31% of those aged 11 to 14 and 38% of those aged 15 to 20, are to physicians in general or family practice.[1] Some general practitioners argue that they are in a better position to manage the healthcare needs of adolescents than pediatricians or physicians in other specialties because they are specifically trained and experienced in managing the health care of all members of the family and in balancing the needs of each family member if conflict should arise. The parent-child conflicts of adolescents match well with this area of expertise. General and family practitioners traditionally manage a wide range of problems, including medical, gynecologic, and mental health concerns; these fit the diverse healthcare needs of the adolescent age group. Hundreds of rural counties in the United States have no pediatricians, gynecologists, or psychiatrists, and the general practitioner must assume responsibility of all adolescent health needs in these areas. Currently, management of adolescent health issues is receiving increased emphasis in general and family practice training, and it is clear that general practitioners will continue to provide a large portion of the medical care to adolescents in future years.

Obstetrics and Gynecology

The number of visits by adolescents to obstetrician/gynecologists increases significantly throughout the adolescent years, from 1% of all visits in the 11- to 14-year-old age group to 11% of visits for those aged 15 to 20.[1] Similar in some ways to the issues faced by pediatricians incorporating specific adolescent healthcare needs into previously established practice styles are the challenges to obstetrician/gynecologists managing the problems of adolescents in settings more conducive to older women. The role of parental involvement and the ability to relate to adolescents in a nonjudgmental manner are two issues increasingly being faced by obstetrician/gynecologists. Because most research and publications in adolescent gynecology emanate from major medical centers, which are often inner-city based, gynecologists in office-based practice must make decisions for rural or suburban adolescents in the areas of contraception, pregnancy, and sexually transmitted disease without an appropriate database. Increasing attention to these issues should result in improved adolescent health care delivery by obstetrician/gynecologists in the future.

Internal Medicine

Visits to internists constitute 4% of office-based visits for 11- to 14-year-old adolescents and 6% of visits for 15- to 20-year-olds. It is estimated that 14% of all visits to internists are by persons under 24 years of age. A position paper by the American College of Physicians has called for better training and more involvement in the care of adolescents by internists.[15] It emphasized the role that internists can play in the interaction between the health behaviors of adolescents and the health status of adulthood, and encouraged internists to participate in efforts devoted to health promotion and disease prevention. The inclusion of adolescent medicine training in internal medicine residency programs is currently being mandated as a first step in ensuring that internists make adolescent health care a new priority.

Psychiatry

Only 2% of all office-based visits by adolescents are to psychiatrists, a surprising figure considering that various studies have demonstrated mental health problems in up to 20% of adolescents.[16,18] Two factors account for the relatively few adolescents seen by psychiatrists. First, pediatricians and other specialists are increasingly developing experience in handling behav-

ioral difficulties in the office setting, limiting the need for referral of mental health issues for specialty care. Second, a large percentage of adolescent referrals are to psychologists, social workers, and other therapists, rather than to psychiatrists. Certainly the small number of psychiatrists relative to other mental health personnel plays a major role in this finding. Some, if not many, psychiatrists do not like working with the adolescent age group, which also may play a role. It has been estimated that less than 2% of all adolescents receive mental health services yearly.[19] An increased availability of community-based mental health services for adolescents has been called for as a priority in the 1990s.[19]

Surgery and Surgical Subspecialties

Although the surgical subspecialties (including dermatology) account for over 20% of all adolescent visits, no evidence from the medical literature indicates that any special attention has been paid to adolescent health care in residency training or surgical practice. Most surgeons generally treat the adolescent's specific problem, paying more or less attention to the context and psychological factors that may be involved. The increased focus on adolescent health issues in the lay press and general medical literature may encourage more surgeons to be more attentive to these issues, but it is unlikely that formal training in adolescent health care will soon be available to surgical residents.

Adolescent Medicine Specialists

With the introduction in 1994 of Board Certification in Adolescent Medicine, the role of adolescent medicine specialists has received increased attention. While adolescent medicine has traditionally been a hospital- or clinic-based specialty, a growing number of adolescent medicine specialists have opened office-based practices available solely to adolescent and young adult patients.[11,12,20,21] These practices, currently one to two dozen nationwide, are generally located in or near major cities. Each practice has a unique way of positioning itself in the medical marketplace: some adolescent medicine private practitioners concentrate on subspecialties such as mental health counseling, substance abuse evaluations, or endocrinologic disorders; others maintain a general medical practice without additional subspecialization. Although specialty certification may encourage more adolescent medicine specialists to open practices in the years ahead, it is unrealistic to expect them to provide care to any but the smallest minority of adolescents. Therefore, efforts directed at improving health care for adolescents seen in office-based settings will continue to be aimed at the practitioners in each medical specialty.

HOSPITAL-BASED HEALTH CARE, HEALTH MAINTENANCE ORGANIZATIONS, AND OTHER SETTINGS

Hospital-Based Health Care

Approximately 30% of outpatient adolescent health care takes place outside office-based practices, mainly in hospital-based clinics, where the issues facing the private sector are further compounded by the effects of poverty and bureaucracy. Some medical centers have specifically designated adolescent clinics, but many large centers and most medium- or small-sized ones do not. Instead, teenagers are allocated to pediatric clinics, medical clinics, family planning clinics, or surgical clinics, with placement often based on arbitrary age cutoffs or diagnostic categories. Even where specific adolescent services are offered, no standard definition exists of what constitutes the adolescent age group: classifications range from ages 13 to 17 at one extreme to ages 10 to 25 at the other. Some adolescent clinics treat teenagers with chronic illnesses; other medical centers assign such patients to specialty clinics. This lack of uniformity creates a wide diversity in the quality of outpatient health services available to adolescents in hospitals throughout the United States.

A similar lack of uniformity extends to inpatient treatment of adolescents.[22] It is estimated that there are approximately 40 to 60 adolescent units in North America, with several others in Europe, Asia, South America, and Australia. A 1994 survey of directors of 25 adolescent units determined that these units have a range of six to 35 beds (mean 19.2); have lower age limits of 10 to 13 years and upper age limits ranging from 17 to 24 years; and have a mean of 60% of admissions for medical conditions, 28% for surgery, and 6% each for gynecologic and psychiatric care.[22] While these units provide an age-appropriate mileau that meets the developmental and psychological needs of adolescents, it is clear that most hospitalized adolescents do not receive the benefits of such units.

Health Maintenance Organizations

With an increasing number of people receiving health care from Health Maintenance Organizations (HMOs), the ability of HMOs to provide age-appropriate care to adolescents takes on ever-increasing importance. Most adolescents are managed in HMOs by procedures similar to those described for other private practice or hospital-based settings (i.e., by a diverse group of medical specialists without specific accommodations for adolescent health care needs).[23,24] In recent years, however, several large staff model HMOs have established adolescent medicine practices within their groups, stipulating the ages at which patients are seen by internists versus pediatricians and arranging special services such as educational programs, evening hours, separate visiting areas, and even hotlines. Initial evaluations of these practices have demonstrated that they are well accepted and quickly grow to full capacity. It is hoped that adolescent issues will be considered by more HMOs as administrators become convinced that the economic advantages they offer in attracting patients and providing preventive care outweigh the expenses necessary to provide the extra services required by adolescents.

School-Based Health Centers

Beginning with three high school–based health centers in the United States in 1980, the numbers of such centers grew to over 300 in 1992, over 600 in 1994, and over 900 in 1996.[25] Most are located in high schools, generally in urban communities, with growing numbers in middle and elementary schools, and some in rural or suburban communities. These health services have been able to overcome the initial controversies about sexuality-related care that accompanied their initial establishment. They are currently struggling with the financial issues necessary for long-term survival, and have demonstrated their ability to meet a wide range of medical and psychological needs for high-risk youth.[26] A fuller discussion of the care provided and the issues faced in school-based health centers can be found in Chapter 130, "School Based Health Care."

College Health Services

There are more than 3400 institutions of higher education in the United States, and about 1500 provide health care to their students.[27] Approximately 10 million students are served by this healthcare system, with an average of two to three visits per year. College health services are organized in many different ways: some serve merely as a triage or referral service and others provide a wide range of comprehensive health services. The larger student health centers include dental, optometric, laboratory, pharmacy, and x-ray services. They may also be responsible for campus-wide health education efforts and complete mental health services. The level of healthcare delivery varies from campus to campus, with the quality of even those that provide excellent care often negatively perceived by both the medical and academic communities. The American College Health Association periodically issues standards for health care in college health services, but few health services are accredited by regulatory bodies that monitor their care. The best of the college health services now consider it their mission to "become integrated into the college community as accountable, responsible, authoritative partners in the academic enterprise."[27]

Health Care in the U.S. Army Medical System

Army military families include about 180,000 teenage dependents, and approximately 184,000 adolescents aged 17 to 19 are enlisted in active military duty. Medical care is provided through an Army healthcare system spread throughout the world. As summarized by the Chief of Adolescent Medicine at William Beaumont Army Medical Center, (Walter K. Imai, MD, personal communication, 1991), the healthcare system provided for these adolescents must be able to care for the general health needs common to all adolescent populations while also paying particular attention to the special problems that may arise for these teenagers because of frequent moves, parental absence, cultural and language diversity, exposure to unusual risks associated with foreign travel, and both peacetime and wartime Army activities. Adolescent dependents are cared for by pediatricians, gynecologists, family practitioners, internists, emergency medicine physicians, and general medical officers; they constitute 20% of dependent children's outpatient visits in the Army healthcare system. Adolescent medicine specialists are taking increasing responsibility for dependent adolescent health care, with adolescent medicine clinics currently available at more than 12 Army installations. In contrast, adolescents enlisted in active duty receive most medical care from emergency medicine and general medical officers (see Chapter 93, "The Military and the Adolescent").

Health Care in Correctional Facilities

The average daily population of juveniles in public detention or correctional facilities nationwide is more than 50,000 and represents approximately 2 per 1000 of the adolescent population.[28] Medical care provided ranges from on-site comprehensive health care to off-site referral services. Adolescents treated in these facilities represent the highest-risk youth in the country from both medical and psychosocial perspectives, and the ability of these facilities to handle most health problems is further limited by the transient nature of their involvement with many of these adolescents. Healthcare standards for correctional facilities have been established by the American Medical Association and the National Commission on Correctional Health Care, but compliance with these standards is voluntary.

MEDICALLY UNDERSERVED ADOLESCENTS

A current growing concern relates to adolescents who do not have access to appropriate health care through any of the available means. Research has determined that 15% of adolescents are uninsured and that adolescents from families with incomes below the poverty level have 13% fewer physician contacts on an annual basis than other adolescents.[29,30] These adolescents are more likely to be described as being in only fair or poor health or to be suffering from a disabling chronic illness than other adolescents. This disparity is especially evident in those who do not receive Medicaid: that is, those from families that are sometimes called "the working poor." Although legislative efforts are attempting to ameliorate this situation, those who provide health care to adolescents will continue to face these economic realities in the future. A report from W. T. Grant Foundation stated that a large percentage of youths who do not attend college enter the ranks of poverty or become the next generation of "working poor."[31] The Society for Adolescent Medicine has developed a position paper that summarizes the barriers to care for youth and outlines the approaches to improving access to health care for adolescents in all settings.[32] This Society has also prepared a position paper on the health needs of homeless and runaway youths, with a series of recommendations aimed at improving the health care of these underserved adolescents[33] (see Chapter 89, "Out-of-Home Living Arrangements").

References

1. Nelson C: *Office visits by adolescents,* DHHS Pub No (PHS) 91-1250, Washington, DC, 1991, U.S. Department of Health and Human Services.
2. Council on Child and Adolescent Health: Age limits of pediatrics, *Pediatrics* 81:736, 1988.
3. Fisher M: Parents' views of adolescent health issues, *Pediatrics* 90:335-341, 1992.
4. Williams RL: The office setting for adolescent care: concerns of physicians, patients and parents, *Adolesc Med: State of Art Rev* 2:381-388, 1991.
5. Bradford J, Lyons W: Adolescent medicine practice in urban Pittsburgh—1990, *Clin Pediatr* 31:471-477, 1992.
6. Nussbaum MP, Shenker IR, Feldman JG: Attitudes versus performance in providing gynecologic care to adolescents by pediatricians, *J Adolesc Health Care* 10:203-208, 1989.
7. Beatty ME, Lewis J: Adolescent contraceptive counselling and gynecology: a deficiency in pediatric office-based care, *Conn Med* 58:71-78, 1994.
8. Blum RW, Bearinger LH: Knowledge and attitudes of health professionals toward adolescent health care, *J Adolesc Health Care* 11:289-294, 1990.
9. Key JD, Marsh LD, Darden PM: Adolescent medicine in pediatric practice: a survey of practice and training, *Am J Med Sci* 309:83-87, 1995.
10. Marks A, Fisher M, Lasker S: Adolescent medicine in pediatric practice, *J Adolesc Health Care* 11:149-153, 1990.

11. Shapiro E: Obstacles to adolescent care in general practice, *Adolesc Med: State of Art Rev* 2:389-396, 1991.

12. Lopez RI: Obstacles to adolescent care: economic issues, *Adolesc Med: State of Art Rev* 2:415-428, 1991.

13. Long WA: Treating teens for fun—and profit, *Contemp Pediatr* 8:31-48, 1991.

14. Jenkins RR, Saxena SB: Keeping adolescents healthy, *Contemp Pediatr* 12:76-89, 1995.

15. American College of Physicians: Health care needs of the adolescent, *Ann Intern Med* 110:930-935, 1989.

16. Kashani JH, Beck NC, Hoeper EW, et al: Psychiatric disorders in a community sample of adolescents, *Am J Psychiatry* 144:584-589, 1987.

17. Brandenburg NA, Friedman RM, Silver SE: The epidemiology of childhood psychiatric disorders: prevalence findings from recent studies, *J Am Acad Child Adolesc Psychiatry* 29:76-83, 1990.

18. McGee R, Feehan M, Williams S, Partridge F, Silva P, Kelly J: DSM-III disorders in a large sample of adolescents, *J Am Acad Child Adolesc Psychiatry* 29:611-619, 1990.

19. Burns BJ: Mental health service use by adolescents in the 1970's and 1980's, *J Am Acad Child Adolesc Psychiatry* 30:144-150, 1991.

20. Grace E: Incorporating adolescent gynecology into a general practice, *Adolesc Med: State of Art Rev* 2:397-404, 1991.

21. Marks A: How to make the most of an adolescent's first visit, *Pediatr Management* December:26-30, 1992.

22. Fisher M: Adolescent in-patient units, *Arch Dis Child* 70:461-463, 1994.

23. Fine JS: The practice of adolescent medicine in staff model HMOs, *HMO Pract* 3:16-21, 1989.

24. Klitsner IN, Borok GM, Neinstein L, MacKenzie R: Adolescent health care in a large multispecialty prepaid group practice: who provides it and how well are they doing?, *West J Med* 156:628-632, 1992.

25. Making the Grade: State and local partnerships to establish school-based health centers, Washington, D.C., 1996, George Washington University.

26. Fisher M, Juszczak L, Friedman SB, Schneider M, Chapar G: School-based adolescent health care: review of a clinical service, *Am J Dis Child* 146:615-621, 1992.

27. Faigel HC: Health care in college, *Adolescent Medicine: State of the Art Reviews* 7:231-238, 1996.

28. Council on Scientific Affairs: Health status of detained and incarcerated youths, *JAMA* 263:987-991, 1990.

29. Newacheck PW: Improving access to health services for adolescents from economically disadvantaged families, *Pediatrics* 84: 1056-1063, 1989.

30. Newacheck PW, McManua MA, Gephart J: Health insurance coverage of adolescents: a current profile and assessment of trends, *Pediatrics* 90:589-596, 1992.

31. Haggerty RJ: Care of the poor and underserved in America. Older adolescents: a group at special risk, *Am J Dis Child* 145:569-571, 1991.

32. Klein JD, Slap GB, Elster A, Schonberg SK: Access to health care for adolescents: a position paper of the Society for Adolescent Medicine, *J Adolesc Health* 13:162-170, 1992.

33. Farrow JA, Deisher RW, Brown R, Kulig JW, Kipke MD: Health and health needs of homeless and runaway youth: a position paper of the Society for Adolescent Medicine, *J Adolesc Health* 13:717-726, 1992.

CHAPTER 11

Interviewing the Adolescent and Family

•

Cynthia R. Pegler and Stanford B. Friedman

Despite the public and private spending on our healthcare system, many adolescents still have difficulty accessing the system. Most teens present annually to the healthcare provider so that a "form for school" can be filled out. The provider should be skilled in dealing with this age group and should have some formal training in adolescent medicine, but regretfully, this is often not the case. As a result, the proper screening of health issues that are germaine to the care of this group are not always met. Furthermore, the provider may not feel comfortable interviewing teenagers and follow-up visits may be thwarted. If there is one rule in dealing with this age group, it is to make them feel comfortable and welcomed.

Ideally, there should be a continuity of care for this population, either in a private office or in a clinic or ambulatory setting. A general pediatric clinic hardly meets the needs of adolescents, and obstacles to their health care immediately surface. To provide a "complete" healthcare package to the adolescent, a comprehensive and empathetic approach is necessary. The guidelines in providing their care can be found in *Guidelines for Adolescent Preventive Services (GAPS)*[1] published by the American Medical Associations and *Bright Futures: Guidelines for Health Supervision of Infants, Children and Adolescents,*[2] which are both aimed at the primary health care provider in the ambulatory setting.

These help the primary care provider with issues of screening, guidance, and immunizations for the adolescents. At the recommended routine annual visit, preventive health measures can be reinforced both to the adolescents and to their parents. The guidelines can help to identify those teens who have behaviors that place them at risk, as well as help the provider to develop a therapeutic plan. For adolescents, the guidelines are developmentally appropriate and apply to the early, middle, and late adolescent years. The health supervision interview includes a series of "trigger questions" for parents and teens. The focus is on the developmental issues, school and vocations performance, and anticipatory guidance.

Both *GAPS* and *Bright Futures* are excellent sources for more efficiently interacting with adolescents. They help the primary care provider to better identify those adolescents at risk, and they provide the structure and necessary guidance appropriate to the adolescent's developmental age. This type of comprehensive screening and care is essential if we are to identify at-risk issues for this age group.

SETTING FOR ADOLESCENT PATIENTS

The initial contact with an adolescent usually sets the tone for future physician-patient relationship and future therapeutic interventions. How the physician interacts with the patient and family at the first visit is critical in giving both the adolescent and the parents a "message" about the physician's style, as well as his or her concern about the teenager's health and well-being. An adolescent's first impression of a physician and the practice will be reflected by the waiting room. Although this may seem of little consequence, one can imagine how teenagers feel in pediatric waiting rooms sitting on a kindergarten-sized chair, surrounded by a jungle-gym and pop-up books, and outnumbered by infants and toddlers. Equally difficult is sitting in a waiting room with older adults who are reading *The Atlantic Monthly* or *U.S. News and World Report.* Because adolescents are struggling with issues of maturity and wish to be treated as grown-up, the office decor should reflect these developmental issues. It is not necessary to cater to the teenagers with posters and "cool" office equipment, but only to provide appropriate seating. Also, the waiting room should have magazines (e.g., on sports, fashion, entertainment), pamphlets that describe the services that the office provides, and literature focusing on adolescent-specific issues. In

practices where adolescents are seen with some regularity, there should be one consultation room with books, brochures, and pamphlets on growth and development, sexuality, contraception, and drugs. The availability of this information demonstrates to the adolescent and the family that these topics are open for discussion, and imparts a sense of importance and legitimacy to these issues. It is best that physicians who also manage younger children have a separate waiting area or separate appointment times established for adolescents. Obviously this may not be practical in all situations, but the office must provide privacy to the adolescent.

In some instances the first contact the physician may have with the adolescent is in the hospital setting. In this hectic environment it may be difficult to find a quiet place to obtain the medical history. The interview should take place in a private area, preferably without the presence of other patients or visitors, with the physician conveying a willingness to listen. Whether in the hospital or office setting, it is important to avoid interruptions (except for emergencies). This communicates to the adolescent and family that their time is valuable and that their concerns are regarded seriously.

It is important that adolescents feel comfortable in the interview setting, but it is more important that they feel comfortable with the interviewer and assured that the physician's primary concern is helping them regardless of the problem. The physician should indicate to the adolescent and family both by words and deeds that the adolescent, not the parents, is the patient. The physician caring for adolescents should feel at ease with this age group and genuinely enjoy caring for teenagers. Otherwise, the adolescent will sense the discomfort and the doctor-patient relationship will be hampered. Adolescents have an amazing capability to read the facial expressions, body language, and overall interest of the physician. An adolescent will quickly decide if the physician is genuinely interested in him or her as a patient.

One should avoid overidentification with the adolescent by adoption of an adolescent style of dress or language; this approach is inappropriate. The adolescent does not wish the physician to be a peer, and such attempts will diminish the physician's value to the teenage patients. To ensure a good working relationship, it is important to be empathetic and nonjudgmental and to convey interest in the adolescent's concerns, especially since the parents typically provide all the judgmental care.

INITIAL VISIT OF A NEW PATIENT

While many teenagers seen by pediatricians "grow up" in the practice, some adolescents present to the physician de novo. This may stem from a move to a new geographic area, a request for consultation by another physician, or the family's wish to change doctors. At this initial visit it is preferable to meet the adolescent and *both* parents. If circumstances do not permit this (e.g., in the case of a working parent who cannot leave or a divorced parent living some distance away), assure the family that the absent parent is also welcome. Note the reported reluctance of the other parent to be present, especially if the visit involves a significant medical or psychological problem, and do not simply accept at face value a statement that the other parent would not want to attend. An absent parent often may not have been informed of the visit, and when contacted later may express the wish to have been present to state his or her concerns and to participate in the adolescent's care. If the spouse is described as uninvolved or disinterested, suspect that the missing parent may well present an important point of view.

After introductions in the waiting room, the physician must decide whether to meet with the adolescent and parents together or separately. This decision generally depends on the particular reasons for the visit, the physician's style, and the time allotted. The physician may first see the parents briefly and explain that the rest of the allotted time will be devoted to the adolescent. The parents can state their concerns, provide a family history, and discuss family dynamics and problems without their teenager being present. This approach may be especially helpful when the adolescent is reluctant to receive or resentful of medical attention, or when parents have significant marital problems. At the subsequent meeting with the adolescent, review the parents' concerns. A disadvantage to this approach is that the adolescent spends time waiting when it is his or her needs that are to be addressed. While the parents are being interviewed, the adolescent's anxiety and resentment may increase and the adolescent may feel that the physician is siding with the parents.

An alternative approach is to interview the parents alone at an initial visit and to see the adolescent at a subsequent visit. Time constraints imposed by an adolescent sitting in the waiting room are nullified, the adolescent is not kept waiting, and the physician has time to examine the parents' concerns. This is somewhat of a luxury in terms of office fees, but at times it may be the best way to understand important and complex issues within the family. Most families will not mind the additional times and associated fees and will welcome appropriate attention directed to a serious problem.

A third approach is to interview the adolescent and family together. This allows them all to state their concerns in each other's presence and enables the physician to observe their interactions. Encourage the adolescent to do most of the talking by saying that since the adolescent is the patient, it is important that he or she

provide as much history as possible. The parents can supply a family history, some of which the adolescent may first learn during this interview. This interview approach provides the best observations of family interactions and dynamics. For instance, when the teenager is directly questioned, a parent may supply the answer; the physician may then further explore issues about the adolescent's needs for independence. This approach also allows the physician to present the ground rules regarding confidentiality to the adolescent and parents together.

VISIT FOR PATIENTS UNDERGOING FOLLOW-UP BY PEDIATRICIAN

The previous discussion focused on the adolescent patient who presents de novo to the physician. However, some adolescents are followed by the same physician from childhood and into puberty and adolescence. In this situation the physician can formally meet with the family when the child is somewhere between the ages of 10 to 12 years to discuss with them the changing relationship that should take place in future visits. This involves direct access to the physician for the adolescent and issues related to confidentiality and payment. It can be explained at this time that the parent should no longer be present for the physical examination, or all of the interview.

Employ anticipatory guidance for both the parents and the youngster regarding the coming changes. Discuss with the parents the goals they have for their child and see if these goals are consistent with the child's interests and talents. Disparities noted in early adolescence may well be a harbinger of problems in later adolescent years.

CONFIDENTIALITY

Whether the adolescent and parents are interviewed separately or together, address the rules of confidentiality and guarantees to both the teenager and parents. Inform the adolescent that what is discussed will not be revealed to anyone else without his or her permission. This may help avoid a situation in which the parents ask the physician to provide confidential details obtained from the adolescent's interview. The one exception is information that would place the adolescent or another individual at risk for serious harm (i.e., potential suicide or homicide, or a significant medical problem not being appropriately managed). The physician must decide if the adolescent is in danger. In such a situation, the family must be notified and other appropriate measures taken. However, the adolescent will have the opportunity to participate in the "telling."

The physician must be familiar with the state laws concerning consent and confidentiality for minors. This includes the freedom the physician has in assessing and treating specified medical problems without parental knowledge or consent. In most states confidentiality laws cover pregnancy, abortion, contraception, treatment for sexually transmitted diseases, and drug counseling. Regardless of whether an issue is being managed with the knowledge of parents or confidentially, it is essential that the physician remain nonjudgmental. As the adolescent's advocate, the physician must inform the adolescent of his or her options and work toward a solution that is in the adolescent's best interest.

FEES

Since visits may be both lengthy and confidential, it is obvious that creative methods of billing must be used in providing health care to adolescents, especially in the private practice setting. Some physicians use an established agreement whereby parents pay for visits that may be initiated by the adolescent without the parents' presence, while others accept a reduced fee from adolescents for "confidentiality visits," assuming that these teenagers will pay full price for most of their visits. Many physicians bill for teenage visits on the basis of time expended, rather than simply using a flat fee for all visits as is customary for children and adults.

CORE OF INTERVIEW

After explanation of the rules of confidentiality and establishment of a fee structure, the core of the interview follows. Although the emphasis will depend both on the reason for the visit and on the style of the physician, the interview may include the following components:
1. Determination of the chief complaint
2. Evaluation of family history
3. Assessment of relationship with peers
4. Determination of school performance
5. Achievement of the psychosocial tasks of adolescence
6. Impressions of parents' views of their adolescent and the adolescent's view of himself or herself
7. Mental status examination

CHIEF COMPLAINT

As traditionally described in medical practice, the chief complaint relates to the reason why the adolescent has come to the office or has been admitted to the hospital. All details concerning the chief complaint, including its duration and any attempts made at remedying the situation, need to be addressed. How others (e.g., family members, friends) have been affected should also be assessed. It is not unusual for the adolescent to perceive a completely different reason for referral for treatment to the physician from that expressed by the parents. In such situations the information presented by the adolescent and family needs to be integrated to establish how the adolescent can best be helped. It is common for many adolescents to indicate that they are being seen for a "check-up." It is crucial in these cases to determine why they require a check-up at this particular time. Although some adolescents receive regular yearly check-ups and others require one for school, sports, or a job, many other so-called check-ups are in fact "a ticket of admission" to address a problem that was not revealed when the appointment was requested.

FAMILY HISTORY

The family history includes a determination of (1) who is in the family, who resides together, and how the adolescent interacts and functions within the family; and (2) the family medical history. Ask the teenager how he or she relates to each parent and to each sibling and about his or her responsibilities in the family. Note if the adolescent has any specific role within the family such as caring for younger siblings or meeting specific needs of either parent. However, the adolescent should not be requested to reveal family secrets or problems (e.g., marital discord, parental alcoholism), since this may well lead to resentment by the patient and ultimately the parents. Such information should come directly from the parents.

RELATIONSHIP WITH PEERS

This area of questioning includes determining how the adolescent functions among his or her peers. Does the adolescent have a best friend? If so, how long has the friendship been in existence? What activities does the adolescent share with his or her friends?

Include an assessment of sexuality in the interview and do not assume a heterosexual preference. Although this issue may be delayed until a firmer doctor-patient relationship has been established, the questioning needs to be open-ended in nature without the physician making any assumptions about sexual behavior. The last thing a male adolescent who thinks he might be gay wants to be asked is: "So, do you have a girlfriend yet?"

Questions related to experimentation with or use of cigarettes, drugs, and/or alcohol need to be answered to obtain honest answers to these questions, as well as those

---

BOX 11-1
Questions for Adolescents

- What do your classmates think of you?
- How would your parents describe you?
- Where do you see yourself 5 years from now?
- What things would you like changed in your life?
- What would you advise your parents if you were in my place?

BOX 11-2
Questions for Parents

- What are your teenager's *strong* points?
- What is the *worst* thing that could happen to your youngster?
- Where do you see your adolescent 5 years from now?
- How *happy* is your teenager now?
- In what situations does your adolescent follow or not follow your requests?

---

regarding sexuality. Inquire without the parents present. This interview may have to be deferred to a later time.

SCHOOL

The school history includes past and present performance. Any changes, especially a decline in grades, may indicate that difficulties are being encounted in school work or in other areas of the adolescent's life. In some situations school records should be obtained for review by the physician. Future goals of the adolescent and parental goals for the adolescent should be compared and any significant discrepancies noted. Unrealistic expectations on either part need to be addressed.

TASKS OF ADOLESCENCE

Classic tasks of adolescence include separating from the family and becoming independent, developing a sexual identity, and determining a sense of one's academic and career goals. These may be briefly evaluated during an initial interview by asking several key questions, or in greater depth for those who seem to be having specific psychosocial difficulties (see Chapter 8).

ADOLESCENT AND PARENT VIEWS

In evaluating an acute problem, especially one of a psychosocial nature, or in establishing a relationship for the future, it is important to develop a concept of how the parents view their teenager and how the adolescent views him- or herself. In the authors' experience, 10 key questions addressed to the adolescent and the parents can provide the avenues of exploring these areas (see Boxes 11-1 and 11-2). The answers to these questions generally provide important information and lead to further questions about the values and priorities, as well as problem areas, of the teenager and the parents. If parents cannot identify any strong points in their teenager, the physician

should strongly suspect parental rejection and low self-esteem in the teenager.

MENTAL STATUS EXAMINATION

The mental status examination incorporates both nonverbal and verbal components of the interview. The appearance of the adolescent, including clothing, posture, and hygiene, should be noted. Does the adolescent look his or her stated age? Observe for eye contact (or lack thereof), facial expression, fidgeting, level of alertness, and other body language signals. Emotional reactions to questions are important. Do certain questions make the adolescent tearful, frightened, angry, or uncomfortable? The quality of the adolescent's speech (e.g., animated or without affect) should be assessed. Appetite, sleep and weight changes, and any concerns about weight should be evaluated, and direct questioning regarding depression and/or suicidal ideation included. Obtain information regarding insight and judgment, if appropriate. Intellectual level can be roughly judged by the teenager's ability to understand and respond to the physician's questions. It is often not possible to obtain all this information in one interview. It may be preferable to gather the information over several meetings, each relatively short, about 20 to 30 minutes per session, spaced about 2 weeks apart. The adolescent may find this approach less threatening and the physician can obtain a more complete history while also establishing rapport. Assessment and treatment are not entirely separate entities; treatment of the complaint starts with the first interview.

INTERVIEW STYLE

Whether adolescents are interviewed over one or several sessions, the interview is best conducted when they are as relaxed as possible. In general, start an interview with nonthreatening questions such as where the adolescent live or go to school. Show genuine interest in the answers and ask for clarification if an answer is not entirely clear. For example, the physician may respond: "I'm not sure I understand your answer. Can you explain it to me again?" The physician must phrase the questions in language and terms understood by the adolescent to facilitate better communication between physician and adolescent. The adolescent should never feel "talked down to" or talked to as a little child. The physician may want to further the interview with "How can I help you today?" instead of "Why are you here today?" Open-ended questions are preferred to those that generate a "yes" or "no" answer. For instance, "What do you like or dislike about school?" yields a better response than "Do you like school?" Answers such as "okay" or "all right" need to be pursued further. Options include simply repeating the answer and giving the adolescent the opportunity to elaborate by asking "What is there about school that makes it okay?" Allow the adolescent sufficient time to answer questions; some brief silent pauses are beneficial and allow him or her not to feel pressured.

Another technique that is frequently helpful in interviewing adolescents is use of the third person. For instance: "I know many teenagers your age have tried alcohol at parties. How do you feel about that?" In this way the adolescent may not feel as if he or she is being accused. The physician must be sensitive and aware of the cues given by the adolescent. The teenager who becomes tearful in response to a certain question can be asked, "It seems that talking about this makes you sad. Why is that?" The angry or hostile adolescent who denies any problems despite parental concerns may respond to the following statement: "I can see that you're very angry about being here today. Sometimes when people get angry it is harder for them to talk. Is that the case with you?" Communication between physician and adolescent can begin even if it is not the most ideal interview situation.

COMMON PITFALLS

Several common pitfalls exist in the assessment of adolescent behavior. First, the physician is often tempted to assess the specific behavior of an adolescent in terms of his or her own previous behavior as a teenager. If an adolescent has been caught shoplifting, the physician may reassure the parents that shoplifting is not a serious offense since he himself once was caught shoplifting. (This of course implies that the physician has "turned out well" and therefore shoplifting is not considered a deterrent to a favorable outcome.) Second, it is often common among some physicians to evaluate, perhaps unconsciously, the behavior of an adolescent patient by their expectations for their own children. A physician opposed to the use of marijuana by his or her own teenagers may assume that the parents of the adolescent patient may share this view of drug use, and counsel them and their teenager accordingly. Last, the physician may judge adolescent behavior with a faulty database. The pediatric literature contains information about normative and abnormal teenage behavior that can guide physicians better than their own (limited) experiences, or in preference to their own outdated and perhaps inaccurate perceptions of adolescent behavior.

CONCLUDING THE INTERVIEW

End the interview with a summary of the session. Give the adolescent the opportunity to respond and ask questions. Admit that certain areas may have been missed and ask, "Did I leave anything out that I should know?" This acknowledges that the physician is limited in helping the adolescent if important information is not elicited, and implies that the patient (and parents) share in the responsibility to inform the physician about important issues. When the parents and adolescent are interviewed separately, it is best to summarize first with the adolescent then to repeat the summary with the parents present. The parents can ask questions, and arrangements can then be made for subsequent appointments.

References

1. Elster A, editor: *AMA guidelines for adolescent preventive services (GAPS) recommendations and rationale,* Baltimore, 1994, Williams & Wilkins.
2. Green M, editor: *Bright futures: guidelines for health supervision of infants, children and adolescents,* Arlington, VA, 1994, National Center for Education in Maternal and Child Health.

Suggested Readings

Felice M, Friedman SB: Behavioral considerations in the health care of adolescents, *Pediatr Clin North Am* 29:399, 1982.

Hammar SL, Holterman V: Interviewing and counselling adolescent patients, *Clin Pediatr* 9:47, 1970.

Nenstein LS: *Adolescent health care: a practical guide,* Baltimore, 1991, Urban & Schwarzenberg.

Smith J, Felice M: Interviewing adolescent patients—some guidelines for the clinician, *Pediatr Ann* 9:88, 1980.

CHAPTER 12

Medical History

•

Andrea Marks

A critical component of the health encounter with any patient is the medical history.[1] A thorough medical history not only elicits information but also gives back a message. In addition to a traditional medical history (past illnesses, hospitalizations, operations, allergies, and immunizations) obtained from the parent(s) and the adolescent, the physical and emotional well-being, the social life, and any health risk behaviors of the adolescent need to be emphasized. Thus, health providers define their purview as inclusive rather than exclusive of the most likely disorders and dysfunctions affecting teenagers today.[2] The thorough medical history demonstrates to adolescents that the health provider has an understanding of their world, enhancing the likelihood that useful, or even critical, information will surface and that a meaningful relationship between them will ensue.

FORMAT

At the initial visit of an adolescent patient (under age 18) accompanied by his or her parent(s), it is recommended that the parent(s) be interviewed alone first to obtain a portion of the medical history. This helps the physician obtain the most thorough and accurate history, because many parents are not comfortable discussing certain information or concerns if their child is present. Before the interview, the adolescent and parents should be informed that the adolescent will be interviewed alone for the second part of the medical history, followed by the physical examination. Early in the adolescent's interview, the physician should explain that most parents appreciate the opportunity to meet with the physician alone one time and that the adolescent is interviewed second to preserve their confidentiality. Most adolescents appreciate such candidness, and this sequence does not alienate them but serves to engender their trust. Some younger adolescents are not ready for a totally independent relationship with their health provider and are relieved that their parents have a relationship with the physician.

HISTORY FROM PARENTS

Medical History

The medical history obtained from parents includes the "chief complaint"; the adolescent's medical history; the family medical history; and the social history pertinent to the adolescent's life at home, in school, and with peers. The chief complaint expressed by the parents is the problem of greatest concern to them. The adolescent may report a chief complaint that is identical to, similar to, or totally different from the primary concerns of the parents. The ensuing scenario is interesting and significant. Parents are usually most familiar with the adolescent's medical history: the perinatal period, early developmental milestones, serious or chronic illnesses, hospitalizations, operations, significant injuries or accidents, allergies, regular use of medications, and immunizations.

Family History

The family history lists the ages and health status of the parents and siblings and notes whether any first-degree relatives (grandparents, aunts, uncles, first cousins) have genetic or familial medical conditions. These conditions include heart disease, hypertension, hypercholesterolemia, major organ system disease, contagious diseases such as tuberculosis or hepatitis. Psychiatric disorders, which may also be genetic, including depression, schizophrenia, alcoholism, drug abuse, or eating disorders are also reviewed. The family medical history provides more than just a list of diseases: it also gives a clue to the residential "health environment." The family history may also include information pertaining to the parents' (and siblings') type of work, level of education, and location (if not residing at home).

Psychosocial History

In the psychosocial (developmental) history, parents are asked to describe their child's personality, strengths, weaknesses, and general adjustment to family life, school, and peer group. If time is limited, the parents may simply be asked whether they have any specific concerns in any of these areas. If time allows, they may elaborate.

Meeting alone with parents for an initial interview is an approach to adolescent health care that may be controversial. This initial time with parents may not be necessary when the adolescent has grown up in a pediatric or family medicine practice.[3] However, in a first visit the physician is in a better position to elicit specific data regarding the adolescent's health and to become acquainted with the parents if they are interviewed alone. Furthermore, all teenagers are not at the same maturity level or ready to assume complete independence with their health provider. Interviewing the parents alone with the full knowledge of the patient, rather than a phone conversation behind the adolescent's back, is an approach that can be enormously helpful and remarkably nonproblematic. Health providers must develop their own style, one that works best for them and their patients.

HISTORY FROM ADOLESCENT

Components of the medical history obtained from the adolescent interviewed alone include the chief complaint, a detailed review of systems that includes items particularly pertinent to adolescents, the patient's version of the psychosocial history, and the crucial medicosocial history that reviews various health risk behaviors. Talking candidly and openly with adolescents about numerous important and sensitive areas of their lives can be a challenging task. The key to a thorough and meaningful interview with adolescents is to put them at ease and to help them to trust you by *sticking to their agenda,* even if this requires modifying your own approach and goals. The "art" of achieving this trust at a first meeting with an adolescent must be cultivated and perfected by the physician. Naturally, it is easier to establish a relationship with some patients than with others. The initial interview sets the tone for future encounters, and the primary goal is to engender adolescents' confidence in the physician as an adult who understands their world, is nonjudgmental, enjoys talking with them, and is committed to responding to their needs.

Chief Complaint

As already noted, the adolescent's chief complaint may be identical to, similar to, or completely different from that of the parents. Some adolescents initially appear to have no complaints at all, but as such adolescents become increasingly comfortable during the course of the initial interview and "trigger" questions are asked, specific concerns may emerge, or at a subsequent visit

they may raise an issue that was not discussed at the first meeting or was not a problem at that time.

Review of Systems

A review of systems includes questions about headaches, breathing, bowel movements, and other traditional subjects. Additional queries pertain to aspects of adolescents' daily routine that affect their health such as physical activity, weight patterns and attitudes, diet and appetite, sleep, and menstruation. Such inquiries frequently disclose areas of concern or dysfunction. A sleep disturbance may signal a serious depression, or the patient may be struggling with an eating disorder. Many girls would benefit from some discussion regarding treatment of menstrual cramps, even if they did not think it was important enough to mention themselves.

Psychosocial History

The psychosocial history aims at assessing the adolescent's progress in tackling the three key tasks of adolescence: establishing a sense of independence or individuation from parents, developing a sexual and gender identity in the peer group, and planning for a future role in society. Offer's[4] studies have shown that normal adolescents follow several possible patterns of psychosocial growth, including continuous, surgent, tumultuous, or other roads to maturity. He concluded that no specific pattern of growth is superior and that each is dependent on a wide range of factors, including genetics, life experiences, childrearing practices, social environment, and individual psychological make-up.

The psychosocial history may begin with a general question such as "How are things going for you these days?" Some adolescents will respond with a detailed description of their life at home, with peers, and at school. Most adolescents, however, require more specific questions such as "How would you describe your relationship with your mother (father, brother, sister)?" "Do you have as many close friends as you want?" "What is it like for you being at school?" Most of the problems described by adolescents relate to conflicts at home, changing friendships, or difficulties at school. The health provider should acknowledge the importance of these concerns, chat briefly about each, and offer to meet again soon for further discussion of significant problems. Very serious matters warrant consultation with the adolescent's parents and/or a mental health professional.

Medicosocial History

The psychosocial history is related to the medicosocial history, which inquires about activities, feelings, or experiences that involve health risks. These activities include smoking cigarettes, drinking alcoholic beverages, using drugs, having sex, driving recklessly, or engaging in other accident-prone behavior. The adolescent should be questioned directly about feelings of intense, frequent, or prolonged depression, with possible suicidal ideation or a history of suicide attempts, or any experiences involving abuse in any form: verbal, physical, or sexual. Most teenagers are aware from their own environments or through the media that these are highly prevalent issues for young people today. Therefore, it is appropriate to begin by stating that these are "routine" questions asked of all patients and to reassure adolescents that they are in no way being singled out. Consider the patient's age, maturity, comfort level during the visit, description of his or her home life, and relationships with peers and at school. Many patients will be unable to answer the questions fully or honestly at a first encounter; therefore, it is important to indicate that they should feel free to return in the future if concerns or health needs related to these matters arise.

CONFIDENTIALITY

A wide-ranging difference of opinions exists among physicians who care for adolescents regarding the limits of confidentiality. What does a physician do if an adolescent does not want the parents to know about a mild depression? What if the depression is severe? What about mild versus severe drug use? Having sex versus being pregnant? The law does not always give the needed or comfortable answers. We must consider and decide how we will respond when faced with such challenging clinical situations.

ANTICIPATORY GUIDANCE

While the medical history is obtained, opportunities arise for providing anticipatory guidance to parents or the adolescent regarding a wide range of health issues. Such discussion must be brief and will depend on the adolescent's age and pubertal and psychodevelopmental maturity. Anticipatory guidance with parents may pertain to school, nutrition, puberty, or relationships at home or with peers; with the adolescent, discussion often centers on menstruation, weight concerns, mood, or various risk behaviors. It may be necessary to schedule a follow-up visit to provide more in-depth counseling on any of these matters.

GUIDELINES FOR ADOLESCENT PREVENTIVE SERVICES

In 1992, *Guidelines for Adolescent Preventive Services (GAPS)* was published by the Department of Adolescent Health of the American Medical Association. The GAPS recommendations are the most comprehensive and creative set of recommendations ever advocated to address the challenging task of incorporating health promotion (anticipatory guidance for parents and adolescents) and disease prevention (screening and immunizations) into *annual* adolescent preventive services visits. GAPS recommends meeting alone with parents at an initial visit during early adolescence, then at least one other time during middle adolescence, and optionally again during late adolescence.[5]

References

1. Marks A, Fisher M: Health assessment and screening during adolescence, *Pediatrics* 80 (suppl):135, 1987.
2. Marks A, Malizio J, Hoch J, et al: Assessment of the health needs and willingness to utilize health care resources of adolescents in a suburban population, *J Pediatr* 102:456, 1983.
3. Neinstein LS: *Adolescent health care, a practical guide,* ed 2, Baltimore, 1991, Williams & Wilkins.
4. Offer D: *The psychological world of the teenager,* New York, 1973, Basic Books.
5. American Medical Association Department of Adolescent Health: *Guidelines for Adolescent Preventive Services (GAPS),* Chicago, 1992, AMA.

CHAPTER 13

Physical Examination

•

Marcie B. Schneider

Adolescents generally require physical examinations for three reasons: evaluation and treatment of an illness, medical clearance for sports or employment, and routine check-ups. This chapter focuses on the general check-up, including discussion of the issues of privacy and confidentiality and description of the actual physical examination of the adolescent—how it differs from the examination of children or adults and why it is particularly important in this age group.

How frequently a physical examination should be performed in well adolescents has been debated. In 1985 the American Academy of Pediatrics recommended that adolescents be seen every 2 years for health maintenance.[1] However, given the complex physical and psychological changes occurring during the adolescent years, many clinicians believe that ideally every adolescent should undergo a yearly physical examination to permit close monitoring of these changes and to provide preventive and anticipatory guidance about medical and psychosocial issues. In 1989 the U.S. Preventive Services Task Force recommended annual comprehensive visits for adolescents, including a physical examination, discussion of behavioral issues, and preventive care.[2]

Since the mid-1980s the focus on preventive services and health promotion has continued to increase. *Bright Futures*, a report sponsored by the Maternal and Child Health Bureau of the U.S. Department of Health and Human Services in 1994, provides guidelines for health supervision of adolescents. These guidelines include a recommendation for yearly health supervision visits, including developmental surveillance, observation of parent-child interaction, physical examination, additional screening procedures, immunizations, and anticipatory guidance for the family.[3] *Guidelines for Adolescent Preventive Services* (GAPS), a healthcare package developed by the American Medical Association in 1992, differentiates between the need for preventive services and the need for a physical examination. The GAPS recommendations include an annual routine health visit for persons aged 11 to 21 years (for developmental monitoring, preventive services, and an-

ticipatory guidance), but only three complete physical examinations during those years (one each in early, middle, and late adolescence).[4] In 1995 the American Academy of Pediatrics published new recommendations for preventive pediatric health care that include yearly visits for a complete physical examinations, developmental and behavioral assessment, and anticipatory guidance.[5]

PREPARATION

Although the physical examination of adolescents is similar to that of children, issues of patient privacy and confidentiality come to the forefront in adolescents. It is the physician's role to ensure that the patient receives comprehensive care in a comfortable manner and that parents' concerns about their teenager are addressed.

It is desirable to examine the adolescent alone for several reasons. Adolescents have an increased need for privacy once puberty begins and are often uncomfortable about bodily changes. Although they may feel embarrassment due to exposure of their bodies, adolescents find the examination tolerable because it serves a necessary purpose: the assurance of good health and normalcy. However, revealing their bodies to more than one person at the time of the examination may be both embarrassing and unwarranted. In addition, the physical examination may provide the only chance for physician and patient to be alone; as such, it offers a time for the patient to express confidential concerns. The physician can address these concerns and pose any confidential questions not previously asked, such as issues related to sexuality. The physical examination may reveal acne, gynecomastia, or breast asymmetry that previously may not have been reported to the physician, possibly because the teenager may have been too worried or too embarrassed. The physician can use this opportunity to mention the finding, inquire about the patient's concerns, obtain a history of the problem, and discuss the evaluation and possible treatment approaches. The physical examination is the time for performing and teaching breast and testicular examinations. The teaching aspect enlists the participation of the adolescent in his or her care and in turn gives the adolescent more responsibility. Finally, examining the adolescent alone delivers the message to patient and family that the "child" is growing up. It acknowledges that certain issues are confidential between physician and patient and that the adolescent has the right to privacy. This is one step in shifting the responsibility of health care from the parent to the adolescent.

Despite the sound reasons presented for examining adolescents alone, certain conditions warrant examining the patient in the presence of a parent or another chaperone. The decision as to who should be present during the physical examination of the adolescent is based on consideration of legal, developmental, and specific medical issues. The needs of the patient, parent, and physician are considered in this decision.

Legally, a physician in the United States can perform a pelvic examination with the consent of the patient alone (i.e., without parental consent). According to the Supreme Court of the United States, minors may seek evaluation and treatment for pregnancy, contraception, sexually transmitted diseases, and abortion.[6] Each state, however, has the right to regulate adolescents' access to such care.[7] Physicians who plan to perform pelvic examinations must familiarize themselves with their state's regulations regarding the rights of minors with respect to sexuality-related issues. In the current medicolegal climate, it is wise to have a female chaperone present for any pelvic examination performed by a male physician. Individual physicians may also opt to have a chaperone present for breast and testicular examinations.

Developmentally, teenagers in their early adolescent years, or those who are older but developmentally immature, may feel comfortable with a parent or other staff member present during the physical examination. Data show that many adolescents (especially during the early adolescent years), when given the choice, opt to have a family member accompany them as a chaperone during the genitalia examination.[8] When the patient is severely mentally handicapped, a parent may interpret the patient's needs to the physician and provide the support necessary to the patient for a successful examination. Family or staff may also be used in situations in which assistance is needed in examining the patient, for example, with a wheelchair-bound patient who needs to be lifted onto a table.

Preparation is necessary for establishing the new routine of examining adolescents without a parent present so that there will be no surprises. The physician continuing to provide care for a patient can begin preparation for examining the patient alone during late childhood by reminding the patient and parents at each routine visit that the structure of the visit will change at a certain point in time, usually the onset of puberty. If the physician is seeing a teenager for a first visit, the structure of the visit can be presented at the onset to both patient and parents. Both patient and parents should be offered the opportunity to express concerns. Examination of the patient alone should not present a difficulty; if it does, psychosocial problems requiring exploration might exist within the family.

PERFORMANCE

For physical examination of the adolescent, the examination room should be equipped with a lockable door so that the patient will be assured privacy. For a complete physical examination, adolescents ideally should wear a hospital gown and underwear. They should be reassured that their privacy will be respected and that only the areas being examined at that moment will be revealed under the gown. It is important to assure patients that while wearing the gown they will receive an adequate physical examination and that all areas of the body will be examined.

Adolescents, especially in the early adolescent years, may be more embarrassed about their bodies than children or adults would be; therefore it is logical to begin the physical examination with the least sensitive and least embarrassing areas. The examiner should start with the vital signs, followed by the head and neck examination, working down to the feet in an orderly fashion. Examination of the genitalia may be uncomfortable for the patient (as well as for some physicians). Talking through the examination and describing various aspects of it as one proceeds may help to delineate the professional boundaries and ease any tension. Breast and testicular examinations should generally be performed as part of the general examination of teenagers. The pelvic examination, if necessary, is reserved for the end, since it is the one time that a chaperone may be needed, and a set-up for laboratory tests is required.

Five major areas in any complete examination of the adolescent are (1) measurement of vital signs and growth parameters; (2) examination of the head and neck; (3) cardiac, respiratory, abdominal, and neurologic examination; (4) musculoskeletal examination; and (5) examination of the genitalia.

Measurement of Vital Signs and Growth Parameters

Vital signs traditionally include measurement of temperature, blood pressure, pulse, and respiratory rate. Blood pressure and pulse are important parameters to check in the routine examination of the adolescent. Because many adolescents are nervous before their

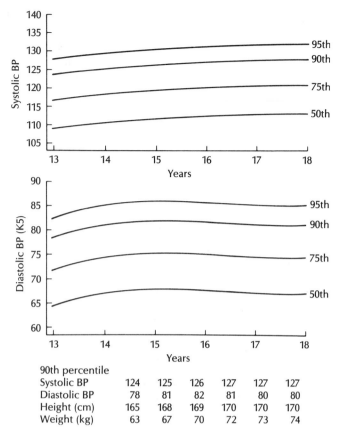

90th percentile						
Systolic BP	124	125	126	127	127	127
Diastolic BP	78	81	82	81	80	80
Height (cm)	165	168	169	170	170	170
Weight (kg)	63	67	70	72	73	74

Fig. 13-1. Blood pressure measurements in females aged 13 to 18 years. (From Report of the Second Task Force on Blood Pressure Control in Children, 1987: *Pediatrics* 79:1-25, 1987. Reproduced by permission of *Pediatrics.*)

physical examination, any elevated blood pressure or pulse should be remeasured at the end of the visit, when the patient feels more comfortable.

Although heart rate significantly decreases in the first few years of life, little change is apparent during the late childhood, adolescent, and adult years. Generally, adolescents have heart rates of less than 80 beats per minute. Routine pulse checks may help identify the occasional adolescent with an irregular heartbeat. Exercise tests that measure the pulse before exercise and 1 to 2 minutes after a 1-minute exercise challenge are performed by some clinicians as part of a sports physical examination in an attempt to uncover the rare teenager with an arrhythmia. The usefulness of this test has been debated among cardiologists, however, and the literature contains no specific recommendations.

Since 1% to 2% of teenagers in the general population are estimated to have hypertension, it is important that adolescents be screened for blood pressure at each check-up.[9] Hypertension is defined as blood pressure greater than the 95th percentile for age when repeated on three separate occasions. As with children, blood pressure changes during the adolescent years necessitate the use of standardized curves to determine whether a particular adolescent has elevated blood pressure for his or her age (Figs. 13-1 and 13-2). Blood pressure ideally should be measured in the right arm, with the patient sitting and the arm raised to the level of the heart. The bladder of the blood pressure cuff should cover two thirds of the upper arm and completely encircle the arm. In an adolescent the Korotkoff sounds recorded are K1 and K5. (K1 is the onset of sound, i.e., systolic blood pressure; K5 is the disappearance of sound, i.e., diastolic blood pressure.) In a child, K1 and K4 (muffling of sound) are used. The reason for this difference is that K5, often difficult to detect in children, may eventually occur simultaneously with K4 and is easier to detect by adolescence.[10] A patient with elevated blood pressure determined on three separate occasions should be evaluated for the cause of the hypertension.

Growth parameters that should be measured regularly during the adolescent years include height and weight. Changes in height take place most dramatically during the early to middle adolescent years. Boys undergo a growth spurt at an average of 14 years of age, while girls undergo their growth spurt approximately 2 years earlier, at an average of 12 years of age. Chronic illnesses (e.g., Crohn's disease, asthma) may adversely affect growth

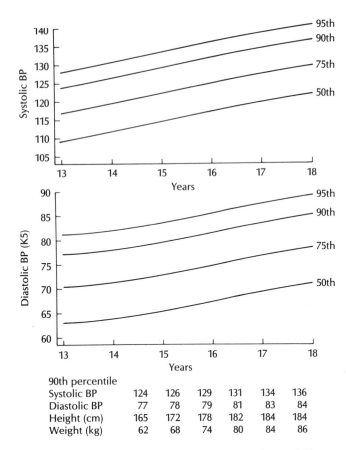

90th percentile						
Systolic BP	124	126	129	131	134	136
Diastolic BP	77	78	79	81	83	84
Height (cm)	165	172	178	182	184	184
Weight (kg)	62	68	74	80	84	86

Fig. 13-2. Blood pressure measurements in males aged 13 to 18 years. (From Report of the Second Task Force Blood Pressure Control in Children, 1987: *Pediatrics* 79:1-25, 1987. Reproduced by permission of *Pediatrics*.)

even before they become apparent, and physiologic delays in growth also affect many youths. Height should be measured at each check-up, with the patient in bare feet and standing straight; ideally a stadiometer attached to the wall should be used, since scale measurements of height are often inaccurate. The patient's height is then plotted on a standardized growth curve (Figs. 13-3 and 13-4). Separate growth curves exist for certain disorders, including Down syndrome, Turner's syndrome, and achondroplasia. The height at each check-up can then be compared with that at previous visits to monitor the progression of the patient's growth. A major change in percentiles on the growth curve requires further evaluation.

Weight changes that occur during early adolescence may be even more dramatic than changes in height. The average teenager gains 30 to 50 pounds during the early adolescent years. Adolescents should be weighed at each check-up, because the incidence of obesity and eating disorders including anorexia nervosa and bulimia increases during adolescence, and patients with chronic illnesses, such as Crohn's disease or diabetes, may present with weight loss. Patients should be weighed in a

hospital gown to obtain accurate and comparable weights from visit to visit. As with height, the weight should be plotted on a standardized weight curve (Figs. 13-3 and 13-4). The weight at each visit can then be compared with previous measurements to check for a normal progression. A significant change in percentiles on the weight curve indicates the need for an evaluation of possibly inappropriate weight loss or gain.

Examination of the Head and Neck

Included in this part of the examination are evaluation of the eyes, ears, nose, throat, teeth, skin, neck, and lymph nodes.

The American Academy of Ophthalmology recommends that primary care physicians evaluate all patients over the age of 5 years on a yearly basis for visual acuity, using the corneal light reflex test, the cover and uncover test, and funduscopic examination.[11] Visual acuity worsens in the teenage years: approximately one in every four 17-year-olds has vision of 20/40 or worse, at which level glasses are recommended. Visual acuity is most easily measured by the Snellen chart. The corneal reflex is tested by touching the tip of a cotton swab to the cornea; a blink is the normal response. The cover and uncover test requires the patient to cover one eye and focus with the other eye on a particular spot. The patient then uncovers the covered eye to check where that eye is focused. If it is not in line with the other eye, strabismus is present. Funduscopic examination of the optic disc and blood vessels can then be performed. Referral to a specialist is recommended if the vision in either eye is worse than 20/40, if the corneal light reflex is not present, if strabismus is found, if results of the funduscopic examination are abnormal, or if any other eye abnormalities are detected.

Evaluation of ear, nose, and throat differs little for teenagers from that for other populations. Many adolescents are routinely tested for hearing problems in school, although the value of auditory screening of adolescents in the school setting has been questioned.[12] Screening for hearing loss in the general medical office, with a high level of ambient noise and little audiologic equipment, is difficult. Patients complaining of hearing loss or with a history of borderline or abnormal school hearing test should be referred for formal audiologic testing.

Adolescents experience changes in dentition (primary teeth change to permanent), facial structures, hormone levels, and personal habits (smoking, snacking)—factors that affect the oral cavity. Decayed, missing, or filled teeth and gingivitis increase with age.[13] From 13% to 50% of teenagers have malocclusion that would benefit from orthodontic treatment.[14] Physical examination of the teeth gives the physician an opportunity to identify any

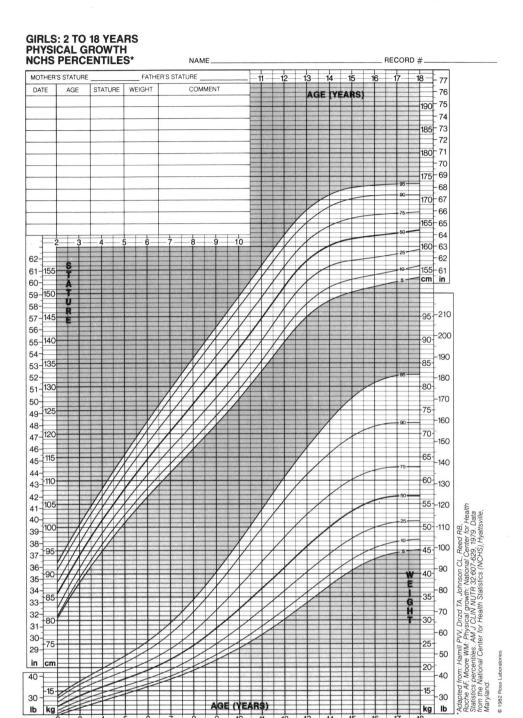

GIRLS: 2 TO 18 YEARS
PHYSICAL GROWTH
NCHS PERCENTILES*

Fig. 13-3. Standardized growth curve for females aged 2 to 18 years. (Modified from Hamill PVV, Drizd TA, Johnson CL, et al: Physical growth, *Am J Clin Nutr* 32:607-629, 1979. Data from the National Center for Health Statistics [NCHS], Hyattsville, MD. Reprinted with permission of Ross Laboratories, Columbus, Ohio. Copyright 1980 Ross Laboratories.)

acute problems and to discuss the need for preventive dental care. Every patient should be referred for a dental check-up at least once a year.

Examination of the adolescent must include evaluation of the skin, especially for acne. Although acne may be most common and bothersome on the face, the chest and back should be evaluated, because acne often affects these areas. Adolescents may have other dermatologic findings, and the skin must also be checked for fungal or bacterial infections, café au lait spots, scars, nevi, or striae (see Chapter 72, "Dermatologic Problems").

The neck should be checked for thyroid size, masses, or tenderness. If an abnormal thyroid gland is present, thyroid function tests should be performed. Lymph nodes

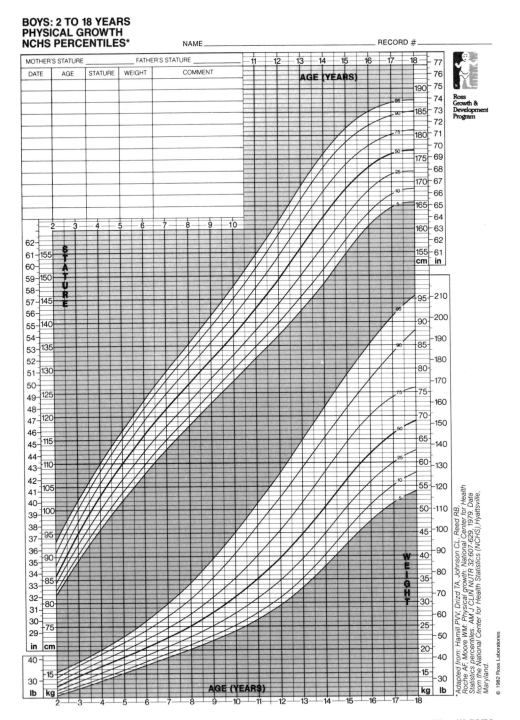

Fig. 13-4. Standardized growth curve for males aged 2 to 18 years. (Modified from Hamill PVV, Drizd TA, Johnson CL, et al: Physical growth, *Am J Clin Nutr* 32:607-629, 1979. Data from the National Center for Health Statistics [NCHS], Hyattsville, MD. Reprinted with permission of Ross Laboratories, Columbus, Ohio. Copyright 1980 Ross Laboratories.)

should be evaluated at each check-up. The cervical (submandibular, submental, preauricular, postauricular, occipital, anterior, and posterior), supraclavicular, axillary, epitrochlear, and inguinal nodes should be checked. If lymphadenopathy is found, the cause should be investigated (see Chapter 53, "Lymphadenopathy and Splenomegaly").

Cardiac, Respiratory, Abdominal, and Neurologic Examination

Examination of the cardiac, respiratory, abdominal, and neurologic systems in adolescents does not differ significantly from that in late childhood or early adulthood. It is the rare teenager who is diagnosed with an abnormality in these systems for the first time during adolescence, and it is equally rare for an asymptomatic teenager to be diagnosed with a chronic disease affecting these organs during the adolescent years. However, anecdotal reports and the case report literature abound with cases of just such adolescents, emphasizing the need for vigilance in performance of the cardiac, respiratory, abdominal, and neurologic examinations in "healthy" adolescents.

Musculoskeletal Examination

Musculoskeletal aches and injuries are common during the adolescent years because of increased involvement in competitive sports during a time of rapid growth. In addition, several musculoskeletal disorders may occur during these years, including Osgood-Schlatter disease and slipped capital femoral epiphyses. Generally, a complete musculoskeletal evaluation is advised for adolescents involved in competitive athletics, and evaluation of specific areas of the musculoskeletal system is required for those with particular complaints. The general practitioner must be comfortable with the musculoskeletal examination of adolescents to avoid both under and overreferral for radiologic procedures and specialty evaluations.

Scoliosis is present in 1% to 2% of adolescents,[15] occurring somewhat more frequently in girls than in boys. Since scoliosis progresses most rapidly during the adolescent growth spurt, and because girls generally enter puberty earlier than boys, scoliosis develops in girls at a younger age than boys. Although it is debatable whether mass screenings of scoliosis in the school setting are worthwhile, all experts agree that screening for scoliosis should be an integral part of the physician's annual check-up for patients of both sexes, beginning in middle childhood.[16]

The complete examination for scoliosis includes evaluation of the spine with the patient in three standing positions.[17] The patient's back is first examined from behind, with the patient standing upright. In this position the patient can be evaluated for shoulder alignment, scapular prominence, hip prominence, asymmetric arm to body distance, and pelvic asymmetry. A string can be dropped from the occiput to the level of the buttocks; if a curvature of the spine is evident, the end of the string will not fall in the crease between the buttocks. The patient is then examined while bending forward 90 degrees, with arms extended and palms together (Adams test). In this position, a rib or lumbar hump can be seen. Finally, the patient is examined from the side while he or she stands in such a way that thoracic or lumbar lordosis may be noted.

It is questioned whether every adolescent with a positive finding on scoliosis screening needs to be referred for further radiographic or orthopedic evaluation.

Mass screenings have revealed large numbers of youths who are found to be positive but whose curves are too small to ever require intervention. Development of a specially designed inclinometer called a Scoliometer, an instrument that measures the angle of trunk rotation, has helped resolve the issue of whom to refer for further evaluation.[16] It has been determined that those with an angle of trunk rotation of less than 5 degrees are extremely unlikely to have a curve that requires any type of treatment. Patients who have scoliosis determined on physical examination and a small angle of trunk rotation can be followed clinically rather than being referred for radiographic and orthopedic evaluation. The frequency of follow-up is guided by the pubertal stage of the patient; more frequent visits are required for those who are prepubertal or in early puberty than for those at the end of their pubertal growth.

Examination of Genitalia

Genitalia change dramatically during adolescence. Tanner staging is the most common method used to follow the pubertal development of the genitalia in adolescents.[18] Tanner and Marshall studied 192 English schoolgirls and 228 English schoolboys throughout puberty. They noted that secondary sex characteristics developed in a consistent pattern in their study population. These characteristics included the development of breasts and progression of pubic hair in girls, and changes in the genitalia (testes, scrotum, penis) and pubic hair in boys. Other secondary sex characteristics such as axillary and facial hair changes are not included in Tanner staging, since their progression varies considerably during puberty.

Tanner stages are depicted in Figures 13-5 and 13-6. Included are five stages for breast development; five stages for female and male pubic hair development; and five stages for testicular, scrotal, and penile development. Tanner stage 1 represents the prepubertal stage, Tanner 2 denotes early pubertal changes, Tanner 3 represents midpuberty, Tanner 4 is the preadult stage, and Tanner 5 represents adult development. Progression through Tanner 4 is noted in all adolescents; progression from Tanner 4 to 5 is not always found and may vary between ethnic groups. Every adolescent should be evaluated for Tanner staging at each check-up so that those with normal development can be reassured and those with abnormalities can be further evaluated.

In girls the course of pubertal events generally progresses from thelarche (breast budding) to pubarche (onset of pubic hair appearance) to the time of the peak height velocity (growth spurt) and, lastly, menarche (Fig. 13-7). Thelarche occurs at a mean age of 10.5 to 11 years, with a wide range of normal, from 8 to 13 years. Pubarche usually follows thelarche within 6 months, although in up to 25% of girls pubarche may precede thelarche. Peak

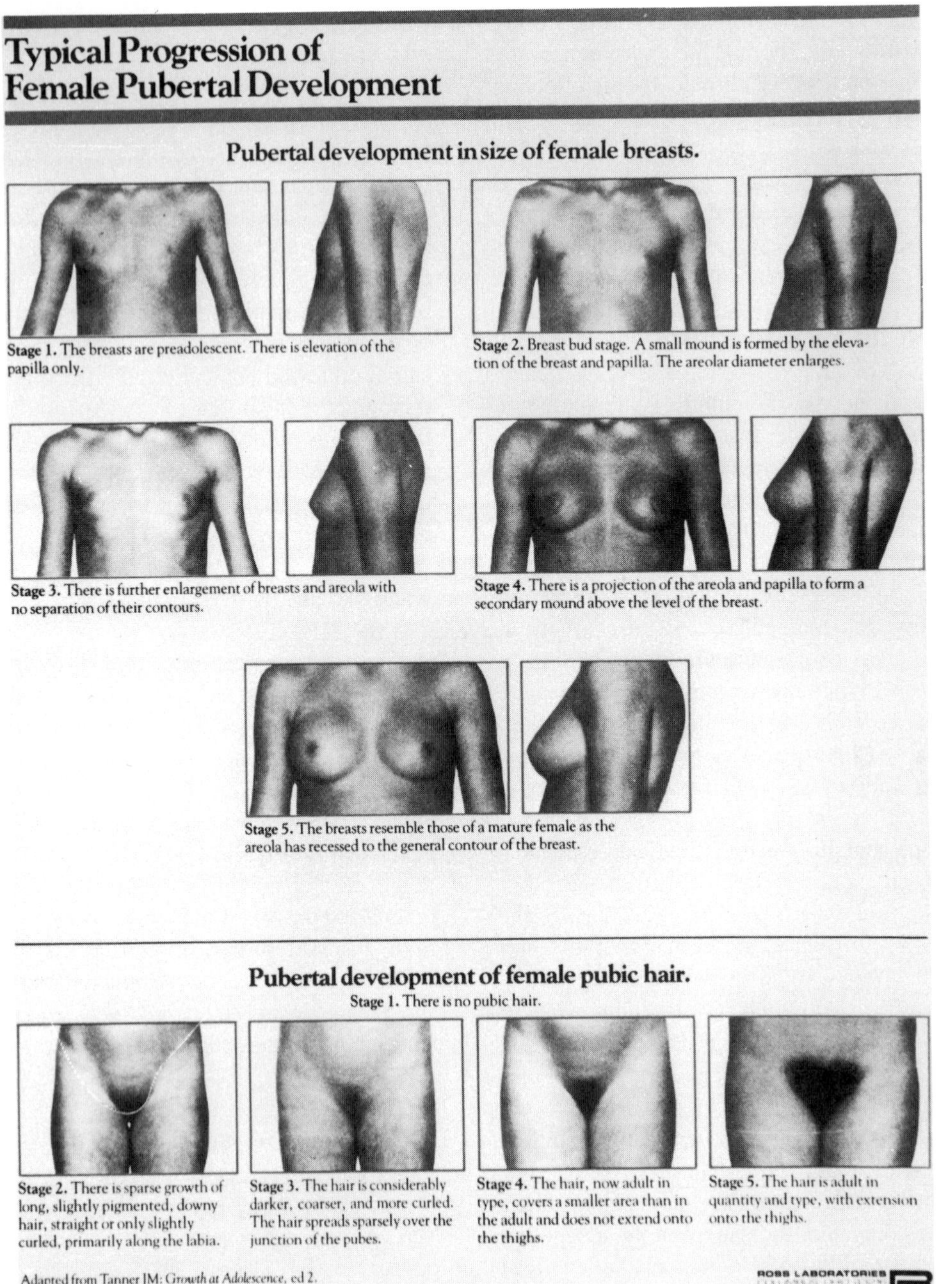

Fig. 13-5. Tanner stages of female pubertal development. (Modified from Tanner JM: *Growth at adolescence,* ed 2, Oxford, 1962, Blackwell Scientific. Reprinted with permission of Ross Laboratories, Columbus, Ohio. Copyright 1962 Ross Laboratories.)

height velocity (PHV) generally occurs as 12.1 ± 0.8 years, when breast and pubic hair development are between Tanner stages 2 and 3 (which is generally 1.5 to 2 years after the onset of puberty). Menarche begins at an average of 12.7 years, with a range from 9 to 16 years[19]; this generally occurs 2.3 ± 1.1 years from the appearance of breast budding (Tanner breast stage 2).[20] Most girls are in Tanner stage 4 of breast and pubic hair development at

the onset of menarche. A girl without breast development by age 13 years or without the onset of menses by age 16 should be evaluated for pubertal or menarchal delay.

The sequence of pubertal events in boys includes testicular enlargement, followed by pubarche and PHV (Fig. 13-8). In a minority of boys, pubarche precedes testicular enlargement. Genital changes in boys begin at a mean age of 11.6 years, with a range from 9.5 to 13.8

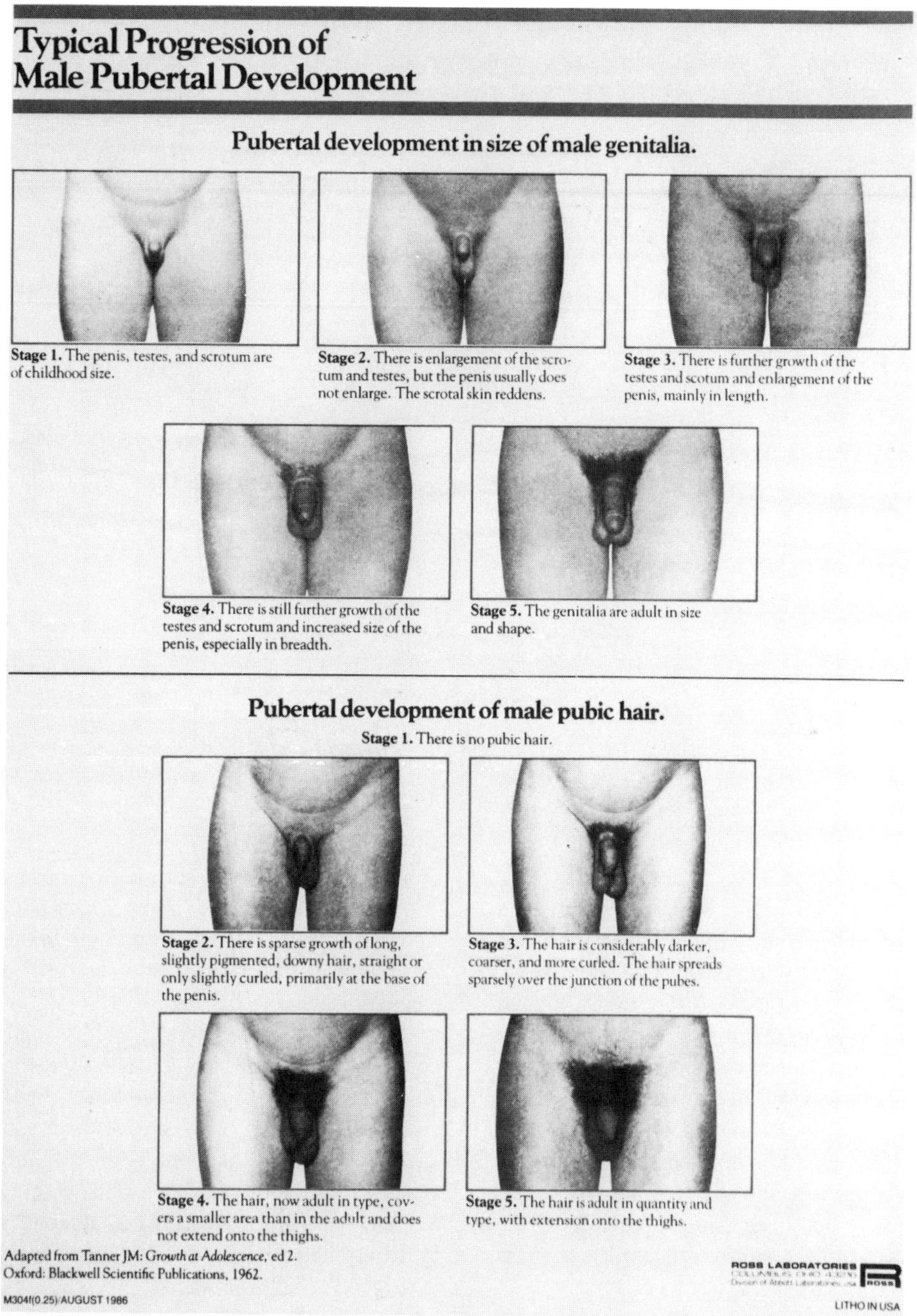

Fig. 13-6. Tanner stages of male pubertal development. (Modified from Tanner JM: *Growth at adolescence,* ed 2, Oxford, 1962, Blackwell Scientific. Reprinted with permission of Ross Laboratories, Columbus, Ohio. Copyright 1962 Ross Laboratories.)

years. Pubarche occurs at a mean of 11.8 years. PHV occurs on average at 14.1 ± 0.9 years, which is generally during genital stage 4 and pubic hair stage 3 or 4.[21] Boys experience their growth spurt at a much later time and in a more advanced sexual maturational stage than girls; this accounts for the height differences of boys and girls in junior high school.

The female breast examination is performed to detect breast masses: most important, those masses that may become or are already malignant. It has been recommended that the breast examination be incorporated into the general check-up of female patients as soon as breast budding appears.[22] Because breast cancer is extremely rare in the teenage years, and since the examination is often embarrassing to an adolescent in the breast-budding stage, it seems reasonable to postpone the examination until she is emotionally more mature (middle adolescence) or has Tanner stage 3 breast development. The

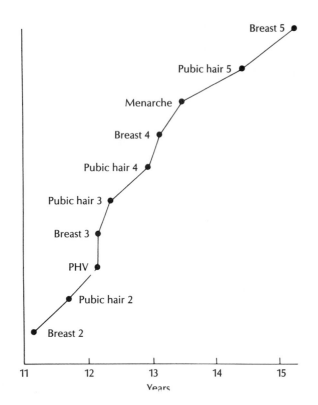

Fig. 13-7. Sequence and mean age of pubertal events in females. (From Root AW: Endocrinology of puberty, *J Pediatr* 83:1-19, 1973.)

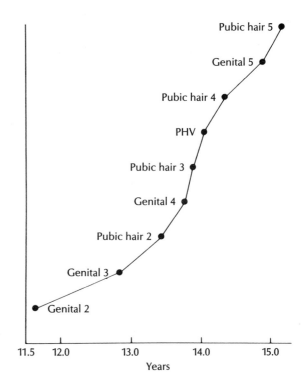

Fig. 13-8. Sequence and mean age of pubertal events in males. (From Root AW: Endocrinology of puberty, *J Pediatr* 83:1-19, 1973.)

breast examination may be done with the patient in a sitting and/or lying position. It is important that the arm be above the head during examination of the breast, because the tail of the breast extends into the axilla and may otherwise be missed. Examination of the breast includes inspection for assessment of Tanner stage; detection of any variations or abnormalities in the configuration of breast, areola, or nipple; and palpation for consistency of breast tissue and the presence of any masses. Palpation begins at the external borders of the breast and progresses in concentric circles toward the nipple. Finally, the nipple is gently squeezed to express any discharge.

Palpation of the breast will reveal fibrocystic disease in approximately 50% of females. Because this condition occurs so frequently, appears to be hormonally modulated, and is not associated with an increased risk of breast cancer, Love et al[23] recommended that fibrocystic disease be renamed "physiologic nodularity" or "lumpy breasts." The finding of physiologic nodularity on breast examination in teenagers is common and cause for reassurance, not alarm.

Discrete breast masses in teenagers are almost always benign; 80% to 90% of these masses are fibroadenomas. On examination, fibroadenomas are firm, mobile, and less than 5 cm in diameter. Cysts account for most nonfibroadenomatous masses; usually they are multiple, spongy and tender and enlarge just before menses.

Fibroadenomas and cysts may be observed for 2 to 3 months before referral to a surgeon, because many resolve spontaneously. Masses requiring immediate surgical referral are hard, nonmobile, or associated with skin changes or nipple discharge.[22]

Any nipple discharge requires evaluation. If the discharge represents galactorrhea, pregnancy, postpregnancy status (abortion, miscarriage, or postpartum), drug use, prolactinoma, or hypothyroidism should be considered as possible diagnoses. If the discharge is due to an abscess, antibiotic treatment and warm soaks are used, with incision and drainage by a surgeon if needed. Lastly, if the discharge is bloody or serous, immediate referral to a surgeon is appropriate.[22]

The physician can use the time during the breast examination to teach the adolescent how to examine her own breasts. Debate exists over the usefulness of teaching breast self-examination to adolescents. Some physicians believe that it causes more anxiety about breast cancer than necessary in an age group that rarely has the disease and is not likely to follow through on appropriate self-examination. Despite these concerns, many believe that teaching breast self-examination to adolescents is worthwhile, if only to stress an important habit that will take on added significance after adolescence.[24,25] The American Cancer Society circulates a pamphlet that teaches women how to examine their breasts in three stages: in the shower, standing before a mirror, and in a prone position.

Gynecomastia develops in many boys during adolescence; approximately two thirds of boys are affected, with the peak occurrence at age 14. Most cases resolve within 2 years, with approximately 7% persisting for 3 years. Gynecomastia occurs bilaterally in approximately three fourths of patients, with the two sides enlarged either sequentially or simultaneously.[26] Embarrassment may prevent many teenage boys from mentioning gynecomastia to their physicians. In examining the male breast, it is essential to differentiate breast tissue from fat tissue. True breast tissue in the 10.5- to 15-year-old age group with an otherwise normal physical examination warrants observation for a period. If the gynecomastia persists or worsens, disorders such as Klinefelter's syndrome, adrenal tumors, alcoholism, or steroid abuse should be considered. Surgical biopsy of breast buds during middle adolescence is rarely indicated. Surgical treatment may be reserved for those males who in late adolescence have persistent gynecomastia without a treatable etiology and who perceive that the gynecomastia interferes with their lives.

Testicular examination is performed to determine the presence of testicular masses, varicoceles, and hernias. The examination includes inspection for size, shape, and Tanner stage; palpation for consistency and masses of the testes, vas deferens, and epididymis; and evaluation for the presence of a hernia by inserting an index finger into the external inguinal ring while the patient coughs. If testicular size is in question, an orchidometer (a string of testicular models marked by size in cubic centimeters) is used to measure testicular volume. Because testicular cancer is the most common cancer in young adult males, the physician may consider teaching patients testicular self-examination. As is the case with breast examination, the value of teaching testicular self-examination remains controversial, since it is argued by some that the anxiety created, combined with the time and money spent to teach the examination, may outweigh the possible benefits.[25]

Pelvic examination is recommended for females who are sexually active, have a vaginal discharge and/or suspicion of a sexually transmitted disease, or have primary or secondary amenorrhea, severe dysmenorrhea, or irregular menses; it should be a routine procedure for those 18 years of age or older.[27] The pelvic examination includes inspection of the external genitalia (for lesions and anatomic abnormalities), vagina (for estrogen effect and discharge), and cervix (for erosion and eversion); and palpation of the cervix (for firmness and tenderness), uterus (for size, tenderness, and position), and adnexa (for size, tenderness, and masses). A Papanicolaou smear and appropriate cultures should be taken. Many adolescents have an erythematous, nonfriable, symmetric ring around the external os of the cervix. This is known as eversion, representing an endocervix that has not yet inverted, as it generally does by adulthood. It is important to recognize eversion of the cervix so that it is not mistaken for an erosion or infection. Issues related to the pelvic examination are discussed in detail in Chapter 135 "The Pelvic Examination."

COMPLETION

On completion of the physical examination, patients can change back into their clothes so that they can feel more comfortable when the findings are presented. Findings, evaluation, and treatment of both confidential and nonconfidential problems can then be discussed. Anticipatory guidance about health issues enlists the patient as an active participant in his or her health care. Finally, the parents can be invited back into the room to discuss nonconfidential findings and health implications.

References

1. Green M, editor: *Guidelines for health supervision,* Elk Grove Village, IL, 1985, American Academy of Pediatrics.
2. Fisher M, editor: *Guide to clinical preventive services: an assessment of the effectiveness of 169 interventions. Report of the U.S. Preventive Services Task Force,* Baltimore, MD, 1989, Williams & Wilkins.
3. Green M, editor: *Bright futures: guidelines for health supervision of infants, children, and adolescents,* Arlington, VA, 1994, National Center for Education in Maternal and Child Health.
4. Elster AB, Kuznets NJ, editors: *AMA guidelines for adolescent preventive services—recommendations and rationale,* Baltimore, MD, 1994, Williams & Wilkins.
5. Committee on Practice and Ambulatory Medicine: *Recommendations for preventive pediatric health care, Pediatrics* 96:373-374, 1995.
6. Morrissey JM, Thorpe JC: *Rights and responsibilities of young people in New York: a legal guide for human service providers,* New York, 1986, New York City Youth Bureau.
7. Markham BF: Legal issues for the practicing pediatrician, *Pediatr Clin North Am* 28:617-625, 1981.
8. Phillips S, Bohannon W, Heald FD: Teenagers' choices regarding the presence of family members during the examination of genitalia, *J Adolesc Health Care* 7:245-249, 1986.
9. Fixler DE, Laird NP, Fitzgerald V, et al: Hypertension screening in schools: result of the Dallas study, *Pediatrics* 63:32, 1979.
10. Report of the Second Task Force on Blood Pressure Control in Children, 1987: *Pediatrics* 79:1-25, 1987.
11. American Academy of Ophthalmology: *At first sight. Ophthalmic problems seen by primary care physicians: children's vision screening,* San Francisco, 1988, American Academy of Ophthalmology.
12. Nietupska O, Harding N: Auditory screening of school children: fact or fallacy?, *Br Med J* 284:717-720, 1982.
13. Casamassimo PS, Castaldi CR: Considerations in the dental management of the adolescent, *Pediatr Clin North Am* 29:631-651, 1982.
14. National Center for Health Statistics: *An assessment of the occlusion of the teeth of youths 12-17 years, United States.* Vital and Health Statistics. Series 11 No. 162. DHEW Publication No. (HRA) 77-1644. Public Health Service. Washington, DC, 1977, U.S. Government Printing Office.
15. Lonstein JE: Natural history and school screening for scoliosis, *Orthop Clin North Am* 19:227-238, 1988.
16. Bunnell WP: Are you overreferring scoliosis?, *Contemp Pediatr* 2:64-76, 1985.

17. Proceedings of the 1976 Annual Meeting of the House of Delegates, resolution 76-5: Spine deformity screening, *J Kansas Med Soc* 77:726, 1976.

18. Tanner JM: *Growth at adolescence,* ed 2, Springfield, IL, 1962, Charles C Thomas.

19. Root AW: Endocrinology of puberty, *J Pediatr* 83:1-19, 1973.

20. Marshall WA, Tanner JM: Variations in pattern of pubertal changes in girls, *Arch Dis Child* 44:291-303, 1969.

21. Marshall WA, Tanner JM: Variations in pattern of pubertal changes in boys, *Arch Dis Child* 45:13-23, 1990.

22. Beach RK: Routine breast exams: a chance to reassure, guide, and protect, *Contemp Pediatr* 70:100, 1987.

23. Love SM, Gelman RS, Silen W: Fibrocystic "disease" of the breast—a nondisease?, *N Engl J Med* 307:1010-1014, 1982.

24. Frank JN, Mai V: Breast self-examination in young women: more harm than good?, *Lancet* 2:654-657, 1985.

25. Goldbloom RB: Self-examination by adolescents, *Pediatrics* 76: 126-128, 1985.

26. Nydick M, Bustos J, Dale JH, Rawson RW: Gynecomastia in adolescent boys, *JAMA* 178:449-454, 1961.

27. Emans SJ, Goldstein DP: *Pediatric and adolescent gynecology,* ed 3, Boston, 1990, Little, Brown, p 21.

CHAPTER 14

Laboratory Testing

•

Martin Fisher

Evaluation of the health status of adolescents generally includes laboratory testing. Findings from the history taking and physical examination determine whether the adolescent requires routine laboratory screening tests, specialized laboratory tests indicated because of the individual's life style or background, or problem-oriented laboratory testing due to a specific complaint or physical finding. The clinician determines which tests belong in each of these three categories; which test results must be interpreted differently in the adolescent compared with patients who are younger or older; and arrangements to be considered in managing special adolescent problems such as the need for confidentiality, limited fees, and fear of needles.

ROUTINE LABORATORY SCREENING

Laboratory tests that should be considered in routine screening of all adolescents include those that will detect problems that are potentially serious if not discovered, are relatively common in the population, and are amenable to treatment acceptable to adolescents.[1] The tests should be simple and convenient, yielding results that are both reliable (i.e., similar on repeated measures) and valid (i.e., both sensitive and specific).[2] According to this definition, few tests should be ordered routinely for adolescent patients, regardless of their apparent health status or health risks. Tests to be considered include hematologic

screening, serum chemistries, urinalysis, lipid profile testing, evaluation of immunity to certain infections, and hormonal testing. Several specialists in adolescent medicine have given their views of which tests to perform, and how often,[1,2] and several national organizations have presented their recommendations in official reports.[3-5] Among the latter are the *Guidelines for Health Supervision* by the American Academy of Pediatrics (AAP) in 1988; the *Guidelines for Adolescent Preventive Services* (GAPS) published by the American Medical Association in 1992; and the *Bright Futures Guidelines for Health Supervision of Infants, Children and Adolescents* produced by the Maternal and Child Health Bureau of the U.S. Department of Health and Human Services in 1994.[3-5] Because there are no specific right or wrong answers in determining the advisability of laboratory screening tests, the recommendations of the various reports do not always agree, and specific subspecialty organizations may present additional recommendations for particular tests. Current recommendations for each laboratory test are summarized in Table 14-1 and discussed in this chapter. Individual tests are discussed further in appropriate chapters and in the references listed at the end of this chapter.

Hematologic Screening

An estimated 8% of adolescent girls and 3% of adolescent boys are anemic, usually as a result of iron

TABLE 14-1
Laboratory Screening Tests Recommended for Adolescents

Routine Screening	Recommendation
Hemoglobin or hematocrit level	Once between ages 12-20 yr (AAP)[3]
	Annual in females with heavy menses, chronic weight loss, nutritional deficit, or athletic activity (Bright Futures)[4]
	Not specifically recommended (GAPS)[5]
Serum chemistries	Not recommended routinely
Urinalysis	Dipstick urine in those who are sexually active
Cholesterol level	Selected screening as follows (NCEP)[9]:
	Total cholesterol value if ≥19 yr of age or parent has cholesterol ≥240 mg/dl
	Fasting lipoprotein analysis if parent or grandparent has heart disease <age 55
	Total cholesterol if family history unknown or adolescent has risk factors (see text), at discretion of physician
Antibody titers (MMR, hepatitis B, varicella)	Not currently recommended
Tuberculin testing	Tuberculin testing in adolescents at risk (GAPS, Bright Futures)[4,5]
Hormonal testing	Not recommended routinely

Special Circumstances

Sexually active adolescents	Pap smear yearly; gonorrhea and *Chlamydia* screening; syphilis serology in high-risk youth
Alcohol and drug use	Drug/alcohol levels when warranted; screening for sequelae (hepatitis, AIDS)
Homosexuality	Screening for STD, hepatitis, and AIDS
Adolescents from foreign countries	Stool examination for ova and parasites, tuberculin testing
Pre-sports evaluation	ECG/CXR only if clinically warranted
Preoperative screening	Blood count, clotting studies, blood bank specimen; ECG/CXR only if clinically warranted

AAP, American Academy of Pediatrics; *CXR*, chest x-ray; *ECG*, electrocardiogram; *GAPS*, Guidelines for Adolescent Preventive Services; *MMR*, measles, mumps, and rubella; *NCEP*, National Cholesterol Education Program; *Pap*, Papanicolaou; *STD*, sexually transmitted disease.

deficiency.[1,2] Several factors characteristic of the adolescent age group, including rapid growth, poor eating habits, and increased menstrual blood loss in some females, are thought to account for these abnormally low levels. The AAP has recommended that all adolescents between the ages of 12 and 20 years have a hemoglobin or hematocrit test at one time during adolescence.[3] The Bright Futures Guidelines recommend annual screening in females who have moderate to heavy menses, chronic weight loss, or nutritional deficit or who undertake athletic activity[5]; the GAPS recommendations do not include any screening for anemia.[4] Hemoglobin and hematocrit values remain unchanged in girls but increase significantly in boys during the adolescent years because of the effects of androgen production on hematopoiesis. Possibly because of the presence of the sickle cell gene in the community, mean hemoglobin levels of black adolescents of both sexes are approximately 1 mg/dl lower than those of their white counterparts. Screening for sickle cell trait (using the sickle prep) and thalassemia (using the mean corpuscular volume) in at-risk populations has been recommended by some authors.[2] Research

in recent years has shown that some adolescents, especially those who participate in sports activities, may have subtle degrees of anemia not detectable by hemoglobin or hematocrit determination, but more sophisticated screening (using ferritin levels) is recommended by only some authors.[2] There is universal agreement that total and differential leukocyte counts serve no purpose in clinically well children and adolescents.[6]

Serum Chemistries

Some clinicians and many hospitals have a policy of determining electrolyte values and other serum chemistries (including liver function tests, albumin levels, blood urea nitrogen, and creatinine levels) in all adolescent patients. However, there is no evidence that these are useful screening tests for this age group. Although abnormalities may be disclosed in the rare teenager with undetected disease or in the adolescent with surreptitious bulimia nervosa or substance abuse problems, the relatively high cost and large number of false-positive results far outweigh the benefits.

Urinalysis

A complete urinalysis that includes either a microscopic or a dipstick evaluation is not currently being recommended by the AAP, GAPS, or Bright Futures Guidelines as part of routine health care for adolescents.[3-5] Problems for which a urinalysis is advocated in younger or older patients, including urinary tract infection, adult-onset diabetes mellitus, and renal disease, do not appear with the same frequency or implications in the adolescent age group. Some clinicians, however, continue to perform routine dipstick urinalyses on their adolescent patients in the belief that the small expense justifies its use in detecting urethritis or a urinary tract infection (which may be indicated by a positive nitrite or leukocyte esterase test), diabetes mellitus (indicated by glycosuria), or renal disease (proteinuria and/or hematuria). Some have recommended urinalysis to screen for eating disorders, since poor eating habits may be indicated by ketonuria and bulimia, possibly indicated by an alkaline pH.[7] Evidence indicates that urinalysis is most useful for detecting urinary tract or urethral infections (specifically those due to *Neisseria gonorrhoeae* or *Chlamydia trachomatis*) in teenagers who are sexually active.[8] Most practitioners continue to perform a dipstick urinalysis in all adolescent patients every 1 to 2 years despite the lack of formal recommendations to do so.

Lipid Profile

No area of screening has engendered more controversy than the question of whether children and adolescents should receive routine screening for cholesterol levels. In 1992, an Expert Panel on Blood Cholesterol Levels in Children and Adolescents of the National Cholesterol Education Program (NCEP) recommended selective, rather than universal, screening in adolescents, and this recommendation has been adopted by both the GAPS and Bright Futures reports.[3,4,9] Recommendations of the Expert Panel include the following: (1) measurement of total cholesterol should be performed in young adults over 19 years of age and in those whose parents have a serum cholesterol level greater than 240 mg/dl; (2) adolescents with an unknown family history or who have multiple risk factors for future cardiovascular disease (e.g., smoking, hypertension, obesity, diabetes mellitus, excessive consumption of dietary fats) may be screened for total serum cholesterol at the discretion of the physician; and (3) those with a family history of cardiovascular disease in a parent or grandparent under the age of 55 should be screened with a fasting lipoprotein analysis. Recommendations based on the results of these screening tests are presented in Chapter 30, "Hyperlip-

idemia and Atherosclerosis." Although many physicians have opted for universal screening of all adolescents, the Expert Panel opted not to recommend universal screening because (1) tracking of values into adulthood is not completely consistent, (2) universal screening could lead to unwarranted labeling of many adolescents, (3) for most individuals it is unnecessary to begin therapy before adulthood, and (4) there is insufficient evidence of the long-term safety and efficacy of drug therapy for hyperlipidemia in childhood and adolescence.[9]

Immunity Status

Ensuring that teenagers are adequately protected against infections for which immunizations or prophylactic antibiotics are recommended (diphtheria, tetanus, poliomyelitis, measles, mumps, rubella, varicella, hepatitis B, and tuberculosis) is an important part of well-adolescent health care. A history of infection or previous immunization is the first step in this process, and laboratory testing sometimes provides additional information. Determination of antibody levels to rubella, mumps, measles, varicella, and hepatitis B can be an adjunct in evaluating susceptibility to these infections, and tuberculin skin testing remains a mainstay in efforts to prevent tuberculosis. Laboratory testing in each of these areas has undergone major changes in the past few years.

Studies in the early and mid-1980s showed that approximately 10% to 15% of adolescents were susceptible to rubella, regardless of their socioeconomic status or immunization history. On the basis of this finding, it was recommended that teenagers, especially females, be tested for rubella antibodies, and that those with negative results be immunized. Although similar numbers of adolescents were found to be susceptible to mumps and measles, routine screening for antibody levels to these diseases was not recommended because, unlike rubella, inexpensive testing for antibody levels to mumps and measles was not available. The upsurge in measles among children and adolescents noted in the late 1980s prompted a Centers for Disease Control and Prevention (CDC) and AAP recommendation that all children and adolescents receive two doses of measles, mumps, and rubella vaccine, preferably by 12 years of age.[10,11] This policy has eliminated the need for antibody testing for immunity to these infections in adolescents on a routine basis.

The recent introduction of varicella and hepatitis B vaccines has raised the question of whether antibody screening should be performed before immunization for these diseases. Specific recommendations for both of these vaccines do not advise antibody screening for either disease. In the case of varicella, it is recommended that adolescents over age 12 who do not have a clinical history of disease receive two shots, 4 to 8 weeks apart, without previous antibody screening.[12] In the case of hepatitis B, it is suggested, although not yet officially recommended, that adolescents receive three shots at times zero, 1 month, and 6 months, also without previous antibody testing.[13] In general, for all of the viral infections it has been determined that the financial and logistic costs of screening outweigh the financial and clinical costs of vaccination.

In contrast, tuberculin testing remains an important part of tuberculosis control efforts in teenagers. However, which teenagers to test, which test to use, how often to test, and how to interpret the results are all questions that have been reevaluated in recent years. The American Thoracic Society and the CDC recommend routine tuberculin testing only in high-risk populations in which the prevalence of tuberculin sensitivity exceeds 1%.[14] Because adolescents seem to be at increased risk for the development of active disease and since any single case found may lead to several patients being treated, the AAP calls for testing during early adolescence in low-risk populations and yearly for those in higher-risk groups.[15] Both GAPS and Bright Futures recommend tuberculin testing in adolescents with specific risk factors (residence in a high prevalence area, exposure to tuberculosis, immigrant status, homelessness, history of incarceration, employment in a health care facility).[4,5] GAPS recommends that the timing of this test be based on individual circumstances, while Bright Futures advises annual testing in adolescents at risk. The Bright Futures Guidelines also recommend one test at 14 to 16 years of age in all adolescents.

Tuberculin testing is performed using an intradermal injection of 5 tuberculin units (e.g., the Mantoux test) of purified protein derivative; multipuncture testing (e.g., the tine test) is no longer considered a sufficient screening mechanism.[16] Although induration of 10 mm or more in the Mantoux test at 48 to 72 hours has traditionally been considered a positive reaction, more recent changes aimed at decreasing both the false-positive and false-negative rate of this test have come into effect.[14,16] The changes promulgated by the American Thoracic Society and the CDC recommend that skin tests be considered positive if indurations are (1) ≥5 mm in persons with recent close contact with tuberculosis, with a positive chest x-ray finding, or who are immunosuppressed; (2) ≥10 mm in persons with known risk factors such as the foreign-born, the homeless, intravenous drug abusers, or those with other diseases associated with tuberculosis; and (3) ≥15 mm in those without other risk factors. Adolescents who have received bacille Calmette-Guérin (BCG) vaccine should also be tested, since BCG vaccination causes an inconsistent tuberculin response that decreases with time,

and these individuals should be treated no differently from those who never received the vaccine.[16]

Hormonal Testing

Hormonal changes are a hallmark of adolescence, but routine testing for hormonal levels is not recommended at any time during the adolescent years. Only patients with findings suggestive of endocrine disorders, such as short stature, delayed development, thyroid disease, or menstrual irregularities, require any hormonal studies.

Conclusion

Certain routine laboratory tests should be used sparingly in adolescent patients. A one-time hemoglobin determination, urinalysis, tuberculin test, and cholesterol screening will suffice for most healthy teenagers, and even these are not considered necessary by all authorities. More frequent use of these tests or the use of additional screening tests should be guided by clinical findings, including special circumstances that may put the adolescent at additional risk.

SCREENING IN SPECIAL CIRCUMSTANCES

Certain adolescents, by virtue of their activities or background, may be considered for additional laboratory screening tests despite the lack of any overt physical findings or complaints. This group includes teenagers, both straight and gay, who are sexually active or involved with drug or alcohol use; those from foreign countries; and those being seen specifically for a pre-sports or preoperative examination. Controversy exists over the specific tests warranted, with a tendency to include more testing in each of these circumstances than for the general population because of the greater risks and smaller numbers of involved adolescents.

Sexually Active Adolescents

All teens who are sexually active risk acquiring several sexually transmitted diseases (STDs). Females are at risk for the development of cellular changes, which may be precursors of cervical neoplastic disease. Screening for the presence of infection in both sexes and performance of a Papanicolaou (Pap) smear in females are recommended.[1-5,8] A Pap smear should be performed yearly in all sexually active adolescent females; the costs are minimal, the benefits are significant, and the risks of cervical cancer are documented to be greater in those who have intercourse at a younger age.[17]

Gonorrhea in adolescents remains a problem; it can be asymptomatic in both males and females. A screening test for gonorrhea is recommended for all sexually active adolescents: yearly in high-risk urban youth and less frequently in lower-risk suburban or rural youth.[18] Chlamydial infection has been found in 10% to 25% of sexually active adolescents in all clinical settings.[18] Infection with *C. trachomatis* is frequently asymptomatic in both sexes and may lead to future fertility problems in females. Testing is recommended as an initial screen in all sexually active adolescents, and annually if there is a change in partners. Culture or one of the more rapid and less expensive antigen detection methods commercially available may be used for both gonorrhea and *Chlamydia* testing.[18] Some clinicians use a dipstick urinalysis to prescreen for evidence of urethritis in symptomatic adolescents, especially males, rather than testing all adolescents for gonorrhea and *Chlamydia* directly.[19]

Syphilis, which decreased significantly among adolescents in the late 1970s to early 1980s, has shown a dramatic resurgence, especially in urban, inner-city youth.[20] Accordingly, serologic testing for syphilis is again being routinely recommended for sexually active adolescents living in high-risk areas. Other STDs for which laboratory screening methods are available include trichomoniasis, bacterial vaginosis, and candidiasis; each may be detected on a saline wet mount of vaginal secretions. There is no screening test for asymptomatic genital herpes, nor is there a readily acceptable screening test for human papillomavirus (different types of which are associated with venereal warts and cervical neoplastic disease).

Homosexuality

Estimates show that homosexual orientation among adolescents may be as high as 10%, especially among males. The male homosexual is at risk for classic STDs, specific intestinal infections, traumatic injuries related to sexual practices, drug abuse, physical assault, and AIDS. Screening tests in these adolescents should include a serologic test for syphilis, a culture for gonorrhea from all appropriate sites (urethra, anus, throat), a culture or antibody test for *Chlamydia,* measurement of hepatitis surface antigen and antibody, and antibody testing for AIDS.[21] Appropriate counseling must be available to explain the testing and prepare for the consequences of any positive results. (See Chapter 67, "HIV Infection and AIDS" and Chapter 99, "Sexual Orientation and Gender Identity.")

Alcohol and Drug Use

Laboratory screening may be considered in two distinct ways when treating adolescents involved with drug and alcohol use. Screening for alcohol or drugs may be useful in monitoring some teenagers suspected of substance abuse, and screening for certain sequelae of substance abuse may be useful in others. Sophisticated laboratory techniques have made the analysis of serum or urine for illicit substances readily available.[22,23] Few advocate these tests in mass screenings of adolescents, except perhaps for those participating in high-level sports or high-risk jobs. While parents or a school may sometimes insist that an adolescent be screened for substance use, many clinicians prefer to offer the test to the patient, using acceptance or refusal as a basis for further decision making and counseling. Urinalysis may be useful in the emergency room setting after an overdose or for ongoing management of an adolescent known to be a substance abuser. These patients, especially if there is a history of intravenous drug use, may also benefit from screening for liver function abnormalities, hepatitis B antigen and antibody, and AIDS, provided that appropriate counseling is available.

Adolescents from Foreign Countries

Adolescents from Asia, Africa, and South America are routinely screened for ova and parasites. Since BCG vaccination is used widely in these continents for prevention of tuberculosis, interpretation of tuberculin testing may be more difficult for foreign-born adolescents. It is recommended, however, that tuberculin testing be interpreted no differently in these adolescents, since the duration of BCG immunity is so variable, and unpredictable from country to country.[16]

Pre-sports Evaluation

The adolescent who plans to join in organized sports activities generally undergoes a specialized evaluation before being allowed to participate.[24,25] Although this evaluation includes several focused areas of questioning on the medical history and some specific aspects of the physical examination, no special laboratory tests are required. Blood counts and urinalyses may be performed as part of routine health care, and an electrocardiogram (ECG) and chest radiograph taken only if findings in the history or physical examination warrant their use. Some thought is being given to the possibility of routine use of sonography in the pre-sports evaluation to detect abnormalities that could put the athlete at risk for sudden death; however, the costs are too prohibitive at the present time for use in routine screening.

Preoperative Screening

Screening for a surgical procedure usually involves a series of blood tests (blood counts, clotting studies, blood bank specimen), a urinalysis, a chest radiogram, and an

ECG. Studies have raised questions about the value of the blood tests and the urinalysis in children and adolescents, but these tests generally continue to be performed.[26-28] Several large-scale studies have shown that neither the chest radiograph nor the ECG need be performed in the "healthy" adolescent with no previous evidence of pulmonary or cardiac disease; many institutions no longer include these tests in the preoperative procedures for children and adolescents.

SPECIAL CONSIDERATIONS IN INTERPRETATION AND PERFORMANCE OF TESTS

Several factors in the interpretation and performance of laboratory tests in adolescents are different from the considerations ordinarily applied to either children or adults. The physical changes of adolescence have an impact on the results expected for certain tests, and several psychosocial issues affecting teenagers require special accommodations in the procedures needed in order to perform testing adequately in this age group.

Laboratory Values

In most laboratory tests the range of the normal standard is no different for adolescents from that for children or adults; however, specific biochemical, hematologic, and hormonal tests have significant differences, often with major clinical implications.[29,30] These differences may be due solely to the effects of growth, they may vary with the Tanner stage, or they may represent a normal progression from childhood values to ultimate adult levels. Specific tests with clinical implications are discussed below.

SERUM ALKALINE PHOSPHATASE. Because of skeletal growth, significantly elevated alkaline phosphatase levels are characteristic of early adolescence, especially at Tanner stages 2 to 4. In a laboratory test with normal childhood or adult values in the low to mid-100s, a value in the mid-300s would be perfectly acceptable in growing adolescents. Such values would *not* call for an evaluation for renal, bone, or liver disease, as might be the case for other age groups.

CHOLESTEROL AND TRIGLYCERIDE LEVELS. Progression in cholesterol and triglyceride levels from childhood to adulthood is reflected in the 95th percentile values for total cholesterol and triglycerides of 200 and 140 mg/dl, respectively, in adolescents. These values would be considered at the lower levels of borderline in the adult. Further work-up and dietary counseling in adolescents must be based on age-appropriate levels.

HEMOGLOBIN OR HEMATOCRIT LEVELS. Because of the hematopoietic effects of testosterone, hemoglobin and hematocrit levels increase significantly in boys, from a mean hematocrit of 39% at Tanner stage 1 to 44% at Tanner stage 5. Similar differences do not occur in girls, who may experience a decrease in hemoglobin or hematocrit levels during adolescence if the onset of menstruation includes prolonged or heavy periods. Research reveals that black adolescents have hematocrit values 1% to 3% lower than those of their white counterparts.

IMMUNOGLOBULIN VALUES. The range of normal values for immunoglobulins of all classes increases from the childhood to adults years because of the increasing load of antibodies developed over time. These differences, also noted during the adolescent years, seldom have clinical significance because of the notable overlap in values for all age groups.

ESTROGEN AND TESTOSTERONE LEVELS. Increasing levels of estrogen in girls and testosterone in boys are hallmarks of the hormonal changes that occur during adolescence, but smaller increases of each also take place in the other sex. These natural increases may have clinical implications in the development of gynecomastia in males and hirsutism in females.

LUTEINIZING AND FOLLICLE-STIMULATING HORMONE LEVELS. Increases in luteinizing and follicle-stimulating hormone mark the onset of puberty in both boys and girls. Evaluation of these levels forms an important part of the testing required for those with pubertal abnormalities.

THYROID HORMONE LEVELS. Although thyroid hormone levels do not change during the adolescent years, pregnant teenagers or those taking oral contraceptives have elevated total thyroid hormone levels because of increases in thyroid-binding globulin. The free thyroxine index should be measured to confirm elevations in such patients.

Office Laboratory Tests

Specific psychological and social issues must be considered in the provision of health care to adolescent patients. Performances of laboratory testing is no exception. Because many adolescents are afraid of needles and may not understand the need for them, and since physical or psychological coercion is generally impossible, it is often necessary to employ a patient but firm approach when drawing blood from teenagers. Confidential healthcare issues often necessitate arrangements of alternative payment options for the teenager who needs a Pap smear, a pregnancy test, or testing for STD. Many routine laboratory tests are now available as rapid, office-based tests. Testing for pregnancy, *Chlamydia*, mononucleosis, strep throat, and anemia may be offered in the office setting without involving an outside laboratory. Advantages include both rapidity of diagnosis, which fits well with the "do-it-now" time frame within which many adolescents function, and avoidance of the large bills often generated by outside laboratories. However, interpretation of these tests and further decision making must be handled with great care, since the sensitivity and specificity of these tests may not be as satisfactory as desired in all cases. Attention to details such as these often distinguishes the successful management of medical concerns in the teenage patient.

References

1. Marks A, Fisher M: Health assessment and screening during adolescence, *Pediatrics* 80:133-158, 1987.

2. Cromer BA, McLean CS, Heald FP: A critical review of comprehensive health screening in adolescents, *J Adolesc Health* 13:1S-65S, 1992.

3. Committee on Psychosocial Aspects of Child and Family Health: *Guidelines for health supervision, II.* Elk Grove Village, IL, 1985-1988, American Academy of Pediatrics.

4. American Medical Association: *Department of Adolescent Health: Guidelines for adolescent preventive services (GAPS),* Chicago, 1992, AMA.

5. Green M, editor: *Bright futures: guidelines for health supervision of infants, children, and adolescents,* Arlington, VA, 1994, National Center for Education in Maternal and Child Health.

6. Moyer VA, Grimes RM: Total and differential leukocyte counts in clinically well children, *Am J Dis Child* 144:1200-1203, 1990.

7. Arden MR, Budow L, Bunnell DW, et al: Alkaline urine is associated with eating disorders (letter), *Am J Dis Child* 145:28-30, 1991.

8. Jenkins RR, Saxena SB: Keeping adolescents healthy, *Contemp Pediatr* 12:76-90, 1995.

9. National Cholesterol Education Program: Highlights of the Report of the Expert Panel on Blood Cholesterol Levels in Children and Adolescents, *Pediatrics* 89:495-501, 1992.

10. Mason WH: Measles, *Adolesc Med: State of Art Rev* 6:1-14, 1995.

11. Ross LA: Rubella, *Adolesc Med: State of Art Rev* 6:15-26, 1995.

12. Committee on Infectious Diseases, American Academy of Pediatrics: Recommendation for the use of live attenuated varicella vaccine, *Pediatrics* 95:791-796, 1995.

13. Centers for Disease Control: Hepatitis B virus: a comprehensive strategy for eliminating transmission in the United States through universal childhood vaccination: recommendations of the Immunization Practices Advisory Committee (ACIP), *MMWR* 40:1-25, 1991.

14. American Thoracic Society: Diagnostic standards and classification of tuberculosis, *Am Rev Respit Dis* 142:725-735, 1990.

15. American Academy of Pediatrics: *Report of the Committee on Infectious Diseases,* Elk Grove Village, IL, 1994, American Academy of Pediatrics.

16. Starke JR: The tuberculin skin test, *Pediatr Ann* 22:612-620, 1993.

17. Roye CF: Abnormal cervical cytology in adolescents: a literature review, *J Adolesc Health* 13:643-650, 1992.

18. Committee on Adolescence, American Academy of Pediatrics: Sexually transmitted diseases, *Pediatrics* 94:568-572, 1994.

19. Shafer M, Schachter J, Moncada J, et al: Evaluation of urine-based screening strategies to detect *Chlamydia trachomatis* among sexually active asymptomatic young males, *JAMA* 270:2065-2070, 1993.

20. Melvin SY: Syphilis: resurgence of an old disease, *Prim Care* 17:47-57, 1990.

21. Bidwell RJ, Deisher RW: Adolescent sexuality: current issues, *Pediatr Ann* 20:293-302, 1991.

22. Woolf AD, Shannon MW: Clinical toxicology for the pediatrician, *Pediatr Clin North Am* 42:317-333, 1995.

23. Schwartz RH: Testing for drugs of abuse: controversies and techniques, *Adolesc Med: State of Art Rev* 4:353-370, 1993.

24. Nelson MA: Medical exclusion from participation in sports, *Pediatr Ann* 21:149-155, 1992.

25. Committee on Sports Medicine and Fitness, American Academy of Pediatrics: Medical conditions affecting sports participation, *Pediatrics* 94:757-760, 1994.

26. Stewart DJ: Screening tests before surgery in children, *Can J Anaesth* 38:693-695, 1991.

27. Lawrence VA, Gafni A, Gross M: The unproven utility of the preoperative urinalysis: economic evaluation, *J Clin Epidemiol* 12:1185-1192, 1989.

28. Roy WZ, Lerman J, McIntyre BG: Is preoperative haemoglobin testing justified in children undergoing minor elective surgery? *Can J Anaesth* 38:700-703, 1991.

29. Tietz NW, editor: *Clinical guide to laboratory tests,* Philadelphia, 1983, WB Saunders.

30. Wallach J: *Interpretation of diagnostic tests: a synopsis of laboratory medicine,* Boston, 1986, Little, Brown.

CHAPTER 15

Psychosocial Intervention

•

Sheridan Phillips

During the course of managing an adolescent's health care, the physician may weigh the advisability of psychosocial intervention. The specific psychosocial issue could be directly related to the adolescent's health status, could be interacting with physiologic factors, or could be relatively unrelated to the adolescent's current physical state. Examples include suicidal ideation, abdominal pain symptomatic of anxiety, noncompliance with a diabetic regimen, high level of conflict with parents or peers, and difficulty with adolescent transitions. The degree of concern about such issues varies; psychosocial intervention may be essential in some instances but not urgent in others.

When considering a psychosocial referral, the physician may be unsure of the therapeutic options available and the nature of the treatment. This uncertainty hampers efforts to make an appropriate and timely referral and provide information to the adolescent and parents. It also makes the physician reluctant to recommend psychosocial treatment for less severe problems. This chapter describes the most common forms of psychosocial interventions, with emphasis on those most frequently used with adolescents; it briefly reviews their efficacy and suggests ways to make the most successful referrals. With this information, the physician can become more comfortable in making referrals in general and be more inclined to make them in marginal instances, when psychosocial intervention may not be essential but could be of substantial assistance.

The many options for intervention reflect the differences in therapists' theoretical orientations and the various modalities of treatment (e.g., family therapy or individual therapy), as shown in Table 15-1. Each theoretical orientation is presented as separate and distinct, but it is important to emphasize that these are artificial divisions. In practice, therapists commonly use

a combination of approaches, depending on individual needs. Although not discussed here, medication is also appropriately used in conjunction with psychosocial intervention for optimal treatment of disorders such as attention-deficit hyperactivity disorder (ADHD) and severe anxiety.

PSYCHODYNAMIC THERAPY

In relation to psychotherapy, the term *dynamic* refers to the concept of force.[1] In the personality theory posited by Sigmund Freud, personality is a system of forces in conflict with one another, which results in the emotions and behavior—both adaptive and pathologic—that constitute personality. These conflicting forces exist at different levels of awareness; however, the concept of unconscious conflict is central to the model. Thus, an individual's "psychodynamics" refers to his or her conflicting conscious and unconscious forces, motives, and fears.

Psychodynamic therapy encompasses a number of approaches, all based on Freud's fundamental assumptions. His daughter Anna Freud, Melanie Klein, and a number of child analysts adapted Freud's theories for the treatment of children.[2-4] This treatment focuses on identifying and resolving underlying conflicts among the adolescent's instinctual urges (id), conscious regulation or reality orientation (ego), and "conscience" or self-evaluative thoughts (superego). If these conflicts are resolved, it is assumed that the adolescent's behavioral disturbances will also resolve.

The psychodynamic therapist must first develop a rapport with the child or adolescent. In this climate the patient may freely verbalize thoughts and feelings, which some therapists feel is inherently therapeutic. For young

TABLE 15-1
Overview of Therapeutic Orientations and Modalities Commonly Employed for Intervention With Adolescents

	Modality				
Orientation	Individual	Parents and Adolescent	Family	Group	Residential
Psychodynamic/analytic	X	Adapted		Adapted	Adapted
Behavioral	X	X	X	X	X
Phenomenologic/humanistic					
Client centered	X			X	
Gestalt	X			X	
Systems		X	X		
Eclectic	X	X	X	X	X

Modified from Hoekelman RA, Friedman SB, Nelson NM, Seidel HM, Weitzman ML, editors: *Primary pediatric care,* ed 3, St Louis, 1997, Mosby–Year Book, p 762.
Xs refer to common therapeutic approaches. "Adapted" refers to a modified form of treatment.

children, most therapists use a playroom setting. The therapist interprets the symbolic meanings revealed in the child's fantasies, dreams, or free play. However, this analytic approach is usually not appropriate for adolescents. Adolescents are generally too old for play therapy and too young for traditional psychoanalytic techniques, such as free association or dream interpretation.

Traditional psychodynamic therapy involves an exclusive patient-therapist dynamic. Anna Freud advocated educating parents about their child's problems, but many therapists consider it inappropriate to incorporate other family members in the therapeutic process. The family of an adolescent who is in psychodynamic therapy may thus have several therapists to avoid transference problems and competition for the therapist's attention. There are clear difficulties inherent in this approach, such as poor coordination of therapeutic strategies and lack of communication with parents. This has prompted some therapists to see the family together or to meet separately with the parents. A group therapy approach has also been used to maximize therapy time and allow adolescents to interact and share experiences with peers. Group activities may include games or arts and crafts that are controlled indirectly by the therapist. With older teenagers, psychodrama and various talk techniques may be employed. Groups may be homogeneous (e.g., victims of sexual abuse) or heterogeneous (both aggressive and withdrawn patients). Residential treatment settings based on this model feature an open and tolerant atmosphere with extensive use of expressive materials such as paint and clay.

Traditional analysis requires four or five sessions a week for 3 to 5 years, which makes it expensive and restricts its application. Thus, shorter-term forms of psychotherapeutic intervention have evolved that typically employ fewer sessions for 2 to 3 years with the more limited goals of increasing capacity for reality testing,

strengthening object relations, and alleviating fixations. Even modified analytic treatment, however, is most appropriate for patients who have many assets and are only moderately disturbed. Some features of analytic therapy have been incorporated in other approaches.

BEHAVIOR THERAPY

Behavior therapy uses empirical methods to identify and alter behavior.[5,6] The therapist gains an understanding of the nature of the problem by observing behavior and determining the patient's responses to triggering events. The therapist looks at the problem in the context of the patient's history, identifies variables that control the problem behavior, and then develops a hypothesis from the functional analysis of the data to serve as a guide during therapy. Data collection is central to testing the working hypothesis and judging the success of treatment. The patient is often involved in monitoring his or her reactions and responses and in planning the course of treatment.

Initially, behavioral analysis used a stimulus-response approach, with the aim of finding the stimuli that provoked a specific reaction. This early model evolved to include the patient's perception of the stimulus and the consequences of the response. In the mid-1970s, behavior therapists began to emphasize the importance of cognition as well as overt behavior (cognitive-behavior therapy). The behavior therapist thus attends to such issues as patients' expectations of themselves and others, how events are labeled, and the nature of self-statements.

Basic research in cognitive and developmental psychology provides a problem-solving framework that has been increasingly employed for interventions emphasizing the cognitive processes that underlie social behavior (e.g., generating and testing alternative solutions). For example, Kendall and Braswell[7] developed and evaluated interventions that focus on altering the ways in which impulsive children think about and work through academic and social problems. Robin and Foster[8] conducted a series of studies demonstrating the efficacy of a problem-solving model for negotiating parent-adolescent conflict, and Spivack and Shure[9] reported success with an interpersonal cognitive problem-solving skills program involving a variety of ages and problems. As attitudinal and perceptual processes were better understood and therapy was directed toward their modification, behavior therapy moved closer to other therapeutic approaches such as ego psychology.[10]

Behavior therapists base therapeutic interventions on the principles and models of experimental psychology: classic and operant conditioning, observational-social learning or modeling, information processing, problem solving, and development of self-control derived from learning theory. The process of attitude change from social psychology was also incorporated. The underlying theory for behavior therapy is social learning theory, in which normal and abnormal behaviors are considered to be on a continuum. It assumes that maladaptive behaviors and normal behavior are acquired through similar processes. The use of adaptive behavior should thus alter patients' self-perception and the way others perceive and react to them. According to Bandura's "self-efficacy" theory,[11] successful therapy results from a variety of interventions that, over time, gradually convince the patient of his or her ability to cope effectively. In cognitive-behavioral interventions, the same empirical approach used to modify overt behavior is used to identify and alter covert behaviors (cognitions) such as irrational beliefs.

The behavioral approach is characterized by interventions specific to an individual patient's needs. Therapy therefore varies for different patients. Standardized treatment "packages," developed primarily for research and demonstration purposes, have been adapted for individual therapy. The actual treatment plan is derived from the functional analysis or behavioral formulation of the problem. For example, one goal of assessment is to determine whether the patient lacks appropriate skills (a behavioral deficit) or whether these skills have been learned but are evidenced in only some circumstances (an inhibition). In the former case, therapy would focus on skill acquisition; in the latter, interventions would be directed toward reducing the inhibition.

The behavior therapist draws from a variety of techniques, ranging from parent training and contingency contracting (typically within a problem-solving/negotiation framework) to relaxation training and desensitization (generally used for specific fears and phobias). Treatment often includes several components. For example, problem-solving skill training would focus on how the adolescent (and/or parents) approaches situations, teaching a step-by-step approach to solving problems through the use of structured tasks (e.g., games, academic activities, and stories), modeling and role playing with the therapist, and applying skills to real-life situations.[8] Similarly, anger control would focus on identifying and changing irrational beliefs and expectations, teaching the patient to detect physical arousal that signals the build-up of anger, generating alternative responses, and implementing these in a variety of anger-producing situations.[12]

Some commonalities exist, regardless of the specific problem. The focus is primarily on the present. Concrete goals are jointly defined and planned to be accomplished in a relatively short time frame; both therapist and patient assess the progress. Therapy is active and includes homework assignments. It is assumed that insight alone does not bring about a satisfactory behavioral change but that gradual learning and new behavioral constructs are the ingredients necessary for change. Because of the interpersonal nature of the therapy, practitioner characteristics are also an important aspect of the therapeutic change. Goldfried and Davison[6] argue that a tough-minded approach to conceptualizing problems does not interfere with a close patient-therapist relationship.

Behavior therapy was initially used with psychotic, retarded, and autistic patients and those with severe phobias. This approach is now used for many age groups with diverse problems. Psychotropic drugs may be used if necessary, but medication withdrawal is typically the eventual goal. Many nonclinical situations have also been subjected to behavioral analysis: for example, political action and change in public opinion. Self-help books[13,14] and video instructional programs[13-17] are other examples of its application to the general education field. It is also possible to examine the contingencies that exist in settings such as pediatric clinics or corporations to determine whether the extant contingencies promote or discourage desired behavior such as keeping appointments or increasing productivity. These efforts are generally considered behavior modification; behavior therapy is reserved for clinical problems.

Behavioral interventions have been widely used in the classroom.[2,4] Residential programs for juvenile delinquents have also been developed to provide an intensive treatment environment and gradual return of adolescents to their homes. In fact, it is now difficult to find residential programs for emotionally disturbed and retarded children that do not make at least some use of behavioral principles. The first inpatient programs were developed to treat antisocial behavior, but intensive behavioral programs have now been designed to address many additional disorders such as substance abuse, anorexia, bulimia, depression, and suicide risk.[18] Most behavioral intervention, however, is conducted in outpatient settings.

In the early years of behavior therapy, treatment focused on conduct disorders and anxiety (fears and phobias). Over the past two decades, however, behavioral and cognitive-behavioral interventions have been applied to a wide variety of problems, ranging from panic disorder and obsessive-compulsive disorder to bulimia and insomnia.[19-23]

In pediatric and mental health settings, behavior therapy typically employs a combination of sessions with the adolescent and parent(s), both individually and together, and with key personnel in the school or other agencies when relevant. The extent to which treatment focuses on the teenager versus the family reflects the nature of the presenting problems. With multiple problems, the therapist may alternate family sessions (e.g., working on communication and problem solving) with individual sessions (e.g., addressing problems with peers). Sessions are scheduled once or twice a week and can continue for four sessions or as long as 2 years. Behavior therapy is also effective for groups of adolescents and/or their parents. This maximizes professional time and allows the patient an opportunity to interact with peers in a therapeutic setting (e.g., engage in role playing). Group therapy generally involves a relatively homogeneous group so that specific problems can be addressed. Group sessions usually do not extend beyond 6 months. Two therapists most often lead the group so that they can offer two models of behavior and model interaction with each other (e.g., a male and a female with a parent group).

PHENOMENOLOGIC THERAPIES

Phenomenologic or humanistic therapies share similarities with psychodynamic therapy, focusing on identifying inappropriate behaviors and altering the pattern by making the patient aware of his or her motivations and needs. Both are thus insight oriented and are based on a free therapeutic milieu, with the patient-therapist relationship being the primary vehicle for patient growth. Humanistic therapy, however, emphasizes free will and the patient's freedom of choice.

Client-Centered Therapy

In Carl Rogers' model the terminology is *client,* not *patient,* to avoid the stigma of "sickness." A subjective rather than an objective view of events is stressed so that perceptions and feelings can be explored by the client, who guides the therapeutic process.[3] The most fundamental concept in client-centered therapy is trust. Rogerians believe that the tendency to strive to actualize or to realize a person's potential is as much a human drive as the reduction of biologic tensions (e.g., hunger) and that this process can proceed unhampered within a trusting and nonjudgmental relationship with the therapist. Demonstrating trust that clients can set their own goals and monitor their progress toward achieving these goals has special meaning for the treatment of children and adolescents, who are often viewed as requiring detailed, constant guidance and/or supervision. In contrast, Rogerians assume that maximal development will occur when the client is not made to struggle for and be concerned about approval by others.

To establish a successful relationship, the therapist must display congruence or genuineness, an unconditional positive regard or warmth, and empathy. The therapist establishes a deeply human, genuine, and open relationship with the client but leaves the responsibility for change with the client. The therapist conveys warmth for and acceptance of the client and expresses confidence in the client's ability to change. Interpretations and value judgments are avoided by the therapist, who only paraphrases the client's views.

Although client-centered therapy was developed for adults, it has also been used with older adolescents and groups such as encounter groups. However, patients with severe pathologic conditions are not appropriate candidates for client-centered therapy. The typical course of intervention is one or two sessions a week for anywhere from a month to several years.

Gestalt Therapy

Gestalt therapy is a phenomenologic-existential therapy founded by Frederick (Fritz) and Laura Perls in the 1940s. As with client-centered therapy, the goal is to promote growth by increasing self-awareness, or insight. In Gestalt therapy, insight is a clear understanding of the situation being studied. Because awareness without systematic exploration is not sufficient to develop insight, Gestalt therapy uses focused awareness and experimentation to achieve insight. It is most easily distinguished from client-centered therapy by its treatment methods, which involve an active, directive therapist and often dramatic techniques. Gestalt therapy teaches therapists and patients the phenomenologic method of awareness, in which perceiving, feeling, and acting are distinguished from interpretation that reflects preexisting attitudes.[1] What is directly perceived and felt is considered more reliable than interpretations. Patients and therapists learn to *dialogue,* that is, communicate their phenomenologic perspectives. Differences in perspectives become the focus of experimentation and continued dialogue. The goal is for clients to become aware of what they are doing, how they are doing it, and how they can change themselves while learning to accept and value themselves. Gestalt therapy's focus is on the present and on process (what is happening) rather than on content (what is being discussed). The emphasis is on what is being done, thought, and felt at the moment rather than on what was, might be, could be, or should be. Language is an important element in getting the patient to take responsibility for his or her feelings. When patients say, "It's really aggravating to hear that," they might be asked to rephrase this as "I am angry with you for saying that to me." Some dramatic exercises help patients externalize conflicts and feelings. In one case a patient may confront an empty chair, imagining that his father is sitting there, and tell him the things he has been unable to say to him directly. In another situation in which a patient may not be able to decide whether to attend a local college and live at home or to go away to school, he may be asked to alternate sitting in two chairs. When sitting in one chair, he supposes that he is staying home and tells how he feels about it; in the other, he experiences the part of himself that wants to go away to college and reflects those feelings. Patients can thus sort out their emotional conflicts as the balance gradually shifts and one side predominates.

Gestalt therapy is generally used with adults and older adolescents who have mild or moderate disturbances. Individual treatment typically involves one or two sessions a week for a period of a few months to several years. Group sessions usually progress from intensive weekend meetings to an evening once a week for 6 months to a year, although some continue much longer.

SYSTEMS THERAPY

Systems therapy is a form of family therapy that views the family as a dynamic system, rather than a collection of individuals, that is maintained or changed by means of feedback, either positive or negative. Intervention attempts to modify the relationships within the family to achieve harmony. The relationships between and among family members are hypothesized to have developed in a specific manner to achieve homeostasis for that family. This relatively stable state may be periodically disrupted by external events, such as geographic relocation, or by change within the family, such as the birth of the first child or new siblings. This disruption triggers changes in the family members' relationships and the subsequent reemergence of a homeostatic state, which may be different from the previous one, in much the same manner that a mobile is affected by a gust of wind. Homeostasis may sometimes be achieved in ways that are not beneficial for all members, as when a "problem child" is distracting attention from an unhappy marriage.[24]

According to systems therapists, the child with behavior problems is the "identified patient," but the entire family must be treated as a unit. Conjoint family therapy is therefore conducted with all family members meeting together as a group, except for infants and toddlers. The therapist redefines the presenting problem as a disturbance in family process and/or poor communication.

Various systems proponents analyze the triangles created either within the nuclear family or within three generations; in either case they observe and seek to assist the family in the modification of maladaptive tactics for gaining closeness or distancing within the family structure.[1] One goal of therapy is to identify covert family "rules" that consistently produce the same maladaptive interactions. For example, a stepfather believes his marriage could be threatened by his stepdaughter who dislikes him. He is thus overly critical of her and encourages conflict between daughter and mother to diminish the daughter's influence with her mother. Through treatment the family members are assisted to develop appropriate communication, such as using direct messages; avoiding the use of a "double bind" (in which the individual receives simultaneous contradictory demands so that any action leads to at least partial failure); and minimizing "scapegoating" of the identified patient.

Minuchin's structural family therapy emphasizes family "sets" (hierarchy of family relations and alliances between members) as the target for change.[24,25] The specific focus of intervention reflects the initial family structure. For example, with an enmeshed, overinvolved family the therapist would attempt to strengthen the parental alliance, establish boundaries, and promote activities outside the family. The goal for a disengaged family would be to restructure appropriate alliances and reestablish the distanced member(s) within the family.

Systems therapy is appropriate for both children and adolescents. In some cases all family members attend; in others the parents may be seen alone for part of the treatment: for example, if marital conflict poses a treatment problem. Once-a-week sessions of 1 to 2 hours, supplemented by homework tasks, may continue for several months or several years.

A systems approach to treating families can be successfully combined with other approaches. For example, Robin and Foster have developed an integrated approach to negotiating parent-adolescent conflict that combines aspects of behavior therapy (behavioral contracting, reinforcement, modeling, skill training, and rehearsal), cognitive behavior therapy (addressing irrational beliefs and expectations), and systems therapy (placing intervention in the context of the family system).[8] This blending and integrating of approaches incorporates specific family-related concepts with an empirical approach to analyzing and altering maladaptive behaviors, both overt and covert.

ECLECTIC THERAPY

Eclecticism refers to a multimodal amalgam of therapeutic approaches rather than to a systematic, delineated theoretical model. Some therapists identify their orientation as eclectic, by which they mean that they meld a number of techniques from several therapeutic modalities. While most approaches have some common features, such as mutual respect for the other person, the need to alter the client's perceptions of self and/or the external world, and gradual reduction of conflict, many therapists find it necessary to borrow precepts and procedures other than those of their original training orientation. Thus, eclectic therapy may be viewed not so much as a school of thought but rather as the absence of an identified school.

Technical eclecticism involves the use of a specific theoretical framework to conceptualize the patient, the patient's problems, and attempts to change, while drawing on techniques from different theoretical orientations, depending on the needs of the patient. For example, a behavior therapist may be guided by the principles of social learning theory and yet employ Gestalt exercises to help overly intellectual patients identify emotional factors that influence their problem solving or decision making. Similarly, behavior therapists might use play materials or games with younger adolescents. These techniques, however, are carefully selected to fulfill a specific purpose that is part of an overall therapeutic strategy; in other words, they use them in their capacity as behavior therapists. In contrast, *theoretical eclecticism* eschews the guidance of any theoretical system. I believe that any theory is better than no theory, since successful therapy requires some purposeful stance on the part of the therapist.

THERAPEUTIC OUTCOME

Beginning in 1952, a series of startling reports suggested that traditional psychotherapy did not yield greater improvement than that which occurred from spontaneous remission in the absence of formal treatment, both for adult and child patients.[26,27] This not only fueled a search for different approaches to treatment but also stimulated interest in documenting the efficacy of psychosocial intervention. Ideally, such outcome research would determine what type of intervention is most effective for a particular disorder evidenced by a child of a specific age and sex. Unfortunately, the field has not yet progressed to this point, especially with regard to adolescents, for several reasons.

First, there have been fewer formal evaluations of psychotherapy with adolescents than with either adults or children. There is no inherent reason for this phenomenon; it merely parallels the general state of knowledge with regard to psychological functions. For both normal and abnormal behavior, the greatest amount of information is typically available for adults, with considerably less for children and even less for adolescents.

Second, the overwhelming majority of outcome research has focused on behavioral and cognitive-behavioral interventions, with relatively little evaluation available regarding humanistic, psychodynamic, family/systems, or eclectic approaches. At least in part, this reflects the attitudes of individuals who are attracted to different theoretical orientations. For example, behavior therapists view treatment as a hypothetical-deductive process that follows scientific principles and thus is entirely amenable to study, whereas many analysts view therapy as an art rather than a science, and are thus relatively disinterested in research.

Third, conducting good outcome research is an extraordinary challenge involving numerous and varied obstacles. Some of these are theoretical. For example, how does one measure or study the "unconscious," which is by definition inaccessible? Some obstacles are conceptual: when goals for therapy are different, how can one determine an acceptable criterion for the "success" of treatment? Similarly, how can comparable outcome measures be developed? Methodologic issues abound, such as determining "success" rates on the basis of the number of patients who began treatment versus the number who completed therapy. Other issues are practical ones, such as ensuring comparable levels of skill and therapist characteristics across different treatment conditions: one can use "switch hitters" who are likely to be differentially skilled in different types of therapy, or one can use a design that confounds individual therapists and therapeutic approaches. Even more basic is the issue of therapeutic integrity: in a large treatment study of antisocial youths 8 to 17 years old,[28] Kazdin[26] observed that 35% of the group therapists in the behavior-modification treatment condition did not implement the behavioral procedures appropriately; only 25% of the group leaders in the social work treatment condition carried out the intervention appropriately, and 44% of the minimal-treatment leaders carried out systematic interventions even though none were supposed to. Under such circumstances the relative efficacy of different treatments is difficult to assess. Finally, it is important to consider the ethical problems occasioned by withholding treatment from a control group or by providing only minimal treatment; since appropriate assessment of outcome should include posttreatment data, treatment for control group patients could be delayed as long as 1.5 to 2 years.

Given the degree of difficulty inherent in outcome research, few studies have systematically compared and evaluated different therapeutic approaches and different presenting problems. In general, the available data indicate that psychotherapy is more effective with adolescents than no treatment and that behavioral and cognitive-behavioral approaches yield treatment effects equal to or greater than those found for nonbehavioral interventions.[29] Consistent effects have also been found for therapist characteristics (e.g., level of training and experience) and the nature of the disorder (e.g., neurotic disorders being more amenable to intervention than conduct disorders).[26,27]

More data are available from research that has focused on a specific problem or disorder and evaluates only one therapeutic approach (or treatment package) together with appropriate control and/or comparison groups. For example, one treatment package that combines problem solving (a cognitive-behavioral approach) and systems therapy has been well documented as an effective intervention for parent-adolescent conflict.[8] The efficacy of behavioral and cognitive-behavioral treatment has been empirically demonstrated for such disparate problems as conduct disorders,[30] depression,[31] panic disorder, obsessive-compulsive disorder, substance abuse, anorexia, bulimia, and insomnia.[19-23] Ultimately, such focused but programmatic research may yield more useful data regarding clinical efficacy than the massive, multivariable outcome study.

SUCCESSFUL REFERRALS

The attempt to refer an adolescent or family sometimes ends in failure even when psychosocial intervention is clearly indicated. Such failures typically occur at two points in the referral process: (1) at the outset, when the adolescent or parents deny that the problem exists or that they need assistance in resolving it; or (2) when, while apparently accepting the recommendation, the adolescent somehow never manages to appear in the therapist's office.

Clinical experience suggests that the probability of a successful referral is increased by eliminating the need for the adolescent to leave the clinical setting that is familiar and comfortable to obtain psychosocial treatment. This can be accomplished by including a mental health specialist on the staff of a general adolescent medicine clinic or as a member of a group practice. The presence of a full-time mental health expert has multiple advantages. First, this conveys the message that psychosocial intervention is clearly part of comprehensive health care rather than being "outside" or something quite different from medical care; it also indicates that such referrals are common rather than being recommended only rarely for

"abnormal" cases. In addition, the fact that this individual is in partnership with the physician implies that he or she is well regarded and respected by the physician. Second, it is easy and natural for the primary health care provider to introduce the adolescent to the therapist personally; even very brief interaction seems to have considerable influence on the adolescent's and parents' willingness to make and keep that first crucial appointment. Physical proximity has other advantages, facilitating coordination and integration of care. Not only is it easy to communicate verbally, but sharing the same patient record guarantees that the physician's notes and findings are immediately accessible to the psychotherapist, and vice versa. Finally, frequent and ongoing interaction with this psychotherapist enables the physician to become very familiar with the therapist's style and level of competence, which hopefully will increase physicians' confidence in the therapist and thereby increase their readiness to refer adolescents for therapy.

The availability of a practice-based mental health specialist can assist with issues other than mental health referrals. This individual can provide consultation regarding how to increase compliance with medical appointments, compliance with treatment regimens, and the efficacy of prevention efforts (e.g., contraception).[32] It has been shown that greater physician knowledge of strategies to increase compliance can significantly improve patient compliance,[33] and the presence of a behavioral specialist can facilitate this process.

In most practice settings it is feasible to include a mental health specialist who can typically generate more than sufficient revenue to cover his or her salary after some 6 months in practice. In fact, many group practices that have done so have added a second individual after 1 or 2 years of experience with the first mental health care provider. In some settings, however, it is not feasible to include a full-time therapist, such as in areas with sparse mental health resources or in solo practices with relatively low patient volume. In such cases one might consider recruiting a therapist who could work on site several days a week. If even that is impossible, it would still be advisable for the therapist to come to the practice site to meet the adolescent and parents and to conduct the first session with them in the primary practice setting.

Even with a full-time therapist on site, it may be necessary to have access to other resources, since even a well-trained individual cannot provide every possible mental health service at a high level of competence. The external specialist should be an individual who can both assess and treat the problem to reduce the number of transitions for the adolescent. As noted earlier, a personal introduction should be arranged.

Discussion thus far has focused primarily on reducing referral failures that occur in transition (for additional details, see Phillips et al[34]). With regard to "resistance" problems, when the adolescent or parents deny the need for psychosocial intervention, the physician should "normalize" the situation. It is interesting that reluctance to use professional assistance is not evident in most other areas of life. Plumbers, accountants, dentists, and lawyers are employed routinely without extensive soul searching. In contrast, even mild deficiencies in interpersonal or parenting skills are often viewed as evidence of personal abnormality. It can be useful to adopt a behavioral/ learning view of personality, noting that one is not born with such skills, that all skills in life are acquired quasi-randomly, and that most individuals possess a collection of stronger and weaker skills in different areas.

Group intervention that focuses on "normal" parenting problems or "normal" issues for adolescents is more likely to appeal to resistant parents and adolescents than is individual intervention. Although the physician must remain firm in instances when he believes that intensive individual intervention is required immediately, resistance in less urgent cases can be lessened by recommending participation in groups for normal teenage problems or targeted groups such as Alateen for children of alcoholic parents.

Group intervention that includes normal adolescents can be highly therapeutic. In fact, one large-scale study that evaluated various interventions for antisocial youths reported the greatest improvement for those treated in mixed groups, which included both referred and nonreferred (normal) adolescents.[28] The advantage of such a mixture is the availability of several models to enable adolescents to learn from one another. Participants also learn that all adolescents have some kind of problem, which makes it less threatening to acknowledge their own.

The other major advantage of group intervention is increased familiarity with the therapist/group leader. As adolescents and parents come to believe that this individual can truly assist them, they become increasingly willing to consider individual treatment. In fact, it is common for the group therapist to be asked if he or she would be willing to see the adolescent and/or parents for additional work; cases often evolve from group to individual or from individual to family to marital therapy.

The multiple advantages of group intervention emphasize the utility of incorporating a mental health specialist in the practice setting. This individual can provide consultation and individual or family therapy and can also conduct a variety of focused groups. Some pediatric practices include group activities as a routine component of health care (e.g., for new mothers).

In summary, compliance with the recommendation for psychosocial intervention can be enhanced by increasing acceptance of intervention and by reducing the difficulty of making the transition to another health care provider.

Resistance can be addressed via several tactics to "normalize" such intervention, and transitions are facilitated by ensuring personal contact with the new provider. Both strategies are best accomplished by formally incorporating mental health as a component of comprehensive health care.

References

1. Corsini RJ, Wedding D: *Current psychotherapies,* ed 4, Itasca, IL, 1989, Peacock Publishers.
2. Gelfand DM, Jenson WR, Drew CJ: *Understanding child behavior disorders,* ed 2, New York, 1988, Holt, Rinehart & Winston.
3. Achenbach TM: *Developmental psychopathology,* ed 2, New York, 1982, John Wiley.
4. Quay HD, Werry JS: *Psychopathological disorders of childhood,* ed 3, New York, 1986, John Wiley.
5. Davison GC, Neal JM: *Abnormal psychology: an experimental clinical approach,* ed 4, New York, 1986, John Wiley.
6. Goldfried MR, Davison GC: *Clinical behavior therapy,* New York, 1976, Holt, Rinehart & Winston.
7. Kendall PC, Braswell L: *Cognitive-behavioral therapy for impulsive children,* New York, 1985, Guilford Press.
8. Robin A, Foster SL: *Negotiating parent-adolescent conflict: a behavioral-family systems approach,* New York, 1989, Guilford Press.
9. Spivack G, Shure MB: The cognition of social adjustment: interpersonal cognitive problem solving thinking, *Adv Clin Child Psychol* 5:323, 1982.
10. Garfield S, Bergin AE: *Handbook of psychotherapy and behavioral change,* New York, 1986, John Wiley.
11. Bandura A: Reflections on self-efficacy. In Franks CM, Wilson GT, editors: *Annual review of behavior therapy: theory and practice,* vol 7, New York, 1979, Brunner-Mazel.
12. Feindler EL, Ecton RB: *Adolescent anger control: cognitive-behavioral techniques,* Des Moines, 1986, Allyn & Bacon.
13. Brigham TM: *Self-management for adolescents,* New York, 1989, Guilford Press.
14. Brigham TM: *Managing everyday problems,* New York, 1989, Guilford Press.
15. Cisek J, George A: *Why is it always me?* Champaign, IL, 1991, Research Press.
16. Cisek J, George A: *The bizarre trial of the pressured peer,* Champaign, IL, 1986, Research Press.
17. Wagonseller BR: *The practical parenting series: adolescence,* Champaign, IL, 1986, Research Press.
18. Van Hasselt VB, Kolko DJ: *Inpatient behavior therapy for children and adolescents,* New York, 1992, Plenum.
19. Beck JG, Zebb BJ: Behavioral assessment and treatment of panic disorder: current status, future directions, *Behav Ther* 25:581-611, 1994.
20. Mattick RP, Andrews G, Hadzi-Pavlovic D, Christensen H: Treatment of panic and agoraphobia: an integrative review, *J Nerv Ment Dis* 178:567-576, 1990.
21. Steketee G: Behavioral assessment and treatment planning with obsessive compulsive disorder: a review emphasizing clinical application, *Behav Ther* 25:613-633, 1994.
22. Smith DE, Marcus MD, Eldredge KL: Binge eating syndromes: a review of assessment and treatment with an emphasis on clinical application, *Behav Ther* 25:635-658, 1994.
23. Lichstein KL, Riedel BW: Behavioral assessment and treatment of insomnia: a review with an emphasis on clinical application, *Behav Ther* 25:659-688, 1994.
24. Zuk G: *Family therapy: a triadic-based approach,* New York, 1981, Behavioral Books.

25. Bernstein DA, Nietzel MT: *Introduction to clinical psychology,* New York, 1980, McGraw-Hill.
26. Kazdin AE: Psychotherapy for children and adolescents, *Annu Rev Psychol* 41:21, 1990.
27. Phillips S, Weist MD: Options for psychosocial intervention with children and adolescents. In Hoekelman RA, Friedman SB, Nelson NM, Seidel HM, Weitzman ML, editors: *Primary pediatric care,* ed 3, St. Louis, 1997, Mosby–Year Book.
28. Feldman RA, Caplinger TE, Wodarski JS: *The St Louis conundrum: the effective treatment of antisocial youths,* Englewood Cliffs, NJ, 1983, Prentice Hall.
29. Weisz JR, Weiss B, Alicke MD: Effectiveness of psychotherapy with children and adolescents: a meta-analysis for clinicians, *J Consult Clin Psychol* 55:542-549, 1987.
30. Wilson GT, Franks CM, Kendall PC, Foreyt JP: *Review of behavior therapy: theory and practice,* vol 11, New York, 1987, Guildford Press.
31. Wilkes TCR, Belsher G, Rush AJ, Frank E: *Cognitive therapy for depressed adolescents* New York, 1994, Guilford Press.
32. Phillips S: Compliance with medical regimens. In Noshpitz JD, et al editors: *Handbook of child and adolescent psychiatry,* New York, 1997, Basic Books.
33. Maiman LA, Becker MH, Liptak GS, Nazarian LF: Improving pediatricians' compliance-enhancing practices: a randomized trial, New York, *Am J Dis Child* 142:773-779, 1988.
34. Phillips S, Sarles RM, Friedman SB: Consultation and referral. In Hoekelman RA, Friedman SB, Nelson NM, Seidel HM, Weitzman ML, editors: *Primary pediatric care,* ed 3, St Louis, 1997, Mosby–Year Book.

Suggested Readings

Goldfried MR, Davison GC: *Clinical behavior therapy,* New York, 1976, Holt, Rinehart & Winston.
    A short classic that briefly highlights the history, theoretical assumptions, and procedures of behavior therapy, illustrated by clinical vignettes and transcripts. A clearly written and very readable contribution by clinical "masters," it promotes understanding of the actual clinical process, which is often absent in scientific reports.

Kazdin AE: Psychotherapy for children and adolescents, *Annu Rev Psychol* 41:21, 1990.
    A review of strategies taken to assess the efficacy of psychotherapy, findings of major studies, and discussion of methodologic issues relevant to outcome research; excellent discussion for the sophisticated reader.

Martin G, Pear J: *Behavior modification: what it is and how to do it,* ed 3, Englewood Cliffs, NJ, 1988, Prentice Hall.
    A practical, detailed guide for the novice.

Phillips S: Therapeutic approaches for behavior problems in childhood and adolescence. In Hoekelman RA, Blatman S, Friedman SB, Nelson NM, Seidel HM, Weitzman ML, editors: *Primary pediatric care,* ed 3, St Louis, 1997, Mosby–Year Book.
    Intended for the pediatrician and other professionals relatively unfamiliar with psychotherapy; discusses evaluation of the efficacy and challenges of outcome research; major approaches to psychosocial intervention, including efficacy; and indications for the use of alternative forms of intervention.

Phillips S, Sarles RM, Friedman SB, Boggs JE: Consultation and referral for behavioral and developmental problems. In Hoekelman RA, Blatman S, Friedman SB, Nelson NM, Seidel HM, Weitzman ML, editors: *Primary pediatric care,* ed 3, St Louis, 1997, Mosby–Year Book.
    Written for the pediatrician and other non–mental health professionals; discusses the process of consultation and referral in inpatient and ambulatory settings and recommends strategies for increasing the efficacy of referrals. Discusses selection of a consultant, including a description of training experiences for different disciplines providing mental health services.

CHAPTER 16

Pharmacologic Considerations

•

Audrey Rogers

The pharmacologic management of adolescents frequently presents a major challenge. The successful clinician employs knowledge from multiple disciplines, since psychosocial developmental theory, pathophysiology, behavioral theory, psychology, and developmental pharmacology all apply (Fig. 16-1).

This chapter presents specific principles of pharmacologic intervention that a clinician should consider in instituting or monitoring drug therapy in an adolescent. The objective of any therapeutic intervention is to maximize drug efficacy while minimizing associated toxicity. Achieving the goal of producing the desired

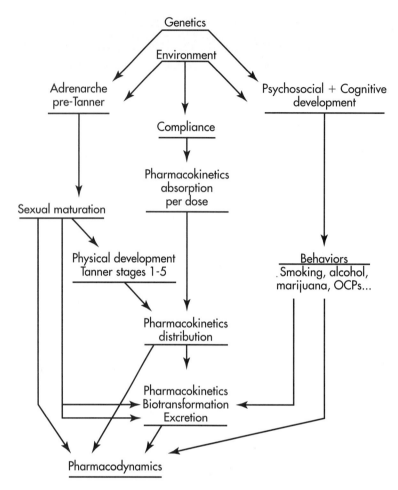

Fig. 16-1. Model for the study of drug effect in adolescents, showing the influence and interaction of genetic, environmental, physical, psychosocial, and behavioral factors to be considered in the monitoring of drug effect in adolescents. *OCPs,* oral contraceptive pills. (Reprinted by permission of Elsevier Science Inc. from "A Research Agenda for the Study of Therapeutic Agents in Adolescents" by Audrey Smith Rogers, JOURNAL OF ADOLESCENT HEALTH, Vol. No. 15 p. 673. Copyright 1994 by the Society for Adolescent Medicine.)

pharmacologic effect with minimal adverse consequences requires both devising a scientifically sound method for objectively and systematically evaluating drug effect and carefully crafting an acceptable regimen in collaboration with the patient.

DESIGNING THE DRUG REGIMEN

All who drink of this remedy recover in a short time, except those whom it does not help: who all die. Therefore, it is obvious that it fails only in incurable cases. Galen (ca. 200 CE)

For most drugs the ability to measure drug concentration in body fluids, relate these levels to drug effect, and titrate dosage to modulate response have provided the capacity for rational drug therapy. However, there is immense variability in human systems; individualization of therapy requires the identification of sources of variability in drug response, the quantification of their impact on drug response, and the modification of drug dose or schedule to compensate for these effects.[1]

Sources of variability in drug response can be divided into two broad categories: those attributed to the therapeutic agent itself and those attributable to the individual for whom the therapy is intended. For the former, factors such as molecular size and shape, solubility at site of absorption, degree of ionization, and relative lipid solubility of the drug's ionized and nonionized forms are critically important for the drug's movement into and out of the systemic circulation. This movement involves passage across cell membranes that are endowed with high electric resistance and relative impermeability to highly polar molecules.[2] Considerable regulatory attention has been focused on identifying the variability and standardization of agents. Data on rates of tablet dissolution, bioavailability, and both bioequivalence and therapeutic equivalence are expected as part of new drug applications.[3] Clinically important information on these

TABLE 16-1
Sources of Variability in Drug Response and Toxicity Profile Attributable to Individual Characteristics

Biologically Endowed	Behaviorally Related	Environmentally Induced
Physical		
Age, gender, Tanner stage, cardiovascular function, gastrointestinal function, immunologic function, hepatic function, renal function, albumin concentration	Exercise, dietary factors, stress, alcohol intake, tobacco or marijuana smoking, starvation	Occupational exposures, other drugs, sunlight, barometric pressure, circadian and seasonal variations
Acquired		
Pregnancy, lactation, disease, infection, immunization		
Pharmacogenetic		
Defects in metabolism of drugs: Slow inactivation of isoniazid, succinylcholine sensitivity, deficient parahydroxylation of phenytoin, bishydroxycoumarin sensitivity, phenacetin-induced methemoglobinemia, deficient *N*-glucosidation of amobarbital, impaired drug oxidation (debrisoquine, nortriptyline, codeine) Altered receptor sites: Warfarin resistance, glucose-6-phosphate dehydrogenase deficiency		

Modified after Vesel E: Pharmacogenetics. In Yaffe S, Aranda J, editors: *Pediatric pharmacology: therapeutic principles in practice,* ed 2, Philadelphia, 1992, WB Saunders, pp 29-44.

factors is therefore available, appearing in the drug labeling for the agent. Recently, however, the drug development, medical, and regulatory science communities have been urged to include the evaluation of human heterogeneity as a means of defining the remaining variation in drug action and potential injury in individuals before the marketing of new drug products.[4] The evaluation of variability induced by the endocrine changes of puberty should be included in this charge.[5]

Sources of variability in drug response and toxicity profile attributable to individual characteristics are listed in Table 16-1. Since all these sources of human heterogeneity in drug response have the potential to influence and alter drug response in various ways, it is important for the clinician to carefully assess their impact.

Clinical Pharmacology

Selected concepts employed in clinical pharmacology are defined in Table 16-2. A full discussion of adolescent-specific pharmacodynamics is beyond the scope of this chapter; nevertheless, it is important to note that the effects of puberty-associated endocrine modifications on receptor sensitivities in certain organ systems have not been systematically evaluated and may be of clinical relevance. For example, a sexual dimorphism in insulin sensitivity in insulin-dependent adolescents with diabetes mellitus has been attributed to sex-related differences in growth hormone; the action of insulin was reduced in adolescent girls compared with adolescent boys.[9] Adolescence is a period of sexual maturation, and reported gender differences in drug response may become apparent in youths for the first time as maturation progresses; differences have been reported for general and local anesthetics, salicylates, imipramine, diazepam, and phenothiazines.[10,11] Certainly, the focus of this chapter on the demonstrated and theoretical pharmacokinetic alterations in adolescents should not obscure the importance of pharmacodynamic evaluation. Indeed, methodologies for effect-controlled clinical trials have been proposed in which drug evaluation is anchored in pharmacodynamic parameters rather than purely pharmacokinetic ones.[12]

However, the larger proportion of adolescent-specific drug research that has occurred is available from

TABLE 16-2
Definition of Pharmacologic Terms

Term	Definition
Pharmacodynamics	Mathematical description of the intensity and time course of drug *effect* as a function of drug concentration
Pharmacokinetics	Mathematical description of the dynamic changes in drug *concentration* as a function of the processes of absorption, distribution, biotransformation, and elimination
Volume of distribution	The fluid volume that would be required to contain all of the drug in the body if the drug concentration found in the blood or plasma was uniform throughout the body
Dose-dependent kinetics (zero-order Michaelis-Menten)	Constant *amount* of drug eliminated per unit of time
Dose-independent kinetics (first order)	Constant *fraction* of drug eliminated per unit of time
Elimination half-life	Time required for the amount of drug in the system to be reduced by one half; the half-life is a derived value that changes as a function of the drug's volume of distribution and its clearance

Data from Benet,[2] Gibaldi,[7] Ross.[8]

pharmacokinetic evaluations (Box 16-1). Pharmacokinetics is the application of mathematical techniques to study and characterize the time course of drug disposition in the body and how disposition is affected by the processes of absorption, distribution, biotransformation (metabolism), and elimination (Table 16-3). A working knowledge of basic pharmacokinetic principles can be used clinically to adjust dosage or schedule at critical adolescent growth and maturational timepoints to achieve therapeutic drug levels for the youth based on the unique rate processes that are exhibited.

ABSORPTION. Absorption is that process through which drug leaves its site of administration and the extent to which this movement occurs; bioavailability designates the extent to which the drug reaches its site of action.[2] The physicochemical properties of the drug and the physiologic barriers it may encounter determine its optimal route of administration (e.g., first-pass effect, in which certain drugs, such as nitroglycerin, are effectively fully metabolized before entering the systemic circulation); an additional consideration is the desired rapidity of drug effect.

Bioavailability from orally administered drugs is affected by gastric acid secretion, gastric emptying time, gastric blood flow and surface area, intestinal transit time, first-pass effect, diet, and concomitant drug therapy.

Adolescent applications. In general, the time required for gastric emptying influences the *rate* of absorption but not the *extent* of absorption. Therefore, unless a rapid onset of drug effect is desired, the consequences of adolescent "grazing" and continuous ingestion of food have little effect on the overall absorption of the drug in most cases. Therefore, a requirement that the adolescent take medications "on an empty stomach" need not be

exacted unless the drug is inactivated by stomach acid (e.g., penicillin G), in which case a delay in gastric emptying can expose the drug to gastric acid for a longer time and decrease bioavailability.[13]

Drug interactions. The potential for chemical and drug interactions does exist in the stomach; for example, the chelation of cations (calcium, magnesium, aluminum, iron) and tetracyclines, which prevents absorption of the cation-tetracycline complex.

DISTRIBUTION. After absorption, depending on its physical characteristics, the drug distributes throughout interstitial and cellular fluids. This distribution occurs at different rates: first, the vascular system and highly perfused organs, and subsequently into muscle, skin, and finally fat. Fat may act as a long-term reservoir of drug, since blood flow to this tissue is limited. Other tissues may accumulate drug in higher concentrations than expected owing to factors such as pH gradients or binding to intracellular constituents (e.g., digoxin, which binds to Na^+, K^+-ATPase in muscle). Drug distribution may also be limited by binding to plasma proteins, which restricts drug access to cellular sites of action and retards its elimination from the body.[2]

The usual apparent volume of distribution (V_d) for a drug is a helpful construct in evaluating these factors. Volumes of distribution fall into four categories:

1. Values equivalent to total body water (0.5 L/kg); e.g., theophylline, which is a small, water-soluble, nonionized molecule distributing evenly and easily throughout most body tissues.
2. Values equivalent to extracellular water only (0.25 L/kg); e.g., gentamicin, which is a water-soluble, larger ionized molecule whose distribution is limited to vascular and extravascular spaces.

BOX 16-1
Clinical Guidelines[10,12]

1. CONFIRM THE DIAGNOSIS BEFORE INITIATING THERAPY IF POSSIBLE.
   Consider that the choice of no therapy is also an intervention with risks and benefits. In the face of uncertainty about the diagnosis and the pressure to treat empirically, delaying therapy until a condition evolves more definitively may be more prudent, offering more benefit than risk.

2. OBTAIN A THOROUGH DRUG HISTORY.
   In a nonjudgmental fashion and with great patience, systematically review all prescription, nonprescription, and illicit drugs that the adolescent may be using. Without this information, evaluation of drug effect and monitoring for toxicity is incredibly more difficult.

3. UNDERSTAND THE PATHOPHYSIOLOGY OF THE DISEASE.
   Without a clear knowledge of the signs, symptoms, and manifestations of the illness, one cannot effectively monitor for drug effect or toxicity.

4. USE THERAPEUTIC AGENTS WHOSE PHARMACOLOGY YOU UNDERSTAND.
   Refrain from prescribing the "drug of the month" or new drug samples left by drug company representatives. Rely on those agents whose labeling information you have studied. Know the drug's pharmacodynamics and pertinent pharmacokinetics, and the mechanisms of important drug interactions, in order to individualize therapy.

5. APPRECIATE THE FULL CONSEQUENCES OF PHARMACOLOGIC THERAPY.
   Adolescent pregnancy is commonly unplanned and unexpected. Clinicians need to be attuned to the possibility of pregnancy in their patients and choose therapeutic agents with regard to their teratogenic potential, carefully weighing the severity of the indication, the likely benefit from therapy, and its attendant potential risk.

6. SET THERAPEUTIC GOALS AND DEFINE THE END POINTS OF TREATMENT IN THE CHART.
   Setting therapeutic end points, particularly for limited regimens, involves an automatic evaluation of the success of the intervention. This is a process too frequently neglected by busy physicians who consequently become too casual with prescriptions and too uncritical of the merits of drug therapy.

7. BE PARTICULARLY VIGILANT IN USING DRUGS WITH NARROW THERAPEUTIC INDICES AND VERY CAUTIOUS IN HIGH-RISK CLINICAL SITUATIONS.
   These are dangerous drugs and difficult medical problems in which clinical parameters change rapidly.

8. ENGAGE THE PATIENT AS A COLLABORATOR IN DESIGNING THE REGIMEN SO THAT THE TREATMENT CAN BE INDIVIDUALIZED SOCIALLY.
   The prescription can be conceptualized as a contract in which the prescriber and the patient agree on schedule, end points, and toxicities, thus enhancing compliance and successful, safe drug treatment.

9. REPORT ADVERSE DRUG EVENTS TO THE SPONTANEOUS REPORTING SYSTEM OF THE FOOD AND DRUG ADMINISTRATION.
   There is little information on adverse drug effects in adolescents. One reason may be that adverse drug effects are indeed rare in this age group because of inherent physiologic resiliency and capacity. Another reason may be that such events are not reported.[34] Prescribers may have a low index of suspicion and fail to recognize the role drugs may play in the face of clinical deterioration. Some may think that, because the event has appeared in the literature, it need not be reported. The adverse drug event reporting system is the fuel that drives the engine of postmarketing drug safety evaluation. Careful monitoring and reporting of adverse drug events will ensure that adolescent-specific evaluation occurs if indicated.

---

3. Values equivalent to that of plasma albumin (0.1 L/kg); e.g., warfarin, which is water soluble, small, and nonionized but 99% protein bound in the plasma.
4. Values far in excess of total body water; e.g., digoxin, which binds to Na^+, K^+-ATPase, an enzyme found in high concentrations in brain, liver, kidneys, and muscle, is found in low concentrations in the serum, yielding a V_d of 7 L/kg.[14]

In general, drugs with a large V_d are lipophilic and frequently bind avidly to tissue sites. They require hepatic biotransformation to be eliminated from the body. Conversely, drugs with a small V_d are composed of large molecules or bind to plasma proteins, are hydrophilic, and are predominantly eliminated unchanged through the kidney.[15]

Adolescent applications. Adolescents undergo remarkable changes in both body size and body composi-

TABLE 16-3
Selected Common Adolescent Conditions and Disease States Affecting the Kinetics of Drugs

Pharmacokinetic Parameter	Condition or Disease State	Mechanism	Clinical Result
Absorption	Bulimia/anorexia nervosa	Erratic intake	Therapeutic failure
		Organ dysfunction and electrolyte imbalance	Possible enhanced toxicity
Distribution	Obesity	Increased fat tissue acts as reservoir for lipophilic drugs	Prolonged clearance
	Malnutrition	Decreased fat, muscle mass, decreased plasma protein	Amplified drug clearance with/without enhanced drug effect or toxicity
	Renal failure	Decreased protein binding	High unbound drug levels in face of low serum levels
	Burns	Massive fluid shifts, cell membrane disruption, decreased serum albumin	Dependent on many factors
Biotransformation	Hepatitis	Impaired metabolism	Toxicity potential depends on drug characteristics
Excretion	Burns	Renal blood flow and GFR decreased acutely	Toxicity potential
	Renal insufficiency	Accumulation of endogenous acids that compete/displace plasma protein-bound drug	For drugs >90% bound, enhanced drug effect/toxicity
	Renal failure	Accumulation of agents, >40% renally eliminated	Toxicity potential depends on drug characteristics

Data from Brater,[25] Bonate.[35]
GFR, glomerular filtration rate.

tion as puberty unfolds. Lean body mass increases in both sexes but substantially more in boys. Boys actually lose some body fat during peak height spurts, while girls always accumulate fat during puberty. In late puberty girls may have 25% of body weight in fat; boys have approximately 12%.[16]

Drug interactions. Many drugs bind to plasma proteins but do so in a rather nonselective manner. Consequently, many drugs with similar physical or chemical characteristics readily compete for the same binding sites with each other and with endogenous substances. Drug that is displaced may be redistributed in higher concentrations to its site of action or be more readily eliminated.[2] For example, when an adolescent with epilepsy whose seizures are well controlled on chronic therapy with phenytoin is treated for musculoskeletal injuries with the nonsteroidal anti-inflammatory drug phenylbutazone, the displacement of phenytoin from plasma protein binding sites by the phenylbutazone will produce increased levels of phenytoin in the plasma.[17] Clinicians who manage chronic conditions must be well acquainted with the pharmacokinetic characteristics of the drugs they employ, and particularly aware of the

binding potential of the drugs. Those highly bound drugs with narrow therapeutic indices must be monitored closely, with attention to whether the assays available for measuring serum concentration distinguish between bound and unbound drug.[18]

BIOTRANSFORMATION. The same characteristics of drugs that ensure their ease of absorption would guarantee their endless recirculation in the body if there were no mechanism for their alteration into more polar (and easily excreted) moieties. The body has developed the capacity to metabolize both endogenous and exogenous substances through a series of chemical reactions, and thus promote their elimination. While the enzyme systems responsible for the metabolism of many drugs can be found in the liver, it is important to remember that these enzymes can be found in other organs (kidney, lung, and gastrointestinal epithelium) and, although in smaller quantities, can sometimes exert clinically important effects (e.g., the first-pass effect).[2]

Biotransformation of a drug frequently does not inactivate the drug nor remove it from the body. The chemical reactions produced by the enzymes involved in biotransformation can be classified as phase I or phase II reactions. Phase I reactions (oxidation, reduction, or hydrolysis) convert the compound into a polar metabolite that may be pharmacologically inactive, one that has less activity, or occasionally one with more activity than its parent compound. Similarly, the toxicity profile of a metabolite may be comparable with or more or less toxic than its parent drug.[2] Phase II reactions couple the compound or its polar metabolite with an endogenous substrate (e.g., glucuronate, glutathione, glucose, sulfate, acetate) that enhances its elimination from the body. Of particular note is the cytochrome P-450 (CYP-450) family of enzymes, the dominant phase I oxidative system that metabolizes, to some degree, most drugs used clinically in humans.

Adolescent applications. Variability in the CYP-450 system can have pronounced consequences by altering kinetics and producing "mechanism-based" toxicities,[19] by altering the activation of "pro-drugs" and causing therapeutic failure, or by shunting metabolism toward other metabolic products with differing activity or toxicity.[1]

Variability in the amount and activity of hepatic drug-metabolizing enzymes can result from a number of factors, including administration of drugs or exposure to environmental toxins, hepatic disease, and large pharmacogenetic differences in individual capacity.[2]

Developmental variability is also a factor. CYP-450 function in newborns is very limited but increases with a great deal of interindividual variation in the first year of life. From toddlers to puberty, drug clearance is often greater, drug half-life is shorter, and daily dosing requirements are larger than in adults. An 8-year-old child may require 24 to 36 mg/kg/day to maintain a theophylline serum level of 15 μg/ml, whereas an adult can be maintained with a daily dose of 16 mg/kg. Little information is available on the functional development during the transition period between these two ages. Recent information employing the caffeine breath test suggests a Tanner-stage dependent decrease in clearance, measuring oxidation demethylation in a specific cytochrome P-450 enzyme, CYP1A2.[20] CYP1A is responsible for the metabolism of caffeine, imipramine, and phenacetin.[21] The correlation with Tanner staging depends on gender: the decrease in clearance was observed in girls at an earlier stage than comparable clearance decreases in boys. Among phase II reactions, there are few comparable data.[22] However, information on differential glucuronidation by gender does exist for certain drugs, namely, oxazepam and temazepam, with decreased rates in women,[23,24] and gender differences for oxidation and sulfation have also been reported.[11]

Drug interactions. The metabolizing capacity of hepatic enzyme systems can be induced (up-regulated) by a number of conditions, including smoking and the administration of drugs. For the P-450 cytochrome system, there are two major types of inducers: aromatic hydrocarbons and phenobarbital-like substances; other agents can induce individual isozymes (e.g., ethanol, rifampin, dexamethasone, clofibrate).[2] For example, the increased plasma clearance of oral contraceptives is directly attributable to the enzyme-inducing properties of rifampicin, leading to contraceptive failure and unintended pregnancy[25]; rifampin also increases the clearance of phenytoin through stimulation of microsomal enzymes.[26]

Conversely, some drugs may inhibit (down-regulate) the metabolism of others; for example, cimetidine inhibits the metabolism of imipramine and desipramine.[26] For some drugs the clinical situation is much more complex. The hepatic metabolism of carbamazepine is inhibited by erythromycin, propoxyphene, cimetidine, and isoniazid, while carbamazepine induces the metabolism of phenytoin, primidone, and valproic acid, among others. In fact, carbamazepine induces its own metabolism, and its serum concentration needs to be reevaluated after 4 to 6 weeks of initiation of therapy to ensure adequate drug levels.[27]

RENAL EXCRETION. The kidney is the primary organ through which drugs and their metabolites are eliminated from the body. This elimination involves three processes: filtration, secretion, and reabsorption. The amount of drug filtered is a function of the integrity of the glomerulus, the glomerular filtration rate (and renal blood flow), the size and charge of the drug molecule, and the extent of protein binding.[2,28] Decreased renal function has serious clinical consequences, and any drug therapy undertaken in such circumstances must be carefully monitored, particularly if the drug's therapeutic index is narrow, if the drug is highly protein bound, or if more than 40% of the drug is excreted unchanged in the urine.[28] In the proximal tubule, certain organic acids and bases are added to the filtrate by active, carrier-mediated tubular secretion; this process is nonselective, and ions of similar charge compete for transport.[2] In the proximal and distal tubules, passive reabsorption of many drugs can occur, depending on urinary flow and urinary pH (which determines the degree of ionization of the drug; only nonionized drug is reabsorbed).

Adolescent applications. There may be maturational changes in the renal elimination of drugs that correlate more closely with sexual maturation (as evidenced by Tanner stage) than with strict chronologic age. This has been suggested for digoxin clearance, in which the enhanced net tubular secretion of digoxin seen in infants appeared to decrease to adult values in subjects categorized as Tanner stages 4 and 5.[29,30]

Drug interactions. Since the secretion process is nonselective, a number of acids may compete for secretion. This can cause clinical problems if the expected elimination of one is impaired by the other; for example, methotrexate toxicity has been reported when this agent is coadministered with salicylates or nonsteroidal anti-inflammatory agents. Conversely, the competitive process can be used to clinical advantage: probenecid interferes with the elimination of penicillin, thereby prolonging therapeutic serum concentrations.[28]

The pH-dependent nature of drug reabsorption has the potential for adverse drug interactions but can be therapeutically advantageous. In overdose situations, such as salicylate poisoning, the pH of urine can be altered to promote drug clearance and reduce toxicity. When tubular urine is more alkaline, weak acids are more ionized and can be eliminated more rapidly; when tubular urine is more acidic, the excretion of weak acids is reduced. The pH of the tubular urine has opposite effects on weak bases.[2] Weak acids include chlorpropamide, salicylates, phenobarbital, trimethoprim, and sulfonamide derivatives; weak bases include amphetamines, ephedrine, and quinine.[28]

CLEARANCE. Clearance is the rate of drug elimination by all routes normalized to the concentration of drug in some biologic fluid; in pharmacology, clearance is generally restricted to the measurement of drug elimination from the plasma. Clearance is expressed as the volume that would have to be completely freed of drug to account for its elimination from the body. Although other organs may contribute substantially for particular drugs (e.g., lungs for paraldehyde), drug clearance is chiefly mediated through the liver and kidney, and thus blood flow to these organs becomes a crucial determinant of the clearance of drug from the body.

Elimination kinetics follow two paths: dose dependent and dose independent. A simple illustration of the difference between these paths is the interstate highway system, which can move a considerable amount of traffic in a steady, efficient, and predictable fashion (dose-independent kinetics). If, however, a toll booth is placed on the highway, the movement of traffic becomes a function of the capacity of the toll booth attendant, and traffic backs up (dose-dependent kinetics).

Dose-dependent kinetics. The elimination kinetics exhibited by some drugs whose metabolism involves a saturable pathway are termed dose-dependent, zero-order, or Michaelis-Menten kinetics. For these drugs, the clearance of the drug and its half-life in the body are determined by the dose administered, and even a small increase in dosage may produce a large increment in plasma concentration as metabolic pathways approach saturation. All drugs can exhibit dose-dependent kinetics in overdose situations. However, commonly used drugs that can exhibit dose-dependent kinetics at their therapeutic serum concentrations include ethanol, aspirin, phenytoin, and propranolol.

Dose-independent kinetics. Most drugs are cleared from the body in a predictable fashion, with a constant percentage of the drug's concentration being lost per unit of time, and exhibit dose-independent or first-order elimination kinetics. For these drugs, an increase in dosage results in a predictable and proportionate increase in serum drug concentration.

Elimination half-life. For drugs exhibiting first-order kinetics, the elimination half-life can be determined by plotting the drug's exponential decay in the plasma as a function of time and determining the two time points at which the concentration is diminished by one half; the difference between these two time points is the elimination half-life for the drug. The elimination half-life is important for three clinical considerations: (1) to determine how much time will be required to achieve the ultimate steady-state concentration of drug in the plasma; (2) to determine the duration of time needed for plasma drug levels to fall once drug administration is discontinued; and (3) to design an appropriate dosing interval.[15] When a given dose of drug is administered on a schedule that approximates the drug's elimination half-life, the drug concentration will rise until a plateau is achieved where the amount of drug entering the system per dosing interval is equivalent to the amount of drug being eliminated from the system; that is, the drug concentration is at steady state. The plateau is achieved incrementally: 50% at the end of the first half-life, 75% by the end of the second, 87% by the third, 93% by the fourth, and 97% at the end of five half-lives. Thus, dosing on the drug's half-life requires a time period equivalent to approximately 5 half-lives to achieve steady-state concentrations. In emergent situations, such as acute asthma and congestive heart failure, waiting the time required to achieve steady-state drug concentrations by dosing on a schedule determined by the elimination half-life is unacceptable, and loading doses of the drug are employed to reach therapeutic serum levels more rapidly.

NEGOTIATING THE DRUG REGIMEN

Doctors pour drugs of which they know little, to cure diseases of which they know less, into human beings of which they know nothing. Voltaire (1694-1778 CE)

The first requirement of any prescribing clinician is a commitment to understanding his or her own practice regarding drug prescribing. Is pharmacologic intervention employed empirically before a working diagnosis is established? Is drug therapy substituted for other time-consuming or uncomfortable psychosocial interventions? Is the prescription used as a signal that the visit is completed? Is some medication given because some medication is expected? Too frequently, the prescription has come to be viewed as an expected and essential transaction that formally concludes the transaction between patient and physician.[31] As many as 75% of all office visits to a physician end with one or more new prescriptions.[32] Too few of these prescriptions represent nothing more than the closure of the medical visit, not the beginning of what should be viewed as a clinical trial with a single subject. If the prescription were conceptualized in this manner, the need for a measurable therapeutic objective, attention to individualized dosing, and a system of continuous measurement becomes apparent.[15]

The need for an informed and collaborative patient is also clear. The negotiation process can provide a critical learning period in which individuals realize the pivotal role they play in assuming responsibility for their own health. This is a particularly crucial responsibility for adolescent primary care providers whose patients are in the process of adopting behaviors that will influence their adult health.

Compliance with or adherence to the therapeutic regimen is the essential condition of successful pharmacologic intervention, and attention to the factors affecting it cannot be overemphasized. The conventional precept of simplifying agents, number, and schedule to fit into the patient's life style is extraordinarily complicated by adolescents' denial of risk and consequences in an attempt to be like everyone else.[33] Compliance is more fully addressed in Chapter 17, "Compliance with Health Recommendations."

References

1. Rogers AS: The role of cytochrome P450 in developmental pharmacology, *J Adolesc Health* 15:635-640, 1994.
2. Benet LZ, Mitchell JR, Sheiner LB: Pharmacokinetics: the dynamics of drug absorption, distribution, and elimination. In Gilman AS, Rall TW, Nies AS, Taylor P, editors: *Goodman and Gilman's the pharmacologic basis of therapeutics,* ed 8, New York, 1990, Pergamon Press, pp 3-32.
3. Myers A, Moore SR: The drug approval process and the information it provides. In Hartzema AG, Porta MS, Tilson HH, editors: *Pharmacoepidemiology: an introduction,* Cincinnati, 1991, Harvey Whitney, pp 47-62.
4. Peck CC, Temple R, Collins JM: Understanding consequences of concurrent therapies, *JAMA* 269:1550-1552, 1993.
5. Rogers AS: A research agenda for the study of therapeutic agents in adolescents, *J Adolesc Health* 15:672-678, 1994.
6. Vesel E: Pharmacogenetics. In Yaffe S, Aranda J, editors: *Pediatric pharmacology: therapeutic principles in practice,* ed 2, Philadelphia, 1992, WB Saunders, pp 29-44.
7. Gibaldi M: *Biopharmaceutics and clinical pharmacokinetics,* ed 2, Philadelphia, 1977, Lea & Febiger, pp vii.
8. Ross EM: Pharmacodynamics: mechanisms of drug action and the relationship between drug concentration and effect. In Gilman AS, Rall TW, Nies AS, Taylor P, editors: *Goodman and Gilman's the pharmacologic basis of therapeutics,* ed 8, New York, 1990, Pergamon Press, pp 33-48.
9. Arslanian SA, Heil BV, Becker DJ, et al: Sexual dimorphism in insulin sensitivity in adolescents with insulin-dependent diabetes mellitus, *J Clin Endocrinol Metab* 72:920-926, 1991.
10. Fletcher CV, Acosta EP, Strykowski JM: Gender differences in human pharmacokinetics and pharmacodynamics, *J Adolesc Health* 15:619-629, 1994.
11. American College of Clinical Pharmacy: ACCP white paper: women as research subjects, *Pharmacotherapy* 13:534-542, 1993.
12. Levy G, Ebling WP, Forrest A: Concentration- or effect-controlled trials with sparse data, *Clin Pharmacol Ther* 56:1-8, 1994.
13. Wright JM: Drug interactions. In Melmon KL, Morrelli HF, Hoffman BB, Nierenberg DW, editors: *Melmon and Morrelli's clinical pharmacology: basic principles in therapeutics,* ed 3, New York, 1992, McGraw-Hill, pp 1012-1021.
14. Holford N: Clinical pharmacokinetics and pharmacodynamics: the quantitative basis for therapeutics. In Melmon KL, Morrelli HF, Hoffman BB, Nierenberg DW, editors: *Melmon and Morrelli's clinical pharmacology: basic principles in therapeutics,* ed 3, New York, 1992, McGraw-Hill, pp 951-964.
15. Nierenberg DW, Melmon KL: Introduction to clinical pharmacology. In Melmon KL, Morrelli HF, Hoffman BB, Nierenberg DW, editors: *Melmon and Morrelli's clinical pharmacology: basic principles in therapeutics,* ed 3, New York, 1992, McGraw-Hill, pp 1-51.
16. Finkelstein JW: The effect of developmental changes in adolescence on drug disposition, *J Adolesc Health* 15:612-618, 1994.
17. Shlotzhauer TL, Lambert RE, McGuire JL: Metabolic and degenerative disorders of connective tissue and bone. In Melmon KL, Morrelli HF, Hoffman BB, Nierenberg DW, editors: *Melmon and Morrelli's clinical pharmacology: basic principles in therapeutics,* ed 3, New York, 1992, McGraw-Hill, pp 486-504.
18. Levine M, Chang T: Therapeutic drug monitoring of phenytoin: rationale and current status, *Clin Pharmacokinet,* 19:341-358, 1990.
19. Murray M: P450 enzymes, *Clin Pharmacokinet* 23:132-146, 1992.
20. Lambert GH, Kotake AN, Schoeller D: The CO_2 breath tests as monitors of the cytochrome P450 dependent mixed function monooxygenase system. In MacLeod S, Okey A, Spielberg S: *Developmental pharmacology,* New York, 1983, Alan R. Liss, pp 119-145.
21. Gonzalez FJ, Idle JR: Pharmacogenetic phenotyping and genotyping: present status and future potential, *Clin Pharmacokinet* 26:59-70, 1994.
22. Capparelli EV: Pharmacokinetic considerations in the adolescent: non-cytochrome P450 metabolic pathways, *J Adolesc Health* 15:641-647, 1994.
23. Greenblatt DJ, Divoll M, Harmatz JS, Shader RI: Oxazepam kinetics: effects of age and sex, *J Pharmacol Exp Ther* 215:86, 1981.
24. Divoll M, Greenblatt D, Harmatz J, Shader R: Effect of age and gender on disposition of temazepam, *J Pharm Sci* 70:1104-1107, 1981.
25. Breckenridge AM, Back DJ, Orme M: Interactions between oral contraceptives and other drugs, *Pharmacol Ther* 7:617-626, 1979.
26. Scott G, Nierenberg DW: Appendix II drug interactions. In Melmon KL, Morrelli HF, Hoffman BB, Nierenberg DW, editors: *Melmon and Morrelli's clinical pharmacology: basic principles in therapeutics,* ed 3, New York, 1992, McGraw-Hill, pp 1073-1083.
27. Pippenger CE: Clinically significant carbamazepine drug interactions: an overview. *Epilepsia* 28 (suppl 3):S71-S76, 1987.
28. Brater DC: Treatment of renal disorders and the influence of renal function on drug disposition. In Melmon KL, Morrelli HF, Hoffman BB, Nierenberg DW, editors: *Melmon and Morrelli's clinical pharmacology: basic principles in therapeutics,* ed 3, New York, 1992, McGraw-Hill, pp 270-308.
29. Linday LA, Drayer DE, Khan MA-Ali, et al: Pubertal changes in net renal tubular secretion of digoxin, *Clin Pharmacol Ther* 35:438-446, 1984.
30. Linday LA: Developmental changes in renal tubular function, *J Adolesc Health* 15:648-653, 1994.

31. Manasse HR: Medication use in an imperfect world: drug mis-adventuring as an issue of public policy, Parts 1 and 2, *Am J Hosp Pharm* 46:929-944, 1141-1152, 1989.

32. Soumerai SB, Avorn J: Principles of educational outreach ("academic detailing") to improve clinical decision making, *JAMA* 263:549-556, 1990.

33. Brooks-Gunn J, Graber J: Puberty as a biological and social event: implications for research on pharmacology, *J Adolesc Health* 15:663-671, 1994.

34. Rogers AS, Israel E, Smith CR, Levine D, McBean AM, Valente C, Faich G: Physician knowledge, attitudes, and behavior related to reporting adverse drug events, *Arch Intern Med* 148:1596-1600, 1988.

35. Bonate PL: Pathophysiology and pharmacokinetics following burn injury, *Clin Pharmacokinet* 18:118-130, 1990.

CHAPTER 17

Compliance with Health Recommendations

•

Barbara A. Cromer

Therapeutic success is limited by the degree of compliance with the prescribed regimen. In all age groups the prevalence of compliant behavior is generally disappointingly low, estimated at 50%.[1] Among selected adolescent populations with different medical and psychosocial conditions, the likelihood of compliance is variable.[2] Compliance tends to be higher in certain clinical situations, for example, treatment of acute illnesses versus the practice of preventive health measures (especially those involving life style changes). Complex personal and environmental influences create unique considerations in each case.

Despite numerous research efforts designed to identify psychosocial factors that are consistently associated with the compliant patient, no such clear profile has been established.[2] The factors considered in this research include demographic background and personality characteristics such as self-esteem and locus of control (a measure of self-determination), as well as family variables such as cohesiveness and level of effective communication. Most of these factors do not lend themselves to expeditious assessment in the office or clinic setting, and they represent personality traits that tend to be resistant to behavioral intervention. In addition, research findings have varied from study to study. Recent attention has been directed toward evaluating other personal and environmental variables that are potentially more responsive to behavioral manipulation.

IDENTIFICATION

Accurate identification of the noncompliant patient is more difficult than it would seem. The most direct approach is to simply inquire as to behavior related to the treatment regimen. However, because of the need of many adolescents to appear in a socially desirable light, they often overstate their level of compliance (as do adults). For example, one study of adolescents with asthma found appreciable discrepancies between self-recorded compliance and prescribed aerosol treatment as measured by Nebulizer Chronolog (an electronic timer device).[3] In all cases the adolescents reported better compliance than that documented by the Nebulizer Chronolog.

Any patient with persistent symptoms, despite prescribed treatment with a known effective regimen, should be suspected of noncompliance. This case scenario is usually easy to interpret when it involves a symptomatic illness such as streptococcal pharyngitis, for which there is definitive treatment and a clearly measurable outcome. It is more difficult to assess the level of compliance in an adolescent with chronic illness whose progress is also influenced by psychosocial factors, such as stress or hypertension, and environmental influences, such as barometric pressure in asthma. Even in these circumstances, however, the index of suspicion for noncompliance should be high.

Despite the wide variability of compliance across different patient populations, it is evident that in the same individual the likelihood of compliant behavior is relatively consistent with the treatment of different clinical conditions. The implication is that behavior related to compliance emanates from a cluster of stable personality constructs. A related observation is that previous compliance predicts future compliance. In one analysis of data from the longitudinal National Survey of Family Health, the strongest prediction of reported noncompliance with the current birth control method was noncompliance with the initially reported method.[4] Adolescents with persistent symptoms who have a history of noncompliance should be suspected of more of the same behavior, and intervention strategies should be implemented early in the treatment schedule.

A common notion held by many physicians is that they can accurately predict which of their patients will comply with their prescriptive advice. This may be true in some patients, especially those whose behavioral history is familiar to the physician. However, several studies have demonstrated that physicians' estimates can err greatly in comparison with more objective measures of compliance.[5]

Bioassays of certain drugs have been developed to aid in the assessment of compliance as well as in adjusting the dosage of medication according to individual responses. Most assays are performed on serum and provide the most helpful information when used with drugs that are taken habitually, have a long half-life, and reach a steady-state level in the blood. Examples include sustained-release theophylline preparations and several anticonvulsants. Although drugs can also be detected in urine, measurement is qualitative and usually applies only to drugs taken in the previous 24 hours. Some bioassays have been adapted to saliva specimens, an attractive alternative for adolescents who dread venipuncture, but these are not yet available in community laboratories. A variety of devices have been developed for electronic monitoring of dosing and self-testing, including the glucometer, which records the time of testing and the blood glucose level, as well as the Medication Event Monitoring System (MEMS), which records the opening of bottles for removal of tablets.[6] Another creative approach that has demonstrated great promise as an accurate objective measure of medication compliance is the use of deuterium oxide, a stable isotope.[7] Tagged to the prescribed drug, it is assayed in urine and, if multiple samples are obtained, a curve of compliance over the interim time period can be established. Objective measurement of behavioral recommendations is even more difficult because direct observation is the only accurate method available. In these circumstances, reports by a family member regarding the adolescent's compliance with a behavioral regimen may be helpful.

DEVELOPMENTAL ISSUES

The level of cognitive sophistication differs from adolescent to adolescent and may be independent of chronologic age; the individual teenager may also exhibit inconsistencies in cognitive understanding within different areas of his or her life. As a result of cognitive immaturity, some adolescents have difficulty understanding the abstract concepts related to disease or appreciating the benefits of preventive health practice.[8] Comprehensive assessment of cognitive maturity is difficult in any setting and actually unnecessary for effective communication between practitioner and adolescent. One can assume that every adolescent can understand disease and its treatment at a concrete level. Compliance in this age group is enhanced by the following strategies: (1) visual aids such as abnormalities displayed on x-ray films; (2) focus on immediate benefit from treatment, such as relief of abdominal pain with appropriate treatment of pelvic inflammatory disease; and (3) when available, starter samples of medication so that the patient experiences beneficial effects and is encouraged to have the prescription filled and to continue treatment. Even adolescents who think mainly on a concrete level can participate in self-management. This is also true for teenagers with a chronic condition whose daily care requires some parental involvement. Adolescent self-management encourages independence from the family, an important developmental task of adolescence. A goal for the adolescent with a chronic condition in the transition to adulthood is the assumption of primary responsibility for his or her care (and that the activities that require another person be assumed by a person outside the family).

Other behavioral strategies of self-management involve self-monitoring and self-reinforcement.[1] The classic example of self-monitoring is home glucose testing in patients with diabetes where immediate feedback is given regarding metabolic control, thereby providing an opportunity for sensible adjustment of insulin and diet. With the provision of initial education and then extended supervision from which the adolescent is eventually weaned, the teenager can learn his or her symptoms of poor control, anticipate certain problems such as hyperglycemia from respiratory infections, make minor adjustments in insulin dosage, and learn the danger signs that need parent and physician attention. Unfortunately, self-monitoring techniques are not available for most chronic disorders. Self-reinforcement can be used in all clinical situations and simply means that the adolescent implements the reinforcement instead of the parent. One such example is recording enuresis in a diary. Although self-management implies that the primary responsibility for daily care lies with the adolescent, negotiating during follow-up visits, particularly if clinical progress is not favorable, is important so that new ideas for self-reinforcement can be discussed. The degree of self-management that the adolescent can attain varies from individual to individual; thus, initial experimentation and slowly graduated assumption of self-care are advised.

The consolidation of body image and sense of identity also occurs during adolescence, and this process is reflected in the adolescent's peer group. When the course of a disease or its treatment affects the adolescent's ability to conform to the peer group, noncompliance may result. The practitioner should be aware of therapeutic regimens that adversely affect cosmetic appearances, such as drugs that cause hirsutism or daily activities that cause excessive fatigue. Conversely, in selected circumstances, interventions focusing on maintenance of a normal appearance and level of activity (e.g., medication to improve acne or control wheezing) may be helpful in improving compliance.

Certain coping mechanisms that adolescents commonly mobilize in response to stress may interfere with their willingness to comply with a treatment regimen.[5] In most teenagers these mechanisms reflect normal development and function by decreasing the anxiety and feelings of dependency that result from internally or externally induced stress. However, excessive use of these mechanisms can cause the adolescent to become dysfunctional and obstruct the progress of a treatment program. For example, denial of the potentially life-threatening nature of cancer protects the patient from excessive anxiety. Problems ensue when the denial is so pervasive that the patient minimizes the seriousness of the disorder and therefore the need for treatment. The same issues apply to other defense mechanisms common to (although certainly not limited to) this age group, which include regression and rationalization. This presents a difficult problem for the practitioner because of the strong need of the patient to defend against unacceptable anxiety. Rather than trying to penetrate these defenses, it may be more advisable to attempt to understand the cause of the stress and to provide pertinent education or counseling.

INTERVENTION STRATEGIES

Education

Educational programs to increase patient compliance have the following basic format: (1) information regarding the skills and correct procedure necessary to carry out a treatment protocol, (2) descriptive comparison of the natural history of the disorder resulting from compliance versus noncompliance, and (3) instruction as to the conceptual basis of the disease and its pathophysiology. Previous research has demonstrated varying levels of success with each of these formats. Behavioral interventions are listed in the accompanying box.

> **BOX 17-1**
> **Behavioral Interventions**
>
> EDUCATION
> Detail correct procedure
> Describe prognosis with noncompliance
> Inform as to conceptual basis of disease
> Orient education directed at clinicians
>
> TAILORING OF TREATMENT REGIMEN
> Minimize number of drugs and dosage frequency
> Choose regimens with least financial cost and social restrictiveness
> Choose regimens with minimal side effects
> Instruct within sociocultural context of patient
>
> ENLISTING FAMILY SUPPORT
> Involve parent(s) in direct supervision of treatment protocol
> Enlist parent(s) in providing general support for compliance
> Enlist peer(s) in providing support to the adolescent in a dysfunctional family

---

A prerequisite for compliance is that the patient comprehend the details of the treatment procedure. Exit interviews with patients generally reveal an inadequate understanding of the prescribed therapeutic regimen. This may be especially true for adolescents, who are often unwilling to admit that they do not fully comprehend the treatment protocol. This type of education includes written directions regarding dosage schedules and instruction in the proper use of ancillary devices such as inhalers or vaginal suppository applicators. Recommendations regarding the optimal circumstances in which to self-treat are also helpful: for example, decreasing insulin before strenuous exercise in patients with diabetes. This educational format has the highest likelihood of success in enhancing compliance in the adolescent patient.

The second educational format commonly employed is "scare tactics"—some dreaded consequence that may occur as the result of noncompliance, such as sterility in pelvic inflammatory disease. This approach has numerous drawbacks. For example, the adolescent female after treatment for pelvic infection may feel a need to test her fertility by stopping contraception. Another interpretation by the patient with recurrent infection is that sterility has already occurred and thus treatment would be of no benefit. An additional problem is that if the dreaded consequence does not result (e.g., hospitalization for failure to maintain minimal weight in anorexia nervosa), the clinician loses credibility, and future warnings carry less importance.

The third educational approach is didactic teaching. This may involve discussing the cause of the disease, its pathophysiology, and the conceptual basis for treatment, as is traditional for patients with chronic conditions such as diabetes. The general assumption of clinicians is that the more patients know about their disorder from an intellectual perspective, the more likely they are to adhere to treatment. Unfortunately, in this age group the individual's level of abstract knowledge is a poor predictor of compliance.

Research suggests that an effective educational approach is physician rather than patient directed. In a study by Maiman et al,[9] virtually all the pediatricians in Rochester, New York received (1) tutorials and mailed instructions regarding compliance strategies, (2) mailed instructions only, or (3) no intervention. They found increased knowledge related to compliance among the physicians, as well as increased compliance in their pediatric patients, in the first two education groups as compared with the group of physicians who received no intervention.

Treatment Regimen Modification

Modification of the treatment regimen as a strategy to enhance compliance is appealing because of its practical applicability and its implied element of negotiation with the patient. The first consideration is to keep the regimen as simple as possible. There appears to be a linear, negative relationship between the number of pills (and behaviors) prescribed per day and the level of compliance. Since noncompliance is associated with frequent dosage schedules, it is prudent to use pharmaceutical preparations that require the fewest number of doses per day and to minimize the number of prescribed drugs. The ultimate solution is to eliminate the potential for noncompliance by administering the treatment in a single dose in the physician's office. Examples include intramuscular medroxyprogesterone acetate (Depo-Provera) for contraception, ceftriaxone sodium (Rocephin) for gonorrhea, and long-acting penicillin G benzathine (Bicillin) for strep throat. Unfortunately, this kind of treatment option is available for only a few medical conditions. If full compliance with a complex medical or behavioral regimen is not realistic, prioritizing the recommendations may enhance compliance with the most important parts of the treatment program. At times, compromise may be appropriate.

Another important consideration in choosing the optimal treatment, particularly in the adolescent, is the cost of the treatment from both a financial and psychosocial perspective.[5] One must balance the positive effect on compliance by administering treatment in a single dose with the relative financial cost. For example, azithromycin, single-dose medication effective in lower genital tract infection with *Chlamydia trachomatis,* costs approximately $20.00, whereas a

7-day course with similarly effective doxycycline is only about $5.00.

Exploration of the intrusiveness of the treatment program on the adolescent's daily life, with appropriate modification when possible, can help avoid potential noncompliance. For example, many adolescents resist taking medication at school, usually because their peers tease them about "taking drugs." In this situation, arrange the dosing schedule so that the adolescent can avoid a dose during school hours. Changes in behavior are always a challenge regardless of age, but therapeutic recommendations modified to the patient's life style may ameliorate the difficulty. An example is the patient with cardiac disease who cannot tolerate running sports such as basketball but who can still be a part of the team by serving as a manager or trainer.

An additional important consideration in the management of adolescents is the explanation of treatment in terms compatible with their cultural background. In some cases the practitioner's advice contradicts folk wisdom and competes with the patient's explanatory model of issues related to his or her health. For example, home remedies and healing by dietary manipulation are practiced by subcultures across the country. To avoid potential noncompliance, it may be wise to incorporate new treatment regimens into traditional practices rather than attempting to replace them. It is also important to explore with adolescents their interpretation of and ideas for management of the disease, including perceptions of family members and friends.[10] This interaction actively involves adolescents in the problem-solving process and prevents them from simply being passive recipients of directive information.

The occurrence of adverse side effects to treatment may result in its discontinuation. Undesirable side effects such as altered cosmetic appearance may outweigh the benefits of treatment from the adolescent's perspective, especially when the side effects occur from treatment for an asymptomatic condition. Although, in many clinical situations, drugs with significant side effects cannot be avoided, preparation of the patient before the initiation of treatment and close follow-up at the beginning may allay fear about anticipated results that exceed realistic expectations and lessen the likelihood of noncompliance.

Enlisting Family Support

Extensive family involvement is expected for the successful completion of treatment protocols prescribed for young children. The age at which children achieve developmental maturity to self-administer medication or direct their own behavioral program has not been clearly established. Clinicians recognize the developmental need of the adolescent to achieve eventual independence from the family, and they frequently limit discussion of therapeutic recommendations to the adolescent. This may be appropriate for some teenagers, particularly older adolescents; however, for others a certain degree of supervision by a parent may be indicated. Several studies have demonstrated that in cohesive families with effective communication the enlistment of family involvement is helpful in enhancing adolescent compliance.[11] This support can be provided in the form of general resources (e.g., payment for medications, transportation to appointments), direct reminders to comply, or other methods of reinforcement. Some adolescents respond to formalized modes of reinforcement termed *contracting*. For example, points may be earned for compliant behavior and exchanged at regular intervals for specified rewards. Parents' cooperation is often required to fulfill the adolescent's contract by administering points or verifying behavior.

In contrast to the positive influence of effective family involvement on adolescent compliance, dysfunctional family interactions are associated with poor compliance. Enlistment of family support in the treatment programs in such cases may be counterproductive to creating a conducive atmosphere for adolescent compliance. In these clinical situations, although behavioral interventions with parental supervision may be attempted, close follow-up assessment is recommended. An alternative approach in dysfunctional families is to enlist the support of a peer; support for this approach can be found in studies reporting the effectiveness of peer counseling in enhancing compliance in adolescents with a variety of health problems.

Indications for Referral

Behavioral interventions instituted by the primary care practitioner to increase compliance in the adolescent do not always meet with success. Referral for mental health consultation is indicated in dysfunctional families when the clinician's intervention has been ineffective. In many situations the mental health professional can provide consultative advice regarding a different behavioral intervention, and the primary care clinician can execute the program. However, in many situations, adjunctive individual or family counseling is helpful and should be conducted in conjunction with medical management.

References

1. Rapoff MA, Barnard MU: Compliance with pediatric medical regimens. In Cramer JA, Spilker B, editors: *Patient compliance in medical practice and clinical trials,* New York, 1991, Raven Press, pp 73-98.
2. Dunbar J, Waszak L: Patient compliance: pediatric and adolescent populations. In Gross AM, Drabman RS, editors: *Handbook of clinical pediatrics,* New York, 1990, Plenum, pp 365-382.
3. Coutts JAP, Gibson NA, Paton JY: Measuring compliance with inhaled medication in asthma, *Arch Dis Child* 67:332-333, 1991.
4. DuRant RH, Sanders JM Jr, Jay S, et al: Analysis of contraceptive behavior of sexually active female adolescents in the United States, *J Pediatr* 113:930-936, 1988.
5. Cromer BA, Tarnowski KJ: Noncompliance in adolescents: a review, *J Dev Behav Pediatr* 10:207-215, 1989.
6. Cramer JA: Methods to measure patient compliance. In Cramer JA, Spilker B, editors: *Patient compliance in medical practice and clinical trials,* New York, 1991, Raven Press, pp 1-10.
7. Rodewald LE, Pichichero ME: Compliance with antibiotic therapy: a comparison of deuterium oxide tracer, urine bioassay, bottle weights, and parental reports, *J Pediatr* 123:143-147, 1993.
8. Brooks-Gunn J: Why do adolescents have difficulty adhering to health regimes? In Krasnegor NA, Epstein L, Johnson SB, et al, editors: *Developmental aspects of health compliance behavior,* Hillsdale, NJ, 1993, Lawrence Erlbaum, pp 125-152.
9. Maiman LA, Becker MH, Liptak GS, et al: Improving pediatricians' compliance-enhancing practices: a randomized trial, *Am J Dis Child* 142:773-779, 1988.
10. Donovan JL, Blake DR: Patient non-compliance: deviance or reasoned decision-making, *Soc Sci Med* 34:507-513, 1992.
11. Falvo DR: *Effective patient education: a guide to increased compliance,* ed 2, Gaithersburg, MD, 1994, Aspen, pp 197-214.

CHAPTER 18

Legal and Ethical Concerns

•

Abigail English

Health care professionals providing services to adolescents frequently encounter legal issues and ethical dilemmas in caring for their young patients. Some of the legal issues may be resolved easily if practitioners are familiar with the basic legal principles that apply to adolescent health care; others may require consultation with legal counsel. The ethical concerns are at least as complex as the legal issues and often may benefit from multidisciplinary consideration. The legal and ethical issues of greatest concern in the field of adolescent medicine are usually related to consent, confidentiality, or payment for care. Basic questions for each category are as follows[1]:

1. Who has authority to give consent for care? Whose consent is required?
2. To what extent are the communications and records involved in the care protected as confidential? Who has the authority to release confidential information? Whose authorization is required?
3. Who is responsible for payment—adolescent, parent, public or private insurer, an alternative source of public or private funding?

The legal principles that govern these questions are based on decisions of the state and federal courts, statutes enacted by the U.S. Congress and state legislatures, regulations issued by federal and state administrative agencies, and the rights guaranteed by the U.S. Constitution and the state constitutions. Since specific legal provisions vary among states, it is important for practitioners to be familiar with local requirements.[2,3] However, certain basic legal principles related to consent, confidentiality, and payment generally apply. Basic principles of medical ethics and the requirements set forth in the professional code of ethics for each of the health care professions are also

critical elements in establishing the framework for providing health care to adolescents.[4,5]

The legal status and the developmental characteristics of adolescents differ from those of both adults and younger children, and directly affect the laws and ethical principles that apply to their health care. For example, minors traditionally do not have the legal capacity to make certain important decisions, in part because the law is based on the presumption that they lack the developmental capacity to do so on an independent basis.[3] Despite significant legal restrictions on the liberty of adolescents as well as younger children, however, adolescents have been permitted greater rights than younger children to participate in their own health care decisions.[2-7]

LEGAL RIGHTS OF PARENTS

Historically, the authority to make most decisions about the lives of minor children, including health care decisions, has been vested by law in their parents. The legal rights of parents were established originally in court decisions and statutes embodying common law principles of parental custody and control over their minor children and more recently in decisions recognizing the constitutionally protected rights of "family privacy" and "family integrity." Since the beginning of the twentieth century, the authority of parents has been subject to state intervention and limitation by juvenile courts and child welfare authorities when parents have abused or neglected their children or abdicated their parental responsibilities.[8] Juvenile courts have specifically been empowered to make medical decisions and to authorize medical care when a child's life would otherwise be endangered.[3] Generally, however, parents are responsible for their children's medical care, including the obligation to pay for the care, as well as the authority to give consent and to make

Supported by the Carnegie Corporation of New York, which is not responsible for the views expressed herein.

decisions about disclosure of confidential medical information.[3,5,8]

LEGAL RIGHTS OF MINORS

The legal rights of adolescents who are minors (in almost every state, those under the age of 18) have been expanded significantly in recent decades, particularly with respect to health care decisions.[5,8] Although the concept of the legally "emancipated minor" was recognized in early court decisions,[9] most expansions in the legal rights of minors occurred in the second half of the century. During the 1960s and 1970s, the U.S. Supreme Court determined that the Constitution protects minors as well as adults and recognized the constitutional rights of minors in the areas of due process (in delinquency proceedings[10]), free speech (in the school setting[11]), and privacy (with respect to contraception[12] and abortion[13,14]). The privacy decisions, in particular, have had a significant impact on adolescents' rights to make health care decisions. During the same period that the Supreme Court was expanding the constitutional rights of minors, many state legislatures enacted statutes enabling minors to consent to their own health care or lifting the requirement of parental consent in specified circumstances.[2,3] These statutes were based on some of the same policy considerations that had been acknowledged by the Supreme Court in its constitutional decisions concerning contraception and abortion: the government's strong interest in encouraging adolescents to seek health care, particularly care related to sexuality and substance abuse; the deterrent effect of parental consent requirements for some minors; and the capacity of "mature minors" to make health care decisions.[2,3,5]

CONSENT

The consent of a person legally authorized to provide it is a basic requirement for the provision of health care to patients of all ages. The failure to obtain a legally valid consent may result in legal liability for battery (the unauthorized touching of another person), negligence, or malpractice.[15] In addition, obtaining consent before providing health care is an ethical obligation designed to ensure respect for patients as persons and for their autonomy.[16]

Consent of Parents

The traditional requirement of parental consent for the health care of minors has rested on a dual presumption in the law: first, that minors do not have the legal capacity to enter into binding contracts (and the relationship between physician and patient is a contractual one); and second, that minors lack the developmental capacity to make health care decisions. In many situations, parental involvement in the health care of adolescents benefits the latter, and the parental consent requirement does not interfere with the adolescent's ability to obtain care. However, some adolescents—for example, those who are seeking care for conditions that they cannot or will not discuss with their parents or those who are living apart from their families—are unable to obtain care if their parents' consent is required. The courts and legislatures have created numerous exceptions that enable many of these adolescents to obtain care independently of their parents.

In addition to provisions enabling minors to consent to their own care, the law in most states provides for a variety of alternatives to parental consent whereby courts or other adults may authorize care. The legal guardian of a minor would almost always be legally authorized to consent to care. Legal guardians include both individuals appointed by the court when parents are deceased or are unable or unwilling to provide proper care for their children, and juvenile or family courts that have assumed jurisdiction of a minor. In every state, juvenile or family courts may provide consent for treatment of minors who are under their jurisdiction, including children and adolescents who are delinquents, status offenders (runaways, truants, children beyond parental control), and abused and neglected children. The authority to provide the consent may be delegated to a social worker or a probation officer, although the parent usually also retains authority to consent unless parental rights have been permanently terminated. Foster parents are usually authorized to give consent, at least for ordinary care, and biologic parents themselves may authorize other adults to provide consent. In addition, most states provide for court authorization of medical care for children and adolescents who are victims of serious medical neglect.[3,8]

Consent of Minors

To facilitate the ability of adolescents to obtain care when a parental consent requirement would pose a significant barrier, the courts and legislatures have created numerous opportunities for minors to consent to their own care. Adolescents are most likely to need independent access to care when they are living apart from their parents; when they have been physically, sexually, or emotionally abused by their families; when they require sensitive services (e.g., related to sexual activity or substance abuse); or when for normal developmental reasons they desire privacy.[6,8] Most of the exceptions to the requirement of parental consent have been developed to address these situations.

Consent Based on Status

Courts and legislatures have recognized the right of minors who have a certain status to consent to their own health care. The categories of minors who may consent on the basis of their own status include mature minors; emancipated minors, including married minors; minors living apart from their parents (including runaways and homeless youths); pregnant minors; minor parents (who may be authorized to consent for themselves, their children, or both); minors older than a specified age; and high school graduates.[2,3,6] Although not every state has adopted each of these exceptions, the right of mature minors and emancipated minors to consent to their own care has been widely recognized.

Mature Minors

The doctrine of the mature minor has been developed by the courts on the basis of common law and constitutional principles. A mature minor is one who can understand the risks and benefits of the proposed treatment and is therefore able to give informed consent for the care.[5,6] As a result of the courts' willingness to rely on the mature-minor doctrine, experts agree that there is minimal risk of liability for failure to obtain parental consent when the care provided is based on the informed consent of a mature minor, when the patient is an older adolescent, when the care is not negligent, and when the treatment is provided for the minor's benefit.[5-7] Although only a few states have enacted mature-minor statutes,[2,3] courts have even been willing to recognize the mature-minor rule in the absence of a specific statute.[2,5-7] The concept of the mature minor has even provided the basis for judicial recognition of the right of an adolescent to refuse lifesaving care, particularly if there is no apparent conflict between the minor and the parent with respect to the decision.[17]

Emancipated Minors

On the basis of long-standing common law tradition dating back to colonial times, minors have been considered legally emancipated if they are married, serving in the armed forces, or living independently of their parents and managing their own financial affairs.[9] The determination that an individual adolescent was an emancipated minor traditionally occurred in the context of a specific legal dispute. More recently, however, numerous states have enacted specific statutes enabling minors to seek a court declaration of emancipation on a prospective basis if they meet statutory criteria.[2,3]

Legal emancipation generally relieves parents of the legal liability for support and grants minors many adult rights such as establishing a separate residence and entering into binding contracts. Although not every state emancipation statute explicitly authorizes emancipated minors to consent to their own health care, courts have recognized the right of emancipated minors to do so even in the absence of a specific statute.[5-7]

Consent for Specific Services

Every state has laws permitting minors to consent to a range of specific health services.[2] These services often include emergency care, contraceptive services, pregnancy-related care, diagnosis and treatment of sexually transmitted diseases (STDs) or venereal diseases, diagnosis and treatment of contagious or communicable diseases, human immunodeficiency virus (HIV) testing or treatment,[18] treatment of drug and/or alcohol problems, inpatient and/or outpatient mental health services, and care related to a rape or sexual assault. Although not every state has statutes covering each of these services, virtually every state provides for emergency care, STD or venereal disease treatment, and substance abuse treatment without parental consent. Most states have provisions covering contraceptive services and pregnancy-related care, and a growing number of states' minor consent laws include mental health services and HIV-related care. Some, but not all, of the statutes address the issues of parental notification and financial responsibility, and a few expressly relieve physicians of any liability for providing care without obtaining consent.[2,3,5,6]

The laws pertaining to reproductive health care—contraceptive care and abortion services in particular—have been the subject of extensive litigation in the state and federal courts, including the U.S. Supreme Court. These decisions have delineated the scope of the minor's privacy rights under the Constitution. Although the scope of these rights is subject to change as the Supreme Court decides new cases, at the present time certain principles have been clearly established. At minimum, minors' access to contraceptive services is protected by the right of privacy,[12] parents may not be given an arbitrary veto power over the abortion decisions of their minor daughters,[13] and a state may require parental consent for abortion only if it also establishes a "judicial bypass" procedure whereby, without parental notification, minors can obtain a court order authorizing them, if they are mature, to give their own consent or, if they are immature, determining whether an abortion would be in their best interests.[14] More than half of the states have enacted parental involvement and/or judicial bypass laws, although some of these have been enjoined by the courts; a few states have enacted alternative laws requiring counseling or consultation with a responsible adult, not necessarily a parent, before an abortion.[19]

Informed Consent

In providing most medical care, the physician has the obligation not only to obtain consent but also to ensure that the consent is informed. The doctrine of informed consent requires the disclosure to the patient of at least the following information[1,16]:

1. Diagnosis
2. Benefits and risks of the proposed procedure or treatment
3. Alternative procedures or treatments with their benefits and risks
4. Consequences of not going forward with the proposed procedure or treatment

The standard for deciding what risks must be disclosed traditionally has been the prevailing practice in the medical community, but an increasing number of states have adopted a "subjective" standard and require disclosure of any information that would be relevant to the patient's decision.[2,5,16]

Although a few of the state statutes enabling adolescents to obtain specific services without parental consent appear to relieve the physician of any liability for failure to obtain consent, many of the minor consent laws explicitly or implicitly require that the minor be capable of giving an informed consent to the care.[2,3,5] Moreover, from an ethical perspective, it is always appropriate for the practitioner who is treating the adolescent on an independent basis to ensure that the adolescent understands the proposed treatment or procedure and is voluntarily agreeing to go forward. Even when parents are providing the informed consent (e.g., for complex surgery or some other high-risk procedure), it is desirable to involve the adolescents in the decision-making process to ensure their understanding and cooperation. This is likely to increase the level of compliance among adolescent patients. It is also consistent with studies that have found adolescents to be capable of giving informed consent and making medical decisions.[3]

CONFIDENTIALITY

Maintaining the confidentiality of information concerning the health care of adolescents serves several important purposes. The assurance of confidentiality encourages adolescents to be more open in providing information about their health histories. Many adolescents are reluctant or completely unwilling to seek care without such assurance. Some live in dysfunctional families and fear hostile or abusive responses from their families; others desire privacy in their health care as part of the normal process of developing autonomy.[6]

Health care professionals are obligated both legally and ethically to maintain the confidentiality of medical information, including both verbal communications and written records.[2,5-7] This obligation is derived from a variety of legal sources and from the codes of ethics of most of the health care professions.[3,4] The legal sources include the constitutional right of privacy, the physician-patient and psychotherapist-patient privileges, and federal and state statutes requiring protection of confidentiality.[20] Many states have enacted medical confidentiality provisions or medical records legislation, and many federal funding statutes contain confidentiality requirements.[1,4,5,20] Moreover, many professional health care organizations have issued specific policy statements addressing confidentiality issues.[21]

Most communications between a health care practitioner and a patient, and most records documenting the health care services provided, are confidential and may be disclosed only with appropriate authorization.[5,22] Parents are usually entitled to have access to information, including written records, concerning their children's health care, and parental authorization is usually necessary to release that information.[3] However, in some situations, particularly if the adolescent has the right to consent to the care, it is the adolescent who has the legal right to disclose or refuse to release confidential medical information.[2,4]

In some cases the decision whether to disclose confidential information is within the discretion of the health care professional, such as when statutes permit but do not require parental notification.[2,3] In other situations the practitioner is mandated by law to disclose information. For example, every state has enacted mandatory child abuse reporting laws, which often include sexual abuse and exploitation as well as emotional abuse. Also, in most states practitioners must reveal serious dangers to the patient (such as suicidal ideation) or to others (such as violent threats against the life of an identifiable victim).[2,4,5] In addition, most states have requirements that certain STDs as well as other infectious, contagious, or communicable diseases must be reported to the local public health authority. Specific legal provisions vary among the states, and specific ethical requirements differ somewhat among the various health care professions. In any case, health care professionals have an ethical responsibility to inform their adolescent patients at the outset about the scope and the limits of confidentiality.

PAYMENT

The financial responsibility of parents for their children, which extends until the children are legally emancipated or reach the age of majority, includes the obligation to provide adequate health care.[2,5] A few of the minor consent statutes relieve parents of financial liability for care to which the minor may consent, or specify that parents may not be notified even for billing purposes; some of these statutes also specify that the minor is responsible for payment.[2,3] Few adolescents are financially capable of paying for their own medical care, even for routine services. Therefore, their access to such care is dependent on insurance coverage or publicly or privately funded sources.[23] One in seven adolescents is not insured at all, either privately or through public programs such as Medicaid, and many others are seriously underinsured.[23,24] Even those who are insured may not be able to use the coverage for care sought on an independent or confidential basis if their parents' involvement is required to access the coverage.

Many public programs provide some funding for adolescent health services or offer direct care. Federally funded programs include Medicaid and its early and periodic screening, diagnosis, and treatment (EPSDT) component; the Maternal and Child Health Block Grant; the Title X Family Planning Programs; the Alcohol, Drug Abuse, and Mental Health Block Grant; the Adolescent Family Life Act; the Community Health Centers; the Migrant Health Centers; the Indian Health Services; the Preventive Health and Health Services Block Grant; and the Hill-Burton program.[2,5] At least one of these programs, the EPSDT component of Medicaid, as amended by Congress in 1989, offers the promise of expanding adolescents' access to preventive care as well as diagnostic services and follow-up treatment if fully implemented at the state level.[25] However, despite the large number of federally funded programs, the level of funding and services is inadequate to meet the health care needs of adolescents. Moreover, the current rapid shift to managed care is having a major impact on the financing of adolescent health care services.[26] Enabling adolescents to obtain appropriate services to treat or ameliorate their health problems is an important ethical concern for practitioners and cannot be achieved without adequate funding sources.

CONCLUSION

To resolve the legal and ethical dilemmas that arise in providing services to adolescents, health care practitioners must develop a familiarity with applicable legal and ethical principles. These principles include the requirements of informed consent, which involve those laws enabling minors to consent to care based on their status or for specific services, and the obligations of confidentiality. In addition, to ensure that adolescents are able to obtain essential health care services, health care professionals must be informed about the various funding sources available for such care. Adolescent health care providers have an ethical obligation not only to treat their patients with respect by involving them in health care decisions and by honoring their need for confidentiality, but also to act as their advocates by working to expand their access to care through increased funding and development of services appropriate for adolescents.

References

 1. English A: Legal aspects of care. In McAnarney ER, Kreipe R, Orr DP, Comerci GD, editors: *Textbook of adolescent medicine,* Philadelphia, 1992, WB Saunders.
 2. English A, Matthews M, Extavour K, Palamountain C, Yang J: *State minor consent statutes: a summary,* Cincinnati, 1995, Center for Continuing Education in Adolescent Health.
 3. Gittler J, Quigley-Rick M, Saks MJ: *Adolescent health care decision making: the law and public policy,* Washington, DC, 1990, Carnegie Council on Adolescent Development.
 4. English A, Tereszkiewicz L: *School-based health clinics: legal issues,* San Francisco, 1988, National Center for Youth Law.
 5. English A: Treating adolescents: legal and ethical considerations, *Med Clin North Am* 74:1097, 1990.
 6. Morrissey JM, Hofmann AD, Thrope JC: *Consent and confidentiality in the health care of children and adolescents: a legal guide,* New York, 1986, Free Press.
 7. Holder AR: *Legal issues in pediatrics and adolescent medicine,* ed 2, New Haven, CT, 1985, Yale University Press.
 8. English A: Overcoming obstacles to care: legal issues, *Adolesc Med: State of Art Rev* 2:429, 1991.
 9. Katz SN, Schroeder WA, Sidman LR: Emancipating our children—coming of legal age in America, *Fam Law Q* 7:211, 1973.
10. *In re Gault,* 387 U.S. 1 (1967).
11. *Tinker v. Des Moines Independent School District,* 393 U.S. 511 (1969).
12. *Carey v. Population Services International,* 431 U.S. 678 (1977).
13. *Planned Parenthood of Central Missouri v. Danforth,* 428 U.S. 52 (1976).
14. *Bellotti v. Baird,* 443 U.S. 622 (1979).
15. Rozovsky FA: *Consent to treatment: a practical guide,* ed 2, Boston, 1990 and 1995 (suppl), Little, Brown.
16. Appelbaum PS, Lidz CW, Meisel A: *Informed consent: legal theory and clinical practice,* New York, 1987, Oxford University Press.
17. *In re EG, a Minor,* 549 NE2d 322 (Ill. 1990).
18. English A: Adolescents and HIV: legal and ethical questions. In Quackenbush M, Clark K, Nelson M, editors: *The HIV challenge: prevention education for young people,* ed 2, Santa Cruz, CA, 1995, ETR Associates.
19. Crosby MC, English A: Mandatory parental involvement/judicial bypass laws: do they promote adolescents' health? *J Adolesc Health Care* 12:143, 1991.
20. Soler MI, Shotton AC, Bell JR: *Glass walls: confidentiality provisions and interagency collaborations,* San Francisco, 1993, Youth Law Center.
21. Gans J, editor: *Policy compendium on confidential health services for adolescents,* Chicago, 1993, American Medical Association.
22. Roach WH, Younger P, Conner C, Cartwright KK: *Medical records and the law,* ed 2, Githersburg, MD, 1994, Aspen Publishers.
23. U.S. Congress: Office of Technology Assessment: *Adolescent health, vol 1. Summary and policy options, OTA-H-468,* Washington, DC, 1991, U.S. Government Printing Office.
24. Newacheck PW, McManus MA, Gephart J: Health insurance coverage of adolescents: a current profile and assessment of trends, *Pediatrics* 90:589, 1992.
25. English A: Early and periodic screening, diagnosis, and treatment program (EPSDT): a model for improving adolescents' access to health care, *J Adolesc Health* 14:524, 1993.
26. Society for Adolescent Medicine: A position paper on meeting the needs of adolescents in managed care. *J Adolesc Health* (in press).

CHAPTER 19

Financing Adolescent Health Services

•

Claire D. Brindis

ADOLESCENT HEALTH CARE: UNIQUE NEEDS AND CHALLENGING BARRIERS

Although they are generally regarded by most health professionals and the public at large as a healthy population, adolescents tend to manifest a set of healthcare needs unique to their age group, needs that for a significant proportion either go unmet or are addressed in a fragmented, inconsistent manner. Access to healthcare services for most adolescents largely depends on whether they have health insurance, whether services are easily accessible, and whether they feel comfortable about receiving care even when it is readily available.

Large numbers of adolescents do in fact face significant barriers to care. These include the fragmentation of health services that results from the categorical structure of public funding, and the bewildering (and sometimes conflicting) diversity of eligibility criteria imposed by categorical funding on adolescents seeking healthcare access. Lack of staff trained to respond to the specific and unique healthcare needs of adolescents, and the lack of multiple access points, are also major systemic problems.[1,2] Moreover, in addition to supplying traditional health services, healthcare providers must deal with the challenge of attempting to provide the counseling and health education services many adolescents desperately need, but for which reimbursements are either inadequate or unavailable.[3]

Many adolescent health problems are medical manifestations of difficulties rooted in social behaviors, and a large number of these health problems may be preventable. Adolescents tend not to be concerned about disease or illness and are particularly reluctant to seek care for potentially embarrassing or personal healthcare needs, especially in cases of suspected pregnancy or sexually transmitted diseases (STDs).[4] Adolescents may also forgo treatment when parental consent is required or when they are concerned about confidentiality. Despite the high incidence of adolescent pregnancy and STDs, as well as high rates of injuries, substance abuse, and psychosocial health problems, adolescents seek care much less frequently than their numbers in the population would suggest. Although they constitute 17% of the U.S. population, adolescents make only 11% of total medical office visits, the lowest visit rate for any age group.[5]

The leading causes of death among adolescents are also different from those in other age groups, with adolescents more likely to die as a result of injuries from accidents or from suicide or homicide. Other common health-threatening behaviors include riding in cars without seat belts, using illicit drugs, driving or riding with drivers under the influence of alcohol and other drugs, smoking, having unprotected intercourse, and using firearms.[6]

Although financial restrictions constitute a significant barrier to healthcare access, it is important to acknowledge that even when financial barriers are removed, other types of obstacles still prevent access in many cases. Even when services are available and adolescents are willing to seek treatment, office hours that conflict with school, social, or work schedules may also serve as barriers to care.

The challenge of adequately financing the many and unique health service needs of adolescents represents a major piece in a troubling puzzle: how to practice good medicine within the fiscal and resource constraints of our existing healthcare system. To achieve the dual goals of (1) improving the health status of adolescents and (2) simultaneously containing healthcare expenditures, the financing of adolescent health care must first be ad-

This work was supported in part by Grant No. MCJ063A80 from the Maternal and Child Health Bureau, Health Resources and Services Administration.

dressed. This chapter describes the financial barriers adolescents experience in obtaining care, as well as the financing challenge that this population represents to healthcare providers.

IMPACT OF HEALTH INSURANCE ON ADOLESCENT HEALTHCARE UTILIZATION

The most important predictor in determining whether an adolescent seeks care is the availability of a viable source of payment. Health insurance coverage plays a major role in determining if, when, where, and how often an adolescent obtains medical services. Of the approximately 30 million adolescents aged 12-17 in the United States in 1992, 4.5 million (14%) lacked reasonable access to health care because they did not have basic health insurance.[7] Uninsured adolescents are more likely than their insured counterparts to be members of poor and minority families, to use fewer health services, to experience significantly longer intervals between visits, to make fewer return visits, and to seek medical care at hospital emergency rooms.[5,7]

Ethnic minority and low-income adolescents represent disproportionately large numbers of those adolescents without health insurance. Analysis of a representative sample of data collected through the child health supplement of the 1988 National Health Interview Survey* showed that African-American and Latino adolescents were twice and three times as likely, respectively, to be uninsured as white adolescents.[5] One in three Latino adolescents reported having no health insurance.[5] Compared with 11% of white teens, 20% of African-American and 34% of Latino adolescents were without health insurance.[5]

Another barrier to care, which interacts with race and ethnicity, is poverty. Again, analysis of data from the 1989 National Health Interview Survey showed that adolescents with family incomes below the federally defined poverty level were three times as likely to be uninsured as those from families above the poverty line.[7] Of adolescents in families below the poverty level, 33% were without health insurance, compared with 10% of those above the poverty line.[5] Controlling for income, although African-American adolescents were not significantly less likely to be insured than were whites, a Latino background remained a significant predictor of insurance status.[5]

Not surprisingly, poverty not only increases the likelihood that an adolescent will lack health insurance,

but it also increases his or her risk for poor health. Because poor and nonwhite adolescents are less likely to be insured, and because they also bear the burden of poorer health status, they are far less likely to obtain care, resulting in a far greater risk for poor health.[1] Indeed, the high correlation of poverty and poor health places these adolescents at greater risk for health morbidity.[7]

Both the availability and the type of health insurance, whether a private commercial plan or a publicly subsidized insurance program such as Medicaid, influence the degree of access to care. Adolescents with private insurance are much more likely to report excellent health, and those with public or no insurance are more likely to report fair or poor health.[7] Although Medicaid coverage significantly reduces barriers to care for poor and low-income adolescents, one of every three (more than 1.7 million adolescents) with family incomes below the poverty level in 1993 had neither Medicaid nor private health insurance coverage. Nearly 1 million others whose families lived just above the poverty level were also without coverage.[5]

Even adolescents with Medicaid coverage encounter barriers to care. Because of low reimbursement levels (as well as delays in receiving reimbursement payments), increasing numbers of pediatricians will not accept Medicaid patients.[3] Because states have some latitude in setting their Medicaid reimbursement rates, the median national reimbursement level for Medicaid patients in 1989 represented only 57% to 70% of private market charges.[8] These low reimbursement rates have traditionally served as a strong disincentive for physicians to accept Medicaid patients. Again, this has racial and ethnic implications: a 1992 study revealed that, of adolescents with health insurance, African-American adolescents were significantly more likely to be insured by Medicaid than were whites, and were consequently less likely to have access to a health provider and more likely to be at risk for health morbidities.[7]

Approximately one in four adolescents have never received the primary care services recommended by professional guidelines for adolescents.[5] Within any given 2 year period, insured adolescents are twice as likely as their uninsured peers to have visited a physician at least once, often for primary care needs.[1,9] Thus, although insurance coverage is not the only factor that determines whether or not an adolescent receives routine, preventive health care, it is certainly a major one.

OTHER BARRIERS TO HEALTHCARE UTILIZATION

In addition to lack of or inadequate insurance coverage, the inability to pay for prescriptions and other medical services also serves as a barrier for adolescents

---

*Surveys conducted by the U.S. Census Bureau for the National Center for Health Statistics.

seeking care. Such financial barriers not only delay entry into the health care system, but also potentially interfere with treatment and medication compliance. Even if adolescents have insurance, when copayments are required there is some evidence that they may be less likely to return for follow-up appointments.[10]

Financial barriers are particularly troublesome for nonwhite adolescents. Not only are minority adolescents less likely to be insured, but in an examination of health-care utilization patterns documented by the 1988 National Health Interview Survey, only 59% of African-American adolescents and 58% of their Latino peers reported that their routine care was provided by a private physician or clinic or a Health Maintenance Organization (HMO), compared with 81% of the white respondents.[5] African-American and Latino adolescents were significantly more likely to identify a neighborhood clinic or a hospital as their source of primary care. According to one study, one in five Latino or other nonwhite teens reportedly had no regular source of routine care.[5] Despite data documenting that African-American and Latino adolescents exhibit poorer health relative to white adolescents, the former made significantly fewer physician visits per year.[5]

Confidentiality of services is also a major issue for adolescents. Providing health services on a confidential basis is essential before many adolescents will seek drug and alcohol counseling, mental health counseling, and services related to sexual activity (e.g., STD screening and treatment, access to contraceptives, and prenatal care). Adolescents must have access to care independent of financial constraints if they are to feel comfortable in seeking healthcare services that they wish to keep confidential. Finding ways to finance confidential services, regardless of family income or health insurance coverage, is therefore a significant challenge. Evidence shows that a great proportion of adolescents will not seek services when parental notification is required. One national survey showed that only 45% of adolescents would seek care for depression if parental consent were mandatory, and less than 20% would seek contraceptive, STD, or drug and alcohol services under the same conditions.[4] These are precisely the types of services that are critical to the overall health and well-being of adolescents as they negotiate a difficult period of life. Such particular healthcare needs can substantially influence the adolescent's general health status and often result in more serious (and expensive) health conditions in later years, if not immediately, when left untreated. These medical problems therefore have distinct financial implications both for the individual and for the public at large. The sequelae of untreated conditions will be more complicated and expensive for the individual, and for the public the costs of treating communicable diseases will be added to the already large burden shouldered by public healthcare systems.

Another obstacle to optimal health care for adolescents is the "perceived invulnerability" typical of most adolescents. Adolescents are typically unwilling to seek care in a timely manner, or do so only when they feel they are in crisis. If access to health care is difficult owing to financial, geographical, or scheduling problems, a reliance on more costly sources of care, primarily hospital emergency rooms, is very often the result. This sense of invulnerability, as well as the desire for confidential care, often means that primary care is not sought through appropriate, less expensive channels, and that the inappropriate reliance on costly emergency room care occurs unnecessarily often. To decrease these unnecessary financial costs, those in charge of health systems need to understand the developmental nuances of their adolescent patients and to develop strategies targeted specifically to adolescents. To obviate the tendency of adolescents to ignore health needs or delay seeking care, more easily accessible services must be available, such as school-based or school-linked services, as well as health education on how to use health systems more effectively. Tracking systems to ensure that adolescents follow up on appointments are also necessary.[11]

FINANCING PREVENTIVE HEALTH SERVICES

Adequate financing of health care for adolescents is contingent upon a health services framework that encompasses the full range of adolescent healthcare needs. The American Academy of Pediatrics,[12] the Institute of Medicine,[13] the American Academy of Family Physicians,[14] and the U.S. Public Health Service[15,16] all recommend that healthy adolescents be given routine preventive healthcare examinations at 2-year intervals, with more frequent examinations for those afflicted by chronic health problems. The American Medical Association (AMA) recommendations for adolescents call for yearly routine examinations as a means of preventing or delaying risk-taking behaviors.[17,18] To prevent the adoption of health-damaging behaviors, the AMA's recommended guidelines for these annual visits specify disease detection, physical growth and psychosocial health assessments, and health education and guidance. The challenge lies in how to pay for these preventive health services.

Out-of-pocket payment requirements would certainly be a deterrent for many families interested in preventive care services. Because many insurance plans do not cover routine, yearly preventive examinations, families who cannot afford out-of-pocket payments will forego annual examinations, and opportunities for early and timely investment in prevention will be missed.

Children and adolescents who are covered by private health insurance tend to enjoy a full scope of covered benefits for traditional, acute care, and inpatient medical services, such as hospital care, physician services, and prescription drugs. However, they are typically not well insured for preventive care services such as immunizations or for the case management services that are proved to be efficacious for adolescents.[19] High copayments, deductibles, and out-of-pocket expenditures can further discourage parents from purchasing health insurance that covers preventive services. This is particularly true for young and low-income families, for whom out-of-pocket expenses represent a greater proportion of total family income. In addition, inadequate reimbursement rates for preventive services usually means that these services are given very low priority by health practitioners, if they are provided at all.[20] Without specific financial incentives to reimburse physicians for providing these kinds of services, adolescents are rarely allotted the time necessary to provide them.

However, as more and more Americans join managed care programs, the incentive to keep people healthy will grow for the provider: the "profit" will not lie in treating the sick so much as in keeping people healthy. Although fee-for-service medical care progressively rewards physicians financially for diagnosing and treating greater numbers of medical conditions, it is unlikely that this situation will continue to exist. On the other hand, adolescent health advocates are concerned that, because they will be receiving a flat capitated payment, physicians with adolescent patients will not put any particular emphasis on outreach to adolescents. Without additional incentives, it is also feared that physicians will not spend the clinical time necessary to adequately respond to the unique health and psychosocial needs of adolescents. Adolescent health advocates are therefore concerned that an under-served group will become even more under-served.

Another issue is the very limited body of knowledge that speaks to the efficacy of preventive visits for adolescents, and many physicians are consequently uncertain about preventive treatment approaches. It is known that physicians are helpful in shaping the health behaviors of adults, but the degree to which they actually or potentially influence health behaviors of adolescents is not well understood.

There is also increasing evidence that rising private health insurance costs are reducing coverage of the adolescent dependents of the working insured. Faced with the challenge of having to pay a greater share of the continually growing cost of family insurance coverage, some families are choosing not to cover their dependents. Some employers have eliminated benefits for dependents altogether, the net result of which is to effectively increase the cost-sharing requirements imposed on the employees. Finally, even those adolescents fortunate enough to have private health insurance may not be covered for the services they need most, such as mental health services

and substance abuse treatment; these services, if covered at all, are often subject to stringent limitations.

SHIFT TO MANAGED CARE: IMPLICATIONS FOR FINANCING ADOLESCENT HEALTH SERVICES

From 1987 to 1990, the proportion of all employees in the United States who were covered by HMO or preferred provider health plans increased from 27% to 33%.[19] By January 1996, approximately 4.7 million Medicaid beneficiaries were enrolled in an HMO (representing almost one in five recipients), an increase of nearly 300% since 1985.

The continuing shift to a managed care health services environment carries with it a host of implications for adolescent health care. As a group, adolescents are in danger of being lost in the shuffle as this massive systemic change takes place because (1) they are under-users of health services, (2) they face a variety of problems in obtaining care, and (3) they are often uninsured or under-insured. As the proportion of adolescents covered by managed care institutions continues to grow, fewer resources may be available to finance the existing network of alternative service delivery providers. These include school-based and community health centers that adolescents have relied on for primary care and other health services in the past, particularly for such sensitive or confidential services as psychological and reproductive health needs. Unless managed care groups recognize that the existing network of providers is more responsive to adolescent health needs, it is likely that the independent community clinics, health departments, and other "safety net" providers will diminish in importance. Financing will be channeled into fewer systems. Although Medicaid billing channels in many states are currently available to school-based and community clinics as well as managed care organizations, there are plans to consolidate most providers into one capitated system of care. Managed care groups will want to be the main providers, since they need the numbers of beneficiaries to keep receiving the capitated rate. It is unlikely that managed care groups will want to share their capitated rate with other providers, unless those providers show that their services are cost effective or that they can do a better job with adolescents. School-based clinics in particular are vulnerable because little outcomes research has been conducted to establish their viability relative to other, more long-standing systems of care. However, the managed care system does hold promise that adolescents will have increased access to comprehensive primary and preventive services, because managed care plans have built-in incentives for cost containment. Preventive services are generally not covered for adolescents unless they belong to an HMO.

Throughout the United States, one prominent sign of the shift to managed care is reflected in the increasingly important role played by individual states in instituting major healthcare reforms, primarily through the implementation of managed care financing and service delivery strategies for Medicaid recipients. The expansion of Medicaid managed care promises to increase access to primary care for many low-income individuals, but at the same time states also expect healthcare providers to control service utilization, and thus expenditures, by relying on a system of fiscal gatekeepers. These primary care physicians serve as the patient's healthcare coordinator, and, in their capacity of gatekeepers, control and monitor the use of expensive specialists. Just how, and with what results, these restraints on expenditures interact with the concurrent efforts of adolescent healthcare proponents to increase access to primary care for adolescents remains to be seen. Providers and policymakers concerned with adolescent health care recognize that adolescents do not use the healthcare system as appropriately as they could and should. They also recognize that health promotion efforts directed toward adolescents must be given greater emphasis. How these goals can be attained against the tide of effort that will most certainly continue to be channeled into cost containment will require careful monitoring by adolescent health advocates and government policymakers.

In this pluralistic environment of competing interests and conflicting priorities, continued and rapid change in healthcare delivery and financing is likely to be the norm in the foreseeable future. The special challenges that adolescents represent will require a system of care that is flexible, user friendly, and comprehensive, and one that provides a variety of service entry points. Managed care systems will need to consider a variety of possible adaptations. These might include capitated or fee-for-service subcontracts with a variety of community-based health programs, such as school-based health centers.

Strong and effective outreach strategies targeted to adolescents, combined with a range of alternative entry points into the healthcare system, will be essential to ensure the equitable availability and use of healthcare resources. However, information that might illuminate the experience of adolescents enrolled in managed care plans is so far extremely limited. This effectively precludes a truly reliable assessment upon which to base plans that would encourage the most appropriate possible use of healthcare services by adolescents. Although the specific configurations of health services and financing that will emerge in the twenty-first century remain to be seen, both financial and nonfinancial barriers to care will have to be weighed and explored if—to the ultimate benefit of the larger society—the delivery of care to adolescents is to be improved to a level that truly meets their unique and complex needs.

References

1. Wood DL, Hayward RA, Corey CR, et al: Access to medical care for children and adolescents in the United States, *Pediatrics* 86:666-673, 1990.
2. Blum RW: Physicians' assessment of deficiencies and desire for training in adolescent care, *J Med Educ* 62:401-407, 1987.
3. Yudkowsky BK, Cartland JDC, Flint SS: Pediatrician participation in Medicaid: 1978 to 1989, *Pediatrics* 85:567-577, 1990.
4. English A: Ensuring access to health care for teenagers: legal and ethical issues concerning consent and confidentiality, *Youth Law News* 6:22-24, 1985.
5. Lieu TA, Newacheck PW, McManus MA: Race, ethnicity, and access to ambulatory care among U.S. adolescents, *Am J Public Health* 83:960-965, 1993.
6. Brindis CD, Irwin CE, Millstein G: U.S. profile of adolescent health. In McEnerey ER, Kreipe RE, Orr DR, Comerciz GD, editors: *Textbook of adolescent medicine,* Philadelphia, 1992, WB Saunders, pp 12-27.
7. Newacheck PW, Hughes DC, Cisternas M: Children and health insurance: an overview of percent trends, *Health Affairs* Spring: 244-254, 1995.
8. McManus M, Flint S, Kelly R: The adequacy of physician reimbursement for pediatric care under Medicaid, *Pediatrics* 87:909-920, 1991.
9. Newacheck PW, McManus MA: Health insurance status of adolescents in the United States, *Pediatrics* 84:699-708, 1989.
10. Gans JE, McManus MA, Newacheck PW: *AMA profiles of adolescent health care: use, costs, and problems of access,* Chicago, 1991, American Medical Association.
11. Brindis CD, Kapphahn C, McCarter V, Wolfe A: The impact of health insurance status on adolescents' utilization of school-based clinic services: implications for health reform, *J Adolesc Health* 16:18-25, 1995.
12. American Academy of Pediatrics Committee on Psychosocial Aspects of Child and Family Health: *Guidelines for Health Supervision II,* Chicago, 1988.
13. U.S. Department of Health, Education and Welfare: *Healthy people: the Surgeon's General's report on health promotion and disease prevention background papers.* DHEW Publication No. 79-55071 A. Washington, DC, 1979, Government Printing Office.
14. American Academy of Family Physicians: Age charts for periodic health examination. Reprint No. 510. Kansas City, MO, 1991, American Academy of Family Physicians.
15. U.S. Preventive Services Task Force: *Guide to clinical preventive services: an assessment of the effectiveness of 169 interventions. Report of the U.S. Preventive Services Task Force,* Baltimore, 1989, Williams & Wilkins.
16. Green M, editors: *Bright futures: guidelines for health supervision of infants, children and adolescents,* Arlington, VA, 1994, National Center for Education in Maternal and Child Health.
17. American Medical Association: *Guidelines for adolescent preventive services,* Chicago, 1992, American Medical Association.
18. Elster AE, Kuznets NJ: *AMA guidelines for adolescent preventive services: recommendations and rationale,* Baltimore, 1994, Williams & Wilkins.
19. Solloway MR: An overview of health insurance coverage and access to child health supervision services. In Solloway MR, Budetti PP, editors: *Child health supervision: analytical studies in the financing, delivery, and cost-effectiveness of preventive and health promotion services for infants, children and adolescents,* Arlington, VA, 1995, National Center for Education in Maternal and Child Health.
20. HMO Industry Report 6.2: *The Interstudy competitive edge,* St. Paul, Minn., 1966, Interstudy Publications.

CHAPTER 20

Assessment and Management of Pain

•

Candace J. Erickson

Since the mid-1980s there has been a surge of interest in pain management for children and adolescents. A growing body of research has begun to provide the theoretical and empirical basis on which to develop sound clinical practice. In addition to the numerous original research articles, three textbooks and a volume of the Pediatric Clinics of North America have been devoted to reviews of pediatric pain.

UNDERTREATMENT OF PAIN

Despite the recent advances in our knowledge of pediatric pain, little change has occurred in clinical practice. Wall and Melzak[1] reported the persistent undertreatment of chronic pain in adults, and numerous investigators have demonstrated that children and adolescents are rarely treated as vigorously as adults with similar problems. In fact, pediatric patients often receive little or no analgesia for postoperative or procedural pain.

Schechter[2] postulated three major reasons for this undertreatment of pediatric pain. The first factor is lack of information about pain management. Most pediatric textbooks contain little on the treatment of pain. Much of the research on pain has been published in journals outside the pediatric field, for example, in anesthesiology or neurology journals. Methodologic and ethical problems in performing pain research in children have also limited the information available. A second factor is a widespread attitude that disparages the treatment of pain and values a stoic response to discomfort. This attitude has both cultural and religious roots and influences the use of medication for relief of pain. A third factor is the number of misconceptions regarding pediatric pain.

One important misconception is that children do not experience the same degree of pain as adults because of the immaturity of their nervous system. A considerable body of evidence demonstrates that even neonates have the anatomic and neurochemical capability to experience pain and to respond to painful stimuli in ways similar to adults. A second important misconception is that a predictable amount of pain is appropriate for a specific type or amount of tissue damage. However, there is *not* a linear relationship between the amount of tissue damage and the amount of pain experienced. Consequently, there is no basis for determining that a patient is experiencing more pain than is "reasonable." Another misconception that has interfered with the provision of adequate analgesia is an exaggerated concern that the use of opioids will lead to addiction. The available research strongly indicates that addiction is rare when opioids are used for medical purposes. In fact, in a study by Porter and Jick,[3] evaluation of 11,000 hospitalized patients treated with opioids demonstrated that addiction developed in only four patients.

FACTORS AFFECTING PERCEPTION OF PAIN

In 1979, the International Association for the Study of Pain defined pain as "an unpleasant sensory and emotional experience associated with actual or potential tissue damage, or described in terms of such damage."[4] The Association stated that "... pain is always subjective. Each individual learns the application of the word through experiences related to injury in early life."[4] As this definition implies, pain is conceptualized as consisting of two components: a sensory component that is neurophysiologically based and a perceptual/experiential component that is cognitively and emotionally based.

Physiology

The sensory component of pain is initiated when tissue injury releases substances such as bradykinin, histamine, and prostaglandins, which activate and sensitize nociceptors in the skin or viscera. These nociceptors give rise to two types of primary afferent sensory neurons: thinly myelinated A-delta fibers, which mediate sharp, well localized pain; and unmyelinated C fibers, which mediate dull, poorly localized pain as well as pain from pressure, heat, or chemical irritation. These neurons enter the spinal cord and synapse with other neurons in the dorsal horn. From there the pain impulses ascend via the spinothalamic tracts; relay through the thalamus and other parts of the brain stem; and eventually terminate in the postcentral gyrus of the cortex, the limbic system, and other areas of the cortex associated with the affective components of pain perception.

In the dorsal horn, mechanisms modulate the flow of pain impulses from the peripheral nociceptors to the higher cortical centers. A-alpha fibers from the periphery can inhibit pain impulses by blocking or modulating transmission from the A-delta and C fibers. Pain transmission can also be modulated by descending inhibitory pathways from higher cortical centers. Enkephalins are important in local modulation of impulses in the dorsal horn, and norepinephrine and serotonin are important in the descending endogenous pain control pathways. In 1965 Melzak and Wall[5] developed the ''gate control theory'' that posited the modulation, or gating, of pain transmission in the spinal cord. Our current understanding of the complex circuitry that regulates pain transmission corresponds well with this concept. The existence of descending inhibitory pathways also provides a plausible biologic explanation for the influence that psychological and cognitive factors have on pain perception.

Psychological and Cognitive Factors

To adequately understand and manage pain, numerous psychological and cognitive factors that influence pain perception must be considered.

Context

The context in which the pain occurs can significantly affect the amount of pain experienced. This phenomenon was first described by Beecher,[6] an anesthesiologist in World War II, who noted that soldiers wounded in battle reported less pain and requested less analgesia than civilians with similar injuries. Injuries were expected

consequences of battle and soldiers were grateful just to be alive. War injuries were also viewed as signs of valor and often provided the soldiers with grounds for discharge. However, for civilians the injuries were unexpected, were not associated with societal accolades, and represented only an uncertain future. Consequently, the civilians felt stronger discomfort associated with injuries. Subsequent studies have confirmed the importance of the psychological meaning of pain in moderating the suffering experienced.

The difference in response to acute versus chronic pain is another example of how context influences perception of pain. Acute pain is usually perceived as an indicator that something is wrong. The individual then mobilizes to resolve the problem and eliminate the pain. This situation entails both anxiety and mobilization to action. The expectation is that once the problem is resolved, the pain will stop. With chronic pain, the pain no longer functions as a useful signal since the patient is already aware of the problem. In fact, the patient anticipates that once the pain begins, it is likely to worsen. This awareness increases the anxiety. Fear that the pain will not be treated adequately may also escalate the anxiety. Even when the pain remits, it is likely to recur, minimizing any sense of relief. Anger about disability caused by the disease and frustration over a continual lack of control can also compromise the patient's tolerance of discomfort. For patients with chronic pain, this spiral of anxiety and despair may greatly magnify the perception of pain. The provision of prompt, adequate pain relief is an important step in breaking this cycle.

Cognitive and Developmental Stages

A child's understanding of the meaning of pain is clearly influenced by his or her cognitive and developmental stages. Very young children may see pain as a random event that has no purpose. Children who are still in the egocentric stage of preschool and young school age (Piaget's preoperational stage) often see pain as a punishment for some misdeed. Older children use their cognitive abilities to understand that pain is associated with illness and that it serves as a warning signal. They can also understand that procedural pain may have a logical purpose or benefit. However, as older children and adolescents develop a greater ability for abstraction (Piaget's stage of formal operations), they may associate pain and other symptoms with tissue damage and potential disability.

The developmental stage of a child influences his or her willingness and ability to report pain experiences. Young children may not report pain because they fear the injection of pain medication. Older children and adolescents are less likely to be distressed by injections. However, even when they are afraid of shots, older youngsters can use their more developed cognitive skills to see the ultimate benefit of the injection. Younger children are less likely to report pain verbally and are more inclined to be irritable or to cry. It can sometimes be difficult to determine that pain is the cause of these symptoms. Most adolescents verbalize reports of pain and are less likely to demonstrate extreme pain behaviors such as crying. This is developmentally appropriate behavior. However, the lack of observable evidence of distress may discourage clinicians from believing a youngster's report of pain.

Previous Experience with Pain

An adolescent's previous experience with pain will affect current expectations. If previous experiences were negative, the individual is likely to be anxious and to feel helpless. An adolescent who emerged from a previous painful experience with a feeling of mastery is more likely to view the current one as a challenge that can be mastered. Reports of painful experiences by those close to the adolescent also influence feelings about and expectations of a painful experience. Therefore, it is important to assess not only the adolescent's previous experiences of pain but also the experiences and attitudes of family members and friends.

Physical and Emotional States

An individual's physical and emotional states can influence that person's tolerance of pain. Fatigue and physical discomfort can decrease pain tolerance. Similarly, anxiety and depression both accentuate pain perception. Conversely, excitement and happiness increase pain tolerance.

Gender and Culture

Research has demonstrated subtle influences of gender and culture on pain perception. Males and females have similar pain thresholds, but males demonstrate greater tolerance of laboratory-induced pain than do females. It is unclear whether this difference in tolerance is biologically based or the result of societal expectations that males be braver and stronger. Some cultures tolerate or encourage open expressions of pain; others demand a stoic acceptance of adversity. However, individual differences in how children experience pain overshadow these gender and cultural differences.

Individual Differences

When confronted with the identical painful stimulus, some adolescents continue their activities, some stop momentarily to acknowledge the discomfort and provide a simple remedy to relieve it, and others abandon their activities and behave as if a catastrophe has occurred. Petrie's study[7] of adolescents and adults described such youngsters as "reducers," "moderates," and "augmentors." Petrie found that members of each group were likely to distort their perceptions in other areas, such as in estimating size, in the same way they distorted their perception of pain. Aspirin and alcohol, both of which are associated with increased pain tolerance, significantly lessened pain for "augmentors" but had little effect on "reducers." It is unclear whether these differences reflect biologic or psychological differences, or both.

Psychological Function

Most adolescents have an emotional reaction to pain, commonly one of anxiety, anger, and/or depression. However, for some patients pain may serve a variety of psychological functions. A few examples of situations in which a youngster might have a psychological investment in experiencing pain include those in which the pain (1) elicits love and attention, especially if the adolescent is ignored when not in pain; (2) allows avoidance of feared or unwanted situations that would be unavoidable if there were no pain; (3) maintains family stability in a family that mobilizes and comes together only when the youngster is in pain; (4) is interpreted as punishment for real or imagined wrongs; (5) permits identification with a loved one who has similar pain; and (6) allows the youngster to control others. When pain serves an important psychological function, psychotherapeutic intervention needs to be directed at the underlying psychological situation.

At this point, a few words about psychogenic pain are appropriate (see Chapter 119, "Psychosomatic Disorders and Conversion Reactions"). The term *psychogenic* usually refers to pain that is not caused by tissue damage but is experienced because it serves some important psychological function. It is often difficult to distinguish pain of physical origin from psychogenic pain. A number of factors are commonly misconstrued as indicating that pain is psychogenic. Patients who are experiencing pain and are depressed or anxious are often labeled "psychosomatic." However, as noted previously, physical pain can cause anxiety and depression. When a patient responds to conversation with a decrease in pain intensity, many healthcare providers assume that the patient has been exaggerating the discomfort. However, most patients respond to conversation or other distractions with a decrease in pain perception. When a patient stages a display of pain behaviors when a caregiver is present but is quiet when alone, the patient's pain is often not believed. However, patients often feel the need to convince their physician of their pain and therefore are more explicit and dramatic about their symptoms in the presence of the physician or nurse. Once no one hears the expressions of pain, most patients conserve their energy and discontinue efforts to elicit help. In addition, when the attitude of the physician or the nurse indicates doubt of patients' self-report of pain, patients often feel compelled to be more forceful in describing their symptoms. Response to a placebo is often misinterpreted as indicating psychogenic pain even though it has been well documented that patients with clearly demonstrable tissue damage respond to placebo and other forms of suggestion. Similarly, the increasing need for a drug in a patient with a steady-state disease is often assumed to mean that the patient is not actually experiencing pain. This assumption occurs despite our knowledge that drug tolerance is a predictable consequence of the use of opioid medication.

Four indicators that pain may have its origin in psychological issues are as follows: (1) psychological factors are identifiable before the onset of pain; (2) when secondary gains are eliminated, the pain disappears; (3) the characteristics of the pain are not consistent with anatomic or neurologic distributions; and (4) a "belle indifférence" to the symptom is noted. It is important to remember that psychogenic pain is different from malingering and that it is truly experienced as pain by the patient. It should therefore be appropriately treated.

ASSESSMENT

Assessment of pain should attempt to discover the cause of the pain, record its quality and intensity, identify factors that modify the pain experienced, and determine the impact of the pain on the patient's life. Stimmel[8] proposed a mnemonic, PQRST, which can be useful in history taking. *Palliative* and *provoking* factors should be identified. The *quality* of the pain (e.g., sharp, burning, or tearing) and its *radiation* should be described. The *severity* should be assessed and followed. *Temporal* factors (e.g., relationship to meals or time of day when worse) should be delineated. Assessment of these factors aids in diagnosis, points to useful therapeutic methods, and provides the means for monitoring the effectiveness of treatment.

The intensity of pain can be measured by physiologic monitoring, observation, and self-reporting. Physiologic changes, such as in heart rate or blood pressure, are often nonspecific. Although observable pain behaviors can be externally verified, they do not allow for the fact that different behaviors may have different meanings to different individuals. Because pain is by definition a subjective experience, self-reporting of pain is essential. Self-report measures have proved reliable across a large age range. Children 7 years of age or older are able to report the intensity of their pain with a visual analog scale.

On this type of scale the youngster draws a line to indicate his or her discomfort level at the appropriate point on a 10-cm horizontal line; the left end of the line is labeled "no pain" and the right end is labeled "the worst possible pain." Tools such as the Varni/Thompson Pediatric Pain Questionnaire[9] and the McGill Pain Questionnaire[10] can be used to obtain a more complete description of the youngster's pain and pain behaviors.

TREATMENT

Several general considerations should be mentioned before specific treatment modalities are discussed. Because pain is a symptom, it is essential to determine the cause and to treat the underlying problem when possible. When the symptom of pain is being treated, the approach should be preventive. Whenever possible, pain should be eliminated and prevented from recurring. Less medication is required to prevent pain than to control it once it has occurred. Because of this principle, prn (as needed) medication orders are not appropriate in the treatment of pain. Such orders often result in the patient experiencing considerable amounts and duration of pain before medication is administered. Finally, pain treatment must be individualized. The specific combination of treatments used should be determined by the patient's needs. Because there is *no* linear relationship between the amount of tissue damage and the severity of pain experienced, each patient should receive whatever intervention is needed to control the pain. Medication should be titrated against the patient's pain, the end point being the effective prevention of pain. Only the emergence of unacceptable side effects should limit the amount of medication given.

Cognitive and Behavioral Approaches

INSTRUCTION. Many youngsters have difficulty tolerating pain because they are frightened. A simple, calm explanation of what is happening and how it is going to feel often soothes anxieties and permits the adolescent to feel some control over the situation. It is particularly useful to anticipate the physical sensations that the patient may experience. When a youngster is anxious, any strange sensation will be startling and may be interpreted as pain. Anticipating the sensation diminishes the startle response, and labeling the sensation (e.g., saying that a tourniquet will be tight) can help reframe it away from pain.

CONTROL. Patients in pain often feel out of control. Therefore, promoting control in any way possible can be helpful. In a study of patients with burn injuries, Kavanagh[11] developed a program that emphasized patient control and predictability of aversive events. Children were encouraged to participate in changing their own wound dressings and were permitted to schedule the dressing changes. The youngsters became increasingly involved in the task and required significantly fewer analgesics for debridement. They also showed fewer of the psychological consequences common among burn patients with long hospitalizations.

DISTRACTION. Providing age-appropriate activities for patients can often help distract them from their pain. The more interesting the activity to the individual, the more effective it will be in distracting him or her and in decreasing the awareness of discomfort. In addition to conversation, video games and music are especially useful distraction techniques for adolescents.

RELAXATION. Multiple techniques are available for eliciting a physiologic relaxation response in adolescents.[12] Progressive relaxation consists of alternate tensing and relaxing of each muscle group in succession. Biofeedback uses physiologic monitoring to help the youngster identify and replicate relaxation responses. In meditation, the patient is asked to focus attention on a specific word or idea or to pay attention to body processes, particularly breathing. The use of relaxation decreases anxiety and diminishes the muscular tension that often accompanies, and may exaggerate, pain. Relaxation has proved particularly useful in the control of tension headaches.

SELF-HYPNOSIS. Self-hypnosis refers to a self-induced state of relaxation accompanied by focused attention and mental imagery. Specific images can be used to suggest analgesia. Pain control usually begins while the subject is in an altered state of consciousness or "trance." However, with posthypnotic suggestion the analgesia can persist for several hours after the subject has emerged from the trance. Multiple studies have demonstrated the successful use of hypnosis for management of procedural pain in children and adolescents.[13] One well-controlled study found hypnosis to be more effective than propranolol in the treatment of juvenile migraine headaches.[14] Self-hypnosis is simple and easy to learn, requiring an average of four sessions for older children to accomplish control of pain. Youngsters are much more adept at learning hypnotic skills than adults, and most children can learn to use hypnosis well.

The advantages of self-hypnosis for control of pain are that (1) it promotes a sense of autonomy and mastery, (2) it has virtually no side effects, (3) it avoids the sedation and other side effects seen with pharmacotherapy, and (4) it can be used for treatment of anxiety and nausea as well as for pain. The only drawbacks to the use of hypnosis are the skepticism and resistance of patients, families, and health professionals and the scarcity of appropriately trained professionals to train the patients in hypnotic skills.

COGNITIVE STRATEGIES. Several studies have demonstrated the effectiveness of teaching children and adolescents techniques for talking themselves through pain. These include having the patient find something good in the situation (e.g., saying "It will be over quickly" or "It will help me get better faster") or reminding the patient of ways to cope with the pain (e.g., saying "I can take deep breaths" or "I can count to ten and it will be over."). It can also be helpful to explore the patient's understanding of pain. Most youngsters see pain as "bad." They often forget that pain is an important warning signal from the body that protects them from harm. Reframing pain as a useful and important part of the body's defense system frequently helps youngsters shift from a negative attitude toward pain to a more neutral stance.

Physical Measures

HEAT AND COLD. The time-honored advice for the treatment of fractures—elevation, immobilization, and application of ice—is still sound. Cold may decrease pain through two mechanisms: by reducing hyperemia and swelling, thus decreasing discomfort; and by directly suppressing neuronal excitability. If pain is caused by problems such as muscle spasm, applying heat may increase perfusion and relax the muscle. Alternating heat and cold can also be effective, especially in deafferentation pain such as stump pain after amputation.

TRANSCUTANEOUS ELECTRICAL NERVE STIMULATION. In transcutaneous electrical nerve stimulation (TENS), a battery-operated signal generator with conductive pads is used to apply a small electrical current to the skin. The electrical current causes a "buzzing" sensation in the dermatomes to which it is applied. According to the "gate control" theory, TENS effects analgesia by increasing the large fiber input to the spinal cord, thereby inhibiting afferent nociceptive transmission. TENS has proved effective for management of acute somatic pain and many forms of chronic neuropathic pain. Its effectiveness depends on positioning the electrodes properly (near the painful site, in corresponding dermatomes, or at acupuncture points), varying the pulse characteristics (frequency and continuous vs. burst modes), and increasing the intensity of the stimulus until discomfort or muscular contractions occur. Although TENS is safe, it should not be used on the anterior neck because of the risk of hypotension as a result of baroreceptor stimulation. Other contraindications include the presence of a demand pacemaker, skin irritation or hypersensitivity, and the patient's (or parents') inability to understand the principles of operation.

ACUPUNCTURE. Acupuncture is an ancient Chinese technique in which very fine needles are placed at specific points, known as acupuncture points, in the skin. These points correspond to trigger points and points of low electrical resistance. Recently, variations of acupuncture have been developed, including acupressure, in which finger pressure is substituted for the needles, and electroacupuncture, in which electrical current is applied through the needles. Although the mechanism through which acupuncture controls pain remains unclear, some reports state that acupuncture analgesia is reversed by naloxone. Although no controlled studies of the use of acupuncture in children have been done, there have been anecdotal reports of its effectiveness in a variety of conditions, including headache, peripheral neuropathic pain, and chronic chest pain in cystic fibrosis. Acupuncture has no serious side effects provided that sterile, disposable needles are used. However, some youngsters reject acupuncture because they fear needles.

Pharmacologic Approaches

Analgesic medication should be viewed as only one component of pain management. Many of the interventions previously described have no significant side effects and can control or substantially diminish pain and suffering. Their use may eliminate or reduce the amount of medication required to treat a patient's pain, thus decreasing potential side effects from the medication. Since the aim of therapy is to eliminate the pain and prevent its return, it is important to prescribe adequate amounts of medication on a regularly scheduled basis. The type and amount of medication needs to be individualized. The World Health Organization's Cancer Pain Initiative developed a three-step model for analgesics.[15] Nonopioid analgesics with or without adjuvants can be used for management of mild pain. A weak opioid is used in conjunction with a nonopioid analgesic and adjuvants for management of moderate pain or persistent mild pain. For management of severe pain, a strong opioid should be used with a nonopioid and adjuvants. It is recommended that analgesics be used in a stepwise fashion in order of increasing potency. However, it is imperative to ensure that the selected frequency and dosage of medication is effective in maintaining adequate analgesia. Administering medication in quantities barely sufficient to control the pain when the medication is at its peak level will result in significant periods of pain.

Drugs such as nonopioid analgesics and codeine, which have a ceiling effect, produce no significant increase in analgesia if the dose is increased beyond the usual therapeutic level. To increase analgesia with such drugs, an additional analgesic or adjuvants must be administered; otherwise, it is necessary to progress to a stronger analgesic. The stronger opioids do not exhibit a ceiling effect, and doses can be increased as needed unless unacceptable side effects result. Tolerance, which is defined as diminished effectiveness of the drug after repeated administration, may develop with the use of opioids and can be managed by increasing the dosage. Physical dependence, which is defined as the need to continue administration of the drug to prevent withdrawal symptoms, often occurs in individuals who have received opioids for 2 weeks or more.

It is postulated that withdrawal symptoms occur because the exogenous administration of opioids decreases the level of normally present endogenous opioids. When the exogenous opioids are withdrawn, insufficient quantities of endogenous opioids remain and withdrawal symptoms occur. Withdrawal can be managed once opioids are no longer required for analgesia by tapering the dosage of the drug over a 5- to 7-day period.

It should be underscored that physical dependence is not the same as addiction. Addiction is a psychological syndrome characterized by compulsive drug-seeking behavior that is usually associated with a desire to achieve euphoria rather than analgesia. No evidence indicates that administration of opioids for control of pain results in addiction. On the contrary, it can be argued that reluctance to treat pain adequately is more likely to lead to obsessive concerns with obtaining medication.

Children often fail to report pain if they think they will receive an injection. Therefore, when parenteral medication is needed, intravenous administration should be considered. Continuous intravenous administration of opioids avoids the peaks and troughs associated with bolus administration and is consequently safer and more effective in providing continuous pain relief. Patients can control analgesia by the use of a computer-driven pump that allows them to titrate the opioids by self-administering regulated amounts of medication. This type of device has been used extensively with teenagers postoperatively. Patients are usually able to maintain an acceptable level of comfort with minimal side effects. They appear to benefit from the control that self-administration affords, and they generally require a smaller total dose of opioids than with other modes of administration. While nonopioids are ordinarily administered orally, clinicians may forget that opioids also can be effective when given orally. If intravenous access is problematic, orally administered opioids should be considered before intramuscular injections. However, it must be remembered that equianalgesic oral doses are considerably higher than the parenteral dose (Table 20-1).

Many analgesic medications have known side effects. The clinician should be familiar with these effects and be prepared either to change the pain management regimen or to treat the side effects. The usual side effects of common analgesic agents are described later. However, effective analgesia can usually be obtained without significant side effects.

NONOPIOID PERIPHERAL ANALGESICS. These medications are thought to act peripherally by decreasing the

TABLE 20-1
Recommended Starting Doses for Analgesic Medication*

Drug	Route	Dose (mg/kg/dose)	Frequency
Acetaminophen	PO	10-15	4 hr
	PR	15-20	4 hr
Aspirin	PO	10-15	4 hr
Ibuprofen	PO	4-10	6-8 hr
Naproxen	PO	5-7	8-12 hr
Tolmetin	PO	5-7	6-8 hr
Ketorolac (Toradol)	PO	0.5-1.0	6 hr
	IM	0.5-1.0	6 hr
Codeine	PO	0.5-1.0	4 hr
Morphine	Continuous IV or SC	0.05-0.06 mg/kg/hr	
	IV bolus	0.08-0.10	2 hr
	IM/SC	0.1-0.15	3-4 hr
	PO	0.2-0.4	4 hr
Morphine (timed release) (MS Contin, Oramorph SR)	PO	0.3-0.6	12 hr
Meperidine (Demerol)	IV	0.8-1.0	2 hr
	IM/SC	0.8-1.3	3-4 hr
	PO	1.0-2.0	4 hr
Methadone	IV	0.1	q 4 hr initially, then q 6-12 hr[†]
	PO	0.1	4-12 hr
Hydromorphone (Dilaudid)	IM	0.02-0.03	2-4 hr
	PO	0.05-0.10	4 hr
Fentanyl citrate	IV	1-2 µg	1-2 hr

PO, by mouth; PR, per rectum; IV, intravenous; SC, subcutaneous; IM, intramuscular.
*These recommendations are for patients who have not had previous repeated or prolonged exposure to opioids. For all medications, doses should be adjusted to the needs of the individual. With severe, ongoing, acute pain or chronic pain, opioid doses should be increased steadily until comfort is achieved, unless limited by side effects.
[†]Methadone requires careful titration. If somnolence occurs, the interval between doses should be increased or the dose should be diminished immediately.

production of prostaglandin, a substance that sensitizes nociceptors to the histamine and bradykinin released at sites of tissue injury. Although it is postulated that these agents may also act centrally, normal therapeutic doses do not affect mood or sensorium. Since these agents exhibit a ceiling effect, there is no clinical usefulness in increasing doses beyond the normal therapeutic range.

Acetaminophen. This is the drug of choice for management of mild pain. It has both antipyretic and analgesic effects. Unfortunately, it does not have antiinflammatory properties. Acetaminophen, which is well absorbed orally, is available as elixir, oral drops, pills, and chewable tablets. To avoid overdosing or undermedicating, parents should be warned that the concentration of acetaminophen, and therefore the volume dose, is different for the two liquid forms. Rectal absorption of acetaminophen is erratic. After oral administration, acetaminophen is detectable in the blood within 20 to 30 minutes, and its peak analgesic efficacy occurs in about 1 hour. Acetaminophen does not cause gastritis or bleeding problems, nephropathy is unlikely with therapeutic doses, and hepatic damage is primarily of concern in cases of overdosage.

Aspirin. Although long the standard with which other peripheral analgesics were compared, aspirin use in children and adolescents has decreased in recent years. Aspirin has both antipyretic and anti-inflammatory properties in addition to its analgesic action. It is rapidly absorbed orally, with an onset of action in 15 to 30 minutes and peak effectiveness in 60 to 90 minutes. It is available in pills and chewable tablets, but no adequate liquid preparation is available. Although suppositories are available, rectal absorption is variable. The most common side effect of aspirin is gastric irritation, which can be diminished by consuming it with food or antacids. Aspirin decreases levels of factor VII and interferes with platelet aggregation, which limits its usefulness in patients with hematologic compromise. Aspirin is contraindicated for patients with varicella or influenza because it has been implicated in the development of Reye's syndrome.

Nonsteroidal antiinflammatory drugs. Like aspirin, nonsteroidal antiinflammatory drugs (NSAIDs) are particularly useful in the treatment of inflammatory pain, bone pain, and pain associated with rheumatoid conditions. NSAIDs exhibit antipyretic and antiinflammatory properties in addition to their analgesic effects. The advantage of these medications[5] over aspirin is that the maximal analgesia attainable is greater; however, NSAIDs have not been extensively studied in children and adolescents and are considerably more expensive than aspirin. They are well absorbed orally. Ibuprofen and tolmetin require administration four times a day, whereas naproxen has a longer duration of action and can be administered twice or three times daily. Because NSAIDs have side effects similar to those of aspirin, they should be consumed with meals and their use should be avoided in patients with bleeding problems. Nephrotoxicity and hepatotoxicity are rare when NSAIDs are used for only several weeks; however, either may occur during long-term use for arthritic conditions. Patients receiving long-term NSAID therapy should have renal and hepatic function monitored twice yearly. Interestingly, an adverse reaction to one NSAID does not indicate that a similar reaction will necessarily occur with administration of a different NSAID.

Ketorolac (Toradol) is a NSAID that can be administered orally or parenterally. It was originally released for oral and intramuscular administration, although there have been reports of intravenous use also. It has advantages over opioids in that it does not cause respiratory depression or nausea and vomiting. It can be combined with acetaminophen or opioids. The starting dose is 0.5 to 1.0 mg/kg every 6 hours. Bioavailability of the drug appears to be equivalent across all routes of administration. As with all NSAIDs, potential adverse effects include decreased renal function, hypokalemia, and bleeding diatheses. There have also been reports of bronchospasm and anaphylactoid reactions in adults.

Combination preparations. A number of over-the-counter preparations that combine caffeine, buffers, antihistamines, or antispasmodics with aspirin or acetaminophen are available. Moertel et al[16] compared a number of these preparations with generic aspirin and found that none were superior to aspirin. Because these combination preparations are more expensive and are not more effective than aspirin, plain acetaminiophen or aspirins remain the drug of choice for mild analgesia.

OPIOID ANALGESICS. Opioid analgesics are thought to work by mimicking endogenous opioids. They bind to the opioid receptors in the brain, brain stem, and spinal cord. One specific receptor, the mu receptor, is generally associated with analgesia, but it is possible that the differences in analgesia and side effects between opioid medications are the results of different receptor specificities with actions at the kappa or sigma receptors. Pain has both a sensory and an affective component, and opioids affect both components of pain. They suppress autonomic responses to noxious stimuli (e.g., tachycardia, hypertension, and sweating) and they also greatly diminish the distress experienced by the patient. Patients often report that the pain is still present but that it no longer bothers them. This effect may be related to the euphoria caused by opioids.

The effective analgesic dose of opioids varies not only from drug to drug but also from person to person.

Because most opioids are pure agonists, they do not have a ceiling effect and the dose can be increased until analgesia is obtained. The doses listed in Table 20-1 are guides for starting doses in patients who have not received opioids previously. The elimination half-life of most opioids is 2 to 3 hours; therefore, in patients with severe pain, the administration of the medication every 4 to 6 hours will lead to extreme fluctuations in plasma levels and alternating periods of comfort and pain.

The various routes of administration for opioids are oral, intravenous, subcutaneous, intramuscular, transmucosal (nasal, buccal, and rectal), transdermal, and neuraxial (epidural and subarachnoid). Oral preparations of all commonly administered opioids are available, and the oral route is recommended if the patient can ingest and absorb pills or elixirs. Orally administered opioids can be effective even in patients with severe pain. However, because the oral/parenteral ratio of equianalgesic doses may be as high as 6:1, oral doses need to be appropriately higher than parenteral doses (see Table 20-1). Intravenous boluses can cause significant fluctuations in plasma level and should be given slowly and at sufficiently short intervals to ensure a constant effect. Continuous intravenous or subcutaneous administration is ideal to provide a constant plasma level; however, both require use of infusion pumps and the former requires intravenous access. Continuous infusions also require that the staff maintain vigilance in monitoring the effects of the medication. Subcutaneous administration may lead to local skin irritation. Intramuscular administration results in less dramatic fluctuations of plasma levels than does a comparable intravenous bolus. However, intramuscular injections should be avoided because of the anxiety and pain caused by the injections. Transmucosal administration results in variable absorption and may not be possible in the presence of mucositis. Transdermal administration also has variable absorption, as well as having a delayed onset of action and residual effect after removal of the patch. Neuroaxial administration requires invasive procedures, but it may be effective even when a patient's pain is refractory to systemic opioids.

Numerous side effects are common to all opioids, with respiratory depression a main concern. Opioids decrease the ventilatory response to hypoxemia and hypercapnia. However, for most patients a wide margin exists between the analgesic dose and a dose that will cause respiratory depression. Patients with respiratory insufficiency, airway compromise, and certain neurologic conditions may be more sensitive to opioid-induced respiratory depression. Therefore, reduced doses and careful monitoring are necessary in these patients. Opioid effects on respiration can usually be monitored through decrements in respiratory rate. Maximal respiratory depression occurs 7 minutes after intravenous administration, 30 minutes after intramuscular administration, and 90 minutes after subcutaneous administration. Naloxone can reverse the actions of opioids; however, a full reversal dose (0.01 to 0.02 mg/kg) can precipitate dysphoria, acute anxiety, nausea and vomiting, and (rarely) pulmonary edema. Therefore, full reversal should be used only in life-threatening situations. If time permits, the dose of naloxone can be titrated in smaller increments (0.002 mg/kg) to secure the return of spontaneous respirations but not effect a full reversal of sedation or analgesia. In less severe cases, oxygen can be administered, and the patient can be stimulated and reminded to breathe until the respiratory depression subsides. Continual observation is required until the patient is breathing spontaneously. The effects of naloxone are short-lived (30 to 45 minutes), so renarcotization is possible and prolonged monitoring of respiratory status is indicated. Naloxone can be readministered as frequently as every 2 to 3 minutes if necessary. Fortunately, tolerance for respiratory depression and sedation parallels tolerance for analgesia; therefore, increasing the dose of medication to effectively control pain is unlikely to lead to respiratory depression.

Tolerance often develops with prolonged use of opioids and can be managed by increasing the dose. Although tolerance for sedation and respiratory depression parallels tolerance for analgesia, this is not true of other side effects such as constipation. Dependence may occur after 1 to 2 weeks of opioid use and requires continued administration of the drug to prevent withdrawal symptoms such as tachycardia, tachypnea, sweating, diarrhea, dysphoria, and agitation. Physical dependence can be managed by tapering the dose of the opioid over a 5- to 7-day period once analgesia is no longer required. As noted previously, dependence is not the same as addiction.

Sedation is another common side effect of opioids. Although sedation may be useful for patients undergoing painful procedures, it is often troublesome for ambulatory patients. A range of doses can produce analgesia without marked sedation; however, if sedation is a problem, it can be treated with stimulants.

Opioids slow intestinal motility and thus frequently cause constipation. This side effect should be anticipated and treated with stool softeners or laxatives to stimulate peristalsis. Nausea and vomiting can also be troublesome side effects of opioids; if extreme, they can be treated with phenothiazines or other antiemetics. Opioids stimulate the release of histamine, causing pruritus, which can be controlled by antihistamines such as diphenhydramine hydrochloride or hydroxyzine. Other side effects of opioids can include cough suppression, miosis, urinary retention, biliary spasm, and vasodilation.

Since opioids are metabolized in the liver and the metabolites are excreted in the urine, patients with hepatic or renal dysfunction may have an exaggerated response to all effects of opioids.

Codeine. Codeine is a weak opioid that is well absorbed orally; it is often used alone or in combination with aspirin or acetaminophen for relief of moderate pain. Like the nonopioid analgesics, codeine has a ceiling effect, so that escalating the dosage above the normal therapeutic range provides little additional analgesia. However, combining codeine with a peripherally acting nonopioid produces more analgesia than either agent would generate independently. Such combinations are recommended because they are more effective without causing additional side effects.

Morphine. Morphine is the standard with which all other opioids are compared. It is inexpensive, has been well studied, and has been used extensively in children and adolescents. For relief of acute pain, the oral/parenteral ratio is 6:1. However, with chronic administration the effect of the enterohepatic circulation and the analgesic properties of a metabolite make the oral/parenteral ratio closer to 3:1. The availability of several new oral time-released preparations allow administration two or three times daily.

Meperidine. Meperidine (Demerol) has little or no advantage over morphine. Its duration of effect is slightly shorter because morphine is trapped across the blood-brain barrier. In the chronic administration of meperidine, accumulation of normeperidine, an active metabolite, has been associated with dysphoria and seizures.

Methadone. Methadone is metabolized slowly and has a prolonged duration of action. It is well absorbed after oral administration. Methadone requires careful titration because its analgesic effects last from 6 to 8 hours and its plasma half-life is 17 to 24 hours. If somnolence occurs, either the dose should be decreased immediately or the interval between doses should be significantly prolonged. After initial loading, a constant clinical effect can usually be maintained by administering the medication every 4 to 6 hours intravenously or every 6 to 8 hours orally. Since methadone cause little euphoria, it is an excellent drug to administer to youngsters with chronic pain because it permits them to engage in their daily activities without an altered sensorium.

Hydromorphone hydrochloride. Hydromorphone (Dilaudid) is similar to morphine in most respects. Its elixir form is reportedly more palatable than morphine elixir.

Fentanyl citrate. Fentanyl is a potent, short-acting opioid that generates far less histamine release than morphine, thus causing less pruritus and vasodilation. Its short duration of effect makes this medication ideal for sedation and analgesia in short, painful procedures. The decreased histamine release also makes this agent useful for continuous infusion in patients in whom other opioids cause pruritus refractory to antihistamines. Fentanyl is highly lipophilic and can be administered mucosally or transdermally. Currently, use of a fentanyl lollipop for procedural analgesia is being investigated.

LOCAL ANESTHETICS. In the hands of an anesthesiologist, local anesthetics can be used quite effectively in nerve blocks or through epidural administration. However, these types of anesthestics are more commonly used for painful procedures, such as various types of punctures and suturing of lacerations. When local anesthetics are used, there are two important considerations to keep in mind. First, for adequate pain control, the anesthetic must be administered sufficiently in advance of the procedure to have time to take effect. Second, it is always important to consider the potential effects of systemic absorption of the anesthetic. Three commonly used local anesthetics are discussed below.

Lidocaine. The term *local anesthetic* usually refers to lidocaine and similar drugs that are administered into the skin or a wound through local infiltration. The potential for systemic toxicity from this use of these drugs is dependent on (1) the dose administered, (2) the vascularity of the site, (3) alterations of the rate of systemic uptake (e.g., use of vasoconstrictors), (4) alterations of the threshold of toxicity (e.g., concomitant administration of diazepam, which increases the seizure threshold), and (5) how the medication is administered (e.g., aspiration before injection to prevent intravenous administration). Systemic toxicity of local anesthetics includes central nervous system excitation with possible seizures, decreased cardiac contractility, and vasodilation. The best way to guard against systemic toxicity is to set a limit on the total dose of anesthetic that will be given. For lidocaine, the maximal dose should be 7.0 mg/kg. A 1% solution of lidocaine has contains 10 mg/ml.

Tetracaine, adrenaline, and cocaine. In recent years, two topical anesthetics have been developed and are now in common use. The first of these is a combination of tetracaine, adrenaline, and cocaine (TAC). There have been several formulations of TAC, but the dilute solution of 1.0% (10 mg/ml) tetracaine, 1:4000 (250 μg/ml) epinephrine, and 4.0% (40 mg/ml) cocaine is just as effective as more concentrated solutions, with less potential for toxicity. Using this concentration of solution, the total dose should be limited to 1.5 ml per 10 kg body weight. The solution is placed in a sponge or pledget, which is then placed in the wound. TAC should not be used on mucous membranes, because enhanced absorption will increase possible systemic toxicity. It should not be used in areas with limited circulation, such as the penis or digits, because of the vasoconstriction caused by both epinephrine and cocaine.

EMLA. A second topical anesthetic is EMLA cream. EMLA is a eutectic mixture of local anesthetics, lidocaine 2.5% and prilocaine 2.5%. A glob of this cream is placed directly on intact skin and covered with an occlusive dressing for 60 minutes (120 minutes may be required for highly pigmented skin). Increasing the duration of application increases both the anesthetic effect and the depth of the anesthesia. However, an anesthetic effect has not been reported below the dermal layers, so EMLA would not be expected to affect any muscular pain from an IM injection. Absorption will vary depending on the thickness of the skin, with onset of action most rapid on areas with thin skin. The site of application can remain anesthetized for up to 2 hours after removal of the cream. Common adverse reactions include blanching, redness, and itching. EMLA should not be used on open wounds, on mucous membranes, or in children under 1 month of age because of the increased potential for systemic toxicity. It can cause severe eye irritation, and it has an ototoxic effect when instilled into the middle ear. EMLA should not be used in patients with methemoglobinemia or in those receiving treatment with methemoglobin-inducing agents.

ADJUVANT MEDICATIONS

Tricyclic antidepressants. The tricyclics imipramine hydrochloride and amitriptyline hydrochloride have been shown to decrease reported pain and pain behaviors and to improve mood and functional parameters, such as sleep and school attendance, in patients with various forms of chronic and neuropathic pain. These agents are thought to work through the monoaminergic pain inhibitory systems in the central nervous system. Generally, analgesia and sleep improvement occur sooner and at lower doses than do the antidepressant effects. A single small dose of a tricyclic taken 1 to 2 hours before bedtime can be effective for analgesia as well as for normalizing sleep. The most common side effects are morning drowsiness and dry mouth, which represent anticholinergic effects. These side effects usually diminish over time and can be minimized by starting with small doses and increasing the dose slowly every few days. Either amitriptyline or imipramine can be started with single evening doses of 0.1 mg/kg; the dose can be advanced as tolerated over 2 to 3 weeks to 0.5 to 2 mg/kg. Tricyclics can cause conduction abnormalities. Therefore, if the patient's history or physical examination indicates possible problems or if large doses are required, electrocardiographic (ECG) monitoring of conduction and repolarization should be performed.

Stimulants. Methylphenidate hydrochloride and dextroamphetamine both enhance analgesia and counteract the sedation caused by opioids. They have been particularly useful in the management of pain in patients with cancer. The use of stimulants for treatment of conditions other than cancer pain should be considered carefully, and they should be employed only on a short-term basis. The starting dose is 0.05 to 0.1 mg/kg given orally early in the morning and again at midday. Evening doses can cause sleep disruption. If necessary, the dose can be advanced to 0.2 to 0.3 mg/kg.

Neuroleptics. Phenothiazines and butyrophenones have been combined with opioids to produce sedation for procedures. However, whether neuroleptics provide any analgesia is a controversial matter. In fact, some phenothiazines, such as promethazine hydrochloride (Phenergan), are probably antianalgesic. Neuroleptics have been useful in the treatment of nausea and vomiting; the dosage required for treating opioid-associated nausea is much lower than that for nausea associated with chemotherapy. These medications can also be useful in the treatment of severe anxiety reactions. However, neuroleptics may produce sedation, aggravate respiratory depression, cause dysphoria, and occasionally lead to extrapyramidal side effects such as dystonic reactions and tardive dyskinesia. The incidence of extrapyramidal symptoms can be diminished by concomitant treatment with antihistaminic/central anticholinergic drugs such as diphenhydramine hydrochloride.

Antihistamines. These medications are used principally to treat opioid side effects such as pruritus or to counteract reactions to neuroleptics. There is little if any analgesic action. The predominant action is sedation, and the margin of safety for the use of antihistamines as sedatives is quite high.

Anticonvulsants. Neuropathic pain may be associated with increased excitability of peripheral nerves, and sometimes it responds to anticonvulsants. Carbamazepine (Tegretol), phenytoin, and clonazepam are the most commonly used anticonvulsants in this context.

Sedatives. It is often useful to provide youngsters with sedation during painful episodes, particularly when dealing with the pain generated by medical procedures. The use of a sedative can substantially decrease the adolescent's anxiety in such situations and can provide both retrograde and anterograde amnesia about the procedure. However, it must be remembered that when a sedative is used alone, it does *not* provide any analgesia. Sedatives, except for those such as morphine and ketamine, which are primarily analgesics, should *always* be used in conjunction with some form of analgesia during painful procedures. A number of other potential problems must be kept in mind when using sedatives. Combining sedatives with narcotic analgesics increases sedation and the risk of respiratory depression. It is difficult to attain just a level of conscious sedation and to avoid slipping into deep sedation. Often a youngster can be at a level of conscious sedation before a procedure begins, but then the stimulus of the procedure arouses the patient to a level where he or she is reacting more forcefully than is desired. Meanwhile, because of the effect of the sedative, the youngster behaves as if drunk and can no longer use intrinsic cognitive abilities to help cope with the procedure. When this happens during a procedure, it is tempting to give more sedative to suppress the youngster's response. Administering more sedative may provide a level of sedation appropriate during the procedure, but it can then cause oversedation once the procedure is completed and the additional stimulation

ceases. This problem can often be minimized by ensuring that sufficient amounts of analgesics are administered in conjunction with the sedation, so that there is good pain control. Absence of pain often decreases the stimulus of the procedure to a level that does not disrupt the sedation. Because of the potential risks of oversedation during medical procedures, the Committee on Drugs of the American Academy of Pediatrics (AAP) in 1992 revised the Academy's guidelines for monitoring and management of pediatric patients during and after sedation for diagnostic and therapeutic procedures.[17] Because these guidelines are now the basis for standard medical practice, all physicians working with children or adolescents should be conversant with them. Therefore, they are reviewed briefly here. Any physician prescribing sedation should first study the complete Committee Guidelines.

The guidelines define *conscious sedation* as "a medically controlled state of depressed consciousness that (1) allows protective reflexes to be maintained, (2) retains the patient's ability to maintain a patent airway independently and continuously, and (3) permits appropriate response by the patient to physical stimulation or verbal command (e.g., 'open your eyes')." At this level of sedation, the guidelines state that an anesthetic-type record must be maintained and that vital signs must be recorded periodically. Pulse oximetry and some type of continuous cardiac monitoring is required. Support staff can assist in the monitoring of the patient. After the procedure is completed, the patient must be monitored in a recovery room setting where he or she can be observed constantly and where vital signs can be monitored and recorded periodically. The guidelines define *deep sedation* as "a medically controlled state of depressed consciousness or unconsciousness from which the patient is not easily aroused. It may be accompanied by a partial or complete loss of protective reflexes, and includes the inability to maintain a patent airway independently and respond purposefully to physical stimulation or verbal command." For patients who are deeply sedated, the following are required both during and after the procedure: (1) an independent observer, i.e., *not* a person involved in performing the procedure, should observe the patient continuously and record vital signs at least every 5 minutes; (2) in addition to pulse oximetry and cardiac monitoring, some method for monitoring ventilatory adequacy, such as capnography or a precordial stethoscope, should be used; (3) a defibrillator and an ECG monitor must be readily available; (4) at least one of the individuals present "must be trained in, and capable of, providing basic life support, and . . . skilled in airway management and cardiopulmonary resuscitation; training in pediatric advanced life support is strongly encouraged"; and (5) intravenous access is necessary. The independent observer and the availability of a defibrillator and an ECG monitor are also required by the Joint Commission on Accreditation of Healthcare Organizations. Conditions necessary for discharge from monitoring when using either conscious sedation or deep sedation are as follows: (1) cardiovascular function and airway patency must be satisfactory and stable; (2) the patient must be easily arousable, with protective reflexes intact; (3) the patient should be able to talk and to sit up unaided, if these are developmentally appropriate; (4) if the patient is too young or too handicapped to talk or sit up, he or she must be as close to the presedation state of consciousness as possible; and (5) hydration must be adequate. Since the publication of these guidelines, it is both ethically and medicolegally necessary that appropriate monitoring be maintained whenever sedation is used.

There are numerous effective sedatives for use in the adolescent population. For a complete review, the reader is referred to Coté's *Sedation for the Pediatric Patient*.[18] Discussion of the most commonly used sedatives follows.

The *benzodiazepines* are by far the most widely used sedatives in adolescents and adults. Diazepam (Valium) has been used for many years with great success. The usual dose for sedation is 0.1 to 0.3 mg/kg given either intravenously or orally. Diazepam should not be administered intramuscularly because it is both painful and poorly absorbed. Even when it is given intravenously, patients often complain that diazepam is painful. The two major problems arising from the use of diazepam as a sedative are its long duration of action (18 hours) and the fact that respiratory depression is likely when diazepam is combined with narcotic analgesics. Because diazepam is metabolized in the liver, it must be used with caution in patients with compromised hepatic function. Diazepam may be useful in very-short-term administration for individuals in whom muscle spasm is a major precipitant of pain. This drug is generally overprescribed for management of anxiety, sleep problems, and chronic pain.

Midazolam (Versed) is a newer benzodiazepine with several advantages over diazepam. It is water soluble, which effectively eliminates pain on intravenous or intramuscular administration. It also has a much shorter elimination half-life (1.5 to 2 hours), which makes it more suitable when shorter duration of sedation is required. Of all sedatives, it also comes closest to producing true conscious sedation, with the youngster being calm, compliant, and receptive to most nonthreatening procedures. In fact, most children do not fall asleep when midazolam is used. The drug is formulated for intravenous administration but can be given by other routes as well. Compared with intravenous administration, the fractions of drug availability by other routes are as follows: 0.9, intramuscular; 0.6, intranasal and sublingual; 0.5, rectal; and 0.3, oral. Appropriate doses of midazolam are IV or IM, 0.05 to 0.15 mg/kg; sublingual or nasal, 0.2 to 0.5 mg/kg; and oral or rectal, 0.5 to 0.75 mg/kg. Nasal and sublingual administration result in sedation in 10 to 15 minutes; 20 to 30 minutes is required

after oral administration. There can be prolonged elimination after intramuscular administration. One problem encountered with oral and sublingual administration is a bitter after-taste, which is difficult to disguise. Coté recommends asking the patient to swallow as much as possible in the first gulp. Respiratory arrest has been reported when combining midazolam with fentanyl.

Chloral hydrate has long been a very popular sedative for younger children, although it is not used as often with adolescents. The usual dose is 20 to 75 mg/kg orally or rectally; 100 mg/kg or 2.0 g, whichever is less, is the highest recommended dose. The onset of sedation is usually about 1 hour after administration. The sedative effects of chloral hydrate can be prolonged, and the peak sedation may occur well after a procedure has been completed. Chloral hydrate has minimal effects on respiration, but there have been instances of severe respiratory depression, particularly when chloral hydrate has been combined with other sedatives or narcotic analgesics. As with any sedative, monitoring according to the AAP guidelines is necessary. Chloral hydrate also has a bitter taste, which can make it difficult to administer.

The *DPT cocktail* is another popular sedative consisting of Demerol (meperidine, 25 mg/ml), Phenergan (promethazine, 6.5 mg/ml), and Thorazine (chlorpromazine, 6.5 mg/ml). It was developed for induction of anesthesia, but after it was successfully used for sedation and analgesia during cardiac catheterizations, it became widely used as a pediatric sedative for medical procedures. There are numerous problems with this combination of medications. It is often used even when a procedure is not painful and a narcotic is not necessary. However, the combination of the narcotic with the phenothiazines greatly increases the risk of respiratory depression. There are reported cases of severe respiratory depression and death both during and after procedures when a DPT cocktail was used for sedation. The phenothiazines are alpha-adrenergic blocking agents and can cause profound hypotension when administered to a patient with a contracted blood volume. They also decrease the seizure threshold and can cause dystonic reactions. The DPT is very long-acting, with a mean "time asleep" of 4.7 ± 1.4 hours and a mean time to "return to normal" of 19 ± 15 hours. This means that prolonged monitoring is essential. In addition, the dosage recommendations vary by a factor of 10, from 0.02 to 0.2 ml/kg, with an upper limit of 4 ml in two divided doses. However, complications have been reported with doses as low as 0.07 ml/kg. At present, with the availability of shorter-acting and effective sedatives, there are few indications for use of this combination of drugs, each of which produces its own set of potential adverse reactions. The DPT mixture should never be given intravenously, as the risk of severe respiratory depression is markedly increased with rapid administration.

CONCLUSION

With the recent advances in pain management, there are now safe and effective ways to significantly reduce the suffering of adolescents who have either acute or chronic pain problems. However, to optimize pain management, the health professional needs not only to correctly diagnose and treat the cause of the pain, but also to understand the factors that influence pain perception, appropriately assess and monitor the patient's discomfort level, and tailor the treatment program to the needs of the individual. As Weisman and Schechter[19] noted, "The skill of physicians should be assessed not only by their cure of illnesses, but by the comfort they provide in the process."

References

1. Wall PH, Melzak R, editors: *Textbook of pain,* New York, 1984, Churchill Livingstone.
2. Schechter NL: The undertreatment of pain in children, *Pediatr Clin North Am* 36:781, 1989.
3. Porter J, Jick H: Addiction rate in patients treated with narcotics, *N Engl J Med* 302:123, 1980.
4. International Association for the Study of Pain: Subcommittee on Taxonomy. Pain terms: a list with definitions and notes on usage, *Pain* 6:249, 1979.
5. Melzak R, Wall PD: Pain mechanisms: a new theory, *Science* 150:971, 1965.
6. Beecher HK: Relationship of significance of wound to the pain experienced, *JAMA* 161:1609, 1956.
7. Petrie A: *Individuality in pain and suffering,* Chicago, 1967, University of Chicago Publishing.
8. Stimmel B: *Pain, analgesia and addiction: the pharmacological treatment of pain,* New York, 1983, Raven Press.
9. Varni JW, Thompson KL, Hanson V. The Varni/Thompson Pediatric Pain Questionnaire. I. Chronic musculo-skeletal pain in juvenile rheumatoid arthritis, *Pain* 28:27, 1987.
10. Melzak R: The McGill Pain Questionnaire: major properties and scoring methods, *Pain* 1:277, 1975.
11. Kavanagh C: Psychological intervention with the severely burned child: report of an experimental comparison of two approaches and their effects on psychological sequelae, *J Am Acad Child Psychiatry* 22:145, 1983.
12. Masek BJ, Russo DC, Varni JW: Behavioral approaches to the management of chronic pain in children: symposium on recurrent pain in children, *Pediatr Clin North Am* 31:1113, 1984.
13. Erickson CJ: Applications of cyberphysiologic techniques in pain management, *Pediatr Ann* 20:145, 1991.
14. Olness K, MacDonald J, Uden D: Prospective study comparing propranolol, placebo, and hypnosis in management of juvenile migraine, *Pediatrics* 79:593, 1987.
15. World Health Organization: *Cancer pain relief,* Geneva, 1986, World Health Organization.
16. Moertel CG, Ahmenn DL, Taylor WF, et al: Relief of pain by oral medications: a controlled evaluation of analgesic combinations, *JAMA* 229:55, 1974.
17. Committee on Drugs of the American Academy of Pediatrics: Guidelines for monitoring and management of pediatric patients during and after sedation for diagnostic and therapeutic procedures, *Pediatrics* 89:1110, 1992.
18. Coté CJ: Sedation for the pediatric patient: a review, *Pediatr Clin North Am* 41:31, 1994.
19. Weisman SJ, Schechter NL: The management of pain in children, *Pediatr Rev* 12:237, 1991.

Suggested Readings

American Pain Society: *Principles of analgesic use in the treatment of acute pain and cancer pain,* ed 3, Glenview, IL, 1992, American Pain Society.

McGrath PM: *Pain in children: nature, assessment, and treatment,* New York, 1990, Guilford Press.

McGrath PJ, Unruh AM: *Pain in children and adolescents,* New York, 1987, Elsevier.

Ross DM, Ross SA: *Childhood pain: current issues, research, and management,* Baltimore, 1988, Urban & Schwarzenberg.

Schechter NL, editor: Acute pain in children, *Pediatr Clin North Am* 36, 1989.

CHAPTER 21

Chronic Illness

•

Susan M. Coupey

Traditionally, health professionals who care for adolescents have been thought of as serving an essentially healthy population. The popular notion is that these professionals care for acute, self-limited illnesses; trauma; and behavioral problems. Therefore, the wide prevalence of chronic health conditions among young people is not often appreciated. Part of the reason for this misperception is that the epidemiology of chronic disease has changed dramatically over the last 30 years. There are now a significant number of adolescents who are living with chronic illness, whereas in the past many would have died in childhood. In addition, the training of physicians for long-term management of chronic illness is often inadequate. Although biomedical treatment for most common chronic diseases is well defined and widely available, healthcare providers have discovered that optimal management of illness in the adolescent age group is complex and not limited to biomedical prescription. Psychosocial, cognitive, and developmental factors all feature prominently in the ongoing care of adolescents with chronic diseases, but these areas are frequently neglected in physician training.

In this chapter, the epidemiology of chronic illness in the adolescent age group is reviewed. In addition, two other psychosocial areas that are particularly relevant to the needs of the chronically ill adolescent population are addressed. The first area is mental health. Chronic diseases that have no cure and therefore must be endured and managed on a daily basis—over months, years, even a lifetime—are a continuing source of stress that can adversely affect the mental health of the individual. Compromised mental health may make management of the physical illness more difficult. Conversely, when chronic disease is present, the preexisting psychological resources and the emotional health of both adolescent patients and their families can become crucial variables influencing physical health. This influence can occur through differential use of the healthcare system and the level of compliance with medical recommendations by dysfunctional as opposed to emotionally healthy adolescents and families. The second psycho-

social issue discussed in this chapter is risk-taking behavior. Risk taking in the areas of sexuality and substance use is an important contributor to morbidity in the adolescent age group. However, when this behavior interacts with chronic illness, the health consequences are often exacerbated. Conversely, chronic illness may offer protection against certain types of risk taking, and this knowledge may be helpful in healthcare management.

EPIDEMIOLOGY

There is little evidence of change in the incidence of the major chronic disorders of childhood.[1] As in the past, a certain number of children are born with or develop conditions such as cystic fibrosis, congenital heart disease, sickle cell disease, diabetes mellitus, chronic renal disease, hemophilia, and epilepsy. The exceptions include cerebral palsy, which has shown a decline, and leukemia and ventricular septal defect, both of which have had an increased incidence. In addition, with newer prenatal diagnostic techniques, selective termination of pregnancy, and dietary prevention, a decline in the incidence of neural tube defects and possibly of Down syndrome can be expected in the future.

What has changed dramatically is the survival of children with chronic illness. For example, recent developments in open heart surgery have allowed many children with previously fatal congenital heart lesions to reach adulthood. Similarly, improvements in cancer chemotherapy have transformed childhood cancer from an almost uniformly acute and fatal condition to one that is often chronic and potentially curable. Therapeutic advances such as organ transplantation, improved respiratory technology, aggressive use of new antibiotics, and home-based parenteral nutrition have all contributed to improved survival of children with many different diseases. It is predominantly this increased survival that has accounted for the dramatic increase in the prevalence of chronic illness in adolescents and young adults.

In the early 1960s, it became clear that the number of "handicapped" children was increasing in most developed countries having sophisticated systems of medical care. In 1971 Pless and Roghmann,[2] comparing three large epidemiologic surveys, two in Britain and one in New York, estimated the prevalence of chronic disorders in childhood. The prevalence differed among the three surveys largely because of methodologic differences, such as the definition of chronic illness and the age range studied. However, the authors concluded that in childhood, from approximately 0 to 16 years, the prevalence of chronic illness ranged from 5% to 20%. Newacheck,[3] analyzing data from the 1984 National Health Interview Survey, reported a 6% prevalence in American adolescents aged 10 to 18 years of some degree of disability or limitation of activity due to a chronic health condition. The leading causes of disability in this study were mental disorders, including retardation, and respiratory diseases. Adolescents living in poverty were 46% more likely to be limited by chronic health conditions than those from families with incomes above the poverty level. Analysis of data from the 1988 survey indicated that 5% of children under age 18 years had a severe chronic condition, and they accounted for 19% of physician contacts and 33% of hospital days related to chronic illness.[4] In addition, data from this 1988 survey indicated that children from poor families in the United States were at higher risk of having severe chronic illness, were 118% more likely to be uninsured, and were 42% more likely to lack a usual source of medical care than children from nonpoor U.S. families.[5]

In 1986 Cadman et al,[6] in a rigorously designed household sample survey of children aged 4 to 16 years living in Ontario, reported a 19.6% prevalence of serious chronic health problems of at least 6 months' duration. In the adolescent cohort aged 12 to 16 years, they found a prevalence of chronic illness without disability of 14.6% in boys and 13.8% in girls; the prevalence of chronic illness with disability (limiting normal function) was 5.8% in boys and 5.2% in girls. The limitation of normal function in this report included restrictions in physical activity, mobility, self-care, school, or play. Overall, boys and adolescents had a slightly higher rate of chronic health conditions than did girls or younger children. Offspring of families whose income was below the poverty line in this Canadian study had a 23.7% prevalence of chronic health problems compared with 18.3% among more economically advantaged children.

Whereas these associations are consistent with the other large epidemiologic surveys, it can be concluded with a reasonable degree of confidence that, despite varying definitions of chronic illness in different surveys, a substantial proportion of adolescents (up to 20%) lives with a chronic health condition, and that about 6% of this population, or nearly 2 million adolescents in the United States, are limited in normal functioning because of such a condition. In addition, adolescents from poverty groups are more likely to have a severe chronic illness than those whose families have adequate resources, and in the United States they are more likely to lack health insurance.

MENTAL HEALTH AND CHRONIC ILLNESS

The relationship between mental health and chronic physical illness has been the subject of much study. Earlier literature is replete with studies describing the psychological attributes that were thought to be specific to particular chronic diseases. Because of the categorization of patients according to disease for biomedical care, psychosocial studies tend to use the same groupings, especially when the samples are drawn from clinic populations. Such studies compare groups of patients who have diabetes, asthma, or cancer with a well population. When psychosocial abnormalities are noted, the findings may be interpreted as if they are specific to the disease entity. For example, a study of the social competence and behavioral adjustment of 7- to 15-year-olds who are long-term survivors of cancer found that school-related problems and somatic complaints were increased fourfold in this group compared with the general population.[7] In addition, the data showed that functional impairments increased the risk of academic and adjustment problems. While these findings are undoubtedly true for cancer survivors, they may also apply to children and adolescents with other chronic conditions. The study also found, however, that having had cranial irradiation for treatment of leukemia was an additional independent risk factor for school-related problems. This finding is clearly a disease-specific effect.

Hurtig et al[8] tested the relationship between illness severity and psychosocial adjustment in 70 patients aged 8 to 16 years with sickle cell anemia. The authors hypothesized that severity of disease would be a significant predictor of the level of psychosocial adjustment, but they found little support for their hypothesis. Instead, individual differences, particularly age and sex, were more important contributors to adjustment than were disease-specific factors. Adolescents with sickle cell disease were less well adjusted and had poorer school performance than younger children with the disease. In addition, limitations imposed by the disease that affect adjustment had a greater impact on boys than on girls. Again, it is likely that these findings are not specific to sickle cell disease and would be found in similar studies of other chronic conditions.

Noncategorical Approach

As health care providers have begun to care for large numbers of chronically ill adolescents, it has become apparent that the traditional biomedical, organ-system approach to management is limited, particularly when mental health is considered. Expanding one's thinking beyond the specific pathophysiology of the disease to include the many generic issues related to chronic illness allows for broader understanding and improved treatment of the adolescent patient. Chronic disease can be associated with changes in mobility, energy level, physical appearance, self-esteem, affective state, cognitive functioning, and social and peer interactions. These changes, in turn, can affect the overall health of the adolescent and the severity of the chronic illness. The mechanisms by which these effects operate within individual patients include mental and emotional health, compliance with medical treatment, risk-taking behaviors, and utilization of health care. In addition, the maturation of the chronically ill adolescent into an independent, functional adult can be impeded if these effects interfere with education and employability.

Pless and Pinkerton[9] and Stein and Jessop[10] advocated a noncategorical model of childhood chronic illness, stating that there are many more commonalities than differences in the experience of youngsters with chronic diseases. Strategies and interventions aimed at improving the overall health of adolescents in the face of a chronic condition are best conceptualized across traditional disease categories. A 1993 article in the journal *Pediatrics* discussing the definition and classification of chronic health conditions recommends "the development of a 'generic' approach, which focuses on elements that are shared by many conditions, children, and families."[11]

Influence of Chronic Illness on Mental Health

Several epidemiologic surveys assessing mental health and using noncategorical groups of chronically ill patients have appeared in the literature. These provide data that help to elucidate which psychosocial problems are disease specific and which are common to patients with various diseases. One study that examined mental health in over 700 adults with one of six different chronic diseases (e.g., arthritis, diabetes, cancer) found that mental health was fundamentally independent of specific physical disease diagnosis and did not differ significantly from the mental health of the general public.[12] The study did provide support for a noncategorical approach, showing that mental health was poorer in newly diagnosed patients and in those with critical illness. Also, in this group of adult patients, older individuals had better

mental health than younger ones. A study of the mental health of young adults (mean age 21.9 years) with chronic illness found that selected noncategorical risk factors (i.e., poor prognosis, restricted activity days, hearing and speech problems, and perceived unpredictability of symptoms) had significant effects on mental health status, heightening the risk for poor mental health.[13]

The pediatric literature and the adolescent literature present somewhat contradictory information about the relationship of chronic physical illness and mental health. Some studies indicate that adolescents with chronic diseases are just as well adjusted as their healthy peers, whereas other studies show poorer mental health in adolescents with illness. Kellerman et al,[14] comparing 168 adolescents having various chronic diseases with 349 healthy adolescents, found no differences in anxiety or self-esteem between healthy and ill groups or between groups with different chronic diseases. Drotar et al[15] studied children aged 3 to 13 years who had cystic fibrosis. They found that these children achieved an age-adequate adjustment at home and at school, and noted that adjustment was largely unrelated to the severity of the disease.

Two large epidemiologic surveys have helped to clarify our thinking in the area of psychiatric and adjustment disorders in relation to chronic disease. Both the Ontario Child Health Study,[16] a Canadian household sample survey, and an analysis of data from a nationally representative sample of over 11,000 children and adolescents in the United States by Gortmaker et al[17] found that children and adolescents with chronic physical health conditions are at increased risk for psychiatric disorders and social adjustment problems. In the Ontario study, children and adolescents with both chronic illness and associated disability, compared with well children, were at more than three times the risk for psychiatric disorders and also were at high risk for social adjustment problems. Those with chronic illness but no associated disability were at considerably less risk, and they were not much different in terms of mental health risk from the well population. Thus, it seems that, although chronic physical illness is certainly a risk factor for psychiatric and emotional disorder, mental-health problems disproportionately affect those who are disabled by their disease. Adolescents with a chronic physical condition but no disability are as likely to be psychosocially healthy as their well peers. Among adolescents with chronic illness and disability, the relationship between severity of handicap and poor mental health may not be direct. Friedman[18] and others have documented that mildly disabled adolescents, who are neither perfectly healthy nor obviously ill, may be more at risk for emotional ill health than their more disabled peers. There is some evidence that this "marginality"—that is, identifying with two groups, ill and healthy, yet not really belonging to either—predisposes the adolescent to social and emotional adjustment problems. This idea is reinforced by a 1995 study evaluating psychosocial adjustment in children with facial port-wine stains and comparing it with the adjustment noted in children with prominent ears.[19] The children with disfiguring facial birthmarks were found to be as well adjusted as or better adjusted than nondisfigured peers, whereas those with prominent ears were less well adjusted. The authors suggest that having a clearly abnormal disfigurement, such as a port-wine stain, elicits uniformity of both opinion and support from family, whereas having a deformity such as prominent ears, which is merely an exaggeration of normal, is not as likely to elicit support and may explain the poorer mental health in that marginally disfigured group.

Orr et al[20] attempted to clarify the specific psychosocial areas of functioning that are problematic for adolescents who have grown up with a chronic disease. They performed a follow-up, from ages 13 to 22, on a cohort of chronically ill children who had been identified in a representative sample of an upstate New York community 10 years earlier. The adolescents with chronic conditions were compared with a matched group of well adolescents drawn from the same population. This study, like that of chronically ill adults described previously,[12] found that most youths, both well and ill, appeared psychosocially healthy. However, among those adolescents who reported some impairment resulting from their illness, specific psychosocial areas appeared most vulnerable to dysfunction. One area related to achieving independence: for example, planning for the future, dating, obtaining a driver's license, and remaining in school. Another area of vulnerability was family relationships: for example, engaging in family activities, talking with parents, and achieving satisfaction with family life. In addition, the overall social adjustment of the more severely ill adolescents, as measured by the California Psychological Inventory, appeared to be less adequate. The authors concluded that "There is no inherent theoretical reason to believe that the impact of illness should be so global or severe as to produce consistent psychiatric disturbance. Instead [our] findings suggest that chronic nonfatal illness most influences youth in planning for their future and in their own feelings of psychological well-being."

Taken together, the results of all these studies allow us to conclude that severe chronic illness is a risk factor for poor mental health. However, most adolescents with chronic physical health conditions, including many with severe illness, are mentally healthy. Some studies suggest that age and sex are important mediating characteristics, adolescence and male sex being associated with a higher risk for poor mental health. None of the studies provides support for specific diseases as independent risk factors for psychiatric disorder.

Risk Factors and Protective Factors

Chronic illness does not occur in a vacuum. It affects particular adolescents and their families, who already have strengths and weaknesses that will influence their adaptation to the illness (Fig. 21-1). Rae-Grant et al,[21] analyzing data from the Ontario Child Health Study, examined risk factors and protective factors for behavioral and emotional disorders in children and adolescents. In the adolescent cohort aged 12 to 16 years, two risk factors significantly predicted the presence of psychiatric disorder: family problems (e.g., severe discord or domestic violence) and parental problems (e.g., psychiatric illness, physical illness, or criminality). The authors also found two protective factors associated with the absence of psychiatric disorder: being a good student and having a confidant. These findings are consistent with other published reports. The article by Rae-Grant et al[21] also provides an excellent review of the literature on risk and protective factors for mental illness in children and adolescents.

Chronic physical "handicap," or chronic illness with disability, is noted to be one of several such risk factors for psychiatric disorder. Other risk factors reported in various published studies include sex (boys are more vulnerable than girls), psychiatric illness in a parent, criminality in a parent, low socioeconomic status, overcrowding or large family size, and severe marital discord. Rutter[22] found that children with only one risk factor were not any more likely to have emotional disorders than those with no risk factors. However, two risk factors in the same child increased the risk for psychiatric disorder fourfold. If more than two factors were present, the risk for mental health problems increased several times further.

In contrast, there are protective factors that foster resilience to psychiatric disorder. Garmezy[23] and Rutter[24] delineated several factors—within the child or adolescent, the family, and the community—that are capable of modifying or ameliorating a person's response to the risk factors described, including the presence of chronic physical illness. Protective factors within the adolescent include positive temperament, above-average intelligence, and social competence (measured by academic achievement, competence in activities such as sports or music, and ability to relate to others easily). Protective family factors include a supportive relationship with at least one parent (even in homes with marital discord), family closeness, and adequate rule setting. Rutter et al[25] studied the school environment and found that good schools can function as protective environments for adolescents and can help to ameliorate other risk factors for poor mental health. Similarly, both community institutions and significant adults in the community can have a positive impact on the mental health of adolescents.

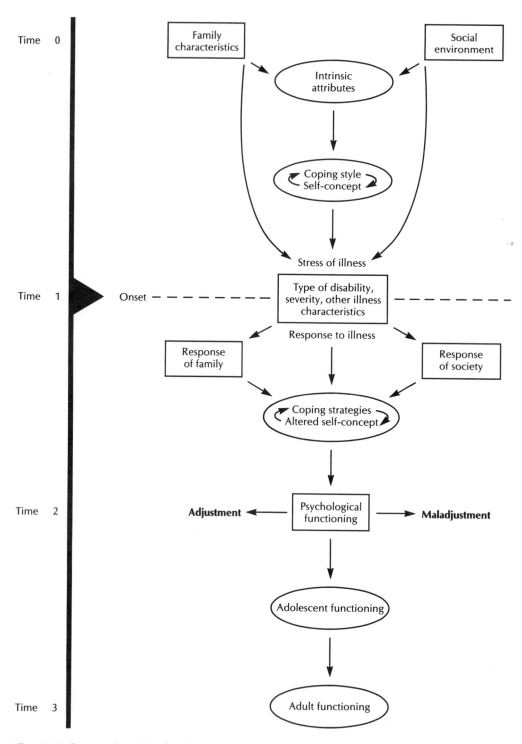

Fig. 21-1. Integrated model of adjustment to chronic physical illness, indicating preexisting psychological, familial, and social conditions at time 0 and response to illness at time 1, both influencing adjustment shown at time 2. All factors continue to affect functioning through developmental stages of adolescence and adulthood shown at time 3. When maladjustment is present, this model can help determine which factors may be amenable to successful therapy. (From Pless IB, Pinkerton P: *Chronic childhood disorder—promoting patterns of adjustment,* London, 1975, Henry Kimpton.)

To summarize, there are two ways of looking at the relationship of mental health and chronic physical illness. Most studies indicate that a chronic physical illness, even with its attendant problems and stresses, does not necessarily lead to emotional dysfunction; in fact, it is associated with good mental health in most of those affected. Adolescents with chronic illness and disability, however, are at increased risk for psychiatric and psychosocial dysfunction. Another, perhaps more fruitful, approach is to view chronic physical illness as one of several important risk factors for poor mental health and to evaluate the total burden of risk factors borne by each individual patient. When balanced by the individual's protective factors, this method of evaluation allows a more accurate prediction of mental health risk. Primary and secondary preventive interventions can then be targeted at individuals with multiple risk factors and should not need to be disease specific.

Significance of Mental Health in Chronic Illness

Why is the mental health of adolescents with chronic physical illness so important? There are several reasons, but perhaps the most compelling one is that poor mental health is associated with poor physical health and even death. Strunk et al[26] conducted a study to determine the clinical characteristics associated with death from asthma in 21 children and adolescents with severe asthma. Patients had died a mean of 1.2 years after discharge from an inpatient psychosomatic unit. Hospital records were examined for 57 physiological and psychological characteristics and analyzed to see which of these could be used to distinguish the group of patients who subsequently died from a matched group of controls. Ten of the 14 differentiating characteristics reflected the psychosocial status of the patient or the family; only four of them reflected physiologic status. The psychological characteristics associated with death from asthma included disregard of perceived asthma symptoms; self-care inappropriate for age; patient-staff, patient-parent, and parent-staff conflict; depressive symptoms; and family dysfunction. The authors concluded that "psychologic risk factors were prominent in severely asthmatic children who subsequently died of asthma." These findings are supported in a clinical report by Fritz et al,[27] who noted that of three adolescents who died of asthma, all had depressive symptoms and dysfunctional families.

It is likely, although not proven by these studies, that the poor mental health of the children and adolescents who suffered fatal asthma attacks, and the prominent dysfunction exhibited by their families, were not primarily a result of the asthma per se but represented preexisting conditions related to other risk factors. However, the fact that these youngsters had asthma along with other risk factors for emotional disorder placed them at much higher risk for death than other children with similar risk factors but no asthma.

Noncompliance with prescribed medical treatment is another problem associated with poor mental health in adolescents who have chronic physical health conditions. Poor compliance often leads to a poor outcome of treatment and thus more severe chronic illness. Korsch et al[28] examined factors associated with noncompliance with immunosuppressive therapy in 14 pediatric patients (13 adolescents) with transplanted kidneys, and compared them with psychosocial indicators in 66 transplant patients without compliance problems. Results showed that noncompliant patients were those whose personality function was deviant before the physical illness intervened. In addition, these patients came from families with lower incomes, were often part of a fatherless household, and had more communication difficulties than did the compliant patients. The physical health of these patients was significantly compromised by their noncompliance; eight patients lost their transplanted kidneys, and the remaining six had impaired renal function. The authors note that if, as their data indicate, noncompliance is related to psychosocial problems that existed before the physical illness occurred, it may be unrealistic to expect psychosocial support during the treatment program to succeed in preventing noncompliance.

A 1989 study focused on investigation of the role of psychosocial variables in predicting compliance with theophylline treatment in a population of 38 children and adolescents with asthma.[29] Analyses indicated that an adequate mean theophylline level over the previous 2 years (indicating compliant behavior) was predicted by a combination of few behavioral problems in the child and little conflict in the family. These results indicate that better psychosocial health of both child and family is associated with good compliance. These data are consistent with other studies of patients with asthma and other chronic illnesses, and provide support for the importance of the relationship between compliance with medical treatment and mental health.

Jacobson et al[30] conducted a longitudinal study of 57 children and adolescents with newly diagnosed diabetes mellitus. The purpose was to identify baseline psychosocial factors, present at onset of disease, that predict diabetes-related compliance 18 months later. Initial measures indicating high self-esteem, high perceived competence, good social functioning, good adjustment to diabetes, and few behavioral symptoms predicted subsequent compliance. The authors noted that their findings highlight the linkage of personality and adjustment with compliance. This study also found that age was a predictor of compliance. Adolescents aged 13 to 15 years were less compliant than preadolescents aged 9 to 12 years. The authors noted that "this and other studies suggest that a purely medical model for treating diabetes in adolescents will not have an impact on critical problems underlying poor outcome." They suggested that family therapy, behavioral approaches, and individual counseling may be needed to improve management and to provide optimal therapy.

If the noncategorical model is applied to these studies, there is no reason to believe that the findings are specific to asthma, renal failure, or diabetes. Poor compliance with medical treatment seems more likely to occur if the patient (1) is an adolescent, (2) has low self-esteem and poor social competence, (3) is depressed or emotionally unstable, (4) has a dysfunctional family, and (5) lives in poverty. Whether the patient has systemic lupus erythematosus (SLE), asthma, sickle cell disease, or diabetes mellitus seems to be less relevant. However, poor compliance is likely to be associated with more frequent exacerbations of illness, doctor visits, and hospitalizations; more physiologic complications of the disease; more days of school or work missed; and more disability. Thus, poor mental health in combination with chronic physical illness can significantly contribute to functional limitation.

Cross-sectional studies, such as those described above, that find a significant association between chronic illness with disability and psychiatric disorder cannot distinguish cause and effect. In all probability, both directions apply; that is, disability causes psychiatric disorder and psychiatric disorder causes disability. Prospective longitudinal studies are needed to determine the relative contribution of these causes and effects within specific illness categories.

Regardless of the causal direction of these associations, however, it is clear that a significant subgroup of the chronically ill adolescent population requires mental health intervention in addition to biomedical treatment. For high-risk adolescent patients, interventions aimed at improving the individual's competence and self-esteem and strengthening the family support system are important. Such interventions could be implemented across diagnostic groups rather than becoming duplicated services for adolescents with different medical diagnoses.

RISK-TAKING BEHAVIORS

Risk-taking behaviors, including unprotected sexual intercourse and substance abuse, are important causes of morbidity in adolescents. Only recently, however, have health care providers begun to document these behaviors in adolescents with chronic illness. Since the mid-1980s, several reports have described the adverse health effects of risk taking. These reports have highlighted complicated pregnancies in young women with cystic fibrosis, illicit drug use by adolescents with various chronic diseases, and sudden death associated with illicit drug use in adolescents who have cardiac or pulmonary diseases.[31-33] It is ironic that risk taking among chronically ill teenagers is probably directly related to the vastly improved management of their diseases. Improved management most often results in normal or near-normal growth, pubertal development, and fertility; better nutritional status; normal energy levels; and age-appropriate opportunities for social interaction that can, and often do, include experimenting with risk-taking behaviors.

Sexual Behavior

Data are sparse concerning the prevalence of all risk behaviors in adolescents with chronic physical health conditions, but sexual behavior has been studied in selected populations. Alderman et al, in a study of inner-city adolescents aged 14 to 17 years with serious chronic medical illnesses, reported that 33% had had sexual intercourse at least once, and this rate of sexual experience was not different from that found among their healthy peers.[34] The authors found a significant interaction effect of chronic illness and gender on age at first intercourse. Chronically ill girls had a significantly earlier age at first intercourse (mean 13.8 years) than their healthy peers (mean 15.3 years), but the opposite was true for boys with a chronic illness. The adolescents in this sample were mostly from poor minority groups and had illnesses such as asthma, diabetes mellitus, sickle cell anemia, and epilepsy.

In Montreal a survey of 14- to 18-year-old boys and girls who had chronic diseases that were somewhat different from those in the study by Alderman et al[34] (diabetes, seizures, arthritis, inflammatory bowel disease, chronic renal failure) and who were mostly white and middle class indicated that only one quarter of these adolescents had had sexual intercourse.[35] Nearly one third of this sample had chronic conditions often associated with delayed puberty: inflammatory bowel disease and chronic renal failure. This fact, along with cultural and psychosocial differences, may account for the difference in prevalence of sexual intercourse found in the two studies. Nevertheless, it is probably correct to assume that a significant proportion of adolescents who have chronic physical diseases initiate sexual intercourse in middle to late adolescence. This timing is similar to that of the population of healthy teenagers.

Several studies report sexual behavior in small samples of adolescents with specific chronic conditions. In a survey of 29 girls and women older than 12 years of age who had cystic fibrosis, about one third had engaged in sexual intercourse.[36] Although none of the girls younger than 18 years was sexually experienced, nine of the 13 women who were older than 18 had had sexual intercourse. This delay in sexual debut is likely to be related to the delayed puberty associated with this illness.

Chamberlain et al[37] studied sexual behavior in mentally retarded girls and found that 45% of mildly retarded 15- to 19-year-old girls were nonvirgins. This is not significantly different from the general population of 15- to 19-year-olds. Fewer moderately and severely retarded girls, 30% and 9% respectively, were sexually active.

Although chronically ill adolescents are a heterogeneous group, and these data reflect small, nonrepresentative samples, some generalizations about sexual behavior can be inferred. First, girls with common chronic disorders such as asthma, diabetes, epilepsy, cancer, and mild mental retardation—which allow for relatively normal pubertal development and peer interaction—are likely to be similar to the general population in their sexual behavior. This means that more than half of them will initiate sexual intercourse in their teenage years, and about one out of every three nonvirgins will become pregnant before the age of 20. Comparable data for chronically ill boys are not available, although in certain population groups they may initiate sexual intercourse at a later age than their healthy peers. For girls with a chronic disease associated with delayed puberty, such as cystic fibrosis, initiation of sexual intercourse is most often delayed until the young adult years. The literature also provides evidence that adolescent girls and boys suffering from conditions that severely limit their mobility and their opportunities for normal peer interactions, such as spina bifida, are less likely to initiate sexual intercourse in their teenage years.[38]

These data make it clear that it is imperative that adolescents with chronic disease be provided with access to sexuality-related health care. Pregnancy, childbirth, and abortion often involve increased risk in the presence of a chronic condition, and pregnancy may exacerbate some diseases. Such risks have been well documented for women with heart disease; there is a high mortality in pregnant and parturient women who have pulmonary hypertension. Pregnancy may exacerbate asthma in the mother, and fetal oxygenation may be compromised during an acute asthmatic episode. Pregnancy in an adolescent with sickle cell disease is associated with increased risk for stroke, pulmonary embolism, pyelonephritis, and pneumonia.[39] Medications taken by the pregnant adolescent who has cancer, epilepsy, SLE, or certain other diseases may harm the fetus. Many girls with a chronic illness are eventually able to bear healthy children, but the management of these complicated, high-risk pregnancies demands a degree of compliance and medical regimentation that is often impossible to achieve during adolescence, particularly since these pregnancies are often unplanned and unintended. The chronically ill pregnant adolescent and her fetus are thus at higher risk for complications than the chronically ill adult pregnant woman and her fetus.

Sexually transmitted diseases (STDs) are a significant cause of morbidity in the general adolescent population and often result in health problems for those with chronic illness.[40] STDs may be more difficult to diagnose in young people who have chronic conditions because the symptoms, such as menstrual irregularity, dysuria, and abdominal pain, may mimic those of the condition itself. Immunosuppression, either from medications or from the disease, may cause STDs to be more severe and more difficult to treat than would be the case with nonimmunocompromised adolescents. For example, it is extremely difficult to eradicate venereal warts in girls who have SLE, and adolescents infected with human papillomavirus are at increased risk for cervical dysplasia and ultimately for cervical cancer. Because of their high risk for cervical disease, adolescents with SLE require specific counseling regarding the use of barrier contraceptives when they become sexually active.

Chronically ill adolescents who are sexually active need to be identified by their healthcare providers and given appropriate contraceptive and STD counseling, with yearly Papanicolaou smears and STD screening. In addition, all chronically ill adolescents, whether sexually active or not, benefit from anticipatory guidance about the optimal timing of pregnancy and childbearing and the genetic implications, if any, of their particular disease.

Substance Use and Abuse

The use of nonprescription or illicit substances by adolescents who have chronic disease has not been studied intensively. Clinical impressions indicate that many chronically ill adolescents, who are often dependent on daily medication for treatment, are less likely than healthy teenagers to use illicit or recreational substances. However, this idea may be wishful thinking on the part of healthcare providers. In the study of inner-city middle adolescents by Alderman et al,[34] no difference in use of cigarettes (one of every seven adolescents smoked daily), alcohol, or illicit drugs was found between those with and those without chronic illness.

A survey by Stern et al,[41] focusing on the recreational use of psychoactive drugs by 173 patients aged 18 years or older with cystic fibrosis, indicated that the use of these drugs was widespread. Of these patients, 11% were regular smokers of tobacco, with a median age of 16 years for beginning smoking; an even greater number, 20%, smoked marijuana; and 60% used alcohol, with nearly 10% of the older teenagers in the sample reporting heavy drinking. Cocaine and other illicit drug use was relatively rare. Only one patient had been an intravenous drug abuser and was undergoing methadone maintenance therapy. This study also brought to light the important interactions of different psychoactive substances with cystic fibrosis. Patients often reported that alcohol use increased their pulmonary symptoms; however, surprisingly, most smokers who had cystic fibrosis noted no pulmonary effect from smoking.

A study examining the social characteristics of adolescents with epilepsy compared substance use in three different groups of adolescents aged 13 to 19 years. The groups included 34 patients with idiopathic epilepsy, 32 with various chronic diseases other than epilepsy, and 50 with no chronic illness.[42] Fewer adolescents with epilepsy had tried cocaine or were daily smokers (3% and 9%, respectively) than adolescents who had other chronic diseases (21% and 19%, respectively) or were well (21% and 30%, respectively). Approximately 15% of the teens in each group reported drinking alcohol once a week or more. About 20% in each group reported that they used marijuana, with fewer than half using it once a week or more. These two studies suggest that substance abuse may not be as rare among chronically ill youths as is often assumed.

Substance use by adolescents with chronic physical illness can contribute significantly to morbidity and mortality. The nonprescribed drugs taken may interact with prescribed drugs to cause deleterious effects. For example, in a case reported by Szefler et al,[32] a 17-year-old severely asthmatic girl developed theophylline toxicity after self-medication with several over-the-counter medications and illicit drugs, including amphetamines and barbiturates. Certain specific chronic conditions, notably cardiac anomalies, put affected individuals at particular risk of death from even one-time use of substances such as cocaine or other stimulants.

Healthcare providers should be alert to the effects of nonprescribed substances used by chronically ill adolescents, because the studies described above indicate that such use may be common. Given the potentially severe adverse health effects, anticipatory guidance and counseling relevant to the particular disease and its interaction with different classes of drugs is warranted.

FUTURE TRENDS IN PATIENT MANAGEMENT

In the coming decades the management of chronic disease in adolescents and young adults is likely to continue to advance and improve. Indeed, many new therapeutic modalities are already known, but they have not been widely implemented for a variety of reasons. As research data continue to indicate the necessity for a biopsychosocial, multidisciplinary approach to achieve optimal management, creative ways of improving the health and functioning of chronically ill young people will undoubtedly be found.

In the biomedical arena the widespread use of technologic devices to manage chronic conditions can be expected. Many individuals with diabetes now have devices that enable them to better monitor their blood glucose at home. Soon, they may have computerized insulin pumps that effectively automate insulin administration. Adolescents with sickle cell anemia may have the frequency of painful crises reduced by newer medical management strategies. Advances in surgery and immunology will almost certainly enable many more adolescents with transplanted organs to live at least long enough to attend high school and college.

Improved nutritional management of adolescents with chronic diseases will result in further normalization of growth in stature and weight and in pubertal development. In particular, adolescents with cystic fibrosis, sickle cell disease, inflammatory bowel disease, or cancer will profit from home parenteral nutrition and newer elemental diets. Better growth and development will in turn result in more normative social behavior, including risk-taking behaviors, which may lead to other medical problems. Longer-acting formulations of medications allowing for once- or twice-daily dosing can be expected to improve compliance and overall health for many chronically ill adolescents.

In the area of mental health, a steady increase in interest and research related to chronic physical health conditions has taken place since the mid-1970s. In the next two decades we are likely to see the fruits of this new knowledge translated into improved medical management. Morbidity and mortality may be related as much, if not more, to the emotional health of the young person as to the physiologic aspects of the chronic disease. Additional noncategorical studies will clarify the psychosocial characteristics of adolescents and their families that predict severe illness and the mechanisms through which they act. These data will form the basis for the design of interventions aimed at preventing adverse outcomes and facilitating healthy development. The need for interdisciplinary collaboration among mental health professionals, physicians, sociologists, educators, and others involved in research and the management of chronically ill adolescents will be increasingly recognized and accomplished.

In the social and developmental arena, the necessity of assisting chronically ill adolescents to become functioning adults must be recognized. This recognition may encourage an emphasis on interventions leading toward employment, healthy sexuality, and marriage. Research areas that also need to be addressed include employment discrimination, stigma, and health insurance coverage.

In recent years, as more adolescents with chronic illnesses mature into adulthood, programs to help them transition from pediatric into adult-oriented healthcare settings have been developed. Growing recognition that most pediatric health care settings do not promote independent decision making or encourage a self-concept of maturity in older adolescent and young adult patients has spurred the development of such programs. In addition, internists are unfamiliar with many childhood chronic diseases such as cystic fibrosis or congenital heart disease and often welcome the opportunity to work alongside pediatricians in a special transition program. Interdisciplinary models for treatment of complex chronic illness that include nutritional and psychosocial support as well as medical care are well developed in pediatrics but only beginning to evolve in internal medicine. Such models seem well suited to young adults with chronic conditions, many of whom have some psychosocial maturational delay as a result of their illness and require more comprehensive services than do most adults. However, funding is a constant source of difficulty for transition programs, since many young adults with chronic illness are uninsured.

At the societal level, improved organization and financing of services for adolescents and young adults are needed. In addition, chronic care issues need to be emphasized in the training of physicians at both primary care and subspecialist levels. Lastly, more interdisciplinary research funds are needed to allow behavioral science researchers to collaborate with clinicians in order to facilitate the development of better theoretical models to explain the complex effects of chronic illness on the adolescent patient.

References

1. Gortmaker SL, Sappenfield W: Chronic childhood disorders: prevalence and impact, *Pediatr Clin North Am* 31:3, 1984.
2. Pless IB, Roghmann KJ: Chronic illness and its consequences: observations based on three epidemiologic surveys, *J Pediatr* 79:351, 1971.
3. Newacheck PW: Adolescents with special health needs: prevalence, severity, and access to health services, *Pediatrics* 84:872, 1989.
4. Newacheck PW: Taylor WR: Childhood chronic illness: prevalence, severity, and impact, *Am J Public Health* 82:364, 1992.
5. Newacheck PW: Poverty and childhood chronic illness, *Arch Pediatr Adolesc Med* 148:1143, 1994.
6. Cadman D, Boyle MH, Offord DR, Szatmari P, Rae-Grant NI, Crawford J, Byles J: Chronic illness and functional limitation in Ontario children: findings of the Ontario Child Health Study, *Can Med Assoc J* 135:761, 1986.
7. Mulhern RK, Wasserman AL, Friedman AG, Fairclough D: Social competence and behavioral adjustment of children who are long-term survivors of cancer, *Pediatrics* 83:18, 1989.
8. Hurtig AL, Koepke D, Park KB: Relation between severity of chronic illness and adjustment in children and adolescents with sickle cell disease, *J Pediatr Psychol* 14:117, 1989.
9. Pless IB, Pinkerton P: *Chronic childhood disorder—promoting patterns of adjustment,* London, 1975, Henry Kimpton.
10. Stein R, Jessop D: A non-categorical approach to chronic childhood illness, *Public Health Rep* 97:354, 1982.
11. Perrin EC, Newacheck PW, Pless IB, et al: Issues involved in the definition and classification of chronic health conditions, *Pediatrics* 91:787, 1993.
12. Cassileth BR, Lusk EJ, Strouse TB, Miller DS, Brown LL, Cross PA, Tenaglia AN: Psychosocial status in chronic illness: a comparative analysis of six diagnostic groups, *N Engl J Med* 311:506, 1984.
13. Ireys HT, Werthamer-Larsson LA, Kolodner KB, Gross SS: Mental health of young adults with chronic illness: the mediating effect of perceived impact, *J Pediatr Psychol* 19:205, 1994.
14. Kellerman J, Zeltzer L, Ellenberg L, Dash J, Rigler D: Psychological effects of illness in adolescence. I. Anxiety, self-esteem, and perception of control, *J Pediatr* 97:126, 1980.
15. Drotar D, Doershuk CF, Stern RC, Boat TF, Boyer W, Matthews L: Psychosocial functioning of children with cystic fibrosis, *Pediatrics* 67:338, 1981.
16. Cadman D, Boyle M, Szatmari P, Offord DR: Chronic illness, disability and mental and social well-being: findings of the Ontario Child Health Study, *Pediatrics* 79:805, 1987.
17. Gortmaker SL, Walker DK, Weitzman M, Sobol AM: Chronic conditions, socioeconomic risks, and behavioral problems in children and adolescents, *Pediatrics* 85:267, 1990.
18. Friedman SB: The concept of "marginality" applied to psychosomatic medicine, *Psychosom Med* 50:447, 1988.
19. Sheerin D, MacLeod M, Kusumakar V: Psychosocial adjustment in children with port-wine stains and prominent ears, *J Am Acad Child Adolesc Psychiatry* 34:1637, 1995.
20. Orr DP, Weller SC, Satterwhite B, Pless IB: Psychosocial implications of chronic illness in adolescents, *J Pediatr* 104:152, 1984.
21. Rae-Grant N, Thomas BH, Offord DR, Boyle MH: Risk, protective factors and the prevalence of behavioral and emotional disorders in children and adolescents, *J Am Acad Child Adolesc Psychiatry* 28:262, 1989.
22. Rutter M: Protective factors in children's responses to stress and disadvantage. In Kent MW, Rolf JE, editors: *Primary prevention of psychopathology: social competence in children,* vol 3, Hanover, NH, 1979, University Press of New England.
23. Garmezy N: Stressors of childhood. In Garmezy N, Rutter M, editors: *Stress, coping and development in children,* New York, 1983, McGraw-Hill.
24. Rutter M: Resilience in the face of adversity: protective factors and resistance to psychiatric disorder, *Br J Psychiatry* 147:598, 1985.
25. Rutter M, Maughn B, Mortimori P, Auston J: *Fifteen thousand hours: secondary schools and their effects on children,* London, 1979, Open Books.
26. Strunk RC, Mrazek DA, Wolfson-Fuhrmann GS, LaBrecque JF: Physiologic and psychological characteristics associated with deaths due to asthma in childhood, *JAMA* 254:1193, 1985.
27. Fritz GK, Rubinstein S, Lewiston NJ: Psychological factors in fatal childhood asthma, *Am J Orthopsychiatry* 57:253, 1987.
28. Korsch BM, Fine RN, Negrete VF: Noncompliance in children with renal transplants, *Pediatrics* 61:872, 1978.
29. Christiaanse ME, Lavigne JV, Lerner CV: Psychosocial aspects of compliance in children and adolescents with asthma, *J Dev Behav Pediatr* 10:75, 1989.
30. Jacobson AM, Hauser ST, Wolfsdorf JI, Houlihan J, Milley JE, Herskowitz RD, Wertlieb D, Watt E: Psychologic predictors of compliance in children with recent onset of diabetes mellitus, *J Pediatr* 110:805, 1987.
31. Palmer J, Dillon-Baker C, Tecklin JS, Wolfson B, Rosenberg B, Burroughs B, Holsclaw DS, Scanlin TF, Huang NN, Sewell EM: Pregnancy in patients with cystic fibrosis, *Ann Intern Med* 99:596, 1983.
32. Szefler SJ, Rogers RJ, Strunk RC: Drug abuse and the asthmatic patient: a case report, *J Allergy Clin Immunol* 74:201, 1984.
33. Dowling GP, McDonough ET, Bost RO: "Eve" and "ecstasy": a report of five deaths associated with the use of MDEA and MDMA, *JAMA* 257:1615, 1987.
34. Alderman EM, Lauby JL, Coupey SM: Problem behaviors in inner-city adolescents with chronic illness, *J Dev Behav Pediatr* 16:339, 1995.
35. Carroll G, Massarelli E, Opzoomer A, Pekeles G, Pedneault M, Frappier JY, Oretto N: Adolescents with chronic disease: are they receiving comprehensive health care?, *J Adolesc Health Care* 4:261, 1983.

36. Neinstein LS, Stewart D, Wang CI, Johnson I: Menstrual dysfunction in cystic fibrosis, *J Adolesc Health Care* 4:153, 1983.
37. Chamberlain A, Rauh J, Passel A, McGrath M, Burket R: Issues in fertility control for mentally retarded female adolescents: sexual activity, sexual abuse and contraception, *Pediatrics* 73:445, 1984.
38. Blum RW, Resnick MD, Nelson R, St Germaine A: Family and peer issues among adolescents with spina bifida and cerebral palsy, *Pediatrics* 88:280, 1991.
39. Morrison JC: Hemoglobinopathies and pregnancies, *Clin Obstet Gynecol* 22:819, 1979.
40. Coupey SM, Alderman EM: Sexual behavior and related health care for adolescents with chronic illness, *Adolesc Med: State of Art Rev* 3:317, 1992.
41. Stern RC, Byard PJ, Tomashefski JF, Doershuk CF: Recreational use of psychoactive drugs by patients with cystic fibrosis, *J Pediatr* 111:293, 1987.
42. Westbrook LE, Silver EJ, Coupey SM, Shinnar S: Social characteristics of adolescents with idiopathic epilepsy: a comparison to chronically ill and non-chronically ill peers, *J Epilepsy* 4:87, 1991.

CHAPTER 22

Potentially Fatal Illness

•

Lynda B. Cooper

Great strides in the treatment of life-threatening illness have forced physicians to change their approach to patient management. New treatments have prolonged life and even led to many cures, forcing health care providers to face new clinical and ethical dilemmas. Patients, families, and health professionals must live with the difficulties of a potentially fatal illness and the rigors of treatment. Whether the teenager survives into adulthood or dies of the disease, he or she must continue to participate in family, school, and community life.

LIFE-THREATENING ILLNESS

The three leading causes of death in the adolescent age group are accidents, homicide, and suicide. However, most pediatric practices have patients with potentially fatal illnesses. These patients may have been born with congenital disorders such as cardiac disease (the fifth leading cause of death in adolescence), cystic fibrosis, or muscular dystrophy. While improved treatment for many disorders has added years of good quality, many patients experience exacerbations and progression during adolescence. For example, children who were infected with the HIV virus prenatally or by transfusion frequently became ill by the time of adolescence. Some patients, formerly healthy, are stricken with a potentially fatal illness such as cancer (the fourth leading cause of death in adolescence) or AIDS before or during adolescence.

EFFECTS ON THE ADOLESCENT

Teenagers who were born with or acquired a potentially fatal illness during childhood enter adolescence with knowledge about their illness. They have learned the routines associated with treatment and self-care; developed relationships with physicians, healthcare staff, and other patients; and formed a "patient identity." If the family has coped well with the illness, the patient has been allowed to take increasing responsibility for his or her care. Most of these patients behave like teenagers with chronic illnesses: they balance their need for independence with their need for compliance with medical care.

The most common potentially fatal illness diagnosed during adolescence is cancer. Pediatric oncology centers have developed knowledge about the management of teenagers with a life-threatening illness. As teams who care for children with cystic fibrosis, neuromuscular diseases, and AIDS confront the problems of their older, sicker patients, they can benefit from the experience of these centers.

The diagnosis of cancer evokes varying degrees of fear, anger, and sadness in every new teenage patient. The patient and the family must quickly master complex medical information and develop relationships with professionals in a hospital that may be a great distance from home. Virtually all families of adolescents with cancer are informed of the diagnosis at a major medical center. To establish trust and ensure compliance, physicians explain the disease and the treatment options as soon as possible. Some adolescents with cancer have a much better outlook than others, but all must live with an uncertain future. In general, teenagers are told that a combination of chemotherapy, radiation, and surgery will be used to fight their disease and that these treatments are aimed at bringing about a remission, which may lead to a cure. However, the cost of remissions, whether they continue indefinitely or end in relapse, is high. Teenagers often endure frequent hospitalizations, nausea and vomiting, and hair loss. Their treatment often requires new technology: indwelling catheters for venous access, hyperalimentation for nutritional support, and sometimes medication pumps for control of pain.

Teenagers stricken with illness experience a major disruption in development. At a time when autonomy is a central issue, they must regress to childlike dependence on adults to provide their care. When physical appearance is of foremost importance, hair is lost, weight is lost or gained, and radical surgery may be necessary. During a period when peer relationships are more important than family, friends are usually sympathetic and supportive but do not incorporate the teenager who is sick and weak into their ongoing activities. When sexual identity is evolving, teenagers with a serious disease are struggling with impaired body image and worries about reproductive capabilities. Realistic concerns about the future may well impair their ability to plan for higher education or consider specific vocational choices.

Most teenagers report surprisingly good adjustment to these problems, especially those who experienced normal development before the illness. As they move through the crisis of diagnosis to periods of remission and less treatment, or of relapses and death, these teenagers employ a variety of coping mechanisms to help them manage stress and disruption. Most life-threatening illnesses, and cancer particularly, is marked by stages.

During the crisis of diagnosis, it is not unusual to see a significant degree of avoidance. Teenagers may refuse to use the word "cancer" and they may reject offers of explanation of treatment. Some may express feelings of fear and anger at the disruption in their lives. They test the team as they try to maintain some control and despair at the loss of life as it was. Others may try to be the "good patient," surprising everyone with cheer and attempts at heroism. Whatever the coping mechanism employed, most teenagers learn to adapt to the difficulties caused by serious illness. They distract themselves with the normal activities of adolescents, such as learning to drive, going to school or working with a tutor, and maintaining relationships with friends. Some sex differences in adjustment are evident: girls are better able to maintain close friendships, which typically revolve around conversations and shared confidences. Boys' relationships, which often involve sports and other physical activities,

may be more disrupted. On the other hand, boys report that their male friends are more accepting of the changes in their appearance, while girls feel that their altered appearance keeps them isolated from the social life of their peers.

As teenagers become more involved in their own care, they no longer need to deny the seriousness of their illness or refuse information. However, they talk of "forgetting" about their disease when they are not in the clinic or hospital, and most are able to maintain hope even when their condition is clinically deteriorating. They identify with survivors they know and point out differences between themselves and those who have died of similar diseases. These cognitive maneuvers are the hallmark of good coping skills among teenagers.

EFFECTS ON FAMILY

To facilitate teenagers' adjustment to their illness and its treatment, the team must assess the family's structure and the resources its members will use to cope with the overwhelming stresses of a potentially fatal illness. In spite of the changing face of the American family, every patient lives with someone: a parent or parents, a sibling or siblings, and often some extended family. A stepparent also may be involved.

The structure of the family needs to be examined. How are decisions made and conflicts solved? How strong are the affectional ties among members? Are roles and responsibilities flexible and generationally appropriate? Are all family members' needs considered important? Are members allowed to be individuals with their own ideas? The pediatrician who has known the family has valuable information to offer the specialized health care staff about how a particular family will respond to the various challenges.

Intellectual Challenges

The family must learn the new language relevant to diagnosis, treatment, and prognosis. Family members must make important decisions about choosing a treatment center and are asked to give informed consent to complex treatment protocols at a time when they are overwhelmed with strong emotions. The team can judge the family's ability to understand the information, and refer them to organizations and self-help groups that can provide appropriate material.

Practical Issues

Family members must cope with financial stresses that result from medical bills and loss of income. They may have to negotiate a complex managed care system. They must arrange for frequent appointments for the patient and any necessary child care for siblings. Many teenagers who can attend school during treatment require additional help, and some must have home instruction, especially during the more intense phases of today's aggressive protocols. Home care services offer an opportunity to leave the hospital sooner, but families must acquire and manage highly technical equipment while they learn to handle the side effects of treatment.

Emotional and Interpersonal Factors

Teenagers and their parents experience the gamut of strong feelings: grief, anger, guilt, and fear. All these emotions are normal, and they are expressed at various times during the illness experience. Friends and extended family can be helpful, but they may also cause stress with questions and unsolicited advice. The marital relationship may be strained during certain crisis points, such as diagnosis, surgery, and relapse, as the couple copes with fear, stress, and fatigue. Siblings may feel isolated and angry when they see the family resources depleted by the demands of the patient's illness. While adolescents with cancer usually freely share their diagnosis with friends, adolescents with AIDS may be reluctant to risk ostracism. Those who have remained well in spite of transfusion-acquired infection must now decide whether to disclose their illness to friends at school.

While most teenagers and families successfully cope with the demands of illness and treatment, often with the help of support networks and community resources, some have adjustment problems that predate or coexist with the illness. Poverty, substance abuse, and psychiatric illness may complicate the management of the teenage patient. Single-parent families and those with poor social contacts often have difficulty meeting the demands of the illness and treatment. Teenagers prenatally exposed to AIDS may outlive other family members.

The Existential Experience

Most family members struggle to find meaning in the tragedy they are facing. They try to maintain hope while being realistic about the possibility of death. They seek relationships with families of other patients to reduce the sense of isolation they feel from extended family and friends. They look for ways to enrich their child's life and improve family spirit when the patient is well enough to participate.

SOURCES OF HELP

After assessing the structure of the family, the strength of each member, the tasks they must face, and the

resources available to them, the team can recommend many sources of help. The social worker in the hospital can guide the pediatrician and the family to numerous organizations that provide services to those with serious illness.

National groups such as the American Cancer Society, Leukemia Society, Hemophilia Foundation, Muscular Dystrophy Association, and Cystic Fibrosis Research Foundation offer families information and referrals to local chapters (see the list of community resources at the end of this chapter). Summer camps are available for children with disabling illnesses who can benefit from the fun, independence, and socialization that a camp experience offers. Wish fulfillment organizations such as the Make-a-Wish Foundation and the Starlight Foundation offer teenagers with life-threatening illness opportunities for trips, shopping sprees, and introductions to popular celebrities.

Many adolescents, parents, and siblings benefit from participation in self-help groups. Various types of medical self-help groups are found in many communities and medical centers and are intended to offer support to patients and families during every phase of the experience from diagnosis to bereavement. These groups sponsor activities that promote mutual support, advocacy, and education.

Most help comes directly from the healthcare team, who try to respect the adolescents' special needs for privacy and accept behavior that ranges from childlike to mature beyond their years. Teenagers with a history of rebelliousness or "acting out" behavior will test the limits of the healthcare team. Their poor ability to tolerate pain and medically related limitations may influence compliance and ultimately their health status. Each of these special problems requires more intense intervention by consultants in social work, psychology, psychiatry, and behavioral pediatrics.

ISSUES FOR SURVIVORS

Adolescents who are cured by modern medical intervention face new challenges. Their families have paid a financial price for their cure that may affect the resources available for education. In addition to medical bills, costs include out-of-pocket expenses for travel, parking, restaurant meals, child care, and special gifts for both patient and siblings. The careers of the parents may have been disrupted by emotional distress and missed work. Frequently, the financial impact is felt long after treatment ends.

Survivors also must cope with the long-term sequelae of treatment such as disfigurement, neurologic problems, and sterility. Disruption in psychological and social development may lead to prolonged dependence on parents and caution in forming intimate relationships.

Survivors may face discrimination in employment and insurance. In addition, the specter of relapse or secondary malignancy always exists. Despite these problems, long-term survivors are psychologically healthier than might be expected. Many patients who return for yearly follow-up visits report that they have actually benefited from having had a potentially fatal illness. They report having a better outlook on life, an increased appreciation of being alive, and a renewed belief that adults are helpful and trustworthy.

TERMINAL ILLNESS

Despite remarkable progress against formerly fatal illnesses, many patients still have poor prognoses, especially after a relapse, or as the disease progresses. This is the worst time for a teenager who has done everything possible to comply with treatment. Most patients and families continue to seek aggressive therapies to prolong life, or they may look for a remote cure. It was common a few years ago to consider the relapsed child to be dying, but new experimental protocols offered in many treatment centers have changed the point at which patients are seen as terminal. Organ and bone marrow transplants are currently offered to patients who just a short time ago would have received only palliative care. Although parents and patients frequently know that the chance of a cure is negligible, their hope is bolstered by the patient's former successful treatment and the successful treatment of other patients. Teenagers with AIDS are encouraged by the progress made against cancer, once a death sentence.

Various ethical dilemmas are associated with these developments. Although it is generally considered appropriate for a competent adult to agree to experimental treatment or to forego it, the ability of a teenager to participate in such a decision is far more ambiguous. Legally, teenagers have no more right to refuse or consent to health care than younger pediatric patients. In reality, however, a teenager is physically, intellectually, and morally more like an adult than a young child. Through good communication and sensitive assessment, the adolescent's decision-making capacity must be evaluated within the context of a particular situation. For instance, the teenager who refuses chemotherapy for newly diagnosed leukemia because of fear of hair loss does not meet the standards for good decision-making capacity. However, the 14-year-old who chooses to forego painful therapy with unproven benefit may fully understand the consequences of that decision. The physician and family must give serious consideration to the adolescent's point of view.

Some families wish to continue treatment in the face of overwhelming odds against success. They believe that they must do everything possible to save their child.

Although such efforts may be seen by some staff members as futile and painful for the patient, they provide hope to the families while their child is alive and peace of mind after the death of the child. Some teenagers may talk about their impending death to family and staff, but many do not. Some are more likely to verbalize their fears about pain, medical deterioration, and isolation. The physician and other staff members can help the patient and the family by management of pain and examination of the alternatives for home and hospital care. Staff members familiar with the patient and the family must continue to stay involved as the child nears death.

Parents may need an opportunity to talk about envisioning the world without their child. They might rehearse the funeral scene and think about how to prepare siblings for the death. Physicians, social workers, nurses, and friends can help to support this anticipatory grief work.

BEREAVEMENT

When a teenager dies after a long illness, the parents are frequently exhausted and depleted. Even when they have acknowledged the inevitability of death, parents may experience loss of control, anger, and guilt as well as shock and despair at the time of death.

Parental bereavement is different from other grief experiences. Contrary to the adage that "time heals all wounds," it has been observed that parental grief intensifies at such times as the anniversary of the child's death, birthdays, and other milestones. Parents commonly describe intense pain at seeing their teenagers' friends go off to college and begin bright futures. They experience the birth of other people's grandchildren as reminders of their loss. Enshrinement of the dead child's bedroom, obsession with the details of the last days, and isolation from family and friends may characterize life for many months or years after the child's death and for periods throughout the lifetime of the parents. Physicians and mental health professionals can refer grieving parents to agency bereavement centers or to self-help groups such as Compassionate Friends.

Schools are becoming more responsive to the needs of students whose lives are affected by the death of a classmate. Teachers are being trained to lead class discussions on the event, and students are encouraged to participate in memorial activities (see Chapter 86, "Mourning").

ROLE OF THE PEDIATRICIAN

The pediatrician (or family physician), who may have considerable knowledge of the patient and the family, can be a valuable member of the staff caring for a teenager with a potentially fatal illness. He or she is able to interpret complicated medical data and explain "high-tech" procedures, can be available to talk to the patient and the family if conflicts arise with the hospital staff, can manage interim care, and may oversee home care. Parents have expressed gratitude to the pediatrician who pronounces their child dead at home so that the body is taken to a funeral chapel instead of a morgue. The pediatrician can also keep in close touch with the parents after the child's death and encourage them to participate in bereavement groups. Whether the adolescent with a life-threatening illness survives or dies, that individual's care requires intense involvement by the pediatrician. The pediatrician who stays closely involved is rewarded with an intimate relationship with both patient and family during a most dramatic struggle.

Suggested Readings

Armstrong-Daily A, Goltzer S: *Hospice care for children,* New York, 1993, Oxford University Press.
A valuable overview of topics related to the hospice environment. Strong chapters on staff reaction to families facing terminal illness.

Chesler M, Barbarin O: *Childhood cancer and the family,* New York, 1987, Brunner/Mazel.
Writers describe the phases and tasks facing families. A well-organized text.

Cincotta N: Psychosocial issues in the world of children with cancer, *Cancer Suppl* 71:10, 1993.
A beautifully written look into the world of the child with cancer.

Koocher G, O'Malley J: *The Damocles syndrome: psychological consequences of surviving childhood cancer,* New York, 1981, McGraw-Hill.
Cancer survivorship issues are highlighted in this classic text.

Lantos J, Miles S: Autonomy in adolescent medicine, *J Adolesc Health Care* 10:460, 1989.
Overview of legal issues associated with consent to treatment.

Lukin S: Role of adolescents in decisions concerning their cancer therapy, *Cancer Suppl* 71:10, 1993.
Excellent discussion of complex ethical dilemmas that arise when there is disagreement among adolescent patients, their families, and caregivers.

Perrin J, Shayne M, Bloom S: *Home and community care for chronically ill children,* New York, 1993, Oxford University Press.
Review of important public policy issues in the care of chronically ill children.

Rando TA, editor: *Parental loss of a child,* Champaign, IL, 1986, Research Press.
Author describes the unique aspects of parental grief. Excellent treatment of the differences among families whose losses follow long and brief illnesses.

Schowalter J, Patterson P, Tallmen M, Kutscher A, Gallo S, Peretz D, editors: *The child and death,* New York, 1983, Columbia University Press.
This classic text describes the child's developing comprehension of death and dying.

Zeitzer LK: Cancer in adolescents and young adults: psychosocial aspects, *Cancer Suppl* 71:10, 1993.
Good treatment of the impact of cancer on identity formation and autonomy in adolescence.

Resources

American Cancer Society
1599 Clifton Road NE
Atlanta, GA 30392
(800) 227-2345
Publications' referrals to local chapter services.

Association for Brain Tumor Research
2720 River Road
Des Plaines, IL 60018
(708) 827-9910
Offers information and computerized referral service.

Candlelighters
7910 Woodmont Avenue Suite 460
Bethesda, MD 20814
(800) 366-2223
Focuses on support and advocacy for families of children with cancer.

Compassionate Friends
P.O. Box 3696
Oak Brook, IL 60522
(312) 323-5010
Supplies list of local chapters of self-help groups for bereaved parents.

Cystic Fibrosis Research Foundation
6931 Arlington Road
Bethesda, MD 20814
(301) 951-4422
Offers information and referral to local groups.

HANDI (Hemophilia and AIDS/HIV Network for Dissemination of Information)
110 Greene Street, Suite 303
New York, NY 10012
(800) 42-HANDI

Make-a-Wish Foundation
2600 N. Central Avenue, Suite 936
Phoenix, AZ 85004
Grants the wishes of children who have a life-threatening illness.

Muscular Dystrophy Association
810 Seventh Avenue
New York, NY 10019
(212) 586-0808
Supplies information and referral to local groups.

National Self-Help Clearinghouse
25 W. 43rd Street
New York, NY 10036
(212) 642-2944
Offers referral to local self-help groups and resources.

SKIP (Sick Kids need Involved People)
990 Second Avenue, 2nd Floor
New York, NY 10022
(212) 421-9160
Supplies case management and advocacy services for families of children with complex health care needs.

PART TWO

Medical Disorders

CHAPTER 23

Pituitary Disorders

•

H. Verdain Barnes and Maria R. Coccia

Pituitary gland disorders are rare in adolescents. In this chapter, discussions are limited to central diabetes insipidus and various pituitary neoplasms that may affect endocrine function.

DIABETES INSIPIDUS

Diabetes insipidus (DI) affects the regulatory mechanism controlling plasma osmolality. Central (neurogenic) DI results from an absolute or relative decrease in arginine vasopressin (AVP), or antidiuretic hormone. AVP is an octapeptide produced by the supraoptic nuclei of the hypothalamus. It is transported to the posterior pituitary via axons, where it is stored until the plasma osmolality increases or extracellular fluid decreases. In patients with posterior pituitary disease, AVP is typically deficient.[1]

Tumors are the most common cause of acquired central DI in all age groups, craniopharyngioma being the most common tumor etiology in adolescents. However, any primary or secondary (metastatic) tumor of the pituitary-hypothalamic area can produce DI, including suprasellar germinoma, juvenile astrocytoma, meningioma, and pinealoma. Of patients with craniopharyngioma, 10% to 30% develop DI, and about 50% of those with a suprasellar germinoma have DI as the presenting symptom.[2]

In the adolescent, trauma is an important cause of DI. This can result from surgical intervention for neoplasms in the hypothalamic-pituitary region or from accidental head trauma. The types of accidental trauma most likely to produce DI are basilar skull fractures and ruptures of the pituitary stalk.[2]

The remaining causes of DI can be categorized as infectious, vascular, or miscellaneous. Acute infectious causes include measles, mumps, basilar meningitis, encephalitis, diphtheria, and scarlet fever. Diabetes insipidus also may result from chronic infections such as tuberculosis, brucellosis, syphilis, and actinomycosis. Any disease process capable of producing intracranial vasculitis, thrombosis, hemorrhage, or aneurysm can, if appropriately located, result in DI. Other known causes include histiocytosis X, sarcoidosis, Sheehan's syndrome, sickle cell disease, amyloidosis, lymphoma, and leukemia.[2]

Familial causes of DI are transmitted as an autosomal dominant or X-linked trait. Diabetes mellitus in association with DI may be a familial autosomal recessive syndrome consisting of concomitant DI, diabetes mellitus, optic atrophy, and nerve deafness (Wolfram's syndrome). In many cases of DI the precise cause is unknown.[1]

Polyuria and polydipsia in the pregnant adolescent presents a clinical challenge. Early during pregnancy there is a decrease in the body's "osmostat," resulting in a decline in the set point for serum osmolality by about 10 mOsm/kg. In addition the placenta produces vasopressinase, an enzyme that inactivates vasopressin. The result is a two- to fourfold increase in the metabolic clearance rate of vasopressin.[2] Partial AVP deficiency is accentuated by these changes. Owing to these and other physiologic changes of pregnancy, the results of standard screening and evaluation for DI cannot be interpreted with confidence. Pregnant adolescents in whom there is a possibility of DI should be referred to a qualified endocrinologist.

Clinical manifestations of DI vary, depending on the cause and the degree of decrease in AVP production. In uncomplicated DI, most patients give a history of abrupt new onset of increasing nocturia and/or enuresis. These patients frequently crave ice water or cold beverages; they complain of thirst during the night and polydipsia and polyuria during the day. Adolescents may repeat chronic fatigue and/or demonstrate poor school or work performance. Despite excessive urination, dehydration does not typically become clinically evident unless there is limited access to fluids or the thirst mechanism is dysfunctional.[1] The polyuria of DI may be masked by concomitant secondary adrenal or thyroid insufficiency; hence, DI may be discovered only when corticosteroids or thyroid hormone are administered. Consequently, corticosteroids should be started early in the preoperative period when surgery is anticipated.

Laboratory data that support a diagnosis of DI include hypernatremia, elevated plasma osmolality, and a dilute urine. Because of considerable overlap, these values do not allow differentiation among nephrogenic DI, psychogenic water drinking, and central DI. A more definitive diagnosis can be made with the water deprivation test and/or a response to AVP administration. The most definitive test is to measure plasma AVP concentration and plasma osmolality before and during an infusion of hypertonic saline. Patients with DI have a subnormal or nonmeasurable AVP concentration compared with their level of plasma osmolality. When the clinical manifestations of DI are accompanied by hypokalemia, hypercalcemia, or azotemia, nephrogenic DI is a primary consideration.

Treatment of DI involves hormone replacement. The current preparation of choice is DDAVP (desmopressin). This synthetic analog of AVP is administered intranasally. The dosage is 0.1 to 0.2 mL once or twice daily. Its duration of action varies between 8 and 24 hours, with a peak serum level at about 4 hours after administration. Disappearance from the plasma generally correlates with the duration of antidiuretic effect.

Nonhormone therapy with vasopressin amplifiers is effective in some patients, but such treatment requires relative vasopressin deficiency. Chlorpropamide, an oral hypoglycemic agent, enhances the response of renal medullary cyclic AMP to vasopressin. Symptomatic hypoglycemia is a rare complication when daily doses of 150 mg/m^2 or less are used. Other drugs of similar action are unproven.

Other pharmacologic agents that have been used with DI include clofibrate and carbamazepine. Both have a central effect that stimulates the release of vasopressin, although by apparently different mechanisms. Carbamazepine is not recommended for adolescents, because its potential side effects tend to outweigh the benefits.

HYPOTHALAMIC/PITUITARY NEOPLASMS

Craniopharyngiomas occur primarily in the first two decades of life and account for 5% to 10% of brain tumors in this age group. Approximately 50% of craniopharyngiomas are discovered before the patient reaches the age of 20 years. Tumor location is usually suprasellar but can be intrasellar. In either case the tumor may produce sellar changes and affect endocrine function. Craniopharyngiomas are benign cystic and/or solid tumors that typically have an embryonic origin from Rathke's pouch. Growth in size often produces signs and symptoms of increased intracranial pressure or endocrine dysfunction or both. The sella turcica is enlarged or distorted in at least 50% of patients.

Symptoms and signs of craniopharyngioma vary with age, size of the lesion, and location, and depend on whether there is tumor encroachment on other cranial structures such as the optic chiasm. In adolescents the most common symptoms and signs are increased intracranial pressure (headache, vomiting, and papilledema) and visual field loss or defects in about 60% of patients. Less frequent are endocrinopathies that result in short stature with a delay in bone age and/or DI. Often the endocrine disturbances are present for months before diagnosis but have been ignored.

Jenkins et al[4] reported the clinical features of 14 children and adolescents aged 5 to 18 years with a craniopharyngioma. Most of the adolescents had chemical hypothyroidism, and three had DI; most also had subnormal luteinizing hormone and follicle-stimulating hormone values for their stage of pubertal development. All had an abnormal response to luteinizing hormone–releasing factor. Hypoglycemia may be seen as a result of growth hormone and/or cortisol deficiency. Deficient growth hormone response to hypoglycemia is characteristic in patients with growth retardation. Precocious puberty secondary to a craniopharyngioma is rare.

Intracranial calcification is commonly seen in youths (>70% compared with about 2% in adults). Calcification may be dense, nodular, flocculent, or curvilinear in the suprasellar or retrosellar region and within the sella. Computed tomography (CT) and magnetic resonance imaging (MRI) are best for identifying calcium and defining the anatomy in and around the tumor, respectively.

The optimal treatment for a craniopharyngioma is controversial. In general, therapy should be based on the patient's symptoms and complications in addition to tumor size. Currently, there is no ideal curative therapy. Some authors advocate total surgical excision if possible. Transsphenoidal microsurgery is probably the procedure of choice for intrasellar and suprasellar tumors. Large tumors should be removed transcranially. A two-stage procedure may be needed: the frontal approach to excise the suprasellar mass and the transsphenoidal approach to remove the intrasellar portion. Since craniopharyngiomas are radiosensitive, a combination of partial excision and radiation is efficacious for some patients, particularly when the entire tumor cannot be removed. The recurrence rate 3 years after surgery with incomplete removal is high (upward of 90%).

Postoperative endocrine deficiencies are common. Diabetes insipidus occurs in about 50% of patients; 50% to 80% have thyroid-stimulating hormone (TSH) deficiency; 50%, adrenocorticotropic hormone deficiency; and 40% to 50%, gonadotropin deficiency. In 10% to 65% of patients, slow linear growth persists; however, catch-up growth occurs in some patients.[3]

THYROID-STIMULATING AND HORMONE-SECRETING PITUITARY NEOPLASMS

Hyperthyroidism secondary to a TSH-producing pituitary neoplasm is rare. Approximately 70 such cases have been reported in the literature. These tumors are basophilic or chromophobic adenomas, males and females are affected in equal numbers. Adolescents with such a tumor may complain of headache and visual changes as well as signs and symptoms of hyperthyroidism. Goiter is usually seen; ophthalmopathy is rare, however, occurring only if the tumor has extended into the orbit. Dermopathy and pretibial myxedema are not seen.

Third-generation TSH is critical in differentiating pituitary hyperthyroidism from Graves' disease. In contrast to Graves' disease, serum TSH is detectable—either normal or elevated—in the presence of a concomitant elevation of the thyroid hormones. Third-generation TSH values may be as low as 1 μU/ml. The TSH alpha-glycoprotein subunit is also helpful in establishing the diagnosis of a TSH-secreting neoplasm; the alpha subunit is secreted in excess of the amount of the intact molecule secreted. The ratio of TSH alpha subunit to TSH is typically greater than 1, while the beta subunit is regularly undetectable. The TSH levels typically do not respond to thyrotropin-releasing hormone stimulation in patients with a TSH-producing neoplasm; however, a response does not exclude a tumor. Computed tomography and MRI can be used to confirm the presence and location of the tumor. Macroadenomas are usually found, but a few microadenomas have been reported.

The treatment of choice is transsphenoidal pituitary surgery, with or without accompanying external irradiation. Because these TSH-producing pituitary tumors are aggressive and may continue to grow, thyroid gland ablation is not recommended. The use of medical therapy to suppress TSH is currently under investigation.[4,6]

References

1. Bacon GE, Spencer ML, Hopwood NG, Kelch RP: *A practical approach to pediatric endocrinology,* Chicago, 1990, Mosby–Year Book, pp 264-272.
2. Moltich ME: Endocrine problems of adolescent pregnancy, *Endocrinol Metab Clin North Am* 22:649-672, 1993.
3. Barnes HV: Diseases of the endocrine system and metabolic disorders: diabetes insipidus. In Spivak JL, Barnes HV, editors: *Manual of clinical problems in internal medicine,* Boston, 1990, Little, Brown, pp 163-230.
4. Jenkins JS, Gilbert CJ, Ang V: Hypothalamic-pituitary function in patients with craniopharyngiomas, *J Clin Endocrinol Metab* 43:394-399, 1976.
5. Styne DM: The therapy for hypothalamic-pituitary tumors, *Endocrinol Metab Clin North Am* 22:631-648, 1993.
6. Beck-Pecooz P, Mariotti S, Guillausseau PJ, Medri G, Piscitelli G, Bertoli A, Barbarino A, Rondena M, Chanson P, Pinchera A, Faglia G: Treatment of hyperthyroidism due to inappropriate secretion of thyrotropin with the somatostatin analog SMS 201-995, *J Clin Endocrinol Metab* 68:208-214, 1989.

CHAPTER 24

Thyroid Disorders

•

H. Verdain Barnes and James V. Hennessey

Thyroid disorders account for a large number of the endocrine problems seen in adolescent patients. The critical role of thyroid hormone in normal growth and development makes these disorders especially important. Generally, females are affected more frequently than males. The insidious onset of clinical symptoms may delay or make diagnosis difficult, and the associated behavioral problems may be difficult to differentiate from adolescent adjustment problems. This chapter focuses on the most clinically relevant conditions associated with thyroid dysfunction in the adolescent.

EVALUATION OF THYROID FUNCTION

Evaluation of thyroid function requires an understanding of the physiologic system involving the pituitary-thyroid axis, which maintains thyroidal homeostasis. Pituitary secretion of thyroid-stimulating hormone (TSH) is regulated by negative feedback of the thyroidal product thyroxine (T_4) and by circulating levels of triiodothyronine (T_3). Most circulating T_3 is generated peripherally in the liver from T_4 by type I monodeiodinase; the remaining T_3 is generated locally in the pituitary by type II monodeiodinase. Circulating T_3 interacts with nuclear thyroid hormone (T_3) receptors of the TSH-producing cells (thyrotrophs) of the anterior pituitary. Circulating TSH, T_4, and T_3 levels may be readily measured with reliable clinical assays. Under normal circumstances, T_4 and T_3 remain fairly constant within their respective ranges of normal throughout the day. TSH levels may demonstrate significant excursions throughout the day but generally remain within a wide range of normal.

Failure of the thyroid to produce sufficient thyroxine results in declining circulating T_4 levels (hypothyroidism), thereby decreasing pituitary exposure to thyroid hormone and resulting in elevations of TSH levels. Overproduction of T_4 and/or T_3 (hyperthyroidism) exposes the pituitary to excessive amounts of thyroid hormone and inhibits TSH synthesis and release, resulting in suppressed circulating levels of THS. Inadequate

production of TSH from the pituitary thyrotroph or deficient stimulation by the hypothalamic releasing factor thyrotropin-releasing hormone (TRH) results in deficient thyroid stimulation and subsequent thyroid hormone deficiency (secondary and tertiary hypothyroidism). Both T_4 and T_3 circulate in the serum bound to thyroxine-binding globulin (TBG). Because total thyroid hormone levels may be significantly influenced by an excess or deficiency of TBG, the estimation of free hormone levels by calculated indexes (using the in vitro T_3 resin uptake test) or direct measurement (equilibrium dialysis) provides a clinically useful approximation of the amount of free thyroid hormone available for biologic activity.

Global thyroid glandular function can be evaluated in vivo by measuring the uptake of radioactive iodine (^{123}I or ^{131}I). The radioactive iodine uptake (RAIU) test provides information different from that obtained from images (scans) of thyroid architecture, which may be taken in a patient 6 to 24 hours after ingestion of ^{123}I. Thyroid scans differentiate between functioning and nonfunctioning areas of the thyroid tissue, thus defining anatomy, whereas the RAIU test estimates the percentage of administered isotope captured by the thyroid over a 6- or 24-hour period, giving significant insight into the differential diagnosis of thyroid function.

Autoantibodies directed against various thyroidal structures or enzymatic components may be measured in the serum and are found to correlate with the degree of various autoimmune-mediated processes. Antibodies directed against the thyroid peroxidase enzyme (anti-TPO), previously referred to as antimicrosomal antibodies, and immunoglobulins specific for thyroglobulin are found in most patients with chronic lymphocytic (Hashimoto's) thyroiditis and spontaneous (silent) and postpartum thyroiditis, and also in many patients with Graves' disease. Stimulatory anti-TSH receptor antibodies (TSIs) are most frequently seen in Graves' disease and are considered to be pathogenic. Blocking antibodies specific for the thyrotropin receptor have been found among patients with so-called atrophic thyroiditis, characterized by primary hypothyroidism without a palpable goiter.

TABLE 24-1
Thyroid Function Tests in Various Clinical Conditions

Condition	TSH	T$_4$	T$_3$RU	F-T$_4$	T$_3$	ATA	RAIU	Scan	TG	PIT MRI	Iodine	ESR
Euthyroidism	NL	NL	NL	NL	NL	NI	NI	NI	NI	NI	NI	NI
Hypothyroid 1°	↑	↓	↓	↓	NI	Pos	NI	?I	NI	NI	NI	NI
Hypothyroid 2°/3°	NL/↓	↓	↓	↓	NI	NI	NI	NI	NI	MASS	NI	NI
Thyrotoxicosis												
Hyperthyroidism												
Graves'	↓	↑	↑	↑	↑↑	Pos	↑	NI	NI	NI	NI	NI
Nodular	↓	↑	↑	↑	↑↑↑	Neg	NL/↑	Pos	NI	NI	NI	NI
TSH tumor	NL/↑	↑	↑	↑	↑↑	Neg	↑	NI	NI	NI	NI	NI
hCG	↓	↑	↑	↑	↑↑	Neg	↑	NI	NI	NI	NI	NI
Nonhyperthyroid												
Subacute thyroiditis												
de Quervain's	↓	↑	↑	↑	↑	Neg	↓	NV	↑	NI	NL	↑
Spontaneous	↓	↑	↑	↑	↑	Pos	↓	NV	↑	NI	NL	NL/↑
Postpartum	↓	↑	↑	↑	↑	Pos	↓	NV	↑	NI	NL	NL
Ectopic tissue	↓	↑	↑	↑	↑↑	±	↓	Pos*	↑	NI	NL	NL
Factitious	↓	↑	↑	↑	↑	Neg	↓	NV	↓↓	NI	NL	NL
Iodine exposed	↓	↑	↑	↑	↑	±	↓	NV	↑	NI	↑↑	NL

ATA, antithyroid antibodies; *ESR*, erythrocyte sedimentation rate; *hCG*, human chorionic gonadotropin; *?I*, may be indicated when nodule palpable; *MRI*, magnetic resonance imaging; *Neg*, negative result; *NI*, not indicated; *Pos*, positive result; *RAIU*, radioactive iodine uptake; *Scan*, thyroid imaging; *T$_4$*, free T$_4$; *TG*, thyroglobulin; *T$_3$RU*, in vitro T$_3$ resin uptake; *TSH*, thyroid-stimulating hormone.
*Ectopic tissue localized by whole body scanning.

These blocking antibodies are also thought to be functional in infants with transient neonatal hypothyroidism who are born to mothers with autoimmune thyroid disease.

The intrathyroidal protein thyroglobulin not only serves as a matrix for thyroxine synthesis and as the principal protein of intrathyroidal colloid, but is also secreted along with thyroxine into the circulation. The principal clinical use of thyroglobulin is as a tumor marker in patients with differentiated thyroid cancer after complete surgical and ^{131}I ablation of malignant and normal thyroid tissue. Thyroglobulin is found circulating in excess amounts in endogenously thyrotoxic patients, but should be suppressed in those with diminished TSH levels due to administered thyroid hormone.

Table 24-1 summarizes the results of thyroid function testing in various thyroid conditions, which are described in the sections that follow.

ADOLESCENT GOITER

Thyroid enlargement in the adolescent is not a normal variant. A goiter in adolescents is an outward sign of many different etiologies. As a rule of thumb, a goiter is present when the superior, inferior, medial, and lateral borders of one or both lobes of the thyroid are distinctly palpable.

The diagnosis is made by palpation rather than by inspection alone. The frequency of goiter in adolescents ranges from 1% to 7% in areas where the diet is sufficient in iodine and from 15% to 90% in areas where iodine is deficient. Thyroid enlargement in adolescents peaks between 10 and 17 years of age, with a female-to-male ratio of 4:1 to 18:1.[1]

Hashimoto's thyroiditis (chronic lymphocytic thyroiditis), is the most frequent cause of goiter among adolescents in the United States. This chronic autoimmune disease accounts for nearly 80% of goiters in euthyroid adolescents.[1] Simple goiter, so named because it is a hyperplastic response to TSH, can be used as a collective term for goiters associated with absolute or relative iodine deficiency. Such goiters are rare in the United States.[2] Simple goiter is most common in areas where less than 100 mg of iodine is ingested daily in the diet. Similarly, there is an increased incidence of goiters in adolescents after administration of iodinated compounds or in areas where the diet includes excess iodine.[2] Other conditions associated with simple goiter include a generalized resistance to thyroid hormone and congenital thyroid hormone enzyme defects. Simple goiter also includes abnormal thyroid growth due to a relatively newly described group of proteins known as thyroid growth-promoting immunoglobulins (TGIs), which may stimulate thyroid growth without directly altering thyroid hormonogenesis.[2] Goitrogens also may lead to thyroid enlargement. In addition, subacute thyroiditis conditions may produce goiter in adolescents (see box).

A diagnosis in the euthyroid adolescent with a goiter is typically based on multiple clinical clues. The patient may complain of pressure or fullness in the neck for weeks or months before seeking care. In both Hashimoto's thyroiditis and simple goiter a family history is common. On physical examination, all anterior thyroid borders are palpable and move in a distinctly cephalad direction during swallowing.[1] Fixation of an enlarged thyroid to the surrounding structures is rare in benign thyroid conditions such as de Quervain's thyroiditis (acute nonsuppurative thyroiditis), acute suppurative thyroiditis, chronic fibrosing thyroiditis, and chronic lymphocytic thyroiditis. Consequently, when fixation is encountered, it should be considered a sign of malignancy until proved otherwise. Diffuse thyroid enlargement with a smooth gland contour and texture is most frequently seen in simple goiter, Graves' disease, and (occasionally) Hashimoto's thyroiditis. Cobblestoning, a pebble-like texture of the thyroid surface, is most frequently seen with Hashimoto's. A rapidly growing, firm-to-hard goiter, especially if asymmetric and/or associated with cervical lymphadenopathy, should always raise the suspicion of thyroid malignancy.

A tender thyroid gland is most frequently encountered in de Quervain's thyroiditis, painful subacute thyroiditis, and the rarely occurring acute suppurative thyroiditis. In general, a painful thyroid is rarely seen with thyroid carcinoma and in less than 5% of chronic lymphocytic thyroiditis cases.[1] Palpable lymph nodes are commonly found in acute suppurative thyroiditis and thyroid carcinoma, often with a classic Delphian node. Lymph node enlargement also has been reported with chronic lymphocytic thyroiditis. A thyroid bruit, if present, is relatively specific for a hypervascular state such as Graves' disease or iodine deficiency.

Laboratory evaluation of the adolescent with a goiter should start with a third-generation TSH or its equivalent (Figs. 24-1 and 24-2). The TSH as measured with a third-generation assay can provide insight into the euthyroid state and subtle hyperfunction (suppressed TSH) or hypofunction of primary hypothyroidism.[3] With hyperthyroidism, the circulating concentration should be below the normal range or nonmeasurable. In a radioimmunoassay for total T_4 and/or (T_3) values, one or both will be normal: however, both may be minimally elevated in subclinical hyperthyroidism or vice versa in hypothyroidism.

An assay for antithyroid peroxidase antibodies is the test of choice for Hashimoto's thyroiditis. Antimicrosomal and antithyroglobulin antibodies have been found in over 50% of adolescents with a goiter, which suggests an autoimmune etiology, primarily Hashimoto's thyroiditis,[1] but also in as many as 60% of patients with Graves' disease. Evaluation for possible iodine deficiency includes plasma iodine (abnormal when <1 ng/dl) and 24-hour urine iodine (<100 mg/day is consistent with deficiency). Low plasma and urine iodine values, when combined with elevated RAIU, confirm an iodine-deficient state. A thyroid scan is useful only if a nodular thyroid is prominent on physical examination. The estimation of RAIU using ^{123}I is helpful only when the differential diagnosis includes hyperthyroidism, subacute thyroiditis, iodine deficiency, or excess inorganic iodine. Fine-needle aspiration biopsy of the thyroid can document a diagnosis of chronic lymphocytic thyroiditis, if present, even when antithyroid antibody titers are low (<1:16) or undetectable. Uninodular thyroid enlargement and multinodular enlargement in those adolescents with risk factors for thyroid carcinoma should warrant a diagnostic fine-needle aspiration biopsy if the lesion is nonfunctional on scan. If the goiter is of recent onset, pregnancy should be considered, since the physiologic changes associated with pregnancy may produce thyroid enlargement and nonspecific symptoms consistent with thyroid overactivity.[1]

Management of the adolescent with a goiter depends on the cause. The euthyroid adolescent who is not iodine deficient can be treated with levothyroxine (L-thyroxine) in doses that maintain the third-generation TSH level within the normal range.[3] For individuals in whom a goitrogen (e.g., lithium) appears to be the cause of the

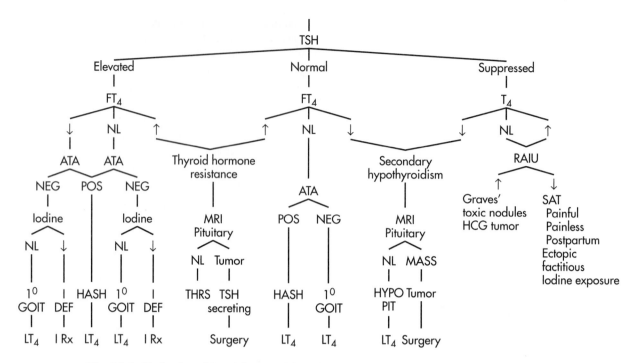

Fig. 24-1. Evaluation of the adolescent with a diffuse goiter. *ATA,* antithyroid antibodies; *FT₄,* free T₄; *HASH,* Hashimoto's thyroiditis; *HYPO PIT,* hypopituitarism; *I DEF,* iodine deficiency; *LT₄,* L-thyroxine; *MRI,* magnetic resonance imaging; *1⁰GOIT,* idiopathic goiter; *RAIU,* radioactive iodine uptake; *SAT,* subacute thyroiditis; *THRS,* thyroid hormone resistance syndrome; *TSH,* thyroid-stimulating hormone.

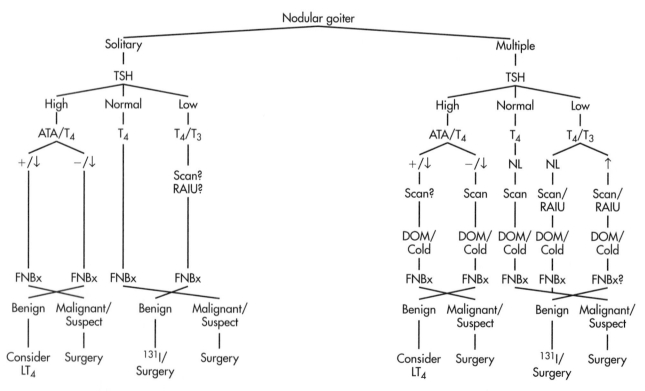

Fig. 24-2. Evaluation of nodular goiter in the adolescent. *ATA,* antithyroid antibodies; *FT₄,* free T₄; *HASH,* Hashimoto's thyroiditis; *HYPO PIT,* hypopituitarism; *I DEF,* iodine deficiency; *LT₄,* L-thyroxine; *MRI,* magnetic resonance imaging; *1⁰GOIT,* idiopathic goiter; *RAIU,* radioactive iodine uptake; *SAT,* subacute thyroiditis; *THRS,* thyroid hormone resistance syndrome; *TSH,* thyroid-stimulating hormone.

goiter, avoiding the goitrogen (if possible) is the therapy of choice. For documented iodine deficiency, administration of 50 to 100 µg of inorganic iodine daily (10 to 15 drops of a saturated solution of potassium iodide [SSKI] weekly) generally returns the thyroid to normal in about 6 months. Definite indications for L-thyroxine suppressive therapy include an elevated third-generation TSH level in an individual who is clinically euthyroid or hypothyroid. Thyroid hormone therapy is also appropriate for patients with progressive thyroid enlargement; pressure symptoms; and/or a large, cosmetically deforming goiter. When L-thyroxine suppression is unsuccessful in reducing goiter size, surgical intervention is a reasonable consideration. Surgery, if performed, should be followed by administration of L-thyroxine sufficient to suppress the TSH level into the low-normal range, which should prevent goiter and/or nodule recurrence.[4]

Prognosis in the adolescent patient depends on the underlying cause. In chronic lymphocytic thyroiditis, shrinkage rates with L-thyroxine replacement vary from 47% to 98%; in simple goiter, rates often approach 90%.[1] Generally, adequate early therapy with L-thyroxine will inhibit further TSH-generated growth. Lifelong treatment may be necessary.

HYPOTHYROIDISM

Hypothyroidism is defined by a constellation of clinical manifestations and decreased levels of circulating thyroid hormone. The typical clinical syndrome is regarded as an early and relatively mild form of thyroid hormone deficiency. The course is usually chronic; if untreated, the condition progresses. Myxedema, the late form of the syndrome, is characterized by essentially no circulating thyroid hormone and clinical progression, which may result in myxedema coma, a medical emergency.

Hashimoto's thyroiditis, the most common cause of adolescent hypothyroidism, is diagnosed in about 1.3% of adolescents aged 11 to 18 years. This condition is more common in females than in males. An increased incidence has been reported among patients with Down and Turner syndromes. The incidence of Hashimoto's thyroiditis also appears to be increased in patients with other autoimmune diseases, such as primary adrenal failure, insulin-dependent diabetes mellitus, and vitiligo.

Hashimoto's thyroiditis is characterized by the presence of active cytotoxic antibodies. The most prominent of these is the complement-fixing antimicrosomal antibody, which, together with an intrathyroidal cell–mediated autoimmune process, eventually leads to cellular necrosis and fibrosis. Polyclonal antibody production is the rule rather than the exception in autoimmune thyroid disease. Antibodies also may be detected against the thyroglobulin components, while others may be directed against the TSH receptors on the cell surface. In Hashimoto's thyroiditis, TGIs are usually associated with a goiter, while blocking antibodies directed at the thyrotropin receptor have been detected in the agoitrous form of the disease.[5]

Other forms of primary hypothyroidism (e.g., hormone underproduction due to defects in hormonogenesis) include iodine deficiency, which is rare in the United States, and congenital enzyme deficiencies. The latter appear to be partial deficiencies if they are first noted during adolescence. Secondary (pituitary) and tertiary (hypothalamic) forms of hypothyroidism are diagnosed most frequently when tumors of the pituitary and/or hypothalamus are present (Box 24-2).

The major reason for establishing an etiology for hypothyroidism is to ensure that therapy is appropriate. Underlying adrenal insufficiency and serious central nervous system pathology should be considered before thyroid hormone therapy is initiated. This is particularly important in patients with hypoadrenalism, since thyroid replacement therapy can precipitate an adrenal crisis. Failure to diagnose a central nervous system lesion that is clinically manifested by hypothyroidism can result in delayed treatment. Assessment of the drug ingestion and diet history may be particularly helpful in identifying the cause of hypothyroidism.

The typical presentation of hypothyroidism in the adolescent includes lethargy or placid behavior in an individual who was previously energetic and active. These symptoms can be confused with those of normal adolescent psychosocial behavior, thus delaying the diagnosis for months or years. Nonspecific complaints, such as dry skin and hair, constipation, and occasional deepening of the voice, are common complaints of the hypothyroid adolescent. A specific abnormality, such as delayed puberty or a retarded linear growth rate, also may be the initial manifestation of hypothyroidism. When questioned, many patients describe noticing an asymptomatic goiter, one that is rarely accompanied by neck soreness or pain radiating to the ears with swallowing. A relatively common manifestation in males is premature testicular enlargement. Pubertal development may be delayed, prolonged, incomplete, or precocious (often with pubic hair growth that is sparse or absent). In some adolescents, hypothyroidism is occult, with few or no overt signs or symptoms. Some patients present with only a chemical manifestation, such as type IV hyperlipidemia.

On physical examination, the dominant sign is a goiter. In Hashimoto's thyroiditis, thyroid enlargement is usually diffuse, with the thyroid two to three times its normal size and firm or pebbly in texture. Especially large goiters that are smooth and symmetric suggest the possibility of an underlying enzyme defect.

BOX 24-2
Etiologic Classification
of Hypothyroidism

I. Primary hypothyroidism
  A. Nongoitrous type
    1. Primary atrophic
    2. Postablative
      a. Iodine 131
      b. External irradiation
      c. Surgical treatment
    3. Postinfectious
      a. Viral
      b. Bacterial
      c. Granulomatous
    4. Infiltrative
      a. Cystinosis
      b. Oxalosis
      c. Sarcoidosis
  B. Goitrous type
    1. Iodine deficiency or excess
    2. Congenital dyshormonogenesis
      a. Trapping defect
      b. Organification defect
      c. Coupling defect
      d. Dehalogenase defect
      e. Proteolysis defect
    3. Thyroid hormone resistance (generalized)
    4. Hashimoto's thyroiditis
    5. Goitrogens
      a. Food (cabbage, turnips)
      b. Drugs (propylthiouracil, methimazole, para-aminosalicylic acid)
  C. Transient type
    1. Following L-thyroxine therapy
    2. Recovery phase of subacute thyroiditis
II. Secondary hypothyroidism (TSH deficiency)
  A. Hemorrhagic type
    1. Pituitary tumor or apoplexy
    2. Postpartum necrosis (Sheehan's syndrome)
  B. Tumorous type
    1. Craniopharyngioma
    2. Pituitary adenoma
  C. Granulomatous pituitary disease
    1. Sarcoidosis
    2. Histiocytosis X
  D. Following pituitary ablation
  E. Isolated TSH deficiency
III. Tertiary hypothyroidism (hypothalamic thyrotropin-releasing hormone deficiency)
  A. Following head trauma
  B. Hypothalamic neoplasm
  C. Granulomatous disease
  D. Following encephalitis

Modified from Greydanus DE, Hofmann AD, editors: *Adolescent medicine*, ed 2, Norwalk, CT, 1989, Appleton & Lange, p 240.

Classic signs and symptoms of hypothyroidism are most frequently found when the hypothyroid state is moderately severe. In this setting pallor may be noted, making the patient appear anemic or jaundiced (carotenemic). Rough, dry skin and dry hair, frequently described as brittle and coarse, are occasionally found. Hoarseness and bradycardia, as well as a narrow pulse pressure, are said to be classic findings, but the incidence is low. Evaluation of the Achilles tendon reflex usually demonstrates a prolonged relaxation phase. If a patient is short in stature for age and family characteristics, occult hypothyroidism must be considered. The electrocardiogram may reveal a sinus bradycardia, low QRS-complex voltage in the standard leads, and in some cases nonspecific ST-T wave changes. Chest radiography may show an enlarged cardiac silhouette, suggesting a pericardial effusion. Pleural effusions also may occur, but usually only with severe hypothyroidism. X-ray examination of the extremities occasionally demonstrates epiphyseal dysgenesis but typically reveals only a delayed bone age. Examination of the sella by computed tomography or magnetic resonance imaging may show pituitary enlargement. This change can occur in primary hypothyroidism but is more common in secondary hypothyroidism. Because secondary hypothyroidism is often associated with pituitary pathology (see Box 24-2), the presence of sellar enlargement requires further diagnostic evaluation.

Laboratory evaluation of the adolescent with hypothyroidism may demonstrate such nonspecific findings as hyponatremia, hypercholesterolemia and/or hypertriglyceridemia, and elevated creatine kinase levels. Anemia (normochromic, hypochromic, microcytic, and occasionally macrocytic) is common in symptomatic patients. Thyroid hormone tests typically reveal low levels of free and total thyroxine (T_4). The test of choice for diagnosing primary hypothyroidism is a third-generation TSH concentration. The level is elevated in primary hypothyroidism and normal or low in secondary or tertiary hypothyroidism, and should alert the clinician to a potential for secondary adrenal insufficiency. Autoimmune hypothyroidism (Hashimoto's thyroiditis) may be confirmed by the presence of antithyroid peroxidase antibodies. Assays directed against the TPO component of the microsome detects anti-TPO antibodies in over 99% of patients with Hashimoto's thyroiditis.[6] Antithyroglobulin and antimicrosomal antibodies are also reported in over 90% of patients.[5] The RAIU test is useful only for the diagnosis of some enzymatic defects. Thyroid fine-needle aspiration cytology, although infrequently necessary, can be diagnostic for lymphocytic thyroiditis as well as helpful in further characterizing the underlying cause.

The differential diagnosis can be confounded by complaints of fatigue and lethargy, which may be confused with adolescent depression, and changes in sexual maturation and growth, which may be confused with constitutional delay of growth and development or with precocious puberty. Since the underlying pathology is important in the adolescent patient, primary hypothyroidism should be differentiated from secondary and tertiary causes. In the critically ill adolescent, caution should be used in the interpretation of routinely obtained thyroid function tests. The "euthyroid sick syndrome" is characterized by the presence of a low total T_4, normal free T_4 (measured by equilibrium dialysis), elevated reverse T_3 (RT_3), and a normal or occasionally depressed third-generation TSH value. In individuals with severe nonthyroidal illness it may be difficult to differentiate secondary or tertiary hypothyroidism from the euthyroid state. This syndrome is usually correctly recognized by the lack of clinical signs of hypothyroidism, absence of a previous pituitary or thyroid history, absence of goiter, and normal deep tendon reflexes. Suppression of serum TSH by dopamine or glucocorticoids may make the interpretation of TSH levels difficult.[3]

Once the diagnosis is confirmed and an etiology established, treatment with synthetic L-thyroxine is started. Given the many nonspecific clinical symptoms of hypothyroidism, long-term thyroid hormone therapy is not warranted solely on empirical clinical grounds. If the patient has documented iodine deficiency, dietary replacement with 50 to 100 µg of iodine daily (10 to 15 drops of SSKI weekly) is usually adequate to reverse hypothyroidism and thyroid gland enlargement. Discontinuing any goitrogen to which the patient is exposed may correct an accompanying hypothyroidism. Treatment of the underlying condition causing secondary and/or tertiary hypothyroidism may result in a recovery of thyroid function, but this is the exception rather than the rule. After careful consideration of potential adrenal insufficiency, L-thyroxine should be cautiously initiated. Replacement in adolescents, at 2 to 2.5 µg/kg/day, may be somewhat higher per kilogram of body weight than in adults.[7] An initial dose of 25 to 50 µg daily is a prudent beginning, with doubling of the initial dose after 3 weeks. Six weeks later a repeat third-generation TSH value should be obtained.[3] If this is at an upper-normal level or minimally elevated, the same dose should be continued and a third-generation TSH level determined again in 6 to 8 weeks. If the TSH remains substantially elevated or has shown only a minimal decrease, the dose should be increased by 25 µg and the TSH measurement repeated in 6 to 8 weeks. The final goal of titration should be a third-generation TSH value in the middle-normal range. In euthyroid individuals the circulating half-life of L-thyroxine is about 1 week, and the TSH level typically reaches equilibrium in about 6 weeks.[3] A satisfactory TSH level can usually be reached within 3 to 6 months.

Adjustment of thyroid hormone dosage on the basis of clinical symptoms is not recommended, since the reso-lution of symptoms often lags behind the pituitary's adjustment to the euthyroid state. Clinical symptoms are notoriously inaccurate for predicting significant hypothyroidism. Chronic overdosing with L-thyroxine (third-generation TSH levels less than normal or undetectable) may be associated with cardiovascular, hepatic, and bone consequences, and should be avoided in settings other than postthyroid ablation for papillary or follicular thyroid carcinoma.[3] Catch-up linear growth and rapid progression of secondary sexual development are common but variable. Pseudotumor cerebri has been reported in children and adolescents treated for primary hypothyroidism, but the condition is rare. The onset of headache after initiation of treatment should prompt further diagnostic assessment.

The ultimate prognosis for adolescents presenting with hypothyroidism depends on the underlying cause. In patients with Hashimoto's thyroiditis, the prognosis for a normal life is good. Evidence suggests that in some patients the ultimate adult height may be less than the predicted height, particularly in those with severe hypothyroidism of prolonged duration before diagnosis and therapy.[8] Finally, from the clinical perspective, it is emphasized that all adolescents with short stature, with or without pubertal delay, and those with type IV hyperlipidemia should be screened for hypothyroidism.

THYROIDITIS

Inflammatory processes involving the thyroid gland in adolescents involve a variety of etiologies (Table 24-2). The most common is chronic lymphocytic (Hashimoto's) thyroiditis. Acute suppurative thyroiditis is rarely encountered, while de Quervain's (giant cell) subacute thyroiditis (acute nonsuppurative thyroiditis) is somewhat more common. In patients with subacute lymphocytic thyroiditis, the painless (silent) form has a female-to-male ratio of up to $3:1$,[5] while the postpartum variety occurs in up to 10% of nondiabetic women after delivery.[9]

Acute suppurative thyroiditis is most frequently caused by infection with streptococcal, staphylococcal, or pneumococcal organisms. Anaerobic organisms that directly invade the thyroid from adjacent structures or by hematogenesis or lymphangitic spread may also be seen. The subacute thyroiditis (SAT) syndromes tend to have specific human lymphocyte antigen (HLA) types, depending on the clinical presentation. Painful (classic de Quervain's) SAT has been associated with HLA-B35 and is thought to be a virus-initiated autoimmune inflammatory response.[10] Painless (silent or sporadic) SAT has been associated with HLA-DR3, HLA-DR4, and HLA-DR5. Similarly, HLA-DR5 and HLA-DR4 have been seen in association with the postpartum variety of SAT. Hashimoto's thyroiditis has been associated with several

TABLE 24-2
Classification of Thyroiditis

Class	Condition	Etiology
Acute thyroiditis	Suppurative thyroiditis	Infectious
Subacute thyroiditis	Lymphocytic (painless)	
	Spontaneous (silent)	Autoimmune
	Postpartum	Autoimmune
	de Quervain's (giant cell/painful)	Postviral/autoimmune
Chronic thyroiditis	Hashimoto's (lymphocytic)	Autoimmune

different HLA-DR types, depending on the population studied. The autoimmune processes found in Hashimoto's thyroiditis include cellular and humoral autoimmune mechanisms characterized by circulating complement-fixing cytotoxic antibodies and intrathyroidal killer T cells, which appear to mediate the inflammatory process.[5]

A diagnosis of acute suppurative thyroiditis is made from a history of a rapidly developing acute febrile illness accompanied by pain and an exquisitely tender enlarged thyroid. Typically, there are overlying erythema, regional lymphadenopathy, high fever, chills, and an elevated sedimentation rate. Aspiration for Gram's stain and culture typically yields one of the causative organisms. The onset of subacute painful (granulomatous) thyroiditis frequently follows 10 to 14 days after a viral upper respiratory infection. The syndrome typically includes fever, chills, malaise, sweats, and weakness in association with a unilateral or diffusely enlarged and tender thyroid, with pain occasionally radiating to the ear. During the acute phase of this disease, the erythrocyte sedimentation rate is typically elevated. Thyroid function tests may yield values ranging from euthyroid to hyperthyroid to hypothyroid, depending on the point in time of the disease's course. Initially, most patients with SAT go through a hyperthyroxinemic phase, which may be associated with thyrotoxic symptoms. At this point 24-hour RAIU values are low (<8%), as is the third-generation TSH value. Circulating thyroglobulin is elevated during this phase, which may help differentiate SAT from factitious thyrotoxicosis. As the inflammatory process continues, thyroid hormone production is interrupted, and thyroxine levels typically decrease into the normal range. This is often followed by a continuing decline to subnormal thyroid hormone levels before a return to normal values after cell recovery. TSH levels correspond physiologically to the circulating free thyroxine. This "roller coaster" course may therefore simulate hyperthyroidism, euthyroidism, secondary hypothyroidism, and primary hypothyroidism before complete recovery occurs. Fine-needle biopsy, if performed, usually reveals giant cells and granulomatous changes, but this is rarely necessary. On the other hand, at presentation, painless (sporadic or silent) lymphocytic SAT may be limited to thyroid enlargement. Postpartum patients and those with silent SAT typically have a goiter

and one or more of thyroid function abnormalities sometime during the first 2 to 3 months after delivery. In contradistinction, those with the painful variety frequently have positive antimicrosomal and/or antithyroglobulin antibodies.

Hashimoto's thyroiditis can present as clinical hypothyroidism, hyperthyroidism, or an asymptomatic euthyroid goiter. Consequently, thyroid function test results may be normal; demonstrate primary hypothyroidism; show an elevated TSH with normal or low-normal total and free T_4 levels; or reveal elevated T_4, T_3, and free thyroxine levels and a suppressed third-generation TSH concentration (Hashitoxicosis).

Management of the thyroiditis syndromes depends on the underlying cause. Aggressive incision and drainage of a thyroid abscess in acute suppurative thyroiditis, and institution of appropriate antibiotic coverage directed by Gram's stain and culture, are important. The patient with painful SAT generally requires only supportive care. Nonsteroidal anti-inflammatory drug administration may be useful for pain control in the acute phase. Severe or persistent cases may respond favorably to a short course of systemic corticosteroids, but this should not be routine. Beta-adrenergic blockers may be useful for symptomatic treatment of the adrenergic manifestations associated with the transient thyrotoxic phase. L-Thyroxine therapy may aid in supporting the hypothyroid patient until full recovery has occurred. The prognosis of acute suppurative thyroiditis is good if diagnosis and therapy have been timely; otherwise, severe soft tissue infection of the neck and mediastinum may result.

Patients with painful SAT have been reported to have an 85% to 90% recovery to normal thyroid function. Rare recurrences have been reported. In both painless and postpartum thyroiditis there is a 70% to 80% recovery to euthyroidism. Painless SAT recurs in 10% to 15% of cases; postpartum thyroiditis is said to have a high rate of recurrence upon subsequent pregnancy.

THYROTOXICOSIS

Thyrotoxicosis is a hypermetabolic state resulting from the exposure of target tissues to excess thyroid

TABLE 24-3
Differential Diagnosis of Thyrotoxicosis

	Mechanism	Serum TSH*	RAIU
Hyperthyroidism	Hyperproduction of T_4/T_3 in thyroid		
TSH Dependent			
Tumorous	TSH secretion	↑ or normal	↑↑
Nontumorous	Selective thyrotrophic thyroid Hormone resistance (PRTH)	↑ or normal	↑↑
TSH Independent			
Abnormal thyroid stimulator			
Graves' disease	Thyroid-stimulating immunoglobulin	↓	↑↑
Trophoblastic disease	Human chorionic gonadotropin	↓	↑↑
Thyroid autonomy			
Toxic adenoma	Benign tumor	↓	↑↑
Toxic multinodular goiter	Foci of functional autonomy	↓	↑↑
Other Causes			
Inflammatory			
Subacute thyroiditis			
Painful (de Quervain's thyroiditis)	Hormone leakage	↓	↓
Painless lymphocytic			
Spontaneous	Hormone leakage	↓	↓
Postpartum	Hormone leakage	↓	↓
Extrathyroidal			
Hormone ingestion	Gastrointestinal absorption	↓	↓
Ectopic thyroid tissue	Functional metastasis/struma ovarii	↓	↓

Modified from Ingbar SH: Classification of the causes of thyrotoxicosis. In Ingbar SH, Braverman LE, editors: *Werner's the thyroid,* ed 5, Philadelphia, 1986, JB Lippincott; p 810.
*TSH, thyroid-stimulating hormone measured with third-generation assay.
†Decreased if patient has been exposed to excessive iodine.
PRTH, pituitary resistance to thyroid hormone; *RAIU,* radioactive iodine uptake.

hormone. Of all the recognized causes of thyrotoxicosis, Graves' disease is the most common in adolescents (Table 24-3), accounting for more than 20% of all thyroid problems seen in some referral centers.[11] A precise diagnosis is essential for appropriate therapy and assessment of prognosis.

Graves' disease is an autoimmune disorder in which the thyroid is stimulated by immunoglobulins that interact with the TSH receptor, thyroid-stimulating immunoglobulin (TSI). The result is an overproduction and release of T_4 and T_3. Half or more of the adolescents with Graves' disease have a positive family history of autoimmune thyroid disease. Graves' disease is associated with other autoimmune diseases, such as pernicious anemia, insulin-dependent diabetes mellitus, autoimmune ovarian failure, and Addison's disease. Genetic predisposition to these autoimmune disorders may have a racial predominance, since the HLA types associated with Graves' disease differ among races. Whites have HLA-B8 and HLA-DR3, Japanese more frequently demonstrate HLA-BW35, and Chinese have HLA-BW46. In whites the presence of HLA-DR3 increases the relative risk of Graves' disease to about 3.7 times that of the population at large. Women

are affected more frequently than men, with at least a 6:1 ratio.[11] Because other forms of thyrotoxicosis are rare among adolescents, their etiologies will not be discussed here. The reader is referred to Table 24-1 as well as to a review.[12]

In 97% to 99% of adolescents the clinical presentation of Graves' disease is typically heralded by a goiter.[11] Nervousness is seen in more than 90% and increased appetite in more than two thirds. A history of weight loss is found in approximately 50% and about 15% experience weight gain. School problems associated with hyperkinesis are common. Palpitations and heat intolerance are noted in approximately one third of patients. Some patients have associated amenorrhea, dyspnea, restless sleeping, fatigue, hyperdefecation, hair loss, neck fullness, and/or vitiligo. Emotional lability—crying, irritability, or intolerance of criticism—is a symptom that may bring the patient to medical attention. On physical examination a resting tachycardia and widened pulse pressures of >50 mm Hg occur in about 80% of patients. Eye manifestations of varying degree are seen in one half to two thirds of patients,[11] but true infiltrative ophthalmopathy of clinical significance is rare (<5%) in adolescents as opposed to adults. Systolic hypertension is present in nearly one half of patients. A thyroid bruit or a systolic ejection murmur has a similar occurrence rate. The goiter associated with Graves' disease is usually symmetric, nontender, without significant nodularity, and firm to rubbery in consistency. A fine tremor of the outstretched fingers occurs in more than two thirds of adolescents. The skin is typically smooth, moist, and warm and appears flushed in about 25% of cases.[11] Rarely, adolescents with Graves' disease have pretibial myxedema, onycholysis, choreiform movements, or anorexia.

The test of choice for diagnosing thyrotoxicosis is a third-generation TSH level. The third-generation TSH value is suppressed below the normal range or nondetectable, which suggests autonomous thyroid function. General laboratory evaluation may demonstrate such nonspecific findings as a moderately reduced white blood cell (WBC) count with relative lymphocytosis and, rarely, thrombocytopenia or hypercalcemia. Adolescents with thyrotoxicosis may rarely have costochondral calcifications on chest radiography, with a frequency inversely related to the age at diagnosis.

Specific thyroid abnormalities include findings that are, at least in part, dependent on the underlying cause. In Graves' disease the serum T_4 and T_3 levels are typically elevated, although a rare patient has only an elevated total T_3. Typically the free T_4 and free T_3 values are elevated. For patients who do not have a high dietary intake of iodine, an RAIU test can be useful. In Graves' disease this test is typically elevated at 1, 6, and 24 hours after oral administration of radioactive iodine.[13] This examination often allows a general differentiation of the two major types of thyrotoxicosis (Table 24-3).

There may be laboratory evidence of thyroid autoimmunity. Antimicrosomal (anti-TPO antibodies) and anti-thyroglobulin antibodies are present in 60% to 80% of adolescents with Graves' disease.[6,11] Adolescents with Graves' disease usually have elevated TSI and thyrotropin-binding inhibitory immunoglobulin (TBII) concentrations. Both of these immunoglobulins are directed against the TSH receptor.[14] A thyroid scan is helpful only in differentiating unusual types of hyperthyroidism in the adolescent with thyroid nodule(s) on physical examination. Solitary or multiple autonomous nodule(s) can be documented by ^{123}I scan in the thyrotoxic patient. In the typical patient with Graves' disease, a scan is not necessary. The bone age of children and adolescents may be advanced for their chronologic age; that is, 1 to 2.5 years advanced in up to 75% of cases.[11]

The differential diagnosis of thyrotoxicosis is shown in Table 24-3. Especially troublesome is the differentiation of the clinically euthyroid patient with elevated thyroid hormone levels who has a generalized resistance to thyroid hormone or protein-binding abnormalities.

Neurologic features may also be confusing, especially in patients with athetoid movements such as those associated with acute rheumatic fever (e.g., mild muscular skeletal pain, low-grade fever, choreiform-like movements) and/or hypokalemic periodic paralysis. Three forms of treatment can be used for patients in the hyperthyroid state of Graves' disease: antithyroid drugs, surgical removal of thyroid tissue, or ablation of the overfunctioning thyroid with radioactive iodine. In the adolescent patient, antithyroid drugs have been used as long-term therapy, and at least 50% of those treated achieved a long-standing remission.[11] In the United States the two principal agents used are propylthiouracil (PTU) and methimazole. PTU inhibits oxidative iodination and coupling, which leads to a decrease in thyroid hormone synthesis and diminishes the peripheral conversion of T_4 to T_3. In addition, there is a modest immunosuppressive effect. Methimazole has a similar effect on the oxidative iodination and coupling process as well as an immune suppressive effect.

PTU and methimazole have similar toxicity profiles. Nonspecific skin rashes, which are often transient, typically occur in the first 3 weeks of therapy. Urticarial eruptions, on the other hand, should be considered serious reactions and usually necessitate a change in therapy. Serious toxicity in the form of agranulocytosis, which occurs as an idiosyncratic, non–dose-dependent reaction to these medications usually appearing within the first 4 to 8 weeks of therapy, may be seen in up to 0.5% of patients, and rarely may occur many months after the initiation of therapy. A baseline WBC count before the start of therapy is useful, given the mild suppressive effect that thyrotoxicosis may have on the granulocyte count. Repeat WBC counts may be indicated at 2- to 3-week intervals for the first 2 to 3 months of therapy, as well as when the patient presents with symptoms of fever or sore throat, to evaluate for major granulocyte suppression.[15] Serious toxicity to one of these agents is an indication to change to an alternative therapy, since substantial overlap exists.

PTU and methimazole may be initiated in high- or low-dose regimens. Alternatively, initial dosages of 150 mg PTU or 20 mg methimazole can be continued twice a day, with L-thyroxine added to maintain euthyroidism during the treatment period.[13] This regimen, in one author's experience (HVB), produces a more stable euthyroid state during therapy than is typically achieved by adjusting the thionamide dose. Owing to its longer half-life, methimazole is more successful in twice- or once-daily doses than PTU. The serum T_4 level should be titrated into the mid-normal range, and ultimately the third-generation TSH value should be maintained within the normal range. The initial duration of therapy can range from months to years, depending on the clinical setting and the patient's wishes.

Various methods have been proposed for predicting the likelihood of remission in patients treated with antithyroid drugs. Adolescents experiencing their first episode of hyperthyroidism, with a small thyroid gland and only mild to moderate hyperthyroxinemia of short duration, appear to be more likely to have a sustained remission. Those with large goiters that increase or fail to decrease in size during therapy have a relapse rate of up to 70% after discontinuation of the antithyroid drug. In general, the duration of treatment affects remission rates: longer treatment periods (18 months or more) appear to be superior to shorter periods (6 months). Adolescent patients treated for longer periods appear to have even higher percentages of remission. Recently, suppression of TBII activity to undetectable levels during treatment has been reported to be predictive of approximately a 90% rate of sustained remission.

For patients who do not take their medications, have serious side effects, or do not want to take a thionamide, ablative therapy should be considered. Subtotal thyroidectomy decreases tissue mass and may result in euthyroidism. An euthyroid state at the time of surgery is desirable to avoid the potential precipitation of thyroid storm. Preoperatively, the patient should be rendered euthyroid with an antithyroid medication. At least 10 to 14 days before surgery the patient should receive 5 drops of Lugol solution three to four times daily, or blocking doses of a beta-adrenergic agent such as propranolol, to decrease intraglandular vascularity. Surgical complications include hypothyroidism in 40% to 65% of patients.[11] The incidence rates for permanent hypoparathyroidism and recurrent laryngeal nerve palsy are lower for subtotal thyroidectomy than reported rates for total thyroidectomy for thyroid cancer. Only surgeons who regularly perform thyroid surgery should undertake these procedures.

Although long experience with radioactive iodine therapy has failed to demonstrate an associated significant increase in the risk of leukemia or other malignancies, and some physicians advocate its use in children and adolescents, a 1990 survey of thyroidologists indicated that only one third of respondents recommended this treatment in younger patients.[13] In our view, for adolescents, radioactive iodine therapy should be limited to cases in which all other measures have failed to control the hyperthyroidism adequately. Certainly those patients in whom recurrent or persistent hyperthyroidism remains after thyroidectomy, and those with serious hematologic toxicity from antithyroid drugs who refuse or are not candidates for surgery, should be treated with radioactive ^{131}I. Before initiation of this therapy, the possibility of pregnancy must be considered in female patients. As a late sequela of radioactive iodine treatment, up to 75% of patients develop hypothyroidism, with a 7% to 25% incidence in the first year and 3% to 5% annually thereafter.

THYROID HORMONE RESISTANCE

The syndrome of thyroid hormone resistance is an important consideration in the differential diagnosis of patients with hyperthyroxinemia. Of the first 70 reported cases, over 50% were children and adolescents.[16] Among these cases, the incidence in males and females was equal. Autosomal dominant inheritance appears to be an operative factor. Proposed defects responsible for the clinical and laboratory manifestations are most likely found at the cellular level. There are three possible subgroupings. The one best described is a generalized resistance to thyroid hormone (GRTH), in which genetically determined abnormalities in thyroid hormone action are present in the periphery and the pituitary. The second form involves pituitary resistance to thyroid hormone (PRTH); in this form, resistance is limited to the pituitary level, and thyroid hormone does not appropriately suppress TSH secretion. A third form is peripheral tissue resistance to thyroid hormone, with normal pituitary sensitivity. This entity has not been documented in adolescents and cannot be diagnosed accurately with currently available clinical laboratory tests.

Diagnosis of the first two forms of thyroid hormone resistance begins with the physical finding of a smooth, symmetric goiter. More than 80% of patients with thyroid hormone resistance have an enlarged thyroid.[16] An overwhelming majority of patients with GRTH are clinically euthyroid (although some are clinically hypothyroid) with a delayed bone age, along with mental retardation, learning disability, emotional disturbance, hearing defect, and nystagmus.[16] In addition, a link between GRTH and attention deficit hyperactivity disorder has been described.[17] There are no signs of Graves' disease. Typically, patients with PRTH present with a combination of thyrotoxic symptoms (without Graves' ophthalmopathy or pretibial myxedema) and a goiter.

The laboratory evaluation of patients with thyroid hormone resistance reveals elevations in total and free T_4 and total T_3. Despite the hyperthyroxinemia, the third-generation TSH values are normal or slightly elevated. The RAIU test shows a higher than normal value. Although this constellation of thyroid function tests may lead to confusion with Graves' disease, therapy for Graves' disease is inappropriate for, and potentially dangerous to, patients with a thyroid hormone resistance syndrome.

A logical diagnostic strategy includes total and free T_4 plus a third-generation TSH evaluation. If the T_4 and free T_4 are high and the TSH value is detectable, and if doubt about the diagnosis still exists (as it should in a clinically euthyroid patient with unexpected T_4 elevation), the performance of a TRH stimulation test to evaluate third-generation TSH responsiveness is appropriate. Finally, a pituitary tumor–producing TSH should be considered, and pituitary imaging may be indicated. Typical findings in thyroid hormone resistance also include a normal T_3-to-T_4 ratio but an elevated reverse T_3 level and an increased thyroglobulin level, both of which are also common in patients with Graves' disease. The sex hormone–binding globulin (SHBG) level, normally elevated in hyperthyroidism, is normal in patients with GRTH.[18] In Graves' disease, typical signs and symptoms are usually present, and the third-generation TSH assay is below the normal range or undetectable. Stimulation with TRH produces no third-generation TSH response in patients with Graves' disease, as compared with those with GRTH, in whom the response is normal or exaggerated. In patients with autoimmune hyperthyroidism, circulating levels of autoantibodies are typically present.

The most difficult differential diagnosis is presented by the two conditions of inappropriate TSH secretion in those patients whose peripheral sensitivity to thyroid hormone is normal. The first of these conditions results from an autonomous secretion of TSH from a pituitary tumor. Characteristically, these patients have no third-generation TSH response to TRH stimulation and an elevated SHBG level.[16,19] Furthermore, in TSH-secreting tumors, the molar ratio of the circulating free alpha subunit glycoprotein to TSH is greater than 1, whereas in PRTH the alpha subunit-to-TSH ratio is less than 1.

Management of patients with thyroid hormone resistance should include genetic counseling. Patients with GRTH, if clinically euthyroid and demonstrating no significant neurologic or growth abnormality, may require no treatment.[16] In severe cases with neurologic, growth, and bone maturation problems, thyroid hormone replacement with two to three times the usual replacement dose may effectively decrease goiter size and return growth and maturation rates toward normal. Special attention must be paid to accurate diagnosis. Among reported cases, most of those requiring intensive long-term thyroid hormone therapy have come to clinical recognition after thyroid ablation for misdiagnosed Graves' disease.

Patients with PRTH present an interesting clinical dilemma. The interruption of thyroid hormone synthesis with an antithyroid drug or thyroid ablation would seem reasonable. Unfortunately, further elevation of the TSH with concomitant pituitary thyrotroph hypertrophy with possible pituitary enlargement may result in an increase in goiter size. Therefore, it is advisable to attempt to directly suppress TSH secretion at the pituitary level, preferably by the use of T_3, a dopamine agonist such as bromocriptine, or 3,5,3′-triiodothyroacetic acid (TRIAC). The prognosis for generalized thyroid hormone resistance syndromes is good. The severity of the defect seems to decrease over time, since infants, children, and adolescents are often more severely compromised than adults.[16]

THYROID CANCER/THYROID NODULES

Although thyroid carcinoma among adolescents is rare, it is the fourth most common cancer found in the 15- to 19-year-old age group. This form of cancer is more prevalent in females than in males, with a ratio of about 2:1.[19] Papillary thyroid carcinoma accounts for up to 69% of tumors in adolescents. Follicular and mixed papillary/follicular carcinomas are common.[19] Medullary carcinoma is seen in approximately 3% to 5% of these patients. Lymphomas of the thyroid gland account for a very small percentage.

Several series suggest an increased frequency of thyroid carcinoma in individuals previously exposed to ionizing radiation to the head or neck for conditions such as thymus, tonsil or adenoid enlargement, hemangiomas, nevi, acne, eczema, cervical adenitis, mastoiditis, sinusitis, allergic rhinitis, and central nervous system tumors. With such a history, the risk may be as high as 700 times greater than that for individuals who are not exposed. The influence of radiation therapy on the development of thyroid carcinoma is inferred from exposure preceding the development of clinical disease by 3 to 40 years, with mean duration of exposure to clinical diagnosis ranging from 7 to 10 years.[19] A history of exposure to ionizing radiation to the head or neck is noted in 50% to 80% of adolescents with thyroid carcinoma.

Patients typically present with a neck mass, a palpable thyroid nodule, or cervical lymphadenopathy. Typically, these findings will have been present for 2 or more years at the time of diagnosis. A clinical history of voice change is infrequent despite the demonstration of laryngeal nerve involvement at surgery in 3% to 7% of adolescents. On physical examination, a thyroid nodule is palpable in 25% to 93% of patients. Palpable cervical lymph nodes are reported at presentation in 7% to 75% of patients, and lymphadenopathy is found at surgery in 75% to 90%.[19] A nontender lymph node in the neck that fails to resolve in a few weeks merits a cervical lymph node biopsy.

Thyroid imaging should be used to further delineate palpable thyroid nodules. A cold, nonfunctional area in the thyroid (i.e., an area of decreased uptake on ^{123}I or technetium-99 [^{99}Tc] scan) is consistent with, but not diagnostic of, thyroid carcinoma. In some surgical series of cold thyroid nodules, a malignancy rate of 20% to 40% has been noted in adolescents, but in adolescent males with a cold nodule the rate is usually above 50%. [123]I is the isotope of choice, since warm, functional areas with use of ^{99}Tc may prove to be cold with [123]I. Recently, malignancy in functional nodular lesions on ^{123}I scanning has been recognized in up to 10% of adolescent patients.[20] Another potentially useful finding on thyroid scan is functional ectopic tissue. Sonographic evaluation of thyroid nodules may help differentiate solid from cystic lesions. A purely cystic thyroid nodule, which is rare, is malignant in 1% to 3% of patients. A mixed solid/cystic lesion yields about 20% malignancy in unselected populations.[20]

Fine-needle aspiration biopsy techniques generally have not been used in adolescents, since higher malignancy rates in this age group support a more aggressive diagnostic procedure. A chest x-ray examination to survey possible metastatic disease is prudent. Lung metastases at presentation are seen in up to 19% of children and adolescents. Results of thyroid function tests are usually normal, but these tests are appropriate for the evaluation of a cold thyroid nodule. In a functional nodule identified with ^{123}I, the possibility of hyperfunction must be evaluated, since an elevation of serum T_3 alone may be seen in over 50% of patients. The third-generation TSH level in patients with hyperfunctioning nodules is typically suppressed.

In medullary thyroid carcinoma, an elevation of serum calcitonin may be seen, particularly in patients with a palpable nodule. The level of carcinoembryonic antigen may be elevated if the disease has spread beyond the thyroid. Calcitonin levels also can be used to detect the C cell hyperplasia phase of medullary thyroid carcinoma—a stage at which high cure rates have been reported. In suspected cases, calcitonin levels are evaluated after stimulation with calcium and/or pentagastrin.

The differential diagnosis of a thyroid nodule includes benign thyroid adenoma and Hashimoto's thyroiditis as well as multinodular goiter. Benign adenomas must also be differentiated from nonthyroid tumors such as lymphoma and from granulomatous disease and cervical hygroma. A pure thyroid cyst or a hemorrhagic thyroid cyst may present as a cold nodule on scan. The differential diagnosis of a functional thyroid nodule includes postsubtotal thyroidectomy, compensatory hypertrophy, and such congenital lesions as hemiagenesis and hemangiomas. Differential diagnosis of solitary thyroid nodules is presented in Box 24-3 and evaluation of solitary thyroid nodules is detailed in Figure 24-3.

In the adolescent with a thyroid nodule, the physician should always consider the possibility of thyroid carcinoma. Because of the high risk of thyroid malignancy in a cold nodule in this age group, we recommend surgical removal. Further therapy should be determined on the basis of the histologic findings. In general, thyroid carcinoma more than 1 cm in diameter or with a positive cervical lymph node or nodes, particularly with a history of head or neck radiation, warrants an ipsilateral thyroidectomy and isthmusectomy with a subtotal thyroidectomy on the contralateral side. This approach is recommended rather than a total thyroidectomy.[21] Surgical complication rates appear to be higher among patients treated with total thyroidectomy, with the incidence of permanent hypoparathyroidism 6% to 8% and that of recurrent laryngeal

---

BOX 24-3
Causes of Solitary Thyroid Nodules

Cysts
  Pure cysts
  Mixed cystic solid lesions
Adenomas
  Autonomously hyperfunctioning
  Nonautonomously functioning
Colloid (adenomatoid) nodules
Thyroiditis
  Acute
  Subacute
  Chronic
    Hashimoto's thyroiditis
    Riedel's struma
Graves' disease
Infections
  Granulomatous infections
  Abscesses
Developmental anomalies
  Unilateral lobe agenesis
  Cystic hygroma
  Dermoid
  Teratoma
Carcinoma
  Primary thyroid
  Secondary (metastatic)
Lymphoma

From Mazzaferri EL: IM for the Specialist, vol 4, 1983; pp 40-52.

---

nerve paralysis 5% to 26%. These rates depend on both the extent of disease and the experience of the surgeon performing the procedure.[21] Lower rates of complications are reported when the recommended ipsilateral lobe and isthmus removal is combined with contralateral subtotal thyroidectomy. Radical or modified radical neck dissection for differentiated thyroid carcinomas is not recommended.

The use of postoperative radioactive ^{131}I therapy for adolescents is controversial. Patients with residual carcinoma after surgical intervention, those with metastatic disease to a cervical lymph node or nodes and lungs, or those with large tumors (>3 cm) appear to benefit from ablative ^{131}I therapy, with diminished recurrence and mortality rates.[19,21] Reported experience with radioactive iodine therapy in children and adolescents with thyroid carcinoma has not shown a significant increase in bone marrow suppression, radiation pneumonitis, or leukemia or an increased incidence of secondary malignancy.[19] Radioactive iodine treatment for medullary thyroid carcinoma is not effective, since the C cells do not concentrate iodine.

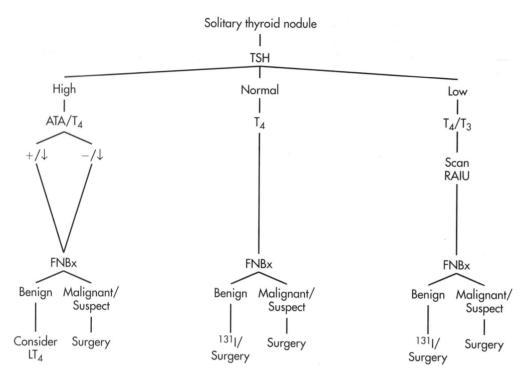

Fig. 24-3. Evaluation of a solid thyroid nodule in the adolescent. *ATA*, antithyroid antibodies; *LT₄*, l-thyroxine; *RAIU*, radioactive iodine uptake; *T₄*, free T₄; *TSH*, thyroid-stimulating hormone.

The final therapy generally used for thyroid carcinoma consists of suppressive doses of l-thyroxine. The dosage should be adjusted so that the third-generation TSH level is below the normal range, thus maximally diminishing thyroid-cell stimulation by thyrotropin.[3] Follow-up surveillance of patients with a differentiated thyroid carcinoma should include measurement of serum thyroglobulin both with and without l-thyroxine; the latter appears to give increased sensitivity in the detection of residual disease. As a marker for residual thyroid tissue, serum thyroglobulin has excellent predictive value in assessment for recurrent or persistent disease.[19] A periodic radioactive ^{131}I scan of the neck, chest, and total body is useful in surveying for metastatic disease and documenting therapeutic ablation.[20] The correlation between a thyroglobulin level and a ^{131}I scan is good. We suggest a follow-up schedule using both thyroglobulin and ^{131}I scan 6 months after radioactive iodine ablation and/or thyroidectomy. Before scanning, l-thyroxine should be discontinued for 6 weeks and T₃ for at least 2 weeks. To maintain a relatively euthyroid state during most of this preparation time, we recommend that patients be treated with triiodothyronine (Cytomel), 25 μg two to three times daily for 3 to 4 weeks after discontinuing l-thyroxine therapy. With this regimen the patient experiences a shorter period of hypothyroidism, since this drug requires discontinuation

for only 2 weeks before isotope administration. Ideally, TSH levels should be more than 40 mIU/ml at the time of ^{131}I scanning. The timing of follow-up scanning is debatable. Some authors recommend scanning at yearly intervals for the first 2 or 3 years after thyroid ablation and then at 3- to 5-year intervals for life.

A routine chest radiography examination for occult lung metastases may enhance detection, because about 10% to 20% of lung metastases do not show a concentration of iodine. Continued surveillance for recurrence and metastases is prudent. One study shows that up to 40% of adolescents undergoing follow-up for as long as 25 years develop lung metastases at some time.[19]

The prognosis for patients who develop differentiated thyroid carcinoma in adolescence is generally very good, with a 5-year survival rate of approximately 99% in 15- to 19-year-olds and a 10-year survival rate of 98%. Despite these encouraging results, the overall estimated excess mortality ratio among adolescents with thyroid carcinoma in comparison with those who do not have this disease is 8:1; the mortality rate also appears to be somewhat higher than that reported in adults.[19] All-age mortality due to thyroid carcinoma, including medullary thyroid carcinoma, has been reported to be 5% to 8%. Unfortunately, relapses are relatively frequent, and most deaths occur during adult life after a "complete cure" at the time of initial therapy. Cumulative risk of relapse in one reported series was the same at 10 to 20 years after initial diagnosis as in the period from diagnosis to 10 years.[19] These mortality rates are comparable with those reported for adults.[21]

The prognosis for medullary thyroid carcinoma is not as predictable as for the differentiated type. The former appears to be curable when detected in the C cell hyperplasia stage. Calcium/pentagastrin stimulation tests are necessary to uncover this subclinical (C cell hyperplasia) stage of medullary thyroid carcinoma, and should be performed in families with medullary carcinoma as well as in families with type 2 multiple endocrine neoplasia syndrome. Once nodular medullary thyroid carcinoma is present, cure rates are highly variable, depending on the extent of the disease. Survival rates range from normal at 10 years for intrathyroidal disease to about 50% when lymph node involvement is present.

References

1. Barnes HV: Goiter in the clinically euthyroid adolescent. In Moss AJ, editor: *Pediatrics update: reviews for physicians,* New York, 1984, Elsevier Biomedical, pp 95-110.

2. Studer H, Ranelli F: Simple goiter and its variants: euthyroid and hyperthyroid multinodular goiters, *Endocr Rev* 3:40-61, 1982.

3. Nicoloff JT, Spencer CA: The use and misuse of the sensitive thyrotropin assays: clinical review 12, *J Clin Endocrinol Metab* 71:553-558, 1990.

4. Fogelfeld L, Wiviott MBT, Shore-Freedman E, Blend M, Bekerman C, Pinsky S, Schneider HB: Recurrence of thyroid nodules after surgical removal in patients irradiated in childhood for benign conditions, *N Engl J Med* 320:835-840, 1989.

5. Dussalt JH, Rousseau F: Immunologically mediated hypothyroidism, *Endocrinol Metab Clin North Am* 16:417-429, 1987.

6. Mariotti S, Caturegli P, Piccolo P, Barbesino G, Pinchera A: Antithyroid peroxidase autoantibodies in thyroid diseases, *J Clin Endocrinol Metab* 71:661-669, 1990.

7. Hennessey JV, Evaul JE, Tseng Y-C, Burman KD, Wartofsky L: L-Thyroxine dosage: a re-evaluation of therapy with contemporary preparations, *Ann Intern Med* 105:11-15, 1986.

8. Rivkees SA, Bode HH, Crawford JD: Long term growth in juvenile acquired hypothyroidism: the failure to achieve normal adult stature, *N Engl J Med* 318:599, 1988.

9. Nikolai TF, Turney SL, Roberts RC: Postpartum lymphocytic thyroiditis: prevalence, clinical course, and long term follow-up, *Arch Intern Med* 147:221, 1987.

10. Farid NF: Immunogenetics of autoimmune thyroid disorders, *Endocrinol Metab Clin North Am* 16:229-246, 1987.

11. Barnes HV, Blizzard RM: Antithyroid drug therapy for toxic diffuse goiter (Graves' disease). Thirty years' experience in children and adolescents, *J Pediatr* 91:313-320, 1977.

12. Loughney MH, Burman KD: Unusual forms of thyrotoxicosis. In Mazzaferri EL, editor: *Advances in endocrinology and metabolism,* vol 5, Chicago, 1994, Mosby–Year Book, pp 349-392.

13. Solomon B, Glinoer D, LaGasse R, Wartofsky L: Current trends in the management of Graves' disease, *J Clin Endocrinol Metab* 70:1518-1524, 1990.

14. Foley TP, White C, New A: Juvenile Graves' disease: usefulness and limitations of thyrotropin receptor antibody determinations, *J Pediatr* 110:378-386, 1987.

15. Tajiri J, Noguchi S, Murakami T, Murakami N: Antithyroid drug-induced agranulocytosis: the usefulness of routine white blood cell count monitoring, *Arch Intern Med* 150:621-624, 1990.

16. Refetoff S: Thyroid hormone resistance syndromes. In Ingbar SH, Braverman LE, editors: *Werner's the thyroid,* ed 5, Philadelphia, 1986, JB Lippincott, pp 1292-1307.

17. Hauser P, Zametkin AJ, Martinez P, Vitiello B, Matochik JA, Mixson AJ, Weintraub BD: Attention deficit-hyperactivity disorder in people with generalized resistance to thyroid hormone, *N Engl J Med* 328:997-1001, 1993.

18. Sarne DH, Refetoff S, Rosenfield RL, Farriaux JP: Sex hormone binding globulin in the diagnosis of peripheral tissue resistance to thyroid hormone: the value of changes after short term triiodothyronine administration, *J Clin Endocrinol Metab* 66:740-746, 1988.

19. Schlumberger M, DeVathaire F, Travogli JP, Vassol G, Lemerle J, Parmentier C, Tubiana M: Differentiated thyroid carcinoma of childhood: long term follow-up of 72 patients, *J Clin Endocrinol Metab* 65:1088-1094, 1987.

20. Vautterle AJ, Rich P, Lsung BME, Achcraft MW, Solomon DH, Keeler EB: The thyroid nodule, *Ann Intern Med* 96:221-232, 1982.

21. Degroot LJ, Kaplan EL, McCormick M, Straus FH: Natural history, treatment, and course of papillary thyroid carcinoma, *J Clin Endocrinol Metab* 71:414-424, 1990.

CHAPTER 25

Insulin-Dependent Diabetes Mellitus

•

Pavel Fort, Jean Corrigan, and Fima Lifshitz

Insulin-dependent diabetes mellitus (IDDM), or type I diabetes, is a leading cause of chronic illness in youth. Its incidence among adolescents surpasses that of many other chronic diseases such as cancer. Each year more than 14 new cases of IDDM per 100,000 population are diagnosed in the United States.[1,2] Most children with IDDM are diagnosed at the beginning of adolescence, with peak incidence earlier in girls than in boys. Unlike adults, in whom diabetes mellitus is not necessarily dependent on insulin treatment (non–insulin-dependent diabetes mellitus [NIDDM], or type II diabetes), most adolescents with diabetes mellitus require insulin injections throughout life to maintain metabolic homeostasis. Children rarely suffer from type II diabetes mellitus. Maturity-onset diabetes of youth (MODY in the former terminology) is a rare genetic form of diabetes usually diagnosed before age 25 years. It is typically responsive to diet and/or hypoglycemic oral agents. It is important to note that diabetes mellitus requiring insulin therapy also may occur in conjunction with other conditions, such as pancreatic disease, steroid use, hormonal and genetic disorders involving insulin resistance, and various syndromes. Types of diabetes mellitus and other categories of glucose intolerance, as well as their diagnostic criteria, are listed in Tables 25-1 and 25-2.

Day-to-day management of patients with IDDM can be one of the most demanding and difficult medical problems encountered in medical practice. This is especially so in the treatment of adolescents with IDDM. Adolescents differ from younger children in their emancipation from parents, their psychosexual orientation, and their search for identity. Although adolescents with IDDM often steer a perilous course between ketosis and hyperglycemia on the one hand and hypoglycemic episodes on the other, the long-term outlook for patients with IDDM has improved significantly with intensified metabolic control of the disease. There are convincing data that the achievement of near-normoglycemia is of paramount importance in ameliorating and postponing chronic complications of diabetes mellitus.[3] Therefore, it is the responsibility of a diabetes team taking care of patients with IDDM to pro-

vide the education and proper, up-to-date management necessary to ensure the best possible short- and long-term outlook for adolescents with IDDM.

The diagnosis of IDDM clearly represents a major challenge for the patient and family and for health professionals. Not only must the adolescent fulfill the tasks of development into adulthood, but he or she also must cope with daily and often very demanding routines of proper care. Since diabetes is a chronic disease with a prognosis that is undoubtedly dependent on the degree of metabolic control, it is necessary for the patient to adhere closely to the prescribed therapeutic regimen. However, some adolescents may not readily accept recommended restrictions imposed by their parents, physicians, and diabetes educators for regulating their disease, especially when such demands interfere with their life style and make them different from their peers.[4] In fact, some adolescents, knowing how important the control of their illness is, use this as a powerful weapon in manipulating their parents. By choosing noncompliance with the prescribed therapeutic regimen or even boycotting the treatment plan to express their independence, these adolescents precipitate serious short- and long-term metabolic consequences.

This chapter focuses on common problems in the management of adolescents with IDDM, including a review of self-management diabetes education. It does not discuss other forms of diabetes mellitus or impaired glucose tolerance, which are different entities with diverse management and treatment and are not commonly seen in general pediatric and adolescent practice. The cause of IDDM is not reviewed here; the reader is referred to another source.[5]

GOALS OF THERAPY AND PATIENT MANAGEMENT

The establishment of clear and reasonable goals for the treatment of IDDM is most important (Box 25-1). In the day-to-day management of patients, every attempt must

TABLE 25-1
Categories of Glucose Intolerance

Clinical Cases	Characteristics
Insulin-dependent diabetes mellitus (IDDM) type I	Usually diagnosed before age 30 yr; insulinopenia; abnormal immune response; certain HLA types; prone to ketoacidosis
Non–insulin-dependent diabetes mellitus (NIDDM) type II (obese or nonobese)	Usually diagnosed after age 30 yr; majority obese; may be asymptomatic; plasma insulin normal or high (insulin resistance); not prone to ketoacidosis
Other types of diabetes mellitus	Pancreatic disease (cystic fibrosis, cystinosis, thalassemia); insulin resistance (leprechaunism, lipodystrophy, ataxia-telangiectasia, acanthosis nigricans); hormonal aberrations (hypercorticolism, acromegaly); genetic syndromes (Down, Turner's, Klinefelter's, Prader-Willi, Laurence-Moon-Biedl, Wolfran's); drugs (e.g., glucocorticoids, growth hormone, L-asparaginase)
Impaired glucose tolerance (IGT) (obese or nonobese)	Usually asymptomatic; plasma glucose higher than normal, but not diagnostic for diabetes mellitus; can be seen in the above listed conditions; prediabetes?
Gestational diabetes mellitus (GDM)	Onset of glucose intolerance during pregnancy; complex metabolic and hormonal changes; insulin resistance may be present

TABLE 25-2
Diagnostic Criteria for Glucose Intolerance in Children and Adolescents

	Diabetes Mellitus	IGT	Normal
Fasting			
Venous plasma	≥140 mg/dl (7.8 mmol/L)	<140	<130
Venous whole blood	≥120 mg/dl (6.7 mmol/L)	<120	<115
Capillary whole blood	≥120 mg/dl (6.7 mmol/L)	<120	<115
2-hr OGTT Value			
Venous plasma	≥200 mg/dl (11.1 mmol/L)	>140	<140
Venous whole blood	≥180 mg/dl (10.0 mmol/L)	>120	<120
Capillary whole blood	≥200 mg/dl (11.1 mmol/L)	>120	<140

Modified from National Diabetes Data Group, 1979.
IGT, impaired glucose tolerance; *OGTT,* oral glucose tolerance test.

be made to achieve near-normoglycemia, regardless of the philosophy of the health care professional, the resources available, and the ability of the patient and family to comply with the rigors of therapy.

The old and still valid goals of therapy for IDDM are easily achievable through conventional diabetes care. The presence of the classic symptoms of diabetes, such as polyuria or polydipsia or even nocturia, is not acceptable. The patient should not be allowed to develop acute complications of diabetes such as ketoacidosis or hypoglycemia. In addition, adolescents with IDDM should exhibit normal growth and sexual maturation and maintain normal serum lipid levels. In view of increasing experimental and clinical evidence suggesting that poor glycemic control of diabetes plays a role in the development of chronic microangiopathic complications, more

rigorous control of the condition must be a desirable goal.[3,6,7] Ideally, blood sugar levels should be maintained in the normal nondiabetic range. However, this is difficult to achieve without imposing a great deal of limitations on the patient's life style and increasing the risk of severe hypoglycemia.[8] Therefore, we and many other pediatric endocrinologists aim to reach preprandial blood sugar levels between 90 and 130 mg/dl (5.0 to 7.2 mmol/L) and postprandial levels below 180 mg/dl (10.0 mmol/L). We strive to keep the urine free of ketones at all times, although ketones may be detectable during an acute illness. There has been a great deal of pressure to attain normal glycosylated hemoglobins, the test that "does not lie." Normal glycosylated hemoglobins are frequently attainable during the early years of diabetes, when some residual function of endogenous insulin production

---

BOX 25-1
Therapy Goals for IDDM

ACHIEVABLE GOALS
Control of symptoms
Avoidance of complications (e.g., ketosis, hypoglycemia)
Maintenance of normal growth and maturation
Maintenance of normal blood lipids
Minimization of urinary glucose losses
Preservation of emotional well-being
Achievement of independence as mature adult

DESIRABLE GOALS
Normal hemoglobin A_{1c} levels
Euglycemia

Modified from Lifshitz F, Fort P: Common problems in the management of children with insulin-dependent diabetes mellitus. In Lifshitz F, editor: *Common pediatric disorders,* New York, 1984, Marcel Dekker, p 4.

remains. However, normal glycosylated hemoglobins are difficult to achieve once total insulin deficiency develops. In fact, even with tight control of diabetes, such as with a continuous insulin delivery system or multiple daily injections of insulin, only 18% of patients reported by the Diabetes Control and Complications Trial (DCCT) study could achieve and maintain normal glycosylated hemoglobins.[3]

Normal glycosylated hemoglobins are rarely achieved in children or adolescents with IDDM. Most of our patients show glycosylated hemoglobins between 7.5% and 9% of total hemoglobin A (normal for our laboratory is 4.1% to 6.4%), which we consider an acceptable level for most children and adolescents undergoing conventional IDDM therapy. The aim is to keep glycosylated hemoglobins as close to normal as possible without risking hypoglycemia and/or emotional maladaption. It is important to keep in mind that different laboratories have established different normal ranges for glycosylated hemoglobins.

A well-informed patient who has a personal, trusting relationship with the physician and other members of the healthcare team is ideally suited to IDDM treatment. Maladaptation for treatment, resulting in worsening of diabetes control, may occur when patients are subjected to excessive demands and to feelings of guilt associated with their difficulty in coping with care. In the management of care for adolescents with IDDM, several specific factors need to be addressed to facilitate adjustment to the disease.[9] The location of the health center or the physician's office should be convenient to the patient. The time of appointments should be flexible, and adolescents should be reminded in writing about their next appointments. Many other factors may interfere with adherence to the therapeutic regimen, including conflicts with parents and teachers, special interests, and alcohol and drug consumption. Such issues should be well known to the medical staff who care for adolescents with IDDM. A willing and experienced medical professional, preferably a pediatric endocrinologist, should be the key person providing care. That individual should possess up-to-date knowledge, enjoy working with teenagers, and be adept at developing a close, nonparental type of relationship with the patient. The professional should also show flexibility and a willingness to compromise when necessary.

INSULIN THERAPY

The administration of insulin represents a mainstay of therapy for IDDM. Insulin is given to correct the metabolism of carbohydrates, protein, and fat and hence to achieve as good a control of diabetes as possible. However, treatment must be individualized. Issues that need to be addressed when insulin therapy is being considered include (1) type and dosage; (2) special problems, such as inadequate insulinization, excessive insulinization, insulin resistance and/or sensitivity, nutrition, exercise, and stress; and (3) mode of treatment, including conventional therapy, intensive therapy, or a continuous insulin delivery system.

Types of Insulin

Major manufacturers of insulin are now producing highly purified insulin from various sources. In addition, the introduction of human insulin produced by DNA recombinant techniques has expanded the availability and choice of insulin preparations. Currently, many physicians routinely start treatment with human insulin or change to that form, claiming that the decreased antigenicity of human insulin as compared with animal products is a major advantage.[10,11] Although certain indications for the use of human insulin have been established (e.g., lipodystrophy, allergy to animal products, gestational diabetes), the precise clinical indications for its routine use are not clear. Moreover, the duration of action of human insulin is shortened; thus, in the case of intermediate preparations, additional insulin injections may be required for treatment. We, and others, have seen frequent morning hyperglycemia in patients receiving evening (before dinner) human intermediate (NPH, Lente) insulin, although this problem can often be ameliorated by moving the insulin injection to bedtime. In addition, it has been reported that in some patients hypoglycemia after administration of human insulin may not be accompanied by symptoms and signs of hypoglycemia, the so-called syndrome of hypoglycemia unawareness,[12] although this issue has been disputed by others.[13]

TABLE 25-3
Insulins by Relative Comparative Action Curves

Insulin Type	Onset (hr)	Peak (hr)	Usual Effective Duration (hr)	Usual Maximum Duration (hr)
Animal				
Regular	0.5-2.0	3-4	4-6	6-8
NPH	4-6	8-14	16-20	20-24
Lente	4-6	8-14	16-20	20-24
Ultralente	8-14	Minimal	24-36	24-36
Human				
Regular	0.5-1.0	2-3	3-6	4-6
NPH	2-4	4-10	1-16	14-18
Lente	3-4	4-12	12-18	16-20
Ultralente	6-10	?	18-20	20-30
Humalog	0.25	0.5-1.5	≤5	?

We routinely begin therapy with pure pork insulin, leaving the use of human insulin to the previously mentioned special circumstances. Management of most patients includes a combination of rapid- and intermediate-acting insulins, which can be mixed in the same syringe. Attempts to introduce Ultralente human insulin as an evening injection to achieve "a better morning glycemia" may not offer any clinical advantage over intermediate-acting insulin.[14] Knowledge of the pharmacokinetics of various insulin preparation is essential for the proper management of IDDM (Table 25-3).

Recently, the Food and Drug Administration approved the clinical use of rapidly acting insulin of rDNA origin under the brand name Humalog. This insulin closely resembles natural pancreatic insulin and thus can be administered immediately before meals. Although Humalog insulin can improve postprandial glycemia, whether this will result in better metabolic control of a patient with IDDM remains to be seen.

Insulin Dosages

The dosages of insulin required by patients with IDDM are fairly constant and predictable despite great variations in many factors that alter insulin action.[15,16] Increased resistance to insulin is noted during puberty, in both nondiabetic and diabetic children. Under normal circumstances, insulin requirements are determined by the patient's age and the duration of diabetes.[16] While prepubertal children with IDDM usually require less than 1 unit of insulin per kilogram of body weight per day, requirements are generally increased in adolescents, often up to 1.5 U/kg body weight daily. However, higher dosages are unusual; they may worsen the control of diabetes and also increase the risk of hypoglycemia. Stress, whether physical or emotional, often leads to increased requirements of insulin. On the other hand, exercise results in more rapid utilization of glucose with

decreasing insulin requirements.[17] However, it is important to be aware that vigorous exercise in the face of hyperglycemia may exert an opposite effect, and ketosis may result.[18] Finally, insulin requirements are directly related to the nutritional intake of the patient. Excessive calorie consumption is associated with an increased need for insulin and an accumulation of fat, leading to undesirable weight gain.

Number of Insulin Injections

The number of insulin injections prescribed per day should depend on the patient's clinical and biochemical status. Patients with IDDM who are growing and developing appropriately, whose glycosylated hemoglobins are maintained in an acceptable range, who have normal serum lipid values, and who are psychologically well adjusted do not, in our opinion, require more than two insulin injections per day. However, there are many situations in which a two-injection insulin regimen may be inadequate to improve the metabolic control of diabetes. Patients who are very young (under 4 years of age), who need total insulin replacement during adolescence, or who require treatment with human insulin may benefit from three or more insulin injections per day. Also, those who have reasonably good blood glucose levels during the day and early evening, but hyperglycemia at night and during the morning hours, may not be receiving adequate insulin throughout the 24-hour period and may do better with multiple insulin injections. In such cases, the clinician must establish rapport with the patient and make sure that he or she needs the split-dosage schedule: that is, that there is evidence of sufficient insulin during the day but insufficient coverage during the night, resulting in nocturnal and early-morning hyperglycemia.

Some patients who report good blood glucose readings may have high levels of glycosylated hemoglobins. If it is assumed that blood glucose levels reflect true values, an attempt should be made to switch the patient to more injections per day. However, the reverse may also be true: changing the patient's treatment from a more complicated to a simpler regimen may be appropriate in some cases. Some patients may be reluctant to accept the split-insulin regimen, and the increased demand on the patient's life style may result in increased stress, which in turn has adverse effects on glucose control. We have seen several patients treated with several insulin injections per day who had frequent blood-glucose monitoring, with glycosylated hemoglobins in the 14% to 15% range, and whose diabetic condition improved dramatically after simplification of the treatment regimen. It must be kept in mind that aiming for strict metabolic control of diabetes should always be balanced with the goal of prevention of maladaptation. Both patient and physician need to accept that the conventional means of diabetes care, consisting of two insulin injections per day, will not always achieve euglycemia on a consistent basis.

Inadequate Insulinization

In practical terms, an adolescent who has had IDDM for several years and is receiving an insulin dosage of less than 1 U/kg body weight per day may be having inadequate insulinization. Regardless of what the patient claims or what is shown on the blood glucose record, it is the physician's responsibility to prove that the patient needs unusually low doses of insulin to maintain good metabolic control. It is possible that in some patients endogenous insulin secretion is partially preserved for many years.[19,20] In these patients, C peptide levels may be measured to ascertain endogenous production of insulin. Adolescents with IDDM who receive insufficient insulin may develop complications such as peripheral neuropathy and hyperlipidemia because of an accumulation of sorbitol and decreased action of lipoprotein lipase, respectively.[21] Moreover, chronic inadequate insulinization may contribute to the development of severe long-term complications of diabetes. When a patient seems to require small doses of insulin or when the insulin requirements decline without an apparent reason, the patient also must be checked for other diseases, particularly hypothyroidism, which is much more prevalent in patients with IDDM than in the general population.[22] Autoimmune thyroiditis (Hashimoto's thyroiditis) is found in up to 25% of patients with IDDM and may be manifested as poor control of diabetes. Finally, the possibility of the surreptitious use of insulin by some adolescents must be kept in mind. Such a situation generally indicates severe psychopathology and must be handled appropriately.[23]

Excessive Insulinization

The use of an insulin dosage of more than 2 U/kg body weight per day in adolescent patients with IDDM should alert the physician to the possibility of excessive insulinization. Excessive insulinization also should be suspected when the glycemic control of diabetes remains poor despite administration of high dosages of insulin. The so-called Somogyi phenomenon denotes a situation in which blood glucose rises after insulin-induced hypoglycemia as a consequence of the sudden release of "antiinsulin hormones," causing a temporary insulin resistance.[24] The Somogyi phenomenon is often used by physicians to explain morning-fasting hyperglycemia. However, others dismiss this phenomenon in many patients who have unexplained hyperglycemia.[25] Patients with IDDM who exhibit hyperglycemia on awakening may be experiencing inadequate insulinization during the early morning hours without having nocturnal hypoglycemia. The Somogyi phenomenon may be suspected when the patient has frequent nightmares, has excessive perspiration during sleep, wakes up irritable, and/or has ketones in the urine on awakening. Body weight usually continues to increase at excessive rates. When the possibility of the Somogyi phenomenon is being considered, the insulin dose should be decreased slowly to an appropriate dosage on a per-kilogram basis. This should be done despite the temptation to counteract hyperglycemia and ketonuria with extra insulin. If the Somogyi phenomenon proves to be the problem, control of diabetes is improved by decreasing the amount of insulin to the recommended level. A 10% decrease in insulin dose every few days and a change to an appropriate ratio (1:3) of rapid- and intermediate-acting insulins are recommended.

Another, perhaps more common cause of early-morning hyperglycemia is the so-called "dawn phenomenon." This is characterized by progressively increasing blood glucose levels after 4 AM and hence greater insulin requirements during that period, without preceding hypoglycemia. The exact mechanism of the dawn phenomenon has not been elucidated, although increased insulin clearance in the face of rising antiinsulin hormones, such as growth hormone and cortisol, may play a role in its development.[26] Prevention of the dawn phenomenon is best achieved by moving insulin administration to the late evening hours.

Insulin Resistance and Sensitivity

In a few instances, when insulin requirements are truly high, the possibility of insulin resistance of various types can be suspected.[27] A change to a less antigenic type of insulin, such as human insulin, may be helpful. Similarly, the administration of insulin by different routes, for example, intraperitoneally or intravenously instead of subcutaneously, will alleviate the problem of insulin resistance to subcutaneously administered insulin.[28] We have seen a few patients who do require higher dosages of insulin on a temporary basis for no apparent reason. An excess of stress hormones cannot be entirely ruled out as a possible cause in such patients.

Insulin sensitivity, causing decreased insulin requirements, is an infrequent occurrence in adolescents with IDDM. As patients grow older, however, the amount of insulin that is needed decreases. Also, a progressive decline in insulin dosage is often seen during the so-called "honeymoon phase" of the disease, which reflects a partial remission of endogenous insulin production. Finally, certain disease states, such as hypothyroidism or hypopituitarism, are accompanied by diminished insulin requirements.[29]

HOME BLOOD-GLUCOSE MONITORING

Assessment of diabetes control through home blood-glucose monitoring (HBGM) is a mainstay of proper diabetes management.[30] Patients and their families must be educated about the importance of such monitoring. They must be motivated and learn how to adjust the dose of insulin according to blood glucose readings. Nowadays, many HBGM devices are on the market. Several sources have credited the contribution of HBGM techniques for the improvement of metabolic control seen in patients given conventional therapy. In some instances, this positive effect may be due to intensive efforts by the patient and healthcare professionals, as well as to other educational and motivational benefits, rather than to HBGM per se. In one study, it was clearly shown that the metabolic condition of patients selected for HBGM improved in the 6 weeks preceding its implementation because of the intense efforts of all involved, including the patient, family, and therapy team.[31] Once the HBGM technique is implemented, an algorithm for multiple dosages of insulin versus multiple blood glucose levels should be followed for more precise metabolic control of diabetes.

It is important to realize that patients may falsify the HBGM records and provide the physician with unreliable data. Such a possibility should be considered whenever the clinical findings and other biochemical parameters, such as glycosylated hemoglobins, are in discordance with reported blood glucose values. Most patients are requested to check their blood glucose four times a day (before breakfast, lunch, dinner, and a bedtime snack) and, once a week, at 2 AM; however, individual adjustments may be made. When blood glucose values are

below or above the desired range, changes in the dose of insulin should be made.

Many patients with IDDM do not adjust their insulin dosage according to blood sugar levels; such patients provide the physician with blood glucose readings but do not use this information for better management of their illness. We have encountered many patients whose use of HBGM has resulted in deterioration rather than improvement of their metabolic status (Table 25-4). These patients were given conventional insulin therapy through twice-daily doses. Insulin dosage changes supposedly were being made according to the blood glucose levels. However, metabolic control was less than desired, and there were complications such as hyperglycemia, hypertriglyceridemia, and/or dermopathy. In no instance could euglycemia be achieved, and there were wide fluctuations in blood glucose levels with high concentrations of glycosylated hemoglobins. This shows that in some cases HBGM may produce information that is highly inaccurate and may be worse than no information at all. Some patients with IDDM provide the physician with results they think that he or she wants to hear rather than giving accurate determinations of blood glucose levels that can be used for effective therapeutic decisions. Furthermore, in many patients the enthusiasm for daily HBGM gradually wanes, and they may eventually stop measuring blood glucose levels completely. In such situations, it may be better to ask them to measure blood glucose once a day at different times of the day rather than insisting on the traditional three to four times per day finger sticks. Obtaining a blood glucose sample is not an entirely painless procedure, even with the latest technical equipment.

Various companies are presently at work on noninvasive meters, although these are currently not available for the general public. An example of the technology presently being explored is a near-infrared light that passes through organic matter, for example, the finger. Some of the light is absorbed, some escapes, and the portion that escapes can be translated into the amount of glucose circulating in the blood. Another technology in progress includes a skin patch that measures glucose with weak, painless electric currents. When this technology is perfected and the noninvasive meters are finally available, this methodology will provide a painless way to obtain accurate information regarding blood glucose measurements. This certainly will help people to achieve and maintain proper control.

INTENSIVE TREATMENT

For patients with IDDM, there has been widespread enthusiasm for intensive insulin therapy, either in the form of multiple daily injections or as a continuous

TABLE 25-4
Home Blood-Glucose Monitoring with Twice-Daily Insulin Administration

Variables	Clinical Findings in Three Patients Who Did Not Do Well		
	Patient 1	Patient 2	Patient 3
Age (yr)	17.5	16.6	10
Duration of diabetes mellitus (yr)	10	14	1
Insulin dosage			
AM	30 NPH	22 NPH	8.5 Lente
	20 regular	12 regular	1.5 regular
PM	20 NPH	16 NPH	5.5 Lente
	10 regular	6 regular	1.5 regular
Weight (kg)	55.0	60.4	28.0
Home blood sugar levels (mg/dl)*			
AM	200-400	80-170	55-400
PM	150-300	70-180	47-400
Hemoglobin A_{1c} (%)	19.9	18.8	10.2
Comments	Fasting triglycerides: 2250 mg/dl; dermopathy	Fasting blood sugar in clinic: 200 mg/dl	Frequent hypoglycemic reactions

From Lifshitz F, Fort P: Common problems in the management of children with insulin-dependent diabetes mellitus. In Lifshitz F, editor: *Common pediatric disorders,* New York, 1984, Marcel Dekker, p 15.
NPH, neutral protamine Hagedorn.
*Measured twice daily, preprandially.
Note: Three children with IDDM presented with poor metabolic control of diabetes despite home blood glucose monitoring and adjustment of insulin dose according to blood glucose levels. Patient 1 developed severe hypertriglyceridemia and dermopathy in spite of an insulin dose close to 1.5 U/kg/day. Patient 2 reported home blood glucose levels much lower than would be expected for the Hgb A_{1c} levels. Patient 3 suffered from frequent clinical hypoglycemic reactions.

insulin delivery system (CIDS). Indeed, some investigators believe that these are highly appropriate routine therapeutic modalities for patients who require insulin therapy.[30] This attitude is based on increasing evidence that poor metabolic control may be an important factor in the genesis of chronic diabetes complications.[3] An increasing variety of CIDS methods are available on the market, and thousands of CIDS devices have been sold. Because intensive insulin therapy requires close monitoring of glycemic control, it is useless to start any of these therapeutic regimens without proper blood-glucose surveillance. Patients undergoing such therapy need intensified overall diabetes management, covering education, nutrition, exercise, and life style. Because intensive treatment requires a high degree of motivation on the part of the patient, it cannot be applied universally.

The possible risks of intensive therapy are (1) failure, (2) hypoglycemia, (3) obesity, (4) accelerated microvascular complications, (5) emotional stress, and (6) special complications of devices, leading to increased frequency of diabetic ketoacidosis, infection, or hyperinsulinemia.[32] Of these, the most dramatic and dangerous are those associated with severe hypoglycemia. The DCCT study reported that up to one third of patients undergoing intensive insulin therapy experienced at least one episode of severe hypoglycemia.[3] Even clinically asymptomatic hypoglycemia could have a deleterious effect on the patient's mental abilities.[33]

There are certain clear-cut indications for the use of intensive insulin therapy, such as before and during pregnancy to reduce the incidence of congenital anomalies.[34] Patients with symptomatic neuropathy or hyperlipidemia and those with growth failure may benefit from such treatment.[35-37] Also, some well-motivated patients who switch from two daily insulin injections to three or four daily injections tend to improve their metabolic control as measured by glycosylated hemoglobins.[3,7] Although it is generally believed that intensive insulin therapy may not be advantageous in patients with poor metabolic control because of nonadherence to the prescribed therapeutic regimen, we have observed several patients with brittle diabetes and recurrent ketoacidosis who have benefited from CIDS treatment. Stabilization of their condition was maintained so that family therapy could be effective.[38]

There is controversy over whether intensive therapy with multiple injections is as effective as CIDS treatment.[39] As already noted, both methods have been effective in temporary situations with specific goals. With rigorous supervision, euglycemia and a normal glycosylated hemoglobin level can be attained on a long-term basis in a highly selected group of patients with IDDM.[3]

In our experience, euglycemia can be attained easily in the first weeks and months of therapy, while the patient is under careful and intensive observation. However, in the ordinary clinical setting, long-term CIDS therapy is fraught with difficulties in maintaining normal blood glucose and glycosylated hemoglobin levels. Improvement in metabolic control is usually short-lived, and a reversal commonly occurs after only several months of treatment. In some instances we, like others, have encountered complications such as dangerous hypoglycemia.[3,8,32] It has been reported that patients with IDDM who are undergoing intensive insulin therapy may be at an increased risk of developing hypoglycemia because of inappropriate release of counterregulatory hormones during hypoglycemic states.[40] Intensive insulin therapy, whether through multiple injections of insulin or through CIDS therapy, requires an extraordinary effort on the part of the patient, the family, and the therapeutic team and is far more demanding than conventional insulin therapy. Intensive insulin therapy may also not be entirely effective in controlling the development or progression of complications in patients with IDDM.[41] For example, in some patients with IDDM who are given intensive insulin therapy, retinopathy not only failed to improve but worsened despite very strict control with insulin infusion therapy for more than 2 years.[42] Similarly, in several patients with IDDM, nephropathy did not improve with intensive insulin treatment.[43] Moreover, even a total reversal of the metabolic derangements of diabetes achieved by pancreas transplantation may fail to reverse the progression of microangiopathic changes in patients with IDDM.[44] It appears that if tight metabolic control is implemented in a patient with IDDM, this should be done as early as possible, well before clinical manifestations of chronic diabetes complications become apparent.

MAJOR COMPLICATIONS OF DIABETES MELLITUS

Diabetic Ketoacidosis

Diabetic ketoacidosis (DKA) is a major emergency in the adolescent patient. DKA is usually defined as hyperglycemia (serum glucose concentration >250 mg/dl [13.9 mmol/L]) and metabolic acidosis (blood pH <7.30 and/or HCO_3 <15 mEq/L). The urine is positive for glucose and ketones. DKA results not only from an actual lack of insulin, but also from a relative deficiency of insulin, which can occur in situations marked by the presence of increased hyperglycemic hormones, such as stress, infection, and inflammation.[45-47]

The initial assessment, generally performed in an emergency room setting, is similar to that for any critically ill patient. Patients with DKA are always dehydrated and the state of dehydration must be carefully assessed. Patients with DKA may continue to have a marked urinary output in spite of severe dehydration and impending renal shutdown. Laboratory studies consist of immediate measurement of serum glucose, electrolytes, ketones, bicarbonate and pH, and serum osmolarity and a complete blood count. In the presence of fever, appropriate cultures of body fluids must be obtained. Monitoring of the serum potassium level is very important, because it may fall precipitously with the initiation of therapy. Often, there is pseudohyponatremia caused by hyperglycemia and hyperlipidemia.[48,49] The serum osmolarity is always elevated, but values above 375 mOsm/L indicate morbid hyperosmolarity, management of which is discussed below.

Intravenous fluid therapy should be started immediately after the initial assessment and blood work are completed. Unless the patient presents with morbid hyperosmolarity, normal saline at a rate of 20 to 40 ml/kg body weight per hour is sufficient for initial therapy. Once the electrolyte status of the patient is known, the composition of fluids should be modified as needed to replace the severe electrolyte losses. Generally, one third of water and sodium replacement is given during the first 8 hours and the remaining two thirds during the next 16 hours. One must be aware of ongoing urinary losses, and proper replacement of these losses must be provided. Potassium salts (half chloride and half phosphate) must be added to the intravenous fluids at once if there is no concomitant hyperkalemia and if the patient has good urinary output. Failure to do so may result in severe hypokalemia, as both correction of acidosis and administration of insulin promote transfer of potassium into the cells.

The acidosis of DKA is due to a combination of mostly ketoacidosis and some lactic acidosis. Since ketoacidosis will respond to the restoration of glycolysis as the principal generator of energy by the administration of insulin, fluid therapy and insulin are the principal agents for the treatment of mild to moderate acidosis (pH >7.15). Bicarbonate administration is generally not necessary if the pH is greater than 7.15. Marked acidosis, however, is life-threatening because of its central nervous system (CNS) effects, which include respiratory depression. The recommended treatment of marked acidosis is as follows:

1. pH 7.15 to 7.00: correct the bicarbonate deficit slowly over 1 hour or more.
2. pH <7.00: 1 mEq/kg $NaHCO_3$ by slow intravenous push.
3. To calculate the bicarbonate deficit: HCO_3 deficit = (15 − serum bicarbonate) × kg body weight × 0.6.

The sodium content of the $NaHCO_3$ should be included in the calculation of total sodium maintenance and replacement. The clinician should remember that overuse of sodium bicarbonate can lead to hypernatremia. Also, as equilibration across the respiratory center of the brain is slow for bicarbonate but rapid for CO_2, the quick correction of metabolic acidosis will be accompanied by retention of CO_2 and paradoxical CNS acidosis. Finally, rapid correction of acidosis may precipitate hypokalemia.

Administration of insulin is an essential component of therapy for DKA. Although there are many theoretical modes of insulin administration in DKA, the intravenous route is best in the early stages.[50] The so-called low-dose insulin infusion has the advantage of supplying a constant steady rate of insulin administration; therefore, a steady serum level of insulin is attained. The usual dose of insulin in adolescents is 0.1 unit of regular insulin per kilogram of body weight per hour. The insulin infusion rate should be governed by a reliable positive-pressure pump. An initial loading blous of insulin is not necessary,[51] but if the blood glucose level at the end of 2 hours of insulin therapy and IV fluids has not fallen by at least 20% of the starting value, an insulin bolus (0.1 U/kg body weight) may be useful, or the rate of insulin infusion may be increased. Once the serum glucose falls below 250 mg/dl (13.9 mmol/L), which usually happens before the correction of acidosis, 5% dextrose is added to the IV fluids. A convenient method for coordinating the glucose with the insulin is to discontinue the insulin infusion and add insulin and glucose in a fixed ratio to the hydration solution. The usual dose in adolescents is 2 units of regular insulin for every 5 g of glucose. In any given patient the insulin/glucose ratio may vary, and proper adjustment of insulin dose may be needed to maintain blood glucose levels in the 100 to 150 mg/dl range (5.6 to 8.3 mmol/L).

Severe Hyperglycemia with Ketonuria

One of the important goals of therapy for IDDM is to avoid acute complications such as DKA. Despite great efforts, DKA remains a real and serious complication of IDDM, especially among patients with poor diabetes control. As with many diseases, the best treatment of DKA is early diagnosis and appropriate therapy. Recognition of impending DKA and institution of extra insulin administration, together with vigorous oral fluid replacement, often aborts DKA, thus avoiding hospitalization. Outpatient management of severe hyperglycemia with or without ketonuria requires a reliable and cooperative patient and family, the ability to stay in close telephone contact with the physician (often on an hourly basis), and an experienced health team.

The typical patient is an adolescent who is going through physical or emotional stress and presents with a blood glucose level over 250 mg/dl (13.9 mmol/L) and positive urinary ketones. Often such a patient is nauseous but has not vomited. If the decision is made

to treat hyperglycemia and ketonuria at home, the patient is instructed to start with a regular insulin dosage of 0.1 U/kg body weight intramuscularly every hour as long as the blood glucose level remains over 250 mg/dl (13.9 mmol/L) and the urine shows moderate or large ketones. In conjunction with insulin administration, the patient is instructed to increase fluid intake. The amount of fluid intake recommended is based on the assumption that the patient is not more than 5% dehydrated and has had no vomiting or diarrhea. Fluid maintenance and replacement are calculated so that one half of the deficit and one third of the maintenance level are replaced in the first 8 hours. Diet (carbonated) soft drinks are a common hydration medium for patients with IDDM, but these vary widely in sodium and potassium content. Resolution of ketonuria and hyperglycemia is equated with therapeutic success. Persistence of mild ketonuria with blood glucose below 250 mg/dl (13.9 mmol/L) is also considered acceptable. We have found that this approach is easy for both patient and family to follow. However, the patient must be in stable condition and able to tolerate oral hydration. If there is any question about the stability of the patient's condition, he or she is instructed to go to the physician's office immediately or to an emergency facility. The details of this approach have been described by Pugliese et al.[52]

Morbid Hyperosmolarity

Morbid hyperosmolarity (MH), defined as serum osmolarity greater than 375 mOsm/L and blood glucose above 1400 mg/dl (77.8 mmol/L) is a life-threatening condition with significant morbidity and mortality.[53] It is seen in situations of near-normal insulin levels and is often precipitated by pneumonia or gram-negative sepsis.[53] Many such patients have been receiving oral hypoglycemia agents. Drugs, such as phenytoin (Dilantin), thiazides, and steroids have also been implicated as precipitating agents.[53] The severe hyperviscosity seen in MH can lead to thromboembolic events, CNS bleeding, acute renal failure, disseminated intravascular coagulation, and shock.[53] Rapid correction of MH, especially in young children, can result in severe cerebral edema.[53] Many such patients are only mildly acidotic or not acidotic at all. Initial evaluation should quickly identify patients with MH, who should be handled in a center where various subspecialties, such as neurology, nephrology, and hematology, are available. Management of patients with MH differs from that of typical DKA. The goals of fluid and electrolyte therapy are resuscitation of the patient from shock, maintenance of adequate perfusion of all vital organs, and a gradual reduction in serum hyperosmolarity. These goals are accomplished by carefully monitoring the interplay of arterial pressure, epidural pressure (when feasible), and urinary output. Hydration must be adequate to maintain the central venous pressure in a normal range. However, overzealous rehydration, especially with hypotonic solutions, can result in cerebral edema.[53] If there is an increase in intracranial pressure, various methods of lowering the pressure, such as hyperventilation, barbiturate coma, and head elevation, should be employed.

It is agreed that isotonic or hypertonic solutions should be used to dilute the glucose in patients with MH.[53] In general, the fluids administered should be only 30 to 40 mOsm/L lower than serum osmolarity. Usually, this can be achieved with normal saline and potassium salts. The osmolarity of standard commercial solutions is as follows: D5W, 252 mOsm/L; normal saline, 308 mOsm/L; $NaHCO_3$, 2000 mOsm/L; and K phosphate, 7000 mOsm/L or 1.7 mOsm/mEq K. As with any hypertonic dehydration, deficits should be replaced slowly over 48 to 72 hours, rather than over 24 hours, as is customary in simple DKA. Patients with MH are in need of insulin therapy. However, there has been some controversy about the dosage of insulin and the best time of administration. The general approach has been to use only half the dose of insulin (i.e., 0.05 U/kg/hr) or even less if there is a precipitous decline in the blood glucose levels. The drop of serum glucose should not exceed 100 mg/dl/(5.6 mmol/L)/hr, especially when the serum glucose level is approaching near normal levels. In fact, it may be preferable to maintain serum glucose levels above 250 mg/dl (13.9 mmol/L) during the first 48 hours of therapy, which can minimize the development of clinically significant cerebral edema.[53]

Hypoglycemia

Hypoglycemia is a common occurrence among patients receiving insulin therapy, especially because recognition of the importance of maintaining blood glucose levels as close to normal as possible to minimize long-term chronic complications of diabetes mellitus.[3] Hypoglycemia is due to the absolute or relative excess of insulin, often precipitated by a lack of food and/or increased exercise. True hypoglycemia is defined as a whole blood glucose concentration less than 50 mg/dl (2.8 mmol/L), although symptoms of hypoglycemia can be seen at much higher concentrations of glucose.[54,55] On the other hand, many patients may remain asymptomatic even at blood glucose levels less than 50 mg/dl (2.8 mmol/L). This has been described as the "hypoglycemia unawareness syndrome."[56]

The symptoms and signs of hypoglycemia have traditionally been divided into neuroglycopenic and adrenergic manifestations.[57] Neuroglycopenia represents a lack of the major fuel (glucose) for the CNS, which can result in cognitive dysfunction, disorientation, seizures, and death when not appropriately treated. Adrenergic

symptoms result from activation of the sympathetic nervous system and are well recognized as anxiety, pallor, headaches, tremor, and increased perspiration. Although most patients can easily recognize the symptoms of hypoglycemia, repeated episodes of hypoglycemia may become asymptomatic, especially at night. It is imperative, therefore, that all patients receiving insulin therapy monitor their blood glucose several times a day, and once or twice a week at 2 to 3 AM also. Teenagers can be at an increased risk of developing hypoglycemia, as they may not comply with dietary recommendations or may experiment with alcohol intake (which aggravates hypoglycemia by blocking neoglucogenesis). Moreover, clinicians should be aware of the surreptitious administration of insulin practiced by some teenagers.[23] Treatment of documented hypoglycemia, with or without symptoms, should be prompt. When symptoms are mild, an extra 5 to 10 g of glucose followed by a protein snack will suffice. More glucose may be needed when symptoms are more severe. If the adolescent is unconscious, 1 mg glucagon should be administered subcutaneously at once, even if a blood glucose level is not immediately available. For that reason, every family with a member having insulin-treated diabetes mellitus should have an emergency glucagon kit at their disposal and be familiar with its use. When the patient is traveling or leaves home for college, there should always be a person capable of administering glucagon to the patient.

Chronic Complications of Diabetes Mellitus

Chronic complications of diabetes mellitus consist of the classic triad of retinopathy, nephropathy, and neuropathy. They remain the main cause of morbidity and mortality in patients with diabetes mellitus, and once established they are usually irreversible. Although the clinical presentation of diabetic complications usually occurs after childhood and adolescence, subclinical manifestations may be encountered at a younger age. The pathogenesis of the chronic complications has not been clearly established, although several theories have been implicated. These include chronic hyperglycemia (the so-called glucotoxic theory), hemodynamic alterations (such as hypertension), hormonal effects, and genetic and environmental factors.[58] Several animal and human studies have shown that the near-normalization of blood glucose levels reduces the frequency and severity of chronic diabetic complications.[3] On the other hand, the clustering of chronic complications among family members with diabetes mellitus points to environmental and genetic factors.[59,60]

DIABETIC RETINOPATHY. Visual impairment is a frequent complication of diabetes mellitus. Among adults, diabetic retinopathy is the leading cause of new cases of blindness.[61] In addition, other eye conditions, such as glaucoma, cataracts, and corneal disease, are more likely to develop in patients with diabetes mellitus. The median duration of diabetes at the onset of retinopathy is reported as 9.1 years, and nearly 100% of patients with type I diabetes mellitus develop detectable eye changes after 15 years.[61] Fortunately, new methods of treatment, such as laser photocoagulation and vitrectomy, have greatly improved the quality of life of such patients. Moreover, the availability and implementation of better metabolic control of diabetes mellitus is expected to significantly reduce all diabetic complications. It is important that all patients with diabetes mellitus receive regular ophthalmologic evaluation so that retinal changes can be detected early.

DIABETIC NEPHROPATHY. Diabetes is the most common cause of end-stage renal disease.[62] Nephropathy can be defined as the presence of clinical proteinuria (>0.5 g of protein per 24 hours). When new sensitive techniques are used, minute amounts of protein (microalbuminuria) can be detected in the urine before the appearance of clinical proteinuria.[63] It is believed that microalbuminuria is an important sign of kidney disease, at least in adults. However, its significance is less clear among children and adolescents with diabetes mellitus.[59] Proteinuria is associated with diabetic glomerulosclerosis, which is characterized by increased basement membrane thickness and expansion of mesangium.[62] Renal hyperfiltration, as evidenced by an increased glomerular filtration rate, is almost always present at diagnosis. Since patients with microalbuminuria have higher mean blood pressures than those without microalbuminuria, antihypertensive treatment has been proposed for such individuals.[63] However, data on the efficacy of such therapeutic approaches in pediatric diabetic populations are not yet available. Similarly, it has not yet been clarified whether intensive control of blood glucose levels and/or diminished protein intake can ameliorate microalbuminuria in pediatric patients. On the other hand, the DCCT study has proved the beneficial effects of improved glycemic control on the long-term renal complications of diabetes mellitus.[3]

DIABETIC NEUROPATHY. Diabetic neuropathy, although not life-threatening, is the most common and troublesome chronic complication of diabetes mellitus.[64] Fortunately, severe forms are rare among children and adolescents with diabetes mellitus, but their incidence increases with duration of disease. The most susceptible nerves are the sensory and motor fibers of the lower extremities. Diabetic neuropathy can be helped by improved glycemic control of diabetes mellitus.[35] Autonomic neuropathy, although a difficult problem in adults with diabetes mellitus, has rarely been observed and clearly diagnosed in diabetic children and adolescents.

Other Complications

Other, usually reversible, complications in children and adolescents with diabetes mellitus include skeletal and joint abnormalities (manifesting as thickening of skin and inability to fully extend the interphalangeal joints, and later on larger joints also), osteopenia, growth failure, and delayed sexual maturation. Diminished growth rates can be seen in poorly control diabetes mellitus.[65] In the past, a common complication of insulin administration was lipoatrophy, most likely an immune-mediated phenomenon. With the introduction of more purified insulins, this condition is seen less often. On the other hand, lipohypertrophy can be observed when there are repeated injections of insulin in the same area. This can result in uneven absorption of injected insulin, leading to wide fluctuations of blood glucose levels. Another, fortunately rare, condition affecting the skin of children and adolescents with diabetes mellitus is necrobiosis lipoidica diabeticorum. This usually presents as round indurated plaques over the anterior aspects of the lower legs. The lesions can become atrophic and ulcerative. The pathogenesis has not been elucidated and treatment has been difficult.[66]

HYPOGLYCEMIC AGENTS

With the exception of maturity onset diabetes of youth, oral hypoglycemic agents are rarely used in adolescents, since most of the patients have type I diabetes mellitus (IDDM). The use of these agents is limited to type II diabetes mellitus (NIDDM), often in combination with various insulin regimens. The most commonly used oral hypoglycemic agents are the sulfonylureas, which have been available since 1955. The hypoglycemic activity of sulfonylureas stems from their ability to stimulate insulin secretion.[67] Therefore, they are of no use in a state of insulinopenia, such as in IDDM. Their pharmacologic effects are exerted by several mechanisms, the details of which are reviewed elsewhere.[68] Commonly used sulfonylurea drugs include tolbutamide, chlorpropamide, tolazamide, acetohexamide, glipizide, glyburide, and gliclazide, each of which differs in its duration of action. The use of these agents should be left to an experienced diabetologist familiar with their side effects, failures, and other drug interactions.

Another group of oral hypoglycemia agents are the biquanides, derivates of quanidine. Unlike sulfonylureas, biquanides do not increase insulin secretion but are thought to (1) reduce hepatic glucose production, (2) increase insulin-mediated uptake of glucose at the periphery, and/or (3) decrease intestinal absorption of glucose.[68] Three biquanides have been available (phenformin, metformin, and butformin), and different issues have been noted for each.

A third class of oral hypoglycemic agents includes inhibitors of α-glucosidase.[68] The representative of these agents is acarbose, which blocks the digestion of starch, sucrose, and maltose; it can be used as an adjunct to sulfonylurea or insulin therapy.

GESTATIONAL DIABETES

Gestational diabetes is defined as diabetes discovered during pregnancy. Although almost any type of diabetes can present during pregnancy, the most common scenario is the unmasking of incipient type II diabetes mellitus by the metabolic demands of pregnancy. After the child's birth, the maternal diabetes usually disappears, although such women are at increased risk for type II diabetes mellitus later in life. Maternal diabetes is known to have profound effects on the fetus, especially when metabolic control is poor. Depending on the onset and severity of maternal diabetes, the fetus may be subjected to a metabolic insult resulting in congenital anomalies, macrosomia, and intellectual impairment. Therefore, it is of the utmost importance that gestational diabetes is recognized early so that effective metabolic control can be implemented as soon as possible. If the mother is known to have diabetes, excellent metabolic control of diabetes before conception is essential. With this approach, the adverse effects of diabetes mellitus on the fetus and child can be minimized.[69]

NUTRITION

The role of proper nutrition in the management of an adolescent with IDDM cannot be overemphasized. Nutrition has been implicated as a factor in increasing the risk of diabetes and contributing to the disease.[70] It may also play a role in the amelioration of complications. Food intake can affect the presence or absence of hypoglycemia, the dosage and timing of injections, and ultimately the prognosis of the patient. Since patients with IDDM have lost the capacity to secrete endogenous insulin, a regular meal pattern is important. Thus, the nutritional requirements of an adolescent with IDDM are similar to those of adolescents without diabetes. In general, the term "diabetes diet" is considered improper because it connotes restriction and denial and may induce unnecessary anxiety in patients with diabetes. Instead, terms such as "meal planning" and "nutritional requirements" are preferable for diabetes patients.[71]

Frequently, patients with hypoglycemia are treated with an overload of carbohydrates. This leads to hyperglycemia, which requires more insulin for treatment. As a result, a vicious cycle of hypoglycemia and hyperglycemia may ensue, leading to poor control of diabetes. The proper treatment for such patients is to avoid hypoglycemic episodes, which require extra carbohydrate intake. Another common problem is increased calorie intake and decreased calorie expenditure. Hyperglycemia may result from overeating, even in those receiving adequate insulin therapy. Some patients gain excessive weight despite marked glycosuria and hyperglycemia. Those who are gaining weight at a rate faster than that expected for height are in a positive nitrogen balance. In such patients, manipulation of insulin dosage or other methods for improving control of IDDM are bound to fail unless treatment includes nutritional rehabilitation.

Rates of ketosis also appear to vary among patients with diabetes in relation to dietary factors; ketonuria may follow the ingestion of a meal with a high fat content and may not be related to insulin treatment. In addition, long-term complications of diabetes may be influenced by nutritional intake and habits.[70] For example, when patients with diabetes having a similar degree of metabolic control are compared, patients in Japan are noted to have gangrene and coronary heart disease less frequently than their Western counterparts. Among Navajo Indians, Nigerians, and certain Pacific populations, there is a lower incidence of microvascular disease among patients with diabetes than in other populations. These differences may be related to variations in genetic factors as well as to nutritional habits.

The key elements of sound meal planning for a person with IDDM are regular timing and consistency of meals and snacks that synchronize with timing of insulin doses. Nutritional recommendations for patients with IDDM have been issued by the American Diabetes Association.[72] These recommendations do not differ substantially from those for the general, or nondiabetic, population. The meal plan should be individualized and based on the usual food intake, with insulin integrated into this established eating and exercise pattern. There is no ideal, but generally 15% to 20% of calories should be provided as protein, and the remaining calories should be contributed by carbohydrate and fat. The total amount of carbohydrate consumed is more important for glycemic control than the source of carbohydrate. Fat intake should include 10% as saturated fats, less than 10% as polyunsaturated fats, and the remainder as monosaturated fats. To achieve this balance, intake of animal fats must be reduced through replacement with vegetable sources. Cholesterol intake should be reduced by limiting the intake of fatty meats and dairy products. The metabolism of both carbohydrates and lipids can be improved further by increased intake of dietary fiber. The protein consumed should be of high biologic quality. Excess protein and fat intake may have adverse effects on both the renal and cardiovascular systems. Indeed, the deleterious effect of high protein intake on kidney function and proteinuria has been described.[73]

It has been reported that different foods exert various effects on blood glucose levels.[74] Substantially different glycemic responses may be noted when even a single food is prepared in a different way. For example, ingestion of whole rice results in a flatter blood glucose curve than does ingestion of rice flour. Also, wheat in flour elicits a lower blood glucose level than does wheat in bread. Jenkins et al[75] suggested the use of a so-called glycemic index to characterize a food according to its blood glucose response. The creation of this index was considered as a possible adjunct to the construction of diets for individuals with diabetes, since it identifies starchy carbohydrate foods with low postprandial glycemic response. However, it has become increasingly apparent that the glycemic response of foods given as mixtures cannot be predicted from the values of the individual foods.

We examined the effects of various carbohydrate foods on postprandial glycemia in 22 children and adolescents with poorly controlled IDDM by giving them a mixed isocaloric diet containing breakfast food of either high or low glycemic index. We found that patients given a high glycemic index meal showed higher serum glucose levels than those who received a low glycemic index meal. However, such differences were not noted when the preprandial dose of regular insulin was adjusted to the amount of carbohydrate feedings. Therefore, as long as proper adjustment of insulin is made, the type of carbohydrate in a single mixed meal does not appear to have a significant effect on the postprandial glycemic response in young patients with long-standing IDDM.[76]

Despite the many new developments in the nutritional management of patients with IDDM, much remains to be learned about optimal nutrition for diabetes patients. Moreover, even when correct recommendations are made, their adoption into an adolescent's life style may not be easily accomplished.

EXERCISE

Exercise is an integral part of the management of patients with IDDM. Better physical fitness and other life style modifications intended to improve the general health of the population (e.g., reduced smoking) have resulted in a decline in the major risk factors associated with atherosclerosis. Regular exercise may benefit patients with IDDM in many ways, such as improved metabolic control of diabetes, better self-image, and amelioration of the chronic complications of the disease.[17,18] If significant weight loss is desired, exercise must be done in conjunction with nutritional modification to achieve maximal results. Even patients who lose only a small amount of weight on an exercise regimen undergo changes in body composition, such as decreased adipose tissue mass and reduced insulin requirements, which may lead to substantial metabolic benefits. For example, it has been reported that both basement membrane thickening and pulse volume improve with better glucose control during physical training.[77] However, caution must be advised for IDDM patients who are undertaking an exercise program. In patients who have had the disease for more than 15 years, ischemic heart disease may be a problem. Moreover, worsening of retinopathy has been reported in patients who have engaged in vigorous exercise.[18] Also, more studies are needed to assess the effects of intensive exercise on microalbuminuria. Post-exercise proteinuria has been documented in patients with IDDM who demonstrate no proteinuria at rest.[78] Because autoimmune neuropathy may predispose a patient with IDDM to orthostatic hypotension, caution must be used when these patients train in a hot environment. Also, orthopedic injuries appear to be more common in patients with IDDM. Patients with degenerative joint disease should avoid jogging. Meticulous attention should be given to foot care, especially in patients with peripheral vascular disease and neuropathy. Properly fitting shoes, often with orthotic aids prescribed by a podiatrist, are essential for safe exercise.

Hypoglycemia is the most frequent and dramatic complication of exercise in an individual with IDDM. In healthy individuals, insulin secretion decreases during exercise, leading to increased hepatic glucose production to compensate for accelerated glucose utilization by muscles.[79] In patients receiving exogenous insulin, such down-regulation does not occur, and relative hyperinsulinism and hypoglycemia ensue. This effect occurs even in patients who are receiving an appropriate amount of insulin and whose disease is well controlled.[80] Not only can patients develop hypoglycemia during exercise, but they may become hypoglycemic several hours after exercise is completed. This phenomenon has been named "late onset of postexercise hypoglycemia," and it should always be kept in mind when the physician is prescribing an exercise program, especially one for the evening hours.[81] Thus, although exercise should be a regular part of the patient's daily routine, it is best that the exercise be planned for the morning, before administration of insulin. Because it is not easy to predict the decrease in insulin requirements that may be needed during a given day's activities, we recommend that patients who have had problems with hypoglycemia take their usual insulin dose and consume an extra 15 to 30 g of carbohydrate before and after every 30 minutes of exercise. Insulin should be administered away from sites of exercised muscle groups, because increased blood flow during exercise results in increased absorption of insulin (in many instances the abdomen may be suitable). A 10% reduction in insulin dosage also may be attempted when physical activities are planned. Under special circumstances, exercise may have an opposite effect on blood glucose. Hyperglycemia rather than hypoglycemia may be seen when blood glucose levels are already high (>250 mg/dl [13.9 mmol/L]), and vigorous exercise in this situation can lead to severe hyperglycemia and even ketosis.

STRESS

Of all chronic diseases, IDDM probably requires the most intense and continuous involvement of the patient. The emotional impact of the unceasing demands of tasks of daily management can be overwhelming under the best of circumstances and even more so during times of stress. On the other hand, not every patient with IDDM experiences emotional disability. In fact, many patients with diabetes are emotionally stronger than their counterparts without this disease. However, when a patient with diabetes is in poor metabolic control, an effort must be made to look for psychosocial stress. The stress may be related to the poor control, but this connection may not be apparent to the physician if the patient does not report it. The physician must explore the psychosocial and physiologic aspects of the patient's condition rather than merely attempting to obliterate the consequences of stress by increasing the dose of insulin. Indeed, the role of a psychiatrist in improving control of diabetes is one of the most readily recognized successes of psychotherapy.[4,82]

EDUCATION

Diabetes self-management education is the key to achieving and maintaining the best possible metabolic control of diabetes mellitus in adolescents. Education provides adolescents and their families with skills to manage diabetes on a day-to-day basis and to incorporate diabetes into the patient's individual life style. Because management of diabetes is complex, especially during the teenage years, the combined efforts of a physician (preferably a pediatric endocrinologist), a diabetes educator, a nutritionist, and an exercise physiologist are essential for designing a successful treatment plan. In other words, a comprehensive education program can be achieved only through the team approach. Diabetes education is not a one-time "fix" but a process that must continue throughout the various developmental stages of adolescence into adulthood. After the diagnosis of diabetes mellitus in an adolescent, the first and most important educational process is assessment of the adolescent and family. The assessment must include cognitive knowledge, skills necessary for care, maturity and developmental level, coping skills, and family relationships and dynamics. The adolescent's schedule, habits, and values must be taken into consideration if a successful outcome is to be expected.

After completion of the initial assessment of the adolescent and family, the diabetes team must assist the family to design initial goals that are realistic, achievable, and measurable. The overall concept is that the goals should be meaningful and the regimen kept simple: the more complex the regimen, the more likely it is to fail. Diabetes education must also be imparted. If the adolescent and the family possess incorrect or inadequate knowledge, inappropriate decisions regarding management may be made based on this lack of information.

It is important to design the educational program in such a way as to be "adolescent friendly." If there is a lack of shared philosophy between the adolescent and the diabetes team, all efforts may prove fruitless. The educational process must also be designed to impart knowledge and develop goals with the adolescent and family in a nonjudgmental atmosphere. Although this is a time when the adolescent is moving toward independence, most adolescents still want to receive approval from their parents and the treatment team and to avoid confrontations. If they believe that they will be "judged," some adolescents may, for example, report false blood glucose values. The educational process should always focus on the "positive," and the adolescent's self-esteem must be promoted whenever possible. Evaluation of the goals set and regimen followed must be performed with the team, adolescent, and family in order to change the regimen and adjust goals when necessary.

Adolescents should be seen at least part of the time on their own, with the parents subsequently brought in to be included in the process. Adolescents may wish to address issues that they may not feel comfortable discussing in front of their parents, and they should always be given that opportunity. The diabetes team must also be available at times convenient for the adolescent so that frequent follow-up can be achieved. A final factor is to encourage telephone follow-up between visits, which provides support for the family and necessary adjustments between visits. The ultimate achievement of diabetes education is to maintain healthy family dynamics while assisting adolescents to develop and grow, and to eventually empower adolescents to assess, educate, motivate, set goals for, and evaluate themselves.

CONCLUSION

Management of IDDM in adolescents is one of the most demanding and perplexing medical problems facing the health care team today. Not only is an adolescent with diabetes prone to acute life-threatening complications, but the unfortunate reality is that the long-term outlook remains problematic. Although a great deal of progress has been made in managing diabetes, much more needs to be done. Despite recent developments, the achievement of euglycemia on a long-term basis is difficult, if not impossible, to accomplish in many adolescents with IDDM. It appears that until implantable mechanical pancreas, isolated beta-cell, or pancreatic transplantations are successful, we may not be able to achieve perfect metabolic control of diabetes. Until better therapeutic methods have been developed, or the prevention of diabetes by specific immunosuppression or early administration of insulin has been achieved, research must continue. This ongoing research requires judicious use of conventional therapy with the proper selection and follow-up of those patients who may benefit from more intensive therapeutic modalities such as the CIDS pump.

Intensive insulin therapy should be limited to those patients who are willing and able to perform accurate and frequent HBGM. Moreover, such patients must have at their disposal highly trained and experienced medical professionals who can provide instructions and make day-to-day adjustments in insulin dosage, nutrition, and exercise. If the above requirements cannot be secured, intensive treatment should not be employed. The intensive treatment of IDDM is also not warranted in patients with advanced microangiopathic changes or those with psychiatric disturbances, including a history of drug abuse. Our present goal for adolescents with IDDM is to provide practical, safe, and effective treatment that is best for the patient, family, and physician.

References

1. U.S. Department of Health and Human Services: *Diabetes in America: diabetes data compiled 1984,* DHHS Publication No. 85-1468 (NIH). Washington, DC, 1985, U.S. Government Printing Office.
2. Pittsburgh Diabetes Epidemiology and Etiology Research Group: Evolution of the Pittsburgh studies of the epidemiology of insulin dependent diabetes mellitus, *Genet Epidemiol* 7:105, 1990.
3. The Diabetes Control and Complications Trial Research Group: The effect of intensive treatment of diabetes on the development and progression of long-term complications in insulin-dependent diabetes mellitus, *N Engl J Med* 329:977, 1993.
4. Drash AL, Becker DJ: Behavioral issues in patients with diabetes mellitus, with special emphasis on the child and adolescent. In Rifkin H, Porte D, editors: *Ellenberg and Rifkin's diabetes mellitus: theory and practice,* ed 4, New York, 1990, Elsevier; p 922.
5. Arslanian S, Becker D, Drash A: Diabetes mellitus in the child and adolescent. In Kappy MS, Blizzard RM, Migeon CJ, editors: *The diagnosis and treatment of endocrine disorders in childhood and adolescence,* ed 4, Springfield, IL, 1994, Charles C Thomas; p 972.
6. Drash AL: The child, the adolescent, and the Diabetes Control and Complications Trial, *Diabetes Care* 16:1515, 1993.
7. American Diabetes Association: Position statement. *Implications of the Diabetes Control and Complications Trial, Diabetes Care* 16:1517, 1993.
8. Santiago JV: Lessons from the Diabetes Control and Complications Trial, *Diabetes* 42:1549, 1993.
9. Goldstein DE, Hoeper M: Management of diabetes during adolescence: mission impossible? In *Clinical diabetes,* Alexandria, VA, 1987, American Diabetes Association; p 1.
10. Fineberg SE, Galloway JA, Fineberg NS, Rathbun MJ, Hufferd S: Immunogenicity of recombinant DNA human insulin, *Diabetologia* 25:465, 1983.
11. Starke Aar, Heinemann L, Hofmann A, Berger M: The action profiles of human NPH insulin preparations, *Diabet Med* 6:239, 1989.
12. Gale EAM: Hypoglycaemia and human insulin, *Lancet* 2:1264, 1989.
13. Patrick AW, Bodmer CW, Tieszen KL, White MC, Williams G: Human insulin and awareness of acute hypoglycaemic symptoms in insulin dependent diabetes, *Lancet* 338:528, 1991.
14. Tunbridge FKE, Newens A, Home PD, Davis SN, Murphy M, Borrin JM, Aliberti KGMM, Jensen I: A comparison of human Ultralente and Lente-based twice daily injection regimens, *Diabet Med* 6:496, 1989.
15. Drash AL: *Clinical care of the diabetic child,* Chicago, 1987, Mosby–Year Book.
16. Drash AL, LaPorte RE, Daneman D, Fishbein H, Goldstein D, Becker D: Insulin requirements in children with diabetes mellitus: changing requirements by age and sex over the initial five years of therapy. In Akerbloom H, editor: *The remission period: pediatric and adolescent endocrinology,* Basel, 1985, A. Karger.
17. Landt KW, Campaigne BN, James FW, Sperling MA: Effects of exercise training on insulin sensitivity in adolescents with type I diabetes, *Diabetes Care* 8:461, 1985.
18. Horton ES: Role and management of exercise in diabetes mellitus, *Diabetes Care* 11:201, 1988.
19. Ikeda Y, Tajima N, Minami N, Ide Y, Abe M: Pancreatic B-cell function of young diabetics assessed by C-peptide immunoreactivity, *Jikeikai Med J* 24:113, 1977.
20. Madsbad S: Prevalence of residual B cell function and its metabolic consequences in type I (insulin-dependent) diabetes, *Diabetologia* 24:141, 1983.
21. Dorchy H, Noel P, Kruger M, deMaertelaer V, Dupont E, Toussaint D, Pelc S: Peroneal motor nerve conduction velocity in diabetic children and adolescents. Relationship to metabolic control, HDL-DR antigens, retinopathy and EEG, *Eur J Pediatr* 144:310, 1985.
22. Drell DW, Notkins AL: Multiple immunological abnormalities in patients with type I (insulin-dependent) diabetes mellitus, *Diabetologia* 30:132, 1987.
23. Orr DP, Eccles T, Lawlor R, Golden M: Surreptitious insulin administration in adolescents with insulin-dependent diabetes mellitus, *JAMA* 256:3227, 1986.
24. Cryer PE, Binder C, Bolli GB, et al: Hypoglycemia in IDDM, *Diabetes* 38:1193, 1989.
25. Tordjman KM, Havlin CE, Levandoski LA, White NH, Santiago JV, Cryer PE: Failure of nocturnal hypoglycemia to cause fasting hyperglycemia in patients with insulin-dependent diabetes mellitus, *N Engl J Med* 317:1552, 1987.
26. Gerich JE: Dawn phenomenon: pathophysiology, diagnosis and treatment, *Clin Diabetes* 6:1, 1988.
27. Cuttler L, Ehrlich RM: Insulin resistance developing in children with IDDM, *Diabetes Care* 5:305, 1982.
28. Schade DS, Eaton RP: Brittle diabetes, subcutaneous insulin malabsorption, and intraperitoneal insulin delivery (abstr), *Diabetes* 32 (suppl 1):4A, 1983.
29. Pittman CS: The effects of diabetes mellitus on thyroid physiology, *Thyroid Today* 4:1, 1981.
30. American Diabetes Association: Consensus statement. Self-monitoring of blood glucose, *Diabetes Care* 17:81, 1994.

31. Daneman D, Siminerio L, Transue D, Betschart J, Drash A, Becker D: The role of self-monitoring of blood glucose in the routine management of children with insulin-dependent diabetes mellitus, *Diabetes Care* 8:1, 1985.

32. Drash AL: Management of the child with diabetes mellitus: clinical course, therapeutic strategies and monitoring techniques. In Lifshitz F, editor: *Pediatric endocrinology,* New York, 1990, Marcel Dekker; p 681.

33. Draelos MT, Jacobson AM, Weinger K, Widom B, Ryan CM, Finkelstein DM, Simonson DC: Cognitive function in patients with insulin-dependent diabetes mellitus during hyperglycemia and hypoglycemia, *Am J Med* 98:135, 1995.

34. Landon MB, Gabbe SG: Diabetes and pregnancy, *Med Clin North Am* 72:1493, 1988.

35. Boulton AJM, Drury J, Clarke B, Ward JD: Continuous subcutaneous infusion in the management of painful diabetic neuropathy, *Diabetes Care* 5:386, 1982.

36. Tamborlane WV, Sherwin RS, Genel M, Felig P: Restoration of normal lipid and amino acid metabolism in diabetic patients treated with a portable insulin-infusion pump, *Lancet* 1:1258, 1979.

37. Rudolf MC, Sherwin RS, Markowitz R, Bates SE, Genel M, Hochstadt J, Tamborlane WV: Effect of intensive insulin treatment on linear growth in the young diabetic patient, *J Pediatr* 101:333, 1982.

38. Noto RA, Ginsberg LJ, Lifshitz F, Pelcovitz D, Kaplan S: Improved management of brittle-psychosocial diabetes by use of portable insulin infusion pump, *J Pediatr* 107:100, 1985.

39. Schiffrin A, Belmonte MM: Comparison between continuous subcutaneous insulin infusion and multiple injections of insulin, *Diabetes* 31:255, 1982.

40. Amiel SA, Tamborlane WV, Sacca L, Sherwin RS: Hypoglycemia and glucose counterregulation in normal and insulin-dependent diabetic subjects, *Diabetes Metab Rev* 4:71, 1988.

41. Tamborlane WV, Puklin JE, Bergman M: Long term improvement of metabolic control with the insulin pump does not reverse diabetic microangiopathy, *Diabetes Care* 5 (suppl 1):58, 1982.

42. Van Ballegooie E, Hooymans JMM, Timmerman Z, Reitsma WD, Sluiter WJ, Schweitzer NMJ, Doorenbos H: Rapid deterioration of diabetic retinopathy during treatment with continuous subcutaneous insulin infusion, *Diabetes Care* 7:236, 1984.

43. Ellis D, Avner ED, Transue D, Yunis EJ, Drash AL, Becker DJ: Diabetic nephropathy in adolescence: appearance during improved glycemic control, *Pediatrics* 71:824, 1983.

44. Ramsay RC, Goetz FC, Sutherland DER, Mauer SM, Robinson LL, Cantril HL, Knobloch WH, Najarian JS: Progression of diabetic retinopathy after pancreas transplantation for insulin-dependent diabetes mellitus, *N Engl J Med* 318:208, 1988.

45. MacGillivray MH, Bruck E, Voorhess ML: Acute diabetic ketoacidosis in children: role of the stress hormones, *Pediatr Res* 15:99, 1981.

46. Schade DS, Eaton RP: Pathogenesis of diabetic ketoacidosis: a reappraisal, *Diabetes Care* 2:296, 1979.

47. Rayfield EJ, Curnow RF, Reinhard D, Kochicheril NM: Effects of acute endototinemia on glucoregulation in normal and diabetic subjects, *J Clin Endocrinol Metab* 45:513, 1977.

48. Hare JW, Rossini AA: Diabetic comas: the overlap concept, *Hosp Pract* 14:95, 1979.

49. Potter JL, Stone RJ: Massive hyperlipidemia in diabetic ketoacidosis, *Clin Pediatr* 14:412, 1975.

50. Tisher JN, Shahshahni MN, Kitabchi AE: Diabetic ketoacidosis: low-dose insulin therapy by various routes, *N Engl J Med* 297:238, 1979.

51. Fort P, Waters SM, Lifshitz F: Low-dose insulin infusion in the treatment of diabetic ketoacidosis: bolus versus non-bolus, *J Pediatr* 96-36, 1980.

52. Pugliese MT, Fort P, Lifshitz F: Treatment of diabetic ketoacidosis. In Lifshitz F, editor: *Pediatric endocrinology,* New York, 1990, Marcel Dekker; p 745.

53. Pugliese MT, Fort P, Lifshitz F: Treatment of diabetic ketoacidosis. In Lifshitz F, editor: *Pediatric endocrinology,* New York, 1990, Marcel Dekker; p 757.

54. Cryer PE, Gerich JE: Hypoglycemia in insulin dependent diabetes mellitus: insulin excess and defective glucose counterregulation. In Rifkin H, Porte D, editors: *Diabetes mellitus,* ed 4, New York, 1990, Elsevier; p 526.

55. Ryan CM, Atchison J, Puczynski S, et al: Mild hypoglycemia associated with deterioration of mental efficiency in children with insulin dependent diabetes mellitus, *J Pediatr* 117:32, 1990.

56. Veneman T, Mitrakov A, Mokan M, et al: Induction of hypoglycemia unawareness by asymptomatic nocturnal hypoglycemia, *Diabetes* 42:1233, 1993.

57. Kappy MS: Carbohydrate metabolism and hypoglycemia. In Kappy MS, Blizzard RM, Migeon CJ, editors: *The diagnosis and treatment of endocrine disorders in childhood and adolescence,* ed 4, Springfield, IL, 1994, Charles C Thomas; p 919.

58. Walker JW, Viberti GC: Pathophysiology of microvascular disease: an overview. In Pickup JC, Williams G, editors: *Textbook of diabetes,* London, 1991, Blackwell Scientific Publications; p 526.

59. Becker DJ: Complications of insulin dependent diabetes mellitus in childhood and adolescence. In Lifshitz F, editor: *Pediatric endocrinology,* ed 2, New York, 1990, Marcel Dekker; p 701.

60. Seaquist ER, Goetz FC, Rich S, Barbosa J: Familial clustering of diabetic kidney disease, *N Engl J Med* 320:1161, 1989.

61. Klein R, Klein BEK: Vision disorders in diabetes. In Hammon R, Harris MWH, editors: *Diabetes in America: Diabetes data compiled 1984,* NIH Publication No. 85-1468, Bethesda, MD, 1985, US Public Health Service; p 1.

62. Vora JP, Anderson S: Diabetic renal disease: an overview with therapeutic implications, *Endocrinologist* 2:223, 1992.

63. Carella MJ, Gossain VV, Rovner DR: Early diabetic nephropathy, *Arch Intern Med* 154:625, 1994.

64. Greene DA, Stevens MJ: Diabetic peripheral neuropathy, *Diabetes Spectrum* 6:234, 1993.

65. Chase HP: Avoiding the short- and long-term complications of juvenile diabetes, *Pediatr Rev* 7:140, 1985.

66. Jelinek JE: Skin disorders associated with diabetes mellitus. In Rifkin H, Porte D, editors: *Ellenberg and Rifkin's diabetes mellitus: theory and practice,* ed 4, New York, 1990, Elsevier; p 838.

67. Malaisse WJ, Lebrun P: Mechanisms of sulfonylurea-induced insulin release, *Diabetes Care* 13 (suppl 3):9, 1990.

68. Lebovitz HE: Oral diabetic agents. In Kahn CR, Weir GC, editors: *Joslin's diabetes mellitus,* ed 13, 1994, Philadelphia, Lea & Febiger; p 508.

69. Becerra JE, Khoury MJ, Cordero JF, Erickson JD: Diabetes mellitus during pregnancy and the risks for specific birth defects: a population-based case-control study, *Pediatrics* 85:1, 1990.

70. Lifshitz F: Nutrition and diabetes. In Lifshitz F, editor: *Pediatric endocrinology,* New York, 1990, Marcel Dekker; p 725.

71. Sperling MA: Diabetes mellitus. In Kaplan SA, editor: *Clinical pediatric endocrinology,* Philadelphia, 1990, WB Saunders; p 127.

72. American Diabetes Association: Position statement. Nutritional recommendations and principles for individuals with diabetes mellitus, *Diabetes Care* 16 (suppl 2):22, 1993.

73. Rudberg S, Dahlquist G, Aperia A, Persson B: Reduction of protein intake decreases glomerular filtration rate in young type I (insulin-dependent) diabetic patients mainly in hyperfiltrating patients, *Diabetologia* 32:878, 1988.

74. Bantle JP, Laine DC, Castle GW, Thomas JW, Hoogwerf BJ, Goetz FC: Postprandial glucose and insulin responses to meals containing different carbohydrates in normal and diabetic subjects, *N Engl J Med* 309:7, 1983.

75. Jenkins DJA, Wolever TMS, Taylor RH, Baker H, Fielden H,

Balwin JM, Bowling AC, Newman HC, Jenkins AL, Goff DV: Glycemic index of foods: a physiological basis for carbohydrate exchange, *Am J Clin Nutr* 34:362, 1981.

76. Weyman-Daum M, Fort P, Recker B, Lanes R, Lifshitz F: Glycemic response in children with insulin-dependent diabetes mellitus after high- or low-glycemic-index breakfast, *Am J Clin Nutr* 46:798, 1987.

77. Peterson CHM, Jones RL, Esterly JA, Wantz GE, Jackson RL: Changes in basement membrane thickening and pulse volume concomitant with improved glucose control and exercise in patients with insulin-dependent diabetes mellitus, *Diabetes Care* 3:586, 1980.

78. Viberti GC, Jarrett RJ, McCartney M, Keen H: Increased glomerular permeability to albumin induced by exercise in diabetic subjects, *Diabetologia* 14:293, 1978.

79. Drash A: Factors affecting metabolic control and insulin requirements (management of the diabetic child). In Podolsky S, editor: *Clinical diabetes: modern management,* New York, 1980, Appleton-Century-Crofts; p 443.

80. Skyler JS: Diabetes and exercise. Clinical implications, *Diabetes Care* 2:307, 1979.

81. Bogardus C, Thuillez P, Ravussin E, Vasquez B, Narimiga M, Azhar S: Effect of muscle glycogen depletion on in vivo insulin action in man, *J Clin Invest* 72:1605, 1983.

82. Gath A, Smith AM, Baum DJ: Emotional, behavioral and educational disorders in diabetic children, *Arch Dis Child* 55:371, 1980.

CHAPTER 26

Adrenocortical Disorders

•

H. Verdain Barnes and Maria R. Coccia

ENZYME DEFECTS IN THE ADRENAL CORTEX

Disorders of the adrenal cortex produce a variety of clinical diseases that may have a devastating impact on the adolescent. Adrenogenital syndrome, which is caused by adrenocortical hyperplasia, is a genetic disorder that may involve several enzymatic defects. These defects in steroidogenesis may not become clinically evident until puberty or later (Table 26-1). Fortunately for the adolescent of today, the clinical course of these disorders is well understood, and most patients can be effectively treated.

21-Hydroxylase Deficiency

Deficiency of the 21-hydroxylase enzyme is the most common form of adrenogenital syndrome, accounting for about 60% of all cases of adrenal disease in adolescents. The estimated general incidence of this deficiency is reported to be 1 in 15,000 in the United States. The defect is variable in expression and produces a wide spectrum of clinical presentations. The four currently defined types of 21-hydroxylase deficiency are (1) the classic virilizing form, (2) a salt-wasting type associated with substantial deficiency in aldosterone synthesis, (3) a symptomatic nonclassic form, and (4) an asymptomatic nonclassic type.[1] Deficiency of this enzyme has a relative effect on the production of both cortisol and aldosterone.

Late-Onset 21-Hydroxylase Deficiency

The 21-hydroxylase deficiency that presents most often in the second decade of life is the nonclassic symptomatic form known as late-onset adrenal hyperplasia. The genetic basis for this form of the disease is controversial. A genetic linkage between the human major histocompatibility leukocyte antigen (HLA) complex and 21-hydroxylase deficiency has been described. Whether the late-onset form is a different disease from classic 21-hydroxylase deficiency or an allele of classic 21-hydroxylase deficiency is not known. Nonetheless,

TABLE 26-1
Adrenogenital Syndromes Caused by Defective Steroidogenesis

Enzyme Deficiency	Altered Step in Hormonogenesis	Serum Hormone Levels	External Genitalia		Typical Age at Diagnosis
			Male	Female	
20, 22-Desmolase	Conversion of cholesterol to pregnenolone	All low	Ambiguous	Normal	Fatal condition at birth; few reported survivors
3β-Hydroxysteroid dehydrogenase	Conversion of pregnenolone to progesterone and 17-OH pregnenolone to 17-OH progesterone	↓ Aldosterone ↓ Cortisol ↓ Testosterone ↑ DHEA	Ambiguous	Mild to moderate virilization	Classic form in infants; late-onset form in adolescents
21-Hydroxylase	Conversion of progesterone to 11-deoxycorticosterone and 17-OH progesterone to 11-deoxycortisol	↓ Cortisol ↓ Aldosterone ↑ 17-OH progesterone	Normal	Virilized	Classic form in infants; late-onset form in adolescents
11-Hydroxylase	Conversion of 11-deoxycorticosterone to corticosterone and 11-deoxycortisol to cortisol	↓ Cortisol ↓ Aldosterone ↑ Deoxycortisol ↑ Deoxycorticosterone ↑ Adrenal androgens	Normal	Virilized	Classic form in infants; late-onset form in adolescents
17-Hydroxylase	Conversion of pregnenolone to 17-OH pregnenolone and progesterone to to 17-OH progesterone	↓ Cortisol ↓ Androgens ↓ Aldosterone ↑ Deoxycorticosterone ↑ Corticosterone	Ambiguous	Normal	Children or adolescents

DHEA, dehydroepiandrosterone.

late-onset disease appears to be transmitted as an autosomal recessive trait, as is true for the classic form of the disease.[2]

The adolescent girl with late-onset adrenogenital syndrome does not have ambiguous genitalia but typically presents with hirsutism and menstrual irregularity. She also may have problem acne that is refractory to oral antibiotics and retinoic acid. Boys with late-onset disease typically have early onset of pubic hair growth, penis enlargement, acne, and beard growth. If the syndrome is uncontrolled, both boys and girls may have an early growth spurt and accelerated epiphyseal closure, which may result in short stature. Without treatment, both sexes may experience infertility.[1] Polycystic ovary syndrome and nonclassic 3β-hydroxysteroid dehydrogenase deficiency can be confused with late-onset adrenogenital syndrome because many of the clinical manifestations are similar.[3,4]

A definite diagnosis of late-onset disease can usually be made by measuring the response of 17α-hydroxy-progesterone (17-OHP) to adrenocorticotropic hormone

(ACTH) stimulation. This test requires a baseline blood sample for 17-OHP followed by the administration of 1 mg of synthetic ACTH (cosyntropin [Cortrosyn]) and a repeat blood sample for 17-OHP 30 and 60 minutes after injection. An exaggerated response signifies late-onset adrenogenital syndrome. Because 17-OHP normally increases during the luteal phase, baseline levels of 17-OHP alone are not useful for diagnosis, particularly in menstruating females. The ACTH stimulation test is currently the most effective means of differentiating late-onset adrenogenital syndrome from the polycystic ovary syndrome,[3] and by adding measurements of dehydroepiandrosterone sulfate (DHEAS), 17-hydroxy-pregnenolone, and cortisol, nonclassic 3β-hydroxysteroid dehydrogenase deficiency can also be differentiated.[4] Adolescents suspected of having late-onset 21-hydroxylase deficiency should be referred to an endocrinologist for comprehensive management.

Treatment for late-onset 21-hydroxylase deficiency consists of glucocorticoid replacement, which may reverse infertility in both sexes. With adequate suppressive therapy, hirsutism may resolve over 1 to 2 years. Early treatment also may prevent short stature if the epiphyses have not yet fused. We recommend that a baseline radiographic bone age be measured at the time of initial treatment. With adequate therapy, the prognosis is good.

Cortisone, 50 to 100 mg intramuscularly daily for 1 week, can be given initially, followed by an oral dosage of cortisone, which may be as high as 25 mg three times daily to achieve optimal control in some adolescents. The dosage guidelines are as follows: hydrocortisone, 15 to 40 mg/m^2/day; prednisone or prednisolone, 5 to 7 mg/m^2/day divided into two or three doses. The amount of steroid given is adjusted on the basis of linear growth, skeletal maturation, and serum 17-OHP levels. The dose of corticosteroid may need to be increased in the morning to achieve optimal control and to more closely approximate the normal diurnal variation. We prefer hydrocortisone therapy for patients with late-onset deficiency.

Classic 21-Hydroxylase Deficiency

The most common form of 21-hydroxylase deficiency is the classic virilizing form, which typically presents during infancy. Three fourths of these cases are "salt wasters" due to accompanying mineralocorticoid deficiency. In girls the classic form is usually obvious at birth because of ambiguous genitalia resulting from excess in utero androgen. During puberty, if inadequately treated, girls develop excessive hair and have amenorrhea. Boys may have normal genitalia, and the condition may not be recognized until sometime during childhood, unless salt wasting is severe. Boys typically present with precocious puberty. If the deficiency is not treated in boys, the testes will remain small for developmental stage. If the condition is uncontrolled, short stature will result in both sexes.[1] A diagnosis of classic 21-hydroxylase deficiency can be confirmed by elevated serum levels of 17-OHP, testosterone, and androstenedione. Patients with significant salt loss have hyponatremia, hyperkalemia, inappropriately high urine sodium excretion, low serum and urine aldosterone, and high plasma renin activity.

In general, therapy includes the use of a glucocorticoid plus a mineralocorticoid for patients with salt wasting.[5] A potential treatment problem during puberty is the development of so-called cortisone resistance. If this occurs, intramuscular treatment is continued until the serum level of 17-OHP is reduced to an acceptable level, and then oral therapy is resumed. An alternative approach is to change to dexamethasone. In some resistant cases, a mineralocorticoid may be helpful, even in patients without salt loss.[5] Because these patients have normal gonads, adequate early treatment usually results in normal cyclic menses and ovulation in girls and adequate spermatogenesis in boys. Adolescent psychosocial adaptation to this condition may be problematic or normal.

Delta^5-3β-Hydroxysteroid Dehydrogenase Deficiency

Delta^5-3β-hydroxysteroid dehydrogenase deficiency (3β-HSD) affects the production of all three classes of adrenal steroids: aldosterone, cortisol, and testosterone. The late-onset or nonclassic form of this autosomal recessive disorder typically becomes noticeable in the peripubertal years. This milder enzyme defect may involve a variety of clinical manifestations. Girls may present with acne, hirsutism, clitoris enlargement without ambiguous genitalia, or postmenarchal menstrual irregularity. Forms that do not include salt loss, and a type in boys that involves a deficiency in the production of glucocorticoids but not androgens, have been reported. In contrast to 21-hydroxylase deficiency, the gonads are involved in this deficiency.[1,5]

ACTH stimulation offers the best current approach to diagnosis. Baseline and 1-hour post-Cortrosyn injection values for DHEAS, 17-OHP, 17α-OH-5 P and cortisol should be measured.[4] In these patients, the baseline ratio of 17α-OH-5 pregnenolone (17α-OH-5 P) to 17-OHP is about 2.8, which is higher than the ratio (1.2) in women without the deficiency. With ACTH stimulation, there is a greater increase in 17α-OH-5 P than in 17-OHP, and thus the ratio increases to between 8 and 14 compared with an increase of up to 5 in women without the deficiency. Serum sampling for 17α-OH-5 P and 17-OHP is done before ACTH stimulation, at the time of stimulation, and 60 minutes later. The diagnosis is made by demonstrating impaired conversion from delta^5 to delta^4 compounds.

Treatment consists primarily of glucocorticoid replacement. In the milder or nonclassic (late-onset) form of this deficiency, glucocorticoid replacement doses may be sufficient.

11β-Hydroxylase Deficiency

Deficiency of the mitochondrial enzyme 11β-hydroxylase occurs in about 10% of patients with adrenogenital syndrome. These patients have a concomitant defect in 18-hydroxylase production in the zona fasciculata, but a normal zona glomerulosa. There is a late-onset form that appears in adolescents and young adults. The clinical manifestations of 11β-hydroxylase deficiency are similar to those of 21-hydroxylase deficiency. Hypertension is an added feature and may dominate the presentation during puberty.[6]

Plasma levels of 11-deoxycortisol (compound S), deoxycorticosterone (DOC), and the adrenal androgens are elevated. An ACTH stimulation test may be helpful in identifying the late-onset form, since plasma renin activity is suppressed as compared with that seen in 21-hydroxylase deficiency.

Treatment of this condition consists of glucocorticoid administration, which may correct the hypertension by suppressing DOC secretion. DOC elevation in the untreated state provides negative feedback to the renin-angiotensin system, and thus adequate therapy results in a rise in plasma renin activity, which then stimulates aldosterone production in the normal zona glomerulosa.

17-Hydroxylase Deficiency

This enzyme defect may present during puberty, although the primary time of diagnosis is the first decade of life. Up to 1994, approximately 50 cases of this rare deficiency have been reported. In 17-hydroxylase deficiency the gonads and adrenals are both affected. The typical clinical manifestation is male pseudohermaphroditism with ambiguous genitalia at birth. Consequently, the gender assignment may be female. At puberty, gynecomastia may develop but without normal secondary sex characteristics. At puberty the female usually presents with amenorrhea and a lack of breast development. The initial presentation commonly includes hypertension and hypokalemia.[1,5-7]

DOC and corticosterone (compound B) concentrations are elevated. Aldosterone levels are low, owing to depressed plasma renin. As with 11-hydroxylase deficiency, renin is suppressed by the negative inhibitory feedback of DOC on the renin-angiotensin-aldosterone system. However, in contrast to 11-hydroxylase deficiency, the biochemical pathway for aldosterone production is not blocked.[1,5-7]

Treatment includes glucocorticoid administration, sex steroid replacement, and reconstructive surgery. In girls, estrogen administration at puberty stimulates breast development and menses. In the pseudohermaphrodite male, the testis is typically located within the abdomen. Consequently, orchiopexy is required, which may save gonadal function and prevent neoplastic changes in the testicles. Glucocorticoid treatment typically reverses the hypertension and hypokalemia. Psychological counseling is required for optimal comprehensive patient management.[1,5,7]

PHEOCHROMOCYTOMA

Pheochromocytoma rarely occurs during the second decade of life. As a cause of secondary hypertension this condition, if undiagnosed and untreated, has significant potential for morbidity and mortality.[8] These tumors arise from chromaffin tissue, typically of the adrenal medulla, but they may develop at any site where chromaffin cells are found. Several characteristics of this tumor differ in adolescents as opposed to adults. In this age group the peak incidence of diagnosis is between 9 and 12 years of age.[7,9] In the series described by Stackpole et al,[9] 65% of patients were 10 years of age or older; most girls were diagnosed between the ages of 11 and 15 years. As girls approach menarche, there is an apparent increase in pheochromocytomas, which suggests a possible correlation between menarche and onset of clinical symptoms.[9] In adolescents, the male-to-female ratio is 2:1, whereas among adults there is a female predominance.[7,9]

Most pheochromocytomas in adolescents are located in one adrenal gland; however, the incidence of multiple tumors is relatively high: 32% compared with 4% in adults.[9] In adolescents, tumors outside the adrenal are usually intraabdominal in the periadrenal area, along the aortic bifurcation, in the organ of Zuckerkandl, along the common iliac artery, or in the urinary bladder.[9]

The symptoms most frequently seen in adolescents often vary from the classic manifestations in adults. In adolescents, sustained hypertension occurs more frequently (approximately 90%) than in adults (50%). On the other hand, adolescents who experience paroxysmal attacks appear to have them more frequently than do adults. The explanation is not clear but may relate in part to a decreased catecholamine response of adrenergic receptors with aging. Headaches and sweating are equally common in youths and adults. Adolescents appear to be more likely to have nausea, weight loss, or visual disturbance; they often appear pale, weak, and anxious and are extremely emotionally labile for their age and stage of development. Tachycardia, chest and abdominal pain, encephalopathy with associated seizures, retinopathy, polydipsia, and polyuria may be seen. Some adolescents have acrocyanosis (puffy red cyanosis of the fingers and tip of the nose) and cool extremities. If the hypertension is long-standing, the adolescent may have cardiomegaly and/or cardiac failure.[9] Some authors consider the general symptoms in adolescents to be more severe than in the adults.

In adolescents the variety of clinical manifestations may delay diagnosis. Diagnosis may be camouflaged by those symptoms that suggest potential renal disease, thyrotoxicosis, emotional disorder, essential hypertension, acute adrenal insufficiency, or acute pancreatitis. Excess catecholamines may produce hyperglycemia, glucosuria, and increased levels of free fatty acids, thus mimicking several features of diabetes mellitus. Persistent hypertension in an adolescent requires careful consideration of the possibility of a pheochromocytoma, since sustained essential hypertension in adolescents is not common.[1,8,9]

Pheochromocytomas occasionally present during pregnancy, and physicians caring for pregnant adolescents should be aware of this as a potential cause of gestation-associated hypertension.[10] The mortality rate for mother and fetus may be as high as 50%.

Pheochromocytomas can be sporadic or inherited as an autosomal dominant trait. They may also be part of the multiple endocrine neoplasia I and II syndromes. This type of tumor is also seen in association with familial neuroectodermal dysplasias such as neurofibromatosis and von Hippel-Lindau disease.

Several tests have been used for diagnosis of pheochromocytoma, but none is ideal. The most specific diagnostic tests currently available are 24-hour urine concentrations of norepinephrine, epinephrine, normetanephrine, and metanephrine.[11] Adolescents with a pheochromocytoma usually excrete more norepinephrine than epinephrine as compared with adults. When urinary epinephrine levels are high, the tumor is more likely to be intra-adrenal or located in the organ of Zuckerkandl.[8] A new test under investigation, which appears to have better sensitivity and specificity, measures the levels of chromogranin A, a compound stored and released by the secretory granules of the tumor.[12] Vanillylmandelic acid, provocative, and blocking tests are no longer recommended.

Some foods (e.g., vanilla, bananas, chocolate, coffee, and citrus fruits) and drugs (e.g., methyldopa, aspirin in high doses, phenothiazines, and tetracycline) may result in spurious elevations of urine catecholamines and their metabolites. Stress and hypoglycemia may also produce elevations in catecholamine levels that are not associated with a pheochromocytoma. In general, excretion of catecholamines and their metabolites is less in adolescents who have not completed pubertal development than in adults. Consequently, the test results should be compared with an age-appropriate reference range.

Once a diagnosis is made, localization of the tumor is paramount. In adolescents this is a challenge, because multiple tumors are common. With the newer imaging methods, arteriography and venous sampling are outdated. Computed tomography (CT) with intravenous contrast is effective. The excellent spatial resolution of the CT scan has been reported to detect about 95% of intra-adrenal tumors; however, tumors less than 2 cm in diameter are often missed. CT imaging is not effective in locating extra-adrenal tumors, nor can it distinguish between cortical and medullary tumors or between functioning and nonfunctioning tumors. The use of an intravenous contrast medium may be a hazard, since administration has been reported to precipitate a hypertensive crisis, albeit rarely.[13]

Magnetic resonance imaging (MRI) has emerged as the preferred method for localizing pheochromocytomas. With this method there are no risks of ionizing radiation or intravenous contrast medium administration. With the aid of signal intensity, a nonfunctioning adrenal mass can often be distinguished from the functioning pheochromocytoma. Metaiodobenzylguanidine (MIBG) scintigraphy is recommended for localizing extra-adrenal pheo-chromocytomas, recurrent or residual disease, and/or a metastasis. MIBG simulates norepinephrine and is taken up and stored by functional adrenal tissue. The ability to perform whole body imaging may make this procedure a cost-effective screening method. MIBG offers superior contrast but inferior resolution compared with MRI or CT scanning. Consequently, MIBG is useful as an adjunct to further substantiate equivocal MRI or CT findings.[13]

Therapy should be referred to an experienced team, including an endocrinologist and an endocrine surgeon who regularly treat this rare tumor. It is impossible to determine whether the surgical specimen is benign or malignant. Histologically, both benign and malignant tumors can show pleomorphic cells, blood vessel involvement, and capsular invasion. Fortunately, malignant pheochromocytomas in adolescents are rare.[8]

HYPERCORTISOLISM

Cushing's syndrome, or hypercortisolism, is rare in adolescents. In adolescents the cause is usually of pituitary origin, with increased ACTH production and secretion, and concomitant adrenal hyperplasia. A pituitary basophilic microadenoma of less than 10 mm is the most common culprit. These pituitary tumors may arise from an increase in corticotropin-releasing factor secreted by the hypothalamus. The adrenal pathology associated with excess pituitary ACTH production (Cushing's disease) includes diffuse adrenocortical and/or micronodular adrenal hyperplasia. The syndrome of ectopic ACTH, or excessive ACTH production by a neoplasm of nonpituitary origin, has rarely been reported in adolescents.[1,5,14]

Primary adrenocortical nodular dysplasia is another rare cause of Cushing's syndrome that merits comment. There are at least four described etiologies: (1) classic macronodular hyperplasia that begins with pituitary ACTH-dependent Cushing's disease; (2) normal or slightly enlarged irregular pigmented adrenal nodularity that in some patients appears to be caused by an IgG subfraction that binds ACTH receptors in the adrenal cortex; (3) bilateral adrenal nodularity associated with an abnormal systhesis of 21-deoxycortisol by the adrenals, resulting in enhanced ACTH production; and (4) adrenal nodular hyperplasia secondary to gastric inhibitory polypeptide (GIP)–dependent cortisol hypersecretion. PPNAD predominantly affects young girls.

Iatrogenic causes of Cushing's syndrome should be considered in the differential diagnosis. For example, an adolescent alcoholic may have elevated ACTH and cortisol levels that return to normal if the alcohol is discontinued. Cushing's syndrome can also be caused by the use of dexamethasone, such as in the liberal use of skin creams or nasal preparations. This type of iatrogenic

Cushing's is typically seen in the adolescent whose underlying disease has been responsive to steroid therapy; the patient receives a high dose from the physician or personally decides to use more glucocorticoid than prescribed, or for a longer time than prescribed. Factitious Cushing's syndrome can occur in adolescents but is very rare.[1]

The adolescent with Cushing's syndrome or Cushing's disease often presents with obesity. Although fat distribution is usually centripetal, it may be generalized. Associated features frequently include a "moon face" and/or "buffalo hump" (dorsocervical fat pad). Muscle wasting of the extremities may be prominent.

If adolescent growth is incomplete, the linear growth rate may be decreased substantially. Other common features seen in adolescents are purple striae, easy bruisability, excessive hair growth, increased acne, and (in prepuberty) premature pubic hair. Virilization per se is rare. Hypertension, poor wound healing, relative osteoporosis, and osteopenia are also common. Compression fractures, congestive heart failure, cerebrovascular accident, and renal calculi are rare in adolescents. The metabolic effects of glucocorticoid excess include impaired glucose tolerance, although overt diabetes mellitus is rare in adolescents with Cushing's syndrome. Psychological problems may dominate the initial presentation.[1,5]

The diagnosis of hypercortisolism is not always easy to establish. The best generally available screening test is a 24-hour collection of urinary free cortisol (UFC). The UFC is elevated in about 90% of patients with Cushing's syndrome. Measurements of urinary 17-hydroxysteroids or 17-ketogenic steroids alone are often not helpful, since many patients with exogenous obesity have borderline or elevated levels. Owing to the variability in cortisol production and release in Cushing's syndrome, testing for a loss of normal diurnal variation is typically not useful, since cortisol levels may lack diurnal variation and may be nonsuppressible in some depressed and obese patients. Low-dose dexamethasone suppression testing produces a substantial number of false-positive and false-negative results. If the UFC level is elevated, further testing is required. The combination of an overnight dexamethasone suppression test (DST) and a 6 day dihydrotestosterone test (DHT) is reported to have a sensitivity of 91% and a specificity of 100% for the diagnosis of Cushing's disease. We recommend that such testing be directed by an endocrinologist.[1,5,15]

The use of simultaneous venous ACTH sampling from the periphery and the inferior petrosal sinus may prove to be the most reliable diagnostic procedure for differentiating pituitary from ectopic Cushing's syndrome. An MRI is currently the best imaging procedure for assessing the pituitary fossa. Both CT and MRI are effective for adrenal gland imaging.[1]

Available treatments for pituitary causes of Cushing's syndrome are transsphenoidal microsurgery and conventional irradiation. Better results with conventional irradiation have been reported in younger patients than in adults. Treatment of adrenal causes, such as an adenoma or carcinoma, consists of surgical excision.[4,16]

HYPOADRENOCORTISOLISM

Addison's disease, or primary adrenal insufficiency, is rare in adolescents. In the classic form of this disease, production of glucocorticoid, mineralocorticoid, and androgen is decreased or absent. In secondary adrenal insufficiency, there is a relative or absolute deficiency of ACTH that leads to decreased stimulation of adrenal steroidogenesis. In secondary disease there is often a deficiency in other anterior pituitary trophic hormones, whereas mineralocorticoid production is affected minimally. Adrenal insufficiency due to inherited enzyme defects is discussed at the beginning of this chapter.

Early in the twentieth century, tuberculosis was the most common cause of Addison's disease in adolescents as well as in adults. Today, autoimmune disease appears to be the most common cause. Two types of polyglandular autoimmune processes may cause Addison's disease. Type I, which is usually diagnosed in childhood, is associated with hypoparathyroidism (76%), mucocutaneous candidiasis (73%), alopecia (32%), malabsorption (22%), gonadal failure (17%), pernicious anemia (13%), chronic active hepatitis (13%), thyroid deficiency (11%), vitiligo (8%), and insulin-dependent diabetes mellitus (4%). Type II is generally seen in midlife, but it can occur in adolescents and is associated with autoimmune thyroid disease (69%), insulin-requiring diabetes (52%), vitiligo (4.5%), gonadal failure (3.6%), pernicious anemia (0.5%), and alopecia (0.5%). In all age groups females are more likely to be affected with either type. Both type I and type II can be familial or sporadic, but only type II is associated with a specific HLA.[1,17]

Adrenomyeloneuropathy, which may present during adolescence, is an X-linked recessive disorder. It is manifested by clinical symptoms of adrenal insufficiency and neurologic signs of weakness, spasticity, and polyneuropathy of the legs. There is often a slow, progressive neurologic deterioration after the onset of adrenal insufficiency.[18]

Tuberculosis currently accounts for approximately 21% of patients with adrenocortical insufficiency. Less common causes of infectious adrenal gland destruction include histoplasmosis, coccidioidomycosis, cryptococcosis, and septicemia, particularly meningococcal and staphylococcal. Infiltrative causes include sarcoidosis, metastases, Hodgkin's or non-Hodgkin's lymphomas, amyloid, hemochromatosis, and adrenal neoplasms such

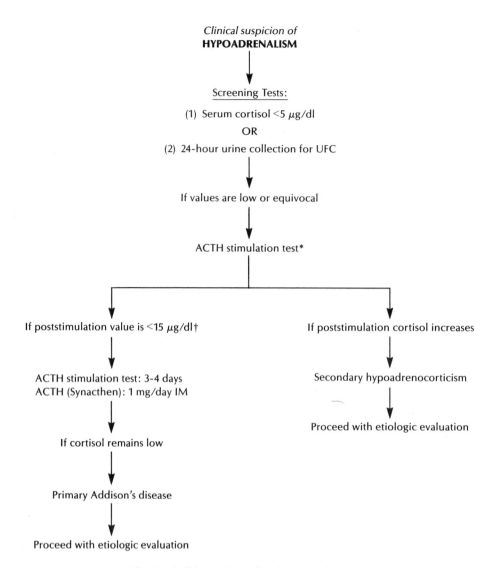

Fig. 26-1. Diagnostic testing for hypoadrenalism.

as pheochromocytoma. Secondary hypoadrenalism can result from neoplasms involving the hypothalamus and/or the pituitary gland. The most common tumor in adolescents is a craniopharyngioma. Other causes include closed head trauma, encephalitis, meningitis, surgical hypophysectomy, and autoimmune hypophysitis.[1]

Adrenal insufficiency can be iatrogenic, specifically after prolonged glucocorticoid therapy and profound suppression of the hypothalamic-pituitary-adrenal axis. Abrupt cessation of steroids in this setting typically causes symptoms of adrenal insufficiency. We recommend a gradual tapering of glucocorticoids over several days when supraphysiologic doses have been administered for 7 days or longer. Recovery of a suppressed hypothalamic-pituitary-adrenal axis may take as little as 2 weeks or as long as 2 years.[1]

Adrenal insufficiency may be subtle. The earliest sign may be nothing more than an increased severity of minor illnesses such as excessive fever with, or prolonged duration of, a common cold. Common symptoms of adrenal insufficiency include fatigue; weakness; anorexia; recurrent nausea, with or without vomiting; constipation, often alternating with diarrhea; intermittent abdominal pain; weight loss; malaise; orthostatic dizziness; irritability; sleeplessness; and, in those with a mineralocorticoid deficiency, salt craving. Any one of these symptoms may dominate the clinical presentation. As the disease progresses, syncope, hypotension, and hypoglycemia may develop and become life-threatening. Hyperpigmentation of the skin in primary adrenal insufficiency may be seen in areas of previous scarring, palmar creases, knuckles, elbows, knees, areolae, and perianal and oral mucosal areas. Hyperpigmentation is not a feature of secondary adrenal insufficiency. Vitiligo may occur as a result of autoimmune destruction of melanocytes in the skin. Pubertal development may be affected if the adrenal insufficiency develops at the onset of puberty. A variety of psychological disturbances has been described, but none is characteristic.

The most severe form of adrenal insufficiency is acute adrenal crisis, characterized by circulatory collapse, severe dehydration, and hypoglycemia.[1,5] This life-threatening combination is rare, but if seriously suspected it should be treated immediately as a true medical emergency.

Laboratory values that support the diagnosis of primary adrenal insufficiency include hyperkalemia, relative hyponatremia, hypoglycemia, and elevated blood urea nitrogen and creatinine levels. Neutropenia, lymphocytosis, and eosinophilia may be seen. Plasma renin activity is elevated in primary Addison's disease but not in secondary disease.[1] None of these tests or the ratios related to these values are diagnostic.

Definitive diagnosis of adrenal insufficiency is made by hormone testing. Measurement of serum cortisol before intravenous ACTH stimulation and 1 hour after stimulation is considered to be the screening test of choice. This is enhanced by also measuring plasma ACTH, aldosterone, and plasma renin activity. Some patients with adrenal autoantibodies have very subtle or no clinical manifestations of adrenal insufficiency. Such patients have chemically evident disease that can be demonstrated by an abnormal response of ACTH and plasma cortisol to ovine corticotropin-releasing hormone.[19] Prolonged ACTH stimulation and metyrapone testing may help differentiate between primary and secondary causes of adrenal insufficiency. Metyrapone testing, however, should be attempted only in a controlled hospital setting, since it may accentuate the glucocorticoid deficiency. ACTH levels in primary Addison's disease are usually more than 200 pg/ml, while in secondary disease ACTH levels are typically low-normal or low (Fig. 26-1).[1,5]

The treatment of primary adrenal insufficiency is with glucocorticoids, and a mineralocorticoid is added if there is combined deficiency. In secondary Addison's disease, glucocorticoid replacement alone is typically all that is required. Replacement therapy with oral hydrocortisone, two to three times daily for a total dosage of 15 to 20 mg/m^2/24 hours, is recommended for adolescents. Prednisone is an alternative: 5 mg in the morning and 2.5 mg in the evening. Dexamethasone is not appropriate treatment for Addison's disease. Fludrocortisone (Florinef), a mineralocorticoid, is recommended in dosages of 0.05 to 0.1 mg/day if there is evidence of mineralocorticoid deficiency after adequate hydrocortisone replacement. If acute illness or other stressful events occur, the dosage of glucocorticoid should be doubled. Adjustments in mineralocorticoid therapy in this setting are not usually needed.

In acute adrenal crisis, hypotension, dehydration, and shock should be immediately and vigorously treated with fluid volume replacement and glucocorticoids. If the patient is in shock, dextrose and normal saline solution should be given at 1.5 to 2 times the maintenance rate. Hydrocortisone is given as an intravenous bolus. For adolescents, the dose is at least 100 to 150 mg. This should be followed by an infusion of 100 mg/m^2 hydrocortisone over 24 hours. As the patient's condition stabilizes, the hydrocortisone dose is tapered toward an individualized replacement dose. Fludrocortisone, if needed, is added to the regimen when the daily dose of hydrocortisone is less than 100 mg/day.

References

1. Barnes HV: Diseases of the endocrine system and metabolic disorders. In Spivak JL, Barnes HV, editors: *Manual of clinical problems in internal medicine,* Boston, 1990, Little, Brown; pp 163-230.
2. Blankstein J, Faiman C, Reyes FI, Schroeder ML, Winter JSD: Adult onset familial adrenal 21-hydroxylase deficiency, *Am J Med* 68:441-448, 1980.
3. Migeon CJ: Diagnosis and treatment of adrenogenital disorders. In DeGroot LJ, Besser GM, Cahill GF, Marshall JC, Nelson DH, O'Dell WD, Potts JT, Rubenstein AH, Steinberger E, editors: *Endocrinology,* Philadelphia, 1989, WB Saunders; pp 1676-1704.
4. Schram C, Jewelewics R, Zarah M, Jaffe S, Mani P, New MI: Nonclassical 3β-dehydrogenase deficiency: a review of our experience with 25 female patients, *Fertil Steril* 58:129-136, 1992.
5. Bacon GE, Spencer ML, Hopwood NJ, Kelch RP, editors: *A practical approach to pediatric endocrinology,* Chicago, 1990, Mosby–Year Book, pp 157-182.
6. New MI, Levine LS: Hypertension and the adrenal cortex. In Kaplan SA, editor: *Clinical pediatric and adolescent endocrinology,* Philadelphia, 1982, WB Saunders; pp 187-198.
7. Voorhess ML: Disorders of the adrenal medulla and multiple endocrine adenomatosis syndromes. In Kaplan SA, editor: *Clinical pediatric endocrinology,* Philadelphia, 1990, WB Saunders; pp 235-258.
8. Bravo EL, Gifford RW Jr: Pheochromocytoma, *Endocrinol Metab Clin North Am* 22:329-341, 1993.
9. Stackpole RII, Melicow MM, Uson AC: Pheochromocytoma in children, *J Pediatr* 63:315-330, 1963.
10. Molitch ME: Endocrine problems of adolescent pregnancy, *Endocrinol Metab Clin North Am* 22:649-672, 1993.
11. Graham PE, Smythe GA, Edwards GA, Lazarus L: Laboratory diagnosis of pheochromocytoma: which analytes should we measure?, *Ann Clin Biochem* 30:129-134, 1993.
12. Hsiao RJ, Neumann HPH, Parmer RJ, Barbosa JA, O'Connor DT: Chromogranin A in familial pheochromocytoma: diagnostic screening value, prediction of tumor mass, and post-resection kinetics indicating two-compartment distribution, *Am J Med* 88:607-613, 1990.
13. Velchik MG, Alavi A, Kressel HY, Engelman K: Localization of pheochromocytoma: MIBG, CT and MRI correlation, *J Nucl Med* 30:328-336, 1989.
14. Trainer PJ, Besser M: Cushing's syndrome—difficulties in diagnosis, *Trends Endocrinol Metab* 1:292-295, 1990.
15. Dichek HL, Nieman LK, Oldfield EH, Pass HI, Malley JD, Cutler GB Jr: A comparison of the standard high dose dexamethasone suppression test and the overnight 8-mg dexamethasone suppression test for the differential diagnosis of adrenocorticotropin-dependent Cushing's syndrome, *J Clin Endocrinol Metab* 78:418-422, 1994.

16. New MI, del Balzo P, Crawford C, Speiser PW: The adrenal cortex. In Kaplan SA, editor: *Clinical pediatric endocrinology,* Philadelphia, 1990, WB Saunders; pp 181-234.
17. Franco-Saenz R: Diseases of the adrenal cortex. In Mulrow PJ, editor: *The adrenal gland,* New York, 1986, Elsevier; pp 284-323.
18. Sadeghi-Nejad A, Senior B: Adrenomyeloneuropathy presenting as Addison's disease in childhood, *N Engl J Med* 322:13-16, 1990.
19. Boscaro M, Betterle C, Sonino N, Volpato M, Paoletta A, Fallo F: Early adrenal hypofunction in patients with organ-specific autoantibodies and no clinical adrenal insufficiency, *J Clin Endocrinol Metab* 79:452-455, 1994.

CHAPTER 27

Growth Disorders

•

Cecilia D. Cervantes and Fima Lifshitz

SHORT STATURE

Since normal growth is evidence of good health, one of the primary concerns of those who care for children and adolescents is the appropriate growth of their patients. Children and adolescents of short stature may face one or more organic or psychologic problem at any time in their lives. Most children become aware of their short stature by the time they enter grade school. However, it is during the teenage years that those who are short experience more adjustment problems than those of normal height. The problems of short stature are often compounded by lack of sexual development and possible withdrawal from social activities. Parents and teachers of children of short stature frequently have difficulty in accepting the child's height and do not treat the child according to actual age level. As a consequence, these individuals need to develop adaptive techniques to cope more effectively with their environment. Most adolescents are able to adapt emotionally, physically, and intellectually to being of small stature.[1] However, some are unable to compensate and develop low self-esteem and various psychological difficulties. Many short children have also been found to have learning problems in school, and a combination of cognitive, physiologic, and psychosocial factors appear to contribute.[2]

To understand growth disorders, it is important to have a unified concept of the various terms used. The terms *dwarfism* and *short stature* are used to describe an individual whose height is below the norm. However, dwarfism connotes a more severe degree of stunting. In general, these terms are derived from the standard growth curves published by the National Center for Health Statistics (NCHS), which are based on healthy, well-nourished Caucasian children of different ethnic backgrounds.[3]

Children and adolescents are described as having short stature if their height falls below 2 standard deviations (SD) from the mean. Dwarfism is present when the height is below 3 SD from the mean. Therefore, children are considered to have normal stature when their height falls within 2 SD of the mean. However, many children and adolescents whose height is below the mean express concerns about their height, and those below the 5th percentile often seek consultation with an endocrinologist.[4]

Short stature, however, is not necessarily a cause for medical concern. It is an abnormal pattern of growth or a deceleration in growth velocity that usually requires investigation by a clinician. A child who has been growing steadily below the 5th percentile parallel to the normal growth curve may be a normal, healthy child with familial short stature or constitutional delay of growth and development, and no further investigation may be needed. However, a child who was previously in the 50th percentile but has fallen to the 10th percentile definitely needs to be evaluated.

In general, most patients of short stature will be considered for evaluation during their childhood years. The clinician who cares for such children during their adolescent years may be called on to manage the psychosocial sequelae, and at times the ongoing medical or endocrinologic care, of these teenagers. Other children, however, may not present for evaluation of their short stature until early adolescence. The clinician who sees these teenagers may perform the initial evaluation in addition to managing the ongoing psychosocial and medical needs. The peak age of presentation for endocrinologic evaluation, especially for boys, is usually between 10 and 12 years. Most causes of short stature are identifiable. In rare instances, however, the reason for stunted growth remains unclear even after extensive investigation. Box 27-1 shows a list of the numerous causes of short stature, divided into nonpathologic and pathologic categories. A third group of patients have idiopathic short stature, in which case no cause for short stature can be demonstrated even after a comprehensive work-up.

NONPATHOLOGIC SHORT STATURE

Familial short stature and constitutional delay of growth and development, which are normal variants of growth, account for about 50% of all children referred to a pediatric endocrinologist for evaluation of short stature.[4]

Familial Short Stature

The diagnosis of familial short stature is given when predicted height falls within a ± 5 cm range of the midparental height.[5] This is sometimes called the target height, which is calculated by using the following formula:

Boys: target height (cm) =
$$\frac{\text{father's ht (cm)} + \text{mother's ht (cm)} + 13}{2}$$
Girls: target height (cm) =
$$\frac{\text{father's ht (cm)} + \text{mother's ht (cm)} - 13}{2}$$

Familial short stature is believed to encompass a heterogeneous group of heritable conditions that can lead to short stature. These may include mild bone development disorders such as hypochondroplasia. In this condition, individuals may present with short stature, mild rhizomelia, fifth metacarpal bone shortening (brachymetacarpia V), and mild shortening of the upper and lower limbs. It is important to identify patients with findings suggestive of bone development disorders or mild skeletal dysplasias. This is best achieved by taking careful anthropometric measurements of every child with short stature to demonstrate or rule out disproportionate shortening of limb segments. Fifth metacarpal bone shortening, rhizomelia, and disproportionate shortening of the arms and legs have been found to be prevalent in families with familial short stature.[6] These findings suggest that abnormalities in endochondral bone devel-

---

BOX 27-1
Causes of Short Stature

NONPATHOLOGIC
Familial/genetic
Constitutional delay of growth and development

PATHOLOGIC
Skeletal dysplasias
Chromosomal abnormalities
   Down syndrome (trisomy 21)
   Turner syndrome
   Prader-Willi syndrome
Genetic syndromes
Intrauterine growth retardation
Nutritional growth failure
Gastrointestinal disorders
   Celiac disease
   Chronic inflammatory bowel disease
Chronic disease
   Chronic renal failure
   Juvenile rheumatoid arthritis
   Malignancy
   AIDS (human immunodeficiency virus infection)
   Thalassemia
   Chronic bronchial asthma
   Sickle cell disease
   Congenital heart disease
   Diabetes mellitus
   Cystinosis
   Chronic liver disease
Endocrine disorders
   Growth hormone-related disorders
   Hypothyroidism
   Glucocorticoid excess
   Hypogonadism
   Precocious puberty

IDIOPATHIC

---

opment may result in not only short stature but also disproportionate shortening of limbs.

In familial short stature the growth rate is normal, the growth curve runs parallel to the normal standards, and the bone age is not more than 2 SD below the mean. Often, however, there is a concomitant constitutional delay of growth and development. In such cases the bone age may be 2 SD below the mean, but these patients have a normal growth rate, with the growth curve remaining parallel to normal standards, and the calculated predicted adult height falling within a 5-cm range of the target height. There may be an apparent deviation from the standard growth curve after the age of 12 years, but this is indicative only of the delay in occurrence of the pubertal growth spurt.

Constitutional Delay of Growth and Development

By definition, patients with familial short stature and/or constitutional delay of growth are characterized by a normal nutritional status, no history or evidence of systemic illness, normal thyroid and growth hormone (GH) levels, and a normal physical examination (including body proportions). The bone age is typically retarded, although rarely below 60% of chronologic age.[7] The insulin-like growth factor 1 (IGF-1) level may be low or normal but usually normal for the bone age. Typically, these children are normal in size at birth but fall at or below the 3rd percentile in height by 2 to 3 years of age. Growth generally progresses at the same percentile until approximately 12 years of age, with annual growth velocity at the lower end of the normal range for age. While peers of the adolescent with constitutional delay of growth and development are beginning to have a growth spurt, the affected individual continues to grow at a much slower rate, resulting in an apparent deviation from the normal growth curve. Later, however, with the onset of puberty, the adolescent experiences a growth acceleration and returns to the normal growth curve, thereby attaining normal height. Some studies have shown that although boys with constitutional delay of growth and development reach their predicted height, they may be short compared with family members and are in the lower range of normal.[8,9]

Regression analyses have shown that final height attainment is influenced negatively by standing height and growth velocity and positively by the degree of segmental body disproportion. Patients who are taller grow at a faster rate. Those who have a major degree of segmental body disproportion, with a short spine and long leg length, attain a final height closer to midparental height irrespective of the delay of epiphyseal maturation.[10]

Constitutional delay of growth and development is probably more common than is generally realized, but most cases of this condition are brought to medical attention in patients with concomitant familial short stature because their short stature is obvious. In contrast, the growth of affected individuals with tall parents may continue to follow a normal curve yet be below that expected for the family, but this discrepancy may not be noticed.

The endocrine findings in children with constitutional delay of growth and development include a decrease in gonadotropin levels, as well as a relative deficiency of GH and IGF-1 for chronologic age. These levels correlate with the delayed bone age and sexual maturation rather than with chronologic age. It is difficult to distinguish constitutional delay of growth and puberty from hypogonadotropic hypogonadism even when the response to luteinizing hormone–releasing hormone (LH-RH) is analyzed. Studies have suggested the use of LH-RH priming before the LH-RH stimulation test. Children with constitutional delay of growth and puberty usually have a greater increment in LH levels than in follicle-stimulating hormone (FSH).[11] The gonadotropin-releasing hormone triptorelin has also been used to differentiate gonadotropin deficiency from constitutionally delayed puberty. In the latter, there are significant increases in gonadotropin and testosterone levels after injection of triptorelin.[12] Growth hormone release after provocative stimuli is usually normal in individuals with constitutional delay, although in some children there is a transient GH deficiency that normalizes during puberty.[13] Some authors would call this a physiologic state of partial GH deficiency. Testosterone, and probably estrogen also, stimulates increased production and secretion of GH. This in turn stimulates IGF-1 production in normal early puberty.

PATHOLOGIC SHORT STATURE

Pathologic short stature is less common than the nonpathologic type, but it deserves more attention and a more detailed investigation because with this condition timely institution of treatment is vital to the attainment of normal height. Pathologic short stature should be suspected in any child or adolescent with abnormal growth velocity (i.e., below the 3rd percentile for bone age) and in those with marked short stature. These patients usually fail to develop sexually. The prognosis for ultimate height is dependent on the specific diagnosis. Pathologic short stature can be the result of primary growth failure due to a genetic abnormality or prenatal damage. Examples are skeletal dysplasia, chromosomal defects, genetic syndromes, intrauterine growth retardation (IUGR), and inborn errors of metabolism with associated skeletal abnormalities. On the other hand, pathologic short stature can be the result of almost any chronic disease. Examples are the abnormal growth associated with nutritional, renal, metabolic, gastrointestinal, endocrine, and other problems. This discussion focuses on the growth problems related to these conditions.

Skeletal Dysplasias

Skeletal dysplasias are inborn errors of bone growth and/or differentiation that may affect either the cartilage or the bone-forming stage of bone development. Over 100 entities make up the skeletal dysplasias.[14,15]

Each condition usually has one or two typical features that would lead one to suspect the diagnosis.[16] Measurement of various limb and body segments, particularly the arm span, sitting height, and upper-to-lower segment ratio, is particularly helpful in distinguishing conditions that affect primarily the spine or long bones. For example, achondroplasia, hypochondroplasia, and pseudoachondroplasia are characterized by short limbs and an increased upper-to-lower segment ratio, whereas spondyloepiphyseal dysplasia is characterized by a short trunk and decreased upper-to-lower segment ratio. The diagnosis ultimately depends on the radiologic findings.[17] One condition that warrants mentioning is hypochondroplasia, which is characterized by a very mild degree of limb shortening and a disproportion of body segments that is less obvious than in achondroplasia. The short stature can be very mild and can very well fall within the lower limits of normal. This is a dominantly inherited trait, and affected individuals can be easily considered in the blanket diagnosis of familial short stature. The typical radiographic finding is a progressive narrowing of the interpedicular distance from L1 to L5.[18]

Many skeletal dysplasias have identifiable metabolic abnormalities that affect various other organ systems.[19] The degree and type of involvement varies among the different conditions. Box 27-2 lists the skeletal dysplasias that have a primary abnormality in carbohydrate, protein, or lipid metabolism, including the mucopolysaccharidoses, the mucolipidoses, and the various lipid storage disorders.

Chromosomal Abnormalities

Down syndrome (trisomy 21 syndrome) is the most common chromosomal disorder that results in short stature. The principal features are usually noted after birth, and the diagnosis is most frequently made in the neonatal period.[20] Stature and growth are reduced from birth to adolescence, but growth deceleration is most marked at first in infancy and again at adolescence. Standard percentile charts for assessment of stature and weight have been devised for children with Down syndrome.[21] In general, children with this syndrome have a tendency to be overweight, beginning in late infancy and continuing through the remainder of the growing years. Their final heights are usually attained by age 15 years. Children with moderate or severe congenital heart disease are about 1.5 to 2 cm shorter and about 1 kg lighter than those without heart disease or with only mild disease.

Turner's syndrome is a second important chromosomal disorder that results in short stature in girls. In some patients short stature may be the only presenting complaint. Turner's syndrome is almost always associated with ovarian dysgenesis; therefore, delayed puberty or amenorrhea is also a common presenting complaint. A component of intrauterine growth retardation may be present, since the mean birth lengths of those with Turner's syndrome are below the normal mean.[22] A deceleration in growth does not occur until about 3 years

---

BOX 27-2
Skeletal Dysplasias with Primary Abnormality in Carbohydrate, Protein, or Lipid Metabolism

MUCOPOLYSACCHARIDE STORAGE DISORDERS
MPS I H (Hurler's syndrome)
MPS I S (Scheie's syndrome)
MPS I H/S (Hurler-Scheie syndrome)
MPS II (Hunter's syndrome)
MPS III (Sanfilippo's syndrome)
MPS IV (Morquio's A and B syndromes)
MPS V (now Scheie's syndrome)
MPS VI (Maroteaux-Lamy syndrome)
MPS VII (Sly's syndrome)

GLYCOPROTEIN STORAGE DISORDERS
Mannosidosis
Fucosidosis
Aspartylglycosaminuria
Sialidosis type II
Combined neuraminidase-β-galactosidase deficiency

GANGLIOSIDE STORAGE DISORDERS
GM$_1$ gangliosidosis

MUCOLIPID STORAGE DISORDERS
Mucolipidosis II (I-cell disease)
Mucolipidosis III (pseudopolydystrophy)

SPHINGOLIPID STORAGE DISORDERS
Gaucher's disease
    Type 1 (chronic, nonneuronopathic type)
    Type 2 (infantile, acute neuronopathic type)
    Type 3 (juvenile, subacute neuronopathic type)
Niemann-Pick disease
    Type A (acute, neuronopathic form)
    Type B (chronic, nonneuronopathic form)
    Type C (chronic, neuronopathic form)
    Type D (Nova Scotia variant)
    Type E (adult neuronopathic form)
Farber's disease (lipogranulomatosis)

HOMOCYSTINURIA

---

of age, and a fall-off in the growth curve becomes most evident after the age of 10 years, a time when the average normal girl is starting to show a pubertal spurt. Patients with Turner's syndrome do not experience a pubertal growth spurt but may continue to grow at a slow rate for several more years. Growth charts for girls with Turner's syndrome have been devised and are illustrated in Chapter 73.[23] The mean adult stature, which ranges from 142.5 to 147 cm,[24,25] can be related to parental height and to the karyotype findings; patients with a mosaic pattern are taller than those with the 45,XO karyotype. Patients with Turner's syndrome have a primary abnormality of the bones, as demonstrated by disproportionately short limbs, cubitus valgus, and metacarpal bone shortening. Scoliosis, genu valgum, and micrognathia also occur commonly in patients with Turner's syndrome.

The growth retardation noted in Turner's syndrome may stem from two possible causes. Although there have been isolated cases of simultaneous GH deficiency and Turner's syndrome, studies have not revealed a strong relationship between the two conditions, except at the age of puberty.[26] However, studies have demonstrated a subnormal GH response before the age of puberty, a growth spurt, and increased GH secretion in patients with Turner's syndrome who are treated with low-dose estrogen before their bone age reaches 10 years.[27] The second possible cause of the short stature is the primary skeletal defect, which is consequent to the chromosomal abnormality.[26] In general, it is recommended that a karyotype be performed in every girl with significant short stature in order to rule out Turner's syndrome.

Prader-Willi syndrome has been the subject of an increased amount of research activity in the last two decades. Although most children with this condition do not present with short stature during childhood, they are typically characterized by a fall-off in growth during adolescence.[28] The adult height, which is approximately an average of 59 inches for girls and 61 inches for boys, is also influenced by the genetic background.[29] The GH dynamics are similar to those of obese controls who do not have Prader-Willi syndrome, including a blunted response to pharmacologic stimuli. Responses to GH treatment have been inconsistent.

The major diagnostic criteria of Prader-Willi syndrome are neonatal and infantile hypotonia, feeding problems during infancy, obesity, hypogonadism, developmental delay, and hyperphagia, in addition to the characteristic facial features of narrow face or bifrontal diameter, almond-shaped eyes, small mouth with thin upper lip, and down-turned corners of the mouth.[28] Approximately 70% of cases have a characteristic deletion of the proximal part of the long arm of chromosome 15[del15(q11 q13)].[30] Those with nondeletion may show maternal disomy for chromosome 15.[31]

Genetic Syndromes

Some of the congenital syndromes associated with primary growth failure but no evidence of skeletal dysplasia are listed in Box 27-3.[32] Among these, Silver-Russell syndrome is probably the most common. Patients with this syndrome generally have small stature, usually of prenatal onset, and asymmetry of the limbs. Clinodactyly (hypoplasia of the fifth finger) is a common feature, and triangular facies (with down-turning of the corners of the mouth) is also seen. Growth-hormone deficiency has been documented in a series of patients with Silver-Russell syndrome who developed growth failure.[33]

BOX 27-3
Congenital Syndromes With Primary Growth Failure and Without Skeletal Dysplasia

Cornelia de Lange's	Seckel's
Rubinstein-Taybi	Hallermann-Streiff
Silver-Russell	Smith-Lemli-Opitz
Mulibrey nanism	Williams'
Dubovitz's	Noonan's
Bloom's	Aarskog's
De Sanctis-Cacchione	Robinow's
Johanson-Blizzard	Opitz's

Cornelia de Lange's syndrome should be suspected in a child who is born small for gestational age with synophrys, down-turned upper lip, and micromelia (small hands and feet). Noonan's syndrome, also called Turner-like syndrome because of the similarity of most features, differs from Turner's syndrome in that there is no chromosome abnormality.[22] Aarskog's syndrome may be suspected in a patient who has mild to moderate short stature with brachydactyly, rounded facies, hypertelorism, cryptorchidism, and cleft scrotum.

In general, the presence of associated dysmorphic features usually leads the clinician to suspect a genetic syndrome as the cause of short stature.

Intrauterine Growth Retardation

Intrauterine growth retardation, which is defined as a birthweight of less than the 10th percentile at a given gestational age, is an important cause of short stature.[34] This condition can result from environmental or genetic influences that limit the intrinsic potential of the fetus to grow or that restrict growth because of a decrease in the amount of available nutrients.[35,36] Studies have shown that infants born small for gestational age, regardless of cause, are at increased risk for short stature in late adolescence.[37] Mean adult height for boys (162 to 170 cm) and for girls (148 to 159 cm) is significantly less than for those born with height appropriate for gestational age.[37,38]

In the typical pattern of growth of children with IUGR,[34] most experience a period of accelerated growth after birth but do not completely catch up in growth, remaining shorter than their peers who were born appropriate in size for gestational age during the first decade of life. They then experience a second growth spurt during adolescence by which they achieve their final adult height.

The final growth pattern of these children into adolescence depends on the severity of the fetal growth retardation, which is generally characterized in infancy by reduction not only of weight but also of length and head circumference. Thus, infants whose weight is reduced at birth but whose length is appropriate for gestational age actually catch up their weight within 3 to 6 months after birth if they are properly fed and cared for and have no medical problem or disease.[35] On the other hand, infants with stunted skeletal growth at birth may follow a variety of courses. Some continue to grow slowly after birth, and their attained growth in height takes a downward course; others have acceptable rates of growth in body length but remain short; in rare instances, others have accelerated increase in body length and catch up in height to normal by the end of the second postnatal year. To evaluate short stature suspected of being due to original IUGR, old measurements of birth length, weight, and head circumference should be obtained. If possible, the cause or factors that contributed to the fetal growth retardation, whether genetic or environmental, should be identified.

Some of the growth-retarding influences that the fetus can be subjected to in utero are listed in Box 27-4. Aside from these extrinsic influences, there may be intrinsic factors that can predispose individuals to IUGR, including race and maternal weight, height, age, and parity.

Nutritional Growth Failure

It is well known that undernutrition is the single most important cause of growth retardation worldwide.[39] Short stature results as an adaptive response to chronic low caloric intake. This growth problem is clearly recognized when it involves poverty-related malnutrition. However, poor growth and delayed sexual development due to poor caloric intake have also been demonstrated among suburban upper-middle-class adolescents in the United States.[40] These adolescents generally demonstrate an inadequate nutrient intake that is related to psychological causes rather than to decreased food availability. Such patients may present difficulties in diagnosis and treatment. They are usually seen because of short stature or delayed puberty. They look healthy and their physical examination is normal, except for delayed pubertal development in some cases. In nutritional growth failure, the patient's weight may be adequate for actual height, masking the nature of the problem. However, when the weight progression in the growth chart is analyzed, the problem becomes apparent. Figure 27-1 shows a 15-year-old boy who had a decreasing growth rate with a fall-off in height percentiles. Review of this patient's weight patterns revealed that his weight stopped increasing after 12 years of age. This cessation appeared concomitantly with his growth deceleration. A careful history will frequently reveal the reasons for the low caloric intake. They may be related to the patient's or parents' beliefs about healthful food, a fear of obesity, or hypercholesterol-

---

> **BOX 27-4**
> **Extrinsic Factors Affecting in Utero Growth**
>
> ENVIRONMENTAL FACTORS
> High altitude
> Toxic agents
>
> MEDICAL/OBSTETRIC COMPLICATIONS OF PREGNANCY
> Toxemia
> Hypertension
> Hemorrhage
> Impaired glucose tolerance
> Malformations of placenta, cord, or uterus
> Anemia
> Severe chronic maternal disease
> Leukemia
> Large ovarian cysts or uterine fibroids
> Long-term maternal medications (e.g., corticosteroids, immunosuppressives, teratogenic or fetal growth–retarding drugs)
> Polyhydramnios or oligohydramnios
> Premature rupture of membranes followed by artificial induction of labor
>
> ADVERSE MATERNAL FACTORS
> Cigarette smoking
> Low weight gain in second and third trimesters
> Low weight for height at conception
> Delivery at ≤16 years of age
> Delivery at ≥35 years of age
> No professional prenatal care
> Use of addictive drugs or consumption of large amounts of alcohol during pregnancy
>
> FETAL FACTORS
> Multiple births
> Fetal infection
> Inborn error of metabolism
> Isoimmunization of fetus

Modified from Miller HC: Prenatal factors affecting intrauterine growth retardation, *Clin Perinatol* 12:307, 1985.

emia, and not necessarily to an overt eating disorder.[41,42]

Excessive exercise is known to suppress the hypothalamic-pituitary-gonadal axis but is more likely to occur when associated with caloric restriction. When puberty is temporarily interrupted by intense physical exercise, stress, and poor nutrition, skeletal maturation often stalls as growth slows and sex steroids fall to low levels.[43] When conditions improve and puberty resumes, later catching up should be possible and final height may not be compromised. However, a study by Thientz et al showed that gymnasts advance through puberty without a normal pubertal growth spurt, particularly of the lower extremities. Thus, they progress through puberty with no accompanying growth spurt, resulting in a compromised

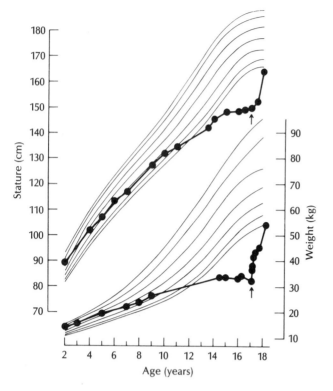

Fig. 27-1. Weight and height curves of a child with growth failure due to prolonged self-imposed caloric restriction associated with fear of becoming obese. After nutritional rehabilitation, catch-up weight gain and growth occur. (From Pugliese MT, Lifshitz F, Grad G, Mark-Katz M: Fear of obesity: a cause of short stature and delayed puberty, *N Engl J Med* 309:513, 1983. Reprinted with permission from the *New England Journal of Medicine.*)

final height.[44] This poor linear growth is probably an adaptive response to an increased energy expenditure in the background of poor intake. An evaluation of the adolescent's diet will demonstrate a low caloric intake for his or her needs. Biochemical nutritional markers and minerals are usually normal except for erythrocyte Na^+-K^+ ATPase activity.[45] The stimulated GH secretion is normal, or even increased, in response to GH-releasing hormone (GH-RH); however, patients with nutritional dwarfism manifest attenuation of spontaneous GH secretion during puberty.[46,47] This may represent a mechanism compensating for energy restriction. When appropriate diets are given to these patients, there is a rapid weight gain followed by increased growth velocity that continues until the patient achieves the previous "channel of growth."

Nutritional growth failure may result not only from a hypocaloric intake but also from a deficiency of micronutrients such as zinc. Zinc deficiency usually occurs in association with caloric or other nutrient deficiencies, but it may also be noted in children whose diets are a poor source of zinc, such as those with specific food idiosyncrasies or strictly vegetarian diets. It may also occur in children with poorly controlled diabetes as well as those

with chronic inflammatory bowel disease (CIBD).[48,49] Mild to moderate zinc deficiency may manifest only as short stature or growth deceleration and can be determined by zinc kinetic studies.[50] Zinc supplementation has been shown to effectively induce growth in short children with zinc deficiency. It is stressed, however, that routine zinc supplementation over the recommended daily allowance should not be undertaken unless zinc deficiency is documented, since excessive zinc intake can induce copper and other mineral deficiencies.[51]

Gastrointestinal Disorders

Any chronic disease of the gastrointestinal tract associated with inadequate absorption of nutrients may lead to impaired growth, delayed puberty, and delayed skeletal age. In some cases the reason for the growth retardation is suspected because of the symptoms of chronic vomiting or diarrhea, as seen in patients with disorders such as infection, dietary intolerances, and cystic fibrosis. In other diseases, poor growth may be the only early manifestation of an occult gastrointestinal problem. However, because the growth failure may evolve gradually, parents may not notice the deceleration until the child appears in the doctor's office for a routine preschool physical and the physician suddenly recognizes it. When untreated, these children may acquire significant short stature in adulthood.

Among the gastrointestinal disorders, diseases that affect the small bowel more commonly affect linear growth, because this organ is the major site of nutrient absorption.[52] Crohn's disease, or regional enteritis, usually manifests in adolescence or early adulthood. Short stature occurs in about 30% of children with CIBD, and it can precede gastrointestinal complaints by up to 3 years.[53] A high sedimentation rate may be a clue to the diagnosis of CIBD in these patients. Many factors may contribute to growth failure in CIBD, the most important of which is believed to be malnutrition. Patients refuse to eat because of anorexia, nausea, vomiting, and abdominal pain. Additionally, there are increased nutrient losses with diarrhea, inflammation, and malabsorption. Fistula formation and surgical resection or bypass procedures, particularly in the terminal ileum, interfere with bile salt and vitamin B_{12} absorption. Finally, with the ongoing inflammatory process, concomitant infection, fever, and rapid growth in puberty, there is an increased nutrient requirement resulting in a negative protein, energy, and mineral balance.[52,54]

There are also non-nutritional causes for the poor growth in adolescents with Crohn's disease. Initial studies suggested that secondary hypopituitarism may be the basis of the retarded growth,[55] but subsequent assessments have not confirmed these findings.[56-58] In some patients, growth retardation can be an undesirable side effect of the steroid therapy often used for this condition. On the other hand, growth may improve with steroid therapy, presumably because disease activity is suppressed.[59] Nutritional rehabilitation is also essential to reverse growth failure and improve the course of the CIBD itself.

Failure to thrive and gastrointestinal symptoms are also present in patients with active celiac disease or gluten-sensitive enteropathy. However, poor growth as the only manifestation of celiac disease also has been reported in patients who are considered to have occult celiac disease.[60] Children diagnosed before 2 years of age have been found to have poor weight gain as the most affected growth parameter, whereas in older children height is more affected.[61] Celiac disease is more common than idiopathic GH deficiency as a cause of short stature.[62] The cause of growth failure in this condition remains unclear but appears to be greatly related to poor nutrition resulting from malabsorption and loss of nutrients, since placing patients on a gluten-free diet can result in improvement in growth velocity.

Although there may be no clinical clues to celiac disease in a child who presents simply with growth failure, a few screening tests can be performed before subjecting the child to a definitive intestinal biopsy. Microcytic anemia is almost always demonstrated.[62] Serum IgA and IgG antigliadin antibodies and serum IgA-endomysial antibodies are sensitive and highly specific tests that are easy to perform.[63,64] Celiac disease should also be suspected in a child who has elevated serum aminotransferase activity.[65] However, in some cases of celiac disease the only diagnostic abnormality associated with short stature is abnormal intestinal mucosa, detected through jejunal biopsy. Confirmation of the diagnosis of celiac disease should be based on documentation of catch-up growth after institution of a gluten-free diet.

Chronic Disease

In addition to the above-mentioned causes of short stature, any chronic illness can result in growth deceleration. This can be due to the disease process itself, the resultant malnutrition, or a complication of treatment. Among the various chronic diseases that may affect an adolescent's growth, chronic renal failure, juvenile rheumatoid arthritis, malignancy, AIDS, thalassemia, asthma, sickle cell disease, congenital heart disease, and insulin-dependent diabetes mellitus will be briefly discussed.

CHRONIC RENAL DISEASE. Growth retardation is a common and serious consequence of chronic renal failure in childhood, particularly when the chronic renal failure has its onset in infancy.[66] The pattern of growth is influenced by the age of the child, the age of onset of chronic renal failure, and the type of treatment given. Growth failure is the result of many factors: poor nutrition associated with unmet caloric demands, chronic acidosis, osteodystrophy due to secondary hyperparathyroidism, hyperphosphatemia, vitamin D deficiency, drug treatment (e.g., steroids), pubertal delay, and functional abnormalities in the GH axis. GH secretion is apparently increased but IGF-1 levels are low, indicating GH resistance.[67,68] Evaluation of the hypothalamic-pituitary-gonadal function of prepubertal boys and girls reveals abnormal hypothalamic-pituitary function. However, testicular and ovarian steroidogenic capacity is not impaired and the biologic response to androgens in boys is preserved.[69] Some patients with end-stage renal disease have also demonstrated evidence of central hypothyroidism.[70]

Treatment of patients with chronic renal failure must include attempts to correct the metabolic and psychosocial abnormalities derived from the disease and to prevent subsequent abnormal growth. The use of alkylating agents, as an alternative to steroid use, has resulted in an increased growth rate in some children with nephrosis who have shown signs of decreased growth velocity with the use of steroids. Finally, there is enough evidence that GH treatment increases the growth rate of prepubertal growth-retarded children with chronic renal failure, making this one of the major recognized indications for GH treatment.[71] Growth hormone treatment is discontinued after renal transplantation, although an increased growth rate during the first 2 years after transplantation occurs mainly in children under 6 years of age.[72]

JUVENILE RHEUMATOID ARTHRITIS. Growth failure is a cause of considerable distress in juvenile rheumatoid arthritis. Multiple factors are involved in the pathogenesis of this growth failure, including steroid treatment, disease activity, and malnutrition, as well as musculoskeletal factors such as flexion contractures, vertebral collapse, and premature epiphyseal fusion. Although the GH status of these patients has not been consistent, IGF-1 levels appear to correlate strongly with growth velocity.[73] Short-term studies show that 25-hydroxyvitamin D treatment improves the bone mineral density of children with active rheumatoid arthritis.[74] However, the effectiveness of treatment does not correlate with growth velocity. Intraarticular corticosteroids appear to be effective treatment of chronic arthritis in children, with no apparent adverse effect on statural growth.[75]

MALIGNANCY. Growth failure is a common finding in children and adolescents with malignancy. This appears to be more of a complication of treatment than of the disease process itself. Cranial irradiation can result in injury to the hypothalamus and pituitary, causing GH deficiency.[76] Spinal irradiation in the treatment of medulloblastoma can injure the vertebral spine, impairing its growth[77]; total body radiation can also destroy the thyroid gland, resulting in hypothyroidism and growth failure if unrecognized and untreated. The gonads can be injured, resulting in hypogonadism and failure to attain a pubertal growth spurt. On the other hand, cranial irradiation can cause central precocious puberty and early epiphyseal fusion. Chemotherapy by itself, without concomitant radiation treatment, does not seem to affect linear growth.[78] Studies in children and adults who had undergone treatment for acute lymphoblastic leukemia have shown that those who did not receive cranial radiation had no significant long-term growth failure.[79] However, those who receive high-dose glucocorticoid treatment for a protracted period, such as those with graft-versus-host disease, may experience steroid-induced growth failure.

AIDS. HIV infection in adolescents is usually acquired after birth, whereas about 90% of children under the age of 13 years with HIV infection in the United States have acquired it before birth.[80] Growth retardation is a major clinical manifestation of HIV infection and is thought to be one of the early signs of AIDS in children with hemophilia who are HIV seropositive.[81] It is almost always associated with a severe delay in bone age and onset of puberty. The cause of the growth failure is multifactorial, with malnutrition the most important factor. Malnutrition is due to inadequate oral intake, gastrointestinal malabsorption, and abnormal energy utilization.[80] Occasionally, a neuroendocrine abnormality is demonstrable, including GH deficiency[82] and secondary hypothyroidism.[83] The characteristic pattern of growth in malnutrition is a decline in weight followed by a decline in height. When abnormalities in height velocity precede weight changes, an altered endocrine function should be suspected and treated accordingly. Intensive nutritional intervention should be undertaken not only with respect to total caloric intake but also with regard to replacement of macro- and micronutrient deficiencies that may affect growth, including iron and zinc.[80] Improvement in growth and weight gain has also proved to be a sensitive predictor of response to antiviral agents.[84]

THALASSEMIA. Short stature and delayed puberty are major clinical manifestations of thalassemia major.[85] Chronic anemia; zinc deficiency; failure of IGF-1 activity; neurosecretory defects of GH; and disturbances of thyroid, hepatic, and cardiac functions all play a role in the development of this problem.[86-89] Starting chelation therapy at an early age has also been implicated in causing growth retardation, since desferrioxamine has been shown to chelate other trace elements aside from iron and to cause toxic effects on iron-dependent enzymes. Thus, patients with thalassemia should be evaluated for endocrine deficiencies as well as nutrient deficiencies, including zinc, at regular intervals and treated promptly.

ASTHMA. Growth retardation and pubertal delay are frequently seen in children with chronic asthma and atopic disease.[90] This problem is exaggerated by the use of pharmacologic doses of glucocorticoids. Inhaled glucocorticoids appear to have less adverse effects on growth than oral or systemic preparations, but they can nevertheless suppress growth velocity, particularly during late prepubertal growth.[91,92] The pathophysiology of this growth failure remains unclear. Doses of beclomethasone up to 0.8 mg/day do not reduce bone mineralization or increase bone resorption.[93] Studies of GH dynamics in children receiving various steroid preparations do not demonstrate major perturbations in GH secretion or IGF-1 levels despite significant retardation of growth velocity.[94] In general, the smallest dose of inhaled corticosteroids to control symptoms should be used. However, since the priority is to treat the asthma, some children with severe disease need a high dose. Growth should therefore be monitored, particularly in those taking systemic preparations or inhaled steroids in dosages over 0.8 mg/day.[95]

SICKLE CELL DISEASE. Long-term follow-up of many children with sickle cell disease, sickle cell trait, and normal children from the newborn period to age 16 years demonstrated a 1.4-year delay in the adolescent growth spurt, a 1.6-year delay in mean age at peak height velocity, and a lower height velocity at the time of onset of the growth spurt in SS patients.[96] Delayed onset of puberty in SS patients has been correlated with delay in peak height velocity. Age at menarche was significantly later than in the AA girls (15.4 versus 13.1 years), but this did not affect final height. The mechanism for this pattern of development is unclear but is similar to that seen in children with constitutional delay of growth and adolescence.

CONGENITAL HEART DISEASE. Growth impairment is frequently seen in patients with congenital heart disease. Cross-sectional studies have suggested that overall, more than 50% of patients with untreated major cardiac malformations will fall below the 16th percentile for height and weight, and about 25% to 30% will fall below the 3rd percentile.[97] Factors contributing to the short stature of these children include low birthweight, extracardiac somatic malformations (musculoskeletal, central nervous, renal, and gastrointestinal), associated genetic syndromes and chromosomal abnormalities, inadequate nutrition, abnormal energy expenditure, and tissue hypoxemia.[98] Early corrective surgery results in a greater improvement in growth than does that performed at an older age.

DIABETES MELLITUS. Before the discovery of insulin in 1922, the insulin-deficient child had a very short life span. A few children lived longer on calorie-restricted diets but became emaciated and stunted in growth. During the early years of insulin treatment, growth stunting and growth delay continued to be a frequent finding. However, with improvement of management techniques, including proper nutrition and education of families, growth failure became an unusual event in diabetic children.[99] One study suggested that accelerated growth, dental age, and pubertal maturation are a common occurrence at the time of diagnosis of insulin-dependent diabetes mellitus.[100] Another study showed that diabetic children 5 to 9 years of age are consistently taller than the national average. However, those diagnosed after 14 years of age tend to be shorter than average.[101] These findings, however, have not been duplicated by other investigators.[102]

What seems very clear is that poor metabolic control results in growth failure.[99] Several mechanisms have been proposed, including the development of zinc deficiency from urinary losses or calcium deficiency from increased calcium excretion in the urine, decreased duodenal calcium absorption, and decreased circulating levels of 1,25-dihydroxyvitamin D. Additionally, diabetic children and adolescents are predisposed to developing frank hypothyroidism (due to autoimmune thyroiditis), which could result in growth failure.[99]

Growth hormone levels are elevated but IGF-1 levels are low in patients with poorly controlled diabetes mellitus, suggesting some degree of GH resistance such as that seen in undernutrition and chronic renal failure. IGF-1 levels have been shown to correlate negatively with hemoglobin A_1C levels.[103] Finally, growth failure observed in diabetes may be due to other coexisting diseases. The prevalence of celiac disease is reported to be 2% to 3% higher among diabetics than in the general population. Treatment with a gluten-free diet results in improvement of linear growth.[102]

MISCELLANEOUS DISORDERS. Almost every chronic illness places a child at risk of developing growth failure. Chronic malnutrition is almost always the major pathogenic factor due to poor oral intake; malabsorption; inability to meet energy demands, such as in congenital heart disease[98]; or altered metabolic state, such as in chronic liver disease and poorly controlled insulin-dependent diabetes mellitus.[102] Nutritional intervention is therefore an important aspect in the management of chronic disease.[104] When multiple organ systems are involved, such as in Gaucher's disease or cystinosis, growth is greatly affected and is almost always accompanied by delayed adolescence.[104,105]

Correction of the underlying disease, if possible, almost always reverses the growth failure but usually does not result in complete recovery of lost height, particularly if treatment is delayed or given at an older age. Furthermore, an underlying endocrine deficiency such as hypothyroidism or GH deficiency should always be sought and treated, as these are not uncommon complications of multisystem diseases.

Endocrine Disorders

GROWTH HORMONE DEFICIENCY. Growth failure due to GH deficiency occurs as a result of specific alterations in the chain of events from the synthesis of GH to its growth-promoting action.[106] A large 1994 study of

American children in Utah revealed a prevalence of 1:3480, most of which cases were idiopathic. Growth hormone deficiency is about three times more common in boys than in girls. In approximately half of all children with GH deficiency the condition may be unrecognized and untreated.[107] GH secretion is regulated by many factors, including somatostatin, GH-RH, insulin, IGF-1, glucose, amino acids, and steroid hormones. Growth hormone is secreted in several discrete bursts throughout the day, most occurring soon after the onset of sleep. Total GH production is greatest during late childhood and adolescence, persisting after full maturation of the skeleton and declining steadily with age.[108] Growth hormone has clear effects on linear bone growth in childhood and adolescence, directly stimulating the differentiation of chondrocyte precursors. Additionally, GH enhances the local production of and responsiveness to IGF-1, which acts to stimulate the clonal expansion of differentiating chondrocytes.[108]

IGF-1 is a growth factor synthesized in the liver and other tissues. Growth hormone, good nutrition, insulin, and (probably) prolactin are necessary for its production.[109] Circulating IGF-1 levels generally correlate well with GH secretion in postnatal life (in well-nourished children with normal GH responsiveness), and hepatic expression of IGF-1 is responsive primarily to GH. Approximately 80% of IGF in the circulation is bound to a binding protein (BP) complex consisting of IGF BP3 and an acid-labile subunit. It is the concentration of this storage form of IGF-1 that is most directly under GH control,[110] increasing with age in children and reaching maximal levels during puberty.[111]

Growth-hormone deficiency can result from decreased secretion of the hypothalamic GH–releasing hormone (GH-RH) or from somatotrope resistance to endogenous GH-RH. The deficiency can be either complete or incomplete, with or without an associated deficiency of other anterior pituitary hormones. Although most cases of GH deficiency are idiopathic, some result from various central nervous system (CNS) disturbances. The presence of a space-occupying intracerebral lesion should be ruled out, particularly tumors that could alter hypothalamic or pituitary hormone secretion. Septooptic dysplasia is one cause of GH deficiency that presents in infancy. It is associated with unilateral or bilateral optic nerve hypoplasia, deficiency of other pituitary hormones, and (in some cases) an absent septum pellucidum.[109]

Acquired GH deficiency can occur in patients who have received cranial and spinal radiation treatment for acute lymphocytic leukemia prophylaxis or as therapy for solid tumors of the brain.[76] Although the pituitary is relatively radioresistant, the hypothalamus can be damaged by as little as 2400 rad.[112] Other conditions that can result in partial or complete hypopituitarism are cerebrovascular accidents involving the hypothalamic/pituitary area in patients with sickle cell anemia or cyanotic heart disease. Not all GH deficiency is permanent, however. It is known that the GH deficiency seen in patients with constitutional delay of growth and development resolves with the onset of puberty or as a result of treatment with sex steroids.

One specific type of GH deficiency is neurosecretory GH dysfunction. Patients with neurosecretory GH dysfunction show evidence of growth deceleration but are able to produce normal levels of GH when given pharmacologic or other provocative stimulation. However, adequate spontaneous GH secretion cannot be demonstrated under physiologic conditions such as sleep.[112] The diagnosis is made after demonstration of inadequate GH secretion in patients whose GH levels are tested at 20- to 30-minute intervals during sleep or for 24 hours. It is generally accepted that a mean GH level of less than 3 ng/ml is abnormally low.[113] During puberty, the levels are expected to be even higher.[114] The measurement of spontaneous GH secretion may provide variable results, and acclimatization to a hospital setting may be necessary in children.[115]

The concept of decreased bioactivity of endogenous GH was originally postulated by Plotnick et al[116] and Rudman et al.[117] This condition was characterized by an attenuated growth pattern associated with normal GH reserves as measured by radioimmunoassay. However, IGF-1 levels are low. There is decreased binding of GH to receptors, which may be caused by a structural abnormality of GH. This possibility has been supported by subsequent findings of structurally abnormal GH polymers with low biologic activity.[118] Children with this GH abnormality manifest an excellent response to GH treatment. Finally, a person can have a receptor or postreceptor defect that results in resistance to both exogenous and endogenous GH treatment. This is best exemplified by Laron dwarfism, a form of hereditary growth failure characterized by a high GH level but low IGF-1 and IGF BP3 levels.[119,120] The defect in this condition lies in the extracellular domain of the GH receptor, as confirmed by the absence of the identically structured GH binding protein in the serum of patients with Laron's syndrome.[121,122] These children respond to IGF-1 treatment.

Rosenbloom et al later described a similar form of GH resistance syndrome in Ecuador with distinctive features of normal to superior intelligence. Molecular studies in these patients revealed a guanine-for-adenine substitution in the third position of codone 180 of exon 6, whereas in Laron's syndrome the genetic defect is a serine substitution to phenylalanine at position 96.[123,124]

Other causes of familial short stature are characterized by either very low or very high levels of GH-binding protein or very high levels of IGF-1.[125-127] These causes of genetic short stature are not yet well elucidated. Resistance to GH can also be secondary to a number of diseases. Somatomedin inhibitors may be responsible for growth failure in uremia and other chronic diseases. Corticosteroids can inhibit the generation of GH and IGF action. This accounts in part for the growth failure in Cushing's syndrome.

The diagnosis of GH deficiency is made when there is a subnormal GH response (usually less than 10 ng/ml) to more than one type of stimulation test. The more common pharmacologic stimuli used are insulin, arginine, levodopa, estrogen, glucagon, beta blockers, and clonidine. Exercise is another common stimulus used to test for GH deficiency. Since each of these tests varies in its sensitivity, more than one test is usually required to confirm a diagnosis.

HYPOTHYROIDISM. Thyroid hormones are essential for normal growth and development. When the diagnosis of hypothyroidism is missed and the condition remains untreated in early life, it is associated with severe mental retardation, neurologic sequelae, and dwarfism. Failure to diagnose and treat hypothyroidism in later childhood can result in permanent stunting of growth and/or learning deficits.[128] Children with acquired thyroid failure commonly have a concomitant acceleration of weight gain. A goiter is usually felt but is not a necessary finding. Bone maturation is delayed, and epiphyseal dysgenesis is demonstrated radiologically. Although the onset of puberty is usually delayed in hypothyroidism, some children develop a paradoxical precocious puberty due to elevation of serum gonadotropin concentrations.[128] The diagnosis is confirmed by demonstrating elevated thyroid-stimulating hormone (TSH) in primary hypothyroidism or a low T_4 (thyroxine) and low TSH in hypothalamic or hypopituitary hypothyroidism. Demonstration of antithyroglobulin and antimicrosomal antibodies confirms the most common cause of acquired hypothyroidism, Hashimoto's thyroiditis. Treatment with thyroid hormone replacement should aim to achieve euthyroidism slowly, since rapid correction may result in psychological and learning difficulties. Neurologic and visual complications, including headaches and visual impairment with papilledema, have been described at the start of levothyroxine therapy.[129]

EXCESS GLUCOCORTICOIDS. Glucocorticoids, whether exogenous or endogenous, are potent inhibitors of linear growth in man and animals.[130,131] The pathogenesis of growth retardation induced by chronic hyperglucocorticoidemia is multifactorial. It can result from (1) inhibited IGF-1 activity, (2) impaired type 1 collagen synthesis, or (3) suppressed GH secretory response to GH-RH.[132] The decreased GH response to GH-RH is possibly because of a hypothalamic somatotropin-release inhibitory factor.[133] Indirectly, GH secretion may be diminished because of the hyperglycemic effect of glucocorticoids. Finally, glucocorticoids are inherently catabolic, thus interfering with both somatic and skeletal growth. To counteract the effect of glucocorticoids on GH secretion, pyridostigmine has been used during provocative tests for GH secretion.[134] The use of a glucocorticoid that has a minimal effect on growth and GH secretion, such as deflazacort, has been recommended.[135] Cushing's syndrome may be caused by hyperplastic functioning tumors of the adrenal cortex, or excessive intake of glucocorticoids for therapeutic purposes. Like that in hypothyroidism, the growth deceleration in Cushing's syndrome is accompanied by excessive weight gain. In patients with no history of systemic steroid intake, a search for an adrenal source is mandatory. The most common cause of hyperadrenocorticism in children and adolescents is nodular hyperplasia, but true tumors do occur.

Usually there are associated virilizing changes and hypertension in Cushing's syndrome. The diagnosis is based on the history, physical examination, and laboratory findings. A 24-hour urinary free cortisol level of more than 125 μg and an elevated serum cortisol level that is not suppressed by dexamethasone confirm the diagnosis of hyperadrenocorticism. Radiologic studies of the adrenal glands, such as computed tomography (CT) and magnetic resonance imaging (MRI), may be used to document an adrenal abnormality. Follow-up studies of patients with Cushing's syndrome reveal inadequate catch-up growth after successful treatment, resulting in significantly compromised final adult height.[136]

HYPOGONADISM. Sex steroids and growth hormone are each important determinants of the adolescent growth spurt.[137] Analysis of GH secretion among normal boys and girls at various stages of development shows that GH secretion increases during pubertal development, coinciding with the normal increase in growth velocity. There is enough evidence to indicate that the pubertal rise in GH secretion is sex steroid dependent.[138,139] Thus, a child with hypogonadism from any cause will manifest an attenuation of growth during adolescence, with a significant deviation from the normal growth curve and failure to achieve an adolescent growth spurt. This deviation from the norm occurs earlier in girls, starting from approximately the age of 9 years, and later in boys, starting from an average age of 12 to 13 years. A similar pattern of growth is seen in children with constitutional delay of growth and development wherein the growth attenuation is transitory and the pubertal growth spurt is only delayed. Primary hypogonadism is characterized by marked elevation of gonadotropin levels in response to low levels of circulating sex steroids during the adolescent years. Pituitary and hypothalamic hypogonadism, however, are difficult to distinguish from normal variant constitutional delay of growth and development. Both LH-RH pulsing and triptorelin have been used to differentiate between these two conditions.[11,12] Pituitary or hypothalamic hypogonadism may be isolated or associated with deficiency of other pituitary hormones. It

may also be associated with a specific syndrome such as Turner's. It is important to look for any suggestion of anorexia nervosa or excessive athletic training, which can result in secondary hypogonadism or delayed adolescence.

PRECOCIOUS PUBERTY. Precocious puberty may be responsible for short stature presenting in an adolescent. The typical pattern of growth is an early acceleration of growth velocity during childhood, with onset of secondary sexual characteristics followed by an early plateau in growth velocity during the adolescent years. When the short adolescent appears more sexually mature than his or her chronologic age and the bone age is significantly advanced (i.e., >14 years for girls and >16 years for boys), untreated precocious puberty with premature epiphyseal fusion is the most likely cause of the decline in growth velocity. There is usually a family history of early puberty and short stature, although a search should be made for CNS lesions as well as functioning gonadal tumors. In addition, McCune-Albright syndrome should be ruled out; this syndrome consists of a triad of physical signs: localized polyostotic fibrous dysplasia, café au lait pigmentation of the skin, and autonomous hyperfunction of multiple endocrine systems (including the gonads).[140] Treatment with LH-RH analogs enables some girls with precocious puberty to achieve their maximal growth potential, particularly those whose predicted adult heights before the start of therapy are below their target heights.[141] On the other hand, girls with precocious puberty whose predicted heights are normal attain a normal final height, comparable with their predicted height even without treatment.[142] These findings suggest that an initial height prediction can be useful in identifying girls with central precocious puberty who are at risk for short adult stature.

EVALUATION OF SHORT STATURE

Box 27-5 outlines the important factors to consider in the evaluation of an adolescent with short stature. A careful history, designed to elicit any significant medical illnesses, must be recorded. Dietary history should be designed to elicit food allergies, idiosyncrasies, faddism, or just poor intake. In addition, a detailed family history must be taken to obtain heights of siblings and other relatives as well as to document any inherited disorders. A thorough physical examination should include accurate anthropometric measurements to detect conditions having particular physical characteristics. Abnormal body segment proportions usually suggest a skeletal dysplasia, which may be either primary or associated with a specific metabolic defect. Actual measurement of the parents' heights will be more helpful than reported heights, since it is known that adults frequently overestimate their

---

BOX 27-5
Evaluation of Short Stature

HISTORY
Birth weight/length
Parental/relatives' heights
Dietary history (allergies, idiosyncrasies, faddism)
Physical activity
Drug intake (steroids, type, dose)
Medical history
Family history
Developmental history
Growth pattern (previous height and weight data)
Headache
Visual disturbance
Psychosocial history

PHYSICAL EXAMINATION
Height/weight/arm span
Sitting height-to-standing height ratio
    (or upper-to-lower segment ratio)
Dysmorphic features
Stage of puberty
Evidence of chronic disease (jaundice, pallor, cyanosis, clubbing)
Skeletal deformity (kyphosis, scoliosis)

BONE AGE

LABORATORY SCREENING TESTS
Complete blood count
Erythrocyte sedimentation rate
Blood urea nitrogen
Creatinine
Serum glutamate pyruvate transaminase
Albumin
Calcium
Phosphorus
Thyroxine (T_4), thyroid-stimulating hormone
Antigliadin/antireticulin antibodies
Insulin-like growth factor 1 (IGF-1)
IGF binding protein 3 (IGF BP3)

GROWTH HORMONE TESTS
Provocative tests
Physiologic: Overnight growth hormone study

---

height. Measurement of parental height will help determine whether the adolescent's stature is within the normal range for the family.

The most important diagnostic tool in the evaluation of the child or adolescent with short stature is the growth chart. Charts based on the NCHS standards illustrate normal growth patterns and whether a patient is deviating from the norm. The growth chart is the most important instrument in helping to differentiate pathologic from nonpathologic growth. Therefore, every effort should be made to obtain growth records from all possible sources: the pediatrician's office, the patient's school, the mother's baby book, and so forth. It cannot be overemphasized that a single height measurement is not nearly as important as the pattern of height progression. An adolescent currently in the 25th percentile may have a more significant pathologic condition than one who falls below the 5th percentile if the former was originally in the 90th percentile. On the other hand, the adolescent who falls below the 5th percentile may be normal if he or she has always followed that particular percentile curve. This is best illustrated in patients with familial short stature or constitutional delay of growth and development. Just as with height, evaluation of progression of weight is essential, especially to detect individuals with nutritional causes of poor growth and short stature. Therefore, it is essential to monitor both height and weight gain regularly.

A radiograph of the left hand and wrist is obtained to determine the patient's bone age. This information is not only a helpful diagnostic tool but also can be used to predict future statural development. Estimating the difference in years and months between chronologic age and bone age can tell the clinician if the patient has advanced, delayed, or appropriate maturation. Advanced maturation is usually associated with shorter than normal adult stature, while delayed maturation may result in either of two possibilities: excessive height or a deficit in adult height.

There are simple laboratory screening tests that can be performed to rule out an organic cause for short stature. A complete blood count may help identify a chronic hematologic condition that can contribute to poor growth, such as thalassemia. A biochemical profile may help identify an adolescent with chronic renal failure or renal tubular acidosis, which may initially be manifested only through poor growth. As noted previously, certain chronic gastrointestinal diseases may be characterized by growth retardation without gastrointestinal symptoms; thus, an elevated sedimentation rate may suggest CIBD, or the presence of antigliadin or antireticulin antibodies may suggest celiac disease.

Thyroid function tests, particularly T_4 and TSH, will help rule out hypothyroidism. Initially, hypothyroidism may be compensated with normal levels of T_4 and detected only by an elevated TSH level.

A karyotype is essential in every girl who presents with significant short stature, to rule out the possibility of Turner's syndrome. A urine metabolic screen may help detect inborn errors of metabolism such as mucopolysaccharidosis, which may significantly affect growth and stature. When there is a significant disproportion between the upper and lower body segment, or between the arm span and standing height, a skeletal survey should be made to rule out skeletal dysplasia. Particular attention should be focused on the lumbar spine, where an abnormal progression of the interpedicular distance from L1 to L5 suggests hypochondroplasia.

When none of the above tests is suggestive of an

etiology for the growth retardation, evaluation of possible GH deficiency is indicated. Since GH secretion occurs in episodic bursts, a random GH level is not helpful unless it is caught at its peak. It is therefore necessary to perform a provocative test for GH secretion using any two stimuli among the following: glucagon, GH-RH, arginine, L-dopa, clonidine, propranolol, estrogen, and exercise.[143] Insulin-induced hypoglycemia is a potent test for GH deficiency but has resulted in devastating complications.[144] Thus, it is no longer a recommended GH provocative test, particularly in children who are highly likely to have GH deficiency or hypopituitarism. A peak GH response below 10 ng/ml after two standard tests is considered diagnostic of classic GH deficiency.[143] Before stimulation tests are performed, screening for GH deficiency can also be done by measuring IGF-1 and IGF BP3 levels. A high level of IGF-1 effectively rules out GH deficiency, whereas low IGF-1 levels may be due to GH deficiency or a state of undernutrition. IGF BP3 levels might therefore be a more helpful screening tool. It should be noted that the GH response may be blunted in obesity because of interference by somatostatin. Also, concomitant use of pyridostiginine or serotonin receptor subtype J-HT$_{1D}$ can be used to improve the GH response to GH-RH.[145-147] It was demonstrated in 1992 that acute administration of glucocorticoids can act as a potent stimulus for GH release, in contrast to the long-term effect of glucocorticoid administration, which results in suppression of GH response to GH-RH.[148] Caloric restriction in preparation for provocative testing has been suggested as a means to potentiate the GH response.[149]

If a child's response to provocative stimuli is normal ($\geq$10 ng/ml) and the growth rate remains poor with no apparent cause, neurosecretory GH dysfunction should be ruled out by measuring spontaneous GH secretion overnight or during a 24-hour period.[150] As noted earlier in this chapter, the results of these tests may be variable and affected by the patient's wakefulness in the hospital setting.[151] Acclimatization to the hospital may be necessary to make this test effective. Markedly elevated levels of GH associated with low IGF-1 are suggestive of GH-resistant states or nutritional dwarfism. The typical weight and height progression in the latter will help differentiate between the two conditions. It should be stressed that any test for GH secretion is helpful only in the child who is not growing at a normal rate.

TREATMENT OF SHORT STATURE

Obviously, the treatment of growth failure and short stature should be directed toward correcting the primary cause. When no treatment is available or when there is no apparent cause, the choice of treatment is complex and difficult. At this time, the use of GH is approved only for children who show clear evidence of GH deficiency

(growth failure, retarded bone age, and abnormal response to at least two provocative tests of GH). It has also been approved for use in short stature due to chronic renal failure.[71] There is evidence that GH is also effective in improving the final height of girls with Turner's syndrome, yet this is not a generally accepted indication for treatment.[152,153]

With the increased availability of biosynthetic GH, there has been mounting pressure to use GH to treat short children who do not have GH deficiency. Many studies have been performed to determine whether GH can increase growth in various conditions associated with short stature, such as Down syndrome,[154,155] achondroplasia,[156] hypochondroplasia,[157] constitutional delay of growth and development,[158] IUGR,[159] Prader-Willi syndrome,[160] and even idiopathic or familial short stature.[161,162] The results have been encouraging for improvement of growth rates, but most long-term studies are either lacking or have failed to show an improvement in final adult height.

In addition to GH, investigators have attempted to delay the progress of puberty in short, normal children who are in puberty with the use of gonadotropin-RH agonists to prolong the period of growth.[163] Results of their studies have shown that inhibiting sexual development in short early-pubertal subjects has no effect on final height, even if GH is added to the treatment regimen.

Aside from concerns about the lack of a long-term benefit of GH treatment in non–GH-deficient subjects, concerns about the potential adverse effects of GH treatment cannot be ignored. In addition to its effects on glucose metabolism, resulting in impaired glucose tolerance or frank diabetes,[164] GH has been implicated as a cause of musculoskeletal complications, including slipped capital femoral epiphyses[165] and scoliosis.[166] Growth hormone has also been shown to increase the peripheral conversion of T$_4$ to T$_3$ or to cause overt hypothyroidism.[167] Other adverse complications include pancreatitis,[168] intracranial hypertension,[169] and prepubertal gynecomastia.[170] Most recently, the possible development of malignancies, particularly leukemia, in patients who have received GH treatment has been a distressing concern. However, close scrutiny of the available data on this issue has resulted in the conclusion that the expected risk for the development of leukemia in patients with idiopathic GH deficiency in the United States is not significantly different from that in the general pediatric population. Children with CNS tumors who have received irradiation therapy, alone or in combination with chemotherapy, may be at increased risk for the development of leukemia regardless of whether they have been treated with GH or not.[171,172]

When the cause of short stature is due to GH insensitivity, the use of IGF-1 appears to be promising.[173,174] Adequate nutritional intake is crucial for the full effect of therapy.[175]

The use of sex steroids in the treatment of growth retardation due to delayed puberty, whether due to constitutional delay of growth and adolescence or to primary or central hypogonadism, has been promoted as a means to cause increased growth and initiation of secondary sexual characteristics and also to prevent the future development of osteoporosis, which this population has been shown to be at risk of developing.[176] However, when considering this form of treatment caution should be exercised to initiate it at an appropriate age (usually 12 years in girls and 14 years in boys) and to use a dose low enough not to result in rapid bone maturation and early epiphyseal closure.[177,180]

There is enough evidence to show that boys with constitutional delay of growth and puberty who are left untreated do not achieve their full genetic potential. It is therefore recommended that active medical treatment of this condition be strongly considered.[181] The most common form of therapeutic intervention employed is low-dose testosterone for about 6 months. Anabolic steroids appear to be a useful alternative.

TALL STATURE

In a society in which height or tallness is a positive physical characteristic, tall stature by itself is a rare complaint, particularly among adolescent males. If it is ever a presenting complaint in an endocrinologist's office, it is usually a female adolescent who has very tall parents and is having adjustment problems in school. Generally, the tall stature does not become of significant concern until the girl starts to have a pubertal growth spurt, when the discrepancy with her peers becomes more apparent. When the concern stems from the pediatrician's office, it is usually due to an observed growth acceleration or associated problems such as precocious pubertal development. In this section the various causes of tall stature and/or rapid and excessive growth outlined in Box 27-6 are discussed.

NONPATHOLOGIC CAUSES OF TALL STATURE

Constitutional or Familial Tall Stature

An individual whose height falls above the 95th percentile of the standard growth chart is considered to be of tall stature. In constitutional or familial tall stature, the height progression follows a steady channel parallel to the normal curve, suggesting the absence of pathology. Moreover, compared with the midparental height, these individuals are appropriate and their growth channels fall within the calculated range of the target height (see

---

BOX 27-6
Differential Diagnosis of Tall Stature

NONPATHOLOGIC
Familial/constitutional tall stature
Obesity

PATHOLOGIC
Genetic syndromes
    Beckwith-Wiedemann
    Sotos'
    Weaver's
    Simpson-Golabi-Behmel
    Marfan's
    Homocystinuria
Chromosome abnormalities
    Klinefelter's
    XYY
Endocrine
    Growth hormone excess
    Estrogen resistance

"Familial Short Stature" at the beginning of this chapter). The bone age may be slightly advanced, or appropriate for chronologic age. In this condition the predicted adult height will significantly determine whether treatment should be instituted or not. Treatment is aimed at decreasing the eventual adult height, and this has been successfully achieved with the use of estrogens that work to hasten epiphyseal closure. Most investigators believe that the effects are greatest when therapy is begun at a bone age below 12 to 13 years and/or a chronologic age below 11 to 12 years.[182] In deciding when estrogen treatment should be initiated, the emotional maturity of the individual is an important factor as well as the patient's psychological readiness to go through menarche.

Obesity

Obesity and excessive weight gain frequently result in rapid growth and tall stature.[183] The rapid growth is accompanied by an accelerated advance in bone age and earlier puberty than in nonobese children. This becomes a presenting complaint in girls who become very tall and grow rapidly as they approach the age of puberty, particularly if they also have genetic tall stature. It is important to rule out genetic syndromes that also cause tall stature and obesity. A more advanced bone age than the individual's chronologic age should reassure the family that final adult height will generally be less than projected. During treatment of obesity the growth rate usually decelerates, bringing the child's height more in line with the heights of the parents but less than that of nonobese peers.[184,185]

PATHOLOGIC TALL STATURE

Genetic Syndromes

BECKWITH-WIEDEMANN SYNDROME. Beckwith-Wiedemann syndrome is probably the most widely recognized of all overgrowth syndromes.[186] It is a genetic condition with generalized overgrowth as a major characteristic. Affected individuals are large at birth in both height and weight. The mean birth length of boys is greater than the 95th percentile for gestational age; thereafter the length parallels the normal curve at or above the 95th percentile throughout childhood and adolescence. In girls the mean birth length is typically at the 75th percentile and increases to the 95th percentile by 18 months; after 9 years, mean height remains between the 75th and 95th percentiles. The bone age advances rapidly during the first 4 years but subsequently slows down. Pubertal development occurs spontaneously at the average time.[187] The distinctive facial dysmorphic features during infancy, including large tongue, round face, prominent cheeks, and narrow forehead, become less prominent as the child grows older, and during adolescence very few clues remain to the original diagnosis.[186]

SOTOS' SYNDROME. Sotos' syndrome, or cerebral gigantism, is characterized by a large size at birth with length frequently greater than the 95th percentile. Growth is excessive during the first 4 years but stabilizes thereafter, resulting in an adult height within the upper limit of normal.[187-189] Although having an advanced bone age, patients enter puberty at approximately the usual time and are taller than expected for their midparental heights. Characteristic dysmorphic features include a large head, a prominent forehead with receding hairline, hypertelorism, a high arched palate, large hands and feet, and low muscle tone. Mental retardation is common. GH and IGF-1 levels are normal. The cause is unknown but there is a possibility of autosomal dominant inheritance.[188]

WEAVER'S SYNDROME. Weaver's syndrome was initially described in 1974.[187] The overgrowth is prenatal in onset. The affected child is large at birth, with subsequent accelerated growth and skeletal maturation during infancy. A minority of patients start to grow rapidly only after birth. Two adults have been reported to have this condition, both above the 97th percentile in height. Characteristic features include a large head, a round face with ocular hypertelorism, down-slanting palpebral fissures, a long philtrum, large ears, and micrognathia. Camptodactyly (flexion of interphalangeal joints) of the hands, clinodactyly (deflection of interphalangeal joints) of the toes, limited elbow and knee extension, and other foot deformities are common. The cause is unknown; X-linked recessive inheritance is possible.[187] No endocrine dysfunction has been specifically identified except in one reported patient who developed hypothyroidism at 6 years of age.[190]

SIMPSON-GOLABI-BEHMEL SYNDROME. This is an X-linked recessively inherited disorder characterized by prenatal onset of overgrowth.[191] The bone age is usually not advanced. Characteristic features include an enlarged head present at birth, a coarse face, ocular hypertelorism, a short broad nose, thick lips, and a large tongue and mouth. The body is plump and stocky and individuals have pectus excavatum, scoliosis, hepatosplenomegaly, umbilical and/or inguinal hernias, broad short hands and feet, postaxial hexadactyly (six digits), and hypoplastic index fingernails. Growth is above the 97th percentile in infancy and childhood. Adolescent and adult patients have well proportioned gigantism of athletic build (192 to 210 cm), a large coarse face, and a deep voice.[192] Mental development can be normal or mildly delayed. Linkage analysis indicates that the gene for this condition maps to the Xq 21.3 region.[187]

MARFAN'S SYNDROME. Marfan's syndrome is a connective tissue disorder inherited in an autosomal dominant pattern with incomplete penetrance.[193] It is one of the most common inherited connective tissue disorders with a prevalence of 4 to 6 per 100,000 persons. Tall stature and dolichostenomelia (extremely long limbs) is the classic phenotype of patients with this condition. Measurement of arm span and sitting height or the upper and lower segment are important aspects of the physical examination. Other skeletal manifestations include arachnodactyly (long fingers and toes), pectus excavatum, and scoliosis. Ocular system involvement includes myopia and dislocation or subluxation of the lenses, which can later result in cataracts or retinal detachment. In contrast to the downward lens dislocation seen in homocystinuria, the lens is usually displaced superiorly. Mitral valve prolapse with regurgitation is the most common cardiac finding. Aortic root dilation with insufficiency, dissection, aneurysm, and rupture are the most serious complications.

The diagnosis of Marfan's syndrome is based on clinical findings. There are no specific laboratory tests to confirm the diagnosis. However, studies have demonstrated mutations in for the fibrillin gene on chromosome 15.[194] Individuals who exhibit some of the skeletal and cardiovascular features of Marfan's syndrome yet do not have ocular abnormalities have been reported. The syndrome in these patients is inherited as an autosomal dominant disorder, but genetic analysis does not show the typical fibrillin gene seen in Marfan's syndrome. It is thought that this may represent a new connective tissue disorder, overlapping but different from classic Marfan's syndrome.[195]

The management of Marfan's syndrome is aimed at the prevention of life-threatening complications and is directed toward the cardiovascular system. Patients with

Marfan's syndrome generally have normal intelligence, although attention deficit disorder and learning disability can occur in almost 50% of affected individuals.

HOMOCYSTINURIA. Homocystinuria is a disorder of amino acid metabolism, most frequently caused by a deficiency of cystathionine β-synthase (CBS), which can result in involvement of the skeletal, neurologic, and vascular systems and the ocular tissues. Thinning and disproportionate lengthening of bones, tall stature, downward optic lens dislocation, and thromboembolic phenomena are the main features of homocystinuria.[196] In contrast to the normal intelligence generally seen in patients with Marfan's syndrome, about 60% of patients with homocystinuria have mental retardation. This could be the result of either accumulation of S-adenosylhomocysteine in the CNS or repeated cerebrovascular thrombotic episodes. Other skeletal findings include osteoporosis, kyphosis, scoliosis, and vertebral collapse.[197] Although most cases are inherited as an autosomal dominant condition, there is genetic heterogeneity. Homocystinuria occurs in about 1 out of every 344,000 live births. Using cDNA, several mutations in the CBS gene have been identified in individuals with CBS deficiency.

The diagnosis is confirmed by demonstrating homocystinuria and a deficiency of cystathionine β-synthetase on liver biopsy, in lymphocytes, or in skin fibroblasts. Treatment includes a high-cystine diet, pyridoxine, and methionine restriction. Pyridoxine-responsive patients usually have milder clinical manifestations. Treatment with betaine, a methyl donor in methionine metabolism, is being evaluated for non–pyridoxine-responsive individuals.[196] By increasing the rate of homocysteine methylation, homocystine levels are lowered, although methionine concentrations may be increased. However, there is compelling evidence that methionine makes a lesser contribution to the pathophysiology of cystathionine β-synthase deficiency than do homocysteine and its derivatives.

Chromosome Abnormalities

KLEINFELTER'S SYNDROME. Tall stature is a frequent finding in children and adolescents with Klinefelter's syndrome. This syndrome is the result of an abnormality in the number of chromosomes. In male patients, two or more X chromosomes are present. The most common karyotype is 47,XXY.[198] The presence of more than one X chromosome results in testicular failure, leading to delayed puberty, impaired testosterone production, and infertility. Other manifestations during adolescence include gynecomastia, small testes in relation to the stage of pubertal development, and impaired sexual functioning. Almost all boys eventually enter puberty and show adequate penile length and pubic hair development, but

oligospermia or aspermia is present. There is an increased frequency of behavioral and psychosocial problems, and verbal IQ scores are lower than expected.[199]

Klinefelter's syndrome should be suspected in an adolescent boy with tall stature, gynecomastia, and small testes who has other evidence of pubertal development, such as penile enlargement and pubic hair. The diagnosis is confirmed by doing a karyotype and demonstrating the presence of more than one X chromosome. Biochemical findings include elevated serum levels of LH and FSH (as a response to the primary gonadal failure) and low-normal serum testosterone levels. Treatment includes replacement therapy with long-acting intramuscular testosterone, 200 to 400 mg every 3 to 4 weeks, which may improve sexual function but does not restore fertility.[199] Gynecomastia may require surgical treatment, since it can be aggravated by testosterone treatment owing to increased peripheral tissue aromatase activity.[200]

XYY SYNDROME. Another chromosomal abnormality that commonly causes tall stature in males is XYY syndrome. Growth acceleration does not become evident until the patient reaches 5 or 6 years of age. In most cases, affected children have behavioral problems and dull mentality.[201] Tall stature is often associated with severe acne, hypospadias and/or cryptorchidism, and radioulnar synostosis. Although XYY syndrome was first described among prisoners, deviant behavior has not been proved to be a necessary finding.[202]

Endocrine Disorders

GROWTH-HORMONE EXCESS. Pituitary acromegaly is extremely rare in childhood and adolescence. It is usually caused by excessive secretion of GH by an adenohypophyseal adenoma arising from somatotroph cells.[203] These are benign epithelial tumors that derive from and consist of adenohypophyseal cells. They are small and slow-growing, and generally confined to the sella turcica. They are diagnosed initially because of the clinical syndrome they create despite their miniature size. Rarely, the tumor spreads outside the sella turcica and invades neighboring tissues, including the sphenoid bone, optic nerve, and brain. Alternatively, the tumor may be ectopic in the sphenoid sinus or parapharyngeal region.

Some pituitary GH-producing adenomas are associated with the syndrome of multiple endocrine neoplasia type I (MEN-I). They can also be part of a rare hypersecretory endocrinopathy, McCune-Albright syndrome, which includes polyostotic fibrous dysplasia, café au lait pigmentations, sexual precocity, hyperthyroidism, GH-secreting pituitary adenomas, and adrenal hyperplasia (see p. 219 in this chapter).

Less frequently, acromegaly may be the result of production of GH-RH by an extrapituitary tumor that results in pituitary hyperplasia and may clinically mimic a pituitary adenoma. The morphologic diagnosis of hyperplasia should prompt a search for a primary lesion. The primary lesion may be found intracranially, as a hypothalamic pituitary gangliocytoma; or extracranially, as a pancreatic islet cell, lung, sympathoadrenergic, adrenal, bronchial, or intestinal tumor.

Aside from GH-secreting microadenomas, GH can be secreted primarily by ectopic GH-secreting tumors. Intracranially, these include somatotropinomas in the sphenoid sinus, sphenoid wings, petrous temporal bone, or nasal cavity. Extracranially, GH secretion can occur in pancreatic islet cell carcinoma or lung tumors.[205]

Growth hormone excess presents clinically as carbohydrate intolerance in up to 50% of patients and as overt diabetes in 10% to 25%. Hypertension is present in 25% to 35% of patients. In about one third of patients, cardiac disease is the presenting problem, including left ventricular wall thickening, asymmetric septal hypertrophy, and decreased ventricular ejection fraction. Patients can also develop neurologic symptoms, including paresthesias and carpal tunnel syndrome, as well as proximal myopathy.[206] Apart from manifestations due to metabolic effects of GH excess, patients also have signs and symptoms attributable to the effects of tumor mass. Up to 89% of patients have visual field defects; headaches are present in 50% to 60%. Hypopituitarism may also occur secondary to the pressure effect of a large GH-secreting tumor mass on other cells, including adrenocorticotropic hormone (ACTH) and TSH deficiency. About 50% to 70% of women with acromegaly develop amenorrhea, and the same percentage of men complain of impotence and decreased libido due to direct pressure on gonadotroph cells by the adenomatous or hyperplastic somatotroph cells.

In a child or adolescent who is growing at an accelerated rate, GH excess should be ruled out. The traditional diagnostic criteria include a failure to suppress GH to less than 2 ng/ml after administration of 50 to 100 g glucose.[204] Frequent sampling of GH can also be used to determine the normal pulsatile character of GH secretion, but this is not practical in most centers. IGF-1 levels should correlate well with GH secretion but do not constitute a highly sensitive test. On the other hand, IGF BP3, which is GH dependent and is an integrated marker of somatotroph function, has proved useful as a biochemical index of GH excess in patients with suspected acromegaly, and also in determining cure after transsphenoidal surgery.[208,209]

The treatment of pituitary acromegaly or gigantism can be difficult. When the lesion seen on MRI or CT imaging is circumscribed, transsphenoidal adenomectomy can be successful.[210] However, when the lesions are less discrete and of long standing, neurosurgical cure may be more difficult. Growth hormone excess may persist, and postoperative hypopituitarism is frequent. Radiation therapy can also cause hypopituitarism[211] and is particularly undesirable in children. Thus, clinicians have resorted to medical treatment. Bromocriptine rarely shrinks GH-secreting adenomas but offers symptomatic relief in 70% to 80% of patients who have headaches, sweating, and joint pains.[212] It is effective in suppressing prolactin secretion but has not always suppressed GH in children.[213]

Somatostatin and its analog, octreotide, appear to be more effective drugs in the treatment of acromegaly.[214] It may be necessary to replace other pituitary hormone deficiencies that have developed because of the growth of the tumor or as a result of its treatment. Therefore, it is important to evaluate every patient with a GH-secreting tumor for other pituitary functions, including antidiuretic hormone, thyrotropin, and gonadotropin secretion.

ESTROGEN RESISTANCE. A mutation in the estrogen-receptor gene was described in 1994 in a young man who presented with tall stature, continued linear growth after adolescence, and incomplete epiphyseal closure at the age of 28 years.[215] He had a decreased upper-to-lower segment ratio as well as disproportionately long arms. He also had progressive genu valgum, axillary acanthosis nigricans, and no gynecomastia. He was normally virilized, but his bone age was markedly delayed and bones were demineralized. The testosterone level was normal, but estradiol, estrone, LH, and FSH levels were elevated. Transdermal estrogen treatment caused no resolution of any of the clinical findings. Genetic studies revealed an autosomal recessive inheritance.

Although patients with estrogen resistance will most likely present with tall stature after adolescence because of failure of epiphyseal fusion, the condition should be considered in the differential diagnosis of tall stature and delayed bone age, particularly during late adolescence in a male who is completely virilized.

EVALUATION OF TALL STATURE

Proper evaluation of an adolescent with tall stature depends on the availability of the following important information: previous growth data; parental heights; family history of tall stature or known genetic disorders such as Marfan's syndrome; accurate anthropometric measurements, particularly height, weight, arm span, lower segment, and sitting height; careful physical examination looking for dysmorphic signs and characteristic features of the various overgrowth disorders; and bone age. An individual who is growing consistently along the same growth channel parallel to the normal curve, with a projected height falling within the range of the midparental or target height, has familial tall stature. The predicted adult height will help decide whether medical intervention is indicated.

On the other hand, an individual who is growing at an accelerated rate away from the normal curve should be investigated for GH excess. An elevated IGF-1, IGF BP3, and random GH level may be strongly suggestive of a pituitary GH-secreting adenoma. Confirmation is generally obtained by an oral glucose load of 50 to 100 g and failure to suppress GH levels to less than 2 ng/ml. A pituitary MRI or CT study will reveal the presence of an adenoma.

It is particularly important to rule out Marfan's syndrome and homocystinuria, as these two conditions can lead to fatal cardiovascular complications. The presence of disproportionate long limbs and arachnodactyly warrants a careful eye examination and cardiac evaluation, including an echocardiogram.

It may be difficult to distinguish Marfan's syndrome from homocystinuria, but a careful history taking and physical examination may help make the distinction. Since Marfan's syndrome is an autosomal dominant condition, a similar characteristic habitus in one parent will most likely be Marfan's syndrome. A valvular cardiac lesion and characteristic upward lens dislocation are features of this syndrome. Homocystinuria is confirmed by demonstrating an elevated level of homocystine in the urine or a deficiency of cystathione β-synthetase on liver biopsy or in skin fibroblasts. Beckwith-Wiedemann syndrome may be difficult to recognize during adolescence, since its distinctive facial features become less prominent at this time. It may be necessary to look at childhood photographs, but demonstration of the characteristic growth pattern, including a large birthweight, will also help in the diagnosis. This condition should be distinguished from tall stature due to simple exogenous obesity. In the latter case, the individual generally has a normal or average size at birth, with rapid growth after the onset of a rapid weight gain sometime during childhood. Furthermore, the distinctive facial features of the overgrowth syndromes are absent in simple obesity. In an obese adolescent whose parents are concerned about extremely tall stature, demonstrating an advanced bone age will help reassure the individual and parents that growth is expected to cease earlier than usual and that the final height attained should be appropriate for the family. Control of weight gain is usually accompanied by a growth deceleration.

Finally, in an older adolescent male who is fully mature sexually but continues to exhibit progressive growth, estrogen resistance should be considered.

Tall stature among males is rarely a presenting complaint, and many overgrowth disorders are frequently overlooked and remain undiagnosed among males. This presents a danger for those with Marfan's syndrome and homocystinuria, who may never be diagnosed until they develop devastating cardiovascular complications. It is therefore essential for clinicians to be familiar with these conditions and to recognize that tall stature should always signal a search for them so that fatal complications can be prevented.

References

1. Sandberg DE, Brook AE, Campos SP: Short stature: a psychosocial burden requiring growth hormone therapy?, *Pediatrics* 94:832, 1994.
2. Siegel PT, Clopper R, Stabler B: Psychological impact of significantly short stature, *Acta Paediatr Scand* (suppl) 337:14, 1991.
3. Hamill PV, Drizd TA, Johnson CL, Reed RB, Roche AF, Moore WM: Physical growth: National Center for Health Statistics percentiles, *Am J Clin Nutr* 32:607, 1979.
4. Lifshitz F, Cervantes CD: Short stature. In Lifshitz F, editor: *Pediatric endocrinology,* ed 2, New York, 1990, Marcel Dekker; p 3.
5. Tanner TM, Goldstein H, Whitehouse RH: Standards for children's height at age 2 to 9 years allowing for height of parents, *Arch Dis Child* 45:755, 1970.
6. Cervantes CD, Lifshitz F: Tubular bone alterations in familial short stature, *Hum Biol* 60:151, 1988.
7. Rosenfeld RG: Constitutional delay in growth and development, *Semin Adolesc Med* 3:267, 1987.
8. Crowne EC, Shalet SM, Wallace WHB, Eminson DM, Price DA: Initial height in boys with untreated constitutional delay in growth and puberty, *Arch Dis Child* 65:1109, 1990.
9. Bramswig JH, Fasse M, Holthoff M-L, von Lengerke HJ, von Petrykowski W, Schellong G: Adult height in boys and girls with untreated short stature and constitutional delay of growth and puberty: accuracy of five different methods of height prediction, *J Pediatr* 117:886, 1990.
10. Albanese A, Stanhope R: Predictive factors in the determination of final height in boys with constitutional delay of growth and puberty, *J Pediatr* 126:545, 1995.
11. Smals AGH, Hermus ARM, Boers GHJ, Pieters GFF, Benraad THJ, Kloppenborg PWC: Predictive value of luteinizing hormone releasing hormone (LHRH) bolus testing before and after 36-hour pulsatile LHRH administration in the differential diagnosis of constitutional delay of puberty and male hypogonadotropic hypogonadism, *J Clin Endocrinol Metab* 78:602, 1994.
12. Zamboni G, Antoniazzi F, Tato L: Use of the gonadotropin releasing hormone agonist triptorelin in the diagnosis of delayed puberty in boys, *J Pediatr* 126:756, 1995.
13. Gourmelen M, Pham-Hur-Trung MT, Girard F: Transient partial hGH deficiency in prepubertal children with delay of growth, *Pediatr Res* 13:221, 1979.
14. Spranger J: Classification of skeletal dysplasias, *Acta Paediatr Scand* (suppl) 377:138, 1991.
15. Shohat M, Rimoin DL: The skeletal dysplasias. In Lifshitz F, editor: *Pediatric endocrinology,* ed 2, New York, 1990, Marcel Dekker; p 147.
16. Pauli RM: Osteochondrodysplasias with mild clinical manifestations: a guide for endocrinologists and others, *Growth Genet Horm* 11:1, 1995.
17. Scott CI Jr: Genetics of short stature. In Steinberg AG, Bearn AG, editors: *Progress in medical genetics,* New York, 1972, Grune & Stratton; p 266.
18. Kozlowski K: Hypochondroplasia. *Pol Rev Radiol Nucl Med* 19:450, 1965.
19. Cervantes CD, Lifshitz F: Skeletal dysplasias with primary abnormalities in carbohydrate, lipid, and amino acid metabolism. In Castells S, Finberg L, editors: *Metabolic bone disease in children,* New York, 1989, Marcel Dekker; p 329.

20. Jones KL: *Smith's recognizable patterns of human malformation,* ed 4, Philadelphia, 1988, WB Saunders; p 11.

21. Cronk CE, Crocker AC, Pueschel SM, Shea AM, Zackai E, Pickens G, Reed RB: Growth charts for children with Down syndrome: 1 month to 18 years of age, *Pediatrics* 81:102, 1988.

22. Lippe B: Turner syndrome: a recognizable cause of adolescent short stature, *Semin Adolesc Med* 3:241, 1987.

23. Lyon AJ, Preece MA, Grant DB: Growth curve for girls with Turner syndrome, *Arch Dis Child* 60:932, 1985.

24. Sybert VP: Adult height in Turner syndrome with and without androgen therapy, *J Pediatr* 104:365, 1984.

25. Brook CGD, Murser G, Zachmann M, Prader A: Growth in children with 45,XO Turner's syndrome, *Arch Dis Child* 29:789, 1974.

26. Rappaport R, Sauvion S: Possible mechanism for the growth retardation in Turner's syndrome, *Acta Paediatr Scand* (suppl) 356:82, 1989.

27. Kastrup KW: Oestrogen therapy in Turner syndrome, *Acta Paediatr Scand* 343:43, 1988.

28. Holm VA, Cassidy SB, Butler MG, Hanchett JM, Greenswag LR, Whitman BY, Grenberg F: Prader-Willi syndrome: consensus diagnostic criteria, *Pediatrics* 91:398, 1993.

29. Bray GA, Wilson WG: Prader-Willi syndrome: an overview, *Growth Genet Horm* 2:1, 1986.

30. Ledbetter DH, Riccardi VM, Airhart SD, Strobel RJ, Keenan BS, Crawford JD: Deletion of chromosome 15 as a cause of the Prader-Willi syndrome, *N Engl J Med* 304:325, 1981.

31. Nicholls RD, Knoll JH, Butler MG, Karam S, Lalande M: Genetic imprinting suggested by maternal heterodisomy in nondeletion Prader-Willi syndrome, *Nature* 16:281, 1989.

32. Jones KL: *Smith's recognizable patterns of human malformation,* ed 4, Philadelphia, 1988, WB Saunders; p 80.

33. Nishi Y, Nakanishi Y, Kawaguchi S, Usni T: Silver-Russell syndrome and growth hormone deficiency, *Acta Paediatr Scand* 71:1035, 1982.

34. Warshaw JB: Perspectives on intrauterine growth retardation, *Growth Genet Horm* 2:1, 1986.

35. Miller HC: Prenatal factors affecting intrauterine growth retardation, *Clin Perinatol* 12:307, 1985.

36. Castillo-Duran C, Rodriguez A, Venegas G, Alvarez P, Icaza G: Zinc supplementation and growth of infants born small for gestational age, *J Pediatr* 127:206, 1995.

37. Paz I, Seidman DS, Danon YL, Laor A, Stevenson DK, Gale R: Are children born small for gestational age at increased risk of short stature?, *Am J Dis Child* 147:337, 1993.

38. Chaussain JL, Colle M, Ducret JP: Adult height in children with prepubertal short stature secondary to intrauterine growth retardation, *Acta Paediatr Suppl* 399:72, 1994.

39. Torun B, Viteri FE: Protein energy malnutrition. In Shils ME, Young VR, editors: *Modern nutrition in health and disease,* ed 7, Philadelphia, 1988, Lea & Febiger; p 746.

40. Lifshitz F, Moses N, Cervantes CD, Ginsberg L: Nutritional dwarfing in adolescents, *Semin Adolesc Med* 3:255, 1987.

41. Pugliese MT, Lifshitz F, Grad G, Mark-Katz M: Fear of obesity: a cause of short stature and delayed puberty, *N Engl J Med* 309:513, 1983.

42. Lifshitz F, Moses N: Growth failure—a complication of dietary treatment of hypercholesterolemia, *Am J Dis Child* 143:537, 1989.

43. Mansfield MJ, Emans SJ: Growth in female gymnasts: should training decrease during puberty?, *J Pediatr* 122:237, 1993.

44. Thientz GE, Howald H, Weiss U, Sizonenko PC: Evidence for a reduction of growth potential in adolescent female gymnasts, *J Pediatr* 122:306, 1993.

45. Lifshitz F, Friedman S, Smith M, Cervantes C, Recker B, O'Connor M: Nutritional dwarfing: a growth abnormality associated with reduced erythrocyte Na^+-K^+ ATPase activity, *Am J Clin Nutr* 54:997, 1991.

46. Pugliese MT: Endocrine function adaptations in undernutrition, *World Rev Nutr Diet* 62:186, 1990.

47. Abdenur JE, Puglese MT, Cervantes C, Fort P, Lifshitz F: Alterations in spontaneous GH secretion and the response to GH-releasing hormone in children with nonorganic nutritional dwarfing, *J Clin Endocrinol Metab* 75:930, 1992.

48. Nakamura T, Higashi A, Nishiyama S, Fujimoto S, Matsuda I: Kinetics of zinc status in children with IDDM, *Diabetes Care* 14:553, 1991.

49. Nishi Y, Lifshitz F, Bayne MA, Daum F, Silverberg M, Aiges H: Zinc status and its relation to growth retardation in children with chronic inflammatory bowel disease, *Am J Clin Nutr* 33:2613, 1980.

50. Nakamura T, Nishiyama S, Futagoishi-Suginohara Y, Matsuda I, Higashi A: Mild to moderate zinc deficiency in short children: effect of zinc supplementation in linear growth velocity, *J Pediatr* 123:65, 1993.

51. Prasad AS, Brewer GJ, Schoomaker EB, Rabbani P: Hypocupremia induced by zinc therapy in adults, *JAMA* 240:2166, 1978.

52. Motil KJ: Gastrointestinal diseases and growth faltering, *Pediatr Rounds: Growth, Nutr Dev* 2:4, 1993.

53. Kanof ME, Lake AM, Bayless TM: Decreased height velocity in children and adolescents before diagnosis of Crohn's disease, *Gastroenterology* 95:1523, 1988.

54. Bresson JL, Schmitz J: Malnutrition in Crohn's disease: substrate deficiency or misuse?, *Horm Res* 38 (suppl 1):76, 1992.

55. McCaffery TD, Nasr K, Lawrence AH, Kirsner JB: Severe growth retardation in children with chronic inflammatory bowel disease, *J Pediatr* 45:386, 1970.

56. Gotlin RW, Dubois RS: Nyctohemeral growth hormone levels in children with growth retardation and inflammatory bowel disease, *Gut* 14:191, 1973.

57. Tenore A, Berman WF, Parks JS, Bongiovanni AM: Basal and stimulated growth hormone concentrations in inflammatory bowel disease, *J Clin Endocrinol Metab* 44:622, 1977.

58. Braegger CP, Torresani T, Murch SH, Savage MO, Walker-Smith JA, MacDonald TT: Urinary growth hormone in growth-impaired children with chronic inflammatory bowel disease, *J Pediatr Gastroenterol Nutr* 16:49, 1993.

59. Whittington PR, Barnes V, Bayless TM: Medical management of Crohn's disease in adolescence, *Gastroenterology* 72:1338, 1977.

60. Rosenback Y, Dinari G, Zahavi I, Nitzan M: Short stature as the major manifestation of celiac disease in older children, *Clin Pediatr* 25:13, 1986.

61. Hernandez M, Argente J, Navarro A, Caballo N, Barrios V, Hervas F, Polanco I: Growth in malnutrition related to gastrointestinal diseases: coeliac disease, *Horm Res* 38 (suppl 1):79, 1992.

62. Ashkenazi A: Occult celiac disease: a common cause of short stature, *Growth Genet Horm* 5:1, 1989.

63. Not T, Ventura A, Peticarari S, Basile S, Torre G, Dragovic D: A new, rapid, non-invasive screening tests for celiac disease, *J Pediatr* 123:425, 1993.

64. Rossi TM, Albini CH, Kumar V: Incidence of celiac disease identified by the presence of serum endomyseal antibodies in children with chronic diarrhea, short stature, or insulin-dependent diabetes mellitus, *J Pediatr* 123:262, 1993.

65. Vajro P, Fontanella A, Mayer M, DeVincenzo A, Terraciano LM, D'Armiento M, Vecchione R: Elevated serum aminotransferase activity as an early manifestation of gluten-sensitive enteropathy, *J Pediatr* 122:416, 1993.

66. Rigden SPA, Rees L, Chatler C: Growth and endocrine function in children with chronic renal failure, *Acta Paediatr* Scand (suppl) 370:21, 1990.

67. Tokieda K, Yi ZW, Chan JCM: *Mechanisms of growth failure in uremia,* Pediatric Nephrology Seminar XXI: Growth Session, 4, 1994.

68. Schaefer F, Hamill G, Stanhope R, Preece MA, Scharer K: Pulsatile growth hormone secretion in peripubertal patients with chronic renal failure, *J Pediatr* 119:568, 1991.

69. Castellano M, Turconi A, Chaler E, Rivarola MA, Belgorosky A: Hypothalamic-pituitary-gonadal function in prepubertal boys and girls with chronic renal failure, *J Pediatr* 122:46, 1993.

70. Pasqualini T, Zantleifer D, Balzaretti M, Granillo E, Fainstein-Day P, Ramirez J, Ruiz S, Gutman R, Ferraris J: Evidence of hypothalamic-pituitary thyroid abnormalities in children with end-stage renal disease, *J Pediatr* 118:873, 1991.

71. Fine RN, Kohaut EC, Brown D, Perlman AJ: Growth after recombinant human growth hormone treatment in children with chronic renal failure: report of a multicenter randomized double-blind placebo-controlled study, *J Pediatr* 124:374, 1994.

72. Tejani A, Fine R, Alexander S, Harmon W, Stablein D: Factors predictive of sustained growth in children after renal transplantation, *J Pediatr* 122:397, 1993.

73. Aitman TJ, Palmer RG, Loftus J, Ansell BM, Royston JP, Teale JD, Clayton RN: Serum IGF-I levels and growth failure in juvenile chronic arthritis, *Clin Exp Rheumatol* 7:557, 1989.

74. Reed A, Haugen M, Pachman LM, Langman CB: 25-Hydroxyvitamin D therapy in children with active juvenile rheumatoid arthritis: short-term effects on serum osteocalcin levels and bone mineral density, *J Pediatr* 119:657, 1991.

75. Huppertz H-I, Tschammler A, Horwitz AE, Schwab KO: Intraarticular corticosteroids for chronic arthritis in children: efficacy and effects in cartilage and growth, *J Pediatr* 127:317, 1995.

76. Shalet SM, Beardwell CG, Morris-Jones PH, Pearson D: Growth hormone deficiency after treatment of acute leukemia in children, *Arch Dis Child* 5:489, 1976.

77. Shalet SM, Gibson B, Swindell R, Pearson D: Effect of spinal irradiation on growth, *Arch Dis Child* 62:461, 1987.

78. Sklar C, Mertens A, Walter A, Mitchell D, Nesbit M, O'Leary M, Hutchinson R, Meadows A, Robison L: Final height after treatment for childhood acute lymphoblastic leukemia: comparison of no cranial irradiation with 1800 and 2400 centigrays of cranial irradiation, *J Pediatr* 123:59, 1993.

79. Katz JA, Pollock BH, Jacaruso D, Morad A: Final attained height in patients successfully treated for childhood acute lymphoblastic leukemia, *J Pediatr* 123:546, 1993.

80. Barnes G: Human immunodeficiency virus infection, *Int Semin Paediatr Gastroenterol Nutr* 3:1, 1994.

81. Brettler DB, Forsberg A, Bolivar E, Brewster F, Sullivan J: Growth failure as a prognostic indicator for progression to acquired immunodeficiency syndrome in children with hemophilia, *J Pediatr* 117:584, 1990.

82. Jospe N, Powel KR: Growth hormone deficiency in an 8-year-old girl with human immunodeficiency virus infection, *Pediatrics* 86:309, 1990.

83. Laue L, Pizzo PA, Butler K, Cutler GB: Growth and neuroendocrine dysfunction in children with acquired immunodeficiency syndrome, *J Pediatr* 117:541, 1990.

84. McKinney RE, Wilfert C: Growth as a prognostic indicator in children with human immunodeficiency virus infection treated with zidovudine, *J Pediatr* 125:728, 1994.

85. Yesilipek MA, Bircan I, Oygür N, Ertug H, Yegin O, Guven AG: Growth and sexual maturation in children with thalassemia major, *Haematologica* 78:30, 1993.

86. Kattamis C, Liakopoulou T, Kattamis A: Growth and development in children with thalassemia major, *Acta Pediatr Scand Suppl* 336:111, 1990.

87. Masala A, Meloni T, Gallisai D, Alagna S, Rovasio PP, Rassu S, Milia AF: Endocrine functioning in multitransfused prepubertal patients with homozygous beta-thalassemia, *J Clin Endocrinol Metab* 58:667, 1984.

88. Saenger P, Schwartz E, Markenson AL, Graziano JH, Levine LS, New ML, Hilgartner MW: Depressed serum somatomedin activity in beta-thalassemia, *J Pediatr* 96:214, 1980.

89. Shehadeh N, Hazani A, Rudolf MC, Peleg I, Benderly A, Hochberg Z: Neurosecretory dysfunction of growth hormone secretion in thalassemia major, *Acta Pediatr Scand* 79:790, 1990.

90. Spock A: Growth patterns in 200 children with bronchial asthma, *Ann Allergy* 23:608, 1965.

91. Hauspie R, Crowley S, Alexander F: Maturational delay and temporal growth retardation in asthmatic boys, *J Allergy Clin Immunol* 59:200, 1967.

92. Balfour-Lynn L: Growth and childhood asthma, *Arch Dis Child* 61:1049, 1986.

93. Konig P, Hillman L, Cervantes C, Levine C, Maloney C, Douglass B, Johnson L, Allen S: Bone metabolism in children with asthma treated with inhaled beclomethasone dispropionate, *J Pediatr* 122:219, 1993.

94. Crowley S, Hindmarsh PC, Matthews DR, Brook CGD: Growth and growth hormone axis in prepubertal children with asthma, *J Pediatr* 126:297, 1995.

95. Price JF: Asthma, growth, and inhaled corticosteroids, *Respir Med* (suppl A) 87:23, 1993.

96. Singhal A, Thomas P, Cook R, Wierenga K, Serjeant G: Delayed adolescent growth in homozygous sickle cell disease, *Arch Dis Child* 71:404, 1994.

97. Weintraub RG, Menahem S: Growth and congenital heart disease, *J Paediatr Child Health* 29:95, 1993.

98. Mehrizi A, Drash A: Growth disturbance in congenital heart disease, *J Pediatr* 61:418, 1962.

99. Levitsky LL: Growth and pubertal pattern in insulin dependent diabetes mellitus, *Semin Adolesc Med* 3:233, 1987.

100. White P: Childhood diabetes. Its course and influence on the second and third generations, *Diabetes* 9:345, 1960.

101. Songer TJ, LaPorte RE, Tajima N, Orchard TJ, Rabin BS, Eberhardt MS, Dorman JS, Cruickshanks KJ, Cavender DE, Becker DJ, Drash AL: Height at diagnosis of insulin dependent diabetes in patients and their non-diabetic family members, *Br Med J* 292:1419, 1986.

102. Vanelli M, deFanti A, Adinolfi B, Ghizzoni L: Clinical data regarding the growth of diabetic children, *Horm Res* 37 (suppl 3):65, 1992.

103. Blethen SL, Sargeant DT, Whitlow MG, Santiago JV: Effect of pubertal stage and recent blood glucose control on plasma somatomedin C in children with insulin-dependent diabetes mellitus, *Diabetes* 30:868, 1981.

104. Pastores GM, Lenz P: Growth and development in children with type 1 Gaucher disease. Gaucher clinical perspectives, *Mol Med Ther* 3:1, 1995.

105. Winkler L, Offner G, Krull F, Brodehl J: Growth and pubertal development in nephropathic cystinosis, *Eur J Pediatr* 152:244, 1993.

106. Schaff-Blass E, Burstein S, Rosenfield RL: Advances in diagnosis and treatment of short stature with special reference to the role of growth hormone, *J Pediatr* 104:801, 1984.

107. Lindsay R, Feldkamp M, Harris D, Robertson J, Rallison M: Utah growth study: growth standards and the prevalence of GH deficiency, *J Pediatr* 125:29, 1994.

108. Inzucchi SE, Robbins RJ: Effects of growth hormone on human bone biology, *J Clin Endocrinol Metab* 79:691, 1994.

109. Costin G, Murphee AL: Hypothalamic-pituitary function in children with optic nerve hypoplasia, *Am J Dis Child* 139:249, 1985.

110. Jones JI, Clemmons DR: Insulin-like growth factors and their binding proteins: biological actions, *Endocr Rev* 16:3, 1995.

111. Juul A, Dalgaard P, Blum WF, Bang P, Hall K, Michaelsen KF, Muller J, Skakkebaek NE: Serum levels of insulin-like growth factor (IGF)–binding protein-3 (IGFBP-3) in healthy infants, children, and adolescents: the relation to IGF-I, IGF-II, IGFBP-1, IGFBP-2, age, sex, body mass index, and pubertal maturation, *J Clin Endocrinol Metab* 80:2534, 1995.

112. Morris AH, Reiter ED: Growth hormone: diagnostic and therapeutic dilemmas, *Semin Adolesc Med* 3:283, 1987.

113. Spiliotis BE, August GP, Hung W, Sonis W, Mendelson W, Bercu BB: Growth hormone neurosecretory dysfunction: a treatable cause of short stature, *JAMA* 252:2223, 1984.

114. Zadik Z, Chalew SA, Kowarski A: Assessment of growth hormone secretion in normal stature children using 24-hour integrated concentration of GH and pharmacologic stimulation, *J Clin Endocrinol Metab* 71:932, 1990.

115. Donaldson DL, Hollowell JG, Pan F, Gifford RA, Moore WV: Growth hormone secretory profiles: variation on consecutive nights, *J Pediatr* 115:51, 1989.

116. Plotnick LP, Van Meter QL, Kowarski AA: Human growth hormone treatment of children with growth failure and normal growth hormone levels by immunoassay: lack of correlation with somatomedin generation, *Pediatrics* 71:324, 1983.

117. Rudman D, Kutner MH, Blackstone RD, Cushman RA, Bain RP, Patterson JH: Children with normal variant short stature: treatment with human growth hormone for six months, *N Engl J Med* 305:123, 1981.

118. Valenta LJ, Sigel MB, Lesniak MA: Pituitary dwarfism in a patient with circulating abnormal growth hormone polymers, *N Engl J Med* 312:214, 1985.

119. Laron Z, Kowadlo-Silbergeld A, Eshet R, Pertzelan A: Growth hormone resistance, *Ann Clin Res* 12:269, 1980.

120. Savage MO, Blum WF, Ranke MB, Postel-Vinay MC, Cotterill AM, Hall K, Chatelain PG, Preece MA, Rosenfeld RG: Clinical features and endocrine status in patients with growth hormone insensitivity (Laron syndrome), *J Clin Endocrinol Metab* 77:1465, 1993.

121. Laron Z: An update on Laron syndrome, *Arch Dis Child* 68:345, 1993.

122. Counts DR, Cutler GB Jr: Growth hormone insensitivity syndrome due to point deletion and frame shift in the GH receptor, *J Clin Endocrinol Metab* 80:1978, 1995.

123. Rosenbloom AL, Guevara-Aguirre J: Prismatic case: bienvenidos a mi tierra de soledad: from poetry to molecular biology in Southern Ecuador, *J Clin Endocrinol Metab* 79:695, 1994.

124. Amselem S, Duquesnoy P, Attree O, Novelli G, Bousnina S, Postel-Vinay MC, Goossens M: Laron dwarfism and mutation of the growth hormone receptor gene, *N Engl J Med* 321:989, 1989.

125. Carlsson LMS, Attie KM, Compton PG, Vitangcol RV, Merimee TJ: Reduced concentration of serum growth hormone binding protein in children with idiopathic short stature, *J Clin Endocrinol Metab* 78:1325, 1994.

126. Rieu M, LeBouc Y, Villares SM, Postel-Vinay C: Familial short stature with very high levels of growth hormone binding protein, *J Clin Endocrinol Metab* 76:857, 1993.

127. Momoi T, Yamanaka C, Kobayashi M, Haruta T, Sasaki H, Yorifugi T, Kaji M, Mikawa H: Short stature with normal growth hormone and elevated IGF-I, *Eur J Pediatr* 151:321, 1992.

128. Blizzard RM: Thyroid hormone and its effect on growth and development, *Pediatr Rounds: Growth Nutr Dev* 2:3, 1993.

129. Rovet J, Daneman D, Bailey J: Psychologic and psychoeducational consequences of thyroxine therapy for juvenile acquired hypothyroidism, *J Pediatr* 122:543, 1993.

130. Blodgett FM, Burgin L, Iezzoni D, Gribetz D, Talbot NB: Effects of prolonged cortisone therapy on the statural growth, skeletal maturation and metabolic status of children, *N Engl J Med* 254:636, 1956.

131. Price JF: Asthma, growth, and inhaled corticosteroids, *Respir Med* 87 (suppl A):23, 1993.

132. Allen DB, Goldberg BD: Stimulation of collagen synthesis and linear growth by GH in glucocorticoid-treated children, *Pediatrics* 89:416, 1992.

133. Wehrenberg PJ, Bergman L, Stagg L, Ndone J, Giustina A: Glucocorticoid inhibition of growth in rats: partial reversal with somatostatin antibodies, *Endocrinology* 127:2705, 1990.

134. Locatelli V, Torsello A, Redaelli M, Ghigo E, Massara F: Cholinergic agonist and antagonist drugs modulate the growth hormone response to growth hormone–releasing hormone in the rat: evidence for mediation by somatostatin, *J Endocrinol* 111:271, 1986.

135. Ferraris JR, Day PF, Gutman R, Granillo E, Ramirez J, Ruiz S, Pasqualini T: Effect of therapy with a new glucocorticoid, deflazacort, on linear growth and growth hormone secretion after renal transplantation, *J Pediatr* 121:809, 1992.

136. Magiakou MA, Mastorakos G, Chrousos GP: Final stature in patients with endogenous Cushing's syndrome, *J Clin Endocrinol Metab* 79:1082, 1994.

137. Cara JF: Growth hormone in adolescence. Normal and abnormal, *Endocrinol Metab Clin North Am* 22:533, 1993.

138. Martha PM Jr, Gorman KM, Blizzard RM: Endogenous growth hormone secretion and clearance rates in normal boys, as determined by deconvolution analysis: relationship to age, pubertal status, and body mass, *J Clin Endocrinol Metab* 74:336, 1992.

139. Rose SR, Kibarian M, Gelato M: Sex steroids increase spontaneous growth hormone secretion in short children, *J Pediatr Endocrinol* 3:1, 1988.

140. Foster CM, Fenillan P, Padmanabhan V, Pescovitz OH, Beitins IZ, Comite F, Shawker TH, Loriaux KL, Cutler GB Jr: Ovarian function in girls with McCune-Albright syndrome, *Pediatr Res* 20:859, 1986.

141. Brauner R, Adam L, Malandry F, Zantleifer D: Adult height in girls with idiopathic true precocious puberty, *J Clin Endocrinol Metab* 79:415, 1994.

142. Bar A, Linder B, Sobel EH, Saenger P, DiMartino-Nardi J: Bayley-Pinneau method of height prediction in girls with central precocious puberty: correlation with adult height, *J Pediatr* 126:955, 1995.

143. Rosenfeld RG, Albertsson-Wikland K, Cassorla F, Frasier SD, Hasegawa Y, Hintz RL, LaFranchi S, Lippe B, Loriaux L, Melmed S, Preece MA, Ranke MR, Reiter EO, Rogol AD, Underwood LE, Werther GA: Diagnostic controversy: the diagnosis of childhood GH deficiency revisited, *J Clin Endocrinol Metab* 80:1532, 1995.

144. Shah A, Stanhope R, Matthew D: Hazards of pharmacologic tests of growth hormone secretion in childhood, *Br Med J* 304:174, 1992.

145. Ghigo E, Mazza E, Imperiale E, Rizzi G, Benzo L, Muller EE, Camanni F, Massara F: Enhancement of cholinergic tone by pyridostigmine promotes both basal and GH releasing hormone–induced GH secretion in children of short stature, *J Clin Endocrinol Metab* 65:452, 1987.

146. Mota A, Bento A, Penalva A, Pombo M, Dieguez C: Role of the serotonin receptor subtype-5-HT$_{1D}$ in basal and stimulated growth hormone secretion, *J Clin Endocrinol Metab* 80:1973, 1995.

147. Cordido F, Dieguez C, Casanueva FF: Effect of central cholinergic neurotransmission enhancement by pyridostigmine on the growth hormone secretion elicited by clonidine, arginine, or hypoglycemia in normal and obese subjects, *J Clin Endocrinol Metab* 70:1361, 1990.

148. Casanueva FF, Burguera B, Alvarez CV, Zugaza JL, Pombo M, Dieguez C: Corticoids as a new stimulus of growth hormone secretion in man, *J Pediatr Endocrinol* 5:85, 1992.

149. Maghne M, Valtorta A, Moretta A, Larizza D, Preti P, Palladini G, Calcante S, Severi F: Diagnosing growth hormone deficiency: the value of short term hypocaloric diet, *J Clin Endocrinol Metab* 77:1372, 1993.

150. Donaldson D, Pan F, Hollowell JG, Stevenson JL, Gifford RA, Moore WV: Reliability of stimulated and spontaneous GH levels for identifying the child with low GH secretion, *J Clin Endocrinol Metab* 72:647, 1991.

151. Spath-Schwalbe E, Hundenborn C, Kern W, Fehm HL, Born J: Nocturnal wakefulness inhibits GH releasing hormone–induced GH secretion, *J Clin Endocrinol Metab* 80:214, 1995.

152. Rosenfeld RG, Frane J, Attie KM, Brasel JA, Burstein S, Cara JF, Chernausek S, Gotlin RW, Kuntze J, Lippe BM, Mahoney PC, Moore WV, Saenger P, Johanson AJ: Six year results of a randomized prospective trial of human growth hormone and oxandrolone in Turner syndrome, *J Pediatr* 121:49, 1992.

153. Rosenfeld RG: Growth hormone therapy in Turner's syndrome: an update on final height, *Acta Paediatr Suppl* 383:3, 1992.

154. Torrado C, Bastian W, Wisniewski KE, Castells S: Treatment of children with Down syndrome and growth retardation with recombinant human growth hormone, *J Pediatr* 119:478, 1991.

155. Guyda HJ: *Growth hormone treatment for children with Down syndrome,* National Cooperative Growth Study, Proceedings from the Eight Annual Investigator's Meeting 1994, p 34.

156. Yamate T, Kanzaki S, Tanaka H, Kubo T, Moriwake T, Inoue M, Seino Y: Growth hormone treatment in achondroplasia, *J Pediatr Endocrinol* 6:45, 1993.

157. Appan S, Laurent S, Chapman M, Hindmarsh PC, Brook CGD: Growth and growth hormone therapy in hypochondroplasia, *Acta Paediatr Scand* 79:796, 1990.

158. Bierich JR, Nolte K, Drews K, Brugmann G: Constitutional delay of growth and adolescence. Results of short term and long term treatment with GH, *Acta Endocrinol* 127:392, 1992.

159. Balsamo A, Tassoni P, Cassio A, Colli C, Tassinari D, Cicognani A, Cacciari E: Response to growth hormone therapy in patients with GH deficiency who at birth were small or appropriate in size for gestational age, *J Pediatr* 126:474, 1995.

160. Connor EL, Rosenbloom A: Effects of growth hormone in Prader-Willi syndrome, *Clin Pediatr* 32:296, 1993.

161. Kaplowitz PB: Effect of growth hormone therapy on final versus predicted height in short twelve to sixteen year old boys without growth hormone deficiency, *J Pediatr* 126:478, 1995.

162. Spagnoli A, Spadoni GL, Cianfarani S, Pasquino AM, Troiani S, Boscherini B: Prediction of the outcome of growth hormone therapy in children with idiopathic short stature, *J Pediatr* 126:905, 1995.

163. Job JC, Toublanc JE, Landier F: Growth of short normal children in puberty treated for 3 years with growth hormone alone or in association with gonadotropin releasing hormone agonist, *Horm Res* 41:177, 1994.

164. Czernichow P: Growth hormone administration and carbohydrate metabolism, *Horm Res* 39:102, 1993.

165. Rappaport EB, Fife D: Slipped capital femoral epiphysis in growth hormone deficient children, *Am J Dis Child* 139:396, 1985.

166. Gruber MA: *Musculoskeletal complications of growth hormone therapy,* National Cooperative Growth Study, Proceedings from the Eighth Annual Investigator's Meeting 1994, p 11.

167. Jorgensen JOL, Moller J, Skakkerbaek NE, Weeke J, Christiansen JS: Thyroid function during growth hormone therapy, *Horm Res* 38 (suppl 1):63, 1992.

168. Malozowski S, Hung W, Stadel BV: Acute pancreatitis associated with growth hormone therapy for short stature, *N Engl J Med* 332:401, 1995.

169. Malozowski S, Tanner LA, Wysowski D, Flemming GA: Growth hormone, insulin like growth factor I, and benign intracranial hypertension, *N Engl J Med* 329:665, 1993.

170. Malozowski S, Stadel BV: Prepubertal gynecomastia during growth hormone therapy, *J Pediatr* 126:659, 1995.

171. Shalet SM: Leukemia in children treated with growth hormone, *J Pediatr Endocrinol* 6:109, 1993.

172. Foley TP Jr: *Growth hormone therapy and leukemia,* Sixth Annual National Cooperative Growth Study, November 1992, Los Angeles, CA.

173. Laron Z: One-year treatment with IGF-I of children with Laron syndrome, *Clin Courier* 11:7, 1993.

174. Savage MO: Therapeutic response to recombinant IGF-I in 32 patients with growth hormone insensitivity, *Clin Courier* 11:9, 1993.

175. Underwood LE, Backeljauw PF: Effect of prolonged IGF-I treatment in children with GH insensitivity syndrome, *Clin Courier* 11:11, 1993.

176. Hergenroeder AC: Bone mineralization, hypothalamic amenorrhea, and sex steroid therapy in female adolescents and young adults, *J Pediatr* 126:5, 1995.

177. Crowne EC, Wallace WHB, Moore C, Mitchell R, Robertson WR, Shalet SM: Degree of activation of the pituitary-testicular axis in early pubertal boys with constitutional delay of growth and puberty determines the growth response to treatment with testosterone or oxandrolone, *J Clin Endocrinol Metab* 80:1869, 1995.

178. Adan L, Souberbielle JC, Brauner R: Management of the short stature due to pubertal delay in boys, *J Clin Endocrinol Metab* 78:478, 1994.

179. Zachmann M, Studer S, Prader A: Short term testosterone treatment at bone age of 12-13 years does not reduce adult height in boys with constitutional delay of growth and adolescence, *Helv Paediatr Acta* 42:21, 1987.

180. Strickland AL: Long term results of treatment with low dose fluoxymesterone in constitutional delay of growth and puberty and in genetic short stature, *Pediatrics* 91:716, 1993.

181. Crowne EC, Shalet SM, Wallace WHB, Eminson DM, Price DA: Final height in boys with untreated constitutional delay in growth and puberty, *Arch Dis Child* 65:1109, 1990.

182. Frasier SD: Excessive growth, *Semin Adolesc Med* 3:275, 1987.

183. Epstein LH, Wing RR, Valaski A: Childhood obesity, *Pediatr Clin North Am* 32:362, 1985.

184. Epstein LH, Reva, RW, Koeske R: Long term effects of family based treatment of childhood obesity, *J Consult Clin Psychol* 1:91, 1987.

185. Merritt RJ: Obesity, *Curr Probl Pediatr* 12:1, 1982.

186. Hunter AGW, Allanson JE: Follow-up study of patients with Wiedemann-Beckwith syndrome with emphasis on the change in facial appearance over time, *Am J Med Genet* 51:102, 1994.

187. Jones KL: The etiology and diagnosis of overgrowth syndromes, *Growth Genet Horm* 10:6, 1994.

188. Jones KL: *Smith's recognizable patterns of human malformation,* Philadelphia, 1988, WB Saunders; p 128.

189. Blizzard RM, Johanson A: Disorders of growth. In Kappy MS, Blizzard RM, Migeon CJ, editors: *Wilkins. The diagnosis and treatment of endocrine disorders in childhood and adolescence,* ed 4, Springfield, IL, 1994, Charles C Thomas; p 425.

190. Amir N, Gross-Kieselstein E, Hirsch HJ, Lax E, Silverberg-Shalev R: Weaver-Smith syndrome: a case study with long term follow up, *Am J Dis Child* 138:1113, 1984.

191. Neri G, Marini R, Cappa M, Borrelli P, Opitz JM: Simpson-Golabi-Behmel syndrome: an X-linked encephalotrophoschisis syndrome, *Am J Med Genet* 30:287, 1988.

192. Behmel A, Plochl E, Rosenkranz W: A new X-linked dysplasia gigantism syndrome: follow up in the first family and report on a second Austrian family, *Am J Med Genet* 30:275, 1988.

193. Manusov EG, Martucci E: The Marfan syndrome. An underdiagnosed killer, *Arch Fam Med* 3:822, 1994.

194. Pyeritz RE, Francke U: Conference report. The second international symposium on the Marfan syndrome, *Am J Med Genet* 47:127, 1993.

195. Boileau C, Jondeau G, Babron MC, Coulon M, Alexandre JA, Sakai L, Melki J, Delorme G, Dubourg O, Bonaiti-Pellie C, Bourdarias JP, Junien C: Autosomal dominant Marfan-like connective tissue disorder with aortic dilation and skeletal anomalies not linked to the fibrillin genes, *Am J Hum Genet* 53:46, 1993.

196. Mudd SH, Levy HL, Skovby F: Disorders of transsulfuration. In Scriver CR, Beaudet AL, Sly WS, Valle D, editors: *The metabolic and molecular bases of inherited disease,* ed 7, New York, 1995, McGraw-Hill; p 1279.

197. Schedewie H, Willich E, Grobe H, Schmidt H, Muller KM: Skeletal findings in homocystinuria: a collaborative study, *Pediatr Radiol* 1:12, 1973.

198. Klinefelter HF, Reifenstein EC, Albright F: Syndrome characterized by gynecomastia, aspermatogenesis without aleydigism and increased secretion of follicle stimulating hormone, *J Clin Endocrinol Metab* 2:615, 1942.

199. Frasier SD: Excessive growth, *Semin Adolesc Med* 3:275, 1987.

200. Mahoney CP: Adolescent gynecomastia. Differential diagnosis and management, *Pediatr Clin North Am* 37:1389, 1990.

201. Court Brown WM: Males with an XYY sex chromosome complement, *J Med Genet* 5:341, 1986.

202. Witkin NA, Mednick SA, Schulsinger F: Criminality in XYY and XXY men, *Science* 193:549, 1976.

203. Melmed S: Etiology of pituitary acromegaly, *Endocrinol Metab Clin North Am* 21:539, 1992.

204. Asa SL, Kovacs K: Pituitary pathology in acromegaly, *Endocrinol Metab Clin North Am* 21:553, 1992.

205. Faglia G, Arosio M, Bazzoni N: Ectopic acromegaly, *Endocrinol Metab Clin North Am* 21:575, 1992.

206. Molitch ME: Clinical manifestations of acromegaly, *Endocrinol Metab Clin North Am* 21:597, 1992.

207. Melmed S: Acromegaly, *N Engl J Med* 322:966, 1990.

208. Grinspoon S, Clemmons D, Swearingen B, Klibanski A: Serum insulin-like growth factor-binding protein-3 levels in the diagnosis of acromegaly, *J Clin Endocrinol Metab* 80:927, 1995.

209. Jorgensen JOL, Moller N, Moller J, Weeke J, Blum WF: Insulin-like growth factors (IGF)-I and -II and IGF binding protein-1, -2, and -3 in patients with acromegaly before and after adenomectomy, *Metabolism* 43:579, 1994.

210. Roelfsema F, vanDulken H, Frolich M: Long term results of transphenoidal pituitary microsurgery in 60 acromegalic patients, *Clin Endocrinol (Oxf)* 23:555, 1985.

211. Eastman RC, Gorden P, Glatstein E, Roth J: Radiation therapy of acromegaly, *Endocrinol Metab Clin North Am* 21:693, 1992.

212. Shalet SM: Endocrine outcome of pituitary and hypothalamic tumors, *Clin Courier* 11:21, 1993.

213. Gelber SJ, Heffez DS, Donohoue PA: Pituitary gigantism caused by growth hormone excess from infancy, *J Pediatr* 120:931, 1992.

214. Ho KY, Weissberger AJ, Marbach P, Lazarus L: Therapeutic efficacy of the somatostatin analog SMS 201-995 (octreotide) in acromegaly. Effects of dose and frequency and long term safety, *Ann Intern Med* 112:173, 1990.

215. Smith EP, Boyd J, Frank GR, Takahashi H, Cohen RM, Specker B, Williams TC, Lubahn DB, Korach KS: Estrogen resistance caused by a mutation in the estrogen-receptor gene in a man, *N Engl J Med* 331:1056, 1994.

CHAPTER 28

Disorders of Puberty

•

Ramin Alemzadeh, Michael Pugliese, and Fima Lifshitz

This chapter focuses on disorders of puberty that involve the timing and tempo of sexual maturation and the quality of that maturation. As a broad rule, with numerous exceptions, sexual precocity tends to be of benign or idiopathic causes in the female but of pathologic causes in the male.[1] Conversely, delayed sexual development tends to have pathologic causes in girls and is usually benign or of nonpathologic causes in boys.[2] In addition, an abnormal tempo (i.e., a rate of sexual maturation that is too fast or too slow) may be caused by various types of underlying pathologic conditions.[3]

SEXUAL PRECOCITY

DEFINITIONS

Sexual maturation is considered precocious if the physical signs of puberty appear before 8 years of age in girls and 9½ years in boys.[4] It is clinically useful to distinguish isosexual from contrasexual precocious sexual maturation. Isosexual precocity denotes the appearance of phenotypically appropriate primary or secondary sex characteristics, whereas physical changes consistent with those of the opposite sex are considered to represent contrasexual precocity (i.e., feminization among boys and virilization among girls).[4] This is caused by estrogen excess in boys and androgen excess in girls. In addition, it is important to distinguish between complete and incomplete (e.g., isolated breast or pubic hair) isosexual pubertal development. Complete, or true, precocious puberty is characterized by premature sustained activation of the hypothalamic gonadotropin-releasing hormone (Gn-RH) pulse generator,[5] whereas incomplete, or pseudoprecocious, puberty is seen in a large group of disorders that are not caused by premature activation of the neuroendocrine reproductive system. In this latter group, the source of sex steroid may be

exogenous or endogenous, gonadal or extragonadal. The hormone may be autonomously produced, independent of gonadotropin stimulation or control.

CENTRAL ISOSEXUAL PRECOCITY

A patient with true precocious puberty must exhibit early activation of gonadotropins (gonadarche)—with release of both follicle-stimulating hormone (FSH) and luteinizing hormone (LH)—to account for the presence of secondary sex characteristics. Such premature activation of the hypothalamic-pituitary axis is about five times more common in girls than in boys.[3] This type of early development, referred to as central precocious puberty, differs from the sexual precocity attributable to excessive androgens or estrogens without release of FSH and LH, which is called peripheral precocious puberty.

In central isosexual precocity, the gonadotropin and steroid concentration in plasma, the LH response to Gn-RH administration, and the amplitude and frequency of LH pulses are in the normal pubertal range.[6,7] Patients with central precocious puberty, who demonstrate a pubertal response of LH to Gn-RH and increased pulsatile LH secretion at night, may (1) revert spontaneously to a more immature pubertal state, (2) persist without further progression, or (3) fluctuate between progression and regression.[1,8]

Progression of secondary sexual maturation in patients with sexual precocity tends to occur more rapidly (fast tempo) than that seen in the normal pattern of pubertal maturation. The rapid growth is associated with increased growth hormone (GH) secretion and elevation of serum insulin-like growth factor 1 (IGF-1, somatomedin-C) levels because of stimulation by gonadal steroids.[9,10] The skeletal (bone) age is advanced to various degrees in these children. The ratio of bone age to chronologic age and the rise of IGF-1 above normal values for age are predictive of outcome. Therefore, mildly affected children progress less rapidly and are more likely to maintain their target height,[11] while those with rapid progression experience loss of predicted final height.[11-13]

A case of early sexual development that is in accord with the sex of the child (i.e., isosexual puberty) is described below to highlight the presentation, evaluation, and differential diagnosis of central isosexual precocity.

S.R. was a 6½-year-old black girl who presented to the pediatric endocrinologist with a history of gradual appearance of breast buds since age 5½ years. At the time of examination the patient had pigmented areolae more than 2 cm in diameter and breast tissue more than 5 cm in diameter (Fig. 28-1). She had growth of pubic hair and moderate vaginal estrogenization without clitoromegaly. The patient also had associated moderate axillary sweating and development of axillary hair during the previous 3 months. Her sexual development was classified as Tanner stage 3.

The history of this patient is typical of the isosexual precocity that follows a fast tempo. Sexual maturation was considered precocious because the physical signs of puberty appeared before 8 years of age. In this patient the tempo of puberty was also accelerated since she developed axillary hair less than 1 year from the beginning of breast enlargement. The early onset of puberty and the rapid tempo of sexual maturation noted suggest a possible underlying pathology (Table 28-1). However, it is well known that the clinical course of patients with idiopathic isosexual precocity can be highly variable, and the rate of pubertal progression does not always follow a normal pattern even in the absence of pathology.[4]

Evaluation and Differential Diagnosis

Premature activation of the hypothalamic-pituitary-gonadal axis is usually of idiopathic nature in most girls with central isosexual precocity. Indeed, a detailed evaluation of patient S.R. revealed no history of brain injury secondary to benign or malignant central nervous system (CNS) tumors, therapeutic irradiation, head trauma, or infection (e.g., meningitis with encephalitis), all of which can lead to neuroendocrine dysfunction and precocious puberty[3] (Table 28-1). Also, there was no history of exposure to topical, parenteral, or oral steroid-containing medications.[14]

A review of S.R.'s growth record showed a rapid acceleration in growth since age 5 years. Her height increased over 18 months from the 75th to the 95th percentile (Fig. 28-2). Weight, however, remained proportional to height both before and after the appearance of pubertal changes. There was no evidence of excessive

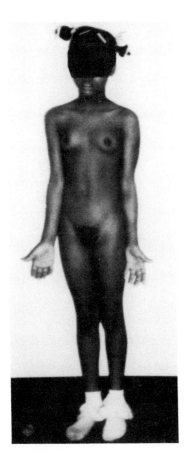

Fig. 28-1. Patient S.R. with signs of central isosexual precocity at age 6½ years.

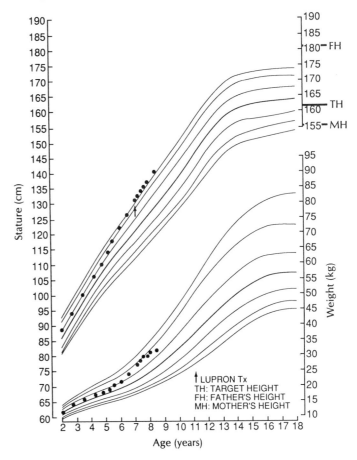

Fig. 28-2. Growth chart of patient S.R. showing central isosexual precocity.

TABLE 28-1
Differential Diagnosis of Precocious Puberty

Type	Pathologic Features	Clinical Characteristics
Central isosexual precocity (complete)	Idiopathic	>90% of female precocity
	CNS disorders	Gonadotropin dependent
	Acquired	Isosexual
	Hypothalamic hamartomas or germinomas	Common cause of male precocity
	Craniopharyngiomas, ependymomas	
	Suprasellar or arachnoid cysts	
	Space-occupying lesion (brain abscess)	
	Brain damage due to chemotherapy, radiotherapy, head trauma, ventriculoperitoneal shunt, hydrocephalus, or infection (e.g., meningitis or encephalitis)	
	Congenital	Isosexual
	Septo-optic dysplasia	Growth hormone deficiency, diabetes insipidus
	Silver's syndrome (Russell's syndrome)	Skeletal anomalies
	Chronic primary hypothyroidism	Growth delay
Peripheral sexual precocity	Ovarian disorders	Ovarian development
	Derived from theca or granulosa cells	
	Cysts or tumors (estrogen secreting)	Isosexual
	Virilizing tumors (arrhenoblastoma)	Heterosexual
	McCune-Albright syndrome	Isosexual
	Testicular disorders	Unilateral or bilateral
	Leydig or Sertoli cell tumor	With or without adrenal rest tissue; high testosterone level; isosexual familial
	Gonadoblastoma/dysgerminoma	Isosexual, common in males
	Testotoxicosis	Isosexual; virilizing effects in females (heterosexual)
	Gonadotropin-secreting tumors	High blood levels of LH-like human chorionic gonadotropin
	Chorioepithelioma	
	Hepatoblastoma	
	Teratoma (sacrococcygeal)	
Pseudoprecocious precocity (incomplete)	Premature thelarche	Normal variant
	Premature adrenarche/pubarche	Normal variant
	Adrenal disorders	Late-onset forms (prepubertal LH/FSH)
	Enzyme defects: congenital adrenal hyperplasia; 21-hydroxylase, 11-hydroxylase, 3β-hydroxysteroid deficiencies	Elevated dehydroepiandrosterone and/or androstenedione
		Isosexual (in boys)
		Heterosexual (in girls)
	Tumors	Isosexual/heterosexual
	Virilizing	Often malignant
	Feminizing	Rare
Pubertal gynecomastia	Exposure to estrogens	Isolated breast development

FSH, follicle-stimulating hormone; *LH*, luteinizing hormone.

weight gain before the onset of puberty, an important consideration, since obesity can be a possible cause of accelerated growth and sexual maturity.[15] The physical examination revealed areas of abnormal skin pigmentation (café au lait patches) on the left shoulder and upper arm as found in patients with McCune-Albright syndrome or neurofibromatosis (Fig. 28-3). Visual fields and fundi were not altered, there was no evidence of papilledema, and the neurologic examination showed no apparent alterations. The thyroid was palpable but not enlarged,

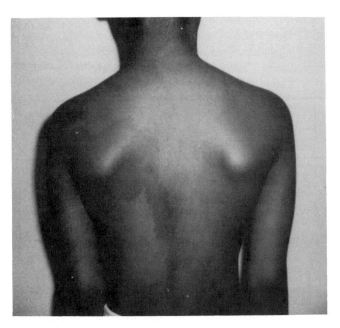

Fig. 28-3. Café au lait pigmentation seen in patient S.R.

with no evidence of hypothyroidism, which is a possible cause of gonadotropin-dependent precocious puberty.[16] There was no evidence of organomegaly or intraabdominal mass, which may be found in patients who have large ovarian cysts or tumors as the cause of premature sexual development.

Radiographic assessment of skeletal maturity (bone age) was advanced by 2 years as compared with chronologic age. In view of the café au lait pigmentation of the skin, radiographs of the long bones and a bone scan of the extremities were obtained, but these did not show any evidence of focal dysplasia characteristic of the bony changes in McCune-Albright syndrome. A vaginal smear for maturation index showed intermediate and superficial squamous cells, a finding consistent with estrogen-induced mucosal maturation. A magnetic resonance imaging (MRI) study of the brain revealed no evidence of pituitary and/or hypothalamic lesions or malformations. This is particularly important, since a Gn-RH–secreting hypothalamic hamartoma[17] is one of the more frequently diagnosed CNS congenital malformations found in girls with precocious puberty. The hamartoma consists of redundant CNS tissue containing Gn-RH neurons that are independent of CNS inhibitory influences and function as an ectopic hypothalamus episodically secreting Gn-RH. The normal MRI picture was consistent with the absence of CNS pathologic conditions noted in most girls with this disorder.[1] Ultrasonography revealed enlargement of the uterus and ovaries with multiple follicles, characteristics consistent with Tanner stage 3 of sexual maturation. Such follicular

cysts may occur in girls with idiopathic precocity and are probably secondary to gonadotropin release. However, pelvic ultrasonography ruled out an isolated estrogen-producing ovarian tumor or cyst as a cause of the premature onset of puberty.[18]

Laboratory data revealed normal levels of serum thyroid hormones, prolactin, testosterone, estradiol, and β-hCG (human chorionic gonadotropin); basal serum levels of LH and FSH corresponded to prepubertal values[19] (Table 28-2). There was a significant overnight pulsatile secretion of gonadotropins along with a rise in the level of these hormones after intravenous administration of synthetic Gn-RH (Table 28-3). These biochemical findings, which are consistent with Tanner stage 3 of sexual development, confirmed the clinical assessment of the pubertal stage observed clinically.[4]

The exhaustive evaluation performed in this patient established the diagnosis of idiopathic sexual precocity that followed a moderately accelerated tempo, and it ruled out the possibility of any underlying pathology. The comprehensive work-up was necessary since the patient's maturational process followed a rapid tempo and she had café au lait spots, which raised the possibility of McCune-Albright syndrome, leading to premature pituitary-hypothalamic activation with development of full central sexual precocity.[20] In most other cases of precocious puberty a clinical decision to observe and follow up without subjecting the patient to such an exhaustive work-up suffices, as long as there is an appropriate progression without any other clinical signs to suggest a specific pathologic condition.

Treatment

Since there was no evidence of underlying pathology as a cause of sexual precocity and since the tempo was accelerated, patient S.R. was treated with a Gn-RH agonist, an analog of Gn-RH [leuprolide (Lupron)]. The mechanism of action of Lupron is based on its competitive inhibition of endogenous gonadotropin release by binding to pituitary receptors. Gn-RH agonist therapy produces complete suppression of gonadotropins and regression of breast tissue.[21] Indeed, 12 months after the initiation of Lupron therapy, S.R. revealed no further maturation of breast tissue, and her growth showed decreased velocity to a prepubertal range (4 to 6 cm/yr) (Fig. 28-1). There are several forms of Gn-RH agonists, including preparations that are effective in single daily subcutaneous injections (4 to 48 μg/kg/day) or long-acting depot preparations to be given once monthly as intramuscular injections (6 to 7.5 mg every 3 to 4 weeks). There are also nasal preparations available for daily administration; however, these may require large doses and are not yet approved for clinical purposes in the United States.

TABLE 28-2
Daytime Basal Level, Peak Amplitude, and Peak Frequency of LH and FSH by Pubertal Stage in Both Sexes

Sex	Hormone	Tanner Stage	Basal Hormone Level	Peak Amplitude (Overnight)	Peak Frequency/ 12 hr (Overnight)
Girls	LH (IU/L)	1	2.9 ± 0.6	4.5 ± 1.4	5.4 ± 2.4
		2	2.1 ± 0.6	7.9 ± 5.3	5.8 ± 2.5
		3	5.7 ± 2.2	14.3 ± 12.2	5.8 ± 1.9
		4	7.9 ± 2.6	14.1 ± 5.5	6.1 ± 1.7
		5	10.2 ± 4.0	14.4 ± 5.0	5.7 ± 2.5
	FSH (IU/L)	1	3.8 ± 1.4	6.4 ± 2.5	3.3 ± 2.4
		2	5.0 ± 3.6	8.0 ± 5.8	4.5 ± 3.1
		3	7.3 ± 2.3	9.2 ± 3.9	4.7 ± 2.0
		4	7.2 ± 1.4	8.9 ± 1.5	3.6 ± 1.9
		5	7.8 ± 2.5	7.5 ± 3.8	4.1 ± 3.2
Boys	LH (IU/L)	1	3.1 ± 0.8	4.8 ± 2.6	4.6 ± 3.0
		2	3.3 ± 1.1	12.8 ± 11.3	5.0 ± 1.7
		3	6.8 ± 2.6	20.4 ± 9.4	6.4 ± 2.4
		4	7.6 ± 3.7	15.6 ± 4.6	4.9 ± 1.9
		5	6.6 ± 1.3	11.5 ± 3.1	6.0 ± 2.1
	Girls	1	2.2 ± 0.7	4.6 ± 4.4	2.8 ± 2.4
		2	3.6 ± 1.9	4.9 ± 2.7	4.3 ± 1.5
		3	5.3 ± 2.6	6.5 ± 2.8	6.0 ± 1.2
		4	5.8 ± 2.3	7.2 ± 2.5	4.7 ± 1.6
		5	5.8 ± 1.4	6.9 ± 5.2	3.5 ± 2.3

Modified from Oerter KE, Uriarte MM, Rose SR, et al: Gonadotropin secretory dynamics during puberty in normal girls and boys, *J Clin Endocrinol Metab* 71:1251-1258, 1990. Copyright © The Endocrine Society.
FSH, follicle-stimulating hormone; *LH,* luteinizing hormone; ±, standard deviation.

TABLE 28-3
Gonadotropin-Releasing Hormone Stimulation Test Results in Both Sexes

Sex	Tanner Stage	Peak LH (IU/L)	Peak FSH (IU/L)	Peak LH/Peak FSH (IU/L)
Girls	1	10.6 ± 3.5	23.3 ± 12.1	0.5 ± 0.2/0.3-0.7
	2	16.7 ± 18.3	15.7 ± 6.9	0.9 ± 0.8/0.3-1.4
	3	38.9 ± 23.7	14.6 ± 4.8	2.9 ± 2.0/0.8-0.6
	4	109.4 ± 62.9	20.4 ± 6.5	5.6 ± 3.2/2.6-12.2
	5	81.7 ± 62.3	14.0 ± 2.8	6.0 ± 5.4/1.1-18.1
Boys	1	13.5 ± 8.8	11.9 ± 6.1	1.4 ± 1.1/0.4-3.6
	2	18.1 ± 9.2	9.3 ± 10.3	6.4 ± 8.2/0.7-12.3
	3	38.5 ± 9.4	7.3 ± 2.6	5.6 ± 1.7/3.5-7.1
	4	55.1 ± 14.8	12.6 ± 3.7	4.5 ± 1.1/2.9-5.4
	5	36.9 ± 6.6	9.6 ± 2.1	4.1 ± 1.5/2.4-6.2

Modified from Oerter KE, Uriarte MM, Rose SR, et al: Gonadotropin secretory dynamics during puberty in normal girls and boys, *J Clin Endocrinol Metab* 71:1251-1258, 1990. Copyright © The Endocrine Society.
FSH, follicle-stimulating hormone; *LH,* luteinizing hormone; ±, standard deviation.

In patients with precocious puberty caused by a brain tumor, the treatment of choice is careful biopsy of the mass followed by radiotherapy (if the tumor is radiosensitive). Neurosurgical experience has shown promising success in resection of some hypothalamic hamartomas, with complete regression of sexual precocity,[22] but successful treatment can usually be accomplished by medical means with gonadotropin agonists. Radiation-induced precocious puberty may be associated with other pituitary problems (e.g., GH deficiency), which should be assessed before the institution of therapy. Patients

affected with a combination of GH deficiency and precocious puberty may demonstrate a normal growth rate for chronologic age but an abnormal growth rate for pubertal stage. This occurs as sex steroids temporarily counter the effects of GH deficiency. However, there are limited data on the long-term pattern of premature activation of gonadotropin release in these patients.

In all children with precocious puberty, the aim of treatment should be considered carefully before therapy is begun. If there is minimal pubertal development with no growth acceleration, clinicians are advised to observe the progression of puberty for 3 to 6 months before initiating treatment. This allows them to avoid unnecessary treatment in children with slow or self-limiting pubertal progression. On the other hand, rapid pubertal progression and growth is a clear indication for therapy. If a pubertal growth spurt has already occurred, only a small percentage of growth potential remains; therefore, treatment cannot be expected to significantly influence ultimate height.

Psychosocial Aspects

Studies on the psychological effects of precocious puberty suggest that these children may be at risk for behavior problems.[23,24] Using the Child Behavior Checklist, Sonis et al[25,26] discovered a higher than expected prevalence of behavior problems and poor social skills among girls with precocious puberty regardless of the cause.

The most important part of therapy involves supportive counseling for both child and parents. This counseling is crucial for a child who may be the focus of ridicule, harassment, or rejection by peers or other family members. The parents may be advised to relate to the child according to chronologic age rather than the age he or she appears to be, and the patient should be counseled about the possibility of becoming a short adult despite being a tall child.

Patient S.R. (described earlier) underwent a comprehensive psychological evaluation and was found to be immature for her chronologic age and to have a low intelligence quotient (IQ = 70). She was referred for special education classes. Her parents initially reacted with fear and confusion regarding the outcome of early puberty and its impact on their daughter's interaction with classmates and the adults in her environment. The parents were counseled that treatment would help delay the pubertal progression and that the child would attain an appropriate final adult height. Moreover, they were reassured that their child's body functioned normally, although they could anticipate some dysphoric adjustment and behavior changes in the months to come.

Although S.R. had a low IQ score, other studies have demonstrated average to high-average IQ scores in girls with idiopathic precocious puberty. It has been suggested, however, that this finding may reflect a referral bias. School acceleration has been recommended for such patients to help them bridge the gap between chronologic age and physiologic age.[27]

PERIPHERAL SEXUAL PRECOCITY

Early development of secondary sex characteristics can occur without maturation of the hypothalamic-pituitary-gonadal axis (i.e., lack of gonadarche). This is called peripheral precocious puberty. In such patients, puberty may be complete or incomplete. In girls, incomplete precocious puberty may be manifested as growth of sexual hair (pubarche) or menstruation (adrenarche) without breast development. For boys, there may be virilization without testicular enlargement. There may be several causes of peripheral sexual precocity, as described below.

Complete Puberty Syndromes

GONADOTROPIN-SECRETING TUMORS. Rarely in boys, and even more rarely in girls, extrapituitary tumors may cause isosexual precocity without gonadarche. In such patients the LH-like activity may be produced by chorioepitheliomas, hepatoblastomas, teratomas, or intracranial germinomas. A gonadotropin-secreting tumor should be suspected in a patient with precocious puberty who presents with elevated baseline LH and FSH levels but in whom there is no rise in serum LH and FSH concentrations after Gn-RH stimulation. Treatment of these tumors may involve complete surgical resection. However, inoperable tumors can be treated with a combination of radiotherapy and chemotherapy.

McCUNE-ALBRIGHT SYNDROME. McCune-Albright syndrome includes a gonadotropin-independent precocious puberty that occurs primarily in girls.[28] The syndrome is characterized by premature onset of puberty, polyostotic fibrous dysplasia, and melanotic cutaneous macules ("coast of Maine" café au lait spots), which are located on the same side of the body as the bone lesions (Fig. 28-3). Other endocrinopathies also may accompany this disorder, including hyperthyroidism, hypercortisolism, GH hypersecretion, acromegaly, and hypophosphatemia. These endocrine disorders are believed to result from autonomous hyperfunctioning of target glands. Gonadotropin-independent precocious puberty due to autoimmune ovarian hyperactivity, without bony lesions and café au lait skin pigmentations, have been described as incomplete forms of McCune-Albright syndrome.[29] Functioning ovarian cysts have been found to be the cause of the precocious puberty in such patients. In some patients only premature thelarche, with little or no pubic hair development, may be seen. Classically, a menstrual period that occurs as the first sign of puberty should alert the clinician to the possibility of McCune-Albright syndrome.

Treatment of McCune-Albright syndrome with Gn-RH agonists or progestational agents has been unsuccessful. However, there is some evidence that patients with this syndrome may respond to cyproterone or testolactone. The long-term effectiveness of these agents is currently under investigation.

OVARIAN CYSTS. An isolated ovarian follicular cyst with autonomous estrogen production may result in the development of peripheral precocious puberty. Such cysts

TABLE 28-4
Premature Thelarche versus Precocious Puberty in Girls

	Premature Thelarche	Precocious Puberty
Growth velocity	Normal	Accelerated
Breasts	Enlargement	Adolescent
Vaginal mucosa	Red or dark pink	2 to 4+ yr pink
Pubic hair	Never	Sometimes
Acne	Never	Sometimes
Bone age	Not advanced	Accelerated after 6 mo

are usually self-limiting in that spontaneous regression of the cyst leads to a fall in estrogen levels; this decrease may be accompanied by withdrawal bleeding. Initial treatment of an isolated follicular cyst should be conservative, with careful monitoring and no surgical intervention, unless a surgical emergency such as torsion is likely. Follow-up sonography and estrogen level testing after 1 to 4 months usually shows regression.

FAMILIAL TESTOTOXICOSIS. This condition is a rare form of premature sexual development that occurs in boys and is inherited as an autosomal dominant disorder.[30] Some authors believe that it is similar to McCune-Albright syndrome in that the gonads are autonomous and continue to function in the absence of gonadotropins. In these patients, a mutation of the LH receptor involving a single base change has been shown to result in increased cyclic AMP production. This provides evidence that the autonomous Leydig cell activity is the result of an activated LH receptor.[31] There is also testicular enlargement with increased production of testosterone (reaching the adult male range), but serum LH response to Gn-RH remains prepubertal. Familial testotoxicosis may be differentiated from McCune-Albright syndrome by the lack of characteristic pigmented skin macules and polyostotic fibrous dysplasia.

Treatment of familial testotoxicosis involves a combination of testolactone (an aromatase inhibitor) and spironolactone, as well as ketoconazole, all of which interfere with testosterone production. However, the long-term efficacy of these has not been determined.

Incomplete Pseudoprecocious Puberty Syndromes

PREMATURE THELARCHE. Isolated premature breast development, or premature thelarche, is a frequent problem in infancy.[32] As early as 6 months of age, breast tissue may appear, usually without areolar development. In most instances the breast tissue resolves spontaneously by 2 years of age. In addition, there may be asymmetric or unilateral breast development, which may occur at any age. Premature thelarche in infancy may be due to persistent physiologic stimulation of the ovaries by gonadotropins and hypersensitivity of breast tissue to modest concentrations of circulating estrogens. Ovarian hormone production is greater during infancy than in later childhood, and breast growth may occur because of increased stimulation or extraresponsive breast tissue. In children older than 6 years, premature thelarche is generally due to increased sensitivity of breast tissue to circulating estrogens or a transient increase in sex-hormone secretion.

The clinician must be able to distinguish premature thelarche from precocious puberty in girls (Table 28-4). In general, growth velocity, bone age, serum estradiol, and LH and FSH levels are normal in the child with premature thelarche, although a vaginal smear may show mild estrogenization. The development of breast tissue in a girl with isosexual precocious puberty is followed by adrenarche and/or pubarche, whereas premature thelarche is characterized by isolated maturation of the breasts. However, since breast development is usually the first sign of sexual precocity, girls with premature thelarche should be followed carefully at regular intervals to assess other early signs of true precocious puberty.

Premature thelarche does not require specific treatment and should involve only observation to monitor whether excessive sex hormones are being secreted episodically. Patients should be evaluated every 3 to 12 months, depending on the rapidity of development of secondary sexual characteristics.

PUBERTAL GYNECOMASTIA. In pubertal boys, unilateral or bilateral breast enlargement, or gynecomastia, is usually a normal variant of pubertal development.[33] This condition usually occurs in association with testicular enlargement and other signs of normal pubertal progression.[34] The most severe form of this disorder, termed *pubertal macromastia,* may persist to adulthood.[35] Pubertal gynecomastia may rarely be caused by an estrogen-producing tumor; exposure to drugs containing estrogen, drugs with estrogen-like actions (e.g., digitalis), or drugs with unknown mechanisms of action (e.g., marijuana); or underlying pathology (e.g., Klinefelter's syndrome). Gynecomastia in a prepubertal boy should always be considered abnormal, even more so if the degree of progression is rapid.[36]

TABLE 28-5
Premature Pubarche/Adrenarche versus Virilization in Girls and Boys

	Pubarche/ Adrenarche	Virilization	Hirsutism	Hypertrichosis
Sexual hair	Present	Present	Present	Absent
Acne	0 to 1+ yr	1+ to 4+ yr	1+ to 4+ yr	0
Clitoral/phallic enlargement	Never	Often	1+ to 4+ yr	0
Growth velocity	Normal	Accelerated	Accelerated	Normal
Bone age	Normal or 1+ accelerated	Accelerated after 6 mo	Normal or 1+ accelerated	Normal

The cause of pubertal gynecomastia is not understood completely. It has been suggested that, as in all other forms of gynecomastia, this condition involves an abnormality in the androgen/estrogen ratio.[37] In middle adolescence the secretion of adrenal androgens may be more pronounced than the secretion of testosterone from the testes. Androstenedione is the major substrate for the peripheral aromatase system in which androgens are converted to estrogens. Therefore, more estrogen than testosterone can be produced during the period of life when gynecomastia develops. In some boys with gynecomastia, estradiol (E_2) levels are found to be elevated. Also, prolactin elevation has been observed in prepubertal boys who later develop gynecomastia.[38] In view of the lack of consistency in hormonal levels, it is possible that pubertal gynecomastia results from both a transient imbalance of testicular and adrenal hormone secretion and an increase in breast-tissue receptor sensitivity to circulating levels of estrogens.

In the presence of a persistently elevated serum estrogen level, an endogenous source of estrogen production (e.g., an adrenal tumor or a testicular Leydig's cell tumor) should be ruled out. In a patient who has a negative history of exposure to medications that contain estrogen or drugs, close clinical follow-up to assess the rate of progression of gynecomastia is generally sufficient.[36]

In adolescent gynecomastia the most important aspect of management is supportive therapy. It should be emphasized to the patient that breast development is a normal part of pubertal development in boys and does not represent evidence of generalized feminization. Mood changes and behavioral manifestations of aggression or depression have been seen in boys with gynecomastia, and are usually related to age of onset, size of breasts, and previous personality adjustment.[39] Formal referral for psychotherapy may be advised in some cases. Drugs such as clomiphene (an antiestrogen), testolactone (an aromatase inhibitor), and dihydrotestosterone[40] in a topical or injectable form have produced some success in reduction of gynecomastia when breast size is below

Tanner stage 3. However, since long-standing gynecomastia may lead to progressive fibrosis of the glandular tissue, medical treatment is often unsuccessful. Surgical management of male gynecomastia is indicated in patients with markedly enlarged breast tissue or those who have significant adjustment problems attributed to the gynecomastia. However, it is advised that surgical resection of breast tissue be undertaken only after completion of puberty, to avoid recurrence of the gynecomastia.

PREMATURE PUBARCHE AND ADRENARCHE. Premature appearance of sexual hair on the pubis is called *pubarche;* early appearance of both axillary and pubic hair is termed *adrenarche.*[41] In patients with pubarche or adrenarche, there is no pubertal maturation of the gonads (gonadarche). These entities are most commonly observed in obese girls between 5 and 8 years of age.[42] The clinician must be adept in distinguishing the premature appearance of sexual hair from generalized hirsutism or hypertrichosis. It is also necessary to identify patients with virilization that is manifested by pubarche and/or adrenarche (Table 28-5). Premature pubarche may be an isolated finding or may be associated with mild acne, body odor, oiliness of the skin, and axillary perspiration and hair. There may also be a slight acceleration of linear growth and advancement of bone age. These changes are accompanied by a mild elevation of plasma adrenal androgens—dehydroepiandrosterone (DHEA), dehydroepiandrosterone sulfate (DHEA-S), and androstenedione—just above the prepubertal range (Table 28-6). However, the child's degree of sexual maturation should be followed, since abnormal progression, excessive virilization (e.g., clitoromegaly), or elevated DHEA and DHEA-S levels may suggest pathologic causes, such as adrenal hyperplasia and adrenal or gonadal tumors.[43]

Premature adrenarche and pubarche do not require specific treatment, but these conditions should be carefully monitored to determine whether excessive sex hormones or androgens are being secreted. These children should be reevaluated every 3 to 12 months.

TABLE 28-6
Baseline and Post–ACTH–Stimulated Adrenal Steroids

Steroid	Prepubertal Age Group			Pubertal Age Group		
	Baseline (0 min)	Post-ACTH (60 min)	Δ	Baseline (0 min)	Post-ACTH (60 min)	Δ
Androstenedione (ng/dl)	32 (5-51)	64 (30-144)	33 (5-111)	82 (53-149)	141 (84-149)	59 (9-130)
Cortisol (µg/dl)	13 (7-20)	29 (22-41)	16 (11-30)	10 (5-19)	24 (15-33)	14 (8-22)
DHEA (ng/dl)	69 (15-140)	125 (34-263)	56 (5-140)	262 (123-474)	559 (210-1068)	297 (50-648)
DHEA-S (ng/dl)	25 (5-114)	31 (5-120)	6 (0-18)	128 (32-305)	139 (33-310)	11 (0-16)
DOC (compound S) (µg/dl)	8 (3-17)	56 (18-119)	48 (14-110)	8 (3-17)	56 (18-119)	48 (14-110)
17-OH-pregnenolone (ng/dl)	56 (15-151)	318 (165-441)	262 (78-400)	118 (44-235)	798 (347-1170)	680 (189-1025)
17-OH-progesterone (ng/dl)	46 (10-110)	185 (83-280)	139 (30-240)	58 (14-169)	154 (88-292)	96 (37-216)
Testosterone (ng/dl)	5 (<3-9)	9 (<3-15)	4 (0-7)	82 (5-310)	89 (5-294)	7 (0-12)
Precursor/Product Ratios*						
$\frac{\text{17-OH-Progesterone}}{\text{Cortisol}}$	3.5 (1.0-6.0)	6.4 (5.0-9.5)		5.5 (1.0-10.0)	6.4 (3.5-9.5)	
$\frac{\text{DHEA}}{\text{Androstenedione}}$	1.8 (1.1-1.5)	1.9 (1.5-4.5)		3.2 (1.5-6.0)	4.0 (2.6-7.0)	
$\frac{\text{17-OH-pregnenolone}}{\text{17-OH-progesterone}}$	1.2 (1.0-6.0)	1.7 (1.2-4.9)		2.0 (1.9-3.5)	5.2 (2.0-8.0)	
$\frac{\text{17-OH-pregnenolone}}{\text{DHEA}}$	0.9 (0.3-1.5)	2.5 (1.5-6.8)		0.45 (0.2-0.7)	1.4 (0.5-2.3)	
$\frac{\text{DOC (compound S)}}{\text{Cortisol}}$	5.5 (3.5-7.5)	7.1 (4.0-12.0)		5.4 (3.5-7.5)	7.2 (4.5-12.0)	

Data supplied by Endocrine Sciences, Tarzana, CA.

Note: Data shown as mean and normal range for adrenal steroids in plasma before and after ACTH stimulation.

*Use of precursor/product ratios is helpful in diagnostic evaluations of children with premature pubarche/adrenarche. In late-onset 21-hydroxylase deficiency, ACTH-stimulated 17-OH-pregnenolone/cortisol ratio is above 6.4 (>2 SD above normal mean), whereas 17-OH-pregnenolone/17-OH-progesterone ratio >8.0 and DHEA/androstenedione above 7.0 (>2 SD above normal mean) can be seen in 3β-hydroxysteroid deficiency. Elevated serum DOC/cortisol ratio (>12.0) in a child with premature adrenarche and hypertension may be consistent with 11-hydroxylase deficiency.

ACTH, adrenocorticotropic hormone; *DHEA,* dehydroepiandrosterone; *DHEA-S,* dehydroepiandrosterone sulfate; *DOC,* deoxycorticosterone.

VAGINAL BLEEDING. Vaginal bleeding in the absence of breast development does not represent the onset of menses. Most commonly it is caused by foreign bodies, trauma (e.g., from masturbation), or sexual abuse. Documentation of a possible hymenal tear or a vaginal opening of more than 5 mm is consistent with vaginal penetration by a foreign body. Occasionally, tumors of the genital tract, such as botryoid sarcoma, may present with vaginal bleeding and discharge. When menarche occurs early without other secondary sexual characteristics, the possibility of McCune-Albright syndrome should be considered.

ADRENAL HYPERPLASIA AND TUMORS. Pseudoprecocious puberty may also be the result of adrenal hyperplasia that leads to excessive androgen production.[44] In boys, adrenal enzymatic defects, such as 21-hydroxylase deficiency, may lead to the appearance of pubic hair, acne, penile enlargement, accelerated growth, and advanced skeletal maturation without testicular enlargement. In girls, this condition is characterized by heterosexual precocity, with the adrenal steroidogenic defects (21-hydroxylase, 11-hydroxylase, and 3β-hydroxysteroid dehydrogenase) producing early appearance of pubic hair, acne, clitoral enlargement, linear growth acceleration, and advanced bone age. Male-pattern baldness and severe cystic acne refractory to oral antibiotics and retinoic acid has been attributed to late-onset 21-hydroxylase deficiency.

Children with adrenal hyperplasia generally have varying degrees of cortisol deficiency with or without mineralocorticoid deficiency. Determination of the specific enzymatic adrenal defect that has led to pseudoprecocious puberty is best accomplished by evaluating the levels of adrenal hormones through an adrenocorticotropic hormone (ACTH) stimulation test (Table 28-6). This test is useful in differentiating late-onset adrenal hyperplasia from polycystic ovarian syndrome. In the late-onset 21-hydroxylase variety of adrenal hyperplasia, the baseline 17-OH-progesterone is sufficiently elevated to obviate the need for a full test. The late-onset, or nonclassic, 3β-hydroxysteroid defect can be established only with a corticotropin test. In patients with pubarche who do not demonstrate acceleration of linear growth, advanced skeletal maturity, and other secondary sex characteristics, the corticotropin stimulation test is not indicated. Mild, late-onset 11-hydroxylase deficiency should be suspected if there is hypertension and laboratory evidence of hyperaldosteronism, hypernatremia, and kypokalemic alkalosis.

Tumors of the adrenal cortex also have been described in pseudoprecocious puberty. These tumors produce excessive androgens or estrogens, resulting in either virilizing or feminizing sexual precocity, and they may be of a malignant nature. Occasionally, these tumors are associated with cushingoid signs, which are secondary to glucocorticoid overproduction, and hypertension. Virilizing tumors also have been associated with Beckwith's syndrome, some hamartomatous lesions, and astrocytomas. Laboratory tests reveal elevated levels of DHEA and androstenedione in children with such tumors. The diagnosis of an adrenal tumor is confirmed by abdominal ultrasonography, computed tomography (CT) scanning, and/or MRI.

Management of adrenal hyperplasia includes glucocorticoid replacement therapy with complete adrenal suppression. Treatment of adrenal tumors involves surgical intervention in combination with chemotherapy and/or radiotherapy based on the histopathologic picture.

OTHER TUMORS. Rare tumors of the testes, such as Leydig or Sertoli cell tumors, dysgerminomas, and gonadoblastomas, may be responsible for premature sexual development in boys. These tumors are characterized by lack of enlargement, or asymmetric enlargement, of the testes along with greatly elevated serum testosterone levels. Testicular sonography and biopsy are essential to establish the diagnosis.

Testicular tumors, such as Leydig or Sertoli cell tumors, usually require surgical therapy with or without chemotherapy; gonadotropin-secreting tumors, such as hepatoblastomas, are often radiosensitive. In girls, surgical resection of large ovarian cysts is indicated because of the risk of torsion and potential transformation to malignancy.

DELAYED PUBERTY

DEFINITIONS

The absence of early physical changes of puberty by age 13 years in girls and 14 years in boys justifies evaluation for causes of delayed puberty. Lack of appropriate pubertal progression also requires diagnostic assessment. Such assessment is needed if there is a 5-year delay between the onset of puberty and menarche (in girls) or completion of genital growth (in boys). Approximately 3% of children have a delay in the development of secondary sex characteristics.[45,46] In contrast to precocious puberty, delayed puberty is noted more often in boys than in girls; most have no underlying pathology. Often, such patients are considered to have constitutional growth delay. However, some children with delayed puberty may present with a wide variety of abnormalities (Box 28-1).

CONSTITUTIONAL GROWTH DELAY

The most common cause of short stature and sexual infantilism in the adolescent period is constitutional growth delay (CGD), accounting for more than one third of growth disorders of children evaluated by pediatric endocrinologists.[47] The total incidence in the population may be even higher, because pediatricians do not usually refer patients with CGD to an endocrinologist. This condition is characterized by short stature as a variant of normal growth. The patients are typical "slow growers" and "late bloomers." Patients with CGD show delayed skeletal maturation, retarded sexual development, and frequently a family history of the same problems. CGD is often recognized long before adolescence, when sexual development is not a concern. As an aid to understanding the evaluation of CGD, a representative case is discussed below (Fig. 28-4).

B.P. was a 14½-year-old white boy who presented to the pediatric endocrinologist with absent pubertal development and short stature. At the time of evaluation, his weight and height were below the 5th percentile, with weight appropriate for height. A review of the patient's growth records demonstrated a deceleration of linear growth before 3 years of age. However, after the third year of life, growth progressed at an appropriate rate below but parallel to the 5th percentile by National Center for Health Statistics standards. Growth followed the 5th percentile for the late maturer according to the chart of Tanner.[48] The patient continued to grow at a prepubertal rate of 4.6 cm per year until the time of evaluation. Weight remained proportional to height throughout, progressing on the 5th percentile until 14 years of age.

Detailed evaluation of this patient revealed no history of chronic illness, dieting, unusual food patterns and aversions, or

BOX 28-1
Differential Diagnosis of Delayed Puberty

I. Normal or low serum gonadotropin levels
  A. Constitutional delay
  B. Chronic systemic illnesses (regional enteritis, cyanotic congenital heart disease, sickle cell anemia, malnutrition)
  C. Gonadotropin deficiency
    1. Kallmann's syndrome (isolated gonadotropin deficiency)
    2. Congenital hypopituitarism
    3. Central nervous system disorders
      a. Tumors (craniopharyngiomas, germinomas, astrocytomas, neurofibromas, pituitary adenomas, histiocytosis X)
      b. Postinfectious brain lesions (encephalitis, meningitis)
      c. Head injury
      d. Radiation injury
      e. Congenital malformations of brain (septo-optic dysplasia)
  D. Endocrinopathies (hypothyroidism, hyperprolactinemia, diabetes mellitus, Cushing's disease)
  E. Anatomic anomalies (absent uterus or vagina, imperforate hymen)
  F. Psychiatric disorders and psychosocial dwarfism
II. Elevated serum gonadotropin levels
  A. Turner's syndrome
  B. Klinefelter's syndrome
  C. Pure gonadal dysgenesis (XX and XY)
  D. Enzymatic defects in steroidogenesis (cholesterol desmolase complex, 3β-hydroxysteroid dehydrogenase, 17α-hydroxysteroid, $C_{20,22}$-desmolase, 17β-hydroxysteroid oxidoreductase
  E. Bilateral gonadal failure
    1. Postinfectious (orchitis, parotitis [mumps], and coxsackie B virus infection)
    2. Autoimmune destruction
    3. Radiation injury (doses in excess of 1500-2000 rad)
    4. Chemotherapy
    5. Galactosemia
    6. Posttraumatic
    7. Postsurgical
    8. Idiopathic (vanishing testis syndrome)
    9. Resistant ovary syndrome
  F. Testicular feminization
III. Miscellaneous disorders
  A. Prader-Willi syndrome
  B. Laurence-Moon-Biedl syndrome
  C. Alström's syndrome
  D. Noonan's syndrome
  E. Germinal cell aplasia (Del Castillo's syndrome)
  F. Myotonic dystrophy

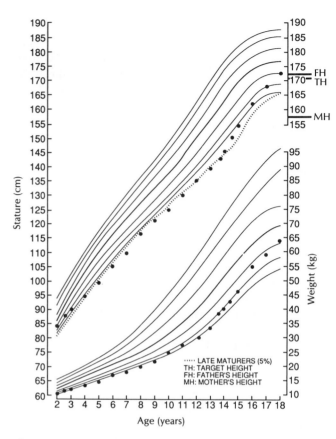

Fig. 28-4. Growth chart of patient B.P. showing constitutional growth delay.

excessive exercise. The family history suggested a delayed onset of puberty in the patient's father, who did not shave until the age of 19 years.

Physical examination revealed a height below the 5th percentile and a weight in the 10th percentile. B.P.'s height age was 11.5 years. He had a normal arm span for height and a normal ratio of upper/lower body segments. Assessment of dental maturation indicated an approximate dental age of 11 to 12 years. There were no apparent dysmorphic features (webbed neck, low hairline, antimongoloid slants of palpebral fissures, cubitus valgus), as may occur in Noonan's syndrome. Visual fields and fundi were normal, with no evidence of papilledema; the neurologic examination showed no deficits, as may be seen in some patients with space-occupying brain lesions. Neurodevelopmental milestones were appropriate for chronologic age. The thyroid was palpable but not enlarged, with no clinical evidence of hypothyroidism, which can also result in delayed sexual development. Abdominal examination revealed no evidence of organomegaly or intraabdominal mass, thus decreasing the likelihood of Crohn's disease, and no other aberrations found in underlying systemic illnesses that could lead to delayed puberty. There was no pubic or axillary hair and the testicles were of Prader 2-ml size (prepubertal); genitalia were Tanner stage 1 and unambiguous.

TABLE 28-7
Principal Features of Constitutional Growth Delay and Nutritional Dwarfism

Feature	CGD	NND	OND (CIBD)
Growth rate	Normal	Subnormal	Subnormal
Weight gain	Normal	Subnormal	Subnormal
Weight/height ratio	Normal	Normal or subnormal	Normal or subnormal
Sexual development	Delayed	Delayed	Delayed
Bone age	Delayed	Delayed	Delayed
Biochemical parameters			
Sedimentation rate	Normal	Normal	Abnormal
Insulin-like growth factor (somatomedin C)	Normal	Normal	Subnormal
Retinol-binding protein	Normal	Normal	Subnormal
Prealbumin	Normal	Normal	Subnormal
Albumin	Normal	Normal	Subnormal
Transferrin	Normal	Normal	Subnormal
Thyroid function tests	Normal	Normal	Normal
Serum folate	Normal	Normal	Subnormal
Na^+/K^+ ATPase	Normal	Subnormal	Not known

CGD, constitutional growth delay; *CIBD*, chronic inflammatory bowel disease; *NND*, nonorganic nutritional dwarfism; *OND*, organic nutritional dwarfism.

Radiologic assessment of bone age (BA) suggested a significant maturational delay of approximately 2 to 3 years compared with chronologic age. This delayed bone age corresponded to a height age (HA) of 12 years, with a BA/HA ratio of 1.0, which is consistent with the diagnosis of CGD. In contrast, delayed skeletal maturity disproportionate to height (BA/HA <1.0) suggests possible pathologic or endocrine causes of delayed growth and sexual development. Complete blood count, erythrocyte sedimentation rate, serum electrolyte levels, liver function tests, and thyroid function tests were within normal limits. Serum gonadotropins, testosterone, and prolactin levels corresponded to prepubertal values (Table 28-2). A Gn-RH stimulation test did not result in a rise of LH and FSH, and results were indistinguishable from the levels of normal prepubertal males (Table 28-3). These biochemical findings correspond to Tanner stage 1 of sexual development and confirm the clinical assessment of pubertal stage. It should be noted that there is great difficulty in using the Gn-RH test to differentiate the patient with CGD from one with hypogonadotropic hypogonadism (Kallmann's syndrome),[49] since both patients have a low LH response after Gn-RH stimulation. However, it has been suggested that the use of a Gn-RH agonist (nafarelin) to assess a 24-hour LH response may help distinguish these two entities.[50] The applicability and validity of using such an agonist in the diagnostic work-up of patients with delayed puberty is yet to be determined. The detailed work-up described here can confirm the diagnosis of CGD and rule out the possibility of underlying pathology. However, longitudinal evaluation of growth progression may suffice in most instances, as this patient grew well and developed sexually. In our index patient with CGD, psychological reassurance

allowed him to follow his natural course. The pattern of linear growth showed gradual acceleration at the onset of puberty around age 15 years. B.P. continued to show pubertal growth acceleration and attained his familial target height by 18 years of age (Fig. 28-4).

Differential Diagnosis

Nutritional dwarfism. It is often difficult to distinguish CGD from nutritional dwarfism (ND).[51] The principal differences between CGD and ND are shown in Table 28-7. Patients with suboptimal nutrient intake may have a healthy appearance with short stature and delayed puberty that resembles CGD. Only a complete dietary history can reveal the underlying nutritional deficiency or suboptimal nutrient intake. The clinician may elicit a history of previous dieting for a variety of reasons, which include fear of obesity, fear of hypercholesterolemia and other unspecified concerns, or dietary beliefs such as vegetarianism.[51-53] A history of compulsive exercising, vomiting, and weight loss should be clues to more severe eating disorders such as anorexia nervosa. Growth failure and delayed puberty may be seen in these patients when the disease starts early, especially before 12 years of age. Patients with ND and delayed puberty demonstrate a different growth pattern than those with CGD (Fig. 28-4). Patients with ND usually have growth (weight and height) that progresses along normal percentiles. However, when the nutrient intake decreases, weight and height increments slow down, and a downward shift across percentiles becomes evident. For instance, the patient with ND shown in Figure 28-5 demonstrates a rate of weight gain that decreased after 3 years of age, paralleled by a slow growth rate, and with height falling to the 10th percentile

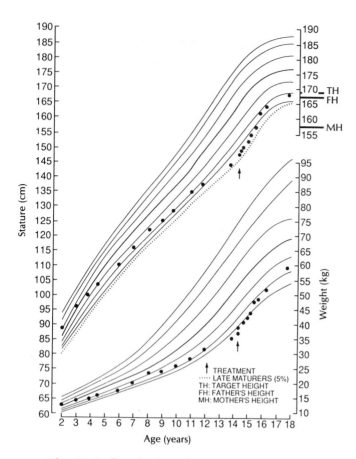

Fig. 28-5. Growth chart of a patient with nutritional, or nonorganic, dwarfism. Institution of appropriate nutritional intake *(arrow)* results in satisfactory weight gain with catch-up growth.

by 6 years of age. Between 6 and 12 years of age, weight and height proceeded along the 10th percentile, but thereafter poor weight gain with corresponding decreased growth was noted. Both weight and height fell below the 5th percentile for age, although the height was at the 5th percentile for late maturers in the Tanner classification. After nutritional rehabilitation, the patient showed satisfactory catch-up growth, with weight and height reaching levels expected for the family. It is important to note that this pattern of growth differs from the pattern of patients with CGD (Fig. 28-4), in whom weight and height progression is appropriate after age 3 years until puberty, which is attained at a later age. Although physicians generally follow growth patterns accurately in the assessment of patients with growth and pubertal development disorders, there is often little consideration given to body weight progression. Normal progression of weight and height in a short child suggests CGD and/or familial short stature; normal weight progression in a patient with slow growth and delayed sexual development is suggestive of an endocrine disorder; poor weight gain associated with poor height increments suggests ND. It is possible for there to be no body weight deficit for height,

just lack of adequate weight gain, in patients with ND.[52] After the institution of appropriate nutritional intake, a satisfactory weight gain with catch-up growth is attained in patients with ND (Fig. 28-5). The bone age delay of ND patients usually corresponds to the time when weight gain slowed or ceased, whereas that of CGD does not correlate with the weight progression of the patient (Fig. 28-4).

Although ND and delayed puberty may be due to nonorganic causes, it may also be associated with other pathologic conditions, particularly Crohn's disease or occult celiac disease.[54,55] In fact, chronic inflammatory bowel disease may be manifested clinically by a growth pattern characteristic of ND (Fig. 28-5) and delayed puberty without any other clinical abnormalities. Decreased growth velocity and weight gain may precede any gastrointestinal manifestations and/or radiologic and biochemical evidence of Crohn's disease for up to 3 years. Asymptomatic, or so-called occult, celiac disease also should be considered in the differential diagnosis of a child with poor growth and delayed sexual development, even when there is no clinical or biochemical evidence of malabsorption.

Organic ND caused by inflammatory bowel disease and celiac disease may be differentiated from CGD and nonorganic ND by alterations in some biochemical indexes. Most patients with Crohn's disease have an elevated sedimentation rate with or without underlying iron, zinc, and/or magnesium deficiencies.[56,57] On the other hand, those with celiac disease usually have antigliadin and antiendomysial antibodies, low serum folate level, low serum ferritin level, and microcytic anemia, and they exhibit typical alterations of the intestinal mucosa. In addition, patients with chronic inflammatory bowel disease have decreased IGF and normal or low serum protein levels. Finally, it has been shown that the only biochemical alteration detectable is a response in red cell Na^+/K^+ ATPase (adenosinetriphosphatase) activity, a marker of nutritional status, in patients with nonorganic ND.[58]

OTHER PATHOLOGIC CAUSES. Patients with CGD also need to be distinguished from patients with other pathologic causes of growth and pubertal delay. The latter usually present with a history of delayed growth and sexual development associated with a subnormal growth rate (<3rd percentile on a growth velocity chart), significant delay in skeletal maturity that exceeds the delay of height age (BA <HA), and/or abnormal arm span/height ratio. Documentation of the above features necessitates additional diagnostic testing to rule out possible underlying pathologic causes. The differential diagnosis of pathologic causes of delayed puberty is shown in Box 28-1.

Many chronic systemic diseases are known to cause growth and pubertal delay or lack of pubertal progression. These include sickle cell anemia, diabetes mellitus, cyanotic heart disease, chronic connective tissue disorders, cystic fibrosis, CNS tumors (as well as their respective modes of therapy, including surgery, chemotherapy, or radiotherapy), any major CNS infection, trauma, and malformations such as optic dysplasia. Additionally, in patients with a history of abdominal pain, diarrhea, or abnormal stools, Crohn's disease or celiac disease should be suspected.

Individuals with CGD may be differentiated from those with delayed puberty secondary to panhypopituitarism or isolated hypopituitarism by the presence in the latter group of subnormal growth rate (2 SD below mean for age), abnormal upper/lower segment ratio less than 1.0 (0.88 in blacks), and abnormal arm span/height ratio (arm span >5 cm more than height). If, however, a hypothalamic or pituitary lesion is suspected, the clinician should look for other clinical characteristics of hypopituitarism, such as hypothyroidism, diabetes insipidus, or hyposmia/anosmia (Kallmann's syndrome). A lateral skull x-ray examination or CT of the brain may reveal pituitary calcification, enlargement of the sella turcica, or a space-occupying lesion.

An abnormal upper/lower segment ratio is also present in primary hypogonadism, such as Klinefelter's syndrome. Testicular location (scrotal, inguinal, or nonpalpable), size, and consistency are important. A testis less than 2.0 cm along the longitudinal axis is prepubertal in size. A testicular size of 1.0 cm or less in a pubertal boy, particularly if unusually firm or soft, is suggestive of a hypogonadal state. A rise in circulating testosterone levels to higher than 300 ng/dl after 5 days of hCG stimulation (3000 $IU/m^2/day$) demonstrates adequate Leydig cell function.

It may be difficult to differentiate the patient with CGD from one with a neurosecretory GH defect. Indeed, some authors believe that this type of defect may be a feature of CGD. However, patients with CGD grow at a normal rate on the 5th percentile for late bloomers and have a mean overnight GH level of 3 ng/ml or more.[59] In contrast, patients with a neurosecretory GH defect have a subnormal growth rate (<3rd percentile on a growth velocity chart) and growth below the 5th percentile for late bloomers, with mean overnight GH levels below 3 ng/ml. Both conditions have a normal GH response to provocative GH tests.

Many endocrine disorders can delay both the onset of puberty and its progression. These include hypothyroidism, Cushing's disease, glucocorticoid excess, diabetes mellitus, and hyperprolactinemia. Anatomic anomalies, such as abnormal development of the müllerian system with absence of the uterus or the vagina, should be suspected in any girl who has not menstruated within 5 years of the onset of breast development.

Psychiatric disorders in later childhood or early adolescence may cause delay in the onset of puberty or its progression. Anorexia nervosa, probably the most common cause of hypogonadotropic hypogonadism in girls, is characterized by amenorrhea and undernutrition secondary to self-induced starvation. Delayed puberty may also be seen in older children with psychosocial dysfunction. Some of these children may display a voracious appetite and excessive thirst, even going so far as to search for food among garbage cans and to drink from toilet bowls. A number of factors have been noted to result in this behavioral pattern, such as institutional care, physical or psychological neglect, poor childrearing practices, socioeconomic deprivation, and emotional stress.[60,61] Clinicians should be aware that the history obtained from the parents or caregivers may not always reveal the true nature of the child's environment. It is necessary for clinicians to be alert to evidence of physical abuse such as bruising and/or fractures. In some cases, older children with psychosocial dwarfism have been found to show evidence of hypopituitarism. Bone age is delayed in these individuals, regardless of whether endocrine abnormalities are present.

Psychological Aspects

Similar to those with precocious puberty, adolescents with delayed puberty face psychosocial problems in dealing with their family and peers. Boys may be worried about their gender identity, the size of their sex organs, and their lack of sex characteristics and may feel out of step with their peers. Like boys, girls with delayed puberty usually avoid heterosexual social activities, seek younger friends, and are concerned about lack of secondary sex characteristics. Therefore, those with delayed puberty are at risk of having (1) poor body image and low self-esteem, (2) emotional reactions, (3) long-term dependency on parents, and (4) deficits in acquisition of appropriate social skills. It also has been reported that many boys with delayed puberty experience academic problems.[62] Psychological counseling can be helpful in the management of delayed puberty in patients with constitutional delay and other forms of hypogonadism, especially if hormonal treatment is being considered. The adolescent and family require continuous counseling and reassurance during hormonal treatment, since the effects of therapy are not immediately evident.

Treatment

Drug treatment of patients with CGD is controversial. Human growth hormone (HGH) is commercially available, and the practicing physician is now under mounting pressure to prescribe it for short children, especially males, even when they are not deficient in this hormone. The medical literature contains reports of improved growth with this treatment in "normal short children" who have constitutional delay and familial short stature.[63,64] However, there is no definite evidence that transient improvements in growth rates with HGH treatment or other growth-promoting agents will produce permanent beneficial effects and improve ultimate stature. Other pharmacologic agents have been used to stimulate growth as well as to promote sexual development.[65,66] Ideally, such agents should accomplish both of these objectives with minimal side effects and without danger of damage to the gonads or a decrease in final adult height. The medical literature contains many descriptions of anabolic compounds that are reputed to prevent induction of skeletal maturation but also have excellent growth-inducing properties. However, a similar number of reports question these claims.

In general, there seems to be a psychological advantage to inducing puberty in patients who might otherwise have very delayed sexual maturation. However, treatment with medications should be reserved for patients who have attained the psychological development appropriate for puberty. Therapy may not be indicated for any patient with a chronologic age less than 12 years or a bone age less than 10 years. It should always be kept in mind that anabolic steroids given for short periods may accelerate growth and bone maturation but will not increase ultimate height.[67]

Despite these concerns, low-dose therapy, 100 to 150 mg testosterone enanthate, may be given to males once every 4 weeks for a total of three doses. Within 1 month after the end of this regimen, most males show signs of penile enlargement and pubic hair growth, and most have a better self-image because of this development. If spontaneous pubertal development does not occur, a second regimen of 3-month testosterone therapy may be started. It is essential to monitor bone age during the course of therapy; if there is any evidence of excessive skeletal advancement, treatment should be discontinued. Oral or sublingual forms of methyltestosterone, 10 to 40 mg daily, may be used for short-term therapy of delayed puberty. The potential risk of the development of hepatocellular carcinoma as a long-term effect of oral testosterone seems remote with a short course of therapy. Once the patient reaches a bone age of 12 to 13 years, he will undergo spontaneous pubertal development, and testosterone should be discontinued. The use of an oral anabolic product (oxandrolone, 0.125 mg/kg/day) has been advocated for the treatment of constitutional pubertal delay. Although oxandrolone does not provide full physiologic replacement, its short-term use has been helpful in initiating puberty without significant bone age advancement.[68] The best course may be reassurance and psychosocial support without drug therapy. The patient described previously, B.P., was reassured that there was no evidence of an underlying pathologic cause for his delayed puberty and that in time he would undergo normal pubertal changes. Indeed, 6 months after his initial visit, he began to demonstrate early signs of puberty (testicular enlargement and pubic hair) that were associated with some linear growth acceleration. During follow-up, B.P. had a pubertal growth spurt (Fig. 28-4) and attained his family target height at 18 years of age.

PRIMARY GONADAL FAILURE

Turner's Syndrome

Patients with Turner's syndrome present with primary hypogonadism, which is characterized by a hypergonadotropic state at the chronologic age at which the onset of puberty is expected in normal girls. Other features of this syndrome include webbed neck (pterygium colli), highly arched palate, ptosis, low-set ears, increased carrying angle of the elbows (cubitus valgus), and lymphedema of the hands and feet (see Chapter 27, "Growth Disorders"). The characteristic karyotype of the patient with Turner's syndrome is 45,XO in females. However, the use of chromosomal analysis has led to the discovery of several other abnormalities of the X chromosome, such as mosaicism, rings, deletions, and rearrangements, each of which can result in one or more of the described features of Turner's syndrome and ovarian dysgenesis.

The incidence of sex-chromosome karyotype abnormalities with complete loss of the X chromosome has been reported to range from 1:2500 to 1:10,000 live-born females.[69,70] However, since the above data were obtained through Barr chromatin body screening techniques, it is highly likely that they underestimate the incidence, because mosaic or other structural abnormalities of the X chromosome may have been missed. The true incidence of Turner's syndrome is not clearly known, since newer chromosome-banding techniques have not been applied to large-population screening programs. In girls with Turner's syndrome, short stature is the most common cause of referral to the pediatric endocrinologist. The osseous abnormality responsible for short stature, affecting vertebrae and long bones, gives the body a stocky appearance with an abnormal upper/lower segment ratio and a shieldlike chest. Scoliosis can occur in up to 12% of patients. Many studies have revealed that GH response to pharmacologic stimuli and physiologic release are similar to that in normal age-matched girls during the prepubertal period. However, GH release is not enhanced after this stage because of lack of onset of puberty in these girls. The abnormal growth in Turner's patients may be secondary to an underlying disturbance of the skeleton, resulting in an abnormal response to GH. Markedly elevated levels of serum gonadotropins, especially FSH, are demonstrated in girls with Turner's syndrome after the age of 10 to 11 years. Use of the

Gn-RH stimulation test to assess the hypothalamic-pituitary axis reveals an exaggerated gonadotropin response in patients with this syndrome.

Klinefelter's Syndrome

The incidence of Klinefelter's syndrome,[71,72] or seminiferous tubule dysgenesis, is approximately $1:600$ to $1:1000$ live births (see Chapter 73, "Congenital and Genetic Disorders"). The most common chromosomal pattern in these patients is XXY. However, multiple X (XXXY) or Y (XXYY) chromosomal patterns or mosaic patterns (XXY/XY) have been reported. Most boys with this disorder are not identified until puberty or early adulthood. However, some patients may present to the pediatrician because of undescended testes, small external genitalia, and/or behavioral problems or mild mental retardation during childhood. Moreover, gynecomastia is a common complaint during puberty. Patients with this syndrome are usually tall and slender, with a decreased upper/lower segment ratio and increased arm span. At the onset of puberty, gonadotropin concentrations in the serum rise. Testicular growth is arrested at midpuberty as a result of progressive hyalinization and fibrosis of the seminiferous tubules associated with adenomatous changes of the Leydig cells and impaired spermatogenesis. Testosterone levels in these patients vary from low to almost normal as a result of variable degrees of Leydig cell function. Therefore, the onset of puberty usually occurs at a normal age, but secondary sex characteristics do not reach that of full maturity. The testes are usually hard and measure less than 5 ml in volume. Gynecomastia results from the increased estrogen/testosterone ratio in patients with Klinefelter's syndrome.

Pure Gonadal Dysgenesis

Gonadal dysgenesis[72] (XX and XY) may be sporadic or familial in incidence. Stature is normal and none of the dysmorphic features of Turner's syndrome are present. These individuals usually have eunuchoid body proportions. Patients with XX gonadal dysgenesis usually have a sexually infantile female phenotype, with or without some virilization, as a result of androgen secretion from the hilar cells of the ovary. An autosomal recessive pattern is the mode of inheritance in the familial type of gonadal dysgenesis. The ovaries are streaked gonads associated with low serum sex steroid levels and elevated gonadotropin levels. Individuals with XY gonadal dysgenesis are taller than those with XX gonadal dysgenesis. The former have an infantile female appearance, with or without some virilization. In XY gonadal dysgenesis patients there is a high incidence of testicular tumors. In familial cases the mode of inheritance is X-linked or male-limited autosomal dominant with genetic heterogeneity. The

testosterone level is lower than in normal males and gonadotropin levels are elevated. Amenorrhea is a major feature of patients with pure gonadal dysgenesis.

Enzymatic Defects in Steroidogenesis

Defects in testosterone biosynthesis, such as 17α-hydroxylase deficiency and 17β-hydroxysteroid oxidoreductase deficiency, are types of familial male hermaphroditism. Also, males with 3β-hydroxysteroid dehydrogenase deficiency present with ambiguous genitalia, while females may appear virilized. Further, patients with cholesterol desmolase deficiency have a phenotypic female appearance regardless of the genotype. Finally, enzyme defects in the female that result in impairment of estrogen biosynthesis by the ovary can produce amenorrhea.

Bilateral Gonadal Failure

Primary gonadal failure can be caused by infection, such as orchitis parotidea associated with mumps; autoimmune destruction, such as oophoritis with or without Addison's disease; chemotherapy and radiation injuries; trauma; and surgical removal. In patients with galactosemia, toxic effects of galactose or its metabolites on the ovary in utero or during the neonatal period have been reported. "Idiopathic vanishing testes syndrome" is a condition characterized by lack of puberty in a healthy male with a 46,XY karyotype and with nonpalpable testes in spite of masculine-appearing external genitalia. It is believed that this syndrome is due to atrophy or destruction of the testes after fetal differentiation of the external genitalia. Patients with resistant ovary syndrome usually present with primary amenorrhea and sexual immaturity. The ovaries are small, containing primordial follicles.

The testicular feminization, or androgen insensitivity, syndrome is secondary to end-organ insensitivity to androgens that can range from that seen in phenotypic females with complete androgen resistance to that seen in phenotypic males manifesting only infertility.[73,74] The prevalence is about $1:20,000$ to $1:64,000$, and it is the third most common cause of primary amenorrhea, after Turner's syndrome and absence of the vagina. At the time of puberty, patients with complete resistance to androgens proceed with feminization, but no menses occur and no pubic or axillary hair develops. The testes are atrophic with arrested sperm formation in the presence of Leydig cell hyperplasia. Gonadotropin concentrations in androgen resistance syndromes reflect the production and response to inhibin but the lack of response to androgens. Therefore, the LH level is elevated and the FSH level is normal in the basal or Gn-RH–stimulated state. On the other hand, partial androgen resistance, or Reifenstein's syndrome, is characterized by a small phallus, hypospadias, small testes, gynecomastia, and azoospermia at puberty. Serum androgen and estrogen levels are elevated, with varying degrees of virilization.

Deficiency in 5α-reductase transmitted as an autosomal recessive condition in genetic males has been classified as an androgen resistance syndrome. However, the disorder is secondary to deficiency of the 5α-reductase enzyme in the scrotal skin, which is responsible for the conversion of testosterone to dihydrotestosterone. Children with this disorder have a blind vaginal pouch and a small phallic structure at birth. During infancy and childhood, they are reared as girls. However, virilization occurs when the testes descend to a labial location at puberty, and these individuals demonstrate deepening of the voice, muscular development, and an increase in phallic size, allowing them to attain a phenotypic male appearance. Full beard growth, acne, and temporary balding do not develop because of the lack of dihydrotestosterone. Patients may be infertile because of blind sperm ducts, despite normal spermatogenesis. Del Castillo's syndrome is characterized by germinal cell aplasia and a moderately increased serum FSH level in patients who are normally virilized. Patients with myotonic dystrophy present with postpubertal seminiferous tubule sclerosis and cataracts.

MISCELLANEOUS DISORDERS

A number of different entities involve delayed or abnormal adolescent development (Table 28-7). Prader-Willi syndrome is a sporadically occurring condition characterized by infantile hypotonia, massive obesity and lack of satiety, short stature, hypogonadism, acromicria (small hands and feet), and mental retardation.[75] Bilateral cryptorchidism and a small, flat scrotum are also characteristic. There is usually a blunted or absent response to Gn-RH stimulation. It is believed that the hypogonadism in Prader-Willi syndrome is due to abnormal hypothalamic function. Boys and girls can be affected in equal numbers.

The Laurence-Moon-Biedl syndrome is inherited as an autosomal recessive condition with intrafamilial variability.[76] It is characterized by polydactyly, obesity, short stature, hypogonadotropic or hypergonadotropic hypogonadism, retinitis pigmentosa, and mental retardation. Alström's syndrome involves hypogonadism, retinitis pigmentosa, diabetes mellitus, and neurogenic deafness.

Noonan's syndrome (pseudo-Turner syndrome) is found in both sexes, with an incidence of 1 in 8000 live births. It is a dominantly inherited condition and the presenting features are similar to those of Turner syndrome (e.g., webbed neck and cubitus valgus).[72] However, there are other characteristic features, such as

triangular-shaped face, pectus excavatum, pulmonic stenosis, and mental retardation. Affected males may have undescended testes that are often functionally impaired in testosterone and sperm production, and these individuals may present with delayed puberty.

TREATMENT OF HYPOGONADISM

Boys

Treatment of the male with hypogonadotropic hypogonadism or testicular defect consists of full androgen replacement to achieve and maintain an adult male state. This includes intramuscular injections of testosterone enanthate or cypionate, at intervals of 2 weeks (200 mg) or 3 weeks (300 mg). Injections of 400 mg every 4 weeks are not recommended because they result in supraphysiologic levels for 7 to 10 days, and then during the fourth week the levels are subnormal. Transdermal scrotal patches may become a substitute for this mode of therapy. The rapidity of the desired pubertal development may be controlled by titrating dosages of androgen upward to full replacement within 3 to 4 years. The dosage of initial therapy depends on the age and maturity of the patient and the rapidity of pubertal development desired. The usual starting dose for intramuscular injections ranges from 50 to 100 mg every 4 weeks.

Ejaculation, as well as semen volume and its appearance, will be normal provided that accessory sex glands are well formed. Induction of spermatogenesis in some males with this condition can be attained by the use of hCG or Gn-RH. This therapy should be provided for adult men at the time that they desire paternity, since it is expensive and cumbersome.

Girls

Initial replacement treatment for young girls with delayed puberty is low-dose estrogen (e.g., 0.3 mg Premarin or ethinyl estradiol, 0.02 mg daily, or the 0.05 mg transdermal patch applied once or twice a week) given for 6 to 12 months. Cyclic estrogen-progesterone can be started if break-through bleeding occurs during this time, with low-dose contraceptive pills used. Cyclic therapy can also be achieved by providing a daily estrogen regimen (ethinyl estradiol, 0.02 to 0.1 mg) for 21 days of the calendar month and by adding progesterone (medroxyprogesterone, 5 or 10 mg/day, or norethindrone, 5 mg/day) for the last 10 of the 21 days (days 12 to 21). The medications are then stopped from day 22 until the first day of the calendar month, at which time the patient should begin estrogen again, even if her period has not stopped. The dosage of estrogen can be varied, adjusted to the rapidity and adequacy of pubertal development.

Ethinyl estradiol (0.02 to 0.10 mg/day), conjugated estrogen (0.03 to 1.25 mg/day), or transdermal treatment to deliver 0.05 mg to 1.0 mg daily can be used. Once full pubertal development has been reached, the estrogen dosage should be the minimum that maintains normal menstrual flow and prevents calcium bone loss, equivalent to 0.625 mg conjugated estrogen. Progesterone in the regimen can be given as medroxyprogesterone, 5 or 10 mg/day, or norethindrone, 5 mg/day.

In some cases of Turner's syndrome, spontaneous menstruation may occur and replacement therapy may not be required. Some cases of fertility in Turner's syndrome have also been reported.[77] In addition, in vitro fertilization can provide a potential opportunity for childbearing in some patients with Turner's syndrome and other causes of gonadal failure who have normally differentiated müllerian structures.[78]

References

1. Kaplan SL, Grumbach MM: Pathogenesis of sexual precocity. In Grumbach MM, Sizonenko PC, Aubert ML, editors: *Control of the onset of puberty,* Baltimore, 1990, Williams & Wilkins; pp 620-660.
2. Reindollar RH, McDonough PG: Etiology and evaluation of delayed sexual development, *Pediatr Clin North Am* 28:267-286, 1981.
3. Lee PA: Disorders of puberty. In Lifshitz F, editor: *Pediatric endocrinology: a clinical guide,* ed 3, New York, 1995, Marcel Dekker; pp 175-195.
4. Lee PA: Normal ages of pubertal events among American males and females, *J Adolesc Health Care* 1:26-29, 1980.
5. Apter D, Butzow TL, Laughlin GA, et al: Gonadotropin-releasing hormone pulse generator activity during pubertal transition in girls: pulsatile and diurnal patterns of circulating gonadotropins, *J Clin Endocrinol Metab* 76:940-949, 1993.
6. Garibaldi LR, Picco P, Magier S, et al: Serum luteinizing hormone concentrations, as measured by a sensitive immunoradiometric assay, in children with normal, precocious or delayed pubertal development, *J Clin Endocrinol Metab* 72:888-898, 1991.
7. Kaplan SL, Grumbach MM: Pathophysiology and treatment of sexual precocity, *J Clin Endocrinol Metab* 71:785-789, 1990.
8. Schwarz HP, Tschaeppeler H, Zuppinger K: Unsustained central sexual precocity in four girls, *Am J Med Sci* 299:260-264, 1990.
9. Ross JL, Pescovitz OH, Barnes K, et al: Growth hormone secretory dynamics in children with precocious puberty, *J Pediatr* 110:369-372, 1987.
10. Harris DA, Van Vliet G, Egli CA, et al: Somatomedin-C in normal puberty and in true precocious puberty before and after treatment with a potent luteinizing hormone–releasing hormone agonist, *J Clin Endocrinol Metab* 61:152-159, 1985.
11. Fontoura M, Brauner R, Prevot C, et al: Precocious puberty in girls: early diagnosis of a slowly progressing variant, *Arch Dis Child* 64:1170-1176, 1989.
12. Bourguignon JP: Variations in duration of pubertal growth: a mechanism compensating for differences in timing of puberty and minimizing their effects on final height. Belgian Study Group for Paediatric Endocrinology, *Acta Paediatr Scand (suppl)* 347:16-24, 1988.
13. Kreiter M, Burstein S, Rosenfield RL, et al: Preserving adult height potential in girls with idiopathic true precocious puberty, *J Pediatr* 117:364-370, 1990.
14. Saenz de Rodriguez CA, Bongiovanni AM, Conde de Borrego L: An epidemic of precocious development in Puerto Rican children, *J Pediatr* 107:393-396, 1985.
15. Merritt RJ: Obesity, *Curr Probl Pediatr* 12:1-58, 1982.
16. Atchison JA, Lee PA, Albright AL: Reversible suprasellar pituitary mass secondary to hypothyroidism, *JAMA* 262:3175-3177, 1989.
17. Mahachoklertwattana P, Kaplan SL, Grumbach MM: The luteinizing hormone–releasing hormone–secreting hypothalamic hamartoma is a congenital malformation: natural history, *J Clin Endocrinol Metab:*118-124, 1993.
18. Wierman ME, Beardsworth DE, Mansfield M J, et al: Puberty without gonadotropins: a unique mechanism of sexual development, *N Engl J Med* 312:65-72, 1985.
19. Oerter KE, Uriarte MM, Rose SR, et al: Gonadotropin secretory dynamics during puberty in normal girls and boys, *J Clin Endocrinol Metab* 71:1251-1258, 1990.
20. Foster CM, Comite F, Pescovitz OH, et al: Variable response to a long-acting agonist of luteinizing hormone–releasing hormone in girls with McCune-Albright syndrome, *J Clin Endocrinol Metab* 59:801-805, 1984.
21. Clemons RD, Kappy MS, Stuart TE, et al: Long-term effectiveness of depot gonadotropin-releasing hormone analogue in the treatment of children with central precocious puberty, *Am J Dis Child* 147:653-657, 1993.
22. Starceski PJ, Lee PA, Albright AL, et al: Hypothalamic hamartomas and sexual precocity. Evaluation of treatment options, *Am J Dis Child* 144:225-228, 1990.
23. Ehrhardt AA: Abnormal puberty: psychological implications and treatment issues. In Shaffer D, Ehrhardt AA, Greenhill LL, editors: *The clinical guide to child psychiatry,* New York, 1985, Free Press, pp 145-160.
24. Ehrhardt AA, Meyer-Bahlburg HF: Idiopathic precocious puberty in girls: long-term effects on adolescent behavior, *Acta Endocrinol (suppl)* 279:247-253, 1986.
25. Sonis WA, Comite F, Blue J, et al: Behavior problems and social competence in girls with true precocious puberty, *J Pediatr* 106:156-161, 1985.
26. Sonis WA, Comite F, Pescovitz OH, et al: Biobehavioral aspects of precocious puberty, *J Am Acad Child Adolesc Psychiatry* 25:674-679, 1986.
27. Money J, Neil J: Precocious puberty, IQ and idiopathic precocious sexual maturation, *Pediatr Res* 1:59-65, 1967.
28. Schwindinger WF, Levine MA: McCune-Albright syndrome, *Trends Endocrinol Metab* 4:238-242, 1993.
29. Kaufman FR, Costin G, Reid BS: Autonomous ovarian hyperfunction followed by gonadotropin-dependent puberty in McCune-Albright syndrome, *Clin Endocrinol* 24:239-242, 1986.
30. Boepple PA, Frisch LS, Wierman ME, et al: The natural history of autonomous gonadal function, adrenarche and central puberty in gonadotropin-independent precocious puberty, *J Clin Endocrinol Metab* 75:1550-1555, 1992.
31. Shenker A, Laue L, Kosugi S, et al: A constitutively activating mutation of the luteinizing hormone receptor in familial male precocious puberty, *Nature* 365:652-654, 1993.
32. Ilicki A, Prager-Lewin R, Kauli R, et al: Premature thelarche—natural history and sex hormone secretion in 68 girls, *Acta Paediatr Scand* 73:756-762, 1984.
33. Nydick M, Bustos J, Dale JH, et al: Gynecomastia in adolescent boys, *JAMA* 173:449-454, 1961.
34. Lee PA: The relationship of concentrations of serum hormones to pubertal gynecomastia, *J Pediatr* 89:212-215, 1975.
35. Marynick SP, Nisula BC, Pita JC Jr, et al: Persistent pubertal macromastia, *J Clin Endocrinol Metab* 50:128-130, 1980.
36. Braunstein GD: Pubertal gynecomastia. In Lifshitz F, editor: *Pediatric endocrinology: a clinical guide,* ed 3, New York, 1996, Marcel Dekker; pp 197-205.

37. Moore DC, Schlaepfer LV, Paunier L, et al: Hormonal changes during puberty. Transient pubertal gynecomastia: abnormal androgen-estrogen ratios, *J Clin Endocrinol Metab* 58:492-499, 1984.

38. Turkington RW: Serum prolactin levels in patients with gynecomastia, *J Clin Endocrinol Metab* 34:62-66, 1972.

39. Schoenfield WA: Gynecomastia in adolescence. Personality effects, *Arch Gen Psychiatry* 5:68-76, 1961.

40. Eberle AJ, Sparrow JT, Keenan BS: Treatment of persistent pubertal gynecomastia with dihydrotestosterone heptanoate, *J Pediatr* 109:144-149, 1986.

41. Ibanez L, Virdis R, Potau N, et al: Natural history of premature pubarche: an auxological study, *J Clin Endocrinol Metab* 74:254-257, 1992.

42. Jabbar M, Pugliese M, Fort P, et al: Excess weight and precocious pubarche in children: alterations of the adrenocortical hormones, *J Am Coll Nutr* 4:289-296, 1991.

43. Siegel SF, Finegold DN, Urban MD, et al: Premature pubarche: etiologic heterogeneity, *J Clin Endocrinol Metab* 74:239-247, 1992.

44. Kohn B, Levine LS, Pollack MS, et al: Late-onset steroid 21-hydroxylase deficiency: a variant of classical congenital adrenal hyperplasia, *J Clin Endocrinol Metab* 55:817-827, 1982.

45. Burstein S, Rosenfield RL: Constitutional delay in growth and development. In Hintz R, Rosefeld RG, editors: *Growth abnormalities: contemporary issues in endocrinology and metabolism,* New York, 1987, Churchill Livingstone; pp 167-185.

46. Rosenfield RL: The ovary and female sexual maturation. In Kaplan SA, editor: *Clinical pediatric endocrinology,* ed 2, Philadelphia, 1989, WB Saunders, pp 259-323.

47. Lifshitz F, Cervantes C: Growth and growth disorders. In Lifshitz F, editor: *Pediatric endocrinology: a clinical guide,* ed 3, New York, 1995, Marcel Dekker, pp 1-18.

48. Tanner JM, Davies PS: Clinical longitudinal standards for height and height velocity for North American children, *J Pediatr* 107:317-329, 1985.

49. Wu FC, Butler GE, Kelnar CJ, et al: Patterns of pulsatile luteinizing hormone and follicle-stimulating hormone secretion in prepubertal (midchildhood) boys and girls and patients with idiopathic hypogonadotropic hypogonadism (Kallmann's syndrome): a study using an ultrasensitive time-resolved immunofluorometric assay, *J Clin Endocrinol Metab* 72:1229-1237, 1991.

50. Ehrmann DA, Rosenfield RL, Cuttler L, et al: A new test of combined pituitary-testicular function using the gonadotropin-releasing hormone agonist nafarelin in the differentiation of gonadotropin deficiency from delayed puberty: pilot studies, *J Clin Endocrinol Metab* 69:963-967, 1989.

51. Lifshitz F, Moses N, Cervantes C, et al: Nutritional dwarfing in adolescents, *Semin Adolesc Med* 3:255-266, 1987.

52. Pugliese MT, Lifshitz F, Grad G, et al: Fear of obesity. A cause of short stature and delayed puberty, *N Engl J Med* 309:513-518, 1983.

53. Lifshitz F, Moses N: Growth failure. A complication of dietary treatment of hypercholesterolemia, *Am J Dis Child* 143:537-542, 1989.

54. Rosenthal SR, Snyder JD, Hendricks KM, et al: Growth failure and inflammatory bowel disease: approach to a treatment of a complicated adolescent problem, *Pediatrics* 72:481-490, 1983.

55. Verkasalo M, Kuitunen P, Leisti S, et al: Growth failure from symptomless celiac disease. A study of 14 patients, *Helv Paediatr Acta* 33:489-495, 1978.

56. Nishi Y, Lifshitz F, Bayne MA, et al: Zinc status and its relation to growth retardation in children with chronic inflammatory bowel disease, *Am J Clin Nutr* 33:2613-2621, 1980.

57. LaSala MA, Lifshitz F, Silverberg M, et al: Magnesium metabolism studies in children with chronic inflammatory disease of the bowel, *J Pediatr Gastroenterol Nutr* 4:75-81, 1985.

58. Lifshitz F, Friedman S, Smith M, et al: Nutritional dwarfing: a growth abnormality associated with reduced erythrocyte Na^+/K^+ ATPase activity, *Am J Clin Nutr* 54:997-1004, 1991.

59. Richards GE, Cavallo A, Meyer WJ 3d: Diagnostic validity of 12-hour integrated concentration of growth hormone, *Am J Dis Child* 141:553-555, 1987.

60. Powell GF, Brasel JA, Blizzard RM: Emotional deprivation and growth retardation simulating idiopathic hypopituitarism. I. Clinical evaluation of the syndrome, *N Engl J Med* 276:1271-1278, 1967.

61. Eisenstein TD, Gerson MJ: Psychosocial growth retardation in adolescence. A reversible condition secondary to severe stress, *J Adolesc Health Care* 9:436-440, 1988.

62. Gold RF: Constitutional growth delay and learning problems, *J Learning Disab* 11:427-429, 1978.

63. Rudman D, Kutner MH, Blackstone RD, et al: Children with normal-variance short stature: treatment with human growth hormone for six months, *N Engl J Med* 305:123-131, 1981.

64. Van Vliet G, Styne DM, Kaplan SL, et al: Growth hormone treatment for short stature, *N Engl J Med* 309:1016-1022, 1983.

65. Zachmann M, Studer S, Prader A: Short-term testosterone treatment at bone age of 12 to 13 years does not reduce adult height in boys with constitutional delay of growth and adolescence, *Helv Paediatr Acta* 42:21-28, 1987.

66. Rosenfeld RG, Northcraft GB, Hintz RL: A prospective, randomized study of testosterone treatment of constitutional delay of growth and development in male adolescents, *Pediatrics* 69:681-687, 1982.

67. Stanhope R, Brook CG: Oxandrolone in low dose for constitutional delay of growth and puberty in boys, *Arch Dis Child* 60:379-381, 1985.

68. Buyukgebiz A, Hindmarsh PC, Brook CG: Treatment of constitutional delay of growth and puberty with oxandrolone compared with growth hormone, *Arch Dis Child* 65:448-449, 1990.

69. Hook EB, Warburton D: The distribution of chromosomal genotypes associated with Turner's syndrome: live birth prevalence rates and evidence for diminished fetal mortality and severity in genotype associated with structural X abnormalities or mosaicism, *Hum Genet* 64:24-28, 1983.

70. Neely EK, Rosenfeld RG: Turner syndrome. In Lifshitz F, editor: *Pediatric endocrinology: a clinical guide,* ed 3, New York, 1996, Marcel Dekker; pp 267-280.

71. Jacobs PA: The incidence and etiology of sex chromosome abnormalities in man, *Birth Defects* 15:3-14, 1979.

72. Grumbach MM, Conte FA: Disorders of sex differentiation. In Wilson JD, Foster DW, editors: *Williams textbook of endocrinology,* ed 8, Philadelphia, 1992, WB Saunders; pp 853-951.

73. Griffin JE, Wilson JD: Syndromes of androgen resistance, *Hosp Pract* 22:159-164, 1987.

74. French FS, Van Wyk JJ, Baggett B, et al: Further evidence of a target organ defect in the syndrome of testicular feminization, *J Clin Endocrinol Metab* 26:493-503, 1966.

75. Knoll JH, Nicholls RD, Magenis RE, et al: Angelman and Prader-Willi syndromes share a common chromosome 15 deletion but differ in parental origin of the deletion, *Am J Med Genet* 32:285-290, 1989.

76. Reinfrank RF, Nichols FL: Hypogonadotrophic hypogonadism in the Laurence-Moon syndrome, *J Clin Endocrinol Metab* 24:48-53, 1964.

77. Kaneko N, Kawagoe S, Hiroi M: Turner's syndrome—review of the literature with reference to a successful pregnancy outcome, *Gynecol Obstet Invest* 29:81-87, 1990.

78. Navot D, Laufer N, Kopolovic J, et al: Artificially induced endometrial cycles and establishment of pregnancies in the absence of ovaries, *N Engl J Med* 314:806-811, 1986.

CHAPTER 29

Nutrition and Eating Disorders

•

Janet Schebendach and I. Ronald Shenker

During adolescence, physiologic, psychological, and social growth and development proceed at varying rates. Therefore, the nutritional needs of adolescents are more accurately associated with physiologic age, as measured by Tanner stages, than with chronologic age. Nutrient requirements during adolescence are affected by growth, changes in body composition, energy expenditure, and other physiologic events that occur during normal maturation. Nutrient intake during adolescence is affected by psychosocial development, self-esteem, and perceived body image.

GROWTH AND DEVELOPMENT

The velocity of physical growth during adolescence is second only to that of infancy but may be preceded by a period of deceleration known as the prepubertal lag. The most rapid phase is the adolescent growth spurt, and although this is a constant phenomenon, it varies in intensity and duration from one adolescent to another. The peak velocity of the adolescent growth spurt averages approximately 9.5 cm per year in males and 8.3 cm per year in females.[1] In boys the growth spurt usually occurs between 12½ and 15½ years of age; in girls it occurs about 2 years earlier. The development of secondary sex characteristics (testicular enlargement) indicates the onset of pubertal growth in boys, with the height spurt occurring toward the end of the growth period. In contrast, the height spurt occurs the beginning of puberty in girls, with menarche occurring at the end of the growth period, approximately 9 to 12 months after peak height is attained.

Total weight gain in the second decade of life is substantial, with sex-determined differences in the rate, amount, and type of tissue gained. Boys gain more rapidly than girls, redistributing body composition by increasing lean body mass and decreasing adipose stores. During their comparable development, girls gain adipose tissue and, to a lesser degree, lean body mass. By age 20, females will have double the amount of adipose tissue but only two thirds as much lean tissue as their male counterparts.[2]

Nutrient requirements increase during the normal developmental process. Consideration of the Tanner stage will alert the health professional to the adolescent's peak height velocity and changes in lean body mass, thus predicting the times of greatest nutrient requirements (see Chapter 6, "Physical Growth and Development" and Chapter 13, "Physical Examination"). Since adolescent development is characterized by increased lean body mass and expanding blood volume, this age group is at risk for iron deficiency. Diagnosis of anemia can be aided by the use of sexual maturity ratings. Normal ranges for hemoglobin levels are dependent on both sex and race.[3] White boys have higher normal values than black boys, while values for black and white girls do not change appreciably with pubertal development.

Longitudinally based height and weight velocity charts for North American children have been developed by Tanner and Davies.[1] These charts are suitable for evaluation of growth throughout the growth period, including puberty. Age standards for pubertal stages and percentiles for early, middle, and late maturers are listed. Lack of normal growth may be indicative of undernutrition.

NUTRIENT REQUIREMENTS

The adolescent's requirements for all nutrients are considerable. However, sex differences in the rate of linear growth, mineralization of the skeleton, and in-

TABLE 29-1
Energy and Protein Requirements in Adolescence: Recommended Dietary Allowances

Age (yr)	Energy		Protein	
	kcal/kg	kcal/day	g/kg	g/day
Male				
11-14	55	2500	1.0	45
15-18	45	3000	0.9	59
19-24	40	2900	0.8	58
Female				
11-14	47	2200	1.0	46
15-18	40	2200	0.8	44
19-24	38	2200	0.8	46

Data from National Research Council: *Recommended dietary allowances,* ed 10, Washington, DC, 1989, National Academy Press.

creases in lean body mass will have significant impact on the individual's needs for energy, protein, iron, calcium, and zinc.

Calories

The adolescent's caloric (energy) requirement is determined by the resting metabolism, growth, and level of physical activity. The resting metabolism reflects the energy needs of the lean body mass, and most age and sex differences in the resting metabolic rate can be attributed to changes in the lean compartment. The greatest caloric need occurs during the adolescent growth spurt.

The energy cost of growth varies with the composition of the tissue gained. In assessing incremental changes in the adipose and lean compartments, it is suggested that the average energy cost of growth over the second decade of life is minimal at 13 calories per day in boys and 7 calories per day in girls.[4] However, at the peak height spurt the energy cost of growth is 66 calories per day in boys and 123 calories per day in girls.[4] The sex difference is attributable to the lower energy cost of relative lean body mass gain in boys versus the adipose gain in girls, which has a higher energy cost.

Although it has been suggested that adolescents in the United States are relatively sedentary, limited data are available on the energy cost of physical activity in this population. Forbes[3] showed that among American adolescents aged 13 and older the ratio of total energy intake to resting metabolism requirements are 2:1 for boys but only 1.5 to 1.7:1 for girls. This difference is attributable to the increased energy cost of physical activity in males.

The Recommended Dietary Allowance (RDA) for energy is indicated in Table 29-1. The total daily recommendation is indicated for either a male or a female reference adolescent of a specified height and weight in three age groups. Because of the great variability in body sizes among adolescents, a more accurate estimate of need may be obtained from the recommended calories per kilogram of body weight rather than from the recommended daily caloric intake for the reference adolescent.

Mean caloric intakes from three consumption studies are indicated in Table 29-2. It appears that males meet the recommended intake more consistently than their female counterparts. The National Research Council[5] acknowledges that reported average intakes for teenage girls are substantially below the RDA; however, it has been suggested that this may be a function of underreporting rather than a true inadequacy.

Protein

Protein requirements for adolescents parallel the growth in lean body mass. The average daily increment of protein gained from age 10 to 20 years is 1.98 g in males and 0.97 g in females. At the peak height spurt the daily increment is 3.8 g for males and 2.2 g for females.[4]

The RDA of protein is expressed in total grams daily for the reference adolescents or in grams per kilogram of body weight per day (Table 29-1). The RDA for protein provides a safety factor and generally exceeds the actual requirements for most adolescents. Despite this safety factor, the RDA is considerably less than the reported intakes summarized in Table 29-2. Teenage boys and girls consume approximately 200% and 150% of the RDA for protein, respectively. The erratic eating habits of the average adolescent often result in parental anxiety over the adequacy of protein consumed. In reality, this is an un-

TABLE 29-2
Mean Intake of Selected Nutrients: Comparison of Three Consumption Studies

	Age (yr)	NHANES I	NFCS	NHANES II
Energy (kcal)				
Male	12-15	2625	2431	2490
	16-19	3010	2629	3048
Female	12-15	1910	1870	1821
	16-19	1735	1721	1687
Protein (g)				
Male	12-15	97	94	92
	16-19	118	106	122
Female	12-15	73	72	66
	16-19	67	69	63
Calcium (mg)				
Male	12-15	1309	1146	1202
	16-19	1310	1144	1370
Female	12-15	940	849	854
	16-19	744	716	725
Iron (mg)				
Male	12-15	14	16	16
	16-19	17	17	18
Female	12-15	10	12	11
	16-19	10	11	10

Data from references 18, 20, 21.
NHANES I, National Health and Nutrition Examination Survey I, 1971-1974; NFCS, Nationwide Food Consumption Survey, 1977-1978; NHANES II, National Health and Nutrition Examination Survey II, 1976-1980.

warranted concern since protein provides approximately 12% to 14% of calories throughout adolescence.[2] The protein content of foods commonly consumed by adolescents is listed in Table 29-3.

Calcium

The skeleton contains approximately 99% of total body calcium. The remaining 1% of body calcium is found in extracellular fluids, intracellular structures, and cell membranes. Approximately 45% of total adult skeletal mass is completed during adolescence, and most of this skeletal growth takes place during pubescence. Although linear growth is less rapid, endochondral bone growth and mineralization of the skeleton still require high amounts of calcium during adolescence, and peak bone mass is probably not attained before age 25.[5]

Calcium retention is highest during the peak height velocity, with estimates varying from 200 mg/day in females to 300 and 400 mg/day in males.[6] The sex difference in stature and its influence on body calcium content is of nutritional importance. A male 186 cm in height can be expected to have almost twice as much calcium (1370 g) as a 154-cm female (730 g).[9]

The RDA for calcium is 1200 mg daily for male and female adolescents aged 11 to 18 years.[5] Consumption studies (see Table 29-2) suggest that male adolescents consume at least 95% of this recommended intake, while females consume only 60% to 78% of the RDA.

The RDAs have been established with a margin of safety for all nutrients except kilocalories. Failure to meet the RDA does not necessarily mean that the adolescent will be deficient in calcium, since calcium absorption is inversely related to dietary content, and the efficiency of absorption is increased during periods of high physiologic requirement. However, a rational approach to reducing the risk of osteoporosis in later life is to ensure an optimal calcium intake for peak bone mass development. Thus, it is prudent to consume amounts of calcium consistent with the RDA throughout childhood and adolescence.

The National Research Council[5] acknowledges the uncertainty about whether there are biologically important differences in the absorption of calcium from different foods or diets. Dietary factors that may favorably affect absorption of calcium include vitamin D and lactose consumption. Factors that may have unfavorable effects on absorption include oxalate and phytate. Those factors having variable effects include dietary protein and

TABLE 29-3
Comparative Protein Content: Adolescent Food Choices

Food Item	Portion	Protein (g)
Entrees		
Cheeseburger on bun	¼ lb	32
Turkey breast sandwich	3 oz	30
Roast beef sandwich	3 oz	28
Chicken nuggets	6 pieces	23
Tuna salad sandwich	3 oz	19
Grilled cheese	2 oz	19
Fried fish filet sandwich	1	16
Hamburger on bun	1 small	15
Cheese pizza	1 slice	14
Roast chicken drumstick	1	12
Taco	1 average	10
Frankfurter on bun	1	9
Scrambled egg (milk added)	1	9
Snack Foods		
Fruit yogurt	8 fl oz	10
Bagel	1 large	10
Peanuts	¼ cup	10
Peanut butter	2 tbsp	8
Sunflower seeds	1 oz wt (edible portion)	7
Ice cream	8 fl oz	5
Cookies (sandwich type)	4 pieces	2
French fries	1 serving	2
Milk chocolate candy	1 oz	2
Beverages		
Milkshake	10 fl oz	10
Milk	8 fl oz	8
Cola	8 fl oz	0

TABLE 29-4
Comparative Calcium Content: Adolescent Food Choices

Food Item	Portion	Calcium (mg)
Entrees		
Grilled cheese	2 oz	396
Cheese pizza	1 slice	367
Cheeseburger on bun	¼ lb	244
Fried fish filet sandwich	1	118
Hamburger on bun	1 small	90
Turkey sandwich	3 oz	66
Tuna salad sandwich	3 oz	63
Roast beef sandwich	3 oz	53
Scrambled egg (milk added)	1	47
Frankfurter on bun	1	39
Taco	1 average	37
Vegetables		
Spinach (chopped)	½ cup	116
Broccoli (chopped)	½ cup	50
Zucchini (green, sliced)	½ cup	23
Snacks		
Fruit yogurt	8 fl oz	345
Cheddar cheese	1 oz	204
Ice cream	8 fl oz	176
Sherbet	8 fl oz	103
Milk chocolate candy	1 oz	65
Peanut butter	2 tbsp	18
French fries	1 serving	10
Beverages		
Hot chocolate (instant)	1 packet/ water	478
Milkshake	10 fl oz	337
Milk	8 fl oz	291
Chocolate milk	8 fl oz	280
Orange juice	8 fl oz	27
Cola	8 fl oz	7

phosphorus. The calcium content of foods commonly consumed by adolescents is listed in Table 29-4.

Iron

The adolescent's need for iron is increased because of changes in lean body mass, expanded blood volume, increased respiratory enzymes, and onset of menses. Individual requirements are variable, being based on sex, race, body size, and athletic performance. In the adolescent male the need for large amounts of iron is secondary to the rapidly enlarging hemoglobin mass. This iron requirement may actually exceed that of a menstruating female for a time.[6] In the adolescent male, increases in body iron content average 0.57 mg/day from age 10 to 20 years, with a peak increment of 1.1 mg/day at the growth spurt. In the adolescent female, increases in body iron content average 0.23 mg/day from age 10 to 20 years, with a peak increment of 0.9 mg/day at the growth spurt.[7]

Sexual maturity ratings are helpful in evaluating when requirements are likely to be the highest.[8,9]

Iron deficiency anemia is cited as the most common nutritional disorder of adolescence. Analysis of data from the Second National Health and Nutrition Examination Survey, 1976 to 1980, indicates a peak prevalence of impaired iron status in males aged 11 to 14 and females aged 15 to 19 (Table 29-5). The RDA for iron is 12 mg for male adolescents aged 11 to 18 and 15 mg for females in the same age group. Consumption studies suggest that adolescent males meet their RDA more readily than do females, whose reported intake is 64% to 79% of the RDA (Table 27-2). The typical American diet contains approximately 6 mg of iron per 1000 kcal consumed.[10] The teenage female's inability to meet her iron requirement may be a function of lower caloric intake.

**TABLE 29-5
Prevalence of Impaired Iron Status
in Adolescence (1976-1980)**

Sex	Age (yr)	Estimated Prevalence Range (%)
Males	11-14	3.5-12.1
	15-19	0.1-0.9
Females	11-14	2.7-6.1
	15-19	2.5-14.2

Data from National Research Council: *Current trends in consumption of animal products. Designing foods: animal product options in the marketplace,* Washington, DC, 1988, National Academy of Sciences, p 58.

In contrast, the teenage male consumes more calories and therefore more iron.

The iron content of many foods commonly consumed by teenagers is indicated in Table 29-6. The absorption of iron is affected by its heme versus nonheme status. Approximately 40% of total iron in animal tissues is classified as heme iron. The remaining 60% of the iron present in animal products, and all of the iron in non–animal products, are classified as nonheme. The absorption of nonheme iron is variable. Dietary factors enhancing absorption include ascorbic acid and the presence of animal tissue in the meal. Factors inhibiting nonheme iron absorption include phytates, bran, and polyphenols in tea. The absorption of heme iron is less affected by other dietary components. Absorption of dietary iron is ultimately affected by the iron status of an individual, with absorption greatest when body stores are low.

Zinc

Zinc retention in male and female adolescents is closely related to pubertal increases in lean body mass and sexual maturation. In the adolescent male, increases in body zinc content average 0.18 mg/day from age 10 to 20 years, with a peak increment of 0.31 mg/day at the growth spurt.[8] Pronounced zinc deficiency, characterized by growth failure and arrested sexual development, has been reported in Middle Eastern adolescent males. Marginal states of zinc nutrition, associated with depressed growth, delayed sexual maturation, and impaired taste function, also have been reported in small segments of the U.S. population.[7,11]

The RDA for zinc is 15 mg for male adolescents aged 11 to 18 years and 12 mg for females in the same age group. However, no conclusions can be reached about the adequacy of zinc intake in this population. Large-scale dietary surveys, such as the Second National Health and Nutrition Examination Survey, 1976-1980, and the Nationwide Food Consumption Survey, 1977-1978, did not

**TABLE 29-6
Comparative Iron Content:
Adolescent Food Choices**

Food Item	Portion	Iron (mg)
Entrees		
Cheeseburger on bun	¼ lb	3.50
Roast beef sandwich	3 oz	2.96
Hamburger on bun	1 small	2.52
Tuna salad sandwich	3 oz	2.25
Chicken nuggets	6 pieces	2.15
Fried fish filet sandwich	1	1.92
Grilled cheese sandwich	2 oz	1.62
Turkey breast sandwich	3 oz	1.60
Taco	1 average	1.46
Frankfurter on bun	1	1.40
Cheese pizza	1 slice	1.05
Scrambled egg (milk added)	1	0.72
Roast chicken drumstick	1	0.57
Snack Foods		
Bagel	1 large	3.81
Sunflower seeds	1 oz (edible portion)	1.92
Raisins	¼ cup packed	1.45
Peanuts	¼ cup	0.66
Peanut butter	2 tbsp	0.60
French fries	1 serving	0.37
Cookies (sandwich type)	4 pieces	0.30
Milk chocolate candy	1 oz	0.30
Fruit yogurt	8 fl oz	0.16
Ice cream	8 fl oz	0.12
Beverages		
Milk shake	10 fl oz	0.66
Milk	8 fl oz	0.12
Cola	8 fl oz	0.12

assess zinc consumption. The Continuing Survey of Food Intakes by Individuals, 1985-1986, did assess zinc intake but only in children aged 1 to 5 years. Dietary data obtained from 267 black and white adolescents surveyed in the Bogalusa Heart Study indicated a mean daily intake of 12.1 mg for those aged 15 years and 14.1 mg for those aged 17 years, suggesting intakes close to the established RDAs.[12]

Data on zinc sources in the U.S. food supply indicate that 71.5% of zinc is provided by animal products.[13] Red meat is the single largest contributor, followed by dairy products, poultry, eggs, and fish. The proportion of dietary zinc from grains has decreased over the past century to the current level of 12.6%.[11] The absorption of dietary zinc is estimated at 20% of intake, with animal sources having superior absorption than that of grain products.[7] The zinc content of foods commonly consumed by teenagers is indicated in Table 29-7.

TABLE 29-7
Comparative Zinc Content:
Adolescent Food Choices

Food Item	Portion	Zinc (mg)
Entrees		
Cheeseburger on bun	¼ lb	5.12
Roast beef sandwich	3 oz	3.99
Turkey breast sandwich	3 oz	3.16
Hamburger on bun	1 small	3.04
Roast chicken drumstick	1	2.96
Taco	1 average	2.19
Chicken nuggets	6 pieces	2.01
Grilled cheese	2 oz	2.01
Cheese pizza	1 slice	1.51
Frankfurter on bun	1	1.29
Fried fish filet sandwich	1	0.97
Tuna salad sandwich	3 oz	0.79
Scrambled egg (milk added)	1	0.70
Snack Foods		
Peanuts	¼ cup	2.40
Fruit yogurt	8 fl oz	1.68
Sunflower seeds	1 oz wt (edible portion)	1.43
Ice cream	8 fl oz	1.41
Peanut butter	2 tbsp	0.80
Bagel	1 large	0.51
Cookies (sandwich type)	4	0.34
French fries	1 serving	0.32
Raisins	¼ cup packed	0.09
Beverages		
Milk shake	10 fl oz	1.52
Milk	8 fl oz	0.52
Cola	8 fl oz	0.10

DIETARY HABITS

Appropriate adolescent development leads to newly acquired independence and decision making, which results in the adolescent spending less time at home. As a consequence, more meals are consumed away from the home, and food choices may be made on the basis of enjoyment and convenience rather than nutrient content. Dietary habits change during adolescence. By age 12 years, almost one third of all adolescents eat only one meal each day with the family, and by age 17 the number of adolescents eating only one meal at home increases to almost one half.[14] In a study of adolescent food intake, Huenemann et al[15] reported that lunch was eliminated more often than breakfast in white children and the reverse in black children. It was found that meal regularity paralleled socioeconomic status, as did nutrient content of the diet.

As more meals are consumed outside the home, intake of "fast food" increases. The nutritional value of these foods is characterized by a high-calorie, high-sodium, and high-fat content, accompanied by a relatively low content of vitamin A, vitamin C, and fiber. In an analysis of a fast-food meal consisting of a quarter-pound hamburger, french fries, and a milkshake, MacLean[16] found the meal to consist of 1027 calories: 49% carbohydrate, 14% protein, and 37% fat. Vitamin C was considered adequate, but vitamin A content was inadequate. The addition of salad bars and low-fat dairy products may increase the vitamin and mineral content and decrease the fat content of such meals.

Snacking is characteristic of adolescent food behavior. Unfortunately, it frequently replaces many of the teenager's traditional meals. There is a concern that the adolescent is snacking on "empty calories." However, food consumption surveys indicate that this may not be so. Data from the Ten-State Nutrition Survey[17] indicated that 78% of teenagers reported snacking on the day of the 24-hour recall. These snacks provided 23% of the daily energy intake and either met or exceeded the RDA for protein, riboflavin, and vitamin C. Nutrients most at risk were calcium, iron, and vitamin A.

Data obtained from the Nationwide Food Consumption Survey[18] indicated that two thirds of 1424 teenagers aged 12 to 18 consumed snacks during the 1-day survey. Peak snacking periods were afternoon and evening. Results indicated that sugar-containing foods, particularly soft drinks, were the most frequently consumed snack foods.[19-21]

Although snacking should not be discouraged, it is evident that snack foods should enhance the nutritional quality of the teenager's diet. Snacks rich in calcium, iron, and zinc should be encouraged (Tables 29-4, 29-6, and 29-7).

NUTRITIONAL ASSESSMENT

Comprehensive nutritional assessment requires three components: a diet history with an estimate of nutrient intake, anthropometric assessment, and laboratory assessment.

Diet History

Information about the adolescent's past and present diet can be obtained by interview and food records. The initial interview should address the teenager's eating habits, attitudes, and health beliefs, as well as socioeconomic and psychosocial factors. A history of fad diets, typical fluid consumption, and use of vitamin and mineral supplements should be obtained. Adolescents often express concern about the size and shape of their bodies. Many over-the-counter products promise weight loss, decreased body fat, and increased muscle mass. These products may contain vitamin and mineral supplements, amino acid supplements, chromium picolinate, herbal diuretics, emetics, laxatives, and ephedrine. Unsupervised use may be hazardous and increase the risk of hypervitaminosis. The diet history should determine use of these products, as well as diet pills, liquid diets, and sports drinks.

During the interview, the adolescent may be queried about typical weekday and weekend food intake, and a recall of food and beverage consumed the previous day may be obtained. Care must be taken not to infer too much from a single one-day recall; however, serial one-day recalls may be reliable for assessment of intake over time. In addition to retrospective methods, prospective 3- to 7-day food records may be useful; however, the teenager must be instructed on proper recording technique. Retrospective tools have considerable respondent burden, and compliance may vary among teens. To supplement or substitute for other methods, a food-frequency questionnaire may be used. This may be self-administered, or reviewed during the interview. This tool determines how often a food is consumed over a specified period. It can be a comprehensive list, or may address particular types of foods or nutrients of interest.

Anthropometric Assessment

Normal physical growth is one of the best indicators of the health and well-being of an adolescent.[22] Growth can be assessed in terms of height and weight gain, as well as changes in body stores of lean and adipose tissue. Anthropometry is the study of these measurements.

Of the many parameters of growth, height and weight are those most routinely obtained. Serial measurements allow the clinician to compare the adolescent's growth with appropriately selected population norms.[23] Height should be measured against a fixed stadiometer or rigid steel rule affixed at a 90-degree angle to the floor. The adolescent should stand without shoes in a nonlordotic position with the eyes and ears in a horizontal plane. A 90-degree angle headboard should be placed firmly on the person's head while the examiner exerts gentle pressure upward on the jaw, reminding the subject to keep heels on the floor. Height should be recorded to the nearest millimeter or ⅛ inch and compared with individuals of the same population, gender, and age, taking sexual maturity rating and parental stature into account. Weight should be recorded to the nearest ¼ pound or kilogram on a tared and zeroed beam balance or electronic scale with the adolescent gowned or in light clothing. Values should be plotted on population and sex-specific growth curves.

Those developed by the National Center for Health Statistics[24] are most typically used; however, values should also be compared with sex-specific tables of weight for height for age, particularly in adolescents at extremes of height percentiles.[25]

Weight for height can also be assessed by body mass index (BMI). This may be calculated (BMI = weight in kilograms/height in meters^2) or read from a nomogram.[26] Sex and age-specific BMI percentiles for U.S. children and adolescents are available,[27] and it is recommended that physicians incorporate the BMI into their health assessment.[28]

Growth and development of the adolescent is accompanied by changes in body composition. While height, weight, and BMI are adequate for assessment of most adolescents, there are times when the physician needs additional information about lean and fat stores.

A variety of techniques are available for measurement of body composition. Many of these have research rather than clinical utility, but an understanding of these methods is essential for interpretation of the literature.

Human body composition can be studied at the atomic, molecular, cellular, tissue-system, or whole body level[29]; however, it is most common to think in terms of fat, lean, and mineral compartments. Fat mass is the quantity of pure fat (triglyceride) in the body, whereas adipose tissue includes the fat (83%) and supporting cellular and extracellular structures (2% protein, 15% water). Lean body mass (LBM) is the part of the body free of adipose tissue; the fat-free mass (FFM) consists of LBM plus the cellular and extracellular supporting structures of the adipose tissue. Extracellular solids (ECS) consist of total body bone mineral, approximately 85% of which is accounted for by the skeleton. Dissection and chemical analyses of human cadavers provide the only means of direct body composition assessment; however, techniques are available for indirect assessment of fat and lean stores.

The "gold standard" for determination of body fat is underwater weighing (densitometry). Although this is a precise, noninvasive research technique, it requires a good deal of cooperation from the subjects, who must exhale completely and then hold their breath for approximately 10 seconds while submerged under water. The procedure is repeated five to 10 times, and residual lung volume must also be measured.

Dual photon absorptiometry (DPA) and dual-energy x-ray absorptiometry (DEXA), used to assess bone mineral content, also provide highly accurate measurements of LBM and body fat. The subject, lying in a supine position, is scanned with photons at two different energy levels. Differential absorption is measured, and total body fat, percentage body fat, regional body fat (trunk, arms, legs, and head plus neck), and fat-free mass are determined. Many institutions are equipped with DPA/DEXA instrumentation; however, testing is expensive, and some radiation exposure does occur, although small. DEXA-derived normative data on sex- and age-related changes in lean tissue, bone mineral content, percentage body fat, and trunk-to-leg fat ratio were obtained in a cross-sectional study of 265 Australian children, adolescents, and young adults.[30] Tanner stage and gender-related changes in body composition have also been assessed by DEXA in the prepubertal and adolescent age group.[31]

Computed tomography (CT) and magnetic resonance imaging (MRI) provide a visual image of adipose tissue and lean tissue within a scanned body section. These methods accurately predict body fat mass, but their cost, long scanning time, and CT radiation exposure limit their use for routine body composition assessment. Their ability to measure regional fat distribution, specifically intraabdominal fat, is a major research advantage. Lean tissue estimated from CT and MRI may be less than FFM estimated by densitometry and DPA/DEXA. Ultrasonography has also been used to measure subcutaneous adipose tissue thickness but is considerably less precise and less accurate than CT and MRI.

Recent advances in body composition methods include impedance techniques: total body electrical conductivity (TOBEC) and bioelectrical impedance analysis (BIA). BIA is rapid, simple, noninvasive, inexpensive, and frequently used in health club settings. BIA values, which are highly correlated with total body water, measure lean tissue more accurately than fat. However, since most electrical resistance occurs in the extremities, BIA may be relatively insensitive to changes in abdominal and/or visceral lean or fat content. A further limitation includes the possibility that changes in electrolyte composition of the body may result in changes in impedance that are independent of changes in lean tissue. TOBEC is a noncontact technique utilizing the same physical properties of the body as BIA. Measurement error is comparable with that of BIA,[32] but this equipment is expensive and nonportable.

Additional techniques for assessment of lean tissue include neutron activation analysis of total body nitrogen; measurement for total body potassium (endogenous 40K or administered 42K); and measurement for intracellular water, which is total body water (measured by isotope dilution) minus extracellular water (measured with bromide, radioactive bromide, or radiosulfate washout technique). These methods, while valuable research tools, are impractical for clinical assessment. Biochemical measures of urinary metabolite excretion include 24-hour creatinine and 3-methylhistidine levels. Although correlation of excretion rates with LBM may be reasonable, the effect of diet,[33] large intraindividual variability in daily urinary creatinine excretion,[34] and

problems inherent in obtaining accurately timed samples may affect the validity of these methods.

A more practical approach to the assessment of body composition is measurement of skinfold thicknesses and body circumferences, obtained at standardized sites by standard techniques.[35]

Skinfolds represent a double layer of subcutaneous tissue, including a small and relatively constant amount of skin and variable amounts of adipose tissue. From 50% to 70% of body fat is located subcutaneously, and selected skinfolds have been found to relate well to body fatness. In a study of 63 male and 81 female adolescents aged 13 to 17.9 years, the highest correlation with percentage of body fat was triceps skinfold (TSF) followed by subscapular skinfold in males, and TSF followed by subscapular and suprailiac skinfolds in females.[36] The sum of triceps, biceps, subscapular, and suprailiac folds can also be used to predict percentage body fat in children and adolescents.[37,38] Estimation of percentage body fat from triceps and calf folds, or triceps and subscapular folds, has been recommended for use in black and white youths aged 8 to 18 years[39]; this method, based on a three-compartment model of body composition, accounts for the chemical immaturity of children. TSF can also be compared with sex- and age-specific population norms.[40]

The midarm muscle circumference, mathematically derived from the midarm circumference and TSF according to the method of Frisancho,[40] can be used to compare lean stores with sex- and age-specific population norms throughout childhood and adolescence. These norms are based on the same samples, age groups, and percentile groups as those published in the U.S. Health Statistics weight-for-height percentiles.[41,42]

Laboratory Assessment

Biochemical assessment of nutritional status includes measurement of visceral protein and iron status. Additional measures of vitamin and mineral stores are available but rarely indicated.

Albumin is the most commonly obtained measure of visceral protein status. Serum levels are determined by the rate of biosynthesis, the rate of catabolism, the volume and nature of the distribution space, abnormal losses, and level of hydration.[43] In states of uncomplicated protein-energy malnutrition in the Western world, the reduction in serum albumin is small. The initial adaptation to semistarvation is a rapid reduction in albumin synthesis; however, catabolism also diminishes, and a shift of albumin from extravascular to intravascular spaces occurs, thereby preserving serum levels. In prolonged semistarvation, such as seen in conditions of famine or in Third World countries, hypoalbuminemia and secondary edema develop. The half-life of albumin ranges from 14 to 20 days, and its slow response to nutritional factors has led investigators to more sensitive indices of visceral protein status. These include serum transferrin, prealbumin, retinol-binding protein, insulin-like growth factor 1, and fibronectin.

Iron deficiency is the most common nutritional disorder of adolescence. Increased requirements during the adolescent growth spurt, decreased dietary intake, and increased menstrual losses all contribute, and biochemical assessment is warranted. The initial state is iron depletion, which progresses to iron deficiency and ends with anemia. A complete blood count (CBC) with erythrocyte indices is effective in detecting the adolescent with moderate anemia; however, a serum ferritin level will detect depleted iron stores before anemia becomes apparent on the CBC (see Chapter 48, "Anemia").

SUMMARY

The nutritional needs of adolescents are determined by sex-related changes in body composition and linear growth. The most rapid change, and thus increased nutritional need, occurs at the adolescent growth spurt. Healthcare practitioners must be particularly aware of growth-related increases in energy, protein, calcium, iron, and zinc requirements for adolescents. Likewise, they must accept that this period of increased need occurs at a stage of psychosocial development that is less conducive to good eating habits. Counseling that enables teenagers to identify and modify their "at-risk" nutrients and eating habits should be the goal of nutritional management in adolescence.

References

1. Tanner JM, Davies PSW: Clinical longitudinal standards for height and weight velocity for North American children, *J Pediatr* 107:317-329, 1985.
2. Marino DD, King JC: Nutritional concerns during adolescence, *Pediatr Clin North Am* 27:125-139, 1980.
3. Forbes GB: Nutritional requirements in adolescents. In Suskind R, editor: *Textbook of pediatric nutrition,* New York, 1981, Raven Press; pp 381-391.
4. Dwyer J: Nutritional requirements of adolescents, *Nutr Rev* 56-72, 1981.
5. National Research Council: *Recommended dietary allowances,* ed 10, Washington, DC, 1989, National Academy of Sciences.
6. Greenwood CT, Richardson DP: Nutrition during adolescence. *World Rev Nutr Diet* 33:1-41, 1979.
7. Forbes GB: Body composition in adolescence. In Tsang RC, Nichols BL Jr: *Nutrition and child health: perspectives for the 1980's;* New York, 1981, Alan R. Liss; pp 55-72.
8. Tanner JM: Growth and maturation during adolescence, *Nutr Rev* 39:43-55, 1981.
9. Daniel WA: Nutritional requirements of adolescents. In Winick M, editor: *Adolescent nutrition,* New York, 1982, John Wiley; pp 19-35.
10. National Research Council: *Recommended dietary allowances,* ed 8 (revised), Washington, DC, 1974, National Academy of Sciences.

11. *Nutrition monitoring in the United States: an update report on nutrition monitoring, 1989,* Baltimore, 1989, U.S. Department of Health and Human Services, U.S. Department of Agriculture.
12. National Research and Demonstration Center: *Arteriosclerosis. Dietary databook: qualifying dietary intakes of infants, children and adolescents, The Bogalusa Heart Study, 1973-1983,* New Orleans, 1986, Louisiana State University Medical Center.
13. National Research Council: *Current trends in consumption of animal products. Designing foods: animal product options in the marketplace,* Washington, DC, 1988, National Academy of Sciences; pp 18-44.
14. Mauer AM: Normal nutrition in the adolescent. In *Pediatric nutrition handbook,* Elk Grove Village, IL, 1979, American Academy of Pediatrics; pp 153-157.
15. Huenemann RL, Shapiro LR, Hampton MC, et al: Food and eating practices of teenagers, *J Am Diet Assoc* 53:17-24, 1968.
16. MacLean D: *Pediatric nutrition in a clinical practice,* Baltimore, 1982, Williams & Wilkins, pp 118-131.
17. Thomas JA, Call DL: Eating between meals: a nutrition problem among teenagers?, *Nutr Rev* 31:137-139, 1973.
18. *Nutrition monitoring in the United States: a progress report from the Joint Nutrition Monitoring Evaluation Committee, 1986,* DHHS Pub. No. (PHS) 86-1255, Baltimore, 1986, U.S. Department of Health and Human Services, U.S. Department of Agriculture.
19. Story M: Adolescent life-style and eating behavior. In Mahan LK, Rees J, editors: *Nutrition in adolescence,* St. Louis, 1984, Times Mirror/Mosby College Publishing; pp 77-103.
20. National Center for Health Statistics: *Dietary Intake Source Data, United States, 1971-74,* DHEW Pub. No. (PHS) 79-1221, Washington, DC, 1979, U.S. Government Printing Office.
21. National Center for Health Statistics: Carroll MD, Abraham S, Dresser CM. *Dietary Intake Source Data. Vital and Health Statistics. Series 11, No. 231,* DHHS Pub. No. (PHS) 83-1681, Washington, DC, 1983, U.S. Government Printing Office.
22. Tanner JM, Goldstein H, Whitehouse RH: Standards for children's heights at ages 2-9 years allowing for height of parents, *Arch Dis Child* 45:755-762, 1970.
23. Luder E, Copperman N: Assessment of nutritional status. In Jacobson MS, editor: *Atherosclerosis prevention: identification and treatment of the child with high cholesterol,* Chur, Switzerland, 1991, Harwood Academic; pp 85-104.
24. Hamil PVV, Drizd TA, Johnson CL, et al: Physical growth: National Center for Health Statistics percentiles, *Am J Clin Nutr* 32:607-629, 1979.
25. Jacobson MS: Nutrition in adolescence, *Annales Nestlé* 53:106-114, 1995.
26. Bray G: Commentary, *Am J Clin Nutr* 54:437, 1991.
27. Hammer LD, Kraemer HC, Wilson DM, et al: Standardized percentile curves for body-mass index for children and adolescents, *Am J Dis Child* 145:259-263, 1991.
28. National Institutes of Health Consensus Development Conference Statement: Health implications of obesity, *Ann Intern Med* 103:1073-1077, 1985.
29. Wang ZM, Pierson RN, Heymsfield S: The five-level model: a new approach to organizing body-composition research, *Am J Clin Nutr* 56:19-28, 1992.
30. Ogle GD, Allen JR, Humphries IRJ, et al: Body-composition assessment by dual-energy x-ray absorptiometry in subjects aged 4-26 y, *Am J Clin Nutr* 61:746-753, 1995.
31. Rico H, Revilla M, Villa LF, et al: Body composition in children and Tanner's stages: a study with dual-energy x-ray absorptiometry, *Metabolism* 42:967-970, 1993.
32. Sjostrom L: Recent methods in the study of body composition. In Tanner JM, editor: *Perspectives in the science of growth and development,* London, 1988, Smith-Gordon; pp 353-366.

33. Jensen MD: Research techniques for body composition assessment, *J Am Diet Assoc* 92:454-450, 1992.

34. Lukasi HC: Methods for the assessment of human body composition: traditional and new, *Am J Clin Nutr* 46:537-556, 1987.

35. Lohman TG, Roche AF, Martorell R, editors: *Anthropometric standardization reference manual,* Champaign, Ill., 1988, Human Kinetics Books.

36. Roche AF, Siervogel RM, Chumlea WC, et al: Grading body fatness from limited anthropometric data, *Am J Clin Nutr* 34:2831-2838, 1981.

37. Durnin JVGA, Rahaman MM: The assessment of the amount of fat in human body measurements from measurements of skinfold thickness, *Br J Nutr* 21:681-689, 1967.

38. Durnin JVGA, Womersley J: Body fat assessed from total body density and its estimation from skinfold thickness: measurements on 481 men and women aged from 16 to 72 years, *Br J Nutr* 32:77-97, 1974.

39. Slaughter MH, Lohman TG, Boileau CA, et al: Skinfold equations for estimation of body fatness in children and youth, *Hum Biol* 60:709-723, 1988.

40. Frisancho AR: New norms of upper limb fat and muscle areas for assessment of nutritional status, *Am J Clin Nutr* 34:2540-2545, 1981.

41. National Center for Health Statistics: *NCHS growth curves for children birth-18 years, United States,* DHEW Pub. No. (PHS) 78-1650, Rockville, MD, 1977, National Center for Health Statistics.

42. National Center for Health Statistics: *Weight by height and age for adults 18-74 years: United States, 1971-1974,* DHEW Pub. No. (PHS) 79-1656, Rockville, MD, 1979, National Center for Health Statistics.

43. Heymsfield SB, Tighe A, Wang ZM: Nutritional assessment by anthropometric and biochemical methods. In Shils ME, Olson JA, Shike M, editors: *Modern nutrition in health and diseases,* ed 8, Philadelphia, 1994, Lea & Febiger; pp 812-841.

CHAPTER 30

Hyperlipidemia and Atherosclerosis

•

Marc S. Jacobson

Screening for risk of atherosclerosis, whether by family history followed by cholesterol and blood pressure measurements (targeted screening) or by universal cholesterol testing, is recommended for all adolescents by the National Cholesterol Education Program expert panel on blood cholesterol in children and adolescents, the Committee on Nutrition of the American Academy of Pediatrics, the American Heart Association, and the American Medical Association Guidelines for Adolescent Preventive Services (GAPS).[1-3] Some physicians, fearing negative effects of low-fat diets on growth or overutilization of medications, argue that no cholesterol testing should be done until adulthood. Others consider that universal treatment with or without screening should be the standard of care and that a concerted effort should be made to lower fat and cholesterol intake, increase habitual physical activity, and prevent smoking for all teenagers.

This debate, until recently, took place with little scientific data available from well-designed studies. This is no longer the case. The relationship of histologic severity of atherosclerotic lesions to measurable risk factors in adolescents has been defined by the Pathobiologic Determinants of Atherosclerosis in Youth (PDAY) study.[4] In addition, the safety and efficacy of low-cholesterol, low-fat dietary treatment has been demonstrated by the Dietary Intervention Study in Children (DISC), a prospective study of growth among early adolescents with moderate hypercholesterolemia, which demonstrated normal growth and development in both treated subjects and controls.[5] Furthermore, the powerful cholesterol-lowering effects of the 3-hydroxy-3-methylglutaryl-coenzyme A (HMG-CoA) inhibitors have shown clear proof of the lifesaving results of cholesterol lowering in both primary and secondary prevention.[6]

Clearly, with new studies documenting the lifesaving effects of cardiovascular disease prevention in adults, the safety of dietary therapy in young adolescents, and the rising prevalence of obesity and cardiovascular risk factors in adolescents, the burden of proof is now on those who state that nothing should be done for adolescents. Therefore, increasing numbers of patients with hyperlipidemia and increased atherosclerosis risk are being identified. Table 30-1 provides normative data for cholesterol, triglycerides, and lipid subfractions for U.S. adolescents.[7] Figures 30-1 and 30-2 provide algorithms for screening and initial evaluation of elevated cholesterol

TABLE 30-1
Lipid Values for Adolescent Atherosclerosis Risk Assessment

		Total Cholesterol				Triglycerides				LDL Cholesterol				HDL Cholesterol			
Percentile		5	50	75	95	5	50	75	95	5	50	75	95	5	50	75	95
Age (yr)	**Sex**																
10-14	M	119	158	173	202	32	66	74	125	64	97	109	133	37	55	61	74
	F	126	164	171	205	32	60	85	105	68	97	109	136	37	52	58	70
15-19	M	113	150	168	197	32	66	88	125	62	94	109	130	30	46	52	63
	F	120	158	176	203	39	75	85	132	59	96	111	137	35	52	61	74
20-24	M	118	159	179	197	44	78	107	165	66	101	118	147	30	45	51	63
	F	121	165	186	237	52	96	126	175	70	98	136	151	37	50	60	73

Data from *Lipid Research Clinics population studies data book,* Pub. No. 80-1527, Bethesda, MD, 1980, National Institutes of Health.
HDL, high-density lipoprotein; *LDL,* low-density lipoprotein.

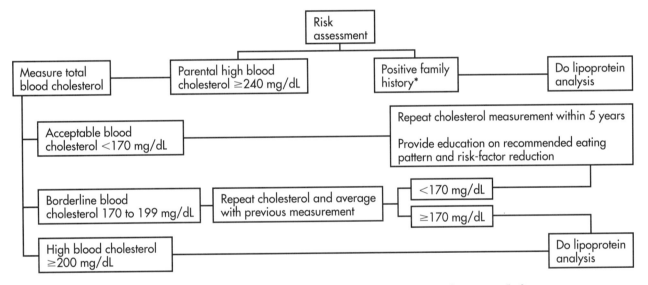

Fig. 30-1. Risk assessment. *Positive family history is defined as a history of premature (before age 55 years) cardiovascular disease in a parent or grandparent. (From *Pediatrics* 89:548-549, 1992.)

levels in adolescents.[3] Optimal treatment requires a comprehensive approach, including nutritional counseling, behavior modification, and medical therapies for the adolescent and family.

DIAGNOSIS

First, the causes of secondary hyperlipidemia should be ruled out in adolescents (Box 30-1). Most of these causes can be eliminated by history and physical examination, but laboratory screening for hypothyroidism, hepatitis, nephrotic syndrome, and pregnancy should be considered. Currently used low-dose oral contraceptives have minimal effects on lipids in the average patient, but adolescents with underlying lipid abnormalities have not been studied thoroughly. A rare form of familial hypertriglyceridemia has been reported to be exacerbated by administration of estrogen, resulting in acute fulminating pancreatitis and death. Smoking in conjunction with the use of oral contraceptives further increases the risk of cardiovascular disease. In general, a lipid profile should be obtained before the initiation of hormone therapy, and repeated periodically thereafter. Although lipid abnormalities are rarely contraindications to oral contraceptive use, screening and appropriate treatment should be part of a comprehensive approach to the patient.

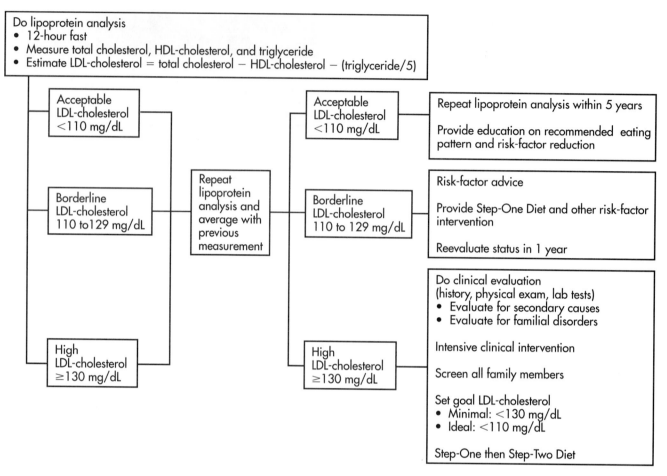

Fig. 30-2. Classification, education, and follow-up based on low-density lipoprotein cholesterol. (From *Pediatrics* 89:548-549, 1992.)

Once secondary causes have been ruled out, hyperlipidemia can be classified as one of three types: (1) familial hypercholesterolemia (FH), a dominantly inherited defect in the gene located on chromosome 19, which codes for the low-density lipoprotein (LDL) cell surface receptor; (2) familial combined hyperlipidemia (FCH), which results from a dominantly inherited excess production of very-low-density lipoprotein (VLDL) from the liver combined with abnormalities in the catabolism of VLDL cholesterol and LDL cholesterol, resulting in increased cholesterol and triglyceride levels[8]; and (3) mixed environmental genetic hyperlipidemia, which may be the result of apolipoprotein phenotype abnormalities or other uncharacterized hereditary defects combined with excessive saturated fat and cholesterol levels in the diet.

Each of the three primary types of hyperlipidemia may involve a family history of early myocardial infarction, stroke, and/or hypercholesterolemia. Only FH is associated with signs of peripheral lipid deposition, such as corneal arcus, xanthomas, or xanthelasmas, which are useful differentiating features. Families with familial combined hyperlipidemia have some members with elevated cholesterol levels, some with elevated triglyc-

eride levels, and some with both.[8] The homozygotes for FH present with total and LDL cholesterol levels in the 700 and 600 mg/dl range, respectively. On average the heterozygotes for FH have a total cholesterol value of 250 to 400 mg/dl and normal triglycerides, while patients with FCH have average total cholesterol levels in the 200 to 250 mg/dl range, with triglycerides above 120 mg/dl. Patients with mixed environmental genetic hypercholesterolemia tend to have lower total cholesterol and triglyceride levels.[1]

INITIAL MANAGEMENT

Treatment of hyperlipidemia in adolescents is important. Extensive autopsy data show the acceleration of lesion formation during this age period. In addition, the direct relationship between the severity of lesions and lipid levels and smoking has been noted in recent years.[4] Treatment should begin if the adolescent's LDL cholesterol level exceeds the 95th percentile for age and sex (Table 30-1). Initial treatment for all types of hyperlipidemia consists of diet modification, weight control, and

---

BOX 30-1
**Causes of Secondary
Hyperlipidemia in Adolescents**

Diet
   Excessive consumption of cholesterol, saturated
      fat, or calories
   Anorexia nervosa
Endocrinologic factors
   Diabetes mellitus
   Hypothyroidism
   Pregnancy, lactation
Renal disease
   Biliary tract obstruction, pancreatitis, hepatocel-
      lular disease
Drugs
   Oral contraceptives
   Corticosteroid administration
   Thiazides
   Beta blockers
   Isotretinoin (Acutane)
Other metabolic disease
   Glycogen storage disease
   Acute intermittent porphyria
   Gout
Connective tissue disease
   Systemic lupus erythematosus
   Juvenile rheumatoid arthritis

BOX 30-2
**Dietary Recommendations for
Management of Hyperlipidemia**

Cholesterol intake: 100 mg/1000 calories
Fat intake: 20%-30% of total calories
   Saturated fat intake <$\frac{1}{3}$ of fat calories
   Polyunsaturated fat intake no more than $\frac{1}{3}$ of
      fat calories
   Monounsaturated fat intake to make up the re-
      mainder
Energy intake sufficient for adequate growth

---

exercise.[1,3] Only those with severe family histories, high levels of serum cholesterol, and failure to respond to diet modifications require pharmacotherapy.[6,9] A significant adjunct to therapy for the lipid abnormality is the prevention and treatment of associated risk factors for atherosclerosis: hypertension, smoking, obesity, and sedentary life style.[10,11]

Dietary modification should be based on the principles of the National Cholesterol Education Program's Step 1 Diet (Box 30-2).[3] Counseling should be focused on reducing the intake of total fat and saturated fat, which is more difficult but also more effective than lowering cholesterol intake per se. Generally the clinician should attempt to modify the adolescent's baseline diet rather than attempt to construct a theoretical diet from general principles. Substituting foods that are low in fat for ones that are high in fat with similar sensory properties has been found to be the most successful approach.[1,11,12] Exercise may be a useful adjunct to a comprehensive diet program because it can help maintain ideal body weight and general cardiovascular and pulmonary function; however, experimental studies of the efficacy of exercise are lacking.

Nutritional counseling by the physician, nurse, or nutritionist should be followed by a repeat lipid profile no sooner than 6 to 8 weeks after diet modification. If the diet

is being followed appropriately, improvement should be seen within this time. If no change or worsening occurs, further investigation of the current diet is indicated. Factors to be explored include the preparation of meals, whether school lunches (generally high in saturated fat and cholesterol) are consumed, and the types and quantities of snacks and fast foods eaten. A nutritionist with expertise in working with adolescents can be invaluable in assessing baseline nutritional status and current diet and in providing education and counseling. Most physicians will need such support to provide comprehensive treatment for hyperlipidemia in adolescents.[1]

PHARMACOTHERAPY

Patients who do not respond adequately to dietary intervention need pharmacotherapy in addition to diet modification. The published data on treatment with medications in the pediatric age group are scanty; thus, pharmacotherapy is reserved for those at very high risk. Medication is indicated for adolescents who have close relatives who experienced early death (age 45 or below) or disability such as myocardial infarct or stroke and LDL cholesterol levels persistently greater than the 95th percentile for age and sex (Table 30-1). In addition, adolescents being considered for medication should have failed to respond with 15% to 20% lowering of LDL cholesterol levels during at least 6 months of intensive diet therapy provided by a nutritionist skilled in working with hyperlipidemic adolescents.[1]

The bile acid–binding resins colestipol and cholestyramine have been used by many specialists with good cholesterol reduction. They are generally agreed to be safe, but their effects on growth and development have not received sufficient scientific attention. The resins are given in a powdered form that must be mixed with water or juice. A new coated tablet (Cholestid) has shown comparable efficacy in adults, and some adolescents find it preferable to the powder. The common side effects of bile acid–binding resins, such as bloating, gas, and constipation, can be avoided by administering low doses initially, with gradual increases from one to three doses per day over the first 4 to 6 weeks. The dose is based on the level of LDL cholesterol rather than on weight or age. In some patients, dosages as high as six packets of resin per day may be needed. If constipation becomes a limiting side effect, the mixing of cholestyramine or colestipol with psyllium powder (Metamucil) can be helpful. Psyllium and other water-soluble fibers have their own mild cholesterol-lowering effects.[1,6]

Niacin (nicotinic acid) acts by reducing the synthesis of VLDL, the precursor of LDL, thereby lowering cholesterol and triglyceride levels. Dosage is in the range of 1 to 3 g per day. The most obvious and frequent side effect of niacin is prostaglandin-mediated flushing of the skin, which may occur within a few minutes of consumption of the oral dose. Pretreatment with aspirin 15 to 30 minutes before the dose is taken can block this side effect. More serious side effects include peptic ulcer disease, gout, and hepatic toxicity, all of which are rare. Administration of the drug with meals and a gradual increase of the dose, beginning with 50 to 250 mg, can minimize side effects.[1,6]

Lovastatin (Mevacor), the first of a new class of cholesterol-lowering drugs that inhibit cholesterol synthesis at the cellular level, can be given in tablet form in a single daily dose. This simplified regimen should significantly improve compliance. The dosage is 20 mg or 40 mg per day based on the LDL cholesterol response. When combined with dietary therapy, lovastatin has been shown to reduce total and LDL cholesterol levels by 25% to 40% in adults with hypercholesterolemia. Two rare, yet major side effects of this drug are myositis, which can progress to myolysis if untreated, and transient elevation of liver enzymes, which is reversible within 2 to 6 weeks of discontinuation of therapy. Periodic monitoring of liver enzymes and creatine kinase is indicated during lovastatin therapy. A placebo-controlled, double-blind clinical trial of the safety and efficacy of lovastatin in pubertal males is in progress. Data from this study will establish the clinical criteria under which this agent may be prescribed for high-risk adolescents.

Probucol, a second drug that works at the cellular level, has had little systematic use in this age group, except for rare adolescents with homozygous FH. Its primary mechanism of action lies in increasing the catabolism of LDL cholesterol levels by a non–receptor-mediated pathway. A secondary mechanism of action, the ability of probucol to act as an antioxidant, may be seen as increasingly important in the prevention of atherosclerotic plaque formation as research in this area progresses. The electrocardiogram must be monitored during probucol therapy, since prolongation of the QT interval may occur; if this is found, or if syncope should occur, probucol should be discontinued. Use of tricyclic antidepressants, phenothiazines, antiarrhythmic agents, digoxin, or beta blockers may potentiate the cardiac toxicity of probucol, as does hypokalemia.

Gemfibrozil is a fibric acid derivative that decreases VLDL levels and is thus most useful in patients with FCH who have elevated triglyceride and LDL cholesterol levels. This agent is not indicated when cholesterol level alone is elevated, and it should not be used when hepatic or renal dysfunction are present. Its use is contraindicated in patients receiving anticoagulants or lovastatin. Major side effects of gemfibrozil occur in the gastrointestinal tract, nervous system, and hematologic system. Periodic monitoring of liver enzymes and complete blood count is advised during gemfibrozil therapy. Adult dosage of gemfibrozil is 600 mg twice a day, taken 30 minutes before mealtime. Gemfibrozil, probucol, and niacin have received no systematic study in adolescents. Their use should therefore be reserved for patients in whom conventional therapy has failed, and then only on an experimental basis.

References

1. Jacobson MS, editor: Atherosclerosis prevention: identification and treatment of the child with high cholesterol, London, 1991, Harwood Academic.
2. Elster AB, Kuznets NJ: *AMA guidelines for adolescent preventive services (GAPS): recommendations and rationale,* Baltimore, 1994, Williams & Wilkins.
3. National Cholesterol Education Program: Report of the expert panel on blood cholesterol levels in children and adolescents, *Pediatrics* 89 (suppl):495-584, 1992.
4. Pathobiologic Determinants of Atherosclerosis Research Group: Relationship of atherosclerosis in young men to serum lipoprotein cholesterol concentrations and smoking: a preliminary report from the Pathobiological Determinants of Atherosclerosis Research Group, *JAMA* 264:3018-3024, 1990.
5. The Dietary Intervention Study in Children Collaborative Research Group: Efficacy and safety of lowering dietary intake of fat and cholesterol in children with elevated low density cholesterol, *JAMA* 273:1429-1435, 1995.
6. Havel RJ, Rappaport E: Management of primary hyperlipidemia, *N Engl J Med* 332:1491-1498, 1995.
7. *Lipid Research Clinics population studies data book,* Pub. No. 80-1527, Bethesda, MD, 1980, National Institutes of Health.
8. Cortner JA, Coates PM, Gallagher PR: Prevalence and expression of familial combined hyperlipidemia in childhood, *J Pediatr* 116:514-519, 1990.
9. Blum CB, Levy RI: Current therapy for hypercholesterolemia, *JAMA* 261:3582-3585, 1989.
10. Walter HJ, Hofman A, Vaughan RD, Wynder EL: Modification of risk factors for coronary heart disease. Five-year results of a school-based intervention trial, *N Engl J Med* 318:1093-1100, 1988.
11. Jacobson MS, Copperman N, Haas MA, Shenker IR: Adolescent obesity and cardiovascular risk: a rational approach to management, *Ann NY Acad Sci* 699:220-229, 1993.
12. Copperman N, Schebendach J, Arden M, Jacobson MS: Nutrient quality of fat- and cholesterol-modified diets of children with hyperlipidemia, *Arch Pediatr Adolesc Med* 149:333-336, 1995.

CHAPTER 31

Anorexia Nervosa

•

Susan M. Coupey

Anorexia nervosa is a clinical syndrome, not a specific disease entity. The syndrome is manifested by the simultaneous occurrence of a variety of physical and psychological signs and symptoms.[1] The most important of these are a significant degree of emaciation accompanied by a firm belief on the part of the patient, most often an adolescent girl, that she is fat. Bruch[2] termed this core symptom of the disorder a "relentless pursuit of thinness." Anorexia nervosa is a classic example of a biopsychosocial illness and, although it is classified as a psychiatric disorder, there are serious physiologic concomitants and complications that warrant intervention by the primary care physician. In addition, consultation by medical or pediatric subspecialists is often needed for seriously ill patients who are hospitalized. The presenting symptom of the disorder is often a physical disturbance such as amenorrhea, hair loss, or weight loss. The primary care physician is frequently the one who makes the diagnosis and provides ongoing health care for young patients with this chronic illness.

Anorexia nervosa is classified among the eating disorders listed in the fourth edition of the *Diagnostic and Statistical Manual of Mental Disorders* (DSM-IV).[3] Bulimia nervosa is classified as a separate disorder. However, there is considerable clinical overlap between the two conditions. Nearly 50% of patients with anorexia nervosa also engage in bulimic behaviors such as binging and purging, and 30% or more of patients with bulimia nervosa have a history of anorexia nervosa. Nevertheless, at our present level of etiologic understanding, there is sufficient difference in the presentation, treatment, and outcome of the two disorders to warrant separation into different diagnostic categories. In particular, the potential physiologic complications are more severe in anorexia nervosa than in bulimia, and the death rate is higher. A single patient may be given the diagnosis of both anorexia nervosa and bulimia nervosa either concurrently or at different points in her history. This dual diagnosis usually indicates the greatest psychopathology.[4]

The DSM-IV criteria for the diagnosis of anorexia nervosa are listed in Box 31-1. The main change from the DSM-III-R criteria is the inclusion of two subtypes, restricting and binge eating/purging, in the new criteria. The diagnostic ability to characterize these subtypes of the disorder has important implications for both treatment and prognosis.

EPIDEMIOLOGY

Most patients diagnosed as having anorexia nervosa are adolescent and young adult women,[5] and over 90% are diagnosed before age 25 years. Approximately 5% to 10% of patients are male, again mostly adolescents, and a smaller percentage are older women. The mean age at onset of anorexia nervosa is usually cited as 14 years, but some authors suggest that the onset may be bimodal, with peaks at 14 and 18 years.[6] Since many patients do not seek treatment for several months to years after symptoms have appeared, the diagnosis is often made in older adolescents or young adults. In a large population-based study, Lucas et al[7] found that the mean age at diagnosis of anorexia nervosa was 22 years for both women and men.

Anorexia nervosa is encountered primarily in adolescents in the middle and upper socioeconomic classes. Traditionally, minority women have been thought to be at low risk for anorexia nervosa. However, there have been several reports in recent years documenting the classic syndrome in African Americans, Hispanics, Asian Americans and Native Americans.[8] Many of these patients were from professional, upper middle-class families and were enrolled in highly competitive schools. Therefore, it appears that upward mobility and higher socioeconomic status are more important than race or ethnicity in determining the risk status for this eating disorder.

There is a general assumption that the incidence of anorexia nervosa has been increasing over the past 40 years, although epidemiologic studies vary in their support of this assumption. The completeness of case finding is in question in many studies because they tend to examine only hospitalized patients, and those seen by

---

BOX 31-1
DSM-IV: Diagnostic Criteria for
Anorexia Nervosa

A. Refusal to maintain body weight at or above a
   minimally normal weight for age and height
   (e.g., weight loss leading to maintenance of
   body weight <85% of that expected; or failure
   to make expected weight gain during period
   of growth, leading to body weight <85% of
   that expected).
B. Intense fear of gaining weight or becoming fat,
   even though underweight.
C. Disturbance in the way in which one's body
   weight or shape is experienced, undue influence of body weight or shape on self-
   evaluation, or denial of the seriousness of
   the current low body weight.
D. In postmenarcheal females, amenorrhea, i.e.,
   the absence of at least three consecutive menstrual cycles. (A woman is considered to have
   amenorrhea if her periods occur only following
   hormone, e.g., estrogen, administration.)

Specify type:

Restricting type: during the current episode of
   anorexia nervosa, the person has not regularly engaged in binge-eating or purging behavior (i.e., self-induced vomiting or the misuse of laxatives, diuretics, or enemas).
Binge-eating/purging type: during the current
   episode of anorexia nervosa, the person has
   regularly engaged in binge-eating or purging
   behavior (i.e., self-induced vomiting or the
   misuse of laxatives, diuretics, or enemas).

American Psychiatric Assoication: *Diagnostic and statistical manual of
mental disorders*, ed 4, Washington DC, 1994, American Psychiatric
Association

---

psychiatrists, and are not usually based on a general
population survey. Thus, any increase in incidence that is
found could be attributed to the greater awareness of the
condition and consequent higher rates of diagnosis
occurring over the past two decades. In one of the few
population-based epidemiologic studies, Lucas et al[7]
studied the incidence of anorexia nervosa for the total
population of Rochester, Minnesota, over a 45-year
period (1935 to 1979). Their records included patients
who had never been hospitalized and had never seen a
psychiatrist. These authors ascertained no significant
long-term trends in the incidence of the disorder.
However, they did document a low point in the incidence
rates in the 1950s, which may account for the findings in
other studies that examined a shorter time span beginning
at this low point. The highest age-specific incidence rate
was found in 15- to 19-year-old girls (56.7 per 100,000
person years). A more recent study of females in primary

care in the Netherlands found an incidence rate for
anorexia nervosa in 15- to 19-year-old girls of 79.6 per
100,000 person years.[9] As in Lucas' study, this was the
highest age-specific incidence rate; the rate for 10- to
14-year-old girls was only 8.6 per 100,000 person years.
A meta-analysis of 29 surveys conducted published between 1973 and 1995 concluded that "anorexia nervosa
remains a rare disorder and there is no evidence of a
secular increase in its incidence."[10] However a 1995
study of the incidence of anorexia nervosa in the female
population of Northeast Scotland over the period from
1965 to 1991 found a mean annual increase in incidence
of 5.3%.[11] The data from this study also suggested,
however, that less severely ill patients were referred for
treatment in the latter part of the study period. There is
fairly good agreement that the incidence of bulimia
nervosa, on the other hand, has increased dramatically
between 1973 and 1995, and some epidemiologic studies
may overlap these two diagnostic categories.

Lucas et al[7] calculated the prevalence rate of anorexia
nervosa on January 1, 1980, in Rochester, Minnesota to
be 204 per 100,000 for female residents and 17 per
100,000 for male residents. For girls in the 15- to 19-year
age range, the prevalence was 1 in 332. Reporting the
prevalence of anorexia nervosa among British schoolgirls
aged 16 to 18 years, Crisp et al[12] noted a rate of 1 in 550
among girls enrolled in state-supported schools and a rate
of 1 in 100 (five times higher) among girls enrolled in
private boarding schools. The boarding school girls were
from families of higher socioeconomic status, which
highlights the importance of sociocultural factors in this
disorder.

These epidemiologic data suggest that physicians
who practice in affluent urban or suburban communities,
or on preparatory school or college campuses, will
encounter numerous cases of anorexia nervosa. One
report from Massachusetts documented a 3.3% prevalence of anorexia nervosa among female medical students.[13] The syndrome is sufficiently common for
reports in the literature to note that girls with some of
the more common chronic illnesses of adolescence have
had coincident anorexia nervosa.[14] This seems to be
especially likely with energy-wasting disorders such as
diabetes mellitus and Crohn's disease. In both of these
disorders the disease process makes it easy for the
individual to lose weight.

ETIOLOGY

The cause of anorexia nervosa remains unclear. In fact,
the syndrome may represent multiple disease entities with
varying etiologies but a similar clinical picture. Consonant with this view is Lucas' description of anorexia
nervosa as a biopsychosocial illness.[15] It implies that

there are vulnerabilities for the illness in all three spheres: biologic, psychological, and sociocultural.

Biologic Factors

In the early years of the twentieth century, anorexia nervosa was thought to result from an organic hypothalamic or pituitary lesion, and for many years it was not differentiated from Simmonds' disease. It is now known that the abnormalities of hypothalamic and pituitary function observed in patients with anorexia nervosa are similar to those noted in other starvation states and are reversible through improved nutrition. Investigation is now being focused on more subtle neurotransmitter abnormalities as a possible predisposing biologic factor. Many neuroendocrine abnormalities have been noted in starved patients with anorexia nervosa, and most of these have been shown to revert to normal with appropriate weight gain. For example, the elevated levels of plasma cortisol, impaired dexamethasone response, and low serotonin levels in cerebrospinal fluid appear to be secondary to malnutrition.[8] Low levels of norepinephrine, the neurotransmitter metabolite, are also found in the cerebrospinal fluid of underweight patients with anorexia nervosa as well as in that of depressed patients. Kaye et al,[16] in a long-term follow-up study of weight-recovered patients with anorexia nervosa, documented persistent decreased levels of this monoamine metabolite. The significance of this finding has yet to be explained, but it may provide a clue to help elucidate the neurobiology of this eating disorder.

The relationship between biologic depression and anorexia nervosa has been studied extensively. Investigators have found an increased prevalence of affective disorders in the families of patients with anorexia nervosa.[8] The converse is not true, however. The relatives of patients with affective disorders do not show an increased prevalence of eating disorders. Severe malnutrition causes depression that is readily ameliorated by refeeding, yet some patients with anorexia nervosa remain depressed even when adequate nutrition has been established, and they are found to have a concurrent major depressive disorder. According to Yates,[8] research seems to indicate that although anorexia nervosa and depression are frequently associated, they are not expressions of a common biologic base. Other studies suggest that patients with eating disorders, including anorexia nervosa, have a high prevalence of co-morbid obsessive-compulsive disorder.[17]

Anorexia nervosa is recognized as a familial disorder with a higher risk for development of the syndrome in female relatives of patients with anorexia nervosa than in female relatives of control subjects.[18] However, the contribution of genetic as opposed to environmental factors is not clear. In a report on a clinical sample of 23 sets of monozygotic twins, 10 sets were concordant for anorexia nervosa and 13 were discordant, which suggests the possibility of a genetic predisposition.[19] A 1995 study of anorexia nervosa in a population-based female twin sample (n = 2163, mean age 30.1 years) found a 0.51% lifetime prevalence of the disorder.[20] In addition, the study found that co-twins of twins with anorexia nervosa were at significantly higher risk for anorexia nervosa, bulimia nervosa, major depression, and low body mass index. Unfortunately, because of the low prevalence of anorexia nervosa in the general population, the numbers of twin pairs concordant for the syndrome were too small to permit any meaningful conclusions about genetic predisposition. Another finding that might suggest a genetic etiologic component is that girls with the chromosomal anomaly resulting in Turner's syndrome appear to be at particular risk for developing anorexia nervosa.[21] All this evidence tends to indicate that some as yet unknown, genetically determined biologic vulnerabilities play an etiologic role in the development of this eating disorder.

Psychological Factors

Psychological factors seem to be important in the etiology of anorexia nervosa. Although the relationship between personality and this syndrome is complex and difficult to study, girls with certain personality traits appear to be at higher risk for the development of anorexia nervosa. These traits include shyness and timidity, social anxiety, obsessiveness, emotional overcontrol, excessive dependency and passivity, compliancy, rigid perfectionism, and self-doubt.[22] It is important to note that malnutrition alone can cause introversion, depression, and obsessiveness and that these traits may improve substantially with weight restoration.

Many girls with anorexia nervosa have experienced separation stresses during early life and have been poorly or inconsistently nurtured. Developmental psychologists view these early losses as contributors to the intense neediness coupled with a poor self-concept that develops in these girls.[8] When such children reach adolescence, they are not well equipped to establish an independent identity and instead attempt to gain some autonomy and control through the manipulation of their diet and exercise regimen.

The families of patients with anorexia nervosa have been the subject of extensive study. As Minuchin et al[23] noted, many show characteristics typical of families with psychosomatically ill children, including enmeshment, overprotectiveness, rigidity, and lack of conflict resolution. Often the child with anorexia nervosa plays a role in the family pattern of conflict avoidance, and this background acts as a reinforcement for the abnormal eating behavior. In some patients a severe form of parenting failure is found that is likely to have played a major role in making the adolescent psychologically vulnerable to the development of anorexia nervosa.[24] For others with this syndrome, although the family may appear distressed over the child's illness, closer study reveals that they function in a reasonably normal manner, and other biologic or sociocultural factors seem to be etiologically predominant in the patient.[25]

Sociocultural Factors

Since the prevailing standard of feminine beauty emphasizes extreme thinness, we are presently experiencing a period of high social vulnerability for the development of anorexia nervosa. This is particularly true for women in the upper social classes and for those who are upwardly mobile. Numerous studies of high school and college student populations have demonstrated that more than half of the young women in these groups are preoccupied with their weight and fearful of becoming fat. Postpubertal young women in the United States express considerable body-image dissatisfaction. Dieting, binging, and purging behaviors are quite common even in nonclinical populations. For example, the national Youth Risk Behavior Survey conducted by the Centers for Disease Control and Prevention on a representative sample of U.S. high school students (grades 9 to 12) found that in 1990, 44% of female students, but only 15% of male students, reported currently trying to lose weight.[26] In addition, 21% of high school girls had a history of using diet pills, and 14% admitted to inducing vomiting for the purpose of losing weight. There is a disturbing trend for this body-image dissatisfaction to filter down into younger age groups, including prepubertal children. A large survey of a middle school population (grades 5 to 8, mean age 12 years) conducted in 1990-1991 in South Carolina found that more than 50% of the girls and 28% of the boys "wanted to lose weight" and/or "felt or looked fat to others."[27] There is considerable evidence that dieting itself is a major risk factor for the development of an eating disorder.[28] Since many more adolescent girls than boys diet, this may explain, in part, why girls are more likely to develop eating disorders.

The young woman who finds herself in a social or occupational environment that encourages excessive thinness, such as ballet dancing or high-fashion modeling, is at high risk of developing anorexia nervosa. Conversely, a young woman with other risk factors for this eating disorder will often choose to become a dancer or a model. Thus, these occupations seem selective for girls with this syndrome. The relationship between athleticism and anorexia nervosa, which is complex and unclear, has only recently been explored in a number of studies. The syndrome is common in both male and female marathon runners and in female gymnasts and dancers. Many of these athletes appear to have less psychopathology than other patients with anorexia nervosa and respond better to treatment, which suggests a predominantly sociocultural etiology. However, intense exercise coupled with strict dieting actually may trigger a biobehavioral response in some individuals that leads to the syndrome of anorexia nervosa.[29] This theory is based on a rat model of an anorexia nervosa type of syndrome that leads to death from "self-starvation." Thus, some of what is considered sociocultural vulnerability for the development of anorexia nervosa may actually have a biologic base that, while not causative, does serve to reinforce the starvation behavior once it begins.

With this biopsychosocial concept of the etiology of anorexia nervosa as a focal point, the important areas of clinical assessment and treatment for patients and their families become clearer. It is helpful to try to determine which areas of vulnerability seem to dominate the onset and persistence of symptoms, and to tailor the therapy accordingly.

CLINICAL FEATURES

General Considerations

The diagnosis of anorexia nervosa can usually be made reliably with a careful history and physical examination.[30] Patients most commonly present because of either excessive weight loss or amenorrhea (primary or secondary). Occasionally, gastrointestinal symptoms predominate and the initial complaint may be abdominal pain and/or vomiting. Younger children may be brought to a physician because of short stature and pubertal delay.[31] Depending on the dominant symptom and the patient's age, the initial contact may be with a gynecologist, pediatrician, internist, family physician, gastroenterologist, endocrinologist, or psychiatrist. Often the adolescent does not acknowledge that she has a problem and is unwillingly brought to the physician by a concerned family member. The adolescent may be hostile and try to minimize her symptoms. The diagnosis may be delayed if the physician follows the patient's lead and focuses exclusively on one of the signs or symptoms without consideration of the full spectrum of the anorexia nervosa syndrome. It is also important, however, that the physician gain the patient's trust and not appear to ignore her concerns. Gentleness, empathy, and understanding, coupled with a firm conviction that the patient does indeed have a problem, will go a long way toward establishing a working relationship. Recently, much attention has been devoted to anorexia nervosa in the media, and many adolescents and some parents will have considered the diagnosis themselves before seeking medical attention. It may be helpful to ask the adolescent if she has wondered whether her symptoms could be due to anorexia nervosa.

The DSM-IV diagnostic criteria listed in Box 31-1 indicate the features that the physician should concentrate on during the history taking and physical examination. Of course, careful weighing and measurement are essential. In addition, a detailed menstrual history, diet history, and body-image history are needed to establish the diagnosis. Laboratory and radiographic procedures may be useful for ruling out other diseases in the differential diagnosis, but they are not helpful in confirming a diagnosis of anorexia nervosa.

Bruch[2] defined the psychological features of the syndrome as consisting of three basic areas: (1) a disturbance of delusional proportions in body image and body concept, (2) a disturbance in the accuracy of the perception or cognitive interpretation of stimuli arising in the body, and (3) a paralyzing sense of ineffectiveness that pervades all thinking and activities of patients with anorexia. Knowledge of these features helps in formulating an approach to the patient and denotes the historical issues that need to be explored when the syndrome is suspected.

Patient History

Although patients with anorexia nervosa are most often brought to the physician by a concerned parent or parents, the bulk of the initial interview is best conducted with the adolescent alone. Since many of the feelings and behaviors that must be inquired about are secret and shameful to the patient, she is unlikely to be frank in the presence of her parents. On the other hand, it is also important to get the parents' point of view on their child's condition, and they should be interviewed separately. Most often this requires an additional office visit so that enough time can be allotted.

At the beginning of the interview with the adolescent, questions designed to determine the amount of weight loss, the time course over which the weight loss has occurred, the patient's estimate of previous high and low weights, and the mechanism of the weight loss are most helpful. Even if the adolescent's chief complaint is that of a symptom secondary to weight loss, such as primary or secondary amenorrhea, the experienced clinician will initially direct the questioning to the weight problem. This can be done easily by saying to the teenager: "I notice that you are very thin. Sometimes the problem you are complaining of can be caused by extreme thinness. How long have you been losing weight?"

Questioning regarding the mechanisms of weight loss should include an accurate assessment of not only energy intake but also energy expenditure through exercise and caloric loss because of vomiting and diarrhea. Energy intake is most easily estimated by instructing the patient to recall every item of food and drink that she had on the previous day for breakfast, lunch, dinner, and snacks. When the diagnosis of anorexia nervosa is being considered, it is important to question the patient in minute detail in order to avoid overestimating the daily caloric intake. If the adolescent reports drinking a glass of milk, she should be asked if it was whole milk or skim. If she had a sandwich for lunch, she needs to be asked if she ate both pieces of bread or removed any of the filling. With this very careful line of questioning, a reliable estimate of the amount of calories consumed by the patient on the previous day can be made. A daily consumption of less than 1500 kcal will lead to weight loss in the normally active teenager. Many patients with anorexia nervosa consume less than 800 kcal per day. Although they do not eat much food, patients with anorexia nervosa are usually very knowledgeable and interested in nutrition, knowing the caloric content of most food items and often becoming involved in shopping and cooking for their families. Sometimes they can make a more accurate estimate of their caloric intake than the physician and are pleased to do so.

One would expect patients with anorexia nervosa to be exhausted and weak from their self-imposed starvation, but they are usually very active, often running, exercising, or dancing several times a day. It is helpful to ask if they have a regular exercise routine at home. What does it consist of? How long is it? How many repetitions do they do? If they take dancing lessons, how frequent are the lessons and how long do they last? If they run or walk regularly, how far do they go and how often? It is also important to establish whether or not these patients feel guilty if they are unable to complete their exercise routine for some reason. Anorexia nervosa is frequently encountered among girls who are serious about ballet study, and in both boys and girls who are distance runners. However, most often the increased exercise—running, bicycling, or aerobic dancing—is a result of the developing eating disorder, not a contributing factor in its cause.

In spite of the name of the syndrome, patients with anorexia nervosa usually have no loss of appetite. They do experience hunger, but they successfully maintain rigid control over their caloric intake and their weight. Sometimes this control weakens and they indulge in binge eating, or bulimia, often followed by self-induced vomiting. Any adolescent suspected of having anorexia nervosa should be questioned about vomiting. She may be quite secretive and embarrassed by this symptom and deny it, even when it has actually occurred. The parents may often be able to offer information about indications of vomiting, such as time spent in the bathroom after each meal or sounds of retching. If the patient responds positively when questioned about vomiting, she should be asked whether she induces the vomiting herself and how she does this. Most patients use mechanical techniques such as placing a finger or a spoon in the back of the throat. Some sophisticated patients consult their home medical encyclopedias and purchase ipecac syrup to induce vomiting. This is a very dangerous practice because the drug is toxic and can induce a myopathy.[32] The thin adolescent also should be questioned carefully about bowel symptoms and habits. Patients with anorexia nervosa are usually constipated and should be asked how often they use laxatives. Since many of these patients believe that laxatives aid in weight loss, laxative abuse is common in this syndrome.

Adolescents with anorexia nervosa perceive themselves as fat even though they appear very thin to others. Several studies have documented this distortion of body image by demonstrating that patients with this syndrome consistently overestimate their body size by 25% to 50%.[33] Inquiries regarding how the patient views her current weight and appearance should be made every time the physician encounters an excessively thin adolescent. Many cachectic girls with anorexia nervosa will say they think they look all right or that they would look better if they lost another few pounds. Most will say that they think their thighs are too big. Some patients with this syndrome, knowing what the physician wants to hear, will acknowledge that they look thin. A useful response by the physician is an empathetic one: "Yes, I agree, but how do you feel?" Most will then break down and respond, "I feel fat."

For all adolescent patients, a careful social and sexual history should be obtained. Teenagers with anorexia nervosa usually have little interest in dating or sexuality. A study of a large group of young adult women with eating disorders found that significantly fewer of those with anorexia nervosa had ever had sexual intercourse compared with those with bulimia nervosa, even after controlling for symptom severity.[34] Also, the women with anorexia nervosa were only half as likely as those with bulimia to report engaging in masturbation, and the degree of caloric restriction was inversely related to having masturbated. Since boys and young men who are homosexual or questioning their sexual orientation may be more at risk than heterosexual boys for developing anorexia nervosa, sensitive questioning about sexual orientation should be made when the diagnosis is being considered in a male.[35,36] It has been widely reported in the popular press that eating disorders result from childhood sexual abuse. Careful studies examining the relationship between anorexia nervosa and previous sexual abuse suggest that although childhood sexual abuse is a vulnerability factor for psychiatric disorder in general, it does not particularly or necessarily lead to an eating disorder.[37,38] Nevertheless, a sexual and physical abuse history should be taken from all patients.

Girls with anorexia nervosa seldom participate in activities with friends; instead, they tend to be loners. They may interact socially with their families, often in activities centered around food. As the condition progresses, however, arguments within the family about her eating behavior frequently cause the adolescent to withdraw and eat alone. Adolescents who have anorexia nervosa are generally excellent students and are very meticulous and obsessive in completing assigned tasks. They are unlikely to smoke or use alcohol or drugs, in marked contrast to patients with bulimia nervosa. However, older patients with a long-standing history of anorexia nervosa, especially when they have the binge-eating/purging subtype, occasionally become alcoholic. A history of depression and suicide ideation and attempts should be obtained, although such attempts are uncommon in patients with anorexia nervosa. In addition, the patient should be asked about psychiatric illness, alcoholism, or drug abuse among her immediate family members.

Careful questioning regarding the timing of the growth spurt and pubertal development is important, since these developmental features are often delayed or abnormal if the eating disorder began at or before puberty.[31] If a girl noted breast budding more than 4 years previously and still has not had menarche, she should be considered to have primary amenorrhea. Absence of breast buds by the age of 13 is consistent with delayed puberty. A careful menstrual history for postmenarchal girls is important. Since the menses often cease prior to any significant weight loss, the duration of amenorrhea should be noted and correlated with the weight history. Some older adolescents with anorexia nervosa who are taking oral contraceptives continue to have monthly withdrawal bleeding. This should not preclude the diagnosis of the syndrome, as noted in the DSM-IV criteria.

Physical Examination

Patients who are emaciated because of anorexia nervosa are usually hypometabolic and hypothermic, and therefore often wear several layers of clothing, which serve to camouflage the degree of their emaciation. The physician can be fooled into thinking that a patient is heavier than she really is, especially if she is not required to undress completely for the physical examination. The patient's hands can provide a clue that she is excessively thin if they are icy cold and a mottled reddish-blue in color (acrocyanosis). The patient should be undressed (wearing a hospital gown) and should have voided before being weighed. Because the formulas for ideal weight for age and height do not correct for skeletal mass and body frame size, some girls with "small bones" look thin but not cachectic at a weight of 25% below the ideal, whereas others with a large frame can appear impressively malnourished with the same degree of weight loss. To assess the severity of the emaciation, the patient should be examined visually for the amount of muscle mass; the presence or absence of an adequate amount of subcutaneous fat; redundant skin folds on the thighs, buttocks, and arms; and bruising or callus formation over the bony prominences of the shoulders and hips (due to lack of subcutaneous padding). Either lanugo or edema of the lower extremities signifies severe malnutrition.

Tanner staging of secondary sexual characteristics is an important factor in assessing pubertal delay or arrest. Since the patient's primary complaint is frequently related to menstrual dysfunction, the question arises regarding the necessity for a pelvic examination. Most adolescent patients presenting with a possible diagnosis of anorexia nervosa are virginal and are usually psychologically unprepared for such an examination at the first visit. It is therefore a good idea to discuss the examination at the initial visit but to defer the actual process until the second or third visit. It is not necessary to insist on a complete speculum and bimanual examination unless the patient has been sexually active. In most instances a careful inspection of the vulva for anatomic abnormalities, and a rectoabdominal bimanual examination to check for the presence of a cervix and the absence of abnormal masses or tenderness, are sufficient. If there has been long-standing hypothalamic suppression, the vaginal epithelium will not be well estrogenized and may be quite atrophic, making any kind of vaginal examination painful.

Most malnourished patients with anorexia nervosa have a resting bradycardia of 60 beats/min or less.[39] Blood pressure is usually in the lower ranges of normal. Severely emaciated, dehydrated patients may have postural hypotension and often experience syncope or dizziness. Since loss of scalp hair is commonly experienced with severe degrees of malnutrition, the hair should be inspected for texture and signs of thinning.

Laboratory Data

In patients with this syndrome, laboratory results are most often surprisingly normal. The hemoglobin level, platelet count, and total protein, albumin, and mineral concentrations are usually within normal limits. The white blood cell count is often low in severely emaciated patients, but it is normal in those who are less malnourished. Despite often severe leukopenia, patients with anorexia nervosa do not appear to have an increased susceptibility to infection.[40] The erythrocyte sedimentation rate is usually very low; if it is elevated even minimally, another diagnosis should be suspected.[39] Although serum electrolyte concentrations are most frequently undisturbed, they may be abnormal in patients who are experiencing dehydration, water intoxication, and vomiting and particularly in those who practice laxative abuse.[41] The blood urea nitrogen concentration also may be elevated in patients who are dehydrated, but creatinine levels remain normal. Serum hepatic transaminase levels are often mildly elevated because of the fatty degeneration of the liver that accompanies starvation. The serum cholesterol concentration is variable and can be either normal or high, whereas the serum carotene concentration is sometimes elevated. The latter finding is specific for anorexia nervosa as opposed to cachexia or other etiologies in which the serum carotene is most often low. The cause of the hypercarotenemia is unclear, but it is probably associated with an acquired defect in the utilization of vitamin A.[42]

Several tests of endocrine function commonly show abnormal results in starved patients, including those with anorexia nervosa. However, many of these hormonal studies need not be performed routinely because they add little to the differential diagnosis or management of this condition. The most frequent findings include minimal elevation of serum cortisol and low serum levels of thyroid hormones and gonadotropins. Twenty-four hour studies of luteinizing hormone (LH) secretion in postpubertal patients with anorexia nervosa have shown that there is a regression of the circadian activity of LH to prepubertal or early pubertal patterns during the acute illness; reversion to the normal adult secretion pattern correlates with physical and psychological recovery.[43]

Vitamin deficiencies are rarely found in patients who have anorexia nervosa, presumably because their diets usually contain sufficient green leafy vegetables and fruits. Trace metals, however, may not be so abundant in the diet. Low plasma and urinary zinc concentrations have been documented in some of these patients.[44] Zinc deficiency may account for the hypogeusia and hair loss reported by some patients and may contribute to the depression associated with starvation. Urinary copper concentrations have also been reported to be subnormal in teenagers with this syndrome.

The urinalysis often shows small amounts of ketones and protein, findings that are consistent with starvation. In addition, the specific gravity may be relatively low, even when the patient is dehydrated because of a renal concentrating defect. Pyuria with negative urine culture, and clearing that occurs spontaneously with hydration and improved nutrition, have been observed in adolescents with anorexia nervosa.[39] One report noted that adolescent girls with eating disorders are significantly more likely than those without such disorders to have alkaline urine, with a pH of 7 or higher.[45]

PHYSIOLOGIC COMPLICATIONS

Hypokalemia and hypochloremic alkalosis occur with some regularity in severely ill patients who are frequent vomiters and laxative or diuretic abusers. These disturbances, if untreated, can lead to serious cardiac complications and even death. In the absence of electrolyte or acid-base derangements, cardiac function at rest is usually normal. Exercise testing of adolescents with anorexia nervosa, however, reveals decreased working capacity and abnormal cardiovascular and sympathetic responses to exercise.[46] Electrocardiographic abnormalities are common in this illness and include bradycardia, decreased QRS amplitude, nonspecific ST-segment and T-wave changes, and prolongation of the QT interval. Some patients develop significant ST-segment depression during exercise, which suggests that myocardial insult has occurred, and these adolescents may be at higher risk for cardiac complications during intense exercise. Echocardiography has demonstrated a reduction in left ventricular muscle mass in some patients. Unexpected sudden deaths do occur, most often in patients who have lost 40% or more of their ideal body weight. These deaths are usually attributed to arrhythmias or degenerative cardiomyopathy secondary to extreme malnutrition.[47]

Gastrointestinal complications are relatively common in anorexia nervosa. Most patients have delayed gastric emptying, abnormal gastric motility, and decreased hydrogen-ion output, leading to symptoms of postprandial fullness, early satiety, and (occasionally) acute gastric dilation when refeeding is done too rapidly. With a judicious refeeding program, these symptoms improve significantly, and prokinetic agents (e.g., metoclopramide, bethanechol) or gastrointestinal radiographic studies are rarely needed.[48] Pancreatic dysfunction is common with anorexia nervosa but is most often asymptomatic. Acute pancreatitis does occur, however, and may be an indication for parenteral nutrition. One study reported that seven of 10 consecutive patients presenting with anorexia nervosa had abnormal pancreatic biochemical test results.[49] All seven had elevated amylase creatinine clearance ratios, but only three patients had elevated serum amylase concentrations, and only one of these was symptomatic. Two of the patients with normal serum amylase levels were also symptomatic with nausea, pain, and/or vomiting. All the symptomatic patients had abnormal pancreatic findings by ultrasound examination that were consistent with pancreatitis. These abnormalities were thought to be due to malnutrition; unlike findings with primary pancreatitis, food intake did not adversely affect these pancreatic study results. The common occurrence of pancreatic dysfunction is also associated with elevated sweat chloride concentrations in up to 75% of patients with anorexia nervosa and should not prompt a diagnosis of cystic fibrosis.[50] An unusual cause of intractable vomiting in anorexia nervosa is the superior mesenteric artery syndrome.[51] This results from vascular compression of the duodenum in cachectic patients who are kept at bed rest.

One of the most worrisome physiologic complications of anorexia nervosa is osteoporosis. A 1991 study indicates that the reduced bone mass noted in these patients may not be completely reversed by recovery from the disorder, and patients may be at higher risk of fractures throughout their lives.[52] Vertebral compression fractures, rib fractures associated with vomiting, and other fractures are not rare in patients with long-standing anorexia nervosa. Bachrach et al[53] studied bone mineral density in adolescent girls with anorexia nervosa in comparison with their healthy peers, and found that patients with eating disorders had significantly lower lumbar vertebral bone density and significantly lower whole body bone mass than normal girls. Two thirds of these young patients had marked deficits in bone mineral density, and in one half of these patients the interval since diagnosis of anorexia nervosa was 1 year or less. Factors related to the development of osteopenia in anorexia nervosa include hypoestrogenemia, glucocorticoid excess, and inadequate calcium and protein intake. In addition, adolescent girls with this eating disorder evidence marked abnormalities in mineral metabolism. Calcium kinetic studies show an increased rate of bone resorption and decreased rate of bone formation.[54] Decreased estrogen secretion is thought to be the most significant factor contributing to osteopenia, and there is some evidence to suggest that estrogen deficiency may have the most profound deleterious effect on bone mineral density if it begins at an earlier age.[55] Malnutrition with low estrogen levels during adolescence may lead to the attainment of a lower peak skeletal mass that persists for life. The effect of exercise on bone mineral density in this disorder remains unclear; some authors found a protective effect against bone loss and others did not.

Partial nephrogenic diabetes insipidus occurs in some patients with anorexia nervosa. They frequently have polyuria and produce a relatively dilute urine even when dehydrated. One study has documented deficient or inappropriate secretion of the antidiuretic hormone arginine vasopressin in response to the infusion of hypertonic saline in four emaciated patients with anorexia nervosa when compared with four age-matched controls.[56] The abnormal vasopressin secretion persisted in these patients when they were restudied after short-term recovery, but it tended to normalize after long-term recovery (defined as 6 months or more of normal weight).

Abnormal neurologic signs are rare in anorexia nervosa; if found, they should prompt a search for another diagnosis. However, findings of cortical atrophy and/or ventricular dilation by computed tomography appear to be common.[57] These abnormalities are found more frequently in patients who have lost a large amount of weight in a short time. These findings appear to be reversible with weight gain, but their clinical significance is unknown.

MANAGEMENT

General Considerations

Anorexia nervosa has physiologic as well as behavioral manifestations, and any treatment plan must address both these concerns.[58] To be most effective and to minimize potential life-threatening complications, the management of patients with this disorder is often conducted jointly by a primary care physician and a psychotherapist. Other healthcare professionals such as nutritionists, social workers, or nurses frequently become valued members of a treatment team, particularly in inpatient settings. During the course of the prolonged treatment usually required for patients with anorexia nervosa, many therapeutic decisions need to be made that take into consideration both physiologic and psychological features of the patient's illness. Frequent communication among members of the healthcare team is critical to avoid giving mixed messages and further confusing an often complex treatment regimen. When it works well, joint therapy by two clinicians with different but complementary skills, or by a team of professionals, serves as a problem-solving model for the patient and her family and presents a unified therapeutic front that addresses the biopsychosocial nature of the illness.

The role of the primary care physician in this partnership includes diagnosis and referral for psychiatric assessment, and encompasses nutritional monitoring and counseling. The primary care physician also must manage the complications of starvation, vomiting and laxative abuse, pubertal delay, menstrual dysfunction, and intercurrent illnesses. In addition, as with any complex chronic illness treated in conjunction with other specialists, the primary care physician may serve as a coordinator of care and as a support to the family. The primary care physician who makes the diagnosis often has a long-standing relationship with the family and is in the best position to explain the seriousness of the illness to the patient and her parents and to convince them of the need for psychiatric referral. Assurance of the physician's continuing concern and involvement with the management of the somatic sequelae of the syndrome helps the patient and family to accept the necessity for psychiatric assessment and treatment.

Indications for Hospitalization

Most physicians would agree that if the patient is 40% or more below ideal body weight, she should be hospitalized immediately in an acute care medical, pediatric, or adolescent unit for emergency nutritional rehabilitation. The risk of death is substantial with this degree of malnutrition. If the patient's weight is 30% to 40% below the ideal, a choice must be made between immediate hospitalization and a short trial of outpatient therapy.[30] If the patient is closer to 40% below ideal weight, if she is losing weight rapidly, if she vomits excessively or uses significant amounts of laxatives/diuretics, or if the physician believes the patient or the family will not be able to cooperate with outpatient therapy, hospitalization is preferable.

A period of outpatient assessment and treatment by a psychotherapist experienced with eating disorders in conjunction with the primary care physician may be a useful option even if the patient ultimately needs to be hospitalized. This approach should be attempted for those who have lost less than 30% of ideal body weight and who have no other indication for hospitalization. This adjustment period allows the patient to develop trust in both of her treating clinicians and will facilitate a smooth transition to postdischarge care, which will be necessary after any inpatient stay. The parents also will have time to adjust to the knowledge that their child has a chronic, life-threatening condition and therefore may be more willing to accept hospitalization at a later date.

Other indications for hospitalization include severe metabolic or cardiovascular disturbance, for example, orthostatic hypotension or systolic blood pressure less than 70 mm Hg; cardiac arrhythmia or pulse less than 40 beats/min; significant hypokalemia or other electrolyte disturbance; and hypothermia with temperature less than 36°C.[59] Additional medical indications include significant infection in a compromised host, such as pneumonia, or an unusual presentation requiring confirmation of the diagnosis.[60] Adolescent boys in whom the diagnosis is being considered may have more co-morbid psychopathology than girls and often benefit from early hospitalization for diagnosis and initiation of treatment.

Psychiatric indications for hospitalization include severe depression or suicide risk, psychosis, out-of-control binging and purging, and family crisis. Sometimes a period of hospitalization is advisable for a patient who has reached a plateau stage in outpatient therapy; although she may have none of the above indications for hospitalization, she may be unable to gain any weight for several months and needs a more structured environment to break her eating patterns.

Inpatient Management

Adolescents whose weight is 40% or more below the ideal for age and height often have altered mental status and are usually not receptive to behavioral modification aimed at encouraging them to eat. These patients probably should have the responsibility for eating removed from them temporarily, and be given either parenteral nutrition or a nutritionally complete liquid diet via nasogastric or nasoduodenal tube. This degree of malnutrition is rarely encountered, but it does occur. One paper reported a 22-year-old woman with an 8-year history of anorexia nervosa who died in hospital after a clinical decision had been made not to pursue aggressive forms of nutritional support.[61] Most hospitalized patients with anorexia nervosa are not in such extreme states and will respond to a structured, well-supervised behavioral modification program of refeeding. Most programs use positive reinforcement, including social activities, visiting privileges, and physical activity, but sometimes negative reinforcement, such as bed rest or isolation, is necessary.[62] The reinforcement should be made contingent on weight gain, an objective measurement, rather than on eating behavior. This approach avoids conflicts with the staff over the amount of food eaten, and discourages patients from hiding food. The behavioral modification program should be individualized for each patient so that the reinforcers chosen are meaningful to the adolescent.

It is difficult to establish a psychotherapeutic relationship with the adolescent while she is severely malnourished, and the initial phase of hospitalization is primarily concerned with improving nutritional status. After 7 to 10 days of adequate intake, a marked improvement in the patient's mood, verbalization, and sociability is usually strikingly apparent, and psychotherapeutic work can then begin. Most treatment programs offer individual supportive therapy and group and family therapy. The goals of individual therapy include providing understanding and empathy for the patient's fear of losing control and becoming fat, while simultaneously offering the patient firm encouragement to gain weight and get better.[63] Helping the patient to see how her emotions are reflected in her weight and her eating behavior can be useful. Group therapy can help patients to become more assertive and to express their feelings. Family therapy, which has been shown to be especially important for younger adolescents with anorexia nervosa, may be started during hospitalization. Often, however, family therapy is used as a form of outpatient treatment.[64] During inpatient treatment, the parents should be kept informed of the patient's progress. It is also helpful to have regular meetings with the parents and all members of the treatment team.

There is considerable individual variation in caloric requirements for weight gain in patients with anorexia nervosa, but general guidelines that can be modified for individual patients are useful. Beginning in hospital with a diet of 1200 to 1500 kcal/day and increasing gradually by 500- to 750-kcal increments per week to 3500 to 5000 kcal/day usually results in the desired weight gain. A reasonable weight goal for a hospitalized patient who is severely emaciated is 1 kg, or 2 pounds, per week. Some treatment programs aim for 3 to 4 pounds/week after an initial period of stabilization, and this seems to be a safe

and attainable goal.[65] Very rapid weight gain is associated with potentially severe complications, including congestive heart failure, pancreatitis, and acute gastric dilation. The clinician who is setting the weight goals should not ignore the role of exercise in expenditure of calories. Some restriction needs to be placed on the amount of exercise the patient is permitted. In the past, treatment programs initially confined the patient to bed and gradually allowed more exercise as weight gain proceeded. This practice is no longer recommended because it may lead to accelerated bone resorption and contribute to the complication of osteoporosis. Nevertheless, exercise should be limited to "activities of daily living" for the first few weeks.

As improvement occurs, patients, and sometimes parents, may ask the physician to adjust the goal for a smaller weight gain per week, especially if the patient has found it impossible to meet a particular goal. The parents often argue that the patient appears to be eating very well, certainly much better than before coming to the hospital, and that the physician must be setting the goal too high. The temptation to accede to this request should be resisted. Sometimes it is illuminating to look closely at the numerical value of the weight when this request is made. Often the patient's weight will plateau when it has almost increased by 5 or 10 pounds, for example, from 80 to 89 pounds. Patients with anorexia nervosa commonly develop self-imposed weight goals that are usually different from the physician's goals. They may become very anxious when their weight is approaching a new decile. Almost all patients with this syndrome have a hard time crossing the 100-pound mark, and many will plateau at 98 or 99 pounds for months if this is allowed.

From a physiologic point of view, most patients can be discharged from the hospital and treated as outpatients when they have gained to the point where they are about 20% below ideal body weight (Fig. 31-1). This allows them a 10% to 15% leeway before having to be rehospitalized. From a psychological perspective, however, it may be advantageous to keep the patient in hospital until she is within 90% to 95% of ideal weight. This may avoid having her plateau at a low weight for long periods during outpatient treatment. Practical considerations, such as insurance reimbursement, may prompt earlier discharge than would be optimal. A 5-foot 3-inch, 16-year-old girl whose ideal weight is 115 pounds and who has lost 35% of this amount and currently weighs 75 pounds must gain 40 pounds. At a rate of gain of 2 pounds/week, this will take a minimum of 20 weeks or about 4½ months. If the patient can gain at a rate of 3 pounds/week, she can be discharged in about 13 weeks. In reality, most patients are hospitalized for 2 to 3 months and then discharged to outpatient follow-up. There is some evidence that patients who are discharged when still

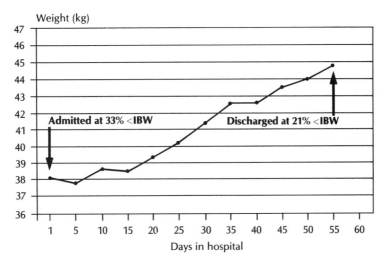

Fig. 31-1. This 16-year-old girl with anorexia nervosa was an honor student at an exclusive preparatory school and a serious and talented ballet student. Requiring 8 weeks' hospitalization, she gained 7 kg (15½ pounds) for an average weight gain of almost 2 pounds per week. Her weight gain was minimal during the first 15 days of hospitalization until a crisis was precipitated by the consideration of tube feeding. The patient never required the tube since her weight began to increase steadily at that point. She was discharged at 21% below ideal body weight (IBW) for age and height.

significantly underweight have higher rates of rehospitalization than those discharged at normal weight.[66]

Outpatient Management

When the diagnosis of anorexia nervosa is made early, patients are less malnourished and often less refractory to treatment. They may do well with outpatient therapy alone. When the illness has been only recently diagnosed, the primary care physician may begin by seeing the adolescent weekly for weighing and brief nutritional counseling. At each visit a weight goal should be set for the following week, and specific methods of attaining that goal should be worked out with the patient.

In the acute phase of illness, most patients with anorexia nervosa eat very limited diets and define many "forbidden foods." Often their daily caloric intake is as low as 600 to 800 kcal and they are eating only three or four different foods. The first task is to increase caloric intake. The patient might go home with a prescription to eat one muffin a day in addition to her usual diet or two containers of yogurt instead of one—whatever appeals to her. Her first weight goal may be simply not to lose any more weight in the following week. A reasonable weight gain goal for outpatient management is 1 pound/week, but it may take a few weeks to attain this. If the adolescent continues to lose weight, the weight at which she will be hospitalized should be clearly understood by both patient and parents. Some physicians advocate written contracts to clarify these goals.[60] The need to hospitalize can be interpreted to the family not as a failure of outpatient treatment but as an indication of the seriousness of the illness.

A daily multiple vitamin and mineral supplement should be recommended until adequate nutrition is established. Diets of less than 1200 kcal/day do not contain adequate amounts of trace elements or vitamins. As the patient gains weight and feels more confident, she should be encouraged to broaden the range of her food choices and eat a more balanced diet. The ultimate weight goal should be close to the ideal weight, but the adolescent can be allowed some input in this decision. She will need a lot of reassurance that she will not be allowed to become fat, and that even after she has reached the target weight the physician will continue to monitor her weight to make sure that she does not gain too much.

When each weight goal is set, it should be clearly understood what will happen if the goal is not met. Usually some type of restriction of exercise (e.g., discontinuing dance lessons or gym class) can be imposed. Such restriction can be explained to the adolescent as a way of helping her to build new muscle tissue (not fat) and become healthier so that later she will be able to participate fully in these activities. It is better not to categorize the restriction as a punishment, although many patients will interpret it as such; if the restriction is imposed, these patients will cry and bargain to be allowed just one more try. If the restriction is to be imposed, it is important to inform the parents and to elicit their support in helping to enforce it. Weight goals and restrictions should be reasonable, fair, and clearly articulated. The physician should not back down in the face of a patient's tantrum.

It is also very helpful for the primary care physician, in the counseling sessions, to interpret physical signs and symptoms for the patient in order to provide accurate, undistorted biologic feedback. Bruch[2] pointed out that one of the core problems in anorexia nervosa is a disturbance in the cognitive interpretation of stimuli arising in the body. Statements such as "Your hair is falling out because you are malnourished, not because you brush it too much" or "It hurts you to sit in school for long periods of time because you haven't enough tissue covering the bones of your pelvis" often need to be repeated over and over again.

Patients with anorexia nervosa usually require outpatient psychotherapeutic treatment for a long time, often 1 to 2 years or more. The psychotherapist has the overall responsibility for the psychological and behavioral management of the patient and her family. The therapist's first task is to engage the patient in treatment, since most of these adolescents are initially resistant and do not acknowledge the need for behavioral intervention. The psychological assessment should begin as soon as possible after the diagnosis is entertained. The psychotherapist conducts an initial assessment of the patient and her family to confirm the diagnosis and to develop a treatment plan. Many therapists choose to see the adolescent individually twice a week, at least initially, and have sessions with the parents once a month. The therapeutic timetable can be modified, of course, as the illness improves or stabilizes. Some psychotherapists recommend treating anorexia nervosa exclusively in a family therapy mode without individual sessions for the patient, and this seems to work well in capable hands, especially for younger patients.[64] Some reliable evidence from a randomized controlled trial comparing family therapy with individual therapy indicates that family therapy was more effective for those patients whose illness was not chronic and had begun before the age of 19 years.[67] This would include most adolescent patients.

During outpatient treatment, it is necessary for the primary care physician and the psychotherapist to communicate frequently and come to an agreement on their approach to the patient and the family so that they can avoid working at cross-purposes.[64] Recovery from anorexia nervosa usually proceeds in a stepwise fashion, with alternating periods of progression and plateaus often punctuated by intervening crises (Fig. 31-2). When the crisis is physical (e.g., weight loss to a point of danger), the primary care physician must take a firm stance with the patient and insist on weight gain. The patient usually will not be pleased with this approach; however, the blow can be softened by an empathetic psychotherapist who upholds the basic treatment goal of weight gain. Alternatively, when the crisis is psychological and the patient

is being urged by the psychotherapist to face issues she would rather avoid, the primary care physician can assume the role of comforter while still stressing the need to work through the psychological issue.

Pharmacologic Therapy

A variety of pharmacologic agents have been employed in the treatment of anorexia nervosa, but to date no single class of drug has proved effective in a majority of patients.[8] Most reported drug trials have been conducted in hospitalized, severely emaciated patients who were also undergoing other forms of treatment. In addition, most reports have included only a small number of patients, have involved no control group, and have not been double blind.[68] Thus, the use of adjuvant pharmacotherapy for this syndrome must be approached with a degree of skepticism.

Phenothiazines were the first class of drug used for treatment of patients with anorexia nervosa, mainly by investigators in the United Kingdom. Chlorpromazine occasionally appears to have some beneficial effects, especially in severely obsessive-compulsive patients with this syndrome, but it is not commonly used for this disorder in the United States. Antidepressants may be helpful if a concurrent diagnosis of major depression is made. However, it is important that severe malnutrition be reversed before this diagnosis is entertained. Cyproheptadine, the serotonin antagonist, has been studied more rigorously than any of the other drugs used for treatment of anorexia nervosa. Several double-blind, placebo-controlled trials have been published. A well-designed study by Halmi et al[69] showed that cyproheptadine was useful for increasing weight gain and decreasing depressive symptoms in patients with the restricting subtype of anorexia nervosa. The drug appears to be relatively safe and well tolerated.

Other drugs that have been used include levodopa, phenytoin, lithium carbonate, and naloxone, all of which have been reported to induce weight gain in a few patients, most of whom were very emaciated. Metoclopramide, domperidone, and bethanechol also have been used as antiemetics and to control the symptoms of flatulent dyspepsia so frequently experienced by patients with anorexia nervosa. These drugs enhance gastric emptying, which is known to be delayed in patients with anorexia nervosa. Metoclopramide has central dopamine-blocking properties, however, and can precipitate depression.

Vomiting and Laxative Abuse

Approximately one third to one half of patients with anorexia nervosa exhibit self-induced vomiting and/or laxative abuse during the course of their illness. These symptoms are difficult to treat. The management of

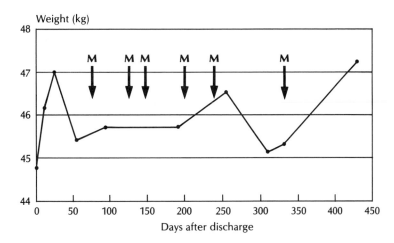

Fig. 31-2. Same patient as in Figure 31-1. The graph indicates weight changes as documented in outpatient treatment for more than 1 year after discharge from hospital. The patient gained rapidly for the first month after discharge, then stabilized at 45.5 kg (100 pounds exactly) for about 6 months. Although this weight was 18% below ideal body weight, menses resumed after 1 year of amenorrhea. The patient had 6 menstrual periods in the year following hospitalization. The precipitous weight loss noted from 275 to 325 days was related to high school graduation and anxiety about going to college. This patient has had an excellent outcome; 8 years after hospitalization, she was free of all symptoms of eating disorder. *M,* menstrual period.

vomiting is best approached by strategies designed to avoid binging. If the patient can control her intake by having frequent small snacks so that she does not become ravenous, she is less likely to binge and hence to vomit. Helping her to identify the foods she is most likely to binge on (usually sweets such as cake and ice cream) and finding ways for her to avoid being tempted by those foods is a useful strategy. Since most girls are ashamed of their vomiting and quite secretive about it, they usually stop the behavior while in hospital, especially if they are prohibited access to a private place for vomiting for approximately 2 hours after eating. Hospitalization may be indicated to help break the cycle of binging and vomiting.

Almost anyone who consumes 800 kcal/day or less will become constipated, and this is the norm for patients with anorexia nervosa. These patients tolerate constipation poorly because it makes the abdomen protrude; with the distorted body image characteristic of this illness coupled with misunderstanding of signals from the body, they interpret this protrusion as a sign of being fat. It is no surprise, therefore, that many of these patients resort to taking laxatives. There is also a widespread, but erroneous, belief that taking laxatives causes less food to be absorbed. Most patients will not tolerate stopping the laxatives abruptly, especially if they have been taking them for a long time. One strategy is to replace cathartic-type laxatives with docusate sodium (Colace), 100 mg three or four times a day, and then to try to gradually taper this stool softener as the patient's diet improves and she gains weight. It is important to monitor

serum electrolyte concentrations in all patients who are vomiting or abusing laxatives.

Menstrual Dysfunction

Amenorrhea is a necessary condition for the diagnosis of anorexia nervosa. Depending on the age and pubertal stage of the patient at the onset of the illness, the amenorrhea may be primary or secondary. Frisch and McArthur[70] demonstrated that menarche occurs when a certain weight for height, or more accurately a certain percentage of body fat, is achieved. Significant malnutrition that results in either failure to accumulate a critical amount of body fat or loss of that critical amount will produce amenorrhea in most girls. In addition, strenuous exercise, even without loss of weight to the critical point, may result in delayed puberty or secondary amenorrhea in some girls.[71] This is due partly to a change in the lean body mass–to–fat ratio and partly to other factors that are probably neurochemically mediated. Psychological stress also will produce amenorrhea in susceptible girls and women. All three of these mechanisms are probably operative in patients with anorexia nervosa. In some patients the weight factor seems to be primary, and they resume menstruation shortly after achieving a weight that is close to ideal (Fig. 31-2). In other patients stress, exercise, or other undetermined neuroendocrine factors predominate. These girls may stop having their menstrual periods prior to any significant weight loss and/or fail to regain menstrual function for months to years after achieving a normal weight. For those girls who do regain regular menstrual function, successful pregnancy with delivery of healthy infants has been reported.[72]

The pathway for all of these causes of amenorrhea is reversible hypothalamic suppression.[59] However, the mechanism of suppression is unclear, and in some patients it may be related to changes in endogenous opioid activity. Clinically, the measurement of serum gonadotropins—follicle-stimulating hormone (FSH) and luteinizing hormone—can be very useful. Since amenorrhea is often the primary symptom that brings the patient to medical attention, it is reassuring if the physician addresses this symptom in as scientific a manner as possible. When the history and physical examination are consistent with the diagnosis of anorexia nervosa, it is not necessary to undertake an extensive hormonal investigation for the amenorrhea. However, measurement of baseline serum concentrations of FSH and LH are helpful and should indicate hypothalamic suppression. The FSH is usually in the low-normal range for the follicular phase of the menstrual cycle, and the LH, a more sensitive indicator, is usually very low. As the patient improves psychologically and gains weight, measurement of LH, in association with physical signs, can help to predict resumption of menses. One of the first physical signs of reversal of hypothalamic suppression noticed by the patient is the appearance of a physiologic vaginal discharge, often accompanied by some mild breast tenderness. If serum LH concentration is measured at this time, it is usually in the intermediate range of 5 to 15 mIU/ml. These physical and biochemical changes can be taken as encouraging signs indicating that menses may resume within 6 months, barring further exacerbations of the syndrome. Serial studies of vaginal cytology focusing on estrogenic effects is another objective method used to predict resumption of menses, although the sampling procedure for this test is often perceived as more invasive and embarrassing to the young virginal patient than taking a blood sample.

The ultrasonographic appearance of the ovaries has been shown to change over the course of nutritional rehabilitation in patients with anorexia nervosa.[73] During the emaciation phase, the ovaries are small, equivalent in size to those of a child of 8 or 10 years. With a moderate but still suboptimal degree of weight restoration, the ovaries increase in size and become multicystic in appearance. As body weight normalizes, a dominant cyst may be noted, and this is often followed by menstruation. Serial ultrasound studies are an expensive way of following ovarian function in girls who have anorexia nervosa and in general are not recommended. However, if a patient undergoes a pelvic ultrasonographic study for some other reason, such as unexplained abdominal pain, it is important to realize that multicystic ovaries are an expected and regular feature of recovery in this disorder.

It should be kept in mind that there is an association between anorexia nervosa and Turner's syndrome. If patients with anorexia nervosa also have primary amenorrhea and exhibit short stature, careful physical examination for other stigmata of gonadal dysgenesis should be conducted, and a karyotype may be indicated. The serum gonadotropin levels are not always elevated when starvation is superimposed on ovarian failure.

Adolescent girls who present to a physician complaining of secondary amenorrhea and are found to have anorexia nervosa probably should not be given hormonal therapy to induce menses, at least initially. In the short term, amenorrhea that is caused by hypothalamic suppression is not dangerous to their health. Medroxyprogesterone (Provera) usually does not induce a menstrual flow because of the lack of priming of the endometrium with estrogen; if this drug is prescribed, it only serves to produce another failure for the patient. Treating the symptom of amenorrhea is not helpful; in fact, it may delay acceptance of the diagnosis of anorexia nervosa by the patient and her family as they continue to focus on an organic rather than a psychiatric cause for the symptom.

In chronic cases of anorexia nervosa, after a year or more of amenorrhea, it may be helpful to prescribe oral contraceptives as a source of estrogen to help prevent osteoporosis; however, this treatment has yet to be proved effective. Measurement of bone mineral density is helpful in making this type of therapeutic decision. Estrogen therapy is not recommended for peripubertal girls who have not yet completed their growth, although this group may be at higher risk for later development of osteoporosis. Rapid reversal of malnutrition is especially important in very young, growing girls.

OUTCOME

As noted earlier, anorexia nervosa is not a benign condition. The literature indicates that for all ages a fatal outcome occurs in 5% to 18% of patients.[74,75] The difference in reported outcome among studies depends partly on the length of follow-up. Many of the deaths occur not in patients in the acute phase of the illness but in those patients who remain chronically ill for years. Sullivan[76] conducted a meta-analysis of 42 published studies to estimate mortality from anorexia nervosa over time. The aggregate mortality rate was 0.56% per year, or 5.6% per decade. This rate is much higher than that of the general female population. The patients may die suddenly from cardiac arrest related to a degenerative cardiomyopathy caused by chronic malnutrition. Some patients with long-standing anorexia nervosa commit suicide. However, even in the 1990s some patients in the acute phase of anorexia nervosa succumb to arrhythmias caused by electrolyte imbalance, overwhelming sepsis, and severe malnutrition, and many of these deaths may be preventable.

Follow-up studies of patients with anorexia nervosa generally include measurements of eating behaviors, body weight, sociosexual adjustment, occupational record, and family relationships. Despite varying nuances of therapy, most studies report similar results.[77] Nearly half of the patients are classified as having a good outcome in all the above-mentioned areas. However, at least one third continue to show some manifestations of both dysfunctional eating habits and psychopathology for many years after onset of the disorder, despite satisfactory weight restoration. These women tend to function well in academic and occupational spheres, but they report continuing depression, loneliness, and impaired social relationships, as well as ongoing body-image distortion. Between 15% and 20% of patients with anorexia nervosa continue to do poorly in spite of intensive medical and psychiatric intervention. They need to be hospitalized repeatedly and remain markedly impaired in all areas of functioning. Factors that correlate with poor outcome include longer duration of illness; older age at onset; the presence of other symptoms such as bulimia, vomiting, or laxative abuse; poor social adjustment during childhood; and a poor relationship with parents. The 40% to 50% of patients with the binge-eating/purging subtype of anorexia nervosa generally have a poorer prognosis than those with the restricting subtype. Over time, patients who receive concurrent diagnoses of anorexia nervosa and bulimia nervosa may exhibit a variety of other impulsive behaviors, including alcoholism, illicit drug use, kleptomania, self-mutilation, and suicide attempts, and these behaviors contribute to the high morbidity and mortality among such patients.

Despite all that is known about the syndrome of anorexia nervosa, it remains a chronic condition with an uncertain and potentially fatal outcome. Because of the biopsychosocial nature of the pathophysiology of this syndrome, further elucidation of its etiology, optimal management, and prognosis demands cooperation among clinicians and investigators from many different areas of medicine.

References

1. Crisp AH, Hsu LKG, Harding B, Hartshorn J: Clinical features of anorexia nervosa, *J Psychosom Res* 24:179-191, 1980.
2. Bruch H: Psychological antecedents in anorexia nervosa. In Vigersky RA, editor: *Anorexia nervosa,* New York, 1977, Raven Press; pp 1-10.
3. American Psychiatric Association: *Diagnostic and statistical manual of mental disorders,* ed 4, Washington, DC, 1994, American Psychiatric Association.
4. Mickalide AD, Anderson AE: Subgroups of anorexia nervosa and bulimia: validity and utility, *J Psychiatr Res* 19:121-128, 1985.
5. Pyle RL: The epidemiology of eating disorders, *Pediatrician* 12:102-109, 1985.
6. Halmi K, Casper R, Eckert E, Goldberg S, Davis J: Unique features associated with age of onset of anorexia nervosa, *Psychiatry Res* 1:209-215, 1979.
7. Lucas AR, Beard CM, O'Fallon WM, Kurland LT: Anorexia nervosa in Rochester, Minnesota: a 45-year study, *Mayo Clin Proc* 63:433-442, 1988.
8. Yates A: Current perspectives on the eating disorders: Part I. History, psychological and biological aspects, *J Am Acad Child Adolesc Psychiatry* 6:813-828, 1989.
9. Hoek HW, Bartelds AIM, Bosveld JJF, et al: Impact of urbanization on detection rates of eating disorders, *Am J Psychiatry* 152:1272-1278, 1995.
10. Frombonne W: Anorexia nervosa: no evidence of an increase, *Br J Psychiatry* 166:462-471, 1995.
11. Eagles JM, Johnston MI, Hunter D, et al: Increasing incidence of anorexia nervosa in the female population of Northeast Scotland, *Am J Psychiatry* 152:1266-1271, 1995.
12. Crisp AH, Palmer RL, Kalucy RS: How common is anorexia nervosa? A prevalence study, *Br J Psychiatry* 128:549-554, 1976.
13. Herzog DB, Pepose M, Norman DK, Rigotti NA: Eating disorders and social maladjustment in female medical students, *J Nerv Ment Dis* 173:734-737, 1985.
14. Sreenivasan U: Anorexia nervosa associated with energy-wasting disorders, *Can Med Assoc J* 130:45-46, 1984.
15. Lucas AR: Toward the understanding of anorexia nervosa as a disease entity, *Mayo Clin Proc* 56:254-264, 1981.
16. Kaye W, Ebert MH, Raleigh M, et al: Abnormalities in CSF monoamine metabolism in anorexia nervosa, *Arch Gen Psychiatry* 41:350-355, 1984.
17. Thiel A, Broocks A, Ohlmeier M, et al: Obsessive-compulsive disorder among patients with anorexia nervosa and bulimia nervosa, *Am J Psychiatry* 152:72-75, 1995.
18. Strober M, Lampert C, Morrell W, et al: A controlled family study of anorexia nervosa: evidence of familial aggregation and lack of shared transmission with affective disorders, *Int J Eat Disord* 9:239-252, 1990.
19. Nowlin NS: Anorexia nervosa in twins: case report and review, *J Clin Psychiatry* 44:101-105, 1983.
20. Walters EE, Kendler KS: Anorexia nervosa and anorexic-like syndromes in a population-based female twin sample, *Am J Psychiatry* 152:64-71, 1995.
21. Doughterty GG Jr, Rockwell K, Sutton G, Ellinwood EH Jr: Anorexia nervosa in treated gonadal dysgenesis: case report and review, *J Clin Psychiatry* 44:219-221, 1983.
22. Strober M: Personality factors in anorexia nervosa, *Pediatrician* 12:134-138, 1985.
23. Minuchin S, Baker L, Rosman BL, Liebmen R, Milman L, Todd TC: A conceptual model of psychosomatic illness in children, *Arch Gen Psychiatry* 32:1031-1038, 1975.
24. Harper G: Varieties of parenting failure in anorexia nervosa: protection and parentectomy, revisited, *J Am Acad Child Psychiatry* 22:134-139, 1983.
25. Yager J, Strober M: Family aspects of eating disorders. In Hales RE, Frances AJ, editors: *American Psychiatric Association annual review,* vol 4, Washington, DC, 1985, American Psychiatric Press.
26. Centers for Disease Control: Body weight perceptions and selected weight-management goals and practices of high school students—United States, 1990, *MMWR* 40:741-750, 1991.
27. Childress AC, Brewerton TD, Hodges EL, Jarrell MP: The kids eating disorders survey (KEDS): a study of middle school students, *J Am Acad Child Adolesc Psychiatry* 32:843-850, 1993.
28. Patton GC, Johnson-Sabine E, Wood K, et al: Abnormal eating attitudes in London schoolgirls—a prospective epidemiological study: outcome at twelve month follow-up, *Psychol Med* 20:383-394, 1990.

29. Epling WF, Pierce WD: Activity based anorexia, *Int J Eat Disord* 7:475-485, 1988.

30. American Psychiatric Association: Practice guideline for eating disorders, *Am J Psychiatry* 150:209-228, 1993.

31. Root AW, Powers PS: Anorexia nervosa presenting as growth retardation in adolescents, *J Adolesc Health Care* 4:25-30, 1983.

32. Palmer EP, Guay AT: Reversible myopathy secondary to abuse of ipecac in patients with major eating disorders, *N Engl J Med* 313:1457-1459, 1985.

33. Garfinkel PE, Moldofsky H, Garner DM, Stancer HC, Coscina DV: Body awareness in anorexia nervosa: disturbances in "body image" and "safety," *Psychosom Med* 49:487-498, 1978.

34. Wiederman MW, Pryor T, Morgan CD: The sexual experience of women diagnosed with anorexia nervosa or bulimia nervosa, *Int J Eat Disord* 19:109-118, 1996.

35. Fichter MM, Daser C: Symptomatology, psychosexual development and gender identity in 42 anorexic males, *Psychol Med* 17:409-418, 1987.

36. Siever MD: Sexual orientation and gender as factors in socioculturally acquired vulnerability to body dissatisfaction and eating disorders, *J Consult Clin Psychol* 62:252-260, 1994.

37. Vize CM, Cooper PJ: Sexual abuse in patients with eating disorder, patients with depression, and normal controls: a comparative study, *Br J Psychiatry* 167:80-85, 1995.

38. Kinzl JF, Traweger C, Guenther V, Biebl W: Family background and sexual abuse associated with eating disorders, *Am J Psychiatry* 151:1127-1131, 1994.

39. Palla B, Litt IF: Medical complications of eating disorders in adolescents, *Pediatrics* 81:613-623, 1988.

40. Bowers TK, Eckert E: Leukopenia in anorexia nervosa: lack of increased risk of infection, *Arch Intern Med* 138:1520-1523, 1978.

41. Greenfeld D, Mickely D, Quinlan DM, Roloff P: Hypokalemia in outpatients with eating disorders, *Am J Psychiatry* 152:60-63, 1995.

42. Robboy MS, Sato AS, Schwabe AD: The hypercarotenemia in anorexia nervosa: a comparison of vitamin A and carotene levels in various forms of menstrual dysfunction and cachexia, *Am J Clin Nutr* 27:362-367, 1974.

43. Katz TL, Boyar R, Roffwang H, Hellman L, Weiner H: Weight and circadian luteinizing hormone secretory pattern in anorexia nervosa, *Psychosom Med* 40:549-567, 1978.

44. Casper RC, Kirschner B, Sandstead HH, Jacob RA, Davis JM: An evaluation of trace metals, vitamins and taste function in anorexia nervosa, *Am J Clin Nutr* 33:1801-1808, 1980.

45. Arden MR, Budow L, Bunnell DW, Nussbaum MP, Shenker IR, Jacobson MS: Alkaline urine is associated with eating disorders, *Am J Dis Child* 145:28-30, 1991.

46. Nudel DB, Gootman N, Nussbaum MP, Shenker IR: Altered exercise performance and abnormal sympathetic responses to exercise in patients with anorexia nervosa, *J Pediatr* 105:34-37, 1984.

47. Isner JM, Roberts WC, Heymsfield SB, Yager J: Anorexia nervosa and sudden death, *Ann Intern Med* 102:49-52, 1985.

48. Waldholtz BD, Anderson AE: Gastrointestinal symptoms in anorexia nervosa. A prospective study, *Gastroenterology* 98:1415-1419, 1990.

49. Cos KL, Cannon RA, Ament ME, Phillips HE, Schaffer CB: Biochemical and ultrasonic abnormalities of the pancreas in anorexia nervosa, *Dig Dis Sci* 28:225-229, 1983.

50. Beck R, Goldberg E, Durie PR, Levison H: Elevated sweat chloride levels in anorexia nervosa, *J Pediatr* 108:260-262, 1986.

51. Pentlow BD, Dent RG: Acute vascular compression of the duodenum in anorexia nervosa, *Br J Surg* 68:665-666, 1981.

52. Rigotti NA, Neer RM, Skates SJ, Herzog DB, Nussbaum SR: The clinical course of osteoporosis in anorexia nervosa: a longitudinal study of cortical bone mass, *JAMA* 265:1133-1138, 1991.

53. Bachrach LK, Guido D, Katzman D, Litt IF, Marcus R: Decreased bone density in adolescent girls with anorexia nervosa, *Pediatrics* 86:440-447, 1990.

54. Abrams SA, Silber TJ, Estaban NV, et al: Mineral balance and bone turnover in adolescents with anorexia nervosa, *J Pediatr* 123:326-331, 1993.

55. Kreipe RE, Forbes GB: Osteoporosis: a "new morbidity" for dieting female adolescents, *Pediatrics* 86:478-480, 1990.

56. Gold PW, Kaye W, Robertson GL, Ebert M: Abnormalities in plasma and cerebrospinal-fluid arginine vasopressin in patients with anorexia nervosa, *N Engl J Med* 308:1117-1123, 1983.

57. Nussbaum M, Shenker IR, Marc J, Klein M: Cerebral atrophy in anorexia nervosa, *J Pediatr* 96:867-869, 1980.

58. Comerci GD: Eating disorders in adolescents, *Pediatr Rev* 10:1-10, 1988.

59. Herzog DB, Copeland PM: Eating disorders, *N Engl J Med* 313:295-303, 1985.

60. Joffe A: Too little, too much: eating disorders in adolescents, *Contemp Pediatr* 7:114-135, 1990.

61. Herbert PC, Weingarten MA: The ethics of forced feeding in anorexia nervosa, *Can Med Assoc J* 144:141-144, 1991.

62. Halmi KA: Treatment of anorexia nervosa: a discussion, *J Adolesc Health Care* 4:47-50, 1983.

63. Yates A: Current perspectives on the eating disorders. Part II. Treatment, outcome, and research directions, *J Am Acad Child Adolesc Psychiatry* 29:1-9, 1990.

64. Liebman R, Sargent J, Silver M: A family systems orientation to the treatment of anorexia nervosa, *J Am Acad Child Psychiatry* 22:128-133, 1983.

65. Andersen AE: *Practical comprehensive treatment of anorexia nervosa and bulimia,* Baltimore, 1985, Johns Hopkins University Press.

66. Baran SA, Weltzen TE, Kaye WH: Low discharge weight and outcome in anorexia nervosa, *Am J Psychiatry* 152:1070-1072, 1995.

67. Russell GFM, Szmukler GI, Dare C, Eisler I: An evaluation of family therapy in anorexia nervosa and bulimia nervosa, *Arch Gen Psychiatry* 44:1047-1056, 1987.

68. Herzog DB: Pharmacotherapy of anorexia nervosa and bulimia, *Pediatr Ann* 13:12, 1984.

69. Halmi KA, Eckert E, Falk J: Cyproheptadine: an antidepressant and weight inducing drug for anorexia nervosa, *Psychopharmacol Bull* 1:103-105, 1983.

70. Frisch RE, McArthur JW: Menstrual cycles: fatness as a determinant of minimum weight for height necessary for their maintenance or onset, *Science* 185:949, 1974.

71. Fears WB, Glass AR, Vigersky RA: Role of exercise in the pathogenesis of the amenorrhea associated with anorexia nervosa, *J Adolesc Health Care* 4:22-24, 1983.

72. Kreipe RE, Churchill BH, Strauss J: Long-term outcome of adolescents with anorexia nervosa, *Am J Dis Child* 143:1322-1327, 1989.

73. Treasure J, Wheeler M, Russel GFM: *Cystic ovaries: a phase of anorexia nervosa,* Presented at the Third International Conference on Eating Disorders, New York, April 1990.

74. Theander S: Outcome and prognosis in anorexia nervosa and bulimia: some results of previous investigators compared with those of a Swedish long-term study, *J Psychiatr Res* 19:493-508, 1985.

75. Schwartz DM, Thompson MG: Do anorectics get well? Current research and future needs, *Am J Psychiatry* 138:319-323, 1981.

76. Sullivan PF: Mortality in anorexia nervosa, *Am J Psychiatry* 152:1073-1074, 1995.

77. Nussbaum M, Shenker IR, Baird D, Saravay S: Follow-up investigation in patients with anorexia nervosa, *J Pediatr* 106:835-840, 1985.

CHAPTER 32

Bulimia Nervosa

•

Marjorie A. Boeck

The word *bulimia,* from the Greek meaning "ox-hunger," refers to an eating pattern in which a large quantity of food is consumed over a brief time. In bulimia nervosa, individuals maintain their weight, despite eating binges, by engaging in a variety of behaviors: purging behaviors such as self-induced vomiting and/or use of laxatives, diuretics, or diet pills; periods of starvation; or excessive exercise. Although binging behavior was practiced by the ancient Greeks and Romans, clinical descriptions of such behavior followed by activity designed to prevent weight gain were first published in the early 1900s. More detailed accounts of the binge-purge phenomena appeared in the 1940s in association with anorexia nervosa, and in the 1970s associated with normal weight.

In 1980, bulimia nervosa became a clinical diagnostic entity for the first time with the publication of the third edition of the American Psychiatric Association's *Diagnostic and Statistical Manual of Mental Disorders* (DSM-III).[1] The criteria were considerably refined on the basis of increased clinical experience in a revised edition published 7 years later (DSM-III-R). The current diagnostic criteria for bulimia nervosa were published in 1994 in the fourth edition of the manual (DSM-IV) and are listed in Box 32-1.[2]

The criteria for bulimia nervosa still include recurrent episodes of rapid consumption of a large amount of food in a discrete period (binging), a feeling of lack of control over eating during this binging period, regular engagement in behaviors to prevent weight gain due to the binging, and a fear of being overweight. In addition, patients must engage in an average of at least two binge-eating episodes a week for a minimum of 3 months to meet the criteria.

The new diagnostic criteria divide both anorexia and bulimia nervosa into "purging" and "nonpurging" subtypes. This eliminates the necessity for many patients with eating disorders to carry both the diagnoses of anorexia nervosa and bulimia nervosa successively or concurrently.

A psychiatric disorder involving a subgroup of obese individuals who binge without effective compensatory behaviors (binge-eating disorder [BED]) has been tentatively defined and appears in DSM-IV as a set of research criteria. This new disorder is discussed in Chapter 33, "Obesity."

EPIDEMIOLOGY

Bulimia nervosa affects primarily women (90%) and has its onset most often between middle and late adolescence. Incidence and prevalence studies of bulimia nervosa have primarily involved questionnaires given to student populations. The incidence has varied greatly, depending on the stringency of the criteria used. Current estimates, again primarily based on studies of specific high school and college student populations, are that 1.7% to 5% of females and less than 1% of males meet the DSM-III-R criteria for bulimia nervosa.[3] An incidence and prevalence study for the general population, which would include both urban and rural subsamples as well as various racial and ethnic backgrounds, is still needed.

It is not entirely clear to what extent the continued increase in, and younger age of onset of, bulimia nervosa represents an actual increase in this behavior or more individuals presenting for treatment. Factors include increased publicity about the disorder among the famous; continued emphasis on slimness as a cultural ideal; and increased awareness of the disorder not only among children and adolescents, but also among parents, teachers, and health professionals.

ETIOLOGY

The exact cause of bulimia nervosa is unknown, but biologic, psychologic, and societal factors all have been implicated, as for anorexia nervosa. The diagnosis reflects a behavioral spectrum that, in its mildest form, does not

---

BOX 32-1
DSM-IV: Diagnostic Criteria
for Bulimia Nervosa (307.51)

A. Recurrent episodes of binge eating. An episode of binge eating is characterized by both of the following:
1. Eating, in a discrete period of time (e.g., within any 2-hour period), an amount of food that is definitely larger than most people would eat during a similar period of time and under similar circumstances
2. A sense of lack of control over eating during the episode (e.g., a feeling that one cannot stop eating or control what or how much one is eating)

B. Recurrent inappropriate compensatory behavior in order to prevent weight gain such as self-induced vomiting; misuse of laxatives, diuretics, enemas, or other medications; fasting; or excessive exercise.

C. The binge eating and inappropriate compensatory behaviors both occur, on average, at least twice a week for 3 months.

D. Self-evaluation is unduly influenced by body shape and weight.

E. The disturbance does not occur exclusively during episodes of anorexia nervosa.

Specify type:

Purging type: during the current episode of bulimia nervosa, the person has regularly engaged in self-induced vomiting or the misuse of laxatives, diuretics, or enemas.

Nonpurging type: during the current episode of bulimia nervosa, the person has used other inappropriate compensatory behaviors, such as fasting or excessive exercise, but has not regularly engaged in self-induced vomiting or the misuse of laxatives, diuretics, or enemas.

From American Psychiatric Association: *Diagnostic and statistical manual of mental disorders,* ed 4, Washington, DC, 1994, American Psychiatric Association.

---

impinge on functioning in aspects of life not connected with food and that may be self-limited. At the other end of the spectrum is an extremely severe disorder in which the individual spends all waking hours eating and purging, with significant dysphoric moods, suicide attempts, stealing, and abuse of alcohol and other drugs. The prognosis in this case is guarded, despite treatment.

Biologic Factors

It has been hypothesized that patients with bulimia nervosa have a dysregulation of serotonin that results in a loss of normal serotinergic inhibition of carbohydrate intake, and inadequate serotonin input into hypothalamic regulatory mechanisms.[4]

Dramatic increases in cerebrospinal fluid levels of pancreatic polypeptide Y (PPY) were reported in patients with bulimia who had abstained from binging.[5] This finding has led to the hypothesis that patients with bulimia may be responding to heightened levels of PPY when they initiate a binge. The endogenous peptide neuropeptide Y (NPY) has also been implicated because it stimulates feeding when administered in various hypothalamic areas.[6] Opiates have also been implicated, especially as they increase the hedonistic effects of sweets and chocolate.[7]

In patients with bulimia nervosa, there is frequently a history of psychopathology in first-degree relatives, most often depression and alcoholism.[8]

Psychologic Factors

Individuals with bulimia nervosa usually feel a lack of self-control and manifest poor self-esteem. They are often compulsive, depressed, and anxious and feel a lack of control over their lives. Although in one study they scored significantly higher than normal controls on measures of impulsivity, this was not related to the severity or frequency of binging behavior.[9]

Family interactions are often problematic. The specific problems vary from parental absence to enmeshment. In one reported 10-week cognitive treatment program, no factors predicted a positive outcome, while a negative prognosis was predicted by a dysfunctional family.[10]

Despite some controversy in the research literature, it appears that the incidence, severity, and/or duration of physical and/or sexual abuse is not greater among bulimic patients than in the female population as a whole.[11-13] Such a history, however, may have a negative impact on therapy and perhaps on prognosis.

The binge-purge cycle has been viewed as a mechanism for regulating tension states. It has been postulated that the binging behavior is maintained because these individuals attempt to maintain a weight lower than what is constitutionally comfortable for them ("set point") by habitually fasting and feeling hungry during the day.

Societal Factors

Patients with bulimia nervosa usually report dissatisfaction with their body and a strong awareness of societal pressure to be thin. Obesity may exist in other family members. The patient also may be overweight to some degree, with the disorder beginning after a period of dietary restriction.

CLINICAL FEATURES

Most research on patients with bulimia nervosa has involved females over the age of 18 years, primarily because it has been conducted within adult psychiatry programs and also because it is easier to use subjects who do not require parental consent.

The typical young adult patient with bulimia nervosa has been described as a middle- to upper-middle-class, intelligent white female who appears socially well adjusted. She begins bulimic behavior in middle to late adolescence, often after a period of voluntary dieting and weight loss, without the knowledge of family members or peers. If she seeks medical attention at all for such symptoms as fatigue, bloating, or irregular menses, she usually does not mention her binge-purge behavior. If the individual seeks psychological treatment, this usually is not for a number of years. She is aware that her pattern of eating is abnormal and fears that she will not be able to stop eating voluntarily.

Most adult binging occurs in private. The eating process itself is frequently not pleasurable, and the individual often swallows the food without thorough mastication. The episode is terminated by gastric discomfort, self-induced vomiting, fear of being caught, or sleep. When the binging episode is over, the individual frequently feels repulsed by her behavior. She may be depressed or angry with herself. If the binge is followed by vomiting or use of a cathartic agent, she may feel a sense of relief and control.

In contrast to adult patients, who are self-referred, many teenagers are brought to treatment after being "discovered" by their parents. Some of these adolescents wish to receive help with their behavior and have deliberately left obvious "clues." Other teenagers view purging as a weight control technique and have no desire to change. Unlike the solitary binging of adults, teenagers may binge and vomit within a group setting. A preoccupation with weight, food, and eating is common, and in rare cases it may ultimately interfere with school performance and peer relationships.

Binging episodes vary in frequency. Most individuals binge at least several times each week, but others binge and purge at least once daily, and some as often as seven times a day. One study reported a mean frequency of binges of 11.7 per week (range, 1 to 46).[14] The mean binge duration was 1.18 hours (range, 15 minutes to 8 hours) with approximately 3500 calories consumed per binge.

Binge eating, as well as the eating of regular meals, has been successfully reproduced in the research laboratory. Contrary to previous thinking, the relative proportions of macronutrients did not differ between the two types of eating.[15] It was also noted that the rate of eating accelerated as a binge progressed, whereas in normal eating the rate slows down as the individual gradually becomes filled.

In a comparison of normal-weight bulimic patients with normal-weight controls, the patients with bulimia showed significantly more impulse buying, stealing, drug use, and suicide attempts.[16] On self-report scales, bulimic patients rated themselves as more compulsive, depressed, and anxious than matched controls; they also saw themselves as having lower self-esteem and less mastery over their lives than the controls. There were no significant differences in the frequency of life-change events during the previous year or in the number of physician contacts between the two groups. Although there were no significant differences in the number of intimate friendships reported, the patients with bulimia reported spending more time alone, having fewer close relatives, and having a negative relationship with parents. They also spent more time involved with food (thinking about it, preparing it, or eating it) than the controls.[17]

PHYSIOLOGIC COMPLICATIONS

The teenager who engages in frequent episodes of binging followed by self-induced vomiting often complains of sore throat and hoarseness. Other complaints include weakness, dizziness, headache, chest pain, muscle cramps, and a general sense of "not feeling well." Approximately 50% of females with bulimia nervosa report at least one episode of secondary amenorrhea despite appropriate weight for height. One study reported such patients to have normal levels of luteinizing hormone, estradiol, and progesterone. There was, however, an abnormality in 24-hour luteinizing hormone secretion if their weight was less than 85% of their previous high weight.[18]

The physical examination is usually entirely normal. Benign bilateral swelling of the parotid glands may occur with frequent purging behavior and is reversible. There may also be characteristic superficial ulcerations, hyperpigmented calluses, or scars on the dorsum of the hands of individuals who use their fingers to induce vomiting. With repetitive emesis, the acidic vomitus causes a loss of tooth enamel, which affects the palatal side of the upper teeth, beginning first with the molars and moving centrally. This may result in dental caries and significant abnormalities of occlusion. Other medical complications include reflux esophagitis, esophageal tears, and aspiration pneumonia. Life-threatening complications, such as ventricular fibrillation due to hypokalemia, renal failure, gastric rupture, toxic megacolon after prolonged laxative abuse, seizures, and tetany, have also been reported. The use of syrup of ipecac to induce vomiting has been associated with death in individuals with bulimia because of this agent's cardiotoxic effects.

Results of laboratory studies are frequently entirely normal in patients with bulimia nervosa. Many teenagers are careful not to engage in purging behavior for 1 or 2 days before a physician visit. It is important for the physician to determine when the last purging episode took place in order to interpret the results correctly. The most common electrolyte abnormality is an elevated serum bicarbonate level indicative of a metabolic alkalosis. Other abnormalities include hypochloremia, hypokalemia, and hypomagnesemia. Occasional patients may require daily oral potassium supplementation. In addition, patients may have an elevated serum amylase level that, in many cases, results from an elevation of the salivary (not pancreatic) isoenzyme.[19]

TREATMENT

Most individuals with bulimia nervosa are treated as outpatients. Occasionally, an inpatient setting utilizing a therapeutic approach similar to that used for anorexia nervosa is indicated. Hospital-based day treatment programs, and programs in which patients eat lunch and/or dinner in a structured setting followed by group therapeutic sessions, are other alternatives. These are particularly useful for patients who have been hospitalized and require continued close monitoring, or for patients beginning to relapse. Unfortunately, state health legislation and the insurance industry have made the establishment of such programs difficult in the United States.

Treatment of patients with bulimia nervosa often benefits from a therapeutic team approach. The team may include some or all of the following members who need to maintain contact with one another: medical physician, nutritionist, and therapist(s). Adolescents may particularly benefit from family therapy.

The physician needs to monitor physiologic complications. Patients with bulimia nervosa who actively seek medical care are aware that they have an eating disorder and are often receptive to education. The physician needs to explain the potential medical complications of purging behavior, reminding the patient that normal laboratory values in the office should not be taken as reassurance because their perceived normalcy may not reflect the true situation and serious danger immediately after purging. Such knowledge has occasionally been sufficient to stop some teenagers from purging.

The role of the nutritionist (who may be a physician or a therapist) is to educate the patient about nutrition and the role of starvation in binging behavior, to set goals for achieving an appropriate dietary intake (he or she may prescribe specific foods, portion sizes, or meals), and to monitor ongoing progress. The patient will require considerable psychologic support, as weight gain often occurs in the process of normalizing eating patterns.

Time-limited outpatient psychotherapy programs conducted for adults with bulimia nervosa have had generally good short-term results. Although the details of the programs vary, some programs offering individual therapy while others use group therapy or a combination of individual and group therapy, they have certain basic

elements in common. The symptoms of binging and purging need to be addressed directly, as they will not necessarily improve along with the improvements in mood or self-esteem that result from psychotherapy. There also needs to be direct attention paid to the establishment of normal eating patterns.

Almost all programs place an emphasis on self-monitoring. Many emphasize specific behavioral paradigms, such as stimulus control, response delay, and problem-solving techniques. Several programs include assertiveness training and/or relaxation training.

Pharmacotherapy plays an important adjunctive role in the treatment of bulimia nervosa. The major drug treatment trials have all involved only adults above age 18. There is considerable anecdotal evidence that pharmacotherapy may be extremely useful in selected adolescents. Because the binging process has been described as occurring in a fuguelike state, phenytoin was one of the first drugs employed and resulted in some success. As bulimia nervosa has been linked to major affective disorders, it was hypothesized that antidepressant medications might be an effective treatment, and their use has completely supplanted that of antiseizure medications. Pope et al[20] reported the first successful treatment of bulimia with an antidepressant, using imipramine in both uncontrolled and controlled trials. Controlled double-blind placebo trials have since been carried out with a variety of tricyclic antidepressants.[21] A patient who initially has a good response to imipramine may later experience tachyphylaxis and respond well to a different tricyclic.

Walsh et al[22] noted that the mood disturbance of some patients with bulimia seemed similar to that of patients with "atypical depression." This term is used to describe patients who, when depressed, retain reactivity to environmental events and experience two or more of the following: increased appetite or weight gain, oversleeping, severe fatigue, and extreme sensitivity to personal rejection. Data suggest that patients with atypical depression respond better to monoamine oxidase inhibitors (MAOIs) for both depressive and bulimic symptoms than to tricyclic antidepressants.[23] The use of these agents requires strict adherence to a tyramine-free diet. This can be a difficult task for adolescents who tend to have a problem with compliance in general and, with bulimia, also have problems controlling food intake.

In the late 1980s, there has been interest in and success with the specific serotonin agonists, especially fluoxetine, for patients who had previously responded to either tricyclic depressants or MAOIs. Fluoxetine is not only an antidepressant but also produces a decrease in appetite, particularly for carbohydrates, as a side effect. It has the advantage of a safer and better tolerated side-effect profile (no dry mouth or constipation and little, if any, cardiotoxicity). A 1994 open trial of fluvoxamine showed similar positive results.[24]

After reports of elevated beta-endorphin levels in obese individuals, it was postulated that the use of narcotic antagonists, such as naltrexone, might reduce binging behavior. Although there have been some positive treatment results, including those from naloxone administration in an adolescent girl, this approach is still highly experimental.[25]

As some bulimic women seem to have seasonal fluctuations of binging, consistent with seasonal affective disorder, light therapy has been tried with some success.[26]

OUTCOME

In a published follow-up study of bulimic adolescents treated in the same medical center–based eating disorders clinic,[27] 56% of the adolescents reportedly recovered from their index episode of bulimia nervosa, but by 18 months all but 6% had relapsed. In interpreting these disappointing results, it is important to note that, although all treatment took place at the same center, the patients did not receive a common program utilizing a treatment team approach. It is likely, however, that this does represent the usual treatment given to adolescents.

Results of long-term follow-up studies (10 years) in bulimic patients are now appearing, mostly from adult inpatient treatment programs in Europe. In most studies, about 45% to 55% were defined as recovered, 30% to 40% still had some symptoms, and the remainder showed no improvement, with a mortality rate as high as 6%. A positive prognosis was associated with younger age at treatment, higher socioeconomic status, and a positive family history of alcohol abuse.[28] Others found a poorer response in adults when "borderline personality" was a co-morbidity.[29]

These studies frequently use small sample sizes, very specific treatment programs, and unique samples that do not allow for generalization. It is not possible to make a realistic statement about treatment prognosis in adolescents at this time.

SUMMARY

Bulimia nervosa is a disorder that primarily affects women and has its onset during middle to late adolescence. Initially, the teenager appears to be well adjusted, since the binging and purging behaviors occur in secret. The primary care physician for adolescents is the healthcare provider most likely to make an early diagnosis of an eating disorder. It is rare for a teenager to voluntarily admit to binging and purging episodes. For

this reason, it is recommended that a dietary history be obtained from all adolescents. Weight fluctuation or weight loss and complaints of fatigue, headaches, dizziness, and vague abdominal pain should raise the level of suspicion for bulimia nervosa. Laboratory findings are likely to be normal because most teenagers are careful not to engage in purging behavior within several days of seeing a physician. Therapeutic strategies include individual and/or family and/or group psychotherapy that uses behavior modification and cognitive restructuring techniques, and offers nutrition education. Pharmacotherapy is helpful in selected patients. Although there are few long-term follow-up studies of patients with bulimia nervosa, the disorder appears to be chronic, with remissions and exacerbations.

References

1. American Psychiatric Association: *Diagnostic and statistical manual of mental disorders,* ed 3, Washington, DC, 1980, American Psychiatric Association.
2. American Psychiatric Association: *Diagnostic and statistical manual of mental disorders,* ed 4, Washington, DC, 1994, American Psychiatric Association.
3. Fairburn CG, Beglin SJ: Studies of the epidemiology of bulimia nervosa, *Am J Psychiatry* 147:401-408, 1990.
4. Saminin R, Garattini S: Serotonin and the pharmacology of eating disorders, *Ann NY Acad Sci* 575:194-208, 1989.
5. Leibowitz SF: Hypothalamic neuropeptide Y, galanin, and amines, *Ann NY Acad Sci* 575:221-233, 1989.
6. Geracioti TD Jr, Liddle RA: Impaired cholecystokinin secretion in bulimia nervosa, *N Engl J Med* 319:683-688, 1988.
7. Drewnowski A, Krahn DD, Demitrack MA, Nair K, Gosnell BA: Naloxone, an opiate blocker, reduces the consumption of sweet high-fat foods in obese and lean female binge eaters, *Am J Clin Nutr* 61:1206-1212, 1995.
8. Hatsukami DK, Mitchell JE, Eckert ED: Eating disorders: a variant of mood disorders?, *Psychiatr Clin North Am* 7:349-365, 1984.
9. Wolfe BE, Jimerson DC, Levine JM: Impulsivity ratings in bulimia nervosa: relationship of binge behaviors, *Int J Eat Disord* 15:289-292, 1994.
10. Blouin JH, Carter J, Blouin AG, Tener L, Schnare-Hayes K, Zuro D, Barlow J, Perez E: Prognostic indicators in bulimia nervosa treated with cognitive-behavioral group therapy, *Int J Eat Disord* 15:113-123, 1994.
11. Welch SL, Fairburn CG: Sexual abuse and bulimia nervosa: three integrated case control comparisons, *Am J Psychiatry* 151:402, 1994.
12. Rorty M, Yager J, Rossotto E: Childhood sexual, physical, and psychological abuse in bulimia nervosa, *Am J Psychiatry* 151:1122-1126, 1994.
13. Pope HG Jr, Mangweth B, Negrao AB, Hudson JI, Cordas TA: Childhood sexual abuse and bulimia nervosa: a comparison of American, Austrian, and Brazilian women, *Am J Psychiatry* 151:732-737, 1994.
14. Mitchell JE, Pyle RL, Eckert ED: Frequency and duration of binge-eating episodes in patients with bulimia, *Am J Psychiatry* 138:835-836, 1981.
15. Walsh BT, Kissileff HR, Hadigan CM: Eating behavior in bulimia, *Ann NY Acad Sci* 575:446-454, 1989.
16. Mitchell JE, Pyle RL: The bulimic syndrome in normal weight individuals: a review, *Int J Eat Disord* 1:61-73, 1982.

17. Johnson C, Larson R: Bulimia: an analysis of moods and behavior, *Psychosom Med* 44:341-351, 1982.

18. Weltzin TE, Cameron J, Berga S, Kaye WH: Prediction of reproductive status in women with bulimia nervosa by past high weight, *Am J Psychiatry* 151:136-138, 1994.

19. Humphries LL, Adams LJ, Eckfeldt JH, Levitt MD, McClain CJ: Hyperamylasemia in patients with eating disorders, *Ann Intern Med* 106:50-52, 1987.

20. Pope HG, Hudson JI, Jonas JM, Yurgelun-Todd D: Bulimia treated with imipramine: a placebo-controlled, double-blind study, *Am J Psychiatry* 140:554-558, 1983.

21. Mitchell JE: Psychopharmacology of eating disorders, *Ann NY Acad Sci* 575:41-48, 1989.

22. Walsh BT, Stewart JW, Wright L, Harrison W, Roose SP, Glassman AH: Treatment of bulimia with monoamine oxidase inhibitors, *Am J Psychiatry* 139:1629-1630, 1982.

23. Rothschild R, Quitkin HM, Quitkin FM, Stewart JW, Ocepek-Welikson K, McGrath PJ, Tricamo E: A double-blind placebo-controlled comparison of phenelzine and imipramine in the treatment of bulimia in atypical depressives, *Int J Eat Disord* 15:1-9, 1994.

24. Ayuso-Gutierrez JL, Palazon M, Ayuso-Mateos JL: Open trial of fluvoxamine in the treatment of bulimia nervosa, *Int J Eat Disord* 15:245-249, 1994.

25. Chatoor I, Herman BH, Hartzler J: Effects of the opiate antagonist, naltrexone, on binging antecedents and plasma beta-endorphin concentrations, *J Am Acad Child Adolesc Psychiatry* 33:748-752, 1994.

26. Lam RW, Goldner EM, Solom L, Remick RA: A controlled study of light therapy for bulimia nervosa, *Am J Psychiatry* 151:744-750, 1994.

27. Herzog DB, Keller MB, Lavori PW, Bradburn IS: Bulimia nervosa in adolescence, *J Dev Behav Pediatr* 12:191-195, 1991.

28. Collings S, King M: Ten-year follow-up of 50 patients with bulimia nervosa, *Br J Psychiatry* 164:80-87, 1994.

29. Steiger H, Stotland S, Houle L: Prognostic implications of stable versus transient "borderline features" in bulimic patients, *J Clin Psychiatry* 55:206-214, 1994.

CHAPTER 33

Obesity

•

Marjorie A. Boeck

Obesity is the most common nutritional disorder in the developed countries of the world. Ironically, while the United States has become a nation obsessed with "dieting," the percentage of obese individuals has increased in both sexes and in all age and ethnic groups. Using age- and sex-specific height and weight percentile cutoffs from national probability samples to define obesity, the percentage of overweight adolescents (12 to 19 years old) increased from 15% at the second National Health and Nutrition Examination Survey (NHANES II, 1976-80) to 21% at NHANES III, 1988-91.[1]

Puberty is a high-risk period for the development of obesity, especially in girls. In boys, puberty is associated with large gains in fat-free mass; in girls, there is a significant deposition in body fat along with a much smaller increase in fat-free mass. In both sexes, there is an increase in central fat and decrease in peripheral fat. The influence and nature of changes in energy expenditure during puberty remains an important area for future investigation.

Unfortunately, 75% to 80% of obese adolescents become obese adults.[2] Longitudinal studies indicate that overweight and fatness during adolescence, even if individuals are of normal weight as adults, result in increased adult morbidity and mortality.[3] Medical complications can begin before puberty if the individual is extremely obese. The social, psychologic, and economic consequences of obesity, although less often stressed, are of equal or greater magnitude.

DEFINITION

Obesity may be defined as a maladaptive increase in the amount of energy stored as fat. There is currently no method to accurately determine the optimal amount of body fat stores or the ideal body weight for a given individual. The method most commonly used in an office setting to determine the degree of overweight is the nomogram that relates weight to age, sex, and height. The shortcomings of this method include a failure to take into account ethnic differences and variations in body frame, an inability to distinguish weight due to muscle from that due to fat, and the inclusion of obese children in the sample of children and adolescents studied to create the nomogram. This is also true for published weight tables, such as those of the Metropolitan Life Insurance Company, which do not reflect ideal body weight but the actual weight of insured adults.

The most accurate office measure of body fat is the direct measurement of subcutaneous fat mass at various anatomic sites, usually the triceps and subscapular skinfolds, using skinfold calipers. The mean of three measurements made on the right side of the body is then compared with standards for age and sex.[4] A major problem with this procedure is that the measurements become increasingly difficult as the degree of adiposity increases, and cannot be done at all if the skinfold exceeds the caliper opening (70 mm).

Other methods for measuring body fat include hydrostatic weighing, bioelectrical impedance analysis (four-electrode plethysmography used to determine total body water), total body potassium, total body dual-photon densitometry, computed tomography (CT), and magnetic resonance imaging (MRI).

The Expert Committee on Clinical Guidelines for Overweight in Adolescent Preventive Services[5] was established to provide a protocol "to identify those at greatest risk of obesity and its adverse sequelae." They proposed that a body mass index (BMI), a method of expressing the relationship between height and weight, be determined for each adolescent seen. The BMI they chose, the Quetelet index, is defined as the weight in kilograms divided by the height in meters squared ($BMI = kg/m^2$). Adolescents with a BMI ≥95th percentile for age and sex or whose BMI is >30 (whichever is smaller) would be defined as "overweight" and be

followed or referred for further in-depth medical assessment. Adolescents whose BMIs are ≥85th percentile but <95th percentile or equal to 30 (whichever is smaller) are considered "at risk" for obesity and should be referred for a second level screening. Cutoff values are given in Table 33-1. The second level screen includes five items: (1) a family history of cardiovascular disease, parental hypercholesterolemia, diabetes mellitus, or parental obesity or that is unknown; (2) blood pressure; (3) total cholesterol; (4) a large increment in BMI (two BMI units in 1 year); and (5) concern about weight. If any of the items in the second-level screen are positive, the adolescent should be followed or referred for in-depth medical assessment. If the screen is negative, the individual should be screened on a yearly basis.

These definitions are considerably more conservative than some previously used and do not include such terms as *obese, superobese,* or *morbidly obese.* Although it is not explicitly stated, this represents an effort to lessen the psychological trauma of being identified as obese. It also switches the emphasis onto screening the entire population for overweight and its physiologic complications.

ETIOLOGY

Obesity is a heterogeneous group of disorders that can result from a variety of pathophysiologic mechanisms. Although it is the result of long-term caloric intake greater than metabolic demand, it is oversimplistic to blame the adolescent for eating too much.

Since 1900, obesity has been divided into two types: *exogenous,* in which food intake exceeds caloric output,

TABLE 33-1
Recommended Cutoff Values for Body Mass Index (BMI, in kg/m²) for Adolescents Who Are Overweight or at Risk of Overweight During Adolescence

	At Risk of Overweight		Overweight	
	BMI <30		BMI >30	
Age (yr)	Males	Females	Males	Females
10	20	20	23	23
11	20	21	24	25
12	21	22	25	26
13	22	23	26	27
14	23	24	27	28
15	24	24	28	29
16	24	25	29	29
17	25	25	29	30
18	26	26	30	30
19	26	26	30	30
20-24	27	26	30	30

From Himes JH, Dietz WH: Guidelines for overweight in adolescent preventive services: recommendations from an expert committee, *Am J Clin Nutr* 59:313, 1994.

and *endogenous,* in which obesity is related to a defined defect in metabolism. Exogenous obesity still accounts for more than 99% of all current obesity.

Genetic and Environmental Influences

The familial nature of obesity has been noted for generations. When both parents are obese, approximately 70% of their children will be obese.[6] When one parent is obese, this incidence drops to 40% to 50%, and when neither parent is obese, it falls to less than 10%. Studies comparing heights and weights of adult adoptees with those of their adoptive and biologic parents,[7] as well as studies of monozygotic twins reared together and apart[8] and of pairs of monozygotic twins deliberately overfed,[9] have indicated a larger role for genetics than previously thought. These studies indicate the importance of genetics but do not tell us what precisely is inherited.

Genes may be associated with basal metabolism, dietary thermogenesis, appetite, satiety, endocrine function, and fat storage. Several rodent models of autosomal recessive obesity (mouse *db,* rat *fa,* mouse *tub*) have been identified, and obesity traits have been mapped to rodent chromosomal regions that are homologous with regions on human chromosomes 1p, 7q, and 11p. Sib-pair linkage analysis is being used on school-age siblings in Muscatine, Iowa, in an attempt to find human genes of DNA sequences on chromosomes 1p, 7q, and 11p that have measurable effects on quantitative indices of obesity or on quantitative traits that are associated with obesity.[10]

Mutation of the obese (*ob*) gene in the mouse results in profound obesity and type II diabetes as part of a syndrome that resembles morbid obesity in humans. The *ob* gene may function as part of a signaling pathway from adipose tissue that acts to regulate the size of the body fat depot. Both the mouse and the homologous human gene have been cloned.[11] Although the level of the secreting factor in humans is highest in the obese, no mutations in the human gene were found in obese people.[12] None of these studies have been carried out in obese children.

An individual may have hypertrophic obesity, due to an increase in fat cell size; hyperplastic obesity, due to an increase in cell number; or a combination of both. In certain individuals, new fat cells may develop during any period of weight gain throughout life. This is probably genetically determined. It is hypothesized that weight reduction does not decrease the number of fat cells, and that once individual fat cells reach a normal size, weight reduction stops.

Set-Point Theory

The set-point theory states that each individual has a genetically determined biologic weight (the set point). The organism will defend its body weight (much like a thermostat) against pressure to change even if the weight is far above the culture's ideal. In human studies, individuals who were supposed to increase their weight by a certain percentage[13] either found it impossible to do so, or had to eat more calories than expected to gain and/or maintain the heavier weight, and in the process had lowered appetite and less interest in food.

Neurochemical Factors

Historically, investigators believed there was a discrete "hunger center" located in the lateral hypothalamus and a "satiety center" located in the ventromedial hypothalamus. It is now recognized that the process of feeding is considerably more complex, and that these "centers" are more like "systems" that regulate feeding behavior by way of an interplay of central and peripheral pathways that include other brain areas, neurotransmitters, circulating metabolites, and hormones. These include neuropeptide Y (NPY), dopamine, norepinephrine and epinephrine, and serotonin.[14]

Dietary Obesity

At least in part, the high prevalence of obesity in the United States may be a result of unlimited access to palatable foods. In taste tests of cream, in which the amounts of sugar and fat varied, obese subjects, in comparison with lean subjects, preferred a high-fat, low-sugar combination.[15] High-fat diets give rise to less intense satiety than high-carbohydrate diets of equal caloric value. Another factor implicated in the current rise of obesity is variety in foods. This is illustrated by studies of genetically normal and obese rats that used a "supermarket diet" consisting of such foods as chocolate-chip cookies, salami, cheese, bananas, marshmallows, and peanut butter given in rotation instead of laboratory chow.[16] Both normal weight and genetically obese adult rats raised on laboratory chow gained 269% more weight than normal controls when fed this supermarket diet for 2 months. Weight gain was even greater in rats fed the diet from the time of weaning, and was often irreversible despite a return to laboratory chow.

Exercise

It remains unclear whether physical inactivity is a cause or a consequence of obesity. Studies of children and teenagers that involved the use of movies to document the extent of physical activity indicated that obese youngsters were less active than their peers. However, obese boys actually expended more calories through activity than nonobese boys when caloric expenditure was measured by oxygen consumption. It has been hotly debated whether television viewing plays a causal role in obesity and whether or not this might be related to an actual decrease in metabolic rate.[17] This sedentary activity involves exposure to many high-calorie foods seen both in television commercials and in the actual programming.

Endogenous Obesity

Only a small fraction of obese adolescents have endogenous obesity as a result of defined genetic syndromes or endocrine abnormalities. These few patients usually can be readily identified by history and physical examination. Endogenous obesity is characterized by growth failure. Patients with this condition are short, have a delayed bone age, and will have an adult height less than that predicted by midparental height. The major causes of endogenous obesity include hypercortisolism, hypothyroidism, genetic syndromes, and hypothalamic lesions.

HYPERCORTISOLISM. Adolescents with hypercortisolism, or Cushing's syndrome, are short, with truncal obesity and moon facies. They may have characteristic purplish striae of the skin resulting from thinning of dermal connective tissue, and they may be hypertensive. The excessive cortisol may result from prescription of exogenous hormone, malignant or benign adrenal tumors, or primary overproduction of adrenocorticotropic hormone (ACTH) (Cushing's disease).

HYPOTHYROIDISM. The adolescent with hypothyroidism may be plump and have myxedema. Hypothyroidism is characterized by a dull facial expression, dry skin, constipation, short stature, and retarded bone age. Hypothyroidism by itself, however, seldom causes massive weight gain.

GENETIC SYNDROMES. A number of genetic syndromes include obesity as a component. It is likely that in future years the number of such syndromes will increase, as will our knowledge of the exact chromosomal abnormalities involved in each one. The clinical features of the most common genetic syndromes are presented in Table 33-2.

HYPOTHALAMIC LESIONS. Hypothalamic lesions, which result in hyperphagia and obesity, may be the result of vascular malformations, neoplasms (Fröhlich's syndrome), or trauma. These lesions may also result from inflammatory processes such as sarcoidosis, tuberculosis, arachnoiditis, meningitis, and encephalitis. The associated obesity is characterized by fat-cell hypertrophy with little hyperplasia. There may be other symptoms related to abnormalities in the hypothalamus, such as increased finickiness, abnormal temperature regulation, visual disturbances, an increase in thirst, and sleepiness. Lesions in the region of the hypothalamus are frequently not detected on high-resolution MRI. Parents usually note a marked change in their child's eating behavior soon after the illness or surgery. Such behavior is similar to that noted in the genetic forms of hypothalamic obesity. Adolescents with this condition have a voracious appetite that never seems to be satisfied. If it is a "satiety" and not an "appetite" disorder, they usually do not consume nonfood items but may eat selectively, rejecting foods that they dislike, such as lettuce or meat. The foraging and stealing of food may require the locking of cabinets and refrigerators. Adolescents with this disorder may engage in negative behaviors, including tantrums, if food is withheld. Some of these patients do well as long as they do not see food and are kept occupied. Weight control in such patients, which is very difficult to regulate, is best accomplished through close supervision in a highly structured setting.

TABLE 33-2
Genetic Syndromes That Include Obesity

Syndrome	Clinical Features
Alström's	Childhood blindness due to retinal degeneration, nerve deafness, acanthosis nigricans, chronic nephropathy, primary hypogonadism (males only), insulin-resistant diabetes, infantile obesity (may diminish in adulthood)
Carpenter's	Mental retardation and acrocephaly, polydactyly and/or syndactyly, male hypogonadism
Cohen's	Microcephaly and mental retardation, short stature, dysmorphic facies
Laurence-Moon-Bardet-Biedl	Retinitis pigmentosa and mental retardation, polydactyly, central (hypothalamic) hypogonadism; rarely: glucose intolerance, deafness, renal disease
Prader-Willi	Short stature with small hands and feet, mental retardation and neonatal hypotonia, cryptorchidism, almond-shaped eyes and "fish mouth"

PHYSIOLOGIC COMPLICATIONS

Many epidemiologic studies, prospective, cross-sectional, and retrospective, have shown that the risk of developing certain health problems and a shortened life span is higher among overweight individuals than among the nonoverweight of the same sex, race, age, and socioeconomic status.[18] The risks increase as the degree of obesity increases. They also increase depending on the patterns of fat distribution, with the upper-segment obesity pattern ("abdominal," "apple," or "android") associated with a higher risk of developing physiologic complications than the lower-segment pattern ("femoral-gluteal," "pear," or "gynoid"). The pattern of fat distribution can be determined either visually or by measuring the circumferences of waist and hip. A waist-hip ratio (WHR) ≥0.8 in females and ≥1.0 in males is high enough to provide that risk.[19] There is new evidence that the body's content of visceral fat as determined by CT or MRI is a better predictor of risk than the WHR.[20]

The physiologic complications of obesity include hyperinsulinism, insulin resistance, acanthosis nigricans, non–insulin-dependent diabetes mellitus (NIDDM), cholesterol gallstones, hypertension, atherogenic lipid profile, coronary vascular disease, stroke, gout, exacerbation of arthritis, obstructive sleep apnea, menstrual abnormalities, and the complications of anesthesia, surgery, and pregnancy. The types of cancer associated with obesity include gallbladder and biliary passages, breast, cervix, endometrium, ovary, and prostate cancer.

It has been estimated that between 10% and 30% of obese children have elevated blood pressure. There is no correlation with age, sex, or duration of obesity.

The insulin response to oral glucose is greatly elevated in obese individuals. Insulin increases both subjective feelings of hunger and lipogenesis while inhibiting lipolysis. Abnormalities in the glucose tolerance test results are observed more commonly if there is a family history of diabetes. A normal fasting insulin is not sufficient to rule out hyperinsulinism or insulin resistance. Common markers for insulin resistance are hyperandrogenism, usually manifested as hirsutism, and acanthosis nigricans. Acanthosis nigricans is a velvety darkening of the skin, especially in black and Hispanic adolescents, caused by melanocyte deposition in the dermis that is found at the neck and often in the axillary and inguinal regions. Both of these conditions are frequently cosmetic problems, especially for females.

Obese teenagers tend to have higher levels of triglycerides, very-low-density lipoprotein (VLDL), low-density lipoprotein (LDL), and total serum cholesterol (TC), and lower levels of high-density-lipoprotein (HDL) than their lean counterparts. A complete 12-hour fasting lipid profile needs to be measured in the overweight adolescent, because the low HDL often results in a total cholesterol value well within the normal range, yet the TC/HDL ratio is very high. This low HDL responds to both weight reduction and exercise.

Obese girls tend to experience menarche at an early age, often by age 10 years, but may develop oligomenorrhea, dysfunctional uterine bleeding, or secondary amenorrhea several years later. The most common cause for this is polycystic ovary syndrome (PCOS), which combines hirsutism, obesity, menstrual irregularity, and infertility associated with enlarged sclerocystic ovaries. The extent to which obesity plays a causative role is still not determined. Necessary diagnostic studies include measurement of serum luteinizing hormone (LH), follicle-stimulating hormone (FSH), estrone, dehydroepiandrosterone (DHEA), androstenedione, and testosterone. Imaging studies of the ovary, such as pelvic ultrasonography, are needed to assess ovarian size and function.

Adolescent obesity is also related to such orthopedic disorders as slipped capital femoral epiphysis and Blount's disease (tibia vara). These disorders are most common in black males. Surgical correction of Blount's disease is most successful if done before the end of the growth spurt and after a weight loss that is then maintained postoperatively.

Morbidly obese adolescents are at risk for obstructive sleep apnea, which may ultimately develop into hypersomnia and the Pickwickian syndrome. Parents usually report that the adolescent snores loudly and sometimes seems to stop breathing. The resultant daytime somnolence often has been overlooked as a symptom because it has been erroneously attributed to late-night television viewing. Such patients warrant polysomnography for diagnosis and subsequently to monitor treatment effectiveness. Continuous positive airway pressure (CPAP) while the patient is asleep is often an effective alternative treatment to tonsillectomy, adenoidectomy, and uvulectomy or tracheostomy while the adolescent is losing weight.

Psychologic Complications

There is no specific "obese personality" and it has been hypothesized that psychopathology in obese individuals is a consequence and not a cause of obesity. In today's culture, with its emphasis on slimness, the adolescent who is obese may have difficulty with self-image and peer relations. This is especially true, even at a lesser degree of overweight, for white girls. Several studies have shown that children and adolescents, when offered a choice of friends, prefer an individual with a physical handicap to one who is obese.[21] Other studies have found a striking similarity between the psychologic traits of obese adolescent girls and those of racial minorities who have been victims of prejudice.[22] Discrimination against the obese in both education and employment has been well documented.[23,24]

Although most obese adults do not have a poor self-image, a severe body-image disturbance may develop during a critical period of adolescence, when negative views of peers and significant adults are incorporated into the adolescent's developing self-concept.[25] Such persons view themselves as being disgusting and having a loathsome body. They will not look into a store display window because they see their own reflection. They divide the world into fat people, who are bad, and thin people, who are good. Such body-image disturbances persist with remarkably little change over long periods and often remain unchanged even after weight reduction. Obese adolescents should be interviewed to identify poor self-image, poor self-esteem, and depression. These adolescents require appropriate psychologic evaluation and treatment.

It has recently become apparent that a subgroup of obese individuals engage in binging behaviors, but without the compensatory behaviors to maintain weight within a normal range. This newly described binge-eating disorder (BED) is discussed in more detail later in this chapter.

MANAGEMENT

The basis for the treatment of obesity is to lower energy intake below that of energy expenditure. The physician specializing in adolescent medicine is in an excellent position to design and monitor an obesity treatment program for the mildly obese. Emphasis should be placed on developing healthy eating patterns with a reduction in health risks rather than achieving an "ideal body weight." Studies in adults indicate that the amount of weight required to reverse physiologic problems is about 10%.[26] Much effort needs to be directed toward making adolescents feel good about their bodies even though they may be larger than the cultural norm or ideal. In adolescents who have not completed their growth spurt and are mildly obese, weight maintenance to grow into their height is an appropriate goal. One must be extremely careful in treating individuals who wish to lose weight but are not overweight or who are particularly successful with their dieting, because some may be at risk for the development of anorexia or bulimia nervosa. (See Chapters 31 and 32, "Anorexia Nervosa" and "Bulimia Nervosa.")

A variety of treatment approaches for obesity exist, including diet counseling, behavior modification, exercise, commercial or self-help programs, school-based programs, very-low-calorie diets, pharmacotherapy, and surgery. None of these approaches has proved particularly successful for long-term maintenance of weight loss, if achieved.

The most recent approach to the treatment of adult obesity is to classify patients by BMI into "mild," "moderate," "severe," or "morbid" obesity. Mild obesity is defined as a BMI of 27 to 30 (25 for women); "moderate obesity" as a BMI of 30.1 to 35; and severe obesity as a BMI >35.

Ninety percent of all obese adults have mild obesity and may not have any physiologic problems for which weight loss would be indicated, depending on their pattern of fat distribution. Mild obesity should be treated, if at all, with conservative methods such as nutrition counseling, exercise, and behavior modification. The subgroup with moderate obesity (9.5%) and severe obesity (0.5%) usually do require treatment, including very-low-calorie diets, pharmacotherapy, and surgery.

There have been reports that individuals who cycle between weight loss and regain might actually be doing themselves more harm than if they remained obese.[27] Newer evidence indicates that this is not true for the moderately and extremely obese.[28]

Role of Parents

Parents exert a powerful influence on the eating and physical activity patterns of their children. They may help their adolescent by purchasing sugar-free drinks or having the entire family alter cooking habits: for example, baking rather than frying chicken. On the other hand, the family may appear to deliberately sabotage the adolescent's dieting efforts. For example, freshly baked cakes may be left on the kitchen counter instead of being stored away. Well-intentioned parents may make adherence to a diet more difficult by constantly nagging their child. Studies have shown that adolescents experienced better short- and long-term weight losses if they and their mothers attended separate weight loss groups than if they attended a group with their mother or if the mother attended no group.

Diet Counseling

Many adolescents do not exhibit an orderly pattern of eating. It is common for them to skip both breakfast and lunch and then eat almost continuously from after school until bedtime. Their diet is frequently high in fat and concentrated sweets and low in fruits, vegetables, and fiber. (See Chapter 29, "Nutrition and Eating Disorders.")

Diets are most likely to succeed if they are highly individualized according to current eating patterns, degree of motivation, intellect, amount of family support, and monetary considerations. For an adolescent boy who is currently consuming over 2 L of regular soda or fruit

---

BOX 33-1
"Free" Foods for Dieters

Artichokes	Greens	Diet soda/
Asparagus	Lettuce	seltzer
Broccoli	Mushrooms	Tea/coffee
Brussel sprouts	Peppers	Broth
Cabbage	Radishes	Mustard
Cauliflower	Spinach	Herbs
Celery	Sprouts	Spices
Cucumbers	Summer squash	Lemon
Eggplant	Tomatoes	Vinegar
Green beans	Zucchini	Soy sauce
Green onions	Water	Sour pickles

---

punch daily, the initial plan might be simply to alter the nature of his fluid intake. An adolescent girl who snacks constantly on soda and candy while studying after dinner might initially substitute a cup of unbuttered popcorn for her usual snacks. Many teenagers claim that they eat very little. They are often correct that the quantity they consume is small, but their choices are often very high in calories. For such individuals a list of "free" foods, which essentially provide no calories, is invaluable (Box 33-1). Some adolescents prefer to be given food exchange lists or calorie counters in order to devise their own diets. Others prefer to be given a diet plan that details the foods and portions to be eaten at each meal. Vitamin and mineral supplementation should be used with any diet that provides fewer than 1200 calories per day.

Before the diet program begins, it is very important that adolescents understand that losing weight is a slow process and that they are learning to eat in a new way for the remainder of their lives. In addition, it is essential that they have a realistic expectation about the rate of weight loss. Since it takes an energy deficit of 3500 to 3600 kcal to lose 1 pound, adolescents need to take in 500 calories a day less than they use to lose 1 pound a week. They should be encouraged to use the concept of "calorie banking," which involves planning ahead and saving some calories in advance to be used at a later date for special parties or holidays. Because compliance with new dietary habits for a prolonged period will present a major difficulty for many adolescents, weigh-in and counseling sessions on a weekly or biweekly basis are essential initially; biweekly or monthly visits may be necessary indefinitely for many patients.

A rational, nutritionally sound dietary approach is to use food exchanges, such as those devised by the American Diabetic Association. In this system, foods are divided into six categories: milk, vegetable, fruit, fat, meat, and bread (Box 33-2). Each food in a given category has an equal amount of carbohydrate, protein, fat, and calories and thus may be substituted for any other food in the same category. This allows flexibility in the

choice of foods eaten without counting calories. The distribution of protein, fat, and carbohydrate is important in order to lose the maximal amount of adipose tissue with a minimal loss of nitrogen. The distribution also conforms to that suggested by the American Heart Association in its step I diet: 20% of calories from protein; 30% of calories from fat (less than one third from saturated, more than one third from monounsaturated, and one third from polyunsaturated); and 50% of calories from carbohydrates, preferably complex carbohydrates, which are high in fiber. A complete distribution of food exchanges for diets of different calorie levels is given in Box 33-3.

Behavioral Treatment

Behavioral programs focus on "how to eat." They are based on the assumption that eating habits must change for the person to achieve and maintain weight loss. Adolescents are asked to keep a diary of all food eaten and the circumstances surrounding its consumption: time, place, activity, and mood. This method identifies specific behaviors to be targeted for change by the program. Programs may focus on slowing down the rate at which food is eaten, using smaller plates, eating mainly in certain areas, and avoiding other activities while eating (e.g., watching television). Various studies on the effectiveness of behavioral treatment indicate that its advantage lies not in the amount of weight lost but in the maintenance of weight once loss has occurred.

Exercise

An exercise program should be a part of every weight-reduction plan. In fact, weight loss after exercise is generally greater than would be expected through the direct expenditure of energy alone. There is some evidence that increased activity in obese individuals may decrease appetite while it increases metabolic rate.

Compliance with exercise programs in the adolescent age group is poor, with various studies reporting a 25% to 75% dropout rate. Reasons for poor compliance include embarrassment, lack of transportation or money, and time pressures. Buddy systems and rewards for attendance at exercise sessions may be of help. It is important to recommend those kinds of exercise that do not require expensive equipment facilities (e.g., walking and climbing stairs). Obese teenagers might benefit from special physical education classes within the school curriculum. In this way they could participate with others having similar skills and stamina, which might be less embarrassing for them.

School-Based Programs

The school as a setting for an adolescent weight-reduction program would seem to have several advan-

BOX 33-2
Sample Food Exchanges

MILK EXCHANGE		
Evaporated milk	½ cup	
Skim milk	1 cup	
Yogurt, plain	1 cup	

VEGETABLE EXCHANGE		
Broccoli	1 cup	
Green beans	1 cup	
Mushrooms	1 cup	
Summer squash	1 cup	
Tomato	1	
Beets	½ cup	
Carrots	½ cup	
Peas, green	½ cup	
Winter squash	½ cup	

FRUIT EXCHANGE		
Apple	1 small	
Banana	½ small	
Grapes	12	
Orange	1 small	
Raisins	2 tbsp	
Strawberries	1 cup	
Apple juice	⅓ cup	
Orange juice	½ cup	

MEAT EXCHANGE		
Beef, lamb, chicken, fish	1 oz	
Egg	1	
Tuna	¼ oz	
Shrimp	5 small	
Peanut butter, smooth	2 tbsp	
Cottage cheese	¼ cup	
Cheddar cheese, American	1 slice	

FAT EXCHANGE		
Butter or margarine	1 tsp	
Mayonnaise; oil	1 tsp	
Almonds	6 small	

BREAD EXCHANGE		
Muffin	1	
Cereal, dry	¾ cup	
Rice, cooked	½ cup	
Noodles, cooked	½ cup	
Crackers, saltine	5	
Corn, sweet	⅓ cup	
Vegetable soup	½ cup	

BOX 33-3
Food Exchanges for Different Calorie Levels

1000 CALORIES
8 oz skim milk or skim milk yogurt
2 vegetable
4 fruit
4 bread
5 meat
2 fat

1200 CALORIES
16 oz skim milk or skim milk yogurt
3 vegetable
4 fruit
4 bread
5 meat
3 fat

1500 CALORIES
16 oz skim milk or skim milk yogurt
3 vegetable
5 fruit
7 bread
5 meat
4 fat

1800 CALORIES
24 oz skim milk or skim milk yogurt
3 vegetable
5 fruit
9 bread
6 meat
5 fat

tages over the physician's office. It encompasses much of the adolescent's waking hours, can provide both adult and peer support, places the problem in an educational rather than a medical setting, allows treatment of individuals whose families cannot financially support individual medical treatment, and makes more efficient use of nutritionist and physician time. There is some evidence that significant weight losses can occur in school-based programs that combine behavior modification, nutrition education, and psychological support, along with the support of food services, and physical education. Such programs are currently not a high priority within the school curriculum. Without increased federal and state support for materials and the training of personnel, the potential for the development and dissemination of such programs will not be realized.

Self-Help and Commercial Programs

Self-help groups include Overeaters Anonymous (OA) and Take Off Pounds Sensibly (TOPS). The success of such peer self-help groups parallels that of similar groups, such as Alcoholics Anonymous in the treatment of alcoholism. Commercial diet programs include Weight Watchers International (both the oldest and the largest, claiming a yearly membership of 3 million members), Nutri-System, Jenny Craig, and Diet Center. Commercial diet programs tend not to collect and/or release data on attrition and success rates. A study of a commercial weight-reduction program in the United States, however, found an attrition rate of 50% at 6 weeks and 70% at 12 weeks.[29] Similar high attrition rates were reported in five other programs on three continents. Commercial programs usually do not accept younger adolescents who might still be actively growing and often require medical clearance before enrollment of those who are extremely overweight. These programs can be beneficial to older teenagers if they attend regularly and follow the program as directed. However, this is unlikely to happen if the program has few teenage participants, because the teenager feels out of place. Teenagers who are very overweight tend to look a great deal older than their chronologic age, and they dislike being mistaken for an adult. Many dislike the public weigh-in aspect of the program. In my experience, attendance at such programs with a parent has been uniformly unsuccessful.

Very-Low-Calorie Diets

Weight loss can be achieved through a very-low-calorie diet (VLCD). While there is no universally accepted definition of a VLCD, it is usually a diet providing only 400 to 800 calories per day (a protein-sparing modified fast), but formulated to provide all essential nutrients and result in positive nitrogen balance. VLCDs should not be confused with the liquid protein diets of the 1970s, which contained poor-quality protein and resulted in deaths related to cardiac atrophy. The current diets provide protein from meat, fish, or fowl (served as food) or from egg and milk sources in liquid form. The amount of carbohydrate to be included, if any, is still controversial.

There are considerable data on the use of VLCDs with adult outpatients for periods of 3 months without complications. Complications associated with VLCD include gallstones, elevated uric acid, and anemia. Symptoms are usually confined to the first few days and include fatigue, dizziness, muscle cramping, headache, gastrointestinal distress, cold intolerance, dry skin, and hair loss. Most patients do not report hunger, probably because of ketosis. Attrition rates vary considerably from 15% to 68%. Treatment by VLCD usually involves four distinct phases: (1) a 1- to 4-week introductory phase in which patients are placed on a traditional 1200- to 1500-calorie diet with increased exercise, (2) the VLCD itself for a period of 8 to 16 weeks, (3) a 4- to 8-week refeeding period in which conventional foods are gradually reintroduced, and (4) a maintenance phase during which time patients are instructed in methods of maintaining their weight loss. The return to eating solid food is frequently a time of very high anxiety for the patient. Although resting metabolic rate is depressed during the dieting process, studies show that it rises to a level appropriate for the individual's new body weight. The average weight loss on a VLCD for 12 to 16 weeks is 20 kg. The weight loss is usually less for women, especially those who are very short, because they have lower caloric needs. Patients tend to regain most of their weight within 1 to 5 years.[30] It is not known whether participation in a formal weight maintenance program would improve these findings. Unfortunately, fewer than one third of patients participate in formal weight maintenance programs.[31] Studies have shown that patients retain some of the health benefits despite regaining much of the weight.[32]

Initially these diets were used successfully in small numbers of adolescents who were monitored carefully as inpatients. More recently, they have been used for periods of 3 months in outpatients in both individual and group settings. No published data are available on the long-term maintenance of weight loss in adolescents.

Pharmacotherapy

Many short-term trials of 4 to 12 weeks have shown that appetite-suppressant drugs produce weight losses two to four times that from a placebo. The effectiveness of the drugs is maintained only while they are taken. According to most current licensing regulations, the pharmacologic treatment of obesity is limited to short periods, usually 12 to 16 weeks. This is based on a belief that obesity can be treated as a short-term disorder, similar to pneumonia, rather than as a chronic disease such as diabetes. Recently, the question has been raised of longer-term/lifelong administration of drugs for the management of obesity.

Currently used medications include phenylpropanolamine, fluoxetine, fenfluramine, and phentermine. Medications should be used in conjunction with a total program of nutritional counseling, exercise, and behavior modification.

The serotonin agonist fluoxetine has proved useful as an adjunct in weight loss programs for adults in comparison with placebo. This drug seems to reduce appetite in general as well as carbohydrate craving. The effect appears to be similar in adolescents, although long-term efficacy has not been established in any age group.[33]

Dexfenfluramine, the active isomer of fenfluramine, has been studied most (although not approved for use in the United States), including a 1-year randomized double-blind placebo trial known as INDEX (International Dexfenfluramine Study) that involved 822 patients from 24 centers in nine countries.[34] Results indicate that such a drug might aid in extended weight loss over time or be an aid in maintenance of weight loss once achieved.

Weintraub et al, in a National Institutes of Health–funded study, enrolled 121 people in a 34-week trial of a combination of phentermine and fenfluramine versus placebo added to a program of behavior modification, caloric restriction, and exercise.[35] At the end of 34 weeks, only nine subjects had dropped out of the study, the active medication groups had lost significantly more weight ($p < .001$), there were no bothersome side effects, and the medication continued to be efficacious.

Although published treatment trials do not involve children or adolescents, there are anecdotal reports of long-term drug effectiveness in these age groups, often at much smaller dosages than used in adults and with no short-term adverse consequences. Under these circumstances, informed consent should be obtained, preferably as part of a research protocol.

Surgery

Criteria for the selection of adults for surgical treatment of obesity include individuals who: are more than 100 pounds above ideal body weight; have a serious illness responsive to weight loss for which no previous treatment has been successful; have an understanding of the surgery and a commitment to lifelong post-operative care; and possess emotional stability without any tendency toward self-destructive behavior.[36] Surgery should be considered only for carefully selected older adolescent patients with significant medical complications who have failed in all other methods of weight reduction.

There are two generic surgical techniques that are reasonably safe and effective: gastric restriction and gastrointestinal bypass. With gastric restriction, patients decrease their food intake to avoid the intense discomfort and vomiting that occur when small additional amounts of food are eaten. The greatest flaw with the procedure is that liquids and semisolids of high caloric density can pass through the pouch in excess (potato chips, chocolate) and that overdistention can cause the pouch to distend. Gastrointestinal bypass surgery may result in diarrhea or the "dumping" syndrome and requires the patient to take vitamin and mineral supplements. These patients also report changes in eating patterns, consuming fewer fats, sweets, milk, and milk products. Studies have shown less depression, anxiety, irritability, and preoccupation with food during weight loss subsequent to gastric bypass procedure than had occurred during previous nonsurgical attempts at weight reduction.[37]

Soper et al[38] studied 25 morbidly obese adolescents, seven of whom had Prader-Willi syndrome, who underwent gastric bypass. They had a mean preoperative weight of 147 kg. The average weight loss of the 18 adolescents with Prader-Willi syndrome was 15% after 6 months and 25% after 36 months. Those patients with Prader-Willi syndrome were less successful, with one patient not losing any weight. There were no interruptions of height growth, no metabolic problems, and no mortality. Four of the patients required subsequent revision of their bypass.

Perioperative mortality in severely obese patients undergoing a primary operation to control obesity is below 1% in centers specializing in this type of surgery. About 50% of severely obese adults maintain a weight loss of more than 50% of excess weight 5 years after surgery. This exceeds the success of any other treatment.[39]

BINGE-EATING DISORDER

Stunkard was the first to identify binge eating among the obese in 1959 and believed it to be a very rare phenomenon.[40] The new binge-eating disorder (BED) appeared for the first time, as a set of research study criteria, in the appendix of the fourth edition of the *Diagnostic and Statistical Manual* of the American Psychiatric Association (DSM-IV) in 1994 (Box 33-4). BED is currently defined as recurrent episodes of binge eating in the absence of regular use of inappropriate

---

BOX 33-4
DSM IV: Research Criteria
for Binge-Eating Disorder

A. Recurrent episodes of binge eating. An episode of binge eating is characterized by both of the following:
   1. Eating, in a discrete period of time (e.g., within any 2-hour period), an amount of food that is definitely larger than most people would eat in a similar period of time under similar circumstances
   2. A sense of lack of control over eating during the episode (e.g., a feeling that one cannot stop eating or control what or how much one is eating)
B. The binge-eating episodes are associated with three (or more) of the following:
   1. Eating much more rapidly than normal
   2. Eating until feeling uncomfortably full
   3. Eating large amounts of food when not feeling physically hungry
   4. Eating alone because of being embarrassed by how much one is eating
   5. Feeling disgusted with oneself, depressed, or very guilty after overeating
C. Marked distress regarding binge eating is present.
D. The binge eating occurs, on average, at least 2 days a week for 6 months.
   Note: the method of determining frequency differs from that used for bulimia nervosa; future research should address whether the preferred method of setting a frequency threshold is counting the number of days on which binges occur or counting the number of episodes of binge eating.
E. The binge eating is not associated with the regular use of inappropriate compensatory behaviors (e.g., purging, fasting, excessive exercise) and does not occur exclusively during the course of anorexia nervosa or bulimia nervosa.

From American Psychiatric Association: *Diagnostic and statistical manual of mental disorders,* ed 4, Washington, DC, 1994, American Psychiatric Association.

compensatory behaviors characteristic of bulimia nervosa. Patients believed to have this disorder currently may be given the diagnosis of DSM-IV: 307.50; "Eating Disorder Not Otherwise Specified." This category is for disorders of eating that do not meet the criteria for any specific eating disorder, and BED is given as an example. Current estimates of the prevalence of "moderate" binge eating range from 23% to 87%.[41] This eating is usually done secretly. Some individuals report unsuccessful attempts to purge.

Some of the obese bingers may be "carbohydrate cravers" who display a high demand for carbohydrate because of its ultimate action on brain neurotransmitter metabolism. Carbohydrate cravers have been noted to ingest an amount of food similar to that eaten by lean controls during three daily meals but to binge on high-carbohydrate foods during the early evening and night. Such individuals are described as having more rigid and extreme dieting attitudes and substantial psychological distress.

Several studies conducted before the development of the new DSM-IV research criteria indicated that obese bingers had less psychopathology and dietary restraint than did patients with bulimia nervosa. Obese binge eaters as compared with obese nonbingers had greater lifetime rates of affective disorder and more often had histrionic, borderline, or avoidant personality disorders.[42]

Obese individuals who binge have a higher dropout rate from weight reduction programs and a higher recidivism rate than those who do not binge. It has been suggested that such individuals need to be identified and enrolled in a treatment program specifically designed for their needs. This is currently a very active research area.

SUMMARY

Obesity is an increasingly common problem in adolescents. The greatest likelihood of success in treating mild to moderate obesity is a program that includes nutritional education and dietary change, behavior modification strategies, and exercise individually tailored to each patient. An effort should be made to diagnose patients who have binge-eating disorder. Because obesity is a chronic illness, long-term monitoring of progress in a group or individual setting is of great importance. The physician should pay special attention to dieting teenage girls who are only mildly overweight; this may signal the onset of anorexia or bulimia nervosa. Carefully selected, morbidly obese adolescents may be candidates for very-low-calorie diets, pharmacotherapy, or surgery when all other efforts to lose weight have failed. Although current therapeutic modalities fall far short of success, it is hoped that the results of basic and clinical research will lead to more promising strategies for the future. Any physician providing care to adolescents should play a major role in addressing the psychologic and sociocultural issues that affect the obese teenager.

References

1. Centers for Disease Control: Prevalence of overweight among adolescents—United States, 1988-1991, *MMWR* 43:818-824, 1994.
2. Stunkard AJ, Burt V: Obesity and the body image. II. Age at onset of disturbances in the body image, *Am J Psychiatry* 123:1443-1447, 1967.
3. Must A, Jacques PF, Dallal GE, Bafema CJ, Dietz WH: Long-term morbidity and mortality of overweight adolescents: a followup of the Harvard Growth Study of 1922-35, *N Engl J Med* 327:1350-1355, 1992.
4. National Center for Health Statistics: *Skinfold thickness of youths 12-17 years, United States,* DHEW Pub. No. (HRA) 74-1614, Washington, DC, 1974, U.S. Government Printing Office.
5. Himes JH, Dietz WH: Guidelines for overweight in adolescent preventive services: recommendations from an expert committee, *Am J Clin Nutr* 59:307-316, 1994.
6. Gurney R: Hereditary factor in obesity, *Arch Intern Med* 57:557-561, 1936.
7. Stunkard AJ, Sorensen TI, Hanis C, Teasdale TW, Chakraborty R, Schuall WJ, Schunlsinger F: An adoption study of human obesity, *N Engl J Med* 314:193-198, 1986.
8. Stunkard AJ, Harris JR, Pedersen NL, McClearn GE: The body-mass index of twins who have been reared apart, *N Engl J Med* 322:1483-1487, 1990.
9. Bouchard C, Tremblay A, Depres J, Nadeau A, Lupien PJ, Theriault G, Dussault J, Moorjani S, Pinault S, Fournier G: The response to long-term overfeeding in identical twins, *N Engl J Med* 332:1477-1482, 1990.
10. Burns TL: The role of genetic epidemiology in the prediction of childhood obesity. In *Workshop on prevention and treatment of childhood obesity: research directions,* Bethesda, MD, 1995, National Institutes of Health; pp 22-23.
11. Zhang Y, Proenca R, Maffei M, Barone M, Leopold L, Friedman JM: Positional cloning of the mouse obese gene and its human homologue, *Nature* 372:425-432, 1994.
12. Considine RV, Considine EL, Williams CJ, Nyce MR, Magosin SA, Bauer TL, Rosato EL, Colberg J, Caro JF: Evidence against either a premature stop codon or the absence of obese gene mRNA in human obesity, *J Clin Invest* 95:2986-2988, 1995.
13. Sims EAH, Danforth E, Horton ES, Bray GA, Glennon JA, Salans LB: Endocrine and metabolic efforts of experimental obesity in man, *Recent Prog Horm Res* 29:457-496, 1973.
14. Blundell JE: Impact of nutrition on the pharmacology of appetite: some conceptual issues, *Ann NY Acad Sci* 575:163-170, 1989.
15. Drewnowski A, Greenwood MRC: Cream and sugar: human preferences for high-fat foods, *Physiol Behav* 30:629-633, 1983.
16. Sclafani A: Animal models of obesity: classification and characterization, *Int J Obes* 8:491-508, 1984.
17. Dietz WH, Gortmaker SL: Do we fatten our children at the T.V. set? Television viewing and obesity in children and adolescents, *Pediatrics* 75:807-812, 1985.
18. VanItallie TB, Lew EA: Overweight and underweight. In Lew EA, Gajewski J, editors: *Medical risks 1987: mortality trends by age and time elapsed,* New York, 1990, Praeger; pp 13.1-13.22.
19. Bjorntorp P: Classification of obese patients and complications related to the distribution of surplus fat, *Am J Clin Nutr* 45:1120-1125, 1987.
20. Fujioka S, Matsuzawa Y, Tokunaga K, Tarui S: Contribution of intraabdominal fat accumulation to the impairment of glucose and lipid metabolism in human obesity, *Metabolism* 36:54-59, 1987.

21. Staffieri JR: A study of social stereotype of body image in children, *J Pers Soc Psychol* 7:101-104, 1967.

22. Monello LF, Mayer J: Obese adolescent girls: an unrecognized "minority" group?, *Am J Clin Nutr* 13:35-39, 1963.

23. Canning H, Mayer J: Obesity—its possible effect on college acceptance, *N Engl J Med* 275:1172-1179, 1966.

24. Gortmaker SL, Must A, Perrin JM, Sobol AM, Dietz WH: Social and economic consequences of overweight in adolescence and young adulthood, *N Engl J Med* 329:1008-1012, 1993.

25. Stunkard A, Mendelson M: Obesity and the body image: I. Characteristics of disturbances in the body image of some obese persons, *Am J Psychiatry* 123:1296-1300, 1967.

26. VanItallie TB, Lew EA: Assessment of morbidity and mortality risk in the overweight patient. In Wadden TA, VanItallie TB, editors: *Treatment of the seriously obese patient,* New York, 1992, Guilford Press; pp 3-32.

27. Lissner L, Odell PM, D'Agostino RB, Stokes J, Kreger BE, Belanger AJ, Brownell KD: Variability of body weight and health outcomes in the Framingham population, *N Engl J Med* 324:1839-1844, 1991.

28. Brownell KD, Rodin J: Medical, metabolic, and psychological effects of weight cycling, *Arch Intern Med* 154:1325-1330, 1994.

29. Volkmar FR, Stunkard AJ, Woolston J, Bailey RA: High attrition rates in commercial weight reduction program, *Arch Intern Med* 141:426-430, 1981.

30. Wadden TA, Bartlett SJ: Very low calorie diets: an overview and appraisal. In Wadden TA, VanItallie TB, editors: *Treatment of the seriously obese patient,* New York, 1992, Guilford Press; pp 44-79.

31. Palgi A, Read JL, Greenberg I, Hoffer MA, Bistrian BR, Blackburn GL: Multidisciplinary treatment of obesity with a protein-sparing modified fast: results in 688 outpatients, *Am J Public Health* 75:1190-1194, 1985.

32. Wing RR, Marcus MD, Salata R, Epstein LH, Miaskiewicz S, Blair EH: Effects of a very-low-calorie diet on long-term glycemic control in obese type II diabetics, *Arch Intern Med* 151:1334-1340, 1991.

33. Boeck MA: Safety and efficacy of fluoxetine in morbidly obese adolescent females, *Int J Obes* 15 (suppl 3):60, 1991.

34. Guy-Grand B, Apfelbaum M, Crepaldi G, Gries A, Lefebvre P, Turner P: International trial of long-term dexfenfluramine in obesity, *Lancet* 2:1142-1144, 1989.

35. Weintraub M, Sundaresan PR, Madan M, Schuster B, Balder A, Lasagna L, Cox C: Long-term weight control study I (weeks 0 to 34), *Clin Pharmacol Ther* 51:586-594, 1992.

36. Task Force of the American Society for Clinical Nutrition: Guidelines for surgery for morbid obesity, *Am J Clin Nutr* 42:904-905, 1985.

37. Saltzstein EC, Gutmann MC: Gastric bypass for morbid obesity: preoperative and postoperative psychological evaluation of patients, *Arch Surg* 115:21-28, 1980.

38. Soper RT, Mason EE, Printen KJ, Zellweger H: Gastric bypass for morbid obesity in children and adolescents, *J Pediatr Surg* 10:51-58, 1975.

39. Kral JG: Surgical treatment of obesity. In Wadden TA, VanItallie TB (eds): *Treatment of the seriously obese patient,* New York, 1992, Guilford Press; pp 496-506.

40. Stunkard AJ: Eating patterns and obesity, *Psychiatr Q* 33:284-292, 1959.

41. Gormally J, Black S, Daston S, Rardin D: The assessment of binge eating severity among obese persons, *Addict Behav* 7:47-55, 1982.

42. Marcus MD, Wing RR, Ewing L, Kern E, Gooding W, McDermott M: Psychiatric disorders among obese binge eaters, *Int J Eat Disord* 9:69-77, 1990.

CHAPTER 34

Chest Pain

•

Rubin S. Cooper

EVALUATION

Chest pain is a common complaint in the adolescent.[1-3] In a society with a high prevalence of atherosclerotic heart disease and hypertension, as well as increased media coverage of sudden death in young athletes, physicians are aware of the concern of patients, parents, and coaches when an adolescent complains of chest pain. An evaluation of chest pain provides a framework for the primary care physician to distinguish between noncardiac and cardiac causes of chest pain.

The initial concern with a patient complaining of chest pain is that the pain may represent myocardial ischemia, which could lead to ventricular dysfunction, arrhythmia, myocardial infarction, and sudden death. Sudden cardiac death affects 200,000 to 400,000 Americans annually and accounts for 15% to 20% of deaths in adults. In the pediatric population, aged 1 to 20 years, sudden cardiac death accounts for 2% to 20% of deaths.[4] Relatively few studies examining sudden death in the pediatric population are available, but a 1990 review notes several cardiac diagnoses in particular, including myocarditis, hypertrophic cardiomyopathy, and congenital coronary artery anomalies.[5] Chest pain due to one of these causes must be taken very seriously.

Chest pain caused by cardiac abnormalities can be divided into three categories: structural abnormalities, acquired myocardial and coronary artery disease, and arrhythmia (Box 34-1). To cause chest pain, these disorders either must produce an imbalance between oxygen demand and delivery to the myocardium, or must cause an irritation of the pericardial or pleural surfaces. Pain may occur with exertion or with positional changes when inflammation is present.

Although cardiac causes of chest pain are of significant concern, most chest pain in adolescents will be found to be noncardiac in origin or to have no discernible cause (Box 34-2). A cardiac origin for chest pain is relatively uncommon in the standard pediatric practice or the pediatric emergency room in comparison with the adult population.

Recurrent chest pain often challenges the physician's skills because there tend to be few physical findings and few helpful laboratory data. Therefore the history is critical, and careful empathetic communication with both the patient and the parents is important. Assessment of the adolescent's and the parents' personalities, their interactions, and the parents' responses to the patient's pain is helpful. Questioning the patient alone is suggested. The adolescent should be asked to describe (1) how long the pain lasts (seconds, minutes, hours, days), (2) how often the pain is felt (times per day, week, and month), (3) the location of the pain (superficial, localized, diffuse, substernal, epigastric), (4) factors that exacerbate or relieve the pain (position, exercise, sleep), (5) the quality of the pain (sharp, aching, burning, or deep), (6) the severity of the pain (mild, moderate, severe, variable), (7) the time of day when the pain is likely to occur (morning, afternoon, evening), and (8) any environmental stresses that may play a role (family fights, school pressures).

The answers to these questions are invaluable and offer the key to proper diagnosis and management of pain from both cardiac and noncardiac causes. Chest pain that occurs with exercise or in association with syncope or "heart palpitations" should raise the greatest suspicion of cardiac disease. Conversely, pain lasting either "one second" or "several hours" and recurrent pain that occurs during quiet activities are less likely to have a cardiac origin.

Physical examination may be helpful in certain circumstances. Chest wall pain is usually reproducible.

BOX 34-1
Causes of Cardiac Chest Pain
in Adolescents

STRUCTURAL ABNORMALITIES
Left ventricular outflow obstruction
    Aortic stenosis, idiopathic hypertrophic subaortic stenosis
    Mitral valve prolapse
    Marfan's syndrome (aortic aneurysm)
    Coronary artery anomalies

ACQUIRED MYOPERICARDIAL AND
CORONARY ARTERY DISEASE
Primary pericarditis
    Infections: bacterial, viral, rickettsial
    Immunologic: rheumatic fever, juvenile rheumatoid arthritis, systemic lupus erythematosus
    Metabolic: uremia
    Tumor: acute lymphocytic leukemia, Hodgkin's and non-Hodgkin's lymphoma
Myocarditis
    Bacterial, viral, rheumatic
    Anemia: sickle cell anemia with angina
Coronary artery disease due to atherosclerosis
    Familial hyperlipidemia
    Prolonged use of steroids

ARRHYTHMIA
Supraventricular tachycardia
Ventricular ectopy
Prolonged QT syndrome

BOX 34-2
Noncardiac Causes of Chest Pain
in Adolescents

Thoracic
    Costochondritis
    Tietze's syndrome
    Muscle strain, spasm
    Blunt trauma
    Hypersensitive xiphoid
    Precordial catch
    Slipping rib syndrome
    Bone (infiltrative tumor—leukemia)
    Breast (trauma, mastitis)
Pulmonary tree
    Reactive airway disease (asthma)
    Pneumothorax
    Diaphragmatic irritation
Gastrointestinal
    Esophageal (reflux, spasm, esophagitis)
    Hiatal hernia
Psychogenic
    Hyperventilation
    Conversion symptoms
    Somatization
    Depression

The dermatomes of T2 to T8 form an inclusive band that covers most of the thorax from the clavicle to just below the xiphoid process. Pain in the T1 to T4 dermatome generally arises from the thoracic viscera (myocardium, pericardium, aorta, pulmonary arteries, esophagus, and mediastinum) and is maximal in the retrosternal and precordial areas. Pain in the T5 to T8 dermatome suggests an origin in the lower thoracic wall, diaphragm, or abdominal viscera (peritoneal surfaces, gallbladder, liver, pancreas, duodenum, and stomach) and tends to be maximal in the xiphoid region and in the back. Pain of cardiac origin is carried by several different nerve chains and thus may be sensed as deep, crushing, and substernal; alternatively, it may be peripheral and sharp, in the arm, shoulder, or neck. Any signs of trauma (bruising and swelling) should be noted. Percussion and palpation over costochondral junctions often localize and reproduce the pain in adolescents with costochondritis. Auscultation with the patient in supine, sitting, and standing positions is key to assessing the presence of pericardial friction rubs, ejection and nonejection clicks, and significant cardiac murmurs.

Laboratory tests should be performed sparingly in the adolescent with chest pain and should be aimed at confirming likely noncardiac causes or detecting important cardiac etiologies. The 12-lead electrocardiogram (ECG) helps assess the rate and rhythm of the heart, detect hypertrophy, and provide evidence of preexcitation syndrome (short PR interval and delta wave) or a prolonged QT interval. Chest radiograph films may be useful in assessing heart size, pericardial and pleural effusions, bony fractures, or pulmonary disease. An echocardiogram with two-dimensional and Doppler evaluation is helpful in the diagnosis of effusion, left ventricular outflow tract obstruction, mitral valve prolapse, and myocarditis. To detect and quantify supraventricular tachycardia, ventricular ectopy, or other arrhythmias, 24-hour ambulatory electrocardiography (Holter) recordings, or event monitors, are helpful.

In general, the primary care physician must determine whether chest pain is cardiac in origin (a small minority of adolescents) or whether it has other causes (the large majority) in order to diagnose noncardiac causes and evaluate cardiac causes before referring the patient to the cardiologist. Chest pain is the second leading cause of referral to pediatric cardiology clinics (heart murmurs are the first).[3] Cardiac causes of chest pain in children and adolescents are most commonly diagnosed in these clinics.

CARDIAC CAUSES

Structural Abnormalities

LEFT VENTRICULAR OUTFLOW TRACT OBSTRUCTION. Chest pain in adolescents may be caused by several types of left ventricular outflow tract obstruction, including most importantly aortic valve stenosis and idiopathic hypertrophic subaortic stenosis. These lesions produce chest pain when the obstruction increases left ventricular wall stress, leading to inadequate perfusion and ischemia.[3]

Aortic valve stenosis occurs in 3% to 6% of children with congenital heart disease. The natural history of aortic stenosis is that its severity is progressive yet often silent. Physical examination reveals a systolic thrill in the suprasternal notch and a systolic ejection click, as well as a systolic ejection murmur in the aortic area. Left ventricular hypertrophy, with or without strain, may be demonstrated by ECG, but as many as 50% of patients with severe valvular obstruction may have a normal ECG result.[6] Chest radiography is not generally helpful in assessing the severity of the obstruction. However, two-dimensional echocardiography and Doppler examination may provide estimations of the systolic gradient to help predict the level and severity of the obstruction. Electrocardiography performed during exercise or stress testing also may aid in functional assessment of the obstruction. Reports in the literature have been conflicting, with questions raised regarding the prudence of performing stress tests in patients with moderate to severe obstruction. Clearly, however, patients with moderate or severe (gradient >50 mm Hg) aortic stenosis who experience chest pain need to have further evaluation and intervention, often including balloon angioplasty and/or cardiac surgery.

The murmur of idiopathic hypertrophic subaortic stenosis may vary considerably and is dependent on the degree of left ventricular filling. The murmur is softer and the gradient diminished with maximal left ventricular filling or increased afterload. The latter occurs when the patient is in a supine position, squatting, or doing isometric exercise. The murmur increases in intensity with maneuvers that impede left ventricular filling, such as standing or performing a Valsalva maneuver.

MITRAL VALVE PROLAPSE. Considerable controversy still exists regarding the diagnosis and management of mitral valve prolapse and the mitral valve prolapse syndrome.[7,8] Patients with mitral valve prolapse should be evaluated for Marfan's syndrome and other connective tissue disorders. The cardiac examination should be performed with the patient in all positions to elicit the findings of a middle to late nonejection systolic click and a middle to late systolic murmur. The ECG picture is often normal but may demonstrate T-wave abnormalities in the inferior leads and/or prominent U waves. The two-

dimensional ECG may help confirm the diagnosis (see Chapter 37, "Mitral Valve Prolapse"). Care should be taken to avoid the overdiagnosis of this entity. The etiology of chest pain associated with mitral valve prolapse is unclear and may represent altered autonomic function and increased responsiveness that is mediated by catecholamine release.

MARFAN'S SYNDROME. The morbidity and mortality noted in patients with Marfan's syndrome are invariably due to aortic aneurysm and rupture. Careful and serial assessment of aortic root diameter by two-dimensional echocardiography and magnetic resonance imaging (MRI) is critical. The prophylactic use of beta blockers in these patients has been recommended, although long-term studies regarding their efficacy are not available.

CORONARY ARTERY ANOMALIES. The congenital anomaly of the coronary artery system most commonly reported in association with sudden unexpected death in adolescents is an anomalous origin of the left coronary artery arising from the right (anterior) sinus of Valsalva.[9] In this rare anomaly the left coronary artery crosses between the aorta and the pulmonary artery and is susceptible to compression of the coronary ostium between the two great vessels. Compression leads to ischemia and sudden death. The physical examination results are normal. On occasion the patient may have a history of exercise-induced syncope. The two-dimensional echocardiogram may not be helpful and angiography is required for diagnosis.

ANOMALOUS ORIGIN OF LEFT CORONARY ARTERY FROM PULMONARY ARTERY. This entity often presents in infancy with cardiogenic shock and/or myocardial infarction and death.[10] It may appear in older children, adolescents, or adults if adequate collateral vessels are present and myocardial perfusion is adequate. Chest pain may develop at any time. The ECG may demonstrate abnormal Q waves consistent with a previous infarction. A two-dimensional echocardiogram may be helpful, although angiography is definitive. The assessment of myocardial perfusion can be accomplished by thallium or positron emission tomography scanning.

CORONARY ARTERIAL FISTULA. Adolescents with a coronary arterial fistula may have chest pain and a continuous heart murmur. This entity rarely produces symptoms but may "steal" blood flow from the normal left coronary artery circulation and result in myocardial ischemia. Two-dimensional echocardiography may demonstrate a dilated coronary artery with diastolic flow at the distal fistulous end.

PULMONARY ARTERY HYPERTENSION. When due to pulmonary vascular disease, this entity may account for up to 15% to 70% of sudden deaths. Usually, recurrent syncope, progressive dyspnea, and hemoptysis are the clinical hallmarks, but chest pain due to hypoxemia and/or a dilated pulmonary artery compressing the posterior aorta may occur. On physical examination there is evidence of cyanosis, clubbing, and a loud pulmonic component with the second heart sound. The ECG demonstrates right axis deviation and right ventricular hypertrophy.

Acquired Myopericardial or Coronary Artery Disease

Patients with myocarditis have fever, tachycardia, tachypnea, and signs of congestive heart failure, including a gallop rhythm, cardiomegaly, and hepatomegaly. The diagnosis of myocarditis should always be entertained if these findings are present in a previously healthy adolescent without known heart disease. Progression to cardiogenic shock and death may be rapid. The ECG typically shows low voltage, low-voltage QRS complexes (5 mm total amplitude or less in the limb leads), flat T waves, and ST-segment depression. A two-dimensional echocardiogram often helps confirm the diagnosis, showing evidence of a dilated and poorly contractile left ventricle.

Pericarditis can present concurrently with myocarditis or as an isolated entity. Chest pain caused by pericarditis is often relieved when the patient is in a sitting or forward position and is made worse in the supine position. A pericardial friction rub is often audible at the apex in the absence of a moderate pericardial effusion. The ECG will show pericardial fluid and pericardial thickening.

Anginal pain with ECG changes of ST-segment and T-segment wave depression has been described in sickle cell anemia.[11] After hypertransfusion, the ST-segment and T-wave depression improves and the angina is relieved.

KAWASAKI'S DISEASE. Coronary artery lesions in Kawasaki's disease (mucocutaneous lymph node syndrome) may take on increasing significance in the future as a cause of chest pain in adolescents.[12] Coronary artery involvement occurs in 15% to 20% of children with Kawasaki's disease. The use of intravenous gamma globulin has decreased the prevalence of coronary artery abnormalities, which previously carried a 1% to 3% mortality rate owing to myocardial ischemia and/or infarction.[13] The long-term sequelae of Kawasaki's disease for patients with aneurysms, as well as for those without apparent cardiac disease, are yet to be established. The natural history of coronary artery disease in adolescents and adults who had Kawasaki's disease as children is still unknown.

ATHEROSCLEROSIS. Although it is the number one diagnostic consideration in adults, angina is an uncommon cause of chest pain in adolescents. In adolescents with a history of familial hyperlipidemia or prolonged use of steroids (a requirement for transplant patients), angina secondary to atherosclerosis must be considered.

DRUG USE. The use of cocaine has been increasingly implicated as a cause of life-threatening cardiac events in adolescents and young adults.[14] Oral and intranasal "recreational" use has been temporally related to acute myocardial infarction, ventricular tachycardia and fibrillation, myocarditis, and sudden death.[15] Unfortunately, the pathogenesis of the cardiac toxicity of cocaine remains incompletely defined. Urine toxicology tests should be obtained for patients with chest pain and/or arrhythmia in the emergency setting.

Arrhythmia

Patients with arrhythmias, whether with structurally normal hearts or with cardiac lesions, may complain of presyncope, syncope, palpitations, weakness, diaphoresis, and chest pain. Palpitations and premature beats are sometimes perceived as chest pain. The chest pain that results from rhythm abnormalities is based on changes in cardiac output, with a resultant increase in subendocardial wall stress and diminished diastolic coronary perfusion. Any sustained tachyarrhythmia can lead to poor coronary perfusion. In patients with a healthy myocardium, sustained supraventricular tachycardia is well tolerated for several hours before producing ventricular dysfunction. Symptoms are more likely to appear with left ventricular dysfunction.

SUPRAVENTRICULAR TACHYCARDIA. In adolescents, supraventricular tachycardia generally produces a regular rate of 150 to 200 beats per minute. It tends to have a rapid onset and offset, may occur at any time during the day, and may last seconds or hours. The paroxysmal nature of the tachycardia may cause atypical chest pain not related consistently to exercise. Hyperthyroidism should be ruled out. If the pain is associated with dizziness and palpitations, a resting ECG and a 24-hour ambulatory ECG (Holter) recording should be obtained. Occasionally, an event recorder will note these episodes if the 24-hour Holter recording is normal. A preexcitation syndrome, such as Wolff-Parkinson-White, may be evident on the resting ECG, as demonstrated by a short PR interval and bundle branch block pattern over the right or left precordial leads. Medical therapy is often successful. If medical therapy is refractory, electrophysiologic studies are available to map or possibly ablate the accessory pathways.

PROLONGED QT INTERVAL SYNDROME. This entity may be associated with chest pain, palpitations, syncope, or even sudden death. Since the condition may be familial, the family history should be examined for sudden death, deafness, and unexplained seizure activity. The corrected QT interval should be calculated by the following equation: QT (in seconds) divided by the square root of the RR interval (in seconds). A corrected QT interval greater than 0.44 seconds is abnormal. The arrhythmia associated with this syndrome is a rapid form of ventricular tachycardia referred to as torsades de pointes. Treatment with beta blockers improves survival rates.

VENTRICULAR ECTOPY. Chest pain is an unusual feature of underlying ventricular arrhythmias. Most children and adolescents with isolated unifocal premature ventricular contractions, and even brief episodes of nonsustained ventricular tachycardia, generally remain asymptomatic. If symptoms are present, ventricular ectopy should be confirmed by Holter recording. Exercise stress testing also is useful in distinguishing benign from malignant rhythms, as well as the rare but potentially lethal catechol-induced ventricular tachycardia.

References

1. Brenner JI, Rengel RE, Berman MA: Cardiologic perspective of chest pain in childhood: a referral problem? To whom?, *Pediatr Clin North Am* 31:1241-1257, 1984.
2. Coleman WL: Recurrent chest pain in children, *Pediatr Clin North Am* 31:1007-1026, 1984.
3. Brenner JI, Berman MA: Chest pain in childhood and adolescence, *J Adolesc Health Care* 3:271-276, 1983.
4. Maron BJ, Roberts WC, McAllister HA: Sudden death in young athletes, *Circulation* 62:218, 1980.
5. Denfield S, Garson A: Sudden death in children and young adults, *Pediatr Clin North Am* 37:215-231, 1990.
6. Alpert BS, Moses DM, Durant MA: Hemodynamic responses to ergometer exercise in children and young adults with left ventricular pressure or volume overload, *Am J Cardiol* 52:563-567, 1983.
7. Bissett GS, Schwartz DC, Metyer RA: Clinical spectrum and long term follow up of isolated mitral valve prolapse in 119 children, *Circulation* 2:423-429, 1980.
8. Boudoulas H, Kolibash AJ, Wooley CF: Mitral valve prolapse: a heterogeneous disorder, *Prim Cardiol* 17:29-43, 1991.
9. Cheitlin D, DeCastro CM, McAllister HA: Sudden death as a complication of anomalous left coronary artery origin from the anterior sinus of Valsalva, *Circulation* 50:780, 1974.
10. Moodie DS, Fyfe D, Gill CC: Anomalous origin of the left coronary artery from the pulmonary artery in adult populations. Long term follow up after surgery, *Am Heart J* 106:381-388, 1983.
11. Hamilton W, Rosenthal A, Berwick D: Angina pectoris in a child with sickle cell anemia, *Pediatrics* 6:911, 1978.
12. Melish ME: Kawasaki syndrome, *Pediatr Ann* 11:255-268, 1982.
13. Newburger JN, Takahashi M, Burns JC: The treatment of Kawasaki syndrome with intravenous gamma globulin, *N Engl J Med* 315:341, 1986.
14. Isner JM, Estes M, Thompson PD, Costanzo-Nordin MR, Subramanian R, Miller G, Kostas G, Sweeney K, Sturner W: Acute cardiac events temporally related to cocaine abuse, *N Engl J Med* 315:23, 1438-1443, 1986.
15. Choi YS, Pearl WR: Cardiovascular effects of adolescent drug abuse, *J Adolesc Health Care* 10:332-337, 1989.

CHAPTER 35

Congenital Heart Disease

•

Michael A. LaCorte

HEART MURMUR IN HEALTHY ADOLESCENTS

It is not uncommon to detect a heart murmur for the first time during a routine examination of a healthy adolescent. Such a finding often creates anxiety on the part of the physician, the adolescent, and the family. However, most heart murmurs detected for the first time during adolescence are innocent heart murmurs that have no significance. Typically these functional heart murmurs are the vibratory (or musical) murmur and the pulmonary ejection murmur.

Vibratory (musical) murmurs are usually heard in early infancy and childhood. This murmur, however, can also be detected during adolescence and is believed to be caused by high-velocity, nonturbulent flow in the left ventricular outflow tract. It is typically described as vibratory or musical, is best heard at the lower left sternal border, and radiates well both to the base and the apex. The quality of the murmur is typical and, once recognized, should not be confused with an organic murmur.

The more important and common murmur heard in adolescence is the pulmonary flow murmur. This murmur is related to turbulence in the main pulmonary artery and appears to be commonly heard in an adolescent during the growth spurt. The pulmonary artery is anterior and close to the chest wall, so turbulence in the main pulmonary artery is easily detected with a stethoscope. These murmurs are ejection in timing, are somewhat harsh in quality, usually do not exceed grade 2 in intensity, and are well localized to the pulmonic area. They are not associated with a pulmonic ejection click, which distinguishes them from the murmur of valvar pulmonic stenosis. In addition, the second heart sound in these patients is normally split and varies, as usual, with respiration, which distinguishes this murmur from the pulmonary flow murmur that is detected in an atrial septal defect.

These two types of innocent heart murmur are completely benign, and the adolescent and family should be reassured that they do not represent significant heart disease. No prophylaxis for dental extractions or minor surgery is required. Follow-up with a pediatric cardiologist is not indicated. By and large, the clinician who is comfortable with the diagnosis of an innocent murmur does not need to refer the adolescent to a cardiologist. At times, however, a youngster with a pulmonary flow murmur may indeed have an atrial communication, and this should always be kept in mind when a pulmonary flow murmur is diagnosed. Therefore, in some instances echocardiography will be necessary, especially with questions concerning splitting of the second heart sound or interpretation of the electrocardiogram (ECG).

EXTRA HEART SOUNDS IN THE ADOLESCENT

It is not uncommon to hear an extra heart sound during a routine cardiac examination in an adolescent. It is quite common to appreciate a third heart sound (S_3) in diastole at the apex of a healthy teenager. Fourth heart sounds (S_4) are less common but can also be a normal finding. A split S_1 is often noted on the cardiac examination and must be differentiated from a click. Clicks have a more "snappy" quality and occur later in systole. Clicks at the base of the heart usually are secondary to thickening of the aortic valve (a fixed click at the upper right sternal border and apex) or the pulmonic valve (variable in respiration and heard at the upper left sternal border).

An important finding is a click (or clicks) at the lower left sternal border, which may be associated with a late systolic murmur, especially in the sitting or standing position. This is the hallmark of mitral valve prolapse. This condition occurs in many otherwise healthy teenagers, especially thin girls. These adolescents often have vague complaints of palpitations, atypical chest pain, and dizziness. In addition to the click and late systolic murmur found on examination, an echocardiogram will be diagnostic. An additional work-up (stress test and Holter monitor) should be performed in significantly symptomatic individuals or those with any arrhythmias (atrial or

ventricular premature contractions noted on the ECG). In almost all cases, reassurance is effective in ameliorating symptoms. In a few cases, beta blockers are required. Endocarditis prophylaxis is not needed for patients with an isolated mitral valve prolapse click but should be recommended when significant mitral insufficiency is present. No physical restrictions are necessary and yearly follow-up is indicated.

LESIONS COMMONLY REQUIRING THERAPY IN ADOLESCENCE

Atrial septal defects often do not come to medical attention until adolescence. There are two major reasons that they may go undiagnosed for many years. The first is that children and adolescents with such defects are almost always asymptomatic. The pathophysiology of an atrial septal defect is that of a volume overload of the right ventricle that is well tolerated for many years. Therefore, symptoms of heart failure, such as shortness of breath, easy fatigability, and exercise intolerance, are not usually seen. The second reason is the paucity of physical findings even when there are large defects. The heart murmur of an atrial septal defect is actually a flow murmur caused by increased flow into the pulmonary artery. Thus, the murmur of an atrial septal defect is not secondary to flow across the defect itself but is essentially a functional murmur, that is, a function of increased pulmonary blood flow. Since the murmur of an atrial septal defect resembles that of a pulmonary flow murmur often heard in adolescence, it may be interpreted as an innocent murmur. The most important physical finding on cardiac examination, albeit subtle, is the fixed splitting of the second heart sound (S_2). In normal persons, the S_2 splits in inspiration and becomes single in expiration. The presence of an atrial communication of significant size results in the absence of the respiratory variation of S_2; therefore, S_2 is widely split and fixed. Primary care providers must be aware of these subtleties of the examination. The ECG can be a valuable tool in the diagnosis of an atrial septal defect. Right ventricular volume overload pattern is typical of this defect, although in some adolescents the ECG may be essentially normal. Employing two-dimensional echocardiography with color flow Doppler, one can easily visualize the defect and document the left-to-right shunt.

Although individuals with atrial septal defects generally remain asymptomatic throughout early adult life, the consequences of the volume overload take their toll as an adult. Surgical closure of atrial septal defects should be performed whenever these are recognized in adolescence. Surgery for atrial septal defects involves either direct suture closure or patch closure with pericardium. Individuals need not receive endocarditis prophylaxis after atrial septal defect closure by these techniques. A new nonsurgical technique currently under investigation involves the use of a "clamshell" device, which was developed at Boston Children's Hospital. This device can be safely placed during a cardiac catheterization. Currently, large clam-shell devices are being developed to accommodate older patients with large atrial communications. Over the next few years it is anticipated that most atrial septal defects will be closed nonsurgically. This will be of great benefit to adolescents who can avoid the medical and psychological effects of open heart surgery.

Another lesion commonly undiagnosed until adolescence is subaortic stenosis, the most common form of which is a membrane beneath the aortic valve. Unlike an atrial septal defect, which clearly must be present from birth, subaortic stenosis can develop during childhood and adolescence and often does not become manifest until later childhood and adolescence. The murmur of subaortic stenosis is generally a harsh systolic murmur, which is heard both at the left lower sternal border and at the right upper sternal border. The murmur is often mistaken for a small ventricular septal defect; prior to two-dimensional echocardiography, many individuals with subaortic stenosis had a diagnosis of small ventricular septal defects. Thus, it is imperative that the teenager with the diagnosis of ventricular septal defect undergo a two-dimensional echocardiogram to make certain that a subaortic membrane is not present. Subaortic stenosis caused by a subaortic membrane is a progressive disease, and turbulence below the aortic valve will ultimately cause damage to the aortic valve and aortic insufficiency. Surgery before the development of aortic insufficiency is recommended. Currently, the recommendation is removal of any subaortic membrane with a pressure gradient of more than 30-40 mm Hg. Cardiac catheterization is no longer required in the management of subaortic stenosis. Two-dimensional Doppler echocardiography is diagnostic, and surgery can be performed on the basis of this noninvasive technique. After recovery from surgery, the adolescent may participate in all activities as long as the pressure gradient across the subaortic region is less than 20 mm Hg. Yearly follow-up must be performed, since there is an incidence of recurrence of subaortic stenosis. Endocarditis prophylaxis is lifelong in these individuals.

Congenital valvar aortic stenosis is a lesion diagnosed early in life. However, it is not unusual for this lesion to progress during adolescence, especially in the period of rapid growth. Often, it is not until adolescence that the pressure gradient across the aortic valve becomes significant and therapy is indicated. The murmur of classic valvar aortic stenosis is a harsh systolic ejection murmur heard best in the aortic area at the right

upper sternal border. A hallmark of valvar aortic stenosis is a thrill that is palpable in the suprasternal notch. A suprasternal notch thrill is present even in individuals with a relatively mild obstruction. In addition, a constant ejection click is usually audible at the apex. The adolescent with aortic stenosis is almost always asymptomatic and may want to participate in competitive sports. A pressure gradient of more than 20 mm Hg warrants restriction from competitive athletics; in individuals with pressure gradients of more than 50 mm Hg or in instances with ST-T wave abnormalities on an exercise stress test, therapy is indicated. Until recently, open surgical valvotomy was the treatment of choice as an initial form of therapy. However, balloon valvuloplasty has become an accepted mode of therapy in individuals requiring treatment for valvar aortic stenosis. This procedure is performed as part of cardiac catheterization and angiography and has proved quite effective as an initial stage of therapy. Valvar aortic stenosis, however, is a progressive lesion, and ultimately a valve replacement is required in most individuals with significant disease. Therefore, adolescents with valvar aortic stenosis must be counseled concerning athletic restriction and should be discouraged from participating in highly competitive athletic endeavors. Endocarditis prophylaxis is a lifelong requirement.

MINOR CONGENITAL HEART DEFECTS IN ADOLESCENCE

The most common congenital heart defect, the ventricular septal defect, often persists into adolescence. This small defect does not require surgical intervention in early childhood. It would be unusual for a ventricular septal defect to be discovered for the first time during adolescence. Such defects are usually followed by a pediatric cardiologist for some time. They generally have little hemodynamic consequence other than creating a fairly harsh and loud murmur. The significance of these defects centers around the need for endocarditis prophylaxis. The adolescent with a small ventricular septal defect should be allowed full activities, with no restrictions involving athletic endeavors.

Another common minor defect followed into adolescence is valvar pulmonic stenosis. Unlike aortic stenosis, which is a progressive lesion, pulmonic stenosis is usually stable from childhood to adult life. The teenager with pulmonic stenosis who has not required either surgical intervention or balloon angioplasty obviously has a minor obstruction, no more than a 30 to 40 mm gradient as measured by Doppler techniques. Other than endocarditis prophylaxis; there are no restrictions, and participation in all sports is permitted.

Minor valvular insufficiency, either secondary to congenital abnormalities of the mitral or aortic valve or secondary to a previous attack of rheumatic fever, is not uncommon in adolescents. Those with hemodynamically insignificant aortic insufficiency or mitral insufficiency need not be restricted. Endocarditis prophylaxis is mandatory.

CONGENITAL HEART DISEASE IN PREGNANT ADOLESCENTS

Corrective cardiac surgery for congenital heart disease, especially cyanotic congenital heart defects, has enabled more women with these defects to reach childbearing age. Physicians caring for the adolescent girl may be faced with a teenager who has congenital heart disease and becomes pregnant. Much of the data concerning pregnancies in females with congenital heart disease were collected by Whittemore et al at Yale (see Suggested Readings). More than 200 women and almost 500 pregnancies were studied. Overall the study showed an equal distribution of live births in patients who had operations and in those who did not. However, the presence of cyanotic congenital heart disease in the mother who did not have an operation resulted in a significantly decreased incidence of live births compared with mothers with other lesions or in whom cyanotic heart disease had been repaired. With the advent of surgical techniques to repair most forms of cyanotic heart disease, it would be rare today to have a teenager with unrepaired cyanotic congenital heart disease.

In other forms of congenital heart disease, such as left ventricular outflow tract obstruction and left-to-right shunts (ventricular septal defect or atrial septal defect), the proportion of live births appears to be related to the mother's cardiac function. Thus, it is anticipated in a teenager with minor congenital heart disease, such as mild left ventricular outflow tract obstruction or a small ventricular septal defect, that the pregnancy will have a good outcome. Excellent antepartum care must be given and prophylactic antibiotic therapy is mandatory prior to delivery.

Another issue that arises is the incidence of congenital heart disease in the offspring of mothers with congenital defects. There is an approximately 15% chance that the adolescent mother will give birth to an infant with congenital heart disease. In most instances the cardiac defect of the infant is similar to that of the mother.

An issue often raised by the adolescent with congenital heart disease is the use of contraception. It is generally agreed that the safest available means of contraception are the diaphragm and the condom. Owing to the risk of thromboembolism, birth control pills are generally avoided, although progestin-only pills have been used

and low-dose pills are probably safe in females who are not at significant risk for thromboembolic phenomenon. Intrauterine devices should not be used because of the risk of endocarditis in females with lesions such as ventricular septal defects and pulmonic or aortic stenosis.

POSTOPERATIVE CONGENITAL HEART DISEASE IN ADOLESCENCE

Although tetralogy of Fallot is the most common cyanotic defect in adolescence, it would be rare today to find an uncorrected "tet" in the U.S. adolescent population. Therefore, there is an increasing population of adolescents who have had corrective cardiac surgery performed in infancy and early childhood for tetralogy of Fallot. After repair these children are no longer cyanotic and in most instances are asymptomatic. The teenager who has had tetralogy of Fallot repair almost always has a residual murmur. These murmurs are usually secondary to mild residual pulmonic stenosis and pulmonic insufficiency. Murmurs of a ventricular septal defect may also be present. Endocarditis prophylaxis is mandatory in the adolescent with successful tetralogy of Fallot repair. Individuals who have an excellent hemodynamic repair as demonstrated by clinical examination, echocardiography, and exercise stress testing may participate in all activities. However, a small group of individuals, especially those in whom ventricular ectopy develops during exercise, require antiarrhythmia therapy and must have exercise limitations.

A second significant group of adolescents have undergone repair of transposition of the great vessels in infancy. Most common is the group who had an atrial switch–type procedure, such as Senning or Mustard. These adolescents are no longer cyanotic but do have a high incidence of arrhythmias; a small percentage of these teenagers require both antiarrhythmic and pacemaker therapy. Although many of these adolescents lead a relatively normal life, some have restrictions, particularly related to competitive sports. At present the preferred method of repair for transposition is the arterial switch procedure. Since this procedure is new, it will be some time before a substantial number of adolescents have had this procedure. It is hoped that because the switch procedure offers better anatomic repair, these adolescents will lead a completely normal life.

A growing population of adolescents have undergone a modified Fontan procedure for treatment of tricuspid atresia or other forms of complex cyanotic congenital heart disease. This procedure, which is in effect a right atrial to pulmonary artery connection, is a form of physiologic repair. Many youngsters who have had this surgery are asymptomatic but have some degree of exercise limitation because the right ventricle is absent.

The absence of the right ventricle limits cardiac output with exercise and in most instances prevents adolescents who have had this procedure from participating in the more strenuous forms of competitive athletic endeavors.

Lastly, a large group of adolescents have had repair of acyanotic lesions early in life; these include atrial septal defects, ventricular septal defects, and atrioventricular canal defects. In general, individuals who have had good hemodynamic repairs without significant residual defect lead normal lives and participate in all athletic endeavors.

Suggested Readings

Engle MA, Perloff JK: *Congenital heart disease after surgery: benefits, residua, sequelae,* New York, 1983, Yorke Medical Books.

Freed MD: Recreational and sports recommendations for the child with heart disease, *Pediatr Clin North Am* 31:1307-1320, 1984.

Rosenthal A: How to distinguish between innocent and pathologic murmurs in childhood, *Pediatr Clin North Am* 31:1229-1240, 1984.

Whittemore R, Hobbins JC, Engle MA: Pregnancy and its outcome in women with and without surgical treatment of congenital heart disease. In Engle MA, Perloff JK, editors: *Congenital heart disease after surgery: benefits, residua, sequelae,* New York, 1983, Yorke Medical Books, pp 362-388.

CHAPTER 36

Cardiac Infection and Inflammation: Rheumatic Fever, Endocarditis, and Myocarditis

•

Milton J. Reitman

ACUTE RHEUMATIC FEVER

Incidence

Acute rheumatic fever, thought to be on the decline since the 1960s, resurfaced in sporadic outbreaks in the 1980s. The resurgence of rheumatic fever extends from the East Coast to the West Coast. In one study at Columbia Presbyterian Medical Center, the incidence of rheumatic fever in 1986 was second only to its incidence in 1969, and the recurrence of rheumatic fever in the mid-1980s was also higher than at any time during the 20-year period from 1969 to 1988.[1]

Acute rheumatic fever is an inflammatory sequela to infection with group A beta-hemolytic streptococcal pharyngitis. The individuals most commonly affected are those in the age group of 5 to 17 years, with males and females affected in equal numbers. It has generally been reported that the risk of developing rheumatic fever after an untreated bout of group A beta-hemolytic streptococcal pharyngitis is 0.3%, but there are no recent data on this risk. General risk factors include crowding, poor medical care, poor nutrition, and a positive family history of the disease. Chorea, as a part of acute rheumatic fever, occurs most commonly in girls after puberty.

Diagnosis

Clinical manifestations of acute rheumatic fever follow the streptococcal pharyngitis by a latency period of 1 to 2 weeks. Patients develop a low-grade fever along with weakness, malaise, joint pain, occasional abdominal pain, and weight loss. Diagnosis is made on clinical grounds, since there are no specific pathognomonic tests for acute rheumatic fever. In 1944, Jones published criteria for guidelines in the diagnosis of acute rheumatic fever, and these have been modified several times. The most recent modification published by the American Heart Association was in 1984 (Table 36-1). The Jones criteria for rheumatic fever include the presence of two major, or one major and two minor, criteria. Either of these combinations is predictive of a high probability of acute rheumatic fever. The major criteria of migratory polyarthritis, carditis, chorea, erythema marginatum, and subcutaneous nodules are specific for rheumatic fever. The minor criteria, which are nonspecific but helpful,

> ### TABLE 36-1
> ### American Heart Association's Revised Jones Criteria, 1984
>
> | Major Criteria | Minor Criteria | Evidence for Streptococcal Infection |
> |---|---|---|
> | Carditis | History of rheumatic fever | Positive throat culture for group |
> | Arthritis | Arthralgia | A β-hemolytic streptococci |
> | Sydenham's chorea | Fever | Antibody evidence of streptococ- |
> | Erythema marginatum | Positive acute-phase reactants | cal infection (elevated or rising |
> | Subcutaneous nodules | (ESR, ZSR, CRP) | ASO, anti-DNase B, AH titer) |
> | | Prolonged PR interval | Recent evidence of scarlet fever |
>
> From American Heart Association. Jones criteria (revised) for guidance in the diagnosis of rheumatic fever, *Circulation* 69:204A-208A, 1984.
> *AH*, antiheart; *ASO*, antistreptolysin O; *CRP*, C-reactive protein; *ESR*, erythrocyte sedimentation rate; *ZSR*, zeta sedimentation ratio.

include arthralgia, fever, a history of rheumatic fever, the presence of positive acute-phase reactants (e.g., increased sedimentation rate), and prolongation of the PR interval. Evidence of streptococcal infection is also helpful in making the presumptive diagnosis of acute rheumatic fever.

Acute rheumatic fever is a self-limiting disease that usually responds to appropriate antiinflammatory therapy. In rare cases the disease may be severe and fulminating. It is important to note that the disease has a tendency to recur. Taranta[2] reported that a subsequent untreated "strep throat" in a patient with a history of rheumatic fever is associated with a 65% chance of a second bout of acute rheumatic fever. Second attacks tend to mimic the initial attack; therefore, if carditis was present in the initial attack, it is most likely to appear again during the subsequent attack.

Treatment

Modes of treatment for acute rheumatic fever are varied, but the most useful and effective of these include bed rest, salicylates, and adrenal corticosteroids. First, however, the streptococcal infection must be eliminated by an eradicating injection of penicillin G benzathine 1.2 million U administered intramuscularly. A 10-day course of an equally effective antibiotic may be used for adolescents allergic to penicillin.

Acute rheumatic fever with arthritis but without carditis is frequently extremely sensitive to aspirin therapy. Aspirin, 75 to 100 mg/kg/day, is given every 6 hours. The dose is adjusted to keep the serum salicylate level between 15 and 30 mg/dl. These high doses of salicylates are continued until the symptoms of arthritis are gone and the sedimentation rate has returned to normal. The salicylates then may be tapered over a period of several weeks. During salicylate therapy the patient should be kept at bed rest or in a quiet environment.

Patients with carditis and cardiomegaly but without congestive heart failure can be treated with either aspirin or steroids. Most cardiologists reserve the use of steroids for patients in whom carditis is symptomatic or in whom there is at least moderate mitral valve involvement.[3] Prednisone is given in immunosuppressive doses, 1 to 2 mg/kg/day every 6 hours. The steroids are continued until all signs of acute disease activity have been resolved, and then tapered over a 4- to 6-week period. In general, aspirin is added to the regimen as the steroids are decreased in order to maintain an adequate anti-inflammatory level and decrease the incidence of "rebounding" of the disease.[2]

Patients with carditis and congestive heart failure are treated with steroids and cardiovascular drugs. Prednisone, digitalis, diuretics, and oxygen are all used. It is crucial to start digitalis therapy gently because many patients are extremely sensitive to the drug; precautions taken to prevent digitalis intoxication, such as monitoring serum electrolyte levels, using an electrocardiographic (ECG) monitor, and monitoring serum digoxin levels, are all important.[3]

Prophylaxis

Recommendations for prophylaxis against recurrence of acute rheumatic fever have recently undergone major changes, since penicillin G benzathine given every 4 weeks does not appear to provide the level of protection previously thought. The present recommendations call for intramuscular injection of penicillin G benzathine every 3 weeks.[4] The World Health Organization[5] emphasizes that intramuscular penicillin G benzathine must be given this frequently to maintain the appropriate serum penicillin level. Because the intramuscular injection method is not popular among adolescent patients, however, the most common form of prophylaxis in this age group is oral penicillin, 250 mg twice daily. It is commonly accepted practice to continue the administration of intramuscular penicillin G benzathine until the patient is old enough and mature enough to understand the need for twice-daily penicillin. This decision is made on an individual basis.

If the clinician is satisfied that the patient is aware of the risks of not taking penicillin and if there is adequate family support, the change to oral penicillin is made. Prophylaxis should be continued at least until the patient reaches adulthood. For young adults in high-risk environments or occupations, such as the military or teaching, antibiotic prophylaxis should be continued. In those with residual rheumatic heart disease, penicillin prophylaxis is continued lifelong.

INFECTIVE ENDOCARDITIS

Etiology

The occurrence of infective endocarditis in a previously healthy adolescent without congenital or acquired cardiac disease is rare. Hospitalization of patients with infective endocarditis accounts for 1.35 per 1000 children admitted, with underlying congenital heart disease present in 80% of the adolescent admissions.[6] Of the remainder, rheumatic heart disease accounts for 5% of admissions, while in 15% of patients no previous heart disease is noted. Congenital heart diseases associated with infective endocarditis are those that result in the development of significant pressure gradients across the defect or the deformed valve. Thus, ventricular septal defects, aortic and pulmonary stenosis, patent ductus arteriosus, coarctation of the aorta, and tetralogy of Fallot are most frequently associated with infective endocarditis. Secundum atrial septal defects are rarely complicated by infective endocarditis.[7] When endocarditis is superimposed on rheumatic heart disease, the vegetations are usually seen on the atrial surface of the mitral valve or on the ventricular surface of the aortic valve.

Although virtually every bacterium and fungus has been implicated as the causative agent in infective endocarditis, the most common infecting organisms are *Staphylococcus viridans* (31%) and *S. aureus* (20%). In one study, *S. epidermidis* was the infecting microorganism in 5% of cases; its presence in a culture medium should therefore alert one to the possibility of it being the infecting microorganism.[8] Gram-negative bacteria, such as *Haemophilus* spp., *Pseudomonas aeruginosa, Klebsiella* spp., and *Escherichia coli,* account for an additional 5% of cases of infective endocarditis. In the otherwise healthy adolescent, fungal infections are rare: less than 1% of cases. Widespread drug use has led to an increased incidence of *S. aureus* and enterococci as the causative agents of infective endocarditis, and gram-negative bacilli and fungi are also noted with increasing frequency in such patients. The presence of pneumonia or meningitis from *Streptococcus pneumoniae* may provide strong evidence for infective endocarditis having been caused by this organism. In drug abusers, left- and right-sided lesions occur in approximately equal frequency because of the common occurrence of tricuspid valve staphylococcal infections.[9]

Clinical Course

The clinical course of infective endocarditis is dependent on the invading organism, the host reaction, and the nature and severity of the underlying heart disease. In the era before antibiotics, infective endocarditis from *S. viridans* resulted in early findings of fever and anemia, with splenomegaly, skin manifestations (Janeway lesions, Osler's nodes, splinter hemorrhages), and arterial embolization occurring as late manifestations. When the disease was caused by *S. aureus* or gram-negative bacilli, the clinical course was always a rapid downhill spiral. The introduction of antibiotics has changed the "unnatural history" of this disease. Today most patients initially do not appear very ill, usually presenting with only unexplained fever and malaise. Pulmonary embolization and neurologic complications may be as high as 8%, however, and additional nonspecific symptoms include anorexia and weight loss, leukocytosis, anemia, and hematuria. An elevated erythrocyte sedimentation rate is an almost universal finding.

Treatment

The goal of antibiotic therapy is to obtain serum antibiotic levels that are greater than the mean bactericidal concentration of the infecting organism.[10] This requires that blood culture levels greater than the mean bactericidal concentration be obtained before instituting therapy. Positive blood cultures are generally reported in 80% to 85% of patients with infective endocarditis. The prognosis for this disorder depends on the type of organism, the duration of the illness before effective therapy is begun, and whether the infecting organism has attacked a native valve or a prosthetic valve. Endocarditis associated with a native valve is much more likely to be cured with antibiotics than is disease involving a prosthetic valve.

Two-dimensional echocardiography can detect valvular vegetations at least 2 mm in diameter. One 1990 study demonstrated that the sensitivity of echocardiograms varies between 40% and 100%.[11] However, the ability to identify vegetations by echocardiography did not alter the prognosis in this series.

Prophylaxis

The recommended standard prophylactic regimen for infective endocarditis has undergone remarkable changes in the past several years. In 1990 the American Heart Association and the American Dental Association finalized recommendations for antibiotic prophylaxis.[12] The standard regimen is 3 g amoxicillin to be given orally before dental and surgical procedures and 1.5 g amoxicillin 6 hours after the initial dose. In small adolescents the initial dose should be calculated as 50 mg/kg of body weight and one half of that amount thereafter. In patients allergic to penicillin, erythromycin ethyl succinate (800 mg) or erythromycin stearate (1.0 g) is given orally 2 hours before the procedure and one half of the initial dose is given 6 hours later. Alternatively, clindamycin (300 mg) may be given orally 1 hour before the procedure and 150 mg 6 hours after the initial dose. Specific cardiac conditions and specific dental and surgical procedures that require prophylaxis have been determined (Box 36-1).

Future Changes

In the future, the prevalence of intravenous drug use among adolescents and the resultant increase in AIDS in this population are likely to change the range of infecting organisms responsible for infective endocarditis, and opportunistic organisms and staphylococci are likely to play more important roles in this disease.

MYOCARDITIS

Etiology

Myocarditis is an inflammatory process of the walls of the heart. The causes of this condition include infectious agents, physical agents, chemicals, drugs, and radiation.[13]

BOX 36-1
Endocarditis Prophylaxis

CARDIAC CONDITIONS IN WHICH ENDOCARDITIS PROPHYLAXIS IS RECOMMENDED
Prosthetic cardiac valves, including bioprosthetic and homograft valves
Previous bacterial endocarditis, even in the absence of heart disease
Most congenital cardiac malformations
Rheumatic and other acquired valvular dysfunction, even after valvular surgery
Hypertrophic cardiomyopathy
Mitral valve prolapse with valvular regurgitation

CARDIAC CONDITIONS IN WHICH ENDOCARDITIS PROPHYLAXIS IS NOT RECOMMENDED
Isolated secundum atrial septal defect
Surgical repair without residua beyond 6 months of secundum atrial septal defect, ventricular septal defect, or patent ductus arteriosus
Previous coronary artery bypass graft surgery
Mitral valve prolapse without valvular regurgitation
Physiologic, functional, or innocent heart murmurs
Previous Kawasaki's disease without valvular dysfunction
Previous rheumatic fever without valvular dysfunction
Cardiac pacemakers and implanted defibrillators

DENTAL AND SURGICAL PROCEDURES IN WHICH ENDOCARDITIS PROPHYLAXIS IS RECOMMENDED
Dental procedures known to induce gingival or mucosal bleeding, including professional cleaning
Tonsillectomy and/or adenoidectomy
Surgical operations that involve intestinal or respiratory mucosa

Bronchoscopy with a rigid bronchoscope
Sclerotherapy for esophageal varices
Esophageal dilation
Gallbladder surgery
Cystoscopy
Urethral dilation
Urethral catheterization if urinary tract infection is present
Prostatic surgery
Incision and drainage of infected tissue
Vaginal hysterectomy
Vaginal delivery in the presence of infection

DENTAL AND SURGICAL PROCEDURES IN WHICH ENDOCARDITIS PROPHYLAXIS IS NOT RECOMMENDED
Dental procedures not likely to induce gingival bleeding, such as simple adjustment of orthodontic appliances or fillings above the gum line
Injection of local intraoral anesthetic (except intraligamentary injections)
Shedding of primary teeth
Tympanostomy tube insertion
Endotracheal intubation
Bronchoscopy with a flexible bronchoscope, with or without biopsy
Cardiac catheterization
Endoscopy with or without gastrointestinal biopsy
Cesarean section
In the absence of infection: urethral catheterization, dilation and curettage, uncomplicated vaginal delivery, therapeutic abortion, sterilization procedures, or insertion or removal of intrauterine devices

From Dajani AS, Bisno AL, Chung KJ, et al: Prevention of bacterial endocarditis, *JAMA* 264:2919-2922, 1990. Copyright © 1990 American Medical Association.

The actual incidence of myocarditis is not known, but it may vary with age, sex, and season of the year. Myocarditis has been found at autopsy in 17% to 21% of adolescents and young adults who have died suddenly.[14] Diphtheria and rheumatic fever were considered to be the two main causes of myocarditis until it was demonstrated that each disease was associated with only about 10% of total cases.[15] It is now commonly believed that many cases of myocarditis follow a viral infection, but in most clinical cases confirmation of a definite viral cause remains difficult. Viruses seldom can be detected in the myocardium even when the course of the disease strongly suggests a viral origin.[16]

A wide variety of organisms have been linked to myocarditis, including viruses, bacteria, protozoa, rickettsiae, and fungi. The most common viruses are coxsackie A and B, echovirus, influenza A and B, and mumps virus. DNA viruses such as Epstein-Barr and varicella zoster have been implicated. The most common virus implicated in acute myocarditis is coxsackie B. However, the link between the virus and myocarditis remains circumstantial, since the virus has rarely been isolated from the myocardium. In addition, myocarditis often remains undiagnosed until scarring has occurred and the patient has been diagnosed as having cardiomyopathy. Nevertheless, the development of dilated cardiomyopathy after a viral infection seems to be more than coincidental.

Clinical Features and Diagnosis

The clinical features of myocarditis are varied and depend on the severity of myocardial involvement. During the acute phase a flulike syndrome that includes fever, pharyngitis, lymphadenopathy, myalgia, and gastrointestinal complaints may occur. The most common cardiac symptom is pericardial pain, which is most often associated with a pericardial friction rub. In more severe cases, cardiac manifestations include signs and symptoms of congestive heart failure, such as a third heart sound, a gallop, rales, jugular venous distention, or peripheral edema. Pericardial effusion, syncope, and ischemic chest pain also may occur. Electrocardiographic changes, including ST-segment elevation, T-wave flattening, inversion in Q waves, and prolongation of the QT interval, all have been described. Complete atrioventricular block is common and ventricular ectopy may occur.

The clinical diagnosis of myocarditis must be confirmed by biopsy. A 1988 study of the value of endomyocardial biopsy showed a positive correlation of only 50% between biopsy findings and clinical suspicion.[17] The variability in the incidence of histologically proved myocarditis depends on the time at which the biopsy is performed (optimally when lymphocytic infiltration and myocyte damage are present); also, a sufficient number of tissue samples must be taken to avoid sampling error. An endomyocardial biopsy performed within 2 weeks of (occasionally even 1 month after) the onset of symptoms may reveal inflammatory changes in the myocardium that are specific to myocarditis. However, attribution of a myocardial lesion to the identified virus still remains circumstantial. A fourfold increase in the titer of virus-neutralizing/complement-fixing or hemagglutination-inhibiting antibodies in paired sera taken at least 2 weeks apart during the course of the disease indicates a recent infection. In light of the clinical findings, a presumptive diagnosis of myocarditis may be made if such an increase occurs.

In the differential diagnosis of acute viral myocarditis, care must be taken to rule out other causes of myocardial inflammation.[18] Street drugs such as cocaine are known to cause coronary artery spasm and also have been implicated in histologic changes consistent with acute myocarditis. Heavy-metal poisoning and alcohol can also cause a cardiomyopathy indistinguishable from the late stages of viral myocarditis (Box 36-2).

BOX 36-2
Etiology of Myocarditis

INFECTIOUS AGENTS
Viral: coxsackievirus (especially group B), echovirus, poliovirus, mumps
Bacterial: diphtheria, tuberculosis, *Salmonella typhi* (typhoid fever), streptococcus (rheumatic fever or direct streptococcal myocarditis), meningococcus
Spirochetal: Lyme disease
Rickettsial
Chlamydial
Fungal: candidiasis, aspergillosis, histoplasmosis
Protozoan: *Trypanosoma cruzi* (Chagas' disease), African trypanosomiasis (sleeping sickness), malaria, toxoplasmosis, amebiasis
Metazoan: schistosomiasis, trichinosis, ascariasis, cysticercosis, echinococcosis

MISCELLANEOUS CAUSES
Metal poisoning: lead, mercury, arsenic
Antineoplastic agents
Antiparasitic agents: emetine, chloroquine, antimony compounds
Psychotropic drugs: phenothiazines, lithium
Animal toxins: snake bite; wasp, spider, scorpion stings
Carbon monoxide
Phosphorus

PHYSICAL AGENTS
Radiation, hypothermia, heat stroke

Treatment and Prognosis

Therapy for acute viral myocarditis has not been well established. Immunosuppression may be beneficial in reducing myocardial inflammation and preventing irreversible myocardial damage.[19] Conventional therapy for congestive heart failure and appropriate antiarrhythmic therapy also are indicated.

The long-term outlook for the patient who has recovered from acute myocarditis depends on the subsequent course of the disease. Patients who show evidence of cardiomyopathy with potential life-threatening arrhythmias are at a 20% risk for sudden cardiac death. Cardiac transplantation is a possibility for patients with refractory congestive heart failure. However, such patients must be assessed in regard to their receptiveness to significant and permanent changes in life style. A multidisciplinary approach to this problem—one that involves the cardiologist and the cardiac surgeon as well as social workers and psychiatrists—is mandatory.

References

1. Griffiths SP, Gersony WM: Acute rheumatic fever in New York City (1969 to 1988): a comparative study of two decades, *J Pediatr* 116:882-887, 1990.
2. Taranta A: Streptococcology for the non-streptococcologist, *Minn Med* 58:585-596, 1975.
3. Ruttenberg HD: Acute rheumatic fever in the 1980s, *Pediatrician* 13:180-188, 1986.
4. Kaplan EL, Berrios X, Speth J, Siefferman T, Guzman B, Quesny F: Pharmacokinetics of benzathine penicillin G: serum levels during the 28 days after intramuscular injection of 1,200,000 units, *J Pediatr* 115:146-150, 1989.
5. World Health Organization Study Group: *Rheumatic fever and rheumatic heart disease.* WHO Technical Report Series No. 764, Geneva, 1988, World Health Organization.
6. Parras F, Bouza E, Romero J, Buzon L, Quero M, Brito J, Vellibre D: Infectious endocarditis in children, *Pediatr Cardiol* 11:77-81, 1990.
7. Blumenthal S: Infective endocarditis. In Moss AJ, Adams FH, Emmanouilides GC, editors: *Heart disease in infants, children and adolescents,* Baltimore, 1977, Williams & Wilkins; p 552.
8. Mansur AJ, Grinberg M, Bellotti G, Jatene A, Pileggi F: Infective endocarditis in the 1980s: experience at a heart hospital, *Clin Cardiol* 13:623-630, 1990.
9. Truxal BA, Murphy RD, Checton JB: *Staphylococcus aureus*–endocarditis in a previously healthy adolescent, *J Adolesc Health Care* 9:325-330, 1988.
10. Weinstein MP: Multicenter collaborative evaluation of a standardized serum bactericidal test as a prognostic indicator in infective endocarditis, *Am J Med* 78:262-269, 1985.
11. Coutlee F, Carceller A, Deschamps L, Kratz C, Lapointe J, Davignon A: The evolving pattern of pediatric endocarditis from 1960 to 1985, *Cardiovasc Med* 6:164-170, 1990.
12. Dajani AS, Bisno AL, Chung KJ, et al: Prevention of bacterial endocarditis, *JAMA* 264:2919-2922, 1990.
13. Rezkalla S, Koner RA: Myocarditis and cardiomyopathy, *Cardiovasc Rev Rep* 48:77, 1991.
14. Kereiakes DJ, Parmley WE: Myocarditis and cardiomyopathy, *Am Heart J* 108:1318-1326, 1984.
15. Gore I, Saphir O: Myocarditis: a classification of 1402 cases, *Am Heart J* 34:827-830, 1947.
16. O'Connell JB, Robinson JA, Gunnar RM, Scanlon PJ: Clinical aspects of virus/immune myocarditis, *Heart Vessels* 1 (suppl 1): 102-106, 1985.
17. Leatherbury L, Chandra R, Shapiro S, Perry L: Value of endomyocardial biopsy in infants, children and adolescents with dilated or hypertrophic cardiomyopathy and myocarditis, *J Am Coll Cardiol* 12:1547-1554, 1988.
18. Billingham ME: The diagnostic criteria of myocarditis by endomyocardial biopsy, *Heart Vessels* 1:133-137, 1985.
19. Mason JW, Billingham ME, Ricci DR: Treatment of acute inflammatory myocarditis assisted by endomyocardial biopsy, *Am J Cardiol* 45:1037-1044, 1980.

CHAPTER 37

Mitral Valve Prolapse

•

Russell J. Schiff

Mitral valve prolapse has been described as the most frequently diagnosed valvular cardiac abnormality in the United States, with prevalence estimates varying from 2% to more than 15%.[1-10] There has been considerable controversy and interest in this diagnosis over the past quarter century because of the lack of unanimity in diagnostic criteria and the association of mitral valve prolapse with cardiac arrhythmias, cerebral embolism, endocarditis, mitral regurgitation, and sudden death. Despite the accumulation of considerable information during that time, much of our knowledge remains incomplete, contradictory, and controversial.[11,12] Also, although abundant information is available regarding adult patients with mitral valve prolapse, there is a paucity of well-controlled studies of children and adolescents with this abnormality.

HISTORY

The midsystolic click and the apical systolic murmur are the auscultatory hallmarks of mitral valve prolapse, but this association was not recognized until the 1960s. In 1913 Gallavardin[13] suggested that pleuropericardial adhesions found at autopsy in four patients were the probable cause of midsystolic clicks and systolic murmurs of variable length. This belief was widely accepted by others.[14,15] It was not until a report by Reid[16] was published in 1961, however, that the association of midsystolic clicks and late systolic murmurs with the mitral apparatus was documented by phonocardiography.

In 1963 Barlow et al.[17] observed mitral valve prolapse with mitral regurgitation on left ventricular angiography in patients with late systolic murmurs on phonocardiography. Five years later Barlow et al[18] first proposed a clinical syndrome associated with mitral valve prolapse.

DIAGNOSTIC CONSIDERATIONS

For many years there was a lack of agreement on diagnostic standards for mitral valve prolapse. In an effort to resolve the dilemma posed by the gray zone between normal and abnormal, it was proposed that the term *mitral valve prolapse* be restricted to a condition in which the leaflet edges fail to appose (i.e., disruption of leaflet edge coaptation).[19] The normal mitral valve bows or billows slightly in a superior and posterior systolic motion into the left atrium. A floppy mitral valve has abnormal, billowing, voluminous leaflets with elongated chordae tendineae, and mitral valve prolapse is usually present. A flail mitral valve is caused by ruptured or grossly

---

BOX 37-1
Guidelines for Diagnosis of Mitral Valve Prolapse

MAJOR CRITERIA
AUSCULTATION
Midsystolic to late systolic clicks and late systolic
   murmur or "whoop" alone or in combination
   at cardiac apex
TWO-DIMENSIONAL ECHOCARDIOGRAM
Marked superior systolic displacement of mitral
   leaflets with coaptation point at or superior to
   annular plane
Mild to moderate superior systolic displacement of
   mitral leaflets with
     Chordal rupture
     Doppler mitral regurgitation
     Annular dilation
ECHOCARDIOGRAM PLUS AUSCULTATION
Mild to moderate superior systolic displacement of
   mitral leaflets with
     Prominent midsystolic to late systolic clicks at
      cardiac apex
     Apical late systolic or holosystolic murmur in
      young patient
     Late systolic whoop

MINOR CRITERIA
AUSCULTATION
Loud first heart sound with apical holosystolic
   murmur
TWO-DIMENSIONAL ECHOCARDIOGRAM
Isolated mild to moderate superior systolic dis-
   placement of posterior mitral leaflet

Moderate superior systolic displacement of both
mitral leaflets
ECHOCARDIOGRAM PLUS HISTORY
Mild to moderate superior systolic displacement of
   mitral leaflets with
     Focal neurologic attacks or amaurosis fugax in
      young patient
     First-degree relatives with major criteria

NONSPECIFIC FINDINGS
SYMPTOMS
"Atypical" chest pain, dyspnea, fatigue, lassitude,
   giddiness, dizziness, syncope
Psychological disturbances
PHYSICAL APPEARANCE
Thoracic bony abnormalities
Hypomastia
ELECTROCARDIOGRAM
T-wave inversions in inferior limb leads or lateral
   precordial leads
Premature ventricular beats at rest, with exercise,
   or on ambulatory ECG
Supraventricular tachycardia
X-RAY EXAMINATION
Scoliosis, pectus excavatum or pectus carinatum,
   or loss of thoracic kyphosis
TWO-DIMENSIONAL ECHOCARDIOGRAM
Mild superior systolic displacement of anterior or
   anterior and posterior mitral leaflets

Modified from Perloff JK, Child JS: Clinical and epidemiologic issues in mitral valve prolapse: overview and perspective, *Am Heart J* 113:1324-1332, 1987.

elongated chordae tendineae with significant mitral regurgitation.

In 1986 Perloff et al[20] established guidelines for the clinical diagnosis of pathologic mitral valve prolapse, using the Jones criteria for acute rheumatic fever as a model (Box 37-1). The objective was to provide clinicians with a more secure basis of judgment so that healthy, asymptomatic persons would not be assigned an inappropriate diagnosis of heart disease. As proposed by Perloff, (1) patients with one or more major criteria can be considered to have mitral valve prolapse beyond reasonable doubt; (2) patients with minor criteria have evidence of possible prolapse and should be advised to undergo periodic reevaluation but not endocarditis prophylaxis; and (3) those with other nonspecific features alone are not likely to have mitral valve prolapse, and they may require evaluation for determination of other possible diagnoses.

The etiologic complex of mitral valve prolapse may be either primary (due to an abnormality of the valve itself) or secondary (in association with a systemic connective tissue disorder, skeletal abnormalities involving a change in left ventricular shape, or cardiac defects involving a reduction of left ventricular cavity size)[21] (Box 37-2).

BOX 37-2
Conditions Associated with Mitral Valve Prolapse

CARDIAC DEFECTS (CONGENITAL HEART DISEASE)
Atrial septal defect
Atrial septal aneurysm
Ventricular septal defect
Patent ductus arteriosus
Tetralogy of Fallot
Membranous subaortic stenosis
Aortic valve prolapse
Bicuspid aortic valve
Valsalva's sinus aneurysm
Coarctation
Tricuspid valve prolapse
Ebstein's anomaly of tricuspid valve
Pulmonary stenosis
Peripheral pulmonary artery stenosis
Idiopathic dilation of pulmonary artery
Anomalous origin of left coronary artery from pulmonary artery
Coronary artery fistulas
Coronary ectasia
Absence of left pericardium
OTHER CONDITIONS
Cardiomyopathy
Idiopathic hypertrophic cardiomyopathy
Endomyocardial fibroelastosis
Left atrial myxoma
Left ventricular aneurysm
Atherosclerotic coronary artery disease
CONDUCTION ABNORMALITIES
Wolff-Parkinson-White syndrome
Lown-Ganong-Levine syndrome
Congenital prolonged QT syndrome
CONNECTIVE TISSUE DISEASES
Marfan's syndrome
Ehlers-Danlos syndrome
Pseudoxanthoma elasticum
Osteogenesis imperfecta
Rheumatoid arthritis

Raynaud's disease
Mixed connective tissue disease
ENDOCRINE DISORDERS
Hyperthyroidism
Chronic thyroiditis
HEMATOLOGIC DISEASES
Sickle cell disease
von Willebrand's syndrome
Platelet hypercoagulability
GENETIC ABNORMALITIES
Turner's syndrome
Noonan's syndrome
Down syndrome
Duchenne's dystrophy and Berger X-linked muscular dystrophy
Myotonic dystrophy
Klinefelter's syndrome
Klippel-Feil syndrome
Fragile X syndrome
THORACIC SPINE AND CHEST WALL ABNORMALITIES
Pectus excavatum
Straight back syndrome
Hypomastia (in women)
Scoliosis
COLLAGEN VASCULAR DISEASE
Polyarteritis nodosa
Kawasaki's syndrome
Rheumatic fever
Systemic lupus erythematosus
METABOLIC DISEASES
Hunter's syndrome
Hurler's syndrome
Homocystinuria
PULMONARY DISORDERS
Pulmonary emphysema
Primary pulmonary hypertension

From Garson A, Bricker JT, McNamara DG: *The science and practice of pediatric cardiology,* Philadelphia, 1990, Lea & Febiger, pp 1973-1986. Reproduced with permission.

Since some of the associated conditions are very common in the general population, with some diseases the question has been raised about whether this association occurs by chance or is a true association.

The normal mitral valve has three histologic layers: the atrialis (facing the atrium), the spongiosa (the middle fibromucoid layer), and the fibrosa (a continuous layer on the ventricular side where the chordae tendineae insert). Microscopic studies in adults with mitral valve prolapse have shown an increase in the mucopolysaccharides of the spongiosa layer with encroachment, disruption, and consequent weakening of the fibrosa.

The familial occurrence of mitral valve prolapse, even without evidence of a generalized connective tissue disorder, has suggested an autosomal dominant pattern with variable expression. The true incidence of this abnormality is unknown at this time because of the varied criteria that have been used in the literature. In an auscultatory survey of 12,050 children aged 2 to 18 years in South Africa, a 1.4% incidence of mitral valve prolapse (based on a midsystolic click with or without a systolic murmur) was noted, with a 1.9:1.0 female-to-male ratio.[22] A study of 3100 children aged 1 month to 18 years (average age, 8 years, 2 months) in California found a 4.97% incidence of clinical auscultatory mitral valve prolapse.[8] In a study of 193 clinically normal children, Warth et al[9] clearly demonstrated the deficiencies of earlier commonly used two-dimensional echocardiographic criteria for mitral valve prolapse. In several studies the overall prevalence by these criteria was 13% (range, 1.3% in 78 children up to 2 years of age to 34.5% in 19 children 10 to 18 years of age). This high prevalence in prescreened "normal" children suggested the need to redefine echocardiographic criteria for mitral valve prolapse. When more stringent criteria were used, overall prevalence of abnormal mitral valve motion detected by Warth et al[9] was 1.5%.

CLINICAL FEATURES

Most children and adolescents with mitral valve prolapse are asymptomatic. The condition is detected because of a click or murmur found on a routine physical examination or during a febrile illness. In Greenwood's study,[8] only 2% of patients in the series had significant symptoms. The Framingham study found no difference in the prevalence of symptoms (i.e., chest pain, dyspnea, or syncope) between the general population and a group with mitral valve prolapse.[23] It is believed that the higher incidence of symptoms in patients with mitral valve prolapse in previous studies was related to inadequate control groups and an ascertainment bias. The most common complaints in symptomatic patients have been atypical chest pain, palpitations, syncope or near-syncope, dyspnea without orthopnea, decreased exercise tolerance, fatigue, and anxiety. As a rule, the chest pain reported by patients with mitral valve prolapse is not typical for any specific complaint and is rarely reproducible on exercise testing. Palpitations occur commonly, but symptoms are often not associated with arrhythmic events noted through 24-hour Holter monitoring. Dyspnea and fatigue are almost always unrelated to myocardial function unless there is significant mitral regurgitation. Near-syncope and syncope, which are rare events, usually are more related to abnormalities of parasympathetic tone. Arfken et al,[24] in a study of 813 children 9 to 14 years of age, found no difference in the level of anxiety between those with mitral valve prolapse and the control group.

The clinical "syndrome of mitral valve prolapse" in adults is characterized by a constellation of auscultatory findings, thoracic wall abnormalities (tall slender habitus, pectus excavatum, pectus carinatum, scoliosis, and kyphosis), low body weight, low blood pressure, and palpitations.[1] These findings are less common in children and adolescents. A highly arched palate, increased joint laxity, or abnormal dermatoglyphic patterns may be present.

The click associated with mitral valve prolapse is best heard at the left sternal border and is typically described as midsystolic or nonejection. However, during systole it may vary anywhere from the first to the second heart sound, and multiple clicks may be present. The timing of the click during the cardiac cycle can be changed by postural and pharmacologic maneuvers (Box 37-3). The click has been thought to originate from sudden prolapsing of the valve leaflets or from tensing of the chordae tendineae.

The murmur of mitral valve prolapse is usually, but not always, preceded by the click and is classically late systolic in timing. Like the click, the murmur varies in timing, intensity, and duration in response to postural and

---

BOX 37-3
"Click" of Mitral Valve Prolapse

EARLIER CLICK/LOUDER, LONGER MURMUR	*LATER CLICK/SOFTER, SHORTER MURMUR*
Decreased left ventricular size, decreased preload or afterload	Increased left ventricular size, increased preload or afterload
Position changes:	Position changes:
• Supine to sitting	• Sitting to supine
• Sitting to standing	• Standing to supine
• Squatting to standing	• Standing to squatting
Tachycardia	Passive leg raising
Amyl nitrite	Phenylephrine
Valsalva maneuver	

pharmacologic maneuvers. The length of the murmur usually corresponds to the severity of mitral regurgitation. It is best heard at the apex with radiation to the left axilla. Occasionally the murmur has been described to have a honking or "whooping" character. The murmur of mitral valve prolapse may be confused with the murmur of obstructive hypertrophic cardiomyopathy because both increase in intensity and duration with standing and decrease with squatting. Mitral valve prolapse cannot be ruled out in any patient until the postural interventions necessary to elicit mitral valve prolapse have been performed.

RADIOLOGIC EXAMINATION

Most patients with mitral valve prolapse have normal cardiac size and contour on chest x-ray examinations unless moderate to severe mitral regurgitation is present (with consequent left atrial and left ventricular enlargement, plus increased pulmonary venous markings). Thoracic skeletal abnormalities such as scoliosis, straight back syndrome, and pectus excavatum may be present.

ELECTROCARDIOGRAPHY

Most children with mitral valve prolapse have a normal electrocardiogram (ECG) reading. However, three types of abnormalities may be observed: abnormalities of rhythm, conduction, or repolarization. Symptomatic cardiac dysrhythmia and conduction disturbances are fairly common (up to a 46% incidence), but serious, high-grade ventricular ectopy (multiform premature ventricular contractions [PVCs], couplets, or ventricular tachycardia) or supraventricular tachycardia is infrequent (4% to 11%) on ambulatory ECG or treadmill exercise.[8,25,26] In the Framingham study, supraventricular tachycardia and complex or frequent PVCs were so common in subjects without mitral valve prolapse that a significant difference from the subjects with mitral valve prolapse was not demonstrated.[27]

Repolarization abnormalities include prolongation of the QT interval and T-wave inversion in the inferolateral leads (II, III, aV_F, V_4 to V_6). Prolongation of the QT interval and prominent U waves have been described in children with mitral valve prolapse.[28] The prevalence of a prolonged QT interval in children and adolescents with mitral valve prolapse varies from 13% to 31%. A prolonged QT interval may be important because of its link with ventricular arrhythmias and sudden death. The Framingham study[27] did not find any differences in the prevalence of a prolonged QT interval in patients with or without echocardiographic mitral valve prolapse. The

incidence of T-wave inversions ranges from 7% to 48%. ST-segment changes are usually absent at rest, are accentuated on standing, and may be induced during exercise. In adults, ST-segment depression occurs early or in the middle of exercise and has a tendency for normalization toward peak exercise.

ECHOCARDIOGRAPHY

The initial diagnosis of mitral valve prolapse was performed with M-mode echocardiography in 1970. This modality was very imprecise, frequently producing false-positive and false-negative results because the M-mode echocardiogram is not spatially oriented and cannot define spatial relationships between the mitral leaflets and the valve annulus. The sensitivity and specificity of mitral valve prolapse improved with the introduction of two-dimensional M-mode echocardiography. Since this type of echocardiography allowed simultaneous visualization of both the valve leaflet and the annulus position from multiple angles, it became the noninvasive modality of choice. With this method the initial definition of mitral valve prolapse was superior systolic motion of the valve leaflets beyond the valve annulus. However, on the basis of these criteria, up to 13% of normal children would be diagnosed as having mitral valve prolapse, and 35% would be so diagnosed in the 10- to 18-year age group.[9] With more stringent criteria, superior systolic motion can be found in only 1.5% of these children from the parasternal long-axis view (Fig. 37-1).

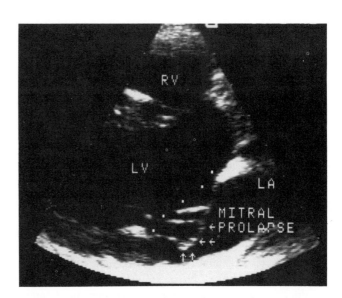

Fig. 37-1. Parasternal long-axis view demonstrating prolapse of both mitral leaflets *(arrows)*. The plane of the mitral annulus is defined by the dotted line. *RV,* right ventricle; *LV,* left ventricle; *AO,* aorta; *LA,* left atrium.

The frequently observed discrepancy between leaflet annular relationships in intersecting views has suggested an underlying geometric property of the mitral apparatus that would produce the appearance of prolapse in one view without actual leaflet distortion. Levine et al[29] found that the mitral annulus had a nonplanar, saddle-shaped configuration rather than the previously assumed euclidean plane. A subsequent study in adults found that patients with leaflet displacement limited to the four-chamber view are no more likely to have associated abnormalities than are patients without displacement in any view, and this implies that these are normal geometric findings without pathologic significance.[30] Instead, restricting the diagnosis of mitral valve prolapse to definite prolapse in at least two echocardiographic planes, or to the parasternal long-axis view with mitral regurgitation demonstrated by Doppler echocardiography, eliminates a large segment of the normal population from being diagnosed incorrectly. Physicians should be reluctant to diagnose mitral valve prolapse on the basis of mild echocardiographic findings (mild leaflet billowing and trace regurgitation by color flow Doppler) in the absence of auscultatory criteria.[31]

CLINICAL COURSE

The prognosis for isolated mitral valve prolapse in adolescence is excellent, and it is a relatively benign condition in most children and adolescents. Rare complications include infective endocarditis, arrhythmias, sudden death, progressive mitral regurgitation, neurologic events, and secondary underlying systemic connective tissue disorders.

In adult studies the risk of endocarditis ranges from 5% to 8%. The group at highest risk includes those with mitral regurgitation and thickened or redundant valve leaflets. Prophylaxis is currently not recommended in those individuals with mitral valve prolapse who do not have thick or redundant leaflets and do not exhibit mitral regurgitation.[32]

In both adults and children with mitral valve prolapse, there is poor correlation between symptoms and arrhythmias. Ambulatory Holter or transtelephonic monitoring can be used to help identify serious arrhythmias.

Sudden death is an extremely rare complication of mitral valve prolapse and is generally thought to be secondary to a lethal arrhythmia. Only a few cases of sudden death have been reported in those under 20 years of age.[12,33] Potential risk factors include complex ventricular arrhythmias, prolonged QT interval, repolarization abnormalities, a history of syncope, or a family history of sudden death. Postmortem studies have shown associated involvement of the conduction system, which could explain sudden death.[34] Many physicians consider that this complication is so rare that it should not be mentioned to the patient or the family for fear of arousing undue anxiety.

Cerebrovascular accidents and brain abscesses have been rare occurrences in children or adolescents with mitral valve prolapse. Studies in adults have shown an association with transient ischemic attacks, acute hemiplegia, cerebellar infarcts, amaurosis fugax, and retinal arteriolar occlusions. Most patients recover from these episodes.

Pregnancy and childbirth are generally safe for women with mitral valve prolapse. In infants born to mothers with mitral valve prolapse, there has not been an increased incidence of congenital heart disease.

MANAGEMENT

Evaluation of adolescents for mitral valve prolapse requires a complete history and physical examination. A resting ECG is recommended to detect evidence of arrhythmias, a prolonged QT interval, and ST-T wave changes. In cases in which the physical findings are positive or equivocal, an echocardiogram is recommended. Ambulatory Holter monitoring or exercise testing is indicated in patients with a history of palpitation, syncope, arrhythmias; a family history of sudden death; or significant mitral regurgitation.

The adolescent with a normal physical examination who has only echocardiographic evidence of mitral valve prolapse without a dysplastic mitral valve does not have pathologic mitral valve prolapse and does not require follow-up by a cardiologist. The typical asymptomatic teenager with uncomplicated mitral valve prolapse requires infrequent cardiac evaluation to ensure that symptoms and physical findings are not changing. These patients need reassurance of the benign nature of mitral valve prolapse, and follow-up with their primary care physicians. The teenager with mitral valve prolapse and valvar regurgitation requires yearly evaluation as well as reinforcement regarding the necessity for prophylaxis against endocarditis.

Ambulatory ECG monitoring is performed in patients who are symptomatic (syncope or palpitations), or if ectopy or a prolonged QT interval is seen on routine electrocardiography.

Criteria for treatment of ventricular arrhythmias in these patients are the same as for other teenagers with ventricular arrhythmias. Patients with isolated uniform PVCs that are eliminated through exercise do not require treatment. Complex ventricular arrhythmias are usually first treated with beta blockers.

SPORTS

A permissive attitude toward participation in all competitive sports is warranted in most patients with mitral valve prolapse on the basis of all evidence available at the present time. This attitude should be modified in patients with any of the following criteria:

1. A history of syncope, documented to be arrhythmogenic in origin
2. A family history of sudden death associated with mitral valve prolapse
3. Repetitive forms of sustained and nonsustained supraventricular tachyarrhythmias or complex ventricular arrhythmias, particularly if exaggerated by exercise
4. Moderate to marked mitral regurgitation
5. A previous embolic event
6. Marfan's syndrome

Athletes with mitral valve prolapse and any of the above criteria can participate in low-intensity competitive sports only. As classified by the American College of Cardiology and American College of Sports Medicine, these include the low-dynamic, low-static, class IA sports of billiards, bowling, cricket, curling, golf, and riflery.[39-41]

PSYCHIATRIC FACTORS

An association between mitral valve prolapse and anxiety disorders, especially panic attacks, has been suggested, but never proved, in the medical and psychiatric literature.[35-37] This association has been evaluated in studies of patients with mitral valve prolapse as well as in studies of those with anxiety disorders; the results of both types of studies showed an inconsistent relationship. Sampling bias, inadequate control groups, and varying diagnostic criteria for mitral valve prolapse are believed to account for the difficulties in proving or disproving the possible association. In some studies of patients with panic disorders, mitral valve prolapse has been reported in up to 25% to 35%, whereas in other studies much lower frequencies have been reported. Most studies of patients with mitral valve prolapse have failed to demonstrate an elevated prevalence of panic disorder compared with a control population.[35-37] Several interesting, albeit theoretical, causal links have been considered. These include the possibility that patients may react to symptoms of mitral valve prolapse with panic, that the physiologic changes associated with anxiety may predispose patients to the development of prolapse, that an unknown intermediary factor may lead to both disorders, and that individuals with the two disorders are more likely to seek treatment than those with either disorder alone. The possibility exists that these explanations also may account for the fact that mitral valve prolapse has been reported to be elevated in other psychiatric disorders, including both bipolar and eating disorders. The latter association has been suggested by one author as accounting for an increased cardiac risk in patients with anorexia nervosa and bulimia, but this has not yet been proved.[38]

References

1. Savage DD, Garrison RJ, Devereux RB, et al: Mitral valve prolapse in the general population. I. Epidemiologic features: the Framingham Study, *Am Heart J* 106:571-576, 1983.
2. Jersaty RM: *Mitral valve prolapse,* New York, 1979, Raven Press; pp 4-7.
3. Procacci PM, Savran SV, Schriter SL, Bryson AL: Prevalence of clinical mitral valve prolapse in 1160 young women, *N Engl J Med* 294:1086-1088, 1976.
4. Markiewicz W, Stoner J, London E, et al: Mitral valve prolapse in one hundred presumably healthy young females, *Circulation* 53:464, 1976.
5. Darsee JR, Nickolic JR, Micoloff NB, Lesser LE: Prevalence of mitral valve prolapse in presumably healthy young men, *Circulation* 59:619, 1979.
6. Sbarboro JA, Mehlman FJ, Wu L, Brooks HL: A prospective study of mitral valve prolapse in young men, *Chest* 75:555, 1979.
7. Wann LS, Srove JR, Hess TR, et al: Prevalence of mitral valve prolapse by two dimensional echocardiography in healthy young women, *Br Heart J* 49:334-340, 1983.
8. Greenwood RD: Mitral valve prolapse: incidence and clinical course in a pediatric population, *Clin Pediatr* 23:318-320, 1984.
9. Warth DC, King ME, Cohen JM, et al: Prevalence of mitral valve prolapse in normal children, *J Am Coll Cardiol* 5:1173-1177, 1985.
10. Levy D, Savage D: Prevalence and clinical features of mitral valve prolapse, *Am Heart J* 113:1281-1290, 1987.
11. Barlow JB, Pocock WA: The mitral valve prolapse enigma—two decades later, *Mod Concepts Cardiovasc Dis* 53:13-17, 1984.
12. Jersaty RM: Mitral valve prolapse: definition and implication in athletes, *J Am Coll Cardiol* 7:231-236, 1986.
13. Gallavardin L: Pseudo dédoublement du deuxième bruit de coeur simulant le dédoublement mitral par bruit extracardique télésystolique surajfoute, *Lyon Med* 121:409, 1913.
14. Mackenzie J: *Disease of the heart,* ed 4, London, 1925, Oxford University Press; p 357.
15. Lewis T: *Disease of the heart,* ed 4, London, 1949, McMillan; p. 154.
16. Reid JV: Midsystolic clicks, *S Afr Med J* 35:353, 1961.
17. Barlow JB, Pocock WA, Marchand P, Denny M: The significance of late systolic murmurs, *Am Heart J* 66:443-452, 1963.
18. Barlow JB, Boxman CK, Pocock WA, Marchand P: Late systolic murmurs and non-ejections ("mid-late") systolic clicks: an analysis of 90 patients, *Br Heart J* 30:203-218, 1968.
19. Barlow JB, Pocock WA: Billowing, floppy, prolapsed or flail mitral valves?, *Am J Cardiol* 55:501-502, 1985.
20. Perloff JK, Child JS, Edwards JE: New guidelines for the clinical diagnosis of mitral valve prolapse, *Am J Cardiol* 57:1124-1129, 1986.
21. Garson A, Bricker JT, McNamara DG: *The science and practice of pediatric cardiology,* Philadelphia, 1990, Lea & Febiger; pp 1973-1986.
22. McLaren MJ, Hawkins DM, Lachman AS, et al: Nonejection systolic clicks and minimal systolic murmurs in black school children of Soweto, Johannesburg, *Br Heart J* 38:718-724, 1976.
23. Savage DD, Devereux RB, Garrison RJ, et al: Mitral valve prolapse in the general population. II. Clinical features: the Framingham Study, *Am Heart J* 106:577-581, 1983.
24. Arfken CL, Lachman AS, McLaren MJ, et al: Mitral valve prolapse: associations with symptoms and anxiety, *Pediatrics* 85:311-315, 1990.
25. Moodie DS: Mitral valve prolapse in children and adolescents, *Cleve Clin Q* 49:181-189, 1982.
26. Webb-Kavey RE, Blackman MS, Sondheimer HM, Byrum CJ: Ventricular arrhythmias and mitral valve prolapse in childhood, *J Pediatr* 105:885-889, 1984.

27. Savage DD, Levy D, Garrison RJ, et al: Mitral valve prolapse in the general population. III. Dysrhythmia: the Framingham Study, *Am Heart J* 106:582-586, 1983.

28. Bisset GS III, Schwartz DC, Meyer RA, et al: Clinical spectrum and long-term follow-up of isolated mitral valve prolapse in 119 children, *Circulation* 62:423-429, 1980.

29. Levine RA, Triulzi MO, Harrigan P, Weyman AE: The relationship of mitral annular shape to the diagnosis of mitral valve prolapse, *Circulation* 75:756-767, 1987.

30. Levine RA, Stathogianis E, Newell JB, et al: Reconsideration of echocardiographic standards for mitral valve prolapse: lack of association between leaflet displacement isolated to the apical four chamber view and independent echocardiographic evidence of abnormality, *J Am Coll Cardiol* 11:1010-1019, 1988.

31. Krivokapich J, Child JS, Dadourian BJ, Perloff JK: Assessment of echocardiographic criteria for diagnosis of mitral valve prolapse, *Am J Cardiol* 61:131-135, 1988.

32. Dajari AS, Bisno AL, Chung KJ, et al: Prevention of bacterial endocarditis, *JAMA* 264:2919-2922, 1990.

33. Edwards JE, Topaz O: Pathologic features of sudden death in children, adolescents, and young adults, *Chest* 87:476-482, 1985.

34. Bharati S, Bauernfeind R, Miller LB, et al: Sudden death in three teenagers: conduction system studies, *J Am Coll Cardiol* 1:879-886, 1983.

35. Margraf J, Ehlers A, Roth WT: Mitral valve prolapse and panic disorder: a review of their relationship, *Psychosom Med* 50:93-113, 1988.

36. Dagger SR, Saal AK, Comess KA, Dunner DL: Mitral valve prolapse and the anxiety disorders, *Hosp Community Psychiatry* 39:517-527, 1988.

37. Gorman JM, Goetz RR, Fyer M, King DL, Fyer AJ, Liebowitz MR, Klein DF: The mitral valve prolapse—panic disorder connection, *Psychosom Med* 50:114-122, 1988.

38. Johnson GL, Humphries LL, Shirley PB, Mazzoleni A, Noonan JA: Mitral valve prolapse in patients with anorexia nervosa and bulimia, *Arch Intern Med* 146:1525-1529, 1986.

39. Mitchell JH, Haskell WL, Raven PB: Classification of sports, *J Am Coll Cardiol* 24:864-866, 1994.

40. Maron BJ, Isner JM, McKenna WJ: Task Force 3: hypertrophic cardiomyopathy, myocarditis and other myopericardial diseases and mitral valve prolapse, *J Am Coll Cardiol* 24:880-885, 1994.

41. Cheitlin MD, Douglas PS, Parmley WW: Task Force 2: acquired valvular heart disease, *J Am Coll Cardiol* 24:874-879, 1994.

CHAPTER 38

Cardiac Rhythm Disorders

•

Sharanjeet Singh

Disorders of cardiac rhythm are becoming increasingly important as a result of the increased application of highly sophisticated monitoring devices in children and adolescents. There appears to be an absolute increase in the prevalence of childhood arrhythmias, especially among late survivors of surgical correction of congenital cardiac anomalies, who remain at risk for cardiac arrhythmias. Long-term survivors of correction of tetralogy of Fallot, for instance, have a 3% to 7% risk of sudden death presumably due to arrhythmias, while children who undergo atrial switch repair for transposition have associated electrophysiologic abnormalities, with less than 30% of long-term survivors displaying normal sinus rhythm.[1]

IRREGULAR HEARTBEAT IN HEALTHY INDIVIDUALS

A variety of cardiac rhythm changes have been documented in apparently healthy children, adolescents, and young adults through long-term monitoring via ambulatory (Holter) electrocardiography. In a group of 100 healthy 14- to 16-year-old boys, heart rates varied from 45 to 200 beats/min during waking hours and 23 to 95 beats/min during sleep.[2] Rhythm changes commonly recorded during Holter monitoring in healthy children and adolescents include sinus block or arrest, first- and second-degree heart block, junctional rhythm, atrial premature beats, and ventricular premature beats. The common occurrence of these "abnormal" rhythm changes in healthy children with no apparent heart disease suggests that such changes are probably not harmful, but long-term studies of their natural history are not currently available.

DIAGNOSIS OF CARDIAC ARRHYTHMIAS

The pediatrician or general physician often may encounter an irregular heartbeat in an adolescent patient who has no symptoms or history of heart disease, during either a routine physical examination or an examination for an unrelated problem. The irregular heart rhythm can be evaluated by a clinical cardiologic examination and documented by a routine ECG with a long "rhythm strip." The ECG can be supplemented with a chest radiograph and/or an echocardiogram if indicated. Episodic arrhythmias may require a 24- or 48-hour ambulatory ECG recording to evaluate the frequency of the irregularity and to document the cardiac rhythm when symptoms such as palpitations, tachycardia, chest pain (discomfort), dizziness, or syncope occur. Relatively infrequent arrhythmias can be documented with a patient-activated or intermittent event recorder. Exercise stress testing is indicated when symptoms or arrhythmias are induced by exertion and for prescribing levels of safe physical activity. Invasive electrophysiologic study may be indicated for determining the mechanism of the arrhythmia or catheter ablation of the responsible focus.

As a broad generalization, the clinical management of cardiac arrhythmias can be divided into the following categories:

1. Arrhythmias that are benign and require no further follow-up.
2. Ones that do not need to be treated but require continued followup. The adolescent with a structurally normal heart and an asymptomatic arrhythmia is usually included in this category.
3. Those that must be treated. Any symptomatic adolescent with syncope or presyncope and a cardiac defect requires cardiac evaluation and treatment. Likewise, the adolescent with a normal heart but a frequent and symptomatic arrhythmia requires therapeutic intervention.

SPECIFIC ARRHYTHMIAS

Premature Atrial Contractions

Premature atrial contractions (PACs) are slightly more common than premature ventricular contractions (PVCs). PACs usually occur in children and adolescents who have an otherwise normal heart. Rarely, PACs are associated with myocarditis, hyperthyroidism, or atrial enlargement or they may represent an adverse reaction in patients receiving sympathomimetic amines.

A premature atrial contraction is defined by a P wave that occurs prematurely and has a contour and axis different from those of a sinus P wave. The PAC may be conducted normally to the ventricle, be aberrantly conducted (resulting in a QRS complex with a shape different from that of a sinus QRS complex), or not be conducted at all (blocked). Blocked PACs cause an inappropriate pause and may mimic sinus bradycardia.

No treatment is indicated for the asymptomatic adolescent with PACs. Frequent PACs that cause brady-

cardia occasionally require treatment with digoxin and/or a beta blocker to abolish the extrasystoles and allow sinus rhythm to prevail.

Premature Ventricular Contractions

Premature ventricular contractions, which may be found on routine ECG examinations in 0.8% to 2.2% of normal children and adolescents, are seen more frequently during ambulatory ECG monitoring.[3] They are commonly found in patients with hypertrophic or congestive cardiomyopathy, myocarditis, arrhythmogenic right ventricle, mitral valve prolapse, and Marfan's syndrome and after surgery for congenital heart disease. PVCs may also be associated with the use of psychotropic drugs, sympathomimetic agents, or anesthetics. A prolonged QT interval, with or without deafness, is an important etiologic factor for PVCs, and a careful measurement of QT interval is indicated when a patient with PVCs is being evaluated.

PVCs, defined as impulses originating in the ventricles, are identified on the ECG as beats having a QRS-complex structure different from those of sinus beats and not preceded by a P wave. The QRS pattern may suggest a bundle branch block pattern with opposite QRS and T-wave inscription. PVCs with left bundle branch structure originate from the right ventricle; those with right bundle branch block pattern arise from the left ventricle. Most PVCs are uniform or unifocal in structure and may occur frequently, sometimes causing a bigeminal or trigeminal rhythm. Multiform or multifocal PVCs suggest a diseased heart, although this is not always the case.

Evaluation of the adolescent with PVCs should include measurement of the QT interval, a 24-hour ambulatory recording, and an echocardiogram to rule out possible causes such as arrhythmogenic right ventricle, myocarditis, cardiomyopathy, mitral valve prolapse, or a tumor. The prognosis of uniform PVCs, especially those occurring without evidence of underlying heart disease, is good. Suppression of uniform PVCs during an exercise test is a reassuring finding, and such patients require no treatment. Patients with PVCs that increase with exercise, or those with multiform or complex PVCs who have no underlying heart disease, require careful follow-up. Patients with mitral valve prolapse, those with various forms of cardiomyopathy, and symptomatic patients with underlying heart disease require antiarrhythmic treatment or ablation of the focus.

Vagal Arrhythmias

The normal heartbeat results from a well-balanced modulation of the sinoatrial and atrioventricular nodes by the autonomic nervous system. Increased vagal tone causes slowing of the rate of depolarization of the sinoatrial node and slowed conduction by way of the atrioventricular node. Sinoatrial slowing allows the subsidiary pacemakers in the atria and ventricles to "escape," that is, discharge spontaneously. Thus, vagus nerve–induced rhythms include sinus slowing, atrioventricular conduction abnormalities, and atrial and ventricular escape rhythms.

Sinus Arrhythmias

Rhythmic variations in the heartbeat occur naturally because of the variations in vagal tone caused by respiration; specifically, the heart rate increases toward the end of inspiration and slows toward the end of expiration. Sinus arrhythmia due to respiratory variations is seen in virtually all normal children and adolescents during ambulatory ECG recording, and frequently even during a routine 12-lead ECG examination. Sinus arrhythmia is more commonly observed when the heart rate is slow, and it tends to disappear with increases in heart rate. The ECG shows a gradual shortening of the PP interval followed by a lengthening of the PP interval. There is usually no significant change in atrioventricular conduction, and the change in PP interval is usually less than 100%.

Sinus bradycardia occurs as a sinus rhythm with a heart rate below the age-specific normal limits. As a broad generalization, sinus bradycardia can be identified on a routine ECG if the heart rate is less than 60 beats/min in a school-age child and less than 50 beats/min in an adolescent. Sinus bradycardia is frequently seen in athletic teenagers and is generally considered to be a normal variant. Sinus bradycardia also may occur in association with hypothermia, hypothyroidism, hypopituitarism, obstructive jaundice, typhoid fever, increased intracranial pressure, or hypertension. In the sick patient with bradycardia, treatment is directed at the primary illness, and the bradycardia is generally not of major importance. Occasionally, marked sinus arrhythmia or bradycardia may be associated with dizziness, near-syncope, or (rarely) syncope. Atropine or other anticholinergic drugs may relieve the symptoms, suggesting mediation by vagotonia. However, the adverse effects of these drugs commonly limit their clinical utility. Reduction of the intensity of physical training may relieve symptoms in the adolescent athlete.

Wandering Atrial Pacemaker

A wandering atrial pacemaker is characterized by a shift in the pacemaker from the sinus node to the atrium or the atrioventricular junction. In this condition, the P-wave structure alternates between positive and negative over several beats. The change usually occurs during periods of bradycardia and is considered to be an escape rhythm due to vagus nerve–induced sinoatrial node suppression. The wandering atrial pacemaker has no significant pathologic importance.

Junctional Rhythm

The junctional rhythm is characterized by a series of QRS complexes without preceding P waves. This rhythm usually originates in the bundle of His, represents an escape rhythm with a rate of 40 to 60 beats/min, and occurs when the sinus node is suppressed because of vagotonia or intrinsic sinus node disease. The junctional rhythm is encountered during periods of sinus bradycardia and frequently may be seen on 24-hour ambulatory ECG recordings in healthy individuals during sleep. Although a nonsustained junctional rhythm has no pathologic importance, a sustained junctional rhythm is usually associated with underlying heart disease.

Supraventricular Tachycardia

Supraventricular tachycardia (SVT) is a rapid, regular rhythm resulting from an abnormal mechanism proximal to the bundle of His. Sinus tachycardia is specifically excluded from this category since it is not caused by an abnormal mechanism. Atrial flutter and fibrillation are identified by routine ECG and are classified as separate entities.

SVT is a common arrhythmia. Adolescent patients recognize the tachycardia or feel discomfort and therefore come to medical attention earlier than would infants or children. Heart failure at presentation is uncommon in adolescents. In one study of 346 patients with SVT, the average heart rate was 235 beats/min (range, 118 to 330 beats/min).[4] In this study, 55% of patients had a normal heart, whereas 45% had one or more factors that could predispose to tachycardia. Congenital heart disease was present in 28% of patients, with Ebstein's anomaly and L-transposition of the great arteries representing important risk factors. Wolff-Parkinson-White syndrome was documented by preexcitation on the ECG in 25% of patients. Reentry, with or without a bypass tract, was the responsible mechanism in 80% of patients with SVT; the remaining patients had an ectopic focus.

The QRS complexes are usually normal (i.e., narrow QRS-complex tachycardia), while SVT resulting in wide QRS-complex tachycardia is rare in children and adolescents.[4] Vagal maneuvers (e.g., the Valsalva), stimulation of the diving reflex by the application of an ice bag or by facial immersion, or carotid massage may be effective in the evaluation and treatment of SVT. Intravenous adenosine (0.1 to 0.25 mg/kg; usual adult dose, 6 to 12 mg), administered as a rapid bolus, has become a treatment of choice for many SVTs. Intravenous verapamil (0.1 to 0.3 mg/kg; usual adult dose, 5 to 10 mg) is an alternative. DC cardioversion is indicated in patients with hemodynamic compromise or who fail to respond to intravenous medication.

Chronic SVT is generally characterized by a slower rate than that of acute SVT, and symptoms are less common. Knowledge of the mechanism underlying the tachycardia is necessary for appropriate treatment in such cases. An electrophysiologic evaluation is helpful for diagnostic purposes. When the underlying mechanism of the tachycardia involves a bypass tract or an ectopic focus, catheter ablation of the pathway or focus is the preferred treatment at most centers.

Ventricular Tachycardia

Ventricular tachycardia is defined as a series of three or more depolarizations originating from the ventricles and resulting in wide QRS complexes on the surface ECG. Other causes of "wide QRS" tachycardia, such as SVT or atrial flutter with aberration, should be differentiated by appropriate electrophysiologic studies. The presence of atrioventricular dissociation, intermittent sinus capture, or fusion beats is helpful in establishing the diagnosis of ventricular tachycardia. The structure of the tachycardia complexes is similar to that found with single PVCs if present. Ventricular tachycardia should also be differentiated from an accelerated ventricular rhythm, which is similar to or slightly faster than the sinus rate. Ventricular escape rhythm consists of wide QRS complexes having a rate slower than the sinus rate.

Ventricular tachycardia commonly results from previous intracardiac surgery. Other causes include cardiomyopathy, intramyocardial tumor, arrhythmogenic right ventricular dysplasia, metabolic disturbances, drug ingestion (e.g., tricyclic antidepressants), and drug toxicity. Prolonged QT syndrome is an important cause of ventricular tachycardia, and a careful measurement of the QT interval is indicated in cases of ventricular tachycardia.

Antiarrhythmic treatment is indicated in patients with postoperative ventricular tachycardia, since hemodynamic compromise is usually present. Symptomatic patients with a normal heart similarly require treatment. Asymptomatic patients with a structurally normal heart, a normal QT interval, and in whom the tachycardia is suppressed by exercise do not appear to have a high risk of sudden death and therefore can be merely followed up with no intervention.

Syncope

Syncope is characterized by an abrupt, brief loss of consciousness and muscle tone with spontaneous recovery. Mild syncopal episodes may be characterized by only dizziness or lightheadedness. Syncope must be differentiated from other states of altered consciousness, such as vertigo, seizures, and coma. Syncope can be a manifestation of a variety of diseases and may result from any of the following pathophysiologic factors:

1. An inadequate supply of energy substrates delivered through the circulatory system to the brain. Hypoglycemia is a common cause.
2. A fall in systemic arterial blood pressure to a level inadequate for maintenance of cerebral circulation, such as may occur in orthostatic hypotension.
3. A decrease in or loss of intrinsic cerebral circulation. Hyperventilation and the accompanying hypocapnia may cause a decrease in cerebral blood flow that can result in loss of consciousness. The common faint or vasovagal episode (vasodepressor syncope) results from a decrease in cerebral perfusion due to hypotension.
4. A variety of cardiovascular phenomena or cardiac disorders. Low cardiac output, the primary cause of cardiac syncope, is usually attributable to obstructed blood flow, such as occurs in aortic stenosis, hypertrophic cardiomyopathy with left ventricular outflow obstruction, mitral stenosis, pulmonary stenosis, or primary pulmonary artery hypertension. Low cardiac output also may result from myocardial dysfunction, such as myocarditis or cardiomyopathy, and severe aortic or mitral regurgitation also can reduce forward cardiac output to the point of causing syncope.
5. Cardiac arrhythmias. These can cause a serious impairment or cessation of cardiac output, with resultant syncope due to a decrease in or loss of cerebral perfusion. Atrioventricular block, supraventricular tachycardia, ventricular tachycardia, junctional rhythm, and the long QT syndrome have all been associated with syncope. Syncope with exercise or emotion occurs in patients with the long QT syndrome due to torsades de pointes ventricular tachycardia, with most affected individuals becoming symptomatic in the first or second decade of life.

The common faint, or vasodepressor syncope, is often precipitated by environmental stimuli such as anxiety, fright, a hot and stuffy atmosphere, the drawing of blood, or the sight of blood. There may be a prodrome, including dizziness, lightheadedness, pallor, nausea, and diaphoresis, which is followed by a loss of consciousness and postural tone and then gradual recovery. There is no seizure activity or loss of bowel or bladder control associated with vasodepressor syncope.

Careful history taking from the patient and witnesses is necessary to confirm the diagnosis of syncope. The history and a careful physical examination may identify specific entities as possible causes, such as findings of aortic stenosis or complete heart block. An ECG is indicated in the initial assessment of syncope; a normal ECG suggests a low likelihood of arrhythmia as a cause of syncope. A Holter monitor should be considered if episodic arrhythmias are suspected. Further diagnostic testing may be done to rule out neurally mediated syncope by upright tilt testing, with or without the use of isoproterenol.[5] Treatment of patients with neurally mediated syncope with beta-adrenergic blockers, anticholinergic agents, and mineralocorticoids has

been suggested, but such therapy needs further evaluation.

References

1. Hesslein PS: Noninvasive arrhythmia diagnosis. In Garson A Jr, Bricker JT, McNamara DG, editors: *The science and practice of pediatric cardiology,* Philadelphia, 1990, Lea & Febiger; pp 1725-1742.
2. Dickinson DF, Scott O: Ambulatory electrographic monitoring in 100 healthy teenage boys, *Br Heart J* 51:179-183, 1987.
3. Yabek SM: Ventricular arrhythmias in children with apparently normal heart, *J Pediatr* 119:1-11, 1991.
4. Ludmirsky A, Garson A Jr: Supraventricular tachycardia. In Garson A Jr, Bricker JT, McNamara DG, editors: *The science and practice of pediatric cardiology,* Philadelphia, 1990, Lea & Febiger; pp 1809-1848.
5. Kapoor WN: Diagnostic evaluation of syncope, *Am J Med* 90:91-106, 1991.

CHAPTER 39

Sudden Cardiac Death

•

Daniel Silbert

The tragedy of sudden death is rare in adolescents. It has been estimated that among teenage athletes the annual incidence of sudden unexpected death related to physical activity is 1 in 200,000 persons.[1,2] Approximately 10 times this number, or 1 in 20,000 young athletes, have cardiac conditions that render them vulnerable to sudden death.[1] There are numerous possible causes of sudden cardiac death. In some cases, preexisting heart disease had been recognized, but in many patients no heart disease had been previously detected because of the absence of either symptoms or an organic heart murmur.

Frequently, syncopal episodes have been noted to precede sudden death. This finding can therefore provide an opportunity for a diagnosis to be made in some adolescents who are at risk and for preventive measures to be taken.

SINUS NODE DYSFUNCTION AND TACHYARRHYTHMIAS

Sinus node dysfunction often causes severe bradycardia frequently associated with tachyarrhythmias. Most commonly this follows open heart surgery, particularly atrial level repair of transposition of the great vessels[3-5] and repair of tetralogy of Fallot, often years after surgery. A poor hemodynamic result after surgery is associated with a higher incidence of arrhythmias and sudden death.[6,7]

Severe bradycardia or tachyarrhythmia may be infrequent and therefore can be missed even with prolonged electrocardiogram (ECG) monitoring. An exercise ECG may help detect subnormal rate increases or the onset of dangerous tachycardias. Treatment includes the use of a permanent pacemaker or antiarrhythmic medications and has succeeded in lowering the frequency of sudden death in patients with these abnormalities.[8]

PROLONGED QT INTERVAL

This rare syndrome was initially described in 1957 as consisting of congenital nerve deafness associated with a prolonged corrected QT interval, which may be transient.[9] Subsequently a similar ECG pattern has been noted in some patients with normal hearing. In both syndromes, episodes of ventricular tachycardia and fibrillation occur that are often provoked by exercise or a strong emotional response.[10] Since these arrhythmias have frequently led to brain damage or death, prompt treatment is mandatory. The use of a beta-blocking drug, such as propranolol, is often effective. When this treatment fails, a left stellate ganglionectomy may be effective in preventing the onset of ventricular arrhythmias. Dangerous prolongation of the QT interval also may be acquired. Electrolyte disturbances, especially hypokalemia, can prolong the QT interval. This has been associated in persons who use liquid protein diets or who have eating disorders. Many drugs, most importantly tricyclic antidepressants and quinidine, have the same potential.[11] Central nervous system trauma, especially subarachnoid hemorrhage and myocarditis or myocardial ischemia, may also cause a significant prolongation of the QT interval.

CONGENITAL AORTIC STENOSIS

A small percentage of adolescents with congenital aortic stenosis are at risk of sudden death, especially during or after vigorous exercise.[12,13] In the presence of a severely stenotic valve, left ventricular oxygen needs increase markedly with exercise because of sinus tachycardia and a major increase in left ventricular pressure. Even in the absence of coronary artery disease, the oxygen supply may be deficient, particularly in the subendocardial layer, and fatal arrhythmias can develop. Fully half of all deaths that have been reported from valvular aortic stenosis have occurred during exercise or shortly after its cessation.[12]

Cardiac centers differ in their approach to aortic stenosis and in their recommendations regarding limitations on exercise. Some prohibit strenuous competitive sports, such as football or track, if the resting transvalvular gradient is above 20 mm Hg, but permit noncompetitive strenuous activity and less strenuous competitive activity, such as baseball.[14] With resting gradients above 50 mm Hg, most cardiologists prohibit all but moderate noncompetitive activity, and many advise surgery or balloon dilation to reduce the severity of stenosis. Stress tests are frequently used and their results taken into account in recommending exercise levels. It must be remembered, however, that aortic stenosis frequently increases in severity over the years and that a stress test does not accurately mimic playing field conditions in terms of duration of exertion, thermal and emotional stresses, and other significant factors.

HYPERTROPHIC CARDIOMYOPATHY

Adolescents with hypertrophic cardiomyopathy have a high incidence and variety of arrhythmias.[15,16] This contributes to the high sudden death rate in this condition, which in one study was 30%, with an average follow-up of 9 years. Many studies have failed to find a significant correlation between arrhythmias and sudden death in these patients.[15,17] Therefore, even several negative Holter recordings do not remove the risk of sudden death. The absence of symptoms and also a negative family history do appear to be associated with a lower risk of sudden death.

Low-risk patients probably do not need antiarrhythmic therapy. In one survey, many patients at a higher risk were not protected from sudden death by beta-blocking drugs. It is hoped that other drugs, such as verapamil and amiodarone, will lower the incidence of sudden death in this condition.[18,19]

CONGESTIVE CARDIOMYOPATHY

A few patients with congestive cardiomyopathy will die suddenly. No correlation has been found between preceding arrhythmias and sudden death in these patients.[20] Antiarrhythmic therapy, although recommended, has met with little success. The risk of sudden death appears to be greater in patients with the poorest left ventricular ejection fraction.[21]

Acute myocarditis may not be apparent; it may appear as only a mild "viral syndrome" and yet result in sudden death. In other patients, myocarditis will cause clear features of congestive heart failure. Children with a previously unrecognized chronic cardiomyopathy may fail to survive an otherwise mild viral illness. In these cases the true nature of the disease may be determined by myocardial biopsy or autopsy study.

ARRHYTHMOGENIC RIGHT VENTRICULAR DYSPLASIA

Recurrent episodes of ventricular tachycardia in otherwise asymptomatic teenagers may be caused by this unusual entity. In its most severe form, the right ventricle is markedly dilated and functions poorly. In less severe cases, it is difficult or impossible to detect any right ventricular abnormalities by noninvasive means, including echocardiography. In such instances, cardiac catheterization is necessary.[22]

In patients with any recurrent ventricular tachycardia, cardiac catheterization and myocardial biopsy are warranted because of the high risks posed by arrhythmogenic right ventricular dysplasia. There are reports of sudden death in the absence of previous symptoms or of known ventricular tachycardia.[23,24] Several cases of right ventricular dysplasia have been found in athletes dying suddenly during vigorous activity.[25-27]

Therapy should be offered to patients with recurrent tachycardia, especially if it is induced by exercise. Treatment with standard antiarrhythmic drugs has met with only limited success. In the most refractory cases, therefore, attempts have been made to surgically isolate the arrhythmogenic focus.

CORONARY ARTERY ABNORMALITIES

Deaths from congenital coronary anomalies are very rare in the adolescent age group. Either coronary artery, left or right, may arise from the opposite sinus of Valsalva; from its origin it usually courses between the aorta and the main pulmonary artery, where it is in danger of being compressed, especially during exercise.[28-31]

Acquired coronary artery disease has assumed a greatly increased importance in recent years, particularly in association with Kawasaki's disease. Aneurysms of the coronary arteries were common before the use of intravenous gamma globulin during the acute phase of the disease.[32] Gamma globulin has greatly reduced the incidence and severity of coronary artery damage, and in some large series no deaths were reported during the acute phase of the disease.[33] The long-term effects of this therapy on mortality and morbidity rates await further study.[34] Isolated reports have noted late sudden death in asymptomatic adolescents with coronary artery lesions.[35,36]

Rapidly developing obliterative coronary arteritis occurs commonly in heart transplant recipients. Treatment strategies so far have been ineffective.[37]

AORTIC ANOMALIES AND MITRAL VALVE PROLAPSE

After repair of coarctation of the aorta, dissection of the ascending aorta or rupture near the surgical site has been reported.[38] The risk is higher in teenagers with Turner's syndrome.

Marfan's syndrome predisposes patients to aortic dissection or fatal arrhythmias.[39] This syndrome also is associated with mitral valve prolapse, although most adolescents with mitral valve prolapse do not have Marfan's syndrome. Deaths from mitral valve prolapse are rare, but they have been reported in association with previous syncope or documented ventricular arrhythmias.[40-42]

BLUNT CHEST TRAUMA

A 1995 report describes 25 instances of sudden death, presumably due to ventricular fibrillation, after blunt left chest trauma.[43] In most cases the trauma resulted from an unexpected blow to the chest by a baseball or hockey puck during ordinary sports activity. The children described in this report ranged in age from 3 to 19 years. Autopsy failed to reveal any evidence of trauma or of an underlying cardiac abnormality in these children and adolescents.

OTHER CONDITIONS CAUSING SUDDEN CARDIAC DEATH

Severe pulmonary hypertension, whether primary or secondary (Eisenmenger's syndrome), can result in sudden death, presumably due to an arrhythmia.[44]

A high incidence of sudden death occurs in patients with Ebstein's anomaly. This is attributed to frequent episodes of serious arrhythmias, which further compromise an already abnormal cardiac function.[45,46]

Pulmonary atresia may also cause sudden death, possibly as a result of hypoxic spells, which may lead to fatal arrhythmias.[11]

PREVENTION

In Epstein and Maron's report of sudden cardiac death among athletes,[1] only 25% showed previous evidence of a cardiac abnormality. A thorough history taking and physical examination should improve on these unacceptable results. The American Academy of Pediatrics has a screening form for high school athletic competition, which should help uncover potentially dangerous medical conditions and lead to appropriate exercise restrictions.[47] Other reviews contain recommendations for athletic competition in children with cardiovascular abnormalities.[48,49]

It is hoped that earlier surgical repair of congenital cyanotic heart disease and those lesions causing pulmonary hypertension will reduce the incidence of life-threatening arrhythmias. When postoperative arrhythmias are found, electrophysiologic studies have been used to provide more informed and more effective drug therapy and to help determine whether a pacemaker is needed.

Medical, and occasionally surgical, treatment may reduce fatalities from the prolonged QT syndrome and from hypertrophic cardiomyopathy. Appropriate exercise restriction should reduce the incidence of death from severe obstructive lesions and the prolonged QT syndrome.

References

1. Epstein SF, Maron BJ: Sudden death and the competitive athlete: perspectives on preparticipation screening studies, *J Am Coll Cardiol* 7:220-230, 1986.
2. Strong WB, Alpert BS: The child with heart disease: play, recreation, and sports, *Curr Probl Cardiol* 6:1-37, 1981.
3. Yabek SM: Sinus node disease in cardiac arrhythmias in the neonate, infant and child, In Roberts MK, Gelband H, editors: *Cardiac arrhythmias in the neonate infant and child,* New York, 1983, Appleton-Century-Crofts.
4. El-Said GM, Gillette PC, Mullins CE, et al: Significance of the pacemaker recovery time after the Mustard operation for transposition of the great arteries, *Am J Cardiol* 38:448, 1976.
5. Gillette PC, Kugler JD, Garson A, et al: Mechanisms of cardiac arrhythmias after the Mustard operation for transposition of the great arteries, *Am J Cardiol* 45:1225, 1980.
6. Garson A, McNamara DG: Sudden death in a pediatric cardiology population, 1958-1983: relation to prior arrhythmias, *J Am Coll Cardiol* 5 (suppl):134B-137B, 1985.
7. Gatzoulis MA, Till JA, Somerville J, Redington AN: Mechanical electrical interaction in tetralogy of Fallot, *Circulation* 92:231-237, 1995.
8. Garson A, Randall DC, Gillette PC, et al: Prevention of sudden death after repair of tetralogy of Fallot: treatment of ventricular arrhythmias, *J Am Coll Cardiol* 6:221, 1985.
9. Jervell A, Lange-Nilsen F: Congenital deaf mutism, functional heart disease with prolongation of the QT and sudden death, *Am Heart J* 54:59, 1957.
10. Bricker JT, Garson A, Gillette PC: A family history of seizures associated with sudden cardiac deaths, *Am J Dis Child* 138:866, 1984.
11. Clark M, Lazzaraza R, Jackman W: Torsade de pointes: serum drug levels and electrocardiographic warning signs, *Circulation* 66 (suppl II):71, 1982.
12. Lambert EC, Menon VA, Wagner HR, Vlad P: Sudden unexpected death from cardiovascular disease in children, *Am J Cardiol* 34:89, 1974.
13. Glew RH, Varghese PJ, Krovetz W, et al: Sudden death in congenital aortic stenosis. A review of eight cases with an evaluation of premonitory clinical features, *Am Heart J* 78:615, 1969.
14. Freed MD: Recreation for the child with heart disease, *Pediatr Clin North Am* 31:1316-1318, 1984.
15. McKenna W, Deanfield J, Franklin R, et al: Arrhythmia in children and adolescents with hypertrophic cardiomyopathy: incidence and relation to prognosis, *J Am Coll Cardiol* 7:204A, 1986.
16. Frank M, Watkins L, Prisant L: Potentially lethal arrhythmias and their management in hypertrophic cardiomyopathy, *Am J Cardiol* 53:1608-1613, 1984.
17. Kuck K, Kunze K, Dernedde J: Value and limitation of programmed electrical stimulation in hypertrophic cardiomyopathy, *Circulation* 72 (suppl III):158, 1985.
18. Spicer R, Rocchini AP, Crowley DL, et al: Chronic verapamil therapy in pediatric and young adult patients with hypertrophic cardiomyopathy, *Am J Cardiol* 53:1614-1619, 1984.
19. McKenna W, Harris L, Rowland E, et al: Amiodarone for long term management of patients with hypertrophic cardiomyopathy, *Am J Cardiol* 54:802-810, 1984.
20. Magiros E, Guarnieri EP, Reid P, et al: Failure of electrophysiological testing to predict death in congestive cardiomyopathy, *Circulation* 72 (suppl III):159, 1985.
21. Von Olshausen K, Schafer A, Mehmel HC, et al: Ventricular arrhythmias in idiopathic dilated cardiomyopathy, *Br Heart J* 51:195-201, 1984.
22. Dungan W, Garson A, Gillette PC: Arrhythmogenic right ventricular dysplasia. A cause for ventricular tachycardia in children with apparently normal hearts, *Am Heart J* 102:745-750, 1981.
23. Rowland T, Schweiger M: Repetitive paroxysmal ventricular tachycardia and sudden death in a child, *Am J Cardiol* 53:1729, 1984.
24. Belhassan B: Sudden death in a child with ventricular tachycardia, *Am J Cardiol* 54:1172, 1984.
25. Panidis I, Greenspan AM, Mintz GS, et al: Inducible ventricular fibrillation in arrhythmogenic right ventricular dysplasia, *Am Heart J* 110:1067-1069, 1985.
26. Topaz O, Edwards JE: Pathological features of sudden death in children, adolescents and young adults, *Chest* 87:476-482, 1985.
27. Maron B: Sudden death in athletes, *Am J Cardiol* 41:803, 1978.
28. Cheitlin MD, DeCastro CM, McAllister HA: Sudden death as a complication of anomalous left coronary origin from the anterior sinus of Valsalva. A not so minor congenital anomaly, *Circulation* 50:780, 1974.
29. Kimbiris D, Iskandrian AS, Segal BL, et al: Anomalous aortic origin of coronary arteries, *Circulation* 58:606, 1978.
30. Davis J, Green DC, Cheitlin MD, et al: Anomalous left coronary artery origin from the right coronary sinus, *Am Heart J* 108:165, 1984.
31. Barth C, Roberts W: Left main coronary artery originating from the right sinus of Valsalva and coursing between the aorta and pulmonary trunk, *J Am Coll Cardiol* 7:366, 1986.
32. Newburger VW, Iakahaski M, Burns JC, et al: The treatment of Kawasaki syndrome with intravenous gamma globulin, *N Engl J Med* 315:341-347, 1986.
33. Rowley AH, Duffy CE, Shulman ST: Prevention of giant coronary artery aneurysms in Kawasaki disease by intravenous gamma globulin therapy, *J Pediatr* 113:290-294, 1988.
34. Denfield SW, Garson A: Sudden death in children and young adults, *Pediatr Clin North Am* 37(1):221, 1990.
35. Kohr RM. Progressive asymptomatic coronary artery disease as a late fatal sequela of Kawasaki disease, *J Pediatr* 108:256-259, 1986.
36. Burke AP, Farb A, Reno V, Goodin J, Smialek JE: Sports related and nonsports related sudden cardiac death in young adults, *Am Heart J* 121:568-575, 1991.
37. Emmanouilides GC, Reimenschneider TA, Allen HD, Gutgesell HP: *Heart disease in infants, children and adolescents,* ed 5, Baltimore, 1995, Williams & Wilkins; p 503.
38. Farfang K, Rostad H, Sorland S, et al: Late sudden death after surgical correction of coarctation of the aorta, *Acta Med Scand* 206:375, 1979.
39. Luckstead EF: Sudden death in sports, *Pediatr Clin North Am* 29(6):1355, 1982.
40. Anderson RC: Idiopathic mitral valve prolapse and sudden death, *Am Heart J* 100:941, 1980.
41. Jeresaty RM: Sudden death in the mitral valve prolapse click syndrome, *Am J Cardiol* 37:317, 1976.

42. Morady F, Scheinman MM, Hess DS, et al: Clinical characteristics and results of electrophysiological testing in young adults with ventricular tachycardia or ventricular fibrillation, *Am Heart J* 106:1306-1314, 1983.

43. Maron BV, Poliac LC, Kaplan JA, et al: Blunt impact to the chest leading to sudden death from cardiac arrest during sports activities, *N Engl J Med* 333:337-342, 1995.

44. Thilenius OG, Nadas AS, Jockin H: Primary pulmonary vascular obstruction in children, *Pediatrics* 36:75, 1965.

45. Watson H: Natural history of Ebstein's anomaly of tricuspid valve in childhood and adolescence: an international cooperative study of 505 cases, *Br Heart J* 36:417, 1974.

46. Bialostozky D, Horwitz S, Espino-Vela J: Ebstein's malformation of the tricuspid valve. A review of 65 cases, *Am J Cardiol* 29:826, 1972.

47. Hulse E, Strong WB: Preparticipation evaluation for athletics, *Pediatr Rev* 9:1-10, 1987.

48. Committee on Sports Medicine and Fitness: Cardiac dysrhythmias and sports, *Pediatrics* 95:786, 1995.

49. The 26th Bethesda Conference: Recommendations for determining eligibility for competition in athletes with cardiovascular abnormalities, *J Am Coll Cardiol* 24:845-899, 1994.

CHAPTER 40

Respiratory Tract Infections

•

Leonard R. Krilov

Respiratory tract infections are common in adolescents, accounting for up to 60% of days lost from school in this age group.[1] Respiratory syndromes encountered range from upper respiratory tract infections (e.g., the common cold, otitis media, sinusitis, pharyngitis) to lower tract disease (e.g., pneumonia). In general, the incidence of respiratory tract infections in adolescents approximates that seen in adults,[1] although certain infections such as from *Mycoplasma, Chlamydia pneumoniae* (also called TWAR strain), and coronavirus are most common in adolescents.

COMMON COLD

A common cold is a mild, self-limited infection of the upper respiratory tract manifested by nasal congestion and discharge, sneezing, cough, and a mild sore throat. Complications of the common cold are rare in adolescents but can include otitis media, sinusitis, and (very rarely) pneumonia. Although medical attention is rarely necessary during an episode of the common cold, it is a major cause of school absenteeism among adolescents.[2]

Symptomatic treatment, including the use of decongestants, is the accepted therapy. The median duration of symptoms ranges from 7 to 10 days, although illness that lasts 14 days or longer is seen in 25% of adolescents.[3] Because of the self-limited and benign course of the common cold, specific diagnostic studies are rarely performed. When such tests are obtained, a number of viral agents can be isolated in at least 60% of patients, including rhinoviruses, which account for approximately 25% of colds in adolescents and adults, and coronaviruses, which account for an additional 10% to 20%.[4,5] Respiratory syncytial virus, parainfluenza viruses, enteroviruses, and adenoviruses have also been implicated

as causes of upper respiratory tract infections in the adolescent age group.

OTITIS MEDIA

Although far less common in adolescents than in younger children, otitis media is the second leading reason for seeking medical attention in patients up to 15 years of age.[6] In older children and adolescents, the primary presenting symptom of otitis media is acute pain. Etiologic agents include *Streptococcus pneumoniae, Haemophilus influenzae,* group A streptococci, and *Moraxella catarrhalis.* Antibiotic therapy directed against these agents is beneficial, and with proper treatment complications of otitis media are rare (Table 40-1).

PHARYNGITIS

Acute pharyngitis is an inflammatory disease of the mucous membranes characterized by soreness or irritation of the throat. Fever, headache, nausea, vomiting, abdominal pain, and cervical adenitis are frequent associated findings. The diagnosis of pharyngitis requires objective evidence of inflammation (erythema, exudate, ulceration, or a combination of these findings).

In most cases of pharyngitis in adolescents, the aim is to separate group A streptococcal disease from other causes because of the need for antibiotic therapy. Such treatment is aimed at prevention of acute rheumatic fever, poststreptococcal reactive arthritis, and suppurative complications of group A streptococcal infection (e.g., sinusitis, otitis media). In addition, the institution of antibiotic therapy within the first 24 hours of symptoms has been associated with shortening of the signs of fever, tender

TABLE 40-1
Suggested Antibiotic Regimens for Respiratory Tract Infections

Syndrome (likely pathogens)	Drug(s) of Choice	Alternatives
Upper Respiratory Tract Infections		
Otitis media/sinusitis (*Streptococcus pneumoniae, Haemophilus influenzae, Moraxella catarrhalis, Staphylococcus aureus*, group A streptococcus)	Amoxicillin	Amoxicillin-clavulanic acid (Augmentin), erythromycin-sulfa, TMP-/SMX, newer cephalosporin,* newer macrolide†
Pharyngitis		
Group A streptococcus	Penicillin VK (PO) or penicillin G benzathine (IM) or oral cephalosporin	Erythromycin, clindamycin, newer macrolide,† amoxicillin (avoid ampicillin in patients with suspected mononucleosis)
Neisseria gonorrhoeae	Ceftriaxone sodium (250 mg IM × one dose)	Ciprofloxacin (not in children or pregnant women)
Lower Respiratory Tract Infections		
Community-acquired pneumonia in normal host (*Mycoplasma pneumoniae, Chlamydia pneumoniae, S. pneumoniae*)	Erythromycin	Doxycycline (if pneumococci on sputum Grams stain, penicillin G), newer macrolide†
Immunocompromised Host		
Human immunodeficiency virus positive (*Pneumocystis carinii*; bacterial: *S. pneumoniae, H. influenzae, Mycobacterium avium intracellulare*, or *M. tuberculosis*; histoplasmosis, coccidioidomycosis)	TMP/SMX	Pentamadine and third-generation cephalosporin or cefuroxime or amoxicillin-clavulanic acid
Hospital-acquired infection (include coverage for Enterobacteriacae, including *Pseudomonas aeruginosa*)	Multiple acceptable regimens depending on hospital flora, sensitivity patterns (e.g., third-generation cephalosporin, antipseudomonal penicillin, imipenem plus aminoglycoside)	
Neutropenia (<500/mm³) chemotherapy (as above + *Legionella pneumophila*, fungi)	As above; possibly add vancomycin and/or erythromycin	Amphotericin B (if evidence of fungal elements)
Tuberculosis	Isoniazid, rifampin (duration 6 to 9 mo) + pyrazinamide (1st 2 mo)	Additional drugs (e.g., streptomycin or ethambutol) if isoniazid resistance likely or if patient is HIV positive
Influenza A	Amantadine, rimantadine	

TMP/SMX, trimethoprim and sulfamethoxazole (Bactrim, Septra).
*Newer cephalosporins include cefuroxime axetil, cefpodoxime, cefprozil, cefaclor, loracarbef, and cefixime.
†Newer macrolides include clarithromycin and azithromycin.

cervical lymphadenopathy, pharyngeal infection, and symptoms of the disease (sore throat, headache, pharyngitis).[7] It has been suggested, however, that such early therapy may abort host antibody response to the organism, making the individual more susceptible to recurrent infection.[8] This hypothesis has not been borne out in other studies.[9] The diagnosis of streptococcal pharyngitis is accomplished by swabbing the tonsils and culturing the specimen on sheep's blood agar. Rapid diagnostic tests to detect group A streptococcal antigens by enzyme-linked

immunosorbent assay (ELISA) or latex agglutination techniques are also available for office use and enable the practitioner to initiate antibiotic therapy at the time of the initial office visit. The sensitivity of the currently available antigen detection tests may be too low (62% to 96%) to allow exclusion of streptococcal infection, but the high specificity (90% to 100%) permits immediate treatment in a patient with a positive test result.[10] In sexually active adolescents, the less likely entity of gonococcal pharyngitis should be considered. Different culture media, such as Thayer-Martin or other enriched chocolate agar media, and selective conditions (increased carbon dioxide atmosphere) are required to isolate *Neisseria gonorrhoeae.*

Exudative pharyngitis is also frequently a prominent part of the infectious mononucleosis syndrome due to Epstein-Barr virus infection.[11] Diagnosis is based on an increase in circulating atypical lymphocytes and a positive heterophile test. Viruses such as adenovirus and enterovirus cause most other cases of both exudative and nonexudative pharyngitis. Other agents implicated in some cases of acute pharyngitis in adolescents include *Mycoplasma pneumoniae* and *Chlamydia* organisms, but the significance and frequency of these agents in this syndrome, compared with their isolation from asymptomatic individuals, is still to be determined.

Antibiotic therapy is indicated for streptococcal or gonococcal pharyngitis. Suggested regimens are listed in Table 40-1. Complications from acute pharyngitis are rare, the most significant being peritonsillar abscess.[12] This disease is seen primarily in adolescents and young adults and is characterized by dysarthria, trismus, and pain on swallowing. Treatment requires high doses of parenteral penicillin in conjunction with incision and drainage of the abscess; an interval tonsillectomy is generally performed 1 to 2 months later.

SINUSITIS

Bacterial infection of the paranasal sinuses can occur during the course of any upper respiratory tract infection. Adolescents are at significant risk for frontal sinusitis compared with adults because of the relatively recent development of their frontal sinuses.[3] It is believed that during the early stages of aeration their small size and narrow openings may predispose to obstruction and secondary infection. Acute infection is associated with obstruction to the normal drainage of the sinuses, and the patient generally presents with purulent rhinorrhea, postnasal drip, nasal obstruction, cough, facial pain, and headache. Headache may be the primary complaint in the adolescent with acute sinusitis. Such headaches are characterized by dull, nonthrobbing pain that increases with head movement, coughing, sneezing, or bending. Headaches of sinus origin tend to be prominent on awakening because of the overnight accumulation of secretions, which create increased pressure on the mucosae of the affected sinus. Localization of the headache and facial pain in an area overlying a given sinus suggests an underlying infection. Pain in the frontal region suggests frontal sinusitis; between the eyes, ethmoiditis; and in the area of the maxilla, maxillary sinusitis. In pansinusitis the pain may be less localized and associated with a constant sensation of facial pressure. Similar

symptoms with protracted rhinitis also have been observed as a result of cocaine abuse.[13] Thus, a history of substance use may be useful in evaluating adolescents with frequent "sinus" conditions.

Sinus tenderness is a useful clinical finding on physical examination. Opacity of the sinuses on transillumination also may be useful, but this is not a very reliable technique. Definitive diagnosis is made by radiographic examination of the sinuses demonstrating mucosal thickening and/or the presence of air-fluid levels in the sinuses.

The etiologic agents of sinusitis include *S. pneumoniae, H. influenzae, M. catarrhalis, Streptococcus pyogenes, Staphylococcus aureus,* and anaerobic bacteria. Antibiotic therapy directed against these agents is administered in conjunction with topical and/or systemic decongestants for 2 to 3 weeks (Table 40-1). Complications of sinusitis include brain abscess, orbital cellulitis, osteomyelitis, cavernous venous thrombosis, and meningitis. Although these complications are rare in the antibiotic era, many patients reported with these complications are adolescents.[14] Thus, if a prompt response to oral antibiotic therapy does not occur, hospitalization for intravenous therapy and possible surgical drainage should be considered.

Chronic sinusitis likely represents repeated damage to the mucosal lining leading to chronic bacterial colonization. The organisms involved are the same as in acute sinusitis, although some studies suggest an increased role for *S. aureus* and anaerobes.[15] Antibiotics may help in acute exacerbations of chronic disease, but true chronic sinusitis requires evaluation by an otolaryngologist for possible surgery.

BRONCHITIS

Bronchitis is a clinically diagnosed inflammatory disease of the tracheobronchial tree. Acute bronchitis presents as a prominent, persisting cough frequently in association with fever and rhonchi.[16] Substernal pain also may be reported in association with the cough. The peak incidence of this disease is the winter months, and most cases are thought to be of viral origin. Cases of bronchitis are especially common during influenza outbreaks. Rhinoviruses, adenoviruses, and other respiratory viruses have also been associated with this disease. Nonviral etiologies are less frequently considered, but *Bordetella pertussis, Mycoplasma pneumoniae,* and *C. pneumoniae* have all been implicated as occasional causes of acute bronchitis. Treatment of acute bronchitis is aimed at control of the cough. Antibiotics are indicated only when a nonviral cause is strongly suggested. Of note in this regard, during a 1993 pertussis outbreak in Cincinnati, a large proportion of the infected individuals were adolescents despite their having received vaccination.[17]

Chronic bronchitis is a clinical diagnosis applied to patients who report productive cough on most days during at least 3 consecutive months over 2 years.[18] Cigarette smoking, infection, and inhalation of fumes or dust are risk factors for developing chronic bronchitis. The diagnosis is more common in individuals over 40 years of age. When the diagnosis is made in an adolescent, consideration should be given to a defect in pulmonary function (e.g., cystic fibrosis, cilial dysfunction) or an immunodeficiency disorder (e.g., IgG subclass or IgA deficiency).[19]

LOWER RESPIRATORY TRACT INFECTIONS

Adolescents with pneumonia most commonly present with cough and fever. Diagnostic tests for pneumonia include a chest x-ray examination, sputum, Gram's stain and culture, complete blood count, and tuberculin skin test. Even with these diagnostic tests, the etiologic agent for individual cases of pneumonia frequently remains undetermined. In the high-risk adolescent who does not respond to empiric therapy, additional evaluations such as bronchioalveolar lavage, open lung biopsy, or more extensive serologic testing may be warranted. The selection of antimicrobial therapy for specific pneumonia syndromes is outlined in Table 40-1.

Lower respiratory tract infections need to be considered differently in the adolescent who has underlying disease as compared with individuals who have underlying pulmonary, cardiac, or immunodeficiency disorders. In the "healthy" adolescent the pathogens causing pneumonia include *M. pneumoniae, C. pneumoniae, S. pneumoniae, Mycobacterium tuberculosis,* and viruses such as influenza and the adenoviruses. In immunocompromised hosts, a number of opportunistic infections, most notably *Pneumocystis carinii,* can occur in addition to these agents. Of the previously listed etiologic agents, *M. pneumoniae* is generally considered the most common cause of pneumonia in adolescents, accounting for up to 50% of cases in this age range.[20] The disease is generally sufficiently mild to respond to oral antibiotic therapy and hence is frequently referred to as "walking pneumonia." Diagnostic clues include fever with recurrent, multiple chills (nonshaking); absence of leukocytosis; and associated extrapulmonary findings, such as gastrointestinal symptoms (nausea, vomiting, anorexia, and/or diarrhea), myalgias, and arthralgias.[21] Less commonly, central nervous system involvement, ranging from ataxia and confusion to syncope and seizures, and dermatologic lesions in the form of macular, vesicular, or urticarial rashes may be seen. Radiologic examination in the individual with *M. pneumoniae* usually reveals multilobular segmental bronchopneumonia. Involvement of the lower lobe is more common than upper lobe disease;

a streaky pattern spreading from the hilum is often seen.[22] Laboratory diagnosis of *M. pneumoniae* requires demonstration of a fourfold rise in complement fixation titers to the organism; isolation in culture is difficult and is not routinely available. The rise in antibody titers occurs 2 to 4 weeks after the onset of the clinical illness. Cold agglutinin titers of 1:128 are suggestive of mycoplasmal infection, but they may not be detected until the second to third week of illness; at a lower titer they may be found in a number of other viral and bacterial infections.[23]

C. pneumoniae has been identified as an important cause of disease in adolescents. The illness caused by this agent is generally mild and resembles mycoplasmal or viral respiratory infections, although the onset may be more gradual than with the latter agents. Serologic studies indicate that acute infection with this agent occurs primarily in the 5- to 14-year-old age group.[24] In adolescents and young adults, the disease is usually milder than in younger children and older adults. There is no seasonal pattern to *C. pneumoniae* infection and most cases occur endemically, although epidemics have been reported.[25]

The clinical illness associated with chlamydial infection typically begins with a sore throat, hoarseness, and fever. This is followed several days to a week later by the development of cough and abnormal breath sounds on lung examination. Chest radiographs typically demonstrate a single subsegmental infiltrate, although bilateral disease can be seen in more severe cases. Laboratory isolation of *C. pneumoniae* is difficult and is not routinely available. Serologic testing for this organism by a microimmunofluorescence test can be performed, but this method also is not readily available. A widely available complement fixation test can detect antibody response to chlamydial infection but is of limited use because it cannot distinguish between *C. pneumoniae, C. psittaci,* and *C. trachomatis.* In addition, the complement fixation antibody responses do not appear until 2 to 3 weeks after the onset of symptoms and may require acute and convalescent titers to confirm the diagnosis. White blood cell counts are generally normal in this infection, although the sedimentation rate is usually elevated. Thus, diagnosis of this infection is generally made on clinical grounds. Fortunately, the treatment for *M. pneumoniae* is also adequate for *C. pneumoniae* (Table 40-1). An association between *C. pneumoniae* and the onset of asthma has been suggested.[26]

Although less common than *Mycoplasma, Chlamydia,* or viral pneumonia in adolescents, pneumococcal pneumonia is a potentially more serious illness and can be associated with empyema formation and/or bacteremia. The acute onset of fever with a single shaking chill and leukocytosis are clues to the diagnosis of pneumococcal pneumonia. Blood cultures are positive in only one fourth to one third of cases in adolescents and adults.

Patients with primary tuberculosis pneumonia may present with clinical features indistinguishable from those of any other acute pneumonia. In young children, close family members or household contacts are generally responsible for tuberculosis infection, but by adolescence only one third of patients with tuberculosis acquire their disease from such contacts.[27] Less commonly, adolescents may present with reactivated cavitary disease or extrapulmonary manifestations of tuberculosis (e.g., Pott's disease, cervical lymphadenitis). Routine tuberculin screening on entry into high school should help detect these individuals. Tuberculin skin testing during any acute pneumonia also may be worthwhile. If tuberculosis infection is suspected, sputum for acid-fast bacilli stain and culture are indicated. With appropriate antibiotic therapy (Table 40-1), clinical cure should be achievable, although noncompliance with treatment is frequently encountered in adolescents.[28]

Influenza is an acute, self-limited infection typically associated with fever, chills, and nasal congestion, along with the systemic manifestations of headaches, myalgias, malaise, and anorexia. These symptoms can last for 10 to 14 days in the untreated individual. Influenza occurs in winter with outbreaks of varying severity. Adolescents with influenza frequently herald the appearance of influenza in the community, and teenagers are thought to play a major role in the spread of the infection.[29]

Two different strains of influenza, A and B, infect humans. Surface proteins of the virus can undergo gradual change (antigenic drift) or sudden major change (antigenic shift), which enables the virus to escape the host immune system and to reinfect individuals who previously had influenza.

Definitive diagnosis of influenzal infection depends on isolation of the agent from respiratory secretions; however, the clinical illness is typical enough for the diagnosis of influenza to be made by an experienced clinician in the absence of laboratory testing. An increase in lower respiratory tract infections in persons of all age groups during the winter months is a useful clue to the presence of influenza in the community. These findings, plus reports of documented influenza cases from the local health department, are useful adjuncts in the diagnosis of influenza.

Treatment of influenza is generally nonspecific and supportive. Early therapy (within the first 24 hours of symptoms) with amantadine hydrochloride or ximantadine has proved beneficial in shortening the course of influenza A infection. It can also provide effective prophylaxis against influenza A infection, although its use is generally restricted to individuals at high risk for severe influenzal illness. A killed virus vaccine that incorporates the three influenza strains likely to circulate during a given winter also is available each fall, but yearly reimmunization is required to maintain protection and account for antigenic changes in the virus. The vaccine is generally not advised for otherwise healthy adolescents.

Complications of influenza in healthy adolescents are rare but can include bacterial pneumonia or primary viral pneumonia. The latter was the cause of many of the deaths in otherwise healthy adolescents during the 1918-1919 influenza outbreak.[3] The occurrence of Reye's syndrome after influenza infection was seen in adolescents in the 1970s and 1980s, but the occurrence of this potentially fatal complication has decreased dramatically since the recognition of the role of salicylates in causing Reye's syndrome and the subsequent decreased use of aspirin.[30] In the compromised host, lower respiratory tract infections may be much more severe. For instance, influenza can cause significant illness in patients with underlying pulmonary, cardiac, or immunodeficiency disorders.

Consequently, these groups should receive influenza vaccine routinely and should be considered for amantadine prophylaxis during influenza outbreaks. Especially severe *M. pneumoniae* infection has been observed in patients with sickle cell disease.[31] An increased occurrence of extrapulmonary tuberculosis has been reported in individuals with HIV infection.[32] In addition, immunocompromised individuals are susceptible to a number of opportunistic infections: (1) bacteria: *Streptococcus pneumoniae, Mycobacterium avium intracellulare, Legionella* species; (2) protozoa: *Pneumocystis carinii, Toxoplasma gondii;* (3) viruses: cytomegalovirus; and (4) fungi: *Aspergillus* species. Prompt treatment of pneumonia syndromes with broad-spectrum coverage is necessary in these individuals. Failure to obtain a clinical response to empiric therapy should lead to aggressive attempts to obtain a definitive diagnosis (e.g., bronchioalveolar lavage and/or biopsy if needed). The development of *P. carinii* pneumonia or other opportunistic infections, or an unusually severe course in a usual pneumonia syndrome, should prompt consideration of an immunodeficiency syndrome or HIV infection.

References

1. Glezen WP, Denny FW: Epidemiology of acute lower respiratory tract disease in children, *N Engl J Med* 288:498-505, 1973.
2. Gwaltney JM Jr: Rhinovirus. In Mandell GL, Bennett JE, Dolin R, editors: *Principles and practices of infectious diseases,* New York, 1995, Churchill Livingstone.
3. D'Angelo L: Infectious disease problems in adolescents, *J Adolesc Health Care* 7:65S-81S, 1986.
4. Greenberg SB, Krilov LR: Laboratory diagnosis of viral respiratory diseases. In Drew WL, Rubin SJ, editors: Cumulative techniques and procedures in clinical microbiology, vol. 21, Washington, DC, 1986, American Society for Microbiology.
5. Schieble JH: Rhinoviruses and coronaviruses. In Lennette EH, Balows A, Hausler WJ Jr, Shadomy HJ, editors: *Manual of clinical microbiology,* Washington, DC, 1985, American Society for Microbiology.
6. Wiet RJ, DeBlanc GB, Stewart J, Dudley JW: Natural history of otitis media in the American native, *Ann Otol Rhinol Laryngol* 89 (suppl 68):14-19, 1980.
7. Randolph MF, Gerber MA, DeMeo KK, Wright L: Effect of antibiotic therapy on the clinical course of streptococcal pharyngitis, *J Pediatr* 106:870-875, 1985.

8. Pichichero ME, Disney FA, Talpey WB, et al: Adverse and beneficial effects of immediate treatment of group A beta-hemolytic streptococcal pharyngitis with penicillin, *Pediatr Infect Dis J* 6:635-643, 1987.

9. Gerber MA, Randolph MF, DeMeo KK, Kaplan EL: Lack of impact of early antibiotic therapy for streptococcal pharyngitis on recurrence rates, *J Pediatr* 117:853-858, 1990.

10. Gerber MA: Comparison of throat cultures and rapid strep tests for diagnosis of streptococcal pharyngitis, *Pediatr Infect Dis J* 8:820-824, 1989.

11. Schwartz RH, Wientzen RL, Grundfast KM: Sore throats in adolescents, *Pediatr Infect Dis J* 1:443-447, 1982.

12. Fried MP, Forrest JL: Peritonsillitis, *Arch Otolaryngol* 107:283-286, 1981.

13. Schwartz RH, Estroff T, Fairbanks DNF, Hoffman NG: Nasal symptoms associated with cocaine abuse during adolescence, *Arch Otolaryngol Head Neck Surg* 115:63-64, 1989.

14. Rosenfeld EA, Rowley AH: Infectious intracranial complications of sinusitis, other than meningitis, in children: 12-year review, *Clin Infect Dis* 18:750-754, 1994.

15. Wald ER: Microbiology of acute and chronic sinusitis, *Immunol Allergy Clin North Am* 14:31-45, 1994.

16. Greenberg SB, Krilov LR: Laboratory diagnosis of viral respiratory diseases. In Drew WL, Rubin SJ, editors: *Cumulative techniques and procedures in clinical microbiology,* vol 21, Washington, DC, 1986, American Society for Microbiology; pp 1-16.

17. Christie CDC, Marx ML, Marchant CD, Reising SF: The 1993 epidemic of pertussis in Cincinnati, *N Engl J Med* 331:16-21, 1994.

18. Dantzker DR, Pingleton SK, Pierce JA, other Task Force Members: Standards for the diagnosis and care of patients with chronic obstructive pulmonary disease and asthma—American Thoracic Society, *Am Rev Respir Dis* 136:225-244, 1987.

19. Reynolds HY: Respiratory infections may reflect deficiencies in host defense mechanisms, *Dis Month* 35:1-98, 1985.

20. Broughton RA: Infections due to *Mycoplasma pneumoniae* in childhood, *Pediatr Infect Dis* 5:71-85, 1986.

21. Mansel JK, Rosenow EC, Smith TF, Martin JW Jr: *Mycoplasma pneumoniae* pneumonia, *Chest* 95:639-646, 1989.

22. Kirby BD: Community acquired pneumonia, *Emerg Med Clin North Am* 3:179-189, 1985.

23. Feizl T: Cold agglutinins, the direct Coombs test and serum immunoglobulins in *Mycoplasma pneumoniae* infection, *Ann N Y Acad Sci* 143:801-812, 1967.

24. Grayston JT, Kuo CC, Wang SP, Altman J: A new *Chlamydia psittaci* strain TWAR, isolated in acute respiratory tract infections, *N Engl J Med* 316:161-168, 1986.

25. Saikks P, Wang SP, Kleemola M, et al: An epidemic of mild pneumonia due to an unusual strain of *Chlamydia psittaci, J Infect Dis* 151:832-839, 1985.

26. Hahn DL, Dodge RW, Golubjatnikov R: Association of *Chlamydia pneumonia* (strain TWAR) infection with wheezing, asthmatic bronchitis, and adult-onset asthma, *JAMA* 266:225-230, 1991.

27. Nemir RL, Krasinski K: Tuberculosis in children and adolescents in the 1980's, *Pediatr Infect Dis* 7:375-379, 1988.

28. Nemir RL: Perspectives in adolescent tuberculosis: three decades of experience, *Pediatrics* 78:399-405, 1986.

29. Glezen WP, Couch RB, Six HR: The influenza herald wave, *Am J Epidemiol* 116:589-598, 1982.

30. Arrowsmith JB, Kennedy DL, Kuritsky JN, Faich GA: National patterns of aspirin use and Reye syndrome reporting, United States, 1980 to 1985, *Pediatrics* 79:858-863, 1987.

31. Shulman ST, Bartlett J, Clyde WA Jr, et al: The unusual severity of mycoplasma pneumonia in children with sickle cell disease, *N Engl J Med* 287:164-167, 1972.

32. Pitchenik AE, Cole C, Russell BW, et al: Tuberculosis, atypical mycobacteriosis, and the acquired immunodeficiency syndrome among Haitian and non-Haitian patients in South Florida, *Ann Intern Med* 101:641-645, 1984.

CHAPTER 41

Asthma

•

Stephen Commins and Elliot F. Ellis

Although the clinician, the pulmonary physiologist, the immunologist, and the pathologist may all have different perspectives of asthma, a current working definition of the disease would include the following characteristics: (1) airway obstruction that is reversible (but not completely so in some patients with severe disease) either spontaneously or with treatment, (2) airway inflammation, and (3) increased airway responsiveness to a variety of stimuli. Since the mid-1980s, emphasis has shifted away from the long-held focus on bronchospasm as the major element in the airway obstructive process to a new appreciation of the inflammatory nature of the disease.[1]

EPIDEMIOLOGY

Asthma is a common illness, particularly during childhood and adolescence, affecting between 9 and 12 million individuals in the United States. The disease, which is a major cause of morbidity in children, is responsible for 25% of all school days missed due to chronic illness. School absence has a major impact on the academic achievement of children with asthma.[2,3] In the United States the total prevalence of active asthma is about 3%, whereas the cumulative prevalence is about 10.6%.[4] Various studies have shown that during the childhood years the prevalence of asthma in U.S. children is about 4% to 9%. From 1964 to 1980 the prevalence rate for children under 17 years of age was reported to have increased by as much as 50%.[4] During the past decade the prevalence has continued to increase disproportionately in younger individuals. In addition, hospitalizations for asthma are on the rise. From 1979 to 1987 hospitalization of children with asthma, ages 0 to 17 years, increased an average of 4.5% per year.[5] The greatest increase, 5% per year, occurred in children 0 to 4 years. In the latter group, hospitalization of black children increased at a rate 1.8 times that of white children. In 1983 it was reported that asthma and wheezing illness was one of the 10 most frequent reasons for visits to a pediatrician, accounting for 2.2 million visits.[6] By 1985 there were 4.5 million visits by children under 15 years of age to physicians' offices for treatment of asthma.[7] The cost of illness due to asthma in 1990 was estimated to be $6.2 billion; of this, approximately $1.6 billion was for inpatient hospital services, the largest single direct medical expenditure for this chronic disease.[8]

The cost of caring for a child with asthma, especially more severe disease, also may be substantial, consuming up to 33% of a family's income.[9] Asthma is the most common cause of hospitalization of children, responsible for 11% to 17% of all children hospitalized in urban U.S. communities.[10] Even more alarming is the reported increase in the mortality from asthma that has been occurring on a worldwide basis since the mid-1980s. During the 1970s, asthma mortality for both children and adults aged 5 to 34 years decreased by approximately 7.8% per year. However, during the 1980s this trend reversed, and mortality increased by 6.2% per year. The rate of increase was fastest in children aged 5 to 14 years and somewhat slower in individuals aged 15 to 34 years. From 1980 to 1987, total deaths from asthma in the United States increased from 2891 to 4360. This represents a 31% increase in mortality rate from 1.3 in 100,000 to 1.7 in 100,000.[11] Several areas have been identified by small-area geographic analysis to have persistently high mortality rates, including New York City and Chicago's Cook County. Poverty, nonwhite race, and living in an urban area appear to be the major determinants of both increased hospitalization and mortality. Several articles about death from asthma during the pediatric years have focused on adolescents who appear to be at special risk.[12-16] Thus, on the basis of prevalence and mortality, physicians specializing in adolescent medicine should have a substantial interest in and knowledge of this disorder.

During early childhood, asthma is more common in boys than in girls by a ratio of 3:2. As age approaches adolescence, the gender distribution disappears. For a long time, genetic factors have been known to play an important role in asthma. Twin studies have shown a significant concordance for asthma in monozygotic twins compared with dizygotic twins.[17] On the basis of population-based studies, there is ample evidence to show an increased prevalence of asthma in first-degree relatives of individuals with asthma. Atopy, usually defined as an increased predisposition to synthesize specific immuno-globulin E (IgE) antibodies against environmental allergens, and asthma are closely related. The prevalence of atopy in patients with asthma varies from approximately 20% to 80%, depending on the age of the population studied and the manner in which atopy and asthma are defined. A high proportion of children attending asthma clinics show evidence of IgE sensitization to house-dust mite.[18] Furthermore, the concentration of house-dust mite allergen in an infant's home is strongly correlated with the age of the first development of asthma.[19] Pedigree analysis of individuals with asthma with or without IgE-mediated allergy suggests that increased bronchial hyperresponsiveness—a finding characteristic of all patients with active asthma but not limited to such patients—and atopy are genetically determined but inherited independently of each other.

Viral respiratory tract infection plays a major role as a provocateur of asthma, especially in early life but also in adolescence.[20,21] The viral agents most often implicated as precipitants of wheezing illness are respiratory syncytial virus (RSV), parainfluenza virus, and rhinoviruses. RSV and parainfluenza are more important in early life, whereas rhinoviruses are more prevalent in older children and adolescents. The mechanism by which respiratory virus infection provokes asthma is not known. There is some evidence that, in infancy, wheezing that occurs during an RSV infection may be due to IgE-mediated sensitivity to the virus.[22] However, it is more likely, especially in older individuals, that mechanical perturbation of the respiratory tract epithelium by the viral infection, and exposure and stimulation of vagal afferent receptors, are the explanation for the viral effect.

PATHOPHYSIOLOGY

Airway obstruction and hyperresponsiveness of the airways are the cardinal features of asthma that are responsible for the signs and symptoms of the disease. The degree of hyperresponsiveness or hyperirritability of the airways varies according to the severity of the asthma. Children and adolescents with mild asthma may be symptom free, with entirely normal pulmonary function. Even after provocative challenge with methacholine, histamine, or exercise, there may be minimal to no evidence of airway hyperresponsiveness. However, as the degree of asthma increases, airway obstruction becomes evident on pulmonary function testing, and airway responsiveness generally increases. The airway obstruction in asthma is caused by a combination of smooth muscle spasm, increased mucus secretion, and inflammation. Airways of patients are infiltrated with inflammatory cells, particularly eosinophils and lymphocytes. There is disruption of the epithelial lining of the airway, with loss of the so-called epithelial relaxant factor, and mucosal edema due to increased permeability of blood vessels in the airways. Asthma results from a complex interaction that involves various inflammatory cells, their secretory products (chemical mediators—e.g., eosinophil-derived major basic protein, T lymphocyte–derived cytokines), airway epithelial cells, and the autonomic nervous system and its chemical messengers (neuropeptides).[1] Hyperresponsiveness of the airways, the hallmark of the disease, is defined as an exaggerated bronchoconstrictor response to many environmental factors of a physical, chemical, or pharmacologic nature. For example, people with asthma are exquisitely sensitive to environmental irritants such as tobacco smoke, sulfur dioxide, and ozone. Exposure to cold air and exercise also provoke bronchoconstriction in those with asthma but not in healthy individuals. Although the degree of hyperresponsiveness of the airways generally remains stable in a given patient over time, it may increase temporarily after exposure to an allergen to which the patient is sensitive. Studies of patients with asthma have shown a reasonably good correlation between the severity of disease, medication requirements, and degree of airway hyperresponsiveness. Despite much research, the mechanism of airway hyperresponsiveness in asthma is not completely understood, but it is closely linked to airway inflammation.

Assessment of airway hyperresponsiveness is accomplished in the pulmonary function laboratory by provocative inhalation challenges with methacholine (a congener of acetylcholine) or histamine, or by the use of nonpharmacologic stimuli such as cold dry air, hypotonic aerosols, and exercise. Measurement of the degree of diurnal fluctuation in the peak expiratory flow rate, with a peak flowmeter used in the morning on arising and at night, reflects the lability of airway function and serves as an indirect measure of the degree of hyperresponsiveness. The physiologic abnormalities secondary to airway obstruction in asthma include resistance to airflow, gas trapping behind obstructed airways, and mismatching of the normal relationship between ventilation and lung perfusion. As the airway obstruction increases, airways close at increasingly higher lung volumes, the functional residual capacity increases, and the patient breathes closer to total lung capacity. The hyperinflation that occurs enables airways to remain open and gas exchange to occur. However, this is a mechanically disadvantageous

situation, since the work of breathing increases markedly and fatigue ensues.

CLINICAL SPECTRUM IN CHILDHOOD AND ADOLESCENCE

Asthma may be looked upon as a spectrum of illness that begins in early life and in some cases persists throughout the entire life span. In most cases the first signs and symptoms of asthma appear during the first 2 years of life but often go unrecognized.[23] During middle childhood there is a tendency toward improvement that most likely occurs because of changes in airway geometry and development of elastic tissue. In children genetically predisposed to IgE sensitization, allergy skin tests become positive.

During adolescence, asthma presents special problems. There is often continued improvement in the severity of the disease in terms of less frequent or less severe symptoms, but in some instances there is substantial denial of symptoms on the part of the patient. Serious impairment of pulmonary function indicative of significant physiologic abnormalities may be observed in adolescents who claim that they are doing well. Adherence to medication regimens is a special problem at this time of life, when there is great concern about independence, body image, and the effects on physical appearance caused by some of the drugs used in treatment, particularly systemic steroids. In a 1995 study of medication use, adolescents with asthma indicated that they wanted complete responsibility for taking their medication without what they perceived as conflict with adults (parents, teachers, school nurses, and physicians) about medication use.[24] While adolescents with mild asthma do not differ from healthy adolescents in regard to emotional and/or behavioral problems, adolescents with mild and severe asthma were reported in 1995 to score higher on psychological tests that reflect irrational beliefs concerning the control of emotions.[25] Certain conditions occurring during adolescence, such as pregnancy, require special attention to ensure a favorable outcome.[26]

DIAGNOSIS AND EVALUATION

History

Fortunately, by adolescence, the signs and symptoms of asthma are sufficiently distinctive for the disorder to be easily diagnosed. As with other diseases, history taking is the most important element in establishing the diagnosis. Topics to be covered are itemized in Box 41-1. Of particular significance in establishing a diagnosis of asthma are the symptoms of cough, wheezing, and shortness of breath brought on by exercise—a circum-

BOX 41-1
Medical History of Asthma

I. Symptoms
   A. Cough, wheezing, shortness of breath, chest tightness, and sputum production (generally of modest degree)
   B. Conditions known to be associated with asthma, such as rhinitis, sinusitis, nasal polyposis, or atopic dermatitis
II. Pattern of symptoms
   A. Perennial, seasonal, or perennial with seasonal exacerbation
   B. Continuous, episodic, or continuous with acute exacerbations
   C. Onset, duration, and frequency of symptoms (days per week or month)
   D. Diurnal variation with special reference to nocturnal symptoms
III. Precipitating and/or aggravating factors
   A. Viral respiratory infections
   B. Exposure to environmental allergens (pollens, molds, house-dust mites, cockroaches, animal danders or secretory products [e.g., saliva])
   C. Environmental change (e.g., moving to a new home, going on vacation)
   D. Exposure to irritants, especially tobacco smoke and strong odors, air pollutants (ozone, sulfur dioxide, nitrous oxide)
   E. Emotional expressions: fear, anger, frustration, crying, hard laughing
   F. Family dysfunction (e.g., separation, divorce, alcoholism)
   G. Drugs (e.g., aspirin)
   H. Food additives (sulfites)
   I. Changes in weather, exposure to cold air
   J. Exercise
   K. Endocrine factors (e.g., menses)
IV. Development of disease
   A. Age of onset, age at diagnosis
   B. Progress of disease (better or worse)
   C. Previous evaluation, treatment, and response
   D. Present management and response, including plans for managing acute episodes
V. Profile of typical exacerbation
   A. Prodromal signs and symptoms (e.g., itching of skin of anterior neck, nasal allergy symptoms)
   B. Temporal progression
   C. Usual management
   D. Usual outcome
VI. Living situation
   A. Home age, location, cooling and heating (central heating with oil, electric, gas, or kerosene space heating), wood-burning fireplace

   B. Carpeting over a concrete slab
   C. Humidifier
   D. Description of patient's room with special attention to pillow, bed, floor covering, and dust collectors
   E. Animals in home
   F. Exposure to cigarette smoke in home
VII. Impact of disease
   A. Impact on patient
      1. Number of emergency department or urgent care visits and hospitalizations
      2. History of life-threatening acute exacerbations, intubation, or oral steroid therapy
      3. Number of school days missed, academic performance
      4. Limitation of activity, especially sports
      5. History of nocturnal awakening
      6. Effect on growth, development, behavior, peer relationships, school or work achievement, and life style
   B. Impact on family
      1. Disruption of family dynamics or routine, or restriction of activities
      2. Effect on siblings
      3. Economic impact
VIII. Assessment of family's and patient's perception of illness
   A. Patient and parental knowledge of asthma and belief in the chronicity of asthma and in the efficacy of treatment
   B. Ability of patient and parents to cope with disease
   C. Level of family support and patient's and parents' capacity to recognize severity of an exacerbation
   D. Economic resources
IX. Family history
   A. IgE-mediated allergy in close relatives
   B. Asthma in close relatives
X. Medical history
   A. General medical history and history of other allergic disorders (e.g., chronic rhinitis, atopic dermatitis, sinusitis, nasal polyps, gastrointestinal disturbances, adverse reactions to foods, drugs), history of early-life injury to the airways (e.g., bronchopulmonary dysplasia or severe pneumonia), viral bronchiolitis, recurrent croup, symptoms of gastroesophageal reflux, passive exposure to cigarette smoke
   B. Detailed review of symptoms

Modified from *Guidelines for the diagnosis and management of asthma*, NIH Publ. No. 91-3042, Bethesda, MD, 1991, National Institutes of Health.

stance unique to asthma and only a few other childhood lung disorders. For reasons that are unclear, some adolescents experience exercise-induced bronchoconstriction and a feeling of tightness without any coughing and wheezing, and this may be the only presenting symptom of the disease. Generally there is a relationship between the degree of exercise-induced bronchoconstriction and the severity of the disease. Adolescents who have moderate to severe asthma are often very limited in terms of exercise tolerance. The nocturnal symptoms of coughing and wheezing, which also are related to the severity of disease, are present in a high proportion of individuals who suffer from asthma.

Persistent cough (in the non–cigarette smoking adolescent), particularly that brought on by exercise and occurring at night or during the early hours of the morning, is characteristic of asthma. Chronic bronchitis, part of the chronic obstructive pulmonary disease clinical spectrum in adults, is not a recognizable entity during the adolescent years in the absence of underlying disease, such as cystic fibrosis, ciliary dyskinesia, or B-cell immunologic deficiency disease. Cough tic typically occurs in boys beginning in late childhood and early adolescence. The cough that is "honking" in nature has been compared to the cry of Canadian geese and is very distressing to the patients and those around them. The clue to diagnosis is the fact that the cough disappears during sleep. Cigarette smoking is a well-known airway irritant causing coughing, particularly in individuals with asthma.

Physical Examination

The physical examination focuses on the upper respiratory tract and the chest. Evidence of chronic rhinitis and sinusitis should be sought, since either could have an adverse effect on the course of the asthma. Lung findings depend on the activity of the asthma and its chronicity. During an acute exacerbation the examiner assesses the patient's ability to talk (i.e., complete sentences or only a few words at a time), the presence of cyanosis, the use of accessory muscles, pulsus paradoxus, and air exchange. If the adolescent is examined when free of symptoms, chest findings may be entirely normal. However, the finding of a hyperinflated thorax with an increase in the anteroposterior diameter of the chest always indicates chronic asthma or another severe obstructive airway problem (e.g., cystic fibrosis) with air trapping. Other stigmata of chronic severe asthma include a square configuration of the chest, a prominent Harrison's groove, and distant breath sounds. True clubbing of the fingers is extremely rare in patients with asthma. When clubbing is observed in a patient suspected of having asthma, other chronic lung disorders, such as cystic fibrosis or other suppurative lung disorders, must be excluded.

Radiographic Examination

A chest radiograph, including both posteroanterior and lateral views, is always indicated in the initial evaluation of an adolescent with asthma. According to the severity of the disease, the radiographic findings may vary from being entirely normal to showing increased lung markings or signs of air trapping (hyperlucency, flattening of the diaphragm, increased anteroposterior diameter, horizontal position of the ribs). Atelectasis, particularly involving the right middle lobe of the lung, is common during early life but rarely seen in adolescence. If concomitant sinusitis is suspected (common in individuals with allergies), sinus radiography or (preferably) a computed tomographic scan of the sinuses should be obtained. Symptoms indicative of gastroesophageal reflux, which may worsen asthma, suggest the need for a barium swallow as an initial procedure.

Pulmonary Function Testing

Pulmonary function testing, which most often consists of only simple spirometry, is an essential part of the evaluation of an adolescent with suspected asthma. If the results show impairment of expiratory airflow, the test should be repeated 15 or 20 minutes after administration of an aerosolized bronchodilator. Measurement of forced vital capacity (FVC), forced expiratory volume in one second (FEV-1), and forced expiratory flow between 25% and 75% of the vital capacity (FEF^{25-75}), together with inspection of the expiratory flow volume curve, provides all the necessary information, except for patients with severe disease, who may require more sophisticated tests to measure lung volumes and gas mixing. Particularly valuable for the day-to-day monitoring of pulmonary function at home is the use of a peak flowmeter, which measures expiratory flow rate and provides a longitudinal assessment of the diurnal degree of airway obstruction and airway stability.

Bronchial Provocation Testing

Bronchial provocation testing, involving the use of either an allergen or pharmacologic agents such as methacholine or histamine, is rarely indicated for the diagnosis of asthma in adolescents. Occasionally, an adolescent is seen who has atypical signs and symptoms of asthma (e.g., a persistent cough) with a normal physical examination and normal spirometric reading. A methacholine or histamine challenge is useful to determine whether such a patient has bronchial hyperresponsiveness, a cardinal finding in all patients with active asthma.[27]

Laboratory Evaluation

A total blood eosinophil count and measurement of serum IgE are often useful in establishing an adolescent's atopic predisposition. Increased serum IgE concentrations or eosinophilia are considered to be markers of an atopic constitution. Cytologic study of nasal secretions is useful for the diagnosis of allergic rhinitis and sinusitis. In allergic rhinitis the nasal smear shows predominantly eosinophils, whereas in sinusitis neutrophils and bacteria predominate, with few (if any) eosinophils noted.

Determination of Specific IgE Antibodies

Adolescents with asthma should undergo an evaluation to determine the role that IgE-mediated allergy plays in their disease. This is most conveniently done by allergy skin testing, using the prick (puncture) technique, with a reasonable number of common inhalant allergens. Skin testing of reactions to foods is rarely indicated. An alternative to allergy skin testing is the determination of specific IgE antibodies by an in vitro technique. Many such techniques are available, but the radioallergosorbent test (RAST) is best known. There is a consensus among allergists that a properly performed and correctly interpreted skin test is preferable to any of the in vitro tests. The results of both the allergy skin test and the in vitro tests must be interpreted in light of the patient's clinical history.

Differential Diagnosis

The differential diagnosis of asthma during adolescence is relatively limited compared with that during early life. There are very few lung conditions that can be confused with asthma. Chronic bronchitis rarely exists as a primary diagnosis during the pediatric years, except in the presence of an underlying disease such as cystic fibrosis, humoral antibody deficiency syndrome, or ciliary dyskinesia. Although it is unlikely, it is conceivable that an adolescent who smokes cigarettes or marijuana excessively could develop a degree of bronchitis with coughing that might be confused with asthma. However, this would be distinctly unusual. Similarly, gastroesophageal reflux as a cause of persistent coughing is rare during the adolescent years. However, in an older child who complains of dysphagia or heartburn, a gastroesophageal reflux study is indicated.

MANAGEMENT

The goal of asthma management is to achieve a degree of control of symptoms that will allow the adolescent to enjoy as normal a life style as possible. This goal can be reached by (1) reducing the number of acute episodes of coughing and wheezing, (2) improving the capacity to engage in exercise and even competitive sports unrestricted by exercise-induced bronchoconstriction, (3) enabling attendance at school on a regular basis, (4) providing uninterrupted sleep through the night (i.e., by control of coughing and wheezing), and (5) minimizing use of the hospital and other urgent care facilities. Reduction of the degree of bronchial hyperresponsiveness and normalization of pulmonary function as much as possible are also important goals. In most cases, these goals can be accomplished without causing significant adverse effects from the therapeutic agents prescribed.

Since all individuals with active asthma have "irritable" airways, treatment of this condition begins with avoidance of irritants such as tobacco smoke, strong odors, and irritant fumes, and exposure to cold air and allergens. In particular, avoidance of house-dust mite exposure by implementation of strict environmental control measures, particularly in the adolescent's bedroom, has been shown to have a very significant effect in reducing both specific and nonspecific bronchial hyperresponsiveness.[18] Immunotherapy, formerly known as hyposensitization or desensitization, plays a role in the management of an adolescent with asthma when allergens cannot be avoided easily.

Pharmacotherapy is the main modality utilized in the treatment of asthma, and a rational approach to pharmacotherapy requires that the physician attempt to match treatment with severity of disease. Therefore, a method of classifying asthma according to the severity of illness needs to be used. One such method, generated by the Expert Panel of the National Asthma Education Program (NAEP), has proved very useful (Table 41-1). The modern approach to asthma therapy focuses on the important role that inflammation plays in the obstructive airway process, particularly in patients with significant disease. Asthma medications are viewed according to their function—as bronchodilators or as antiinflammatory agents. Unfortunately, except possibly for theophylline, no agents available have both antiinflammatory and bronchodilating functions. Figure 41-1 shows an overview of the therapy described in the NAEP report.[28]

Treatment of Acute Asthma

Treatment of acute asthma is directed toward reversing the obstructive airway process as quickly as possible. The drug of choice for this purpose is an inhaled beta$_2$-agonist bronchodilator. Albuterol is most widely used because of its efficacy and safety. An outline for the home management of an acute exacerbation developed by the Expert Panel of the NAEP is seen in Figure 41-2. The management protocol makes use of

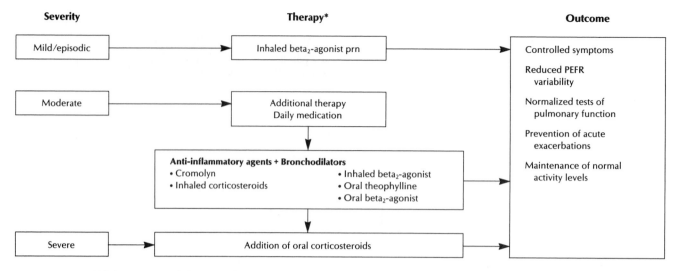

Severity	Therapy*	Outcome
Mild/episodic	→ Inhaled beta₂-agonist prn →	Controlled symptoms

*All therapy must include patient education about prevention (including environmental control where appropriate) as well as control of symptoms. PEFR, peak expiratory flow rate.

Fig. 41-1. Overview of therapy for management of asthma. (Modified from *Guidelines for the diagnosis and management of asthma,* NIH Publ. No. 91-3042, Bethesda, MD, 1991, National Institutes of Health.)

TABLE 41-1
Classification of Asthma by Severity of Disease

Characteristics	Mild	Moderate	Severe
Before Treatment			
Frequency of exacerbations	Exacerbations of cough and wheezing no more often than 1-2 times/wk.	Exacerbation of cough and wheezing on more frequent basis than 1-2 times/wk. Could have history of severe exacerbations, but infrequent. Urgent care treatment in hospital emergency department or doctor's office <3 times/yr.	Virtually daily wheezing. Exacerbations frequent, often severe. Tendency to have sudden severe exacerbations. Urgent visits to hospital emergency departments or doctor's office >3 times/yr. Hospitalization >2 times/yr, perhaps with respiratory insufficiency or (rarely) respiratory failure and history of intubation. May have had cough syncope or hypoxic seizures.
Frequency of symptoms	Few clinical signs or symptoms between exacerbations.	Cough and low-grade wheezing between acute exacerbations often present.	Continuous low-grade cough and wheezing almost always present.
Degree of exercise tolerance	Good exercise tolerance but may not tolerate vigorous exercise, especially prolonged running.	Exercise tolerance diminished.	Very poor exercise tolerance with marked limitation of activity.
Frequency of nocturnal asthma	Symptoms of nocturnal asthma occur no more often than 1-2 times/mo.	Symptoms of nocturnal asthma present 2-3 times/wk.	Considerable, almost nightly sleep interruption due to asthma; chest tight in early morning.
School or work attendance	Good school or work attendance.	School or work attendance may be affected.	Poor school or work attendance.

TABLE 41-1
Classification of Asthma by Severity of Disease—cont'd

Characteristics	Mild	Moderate	Severe
Pulmonary Function			
PEFR	PEFR >80%, predicted variability† <20%.	PEFR 60% to 80% predicted. Variability 20% to 30%.	PEFR <60% predicted. Variability >30%.
Spirometry	Minimal or no evidence of airway obstruction on spirometry. Normal expiratory flow volume curve; lung volumes not increased. Usually a 15% response to acute aerosol bronchodilator administration, even though baseline near normal.	Signs of airway obstruction on spirometry are evident. Flow volume curve shows reduced expiratory flow at low lung volumes. Lung volumes often increased. Usually a >15% response to acute bronchodilator administration.	Substantial degree of airway obstruction on spirometry. Flow-volume curve shows marked concavity. Spirometry may not be normalized even with high-dose steroids. May have substantial increase in lung volumes and marked unevenness of ventilation. Incomplete reversibility to acute aerosol bronchodilator administration.
Methacholine sensitivity	>20 mg/ml	2-20 mg/ml	<2 mg/ml
After Optimal Treatment			
Response to and duration of therapy	Exacerbations respond to bronchodilators without use of systemic corticosteroids in 12-24 hr. Regular drug therapy not usually required except for short periods.	Periodic use of bronchodilators needed during exacerbations for 1 wk or more. Systemic steroids may be needed for exacerbations. Continuous (around-the-clock) drug therapy required. Regular use of antiinflammatory agents may be needed for prolonged periods.	Requires continuous (around-the-clock) multiple drug therapy, including daily steroids, either aerosol or systemic, often in high doses.

Modified from *Guidelines for the diagnosis and management of asthma,* NIH Publ. No. 91-3042, Bethesda, MD, 1991, National Institute of Health.
PEFR, peak expiratory flow rate.
†Variability means the difference either (1) between a morning and evening measure or (2) among morning peak flow measurements.

peak expiratory flow measurements to guide parents in management of the attack. The importance of early administration of corticosteroids for the adolescent who is incompletely responsive to repeated administration of aerosolized beta$_2$-agonists is well documented in the medical literature and must be emphasized.[29,30] It is abundantly clear that early use of steroids reduces the need for emergency department visits and hospitalization, shortens the duration of illness, and prevents relapses in individuals with acute asthma. Physicians who treat children and adolescents need to overcome their "steroidophobia."

A protocol for emergency department management is outlined in Figure 41-3, and another for hospital management is presented in Figure 41-4. In each instance there is escalation of therapy in a stepwise manner according to the severity of asthma. Reports have shown that intravenous aminophylline, for years part of the acute management protocol in hospital emergency departments, adds little but adverse effects to patients who receive optimal inhaled bronchodilator therapy.[31] However, for the patient who is relatively unresponsive to aerosol therapy and needs to be hospitalized for more intensive treatment, intravenous aminophylline should still be tried, although the final word is not in yet. Continuous nebulization of albuterol in higher-than-usual

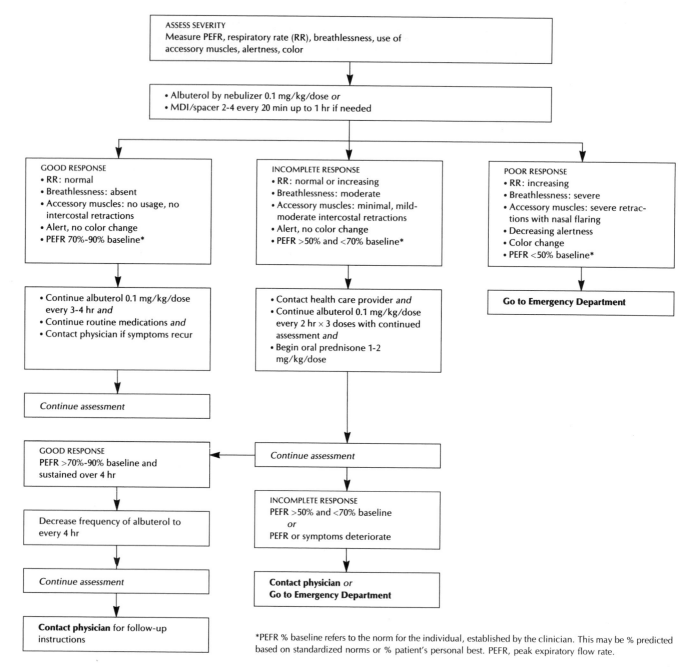

Fig. 41-2. Home management of acute exacerbations of asthma in children and adolescents. (Modified from *Guidelines for the diagnosis and management of asthma,* NIH Publ. No. 91-3042, Bethesda, MD, 1991, National Institutes of Health.)

doses—up to 0.5 mg/kg/hr to a maximum of 15 mg/hr—is often successful in relieving bronchoconstriction. (The usual dose is 0.15 mg/kg every 1 to 2 hours.) In addition, the administration of high doses of corticosteroids (1 to 2 mg/kg/day initially, in divided doses) is essential.

Day-to-Day Management

It is the day-to-day management of adolescents with asthma that keeps them out of the emergency department and the hospital. There have been several excellent reviews of the management of asthma.[1,32-36] Today the need for hospitalization for an acute exacerbation of asthma almost always (except in adolescents with the most severe disease) represents failure of ambulatory management. Since acute asthma is the most common cause of admission to most children's hospitals, enormous savings can be achieved by the application of established asthma management principles.[10]

Protocols from the NAEP report for management of children and adolescents with mild, moderate, and severe

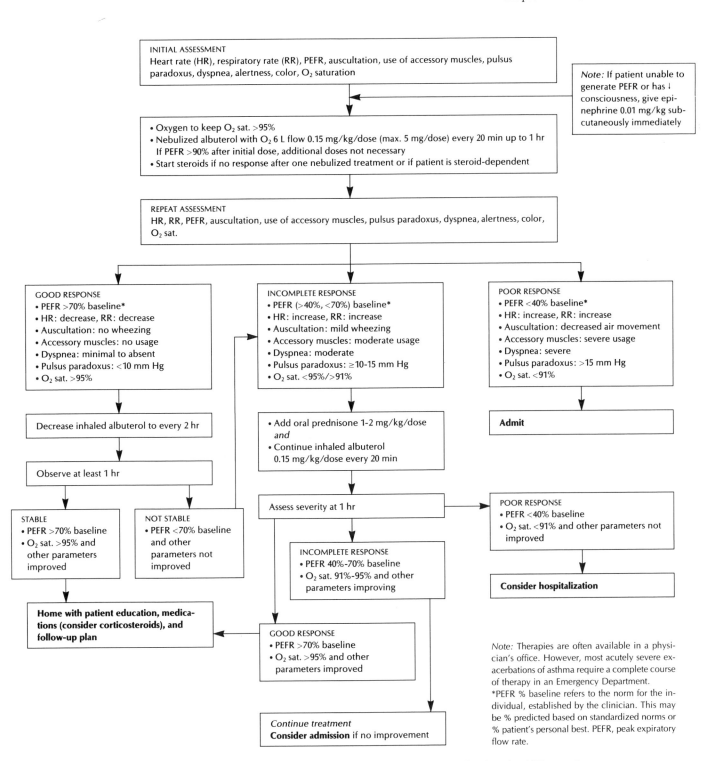

Fig. 41-3. Emergency department management of acute exacerbations of asthma in children and adolescents. (Modified from *Guidelines for the diagnosis and management of asthma*, NIH Publ. No. 91-3042, Bethesda, MD, 1991, National Institutes of Health.)

asthma, as defined in Table 41-1, are shown in Figures 41-5 to 41-7. Essentially, pharmacotherapy involves a stepwise approach according to the severity of disease (Table 41-1). Many adolescents with mild, intermittent asthma can be treated simply via inhalation of an aerosolized adrenergic bronchodilator, such as albuterol, as needed. The aerosol route of administration is greatly

preferred to the oral route because of the more rapid onset of action, better efficacy at a substantially lower dose, and hence fewer adverse effects.

For patients with more persistent symptoms, impaired exercise tolerance, and nocturnal symptoms of cough and wheezing, additional therapy may be needed in the form of a sustained-release theophylline product administered

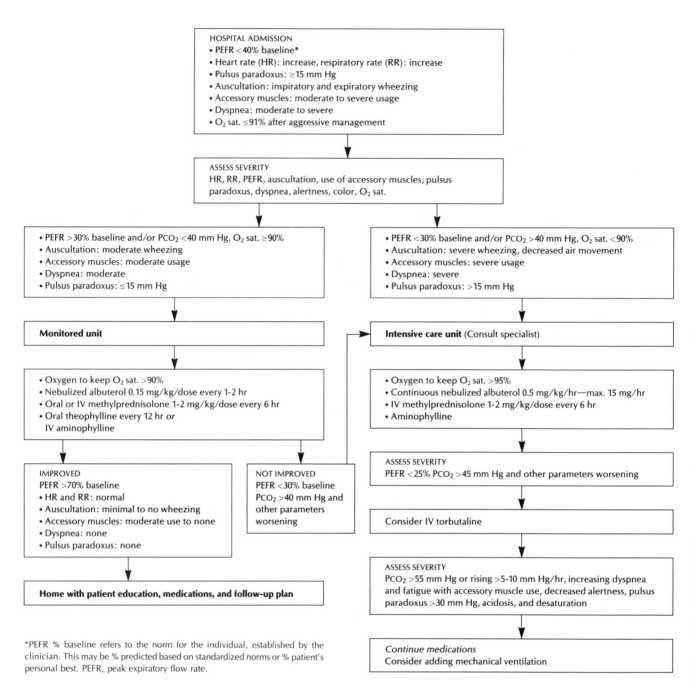

HOSPITAL ADMISSION
• PEFR <40% baseline*
• Heart rate (HR): increase, respiratory rate (RR): increase
• Pulsus paradoxus: ≥15 mm Hg
• Auscultation: inspiratory and expiratory wheezing
• Accessory muscles: moderate to severe usage
• Dyspnea: moderate to severe
• O₂ sat. ≤91% after aggressive management

ASSESS SEVERITY
HR, RR, PEFR, auscultation, use of accessory muscles, pulsus paradoxus, dyspnea, alertness, color, O₂ sat.

• PEFR >30% baseline and/or PCO₂ <40 mm Hg, O₂ sat. ≥90%
• Auscultation: moderate wheezing
• Accessory muscles: moderate usage
• Dyspnea: moderate
• Pulsus paradoxus: ≤15 mm Hg

• PEFR <30% baseline and/or PCO₂ >40 mm Hg, O₂ sat. <90%
• Auscultation: severe wheezing, decreased air movement
• Accessory muscles: severe usage
• Dyspnea: severe
• Pulsus paradoxus: >15 mm Hg

Monitored unit

Intensive care unit (Consult specialist)

• Oxygen to keep O₂ sat. >90%
• Nebulized albuterol 0.15 mg/kg/dose every 1-2 hr
• Oral or IV methylprednisolone 1-2 mg/kg/dose every 6 hr
• Oral theophylline every 12 hr or IV aminophylline

• Oxygen to keep O₂ sat. >95%
• Continuous nebulized albuterol 0.5 mg/kg/hr—max. 15 mg/hr
• IV methylprednisolone 1-2 mg/kg/dose every 6 hr
• Aminophylline

IMPROVED
PEFR >70% baseline
• HR and RR: normal
• Auscultation: minimal to no wheezing
• Accessory muscles: moderate use to none
• Dyspnea: none
• Pulsus paradoxus: none

NOT IMPROVED
PEFR <30% baseline
PCO₂ >40 mm Hg and other parameters worsening

ASSESS SEVERITY
PEFR <25% PCO₂ >45 mm Hg and other parameters worsening

Consider IV torbutaline

Home with patient education, medications, and follow-up plan

ASSESS SEVERITY
PCO₂ >55 mm Hg or rising >5-10 mm Hg/hr, increasing dyspnea and fatigue with accessory muscle use, decreased alertness, pulsus paradoxus >30 mm Hg, acidosis, and desaturation

*PEFR % baseline refers to the norm for the individual, established by the clinician. This may be % predicted based on standardized norms or % patient's personal best. PEFR, peak expiratory flow rate.

Continue medications
Consider adding mechanical ventilation

Fig. 41-4. Hospital management of acute exacerbations of asthma in children and adolescents. (Modified from *Guidelines for the diagnosis and management of asthma,* NIH Publ. No. 91-3042, Bethesda, MD, 1991, National Institutes of Health.)

twice a day (Slo-bid and Theo-Dur are the most widely prescribed), cromolyn (Intal), or nedocromil (Tilade) three or four times a day. Salmeterol, a long-acting β₂ agonist or Volmax, an extended release albuterol tablet may be used advantageously for nocturnal asthma. The availability of a new generation of inhaled corticosteroids has simplified the treatment of adolescents with more significant asthma signs and symptoms. These inhaled agents are very effective in suppressing the inflammatory component of asthma and are indicated in the drug

regimen of all adolescents who have moderate to severe asthma. Growth retardation, which may be observed in adolescents with asthma, is most commonly due to a delay in onset of puberty, rather than aerosol corticosteroid administration. Budesonide, in a dose of 600 µg/day, has not been shown to affect linear growth in adolescents with asthma.[37] Adolescent girls, for unknown reasons, are often the most challenging to treat. With individualization of therapy and the use of home monitoring of peak flow rate, most of these patients can be successfully managed.

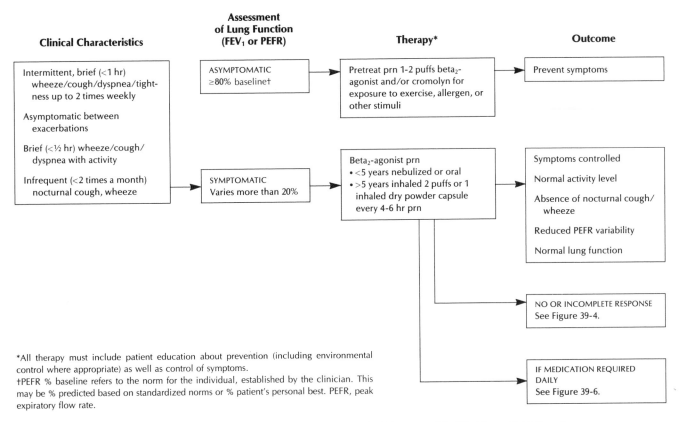

| Clinical Characteristics | Assessment of Lung Function (FEV$_1$ or PEFR) | Therapy* | Outcome |

Fig. 41-5. Management of mild asthma in children and adolescents. (Modified from *Guidelines for the diagnosis and management of asthma,* NIH Publ. No. 91-3042, Bethesda, MD, 1991, National Institutes of Health.)

ASTHMA EDUCATION

Since the mid-1980s, there has been considerable interest in the development of programs designed to teach families about asthma and to help them develop the skills and confidence to manage the disease in cooperation with their physician.[38,39] There is a consensus among health care providers who treat children and adolescents with asthma that the more the family and the child (or adolescent) know about the disease, the better will be the outcome. Fundamentally, the programs, most of which have been developed under the auspices of the National Heart, Lung, and Blood Institute, have a number of common elements. Topics covered during the 4- to 8-hour learning sessions include (1) the pathophysiology of asthma, (2) environmental control, (3) proper use of medication, (4) management of physical activities, and (5) communication with health care providers and school personnel. Although these are often referred to as self-management programs, close cooperation with the child's physician is encouraged.

The programs all seek to increase adherence to prescribed medical regimens and thus reduce morbidity. Families are taught skills to increase their confidence in making judgments about the severity of an acute attack and when to initiate appropriate intervention. Use of the peak flowmeter at home is emphasized as a tool for assessing the severity of an attack and for following the day-to-day course of the illness. Outcome evaluation of the success of asthma education programs suggests that families benefit by acquiring knowledge about asthma that better enables them to handle the illness with less fear and stress and with greater confidence in their skills to manage various aspects of the disease. For the most part, in children and adolescents enrolled in the programs, there have been decreased morbidity, less utilization of emergency department and hospital resources, and improved school attendance and achievement.*

PROGNOSIS

The prognosis for asthma that occurs during the childhood years is excellent. However, long-term studies of airway responsiveness in patients with asthma, some of

---

*Further information about asthma education programs can be obtained by writing to Asthma Programs, National Heart, Lung, and Blood Institute, Building 31-4A-21, Bethesda, MD 20892.

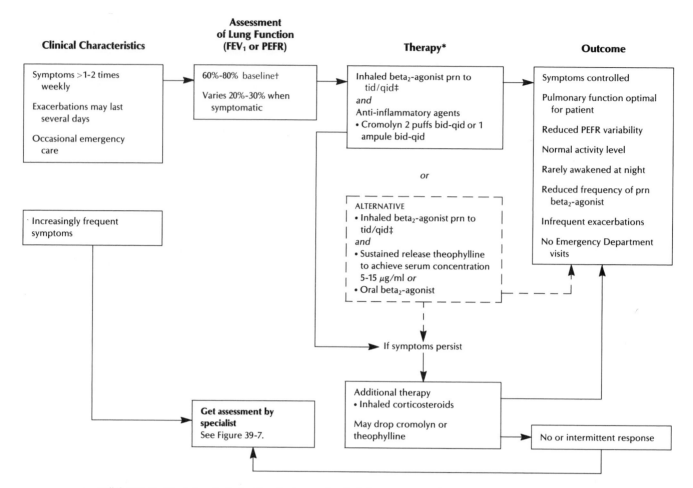

Fig. 41-6. Management of moderate asthma in children and adolescents. (Modified from *Guidelines for the diagnosis and management of asthma*, NIH Publ. No. 91-3042, Bethesda, MD, 1991, National Institutes of Health.)

whom have been asymptomatic for many years, show that airway hyperresponsiveness, as reflected by heightened methacholine responsiveness, remains abnormal for indefinite periods.[40] A number of prospective studies have provided insight into the natural history of asthma in childhood.[41-43]

In a child health and education study conducted in Great Britain, which included 2345 children who had had at least one wheezing episode before their fifth birthday, 80% were free of wheezing by 10 years of age. Only 8% of children who had a single attack of wheezing by 5 years of age continued to wheeze into their tenth year.[42] The more episodes of wheezing the child had by age 5 years, the greater was the risk of continuing wheezing at the age of 10.

The most noteworthy longitudinal study on the natural history of asthma was reported by investigators at the Royal Children's Hospital in Melbourne.[43] In a prospective study of 331 randomly selected children between the ages of 7 and 21 years who were examined both clinically and physiologically, the authors showed that most children with asthma tended to improve during adolescence. Over 50% of subjects whose wheezing began before 7 years of age, and then ceased before adolescence, remained free of wheezing. Of the subjects who seemingly ceased wheezing at 14 years, 45% had minor occurrences between ages 14 and 21 years. Fewer than 20% of children who wheezed persistently during childhood became totally free of wheezing during adolescence. Thus, persistent wheezing during the childhood years is a marker of unfavorable prognosis. It is among this group that will be found a small number of adolescents who have persistent peripheral airway obstruction that is not reversible even after several weeks of high-dose systemic corticosteroid therapy.[44]

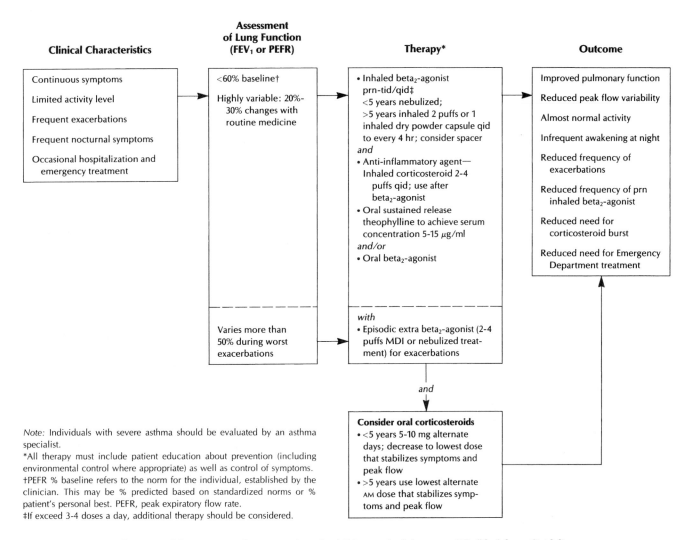

Clinical Characteristics

Continuous symptoms

Limited activity level

Frequent exacerbations

Frequent nocturnal symptoms

Occasional hospitalization and emergency treatment

Assessment of Lung Function (FEV$_1$ or PEFR)

<60% baseline†

Highly variable: 20%-30% changes with routine medicine

Varies more than 50% during worst exacerbations

Therapy*

• Inhaled beta$_2$-agonist prn-tid/qid‡
  <5 years nebulized;
  >5 years inhaled 2 puffs or 1 inhaled dry powder capsule qid to every 4 hr; consider spacer
  and
• Anti-inflammatory agent— Inhaled corticosteroid 2-4 puffs qid; use after beta$_2$-agonist
• Oral sustained release theophylline to achieve serum concentration 5-15 μg/ml
  and/or
• Oral beta$_2$-agonist

with
• Episodic extra beta$_2$-agonist (2-4 puffs MDI or nebulized treatment) for exacerbations

and

Consider oral corticosteroids
• <5 years 5-10 mg alternate days; decrease to lowest dose that stabilizes symptoms and peak flow
• >5 years use lowest alternate AM dose that stabilizes symptoms and peak flow

Outcome

Improved pulmonary function

Reduced peak flow variability

Almost normal activity

Infrequent awakening at night

Reduced frequency of exacerbations

Reduced frequency of prn inhaled beta$_2$-agonist

Reduced need for corticosteroid burst

Reduced need for Emergency Department treatment

Note: Individuals with severe asthma should be evaluated by an asthma specialist.
*All therapy must include patient education about prevention (including environmental control where appropriate) as well as control of symptoms.
†PEFR % baseline refers to the norm for the individual, established by the clinician. This may be % predicted based on standardized norms or % patient's personal best. PEFR, peak expiratory flow rate.
‡If exceed 3-4 doses a day, additional therapy should be considered.

Fig. 41-7. Management of severe asthma in children and adolescents. (Modified from *Guidelines for the diagnosis and management of asthma,* NIH Publ. No. 91-3042, Bethesda, MD, 1991, National Institutes of Health.)

References

1. Barnes PJ: A new approach to the treatment of asthma, *N Engl J Med* 321:1517-1527, 1989.
2. Mak H, Johnston P, Abbey H, et al: Morbidity and school absence caused by asthma and wheezing illness, *J Allergy Clin Immunol* 70:367-372, 1982.
3. Parcel GS, Gilman SC, Nader PR, et al: A comparison of absentee rates of elementary school children with asthma and non-asthmatic schoolmates, *Pediatrics* 64:878-881, 1979.
4. Gergen PJ, Mullally DI, Evans R III: National survey of prevalence of asthma among children in the United States, 1976-1980, *Pediatrics* 81:1-7, 1988.
5. Gergen PJ, Weiss KB: Changing patterns of asthma hospitalization among children, 1979-1987, *JAMA* 264:1688-1692, 1990.
6. Cypress BK: Patterns of ambulatory care in pediatrics: The National Ambulatory Care Survey, *Vital Health Stat* 75:1-60, 1983.
7. National Center for Health Statistics: *Economic costs of respiratory diseases,* Washington, DC, 1986, U.S. Government Printing Office.
8. Weiss KB, Gergen PJ, Hodgson TA: An economic evaluation of asthma in the United States, *N Engl J Med* 326:862-866, 1992.
9. Creer TL, Lewis PD, Cottrell C, Marion PJ: The prevalence and cost of childhood asthma, *Am J Asthma Allergy for Pediatricians* 3:90-96, 1990.
10. Parent JM, Homer CJ, Berwick DM, Woolf AD, Freeman JL, Wennberg JE: Variations of rates of hospitalizations of children in three urban communities, *N Engl J Med* 320:1183-1187, 1989.
11. Centers for Disease Control. Asthma—United States, 1980-1987, *MMWR* 39:493-497, 1990.
12. Rubinstein S, Hindi RD, Moss RB, Blessing-Moore J, Lewiston N: Sudden death in adolescent asthma, *Ann Allergy* 53:311-318, 1984.
13. Strunk RC, Mrazek DA, Fuhrmann GS, LaBrecque JF: Physiologic and psychological characteristics associated with deaths due to asthma in childhood, *JAMA* 254:1193-1198, 1985.
14. Chandler MJ, Grammer LC, Patterson R: Noncompliance and prevarication in life threatening adolescent asthma, *NER Allergy Proc* 7:367-370, 1986.
15. Strunk RC: Workshop on identification of the fatality-prone patient with asthma: proceedings of the Allergy Mortality Task Force, *J Allergy Clin Immunol* 50:455-457, 1987.
16. Niggemann B, Wahn U: Three cases of adolescent near-fatal asthma: what do they have in common?, *J Asthma* 29:217-220, 1992.
17. Edfors-Lubs ML: Allergy in 7000 twin pairs, *Acta Allergol* 26:249-285, 1971.

18. Murray AB, Ferguson AC: Dust-free bedrooms in the treatment of asthmatic children with house dust or house dust mite allergy: a controlled trial, *Pediatrics* 71:418-422, 1983.

19. Sporik R, Holgate S, Platts-Mills TA, Cogswell JJ: Exposure to house dust mite allergen (Der p I) and the development of asthma in childhood, *N Engl J Med* 323:502-507, 1990.

20. McIntosh K, Ellis EF, Hoffman LS, et al: The association of viral and bacterial respiratory infections with exacerbations of wheezing in young asthmatic children, *J Pediatr* 82:578-590, 1973.

21. Minor TE, Dick EC, DeMeo AN, et al: Viruses as precipitants of asthmatic attacks in children, *JAMA* 227:292-298, 1974.

22. Welliver RC, Wong DT, Sum M, et al: The development of respiratory syncytial virus–specific IgE and the release of histamine in nasopharyngeal secretions after infection, *N Engl J Med* 305:841-846, 1981.

23. Speight AN, Lee DA, Hey EN: Underdiagnosis and undertreatment of asthma in childhood, *Br Med J* 286:1253-1256, 1983.

24. Bussing R, Halfon N, Benjamin B, et al: Prevalence of behavior problems in U.S. children with asthma, *Arch Pediatr Adolesc Med* 149:565-572, 1995.

25. Slack MK, Brooks AJ: Medication management issues for adolescents with asthma, *Am J Health-Syst Pharm* 52:1417-1421, 1995.

26. Apter AJ, Greenberger PA, Patterson R: Outcomes of pregnancy in adolescents with severe asthma, *Arch Intern Med* 149:2571-2575, 1989.

27. Shapiro G: Bronchial provocative challenge in children with lower respiratory disease, *Pediatrician* 18:269-279, 1991.

28. *Guidelines for the diagnosis and management of asthma,* NIH Publ. No. 91-3042, Bethesda, MD, 1995, National Institutes of Health.

29. Harris JB, Weinberger MM, Nassif E, Smith G, Milavetz G, Stillerman A: Early intervention with short courses of prednisone to prevent progression of asthma in ambulatory patients incompletely responsive to bronchodilators, *J Pediatr* 110:627-633, 1987.

30. Chapman KR, Verbeek PR, White JG, Rebuck AS: Effect of a short course of prednisone in the prevention of early relapse after the emergency room treatment of acute asthma, *N Engl J Med* 324:788-794, 1991.

31. Littenberg B: Aminophylline treatment in acute severe asthma, *JAMA* 259:1678-1684, 1988.

32. Ellis EF: Asthma: current therapeutic approach, *Pediatr Clin North Am* 35:1041-1052, 1988.

33. Warner JO, Gotz M, Landau LI, Levison H, Milner AD, Pedersen S, Silverman M: Management of asthma: a consensus statement, *Arch Dis Child* 64:1065-1079, 1989.

34. Hargreave FE, Dolovich J, Newhouse MT: The assessment and treatment of asthma: a conference report, *J Allergy Clin Immunol* 85:1098-1111, 1990.

35. Treatment of pediatric asthma: a Canadian consensus, The Medicine Publishing Foundation Symposium Series, 29, Toronto, September 1990.

36. Isles AF, Robertson CF: Treatment of asthma in children and adolescents: the need for a different approach, *Med J Aust* 158:761-763, 1993.

37. Merkus PJFM, van Essen-Zandvliet, Duiverman EJ, van Houwelingen HC, et al: Long-term effect of inhaled corticosteroids on growth rate in adolescents with asthma, *Pediatrics* 91:1121-1126, 1993.

38. Evans D, Mellins R: Educational programs for children with asthma, *Pediatrician* 18:317-323, 1991.

39. Tehan N, Sloane BC, Walsh-Robert N, et al: Impact of asthma self-management education on the health behavior of young adults. A pilot study of the Dartmouth College "Breathe Free" program, *J Adolesc Health Care* 10:513-519, 1989.

40. Townley RG, Ryo RG, Kolothin BN, Kang B: Bronchial sensitivity to methacholine in current and former asthmatic and allergic rhinitis patients and controlled subjects, *J Allergy Clin Immunol* 56:429-442, 1975.

41. Kelly WJ, Hudson I, Phelan PD, et al: Childhood asthma in adult life: a further study at 28 years of age, *Br Med J* 294:1059-1062, 1987.

42. Park ES, Golding J, Carswell F, Stewart-Brown S: Preschool wheezing and prognosis at 10, *Arch Dis Child* 61:642-646, 1986.

43. Martin AJ, McLennan LA, Laudau LI, Phelan PD: Natural history of childhood asthma to adult life, *Br Med J* 280:1397-1400, 1980.

44. Akhter J, Gaspar MM, Newcomb RW: Persistent peripheral airway obstruction in children with severe asthma, *Ann Allergy* 63:53-58, 1989.

CHAPTER 42

Cystic Fibrosis

•

Jack D. Gorvoy and Lynn J. Bonitz

Cystic fibrosis is the most common lethal or potentially lethal autosomal recessive disease affecting Caucasians, with a well-documented estimated incidence among the white U.S. population of 1 in 2500 to 3500 live births.[1-3] The carrier frequency of a little over 3% in the white population also makes this entity the most common lethal trait among Caucasians.[2] Cystic fibrosis occurs wherever Europeans have settled and is extremely rare among Asians (1:32,000) and African-Americans (1:15,000).[1]

Cystic fibrosis is characterized by the following major clinical and laboratory findings:

1. Chronic mucous obstruction of the airways coexisting with recurrent infections of the respiratory system, affecting almost 100% of patients.
2. Insufficient function of the exocrine portion of the pancreas occurring in 85% to 90% of patients, leading to steatorrhea and azotorrhea, and resulting in nutritional consequences of malabsorption.
3. Reproductive complications leading to a fertility rate of less than 2% in males and approximately 25% in females.
4. Two positive sweat chloride values of ≥60 mEq/L obtained by the quantitative pilocarpine iontophoresis test (QPIT), as per the guidelines of the Cystic Fibrosis Foundation of Bethesda, MD. These elevated levels of sweat electrolytes are noted in almost 100% of patients with the disease.
5. Two alleles consistent with a diagnosis of cystic fibrosis. Since identification of the gene for cystic fibrosis and its most frequent mutation (delta F508, which is identified in approximately 75% of patients), more than 600 mutations have been identified. Mutations beyond the most commonly identified 32 mutations are very rare and their distribution is largely dependent on geographic and ethnic origin.[4]

A preliminary draft issued by the National Cystic Fibrosis Foundation defines a diagnosis for cystic fibrosis as the identification of at least two of the clinical criteria (1 to 3) and one of the two positive laboratory criteria (4 and 5).

The ever-increasing awareness of this multisystem disease by clinicians has resulted in a growing patient population identified as having cystic fibrosis. With better recognition of the likely pathogenesis and marked improvement in therapy, the life span of patients with this disease has shifted dramatically to encompass an older age group. What was previously considered the most common fatal genetic disease of Caucasian children has become recognized as a chronic, progressive disease of adolescents and adults. There are now over 5000 individuals over the age of 18 years in the United States with cystic fibrosis, representing approximately one third of all patients known to the Cystic Fibrosis National Registry. The medical and psychosocial needs of these adolescents and young adults, which are numerous and complex, are reviewed in this chapter, along with a brief history of the disorder and an overview of the exciting genetic and therapeutic developments currently taking place in the field.

HISTORY AND RECENT ADVANCES

Since cystic fibrosis is the most recently identified of man's major chronic life-threatening diseases, the his-

torical landmarks of this disorder are of interest. The first comprehensive description of the disease was presented in 1938 by the clinicopathologist Dr. Dorothy Andersen, who referred to it as "cystic fibrosis of the pancreas."[5] In 1945, clinicians in Boston suggested that this entity was a disease of the exocrine glands, the defect being one of inadequate clearance of mucus, and they popularized the term *mucoviscidosis*.[6,7] In the early 1940s, chronic pulmonary infection was recognized as being critical and responsible for the progressive deterioration noted in the illness. At that time, therapy was focused on the prolonged use of antibiotics, which was a turning point in achieving longer survival.

The next important historical event was the recognition that sodium and chloride levels in the sweat of patients were elevated in virtually all of those with cystic fibrosis. This recognition and its diagnostic application were described by Dr. Paul di Sant'Agnese et al in 1953.[8] These authors noted that patients with cystic fibrosis suffered severe hyponatremia and dehydration during heat waves and that some deaths were reported under such conditions. Initially, the diagnostic sweat test was performed by placing the patient in a plastic bag and thermally inducing sweating. The hazards of this method were documented, and the procedure was subsequently abandoned.[9] A more accurate and nonhazardous method, QPIT, was devised by Gibson and Cooke[10] in 1959, and this remains the standard diagnostic sweat test for electrolytes today.

The most recent and most important landmark occurred in 1989 with the discovery of the identity of the cystic fibrosis gene.[2,3] This gene, located on the long arm of chromosome 7 and referred to as delta F508, represents a three-base-pair deletion that results in the loss of a phenylalanine residue at the amino acid position 508 of the gene. In the original report, delta F508 was found to represent about 70% of the cystic fibrosis mutations in a sample of Canadian patients. However, screening of patients in other populations has revealed that the frequency of this mutation varies. Most non–delta F508 mutations are rare, occurring in less than 5% of screened populations.[11]

We are indeed in the midst of a most important era in the history of cystic fibrosis. Advances during the past two decades with the earlier diagnosis and treatment of affected individuals have resulted in improved survival time. The Cystic Fibrosis Foundation's Patient Registry of 1995 indicates a median survival age of 30.1 years.[12]

PATHOPHYSIOLOGY

It has been recognized that cystic fibrosis is associated with a defect in epithelial chloride ion transport caused by mutations in a membrane protein called the cystic fibrosis transmembrane conductance regulator (CFTR).[13,14] In a 1991 study, the suggested explanation for the alteration in the chloride ion channel that is associated with the most common mutation (delta F508) is a failure in maturation of the CFTR glycoprotein. This results in limited transport of the protein to its normal cellular location for membrane insertion and abnormal kinetics in mediation of chloride transport.[15] Concurrent with these findings, other researchers have also demonstrated increased chloride activity in response to raising the levels of cyclic AMP (adenosine 3′,5′-monophosate) by adding the pharmacologic agents forskolin and methylxanthine (IBMX).[16] Thus, the possibility exists that the activity of mutant CFTRs in epithelial cells may be altered by appropriate pharmacologic interventions. Since it is estimated that 92% of patients with cystic fibrosis have at least one delta F508 allele, pharmacologic activation of this mutant protein would be of major benefit.[17] However, other regulating chloride channels have now been identified that may also affect the outcome of pulmonary status.[18,19]

GENOTYPE-PHENOTYPE CORRELATIONS

Whether correlations exist between specific gene mutations and manifestations of cystic fibrosis in different tissues and organs is difficult to establish, since variations in disease expression may be due to both genetic and environmental factors that vary from one organ system or individual to another. There is a current hypothesis that "dominant" mild mutations exist and that their presence confers a pancreatic-sufficient (PS) phenotype. Specifically, a number of relatively uncommon mutations have been reported with pancreatic sufficiency and in some cases nondiagnostic sweat tests.[20] Conversely, a number of mutations other than delta F508 associated with pancreatic insufficiency have been identified.[21] As yet, no genotype-phenotype correlations for the respiratory manifestations of cystic fibrosis have been identified. Reports in recent years identify the missence mutation R117H, considered to be rare in the classic phenotype of cystic fibrosis patients. It is more often associated with a mild form of the disease and pancreatic sufficiency.[22] Many observations have also associated the R117H mutation with congenital bilateral absence of the vas deferens (CBAVD).[23]

The dominant pathogenetic mechanism in cystic fibrosis is a dysfunction of all exocrine glands. Abnormal secretions from the glands, resulting in thickened and tenacious mucus, give rise to obstruction of organ passages and result in a broad array of clinical manifestations and subsequent complications.[24] Abnormalities of sodium and chloride transport across cell membrane surfaces are believed to be responsible for removal of water from glandular secretions, resulting in a dehydrated mucus that initiates a sequence of events leading to the pathologic manifestations seen in cystic fibrosis. As noted above, studies have determined that the gene associated with cystic fibrosis encodes the membrane-associated glycoprotein CFTR, which is responsible for the transport of ions that are defective in patients with cystic fibrosis.[25,26]

Cystic fibrosis presents with a heterogeneous group of clinical findings. Often considered a "disease of complications," cystic fibrosis has been referred to as one of the "great mimickers" in clinical medicine. The protean manifestations of cystic fibrosis are highlighted in Figure 42-1, which presents an overall view of the disease. As noted, the adolescent and young adult years in most patients are marked by the development of significant symptoms and complications resulting from the chronic pulmonary and intestinal abnormalities, as well as concerns about defective reproductive potential. These issues are highlighted in the sections that follow.

PULMONARY DISEASE

Pathogenesis

The major life-threatening process in cystic fibrosis involves the pulmonary system. Until recently, patients with cystic fibrosis were characteristically considered to have normal lungs at birth. However, recent studies have identified the presence of early pulmonary inflammation in many infants as young as 4 weeks of age.[27] Bronchoalveolar lavage (BAL) performed in infants has revealed neutrophils, interleukin 8 (IL-8, a neutrophil chemokine), increased free elastase activity, and other inflammatory indices. In addition, inflammation may be present in the absence of common cystic fibrosis–related pathogens at the time of BAL.[27] Subsequently, progression of lung disease evolves at various ages and with differing degrees of bronchopulmonary obstruction. Initially, obstruction at the bronchiolar level produces air trapping, with abnormal mucus acting as the critical feature compromising the mucociliary approaches and clearance of the airways. Extensive bronchiectasis is the usual finding during the adolescent years. Bronchiectatic cysts, usually most prominent in the upper lobes, may occupy as much as 50% of the cross-sectional area of the lungs.[28] With progression of the obstructive process, peribronchial fibrosis follows, along with a restrictive pattern of lung function. With advanced lung disease, subpleural blebs or cysts may occur, usually in the upper lobe, and these may be the prelude to a complication of spontaneous pneumothorax. Anatomic distortions of the bronchiectatic airways create pools for the large, tortuous, and thin-

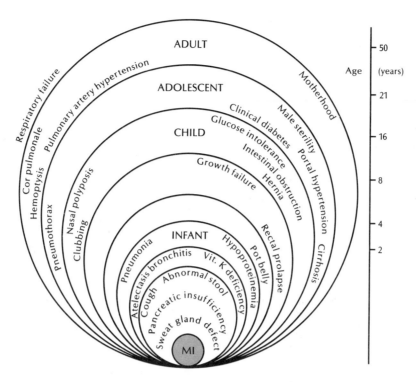

Fig. 42-1. Diagram of the complications noted in cystic fibrosis and the ages at which they are manifested. MI, meconium ileus. (From Schwachman H: *Cystic fibrosis: current problems in pediatrics,* vol 8, St. Louis, 1978, Mosby–Year Book.)

walled bronchial arteries that provide the potential for hemoptysis.[29]

Bacteriologic Findings

Although mucous obstruction is likely to be the primary pathophysiologic event, the more destructive process is chronic infection in the airways. The initial pathogen is usually *Staphylococcus aureus,* and patients with cystic fibrosis have an affinity for this organism throughout life. Along with *S. aureus, Haemophilus influenzae* and *Pseudomonas aeruginosa* (mucoid strain) are the most common offending pathogens. Other gram-negative rods (e.g., *Escherichia coli, Proteus mirabilis,* and the mucoid strain of *Klebsiella pneumoniae*) also may be recovered, especially from the sputum samples of adolescents and adults.[30] It is possible that respiratory viruses are the triggering agents for bacterial colonization. Pulmonary exacerbations associated with influenza A and B, parainfluenza virus, and respiratory syncytial virus are commonly seen. Infections with *Mycoplasma pneumoniae* or atypical *Mycobacterium* species may occur, while anaerobes have been recovered from lung tissue but not detected in the sputum.

The most common clinical course is characterized by progressive suppurative airway disease, with *P. aeruginosa* as the predominating bacterial pathogen.[31] Although

Pseudomonas organisms may be found in newly diagnosed patients, it is most prevalent in adolescents and young adults. The *P. aeruginosa* found in patients with cystic fibrosis is unique, being usually of the mucoid variety and producing copious amounts of alginate. Alginate production is found almost exclusively in the *Pseudomonas* strains isolated from patients with cystic fibrosis. Alginate not only protects the bacteria against phagocytosis but also interferes with mucociliary efficiency. In addition, *P. aeruginosa* produces elastases and proteases that can contribute to tissue damage, especially in early stages of the disease, and may contribute to bronchial vessel erosion and hemoptysis.[32,33] A study in which lower respiratory tract secretions were obtained by bronchoscopic suction identified an incidence of pseudomonads in 42% of nonexpectorating patients with a median age of 4.5 years and in optimal respiratory status.[34] The postpharyngeal gag swab, of course, does not provide such a yield. Once a mucoid *Pseudomonas aeruginosa* organism is established in the airways, it is not eradicated.

P. aeruginosa (mucoid) accounts for up to 90% of morbidity and mortality in cystic fibrosis patients. However, since the mid-1980s, there has been a growing concern over increases in the isolation of *Burkholderia* (formerly *Pseudomonas*) *cepacia* in the respiratory tracts of cystic fibrosis patients.[35,36] While the significant increases noted in *Burkholderia cepacia* infections suggest epidemic spread, the source and transmissibility remain controversial.[37] Susceptibility is more evident in young adult patients, and ribotyping now strongly implicates person-to-person spread.[38] The organism often displays resistance to most antibiotics along with rapid deterioration in lung function. An acute fulminating disease process, resulting in death within months, may ensue.[39] However, the pathogenicity of this organism in man is poorly understood, and some authors have questioned its ability to cause disease. Preexisting lung damage and the effects of other pathogens, may enhance its pathogenic potential.[40] Patients with *B. cepacia* may contaminate the immediate environment, resulting in indirect transmission. The finding that *B. cepacia* may contaminate room air suggests that segregation of infected patients is necessary in the hospital.[41] A low incidence with respect to erratic reappearance on culture of this organism has been reported;[42] and in these cases with doubtful pathogenicity. In conducting laboratory cultures for such isolates, the sputum sample should be innoculated on a *B. cepacia*–selective medium. Aids to its identification include resistance to polymyxin B, production of cytochrome oxidase, and an ability to grow on a citrate medium.

Radiographic Findings

The initial radiographic pattern in cystic fibrosis is usually one of hyperinflation due to the early onset of air trapping. With progression and the appearance of peribronchial cuffing, linear densities become prominent. Predisposition of changes involving the upper lobes, especially on the right, is recognized. Almost all adolescents and adult patients eventually demonstrate interstitial markings and/or cystlike changes. These markings tend to become irregular and eventually appear as reticulonodular lesions. Bronchiectasis, which is present in almost all cases by puberty, is characteristically noted as clustered, small, cystlike areas that represent ectatic bronchi on end and give the appearance of a honeycomb. Atypical bullae or subpleural blebs are present after about 10 years of obstructive bronchopulmonary disease. Lucencies correlating with abscesses may replace the nodular densities. Radiographic improvement with intense treatment is not readily appreciated because of the fixed nature of airway changes. The most striking radiographic evidence of improvement is the diminished inflation of the lungs, which tends to make the fixed markings more prominent. The appearance of branching, finger-like shadows represents mucoid impaction. Computerized tomography of the lungs, performed to delineate central bronchiectasia, adds to the criteria for diagnosis of allergic bronchopulmonary aspergillosis in patients with cystic fibrosis.[43]

Pulmonary Function Testing

Patients with cystic fibrosis eventually develop two major changes in pulmonary function, obstructive and restrictive. Obstruction of the small airways initially can be recognized by reduced maximum midexpiratory flow rates (MMEFR) and elevation of the ratio of residual volume to total lung capacity (RV/TLC).[44] In general, patients progress from initial reductions in MMEFR to reductions in forced expiratory volume (FEV_1) and forced vital capacity (FVC), and then to diminished vital capacity and total lung volumes. FEV_1 is considered one of the most reliable pulmonary function indicators for progression of disease and projection of survival.[45] Oxygenation declines slowly throughout life. When arterial oxygen pressure (PaO_2) values dip below 55 mm Hg on a sustained basis, symptomatic pulmonary hypertension should be expected.[46]

Spontaneous Pneumothorax

The incidence of pneumothorax requiring chest tubes in cystic fibrosis is approximately 20% in adolescent and adult populations; the incidence increases with advancing age and severity of disease.[47] The mechanism is one of spontaneous rupture of apical bullae or blebs. It is estimated that these subpleural blebs are present in approximately 60% of patients with cystic fibrosis after 10 to 12 years of obstructive bronchopulmonary disease. In such cases the FEV_1 is likely to register values of less than 50% of those predicted.

Symptoms suggestive of pneumothorax are chest pain and sudden onset of dyspnea in a patient with chronic obstructive pulmonary disease (COPD). At times there may be concurrent minimal hemoptysis. In addition, a life-threatening tension pneumothorax may be present; this critical event requires prompt recognition. The usual presentation is sudden onset of unilateral chest pain, tachycardia, and cyanosis. Absent breath sounds on one side of the lungs, hyperresonance on the same side, tracheal shift, and displacement of the point of maximal impulse of the cardiac apex are associated findings. Prompt evacuation of the trapped air by syringe aspiration and supplemental oxygen are lifesaving measures. Although a chest x-ray examination should be performed, prompt treatment should not be delayed while this procedure is awaited.

Small pneumothorax collections may be absorbed spontaneously, but it is generally recommended in patients with cystic fibrosis that all pneumothorax incidents be treated by insertion of a chest tube attached to a Pneumovac for underwater drainage. When the air leak has proved to be sealed, instillation of a pleural sclerosing agent is undertaken to decrease the incidence of recurrence. The recurrence rate in untreated patients is approximately 50%. Chemical pleurodesis utilizing tetracycline, quinacrine, or surgical talcum had been used with reasonably good results in reducing the oft-seen recurrences. To reduce the incidence of recurrence even further, some centers proceed initially with an open thoracotomy and perform a partial pleurectomy of the upper portion of the chest, rupturing the blebs and then sewing or stapling the margins of the blebs. The lower portion of the pleural surface is abraded with gauze to secure optimal pleural adhesion.[48] However, with lung transplantation becoming a viable option for patients with advanced disease, a history of pleurectomy and pleural abrasion may disqualify patients as candidates for the procedure in some lung transplantation centers.[49] In addition, chemical pleurodesis can make lung transplantation technically troublesome. However, pleurodesis is not an absolute contraindication for transplantation of lungs.

The complication of pneumomediastinum may occur with or without pneumothorax. This usually presents with subcutaneous emphysema at the neck. Since this serves as a safety valve exit for the air leak, nonsurgical conservative management is generally appropriate.

Hemoptysis

The complication of hemoptysis is a common occurrence in adolescent and adult patients. The degree varies from blood-streaking of sputum, which occurs intermittently in about 60% of patients, or episodes of minor hemoptysis, during which about 2 to 4 oz of blood may be expectorated, to massive, life-threatening hemoptysis, which occurs in approximately 3% of patients. Since episodes of minor hemoptysis may be a prelude to life-threatening major events, in-hospital observation is a prudent course. There may be a need to revise antimicrobial therapy to address the presence of *P. aeruginosa* and *S. aureus* organisms, which may have become more active. Postural drainage is discontinued for the active phase of massive hemoptysis. Empiric use of vitamin K is generally advised, although prothrombin levels are often within the normal range.

The mean age of onset for serious, life-threatening hemoptysis is 18.8 years. By definition, massive hemoptysis involves a blood volume loss of 200 to 300 ml daily for 2 to 3 days or a single loss of about 500 ml. This complication is usually preceded by obstructive bronchopulmonary disease, with inevitable diffuse bronchiectasia. Recurrences may be in the range of 30% to 40%. Release of proteolytic enzymes from neutrophils contributes to the erosion of exposed, tortuous, thin-walled, enlarged, and aneurysmal bronchial arteries, with subsequent rupture into the bronchi. Deaths from contralateral aspiration with asphyxia have been reported.[50]

Treatment of this major complication includes appropriate antimicrobial therapy and, if necessary, blood replacement. Clinical judgment may dictate the need to proceed with bronchial artery embolization via a femoral percutaneous catheter. This may be the treatment of choice for many patients. Unfortunately, effective bronchial artery embolization may improve the quality of life but not necessarily lead to prolongation of life.[51] Before using embolization, we had used an endobronchial balloon tamponade as a temporary procedure, only to recognize the efficacy of embolization.[52] While embolization often produces acute cessation of bleeding, the bleeding has potentially major complications including paralysis, organ infarction and death. Rarely, where bleeding cannot be stopped by embolization, local pulmonary resection may be indicated.

Cor Pulmonale

This complicating event, an end-stage process, is defined as right ventricular hypertrophy secondary to the pulmonary hypertension associated with chronic hypoxemia. Studies of adolescents and adults with COPD demonstrate intermittent pulmonary hypertension during episodes of nocturnal desaturation that occur on the basis of vasoconstriction in patients with cystic fibrosis. Cor pulmonale is associated with advanced COPD, although cardiac findings may be masked by the advanced pulmonary signs. With the advent of right-sided heart failure, the liver may become palpably tender, and peripheral edema may be present. A sudden weight gain in patients with cystic fibrosis and advanced COPD usually denotes right-sided heart failure. Unless associated with a reversible event, such as influenza virus infection, hypercapnia and cor pulmonale generally persist once they have been established.[53] Long-term oxygen therapy may be used to help prevent the development of cor pulmonale. Studies have demonstrated that supplemental oxygen management in adolescent patients with significant hypoxia can effectively decrease mortality.[54]

Upper Airway Complications

Almost all patients with cystic fibrosis reveal opacification of the paranasal sinuses, although clinically acute sinusitis is uncommon. Approximately 20% of adolescent and adult patients may have nasal polyps. Indeed, recurrent nasal polyposis may be a presenting feature for the diagnosis of cystic fibrosis in adolescents or adults, and therefore warrants a sweat test. If nasal polyps become pendulous and obstructive, polypectomy is performed, although there may still be a significant incidence of recurrence. Although rare, progressive unilateral exophthalmos, caused by a pyocele of the ethmoid, may be an early or presenting sign of cystic fibrosis.[55,56]

Antibiotic Therapy

Indications for antibiotic use include virtually any set of symptoms, signs, or radiographic changes that may indicate increased pulmonary infection. Increased cough with more productivity, the appearance or wider dispersion of rales, an increased respiratory rate, and weight loss are all indications for initiation or revision of antimicrobial therapy. A signal for more aggressive management is a deterioration in pulmonary function and arterial blood gas test results.

There are proponents for the initiation of antibiotic therapy prophylactically, even when respiratory symptoms are minimal. In the large number of adolescents and adults who manifest chronic infection with persistent, nonacute respiratory symptoms and chronic auscultatory findings, oral antibiotic therapy, either continuous or intermittent, may be indicated, although there is no general agreement for this approach. With acute and more fulminant episodes, intravenous use of aminoglycosides, semisynthetic penicillins, Imipenem, and cephalosporins (usually in combination) is recommended for at least 10 to 14 days. It is important to note that doses in patients with cystic fibrosis need to be higher than in those with other lung infections. This variation in pharmacokinetics is explained on the basis of greater total body clearance and volume distribution in these patients.[57]

Administration of Aminoglycosides

Since aminoglycosides do not penetrate all membranes, there is a poor correlation between serum levels and sputum concentrations. Strong supportive evidence indicates that aerosolization of an aminoglycoside in the patient with cystic fibrosis will achieve an effective concentration to the lower respiratory tract without risking ototoxicity or nephrotoxicity. Our own studies of gentamycin aerosolization have shown that there are negligible systemic levels of this drug and that the quantitative disposition is largely dependent on the patient's pulmonary function.[58] It has been demonstrated that the median density of *P. aeruginosa* is reduced and that a significant improvement in FEV_1 and FEV_{25-75} can be achieved by means of aerosol administration.[59,60]

Administration of Bronchodilators

Many patients manifest bronchial lability, requiring the administration of bronchodilators, especially beta-adrenergic agonists. Indications for use are audible wheezing, increased respiratory rate, and at least a 15% improvement in FEV_1 after use of the beta agonist. Modes of administration include nebulization, metered-dose inhalers, and the oral route. It is important to recognize that bronchodilators may increase airway resistance in some patients; pulmonary function tests may be necessary to determine this effect. In addition, theophylline derivatives may be effective in some circumstances in which other agents may fail, although tolerance in patients with cystic fibrosis may be reduced. Combining beta agonists and theophylline may not increase the individual effect and may even destabilize the airways. When bronchoconstriction is provoked by cold air or induced by exercise, adding cromolyn sodium to the beta agonists may provide an additive response.

Chest Physiotherapy

The rationale for employing physiotherapy has been to reduce the mechanical consequences of obstructive secretions in patients with cystic fibrosis. Mobilization of mucopurulent secretions leads to reduction in the antigenic bacterial pool, reduced proteolytic activity, and consequently reduced endobronchial tissue damage.[61] Conventional modes of chest physiotherapy include gravity-assisted drainage, percussion, vibration, and coughing; in addition, there are many newly developed methods awaiting evaluation in early clinical trials. It should be recognized that not all techniques are effective for all patients. If there is airway-wall instability, airway collapse can occur with coughing and forced expirations. Some physiotherapy procedures may lead to bronchospasm, increase the risk of hemoptysis, or cause transient elevations of pulmonary artery pressure.

There is a mounting interest in autogenic (self-) drainage. In essence, the efficacy of this approach is based on a breath-stimulating position that keeps the bronchial tree and upper airways open so that during expirations the flow can reach the highest possible speed from the periphery to the mouth or nose. The respiratory rate, amplitude, and effort are adjusted to mobilize the secretions. Conventional drainage techniques, in contrast, achieve localized accelerations of the flow rates, thus mobilizing only a segmental part of the mucus.[62] Adjuncts to physiotherapeutic techniques may include forced expiratory techniques, positive-expiratory pressure, a mechanical vest, and exercise. When exercise is used, careful monitoring and assessment are crucial, and the program must be tailored to individual capabilities.

The Flutter is a hand-held device designed to facilitate mucus clearance in patients with cystic fibrosis. It consists of a hardened plastic mouthpiece at one end and a plastic perforated cover at the other end. A high-density stainless steel ball rests in a plastic circular cone on the inside. As the patient exhales through the Flutter, the ball is displaced and then rolls back into place. This cycle occurs many times during each exhalation, resulting in oscillations that accelerate in accord with expiratory airflow, thus facilitating the upward movement of mucus through the airways.[63]

Administration of Corticosteroids

In 1985, interest was generated in the possibility that steroids might alter the immune-mediated inflammatory pulmonary process.[64] This theory led to double-blind, placebo-controlled trials of alternate-day administration of prednisone for patients with mild to moderate pulmonary disease. The recommendations, although still preliminary, suggest that corticosteroids may be beneficial in selected patients with cystic fibrosis. It must be emphasized that possible complications include increased incidence of cataracts, growth retardation, and (above all) glucose abnormalities among patients receiving high-dose prednisone (2 mg/kg) on alternate days for 2 to 3 years. However, no significant increase in frequency of these complications has been found among patients receiving low-dose prednisone (1 mg/kg) on alternate days, when compared with a placebo group.[65] Follow-up studies will continue to evaluate (1) pulmonary function, FVC and FEV_1; (2) growth velocity; (3) immune function (especially immunoglobulin E); and (4) glucose intolerance. As noted above, corticosteroids are the treatment of choice for aspergillosis, which may occur in cystic fibrosis patients after airway colonization with the pathogenic fungus *Aspergillus fumigatus*.[66]

Aerosolized Recombinant Human DNase I

Cystic fibrosis airway disease is associated with purulent secretions that contain high concentrations of extracellular DNA, a viscous material released by leukocytes. Aerosolized rh DNase (dornase alfa [Pulmozyme]) reduces the viscoelasticity and aids the clearance of airway secretions. Three phases in clinical trials have demonstrated that rh DNase is well tolerated, spirometry is improved, and there is a reduced risk of pulmonary exacerbation. Approved by the Food and Drug Administration in 1993, rh DNase's long-term effects are currently being studied.[67] It is emphasized that patients gain optimal benefit from continued daily use of rh DNase, for when therapy is interrupted, pulmonary function test results return to baseline. There are relatively insignificant adverse events associated with this aerosolization, including voice alterations, pharyngitis, laryngitis, fleeting rash, chest pain, and conjunctivitis. The recommended dose of dornase alfa is one 2.5-mg ampule daily using a recommended jet nebulizer cup (Marquest Acorn II, Hudson T updraft II, Pari LC jet) in conjunction with the Pari Pro Neb compressor. Dornase alfa should not be diluted or mixed with other drugs in the nebulizer cup, as this may lead to adverse structural or functional changes of the dornase alfa in the admixed compound.[68]

Aerosolized Amiloride and Uridine Triphosphate

The airway epithelia of patients with cystic fibrosis have two abnormal ion transports: an inability to secrete liquid by way of the mutated CFTR chloride channel, and excessive reabsorption of salt and water driven by active sodium transport.[69] Current ongoing trials with the use of aerosolized amiloride, a sodium channel blocker, and uridine triphosphate (UTP) aim to activate chloride secretions via an alternative non-CFTR population of chloride channels. It is hoped that the above combination may offer improvement in the rheology and clearance of airway secretions by correcting the ion transport defects pharmacologically.[70]

Ibuprofen

The nonsteroidal antiinflammatory drug ibuprofen is being studied as an alternative to corticosteroids in patients with mild lung disease ($FEV_1 \geq 60\%$ predicted). Initial clinical trials have shown blunting of the inflammatory response in the lungs and a reduction in the rate of decline in lung function.[71] The choice of a study group who initially had mild lung disease was based on the recognition that even though this group appeared to be clinically stable, there would nevertheless be substantial airway inflammation. In high doses, ibuprofen inhibits migration, adherence, swelling, and aggregation of neutrophils, as well as release of lysosomal enzymes.[72] Gastrointestinal complications are possible side effects during an ibuprofen regimen. In addition, ibuprofen may interfere with platelet aggregation, which may increase bleeding tendencies. The drug also decreases blood flow to the kidneys; thus, the ability to clear other drugs from the system is slowed, so that dosage adjustments for concomitant use of other drugs may be necessary.[73]

Lung Transplantation

With improved results from aggressive medical management, there has evolved a patient population with longer survival. Unfortunately, most of these patients still die of progressive pulmonary disease in the third or fourth decade of life. Many of these patients may well be considered ideal candidates for lung transplantation. Indeed, lung transplantation and heart-lung transplantation (HLT) now represent realistic therapeutic options for selected patients with otherwise unresponsive end-stage respiratory disease. Since the first successful HLT procedures for cystic fibrosis were performed in England in 1985, other options for lung transplantation have been developed (e.g., double-lung or sequential bilateral single-lung procedures).[74] For technical reasons, sequential bilateral lung transplantation has become the procedure of choice worldwide. Selection of candidates for transplantation is based on stringent criteria. The major indications are (1) deteriorating chronic respiratory failure in spite of maximal medical treatment—FEV_1 is the major predictor value for survival[75]; (2) severely impaired quality of life; and (3) a positive patient attitude and commitment.[76]

Contraindications and risk factors may be variable in their interpretation at different highly qualified transplant centers. At present, a major problem relating to transplantation is a severe shortage of donor lungs along with increasing numbers of patients with end-stage disease (especially with the longer-surviving population of cystic fibrosis patients). The donor shortage is especially significant in the pediatric population with the need for smaller lungs. This has led to the development of bilateral lobar transplantation in which each donor lung is transected to provide two viable lobar grafts. Some lung transplantation centers are accepting parents or other close relatives as live donors for bilateral lobar transplantation. This is certainly a controversial approach, since three people are placed at surgical risk, but early results suggest that it may be a viable option.[77]

A significant deterrent for transplantation is currently surfacing. The presence of *Burkholderia cepacia,* a virulent multidrug-resistant strain, is associated with a very high incidence of postoperative morbidity and mortality, so that the major U.S. lung transplantation centers have listed patients with this organism as unacceptable candidates at this time.[78]

The actual survival at 1, 2, 3, and 4 years after transplantation is 82%, 70%, 61%, and 61%, respectively, as reported by the University of North Carolina.[79] Bronchiolitis obliterans syndrome (BOS) is the predominant cause of death beyond 1 year.[79] To quote the late Dr. Norman Lewison of Stanford University, "Lung transplantation never will be a panacea for pulmonary ills, but it will be available for selected patients when other treatments have failed."[80]

Nasal Intermittent Positive-Pressure Ventilation

Noninvasive mechanical ventilation for cystic fibrosis patients in end-stage disease awaiting lungs for transplantation appears to be a useful bridge pending the arrival of donor lungs. Nasal intermittent positive-pressure ventilation (NIPPV) delivered noninvasively through a well-fitted nasal or face mask has been shown to be of value in chronic respiratory failure and more recently in acute respiratory failure.[81,82] The use of a conventional ventilator is not without risk in patients who are heavily infected with *P. aeruginosa* and have severe

airflow obstruction. Episodes of hypotension and toxemia may occur, and these may damage other vital organs and render patients unsuitable for lung transplantation. The NIPPV is a flow-generated, time-cycled machine that delivers a predetermined tidal volume either in response to the initiation of a spontaneous breath by the patient or automatically. Oxygen is added through a port in the nasal mask. Expiratory pressures are set at 4 to 8 cm H_2O and inspiratory pressures at 8 cm H_2O, with gradual increases of 2 cm until comfort is achieved (but not to exceed 20 cm H_2O). For patients awaiting lungs for transplantation who are deteriorating rapidly, especially those with hypercapnia and hypoxia, the use of NIPPV until organs are available may be lifesaving as well as cost effective.

GASTROINTESTINAL COMPLICATIONS

Pancreatic Insufficiency

Pancreatic insufficiency affects 85% to 90% of patients with cystic fibrosis, and these individuals require exogenous pancreatic enzyme therapy. The remaining 10% to 15% have enough residual pancreatic function to permit normal digestion, although enzyme secretion ranges from normal to 1% of the mean normal value.[83] Those with reduced pancreatic function may develop symptomatic insufficiency with advancing age. These patients are believed to have a heterozygous genotype, possibly with one of the common mutations, such as delta F508, and one of the rarer ones. Data suggest that many patients without pancreatic insufficiency are diagnosed at a later age and have lower sweat chloride levels, milder respiratory disease, good growth, and a better overall prognosis.

Intestinal Obstruction

Meconium ileus, an intrauterine event, is the initial presentation in approximately 10% of patients with cystic fibrosis. Approximately 17% of adolescents and adults with cystic fibrosis have episodes of intestinal obstruction.[47] Maldigestion associated with pancreatic insufficiency and abnormal secretions from intestinal glands combine to make the fecal contents semisolid, thus leading to high fecal impaction, usually at the ileocecal zone. The clinical findings for this meconium ileus equivalent, also designated distal intestinal obstruction syndrome (DIOS), are abdominal cramps and a palpable doughy, generally nontender mass in the right lower quadrant of the abdomen.[84] DIOS occurs in 2% of cystic fibrosis patients per year.

There is a male preponderance for intestinal obstruction. Although usually presenting in adolescents, it has been reported in patients as young as 10 years of age. It should be recognized that right lower quadrant pain with a mass occurring in a patient taking antimicrobial agents as part of pulmonary therapy may be masking a periappendiceal abscess. Management of DIOS is generally conservative, ensuring compliance with the proper dose of pancreatic enzymes in addition to mineral oil on a daily basis until relief is achieved. If symptoms persist and there is radiographic evidence of intestinal obstruction with fluid levels, a Gastrografin or Hypaque enema may be used, while hydration is ensured via intravenous fluids.[85]

Liver Disease

Focal biliary cirrhosis is a frequent necropsy finding, with a reported incidence of 10% to 27%. Approximately 2% to 5% of patients develop multilobular biliary cirrhosis. Clinically, this complication becomes manifest with hepatosplenomegaly, which may progress to hypersplenism, ascites, and esophageal varices with hematemesis. Hepatic failure accompanied by gastrointestinal hemorrhage accounts for nearly all nonpulmonary deaths due to cystic fibrosis beyond infancy. Of interest, and observed in our own center over more than 30 years, is the fact that a significant number of patients with hepatosplenomegaly have lesser degrees of respiratory difficulties than might be expected, for reasons that are unclear at this time. In total, the reported complication of cirrhosis of the liver with hypersplenism and/or esophageal varices is estimated at 1.5%.

Patients with acute esophageal variceal bleeding require immediate intervention. Currently, the primary treatment is endoscopy and sclerotherapy.[86] The patient who has a recurrent episode of bleeding in which sclerotherapy has failed to eradicate the varices may then be considered as a candidate for portacaval or splenorenal shunting. The predictive data for bleeding varices are controversial. The most widely proclaimed predictive index includes the endoscopic findings and coagulation data. The liver function abnormalities are intermittent, and the histologic lesions are heterogeneous and may lead to sampling error.[87] Currently, it is considered unusual for patients to succumb to active variceal bleeding because of the early initiation of sclerotherapy.

The use of ursodeoxycholic acid (UDCA [Actigall]) therapy has been studied.[88] The beneficial effect of UDCA has been related to the enrichment of the bile acid pool with nontoxic bile acid, which may produce a bicarbonate-rich choleresis. It has been suggested that the therapeutic effects of UDCA in cystic fibrosis patients with liver disease have been demonstrated sufficiently for this agent to be initiated early to avoid severe liver involvement.

As therapy for the pulmonary manifestations of cystic fibrosis has improved, life expectancy has increased and therefore morbidity and mortality from liver disease have been, and will continue to be, more prevalent.

Since liver transplantation is accepted as a choice for end-stage liver disease, several cystic fibrosis patients have undergone orthotopic liver transplantation.[89,90] However, the data for these patients are still too limited to permit determination of the appropriate candidate.

Gallbladder Complications

Abnormalities associated with the gallbladder occur in approximately 33% of patients with cystic fibrosis. Structural variations, including "micro-gallbladder" and multilocated mucus-containing cysts in the submucosa, are present in many patients and are of no clinical consequence. Patients with steatorrhea have up to a sevenfold increase in fecal bile acid excretion.[91] Along with the thickened mucus, this increase leads to the formation of gallstones, often silent, which are found in 5% to 10% of adolescents and adults. Contributing further to cholestasis are drugs such as sulfonamides and oral contraceptives. If the cystic duct is obstructed, cholecystitis may occur.

Gastroesophageal Reflux

The symptoms and signs of gastroesophageal reflux bear an impressive resemblance to those identified with the clinical events that evolve in patients with cystic fibrosis. These include chronic cough, wheezing, recurrent pulmonary infections, vomiting, and growth failure. It has been demonstrated that there is a statistically significant correlation between lower esophageal sphincter pressure and pulmonary function in patients with cystic fibrosis. Factors that may predispose to this complication are the increased intra-abdominal pressures achieved during bouts of paroxysmal coughing and the presence of a flattened diaphragm.[92]

Pancreatitis

In adolescents or adults with residual pancreatic function, recurrent episodes of acute pancreatitis may be noted. The presumed cause is spillage of proteolytic enzymes into the pancreatic parenchyma secondary to blockage of the pancreatic ducts. Clinically, the patient experiences abdominal pain associated with a rising serum amylase level. Eventually, with repeated attacks, the pancreas "burns itself out," with pancreatic achylia the final outcome.

Malnutrition

Malabsorption, decreased oral intake, and hypermetabolism all contribute to an overall energy deficit and poor nutritional status during the preadolescent and adolescent years. At this age, poor compliance also may be a factor and the daily needs for some medications are sacrificed, especially the substitute pancreatic enzymes. A decline in weight, especially during adolescence, may precede the onset of pulmonary deterioration. To help restore an appropriate nutritional state, the goal should be to reach 100% to 130% of recommended daily caloric intake. Aggressive measures to achieve caloric enhancement should be employed, including supplementary elemental food administered by nocturnal tube feeding, if necessary. Supplemental fat-soluble vitamins (A, D, E, and K) are daily needs.

Diabetes Mellitus

Diabetes mellitus is 25 times more common in individuals with cystic fibrosis than in the general population. This complication is present in up to 13% of patients during adolescence and adulthood, and the incidence of glucose intolerance is about 45%. Although hyperglycemia can occur at any age, it is generally a problem in the second and third decades. If the hyperglycemia is intermittent and no glycosuria is present, only dietary adjustment may be necessary. Ketoacidosis is rarely encountered in patients with cystic fibrosis. This may be because the pancreas of these patients does not secrete glucagon in amounts great enough to be associated with ketosis.

Vascular disease affecting the retina, along with arteriovascular calcifications and cataracts, has been reported in a 27-year-old man from our center.[93] Other reports of vascular retinopathy have been documented with prolonged hyperglycemia. Insulin therapy should be handled with caution, because patients with cystic fibrosis frequently become hypoglycemic. Insulin dependence occurs in only 1% of patients, but this exceeds the percentage expected in a normal population of equal age. A familial incidence, although the possibility has been considered, has not been established.

Fibrosing Colonopathy

In addition to the well-documented gastrointestinal manifestations of cystic fibrosis,[94] a 1994 report from the United Kingdom described five children who had strictures of the ascending colon associated with symptoms typical of the meconium ileus equivalent syndrome.[95,96] The term *fibrosing colonopathy* has been proposed to include the pre-stricture state as well as the presence of true strictures. This term applies to patients with cystic fibrosis who show evidence of obstruction, bloody diarrhea, and possibly chylous ascites. In addition, these patients may have abdominal pain, intermittent diarrhea, and poor weight gain. Patients with a history of meconium ileus or DIOS who have undergone intestinal

surgery are at highest risk. This complication occurs most commonly in patients under 12 years of age who have taken more than 6000 lipase units/kg per meal for more than 6 months.[96,97] To establish the diagnosis of fibrosing colonopathy, a contrast enema is the most reliable method. The demonstration of colonic shortening, focal or extensive narrowing, and a lack of distensibility is highly suggestive. Patients with fibrosing colonopathy in the recent state of our interpretation should have the enzyme dosage reduced to within the recommended range of 500 to 2500 lipase units/kg per meal. Patients whose nutritional status cannot be maintained and who show evidence of obstruction, along with uncontrollable bloody diarrhea or chylous ascites, may need to be considered as candidates for surgery.[98,99] Clinicians should be aware that unresponsive diarrhea in patients with cystic fibrosis may be due to problems other than pancreatic insufficiency. More studies are needed to define the recommended dosage schedule for pancreatic enzymes, and caution should be exercised in their empiric use for unresponsive diarrhea. Colonic strictures in children with cystic fibrosis have been identified even on low-strength pancreatic enzymes.[100] Further guidance on the prevention of colonic strictures by the appropriate formulation and dosage of pancreatic enzymes awaits the results of additional epidemiologic studies. The precise etiology remains uncertain.[95]

Crohn's Disease Complicating Cystic Fibrosis

There are several published case reports of the coexistence of cystic fibrosis and Crohn's disease.[101] In patients with cystic fibrosis who have severe gastrointestinal disease; recurrent meconium ileus equivalent; unexplained fevers; an elevated erythrocytic sedimentation rate; rectal bleeding; or ocular, cutaneous, hepatic, or skeletal manifestations suggestive of Crohn's disease, upper and lower endoscopic evaluation should be pursued.[102] Symptoms of Crohn's disease may be easily confused with those of cystic fibrosis. The prevalence of Crohn's disease in the cystic fibrosis population may exceed the worldwide prevalence of Crohn's disease, 9 to 75 per 100,000.[103]

Cancer Risk in Cystic Fibrosis

With improved survival, an increase in late complications, including intestinal cancer, needs to be considered. Several intriguing associations have become apparent in two relatively common disorders, cystic fibrosis and Crohn's disease, that may share many features. Of interest, the metoncogene (associated with some forms of intestinal cancer) resides on chromosome 7, though separated by several hundred kilobases from the cystic fibrosis gene. The question arises as to whether new cystic fibrosis mutations may be more closely related.[104] As the life span of patients with cystic fibrosis increases, more digestive cancers will undoubtedly occur. Although cancer will continue to be an uncommon diagnosis for patients with cystic fibrosis, the increased risk of digestive tract cancers in these patients suggests that persistent or unexplained intestinal symptoms deserve careful investigation.[105] Digestive tract cancers noted in patients with cystic fibrosis include cancers of the esophagus, stomach, small and large intestines, colon, liver, biliary tract, pancreas, and rectum. Many of the cystic fibrosis patients who have developed these cancers have been in only their third decade of life at the time of cancer diagnosis.

GENE THERAPY

As already mentioned, the cystic fibrosis gene, because of its apparent role in chloride conductance and other ion transporters, has been named the CFTR. Confirmation that this indeed has been the correct gene came from studies of epithelial cells in which cAMP-regulated chloride permeability was restored by transfer of normal CFTR complementary DNA (cDNA).[106,107] The discovery of the CFTR gene quickly led to a better understanding of the basic cellular defect and set the stage for an intensive effort to bring gene therapy for cystic fibrosis to the forefront.[108,109] The first clinical trials began in 1993, less than 4 years after identification of the CFTR gene.[110] The CFTR gene covers 250 kilobases (kb) on chromosome 7q.31-32.[111] It encodes for a large protein that functions as a cAMP-regulated chloride channel, with other potential roles in epithelial cell biology.[108] Mutations in the CFTR gene result in insufficient CFTR function in the apical membrane of epithelial cells, which leads to clinical consequences primarily in the respiratory and gastrointestinal epithelium. More than 500 different cystic fibrosis–associated mutations have been identified since 1991.[112] Recombinant human CFTR cDNA, the established genetic material used for gene therapy, can be delivered to airway epithelial cells of the recipient using biologic (viral) or physical/chemical (nonviral) vectors. Among viral vectors, the replication defective adenovirus (Ad) is best studied.[113,114] For more stable, long-term expression in airway epithelium, recombinant adeno-associated virus (AAV) vectors have been developed for CFTR gene transfer.[115] The vector shows encouraging data, with longer-lasting expression and less toxicity than the adenovirus.[116] However, there remain several obstacles to AAV gene therapy, including the potential for mutagenesis.[115]

Liposomes (Lipid:DNA Complexes)

Animal experimentation data have led to clinical trials using cationic lipid-mediated gene transfer. These lipid:DNA complexes are minimally toxic, but efficiency is much lower than with AAV therapy. These complexes mediate gene transfer by an unknown mechanism.[117] There have been promising initial results showing that lipid:DNA complexes can correct the cystic fibrosis genotype in the airways of mice. Thus, human trials using liposomes have been initiated for gene transfer.[118] The lipid:DNA (liposome) complexes are easy to prepare and can deliver genes of unlimited size. They are minimally toxic, although their stability is in question.[117]

Vectors known as molecular conjugates are another method tailored to bring DNA molecules into cells. This strategy is attractive because it could result in cell specificity. Both of the nonviral approaches (lipid:DNA complexes and molecular conjugates), however, present potential difficulties with respect to antigenicity and the feasibility of repetitive administration.[119]

Gene therapy is still in its infancy despite the intense work that is taking place. Transfer of CFTR cDNA has been demonstrated in humans by both molecular and functional evidence. Results are variable, however, with low efficacy and transient expression. The question of toxicity is crucial, especially with the adenovirus vectors.[110] In contrast, the lipid:DNA complexes appear less toxic but with lower efficiency and variable results. As stated by Rosenfield and Collins, "While much has been learned about the feasibility of the current approaches, there are substantial challenges ahead before gene therapy for cystic fibrosis can be considered a proved therapeutic option—in counseling patients and families, convey the hope of success without overstating its imminence."[113]

PSYCHOSOCIAL FACTORS

The personnel who provide psychosocial support to patients with cystic fibrosis are important contributors to the patients and family involved in this chronic, genetic, life-threatening disease. Like all adolescents, teenagers with cystic fibrosis face tasks related to the development of their identity, and this may involve a self-evaluation that is more difficult for the physically handicapped. Adolescents with cystic fibrosis often may be considered "invisibly handicapped" since many patients have no stigmata of the disease.

A high incidence of emotional disturbance is found among adolescents and adults with this disorder. In comparison with the general population, one study demonstrated a high degree of anxiety, unexpressed anger, poor self-image, and inadequate peer relationships in patients with cystic fibrosis.[120] Although studies have shown a greater tendency toward depression among adolescents with cystic fibrosis than among those who are healthy, the differences are generally not greatly pronounced. In one study, girls did seem to show more sadness than boys, but they also tended to have more illness. The patients in this study did not appear to be socially isolated; they usually chose to belong to groups that would accept them.[121]

Young patients with cystic fibrosis generally tend to participate in routine school activities, but girls perform less well than boys in physical education. We have observed that many boys with cystic fibrosis participate in games with considerable enthusiasm, giving themselves an extra interest in life. For most teenage patients, interaction with the rest of the family has been good; if anything, there are fewer disagreements, which may indicate an inability to demonstrate independence. In a study by Troupauer et al,[120] the point was made that the patient's method of coping often closely reflects that of the parents. This study, in common with others and our own observations, also indicated that the major part of the burden of coping with the illness is carried by the mother and that it usually has a significant impact on her well-being. It is common for adolescents with cystic fibrosis to be overprotected and infantilized by their mothers.

The coping methods of patients with cystic fibrosis are a matter of interest. For example, many patients deny the ultimate outcome of the disease but not the disease itself. With recent advances in management and increased understanding by patients and families, it would be of interest to reassess the attitudes and projected plans of those with cystic fibrosis. Since more patients are undergoing lung transplantation, and in view of the rapid progress being made in altering the basic biochemical defect of cystic fibrosis, it is likely that some of the past psychodynamics have changed.

Studies in sexual functioning in patients with cystic fibrosis are limited. One group of authors concluded that patients with this disorder can be assured that they have a reasonable chance for normal sexual functioning.[122]

Career choices are critical for patients with this disorder; some express concern about making realistic choices. Appropriate vocational counseling, which should be incorporated into the entire secondary school years, can help individuals develop sound career goals. The degree of clinical expression of the disease process is, of course, a major determinant of the career paths available. However, physicians who treat adolescents with cystic fibrosis have observed that an increasing number of patients have been pursuing rewarding careers in recent years.

Unfortunately, since the prognosis for cystic fibrosis remains uniformly fatal at this time, the final and ultimate crisis for patients and their families comes as death becomes imminent. With a lingering death, as often occurs in cystic fibrosis, there is intensified anger, confusion, and guilt for the family trying to cope with the situation.

REPRODUCTIVE COMPLICATIONS

Female Reproduction

Menarche may be delayed by about 2 years in females with cystic fibrosis, with anovulatory cycles and secondary amenorrhea common during pulmonary exacerbations. The cervical mucus is thick and desiccated and does not pull into a thread at midcycle. This altered mucus may act as a mechanical barrier to sperm penetration, thus contributing to reduced fertility. Estimated fertility in females with cystic fibrosis is about 25%, in contrast to the 85% fertility rate reported for the normal female population.[123] With chronic exposure to antibiotics and a predisposition to glucose intolerance, *Candida* vaginal infections may be common. In addition, cervicitis and cervical erosion are common pathologic findings. Therefore, regular gynecologic examinations should be scheduled.

For adolescents who are sexually active but not interested in pregnancy, and for those adults who have valid concerns about the risks of pregnancy, contraception is an option. The barrier methods (e.g., condoms and diaphragms) are considered most suitable, since oral contraceptives may cause pulmonary exacerbations and may be responsible for polypoid cervicitis. Data indicate, however, that low-dose oral contraceptives may be used.[124]

Pregnancy in Females with Cystic Fibrosis

It is not surprising that the onset and progression of sexual development in patients with cystic fibrosis is often delayed in a manner dependent on their underlying nutritional and pulmonary status. Currently, more than one third of patients within cystic fibrosis centers are adolescents and adults. This enlarging population is increasingly confronted with matters related to reproductive potential. The occurrence of pregnancy in the course of cystic fibrosis has recently surfaced as a major issue, although the first documented case was reported in 1960. Since that time, there has been a dramatic increase in the number of pregnancies concomitant with the steadily increasing life expectancy and improved quality of life of affected patients.

Until recently, there was a general bias toward not recommending pregnancy for most patients with cystic fibrosis. The most recent studies, however, have shown that the rate of decline in pulmonary function in the 2 years after pregnancy is not significantly greater than in nonpregnant women with cystic fibrosis. Indeed, the 3-year survival for pregnant women was 94% compared with 91% for controls. These encouraging data support the concept that patients with mild disease (i.e., with relatively mild airway obstruction and excellent nutritional status) tolerate pregnancy well, and their efforts to conceive may well be supported. Those whose overall medical status is severely compromised, as evidenced by hypoxemia, cor pulmonale, and marked malnutrition, place both themselves and the fetus at an unacceptably high risk for an adverse outcome, and should be actively discouraged from consideration of pregnancy.

Genetic counseling should be offered to all women contemplating pregnancy. Couples should be informed of the advisability of genetic evaluation of the prospective father and that all clinically unaffected offspring will carry the cystic fibrosis gene. When the father is identified as being a carrier, or remains unidentified as a possible carrier of a rarer mutation, advice should be offered regarding the availability of prenatal diagnostic measures.

Male Reproduction

Males with cystic fibrosis often have delayed growth and sexual maturation. Secondary sex characteristics do develop and the libido is normal. About 98% of males have atretic vasa deferentia with absent or abnormal bodies and tails of the epididymis and seminal vesicles. Although active spermatogenesis is present, no sperm appears in the ejaculate because of the fibrotic or atretic duct. Taussig et al[125] reported a few men who had fathered children and were noted as having intact male reproductive tracts at autopsy. These subjects would be categorized as having mild clinical expression of the disease.

Men with classic cystic fibrosis can have normal testicular spermatogenesis, and epididymal sperm can fertilize eggs in vitro. Their wives should undergo DNA analysis to rule out carrier status to prevent transmission of disease to the offspring.[126]

SCREENING RECOMMENDATIONS

With the recent identification and isolation of the gene responsible for cystic fibrosis, screening is now offered. However, the identification of multiple rare mutations (over 500) along with the one very common mutation makes population screening more difficult. Population screening implies offering a program of carrier testing, with informed consent and genetic counseling, to millions of healthy people. Unlike testing in the general popula-

tion, however, testing for carriers in families in which the disease has occurred is nearly 100% informative. This is because such testing can be performed by the direct method of mutation analysis (when there is a DNA sample available from an affected person in the family), or by an indirect linkage method. The direct method of testing specifically identifies the DNA mutation responsible for cystic fibrosis; this is the most straightforward and definitive method of testing. Currently, direct mutation analysis can identify 80% to 85% of carriers in individuals of Western European origin, 60% of carriers in those of Italian-American descent, and 50% of carriers in Ashkenazi Jews and African-Americans. The indirect method involves the identification of DNA markers that are closely linked to the cystic fibrosis gene. This technique, called linkage analysis, permits tracking of the gene within a family even when the exact mutation cannot be identified. It is now recommended that testing be offered to all individuals and couples with a family history of cystic fibrosis.

Osteopenia

The skeletal health of children with cystic fibrosis is more controversial because some studies have reported normal bone mass, while others have observed that the bone mineral density of children with cystic fibrosis is 10% less than that of age-matched healthy children.[127,128] The most recent study on correlates of osteopenia in patients with cystic fibrosis concluded that peak bone mineral content is significantly reduced in patients with cystic fibrosis.[129] Osteopenia has been identified in children as well as adults, suggesting that inadequate bone mineral acquisition during the first two decades is a major contributor. Several potential risk factors for osteopenia have been considered, including low body mass, inactivity, vitamin D and/or calcium deficiency, glucocorticoid use, disease severity, hypogonadism, and delayed puberty. Bone mass is decreased and the incidence of pathologic bone fractures is increased in adults.[130]

SUBTLE AND ATYPICAL CLINICAL PRESENTATIONS

The subtle and atypical clinical presentations of cystic fibrosis add to the need for recognition that the classic clinical triad may not surface early nor with full clinical expression. There follows a list of those isolated clinical presentations that should be recognized and included in the differential diagnosis for cystic fibrosis:

1. An unexplained chronic cough, especially during the first few years of life, which may not reveal significant radiographic changes.

2. Recurrent pneumonia without pancreatic insufficiency or malnutrition.
3. Intermittent episodes of "wheezing" or "bronchiolitis" during infancy.
4. Right upper lobe atelectasis/pneumonia without significant other contributory symptoms and with no cough.
5. Allergic bronchopulmonary aspergillosis.
6. Panopacification of the paranasal sinuses.
7. Unexplained digital clubbing.
8. Prolonged neonatal jaundice.
9. Hemolytic anemia and edema in infants.
10. Hemorrhagic manifestations, especially in the first year of life. (Abnormalities in prothrombin time and partial thromboplastin time are often but not always present; factors II, VII, and X are involved in about 20%.)
11. Rectal prolapse between the ages of 6 months and 3 years.
12. Right lower quadrant fecal impaction.
13. Recurrent intussusception.
14. Recurrent pancreatitis.
15. Hypoproteinemia and hypoalbuminemia with edema in infancy. (Usually associated with use of soy milk formula, which has inappropriate protein levels for those with pancreatic insufficiency, or breast milk, which has a lower protein content.[131])
16. Metabolic alkalosis in infants over 3 to 4 months of age. (Incidence higher during warmer weather, associated with looser stools and possibly vomiting.)
17. Hepatobiliary disease, focal biliary cirrhosis, multilobular biliary cirrhosis with hypersplenism, or cholestatic jaundice.[132]
18. Gastroesophageal reflux with or without aspiration.
19. Vitamin A deficiency (which may present with bulging anterior fontanelle in infancy).
20. Vitamin E deficiency with possible neuromuscular developmental lag.
21. Congenital bilateral absence of the vas deferens (atretic), along with abnormalities in the epididymis and absence of seminal vesicles.

Congenital Bilateral Absence of the Vas Deferens

Congenital bilateral absence of the vas deferens (CBAVD) is a form of male infertility in which the CFTR mutation has been identified in many infertile males. It has been well documented that males with cystic fibrosis are infertile because of CBAVD. Perhaps 1 in 1000 males in the general population present a similar pathologic problem with infertility.[133] Although patients with cystic fibrosis have mutations in both copies of the CFTR gene, most patients with CBAVD have mutations in only one copy of the gene. Many of those presenting with CBAVD may not appear to have other features of cystic fibrosis, while some have mild pulmonary disease or mildly elevated sweat chloride levels.[134] A DNA variant has been identified in a noncoding region of the CFTR. This variant, labeled as the 5T allele, is found in many patients presenting with CBAVD. It is believed that the 5T allele generates low levels of the normal CFTR protein. A 1995 study demonstrated that the combination of the 5T allele in one copy of the normal CFTR gene with a cystic fibrosis mutation in the other copy is the most common cause of CBAVD.[135] Not all patients with the 5T CFTR genotype have CBAVD, however, as confirmed by the fact that some fathers of children with cystic fibrosis have this genotype and are able to reproduce. Other studies have identified that many CBAVD patients may be compound heterozygotes for CFTR mutations.[136] Further, a second mutation, R117H, known to lead to a mild phenotype in cystic fibrosis patients, was found to occur at high frequency in these male patients.[137]

HOME CARE

Home Oxygen Therapy

When supplemental oxygen is required, effective delivery systems are available for use in the home. In 1995, 6.7% of adults and children with cystic fibrosis required home oxygen therapy.[138] The delivery method (oxygen mask versus nasal cannula), the flow rate, and the expected hours per day of usage determine the oxygen system utilized. Portable oxygen systems are available to give oxygen-dependent patients the ability to travel away from their stationary oxygen delivery system, providing improved quality of life; the ability to continue with their daily routine; and uninterrupted delivery of oxygen.

Home Supplemental Feedings

Supplemental feedings for children and adults with cystic fibrosis provide additional support for patients with greater nutritional deficits. Home supplemental feedings may be accomplished via nasogastric tube, gastrostomy tube, or button. Generally, supplemental feedings at home are provided nocturnally to increase caloric intake while affording normal daytime functioning. In those with severe malnutrition or who are not candidates for enteral feedings, total parenteral nutrition is available at home.

Home Intravenous Antibiotic Therapy

Historically, most of the care for children or adults with cystic fibrosis occurred in the home, with periodic hospitalizations to receive high-tech care, such as intravenous (IV) antibiotic therapy. Since the mid-1980s, IV infusions at home have become a viable alternative to hospitalization for stable patients with cystic fibrosis. Over the past decade, the cystic fibrosis population has become the fourth largest user of home care services. The trend toward using the home care system has been driven by patient demand, as well as economics.[139]

The home infusion/care system is initiated when a patient requires treatment for an exacerbation of the illness. Initially, patients may be hospitalized for stabilization of their condition, determination of therapeutic drug levels, aggressive chest physiotherapy, and daily contact with their physicians. However, there is a growing trend toward having patients enter directly into the home-care system without first admitting them to the hospital if they are medically stable, have appropriate support systems in the home, have access to aggressive chest physiotherapy, and live in close proximity to the cystic fibrosis center for frequent evaluations. Laboratory work, including drug levels, can be obtained at home via the home infusion company.

One important consideration for home infusion, as well as for the hospitalized patient, is proper venous access. Peripheral IV catheters are not the first choice for long-term therapy (i.e., that of more than 1 week's duration) owing to frequent infiltration. Loss of a peripheral IV line in the home can lead to missed dosages of medication while the patient awaits the arrival of a home care nurse to restart the IV. PICC (peripherally inserted central catheter) lines, midline catheters, and Infuse-A-Ports are therefore the recommended access routes for any long term therapy at home.[140] An access route with distribution into the central venous circulation, such as the PICC line or Infuse-A-Port, is always required to provide total parenteral nutrition.

The mode of delivery for medication at home is individualized to meet patient needs, considering cost effectiveness and patient convenience. The choice of delivery system should take into consideration the ease of use, accuracy of infusion rate, and capability for the patient to be ambulatory. Selection of the most appropriate delivery device leads to improvements in quality of life, compliance, and therapeutic outcomes. For patients who plan to infuse their medication at work or school, an elastomeric ambulatory administration pump is most desirable. This device allows for mobility and privacy during infusion as the medication is administered via a premixed, preregulated, hand-held device (such as the Homepump or Intermate) that does not require the use of gravity for infusion. A traditional delivery system of a minibag system using gravity and an IV pole continues to be utilized. With any of the delivery systems, the patient's IV line is maintained by a heparin or saline lock between dosages and used only when medication is needed, generally every 6 or 8 hours.

Patient and family capabilities are one main factor in determining a patient's candidacy for home infusion; other factors include availability of support systems; adequate venous access; and the patient's ability to meet all activities of daily living, as well as medical needs, while ill. The home environment must be suitable for home infusion, including availability of electricity, refrigeration, and telephone access. Home infusion must be compatible with the life style of the patient and family to ensure compliance.[139]

Determining that the patient and family are amenable to the choice of home care system improves compliance with home therapy. The time demands of home infusion, in addition to the other medical needs of the patient with cystic fibrosis, can affect compliance. The patient and family must be informed of the 24-hour demands of home infusion, as well as all that is involved in caring for the patient at home. Noncompliance, as demonstrated by deviation from the prescribed regimen, may reflect stress, a sense of being overwhelmed, or patients' attempts to exert control over their lives.

One major advantage of home infusion is decreased length of hospitalization for the chronically ill population. The effects of decreased length of stay include decreased absences from school and/or work, reduced stress on the family system, decreased risk of nosocomial infection, and (most important) improved quality of life for the chronically ill patient.

The goals of all of the aspects of home care are to improve quality of life, quality of care, and compliance and to meet all of the patient's needs within today's changing healthcare system.

CONCLUSIONS

The overwhelming advances in research into cystic fibrosis since the mid-1980s have provided dramatic opportunities for improved intervention. Many more children with cystic fibrosis are living into adolescence, and many more adolescents with cystic fibrosis are reaching adulthood. Concomitant improvements in quality of life are allowing many of these adolescents and adults to live full, active lives for an increasing number of years. Unfortunately, cystic fibrosis remains uniformly fatal. Therefore, many patients experience significant morbidity or mortality during their adolescent and early adult years, and all patients must live with that reality. It is hoped that new treatments and genetic findings will significantly alter that reality in the near future.

References

1. Boat TF, Welsh MJ, Beaudet AL: *The metabolic basis of disease,* New York, 1989, McGraw-Hill, pp 2649-2680.
2. Wilford BS, Fost M: The introduction of CF carrier screening into clinical practice, *Mitibank Q* 70:629-659, 1992.
3. Fitzsimmons SC: The changing epidemiology of cystic fibrosis, *J Pediatr* 122:1-8, 1993.

4. Tsui LC: Mutations and sequence variations. A report from the Cystic Fibrosis Genetic Analysis Consortium, *Hum Mutat* 1:197-203, 1992.

5. Andersen DH: Cystic fibrosis of the pancreas and its relation to celiac disease. A clinical and pathologic study, *Am J Dis Child* 56:344, 1938.

6. Farber S: Some organic digestive disturbances in early life, *J Mich Med Soc* 44:587-594, 1945.

7. Farber S: Pancreatic function and disease in early life. Pathological changes associated with pancreatic insufficiency in early life, *Arch Pathol* 37:238-250, 1944.

8. di Sant'Agnese PA, Darling RC, Perera GA, Shea E: Abnormal electrolyte composition of sweat in cystic fibrosis of the pancreas, *Pediatrics* 12:549, 1953.

9. Gorvoy JD, Acs H, Stein ML: The hazard of induction of sweating in cystic fibrosis patients, *Pediatrics* 25:977, 1960.

10. Gibson LE, Cooke RE: A test for concentration of electrolytes in sweat of cystic fibrosis utilizing pilocarpine iontophoresis, *Pediatrics* 23:545, 1959.

11. Welsh MJ, et al: In Scriver C, et al, editors: *The molecular and metabolic basis of inherited disease,* ed 7, New York, McGraw-Hill (in press).

12. Fitzsimmons SC: Patient Registry Annual Report. Cystic Fibrosis Foundation, 1995.

13. Riordan JR, Rommens JM, Kerem B, et al: Indentification of the cystic fibrosis gene: cloning and characterization of complementary DNA, *Science* 245:1066-1073, 1989.

14. Rommens JM, Iannuzi MC, Kerem B, et al: Identification of the cystic fibrosis gene: chromosome walking and jumping, *Science* 245:1059-1065, 1989.

15. Dalemans W, Barbry P, Champigny G, et al: Altered chloride ion channel kinetics associated with delta F508 cystic fibrosis mutation, *Nature* 354:526-528, 1991.

16. Drumm ML, Wilkinson DJ, Smit LS, et al: Chloride conductance expressed by delta F508 and other mutant C.F.T.R.s in *Xenopus* oocytes, *Science* 254:1797-1799, 1991.

17. Kerem E, Corey M, Kerem B, et al: The relation between genotype and phenotype in cystic fibrosis—analysis of the most common mutation (F508), *N Engl J Med* 323:1517-1522, 1990.

18. Santis G, Osbore L, Knight RA, et al: Independent genetic determinants of pancreatic and pulmonary status in cystic fibrosis, *Lancet* 336:1081-1084, 1990.

19. Guggino WB: Outwardly rectifying chloride channels and cystic fibrosis, *J Bioenerg Biomembr* 25:27-35, 1993.

20. Knowles MR, Moore P: Evaluation of the patient with borderline sweat test results, *Pediatr Pulmonol* 10(suppl):141-142, 1994. (abstract)

21. Cutting GR: Genotype defect: its effect on cellular function and phenotypic expression, *Semin Respir Crit Care Med* 15:356-363, 1994.

22. The Cystic Fibrosis Genotype-Phenotype Consortium: Correlation between genotype and phenotype in patients with cystic fibrosis, *N Engl J Med* 329:1308-1313, 1993.

23. Gervais R, Dumur V, Rigot JM, et al: High frequency of the R117H cystic fibrosis mutation in patients with congenital absence of vas deferens, *N Engl J Med* 328:466-47, 1993.

24. Sturgess J: Morphologic characteristics of the bronchiolar mucosa in cystic fibrosis. In Quinton P, Martinez R, Hopfer U, editors: *Fluid and electrolyte abnormalities in exocrine glands in cystic fibrosis,* San Francisco, 1982, San Francisco Press; p 254.

25. Frizzel RA, Rechkemmer G, Shoemaker RL: Altered regulation of airway epithelial cell chloride channels in cystic fibrosis, *Science* 233:558-560, 1986.

26. Knowles M, Gatzy J, Boucher R: Increased bioelectric potential differences across respiratory epithelia in cystic fibrosis, *N Engl J Med* 305:1489-1495, 1981.

27. Khan TZ, Wagener JS, Bost T: Early pulmonary inflammation in infants with cystic fibrosis, *Am J Respir Crit Care Med* 151:1075-1082, 1995.

28. Tomashefski JF Jr, Bruce M, Goldberg HI, Dearhorn DG: Regional distribution of macroscopic lung disease in cystic fibrosis, *Am Rev Respir Dis* 133:535, 1986.

29. Mack JF, Moss F, Haper WE, et al: The bronchial arteries in cystic fibrosis, *Br J Radiol* 38:422, 1965.

30. di Sant'Agnese PA, Davis PB: Research in cystic fibrosis, *N Engl J Med* 295:481-485, 1976.

31. Zierdt CH, Williams RL: Serotyping aeruginosa isolates from patients with cystic fibrosis, *J Clin Microbiol* 1:521-526, 1975.

32. Doring G, Obernesser HJ, Botzenhert K, et al: Proteases of *Pseudomonas aeruginosa* in cystic fibrosis patients, *J Infect Dis* 147:744-750, 1983.

33. Bruce MC, Poncz L, Klinger J, et al: Biochemical and pathologic evidence for proteolytic destruction of lung connective tissue in cystic fibrosis, *Am Rev Respir Dis* 132:529-535, 1985.

34. Ramsey BW, Wentz KR, Smith AL, et al: Predictive value of oropharyngeal cultures for identifying lower airway bacteria in cystic fibrosis patients, *Am Rev Respir Dis* 144:331-337, 1991.

35. Govan JRW, Nelson JW: Microbiology of lung infection in cystic fibrosis, *Br Med Bull* 48:912-930, 1992.

36. Isles A, MacKlusky I, Corey N, et al: *Pseudomonas cepacia* colonization inpatients with cystic fibrosis: an emerging problem, *J Pediatr* 194:204-210, 1984.

37. Steinbech S, et al: Transmissibility of *Pseudomonas cepacia* infection in clinic patients and lung transplant recipients with cystic fibrosis, *N Engl J Med* 331:981-987, 1994.

38. Li Pumma JJ, Densen SE: Person to person transmission of pseudomonas cepacia between patients with cystic fibrosis, *Lancet* 336:1094-1096, 1990.

39. Tablon OC, Martone WJ, Jarvis WR: The epidemiology of *Pseudomonas cepacia* in patients with CF, *Eur J Epidemiol* 3:336-342, 1987.

40. Gladman G, Conner PJ, et al: Controlled study of *Pseudomonas cepacia* and *Pseudomonas maltophilia* in cystic fibrosis, *Arch Dis Child* 67:192-195, 1992.

41. Humphreys H, Peckman D, et al: Airborne dissemination of *Burkholderia cepacia* from adult patients with CF, *Thorax* 49:1157-1159, 1994.

42. Teo C: *Pseudomonas cepacia* in patients with cystic fibrosis attending the Royal Prince Alfred Hospital, *Pathology* 100:25, 1993.

43. Stiglbauer R, et al: High resolution CT in children with cystic fibrosis, *Acta Radiol* 34(5):533, 1993.

44. Levison H, Godfrey S: Pulmonary aspects of cystic fibrosis. In Mangos J, Talamo R, editors: *Cystic fibrosis: projection into the future,* 1976, Stratten Intercontinental, p 3.

45. Wagener JS, Taussig LM, Burrows R, et al: Comparison of lung infection and survival patterns between cystic fibrosis and emphysema or chronic bronchitis patients. In Sturgess JM, editor: *Perspectives in cystic fibrosis,* Toronto, 1980, Imperial Press; p 236.

46. Siassi B, Moss AJ, Dooley RR: Clinical recognition of cor pulmonale in cystic fibrosis, *J Pediatr* 78:794, 1971.

47. di Sant'Agnese PA, Davis PB: Cystic fibrosis in adults, *Am J Med* 66:121-132, 1979.

48. Stowes S, Boat TF, Mandelson H, et al: Open thoracotomy for pneumothorax in cystic fibrosis, *Am Rev Respir Dis* 111:611-617, 1975.

49. Cooper JD, Knight S, Truloch T, et al: Early experience using a simplified technique for bilateral lung transplant in cystic fibrosis patients, *Pediatr Pulmonol* 6(suppl):1991, Cystic Fibrosis Conference, Dallas, Wiley-Liss.

50. Holsclaw DS, Grand RJ, Schwachman H: Massive hemoptysis in cystic fibrosis, *J Pediatr* 76:829-837, 1970.

51. Sweezey HB, Fellows KE: Bronchial artery embolizations for severe hemoptysis in cystic fibrosis, *Chest* 97:1322-1326, 1990.

52. Swersky RB, Gorvoy JD: Endobronchial tamponade for massive hemoptysis in patients with cystic fibrosis, *Ann Thorac Surg* 27:262-264, 1979.

53. Stern RC, Borkat G, Hirschfeld SS, et al: Heart failure in cystic fibrosis, *Am J Dis Child* 134:267, 1980.

54. Groves RH Jr, Bailey WC, Buchalter SE: Long term oxygen therapy, *Chest* 100:544-549, 1991.

55. Gorvoy JD, Abramson A: Unilateral exophthalmos in cystic fibrosis (abs). Cystic Fibrosis Annual Meeting, vol 22, p 118. San Francisco: May 1, 1981, Wiley-Liss.

56. Stool S, Kertecz E, Sibinga M, et al: Exophthalmos due to pyocele of the sinus in cystic fibrosis, *Trans Am Acad Ophthalmol Otolaryngol* 70:311, 1966.

57. Bosso JA, Townsend PL, Herbst JJ, et al: Pharmacokinetics and dosage requirements in cystic fibrosis, *Antimicrob Agents Chemother* 28:829, 1985.

58. Ilowite JS, Gorvoy JD, Smeldone GC: Quantitative deposition of aerosolized gentamycin in cystic fibrosis, *Am Rev Respir Dis* 136:1445-1449, 1987.

59. Smith AL: Aerosol aminoglycoside administration, *Pediatr Pulmonol* 6(suppl):79-80, 1991.

60. Hodson ME: Aerosol antibiotic therapy, *Pediatr Pulmonol* 6(suppl):76-77, 1991.

61. Reisman JJ, Rivington-Law B, Corey M, et al: Role of conventional physiotherapy in cystic fibrosis, *J Pediatr* 113:632-636, 1988.

62. Schoni MH: Autogenic drainage: a modern approach to physiotherapy in cystic fibrosis, *J R Soc Med* 82:32-37, 1989.

63. Konstan MW, Stern RC, Doerschuk CF: Efficacy of the Flutter device for airway clearance in patients with cystic fibrosis, *J Pediatr* 124:689-693, 1994.

64. Auerbach HS, Williams M, Kirkpatrick JA, Colten HR: Alternate-day prednisone reduces morbidity and improves pulmonary function in cystic fibrosis, *Lancet* 2:686-688, 1985.

65. Rosenstein BJ, Eigen H: Risks of alternate-day prednisone in patients with cystic fibrosis, *Pediatrics* 87:245-246, 1991.

66. Hudson ME, Warner JO: Respiratory problems and their treatment, *Br Med Bull* 48:931-948, 1992.

67. Fuchs HJ, Borwitz DS, Christiansen DH, et al: Effect of aerosolized recombinant DNase on exacerbations of respiratory symptoms and on pulmonary function in patients with cystic fibrosis; the pulmoenzyme study group, *N Engl J Med* 331:637-642, 1994.

68. Ramsey BW, Dorkin HL: For the consensus conference: practical applications of Pulmozyme, *Pediatr Pulmonol* 17:404-408, 1994.

69. Knowles MR, Olivier KM, et al: Pharmacologic treatment of abnormal ion transport in the airway epithelium in cystic fibrosis, *Chest* 107(suppl):715-755, 1995.

70. Bennett W, Olivier K, et al: Acute effect of aerosolized uridine 5-triphosphate (UTP) +/- amiloride on mucociliary clearance in cystic fibrosis, *Am J Respir Crit Care Med* 149:A670, 1994.

71. Konstan MW, Berger M: Infection and inflammation of the lungs in cystic fibrosis. In David PB, editor: *Cystic fibrosis,* New York, 1993; Marcel Dekker, pp 219-276.

72. Konstan NW, Hillard KA, Davis PB: Effect of ibuprofen on neutrophil (PMN) delivery to mucosal surfaces, *Pediatr Pulmonol* 4(suppl):152-153, 1989.

73. *Physician's desk reference,* Montvale, NJ, 1995, Medical Economics Data Protection Co.

74. Tamm M, Higenbottom T: Heart-lung and lung transplantation for cystic fibrosis: world experience, *Semin Respir Crit Care Med* 15:414-425, 1994.

75. Kotloff RM, Zuckerman JB: Lung transplantation in cystic fibrosis, *Chest* 109:787-798, 1996.

76. Tsang T, Holson ME, Yacoub MH: Lung transplantation for cystic fibrosis, *Br Med Bull* 48:949-971, 1992.

77. Starnes VA, Barr ML, Cohen RG, et al: Living related lung transplantation in cystic fibrosis, *Pediatric Pulmonol* 10(suppl):128-129, 1994 (abstract).

78. Ramirez JC, Patterson GA, et al: Bilateral lung transplantation for cystic fibrosis, *J Thorac Cardiovasc Surg* 103:287-294, 1992.

79. Egan T, Detterbeck F, Mill M, et al: Intermediate term results of lung transplant for cystic fibrosis, *Pediat Pulmonol* 12 (suppl): Sept, 1995.

80. Theodore J, Lewiston N: Lung transplantation comes of age, *N Engl J Med* 322:772-774, 1990.

81. Carrol M, Branthwaite MA: Control of nocturnal hypoventilation by nasal intermittent positive pressure ventilation, *Thorax* 43:349-353, 1988.

82. Caronia C, Silver P, Gorvoy JD, Saigy M: The use of bi-level positive airway pressure [Bi-PAP] in end stage cystic fibrosis patients awaiting lung transplantation, *Chest Crit Care Med* 22(suppl 1):143, 1994 (abstract).

83. Gaskin KJ, Durie PR, Lee L, et al: Colipas and lipase secretion in childhood: onset of pancreatic insufficiency, *Gastroenterology* 86:1-7, 1984.

84. Ojeda VJ, Levitt S, et al: Crohn's colitis and adult meconium ileus equivalent, *Dis Colon Rectum* 29:567-571, 1986.

85. Dalzell AM, Heaf DP, Canty H: Pathology mimicking distal intestinal obstruction syndrome in cystic fibrosis, *Arch Dis Child* 65:540-541, 1990.

86. Terblanche G: Has sclerotherapy altered the management of patients with variceal bleeding?, *Am J Surg* 169:37-41, 1990.

87. Balistreri W: Spectrum of liver disease in patients with cystic fibrosis. North American Cystic Fibrosis Conference, Suppl 5:272, 1990.

88. Colombo C, Castellani MR, Assaisso ML: Ursodeoxycholic acid therapy in cystic fibrosis, *Pediatr Pulmonol* 5(suppl):76-78, 1990.

89. Cox L, Ward RE, Furgiuele TL, et al: Orthotopic liver transplantation in patients with cystic fibrosis, *Pediatrics* 80:571-574, 1987.

90. Mieles L, Orensten D, et al: Liver transplantation status in cystic fibrosis, *Lancet* 1:1073, 1989.

91. Weber A, Roy CC, Morris CL, et al: Malabsorption of bile acids in children with cystic fibrosis, *N Engl J Med* 289:1001-1005, 1973.

92. Davidson AGF, Wong LTK, Schoni H: Gastroesophageal reflux and pulmonary disease in cystic fibrosis patients, *Pediatr Pulmonol* 2(suppl):136, 1988.

93. Gorvoy JD: *Cataracts, arterio-vascular calcification and retinopathy in a patient with cystic fibrosis and diabetes mellitus.* Presented at the Twenty-sixth Annual National Cystic Fibrosis Meeting, Anaheim, CA, May 1985.

94. Park RW, Grand RJ: Gastrointestinal manifestations of cystic fibrosis: a review, *Gastroenterology* 81:1143-1161, 1981.

95. Smyth RL, Van Velzen D, Smyth AR, et al: Strictures of ascending colon in cystic fibrosis and high-strength pancreatic enzymes, *Lancet* 343:85-86, 1994.

96. Oades PJ, Busch A, et al: High strength pancreatic enzymes, *Lancet* 343:109, 1994.

97. Freidman J, FitzSimmons SC: Colonic strictures in patients with cystic fibrosis, *J Pediatr Gastroenterol Nutr* 22(2):153-156, 1996.

98. Zerin JM, Kuhn-Fulton J, White SJ, et al: Colonic strictures in children with cystic fibrosis, *Radiology* 194:223-226, 1995.

99. Pettei MJ, Leonidas JC, Levine J, Gorvoy JD: Pancolonic disease in cystic fibrosis and high-dose pancreatic enzyme therapy, *J Pediatr* 125:587-589, 1994.

100. Jones R, et al: Colonic stricture in children with cystic fibrosis on low strength pancreatic enzymes, *Lancet* 346:499, 1995.

101. Lerner A, Gal N, Mares AJ, et al: Pitfall in diagnosis of Crohn's disease in a patient with cystic fibrosis, *J Pediatr Gastroenterol Nutr* 12:369-371, 1991.

102. Cloney DL, Sutphen JL, Browitz SM, et al: Crohn's disease complicating cystic fibrosis, *South Med J* 87:81-83, 1994.

103. Garland CF, Lilienfeld AM, et al: Incidence rates of ulcerative colitis and Crohn's disease in 15 areas of the US, *Gastroenterology* 81(6):1115-1124, 1981.

104. Lloyd-Still JD: Cystic fibrosis, Crohn's disease, biliary abnormalities, and cancer, *J Pediatr Gastroenterol Nutr* 13:293-297, 1991.

105. Neglia JP, Fitzsimmons SC, Maisonneve P, Schoni MH, et al: The risk of cancer among patients with cystic fibrosis, *N Engl J Med* 332:494-499, 1995.

106. Drumm ML, Pope HA, et al: Correction of the cystic fibrosis defect in vitro by retrovirus-mediated gene transfer, *Cell* 62:1227-1233, 1990.

107. Rich DP, Anderson MP, et al: Expression of cystic fibrosis transmembrane conductance regulator corrects defective chloride channal regulation in cystic fibrosis airway epithelium cells, *Nature* 347:358-363, 1990.

108. Welsh MJ, Anderson MP, Rich OP, et al: Cystic fibrosis transmembrane regulator: a chloride channel with novel regulation, *Neuron* 8:821-829, 1992.

109. Korst RJ, McElvaney NG, Chu CS, et al: Gene therapy for the respiratory manifestations of cystic fibrosis, *Am J Respir Crit Care Med* 151:575-587, 1995.

110. Crystal RG, McElvaney NG, Rosenfeld MA, et al: Administration of an adenovirus containing the human CFTR cDNA to the respiratory tract of individuals with cystic fibrosis, *Nature Genet* 6:42-51, 1994.

111. Rommens JM, Iannuzi MC, Kerem BT, et al: Identification of the cystic fibrosis gene: chromosome walking and jumping, *Science* 245:1059-1065, 1989.

112. Zielenski J, Markiewicz D, Chen HS, et al: Identification of six new mutations in the CFTR gene, *Hum Mutat* 5:43-47, 1995.

113. Rosenfield MA, Collins FS: Gene therapy for cystic fibrosis, *Chest* 109:241-252, 1996.

114. Rosenfield MA, Chu CS, Seth P, et al: Gene transfer to freshly isolated human respiratory epithelial cells in vitro using a replication-deficient adenovirus containing the human cystic fibrosis transmembrane conductance regulator cDNA, *Hum Gene Ther* 5:331-342, 1994.

115. Flotte TK, Conrad C, et al: Pre-clinical evaluation of AAV vectors expressing the human CFTR cDNA, *J Cell Biochem* 21A(suppl): 364, 1995 (abstract).

116. Flotte TK: A phase I study of an adeno-associated virus CFTR vector in adult patients with mild CF lung disease. RAC approved, NIH approval 11-25-94.

117. Zhong W, Leggett D, et al: Cationic liposomes-mediated in vivo gene transfer and expression, *Cell Biochem* suppl 21A:358, 1995.

118. Sorscher EJ, Logan J, Frizzel RA, et al: Gene therapy for cystic fibrosis using catonic liposome mediated gene transfer: a phase I trial of safety and efficacy in nasal airway, *Hum Gene Ther* 5:1259-1277, 1994.

119. Alton EW, Middleton FW, Caplen PG, et al: Non-invasive liposome mediated gene delivery can correct the ion transport defect in cystic fibrosis in mutant mice, *Nature Genet* 5:135-142, 1993.

120. Tropauer A, Franz MM, Dilgard VW: Psychological aspects in the care of patients with cystic fibrosis, *Am J Dis Child* 119:424-432, 1970.

121. Bywater M: Adolescents with cystic fibrosis: psychosocial adjustment, *Arch Dis Child* 56:538-543, 1981.

122. Levine SB, Stern RC: Sexual function in cystic fibrosis. Relationship to overall health status and pulmonary disease severity in 30 married patients, *Cystic Fibrosis Club Abstracts* 122-130, 1981.

123. Oppenheimer EA, Case AL, Esterly JR, et al: Cervical mucus in cystic fibrosis: a possible cause for infertility, *Am J Obstet Gynecol* 108:673-674, 1970.

124. Dooley RB: Polypoid cervicitis in cystic fibrosis patients receiving oral contraceptives, *Am J Obstet Gynecol* 118:972-974, 1974.

125. Taussig LM, Lobeck CL, di Sant'Agnese PA, et al: Fertility in males with cystic fibrosis, *N Engl J Med* 287:586-589, 1972.

126. Mellinger BC, Gorvoy JD, Brenner S, et al: *Sperm from patients with cystic fibrosis and bilateral absence of vas deferens can fertilize human eggs in vitro* (abstr) 11th International Cystic Fibrosis Congress, Dublin, Ireland, August 1992.

127. Mischler EH, Chesney PJ, et al: Demineralization in cystic fibrosis, *Am J Dis Child* 133:632-635, 1979.

128. Gibbens DT, Gilsanz V, et al: Osteoporosis in cystic fibrosis, *J Pediatr* 113:295-300, 1988.

129. Bachrach LK, Loutit CW, et al: Osteopenia in adults with cystic fibrosis, *Am J Med* 96:27-34, 1994.

130. Bhudhikanok G, Lim J, Marcus R, et al: Correlates of osteopenia in patients with cystic fibrosis, *Pediatrics* 97:103-111, 1996.

131. Ivker C, Gorvoy JD: "Lest we forget": a retrospective on a major pitfall in the diagnosis of cystic fibrosis, *Schneider Children's Hosp Q* 5:90-92, 1993.

132. *Gastrointestinal and hepatobiliary complications: changing pattern with age,* Proceedings of 8th International Cystic Fibrosis Congress, Toronto, Canada, 1980, pp 190-193.

133. Collins FS: Ninth Annual North American Cystic Fibrosis Conference, Dallas, TX, October 1995.

134. Casals T, Bassas LL, et al: Extensive analysis of 40 infertile patients with congenital absence of the vas deferens: in 50% of cases, only one CFTR allele could be detected, *Hum Genet* 95:205-211, 1995.

135. Chillon M, Casals T, Bassas L, et al: Mutations in the cystic fibrosis gene in patients with congenital absence of the vas deferens, *N Engl J Med* 332:1475-1480, 1995.

136. Osborne LR, Lynch M, et al: Nasal epithelium transport and genetic analysis of infertile men with CBAVD, *Hum Mol Genet* 2:1605-1609, 1993.

137. Gervais R, Dumur V, Rigot JM, et al: High frequency of the R117H cystic fibrosis mutation in patients with congenital absence of vas deferens, *N Engl J Med* 328:446-447, 1995.

138. Fitzsimmons SC: Cystic Fibrosis Registry updates, Bethesda, Md, 1995, Cystic Fibrosis Foundation.

139. Wong D: Transition from hospital to home for children with complex medical care, *J Pediatr Oncol Nurs* 8:3-9, 1991.

140. Harwood I, Greene L, et al: New peripherally inserted midline catheter: a better alternative for intravenous antibiotic therapy in patients with cystic fibrosis, *Pediatr Pulmonol* 12:233-239, 1992.

CHAPTER 43

Chronic Abdominal Pain

•

Mervin Silverberg

Abdominal pain is one of the most troublesome enigmas facing practitioners who care for children and adolescents. Although patients in preteen years with abdominal pain have been reviewed and closely scrutinized in the literature,[1,2] there is still little scientific explanation for the various presentations of abdominal pain in adolescents. The health care provider faced with an adolescent who has nonacute abdominal pain is likely to think in terms of adult presentations, and this often causes some discomfort to the pediatrician. More often than not, an organic cause of such pain is pursued without adequate indications, and diagnoses are made by exclusion. From the standpoint of healthcare use and costs, functional bowel complaints and related nongastroenterologic symptoms in adults are a major clinical and financial burden in the United States.[31]

CLASSIFICATION

For all practical purposes, chronic abdominal pain (CAP) refers to recurrent or persistent bouts of pain that occur over a minimum period of 3 months, involving at least three episodes, with or without compromising the daily activities of the patient.

Three major categories can be recognized:

1. *Dysfunctional abdominal pain.* More than 90% of adolescents with CAP fall into this subdivision, and two subtypes can be defined. The larger group involves alteration of bowel motility and is referred to as the irritable bowel syndrome (IBS), some- times called irritable colon, spastic colon, mucous colitis, or nervous stomach. The smaller group involves upper abdominal complaints and is known as nonulcer dyspepsia. The latter group has emerged during the past decade and has been variously called pseudoulcer syndrome, functional dyspepsia, and pyloroduodenal irritability.

2. *Psychogenic chronic abdominal pain.* Patients with CAP who have no disorder of bowel habits fall into this category. There is an apparent or subtle association with psychosocial events.

3. *Organic chronic abdominal pain.* This subdivision includes CAP due to a variety of disorders, which may number up to 100, and for which there is a diversity of presentations.

PATHOPHYSIOLOGY

The variability and poor localization of the pain is frequently frustrating. This is not unexpected from neuroanatomic and neurophysiologic points of view. Pain originating in the abdomen, except from the parietal peritoneum, is usually called visceral pain, which, in contrast to somatic pain, is often poorly described and poorly localized.[4,5] Additionally, stimulation of afferent visceral nerves occurs primarily with changes in muscle tension and organ size as seen with stretching, tension, distention, and contraction, along with inflammation and ischemia.

It has been shown that both perception and discomfort thresholds are lower in many patients with IBS or nonulcer dyspepsia than in people without these conditions.[6] The interaction between mind and gut is critical in the understanding of abdominal pain.

Adapted from Silverberg M: Chronic abdominal pain in adolescents, *Pediatric Ann* 20:179-185, 1991.

Dysfunctional Chronic Abdominal Pain

IRRITABLE BOWEL SYNDROME. IBS is characterized by alterations in bowel habits; that is, constipation or diarrhea with abdominal pain. The condition is well defined clinically in children and adults, and an impressive number of adult studies allude to a variety of abnormalities involving motor function of the small and especially the large bowel.[7-9]

The young adolescent, up to 14 years of age, may have the typical features of IBS of childhood[2] or recurrent abdominal pain (RAP) syndrome.[10] This group of patients may have mild changes in bowel habits or alternating diarrhea and constipation, with CAP.

The adolescent over 14 years of age presents with a condition more like adult IBS, with either constipation-predominant or diarrhea-predominant pain. Hereditary and familial factors appear to have some causal relationship; however, the link to altered bowel motility is poorly understood. Abnormal motility patterns have been noted by many investigators, although very few of the individuals studied have been in the adolescent age group. Studies of patients with adult IBS suggest that the colon is hyperreactive to a variety of stimuli,[6] including mechanical distention of the bowel with a balloon, food stimulation, and emotional arousal. To date, there is no evidence to link stress to any specific patterns of intestinal motility. Most reports of common neurotransmitters, such as serotonin and catecholamines, have been unrevealing. Also, attempts to relate the motility disorders to autonomic nervous system dysfunction have provided equivocal results. This is an attractive hypothesis, since so many of the associated clinical manifestations of CAP, such as headaches, limb pains, and dizziness, may be easily explained by autonomic dysfunction. In general, all of these motility studies are vulnerable to close scrutiny; for example, no differences in patterns of diarrhea or constipation have been noted and most have lacked adequate age-matched controls.

NONULCER DYSPEPSIA. This category of CAP is characterized by "peptic ulcer" symptoms with chronic or recurrent upper abdominal pain.[11] Attempts to differentiate these patients from those with IBS on the basis of psychopathology reveal that the distribution of abnormal personality traits is very similar in both conditions. A variety of etiologic factors have been investigated, but most of those investigations have been negative, unclear, or inconclusive. The etiologic factors studied include gastroduodenal dysmotility; food, substance, or medication abuse; and heredity. Chronic gastritis, particularly when associated with *Helicobacter pylori,* and chronic duodenitis are often coexistent, but the cause-and-effect relationship is still controversial.[12,13] Confounding issues include the sensitivity of different tests and differences in study populations, in,

for example, severity of pain, ethnicity, and socioeconomic factors.

Psychogenic Chronic Abdominal Pain

Psychogenic CAP does not originate from intra-abdominal primary processes. The causal relationship to psychophysiologic factors is usually present, but not always evident: for example, stress or the presence of an obvious psychiatric disorder.

Organic Chronic Abdominal Pain

Organic CAP is usually associated with specific structural, inflammatory, and biochemical abnormalities that can be demonstrated directly, by biopsy, or indirectly, by hydrogen breath analysis. The complaints of pain arise from changes in a specific abdominal organ system. Most cases in adolescents are due to disorders in the gastrointestinal tract, with genitourinary diseases not too far behind. This group of diseases is frequently accompanied by constitutional abnormalities, such as fever, weight loss, impaired growth rate, and delayed sexual development. Laboratory studies, although often not specific, point to active inflammatory processes by demonstration of anemia, leukocytosis, an elevated sedimentation rate, and a high serum immunoglobulin G level.

CLINICAL PRESENTATION

Dysfunctional Chronic Abdominal Pain

IRRITABLE BOWEL SYNDROME. The RAP syndrome is said to affect 10% to 15% of unselected schoolchildren between the ages of 5 and 15 years. The median age is 9 to 10 years for girls and 10 to 11 years for boys. The syndrome is usually more prevalent in girls than in boys, ranging up to a ratio of 2:1.

An accurate and detailed history and physical examination is essential for the initial diagnosis. If these are thorough, few studies may be required for confirmation. The pain is described as episodic with few or no signs or symptoms during pain-free intervals. Usually, there are at least three episodes of pain during any 3-month period,[1] the duration varying between 1 and 3 hours in over two thirds of the patients. The pain is usually in the periumbilical area but is often diffuse and poorly localized. There is no relationship between the occurrence of pain and the time of day, meals, or activities, and it rarely wakes the patient from sleep. More than half of the patients describe the pain as crampy. Associated complaints of fatigue, headache, limb pains, dizziness, and nausea are reported in two thirds of the patients; weight gain and growth are rarely affected, except when

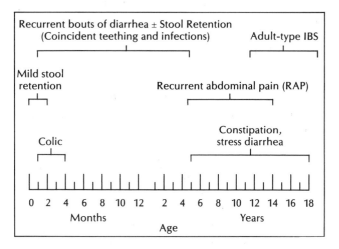

Fig. 43-1. Clinical spectrum of chronic abdominal pain. The child may demonstrate each of the clinical features in an orderly progression or may experience only part of the spectrum, most commonly recurrent abdominal pain. The older adolescent usually presents with stress-related pain and altered bowel habits.

overzealous dietary restrictions are implemented. A history of other functional gastrointestinal disorders may be found in the patient (50%) or in the immediate family (75%) (Fig. 43-1).

The physical examination in these patients is usually unrevealing. The patient looks well but is nervous and often claims to be in pain without showing commensurate pain reactions. Abdominal tenderness, without guarding, is often diffuse but maximal in the periumbilical region. Tenderness over the entire colon can frequently be demonstrated. Diagnostic study results are usually within normal limits; however, excess stool retention can usually be seen in abdominal roentgenograms. Abdominal ultrasonography and gastroduodenal endoscopy should be considered only when there are subtle or obvious reasons for invasive studies.[4] In three reports, although 16 of 215 IBS cases evaluated with abdominal ultrasound revealed abnormalities, none of these accounted for the abdominal pain or affected its management.[14-16] The value of upper endoscopy is controversial. Box 43-1 lists the characteristics of nonorganic CAP.

Adult IBS is seen in the adolescent over 14 years of age and is the most common reason for visits to a gastroenterologist's office by adolescents. Its frequency in adolescents is not documented, but it is said to affect close to 5 million adults in the United States.[17] The abdominal pain is usually in the lower abdomen and associated with at least three of the following:

Abdominal pain relieved by defecation
Increased frequency of stools with the onset of pain
A feeling of incomplete evacuation after defecation
Looser stools with the onset of pain
Abdominal distention
Mucus in the stool

Constipation is more common than diarrhea. Females predominate in a ratio of 2:1, and the disorder is less common in blacks than in other races. The patients tend to be high achievers, to be obsessive-compulsive, to be not very affectionate, and to do well in school, often working hard to achieve good grades. They tend not to be confrontational and are often upset by separation phenomena of all varieties. Many have undue fears, for example, about the safety of their parents.

NONULCER DYSPEPSIA. Nonulcer dyspepsia, a frequently abused and misunderstood term, in the present context is defined as chronic or recurrent upper abdominal pain or nausea of at least 1 months' duration that may or may not be related to meals or exertion. The full-blown syndrome includes bloating, early satiety, eructation, and anorexia. No discernible pathology or laboratory abnormalities have been consistently associated with this disorder, including *H. pylori* infection. Upper endoscopy may be cost effective.[18] The prevalence in the adult population is said to be more than twice that of peptic ulcer disease. The differential diagnoses includes gastroesophageal reflux, gastric motility disorders, biliary dyskinesia, and gallbladder disease. Biliary dyskinesia is a motor disorder of the biliary tract that should be considered in patients with typical biliary pain in whom all traditional evaluations are negative. Chronic pancreatitis is a rare condition that also may be confused with nonulcer dyspepsia.

Psychogenic Chronic Abdominal Pain

Chronic psychogenic pain is easier to diagnose when it accompanies a psychiatric syndrome such as a conversion reaction or depression. It may provide an important secondary gain whereby it diverts attention or provides relief from a more serious affective disorder. It is seen relatively infrequently in clinical practice, and patients who suffer from it may have psychological profiles and abnormal family constellations that are difficult to differentiate from those observed in many of the dysfunctional syndromes. Helpful diagnostic features include the following:

A personality disorder such as hysteria

A strong family history of psychiatric illness

An obvious unresolved emotional or stressful situation

Organic Chronic Abdominal Pain

With the exception of appendicitis, almost all organic intra-abdominal disease may initially present with an acute severe episode, a low-grade chronic pattern, or a combination of the two. Organic disease is also more likely to have chronic continuous pain as opposed to the nonorganic group, which usually has a chronic recurrent pain cycle. The list of organic conditions presenting with CAP is long and impressive, and it is possible to highlight here only the more common specific entities that may be confused with the most common dysfunctional syndromes. It should be kept in mind that these organic disorders and dysfunctional syndromes may coexist in selected cases.

CHRONIC INFLAMMATORY BOWEL DISEASE. Over 20% of patients with Crohn's disease and ulcerative colitis (see Chapter 46, "Disorders of the Small Intestine and Colon") present in the adolescent age group.[19] CAP occurs in more than 50% of these patients, and it is the predominant complaint in 75% of those with Crohn's disease. Typically, the pain in Crohn's disease is postprandial and maximal in the right lower quadrant. Perianal disease such as fissure, fistula, and abscess occurs in more than 75% of patients, occasionally preceding other complaints. Other common features associated with Crohn's disease are fever, weight loss, sexual immaturity, and a variety of extraintestinal manifestations involving the skin, joints, and eyes. There is a higher incidence in patients of Jewish descent, and a family history may be elicited in 30%.

Ulcerative colitis is somewhat less common and is usually associated with bloody diarrhea and signs and symptoms of rectosigmoid disease. Box 43-2 lists some common characteristics of organic CAP.

ACID PEPTIC (ULCER) DISEASE. Peptic ulcer in adolescents is usually primary in nature and duodenal in location (see Chapter 45, "Disorders of the Stomach and Duodenum"); recurrences are noted in over 50% of patients.[20] Pain and tenderness are localized to the epigastric region, often occurring more than 1 hour postprandially, particularly during the night; in older adolescents, it tends to be characterized by the pain-food-relief cycle. A positive family history and occult blood loss are noted in 20% to 25% of patients. Although the exact sensitivity and specificity are unknown, gastroduodenoscopy is the diagnostic gold standard because

---

> ### BOX 43-2
> ### Characteristics of Organic
> ### Chronic Abdominal Pain
>
> Consistently localized at a distance from umbilicus
> Association with vomiting, fever, weight loss, and delayed sexual development
> Frequent nocturnal episodes, particularly with concurrent diarrhea
> Association with hematochezia/melena
> Abnormal laboratory studies

it allows for direct visualization and biopsy of the ulcer; radiographic studies are less revealing. The association with *H. pylori* infection appears to be true for children as well as adults.[21]

CARBOHYDRATE INTOLERANCE. Lactose intolerance is the most common of the carbohydrate intolerances.[22] Chronic abdominal pain due to lactose intolerance is commonly associated with bloating, flatulence, and diarrhea and may be difficult to differentiate clinically from IBS. The syndrome is more prevalent in adolescents who are black, peri-Mediterranean, Native American, or Asian in origin. Sorbitol, a nonabsorbable, common sugar substitute in diets, is also a frequent offender.

DYSMENORRHEA AND PELVIC INFLAMMATORY DISEASE SYNDROMES. In the adolescent female, dysmenorrhea and pelvic inflammatory disease (PID) are two common causes of CAP that must be considered.[23] With dysmenorrhea, the pain typically begins before or close to the onset of menses, lasts up to 3 or 4 days, and is suprapubic and bilateral in location.

Most of these cases are due to primary dysmenorrhea; however, secondary dysmenorrhea should be suspected when there is associated fever, weight loss, or the presence of an intrauterine device. This periodic pain may also be part of endometriosis and PID. Menses may exacerbate the signs and symptoms of IBS. Patients with IBS may show an exaggerated bowel motility response due to prostaglandins or other mediators released during menstruation.

Pelvic inflammatory disease syndrome is the most serious complication of sexually transmitted diseases, which are increasing in frequency because of adolescent sexual behaviors. The risk is greater when the patient is promiscuous and when intrauterine contraceptive devices are used. The PID syndrome may cause recurrent lower abdominal pain, dyspareunia, dysmenorrhea, and occasionally perihepatitis (Fitz-Hugh-Curtis syndrome).

MISCELLANEOUS. Abdominal epilepsy and abdominal migraine are two rare diagnoses that are occasionally invoked with little objective evidence, and are noted here only because they may be clinically misleading.

BOX 43-3
Management Principles
for Chronic Abdominal Pain

1. Disorders present differently in adolescents than in younger children and adults.
2. Disorders related to the genitourinary tract are more prevalent in the adolescent, e.g., dysmenorrhea.
3. Adolescent life-style and stressful environmental situations are common associated factors, e.g., drugs, sexual activity, and food binges.
4. Adolescent denial and shyness are common defenses and must be dealt with in a sensitive, deliberate manner.
5. When the etiology is not organic, the majority of patients improve over time; medication should be used sparingly.
6. The physician should be accessible and have a positive attitude regarding the resolution of symptoms.

TREATMENT

A number of generalizations can be made when one approaches the problem of chronic abdominal pain (Box 43-3). The physician should try to make the diagnosis of dysfunctional and psychogenic causes in a positive, logical manner rather than by exclusion of organic causes. It is essential to explain the symptoms and signs clearly to the patient and family from a physiopathologic point of view and to convey that the pain and other complaints are really in the abdomen and not in the head. Terms such as "emotional," "psychogenic," and "stress-related" are frequently misinterpreted as "imaginary and manipulative" and may alienate the patient or family. The patient's perception and expectations should be factored into the treatment goals, and this should be discussed openly.

Irritable Bowel Syndrome

In mild cases, reassurance is the cornerstone of treatment, and the patient is encouraged to eat regularly, including only foods that are well tolerated. Dietary manipulation[24] is still controversial, except with suspected or actual nutrient intolerances, such as lactose. Despite the widespread "bran wagon," the efficacy of dietary fiber supplements has been studied in IBS patients in controlled crossover studies, with beneficial effects reported in only four out of 10 reports; a placebo effect is most common.[25] When patients insist on a dietary fiber supplement or diet, it should be prescribed with the caveat that excessive fiber may actually increase pain and also cause excess gas and abdominal distention.

A mild laxative should be used when there is evidence of constipation. A stool softener, such as docusate sodium succinate, 100-300 mg two or three times daily, or a senna preparation given twice a day, may be very effective in about 50% of cases. Senokot granules may be given 1 teaspoon, once or twice a day; tablets may be given two tablets, once or twice a day. Chronic laxative use of any kind should be avoided.

Severe cases of constipation require more aggressive therapy. The recommendations for reassurance, dietary therapy, and laxatives are similar to those for milder cases. A clear plan for effecting a postprandial bowel movement is indicated with diarrhea-prone and constipation-prone patients. It is important to present the goal of learning to live with some discomfort, for example, as with migraine headaches, and to develop a plan to normalize the life style as soon as possible. This requires the cooperation of the family and school officials, and general agreement to decrease the attention paid to the patient's somatic complaints. Other behavior strategies include increasing physical activities, rewarding healthy behaviors, and encouraging patient coping and participation in the treatment. Specific techniques such as biofeedback, relaxation, and stress management require special professional intervention.

Multitreatment pain control centers have recently emerged as a rational and efficient modality to treat difficult cases. Some of these centers have used acupuncture and hypnosis as part of the regimen. Unfortunately, to date, there are few studies to evaluate their work.

Psychiatric or psychosocial referrals are frequently necessary and should be made early in the course of management. Several approaches have been used with success, such as individual psychotherapy, behavior modification, and family and group therapy.

Although many patients appear to improve dramatically after hospitalization, this is only transitory and is frequently rejected for reimbursement by third-party payers. Medications, as a general rule, should be used minimally; these include analgesics, antidepressants, and benzodiazepines. Anticholinergic and antispasmodic drugs are widely used by primary care physicians, but there is no evidence that they produce any consistently good results.

Nonulcer Dyspepsia

These patients also require an individualized treatment plan with emphasis on reassurance, primary care physician availability, and defusion of psychosocial issues. Although there is little evidence that these factors make a difference, patients should be advised to avoid smoking, using analgesics, and drinking alcohol and coffee. While no relationship of symptoms to the eating of specific foods has been established, limited dietary elimination should be tried, based on the patient's recorded experience. Prokinetic drugs, H_2-receptor blockers, and antibiotics directed to *H. pylori* are anecdotally successful but remain controversial and cannot be generally recommended.[18]

Finally, psychogenic CAP patients almost always require appropriate input from mental health professionals, and psychoactive drugs may be indicated. The various psychotherapies as noted above should be recommended early in the management of these patients to enable coping strategies to be developed.

SUMMARY

Although there are very few prospective studies of CAP, organic causes of the problem are misdiagnosed in probably less than 5% of adolescents. Response to treatment seems to be better in males who have had signs and symptoms for less than 6 months and is rather poor for patients with complaints that have lasted longer than 2 years. An organized nomenclature is necessary for classifying dysfunctional disorders, and physicians must recognize that these patients represent a heterogeneous population. In general, adequate data from the numbers of the adolescent population affected by these diseases are not available, so that physicians are still required to depend to a large extent on speculation and anecdotal information in assessing and managing these patients.

References

1. Apley J: *The child with abdominal pains,* ed 2, Oxford, 1975, Blackwell Scientific.
2. Davidson M, Wasserman R: The irritable colon of childhood (chronic nonspecific diarrhea syndrome), *J Pediatr* 69:1027-1038, 1966.
3. Longstreth GF: Irritable bowel syndrome: a multi-billion-dollar problem, *Gastroenterology* 109:2019-2031, 1995.
4. Antonson DL: Abdominal pain. *Gastrointest Endosc Clin North Am* 4:1-21, 1994.
5. Mayer EA, Gebhart GF: Basic and clinical aspects of visceral hyperalgesia, *Gastroenterology* 107:271-293, 1994.
6. Whitehead WE, Holtkotter B, Enck P, et al: Tolerance for rectosigmoid distention in irritable bowel syndrome, *Gastroenterology* 98:1187-1192, 1990.
7. Sullivan MA, Cohn S, Snape WJ: Chronic myoelectrical activity in the irritable bowel syndrome: effect of eating and anticholinergics, *N Engl J Med* 298:878-883, 1978.
8. Kellow JE, Gill RC, Wingate DL: Prolonged ambulent recordings of small bowel motility demonstrate abnormalities in the irritable bowel syndrome, *Gastroenterology* 98:1208-1218, 1990.
9. Kopel FB, Kim IC, Barbero GJ: Comparison of rectosigmoid motility in normal children, children with recurrent abdominal pain and children with ulcerative colitis, *Pediatrics* 39:539-545, 1967.
10. Barbero GJ: Recurrent abdominal pain in childhood, *Pediatr Rev* 4:29-34, 1982.
11. Talley NJ, Phillips SF: Non-ulcer dyspepsia: potential causes and pathophysiology, *Ann Intern Med* 108:865-879, 1988.
12. Crabtree JE, Mahony MJ, Taylor JD, et al: Immune responses to *Helicobacter pylori* in children with recurrent abdominal pain, *J Clin Pathol* 44:768-771, 1991.
13. Hardikar W, Feekery C, Smith A, et al: *Helicobacter pylori* and recurrent abdominal pain in children, *J Pediatr Gastroenterol Nutr* 22:148-152, 1996.
14. Van der Meer SB, Forget PP, Arends JW, et al: Diagnostic value of ultrasound in children with recurrent abdominal pain, *Pediatr Radiol* 20:501-503, 1990.
15. Schmidt RE, Babcock DS, Farrell MK: Use of abdominal and pelvic ultrasound in the evaluation of chronic abdominal pain, *Clin Pediatr (Phila)* 32:147-150, 1993.
16. Shanon A, Martin DJ, Feldman W: Ultrasonographic studies in the management of recurrent abdominal pain, *Pediatrics* 86:35-38, 1990.
17. Sandler RS: Epidemiology of irritable bowel syndrome in the United States, *Gastroenterology* 99:409-415, 1990.
18. Silverstein MD, Patterson T, Talley NJ: Initial endoscopy or empirical therapy with or without testing for *Helicobacter pylori* for dyspepsia: a decision analysis, *Gastroenterology* 110:72-83, 1996.
19. Daum F: Pediatric inflammatory bowel disease. In Silverberg M, Daum F, editors: *Textbook of pediatric gastroenterology,* Chicago, 1988, Mosby–Year Book; pp 392-412.
20. Drumm B, Rhoads JM, Stringer DA, et al: Peptic ulcer disease in children: etiology, clinical findings, and clinical course, *Pediatrics* 82:410-414, 1988.
21. Macarthur C, Saunders N, Feldman W: *Helicobacter pylori,* gastroduodenal disease and recurrent abdominal pain in children, *JAMA* 729-734, 1995.
22. Lebenthal E, Rossi TM, Nord KS, et al: Recurrent abdominal pain and lactose absorption in children, *Pediatrics* 67:828-832, 1981.
23. Barr RG: Abdominal pain in the female adolescent, *Pediatr Rev* 4:281-289, 1983.
24. Nanda R, James R, Smith JR et al: Food intolerance and the irritable bowel syndrome, *Gut* 30:1099-1104, 1989.
25. Cook JJ, Irving EJ, Campbell D, et al: Effect of dietary fiber on symptoms and rectosigmoid motility in patients with irritable bowel syndrome: a controlled crossover study, *Gastroenterology* 98:66-72, 1990.

CHAPTER 44

Disorders of the Esophagus

•

James F. Markowitz

Disorders of esophageal structure and function are common in the adolescent. While primary esophageal diseases are most common, the esophagus is also frequently the site of pathology as a consequence of systemic illness. Classically, adolescents complain of symptoms similar to those expressed by adults: dysphagia (difficulty in swallowing), odynophagia (pain on swallowing), heartburn, eructation, water brash, and vomiting. However, less typical complaints also appear to arise from esophageal dysfunction in the adolescent. Therefore, esophageal dysfunction also should be considered in any patient who complains of nausea, especially if it is sensed in the throat rather than the abdomen, or of an ill-defined "empty" or "gnawing" sensation in the subxiphoid or upper epigastric area.

The prevalence of esophageal dysfunction during adolescence has not been determined. A sampling of any busy medical practice that involves caring for adolescents, however, will reveal that complaints suggestive of esophageal disease are frequent. Most patients with these complaints are found to have symptoms arising from gastroesophageal reflux (GER). The remainder are ultimately shown to have a variety of other gastrointestinal or biliary tract disorders. Although the other disorders of esophageal function discussed in this chapter are much less common than GER, they occur often enough to be important considerations for all physicians who provide care for adolescent patients.

DISORDERS OF STRUCTURE AND FUNCTION

Anatomic Abnormalities

Congenital esophageal lesions rarely evade detection during childhood. Occasionally, however, a congenital lesion such as esophageal stenosis from submucosal thickening of the proximal esophagus can remain undiagnosed until adolescence. While these congenital lesions cause dysphagia from early in life, patients can compensate for their symptoms and escape diagnosis until the second or third decade of life. Other congenital lesions are recognized and treated in infancy, but the consequences of lesions such as tracheoesophageal fistula or esophageal atresia often result in ongoing problems during adolescence. Persistent dysmotility and anastomotic narrowing associated with the repair of these lesions can often lead to dysphagia or food impaction. Acquired membranous webs of the proximal esophagus associated with epidermolysis bullosa or iron deficiency anemia, and obstructing (Schatzki's) rings of the distal esophagus, occasionally occur in adolescence. A traction diverticulum due to a foregut cyst also has been described in an adolescent. These esophageal lesions can cause intermittent dysphagia, food or foreign body impaction, and pain. Treatment includes dilation, endoscopic disruption, and surgery.

Primary Dysmotility

Abnormalities of esophageal motility in an otherwise healthy adolescent are unusual. However, certain disorders should be considered in an adolescent who has dysphagia or unexplained chest pain.[1]

ACHALASIA. Achalasia is characterized by incomplete relaxation of the lower esophageal sphincter (LES) after swallowing.[2,3] Frequently, LES pressure is also markedly elevated, and there is an associated absence of coordinated peristalsis in the body of the esophagus. In affected adults, 5% date the onset of their symptoms to before the age of 15 years. The cause of this condition remains unknown, although in children and adolescents achalasia has been associated with chronic intestinal pseudo-obstruction, chronic granulomatous disease, and Chagas' disease. A heightened response to cholinergic agonists such as methacholine suggests denervation hypersensitivity. It is not surprising, therefore, that histopathologic studies often have demonstrated abnormalities of the enteric neurons within the esophagus. More recent studies have demonstrated loss of nonadrenergic, noncholinergic neurons that appear responsible for secreting vasoactive intestinal peptide (VIP) and nitrous oxide, two known mediators of smooth muscle relaxation.[4,5] Achalasia therefore appears to be the clinical expression of unopposed contractile stimuli to the smooth muscle of the esophagus.

Patients with achalasia complain of intermittent but progressive, painless dysphagia. As the disease advances, the ingestion of liquids and solids is affected, and esophageal retention of ingested food occurs. Undigested food is frequently regurgitated, leading to weight loss or an aversion to eating. Chronic pulmonary aspirations result in recurrent pneumonia, chronic cough, or asthma.

The diagnosis of achalasia is suggested radiographically by an aperistaltic esophagus on barium swallow that is associated with a dilated esophageal body tapering to a narrowed distal esophagus, resulting in the typical "bird's-beak" appearance (Fig. 44-1, A). Retained food is also commonly identified within the esophageal lumen. Esophageal manometry (Fig. 44-1, B) reveals characteristic lack of LES relaxation and nonpropagated pressure

waves in the distal two thirds (smooth muscle portion) of the esophageal body. The upper esophageal sphincter (UES) and the upper third (striated muscle) of the esophageal body are usually normal. Although provocative testing with a cholinergic agonist reveals a characteristic spasm of the distal esophagus and LES, the test is painful and rarely indicated.

Treatment often consists of forceful pneumatic dilation, which may relieve symptoms for 1 or more years in 60% to 80% of adolescents. Many centers prefer esophagomyotomy as initial therapy, which often results in permanent resolution of symptoms. While both approaches are generally effective in relieving symptoms, either can be associated with significant short- and long-term morbidity.[6] In particular, severe GER and its complications can occur after disruption of the LES barrier. Pharmacologic intervention with calcium channel blockers has been advocated but appears to offer only transient resolution of symptoms at best.[7] By contrast, recent reports have demonstrated dramatic resolution of symptoms in adults with achalasia after endoscopic

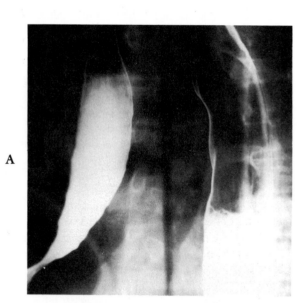

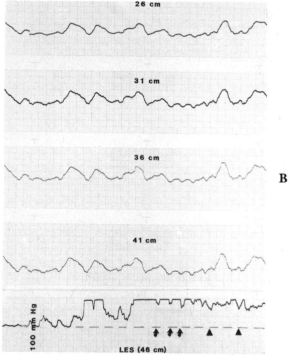

Fig. 44-1. A, Barium esophagram obtained from a 16-year-old boy with achalasia. Note the diffuse dilation of the body of the esophagus with air. The barium level is depicted in the right panel. The left panel demonstrates the typical "bird's-beak" appearance of the distal esophagus. **B,** Esophageal manometry in the same patient. The most distal pressure port is located in the lower esophageal sphincter (LES), 46 cm from the nares. Another four ports are located in the distal and middle esophagus at intervals of 5 cm. Total LES pressure is more than 50 mm Hg (normal = 10 to 20 mm Hg), as evidenced by the cutoff in the recorded signal in the lowermost panel (gastric baseline pressure is indicated by the dashed line). Multiple dry swallows *(curved arrows)* and "wet" swallows of 10 ml of water *(arrowheads)* do not result in relaxation of the LES to baseline gastric pressure. In the middle and distal esophagus, swallowing results in simultaneous rather than peristaltic contractions.

injection of botulinum toxin into the lower esophagus.[8] The toxin directly interferes with smooth muscle contraction, resulting in prolonged reduction of LES tone. Although no reports of the use of this technique in children and adolescents have been published, the method should be as effective in these younger patients as it is in adults.

SPASM. Demonstrated manometrically by high-amplitude, usually nonperistaltic contractions of the body of the esophagus, esophageal spasm causes severe, intermittent chest pain. Patients may or may not also complain of dysphagia. Barium esophagram may reveal a "corkscrew" appearance of the lower two thirds of the esophagus. Results of esophagoscopy are commonly normal. Treatment regimens in adolescents have not been reported extensively. Early studies in adults suggested that calcium channel blockers may be of benefit, but more recent studies have been equivocal. Dilations and long surgical myotomies also have been of some benefit. However, symptoms may be intermittent, and a few adolescents have been reported to be either asymptomatic or having only mild, occasional symptoms 2 years after initial diagnosis despite receiving no specific therapy.[9]

DYSFUNCTION OF BELCH REFLEX. In a few young adults, incapacitating chest pain has been attributed to upper esophageal dysfunction resulting in an inability to belch.[10,11] All these patients had symptoms dating back to adolescence. Reflux of gas from the stomach to the esophagus occurred normally, but the resultant distention of the proximal esophagus failed to trigger appropriate UES relaxation. Manometry confirmed that the tone of the UES always exceeded that of the more distal esophagus, but that the rest of the esophagus had normal manometric characteristics. Pain was relieved by lying down, which minimized gaseous GER, or by passing a nasoesophageal tube through the UES. No other specific therapies have been described.

Secondary Dysmotility

Abnormalities of esophageal motor function also have been described as resulting from a wide variety of systemic disorders (Box 44-1). In addition, toxic injuries to the esophagus—caused by radiation, chemotherapy, injection sclerotherapy, or caustic ingestion—also result in temporary or permanent disruption of normal esophageal motor function. These conditions cause abnormal motor function by different mechanisms that ultimately result in direct injury to either the esophageal smooth muscle or neural elements (Fig. 44-2). Dysphagia and chest pain are common, and the diagnosis is often suggested by the patient's medical history. Treatment varies according to the nature of the underlying illness.

Gastroesophageal Reflux

GER is probably the most common disorder of the esophagus in adolescents.[12,13] Otherwise healthy patients can develop symptoms acutely or can manifest a persistence or exacerbation of symptoms present from childhood. In addition, adolescents with significant neurologic impairment represent a population at particularly high risk for the symptoms of GER and its complications.

ETIOLOGY. Despite the frequency of GER, its cause remains unknown. In contrast to infants with GER who are thought to have reflux because of a relatively immature LES barrier mechanism, adolescents with pathologic GER are unlikely to "grow out" of their symptoms. As in adults, only a small subset of adolescents with GER have a hypotensive LES. Instead, a transient, spontaneous, "inappropriate" relaxation of an otherwise normally functioning LES is the most commonly identified pathophysiologic event precipitating GER in the adolescent. Occasionally, patients have been identified as having GER that appears to be secondary to antropyloric dysfunction, which leads to delayed gastric emptying. The mechanisms underlying these motor disturbances still need to be elucidated.

SYMPTOMS AND SIGNS. Unlike the infant or younger child with GER whose primary presentation is usually effortless regurgitation, the adolescent with GER commonly complains of eructation, water brash, and subster-

---

BOX 44-1
Systemic Disorders Associated with Esophageal Motor Dysfunction

NEUROLOGIC DISORDERS
Familial dysautonomia
Static central nervous system injury secondary to cerebral palsy or cerebrovascular accidents
Multiple sclerosis
Neuropathic forms of intestinal pseudo-obstruction

NEUROMUSCULAR DISORDERS
Myasthenia gravis

MUSCULAR DISORDERS
Muscular dystrophy
Polymyositis, dermatomyositis
Progressive systemic sclerosis
Myopathic forms of intestinal pseudo-obstruction

INFECTIOUS DISORDERS
Chagas' disease

OTHER DISORDERS
Graft-versus-host disease
Chronic granulomatous disease

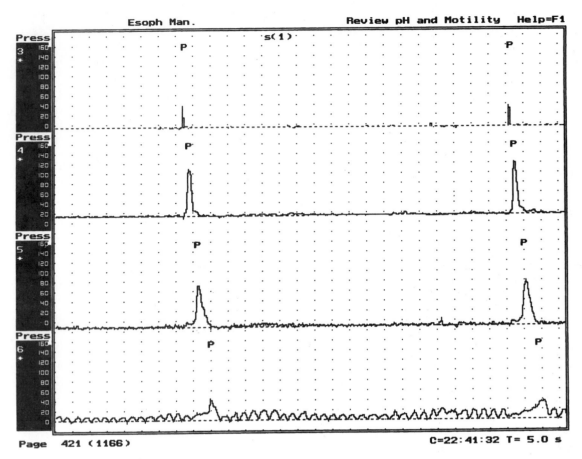

Fig. 44-2. A, Normal esophageal manometry utilizing an ambulatory motility system. An esophageal catheter with four solid-state transducers 10 cm apart was situated so that the most proximal transducer (channel 3) was located in the posterior pharynx and the most distal (channel 6) in the distal esophagus. Two normal esophageal peristaltic waves progress down the esophagus in a coordinated manner, with contraction amplitudes ranging from 60 to 100 mm Hg in the midesophagus. (X axis = 5 seconds/gradation; Y axis = mm Hg).

nal or subxiphoid pain. At times, intermittent dysphagia or odynophagia may be prominent, or hematemesis can cause the adolescent to seek medical evaluation. Occasionally, adolescent patients develop aversions to eating and lose weight, superficially mimicking patients with classic eating disorders. Adolescents with GER are also identified after evaluation of disease processes known to result as complications of GER. These include recurrent aspiration pneumonia, nocturnal asthma, chronic cough or hoarseness, chronic esophagitis, and esophageal stricture.

DIAGNOSIS. In the typical adolescent, a clinical diagnosis of GER can be strongly suspected on the basis of the clinical history. One or more of the following tests may be indicated, however, to differentiate between anatomic abnormalities that might be mimicking GER, to temporally relate episodes of reflux to specific symptoms, or to identify complications of GER.

1. *Contrast radiography* of the esophagus and upper gastrointestinal tract delineates anatomy and to some extent function. Esophageal webs or rings, abnormalities of the gastric outlet, and intestinal malrotation can be identified, as can complications such as esophageal strictures. Careful double-contrast studies are required to delineate esophagitis. Although radiographs can reveal episodes of GER, the false-negative rate can be as high as 50%. In addition, a few uncomplicated episodes of GER during a radiographic study are not necessarily diagnostic of pathologic GER.

2. *Esophageal manometry* can characterize esophageal body and LES motor function. However, in most cases LES pressure correlates poorly with the presence or severity of GER. Therefore, this procedure is not often indicated for routine clinical purposes. Manometry is useful, however, to evalu-

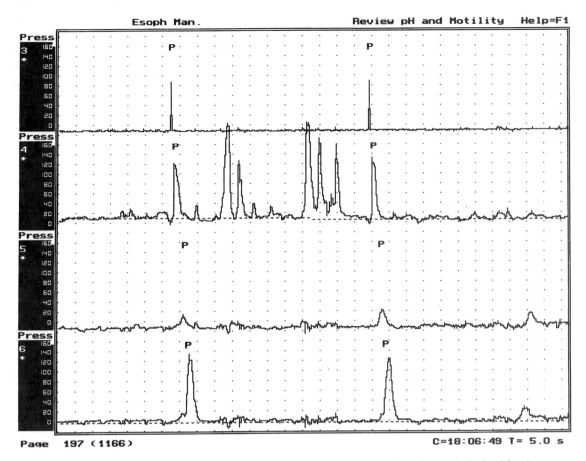

Page   197 (1166)   C=18:06:49 T= 5.0 s

Fig. 44-2, cont'd. B, Abnormal esophageal motility (localized esophageal spasm) obtained from a 17-year-old boy with a neuropathic form of intestinal pseudo-obstruction. The recording device and esophageal catheter placement are identical to that described in **A**. Recurrent spontaneous high amplitude (>150 mm Hg) contractions are noted only in channel 4. These contractions coincided with the subjective experience of chest pain.

ate the adolescent with dysphagia due to GER, primarily by allowing the exclusion of other motility disturbances. It can also be of benefit when performed as a prolonged ambulatory study with a simultaneous pH probe. Such a study can allow the characterization of an episodic clinical symptom such as pain, and clarify the degree to which such a symptom is an "acid" as opposed to a "motor" event.

3. *Radionuclide scanning* can directly demonstrate GER, but this technique generally has been more useful as a means of assessing possible pulmonary aspiration due to reflux. In addition, gastric emptying can be accurately measured with separate labels attached to the liquid and the solid components of a standardized meal.

4. *Flexible esophagoscopy* allows direct visualization and biopsy of the esophageal mucosa. Anatomic lesions of the esophagus such as webs or strictures can be delineated and, at times, treated. Although endoscopy can demonstrate the consequences of

GER such as esophagitis, it cannot directly demonstrate GER itself. It must be remembered that not every patient with symptomatic GER develops esophageal mucosal lesions.

5. *Intraesophageal pH monitoring* is currently the gold standard for diagnosing pathologic GER. Ambulatory 24-hour monitors and sophisticated computer analyses of the tracings are now widely available (Fig. 44-3). When coupled with a careful patient diary, the pH probe is particularly valuable as a means of correlating ill-defined or atypical symptoms with episodes of GER.

6. Reproducing a patient's symptoms by the intraesophageal perfusion of acid, or the *Bernstein test,* is occasionally useful in adolescents with atypical symptoms. However, the subjective nature of the test makes its interpretation difficult. The Bernstein test has been supplanted increasingly by intraesophageal pH monitoring.

TREATMENT. Management of the adolescent with pathologic GER depends on the nature and the severity of

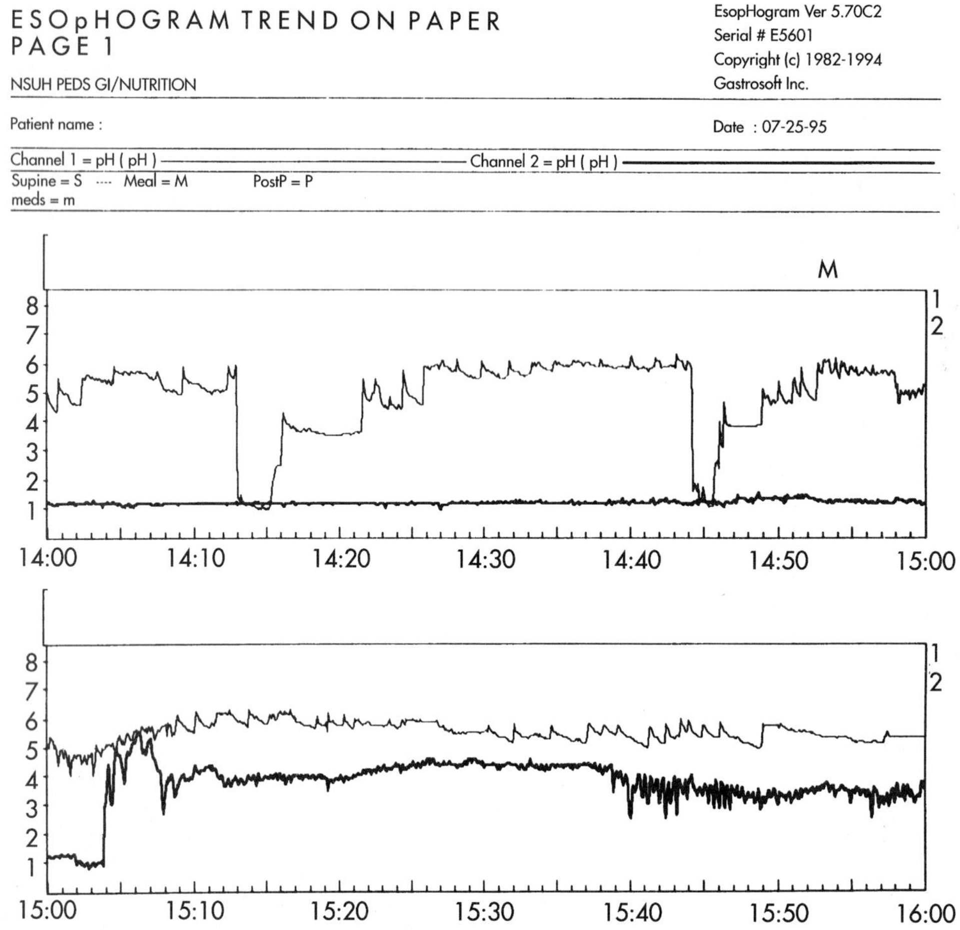
ESOpHOGRAM TREND ON PAPER
PAGE 1
NSUH PEDS GI/NUTRITION
EsopHogram Ver 5.70C2
Serial # E5601
Copyright (c) 1982-1994
Gastrosoft Inc.
Patient name :
Date : 07-25-95
Channel 1 = pH (pH)
Channel 2 = pH (pH)
Supine = S
Meal = M
PostP = P
meds = m
M
1
2
8
7
6
5
4
3
2
1
14:00
14:10
14:20
14:30
14:40
14:50
15:00
15:00
15:10
15:20
15:30
15:40
15:50
16:00

Fig. 44-3. Two-hour segment of a 24-hour ambulatory pH probe recording. Two probes simultaneously record the pH of the distal esophagus (channel 1, top tracing on each panel) and stomach (channel 2, bottom tracing on each panel). Intragastric contents are acid (pH = 1.2) until neutralized by the ingestion of a meal (M). In the time interval before the meal, two distinct, poorly cleared episodes of gastroesophageal reflux (intraesophageal pH drops to <4.0 for >5 minutes) are recorded. (X axis = 1 minute/minor tick; Y axis = pH units).

the symptoms. In general, most patients do well with conservative therapy directed at dietary and life style changes. Patients should be counseled to eat smaller, more frequent meals. Certain foods and medications, smoking, and alcohol intake should be limited or eliminated because of their adverse effects on LES pressure or gastric emptying (see Box 44-2). Raising the head of the bed with blocks or by insertion of a foam wedge under the bedsheet is particularly helpful in patients with nocturnal GER. Coexistent constipation should be identified and treated vigorously, because significant improvement in GER symptoms often occurs as a result of such treatment.

At times, the severity of symptoms or the development of complications such as esophagitis demands more aggressive therapy. In patients with significant pain or esophagitis, acid neutralization with appropriate doses of antacids or the use of H_2-receptor antagonists is beneficial. Ranitidine, famotidine, or nizatidine, with their once- or twice-daily dosage regimens, are often more readily accepted by adolescents than cimetidine, which requires a 6-hour dosing schedule. However, more frequent dosing regimens may be required, even with the newer H_2 blockers. Omeprazole and lansoprazole, potent inhibitors of the parietal cell H^+,K^+ pump, are effective for patients with intractable symptoms or esophagitis. Sucralfate, particularly the liquid preparation, also may be useful. Prokinetic agents, including metoclopramide, domperidone, and cisapride, improve the abnormal esophagogastric motility underlying GER. These agents can be used as adjuncts to, or therapeutic alternatives for, acid suppression, and have proved highly efficacious in the treatment of GER.

In a few patients, GER remains intractable despite aggressive medical therapy. In others, the complications of GER (e.g., esophageal strictures, recurrent aspirations) make trials of medical therapy ill advised. For such patients a surgical antireflux procedure such as the Nissen fundoplication has been beneficial. Short-term benefits have been widely reported, but questions remain as to how long fundoplications will remain effective antireflux barriers.

MUCOSAL DISORDERS

Peptic Esophagitis

ETIOLOGY. Reflux of gastric contents through the LES exposes the esophageal mucosa to hydrochloric acid, pepsin, and (at times) bile salts and pancreatic enzymes. Since the squamous epithelium of the esophagus has a limited ability to protect itself against these noxious agents, inflammation and ulceration can result. Whether esophagitis develops depends on a number of factors, including the nature and concentration of refluxed materials, the frequency of reflux, and the efficiency of esophageal clearance. Clearance is enhanced by both primary and secondary esophageal peristalsis and by the swallowing of bicarbonate-rich saliva, which directly neutralizes refluxed acid. Conversely, clearance is impaired by a hiatal hernia. Although no extensive studies in adolescents have been reported, studies in adults suggest that patients who reflux primarily at night are at greatest risk for developing peptic esophagitis. The infrequent rate of swallowing during sleep predisposes such patients to poor acid clearance and resultant prolonged episodes of acid reflux. Daytime, or so-called upright, refluxers appear to have more discomfort yet less

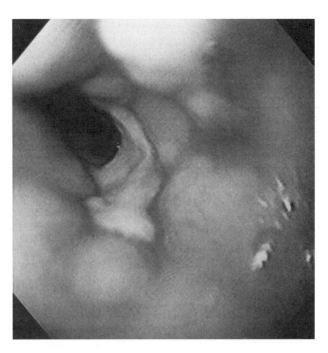

Fig. 44-4. Endoscopic appearance of the distal esophagus of an 18-year-old boy with severe neurodevelopmental retardation. A thick membranous exudate overlies a distal esophageal ulcer. The esophageal lumen distal to the ulceration is somewhat stenotic.

esophagitis than do nocturnal refluxers, possibly because their discomfort results in improved acid clearance through an increased frequency of swallowing saliva, food, or antacid.

Rare patients develop peptic esophagitis from an ectopic patch of gastric epithelium in the distal cervical esophagus. This type of lesion secretes acid and may cause localized esophagitis adjacent to the ectopic tissue.

SYMPTOMS AND SIGNS. The symptoms of peptic esophagitis are not significantly different from those of uncomplicated GER. Odynophagia and dysphagia can range from mild to severe, but patients may also be completely asymptomatic. Pain is described as burning, or crushing, or as a vague, ill-defined sensation. Food impaction or severe dysphagia is unusual unless there is a stricture. Hematemesis or occult gastrointestinal bleeding also can be present. The response to empirically prescribed antacids or dietary manipulations is variable.

DIAGNOSIS. Esophagitis should be suspected whenever a patient with a history of, or symptoms compatible with, GER develops hematemesis, occult gastrointestinal bleeding, or worsening dysphagia or odynophagia. Esophagoscopy is the diagnostic procedure of choice. Visualization of the esophageal mucosa may reveal hyperemia, erosions, or ulcerations with exudate that generally start at the esophagogastric junction and extend proximally for a variable distance (Fig. 44-4). However, there is often poor correlation between endoscopic and histologic severity. Biopsies therefore should be obtained even when the mucosa appears normal.[14]

Barium studies of the esophagus are much less sensitive than endoscopy, but they do offer important information when symptoms suggest that a stricture might be present. However, a normal mucosal contour on a contrast study is not sufficient to rule out the possibility of even moderate degrees of esophagitis.

TREATMENT. Treatment modalities have been outlined in the section on GER. Esophagitis may require vigorous therapy, not only to heal inflammatory changes but also to prevent their recurrence. Often the latter goal is far more difficult to accomplish than the former. Prolonged treatment with a combination of medications designed to suppress acid production and promote more normal esophagogastric motility may be necessary. Elimination of cigarette smoking and cessation of alcohol ingestion remain important adjuncts to therapy.

COMPLICATIONS. Esophageal stricture can occur as a direct result of chronic peptic esophagitis and often heralds significant morbidity. Progressive dysphagia or recurrent food impactions require multiple interventions, including recurrent esophageal dilations. For such adolescents, nutritional intake is often compromised, and growth failure with delayed sexual maturation is not uncommon. Therefore, antireflux surgery, designed to prevent repeated GER after dilation, is frequently indicated.

Another complication of long-standing peptic esophagitis is the development of Barrett's esophagus.[15,16] In this premalignant lesion the normal squamous epithelium of the esophagus is replaced by a gastric type of columnar epithelium. It is well documented in adults that adenocarcinoma arises within the epithelium in Barrett's esophagus. Adolescents with adenocarcinoma of the esophagus and Barrett's esophagus changes have also been described.[17] In our practice the presence of Barrett's esophagus epithelium in an otherwise healthy adolescent is usually an indication for prolonged aggressive medical therapy with omeprazole and/or cisapride or for antireflux surgery. In addition, the premalignant nature of this lesion demands frequent endoscopic surveillance with careful biopsy sampling of the mucosa for the presence of dysplasia or other premalignant markers.[18] Although the literature remains contradictory, there are reports suggesting that Barrett's epithelium can regress if the noxious effects of GER are eliminated.

Caustic Esophagitis

In general, ingestion of caustic agents is not seen in adolescents, except in association with suicide attempts. However, inadvertent ingestions have been reported: for example, Clinitest tablets have been ingested mistakenly.

Although only mildly alkaline, these tablets generate intense heat during hydration, which can result in severe esophageal ulceration and stricture formation. Button batteries also have been inadvertently swallowed. If these objects become lodged in the esophagus, the leakage of their alkaline contents can cause necrosis, perforation, and death. Acid injuries are less common. Patients with strong alkali or acid ingestions may have burns of the oral cavity or respiratory symptoms and varying degrees of dysphagia or odynophagia. The severity of lasting injury is variable, ranging from complete healing without sequelae to intractable, long, and often occlusive esophageal strictures.

Oral medications also can cause acute esophageal damage[19] (Box 44-3). Pills can become impacted within a normal esophagus, especially if they are ingested with little or no fluid. Patients complain of the acute onset of severe odynophagia and the sensation that the pill has become stuck in the esophagus. Esophagoscopy often reveals a highly localized area of ulceration that usually heals rapidly without permanent damage.

There are also a number of iatrogenic causes of esophageal injury in adolescent patients. Radiation and chemotherapy commonly result in esophagitis, which can be aggravated by superimposed peptic or infectious injury. Graft-versus-host disease after bone marrow transplantation also can cause severe esophageal mucosal damage. Injection sclerotherapy for bleeding esophageal varices is another form of treatment producing potentially severe mucosal and submucosal injury, ulceration, and ultimately stricture formation. In general, however, those adolescents who receive sclerotherapy have minimal complaints, and serious strictures have not been reported.

Infection

Infectious esophagitis is a cause of morbidity in both normal and immunocompromised adolescents.[20] Fungal (especially *Candida albicans*) and viral (herpes simplex and cytomegalovirus) agents are most common, but other organisms also have been seen in the immunocompro-

---

BOX 44-3
**Medications Associated
with Caustic Esophagitis**

Tetracyclines
Potassium chloride
Theophylline
Nonsteroidal anti-inflammatory agents
Ascorbic acid
Chloral hydrate

mised patient. Patients complain of severe odynophagia, dysphagia, or chest pain. Diagnosis is best made by endoscopy, at which time brushings and biopsy specimens can be obtained for cytologic and histologic examination and for culture. An esophagram may suggest the diagnosis, but normal or nondiagnostic studies can be seen in 20% to 50% of patients, depending on whether double- or single-contrast studies, respectively, are performed. Treatment is determined by the specific microbiologic cause and the underlying immunocompetence of the patient.

MISCELLANEOUS CONDITIONS

Trauma

Both extraluminal and intraluminal events can injure the esophagus. Penetrating wounds or the effects of externally applied blunt trauma are rare causes of esophageal injury in the adolescent, but intraluminal events are more common causes. Linear tears of the mucosa at the esophagogastric junction (Mallory-Weiss tears) are fairly common after vigorous or prolonged retching or forceful vomiting. Although bleeding can be massive, it usually ceases spontaneously, requires no specific treatment, and leaves no lasting sequelae. By contrast, spontaneous transmural rupture of the esophagus (Boerhaave's syndrome), which is very rare, is associated with a high degree of morbidity and mortality.

Other mechanisms of esophageal injury result in perforations of the esophagus induced by extrinsically applied intraluminal forces. The use of instruments, such as endoscopes, dilators, and nasogastric and orogastric tubes, is the most common reason for perforation injuries, but air-pressure injuries also occur from misplaced endotracheal tubes or purposeful inhalation of materials packaged in high-pressure containers.

Most patients with esophageal perforation have pain, which may be in the neck, chest, or epigastrium, depending on the location of the injury. Dysphagia, fever, and respiratory difficulties can also occur. Subcutaneous emphysema may be palpable in the neck. Plain radiographs of the chest or neck demonstrate mediastinal or subcutaneous air, but the site of perforation is best identified by a water-soluble contrast esophagram. Esophagoscopy is rarely necessary and often ill-advised, except in the case of a suspected Mallory-Weiss tear.

Treatment depends on the site and the cause of perforation and the duration of injury before diagnosis. Surgery is often indicated, but small, noncontaminated leaks can sometimes be treated conservatively (nothing by mouth, antibiotics). Mallory-Weiss tears heal spontaneously once bleeding stops, but basic resuscitative measures applicable to all causes of upper gastrointestinal hemorrhage may be required.

Varices

Submucosal varices arising as a consequence of portal hypertension, in association with either liver disease or prehepatic and (occasionally) posthepatic venous obstruction, are the cause of significant morbidity during adolescence. By one estimate, once varices develop, significant episodes of bleeding will occur in as many as 33% of patients. It is generally accepted that varices do not erode from overlying mucosal ulceration but explode as a consequence of the unequal pressures that exist across the luminal wall of the varix. The current treatment trend avoids surgical intervention as a means of controlling variceal hemorrhage. Instead, endoscopic injection sclerotherapy or rubber band ligation is used to obliterate the varices, thereby preventing further episodes of bleeding.[21] Although these techniques are safe and efficacious in adolescents, sclerotherapy in particular is not without its side effects. Mucosal ulceration (occasionally accompanied by secondary massive hemorrhage), stricture formation, esophageal perforation, pneumonitis, and other less common complications have been described. In addition, these techniques deal only with the consequences of the portal hypertension rather than the cause. Given these realities, adolescents found to have varices are increasingly considered as candidates for the more definitive treatment of liver transplantation.

References

1. Christensen J: Esophageal dysmotility disorders. In Balistreri WF, Vanderhoof JA, editors: *Aspen seminars on pediatric disease,* vol 4, *Pediatric gastroenterology and nutrition,* London, 1990, Chapman & Hall; pp 88-94.
2. Illi OE, Stauffer UG: Achalasia in childhood and adolescence, *Eur J Pediatr Surg* 4:214-217, 1994.
3. Myers NA, Jolley SG, Taylor R: Achalasia of the cardia in children: a worldwide survey, *J Pediatr Surg* 29:1375-1379, 1994.
4. Mearin F, Mourelle M, Guarner F, Salas A, Riveros-Moreno V, Moncada S, Malagelada JR: Patients with achalasia lack nitric oxide synthetase in the gastro-esophageal junction, *Eur J Clin Invest* 23:724-728, 1993.
5. Goldblum JR, Whyte RI, Orringer MB, Appelman HD: Achalasia: a morphologoic study of 42 resected specimens, *Am J Surg Pathol* 18:327-337, 1994.
6. Abid S, Champion G, Richter JE, McElvein R, Slaughter RL, Koehler RE: Treatment of achalasia: best of both worlds, *Am J Gastroenterol* 87:979-985, 1994.
7. Traube M, Dubovik S, Lange RC, McCallum RW: The role of nifedipine therapy in achalasia: results of a randomized, double-blind, placebo-controlled study, *Am J Gastroenterol* 84:1259-1262, 1989.
8. Pasricha PJ, Ravich WJ, Hendrix TR, Sostre S, Jones B, Kalloo AN: Intrasphincteric botulinum toxin for the treatment of achalasia, *N Engl J Med* 322:774-778, 1995.
9. Milov DE, Cynamon HA, Andres JM: Chest pain and dysphagia in adolescents caused by diffuse esophageal spasm, *J Pediatr Gastroenterol Nutr* 9:450-453, 1989.
10. Kahrilas PJ, Dodds WJ, Hogan WJ: Dysfunction of the belch reflex: a cause of incapacitating chest pain, *Gastroenterology* 93:818-822, 1987.

11. Gignoux C, Bost R, Hostein J, Turberg Y, Denis P, Cohard M, Wolf J-E, Fournet J: Role of upper esophageal reflex and belch reflux dysfunctions in non-cardiac chest pain, *Dig Dis Sci* 38:1909-1914, 1993.
12. Orenstein SR: Gastroesophageal reflux. In Hyman PE, Di Lorenzo C, editors: *Pediatric gastrointestinal motility disorders,* New York, 1994, Academy Professional Information Services; pp 55-88.
13. Castell DO, Wu WC, Ott DJ, editors: *Gastroesophageal reflux disease: pathogenesis, diagnosis, therapy.* Mt. Kisco, NY, 1985, Futura Publishing.
14. Dahms B: The histology of reflux esophagitis. In Balistreri WF, Vanderhoof JA, editors: *Aspen seminars on pediatric disease,* vol 4, *Pediatric gastroenterology and nutrition,* London, 1990, Chapman & Hall; pp 95-103.
15. Hassall E: Barrett's esophagus: congenital or acquired?, *Am J Gastroenterol* 88:819-824, 1993.
16. Hassall E: Barrett's esophagus: new definitions and approaches in children, *J Pediatr Gastroenterol Nutr* 16:345-364, 1993.
17. Hassall E, Dimmick JE, Magee JF: Adenocarcinoma in childhood Barrett's esophagus: case documentation and the need for surveillance in children, *Am J Gastroenterol* 88:282-288, 1993.
18. Axon ATR, Boyle P, Riddell RH, Grandjouan S, Hardcastle J, Yoshida S: Summary of a working party on the surveillance of premalignant lesions, *Am J Gastroenterol* 89:S160-S168, 1994.
19. Kikendall JW, Friedman AC, Oyewole MA, Fleischer D, Johnson LF: Pill-induced esophageal injury: case reports and review of the medical literature, *Dig Dis Sci* 28:174-182, 1983.
20. Goff JS: Infectious causes of esophagitis, *Annu Rev Med* 39:163-169, 1988.
21. Stiegmann GV: Endoscopic management of esophageal varices, *Adv Surg* 27:209-231, 1994.

CHAPTER 45

Disorders of the Stomach and Duodenum

•

James F. Markowitz

Disorders of the stomach and the duodenum cause significant morbidity during adolescence. As these disorders result in either mucosal disease or abnormal transport of luminal contents, patients tend to present with either pain and the consequences of ulceration such as bleeding, or with symptoms such as vomiting, bloating, or early satiety. Although adolescents with these complaints are commonly seen in any clinical practice, the true incidence and prevalence of gastroduodenal pathology in the adolescent population has not been clearly defined.

MUCOSAL DISORDERS

Gastritis

Inflammation of the gastric mucosa is associated with a number of important etiologic factors. Gastritis secondary to drugs or other toxins is common, and in the adolescent it occurs principally after ingestion of aspirin, other nonsteroidal anti-inflammatory drugs (NSAIDs), or alcohol.[1] In the severely ill, hospitalized patient, stress-induced pathology is common.[2] Gastritis also occurs as part of the underlying disease process in patients with Crohn's disease and eosinophilic gastroenteritis. Duodenogastric reflux resulting in bile-induced gastritis is rare

in the adolescent, unless there is a concomitant motility disorder or a partial intestinal obstruction, or unless there has been previous gastric surgery. In all these forms of gastritis, pain, vomiting, or upper gastrointestinal bleeding are the primary symptoms. At times, however, patients can be asymptomatic.

Another important cause of both acute and chronic gastritis is infection with *Helicobacter pylori.*[3] This urea-splitting, gram-negative, spiral-shaped bacterium thrives in the mucous layer overlying the gastric epithelium despite the acidic milieu of the stomach, and induces inflammatory changes in the gastric (primarily antral) mucosa. Serologic studies demonstrate increasing rates of infection with age. Intrafamilial clustering has been reported, which suggests either a common environmental source of infection or person-to-person spread. Patients with *H. pylori* may be asymptomatic or may complain of chronic dyspepsia or abdominal pain.

Drug- or alcohol-induced gastritis should be suspected in any previously healthy adolescent who has an acute onset of abdominal pain or upper gastrointestinal hemorrhage. Careful questioning will often uncover a history of a recent ingestion of an NSAID or alcohol. Stress gastritis, by contrast, should be suspected in the severely ill, hospitalized patient with upper, often painless, gastrointestinal hemorrhage. In all cases, however, the definitive diagnosis of gastritis requires direct endoscopic visualization of the stomach in conjunction with mucosal biopsy. Since poor correlation between endoscopic findings and histologic evidence of gastritis has been reported, mucosal biopsies are recommended, especially when the gastric mucosa looks normal. *H. pylori* can be identified histologically by Warthin-Starry, hematoxylin-&-eosin, or other staining techniques. Culture of the mucosal biopsy also can help identify the organism. A rapid method of identifying *H. pylori* makes use of its high urease activity. Embedding a mucosal biopsy specimen within a urea-containing medium that also contains a pH indicator results in a color change arising from the enzymatic degradation of the urea by the bacterial urease. This color change can occur between 1 and 24 hours of the embedding, depending on the density of organisms in the biopsy specimen. Commercially available kits, produced by a number of different manufacturers, have been shown to be highly sensitive and specific. Serologic measurement of *H. pylori*–specific antibodies are also commercially available. Published research documents a high correlation between a positive serologic test and the presence of active gastric infection, but there appears to be a substantial false-positive rate in the routine clinical setting. ^{13}C-urea breath tests eventually may provide a sensitive, specific, and noninvasive diagnostic method of identifying *H. pylori* infection. However, it remains a research tool, as an inexpensive methodology has yet to be made commercially available.

When associated with massive hemorrhage, gastritis is a potentially life-threatening disorder. In such instances, therapy demands appropriate resuscitative measures to maintain intravascular volume regardless of the specific cause of inflammation. In addition, maintaining the intragastric pH level above 4.0 will help minimize ongoing mucosal ulceration from both acid and pepsin. This can be accomplished with H_2 blockers (e.g., cimetidine, ranitidine, famotidine, nizatidine), which are often given by continuous intravenous infusion, or with antacids given via nasogastric tube. If necessary, proton pump inhibitors (omeprazole, lansoprazole) can be used once oral intake has resumed. Parenteral forms of these latter agents have not yet been released in the United States.

Specific treatment for less fulminant symptoms of gastritis depends on the underlying cause. Drug- and alcohol-induced lesions heal rapidly with discontinuation of the offending agent and usually do not require specific therapy. If medication such as an NSAID is required for ongoing therapy, concomitant treatment with a synthetic prostaglandin analog (e.g., misoprostil) has been associated with the prevention of mucosal disease in adults. However, data on the effect of misoprostil on established NSAID gastritis or in preventing NSAID induced mucosal lesions in the adolescent are not available. Stress-related gastritis requires supportive therapies and acid neutralization or suppression until the underlying associated illness improves. Other secondary causes of gastritis often require antacids, H_2 blockers, proton pump inhibitors, or agents such as sucralfate in addition to specific therapies aimed at the underlying disease processes.

The ideal treatment of *H. pylori* infection remains unresolved. Most treatment regimens include either colloidal bismuth subcitrate, which is not available in the United States, or bismuth subsalicylate. However, as a single agent, neither compound eradicates the organism in more than about 20% of patients. The current therapeutic gold standard, a 14-day course of three drugs (bismuth, tetracycline, metronidazole), with or without concomitant acid suppression for symptom relief, results in eradication rates of more than 90%.[4,5] However eradication rates with this regimen are significantly less in environments with metronidazole-resistant bacterial populations, or when patient compliance results in less than 60% of a prescribed drug being consumed. Recent studies suggest that regimens based on two drugs (e.g., omeprazole and clarithromycin) may result in eradication rates approaching that of the triple-drug regimen. However, eradication of the organism does not predictably eliminate dyspepsia or abdominal pain in infected children and adolescents.[6,7] Therefore, the role that *H. pylori* plays in the initiation or perpetuation of these symptoms must be questioned.

Peptic Ulcer Disease

Although the diagnosis of peptic ulcer disease is made routinely in adolescents, neither the incidence nor the prevalence of this condition has been reported for an adolescent population. Males are afflicted more often than females. Nearly three quarters of all peptic ulcers are duodenal, and most occur within the duodenal bulb. When a gastric ulcer is present, it is usually found in the antrum.

Ulcers have traditionally been classified as secondary when they occur in association with other ulcerogenic conditions (Box 45-1). They have been categorized as primary when they occur in patients without predisposing conditions. The literature has suggested that up to 80% of ulcers in adolescents are primary, compared with less than 10% in young children.[8] However, these data were gathered before the recognition of the importance of *Helicobacter* in the pathogenesis of peptic ulceration; so too were the data implicating genetic factors in the pathogenesis of peptic ulcer disease. Previously, it was observed that 20% to 60% of adolescents with primary ulcers had close relatives with ulcer disease, an effect not noted in patients with secondary ulcers. Today it would appear that this familial tendency can largely be explained by a clustering of *Helicobacter* infection rather than

<table>
<tr><td>

BOX 45-1

Conditions Associated with Secondary Peptic Ulcer Disease

Burns
Intracranial trauma or surgery
Sepsis
Collagen vascular disease*
Adult respiratory distress syndrome
Leukemia and lymphoma
Stress associated with systemic disease*

</td><td>

BOX 45-2

Differential Diagnosis of Peptic Ulcer Disease

PRESENTATION: CHRONIC ABDOMINAL PAIN/ VOMITING
Disorders of the esophagus
   Gastroesophageal reflux
   Esophageal stricture, membrane, web
   Esophageal motility disorders
Disorders affecting the stomach and duodenum
   Antral web
   Chronic granulomatous disease
   Crohn's disease
   Eosinophilic gastroenteritis
   Gastroduodenal motility disorders
   Food bezoar
Disorders affecting the intestine
   Obstruction
   Annular pancreas
   Constipation
Other conditions
   Pancreatitis
   Cholecystitis
   Cholangitis
   Bulimia nervosa
   Pregnancy
   Increased intracranial pressure

PRESENTATION: HEMATEMESIS
   Swallowed blood from oropharynx or naso-pharynx
   Mallory-Weiss tear
   Peptic esophagitis
   Esophageal varices
   Hemorrhagic gastritis (drug or stress induced)
   Congestive gastropathy associated with portal hypertension

</td></tr>
</table>

*Ulcerations in these conditions may be the result of common therapies, such as the use of nonsteroidal anti-inflammatory agents, rather than the disease process itself.

intrinsic genetic predispositions. For instance, elevated serum pepsinogen I levels had previously been thought to represent a genetically determined, autosomal dominant trait identifying at-risk members of ulcer-prone kindreds.[9] These studies must now be questioned, as it has been shown that *H. pylori* causes elevated serum pepsinogen levels.[10]

The contribution of *Helicobacter* infection to the development of peptic ulceration of both the gastric and duodenal mucosa continues to be elucidated.[11,12] The gastric mucosa is the exclusive site of *H. pylori* infection. Bacterial urease promotes colonization of the gastric mucosa. Adhesion of the bacteria and the release of various cytotoxins result in induction of humoral, cellular, and local mucosal inflammatory responses. It is therefore not surprising that specific bacterial virulence factors might lead to the development of ulcers. For instance, not all strains produce cytotoxins, which helps to explain why strains differ in their ulcerogenic potential. Despite these observations, many adolescents with peptic ulcer disease cannot be demonstrated as harboring *H. pylori* organisms.[13] The cause of ulceration in these individuals remains to be characterized, but in the adult population surreptitious NSAID abuse, often of over-the-counter products, appears to account for most of these *Helicobacter*-negative ulcers.

Peptic ulcer disease also has been considered a psychosomatic condition. However, few controlled data have been reported to support this contention. The clinical impression exists that the development of acute ulceration or the exacerbation of chronic ulcers is often preceded by a period of high psychological stress. However, controlled studies that have included both adolescent and adult subjects do not reveal significant differences in measures of life stress between ulcer patients and normal controls. Similarly, although specific personality traits have been identified in ulcer-prone individuals, these traits are not exclusive to such patients. Much work remains to be done in this area before the strength of the presumed psychosomatic association can be gauged accurately.

The symptoms associated with peptic ulcer disease in the adolescent are variable. Pain, which is often characterized as sharp or burning, is usually localized in the upper abdomen. The effect that eating produces on the pain is often unpredictable, and at times pain spontaneously disappears for variable periods. Vomiting is generally effortful and may be bilious. However, the effortless regurgitation of gastroesophageal reflux can also be mimicked. Bleeding can occur either as hematemesis or melena, or it can be occult. Although life-threatening hemorrhage occurs in less than 5% of primary ulcers, it can be noted in as many as 25% to 50% of secondary peptic ulcerations. Complications, including perforation or gastric outlet obstruction, also can be seen at initial presentation, but the latter is rare in adolescents. The differential diagnosis of peptic ulceration based on an adolescent's most common presenting symptoms is summarized in Box 45-2.

Adult patients with recurrent ulcers have a frequency of associated *H. pylori* gastritis that approaches 90% to 100%. Corresponding data have not been reported in adolescents, but a similar association seems likely. Before the recognition of the association between *Helicobacter* and peptic ulcer disease, most adolescents with ulcers were thought to have a chronic condition that could be expected to persist into adult life. As many as 50% to 75% of adolescents developed recurrent lesions and/or severe complications if traditional medical therapy was discontinued.[14] Traditional antisecretory therapies induce healing of duodenal ulcers, but after healing with antisecretory medication, ulcer recurrence is the norm rather than the exception. By contrast, drug regimens designed to eradicate *H. pylori* organisms from the stomach not only heal duodenal ulcers, but also result in lower rates of ulcer recurrence than do the traditional antisecretory regimens.[15,16] When ulcers have recurred, persistent or recurrent *H. pylori* infection often has been identified.[17] Therefore, it is currently expected that adolescents infected with *H. pylori* can be cured both of their ulcer and of their potential for ulcer recurrence. Whether adolescents with *Helicobacter*-negative ulcer disease will remain at risk for recurrent ulceration remains to be clarified.

The diagnosis of peptic ulcer is best made endoscopically. The lesion can be visualized, and biopsy material from both the duodenum and the antrum can be obtained. Antral biopsy specimens, examined histologically and embedded in a urea-containing microbiologic medium, are especially important for the identification of *H. pylori* organisms. In cases of severe hemorrhage, endoscopy offers the potential for therapeutic intervention (e.g., with heater probe, bicap laser, injection techniques) as well as diagnosis. Contrast radiography offers an alternative diagnostic approach but is associated with higher false-negative and false-positive rates than endoscopy. When *H. pylori* infection has not been identified or when either multiple ulcers or ulcers in unusual locations are identified, a fasting serum gastrin value should be obtained to rule out the possibility of Zollinger-Ellison syndrome.[18]

The therapy for peptic ulceration in the adolescent is largely extrapolated from studies in adults. The most commonly prescribed medications are listed in Box 45-3. Neutralization of acid and suppression of acid secretion remain the mainstays of therapy, but the use of agents designed to enhance mucosal resistance to ulceration is becoming more widespread. In addition, bactericidal regimens directed at *H. pylori* infection (as outlined in the section on gastritis above) must be considered primary therapy in the infected patient.[5,6] Still to be answered is the question of what type or duration of therapy is

---

BOX 45-3
Medical Therapy for *Helicobacter Pylori*–Negative Peptic Ulcer Disease

AGENTS THAT MINIMIZE INTRALUMINAL ACIDITY
Acid-Neutralizing Agents
  Antacids
Antisecretory Agents
  H₂–receptor antagonists: cimetidine, ranitidine, famotidine, nizatidine
  Prostaglandin analogs: misoprostil, enprostil
  H⁺/K⁺ ATPase inhibitors: omeprazole, lansoprazole
  Anticholinergics: pirenzepine
Agents That Enhance Mucosal Protection
  Prostaglandin analogs: misoprostil, enprostil
  Sucralfate
  Colloidal bismuth subcitrate

---

required to prevent ulcer recurrence in the *Helicobacter*-negative adolescent patient. Although unusual in the adolescent, intractable disease or complications such as uncontrollable hemorrhage or gastric outlet obstruction may necessitate surgical intervention. Parietal cell vagotomy appears to be the best means of preventing ulcer recurrence while also minimizing associated postoperative morbidity. However, chronic medical therapy with proton pump inhibitors can be as effective as surgery in the compliant patient who is not otherwise in need of surgery.

MOTOR DISORDERS

In a state of health, the stomach empties ingested materials by a variety of mechanisms. The proximal stomach acts as a reservoir, relaxing as it receives material to minimize acute increases in intragastric pressure. The smooth muscle of the proximal stomach maintains slow, sustained contractions, which, by regulating the pressure differential between the stomach and the duodenum, control the rate of emptying of liquids into the small intestine. Emptying of digestible solids is controlled by the distal stomach. Regular (three per minute) peristaltic contractions of the antrum occur in response to electrical slow waves arising from a gastric pacemaker. These antral contractions force solids against the closed pylorus, thereby grinding material into particles of approximately 0.1 mm, which then are allowed to pass through the pylorus. By contrast, nondigestible solids that have been ingested do not pass out of the stomach by either mechanism. Instead, they are maintained in the stomach until all digestible material has been emptied, the stomach has resumed a fasting motor pattern, and a migrating motor complex (phase III activity front) has swept the remaining materials through a patent pylorus into the duodenum. Disorders of gastric emptying occur when one or more of these mechanisms is faulty.[19]

DELAYED GASTRIC EMPTYING

Delayed gastric emptying results in the prolonged retention of food in the stomach. It can arise from congenital or acquired anatomic obstructing lesions of the stomach and duodenum, or as the consequence of abnormal gastroduodenal motility. There may be marked gastric distention accompanied by gastric hypersecretion, either postprandially or continuously. As a result, patients complain of a sense of fullness, early satiety, and often dyspeptic symptoms such as nausea, water brash, heartburn, abdominal pain, and vomiting.

Anatomic Obstructions

INTRINSIC CONGENITAL LESIONS. Most congenital anomalies of the stomach and the duodenum are noted during infancy or early childhood. However, partially obstructing webs or membranes can remain asymptomatic until adolescence or adulthood. These rare anomalies occur primarily in the gastric antrum or the prepyloric area, and occasionally in the duodenum. Webs that are noted during adolescence can have either large or quite small central perforations. "Windsock"-shaped lesions also have been described. Why these lesions begin to cause symptoms of obstruction of the gastric outlet or the small bowel after remaining quiescent for years has not been adequately explained. However, it has been postulated that inflammation and edema surrounding the central orifice result in impingement on an already limited opening. Patients may complain of epigastric pain or a sense of fullness. Vomiting or esophageal symptoms suggestive of gastroesophageal reflux are also common. Radiographic studies may reveal a typical translucent line in the antrum that sometimes creates the appearance of a "pseudopylorus" (Fig. 45-1) and causes markedly delayed gastric emptying or enlargement of the stomach and the duodenum proximal to the obstructing lesion. Diagnostic endoscopy often reveals the nature of the lesion. Endoscopy can also be therapeutic, as membranes and webs can be disrupted by "through-the-scope" balloon catheters or cautery. If surgical exploration is required, a deflated balloon catheter should be passed throughout the intestine. The balloon then is inflated and slowly withdrawn to ensure that more distal and less obviously obstructing webs are not missed.

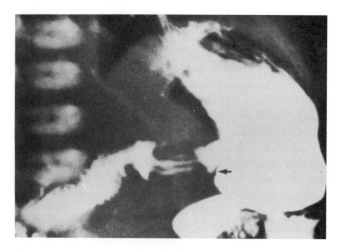

Fig. 45-1. Upper gastrointestinal barium contrast study in a 13-year-old boy with recurrent vomiting. The arrow indicates a negative image of a partially obstructing antral web.

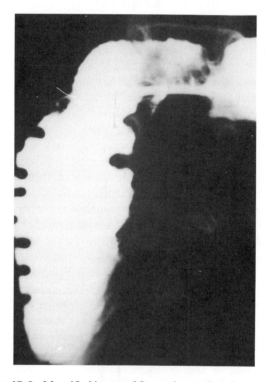

Fig. 45-2. Magnified image of first and second portions of the duodenum (filled with barium by direct instillation) in a 14-year-old girl with a long history of recurrent vomiting and abdominal pain. At surgery, a sharp cutoff in the end of the second portion of the duodenum was found to be caused by extrinsic fibrous bands.

EXTRINSIC CONGENITAL LESIONS. Although extrinsic obstruction of the stomach is rare, duodenal compression syndromes occasionally present during adolescence. The most common abnormality results from extrinsic fibrous bands, which may or may not be associated with malrotation (Fig. 45-2). However, less than 5% of all symptomatic malrotations occur after childhood, and so adolescent cases are limited in number. When the diagnosis of extrinsic obstruction is made in an adolescent patient, the symptoms usually are due to intermittent partial obstruction, frequently occurring after meals. Often, however, evidence of partial obstruction is obtained unexpectedly, when an abdominal radiograph is taken for apparently unrelated symptoms. Generally, the obstruction appears in the third portion of the duodenum. Similar clinical and radiographic findings have been described in adolescents and young adults with compression of the duodenum from the superior mesenteric artery or a preduodenal portal vein.[20]

Extrinsic obstruction of the duodenum also is seen with an annular pancreas. In this situation the obstruction is in the second portion of the duodenum and is commonly associated with underlying duodenal stenosis. Despite its congenital origin, patients with annular pancreas do initially present during adolescence, commonly complaining of pain (often resulting from associated peptic disease), recurrent vomiting, and occasionally hematemesis. Pancreatitis usually does not occur. Diagnosis is aided by barium enema studies, which reveal symmetric narrowing of the second portion of the duodenum that may be associated with proximal dilation. Upper endoscopy often reveals peptic ulceration proximal to the extrinsically narrowed duodenum. Adolescents rarely require surgery for unremitting obstructive symptoms. More commonly, vigorous therapy for the peptic ulcer disease results in marked symptomatic improvement.

Acquired Lesions

A number of other disorders can ultimately result in anatomic obstructing lesions of the stomach or the duodenum. Obstruction of the third portion of the duodenum from the superior mesenteric artery occurs frequently in patients who experience marked weight loss.[20] Adolescents with eating disorders represent a group at high risk for this complication. Although peptic ulcer disease can produce scarring of the duodenum with resultant gastric outlet obstruction, this particular complication is increasingly rare. Another rare cause of anatomic partial obstruction is chronic granulomatous disease, in which a distinctive annular narrowing of the antrum has been described. Other more common entities such as Crohn's disease and eosinophilic gastroenteritis commonly involve the stomach and duodenum. These conditions occasionally delay gastric emptying anatomically by causing a marked narrowing of the gastric antrum and the proximal duodenum (Fig. 45-3). In other cases, however, minimal anatomic abnormality can be identified, yet significant functional impairment of gastric emptying can occur, presumably as a consequence of the

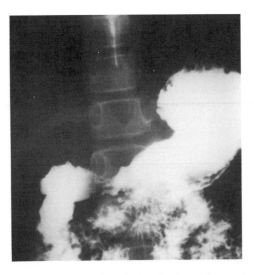

Fig. 45-3. Upper gastrointestinal series in a 15-year-old girl with biopsy-proved gastroduodenal and ileal Crohn's disease. Note the irregularities of the distal stomach and proximal duodenum.

associated inflammation of the gastroduodenal neuromusculature.

Functional Disorders

Impaired gastric emptying due to abnormal gastroduodenal motility can occur acutely or on a chronic basis. Acute gastric atony is common after surgery or when associated with infection. Secretions and any ingested food or drink remain within the stomach for extended periods, resulting in a sense of fullness or bloating, and ultimately vomiting. Symptom resolution is usually rapid without specific therapy.

Chronic "functional" delayed emptying is seen in association with a number of systemic illnesses (Box 45-4). However, occasionally it is seen in adolescents as the consequence of an isolated idiopathic motility abnormality, or as one of a spectrum of abnormalities resulting from one of the neuropathic or myopathic forms of chronic idiopathic intestinal pseudo-obstruction. Decreased antral mechanical activity also can be seen in children with disorders of gastric myoelectrical activity, such as tachygastria or tachyarrhythmia. Symptoms of chronic upper abdominal distention, vomiting, and a sense of bloating (usually associated with anorexia or early satiety) are frequent. Except in unusual circumstances, the emptying of solids is affected earlier and more markedly than that of liquids.

Suspected functional abnormalities of gastric emptying are best confirmed by measurement of the rate of emptying of a standardized meal once anatomic abnormalities have been excluded by radiocontrast studies or endoscopy.[21] With a noninvasive scintigraphic technique in which the liquid and solid phases of a meal are tagged

---

BOX 45-4
Conditions Associated with Chronic Delayed Gastric Emptying

MYOPATHIC CONDITIONS
Muscular dystrophy
Progressive systemic sclerosis
Myopathic intestinal pseudo-obstruction (hollow visceral myopathy)

NEUROPATHIC CONDITIONS
Diabetes mellitus
Multiple sclerosis
Familial dysautonomia
Neuropathic intestinal pseudo-obstruction
Disorders of gastric antral pacemaker activity

MIXED (MYONEUROPATHIC) OR UNKNOWN CONDITIONS
Anorexia nervosa
Gastroesophageal reflux
Malnutrition
Systemic lupus erythematosus
Idiopathic gastroparesis

---

with different radioisotopes, the rate of disappearance of the isotopes from the stomach can be calculated from data obtained from serial gamma-counter measurements. Since gastric emptying is dependent on the caloric density, osmolarity, and nutrient composition of a meal, however, it is especially important that standardized meals be used and emptying rates be interpreted against appropriate controls. Antroduodenal manometric studies can offer insight into the underlying pathophysiologic condition that is giving rise to an abnormal emptying pattern. For instance, myopathic disorders tend to be characterized by low-amplitude or absent contractions, while neuropathic processes result in incoordinated normal or high-pressure contractile waves. Transcutaneous recording of gastric myoelectrical activity is also possible but at present remains a research tool.

The treatment of adolescents with functional delayed gastric emptying requires that careful attention be paid to the nutritional state of the patient. Even moderate degrees of malnutrition can contribute to pronounced gastric dysfunction, and nutritional rehabilitation can improve gastric motility in at least some patients. The subjective sensation of nausea also may need to be suppressed before improvements in emptying can be achieved. Concomitant constipation must be sought, and if present treated, because rectal distention will slow gastric emptying via a cologastric reflex. Adolescents with mild symptoms may respond to dietary manipulation. Decreasing dietary fat and eating smaller, more frequent meals are often effective therapies. In patients who are unable to consume adequate diets, liquid supplements are often better tolerated than solids. Nocturnal enteral or parenteral feedings can be used to supplement oral dietary intake. Patients with more difficult symptoms may respond to prokinetic drugs such as metoclopramide, domperidone, or cisapride.[22] Erythromycin and cefazolin also promote gastric emptying, initiating migrating motor complexes apparently by stimulating motilin receptors. Unfortunately, these medications do not offer permanent solutions, and in many cases tachyphylaxis results in the need to frequently change treatments as clinical efficacy wanes.

DUMPING SYNDROME

Rapid, uncontrolled emptying of a meal into the small intestine results in the dumping syndrome. Dumping can occur as a complication of a gastric surgical procedure such as a Nissen fundoplication or gastrojejunostomy. It can also rarely be seen associated with autonomic neuropathies, as a consequence of uncoordinated gastroduodenal contractions. Early dumping, which occurs within 30 minutes of a meal, is characterized by abdominal discomfort, nausea, weakness, palpitations, diaphoresis, syncope, bloating, and diarrhea. These symptoms are conventionally thought to be caused, at least in part, by rapid fluid shifts into the bowel lumen, resulting in hemoconcentration and tachycardia, associated with an exaggerated release of gut hormones such as vasoactive intestinal polypeptide, enteroglucagon, and neurotensin. Late dumping, which occurs 1 to 3 hours after eating, can result in reactive hypoglycemia (due to hyperinsulinemia induced by an initial rapid rise in blood glucose). Symptoms are often most pronounced after a period of fasting or after hypertonic or high-carbohydrate meals.

When this syndrome is suspected, dumping can be confirmed by an oral glucose tolerance test or by serial measurements of blood glucose after ingestion of a typical meal. Gastric emptying studies, as described above, can be used to analyze both the pattern of emptying and the overall emptying rate (Fig. 45-4).

Dietary manipulation remains the only practical therapy for the dumping syndrome. Meals should be low in simple sugars and relatively high in complex carbohydrates. Increasing dietary fat also may slow emptying. The taking of liquids on an empty stomach or at the start of a meal should be minimized. Smaller, more frequent meals are generally better tolerated. In rare instances, prolonged nasogastric or gastrostomy infusions of an isotonic, nutritionally complete formula may be necessary. Most adolescents do well with dietary manipulations, although a few have persistent, often troublesome symptoms. Experimental therapies for patients with intractable symptoms have included somatostatin or octreotide, or the use of external electrodes for retrograde

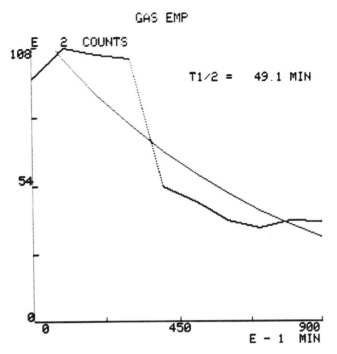

GAS EMP

T1/2 =   49.1 MIN

E - 1 MIN

Fig. 45-4. Gastric emptying study in a 16-year-old boy with neurodevelopmental delay. The patient underwent a Nissen fundoplication and pyloroplasty for severe gastroesophageal reflux 4 years before this study. The jagged line represents emptying of the solid component of a mixed liquid-solid test meal incorporating different radionuclides in various phases of the meal. Time in tenths of a minute is represented on the x axis; the percentage of the solid phase of the meal remaining (indicated by the number of counts for the solid phase of the meal), on the y axis. The smooth curved line represents the mean emptying rate for normal controls having the same test meal. The time required to empty one half of the test meal (T½) is normal, but in a prolonged lag phase after ingestion, no solid material is emptied. This phase is followed by a precipitous rate of emptying, characteristic of the dumping syndrome.

pacing of the proximal small intestine. However, no data have been published on the use of these therapies in adolescents.

References

1. Quinn CM, Bjarnason I, Price AB: Gastritis in patients on non-steroidal anti-inflammatory drugs, *Histopathology* 23:341-348, 1993.
2. Schiessel R, Feil W, Wenzl E: Mechanisms of stress ulceration and implications for treatment, *Gastroenterol Clin North Am* 19:101-120, 1990.
3. Macarthur C, Saunders N, Feldman W: *Helicobacter pylori*, gastroduodenal disease, and recurrent abdominal pain in children, *JAMA* 273:729-734, 1995.
4. Graham DY, Lew GM, Malaty HM, Evans DG, Evans DJ, Klein PD, Alpert LC, Genta RM: Factors influencing the eradication of *Helicobacter pylori* with triple therapy, *Gastroenterology* 102:493-496, 1992.
5. Chiba N, Rao BV, Rademaker JW, Hunt RH: Meta-analysis of the efficacy of antibiotic therapy in eradicating *Helicobacter pylori, Am J Gastroenterol* 87:1716-1727, 1992.
6. Reifen R, Rasooly I, Drumm B, Murphy K, Sherman P: *Helicobacter pylori* infection in children: is there specific symptomatology?, *Dig Dis Sci* 39:1488-1492, 1994.
7. Heldenberg D, Wagner Y, Heldenberg E, Keren S, Auslaender L, Kaufshtein M, Tenebaum G: The role of *Helicobacter pylori* in children with recurrent abdominal pain, *Am J Gastroenterol* 90:906-909, 1995.
8. Dominguez HL, Freston JW: Peptic ulcer disease in adolescence: changing concepts in the age of *Helicobacter pylori, Gastroenterologist* 2:311-314, 1994.
9. Tam PK: Serum pepsinogen I in childhood duodenal ulcer, *J Pediatr Gastroenterol Nutr* 6:904-907, 1987.
10. Wagner S, Haruma K, Gladziwa U, Soudah B, Gebel M, Bleck J, Schmidt H, Manns M: *Helicobacter pylori* infection and serum pepsinogen A, pepsinogen C and gastrin in gastritis and peptic ulcer: significance of inflammation and effect of bacterial eradication, *Am J Gastroenterol* 89:1211-1218, 1994.
11. Ernst PB, Jin Y, Reyes VE, Crowe SE: The role of the local immune response in the pathogenesis of peptic ulcer formation, *Scand J Gastroenterol Suppl* 205:22-28, 1994.
12. Haruma K, Kawaguchi H, Kohmoto K, Okamoto S, Yoshihara M, Sumii K, Kajiyama G: *Helicobacter pylori* infection, serum gastrin, and gastric acid secretion in teen-age subjects with duodenal ulcer, gastritis, or normal mucosa, *Scand J Gastroenterol* 30:322-326, 1995.
13. Chong SKF, Lou Q, Asnicar MA, Zimmerman SE, Croffie JM, Lee C-H, Fitzgerald JF: *Helicobacter pylori* infection in recurrent abdominal pain in childhood: comparison of diagnostic tests and therapy, *Pediatrics* 96:211-215, 1995.
14. Murphy MS, Eastham EJ: Peptic ulcer disease in childhood: long-term prognosis, *J Pediatr Gastroenterol Nutr* 6:721-724, 1987.
15. Hentschel E, Brandstatter G, Dragosics B, Hirschl AM, Nemec H, Schutze K, Taufer M, Wurzer H: Effect of ranitidine and amoxicillin plus metronidazole on the eradication of *Helicobacter pylori* and the recurrence of duodenal ulcer, *N Engl J Med* 328:308-312, 1993.
16. Jaspersen D, Koerner T, Schorr W, Brennenstuhl M, Raschka C, Hammar C-H: *Helicobacter pylori* eradication reduces the rate of rebleeding in ulcer hemorrhage, *Gastrointest Endosc* 41:5-7, 1995.
17. Marshall BJ, Goodwin CS, Warren JR, Murray R, Blincow ED, Blackbourn SJ, Phillips M, Waters TE, Sanderson CR: Prospective double-blind trial of duodenal ulcer relapse after eradication of *Campylobacter pylori, Lancet* 2:1437-1442, 1988.
18. Wolfe MM, Jensen RT: Zollinger-Ellison syndrome: current concepts in diagnosis and management, *N Engl J Med* 317:1200-1209, 1987.
19. Minami H, McCallum RW: The physiology and pathophysiology of gastric emptying in humans, *Gastroenterology* 86:1592-1610, 1984.
20. Marchant EA, Alvear DT, Fagelman KM: True clinical entity of vascular compression of the duodenum in adolescence, *Surg Gynecol Obstet* 168:381-386, 1989.
21. Meyer JH: Invasive (intubation) and noninvasive (radionuclide imaging) techniques for studying gastric emptying. In Dubois A, Castell DO, editors: *Esophageal and gastric emptying*, Boca Raton, FL, 1984, CRC Press; pp 73-82.
22. Grill BB, Flores AF: Treatment of enteric neuromuscular disorders: pharmacotherapy. In Hyman PE, Di Lorenzo C, editors: *Pediatric gastrointestinal motility disorders*, New York, 1994, Academy Professional Information Services.

CHAPTER 46

Disorders of the Small Intestine and Colon

•

Anupama Chawla and Fredric Daum

Although many lesions of the small intestine and colon are common to all age groups, this chapter focuses on certain ones associated more specifically with the adolescent population. Intestinal problems caused by diarrhea, lactose intolerance, inflammatory bowel disease, small bowel obstruction, neoplasms, and other miscellaneous disorders can have a significant impact on the physical and psychosocial health of adolescents.

DIARRHEA IN THE ADOLESCENT

The pathogens that cause infectious diarrhea in adolescents are essentially the same as those found in other age groups. However, with adolescence comes increased mobility, independence, and sexual experimentation, thereby increasing the risk of traveler's diarrhea and of diarrhea from infections acquired by anal intercourse. The incidence of AIDS and opportunistic infections also increases in this age group. Pathogens that may be isolated from adolescent patients with diarrhea are listed in Box 46-1, and an algorithm for evaluation of the adolescent with diarrhea, both infectious and noninfectious, is presented in Figure 46-1. Specific infections, namely enterotoxigenic *Escherichia coli* (ETEC), *Campylobacter jejuni, Shigella, Giardia lamblia, Entamoeba histolytica,* and diarrhea in homosexual males and patients with AIDS, will be discussed in some depth.

Traveler's Diarrhea

One third of persons travelling from developed nations to underdeveloped countries develop traveler's diarrhea from enterotoxigenic ETEC, with the onset usually in the first week.[1] The organism can be found in both water and food. ETEC is a gram-negative bacillus that is motile. It produces a heat-labile or heat-stable toxin. These enterotoxins affect intestinal electrolyte transport through stimulation of adenylate or guanylate cyclase, resulting in diarrhea. In adolescents the usual presentation is a self-limited, watery diarrhea syndrome of mild to moderate severity, most often lasting 3 to 5 days. Diarrhea may or may not be accompanied by fever. The principal treatment is replacement of fluid and electrolytes. There are no indications that antimicrobial agents are effective in the treatment of ETEC in adolescents.

Campylobacter jejuni

C. jejuni is a gram-negative rod and is the most common infectious cause of bloody diarrhea in the pediatric population in developed countries. Untreated water and undercooked chicken have been identified as important vehicles of infection.[2] *C. jejuni* infects either the distal small intestine or the colon causing an inflammatory response, or both. The episode often begins with fever and malaise, followed within 24 hours by nausea, diarrhea, and cramping abdominal pain.[3] The diarrhea can be profuse and bloody. Most cases are self-limited. Complications include fulminant colitis, meningitis, abscesses, pancreatitis, Reiter's syndrome, and Guillain-Barré syndrome.[4,5] Symptomatic individuals may be treated with erythromycin (40 mg/kg/day for 7 days), but most patients have improved significantly by the time of diagnosis and require no specific medical therapy.

Shigella

Shigella is a gram-negative rod that infects the gastrointestinal tract. It is spread through the fecal-oral cycle. The organism is capable of surviving for up to 30 days in foods such as milk, whole eggs, oysters, shrimp, and flour.[6] Toilet paper does not prevent contamination of fingers, so that hand washing is mandatory for infected individuals.

The *Shigella* organism invades epithelial cells of the colonic mucosa, with intraepithelial multiplication leading to destruction of epithelial cells and stimulation of a severe inflammatory response. The organism also produces several toxins, one of which is cytopathic. This toxin most likely assists in the destruction of epithelial cells.

The highest incidence of disease is in children between the ages of 1 and 4 years, but adolescents and adults account for approximately 30% of reported cases. The

---

BOX 46-1
Enteric Pathogens That May Be Isolated from Adolescent Patients with Diarrhea

BACTERIAL
   Enterotoxigenic *Escherichia coli* (traveler's diarrhea) (ETEC)
   Enteroinvasive *E. coli*
   Campylobacter jejuni
   Shigella
   Salmonella
   Clostridium difficile
   Chlamydia trachomatis
   Neisseria gonorrhoae

VIRAL
   Rotavirus
   Herpes simplex

PROTOZOAN
   Giardia lamblia
   Entamoeaba histolytica
   Cryptosporidium
   Isospora belli

---

illness is most commonly characterized by watery stools, which may be bloody. Seizures occur in younger children but are uncommon in adolescents. Isolation of *Shigella* from stool cultures is the definitive laboratory test.

Antibiotics promptly abort the infection but are not needed in patients in whom the diagnosis is made after the acute illness has resolved. Most patients recover without antibiotics. The treatment of choice is trimethoprim-sulfamethoxazole (8 to 10 mg/kg/day trimethoprim and 40 mg/kg/day of sulfamethoxazole in two divided doses for 5 days).[7] Antidiarrheal drugs with antiperistaltic activity are counterproductive in shigellosis as they prolong fever, diarrhea, and excretion of the organism.

Shigella can also present with extraintestinal manifestations. Arthralgia and arthritis have been associated with acute and subacute *Shigella* infection. Reiter's syndrome and hemolytic uremic syndrome have also been reported after acute *Shigella* infection.

Giardia lamblia

This flagellate protozoan infection is found in most countries of the world, its prevalence being highest in the developing world. Age-specific prevalence rates increase throughout infancy and childhood but reach adult levels during adolescence.[8,9] *Giardia* is transmitted by food and water and by direct person-to-person contact. The cyst is the infective form of the parasite.

The mechanism by which *Giardia* causes diarrhea and malabsorption is not clearly understood. Small intestinal

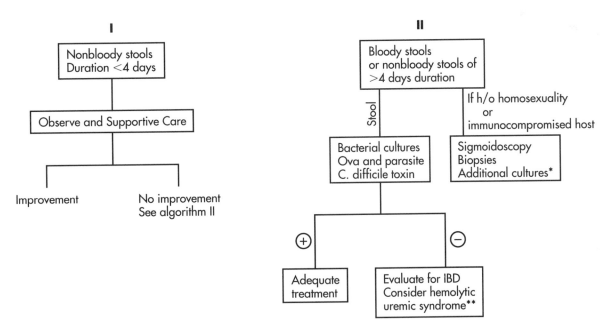

*Outlined in text.
**If accompanied by decreased hematocrit, decreased platelets, and elevated blood urea nitrogen.
IBD, inflammatory bowel disease.

Fig. 46-1. Algorithm for evaluating diarrhea.

morphology can range from normal to partial or even total villous atrophy.[10,11] *G. lamblia* is the most common nonopportunistic protozoan parasite in patients with AIDS, causing acute diarrheal illness similar to that observed in immunocompetent persons.[12] Adults and older children commonly carry *G. lamblia* without symptoms. Infection earlier in life is usually symptomatic. Acute infection often begins with watery diarrhea, which if untreated can progress to abdominal distention, chronic diarrhea with steatorrhea, and weight loss. In the growing adolescent, *G. lamblia* infection may result in growth failure.

Giardia forms can be identified by microscopy of feces or duodenal fluid, or by mucosal biopsy. However, only 80% of positive individuals are detected even after multiple stool examinations. *Giardia* antigen can be detected in the feces, and an enzyme-linked immunosorbant assay (ELISA) is now commercially available. Formalin interferes with this test and therefore should not be used to preserve stool. In a 1995 study, the ELISA sensitivity was 91% and specificity 98%.[13]

The treatment of choice for *Giardia* infections in adolescents is metronidazole (250 mg three times a day for 5 days). Adverse effects include anorexia, nausea, and vomiting. Alcohol ingestion during treatment and for at least 3 days afterward must be avoided, because abdominal cramps, nausea, vomiting, headaches, and flushing may occur. Furazolidone, available in liquid suspension, is an alternative therapy that is 70% to 80% effective. Adolescents should be treated even if they are asymptomatic, to prevent transmission of the organism.

Entamoeba histolytica

E. histolytica causes both the acute and chronic gastrointestinal infection known as amebiasis. Infection is transmitted by the amebic cyst via the fecal-oral route. An increased incidence of amebiasis among homosexual males has been noted for several years.[14,15] The first intestinal lesions are small ulcers about 1 mm in diameter that are indistinguishable from those seen in Crohn's disease or ulcerative colitis. These ulcers subsequently become deeper and may be as large as 1 cm in diameter.[16] Rarely, pseudomembranous colitis may develop. Amebae also disseminate to the liver in as many as 50% of patients with fulminant amebiasis.[17] Dissemination from the liver to the pleura and pericardium has been described. In spite of its potentially invasive character, the most common form of amebic infestation is asymptomatic intraluminal amebiasis. Asymptomatic individuals can serve as a source of infection for the community and should be treated.

Amebiasis in the Western hemisphere is commonly overlooked as it is not considered in the differential diagnosis of chronic or bloody diarrhea. Clinically and endoscopically, amebic colitis can be indistinguishable from inflammatory bowel disease.

Diagnosis can be made from both stool and proctoscopic examination. Characteristically, the mucus is teeming with active trophozoites. If both stool and proctoscopic examinations are negative for amebae, serologic studies should be performed. ELISA assay of both serum and stool is more sensitive than other tests.[18]

In the adolescent population, tetracycline should be used for mild or asymptomatic intestinal amebiasis. Metronidazole is the drug of choice for more severe intestinal and extraintestinal amebiasis.[19] The oral dosage is 50 mg/kg/day in three divided doses for 10 days, to a maximum of 2,250 mg/day. Patients with intestinal amebiasis have an excellent prognosis despite possible relapse. The case fatality rate increases when there is pleural or pericardial involvement. Cerebral amebiasis has been described as having a 96% fatality rate.[20]

Diarrhea in Male Homosexuals and Patients with AIDS

Male homosexuals experience a variety of infections, with diarrheal illnesses particularly common.[21] Common modes of spread include the fecal-oral route and direct rectal inoculation. Agents implicated by the fecal-oral route are similar to those seen in heterosexual populations. Organisms introduced into the rectum by direct inoculation that may cause proctitis or diarrhea include *Neisseria gonorrhoeae*, *Chlamydia trachomatis* (lymphogranuloma venereum [LGV] and non-LGV serotypes), *Treponema pallidum*, and the herpesviruses. A different group of agents should also be considered in persons with altered T-cell immunity, including those with AIDS. These involve *Crytosporidium*, *Isospora belli*, herpesviruses (herpes simplex and cytomegalovirus), *Mycobacteria avium-intracellulare*, and *Salmonella*.[22,23] Diarrhea is a complaint in up to 30% to 60% of patients with AIDS.

LACTOSE INTOLERANCE

In most of the world's non-Caucasian populations, lactase levels decline during adolescence to 5% to 10% of those in infancy.[24,25] Approximately 80% of those who are black or Asian, and 5% to 20% of North American Caucasians, are deficient in lactase.[26] Lactose intolerance due to lactase deficiency should be considered in patients with "idiopathic" diarrhea, irritable bowel syndrome, and recurrent abdominal pain.

In patients with lactase deficiency, lactose not hydrolyzed and absorbed in the small intestine passes into the large intestine and is fermented by colonic microflora with production of hydrogen gas and short-chain fatty acids. These acids produce an acidic stool (pH of <5.0). Fermentation also produces several gases, resulting in increased breath hydrogen, which can be measured by a lactose breath hydrogen (LBH) test.

The symptoms of lactose intolerance include flatus, cramping abdominal pain, and diarrhea. Rectal bleeding is not a symptom of lactose intolerance. When there is superimposed inflammation of the small bowel causing damage to epithelial cells, as seen with bacterial infection or Crohn's disease, rectal bleeding may be seen concomitantly with symptoms of lactose intolerance.

Clinical response to lactose withdrawal from the diet, rather than results of the LBH test, should be used in making decisions about patient management. While LBH analysis may reflect levels of lactose absorption, an abnormal LBH may not always be indicative of lactose intolerance. False-positive results may be seen with inadequate pretest fasting, cigarette smoking, or constipation with fecal impaction. Constipation and fecal impaction, for instance, may delay gastric emptying, leading to stasis and bacterial overgrowth in the small bowel, fermentation of lactose, a state of lactose intolerance, and a positive LBH test even in the presence of adequate lactase. False-negative results are obtained when patients have recently used antibiotics or are non–hydrogen producers (such as occurs in approximately 1% of the population).

Initial treatment of lactose intolerance consists of removing all lactose-containing foods and medications from the diet. Milk pretreated with lactase is available in grocery stores. Over-the-counter replacement enzymes may be added directly to milk (12 to 24 hours before ingestion), or taken in pill form or as chewable tablets with a meal. Considerable variation exists in patient-to-patient ability to tolerate small amounts of lactose. Once improvements in symptoms is documented by exclusion of lactose-containing foods, increasing amounts of these foods can be introduced to assess the individual adolescent's tolerance. Live culture yogurts that contain endogenous beta-galactosidase may be well tolerated by a majority of lactose-intolerant patients and may serve as a good source of calcium in these individuals.

INFLAMMATORY BOWEL DISEASE

Of all the organic, noninfectious, chronic gastrointestinal disorders that occur among adolescents, the idiopathic chronic inflammatory intestinal diseases—nonspecific ulcerative colitis and Crohn's disease—are by far the most common and most perplexing.[27] Despite the endemic nature of these illnesses, especially Crohn's disease, little is known about their underlying causes and pathophysiology. Controversy also flourishes with regard to pharmacologic treatment, operative indications, and the specific nature of surgical intervention.

Ulcerative colitis and Crohn's disease represent distinct pathologic entities, with symptoms and signs that are often indistinguishable. Ulcerative colitis is defined as a chronic inflammatory reaction limited to the mucosa and submucosa of the colon. It is a process isolated to the colon or to the terminal ileum ("backwash ileitis"). In contrast, Crohn's disease is a chronic inflammatory reaction that is transmural. Characteristically, Crohn's disease can affect any portion of the gastrointestinal tract between the mouth and the anus. Despite these clear-cut differences, there is often sufficient overlap when inflammation is restricted to the colon to make differentiation difficult or impossible.

Epidemiology

The incidence and prevalence of ulcerative colitis and Crohn's disease in adolescent populations have not been determined. In the pediatric population as a whole, it appears that the incidence of Crohn's disease has risen steadily.[28] Incidence and prevalence data for Crohn's disease and ulcerative colitis in children are listed in Tables 46-1 and 46-2, respectively.[29] Although there are sharp differences in the reported incidence throughout the

---

TABLE 46-1
Incidence and Prevalence of Crohn's Disease in Children

Location	Years	Ages (yr)	Incidence (per 100,000/yr)	Prevalence (per 100,000)
West, Norway	1984-1985	<15	2.5	12.6
Copenhagen, Denmark	1962-1978	<20	2.2	10.0
Malmö, Sweden	1958-1973	10-15	2.5	
Stockholm, Sweden	1955-1959	0-14	0.14	
Stockholm, Sweden	1970-1974	0-14	1.0	
United Kingdom				10.0

Data from Olafsdottir EJ, Fluge G, Haug K: Chronic inflammatory bowel disease in children in Western Norway, *J Pediatr Gastroenterol Nutr* 8:454-458, 1989.

TABLE 46-2
Incidence and Prevalence of Ulcerative Colitis in Children

Location	Years	Ages (yr)	Incidence (per 100,000/yr)	Prevalence (per 100,000)
West, Norway	1984-1985	<15	4.3	18.1
Copenhagen, Denmark	1970-1978	0-15	6.3	30.0 (1978)
Malmö, Sweden	1958-1973	0-9	1.0	
Malmö, Sweden	1958-1973	10-19	8.0	
Cardiff, Wales	1968-1977	0-20	10.0	

Data from Olafsdottir EJ, Fluge G, Haug K: Chronic inflammatory bowel disease in children in Western Norway, *J Pediatr Gastroenterol Nutr* 8:454-458, 1989.

world, no areas are free of inflammatory bowel disease (IBD). This disease appears to be more common in northwestern Europe and in North America and affects all races. In fact, in the United States the incidence among blacks has increased since the 1970s, and there have been several reports of this disease among other nonwhites in South America, Africa, and Asia. Several studies have confirmed the increased susceptibility of Jews to both Crohn's disease and ulcerative colitis. It does not appear that there is a predominantly urban origin associated with IBD, as once proposed, or that socioeconomic factors are of any significance.

At the Cleveland Clinic, the family histories of 316 patients with ulcerative colitis and 522 patients with Crohn's disease were evaluated.[30] Of patients with ulcerative colitis, 29% had a positive family history of IBD; 35% of those with Crohn's disease had relatives with IBD. Of all first-degree relatives, 15% had IBD. Studies of ABO blood groups, secretor status, and human lymphocyte antigen (HLA) types in patients with IBD have yielded either conflicting results or a negative association with either ulcerative colitis or Crohn's disease.

Etiology

Despite a great number of studies, there is still no evidence to specifically implicate viruses or bacteria in the pathogenesis of IBD. However, viral infections, especially those localized to the upper respiratory tract, may trigger a prolonged exacerbation of intestinal symptoms. In patients with ulcerative colitis, *Aeromonas hydrophila* usually proves to be a bacterial superinfection, not a primary cause. The possible role of unclassified *Mycobacterium* species also remains conjectural. The human gastrointestinal tract provides a critical interface between the individual and a complex mixture of antigens and pathogens in the intestinal lumen. The gastrointestinal immune system is an important component of this interface, generating potent humoral and cellular mucosal responses. Mechanisms that regulate gastrointestinal immune responses may play a role in the pathogenesis of

Crohn's disease. Whether intestinal inflammation is caused by excessive inhibition of immune responses or, conversely, by immune hyporesponsiveness to an undetermined agent in the intestine still needs to be elucidated. The role of eicosanoids in IBD remain a focus of investigative research. There is no evidence to support a role for eicosanoids in the etiology of IBD, but data support their role as mediators in the pathogenesis of IBD. There is no evidence to implicate specific foods or food additives in the pathogenesis of IBD.

The possible impact of the use of oral contraceptives on IBD is still not completely resolved. Logan and Kay[31] reported that women taking oral contraceptives were 1.7 times more likely to develop Crohn's disease and 1.3 times more likely to develop ulcerative colitis than those who had not used contraceptives during the 6 months before disease onset and those who had never used them. Although these differences did not reach statistical significance, the data are consistent with previous reports. Subsequently, Lashner et al[32,33] reported no association between current or former use of oral contraceptives and Crohn's disease or ulcerative colitis. They concluded that there was no evidence to suggest that women who are predisposed to the development of Crohn's disease or ulcerative colitis should be advised to avoid using oral contraceptives.

Cigarette smoking has been shown to be protective against ulcerative colitis but increases the risk for Crohn's disease.[34] In 1996, Cosnes et al showed that patients with Crohn's disease who smoke, particularly women who are heavy smokers, are at a high risk for developing severe disease requiring surgery.[35]

Although there are more than 100 studies suggesting an association between psychiatric illness and ulcerative colitis, these studies have been severely criticized.[36] In seven studies that were considered acceptable, investigators found no evidence of increased psychiatric impairment in patients with ulcerative colitis. In contrast, the frequency of psychiatric disorders in patients with Crohn's disease appears to be significantly higher than in controls. The most predominant psychiatric disturbances are depression and obsessional illness.[37] The severity of

Crohn's disease and that of psychiatric illness appear to be independent of one another, and there is no evidence of a causal relationship between the two.

Crohn's Disease versus Ulcerative Colitis

Initially, it may be impossible to distinguish between Crohn's disease and ulcerative colitis. These two disorders can be differentiated in only 80% of patients on the basis of composite clinical, endoscopic, radiologic, and pathologic findings.

The adolescent with only colonic involvement, and without perianal disease or granuloma detected on biopsy, poses the greatest difficulty in reaching a precise diagnosis. Involvement of the rectum, once considered exclusive to ulcerative colitis, occurs in 80% to 85% of children with Crohn's disease. Conversely, the finding of a normal rectum on sigmoidoscopy, once regarded as inconsistent with ulcerative colitis, may actually be associated with this disease. Biopsy specimens of mucosa that appear to be normal may show varying degrees of inflammation and granulomas, especially if serial sectioning is performed. The use of biopsy findings (i.e., crypt abscess formation, goblet cell populations, patchiness of disease) to distinguish between Crohn's disease and ulcerative colitis may be misleading, especially if the patient has been previously treated. Even in ulcerative colitis, colectomy specimens often show less involvement of the left colon than the right colon after topical steroid therapy has been instituted.

Certain radiologic features are helpful in distinguishing ulcerative colitis from Crohn's disease. However, the distribution of disease (i.e., continuous vs. segmental) as shown by radiographic examination is nonspecific and often does not reflect the extent of inflammation.

Barium enema studies may be misleading, not only in differentiating Crohn's disease from ulcerative colitis, but also in the initial diagnosis of IBD. In our experience, diagnostic barium enema study results have been normal in 25% of children with ulcerative colitis documented endoscopically and histologically. In Crohn's disease the barium enema study rarely reveals rectosigmoid abnormalities despite involvement of this segment in 80% to 85% of affected children. Clearly, to detect inflammation and its distribution and extent, endoscopy and multiple biopsies are preferable to the barium enema study.

Although ulcerative colitis is confined to the colon, Crohn's disease can affect any portion of the digestive tract. Previously, it was thought that among adolescents with Crohn's disease, 30% had ileal involvement, 55% had ileal and colonic involvement, and 15% had disease confined to the colon. More recent data, substantiated by more extensive evaluation of the colon through endoscopy and multiple biopsies sectioned serially, have revealed that about 85% of children with Crohn's disease

have rectosigmoid inflammation. This distribution of disease is similar in those with and those without perianal disease, the ileum being involved in about 85% of children with Crohn's disease.

Symptoms and Signs

In 1979, Hamilton et al[38] studied 148 consecutive, newly diagnosed childhood cases of IBD during an 8-year period (1969 to 1976). All patients were under 19 years of age. In patients with Crohn's disease, the major initial complaints were abdominal pain (39%) and diarrhea (18%). In those with ulcerative colitis, the initial complaints were diarrhea (62%), abdominal pain (12%), and hematochezia (passage of bloody stools) (19%). Most of the patients in this study showed physical signs of chronic disease at the time of diagnosis.

Of the more than 1000 children with IBD seen at North Shore University Hospital–Cornell University Medical College from 1975 to 1996, about 60% were 13 to 18 years of age. Abdominal pain and diarrhea are the most common complaints both at initial diagnosis and during relapse, and these disturbances often awaken the patient. This aspect of pain helps to distinguish IBD from irritable bowel syndrome, which causes discomfort only during awake hours. The pain of IBD is crampy, usually localized in the lower abdomen, and tends to be unrelieved by the passage of flatus or stool. Diarrhea may be of large or small volume. The latter is usually associated with tenesmus, or anorectal urgency, which accompanies the distal left-sided inflammation of either ulcerative colitis or Crohn's disease. Macroscopic blood per rectum, which is characteristic of ulcerative colitis, is also common in Crohn's disease, as is the presence of exudate.

Anorexia is a problem frequently associated with inadequate intake of micronutrients and macronutrients. In Crohn's disease there may be early satiety with solid foods, reflecting upper gastrointestinal disease. How frequently this phenomenon is caused by inflammation, acid or alkaline reflux, or motility disturbance remains to be determined. Increased circulating levels of tumor necrosis factor have been implicated as a cause of the anorexia. Patients with abdominal cramps and diarrhea of an urgent nature may choose not to eat at specific times for fear of having embarrassing accidents. Some adolescent girls also have eating disorders, such as anorexia nervosa or bulimia, that may precede the onset of IBD or appear concomitantly with it.

Delayed growth and sexual maturation is especially common in Crohn's disease. Markowitz et al[39] demonstrated that 31% of adolescents with Crohn's disease show evidence of permanent growth retardation. Growth curves reveal that 60% of adolescents with Crohn's disease drop two standard deviations (SD) or more from their best height percentile for age during adolescence, and 19% remain two SD below their best height percentile at maturity. In comparison, growth retardation in ulcerative colitis appears to be uncommon.

Fever, which occurs in 25% to 50% of adolescents with IBD, may exceed 104°F without a discernible focus of infection (e.g., intra-abdominal abscess). The frequency and severity of anemia in adolescents with IBD are difficult to assess. Studies have not taken into account the fact that hemoglobin and hematocrit levels should reflect pubertal development (Tanner stage), not chronologic age. A hemoglobin level that may be normal for a prepubertal, or Tanner stage 1, adolescent of age 13 years may be significantly abnormal for a pubertal, or Tanner stage 5, adolescent of the same age. Anemia usually results from blood loss, lack of incorporation of iron into erythrocytes in the bone marrow, or both. In the anemia of chronic IBD, erythrocytes are hypochromic and microcytic. However, iron is present in the bone marrow, and normal serum ferritin concentrations reflect normal total body iron stores. The low serum iron levels encountered in adolescents with IBD are probably accounted for by the deposition of available iron in the reticuloendothelial system.

Although arthralgias are common, frank arthritis occurs infrequently among adolescents. Deformities of the joints, resulting from chronic inflammation, are rarely seen with IBD and should alert the clinician to the possibility of a second autoimmune disease, such as rheumatoid arthritis. Several other autoimmune disorders involving the liver, thyroid, and kidney also may be seen in adolescents with IBD.

Radiographs, and in some instances bone scans, should be obtained to determine whether chronic joint discomfort is the result of osteonecrosis. Aseptic necrosis of the hip is rare, even in children or adolescents undergoing chronic steroid therapy. Lower back pain and tenderness may be a nagging clinical problem, especially in older adolescents. Diagnostic studies often reveal no specific skeletal or joint abnormalities, but symptoms and signs remit with nonsteroidal anti-inflammatory medication. Studies have shown the presence of osteopenia in newly diagnosed patients with IBD, especially those with Crohn's disease.[40]

Patients with IBD have increased levels of alpha$_1$-antitrypsin in the stool, which indicates that the hypoalbuminemia noted in IBD likely results from protein loss due to bowel inflammation. Protein intake in adolescents with Crohn's disease is usually adequate despite a deficit in caloric intake. In adolescents with pure malnutrition, such as that caused by anorexia nervosa, hypoalbuminemia is uncommon.

Hydrogen breath tests performed in one study of children and adolescents with IBD demonstrated lactose malabsorption in 21 of 70 patients, with gastrointestinal

---

BOX 46-2
Extraintestinal Manifestations of Inflammatory Bowel Disease

Perianal disease	Hematologic disease
Pancreatitis	Joint disorders
Hepatic abscess	Ocular diseases
Splenic abscess	Pulmonary disorder
Mouth lesions	Nephrolithiasis
Cutaneous lesions	Myocarditis
Vasculitis	Pericarditis
Vascular thrombosis	

Modified from Silverberg M, Daum F, editors: *Textbook of pediatric gastroenterology,* ed 2, Chicago, 1988, Mosby–Year Book; p 398.

---

symptoms present in 14 of the 21.[41] Prevalence did not differ between those with ulcerative colitis and those with Crohn's disease. Patients with diffuse small bowel Crohn's disease had a higher prevalence of lactose intolerance and malabsorption. However, the frequency of lactose malabsorption in children and adolescents with chronic IBD was no greater than in those with chronic abdominal pain of other causes when ethnic differences were accounted for.

Extraintestinal Manifestations

A wide range of extraintestinal manifestations of IBD in adolescents with Crohn's disease or ulcerative colitis have been described (Box 46-2).

Perianal lesions are by far the most common extraintestinal problem and also the most difficult to manage. In one study of 149 children and teenagers with Crohn's disease,[42] a 49% prevalence of perianal disease was noted. Of these 73 patients, 51 patients had fissures and large anal tags (sentinel tags), while 10 had fistulas and 12 had abscesses. Rectal inflammation was present in 94% of patients with fistulas or abscesses, or both, as compared with 63% of all patients without perianal disease (p <.025). Anorectal granulomas were present in 47% of patients with fistulas or abscesses, compared with 9% of patients with nonperianal disease (p >.05). Fifty percent of patients with fistulas and/or abscesses that drained, either spontaneously or after surgical treatment, were healed, while the remainder continued to have chronic drainage.

Differential Diagnosis

The differential diagnosis of IBD must take into account the age of the patient, as well as the signs and symptoms. Box 46-3 provides a list of disorders involving gastrointestinal signs and symptoms that are also common to IBD.

BOX 46-3
Differential Diagnosis of Inflammatory Bowel Disease

UPPER GASTROINTESTINAL TRACT
Reflux esophagitis
Behçet's disease
Acid-peptic disease
Zollinger-Ellison syndrome
Eosinophilic gastroenteritis
Tuberculosis

SMALL AND LARGE BOWEL
Intestinal lymphangiectasia
Celiac sprue
Milk protein allergy
Soy protein allergy
Allergic gastroenteropathy
Eosinophilic gastroenteritis
Irritable bowel syndrome
Tuberculosis
Enteric infections
Colitis (antibiotic-induced)
Hirschsprung's disease with enterocolitis
Stool withholding with encopresis
Acute appendicitis, appendiceal abscess
Neoplasms (lymphoma, carcinoma, adenocarcinoma, [Family Cancer Syndrome])
Radiation
Vasculitis (Henoch-Schönlein purpura, lupus erythematosus, hemolytic uremic syndrome)

MISCELLANEOUS
Anorexia nervosa
Carbohydrate intolerance (lactose, sucrose, xylitol, sorbitol)

Modified from Silverberg M, Daum F, editors: Textbook of pediatric gastroenterology, ed 2, Chicago, 1988, Mosby–Year Book; p 399.

BOX 46-4
Evaluation of Inflammatory Bowel Disease

History
Physical examination
Complete blood count and differential, reticulocyte count, sedimentation rate
Ferritin, serum iron, total iron-binding capacity
Stool: pus cells, Charcot-Leyden crystals, culture and sensitivity, ova and parasites, *Clostridium* toxin
Serum chemistries
Serum folate, vitamin B_{12}
Colonoscopy and biopsies
Esophagogastroduodenoscopy and biopsies
Upper gastrointestinal and small bowel series
Barium enema study
Growth velocity, Tanner stage, bone age
72-hour fecal fat determination
Nutritional assessment
Psychological assessment

Modified from Silverberg M, Daum F, editors: Textbook of pediatric gastroenterology, ed 2, Chicago, 1988, Mosby–Year Book; p 400.

Evaluation

The evaluation of IBD requires a thorough history taking, a comprehensive physical examination, and appropriate laboratory studies (Box 46-4). Special attention should be given to the perianal area. A hemoglobin or hematocrit evaluation may demonstrate anemia, while the serum ferritin level is helpful in assessing total body iron stores. The erythrocyte sedimentation rate (ESR) is often elevated, but normal values are seen even in acute fulminant colitis. If the ESR is elevated, it is more likely to be indicative of IBD than of irritable bowel syndrome, in which laboratory data are normal. Fecal Wright's stains, stool cultures, and examinations for ova and parasites should be obtained to determine whether there are pus cells, Charcot-Leyden crystals, or enteric infection. A low serum albumin concentration indicates protein loss from an inflamed mucosa; a low serum cholesterol concentration often reflects loss of bile salts in the feces due to the presence of significant ileal disease. A low serum folate concentration is indicative of proximal small bowel disease; a low serum vitamin B_{12} concentration points to extensive ileal involvement.

Before the advent of flexible endoscopy, which allows visualization of the entire colon and terminal ileum, it was routine practice to obtain an upper gastrointestinal and small bowel series, a barium enema study, and a rigid proctosigmoidoscopy with biopsies in adolescent patients with possible IBD. Today, it is more common to obtain an upper gastrointestinal and small bowel series and to perform a colonoscopy with multiple biopsies. During colonoscopy, biopsies should be taken even from areas of normal-appearing mucosa, since histologic inflammation may be present in tissue that appears to be normal on endoscopic examination.

In patients receiving corticosteroid therapy, ophthalmologic evaluation, including a slit-lamp examination, on a yearly basis to rule out cataracts is suggested. Adolescents with Crohn's disease may also have asymptomatic anterior uveitis. Growth velocity curves, Tanner staging for sexual maturation, and bone age determination are all useful in assessing the patient's growth and development and potential for future maturation. Although steatorrhea is unusual, even in patients with ileal Crohn's disease, a 72-hour fecal fat study may be warranted in patients with growth failure. Studies of zinc, as well as calcium and vitamin D metabolism, may be helpful in assessing the nutritional status of adolescents with IBD, especially those with growth failure. Before the assumption is made that a patient with IBD is lactose intolerant, it is advisable to perform an LBH test. A glucose breath test also may help determine whether patients, especially those with small bowel Crohn's disease, have bacterial overgrowth.

Pregnancy and IBD

Issues of pregnancy are relevant for adolescents with IBD.[43] Adolescent girls with IBD have many concerns regarding pregnancy: Will pregnancy make the IBD worse? Does IBD interfere with the ability to conceive (fertility), with the pregnancy itself, with a normal delivery, and with the health of the newborn? A study by Baird et al[44] showed no evidence of reduced fertility or increased pregnancy loss in women over 20 years of age with IBD. However, women with Crohn's disease or ulcerative colitis were more likely than control subjects to have preterm births. These data suggest that close obstetric monitoring during the third trimester of pregnancy is advisable.

Nutritional status may well be the most important factor that determines fertility in women with IBD. If the IBD is active, especially when pregnancy begins, spontaneous abortion is more likely. However, most surveys indicate that a woman with IBD has the same overall chance of giving birth to a normal live infant as does a healthy woman. Surgical procedures, including ileostomy and total proctocolectomy with an ileal reservoir, do not pose significant hazards for successful childbirth. Steroids and sulfasalazine, if used judiciously, do not appear to alter the outcome of pregnancy. The use of 6-mercaptopurine or metronidazole during pregnancy is still not advised, although there are no specific data to indicate adverse fetal or perinatal effects from these medications.

Medical Management

Therapy for ulcerative colitis and Crohn's disease in adolescents requires that the clinician focus on issues unique to this population, namely, physical and psychosocial growth and development.[45] With rare exceptions, treatment regimens for adolescents with IBD are extrapolated from adult experience. However, individualized treatment is required because dosages need to be adjusted for patients of a smaller size. Regrettably, there are very few data that deal with either the safety or the efficacy of these "standard" medications.

Treatment is geared toward the suppression of incapacitating symptoms, promotion of normal growth and development, and control of unavoidable complications. Care must be taken to avoid excessive or inappropriate therapy. Treatment requires a careful balance between sufficient intervention to improve the patient's quality of life and avoidance of the deleterious side effects of overtreatment.

NUTRITION AND GROWTH FAILURE. Growth failure and delay in pubertal maturation occur in approximately 30% of children and adolescents with IBD, in particular those with Crohn's disease. Although the specific pathogenesis of this complication needs further elucidation, chronic malnutrition, specifically due to inadequate caloric intake, plays a major role.[46] Nutritional support to provide adequate macronutrients and micronutrients can be provided orally, enterally, or parenterally.

Adolescents with IBD often require 80 to 90 kcal and 3 to 3.4 g of protein per kilogram of ideal body weight per day to achieve their ultimate height potential. Healthy adolescents require only 60 kcal and 2.25 g of protein/kg/day. For patients with quiescent ulcerative colitis or Crohn's disease who are suffering from inadequate weight and height gain and delayed sexual maturation, the use of oral liquid supplements is encouraged. Supplementing the usual diet with liquid formula can result in adequate caloric intake and improved growth. However, the daily volume of formula required to achieve these goals, and the unacceptable taste, often make this approach not feasible.

Data have demonstrated that improved growth can also be achieved with nasogastric infusions of either nonelemental or elemental formulas.[47,48] The use of nocturnal nasogastric infusions requires that the adolescent learn to insert a nasogastric tube at night and remove it the following morning. With this approach, an additional 1500 kcal can be provided per 24 hours, and patients uniformly have significant increases in both weight and height. However, such patients usually become noticeably "fatter" before becoming "taller." Increments in height may not occur for 3 to 6 months after significant weight gain. If patients are compliant with this regimen and their disease remains in remission, they will advance into puberty. Obviously, following the regimen takes motivation on the part of the patient and continuous support by the family and health care providers. The fact that the tube is removed in the morning, thus allowing the patient to pursue normal activities, serves as a motivating factor. Tube feedings permit a certain flexibility because they can be discontinued on weekends and vacations. Percutaneous endoscopic gastrostomy (PEG) was shown in one study to be an alternative to providing nutrition in IBD patients.[49] This approach might not be acceptable to most adolescents, however, because of the disfiguring presence of an abdominal button.

High-calorie intravenous infusion through a central line during sleep hours also provides a possible source of increased calories. The line is capped during the day, making normal activity possible. However, this approach is riskier than tube feedings because it occasionally leads to infection and/or hepatobiliary dysfunction.

ANTI-INFLAMMATORY AGENTS

Sulfasalazine. Although there are data to suggest that sulfasalazine (Azulfidine) is most effective in mild forms of ulcerative colitis or Crohn's colitis, most gastroenterologists also still tend to use sulfasalazine to treat mild to moderate small bowel Crohn's disease. Daily dosages of 50 to 75 mg/kg/day in two or three divided doses often result in lessened disease activity within 10 to 14 days. If no substantial response is seen during this time, the drug is generally discontinued and alternative therapy instituted. Once remission has been achieved with sulfasalazine, the daily dosage usually can be reduced to 30 to 50 mg/kg. Although there are no data on Crohn's colitis or ileitis to indicate that sulfasalazine prevents relapse, this medication is often continued indefinitely in patients with either quiescent ulcerative colitis or Crohn's disease, or at least until puberty is achieved. If relapse occurs, another medication (i.e., a corticosteroid) is probably necessary. Despite the fact that relapse has occurred during previous sulfasalazine therapy, sulfasalazine can be reinstituted at a dosage of 30 mg/kg/day after remission has been induced with the corticosteroids. Sulfasalazine is usually reintroduced when the corticosteroid has been tapered to a dosage of about 0.25 mg/kg/day.

Among adolescents, the incidence of adverse side effects from sulfasalazine is unknown. With 75 mg/kg/day administered in two or three divided doses, complications such as headache, malaise, and hemolysis seem to be infrequent. Non–dose-related (hypersensitivity) reactions, including rashes, fever, aplastic anemia, hepatic necrosis, pulmonary vasculitis, and neurologic complications, are uncommon. Desensitization through incremental administration of 250 mg sulfasalazine every 2 to 3 days until the desired dosage is achieved may be effective in adolescents with mild hypersensitivity reactions, especially rashes. Platelet aggregation is unaffected by the minimal plasma levels of 5-aminosalicylate or sulfasalazine. Renal tubular function also appears unaffected 1 year after inception of sulfasalazine therapy. Sulfasalazine does not appear to have a teratogenic effect on the fetus, although its metabolites readily cross the placental barrier. Despite this, we advise discontinuing the drug in the pregnant teenager who has inactive colitis. Breast milk does contain sulfasalazine and sulfapyridine metabolites, but only small amounts of an infant's bilirubin are displaced from albumin during maternal sulfasalazine therapy. Kernicterus has not been reported as a result of maternal sulfasalazine therapy. To prevent sulfasalazine-induced megaloblastic anemia secondary to the inhibition of folic acid absorption, we prescribe a daily dose of 1 mg folic acid.

Newer 5-aminosalicylic acid compounds. Several newer compounds have been formulated using 5-ASA, the active compound in sulfasalazine (Table 46-3).

Systems have been developed for effective delivery of the 5-ASA moiety in its free form to the distal small intestine and colon.[50] Topical preparations in the form of suppositories, foams, and enemas are also available. A North American multi-institutional study conducted by the Pediatric Gastroenterology Collaborative Research Group was discontinued when interim analysis of the data revealed that sulfasalazine was significantly more effective than olsalazine in children and adolescents with mild to moderate ulcerative colitis.[51] Timed-release 5-ASA has proved to be effective therapy in children and adolescents with Crohn's disease in the small intestine.[52] Data are needed to show whether rectal preparations of 5-ASA in enema suspension, foam preparation, or suppository form are effective and safe in children and adolescents with distal left-sided colitis from Crohn's disease or ulcerative colitis. Rectal 5-ASA offers a good alternative to rectal cortisone, which may have growth-suppressive side effects.

Corticosteroids. *Rectal preparations.* In the adolescent with mild active ulcerative colitis or Crohn's colitis who has predominant symptoms of distal left-sided colitis, such as tenesmus and urgency, rectal corticosteroids, in foam or enema form, are often prescribed concomitantly with sulfasalazine. For some patients, rectal corticosteroids are the key to a diminution in symptoms. Hydrocortisone acetate (Cortifoam) is often better tolerated than a hydrocortisone retention enema (Cortenema) when tenesmus and urgency are particularly severe. Cortifoam is prescribed for one to three times daily, depending on the severity of tenesmus, the urgency, and the frequency of "accidents" or incontinent bowel movements. After the foam preparation has been used for 1 week, the patient can often change to the enema preparation for more extensive local therapy. Insertion of the applicator tip into the anorectum may induce the urge

---

TABLE 46-3
5-ASA Preparations

Agent	Preparation
Oral	
Asacol	5-ASA powder coated with pH-dependent (>7) acrylic resin (Eudragit-S)
Pentasa	5-ASA encapsulated in ethylcellulose micro-granules (pH and time-dependent release)
Claversal/ Salofalk	5-ASA in sodium glycine buffer coated with Eudragit-L
Dipentum	5-ASA dimer linked by an azo bond
Balsalazide	5-ASA linked by an azo bond to 4-amino-benzoyl-β-alanine as an inert carrier
Rectal	
Rowasa	5-ASA enema, suppository

to defecate. Therefore, when the number of daily bowel movements are counted to determine the efficacy of therapy, this must be considered. Once the symptoms of proctosigmoiditis diminish, the daily dose of rectal corticosteroids is reduced by one half, to one application on a weekly basis. When the patient is taking only one foam or one enema preparation each day and is asymptomatic, a tapering therapy schedule may then be utilized (i.e., one full application with one half application every other day followed by one half application daily for 1 to 2 weeks) before the rectal corticosteroid is discontinued completely. An alternative is one rectal application every other day for 1 to 2 weeks, with therapy discontinued if the patient is asymptomatic.

In the asymptomatic adolescent, rectosigmoid pathologic findings alone are not an indication for rectal corticosteroid therapy. Some patients with a significant rectosigmoid pathologic condition remain asymptomatic for several months without any specific topical therapy. There are no data to suggest whether prophylactic corticosteroids prevent recurrent symptoms of proctosigmoiditis or whether steroids minimize the ultimate risk of colon cancer in ulcerative colitis, or of fistula formation in Crohn's colitis.

Oral and parenteral preparations. For the moderately ill patient with ulcerative colitis or Crohn's disease (temperature <38.5°C, moderate to severe cramps, six to 10 loose stools per day with or without blood, and impaired ability to perform normal daily activities), the clinician may prescribe oral prednisone, 0.5 to 1 mg/kg/day, with a daily maximum of 50 to 75 mg. For more severe symptoms, patients may be hospitalized for therapy with intravenous hydrocortisone, 0.5 to 1 mg/kg/dose every 6 to 8 hours. Others have advocated a continuous infusion of hydrocortisone. In patients with severe tenesmus or urgency, rectal corticosteroids may also be used.

After there is clinical evidence of remission, steroids are continued at the same dosage for approximately 2 weeks, and then the daily dose is tapered at a rate of 2.5 to 5 mg of prednisone per week. For example, a dose of 25 mg is reduced to 20 mg over a 7-day period, then to 15 mg, and so on. Steroids are tapered completely, and sulfasalazine is reintroduced when the prednisone dose has been decreased to about 0.25 mg/kg/day. In the adolescent who requires low-dose steroids for the disease to remain in remission, steroids may be given daily in a dosage similar to the steroid concentration that the adrenal gland would produce endogenously. Although oral corticosteroids may be taken on a daily basis in two divided doses, some patients respond better to prednisone in smaller doses taken more frequently throughout the day. Others respond equally well to a single morning dose. Alternatively, if growth suppression due to daily steroid therapy is a matter of concern, steroids may be used on an alternate-day basis, with the dose equal to double that of the daily dose.

If the condition worsens and there are symptoms and signs of acute fulminant colitis, admission to the hospital becomes mandatory. Extreme care should be taken to ensure that the patient has not developed an intestinal perforation or toxic megacolon. The latter, a life-threatening emergency, is unusual in children and adolescents. Medical therapy for acute fulminant colitis includes intravenous hydrocortisone, 1 to 1.5 mg/kg/day every 6 hours, and intravenous antibiotics. A combination of either ampicillin, gentamicin, and clindamycin or one of cefotetan and gentamicin may be prescribed. Seven to 10 days of intensive medical therapy may serve as a cutoff point before determining that a subtotal colectomy and ileostomy is necessary. However, surgical intervention should be made more quickly in the patient who, despite intensive therapy, demonstrates a significant increase in total polymorphonucleocyte count or a "shift to the left," or in the patient who develops signs of peritonitis despite intensive therapy. With this approach, we have not experienced development of a free intestinal perforation or toxic megacolon in any of our adolescent patients. Some patients respond to aggressive medical therapy combined with watchful waiting and slowly move into remission. These patients should receive a full 10-day course of intravenous antibiotics, with slow tapering of prednisone, as would be done for an outpatient with moderately active colitis.

In the adolescent with uncontrollable colonic bleeding from either ulcerative colitis or Crohn's disease, higher doses of intravenous hydrocortisone (up to 80 mg every 6 hours) may be required. Patience may be necessary with a "bleeder," allowing up to 2 to 3 weeks for recovery. This conservative medical approach sometimes demands that patients receive 6 to 8 units of packed red blood cells over this time span. It has been argued that in many instances relapse will occur within 12 to 24 months, requiring surgery, and that the risk of non-A, non-B hepatitis or cytomegalovirus hepatitis from blood products must also be considered. Nevertheless, adolescents with severe colonic bleeding often do well after recovery and do not require colonic surgery.

Side effects. The cosmetic side effects of steroids are disturbing to the adolescent and may lead to poor compliance. Excessive hair growth and acne are transient phenomena that disappear when the dosage is lowered or the medication discontinued. However, the striae, or stretch marks, that result from steroid therapy lead to permanent disfigurement. Although stretch marks lighten in color over time, they do not disappear, even with topical application of cocoa butter or supplemental intake of vitamin E. Plastic surgery is seldom helpful. The dosage of steroids that results in striae is unpredictable. Fortunately, most adolescents who receive steroids do not develop this problem. The puffiness that accompanies steroid therapy can be diminished somewhat by reducing salt intake. Salt should not be added to the diet, and food or beverages that are high in sodium should be avoided. A formal low-salt diet is unpalatable and unnecessary, and often results in diminished caloric intake. Discussing the salt content of the diet with a nutritionist may be helpful.

The long-term complications associated with corticosteroid use, which include osteoporosis and cataract formation, are extremely unusual. Of valid concern is growth suppression resulting from prednisone. Exogenous corticosteroids interfere with linear bone growth, even in the face of adequate dietary intake. Data from Hyams et al[53] revealed that in children and adolescents with IBD, daily intake of prednisone for only 7 to 10 days in commonly prescribed dosages (0.3 to 1 mg/kg/day) can decrease serum procollagen levels, a postulated biochemical marker for linear bone growth. The use of alternate-day dosing regimens has been beneficial in limiting these effects while often maintaining reduced disease activity.

Aseptic necrosis of the hip, although a recognized complication of steroid therapy in adults, is an infrequent complication in children and adolescents. Despite the use of frequent intermittent dosages of corticosteroid preparations, none of our patients has developed this orthopedic problem. One patient with ulcerative colitis did develop osteonecrosis of the left knee and left ankle after receiving a combination of intravenous corticosteroids and Intralipid therapy. One seldom mentioned possible complication of corticosteroid therapy is the risk of overwhelming varicella infection. It is recommended that any susceptible patient who is receiving steroids and is exposed to chickenpox receive an injection of zoster immunoglobulin, to provide passive immunity and the clinical severity of chickenpox. Hospitalization for chickenpox and intravenous acyclovir therapy (25 to 50 mg/kg/day) is unnecessary unless there is bleeding into the skin or eyes, severe mucous membrane involvement, or pneumonia.

Adolescents undergoing steroid therapy appear to be at no greater risk for infection than their healthy counterparts. Similarly, after they have discontinued the steroids, there is no greater risk of adrenal insufficiency from viral or bacterial disorders. However, adolescents undergoing general anesthesia for surgery who have taken steroids for 2 to 4 weeks during the preceding 12 to 24 months should receive steroids before and during the procedure itself and during the next 24 to 48 hours.

Patient compliance. Adolescents are generally more psychologically sensitive to changes in physical appearance than adults. Failure to respond to what appears to be an adequate regimen of corticosteroid therapy, especially in the patient who does not appear to be "cushingoid," suggests a lack of compliance. The need to take medicine

rectally may be particularly disturbing. Patients and families are often confused by the word "enema." In some instances the patient may expel the enema as if it were a cathartic rather than retaining it for therapeutic purposes.

IMMUNOSUPPRESSIVE DRUGS. Two drugs that are available commercially, 6-mercaptopurine (Purinethol) and azathioprine (Imuran), are the most commonly prescribed immunosuppressives for adolescents with intractable Crohn's disease. Clinical trials in adults with Crohn's disease have demonstrated marked improvement in symptoms and lessened disease activity when these agents have been used either alone or in combination with corticosteroids for at least 3 to 6 months. Shorter duration of usage may not result in significant clinical change. Similar data, derived from clinical experience in adolescents with intractable Crohn's disease, have indicated that two thirds of patients experience remission of disease, and 80% are able to completely discontinue corticosteroid treatment when 6-mercaptopurine (1 to 1.5 mg/kg/day with a maximum of 75 mg/day) is used for at least 1 year.[54] Neutropenia, serious infection, and other untoward reactions have not been encountered.

Cyclosporine, originally developed to prevent organ rejection after transplantation, has been used in the management of IBD in recent years. In one study, cyclosporine was found to be effective in achieving clinical remission in 80% of children with acute fulminant colitis refractory to traditional medical treatment.[55] However, within 1 year, most initial responders underwent colectomy because of a flare-up of disease. In most patients the role of cyclosporine therapy is to rapidly ameliorate symptoms, thus mitigating the need for precipitous colectomy, while improving nutrition and allowing psychological adaptation. Benkov et al did not find cyclosporine to be an alternative to surgery in patients with ulcerative colitis.[56]

ANTIBIOTICS

Metronidazole. Only one pediatric study has evaluated the efficacy of metronidazole (Flagyl) in intestinal Crohn's disease. In this study, metronidazole (15 to 20 mg/kg/day) had a steroid-sparing effect in adolescents with active or steroid-dependent Crohn's disease. However, 11 of 13 patients treated for 4 to 11 months subsequently had abnormal sensory examinations.[57] Although the paresthesias and dysesthesias were reversible, the frequency and severity of symptoms limited acceptance of this otherwise effective therapy.

Other antibiotic agents. Oral and/or parenteral antibiotics are indicated for adolescents who have fever and an inflammatory mass or abscess. The combination of cefoxitin or cefotetan with an aminoglycoside is usually effective, although some patients may require coverage with ampicillin, clindamycin, and an aminoglycoside or imipenem. Oral antibiotics such as tetracycline, metronidazole, or erythromycin may suppress symptoms of bacterial overgrowth. However, most broad-spectrum antibiotics have been associated with the development of *Clostridium difficile*–mediated colitis. Patients with an acute onset of bloody diarrhea should be screened for *C. difficile* toxin whether or not antibiotics, including sulfasalazine, have been prescribed in the previous 3 to 6 months.

ANTIDIARRHEAL AGENTS. Of the various antidiarrheal, antispasmotic medications available, only loperamide hydrochloride (Imodium) is not potentially addictive and has not been associated with the onset of toxic megacolon. The response to loperamide varies, but it seems to be most dramatic in reducing ileostomy effluent. Opiates and codeine may reduce abdominal cramps and/or diarrhea, but these agents should be used infrequently (i.e., for special social occasions) and with caution because they may precipitate toxic megacolon.

Ulcerative Colitis

SURGICAL INTERVENTION. In ulcerative colitis, emergency surgical intervention may be necessary because of acute fulminant colitis, massive intestinal bleeding, free perforation, or toxic megacolon. The only current reasons for elective surgery are dependence on growth-suppressive steroids or continuous debilitating symptoms despite medical therapy. Growth and pubertal retardation are no longer primary indications for colectomy. Normal growth and sexual maturation usually can be achieved if the patient receives adequate calories and is not taking high doses of steroids. Colectomy should be performed for growth failure only if the condition is complicated by unremitting symptoms and/or steroid dependence. Increments in height velocity and possible catch-up growth will occur if surgery is performed in puberty, before closure of the epiphyses.

Prophylactic surgery for colonic carcinoma seems unwarranted, even in adolescents who have had ulcerative colitis for more than 10 years. Possible exceptions include the presence of dysplasia in noninflamed tissue, or a colonoscopy or barium enema study suggestive of malignancy. Surveillance colonoscopy with biopsies should be performed every 24 to 30 months in all patients who have had ulcerative colitis for more than 8 years, and is now being recommended by many authorities for patients with Crohn's colitis of similar duration. We have encountered three cases (2 ulcerative colitis and one Crohn's colitis) of adenocarcinoma of the colon in patients in their early twenties with onset of disease of childhood.

SURGICAL TECHNIQUE. The initial surgical approach in the adolescent with presumed ulcerative colitis consists of a subtotal colectomy and ileostomy. The distal sigmoid, rectum, and anus are left intact. The subtotal colectomy specimen is evaluated by an experienced pathologist to confirm the clinical impression of ulcerative colitis. Six to 12 months later, most adolescents opt to have their traditional ileostomy converted to an endorectal pull-through or ileoanal anastomosis. A new ileostomy is created and left intact for 6 to 8 weeks to allow for healing. The ostomy is then closed. Antidiarrheal therapy is offered as soon as symptoms require. Various combinations of loperamide hydrochloride and/or codeine sulfate usually decrease the frequency of stools so that the adolescent can attend school without trepidation. Some adolescents take as many as three loperamide hydrochloride tablets three times a day; while others take somewhat fewer along with 15 mg codeine sulfate two or three times a day. Some also require a bulk-forming agent (e.g., Metamucil or FiberCon) to provide more substance to their stools.

ANTIDIARRHEAL THERAPY. For postsurgical patients with diarrhea, a diet is prescribed consisting of three meals per day and a limited number of snacks to try to minimize the number of daily bowel movements. Despite having an increase in the frequency of stools during the first 6 to 12 months, patients ultimately report that their stools are firm. During school hours, when a bathroom is not easily accessible, the degree of control achieved becomes evident. None of our patients has verbalized regret about having gone through the surgical procedure, despite having to adjust to a significant change from the normal stool pattern for 6 to 12 months.

Crohn's Disease

SURGICAL INTERVENTION. Surgical intervention is recommended only to deal with complications unresponsive to medical therapy. Resection of a localized diseased segment may be preferable to chronic administration of medications, especially corticosteroids. At times, Crohn's colitis is particularly refractory to medical therapy, and 18 of our patients have had elective surgery consisting of a colonic resection (subtotal or total proctocolectomy) and ileostomy. Although some authors may view this approach to colonic Crohn's disease as heresy, fearing the risk of small bowel recurrence, all patients have achieved normal growth and pubertal maturation. Given the available options, including corticosteroids, frequent hospitalizations, and delayed growth and development, this approach is appropriate for certain adolescents with incapacitating colonic Crohn's disease.

The diagnosis of ileostomy dysfunction, which may be made after surgery, is not always obvious from routine digital examination, a small bowel series, or a retrograde stomal study. Therefore, a deflated balloon catheter should be inserted through the stoma, retrograde 15 to 20 cm. The balloon is then inflated with 3 to 4 ml of air, and the catheter is withdrawn under fluoroscopic visualization. If resistance to removal of the catheter is noted, a stenotic lesion must be considered as the primary cause of the ileostomy dysfunction, and surgical correction is necessary.

As in ulcerative colitis, growth failure in Crohn's disease is not considered an indication for surgery unless it is associated with intractable disease activity or corticosteroid dependence. Intestinal strictures leading to recurrent partial obstruction often require resection, but multiple resections may lead to creation of a short bowel, with consequent malabsorption and inadequate gastrointestinal function. Recently, strictureplasty of the small intestine has been advocated as a bowel-sparing technique for such a situation. A longitudinal incision is made through the stenotic bowel wall, and the bowel is then sutured transversely, creating a patent lumen. Careful inspection for malignancy is mandatory.

COURSE AND PROGNOSIS

Physical consequences. Despite the often debilitating effects of IBD, affected children and adolescents eventually reach full sexual maturation. However, if the onset of IBD occurs before puberty, patients often have delayed onset of sexual maturation compared with their parents and siblings. Girls who develop IBD before puberty may reach menarche significantly later than their sisters and mothers.[58] Adolescents may also not reach their calculated ultimate height potential, although most will grow sufficiently so that their height falls within the normal height curves for healthy adults.[59]

Psychosocial consequences. The psychosocial burden of any chronic illness on normal adolescent function can be significant. Studies of children and adolescents with cystic fibrosis and diabetes mellitus have demonstrated high prevalence rates for various forms of psychiatric illness in these groups. Similar findings have been reported in adolescents with IBD. In one study,[60] 60% of children and adolescents with either Crohn's disease or ulcerative colitis had some identifiable psychiatric disorder. Patients with IBD who are of short stature and experience sexual delay often display maladaptive behavior similar to that noted in children with familial short stature.

Although adolescents with IBD may be more compulsive than normal controls and may have psychological states characterized by depression, withdrawal, anxiety, and frequent sleeping, these traits appear to be at least partly due to having a chronic intestinal condition. Studies from our own patient population suggest that, as a group, adolescents with IBD have abnormal styles of coping with stressful life events.[61] In fact, adolescents with IBD are more likely to report that they have experienced fewer stressful life events than would normally occur. This suggests that these patients may have difficulty recognizing and reporting stressful events, or that they tend to use denial to cope with such stresses.

Their coping styles tend to be more rigid and constricted than those of healthy controls.

Team approach to care. To provide adequate care for this group of chronically ill adolescents and their families, our team consists of pediatric gastroenterologists, a pediatric psychiatrist, a nurse clinician, a pediatric nutritionist, and a pathologist with special interest in the gastrointestinal tract. Pediatric surgeons and radiologists are available, as is an enterostomal therapist.

Education for patients and their families involves a variety of modalities, including audiovisual presentations. Adolescents who have learned the technique of inserting a nasogastric tube for nutritional supplementation meet with others about to embark on such a program. Similarly, those who have undergone surgery are asked to counsel their peers who are in need of surgery. Seminars on subjects such as self-image, quality of life, sexuality, and marriage are helpful.

Self-help support groups for parents and other family members of adolescents with IBD can be of enormous benefit. Volunteers whose children suffer from IBD help counsel other parents, especially when their child is first diagnosed. They also visit children who are hospitalized. Finally, educational programs for the lay public can help to define issues about ulcerative colitis and Crohn's disease as they relate to children of all ages.

SYSTEMIC LUPUS ERYTHEMATOSUS

In systemic lupus erythematosus, nausea, vomiting, and anorexia are common signs, and diarrhea occurs less frequently.[62,63] Although ascites and abdominal pain is frequently noted with abdominal vasculitis, painless ascites also has been reported. In most patients the underlying lesion is small vessel arteritis. Jejunal ulcers and perforated colonic diverticula also have been described in association with systemic lupus erythematosus. Arteritis, which leads to local ischemia, has consequences similar to those of mesenteric insufficiency of atherosclerotic origin. Clinically, a cutaneous vasculitis frequently is noted in association with abdominal vasculitis. Radiographically, there may be evidence of pseudo-obstruction, ileus, and thumbprinting, with scalloping of the border of the bowel secondary to submucosal edema and hemorrhage. Pneumatosis cystoides intestinalis (intestinal emphysema) also has been reported. In addition to gastrointestinal hemorrhage, protein-losing enteropathy and malabsorption may occur.

Pathologically, mononuclear cell infiltration of the lamina propria is an almost universal finding in systemic lupus erythematosus, and most patients have one or more lesions suggestive of ischemic bowel disease. Deep colonic ulcers may be seen throughout the colon. Secondary infection, involving *Candida* organisms, cytomegalovirus, herpesvirus, and *Cryptococeus neoformans,* is common.

SCLERODERMA

Although intestinal symptoms and signs of scleroderma are unusual in childhood, adolescents may develop significant motility disturbances of the small bowel with bacterial overgrowth. Abdominal cramps, diarrhea, and bloating with weight loss may result. If such disturbances occur before puberty, a significant delay in growth and sexual maturation may result. Caloric intake may be compromised, and maldigestion and/or malabsorption may result in nutrient wasting.

SMALL BOWEL OBSTRUCTION

Small bowel obstruction due to a membrane encasing the small intestine has been described in a group of girls 13 to 18 years of age.[64] It has been called the "abdominal cocoon." The cause and pathogenesis of this disease are obscure, but it has been postulated that menstrual blood that flows into the peritoneal cavity in a retrograde direction might provide the initial stimulus for chemical peritonitis, with the possibility of a superimposed viral infection. Therapy consists of freeing the adhesions and excising the constricting fibrous membrane surrounding the small intestine.

NEOPLASMS

It is important to note that in the Family Cancer Syndrome and in the multiple polyposis coli syndromes (e.g., familial polyposis coli, Gardner's syndrome), adenomas may undergo malignant transformation during adolescence.[65] An adenocarcinoma of the small bowel has been reported in an 8-year-old with Peutz-Jeghers syndrome, and malignancies of the small intestine also have been described in young adults with this disease. A 15-year-old boy with a paraganglioneuroma of the duodenum has been described as having abdominal pain and massive upper gastrointestinal hemorrhage. This type of tumor causes symptoms similar to those of peptic ulcer disease, but it is histologically benign and may be treated by simple excision.

Malignant transformation in the small or large intestine with Crohn's disease and in the colon with ulcerative colitis is exceedingly rare in adolescence, but it may occur early in the third decade of life. Markowitz et al studied 35 adolescents and young adults who had colitis of 8 years' duration or more with colonoscopy and flow cytometry. Seven patients had aneuploidy (premalignant

DNA changes); one patient had a Dukes C adenocarcinoma. This study emphasizes that adolescents and young adults with childhood-onset IBD are at risk for premalignant DNA changes and colon cancer.[66]

MISCELLANEOUS DISORDERS

Chronic ingestion of irritant laxatives, a behavior sometimes noted in adolescents with anorexia nervosa, may result in the so-called cathartic colon. The radiologic characteristics of this condition are similar to those of advanced ulcerative colitis, with the most extensive changes usually occurring in the right colon. The adolescent may complain of severe constipation; the patient often does not have a bowel movement for as long as 7 to 10 days. Most likely, the cause is a dysmotility.

Adolescents tend to ingest a significant volume of sugar-free products. Sorbitol, the sweetener used in many of these products, is poorly absorbed by the small intestine and may produce an osmotic diarrhea if ingested in large amounts, such as 20 to 50 g.[67] Smaller amounts of ingested sorbitol, such as 5 g, may also cause mild clinical symptoms. Therefore, a careful diet history should be taken in adolescents with gastrointestinal complaints.

References

1. Ryder RW, Sack DA, Kapikian Az et al: Enterotoxigenic *Escherichia coli* and reovirus-like agent in rural Bangladesh, *Lancet* 1:659-633, 1976.
2. Taylor DN, McDermott KT, Little JR, et al: *Campylobacter* enteritis from untreated water in the Rocky Mountains, *Ann Intern Med* 99:38, 1983.
3. Bishop WP, Wishen MH: Bacterial gastroenteritis, *Pediatr Clin North Am* 35:69-87, 1989.
4. Blaser MJ: Bacterial gastrointestinal infections, *Gastroenterol Ann* 3:317-340, 1986.
5. Rees JH, Soudain SE, Gregson NA: *Campylobacter jejuni* infection and Guillain-Barré syndrome, *N Engl J Med* 333:1374-1379, 1995.
6. Merson MH, Goldmann DA, Boyer KM, et al: An outbreak of *Shigella sonnei* gastroenteritis on Colorado River raft trips, *Am J Epidemiol* 100:186-196, 1974.
7. Nelson JD, Kusmiesz H, Jackson L, et al: Trimethoprim-sulfamethoxazole therapy for shigellosis, *JAMA* 235:1239-1243, 1976.
8. Farthing MJG: Giardiasis. In Pounder RE, Chiodini PL, editors: *Advanced medicine 23,* London, 1987, Bailliere Tindall, p 287.
9. Farthing MJG: Host-parasite interactions in human giardiasis, *Am J Med* 70:191-204, 1989.
10. Ament ME, Rubin CE: Relation of giardiasis to abnormal intestinal structure and function in gastrointestinal immunodeficiency syndrome, *Gastroenterology* 62:216-226, 1972.
11. Levinson JD, Nastro LJ: Giardiasis with total villous atrophy, *Gastroenterology* 74:271-275, 1978.
12. Janoff EN, Smith PD, Blaser MJ: Acute antibody responses to *Giardia lamblia* are depressed in patients with AIDS, *J Infect Dis* 157:798-804, 1988.
13. Aldeen WE, Hale D, Robinson AJ, Carroll K: Evaluation of a comercially available ELISA assay for detection of *Giardia lamblia* in fecal specimens, *Diagn Microbiol Infect Dis* 21:77-79, 1995.

14. Mildvan D, Gelb AM, William D: Venereal transmission of enteric pathogens in male homosexuals, *JAMA* 238:1387-1389, 1977.

15. Schmerin NJ, Gelstron A, Jones TC: Amebiasis—an increasing problem among homosexuals in New York City, *JAMA* 238:1386-1387, 1977.

16. Brandt H, Tamayo RB: Pathology amebiasis, *Hum Pathol* 1:351-385, 1970.

17. Adams EB, MacLeod IN: Invasive amebiasis. II. Amebic liver abscess and its complications, *Medicine* 56:325-334, 1977.

18. Tandon A: Use of enzyme linked immunosorbent assay in intestinal and extraintestinal amoebiasis, *Trans R Soc Trop Med Hyg* 75:574-575, 1981.

19. Wolfe MS: The treatment of intestinal protozoin infections, *Med Clin North Am* 66:707-720, 1982.

20. Hughes FB, Faehnle, ST, Simon JL: Multiple cerebral abscesses complicating hepatopulmonary amebiasis, *J Pediatr* 86:95-96, 1975.

21. Quinn TC, Stamm WE, Goodell SE, et al: The polymicrobial origin of intestinal infections in homosexual men, *N Engl J Med* 309:576-582, 1983.

22. Andreani T, Modigliani R, Charpentier Y, et al: Acquired immunodeficiency with intestinal cryptosporidiosis: possible transmission by Haitian whole blood, *Lancet* 1:1187-1191, 1983.

23. Whiteside ME, Barkin JS, May RG, et al: Enteric coccidiosis among patients with the acquired immunodeficiency syndrome, *Am J Trop Med* 298:319-321, 1978.

24. Grand R, Mongtomery RK, Buller HA. In Snape WJ, editor: *Consultation in gastroenterology*, Philadelphia, 1995, WB Saunders; pp 362-367.

25. Ransome-Kuti O: Lactose intolerance review, *Postgrad Med J* 53(2):73-83, 1977.

26. Gray GM: Absorption and malabsorption of dietary carbohydrate. In Winick M, editor: *Nutrition & gastroenterology*, New York, 1980, John Wiley; p 50.

27. Daum F. Pediatric inflammatory bowel disease. In Silverberg M, Daum F, editors: *Textbook of pediatric gastroenterology*, ed 2, Chicago, 1988, Mosby–Year Book; pp 392-418.

28. Barton JR, Gillon S, Ferguson A: Incidence of inflammatory bowel disease in Scottish children between 1968-1983; marginal fall in ulcerative colitis, 3-fold rise in Crohn's disease, *Gut* 30:618-622, 1989.

29. Olafsdottir EJ, Fluge G, Haug K: Chronic inflammatory bowel disease in children in Western Norway, *J Pediatr Gastroenterol Nutr* 8:454-458, 1989.

30. Farmer RG, Michener WM, Mortimer EA: Studies of family history among patients with inflammatory bowel disease. *Clin Gastroenterol* 9(2):271-278, 1980.

31. Logan RFA, Kay CR: Oral contraception, smoking and inflammatory bowel disease—findings in the Royal College of General Practitioners oral contraception study, *Int J Epidemiol* 18:105-107, 1989.

32. Lashner BA, Kane SV, Hanauer S: Lack of association between oral contraceptive use and Crohn's disease: a community-based, matched case-control study, *Gastroenterology* 97:1442-1447, 1989.

33. Lashner BA, Kane SV, Hanauer SB: Lack of association between oral contraceptive use and ulcerative colitis, *Gastroenterology* 99:1032-1036, 1990.

34. Lindberg E, Tysk C, Andersson K, Jarnerot G: Smoking and inflammatory bowel disease. A control study, *Gut* 208, 352-357, 1988.

35. Cosnes J, Carbonnel F, Beaugerie Y, et al: Effects of cigarette smoking on the long term course of Crohn's disease, *Gastroenterology*: 424-431, 1996.

36. North C, Clouse R, Spitznagel E, et al: The relation of ulcerative colitis to psychiatric factors: a review of findings and methods, *Am J Psychiatry* 147:974-981, 1990.

37. Helzer J, Chammas S, Horland CC, et al: A study of the association between Crohn's disease and psychiatric illness, *Gastroenterology* 86:324-330, 1984.

38. Hamilton JR, Bruce GA, Abdourhaman M, Gall DG: Inflammatory bowel disease in children and adolescents, *Adv Pediatr* 26:311-341, 1979.

39. Markowitz J, Grancher K, Rosa J, et al: Growth failure in pediatric inflammatory bowel disease (IBD), *Am J Gastroenterol* 85:1267, 1990.

40. Ghosh S, Cowen S, Hannan JW, et al: Low bone mineral density in Crohn's disease, but not in ulcerative colitis, at diagnosis, *Gastroenterology* 107:1031-1039, 1994.

41. Kirschner BS, DeFavaro MV, Jensen W: Lactose malabsorption in children and adolescents with inflammatory bowel disease, *Gastroenterology* 81:829-832, 1981.

42. Markowitz J, Daum F, Aiges H, et al: Perianal disease in children and adolescents with Crohn's disease, *Gastroenterology* 86:829-833, 1984.

43. Sorokin JJ, Levine SM: Pregnancy and inflammatory bowel disease: a review of the literature, *Obstet Gynecol* 62:247-252, 1983.

44. Baird BD, Narendranathan M, Sandler RS: Increased risk of preterm birth for women with inflammatory bowel disease, *Gastroenterology* 99:987-994, 1990.

45. Daum F: Ulcerative colitis and Crohn's disease. In Bayless T, editor: *Current therapy in gastroenterology and liver disease-3*, Philadelphia, 1990, Mosby–Year Book; pp 291-298.

46. Motil KJ, Grand RJ: Nutritional management of inflammatory bowel disease, *Pediatr Clin North Am* 32:447-469, 1985.

47. Aiges H, Markowitz J, Rosa J, Daum F: Home nocturnal supplemental nasogastric feedings in growth-retarded adolescents with Crohn's disease, *Gastroenterology* 97:905-910, 1989.

48. Belli DC, Seidman E, Bouthillier L, et al: Chronic intermittent elemental diet improves growth failure in children with Crohn's disease, *Gastroenterology* 95:603-610, 1988.

49. Israel DM, Hassall E: Prolonged use of gastrostomy for enteral hyperalimentation in children with Crohn's disease, *Am J Gastroenterol* 90:1084-1088, 1995.

50. Leichtner AM: Aminosalicylates for the treatment of inflammatory bowel disease, *Pediatr Gastroenterol Nutr* 21:245-252, 1995.

51. Ferry G, Grand R, Kirschner B, et al: Results of the Pediatric Gastroenterology Collaborative Research Group clinical trial comparing olsalazine with sulfasalazine in mild to moderate childhood ulcerative colitis, *Gastroenterology* 98:A169, 1990.

52. Griffiths A, Koletzko S, Sylvester F, Marcon M, Sherman P: Slow-release 5-aminosalicylic acid therapy in children with small intestinal Crohn's disease, *J Pediatr Gastroenterol Nutr* 17:186-192, 1993.

53. Hyams J, Moore R, Leichtner A, Carey D, Goldberg B: Relationship of type I procollagen to corticosteroid therapy in children with inflammatory bowel disease, *J Pediatr* 112:893-898, 1988.

54. Markowitz J, Rosa J, Grancher K, Aiges H, Daum F: Long term 6-mercaptopurine (6-MP) in adolescents with Crohn's disease, *Gastroenterology* 99:1347-1351, 1990.

55. Treem WR, Cohen J, Davis PM, et al: Cyclosporine for the treatment of fulminant ulcerative colitis in children. Immediate response, long-term results, and impact on surgery, *Dis Colon Rectum*, 38:474-479, 1995.

56. Benkov KJ, Rosh JR, Schwersenz AH, et al: Cyclosporine as an alternative to surgery in children with inflammatory bowel disease, *J Pediatr Gastroenterol Nutr* 19:290-296, 1994.

57. Duffy L, Daum F, Fisher SE, et al: Peripheral neuropathy in Crohn's disease patients treated with metronidazole, *Gastroenterology* 88:681-684, 1985.

58. Daum F: Delayed menarche in girls with early onset Crohn's disease. In Davidson M, editor: *Growth retardation among children with inflammatory bowel disease,* New York, 1983, National Foundation for Ileitis and Colitis; pp 383-390.

59. Daum F: Growth failure and sites of intestinal involvement in children with Crohn's disease. In Davidson M, editor: *Growth retardation among children with inflammatory bowel disease,* New York, 1983, National Foundation for Ileitis and Colitis; pp 338-355.

60. Wood B, Watkins J, Boyle J, Nogueira J, Zimand E, Carroll L: Psychological functioning in children with Crohn's disease and ulcerative colitis: implications for models of psychobiological interaction, *J Am Acad Child Adolesc Psychiatry* 26:774-781, 1987.

61. Gitlin K, Markowitz J, Pelcovitz D, Strohmayer A, Dornstein L, Klein S: Stress mediators in children with inflammatory bowel disease. In Johnson J, Johnson S, editors: *Advances in child health psychology: Proceedings of the Florida Conference,* Gainesville, FL, 1991, University Presses of Florida; pp 98-113.

62. Coleman WP III, Coleman WP, Derbes VJ, et al: Collagen disease in children: a review of 71 cases, *JAMA* 237:1095-1100, 1977.

63. Hoffman BI, Katz WA: The gastrointestinal manifestations of systemic lupus erythematosus: a review of the literature, *Semin Arthritis Rheum* 9:237-247, 1980.

64. Foo K, Ng K, Rauff A, et al: Unusual small intestinal obstruction in adolescent girls: the abdominal cocoon, *Br J Surg* 65:427-430, 1978.

65. Kahn E, Daum F: Gastrointestinal tract tumors in children. In Silverberg M, Daum F, editors: *Textbook of pediatric gastroenterology,* ed 2, Chicago, 1988, Mosby–Year Book; pp 419-445.

66. Markowitz J, McKinley M, Kahn E, et al: Colon cancer surveillance in patients with childhood onset colitis, *J Pediatr Gastroenterol Nutr* 21:325, 1995.

67. Hyams J: Sorbitol intolerance: an unappreciated cause of functional gastrointestinal complaints, *Gastroenterology* 84:30-33, 1983.

CHAPTER 47

Disorders of the Liver and Pancreas

•

Harvey W. Aiges

Fortunately, the adolescent is less likely to develop serious liver disease than the neonate or the geriatric patient. However, the drug use and sexual experimentation of this age group make adolescents vulnerable to liver damage from hepatotoxic agents and at risk for developing acute and chronic hepatitis, both types B and C. In addition, adolescent girls tend to acquire autoimmune chronic active hepatitis more than any other group.

DRUG-INDUCED HEPATOTOXICITY

Adolescents are particularly vulnerable to drug-induced hepatic damage, because this physiologically and psychosocially explosive phase of life introduces many to the use of either prescribed or illicit drugs in therapeutic, recreational, or abusive ways. Recreational use of alcohol and illicit drugs at some time during the adolescent period is extremely common. These agents, even in limited amounts, by inducing the hepatic smooth endoplasmic reticulum and thus enhancing the excretion of substances requiring glucuronidation, may affect the metabolic activity of other drugs and medications. This is important to consider when prescribing medications such as anticonvulsants or estrogen-containing birth control pills, since these agents may be less effective if the patient is using alcohol or illicit drugs.

Most forms of drug-induced hepatic injury spare children (acetaminophen is a good example; aspirin and valproic acid are exceptions). Adolescents are generally more vulnerable to hepatotoxicity than are children, possibly because of decreases in activity and inducibility of the hepatic mixed-function oxidase enzyme system and reductions in the glutathione content of the maturing hepatocyte.

Substance Abuse

Although most illicit drugs are known to affect the central nervous and cardiovascular systems, the liver also can be damaged. Fatal hepatic necrosis in cocaine abuse has been reported, with a pattern of periportal necrosis identical to that seen in rodent models. Ischemic hepatic damage has been observed with "Ecstasy" (methylenedioxyamphetamine). Hepatic enzyme levels are often increased in heroin users, but this may be related to the fact that many of these individuals show evidence of hepatitis B and/or exposure to human immunodeficiency virus (HIV). Contaminants, such as talc or mannose in the diluent used to inject drugs intravenously, may cause a granulomatous hepatitis. Inhalation of halogenated hydrocarbons (carbona, carbon tetrachloride) and sniffing of airplane glue (toluene) have been associated with centrilobular necrosis that can lead to severe liver damage, hepatic coma, and even death.

Alcohol use and abuse is common among many adolescents. Ethanol is metabolized by the liver through a primary pathway that converts alcohol to acetaldehyde. This process causes an impairment of triglyceride secretion from the hepatocyte, which can cause development of a fatty liver even in the well-nourished adolescent. Other early changes associated with alcohol use may include enlargement of hepatocytes, which can lead to hepatomegaly and induction of microsomal enzymes. This change is manifested by an elevated γ-glutamyltransferase level and mild increases in aminotransferase levels. The induction of the microsomal system also may interfere with the metabolic activity of other illicit drugs, resulting in potentiation of the effects of those drugs when combined with alcohol. More chronic or severe alcohol use can lead to alcoholic hepatitis and cirrhosis, which, fortunately, are exceedingly uncommon in adolescents. Alcoholic hepatitis, which develops in about 20% of chronic alcoholics, is associated with a high mortality rate. Alcoholic hepatitis is the intermediate step for about 75% of those who develop cirrhosis, although some alcoholics develop cirrhosis without ever manifesting overt hepatitis. The mechanisms for development of alcoholic hepatitis are still unknown.

Anabolic Steroids and Oral Contraceptives

The extremely competitive aura surrounding high school and college sports, and a desire on the part of many adolescents to enhance their appearance, have fostered the abuse of anabolic steroids as a way of markedly increasing muscle mass. If such abuse occurs during the pubertal growth phase, premature closure of the epiphysis and ultimate shorter stature (than without steroid use) are likely. In addition, 17α-alkyl androgens—the oral form of anabolic steroids—are hepatotoxic, causing a cholestatic hepatitis in 2% to 3% of adolescents who ingest these agents. Adolescent girls who take oral contraceptives are at a slight risk (<0.01%) of developing cholestatic hepatopathy. In both cases the abnormality is canalicular rather than parenchymal, resulting in elevations of alkaline phosphatase and bilirubin levels that are greater than the elevations in transaminase levels. Patients who abuse anabolic steroids for prolonged periods also may develop hepatic adenocarcinoma later in life.

Miscellaneous Drugs

Cyproheptadine (Periactin) is used as an appetite stimulant in thin or growth-retarded children and adolescents. Prolonged cholestasis has been reported with the use of this agent. Even after the clinical signs and symptoms of cholestatic hepatitis have disappeared in such cases, elevated levels of alkaline phosphatase and γ-glutamyltransferase may remain for up to 3 years, and liver biopsy reveals progressive portal fibrosis and decreased numbers of interlobular bile ducts. Similar findings have been reported with the use of certain psychotropic drugs, such as chlorpromazine and imipramine. Like these medications, cyproheptadine has a tricyclic ring, and that structure may be involved in the hepatotoxicity of these agents. The potential hepatic damage is important in light of the recently noted tendency toward prescription of cyproheptadine, tricyclic antidepressants, and other psychotropic drugs for adolescents with psychiatric disorders.

ACUTE HEPATITIS

In the last few years a great deal of knowledge has been gained about the viruses that cause hepatitis. There are at least five such viruses, causing hepatitis A, B, C, D, and E. These are distinguished from other viruses that cause hepatic inflammation (e.g., Epstein-Barr virus, herpesvirus, and cytomegalovirus) by the fact that in general they cause hepatitis itself rather than a wider clinical illness that may include hepatitis. The relative prevalence of hepatitis caused by these five agents in U.S. adults is as follows: hepatitis B, 50%; hepatitis A, 30%; and hepatitis C, 20%. Hepatitis D viral infection, which occurs only in conjunction with hepatitis B infection, is very infrequent in the United States; hepatitis E has been found only in Americans who have traveled to endemic areas. Although the prevalence rate of acute hepatitis in adolescents has not been studied, it is believed to be close to adult levels. Details of the clinical features of the hepatitis viruses are presented in Table 47-1 and described in the sections that follow.

Hepatitis A Virus

The incidence of infection with hepatitis A virus (HAV), a RNA picornavirus, has been declining steadily in the last 20 years as sanitary conditions have improved. However, the exact incidence is difficult to determine, since so many cases are subclinical or anicteric and therefore are not reported. It has been estimated that 30% of the adult U.S. population show serologic evidence of previous HAV infection. The transmission of HAV is almost always by the fecal-oral route; very infrequently, transmission can occur percutaneously. The incubation period of the virus is about 25 days.

DIAGNOSIS AND CLINICAL FEATURES. The diagnosis of HAV infection is made on serologic grounds. Liver

TABLE 47-1
Features of the Hepatotrophic Viruses

	HAV	HBV	HCV
Incubation	2-6 wk	1-6 mo	2 wk-6 mo
Transmission	Fecal/oral	Blood/sexual	Sporadic
	?Blood/sexual	Perinatal	Blood/sexual
			Perinatal
Diagnosis			
Acute	Anti-HAVIgM	HBsAg	Clinical
		Anti-HBc (IgM)	
Chronic	N/A	HBsAg	HCVAg
		Anti-HBc (total)	PCR (HCV RNA)
Sequelae			
Fulminant	0.1%	<5%	<5%
Carrier	No	Yes	Yes
Chronic	No	Yes	Yes

HAV, hepatitis A virus; *HBV,* hepatitis B virus; *HCV,* hepatitis C virus; *PCR,* polymerase chain reaction.

biopsy is rarely indicated. The diagnosis is based on an immunoglobulin M (IgM) antibody that is first seen at the onset of clinical symptoms (about 5 weeks after exposure) and is evidence of acute infection. This antibody remains positive for 4 to 12 months. The anti-HAV antibody develops at the end of the infection and remains positive for many years; it is evidence of previous HAV infection.

Symptoms of HAV are increasingly apparent in accordance with the age of the host. Eighty-five percent of children under 2 years of age who are infected with hepatitis A are asymptomatic (or have a viral upper respiratory illness), as are 50% of 2- to 4-year-olds with the disease. Adolescents are usually symptomatic, with 75% to 97% of infected patients ill and 40% to 70% icteric. The symptoms of nausea, vomiting, malaise, anorexia, and cholestatic jaundice with pruritus (bilirubin >10 mg/ml) can be severe. However, almost all individuals with HAV infection, regardless of age, will recover. Fulminant hepatitis A is very rare, and chronic hepatitis A does not seem to occur.

TREATMENT AND PREVENTION. Because of the usually benign clinical course of acute hepatitis A, no therapy is indicated. However, immune serum globulin given before exposure or during the incubation period of HAV is protective against the clinical illness. Close personal contacts and household members of patients with acute hepatitis A should receive immune serum globulin (2 ml intramuscularly) within 2 to 4 weeks of exposure. Treatment of casual contacts, such as schoolmates, is not indicated. Travelers unexposed to HAV who visit developing countries where hepatitis A is prevalent should receive the same dose of immune serum globulin 2 weeks before they travel.

A vaccine against HAV is available. It can be given with immune serum globulin for postexposure prophylaxis (use at separate sites). It is unclear who should receive the vaccine. Certainly, high-risk groups such as frequent travelers and day care workers should consider getting vaccinated. Universal childhood HAV vaccination needs further considerations.

Hepatitis B Virus

Hepatitis B virus (HBV) is a DNA hepadnavirus that is most often transmitted parenterally and through sexual contact. The virus has an incubation period of about 45 to 75 days. The disease has a very high prevalence rate in the Orient, Southeast Asia, and the Pacific Rim (including the Eskimo population of Alaska). The large number of people from these areas who become immigrants to the United States should make physicians aware of the possible consequences of hepatitis B (e.g., in adults, cirrhosis and hepatocarcinoma; in infants, risk of perinatal exposure through an HBsAg-positive mother).

DIAGNOSIS AND CLINICAL FEATURES. The HBV consists of an inner core (containing HBcAg, HBeAg, and DNA polymerase) and an outer surface shell (containing HBsAg). These antigenic markers have provided a serologic pattern to the diagnosis and various forms of the disease (Table 47-2). Routine screening for hepatitis B requires at least two serologic markers for maximal certainty. Hepatitis B surface antigen (HBsAg), is found in almost all patients who acquire the infection, and its rise coincides closely with the onset of symptoms. However, the surface antigen usually diminishes before the symptoms are gone, so that a second marker, hepatitis B core antibody (anti-Hbc) is usually needed to confirm the diagnosis. Although the hepatitis B e antigen (HBeAg) is not necessary for the diagnosis, it is an important marker, indicating viral infectivity in the patient.

More patients with hepatitis B are symptomatic than are those with hepatitis A. The asymptomatic patients tend to be infants and children, while adolescents

TABLE 47-2
Hepatitis B Virus: Serologic Findings

Marker	Immunized	Acute	Recovered	Chronic
HBsAg	−	+	−	+
Anti-HBs	+	−	+	−
Anti-HBc	−	+	+	+
eAg	−	+	−	±
Anti-e	−	−	+	−

commonly have clinically evident disease with symptoms of fever, malaise, anorexia, nausea, and vomiting. Twenty-five percent of adolescents with acute hepatitis B are icteric. In up to 10% of cases, extrahepatic (immune complex) symptoms predominate. A common presentation is a serum sickness–like illness with urticaria, arthritis (small joints), angioedema, and a maculopapular rash. Other presentations include nephritis, nephrosis, myocarditis, and pancreatitis. Children may present with Gianotti-Crosti syndrome (papular acrodermatitis), an entity consisting of nonpruritic papules on the face, extremities, and buttocks associated with lymphadenopathy and anicteric hepatitis.

Fulminant, life-threatening hepatitis, although rare, can occur with hepatitis B. An asymptomatic carrier state (HBsAg positive, anti-HBs negative for more than 6 months) occurs in less than 0.1% of Caucasian Americans but in 10% to 15% of Asians and Eskimos. Carriers (especially males) are at risk of developing cirrhosis and hepatocarcinoma, making hepatitis B an enormous worldwide epidemiologic problem. The chronic active form of hepatitis B also can result in cirrhosis and hepatocarcinoma.

TREATMENT AND PREVENTION. The prevention of hepatitis B is critical because of the high incidence of chronic hepatitis and the chronic carrier state with its subsequent risks. More than 90% of infants who acquire the infection perinatally become chronic carriers, as do 10% to 50% of adolescents.

Prevention can be accomplished by two approaches, the most important of which is hepatitis B vaccine. A recombinant DNA–synthesized vaccine has been produced that induces an antibody response to HBsAg. Certainly, all neonates of HBsAg-positive mothers, intimate contacts of patients with acute or chronic hepatitis B, and those with needlestick exposure to HBsAg-positive blood should receive the vaccine. In addition, these groups should receive hepatitis B immunoglobulin for its synergistic effect with hepatitis B vaccine. The HBV vaccine should be incorporated into the current childhood immunization schedule of all neonates and should probably be given to all adolescents. The safety of the recombinant vaccine and its potential for

preventing this serious disease make it imperative for healthcare workers and others at risk to receive the vaccine before exposure may occur. There is no specific treatment for acute hepatitis B. If the infection becomes fulminant, liver transplantation is now considered a therapeutic option. Treatment of chronic active hepatitis B with interferon alfa is becoming more commonplace, but the appropriate dosage and duration of therapy are still unclear.

Hepatitis C Virus

In the United States most non-A, non-B hepatitis (about 85%) is caused by hepatitis C virus (HCV). Hepatitis C is an RNA flavivirus transmitted primarily by parenteral exposure. The most important risk factors are use of intravenous drugs, transfusions, occupational exposure, and sexual exposure. Adolescents are therefore at risk of developing hepatitis C infection, although the prevalence rate in this age group has not yet been determined. It is believed that the peak incidence of hepatitis C occurs between 15 and 36 years of age. About 0.5% to 1% of U.S. adults show evidence of previous hepatitis C infection. Another non-A, non-B hepatitis that has been described is hepatitis E. This RNA virus is transmitted enterally through epidemics in parts of the world where sanitary conditions are poor. In contrast to hepatitis C, hepatitis E is not a significant problem in the United States.

DIAGNOSIS AND CLINICAL FEATURES. The current diagnosis of hepatitis C infection is made by detection of an anti-HCV antibody, which in most laboratories is obtained by the enzyme-linked immunosorbent assay (ELISA) test. Unfortunately, in middle-class populations, there is a very high false-positive rate with this method. If a patient shows a positive antibody titer by ELISA, confirmation should be made by either a radioimmune blot assay or a polymerase chain reaction, which tests for infectivity in addition to antibody production. Other sources of false-positive HCV antibody test results are elevated serum immunoglobulin levels, active autoimmune chronic active hepatitis, and positive rheumatoid factor. False-negative tests can occur with immunodeficient conditions. Anti-HCV antibody is not protective. It can be positive while the virus is present.

Fifty to seventy percent of patients with hepatitis C develop chronic hepatitis. This is usually manifested by a fluctuating pattern of aminotransferase elevation, which occurs in approximately 80% of chronic cases. Most patients with chronic disease have a pattern of chronic active (aggressive) hepatitis, and 50% of them develop cirrhosis within 5 to 10 years. Primary hepatocellular carcinoma has been associated with chronic hepatitis C and cirrhosis.

TREATMENT AND PREVENTION. At present there is no evidence that immunoglobulin is effective in preventing hepatitis C, and there is no vaccine currently in general use. Antiviral therapy (interferon) for acute hepatitis C is still experimental and its use controversial. However, the use of interferon alfa in patients with chronic active hepatitis C has been associated with improvement in approximately 50% of cases, although relapse is common after treatment has been discontinued. Current studies seem to indicate that very-long-term or recurrent treatment may be necessary and will prove to be of greater benefit.

CHRONIC HEPATITIS

Chronic hepatitis is defined as an inflammatory reaction of the liver that continues for at least 6 months without improvement. This definition has been used to avoid mislabeling protracted cases of acute hepatitis, which may show evidence of biochemical and histologic aggressiveness for several months and then remit completely. The two types of chronic hepatitis found in the adolescent age group are chronic persistent hepatitis (CPH) and chronic active hepatitis (CAH).

Chronic Persistent Hepatitis

CPH is a benign form of hepatitis. It is most often associated with a bout of acute viral hepatitis, and its early manifestations are indistinguishable from that entity. However, for reasons that are still unclear, but probably related to the interaction of host immunity factors and the etiologic agent, the acute hepatitis does not clear, and biochemical and histologic abnormalities continue. Persistence of the virus alone does not appear to explain the CPH. CPH has also been seen in association with chronic ulcerative colitis, Crohn's disease, and infections with *Entamoeba histolytica* or *Salmonella* organisms.

CLINICAL ASPECTS. The adolescent with CPH may be asymptomatic or may complain of fatigue, poor appetite, pain in the right upper quadrant, or intolerance of fatty foods. This picture may be seen after a bout of acute viral hepatitis or without an apparent antecedent illness.

Physical examination results may be normal or there may be mild hepatomegaly. Signs of chronic liver disease, such as splenomegaly, cutaneous vascular spiders, palmar erythema, and clubbing of the nails, are absent.

Serum aminotransferase levels are elevated, reaching two to four times normal levels, and may remain elevated for many years. Serum alkaline phosphatase levels are normal, and the bilirubin level is either normal or minimally elevated. The serum immunoglobulin G (IgG) level is normal or just slightly increased. This is an important distinction from CAH. Occasionally, a patient with CPH will have a positive autoimmune marker, such as antinuclear antibodies, smooth muscle antibodies, or antimitochondrial antibodies, but these do not occur in as clear a pattern as in CAH.

DIAGNOSIS. The diagnosis of CPH is confirmed by a needle biopsy of the liver, which should be performed after abnormal liver function tests have persisted for at least 6 months. On biopsy, CPH is noted by expansion of the portal area by mononuclear cells with minimal fibrosis. The limiting plate between the portal area and the lobule is intact, and piecemeal (individual) necrosis of hepatocytes is not seen.

PROGNOSIS AND TREATMENT. Confirmation of CPH through liver biopsy is most helpful in allowing the physician to reassure the patient and family that therapy is not indicated and that the prognosis is excellent. The adolescent should be placed on a normal diet and allowed regular activities as tolerated.

In a review of 99 patients with CPH of various etiologies followed up for an average of 7 years, none of the patients showed evidence of chronic liver disease or cirrhosis. Very rarely, patients initially diagnosed as having CPH may show histologic progression to very mild CAH. These patients are most often HBsAg positive and frequently HBeAg positive.

Chronic Active Hepatitis

CAH is often referred to as chronic aggressive hepatitis. Both are apt terms for a continuing inflammatory process of the liver that often progresses to severe, irreversible destruction (cirrhosis) and death. CAH has been associated with several etiologic agents, the most common being hepatitis C and hepatitis B infections. Autoimmune hepatitis is also seen relatively frequently in the adolescent population. Hepatitis D (delta) hepatitis also can evolve into CAH. In the immunosuppressed teenager, other viral agents, such as cytomegalovirus, rubella, and Epstein-Barr virus, have been implicated in CAH. The same histologic and clinical picture of CAH has been described with isoniazid and methyldopa, as well as in Wilson's disease and α_1-antitrypsin deficiency.

The mechanisms involved in the evolution and continuation of CAH have not been totally clarified. The appearance of hepatic plasma cell infiltrates, hypergammaglobulinemia, and multiple immunogenic disturbances in patients with CAH, and the favorable response to anti-inflammatory and immunosuppressive medications in some forms of the disease, suggest that immunologic factors are involved. It is assumed that various insults to the hepatocytes can create an antigenicity of the cells that may lead to a self-perpetuating antigen-antibody process with subsequent chronic damage. Cell-mediated immune reactions to liver cell antigens occur, and they involve sensitized lymphocytes and mononuclear cells. In vitro assays have shown that peripheral lymphocytes from patients with CAH can destroy hepatocytes, and it is still unclear whether this is a primary or secondary event.

Autoimmune hepatitis. Autoimmune hepatitis (AH) (the new nomenclature for autoimmune CAH) is a disease most frequently seen in adolescent and young adult females. It was first described in 1950 as an adolescent liver disease associated with acne, amenorrhea, and hyperglobulinemia. The disease has also been called lupoid hepatitis, plasma cell hepatitis, active juvenile cirrhosis, and HBsAg-negative CAH.

Clinical features. The initial clinical presentation of AH is variable but usually falls into one of three forms: (1) prolonged typical attacks of presumed acute viral hepatitis, (2) insidious onset of malaise with or without jaundice, and (3) a finding of hepatosplenomegaly on routine physical examination. It is likely that the AH may have been present for months or years before the diagnosis is made in many patients. Amenorrhea is almost universal and should alert the physician to the possibility of chronic liver disease. Girls who are intrapubertal experience arrest of sexual development and may remain at Tanner stage 2 or 3 for a protracted time with primary amenorrhea. Girls who have reached menarche invariably develop secondary amenorrhea. The relationship between activity of liver disease and menses is so strong that physicians may use the return of menstrual flow as a marker of disease remission, especially during treatment.

Physical examination usually reveals a healthy-looking adolescent of normal size. Cutaneous vascular spiders, palmar erythema, acne, and striae may be apparent. Abdominal examination usually shows a very firm, nontender liver below the right costal margin. If the disease has progressed to cirrhosis, however, the liver may not be palpable at all. The spleen is frequently very enlarged. This splenomegaly may be secondary to reticuloendothelial hyperplasia, and the spleen may shrink with therapy, or the condition may be the result of cirrhosis and portal hypertension, and therefore will persist.

Extrahepatic manifestations. Extrahepatic manifestations of this systemic autoimmune disease are common. Several of these are nonspecific, including fever; urticaria; erythema nodosum; generalized lymphadenopathy; and recurrent, nondeforming, migrating polyarthritis of the large joints. Specific extrahepatic disorders associated with AH include renal diseases such as nephritis, nephrosis, and renal tubular acidosis; pulmonary diseases such as pneumonitis and fibrosing alveolitis; a large variety of endocrinopathies; inflammatory bowel disease; and Coombs' test–positive hemolytic anemia. These extrahepatic disorders may precede the clinical onset of AH, or they may appear during the course of the liver disease.

Laboratory findings. Serum aminotransferase (transaminase) levels are often elevated to five to 10 times the normal value. Bilirubin levels are often 2 to 10 mg/ml, although values may be normal. The serum albumin level is usually in the low-normal range at the time of diagnosis, indicating that hepatic synthetic function has been preserved. Similarly, prothrombin and partial thromboplastin times should be normal. However, a patient occasionally presents with abnormal prothrombin and thromboplastin values; in such cases the ability to synthesize coagulation factors is usually normal, but an autoimmune circulating anticoagulant is present.

Serum globulin levels are markedly increased in AH. Serum IgG levels are almost always greater than 2000 mg/ml and most often range between 2500 and 4500 mg/ml. The erythrocyte sedimentation rate is usually elevated. Most patients have markedly elevated titers of anti–smooth muscle antibody (SMA). A type 2 AH has been described (rare in North America) characterized by the presence of anti–liver/kidney microsomal antibodies rather than SMA. Patients with type 2 AH are usually younger and have a more fulminant course than those with type 1 AH (SMA positive).

Diagnosis. The diagnosis of autoimmune hepatitis is made by liver biopsy. This procedure is indicated in the presence of prolonged abnormalities of liver function, elevated IgG levels, and positive SMA titers. The hepatic histology in this disorder is marked by the presence of an inflammatory infiltrate, usually made up of plasma cells and lymphocytes, that markedly expands the portal area. This inflammatory infiltrate extends beyond the portal area and erodes the limiting plate of the hepatocytes, causing individual hepatocellular, or piecemeal, necrosis. If the cellular necrosis is more advanced, areas of necrosis are replaced by fibrosis, and "bridging" of fibrous connective tissue may be seen from portal area to portal area, or from portal area to central vein.

In view of the favorable response to medical therapy for this disease, it seems reasonable to evaluate any adolescent for AH if (1) acute hepatitis is apparent or liver function test results are abnormal, (2) serologic test results for infectious agents are negative, and (3) α_1-antitrypsin deficiency and Wilson's disease have been ruled out. In these cases, if the IgG level is elevated and the SMA positive, a liver biopsy should be performed so that therapy can be initiated if a consistent histologic appearance is noted.

Treatment and prognosis. The drugs of choice for treatment of AH are prednisone (1 to 2 mg/kg/day), azathioprine (1 to 1.5 mg/kg/day), or its metabolite, 6-mercaptopurine (1 to 1.5 mg/kg/day). Treatment often induces biochemical, immunologic, and histologic improvement or remission, and there is no doubt that appropriate use of these agents can increase 10-year survival rates, even if cirrhosis develops.

Many centers begin therapy with prednisone and continue the initial dose until a biochemical and immunologic remission is achieved. Prednisone is then tapered to a dose of less than 20 mg/day. 6-Mercaptopurine is then added and used as a prednisone-sparing agent, allowing a lowering of the prednisone dose to 10 mg every other day. This dose is low enough to avoid the growth-retarding and cosmetic problems associated with steroid use that are so upsetting to adolescents. Daily administration of 6-mercaptopurine and alternate-day use of steroids are continued for 2 years, at which time they are discontinued if liver function tests, serum IgG levels, and SMA are close to or at normal levels. Experience suggests that most patients will need reinstitution of alternate-day steroids to maintain remission or stabilization of the disease.

Many adolescents with AH present with or progress to cirrhosis despite a good biochemical response to therapy. Even with cirrhosis, long-term survival is very likely and a good quality of life possible.

HBsAg-positive chronic active hepatitis. Although most patients with a hepatitis B virus infection have a complete recovery, 5% to 10% either become chronic carriers or develop CPH or CAH. Infections that progress to HBsAg-positive CAH seem to be dependent on the host's immune status and the ability of the HBV to continue replicating in the liver. It is possible that patients who contract HBV infection and have an impaired cell-mediated immune response will fail to clear the virus, and continued hepatocellular necrosis may ensue. It has also been noted in some patients that association of the delta agent (delta hepatitis) with HBV may increase the risk of development of chronic liver disease.

Clinical features. HBsAg-positive CAH occurs predominantly in males 15 to 50 years of age, most commonly in intravenous drug abusers and/or homosexuals. In most cases CAH is not preceded by an obvious case of acute hepatitis B. However, in some patients a mild acute hepatitis may progress to chronicity, or the patient may have CAH at the apparent onset of the acute illness. It is interesting that patients who develop severe hepatitis B infection or survive an attack of fulminant viral hepatitis rarely develop chronic progressive disease. The condition may be recognized as unresolved acute viral hepatitis by prolonged elevation of the aminotransferase levels or by variable jaundice. The patient may be totally asymptomatic. However, most patients with HBsAg-positive CAH show signs of chronic liver disease, such as ascites, vascular spiders, and splenomegaly.

Laboratory data. The aminotransferase and bilirubin levels are mildly elevated in patients with HBsAg-positive CAH. The IgG level is only moderately increased compared with the levels seen in autoimmune hepatitis. Likewise, SMA titers are normal or minimally elevated.

HBsAg is present in the blood, and the antigen and anti-HBc antibody also may be present. The diagnosis is made by the presence of HBsAg and a liver biopsy consistent with CAH. The biopsy picture is similar to that of AH, except that HBsAg may be demonstrated as hepatic cells having a "ground glass" appearance on orcein staining of the tissues.

Treatment and prognosis. The therapeutic approach to HBsAg-positive CAH is very controversial. Corticosteroid therapy may improve liver function and diminish the levels of HBV markers, but the treatment may increase viral replication and unfavorably affect the relapse and death rate. Recombinant interferon alfa may have therapeutic potential in the patient with chronic hepatitis B infection. This medication seems to be associated with loss of hepatitis B DNA, seroconversion, and biochemical and histologic improvement in about one third of patients. This approach needs further evaluation.

In most patients who do not respond to therapeutic interventions, the progression of the disease is slow and insidious. Patients with HBsAg-positive CAH may spontaneously go into remission, unlike patients with AH, who have a very high mortality rate in the first 2 years of disease if therapy has not been instituted. However, many patients with CAH that is associated with HBV will slowly progress to cirrhosis and hepatic decompensation. A recent study has suggested that a poor prognosis may depend on the presence of e antigen. In addition, patients with HBsAg-positive CAH are at risk of developing primary hepatocarcinoma.

OTHER LIVER DISORDERS

Gilbert's Syndrome

Gilbert's syndrome is a common form of mild unconjugated hyperbilirubinemia. It is often first noticed or diagnosed in the adolescent because the jaundice may be noted during stress, illness, fasting, or menstrual periods. The serum bilirubin levels are usually less than 3 mg/dl but occasionally may increase to as high as 7 to 8 mg/dl. The diagnosis is predicated on a mild, fluctuating indirect hyperbilirubinemia in the presence of normal liver function test results and absence of hemolysis.

Hepatic glucuronosyltransferase activity is diminished and there is an increased amount of monoglucuronides in the bile. These abnormalities are also seen in the neonate during the first few days of life and in patients with Crigler-Najjar syndrome (i.e., total absence of glucuronosyltransferase leading to kernicterus). Serum bilirubin levels in Gilbert's syndrome decrease with phenobarbital treatment. However, the benign nature of this entity makes therapy superfluous.

Wilson's Disease

Wilson's disease (hepatolenticular degeneration) is a rare autosomal recessive disorder of copper metabolism first described in 1912 and considered to be a degenerative disorder of the central nervous system associated with cirrhosis. The clinical symptoms are related to excessive accumulation of copper in the liver, central nervous system, kidneys, cornea, skeletal system, and other organs. The reversal of abnormal copper metabolism in patients who receive liver transplantation strongly suggests that the primary defect for this disease is located in the liver. The abnormal gene responsible for this entity has recently been mapped and is located on chromosome 13. The precise biochemical defect responsible for Wilson's disease is unknown, but it is clear that biliary excretion of absorbed copper is inadequate. Although the accumulation of copper in tissues begins in infancy, clinical disease rarely appears before age 6 years and more often in early adolescence. About 50% of patients develop symptoms by age 15 years.

CLINICAL MANIFESTATIONS. Most of the clinical manifestations of Wilson's disease are related directly to copper deposition in specific organs. Most patients present with liver disease, but neuropsychiatric findings are common, especially in the adolescent age group.

HEPATIC SYMPTOMS. The hepatic symptoms, which usually appear first, can be nonspecific, mimicking a variety of acute and chronic liver diseases. In the early asymptomatic phase, or in the presence of inactive cirrhosis, liver function test results may be normal, or serum aminotransferase levels may be only minimally elevated. Wilson's disease may present with clinical, biochemical, and histologic features of CAH, again more commonly in the adolescent. It is certainly mandatory that Wilson's disease be considered and evaluated in any adolescent with chronic liver disease. Occasionally, Wilson's disease presents as fulminant hepatic failure, which is indistinguishable from massive hepatic necrosis and is usually rapidly fatal unless a liver transplantation can be performed.

NEUROPSYCHIATRIC BEHAVIOR. Adolescent patients with Wilson's disease commonly show behavioral changes that are aggressive in nature or a psychotic disorder such as manic-depression or schizophrenia. An organic dementia also can be seen in teenagers with this disorder. The neurologic symptoms are subtle early in the course of the disease, but they progress if treatment is not begun. Lack of coordination and parkinsonian symptoms (e.g., tremors and masklike facies) are most commonly seen.

MISCELLANEOUS EFFECTS. Kayser-Fleischer rings (golden discoloration in the limbic region of the cornea) consist of granules of copper and are usually seen in patients with Wilson's disease. Acute, Coombs' test–negative hemolysis is the presenting symptom of Wilson's disease in up to 15% of patients. The hemolysis is believed to be secondary to an oxidative injury to red blood cell membranes from excess copper. This hemolysis is usually transient and self-limiting. Renal tubular dysfunction, presenting as aminoaciduria, glycosuria, uricosuria, hyperphosphaturia, and hypercalciuria, commonly may be seen. The loss of calcium and phosphate may lead to bony demineralization. D-Penicillamine, the primary mode of therapy, also can cause renal damage. Recently, cardiac dysfunction has been recognized in Wilson's disease as a consequence of copper deposition in the myocardium, and it may present with arrhythmias, cardiomyopathy, and/or autonomic dysfunction.

DIAGNOSIS AND THERAPY. The diagnosis of Wilson's disease is easy when the classic triad of hepatic disease, neuropsychiatric involvement, and Kayser-Fleischer rings is seen. However, in the absence of this triad, the clinician must have a high index of suspicion to make the diagnosis so that therapy can be instituted immediately. No single test is diagnostic and the work-up may be frustrating. The serum ceruloplasmin level may be normal in 10% to 20% of homozygotes for Wilson's disease and may be low in 10% of heterozygotes who do not have the disease. A slit-lamp examination for Kayser-Fleischer rings is mandatory, but the rings may not always be present. The urinary copper level, which is usually very high (>100 μg/24 hours) in this disorder, is probably the best screening test in association with a slit-lamp examination. If the diagnosis is still unclear, a liver biopsy should be performed for a histologic study and for hepatic copper levels. Once the diagnosis has been made, the patient should be treated with D-penicillamine (a copper chelator). The usual adolescent dose is 250 mg administered orally four times a day. Usually there is impressive improvement in symptoms within several weeks. Patients should also receive pyridoxine three times a week to counteract the potential antipyridoxine effects of the chelator. In patients who have very serious side effects from penicillamine, an alternative chelating agent, trientine, has proved effective. The key to a successful outcome with either medication is early diagnosis, continuous maintenance of therapy, and a compliant patient.

Uncommon Liver Disorders

Homozygous α_1-antitrypsin deficiency is an autosomal recessive disorder associated with neonatal cholestasis and childhood liver disease and/or early adult-onset emphysema. The adolescent usually is not symptomatically affected by either the liver or the lung problems, although liver or pulmonary function test results may be abnormal. This diagnosis should be considered in any adolescent who shows biochemical or clinical evidence of chronic liver disease.

An adolescent with no history of liver disease and/or with normal liver function test results who presents with hematemesis secondary to bleeding esophageal varices may have had silent hepatobiliary disease for many years. Cystic fibrosis, which can cause biliary cirrhosis, may be noted with signs of portal hypertension but without evidence of liver disease. Other diseases that may manifest portal hypertension in the adolescent include congenital hepatic fibrosis/polycystic kidney disease, a heritable condition that can cause massive portal tract fibrosis with or without hepatocellular damage; and nodular regenerative hyperplasia, a noncirrhotic disease with regenerative nodules in the hepatic architecture. This entity may be an early manifestation of a collagen vascular disease.

PANCREATIC DISEASE

Diseases of the exocrine pancreas are relatively uncommon in adolescents. Many of the pediatric diseases that affect the pancreas are the result of inborn errors of metabolism: for example, cystic fibrosis, Shwachman-Diamond syndrome, and exocrine enzyme deficiencies, which are almost always diagnosed and first treated before the patient reaches adolescence. In patients with cystic fibrosis (see Chapter 42, "Cystic Fibrosis"), the pancreatic problems stabilize in adolescence, but the hepatobiliary and pulmonary problems usually worsen. In Shwachman-Diamond syndrome, which is characterized by pancreatic insufficiency, cyclic neutropenia, and growth retardation, the steatorrhea improves when the patient reaches adolescence. Pancreatitis can affect the patient during adolescence, but its effects are more significant in adulthood, when alcohol abuse and hepatobiliary disease, especially cholelithiasis or choledocholithiasis, play an important role. Most adolescents with pancreatitis develop the entity secondary to viral infections (e.g., mumps, Epstein-Barr virus, coxsackie B4), trauma, or alcohol abuse. Other less common etiologies include hyperlipidemias, biliary tract obstructions, and drugs (e.g., steroids, 6-mercaptopurine, sulfasalazine, thiazides). Signs and symptoms of acute pancreatitis include abdominal pain and tenderness as well as fever and vomiting. A large amount of fluid may be lost from the vascular compartment. Laboratory evaluation usually reveals elevated serum amylase and lipase levels as well as an increased amylase clearance. Treatment is directed at relief of pain and reduction of exocrine pancreatic secretion (nothing by mouth, nasogastric drainage, intravenous hydration), as well as correction of fluid and electrolyte abnormalities. Acute pancreatitis may cause the development of a pseudocyst or a pancreatic abscess, or may lead to chronic pancreatitis or pancreatic insufficiency.

Suggested Readings

Aggett PJ, Cavanaugh PC, Matthew DJ, et al: Shwachman's syndrome: a review of 21 cases, *Arch Dis Child* 55:331-338, 1980.

Aiges HW: Chronic hepatitis, *Pediatr Ann* 6:439-445, 1985.

Alter MJ, Mast EE: The epidemiology of viral hepatitis in the United States, *Gastroenterol Clin North Am* 23:437-455, 1994.

Ballistreri WF: Viral hepatitis, *Pediatr Clin North Am* 35:637-669, 1988.

Biscelgie AM: Interferon therapy for chronic viral hepatitis, *N Engl J Med* 330:137-138, 1994.

Bortolotti F, Cadrobbi P, Crivellaro C, et al: Long term outcome of chronic hepatitis B in patients who acquire hepatitis B infection in childhood, *Gastroenterology* 99:805-810, 1990.

Bortolotti F, Calzia R, Vegnente A, et al: Chronic hepatitis in childhood: the spectrum of the disease, *Gut* 29:659-664, 1988.

Johnson PJ, McFarlane IG: Meeting Report: International Autoimmune Hepatitis Group, *Hepatology* 18:998-1005, 1993.

Jordan SC, Ament ME: Pancreatitis in children and adolescents, *J Pediatr* 91:211-220, 1977.

Lai CL, Lok ASF, Lin HJ, et al: Placebo-controlled trial of recombinant alpha-interferon in Chinese HBsAg carrier children, *Lancet* 2:877-880, 1987.

Lee WM: Drug-induced hepatotoxicity, *N Engl J Med* 333:1118-1127, 1995.

Maddrey WC, Zimmerman HJ: Toxic and drug-induced hepatitis. In Schiff L, Schiff ER, editors: *Diseases of the liver*, ed 6, Philadelphia, 1987, JB Lippincott; p 591.

Werlin SL, Grand RJ, Perman JA, Watkins JB: Diagnostic dilemmas of Wilson's disease: diagnosis and treatment, *Pediatrics* 62:47-51, 1978.

SECTION 6

Hematology and Oncology

CHAPTER 48

Anemia

•

Mark E. Weinblatt

Anemia, the most common hematologic abnormality of adolescence, is best characterized as reduced concentration of circulating hemoglobin. Since the primary function of red blood cells (RBCs) is to transport and release oxygen, any reduction in this capacity may in turn result in varying degrees of tissue hypoxia, the extent of which may be related to the level of anemia, the rapidity of onset, the underlying pathogenesis, and other associated conditions. It is important to remember that anemia is not only a diagnosis in its own right but often a consequence of an underlying condition that requires explanation.

As with most diseases, there is no substitute for a detailed history and a careful physical examination, both of which often yield sufficient clues to rapidly identify the underlying process (Table 48-1). However, although the presenting signs and symptoms vary, several findings can be attributed directly to the degree of anemia and the compensatory mechanisms that are called upon to satisfy the body's needs for oxygen delivery rather than to the primary disorder. Shunting of blood from nonvital structures, most notably the skin and subcutaneous tissues, directs more oxygen to the heart, brain, and muscles, resulting in the pallor found in most patients with anemia. Increased cardiac output, with tachycardia and associated murmurs, is routinely found in moderately severe anemia. With increasing severity of the condition, signs of failure of this cardiac compensation may include dyspnea, cardiomegaly, and ultimately heart failure, pulmonary edema, and respiratory distress.

Any decrease in the normal levels of circulating RBCs can be a consequence of four different pathologic mechanisms: decreased marrow production, ineffective marrow production, decreased RBC life span, and sequestration and lack of availability of RBCs to the general circulation. In many disorders, such as infection, the anemia is a result of more than one of these functional abnormalities. Although a differential diagnosis can be organized into etiologic and pathophysiologic categories, a functional classification that is more effective in narrowing the spectrum of diagnoses is based on the size and degree of hemoglobinization of the cells (Table 48-2). Disorders associated with quantitative or qualitative abnormal hemoglobin production, such as iron deficiency anemia (IDA) or thalassemia, share a hypochromic and microcytic morphology. Conversely, arrest of nuclear maturation, as seen with the megaloblastic anemias, characteristically produces macrocytic erythrocytes. Finally, acquired failure of production, shortened RBC life span due to extrinsic causes, and many intrinsic cell defects that cause hemolysis are usually associated with normal-sized cells. With this type of schema, initial laboratory evaluation should include a complete blood count with RBC indices, an examination of the peripheral blood smear, and a reticulocyte count to evaluate bone marrow response to anemia. Normal range of hemoglobin for younger teenage boys and girls is 12.5 to 15 g/dl and 12 to 14 g/dl, respectively; for older adolescents, normal adult ranges of 14 to 16 g/dl and 12 to 14 g/dl for boys and girls, respectively, should be used for reference. Further testing is contingent on the results of these simple screening tests.

Differences between boys and girls are likely related to the testosterone level, which increases in male adolescents with age and is a well-known potent stimulator of erythrocyte production. In addition, menstrual blood loss plays some role in the decreased hemoglobin levels in girls. Along with the changes in hemoglobin levels, erythrocyte size increases during adolescence, as reflected by a rising mean corpuscular volume (MCV), until adult levels are reached in older adolescents.

TABLE 48-1
Historical and Physical Findings in Adolescents with Anemia

Finding	Diagnosis
Ethnic and Racial Background	
African-American	Sickle cell disease; G6PD deficiency
Northern European	Hereditary spherocytosis
Mediterranean	Thalassemia, sickle cell disease
Family History	
Gallstones, anemia	Spherocytosis, hemoglobinopathies
Transfusion-dependent anemia	Thalassemia, pyruvate kinase deficiency
Infections	
Pharyngitis, adenopathy	EBV infection with hemolytic anemia
Hepatitis	Aplastic anemia
Travel to endemic area, high fevers	Malaria, babesiosis, leishmania
Pneumonia, "macrocytosis"	*Mycoplasma* infection with hemolysis
Opportunistic infections	HIV infection with hemolysis or marrow suppression
Drugs	
Sulfonamide, quinidine	G6PD deficiency
Phenytoin, trimethoprim	Megaloblastic anemia
Chloramphenicol, phenothiazines	Aplastic anemia
Life Style	
Violent or physical sports	Mechanical hemolysis
Drug abuser, homosexual	HIV infection with hemolysis or marrow suppression
Symptoms	
Melena, hematuria	Blood loss
Chronic diarrhea	Malabsorption of vitamin B_{12} or folate, anemia of chronic disease
Diet	
Vegetarian	Iron or folic acid deficiency
Anorexia nervosa	Anemia of chronic disease, nutritional anemia
Physical Findings	
Jaundice, scleral icterus	Hemolytic anemia
Café au lait spots	Fanconi's anemia
Petechia, adenopathy, hepatospleno- megaly	Leukemia
Glossitis	Iron or vitamin B_{12} deficiency
Triphalangeal thumb	Diamond-Blackfan syndrome
Abnormal thumb, radius	Fanconi's anemia
Hypersplenism	Hemolysis or ineffective erythropoiesis
Lower extremity ulcers	Sickle cell disease

EBV, Epstein-Barr virus; *G6PD,* glucose-6-phosphate dehydrogenase.

HYPOCHROMIC MICROCYTIC ANEMIA

Iron Deficiency Anemia

Iron deficiency anemia is a relatively common problem in adolescence, with 2% to 10% of U.S. teenagers affected. Decreased body iron content can vary in severity, ranging from a state of iron depletion (low body stores) to iron deficiency (low storage and serum iron levels) and, finally, to IDA, in which iron levels are too low to fully support the body's needs for synthesis of hemoglobin. Although decreased dietary intake is the most common cause of IDA in young children, iron depletion in adolescents is often due to a combination of chronic blood loss and inadequate intake.

Only about 1 mg of iron is required daily to maintain normal balance because of the body's excellent conservation and reutilization of iron from senescent erythro-

TABLE 48-2
Classification of Common Adolescent Anemias

Microcytic	Macrocytic	Normocytic
Iron deficiency	Folate deficiency	Autoimmune hemolysis
Thalassemia	Vitamin B_{12} deficiency	Sickle cell disease
Sideroblastic anemias	Hypothyroidism	Spherocytosis
Anemia of chronic disease	Liver disease	Unstable hemoglobins
	Diamond-Blackfan syndrome	Acute blood loss
	Fanconi's anemia	G6PD deficiency
	Congenital dyserythropoietic	Pyruvate kinase deficiency
	anemias	Microangiopathic hemolysis
		Acute infections
		Sports anemia
		Hypersplenism
		Myelophthisic anemia
		Chronic renal disease

G6PD, glucose-6-phosphate dehydrogenase.

cytes. Despite this small requirement, most dietary iron exists in a poorly absorbable form (inorganic or bound to iron chelates). Sources rich in available iron include liver and red meats; all vegetables other than legumes are poor sources of this vital mineral. The recommended daily allowance of dietary iron for the adolescent age group, which is undergoing accelerated growth, is 18 mg. The average male successfully takes in 96% of this amount, making the diagnosis of IDA very uncommon among healthy males. Females ingest only about 60% of the required amount. When this precarious iron balance is associated with heavy menstrual bleeding or the increased requirements of pregnancy, the adolescent girl is at particularly high risk for developing IDA.

Blood loss is often unsuspected and inapparent, with the most common primary sources the gastrointestinal, genitourinary, and respiratory tracts. Menstrual bleeding is a very common cause of iron deficiency. Although average losses are approximately 40 ml/cycle,[1] as much as 500 ml/cycle has been reported. Gastrointestinal bleeding commonly accompanies gastritis, inflammatory bowel disease, diverticulitis, peptic ulcers, polyps, esophageal varices, and roundworm infestations. Hematuria from nephritis, sickle cell disease, and nephrolithiasis can range from microscopic to gross hematuria with clots, frequently requiring transfusion. Recurrent or prolonged epistaxis can produce deceptively large amounts of blood loss, particularly if an anatomic abnormality such as an angiofibroma is involved, or if the bleeding originates in the posterior nasopharynx, with most of the blood swallowed. Any bleeding diathesis—congenital or acquired (particularly those caused by medications)—can further exacerbate bleeding from any anatomic site.

The severity of anemia may not correlate with the clinical symptoms. Many patient complaints, such as fatigue, headache, and decreased attention span, precede any significant anemia and are believed to be related to

impaired function of several iron-dependent enzymes. These symptoms, as well as unusual complaints such as pica and pagophagia, rapidly disappear after the initiation of iron therapy, before any improvement in hemoglobin levels is noted. Besides pallor and cardiovascular signs, findings from physical examination may include glossitis and stomatitis, koilonychia, and (rarely) retinal hemorrhages and exudates.

As iron deficiency progresses, characteristic laboratory features appear. The earliest finding is a lack of stainable iron in the bone marrow, which is accompanied by a falling serum ferritin level. Decreasing serum iron levels and rising total iron-binding capacity (TIBC) account for decreased saturation. When iron is no longer available for erythropoiesis, anemia develops, with a decreased MCV, RBC count, mean corpuscular hemoglobin content, and reticulocyte count. The peripheral blood smear shows typical hypochromic microcytic cells; occasionally, target cells or teardrop-shaped cells are found. Thrombocytosis often accompanies IDA and is sometimes pronounced.

Primary considerations in the differential diagnosis of IDA are other hypochromic microcytic anemias, specifically thalassemia minor and the anemia of chronic inflammation. β-Thalassemia, prevalent in the black population and among individuals of Mediterranean background, and α-thalassemia, prevalent among blacks and Southeast Asians, cause similar abnormalities of the MCV and blood smear, but the abnormalities are far out of proportion to the level of anemia. A widely used method of differentiating iron deficiency from thalassemia trait makes use of this finding, with an (MCV) ÷ (red blood cell count) greater than 13.5 suggestive of iron deficiency, and one less than 11.5 more likely to be thalassemia minor. Patients with thalassemia have normal iron, ferritin, and free erythrocyte protoporphyrin levels; anemia, if present, is mild. Hemoglobin electrophoresis typically reveals an elevated hemoglobin A_2 in patients with β-thalassemia trait, while carriers of α-thalassemia have normal electrophoretic patterns, except with a more severe form, hemoglobin H disease. Other hemoglobinopathies seen with increasing frequency, such as hemoglobin E and hemoglobin Lepore, can also be differentiated from IDA on the basis of normal iron stores. Anemia of chronic inflammation may be either microcytic or normocytic. This condition generally carries normal or elevated ferritin levels with a low TIBC. Another erythrocyte parameter, the red cell distribution width (RDW), a quantitative measure of the degree of anisocytosis, has been believed to be helpful in differentiating iron deficiency (in which the RDW is elevated) from thalassemia (normal RDW), but recent studies have cast doubt on the reliability of this test.

Given the frequency of IDA in adolescents, the question arises as to the best screening test to diagnose the disorder. A complete blood count with erythrocyte indices is very effective in detecting the patient with moderate anemia. Subsequent confirmatory testing for body iron stores is best achieved with serum ferritin assay (<10 μg/L); tests for serum iron and TIBC are less reliable and more predisposed to give misleading results. As an alternative to expensive testing, a therapeutic trial of oral iron therapy can be useful in establishing the diagnosis of IDA, with a rise in the reticulocyte count and hemoglobin content expected within 1 to 2 weeks. In patients who have received iron supplementation before confirmatory testing, an elevated level of free erythrocyte protoporphyrin will help differentiate the patient with IDA from one with a hemoglobinopathy, but not from one with the anemia of chronic disease. Bone marrow examination is rarely necessary to diagnose IDA in adolescents.

Therapy with iron preparations should begin when (1) the diagnosis of IDA is suspected in a patient with a low hemoglobin count or (2) the diagnosis has been confirmed through laboratory testing. Oral preparations are preferred and are the most economical type of treatment. Ferrous sulfate tablets (325 mg) containing 65 mg of elemental iron should be taken three times daily, although smaller doses can be administered if unpleasant side effects occur. Occasional adverse effects include mild gastrointestinal complaints such as a metallic taste, constipation, or diarrhea. Oral supplementation should continue for at least 2 to 3 months after correction of the anemia, and longer for patients with ongoing blood losses. In patients unable to tolerate or absorb an oral preparation for medical reasons, parenteral treatment with intramuscular or intravenous iron dextran can be used, but several observed or potential adverse effects must be considered. Intramuscular injections are often painful and can stain the skin. Intravenous administration can lead to phlebitis and hypotension. Both routes have been associated with systemic reactions, including fever, arthral-

gias, anaphylaxis, headache, nausea, and lymphadenopathy, although newer preparations are associated with a lower incidence of these complications, particularly when lower doses are administered. Transfusions are the most rapid means of replacing depleted iron stores and correcting anemia, but the potential adverse effects make this type of therapy the least desirable, except in the most severely anemic patient. Finally, in addition to treating the iron deficiency, it is very important to determine the underlying cause, whether it be blood loss or inadequate intake, and to make every attempt to achieve correction.

Thalassemia

Although thalassemia trait is a consideration in the differential diagnosis of IDA, it is uncommon for adolescents with this inherited abnormality of globin chain synthesis to have a low hemoglobin level. Characteristic laboratory findings include a very low MCV with hypochromia, microcytosis, and abnormal red cell morphology on the peripheral smear, as well as an increased RBC count; an elevated hemoglobin A_2 level is also found in patients with β-thalassemia trait. On occasion, pregnant patients with heterozygous thalassemia develop some degree of megaloblastic anemia, particularly if they do not receive folic acid supplementation.

Patients with α-thalassemia may have a more variable picture, although most of these patients have normal hemoglobin levels with a low MCV and abnormal blood cell morphology. Confirmation often requires sophisticated globin-chain analysis or family studies. The exception is the patient with three (out of a possible four) abnormal alpha genes, resulting in hemoglobin H disease, with a characteristic chronic hemolytic anemia accompanied by splenomegaly and bone changes. Diagnosis can be established easily by hemoglobin electrophoresis, which demonstrates the abnormal hemoglobin band.

Major morbidity and mortality in thalassemia occur in patients with homozygous β-thalassemia. Diagnosed early in life, this transfusion-dependent condition can begin to produce significant complications in adolescence despite early institution of iron-chelating treatment. Adequate transfusion therapy can prevent skeletal, growth, and developmental abnormalities in most patients, and splenectomy performed late in the first decade of life can decrease transfusion requirements while eliminating hypersplenism-induced pancytopenia. Although the deleterious effects of iron loading can be delayed with deferoxamine infusions, some complications will be noted in adolescents. One of the earliest problems is delayed pubertal changes and onset of menarche until at least the late teens, primarily related to dysfunction of the hypothalamic-pituitary axis. Other endocrinopathies begin to appear in late adolescence with increasing frequency; these include diabetes mellitus, adrenal insufficiency, parathyroid dysfunction, and subclinical hypothyroidism. Hepatic dysfunction, including fibrosis and cirrhosis, can be retarded by chelation therapy, but it is further aggravated by episodes of infectious hepatitis from exposure to many blood donors. Human immunodeficiency virus (HIV)-associated infections, with development of classic acquired immunodeficiency syndrome (AIDS) symptoms, remain a problem in patients who received transfusions before the widespread use of screening procedures. By far the leading cause of death in this patient population remains cardiac complications due to iron overload. Iron is first deposited in the ventricular myocardium, and this is followed by involvement of the conduction tissue.[2] Early signs of cardiac complications include ventricular wall thickening and dilation and occasional premature beats. Progression leads to palpitations, intractable congestive heart failure, and lethal ventricular arrhythmias.

To forestall the onset of iron-related toxicities, it is important to continually emphasize and monitor deferoxamine infusion therapy, with an attempt made to keep serum ferritin levels below 2000 µg/L. Most patients do well with nightly continuous subcutaneous infusions, although more aggressive, high-dose intravenous regimens have been shown to effectively reverse some of the cardiac dysfunction. Continuous monitoring is necessary for signs of deferoxamine complications, including cataract formation, optic neuritis, tinnitus, and renal dysfunction. Effective oral chelators are still unavailable, although clinical trials are in progress.

Although patients can live with transfusion and chelation therapy for many years, a shortened life span from iron-induced complications is still the ultimate result in most patients. There is increasing experience with bone marrow transplantation to replace the abnormal hematopoietic cell line with that of a matched donor. For patients who underwent a transplant before the onset of significant hepatic or cardiac dysfunction, results have been very promising, with more than 85% of patients surviving. At the same time, significant progress is being achieved with fetal hemoglobin stimulation and gene transfer therapy, which holds the possibility of cure for all patients afflicted with this disorder (see also Chapter 49, "Sickle Cell Disease").

Anemia of Chronic Inflammation

Several chronic inflammatory disorders of adolescence are associated with a characteristic anemia that is ameliorated only through improvement of the underlying condition. Typically found in patients with rheumatoid arthritis, systemic lupus erythematosus, inflammatory bowel disease, chronic infection, and lymphomas, this type of anemia is usually moderate, with a hemoglobin level between 7 and 11 g/dl, and rarely symptomatic. Most commonly, the blood smear and indices exhibit a hypochromic microcytic picture, although normochromic normocytic parameters also can be seen.

The pathophysiologic mechanism of this disorder is somewhat complex, with anemia resulting from a combination of decreased RBC survival, disturbed iron metabolism, and deficient bone marrow response. Evaluation typically yields a low serum iron level and TIBC, increased tissue stores of iron with elevated serum ferritin levels, and abundant stainable bone marrow iron. Many studies have found an impairment of iron release from the reticuloendothelial system, resulting in poor reutilization of iron removed from senescent cells and a scenario of "starvation in the midst of plenty." At the same time, there is a poor bone marrow compensatory reaction to the lower hemoglobin levels, owing to abnormal erythropoietin stimulation. Erythropoietin, normally produced in the kidney, induces the transformation of committed RBC precursors into proerythroblasts and ultimately into mature erythrocytes. It also decreases the marrow transit time to enhance early release from the bone marrow into the circulation. Patients with chronic inflammation have a decreased response to erythropoietin, and some patients also have abnormal release of the hormone. The result is bone marrow that does not produce the expected erythroid hyperplasia necessary to correct the anemia.

If no additional cause of anemia, such as blood loss, marrow replacement, or an increased requirement for oxygenation, is superimposed on the preexisting situation, the patient with chronic disease usually does not require transfusion therapy, and the anemia will resolve concurrently with improvement in the underlying problem. As a result of successful correction of anemia and virtual elimination of transfusion requirements in most patients with chronic renal failure, clinical trials that involve the administration of erythropoietin are currently in progress to determine whether elevated levels of this hormone might be able to overcome the poor marrow response to endogenous levels in other conditions such as malignant disorders.

MACROCYTIC ANEMIA

Megaloblastic Anemia

The best-described type of macrocytic disorder is megaloblastic anemia, the most common forms of which result from folic acid or vitamin B_{12} deficiency. A consequence of impaired DNA synthesis, these disorders feature both ineffective erythropoiesis (with intramedullary cell destruction) and hemolysis, with an RBC life span one third to one half of normal. The hallmark of megaloblastic anemia is the presence of very large,

TABLE 48-3
Etiology of Megaloblastic Anemia in Adolescents

Folate Deficiency	Cobalamin Deficiency	Miscellaneous
Inadequate Intake	**Inadequate Intake**	**Drugs**
Malnutrition	Malnutrition	6-Mercaptopurine
Poverty	Vegetarianism	Azathioprine
Overcooked food		5-Fluorouracil
Hyperalimentation	**Decreased Absorption**	Cytosine arabinoside
Synthetic diets		Hydroxyurea
Liver disease	Gastrectomy	Acyclovir
	Pernicious anemia	AZT (azidothymidine)
Decreased Absorption	Zollinger-Ellison syndrome	Nitrous oxide
	Crohn's disease	
Sprue	Ileal resection	**Miscellaneous**
Celiac disease	Lymphoma	
Blind loop syndrome	Tuberculosis	Arsenic
Chronic diarrhea	Pancreatic insufficiency	Orotic aciduria
Crohn's disease	Blind loop syndrome	Congenital dysery-
Gastrectomy	Diverticulosis	thropoietic anemia
Whipple's disease	Intestinal fistulas	Erythroleukemia (M6)
Small bowel resection	*Diphyllobothrium latum*	
Lymphoma	Neomycin	
Anticonvulsants	Para-aminosalicylic acid	
Oral contraceptives	Colchicine	
	Imerslund-Gräsbeck syndrome	
Increased Requirements	**Miscellaneous**	
Pregnancy	Alcohol	
Chronic hemolytic	Transcobalamin deficiency	
anemia	Liver disease	
Hyperthyroidism	Homocystinuria	
Exfoliative dermatitis	Disorders of cobalamin metabo-	
Malignancy	lism	
Cirrhosis		
Folate Antagonism		
Methotrexate		
Trimethoprim		
Pyrimethamine		
Sulfasalazine		
Triamterene		
Pentamidine		
Miscellaneous		
Hemodialysis		
Alcohol		
Cycloserine		
Vitamin B_{12} deficiency		
Inborn errors of folate		
metabolism		

well-hemoglobinized erythrocytes (MCV between 105 and 160), enlarged hematopoietic precursors, and a marked nuclear/cytoplasmic dyssynchrony. In addition to the large RBCs, the peripheral blood smear often contains hypersegmented granulocytes, basophilic stippling, and Howell-Jolly bodies.

The etiologic range of megaloblastic anemias is broad and includes decreased intake, decreased absorption, increased requirements, inborn errors of metabolism, and drug-induced antagonism (Table 48-3). Absorption of folate and cobalamin is frequently altered in diseases of the small intestine, particularly in inflammatory conditions such as Crohn's disease, and in conditions associated with small bowel bacterial overgrowth, such as blind loops and strictures. Levels of vitamin B_{12}, whose absorption from the gastrointestinal tract entails a combination of gastric parietal cell intrinsic factor production as well as a healthy distal ileum, can be dramatically decreased in various gastric disorders, such as gastrectomy or pernicious anemia. Poor or unusual diets can significantly reduce the intake of both folate and cobalamin. Several medications can induce megaloblastic changes by altering and impairing absorption or utilization of folic acid and vitamin B_{12}, by directly inhibiting dihydrofolic acid reductase (particularly methotrexate), or without affecting levels of either folate or cobalamin. In particular, alcohol abuse, chronic anticonvulsant and antimycobacterial medications, and oral contraceptive use are all associated with folate deficiency. Lack of appropriate supplementation in situations characterized by increased folate requirements, including pregnancy and hemolytic anemias, can lead to megaloblastic anemia. Although many of these conditions are very uncommon, as many as 9% of healthy adolescent boys and 4.7% of adolescent girls have only marginal folate levels, which predisposes them to folic acid deficiency.[3]

While symptoms of insufficient folic acid levels correlate with the degree of anemia, vitamin B_{12} deficiency commonly induces neurologic dysfunction, including paresthesias, loss of position sense, and subacute degeneration of the dorsolateral spinal cord. If they are of long standing, many of these changes are irreversible. Other physical findings include yellow skin, glossitis, and papillary atrophy.

The diagnosis of megaloblastic anemia is suspected from the typical hematologic findings, with confirmation dependent on serum folate and vitamin B_{12} assays. Additional work-up, including a bone marrow examination, Schilling test, and deoxyuridine suppression test, is usually necessary to characterize further the pathophysiologic mechanism. More severe deficiencies often result in neutropenia and thrombocytopenia, although these conditions are rarely life-threatening. Elevated levels of serum iron, lactic dehydrogenase, indirect bilirubin, and serum muramidase also may be found in patients with megaloblastic anemia.

After completion of the diagnostic evaluation, therapy should be started expeditiously. Folic acid often can be easily replaced, with 5-mg daily supplementation for 1 to 2 weeks followed by daily administration of 1 mg. Megaloblastic anemia resulting from folate antagonists may require treatment with folinic acid, which is particularly useful in reversing methotrexate toxicity.

Most patients who have cobalamin deficiency require parenteral replacement therapy, particularly if severe gastric disease, ileal disease, or intrinsic factor disorders are involved. Initial treatment usually requires 1 to 2 weeks of daily 1-mg intramuscular injections. This treatment is followed by weekly and finally monthly administrations.

Aplastic Anemias

Marrow failure syndromes are a diverse group of inherited and acquired disorders that can be restricted to the RBCs or can affect all hematopoietic cell lines. Often associated with an elevated fetal hemoglobin level as a compensatory mechanism, these disorders have presenting symptoms of either a normochromic or macrocytic anemia. Depending on the underlying condition, clinical manifestations can be mild or life-threatening.

In teenagers, acquired pure RBC aplasia can be a consequence of medications, infection, inheritance, chemicals, or association with thymoma; idiopathic cases also have been reported. Some of the drugs implicated in transient erythrocyte suppression include azathioprine, chloramphenicol, hydantoins, isoniazid, penicillin, and valproic acid. Reversal rapidly follows discontinuation of the drug in most instances. Many of the infection-related aplasias have been induced by parvoviruses in patients with chronic hemolytic disorders such as sickle cell disease and hereditary spherocytosis. The virus prevents mature erythroid progenitors from replicating. Again, rapid resolution of the anemia occurs as the infection subsides, although transfusions are often required because of the decreased erythrocyte life span characteristic of the underlying hemolytic condition. Nearly all patients with congenital RBC aplasia, the Diamond-Blackfan syndrome, are diagnosed in childhood. While some remain responsive to low-dose prednisone therapy, many develop a resistance to corticosteroid therapy as teenagers and become transfusion dependent. Patients with this syndrome also have an increased risk of developing leukemia as adolescents.

Aplastic anemia, a disorder characterized by a global bone marrow failure, affects all cell lines, resulting in a pancytopenia that places patients at risk for serious hemorrhagic and infectious complications in addition to the anemia. Most constitutional aplasias are diagnosed before the teenage years, but clinical deterioration usually first occurs in adolescence. Patients with Fanconi's anemia, recognized by numerous orthopedic, renal, growth, and cytogenetic abnormalities, often become refractory to androgen and corticosteroid therapy during the adolescent years, with a progression of pancytopenia-related complications. These patients, like those with Diamond-Blackfan syndrome, have a substantially higher risk of acute monoblastic leukemia in addition to hepatocellular carcinoma. Other associations with aplastic anemia include infections (particularly viral hepatitis and Epstein-Barr virus infection), autoimmune disease, pancreatitis, radiation, and various chemicals and drugs (e.g., chloramphenicol, benzene, insecticides, phenothiazines, antimalarials, and hydantoins). However, in most patients with aplastic anemia, no underlying cause is found. Although the exact pathophysiologic mechanism in the evolution of aplastic anemia is unknown, suggestive evidence has pointed to different combinations of pluripotent stem-cell damage, hostile marrow microenvironment, immunologic rejection, and altered activity of hematopoietic growth factors.

The onset of symptoms in acquired aplastic anemia is usually insidious and the physical examination is frequently unrevealing. Infection, pallor, fatigue, and cutaneous bleeding are the most common presenting features. The absence of lymphadenopathy, splenomegaly, and other masses is more suggestive of aplastic anemia, as opposed to the pancytopenia of malignancy. The complete blood count invariably shows some degree of pancytopenia, with macrocytosis a common finding; this is usually a consequence of an elevated fetal hemoglobin level, a manifestation of "stress" erythropoiesis. Platelet and granulocyte counts are decreased, serum iron levels are elevated with saturation of TIBC, and ferritin and erythropoietin levels are elevated. Differential diagnosis includes hypersplenism, which is usually apparent on physical examination; systemic infections that temporarily depress bone marrow production or destroy blood cells in the periphery; myelofibrosis; and marrow replacement with malignant or storage cells. Diagnosis is confirmed through aspiration and biopsy of the bone marrow, typically revealing decreased cellularity, increased fat content, and a predominance of lymphocytes.

For patients with untreated severe aplastic anemia, the prognosis is extremely poor, and most succumb to hemorrhage or overwhelming infection. The outlook has changed dramatically for patients who undergo bone marrow transplant with human leukocyte antigen (HLA)-compatible donor marrow to restore normal hematopoiesis. Patients with no major organ dysfunction who undergo transplantation before heavy transfusion exposure have a cure rate as high as 80%. Graft-versus-host disease has been better controlled with the advent of prophylactic cyclosporine and methotrexate combinations, and graft rejection has decreased with more powerful and selective immunosuppressive therapy. Many patients who have no suitable donor candidates for marrow transplant have attained permanent remission through the use of antithymocyte globulin, cyclosporine, and prednisone, which gives further credence to the immunologic mechanism underlying marrow failure in many patients. The increasing availability of hematopoietic growth factors offers additional hope for further improvements in the therapy for these disorders.[4]

NORMOCYTIC ANEMIA

Intrinsic Erythrocyte Defects

Although no longer possessing a nucleus, the circulating RBC is a dynamic structure that contains a large number of metabolic components necessary to maintain hemoglobin and membrane integrity. To preserve the characteristic biconcave shape of the cell, sufficient membrane is necessary to give the cell optimal deformability, which is important for proper viscosity and blood flow. An electrolyte gradient must be constantly maintained, and hemoglobin iron must be kept in the reduced divalent form for proper functioning. Each of these processes can be affected by many acquired and inherited conditions.

Inherited membrane disorders, spherocytosis being the most common, can dramatically shorten the RBC life span. The erythrocyte in this disorder lacks the normal amount of functioning spectrin, the predominant membrane protein, with a resultant decrease in membrane surface area and cell deformability and shortened RBC half-life. By the teenage years, patients often have significant splenomegaly and compensated hemolytic anemia, with a propensity toward periodic aplastic crises that can necessitate transfusions. Rarely, splenic sequestration with sudden massive splenomegaly and pooling of substantial blood volumes can occur after infection, especially that from Epstein-Barr virus, resulting in severe anemia and even hypovolemic shock. The chronic hemolysis and elevated bilirubin levels predispose older patients to biliary tract disease with cholelithiasis. To avoid these problems, most patients are advised to undergo splenectomy, which removes the primary site of hemolysis, increases the RBC life span and hemoglobin level, and mitigates the risk of biliary tract disease. Although the absence of a functioning spleen can increase the potential risk of overwhelming pneumococcal sepsis, most teenagers possess adequate antibody protection against most strains of *Pneumococcus,* and so the risk of infection is small. However, immunization with Pneumovax vaccine before splenectomy is advised. Many hematologists recommend prophylactic penicillin therapy in addition to Pneumovax immunization, although most discontinue the antibiotic late in the teenage years, when the risk of sepsis is low.

Other RBC skeletal disorders produce characteristic abnormal erythrocyte shapes with varying degrees of hemolysis and anemia. Hereditary elliptocytosis and pyropoikilocytosis are uncommon conditions that also result from an abnormal amount of spectrin. Increased osmotic fragility is not always part of the pathophysiologic mechanism, and despite the dramatic findings on peripheral blood smear, anemia is usually mild. Patients with severe hemolysis often benefit from splenectomy. Stomatocytosis, whether inherited or acquired through such conditions as malignancy or hepatobiliary disease, also results in increased osmotic fragility and electrolyte permeability, with variable hemolysis. Finally, acanthocytosis, found in patients with severe liver disease, malnutrition, anorexia nervosa, and lipid disorders such as abetalipoproteinemia, results in a mild to moderate hemolytic anemia because of the defective outer lipid layer of the cell membrane.

A deficiency in any of several intrinsic erythrocyte enzymes can have serious deleterious effects on cell survival. One of the most prevalent inherited disorders, glucose-6-phosphate dehydrogenase (G6PD) deficiency, renders the RBC susceptible to oxidation during infection and after ingestion of many drugs and foods (most notoriously, fava beans), with subsequent irreversible hemoglobin denaturation, Heinz body precipitation, and cell death. More than 350 variants of this abnormality have been documented.[5] The most severe form is the Mediterranean variant, which has barely detectable levels of the enzyme in all RBCs, regardless of red cell age. In the United States the disorder is found predominantly in the black population, which generally has a milder variant and subsequent clinical course. Reticulocytes and other young RBCs often have normal levels of the enzyme, which affords some protection against hemolysis. Patients are usually asymptomatic, with normal hemoglobin levels until subjected to oxidant stress, which can induce rapid hemolysis, dark urine, jaundice, and anemia. Although only a few commonly administered medications, including sulfonamides, nitrofurantoin, and antimalarials, should be avoided, if possible, in these patients, the list of drugs associated with hemolytic crises in G6PD deficiency is extensive.[6]

Unlike G6PD deficiency, a chronic severe hemolytic anemia often results from a deficiency of pyruvate kinase, the most common enzymopathy of the glycolytic pathway. Believed to be related to decreased adenosine triphosphate levels and interference of cellular synthesis by intermediate metabolites, this deficiency is characterized by brisk hemolysis with hyperbilirubinemia, splenomegaly, and a striking reticulocytosis. Many affected patients require maintenance transfusion therapy. However, splenectomy alleviates transfusion requirements in most patients.

Point mutations in the α- or β-globin chains can significantly alter the conformation and behavior of the hemoglobin molecule, with major clinical consequences. Sickle cell disease (see Chapter 49) is the best-described hemoglobinopathy, with substantial morbidity and mortality. Hemoglobin C, another β-chain mutant, is usually associated with mild anemia and splenomegaly in adolescents. It is symptomatic only when inherited as a double heterozygote with the sickle hemoglobin. Hemoglobin E, common in patients from Southeast Asia, produces mild to moderate hemolysis. As a double heterozygote with β-thalassemia, it behaves like a classic Cooley's anemia. Finally, many unstable hemoglobinopathies are associated with variable hemolysis and splenomegaly and usually require minimal supportive care.

Extrinsic Hemolysis

Antibody-mediated hemolysis in adolescents is an uncommon but potentially serious disorder. Autoimmune hemolytic anemia (AIHA) is typically idiopathic but can be associated with infections (*Mycoplasma pneumoniae,* Epstein-Barr virus, cytomegalovirus, tuberculosis, and respiratory infections), malignancies (primarily lymphomas and leukemias), inflammatory diseases (systemic lupus erythematosus, rheumatoid arthritis, ulcerative colitis, and chronic active hepatitis), and immunodeficiencies. Medications can evoke production of antibodies after attaching themselves to the RBC membrane (e.g., penicillin and cephalosporins) or by forming immune complexes that adhere to the RBCs (e.g., quinidine). The list of agents associated with hemolysis is extensive, with resolution expected after cessation of the drug. The mechanism of development of erythrocyte autoantibodies is unknown, although possibilities include alteration of the cell membrane by an extrinsic agent or proliferation of immunologically aberrant cells that do not recognize host antigens.

Acute AIHA can present in an aggressive fashion, with severe pallor, jaundice, hemoglobinuria, and splenomegaly. Most of these conditions are caused by warm antibodies, IgG proteins that react at 37°C, do not require complement activation, and result in trapping with destruction of RBCs, primarily in the spleen. Patients with warm antibody AIHA usually respond well to corticosteroids, have full recovery within a few months, and have a low mortality rate, mostly from severe anemia or hemorrhage due to associated immune thrombocytopenia. Adolescent patients, however, have a greater likelihood of presenting with an insidious onset characterized by slowly progressive fatigue and pallor. These patients usually have an IgM cold agglutinin that reacts best below 31°C and requires complement activation to produce hemolysis. Many such episodes are associated with Epstein-Barr virus or *M. pneumoniae* infections and exhibit specificity to i or I antigens, respectively. Response to steroids is more variable, and a tendency toward chronicity with a higher mortality is the rule.

Laboratory features in patients with AIHA usually include profound anemia, brisk reticulocytosis (although initially very low), decreased serum haptoglobin level, elevated white cell counts, and elevated bilirubin levels. Erythrocyte agglutination and nucleated RBCs may be evident on the peripheral smear, but the hallmark of the disease is a positive Coombs' antiglobulin test. Further characterization of the antibody often can be helpful in detecting an underlying condition. Because of the often brisk hemolysis, expeditious treatment is indicated. High doses of corticosteroids (2 to 5 mg/kg/day of prednisone) can dramatically slow the rate of cell destruction within 1 to 3 days, as a result of suppressing sequestration by splenic macrophages and, to a lesser extent, decreasing production of the abnormal antibody. If the hemoglobin level continues to drop with increasing symptoms, transfusion with the most compatible units of blood should be performed, with a small test dose given slowly, followed by infusion of the remainder. Preparations should be made to treat possibly severe hemolytic transfusion reactions. Patients with cold agglutinins usually obtain some measure of clinical relief by being kept warm. Many more adolescents than children develop chronic AIHA, and splenectomy is often necessary to achieve a prolonged response. Other treatment modalities currently in use, and yielding variable degrees of success, include immunosuppressive medications (e.g., azathioprine, cyclophosphamide, cyclosporine, and 6-mercaptopurine), high-dose intravenous gammaglobulin, danazol, and plasmapheresis. Patients with chronic AIHA are more likely to have underlying disorders, such as systemic lupus erythematosus, which contribute to a much higher mortality rate.

Miscellaneous Hemolytic Anemias

Although the RBC normally can withstand and recover from continuous trauma as it travels throughout the bloodstream, an estimated 175 miles during its lifetime, a number of different mechanical and physical agents can sufficiently damage the cell to hasten its removal from the circulation. These extrinsic factors are varied, as is the mechanism of hemolysis.

Microangiopathic hemolysis, resulting from pathologic strands of fibrin within arterioles that cause fragmentation of erythrocytes traversing the blood vessels, can range from hemolytic-uremic syndrome (HUS), more commonly seen in young children, to a fulminant disseminated intravascular coagulation. The classic picture of lethargy, pallor, bruising, and decreased urinary output seen in HUS occasionally appears in adolescents, with the kidney the primary organ of concern; renal failure usually is the overriding problem. Adolescents may develop the adult analog of HUS, thrombotic thrombocytopenic purpura, which often presents with more diffuse symptoms. These patients have a higher incidence of central nervous system dysfunction and, as with HUS, have associated schistocytes on peripheral smear, uremia, anemia, thrombocytopenia, and elevated von Willebrand factor. Many patients respond to plasma infusion or plasmapheresis. The most severe microangiopathic hemolysis occurs in disseminated intravascular coagulation (see Chapter 52, "Hemorrhage and Thrombosis").

Infections can shorten RBC life span through many mechanisms, including immune destruction, increased trapping in an enlarged spleen, blood loss, and direct erythrocyte destruction. Brisk hemolysis accompanies malaria and babesiosis, protozoan infections that mediate cellular destruction through intracellular damage, along with recruitment of a host of immunologic mechanisms. *Clostridium perfringens,* which has been reported in teenagers undergoing septic abortion and in some patients with cholecystitis, can release potent hemolytic substances that can induce fatal hemolytic reactions. Many viral infections, including Epstein-Barr virus, rubeola, varicella, and HIV, can be associated with significant hemolysis during or after the acute infection.

Anemia, which is characteristic of most patients with serious renal disease, is a result of decreased production of RBCs combined with a shortened survival. The less functioning renal tissue present, the less erythropoietin will be produced to stimulate compensatory bone marrow production. Although transfusion was formerly part of the mainstay of treatment for the anemia of renal disease, the availability of abundant supplies of recombinant erythropoietin has dramatically reduced or eliminated the need for transfusion therapy in such patients, with concomitant reduction of exposure to blood-transmitted infections.

Hypersplenism from any cause will trap and destroy RBCs, sometimes requiring splenectomy (see Chapter 53, "Lymphadenopathy and Splenomegaly"). Strenuous, repetitive, and sustained physical activities, particularly those that entail physical trauma to various limbs (e.g., karate, marching, running, and hand drumming), all have been associated with mild anemia, partially attributed to localized intravascular hemolysis. Finally, many cardiac conditions, including aortic stenosis, coarctation of the aorta, ball valve replacement, and artificial prosthetic surfaces, can induce sufficient mechanical damage to the RBC membrane to cause hemolysis, occasionally severe enough to require transfusion therapy or replacement of the dysfunctional surface.

Risks of Transfusion Therapy

Bleeding diatheses, surgical losses, and many of the anemias discussed in this chapter can be indications for transfusion therapy. In some instances, replacement is performed on a short-term basis with minimal risks to the patient. Patients who require prolonged or lifetime transfusion therapy often have serious complications resulting from exposure to many donors and intake of large amounts of iron.

A potentially serious immediate complication is a hemolytic transfusion reaction—manifested by fever, backache, nausea, and hypotension—that is usually the result of intravascular hemolysis. If this reaction occurs, the transfusion should be stopped and fluids administered to induce diuresis, increase renal flow, and correct hypotension. This more serious reaction should be differentiated from a febrile response, which is usually mediated by white blood cells and should be treated symptomatically. Other immediate complications, including bacterial contamination, volume overload, air embolism, and bleeding, are rare.

More common problems are encountered long after the transfusion has been administered. Delayed transfusion reactions with hemolysis and posttransfusion purpura are uncommon, appear within 2 weeks of transfusion, and are usually self-limited. Of greatest concern regarding transfusion is the risk of transmitted infections. Hepatitis continues to be a significant problem in patients who undergo long-term transfusion therapy, although the incidences of hepatitis A, B, and C have all been declining through the advent of effective donor screening. Likewise, screening for HIV infection has reduced the risk to approximately 1 in 250,000. Screening also has been instituted for HTLV-1 virus, a cause of T-cell lymphoma in Japan and elsewhere. Rare graft-versus-host disease, which is lethal in immunocompromised patients, can be eliminated through radiation of donor blood.

References

1. Jacobs A, Butler EB: Menstrual blood-loss in iron deficiency anaemia, *Lancet* 2:407-409, 1965.
2. Buja LM, Roberts WC: Iron in the heart: etiology and clinical significance, *Am J Med* 51:209-221, 1971.
3. Daniel WA, Gaines EG, Bennett DL: Dietary intakes and plasma concentrations of folate in healthy adolescents, *Am J Clin Nutr* 28:363-370, 1975.
4. Young NS, Barrett AJ: The treatment of severe acquired aplastic anemia, *Blood* 85:3367-3377, 1995.
5. Beutler E, Yoshida A: Genetic variations of glucose-6-phosphate dehydrogenase: a catalog and future prospective, *Medicine* 67:311-334, 1988.
6. Beutler E: *Hemolytic anemia in disorders of red cell metabolism,* New York, 1978, Plenum Publishing; pp 75-92.

Suggested Readings

Miller DR, Baehner RL: *Blood diseases of infancy and childhood,* ed 7, St. Louis, 1995, Mosby–Year Book.

Nathan DG, Oski FA: *Hematology of infancy and childhood,* ed 4, Philadelphia, 1993, WB Saunders.

Oski FA, editor: *Hematol Clin North Am* 1:381-544, 1987.

Williams WJ, Beutler E, Erslev AJ, Lichtman MA: *Hematology,* ed 4, New York, 1990, McGraw-Hill.

CHAPTER 49

Sickle Cell Disease

•

Mark E. Weinblatt

The biochemical abnormality and clinical pathophysiology of few diseases are as well described as those of sickle cell disease. Although therapeutic results have not kept pace with basic understanding of the hemoglobinopathies, studies of the molecular biology of the sickling phenomenon have yielded many clues that may lead to a cure for this and other hemoglobinopathies.

Sickle cell anemia is the most common heritable hematologic disease in humans. It is a chronic, incurable disorder, the symptomatology of which is the result of expression of a mutant globin gene found on the short arm of chromosome 11. The disease is characterized by a varying degree of hemolysis with sporadic major "crises" that cause significant morbidity and mortality. Complications of this disorder can be relatively mild or life-threatening, affecting every organ system of the body (Table 49-1). Although many crises occur in an obvious, clinically apparent fashion, some potentially devastating situations arise insidiously. Therefore, medical staff who provide care for adolescents with sickle cell disease must be well versed in the multifaceted clinical situations confronting this patient population.

EPIDEMIOLOGY

The sickle cell abnormality is a common mutant that is believed to have originated spontaneously in a multicentric fashion in central Africa, the Middle East, the Mediterranean area, and the Indian subcontinent.[1] Slave trade brought the sickle gene to the Western hemisphere, with a predominance of the Benin and Bantu haplotypes from central West Africa.

The incidence of sickle cell anemia varies in different parts of the world, with 4% of American blacks carrying the gene, as opposed to 14% of the population in Africa. Sickle cell syndromes resulting in significant morbidity and mortality require either a homozygous inheritance of the gene for the β^s polypeptide from each parent (SS) or a doubly heterozygote state with a contribution from a

TABLE 49-1
Sickle Cell Disorders in the Adolescent

Syndrome	SA	SS	SC
Hematocrit	36%-46%	17%-27%	30%-36%
Reticulocyte	1%-4%	12%-25%	5%-10%
Morphology	Normal	ISC, target, poly-chromasia, HJ bodies	Few ISC, mild target and polychromasia
MCV (fl)	82-88	84-88	75-80
Spleen	Absent	Absent	Enlarged
Symptoms	Rare	Severe	Moderate/severe
Hgb Electrolytes	20%-40% S, 55%-80% A, 0%-5% F; 0%-2% A2	80%-100% S, 0%-20% A	50% S, 50% C
Most common features	Hyposthenuria, hematuria	Bones, lungs; biliary tree; growth delay; infection; CNS; placenta; renal	Heads of femur, humerus; eye; sequestration; placenta; renal

Syndrome	S-β^0-thal	S-β^+-thal	S-HPFH	SS-α-thal
Hematocrit	20%-30%	30%-36%	35%-40%	25%-30%
Reticulocyte	10%-15%	2%-6%	1%-4%	5%-10%
Morphology	ISC, target, hypochromia, baso. stippl.	Few ISC, target, hypochromia, baso. stippl.	Target	Few ISC, target, hypochromia
MCV (fl)	62-70	62-70	85-98	68-72
Spleen	Enlarged	Enlarged	Absent	Absent
Symptoms	Severe	Moderate/severe	Absent/mild	Moderate
HgB Electrolytes	75%-100% S, 0%-20% F, 3%-6% A2	50%-80% S, 10%-30% A, 0%-20% F; 3%-6% A2	70%-80% S, 20%-30% F, 0%-3% A2	80%-100% S, 0%-20% F
Most common features	Bones, lungs; biliary tree; growth delay; placenta; CNS sequestration	Sequestration; bones	Bones; renal	Same as SS, usually mild

baso. stippl, basophilic stippling; *CNS,* central nervous system; *Hgb,* hemoglobin; *HJ,* Howell-Jolly; *ISC,* irreversibly sickled cells; *MCV,* mean corpuscular volume; *target,* target cells.

parent carrying a gene that produces either hemoglobin C (SC) or β-thalassemia (S-thalassemia). The incidence of the carrier states for these two additional gene mutations in American blacks is 2.3% for the C gene and 0.8% for β-thalassemia.[1] Since the inheritance of two abnormal β genes is necessary to produce significant clinical symptoms, the overall incidence of affected individuals in the United States is 1 in 650 for the homozygous state, 1 in 1120 for the SC double heterozygote, and 1 in 3200 for sickle-thalassemia.[2] Because of the greater mortality in the homozygous state that occurs at an early age, only half the U.S. adolescent and adult sickle cell disease population is SS, which is an important consideration for genetic counseling.

There has been much speculation about the geographic distribution of the sickle gene in areas where malaria is prevalent. Since homozygous individuals succumb to complications of the malaria parasite at an early age, some advantage must be present to maintain the gene frequency at a constant rate. When the patient with the sickle trait is infected with the parasite, the infected red blood cells sickle more easily and are subsequently removed from the circulation, predominantly in the splenic sinusoids. After additional sickling has taken place in the hypoxic splenic environment, the rigid crystalline hemoglobin structure formed in the red blood cells (RBCs) can directly damage the parasite, leading to its death. In addition, sickling results in a loss of intracellular potassium, which is normally necessary for parasite viability and proliferation.

MOLECULAR BASIS OF SICKLING

Much of the unique functioning of the hemoglobin molecule is related to the special conformation of this tetramer, composed of two α- and two non-α-globin chains. Shortly before birth, gamma chain production begins to fall, resulting in a steady decrease in the formation of fetal hemoglobin. A concomitant increase in β-globin chain formation occurs with the appearance of adult hemoglobin tetramers composed of two α and two β chains ($α^2β^2$). By 6 months of age, more than 90% of hemoglobin is hemoglobin A. Studies of the hemoglobin of patients with sickle cell disease have revealed the presence of a mutant β-polypeptide chain, with the substitution of a hydrophobic valine for hydrophilic glutamic acid in the no. 6 position. The resultant tetramer is designated $α^2β^{s2}$. Conformational changes in the altered molecular structure account for the pathophysiologic shape, and modifications in molecular charge result in different electrophoretic mobility, enabling diagnosis of the abnormal hemoglobin by electrophoresis.

When fully oxygenated in dilute solution, hemoglobins A and S exhibit equal oxygen affinities and solubilities. However, with deoxygenation the sickle hemoglobin forms polymers consisting of long, parallel, rodlike structures that band together to form a spiral shape. This insoluble, firm gel forms a characteristic liquid crystal (tactoid) whose rigid structure distorts the RBC shape and increases the viscosity of blood in an exponential fashion. The sickling phenomenon occurs in a well-defined manner. First, small precipitates are formed and act as nuclei for longer strand formation. Then, more uncommited sickle hemoglobin molecules are joined to the precipitate to form the characteristic sickle cell shape. The time frame is most critical in determining the clinical outcome: the high oxygen content in the lungs transforms the hemoglobin S gel into soluble form in less than 0.5 seconds, and it will remain in solution until it enters the capillary bed. Red blood cells reside in this low oxygen environment for about 1 second; if the time delay for sickling is less than 1 second, sickling and occlusion will occur; if longer than 1 second, blood flow will be unimpeded.[3] This time delay from the beginning of gel formation to the final rigid cell shape is affected by the following parameters, each of which plays a major clinical role:

1. Oxygen is the most important factor, since polymerization will occur only in the deoxygenated state. As the RBC deoxygenates, the oxygen affinity of hemoglobin S falls, thus stabilizing the deoxygenated state. Any additional factor, such as acidemia or increased 2,3-diphosphoglycerate (which binds with hemoglobin and decreases oxygen affinity), that shifts the oxygen dissociation curve to enhance oxygen unloading to the tissues further lowers the intraerythrocytic oxygen levels and increases the degree of sickling. Any clinical situation resulting in hypoxia further potentiates the sickling process.

2. The intracellular concentration of sickle hemoglobin is another important variable that determines the equilibrium between liquid and solid phases. The sickle cell carrier has concentrations of hemoglobin S that are low enough to be virtually symptom free. The presence of α-thalassemia genes also lessens the degree of sickling, possibly by lowering the mean corpuscular hemoglobin concentration of the cell. Any condition resulting in cellular dehydration increases the concentration of intracellular hemoglobin S.

3. Interaction with other hemoglobins can have important clinical effects. Both hemoglobins A and F interact poorly with sickle hemoglobin, increase the delay time, increase the solubility of hemoglobin S, and inhibit the sickling process. This explains the paucity of clinical symptoms in the patient with a high fetal hemoglobin concentration. On the other hand, hemoglobins C and D interact readily with sickle hemoglobin and result in a clinical picture often as severe as the homozygous condition.

Small changes in any of these parameters can have profound effects on the degree of sickling by shortening or lengthening the delay time, which is normally long enough to prevent sickling in 80% of cells in a typical passage throughout the body's circulation.

As a consequence of the initial sickling event, the distortion of the RBC damages the cell membrane proteins. Although the cell can revert to its normal biconcave shape when the sickle hemoglobin returns to a soluble form after reoxygenation, repetitive bouts of sickling permanently damage the membrane structure, ultimately forming an irreversibly sickled cell in a fixed configuration, a cell that can no longer negotiate the tortuous capillary pathways. The damaged membrane leads to leakage of intracellular potassium and an increase in sodium, a consequence of partial failure of the sodium-potassium ATPase pump. Increased permeability of calcium leads to a Ca^{++} influx, resulting in a more rigid cell. The polymerization process, in combination with the increased membrane rigidity and increased adherence of the cell membrane to the endothelial lining, contributes to the final common pathophysiologic pathway, that of hyperviscosity and microvascular stasis. The stagnation of cells leads to localized hypoxia, further sickling, and a vicious cycle that culminates in vascular obstruction, infarction, necrosis, and fibrosis. This process can occur in tissue of any organ, with particular predilection for vascular beds with slow flow and high oxygen extraction, such as the spleen, bone marrow, and placenta. Potentiating factors such as acidemia and dehydration worsen the sickling process; these are often encountered in sites of vasoconstriction (as with cold exposure) and in febrile episodes. Finally, the increased adhesion of cells to the endothelial surface damages the vascular endothelium, exposing the underlying collagen layer that initiates platelet aggregation, coagulation, and thrombosis, which in turn further aggravates the stasis.

CLINICAL FEATURES

Because of the nature of the sickling process, sickle cell disease is characterized by long periods of relative stability interrupted by so-called clinical crises. These crises are traditionally described as vasoocclusive, megaloblastic, aplastic, hyperhemolytic, and sequestration, with most symptoms in adolescents resulting from vasoocclusion or infection. The severity of symptoms usually correlates with the type of sickle cell disorder, with the homozygous SS type typically experiencing more frequent and more debilitating symptoms than the SC or S-thalassemia double heterozygotes. Triggering events heralding the onset of sickle crises are rarely identified in adolescents, unlike children, who frequently have a history of antecedent infection with fever and dehydration.

Vasoocclusive Crises

The sickling phenomenon, with resultant obstruction and infarction, affects all organs of the body in varying degrees. There is usually no change in the hemoglobin level, reticulocyte count, or number of sickle cells present on the peripheral smear, and crises are unpredictable in most circumstances. The most common complaint is pain and tenderness at the site of infarction, with additional symptoms related to the degree and site of end-organ damage.

Skeletal involvement is one of the most frequent causes of pain, resulting most often from sickling and infarction in the sinusoids of bone marrow but also from ischemia of bone and periosteum. In adolescents and adults the most common sites are the lumbosacral spine, knee, shoulder, and thigh, although any bone can be affected. In contrast, young children are prone toward involvement of the smaller tubular bones of the hands and feet. Chief complaints include deep throbbing pain, point tenderness, swelling, fever, and increased warmth overlying the site. Radiographic examination may reveal periosteal elevation in healing infarcts, and radiotechnetium bone scans can yield either "cold spots" at sites of decreased blood flow or "hot spots" in healing infarctions. The typical course of bony infarction runs between 3 and 7 days before resolution, and it frequently requires hospitalization for pain management. This spectrum of symptoms often creates difficulty in differentiating a crisis from osteomyelitis, although migratory pain usually implies infarction as opposed to infection. While traditional radiographic techniques often have not helped in the differential diagnosis, magnetic resonance imaging

(MRI) is becoming a more promising tool for the clinician.[4] Although the ratio of osteomyelitis to bone infarction in the adolescent is approximately 1:50, the appreciable risk of this serious, debilitating, and potentially life-threatening infection in patients with sickle cell disease, and the unreliability of the diagnostic tools, often necessitate performance of a needle biopsy to differentiate the two and to isolate the organism for proper antibiotic therapy.

More serious orthopedic sequelae are seen with infarction of the head of the femur or humerus. Vascular access to these sites is normally tenuous, and obstruction of blood flow can be particularly devastating, with resultant aseptic necrosis and loss of function of the joint. This is more common with the SC subtype and often progresses to the point that prosthetic replacement of the joint becomes necessary.

The vertebrae often exhibit a characteristic "fishmouth" appearance on radiographs. This abnormality is the result of recurrent infarction of the main vertebral arteries, leading to ischemic damage of the central portion of the growth plate with sparing of the outer portions. A weakening of the entire structure can lead to compression fractures. This always must be a consideration in the patient who complains of back pain, and it may be the first sign of impingement of nerve roots or the spinal cord, which requires immediate attention to prevent irreparable neurologic damage.

Pulmonary problems are the most frequent cause of hospitalization in older adolescents and adults, in contrast to the more common admissions for fever or bone pain in children and younger adolescents. Pulmonary infarctions are often indistinguishable from or coexistent with pneumonia, and they can induce localized hypoxia and exacerbation of sickling. Typical findings include chest pain, fever, cough, tachypnea, leukocytosis, and an infiltrate on radiographic examination. Constantly changing pulmonary auscultation favors the diagnosis of infarction over pneumonia; adolescents are less likely to have bacterial infection. A consequence of repeated infarctions is chronic pulmonary disease, with decreased vital capacity and compromised gas exchange. Poorly aerated segments of lung cause shunting and ventilation/perfusion disparity, leading to decreased oxygen tension, desaturation, and further sickling. Although the most commonly encountered pulmonary events are infection or infarction, the acute chest syndrome sometimes can be the result of bone marrow fat emboli released into the circulation after bone marrow infarction and necrosis. This type of respiratory complication is often acute in onset and can cause rapid deterioration in an already compromised organ.

Central nervous system involvement is potentially the most devastating event in patients of all ages with sickle cell disease. Strokes account for approximately 12% of sickle cell mortality; survivors often have hemiplegia, aphasia, cranial nerve palsy, and seizures. There is a 67% risk of recurrence within 1 year if no prophylactic transfusion program is instituted. Unlike the vaso-occlusive targets in other parts of the body, the medium-sized and larger blood vessels are typically affected. On pathologic examination, the larger arteries usually are found to have smooth muscle and intimal proliferation, with stenosis and aneurysmal dilation, which places the arteries at high risk for occlusion and hemorrhage. Possible mechanisms include occlusion of the vasa vasorum, with resultant injury to the arterial wall, repeated endothelial damage from adherent ("sticky") sickle cells, and thrombosis of the narrowed passage. After infarction, hemorrhage can further increase the extent of damage and mortality. For unknown reasons, the incidence of cerebrovascular accidents decreases with age in older adolescents and adults, and hemorrhage becomes a more common event than infarction.[5] Presenting complaints include severe headache, photophobia, and meningismus. Clinical deterioration is rapid and mortality high, making it imperative to obtain an early computed tomography (CT) or MRI scan in an attempt to diagnose any surgically amenable lesions, for example, subdural hematoma. Magnetic resonance angiography can often reveal stenosis of the internal carotid and cerebral vessels, helping to identify those patients at increased risk for stroke. Meningitis, which has a much greater incidence rate in patients with sickle cell disease than in other populations, is another complication that can cause significant brain damage.

The kidneys are very common sites of damage by sickle cells, and this occurs even in the patient with sickle trait. The hypoxic, acidotic, and hyperosmolar environment is especially conducive to the sickling process. Virtually all patients with sickle cell disease have hyposthenuria, a defect that readily leads to dehydration and potentiation of sickling. Fifty percent of patients have enlarged kidneys, and gross hematuria and acute papillary necrosis may accompany infarction. The nephrotic syndrome, another renal complication seen primarily in adolescents with sickle cell disease, is typified by hypertension, hematuria, proteinuria, progressive renal insufficiency, and renal failure. Pathologic findings include membranoproliferative glomerulonephritis with mesangial proliferation, interstitial fibrosis, fusion of the foot processes, and tubular atrophy.[6] Some of these findings may be due to the deposition of immune complexes.

Abdominal pain, a frequent component of vaso-occlusive crises, can imitate emergency surgical disorders, with signs such as guarding, fever, tenderness, rebound, and leukocytosis. This pain can follow infarction of the mesentery or the bowel wall, but consideration must be given to involvement of the liver and biliary tree.

Chronic hemolysis and hyperbilirubinemia contribute to the high incidence of cholelithiasis seen in 50% to 70% of adolescents by the age of 15. Biliary stones in sickle cell patients are soft, accompanied by "sludge" visualized on sonography, and are usually asymptomatic, often found incidentally on radiographic evaluation. The soft, friable consistency of these stones accounts for the somewhat lower than expected occurrence of cholecystitis and the infrequent necessity for cholecystectomy. The presence of cholelithiasis should therefore not by itself be an indication for cholecystectomy. However, when gallstones are symptomatic, laparoscopic cholecystectomy has considerably shortened the morbidity surrounding the surgical procedure. Another cause of right upper quadrant abdominal pain is hepatic infarction, recognized by the appearance of tender hepatomegaly, rising transaminase levels, and greater than usual hyperbilirubinemia. On rare occasions, severe cholestasis and extensive biliary pooling occur in the liver; these conditions are accompanied by dramatic rises in bilirubin (as high as 100 mg/dl) with hepatic necrosis and failure. Patients who have undergone transfusion therapy are also at risk of contracting infectious hepatitis, which is often very difficult to distinguish from infarction. Only about one third of patients exhibit signs of chronic liver dysfunction, yet these multiple, varied insults to the liver lead to a common, usually subclinical, hepatic necrosis and fibrosis or cirrhosis, which is found in many patients at autopsy.

Surprisingly, in patients with sickle cell disease, the heart rarely develops clinical problems. Chronic anemia contributes to tachycardia, cardiac enlargement, and left ventricular hypertrophy, but decreased cardiac function at rest is rarely detected. In the adolescent, cardiomegaly typically causes an exaggerated apical impulse that is displaced to the left side, and the patient occasionally complains of exertional dyspnea, palpitations, and chest pain. However, despite the pronounced deoxygenation of blood passing through the coronary circulation, myocardial infarction is an extremely uncommon event. The rapid transit time through the coronary vessels is shorter than the sickle delay time, which spares the myocardium. In addition, on postmortem examination, patients with sickle cell disease have been found to have surprisingly little atherosclerosis and a larger than normal caliber of the coronary arteries, both of which confer added protection against a devastating infarction.[7] Incidental myocardial fibrosis of varying degrees is a common finding at autopsy.

In sickle cell disease the eye can exhibit a broad range of clinical symptoms. Most patients are found to have increased tortuosity of the retinal vasculature, which is usually of no clinical relevance. However, proliferative retinopathy can develop and progress as a result of constant cycles of sickling and vascular occlusion. The spectrum of findings includes arteriolar occlusion, arteriovenous anastomosis and aneurysm, vascular leaks and neovascular patches, vitreous hemorrhage, and finally retinal detachment. Although these lesions sometimes regress spontaneously, ophthalmologic management, often including laser photocoagulation, is necessary to prevent serious visual impairment. Patients with the SC subtype are most prone to serious ocular complications, including sudden blindness from central retinal artery occlusion. A greater incidence of hyphema in the anterior chamber is also observed in the sickle cell patient, and progressive sickling in this low-oxygen environment often necessitates emergency evacuation of the clot to prevent glaucoma and blindness.

Growth and development abnormalities after the first decade of life are common, with SS homozygotes and sickle-β^0-thalassemia affected to a greater degree than SC or S-β^+-thalassemia. After nearly normal growth in early childhood, the adolescent characteristically experiences slowed height and weight gains and delayed development of secondary sexual characteristics. Patients ultimately achieve normal height after a late adolescent growth spurt, which is made possible by retarded closing of the growth plates associated with the delay in puberty; two thirds of patients between the ages of 10 and 16 have bone ages more than two standard deviations below normal.[8] Menarche is usually delayed an average of 3 years, and this delay is commonly attributed to faulty gonadal steroidogenesis.[9] However, in some patients this delay may be constitutional. Males often have decreased fertility, with lowered sperm count and decreased motility. At the completion of growth, patients are typically underweight for height and have long extremities.

Priapism in males is an uncommon but painful event with potential long-term adverse effects. A result of obstructed venous flow in the corpus cavernosum, this condition can be extremely painful and relatively unresponsive to medical management. Vigorous hydration, avoidance of temperature extremes, liberal use of pain medications and sedation, and transfusions are often successful in treatment. However, priapism is usually a very difficult management problem, particularly in postpubertal patients, frequently resulting in permanent impotence. Surgical procedures usually have been ineffective (sometimes causing impotence while relieving the obstruction), although some success has been obtained by constructing a fistulous tract between the glans and the corpus cavernosum.[10]

Another problem germane to adolescents and adults with sickle cell disease is that of leg ulcers, which often begin as small vesicles or abrasions. As a result of increasingly poor venous flow and stasis in the lower extremities accompanying advancing age, breakdown of surrounding tissues ensues, followed by extension into painful indolent ulcerations. The ulcers are prone to infection and can enlarge to encompass a large area encircling the midtibial region. Because of poor spontaneous healing, ulcers usually require strict bed rest with frequent dressing changes, antibiotic therapy, transfusions, and sometimes skin grafting. If a deficiency is documented, zinc therapy may be of some benefit to accelerate healing.

The pregnant patient with sickle cell disease may develop special problems relevant to herself and to the fetus. During pregnancy the baseline anemia usually is exaggerated by hemodilution and further worsened by folate deficiency. In the last trimester, women are at increased risk for toxemia, heart failure, and postpartum endometritis. Numerous organs are prone toward vasoocclusive crises and infections during the late stages of pregnancy, yielding a higher incidence of life-threatening pyelonephritis, pneumonia, phlebitis, and pulmonary infarctions. The slow blood flow and hypoxic environment in the placenta that follows the transfer of oxygen to the fetal circulation results in a strong inducement to sickling and infarction. This in turn leads to frequent stillbirths, prematurity, and small-for-gestational-age newborns. Although the overall mortality rates for the mother and fetus having optimal care are now about 1% and 15%, respectively, unsupervised pregnancies have yielded rates as high as 20% for the mother and 50% for the fetus. With teenage pregnancy normally a higher risk factor, it is even more important to stress to patients the need for close medical supervision during the entire period of gestation. Folic acid supplementation should be started early in the pregnancy. If vasoocclusive complications begin to appear, usually in the third trimester, conservative management generally includes prophylactic transfusion therapy. Prenatal identification of the hemoglobin status of the fetus can be available as early as 8 to 11 weeks of gestation if desired for consideration of termination of pregnancy. Polymerase chain reaction amplification of specific DNA sequences can yield enough DNA from just a few fetal cells obtained by chorionic villus biopsy, enabling a diagnosis in the first trimester of pregnancy.

Aplastic Crises

To accommodate the shorter RBC life span in sickle cell disease and to maintain a stable hemoglobin level, the bone marrow production is normally 6 to 8 times that of the baseline output. If the marrow production is temporarily inhibited, the 10% to 15% daily fall in hematocrit will cause a profound anemia within a few days. The patient is often pale and easily fatigued, with noticeable pallor. The peripheral blood smear is noteworthy for its lack of the usual polychromasia, reticulocytes, and normoblasts, and bone marrow aspiration shows selective absence of erythroid activity. Within a few days recovery is made evident by brisk reticulocytosis, often mistaken as an episode of increased hemolysis. Aplastic crises, which occasionally have been seen in mini-epidemics, have been linked to parvovirus infections, which cause temporary erythroid aplasia by specific inhibition of the primitive RBC precursor in the marrow (CFU-E).[11] Transfusions are often necessary to keep the patient's condition stable until the bone marrow recovers. A possible role for synthetic erythropoietin or high-dose intravenous gammaglobulin in this setting remains to be established.

Megaloblastic Crises

A frequent problem in regions of poor nutrition, megaloblastic crisis due to folic acid deficiency is now a rare event. The increased RBC turnover in sickle cell disease increases the normal daily requirements of folate to support erythropoietic activity. While most sickle cell patients take supplements of 1 mg folic acid daily, it is unclear whether this is necessary, since a normal diet of folate-fortified foods is the rule rather than the exception in the United States. As noted earlier, the one situation in which daily supplementation is mandatory is adolescent pregnancy.

Sequestration Crises

A serious complication in the very young child, splenic sequestration is a rare event in the adolescent, whose spleen is likely atrophic and fibrotic from years of infarction. Older patients still at risk for this crisis are those with SC or S-β-thalassemia, who have persistent splenomegaly late in life. Typically having no prodrome, the patient is found to be extremely pale, weak, nauseated, and dyspneic and to have tachycardia, severe hypotension, abdominal distention, and cardiac decompensation. The underlying pathophysiologic mechanism is sudden, massive enlargement of the spleen, with trapping of the bulk of circulating RBCs and a life-threatening fall in hemoglobin level. If the condition remains untreated, death often follows within hours from vascular collapse and heart failure. Therefore, the need for early recognition and expeditious institution of therapy is paramount. Rapid correction of shock with plasma expanders and RBC transfusions prevents cardiac decompensation, and within days the spleen returns to normal after mobilization of the pooled blood. In the adolescent who has persistent splenomegaly, one episode of sequestration probably warrants splenectomy because of the risk of recurrence. Another indication for splenectomy in such patients is repeated episodes of splenic infarction.

Infection

Although not a true "crisis," infection remains the single most common cause of mortality in sickle cell disease, accounting for approximately 40% of deaths. In adolescents and adults, the death rate is less often from infection and more often a result of the acute chest syndrome and chronic organ failure, but infections are still an important cause of morbidity, hospitalization, and mortality. The absence of a functioning spleen, with its normal clearing of particulate matter and antibody production, places patients at great risk for overwhelming sepsis, meningitis, and other infections. Defects in the alternate pathway of complement activation; tissue hypoxia from obstructed blood flow; and a deficiency of "tuftsin," a protein that normally promotes phagocytosis, are all additional factors that contribute to the increased incidence of infection. Unlike the situation in younger children, the site of infection in adolescents is frequently evident and the duration often protracted. *Pneumococcus* and *Haemophilus influenzae* bacteria are of greatest concern in the young but are less of a problem in adolescents, who are more often infected with gram-negative organisms. In the adolescent patient with pneumonia accompanied by pleural effusion, *Mycoplasma* infection should be considered as a possibility. *Salmonella* and *Pneumococcus* organisms are the most common identifiable bacterial causes of osteomyelitis and meningitis, respectively.

Although prophylaxis with pneumococcal and *H. influenzae* vaccine boosters should be given in the adolescent years, close observation and early institution of empiric antibiotic therapy in the febrile patient are the mainstays of therapy. Clues differentiating the fever of infection from that of vasoocclusive crisis may include elevated sedimentation rate (usually very low in sickle cell disease), high fever, toxic appearance, and high band count in peripheral blood. However, when the situation is doubtful, antibiotics always must be administered while cultures are pending.

DIAGNOSIS

It is a rare patient with sickle cell disease whose diagnosis has not been established early in life, particularly with newborn screening in effect in most of the United States and other countries. Although establishing the diagnosis is not difficult—requiring only a blood count, a peripheral smear, and hemoglobin electrophoresis—it is important to define the specific subtype of sickle cell disease in order to provide appropriate genetic counseling and to be aware of specific complications associated with each variant. Table 49-1 lists the different laboratory and clinical features of the various forms of sickle cell disease. Besides those listed, common laboratory findings include leukocytosis (white blood cell count, 12,000 to 18,000 cells/mm^3) with a "shift-to-the-left"; thrombocytosis (usual range, 400,000 to 600,000/mm^3) from decreased splenic pooling; low erythrocyte sedimentation rate; and elevated levels of factor VIII, lactic dehydrogenase, and indirect bilirubin. High serum ferritin and low zinc levels are common.

TREATMENT

Patient education and prevention of crises are essential in the management of sickle cell disease. The pathophysiology of sickling should be explained and avoidance of potential sickling triggers emphasized. Specifically, patients should avoid dehydration and temperature extremes, if possible. Prompt attention to fever and infection needs to be stressed continually. Folic acid should be administered, especially for the pregnant patient. With proper education and medical care, survival into middle age can be expected. While the adolescent with sickle cell trait usually only requires genetic counseling regarding the risks of having children with sickle cell disease, information should be supplied regarding some of the infrequent complications seen in people with sickle trait, including hyposthenuria, painful crises in hypoxic environments or dehydrated states, and exaggerated anemia during pregnancy.

Unfortunately, innumerable attempts to develop anti-sickling agents have been unsuccessful. A list that includes urea, low-molecular-weight dextran, anticoagulants, sodium bicarbonate, carbonic anhydrase inhibitors, carbamylating agents, hyperbaric oxygen, cyanate, and cetiedil attests to the varied approaches sought to prevent the sickling process. Attempts to dilute the intracellular sickle hemoglobin with hypotonic intravenous solution and vasopressin, while initially efficacious, proved too toxic and difficult to administer.[12] Therapy for the patient with vasoocclusive crisis remains predominantly symptomatic, with vigorous hydration, bed rest, and correction of the significant electrolyte abnormalities that may be incurred from renal salt wasting. Pain medication, including narcotics, is usually necessary. Such medication is better utilized when given on a fixed schedule rather than an "as needed" basis. Sodium bicarbonate is required only in the event of severe acidosis. Routine use of oxygen should be discouraged because of a lack of efficacy and its potential adverse effects, including suppression of reticulocytosis and rebound erythropoiesis on cessation, which might precipitate another vasoocclusive crisis.

Transfusion therapy plays an important role in several clinical situations. The administration of packed RBCs improves oxygenation, dilutes cells containing sickle hemoglobin with hemoglobin A, suppresses production of new sickle hemoglobin, and decreases blood viscosity. Maintaining hemoglobin S levels at less than 40% is all that is necessary to decrease the blood viscosity more than 50%.[13] Despite many benefits, the risks of infection, RBC sensitization with antibody formation, and hemochromatosis all must be considered before institution of a transfusion program. Indications include sequestration and aplastic crises with profound anemia; severe pneumonia, pulmonary infarction, or other hypoxic situations; central retinal artery occlusion; progressive organ damage (e.g., aseptic necrosis of the femoral or humeral heads, severe renal disease, proliferative retinopathy, chronic skin ulceration, and priapism); complicated pregnancy; and cerebral infarction (to prevent recurrence). Sickle cell disease presents a high risk for anesthesia and surgical complications because of potential acidosis, hypotension, hypoxia, immobilization, and cooling, each of which can trigger sickling. Preoperative transfusions should be administered to lower the sickle percentage to less than 40%. Finally, the patient with recurrent, incapacitating vasoocclusive crises that incur repeated, prolonged hospitalizations is a candidate for a hypertransfusion program. Any patient entering such a program should be treated with nightly subcutaneous deferoxamine to chelate iron and delay the onset of hemochromatosis and further organ damage. In some of these clinical situations, including evolving or acute cerebral infarctions, severe pulmonary infarcts, and severe splenic sequestrations, exchange transfusion can give rapid relief, with expeditious amelioration of the emergency.

FUTURE TRENDS

Although there has been slow progress in the treatment of sickle cell disease during the past few decades, a thorough understanding of the pathophysiologic characteristics of the sickling process, coupled with advances in genetic engineering and other techniques, has yielded some promising new approaches to overcoming the many complications of sickle cell anemia. There are currently three encouraging avenues of exploration that are undergoing further research and trials, as detailed below.

Bone Marrow Transplantation

There have been increasing reported cases of permanent cure in patients with homozygous sickle cell disease who received allogeneic bone marrow transplants.[14] Transplantation (see Chapter 50, "Leukemia") affords the opportunity to eradicate or substantially reduce the abnormal hematopoietic cell line by replacing it with that of a healthy HLA-compatible donor. This has been successful and has been used more extensively for patients with another hemoglobinopathy, thalassemia major, but the treatment still entails a great deal of morbidity and mortality. It probably will not be routinely applied because of preexisting organ damage, which makes the transplant procedure more dangerous for the patient with sickle cell disease. In addition, the enormous cost and manpower involved does not encourage widespread application in its present form. Nevertheless, transplantation has found increased use in several clinical situations, and encouraging reports of transplanted cord-blood stem cells hold promise of another source of donor cells for this patient population.[15]

Stimulation of Fetal Hemoglobin Production

Since fetal hemoglobin interferes with the formation of the sickle polymer, and since patients with hereditary persistence of fetal hemoglobin generally have a much milder clinical course, pharmacologic agents have been used in an attempt to induce greater production of hemoglobin F. After initial limited success with a variety of cancer chemotherapeutic agents, including cytosine arabinoside, 5-azacytidine, and hydroxyurea, several clinical trials have demonstrated a significant reduction in the number of vasoocclusive crises in patients treated with hydroxyurea, resulting in a recommendation for its use in older patients who have had significant sickle-related morbidity.[16-18] Possible mechanisms of this treatment include the recruitment of early RBC precursors during recovery from drug-induced suppression and "hypomethylation" of the DNA template to enhance γ-chain production. Toxicity from the long-term use of these agents is of concern, and safer analogs are being sought. One such group of compounds, the butyric acid family, has shown initial promise in stimulating fetal hemoglobin production,[19,20] but a later study failed to show any sustained clinical response.[21] Further studies need to be done to find optimal compounds and dosing strategies that will have a meaningful effect in patients with sickle cell disease.

Direct Gene Transfer

Another promising approach is direct gene transfer, with insertion of normal DNA, which possesses the ability to produce hemoglobin A, into the patient's erythroid progenitor cells. Recombinant DNA techniques using viral reverse transcriptase have already yielded some success in correction of β-thalassemia[22] and expression of the human β-globin gene in mice.[23,24] Although clinical application of gene transfer on a large scale is still in the future, and there are large hurdles yet to be overcome, these techniques hold much promise for the cure of sickle cell disease, entailing lower morbidity than that from transplantation.

References

1. Pagnier J, Mears JG, Dunda-Belkhodja O, et al: Evidence for the multicentric origin of the sickle hemoglobin in Africa, *Proc Natl Acad Sci* 81:1771-1773, 1984.
2. Heller P, Best WR, Nelson RB, Becktel J: Clinical implications of sickle-cell trait and G6PD deficiency in hospitalized black male patients, *N Engl J Med* 300:1001-1005, 1979.
3. Eaton WA, Hofrichter J, Ross PD: Delay time in gelation: a possible determinant of clinical severity in sickle cell disease, *Blood* 47:621-627, 1976.
4. Rao VM, Fishman M, Mitchell DG, et al: Painful sickle cell crisis: bone marrow patterns observed with MR imaging, *Radiology* 161:211-215, 1986.
5. Van Hoff J, Ritchey AK, Shaywitz BA: Intracranial hemorrhage in children with sickle cell disease, *Am J Dis Child* 139:1120-1123, 1985.
6. Walker BR, Alexander F, Birdsall TR, et al: Glomerular lesions in sickle cell nephropathy, *JAMA* 215:437-440, 1971.
7. O'Neill B, Saunders DE, McFarland DE: Myocardial infarction in sickle cell anemia, *Am J Hematol* 16:139-147, 1984.
8. Platt OS, Rosenstock W, Espeland MA: Influence of sickle hemoglobinopathies on growth and development, *N Engl J Med* 311:7-12, 1984.
9. Alleyne SI, Rausea RD, Serjeant GR: Sexual development and fertility of Jamaican female patients with homozygous sickle cell disease, *Arch Intern Med* 141:1295-1297, 1981.
10. Noe HN, Wilimas J, Jerkins GR: Surgical management of priapism in children with sickle cell anemia, *J Urol* 126:770-771, 1981.
11. Mortimer PP, Humphries RK, Moore JG: A human parvovirus-like virus inhibits haematopoietic colony formation in vitro, *Nature* 302:426-429, 1983.
12. Charache S, Walker WG: Failure of desmopressin to lower sodium or prevent crises in patients with sickle cell anemia, *Blood* 58:892-896, 1981.
13. Anderson R, Cassell M, Mullinax GL, et al: Effect of normal cells in viscosity of sickle cell blood, *Arch Intern Med* 111:286-294, 1963.
14. Ferster A, Devalck C, Azzi N, et al: Bone marrow transplantation for severe sickle cell anaemia, *Br J Haematol* 80:102-105, 1992.
15. Issaragrisil S, Visuthisakchai S, Suvatte V, et al: Brief report: transplantation of cord-blood stem cells into a patient with severe thalassemia, *N Engl J Med* 332:367-369, 1995.
16. Rodgers GP, Dover GJ, Naguchi CT, et al: Hematologic responses of patients with sickle cell disease to treatment with hydroxyurea, *N Engl J Med* 322:1037-1045, 1990.
17. Goldberg MA, Brugnara C, Dover GJ, et al: Treatment of sickle cell anemia with hydroxyurea and erythropoietin, *N Engl J Med* 328:73-80, 1993.
18. Charache S: Experimental therapy of sickle cell disease. Use of hydroxyurea, *Am J Pediatr Hematol Oncol* 16:62-66, 1994.
19. Perrine SP, Ginder GD, Faller DV, et al: A short-term trial of butyrate to stimulate fetal-globin-gene expression in the β-globin disorders, *N Engl J Med* 328:81-86, 1993.
20. Perrine SP, Olivieri NF, Faller DV, et al: Butyrate derivatives. New agents for stimulating fetal globin production in the beta-globin disorders, *Am J Pediatr Hematol Oncol* 16:67-71, 1994.
21. Sher GD, Ginder GD, Little J, et al: Extended therapy with intravenous arginine butyrate in patients with β-hemoglobinopathies, *N Engl J Med* 332:1606-1610, 1995.

22. Constantini F, Chada K, Magram J: Correction of murine β-thalassemia by gene transfer into the germ line, *Science* 233:1192-1194, 1986.
23. Bender MA, Gelinas RE, Miller AD: A majority of mice show long-term expression of a human β-globin gene after retrovirus transfer into hematopoietic stem cells, *Mol Cell Biol* 9:1426-1434, 1989.
24. Ryan TM, Townes TM, Reilly MP, et al: Human sickle hemoglobin in transgenic mice, *Science* 247:566-568, 1990.

Suggested Readings

Nathan DG, Oski FA: *Hematology of infancy and childhood,* ed 4, Philadelphia, 1993, WB Saunders.

Vichinsky E, Lubin BH: Suggested guidelines for the treatment of children with sickle cell anemia, *Hematol Clin North Am* 1:483-501, 1987.

CHAPTER 50

Leukemia

•

Mark E. Weinblatt

Leukemia is the most common malignant disease diagnosed during the adolescent years. While dramatic improvements in long-term survival have been effected during the past four decades, the greatest success has been achieved with young children. A significant increase in cure rate also has been demonstrated among adolescents, but this has not been as great as with younger children, and it usually has been at the price of more intensive therapy and increased adverse effects.

ACUTE LEUKEMIA

Epidemiology

Acute leukemia accounts for approximately 20% of cancers among adolescents. Unlike younger children, in whom acute lymphoblastic leukemia (ALL) is approximately four times more common than acute nonlymphoblastic leukemia (ANLL), ALL in adolescents comprises approximately 50% of the total number of leukemia patients. Although males have a significantly higher incidence of ALL than females, no association with androgenic hormone production has been established. As with younger children, chronic myelogenous leukemia (CML) is a rare disorder among adolescents, accounting for less than 3% of all patients with leukemia.

Etiology

Although the cause of ALL in most patients is unknown, several different factors have been shown to be

associated with the development of this malignancy. The occurrence of leukemia "clusters" and the identification of numerous oncogenic viruses in animals have led many investigators to seek an infectious cause of leukemia.[1] Even though evidence has been scant for most leukemic patients, some success has been obtained with the study of retroviruses. These agents are capable of inserting their genetic code into the germ-line DNA, thus changing the nature of the host cell. The human T-cell lymphotropic virus type I (HTLV-I) has been firmly established as the etiologic agent of cases of T-cell ALL in different parts of the world, and further work is under way to attempt to identify other viruses with similar oncogenic capability. The Epstein-Barr virus (EBV) has been associated with lymphoma, particularly Burkitt's lymphoma in Africa, but no such link has been established in patients with leukemia. It has been suggested that most cases of childhood ALL result from an abnormal immunologic response to a common infection.[2]

Much information has accumulated during this century that implicates radiation in leukemogenesis. Ionizing radiation can damage genetic material in human cells, and, depending on the dose and rapidity of cellular repair, the risk of leukemia is variable. The strongest evidence has been the data collected in Japan after the release of radiation from atomic explosions at Hiroshima and Nagasaki. Three to 10 years after the atomic bombs were detonated, an increased incidence of leukemia was noted in survivors, with children apparently more susceptible than adults. Younger children exposed to radiation were more likely to develop ALL, while postpubertal adolescents and adults had a greater likelihood of contracting acute and chronic myelogenous leukemia. This underscores the complex nature of leukemogenesis, the requirement for whole body irradiation, and the varying susceptibilities of different hematologic cell lines at different ages. Articles describing an increased incidence of childhood leukemia in areas near nuclear power plants and those where weapons are tested often appear in the media, but reports in the scientific literature have been inconclusive.[3-9] There has been no firm evidence of increased risk of leukemia in children who undergo diagnostic radiographic examination or localized radiation therapy for other diseases, or in adults who have had occupational exposure to radiation, but a variety of solid tumors have been linked to radiation exposure.

Substantial exposure to toxic chemicals that cause damage to bone marrow, such as benzene and toluene used in the leather, shoe, and dry cleaning industries, has been associated with leukemia in adults, but direct evidence of this effect in children has not been established. Likewise, proximity to electromagnetic waves associated with high-tension wires has been the subject of several conflicting reports, but to date the association with leukemia remains unconfirmed and increasingly doubtful. A more compelling association has been demonstrated with exposure to antineoplastic cytotoxic agents, particularly alkylating agents such as procarbazine, the nitrosoureas, cyclophosphamide, melphalan, and (most recently) the epipodophyllotoxins etoposide and teniposide. Patients treated with these agents for diseases such as Hodgkin's lymphoma, especially if the agents are administered in conjunction with radiation therapy, have a significantly greater risk of developing a preleukemic syndrome that ultimately transforms into overt leukemia, usually ANLL. Additional associations have been made with immunosuppressive therapy for nonneoplastic conditions such as renal disease, renal transplantation, rheumatoid arthritis, and other autoimmune disorders; however, the risk is still very small and is far outweighed by the benefits of these treatments.

Genetic factors have been shown to play a role in the etiology of pediatric leukemia. Children with Down syndrome (trisomy 21) have a greater than fifteen-fold risk of developing leukemia over the normal population. Approximately 8% of children with Fanconi's anemia, a constitutional aplastic anemia that is usually first manifested in the first decade of life, develop acute myelomonoblastic leukemia in their adolescent years. Patients with other inherited disorders, such as Bloom's syndrome, characterized by a deficiency of DNA ligase 1 needed for DNA repair, and Diamond-Blackfan syndrome, also have been established as having a greater risk of leukemia. These syndromes share features of poor DNA repair that are believed to predispose affected individuals to leukemogenic stimuli. Immune disorders, including severe combined immunodeficiency disease,

Wiskott-Aldrich syndrome, and ataxia telangiectasia (a syndrome characterized by the clinical triad of cerebellar ataxia, ocular telangiectasia, and immunodeficiency), have been linked to higher incidences of leukemia. Increased risks also have been confirmed in children with neurofibromatosis and those in families with siblings who have leukemia or central nervous system tumors.[10] The identical twin of a young child with leukemia has a greater risk of developing that disease than any other population group in early childhood; by adolescence, the relative risk is no greater than that of the average population.

Pathogenesis and Clinical Presentation

Acute leukemia begins in a single somatic hematopoietic progenitor that has undergone transformation to a cell that is no longer capable of normal differentiation and cannot proceed with the normal cellular functions characteristic of the original cell line. Many of these cells no longer possess the normal property of apoptosis, or programmed cell death, thus resulting in a cell that has a dramatically prolonged life span. This new primitive cell can arise from any stage of maturation of hematopoietic differentiation and will undergo clonal proliferation in an unrestricted fashion. The homogeneous features of leukemic cells, as demonstrated by antigenic and isoenzyme analysis, provides abundant proof of the clonal origin of leukemia and has given investigators many clues to the behavior and natural history of this disease. New molecular biology and chromosomal banding techniques have shown that leukemogenesis is frequently associated with chromosome abnormalities and gene translocations, and possibly with the abnormal expression of proto-oncogenes, many of which are human homologues of known viral oncogenes. Many translocations are characteristic of a particular subtype of acute leukemia, and they often convey additional prognostic information to the clinician.

The transformed cell shares many of the antigenic features of the cell of origin, but it lacks the usual regulatory and growth constraints. This constitution enables it to proliferate in a favorable competitive environment at the expense of the normal hematopoietic cell. The decrease in normal cell production in the bone marrow, however, is not a simple matter of competition for nutrients and space. Leukemic cells are able to produce growth factors that can confer longevity to the cell, while secreting other substances that inhibit the maturation and replication of normal hematopoietic cells.

The clonal expansion of the abnormal cell results in a massive accumulation of abnormal cells with qualitative defects. Although this proliferation usually leads to predictable signs and symptoms, the major cause of morbidity and mortality is the paucity of normal functioning, mature hematopoietic cells rather than the presence of malignant cells. Anemia, which is characterized by pallor, fatigue, tachycardia, and headache, is a common finding at diagnosis. While the major pathophysiologic mechanism is related to decreased production in the infiltrated marrow, other contributory factors include decreased red blood cell life span due to sequestration in an enlarged spleen or liver, blood loss resulting from a bleeding diathesis, and hemolysis from infection. A bleeding tendency is another common presenting sign, manifested by skin findings (petechiae and ecchymoses), epistaxis, gingival oozing, and gastrointestinal hemorrhage. This hemorrhagic tendency is usually secondary to thrombocytopenia, again a result of decreased marrow production and decreased platelet life span. Other hemostatic defects may contribute to bleeding, the most serious of which is disseminated intravascular coagulation. This problem occurs in some patients with sepsis and in most patients with acute promyelocytic leukemia when malignant cell destruction releases enormous amounts of procoagulant material contained in the cytoplasm of the cell.

Fever is a common presenting complaint in acute leukemia, and for therapy considerations it must always be presumed to be caused by infection. Predisposition to infection is a consequence of granulocytopenia, with the greatest risk for sepsis present when the absolute granulocyte count is below 200 cells/mm^3. Additional factors that increase the risk of infection include a breach of normal anatomic mucosal and surface barriers (by mucositis, gingivitis, esophagitis, or indwelling tubes and catheters), decreased immunoglobulin production, and the immunosuppressive effects of chemotherapy, particularly corticosteroids and cyclophosphamide. Treatment with broad-spectrum antibiotics encourages overgrowth with opportunistic and resistant organisms that further complicate management.

Other signs and symptoms in adolescents are caused by the proliferation and accumulation of abnormal cells and are similar to those seen in young children and adults. Lymphadenopathy, particularly in the cervical region, is a very common finding in patients with ALL, but less so in those with ANLL. Leukemic cell proliferation usually leads to hepatosplenomegaly. Respiratory distress may result from bronchial compression by mediastinal adenopathy, a common finding in T-cell ALL. The same mediastinal mass also can cause compression of the low-pressure, thin-walled vena cava, which leads to superior vena cava syndrome, manifested by plethora, swelling of the upper torso, neck distention, and headache. A variety of orthopedic symptoms can be seen at presentation. Most commonly in ALL, patients complain of bone pain, a result of periosteal elevation by leukemic cell infiltrates or bone infarctions. Radiographic examination may show typical findings that include metaphy-

seal bands at the distal femurs (not as frequently seen as in early childhood), periosteal new bone formation, and focal lytic lesions. Occasionally the weakened bony cortex leads to pathologic fractures of the extremity or vertebral compression fractures after minimal trauma. Joint swelling, resembling rheumatoid arthritis and unresponsive to nonsteroidal antiinflammatory therapy, is a frequent presentation of acute leukemia.

Central nervous system (CNS) involvement is uncommon at initial diagnosis, but it can appear at any time during follow-up and is associated with a variety of symptoms. Central nervous system disease is believed to result from direct spread of leukemic cells from marrow in the cranium to the leptomeninges and then to the cerebrospinal fluid. The most common complaints are related to signs of elevated intracranial pressure; these include headache, nausea and emesis, lethargy, irritability, and papilledema. Cranial nerve involvement, most often facial (Bell's palsy) and abducens (esotropia), may appear as an isolated finding or in combination with other manifestations. Severe thrombocytopenia can lead to subdural or subarachnoid hemorrhage, often with devastating consequences. A unique, rarely seen "hypothalamic syndrome," characterized by hyperphagia, weight gain, irritability, and diabetes insipidus, is a result of selective involvement of the satiety center of the brain. Spinal lesions rarely have been reported, although in ANLL blast cells periodically form large aggregates leading to epidural compression. Although parenchymal involvement of the brain is rare, extreme leukocytosis with white blood cell (WBC) counts of more than 200,000 cells/mm^3 is often associated with hyperviscosity, intracerebral leukostasis, and intracerebral hemorrhage early in the course of the disease. This condition must therefore be dealt with as an emergency. Cerebrovascular accidents also can be a consequence of infection, particularly with fungi such as *Candida* and *Aspergillus* species.

Unlike the situation in adults, weight loss and cachexia are unusual findings in adolescents with leukemia. These effects can result from a combination of increased catabolic nutritional state and decreased caloric intake from anorexia. Metabolic complications, including hyperkalemia, hypocalcemia, hyperuricemia, and lactic acidosis, are commonly experienced in patients presenting with large leukemic cell burdens. Different subtypes of acute leukemia often have additional characteristic sites of involvement that may present special problems. Soft tissue masses known as chloromas are occasionally seen in ANLL; these masses can appear around the orbit, breast, or spinal cord. Purple papular skin lesions called leukemids are characteristic of monoblastic leukemia subtypes. The monoblastic leukemias are also often associated with gingival hyperplasia, a sanctuary site in which blast cells are often very difficult to eradicate. Testicular involvement, rare at presentation but a persistent problem in patients with ALL, usually presents as a painless, unilateral, firm swelling. Ocular manifestations are infrequent, but leukemic cells can infiltrate all parts of the eye, with the retina and iris most commonly affected. Iritis often causes photophobia, pain, and increased lacrimation, whereas retinal involvement, often accompanied by hemorrhage, can lead to loss of vision. Although many organs such as the kidneys, intestines, and liver may be infiltrated by leukemic cells, it is very uncommon to see dysfunction resulting from this involvement. Weakening of the intestinal wall accompanied by bacterial overgrowth can lead to typhlitis, a devastating inflammation and perforation of the cecum that is often fatal.

Diagnosis and Evaluation

The differential diagnosis of leukemia includes many disorders that can cause hematopoietic cytopenia or hypertrophy of organs of the reticuloendothelial system. Numerous infections can mimic leukemia, with the most ubiquitous caused by EBV. Symptoms of EBV infection may include fever, lymphadenopathy, hepatosplenomegaly, selective cytopenias, or pancytopenia, all similar to those in a child presenting with leukemia; examination of the bone marrow may sometimes be necessary to establish the correct diagnosis. Cytomegalovirus infection, tuberculosis, and AIDS all can present with features similar to those of leukemia. Other malignancies (e.g., lymphoma, sarcoma, and neuroblastoma) and autoimmune disorders (e.g., systemic lupus erythematosus) need to be considered in the patient with organomegaly and cytopenia. Marrow failure syndromes and immune cytopenias (e.g., immune thrombocytopenia purpura) can produce similar symptoms, although usually without enlarged lymph nodes or spleen. Finally, storage disorders (e.g., Gaucher's disease) can cause organomegaly, with associated symptoms of pancytopenia, as hematopoietic cells are sequestered and destroyed. In addition to the disturbances in blood count and the identification of blast cells on blood-smear examination, supportive evidence for the diagnosis of leukemia can readily be found in other blood tests. Both serum uric acid and lactic dehydrogenase levels are frequently elevated as a consequence of increased cell proliferation and destruction. Serum muramidase levels are usually increased in patients with monocytic leukemias.

Persistent neutropenia is a common hematologic abnormality that is often a presenting feature of leukemia, but it is more frequently a result of other processes. Confusing the picture further are neutropenia-related infections, including cutaneous cellulitis, abscesses, pneumonia, septicemia, and perirectal inflammation, features often seen in a child presenting with leukemia, but also associated with granulocytopenia of other causes.

The risk of pyogenic infections is inversely proportional to the level of neutropenia, with mild neutropenia (absolute neutrophil count of 1000 to 1500/mm^3) conferring no increased risk of infections, while severe neutropenia, with a neutrophil count below 500/mm^3, substantially increases the likelihood of contracting bacterial or fungal infections. The underlying pathophysiology of the neutropenia often further contributes to the threat of infection. Those adolescents who develop antibody-mediated neutropenia after viral infections are much less likely to develop serious infections. This picture is not an uncommon finding after infection with hepatitis, measles, rubella, varicella, or EBV. As opposed to children with leukemia, these patients usually have normal platelet and erythrocyte counts, and frequently have associated monocytosis that provides some protection against pyogenic infections. Diagnosis can be established by detecting elevated levels of antineutrophil antibodies. Although the low granulocyte count may persist, special precautions and restrictions are usually not warranted. Other antibody-mediated neutropenias that are secondary to underlying immune disorders, including systemic lupus erythematosus and Felty's syndrome (splenomegaly, rheumatoid arthritis, leukopenia), more commonly present with other physical findings and laboratory abnormalities. Cyclic neutropenia in teenagers will nearly always have been diagnosed earlier in life, having established a typical pattern of oral ulcers, stomatitis, and adenitis during periods of neutropenia, and are not typically confused with leukemia. This disorder is caused by a regulatory defect within the hematopoietic stem cell present from birth and can be easily diagnosed by following twice weekly blood counts for several weeks. Another chronic neutropenia is seen in Shwachman's syndrome, an autosomal recessive disorder characterized by pancreatic exocrine deficiency, neutropenia, and dwarfism, again nearly always diagnosed early in life. An important part of the initial investigation includes a drug history, since many medications can cause neutropenia. Some of the more well-known examples include the sulfa and penicillin families, chloramphenicol, indomethacin, antithyroid medications, the phenothiazines, barbiturates, and anticonvulsants (especially phenytoin and carbamazepine)—the mechanism of action can be either direct marrow suppression or an immune response. Many serious infections, including typhoid fever, tuberculosis, rickettsial infections, and bacterial sepsis, can cause neutropenia and can sometimes mimic leukemia, which can be associated with the same infection—failure to recover a normal granulocyte count after appropriate clinical response to antibiotics should raise concerns about possible marrow infiltration. Finally, other disorders associated with neutropenia, including megaloblastic anemia, anorexia nervosa, copper deficiency, and pronounced splenomegaly, usually can be differentiated from

TABLE 50-1
Associated Findings in Leukemia Cell Subtypes

Characteristics	Subtype
Clinical	
Mediastinal mass	T-cell ALL
Gingival hypertrophy	ANLL: M4, M5
Disseminated intravascular coagulation	APML: M3
Chloroma	ANLL
Syndromes	
Fanconi's anemia	ANLL: M4, M5
Klinefelter's syndrome	ANLL
Shwachman's syndrome	ANLL
Morphologic	
Auer bodies	ANLL: M1-M3
Hypergranulation	APML: M3
Vacuolated basophilic cytoplasm	ALL: L3 (Burkitt's)
Membrane Related	
Common ALL antigen (CALLA)	Common ALL
Surface immunoglobulin	B-cell ALL
T antigens	T-cell ALL
B antigens	B-cell ALL
Cytoplasm	
Leukocyte alkaline phosphate	Low in CML
Periodic acid–Schiff (PAS)	ALL
Myeloperoxidase	ANLL
Chloroacetate esterase	ANLL: M1-M4
Terminal deoxynucleotidyl transferase (TdT)	Common ALL, T-cell ALL
Cytogenetics	
t(9;22)-Ph[1]	CML
t(15;17)	ANLL: M3
t(4;11)	ALL in infants
t(8;14)	ALL: L3 (Burkitt's)
Serum	
Muramidase	ANLL: M4, M5
Lactic dehydrogenase	Elevated with hyperleukocytosis

leukemia with a good history and physical examination and routine screening laboratory studies.

Even when the patient presents with classic signs and symptoms and with many abnormal biochemical values, the definitive test for the diagnosis of leukemia is the demonstration of an abnormal proliferation of the primitive cell line at the expense of normal hematopoietic cells in the bone marrow. After initial confirmation of the diagnosis of leukemia, determining the leukemic subtype is of paramount importance, since the behavior of each one can vary and the treatment must take into consideration the behavior and natural history of that particular leukemia. In the past, morphologic and histochemical tests were the only tools available to the clinician.

Currently, the diagnosis of leukemia in childhood cancer centers is aided by sophisticated cytogenetic and immunophenotyping technologies that allow an extensive characterization of leukemic cell subtypes (Table 50-1). The first step in identification of the leukemia subtype rests with the morphologic description of the leukemic blast cell. Classification of leukemias follows the modified French-American-British (FAB) system, which separates the lymphoid leukemias into three groups (L1-3) and the nonlymphoblastic varieties into seven major subtypes (M1-7). This classification system, which is based on both nuclear and cytoplasmic characteristics, has been found to yield prognostic information regarding the patient. The L1 cell, also known as the "common ALL" cell type, is usually small and homogeneous, with scanty cytoplasm and rare nucleoli. L2 cells, the "undifferentiated leukemia" cell type, are noteworthy for more abundant cytoplasm, heterogeneous size distribution, and prominent nucleoli. This cell type is more common in adolescents than in young children with ALL and is often indicative of a poorer outcome. Finally, L3 cells, or Burkitt's cells, are unique, with their deeply basophilic and highly vacuolated cytoplasm; these cells nearly always demonstrate B-cell characteristics and are pathognomonic of "Burkitt's leukemia." The nonlymphoblastic leukemias include myeloblastic (M1, M2), promyelocytic (M3), myelomonoblastic (M4), monoblastic (M5a, M5b), erythroleukemia (M6), and megakaryoblastic (M7). Each has characteristic findings that are often related to the cell line from which they arise. For instance, cytoplasmic granulation and the presence of Auer bodies are the hallmark of the M1-3 cell types, while monocytic nuclear convolutions are found in M4 and M5. The M6 subtype exhibits prominent erythroid hyperplasia with megaloblastic and dyserythropoietic features, while megakaryoblastic leukemia is characterized by extensive marrow fibrosis and a positive factor VIII antigen.

Complete evaluation of the marrow sample requires a combination of histochemical, immunologic, and cytogenic techniques. Cytochemical testing usually offers further support for the morphologic impression. The periodic acid–Schiff (PAS) reaction is the only consistently positive one to be expected in the lymphoid leukemias. Sudan black and myeloperoxidase are usually strongly positive in ANLL cells, with further differentiation aided by reactions to nonspecific esterase and chloroacetate esterase, positive in monoblastic and myeloblastic subtypes, respectively.

The advent of monoclonal antibody technology has allowed further characterization of the leukemic cell by providing an abundant source of antibodies directed against surface and cytoplasmic antigens, thus enabling the identification of the cell line and the stage of differentiation from which the leukemic clone arose. The most important immunophenotyping in ALL includes the use of B-cell and T-cell markers, in addition to the common ALL antigen (CALLA) antibody test. This classification into immunophenotypic subtypes yields further prognostic information. The presence of T-cell features, more common in adolescents than in younger children, is a poor prognostic finding. Although similar differentiation can be obtained in ANLL by testing the cells against a monoclonal panel of antibodies directed against myeloid and monocytoid surface markers, prognostic information is less evident.

Improved cytogenetic techniques provide additional insight into the nature of the leukemic cell. Abnormal chromosome markers, which are found in most patients with ANLL and in increasing numbers of ALL patients, can be used for diagnostic corroboration, detection of residual disease during treatment, and diagnosis of relapse. The most common findings are translocations, several of which are specific for a particular leukemic subtype. Typical ALL translocations include t(9;22) (q34;q11), t(1;19) (q23;p13.3), and t(8;14) (q24;q32) in Burkitt's leukemia. Frequent AML translocations include t(8;21) (q22;q22), inv(16) (p13;q22), t(9;11) (p21-22; q23), and (in most patients with acute promyelocytic leukemia) t(15;17) (q22;q11-21). In patients with ALL, chromosomal ploidy is a more important prognostic factor, with cells exhibiting hyperploid karyotypes (>50 chromosomes) having a more favorable outcome while a hypodiploid pattern (<45 chromosomes) confers a high-risk, poor prognostic feature. The presence of the Philadelphia chromosome is considered a poor prognostic factor found in only a small percentage of acute leukemia patients, many of whom are diagnosed as they are entering a blast crisis of previously undetected CML.

In addition to an evaluation of the patient's hematologic and biochemical parameters and an assessment of leukemic cells in the bone marrow, certain procedures are necessary to complete the patient work-up at the time of diagnosis. Cerebrospinal fluid must be obtained to detect the presence of leukemic cells in the CNS. A chest radiograph examination is required to detect a mediastinal mass. Baseline function studies of the heart and kidneys usually are necessary before treatment with potentially hazardous medications is begun. Only after such a thorough evaluation is the patient ready to begin therapy.

Prognosis and Treatment

Acute lymphoblastic leukemia. The substantial progress made in the treatment of ALL during the past three decades has primarily been the result of the efforts of national and international collaborative cancer treatment groups that have participated in cooperative studies to better understand the biology and natural history of leukemia, while devising treatment strategies building on the results of earlier therapeutic trials. Part of this progress includes the identification of risk factors that determine a patient's outlook at diagnosis and in some cases by initial response to treatment; it also involves the accrual of patients into treatment groups to compare the effects of different therapeutic regimens. As mentioned earlier, age itself is an important prognostic factor, with adolescence clearly a poorer determinant of outcome than childhood, yet far better than adulthood. Besides age, adolescents have a greater incidence of other poor risk factors indicative of a greater "leukemic burden," including higher WBC count, hepatosplenomegaly, massive lymphadenopathy, mediastinal mass, elevated hemoglobin levels, T-cell markers ("lymphomatous presentation"), and a greater male-to-female ratio. Other high risk

TABLE 50-2
Common Chemotherapeutic Agents Used in the Treatment of Malignancy

Drug	Mechanism of Action	Major Adverse Effects
Actinomycin-D	Intercalation	A, B, E, M, mucositis
Amsacrine*	Intercalation	E, GI, H, M
L-Asparaginase	L-asparagine depletion	E, Anaphylaxis, pancreatitis, coagulopathy
5-Azacytidine*	Inhibition of DNA synthesis	E, GI, H, M
Bleomycin	DNA strand breaks	E, Anaphylaxis, pneumonitis and pulmonary fibrosis
Busulfan	Alkylation	A, E, M, pulmonary fibrosis
Carboplatinum	Platination and cross-linking	E, M, nephrotoxicity, ototoxicity
Carmustine (BCNU)	Alkylation and cross-linking	E, M, pulmonary fibrosis
Chlorambucil	Alkylation	H, M, pulmonary fibrosis
Cisplatin	Platination and cross-linking	E, nephrotoxicity, ototoxicity
Cyclophosphamide	Alkylation	A, M, E, SIADH, hemorrhagic cystitis
Cytosine arabinoside	Inhibition of DNA polymerase	A, M, E, GI, H, fever, neurotoxicity
Dacarbazine (DTIC)	Alkylation	A, E, GI, H, M, pain on administration
Daunomycin	Intercalation and free radicals	A, B, M, E, cardiotoxicity, mucositis
Dexamethasone	Lympholysis	Weight gain, hypertension, hyperglycemia
Doxorubicin	Intercalation and free radicals	A, B, M, E, cardiotoxicity, mucositis
Etoposide (VP-16)	DNA strand breaks	A, E, GI, H, M, hypotension
5-Fluorouracil	Inhibits thymidine synthesis	A, E, GI, M, mucositis, neurotoxicity
Hydroxyurea	Inhibition of DNA synthesis	E, M, mucositis
Idarubicin	Intercalation and free radicals	A, B, M, E, cardiotoxicity, mucositis
Ifosfamide	Alkylation	A, M, E, hemorrhagic cystitis, nephrotoxicity
Lomustine (CCNU)	Alkylation and cross-linking	E, M, phlebitis, pulmonary fibrosis
Melphalan	Alkylation and cross-linking	M, pulmonary fibrosis
6-Mercaptopurine	Purine synthesis inhibition	M, H
Methotrexate	Folate antagonist	E, GI, H, M, mucositis, neurotoxicity
Mitoxantrone	Inhibition of DNA synthesis	A, E, GI, M, cardiotoxicity
Nitrogen mustard	Alkylation	A, B, E, GI, M, mucositis, pulmonary fibrosis
Paclitaxel	Antimicrotubule	M, A, E, anaphylaxis, hypotension, neuropathy
Prednisone	Lympholysis	Weight gain, hypertension, hyperglycemia
Procarbazine	Alkylation and free radicals	E, M, rash, neurotoxicity
6-Thioguanine	Purine synthesis inhibition	M, H
Thiotepa	Alkylation and free radicals	E, M, pulmonary fibrosis
Vinblastine	Mitotic inhibition	A, B, E, M, peripheral neuropathy
Vincristine	Mitotic inhibition	A, B, peripheral neuropathy

A, alopecia; *B*, burn on extravasation; *E*, emesis; *GI*, gastrointestinal; *H*, hepatotoxicity; *M*, myelosuppression; *SIADH*, syndrome of inappropriate antidiuretic hormone secretion.
*Investigational.

factors at presentation include L2 and L3 morphology, CNS involvement, hypoploidy, the presence of translocations, and slow response to therapy. Because of the overall poorer outlook, the Children's Cancer Group (CCG) and others currently treat all adolescents who have ALL with intense regimens that have recently proved effective in overcoming some of these high risk factors.

The numerous chemotherapeutic agents (Table 50-2) used in the treatment of leukemia and other malignancies rely on small qualitative or quantitative differences between normal and malignant cells. Treatment strategies are based on principles of drug synergism, nonadditive toxicity, and cell kinetics. More recent approaches have emphasized vigorous attempts to eliminate the maximal number of abnormal cells in the shortest possible time. Multiagent regimens use intense "pulsed" phases to recruit cells in the resting phase of the cell cycle into a more drug-sensitive phase and to avoid the emergence of a resistant clone.

In more than 95% of adolescents, the initial 4-week phase of treatment is successful in inducing a clinical remission characterized by the virtual disappearance of leukemic cells and a normalization of all blood counts and marrow cell morphology. The subsequent phase of therapy, intensification or consolidation, is aimed at further reducing the number of residual leukemic cells while including prophylactic or therapeutic CNS treatment with a combination of intrathecal chemotherapy and cranial vault radiation. Finally, the maintenance phase of treatment, which lasts from 2 to 3 years, attempts to further eliminate any remaining leukemic cells. The most recent clinical trials from CCG have yielded long-term, event-free survival (and probable cure) in approximately 50% to 60% of adolescents with ALL; there was greater survival in patients without some of the high-risk prognostic features.

ACUTE NONLYMPHOBLASTIC LEUKEMIA. While more dramatic improvements in life expectancy have been achieved in ALL, progress has been much slower in the nonlymphoblastic leukemias. A much larger percentage of patients with this disease never achieve a complete hematologic remission, often succumbing during the first few weeks to serious infections or bleeding. This is a direct result of the much longer period of pancytopenia that these patients usually must endure during the intense induction therapy that is necessary to achieve hematologic recovery. Patients with acute promyelocytic leukemia must contend with disseminated intravascular coagulation, which creates difficult hemostatic management problems, although this subgroup of ANLL appears to have a better overall survival. In addition, sanctuary areas peculiar to these subtypes, such as the skin and gingiva, make it difficult to eradicate all sites of disease completely, resulting in reseeding of the bone marrow with malignant cells. On the other hand, CNS and testicular relapses are less common than in ALL.

Current treatment regimens use combinations of an anthracycline and cytosine arabinoside, which are successful in inducing remission in about 80% to 85% of patients. Those patients who have successfully completed induction therapy then undergo a very intense period of consolidation, which has successfully maintained long-term remission in about half of these patients. The best results of consolidation from the 1970s and early 1980s were achieved with bone marrow transplantation, although recent data suggest that almost similar results can be realized with intense chemotherapy, using very-high-dose cytosine arabinoside, without recourse to marrow transplantation. Recent reports also have cast doubt on the value of maintenance therapy in ANLL. Ongoing clinical trials are now in progress comparing chemotherapy with autologous bone marrow transplant for patients who lack a suitably matched marrow donor.

A recent significant addition to the clinician's therapeutic armamentarium shown to be effective against acute promyelocytic leukemia is trans-retinoic acid (TRA). This orally administered, vitamin A derivative has successfully induced more than 90% of newly diagnosed, as well as relapsed, patients into a complete hematologic remission. Rather than act as a cytotoxic agent, TRA induces the promyelocytes to mature into normal granulocytes, thus minimizing some of the undesirable myelosuppresive effects of chemotherapy and the adverse effects of cell lysis, especially disseminated intravascular coagulation and tumor lysis syndrome. Careful attention must be paid to avoid the so-called "retinoic acid syndrome" heralded by a rising WBC count, and manifested by often fatal pulmonary leukostasis and respiratory distress. Once remission is achieved, more traditional consolidation treatment with chemotherapy and/or bone marrow transplantation is necessary to maintain the remission.

Supportive Care

Equally important as chemotherapy in the management of the adolescent with leukemia are issues of supportive care. Prolonged periods of disease or treatment-induced cytopenias render patients at risk for hemorrhagic and infectious complications. Anemia and thrombocytopenia require the availability and judicious use of selective blood products, preferably from limited donor pools, and irradiated to reduce the possibility of graft-versus-host disease (GVHD) in these severely immunocompromised patients. Prophylactic and empiric broad-spectrum antibiotic therapy is mandatory to protect and treat the patient at risk for a host of opportunistic infections. Periods of neutropenia can be shortened by daily administration of granulocyte monocyte-colony stimulating factor (GM-CSF), significantly reducing the risk of infections. The use of indwelling right atrial central catheters facilitates administration of chemotherapeutic agents, blood products, and other medications, but it also serves as an additional source of infection. Indwelling subcutaneous "ports" located beneath the skin, with no external component and no breach in the overlying skin barrier, have decreased the risk of infection while affording adolescents the freedom of showering and swimming without fear of introducing infection. Careful attention to fluid and electrolyte therapy is mandatory in the face of large leukemic cell burdens, and proper nutritional support is necessary to ensure the best possible outlook. In cases of extreme hyperleukocytosis, immediate intervention is mandatory to reduce the WBC count expeditiously with chemotherapy, exchange transfusion, or leukapheresis. Early cranial vault radiation is considered by many to be beneficial for the patient with neurologic deficits associated with high WBC counts.

A number of problems and special situations are often encountered in the adolescent patient. Varicella and rubeola, potentially life-threatening infections in patients with leukemia, are less of a concern in most adolescents, who usually possess immunity to the diseases. Likewise, long-term adverse psychological, neuroendocrinologic, and growth effects resulting from prophylactic cranial vault radiation are less of a problem than in young children. However, adolescents often have more difficulty with some aspects of treatment than do younger children. Intrathecal chemotherapy, a mainstay of CNS prophylaxis, results in a higher incidence of arachnoiditis and post–lumbar tap headache and back pain in adolescents. The postpubertal patient is also more likely to have decreased gonadal function, including a greater risk of sterility as a result of therapy with medications such as cyclophosphamide. The pregnant adolescent poses additional special problems. Although the prognosis and behavior of leukemia is unaffected by pregnancy, there is a significantly increased risk of bleeding and infection in pregnant patients. The fetus is at high risk of the teratogenic effects of chemotherapy during the first trimester, as well as spontaneous abortion and premature delivery at any stage of gestation. Fortunately, it is extremely rare for vertical transmission of leukemia to the infant to occur.

The developmental and psychosocial demands of adolescence often affect the treatment. The cosmetic effects of chemotherapy and radiation (e.g., alopecia, weight gain, cushingoid facies, acne, dermatitis) result in negative feelings in most adolescents, who are concerned about their appearance and wish to conform to that of their peers. Fatigue, nausea, anxiety, loss of control, and forced absence from school and other activities often lead to fear, anger, isolation, and depression. All these feelings can have a significant effect on the patient's willingness to comply with demanding treatment schedules, and poor compliance is another reason for the poorer outcome in adolescents. The clinician's understanding of normal adolescent transitions and being available to support the patient through this particularly trying time is therefore of paramount importance when treating the adolescent with leukemia.

CHRONIC MYELOGENOUS LEUKEMIA

As opposed to acute leukemia, the patient with CML, which represents only a small percentage of the adolescent leukemic population, often presents with minimal symptoms. This reflects the fact that while an abnormal clonal proliferation is present, normal bone marrow function is preserved until late in the course of the disease. This myeloproliferative disorder, which evolves from a multilineage stem cell, involves all the hematopoietic cell lines and some of the lymphoid lines. The abnormal clone that seems insensitive to normal regulatory mechanisms ultimately expands to become the predominant cell in the bone marrow and blood. At initial presentation, patients are often found to have splenomegaly, pallor, and bone pain without the bleeding and infections that are the hallmark of the acute leukemias. Although fever is sometimes noted, this may be due to increased metabolic activity or leukocyte pyrogen release rather than infection. Those patients with more pronounced hyperleukocytosis complain of symptoms related to leukostasis, including respiratory distress, visual complaints, priapism, and neurologic difficulties (including strokes).

At diagnosis, adolescents characteristically have a higher WBC count than adults (median of $250,000/mm^3$), with circulating myeloid cells in all stages of differentiation. Eosinophilia and basophilia are common and frequently pronounced. Anemia is usually mild and significant thrombocytosis is often present. The bone marrow usually exhibits granulocytic hyperplasia, with myelofibrosis appearing only late in the disease. Elevations of vitamin B_{12} and serum lactic dehydrogenase are usually found. A useful marker of this disease is decreased leukocyte alkaline phosphatase activity, which may result from relatively decreased monocyte mass.[11] Granulocytes also have been shown to have diminished phagocytic and chemotactic activity that often worsens with disease progression.

The hallmark of the patient with CML is the presence of the Philadelphia chromosome, a partially deleted no. 22 chromosome, the deleted portion of which has been translocated to the long arm of chromosome no. 9; t(9;22) (q34;q11) translocation is most common, found in 90% of CML patients. The translocated DNA contains the c-abl proto-oncogene (the human homologue of a murine leukemia virus oncogene) that interacts with the breakpoint cluster region (bcr) of the no. 22 chromosome to produce an 8-Kb m-RNA hybrid, which can serve as a marker for this disease.[12,13] Patients with Ph[1]-negative CML tend to have a shorter chronic phase with a poorer response to therapy for blast crisis.

Patients with CML generally experience prolonged asymptomatic survival until there is a "blastic transformation" to an acute leukemia or the development of myelofibrosis with resultant pancytopenia. After an average of approximately 3 years, the chronic phase of CML undergoes a transformation to a far more aggressive form characterized by a higher WBC count, usually with a shift to more primitive cells. As the blast-cell proportion rises, the disease becomes indistinguishable from the acute leukemias, with symptoms and signs related to both increased cell proliferation and decreased normal hematopoietic elements. Usually accompanying, and sometimes preceding, this conversion is the appearance of other abnormal chromosome markers, commonly a hyperdiploid picture that includes other trisomies and duplication of the Ph[1] chromosome. Once the blast transformation has occurred, the disease usually progresses relentlessly, with only temporary remissions to the chronic phase in some patients.

With the improved prognosis due to the development of effective chemotherapeutic regimens for the treatment of acute leukemia, the relative prognosis for the patient with CML has changed from the best among the leukemias to the worst. Although rising blood cell counts in the chronic phase of the disease can be controlled with medications such as hydroxyurea and busulfan, leukapheresis, splenic radiation, or splenectomy (all of which can improve the quality of life by decreasing the degree of splenomegaly and preventing complications such as respiratory distress, neurologic dysfunction, and priapism), none have had any significant influence on the duration of survival. Interferon can induce hematologic remission in chronic-phase CML and has demonstrated increasing promise in this patient population. The median survival with standard chemotherapy has remained about 40 months, with a poorer outlook expected in the patient with enlarged spleen, high WBC count, greater percentage of immature cells, eosinophilia, or basophilia at presentation.

While traditional multiagent chemotherapy has not resulted in an appreciable difference in the outcome of CML, bone marrow transplantation prior to blastic transformation has been used to achieve some measure of success. The best results have been obtained in patients who receive marrow from a human leukocyte antigen (HLA)-matched sibling while they are still in the first chronic phase, with more than half enjoying long-term survival and possibly cure. Adolescents fare better than adults with transplantation but tend to have a greater degree of GVHD than do younger children, resulting in significant morbidity and mortality. For the patient with no histocompatible donor, investigators are having varying success with a number of experimental techniques, including T cell–depleted, mismatched bone marrow transplants and autologous transplants using the patient's hematopoietic stem cells harvested from the peripheral blood.

BONE MARROW TRANSPLANTATION

As more aggressive chemotherapeutic regimens began to yield increasing numbers of remissions and cures during the past two decades, further progress was hindered by the primary limiting factor in chemotherapy dose escalation, myelosuppression. This factor became more important after the demonstration that many malignancies had a dose-related response to antineoplastic drugs. The use of higher doses of bone marrow–suppressive medications became possible with the development of bone marrow "rescue," which allows patients to receive supralethal doses of chemotherapy and radiation that are ablative to their own marrow.

Initially used in patients with aplastic anemia and those requiring immune reconstitution for immunodeficiency diseases, bone marrow transplantation (BMT) now plays an important role in the treatment of a variety of malignant diseases previously refractory to most standard chemotherapeutic regimens. For patients with leukemia and other malignancies involving the patient's own marrow, the bulk of experience has been gleaned with the use of marrow obtained from twins or histocompatible donors, usually siblings. Potential donors are screened for compatibility using the HLA system, and compatibility is then confirmed by mixed lymphocyte culture or DNA analysis. Marrow is harvested by multiple needle aspirations from the healthy donor, with the donor usually under general anesthesia in the operating room. The marrow is mixed with an anticoagulant and then stored in a sterile container after large particulate matter has been filtered. The recipient is treated with ablative doses of chemotherapy, with or without total body radiation, in an attempt to eradicate the last malignant cell and to suppress the patient's immune system so that the marrow graft is accepted. The donor marrow is then infused intravenously. The stem cells "home in" on the patient's marrow, where they proliferate, differentiate, and repopulate the marrow with normal hematopoietic elements. The pretransplant treatment usually renders the patient pancytopenic for several weeks, during which time comprehensive supportive care is mandatory. Severe immunosuppression will persist for many months.

Several special situations still need to be overcome to further the usefulness of BMT. Although graft rejection has not been a significant problem in the adolescent with malignancy, GVHD mediated by T lymphocytes in the marrow graft has been a persistent source of concern. This pathologic process targets specific organs and sites, including the skin, liver, marrow, and intestinal tract, and occurs in 30% to 70% of patients receiving HLA-identical bone marrow. Acute GVHD appears in the first 3 months after marrow infusion. It usually is manifested by skin rash (progressing from a maculopapular eruption to a confluent, erythematous rash with desquamation and bullae), liver dysfunction, diarrhea, and pancytopenia. Chronic GVHD, occurring after 100 days from the day of transplant and usually seen in patients who also sustained the acute form, is often more generalized, resulting in thickening of the skin or scleroderma, jaundice, weight loss, dystrophic ophthalmologic changes, pulmonary dysfunction, and Coombs'-positive hemolytic anemia. Prophylaxis with methotrexate, antithymocyte globulin, and (more recently) cyclosporine has been effective in decreasing the incidence and severity of GVHD. Prednisone, cyclosporine, azathioprine, and thalidomide are used to treat chronic GVHD, a potentially debilitating and often lethal development in transplant patients. One beneficial result of mild GVHD is a graft-versus-leukemia effect, with fewer relapses observed in patients with mild cases of GVHD. Attempts to completely eradicate GVHD by T-cell purging of donor marrow before infusion have resulted in increased engraftment failures and increased incidence of leukemic relapses, suggesting a beneficial role of donor T cells.

Interstitial pneumonitis is one of the most important transplant complications, with a very high mortality rate. Although the incidence has decreased with the use of hyperfractionated total body radiation, this disorder is seen frequently in patients with severe GVHD. Interstitial pneumonitis is often related to infections such as cytomegalovirus, *Pneumocystis carinii,* herpesvirus, and adenovirus. Prophylactic administration of ganciclovir and acyclovir has effected a decrease in the incidence of cytomegalovirus and herpes simplex infections, respectively. High-dose intravenous gammaglobulin also seems to be beneficial in preventing viral disease. Fungi remain important pathogens in transplant patients, with a somewhat lower incidence observed in laminar airflow units. More intense preconditioning regimens also have led to an increasing incidence of venoocclusive disease of the liver as well as severe renal dysfunction. Parenteral nutrition is usually necessary because of the mucositis and anorexia that result from therapy. Other late effects of transplantation include thyroid and gonadal dysfunction, sterility, cataracts, and secondary malignancies.

Because of progress made in overcoming the many acute and chronic complications of transplantation, therapeutic results in different malignancies have become more encouraging, and BMT is being used for an ever-widening range of diseases. BMT is currently used in several leukemic situations especially pertinent to adolescents, including first-remission ANLL; second-remission and select first-remission, high-risk ALL; and CML in its chronic or early accelerated phase. A further broadening of application has come with the use of autologous BMT, in which the patient's own marrow (and in some instances peripheral stem cells harvested from the blood) is used, thus eliminating GVHD and marrow rejection and decreasing the need for immunosuppressive therapy. This approach is particularly useful for disorders such as brain tumors, lymphomas, and sarcomas, in which marrow involvement is less common. Marrow-purging methods using chemotherapeutic agents, physical techniques, and monoclonal antibodies are more generally available and allow autologous transplants in leukemia and neuroblastoma patients with minimal residual disease. National and international donor registries are helping to locate unrelated HLA-matched donors, thus offering additional options for BMT. The use of more specific T-cell depletion and marrow conditioning in combination with more effective GVHD prophylaxis is permitting more BMTs across the HLA barrier without severe GVHD or marrow failure, thus further expanding the pool of potential marrow donors. Finally, the availability of biologic-response modifiers such as erythropoietin, GM-CSF, and the interleukins is allowing more rapid recovery from severe pancytopenia, thus shortening the period of infection risk. The more widespread use of these hematopoietic enhancers should make BMT an increasingly successful and useful modality in the treatment of malignancy in adolescents.

References

1. Heath CW, Hasterlik RJ: Leukemia among children in a suburban community, *Am J Med* 34:796-812, 1963.
2. Greaves M: A natural history for pediatric acute leukemia, *Blood* 82:1043-1051, 1993.
3. Machado SG, Land CE, McKay FW: Cancer mortality and radioactive fallout in southwestern Utah, *Am J Epidemiol* 125:44-61, 1987.
4. Black D: New evidence on childhood leukaemia and nuclear establishments, *Br Med J* 294:591-592, 1987.
5. Narod SA: Radiation, genetics and childhood leukemia, *Eur J Cancer* 26:661-664, 1990.
6. Urquhart JD, Black RJ, Muirhead MJ, et al: Case-control study of leukaemia and non-Hodgkin's lymphoma in Caithness near Daunreay nuclear installation, *Br Med J* 302:687-692, 1991.
7. Morris JA: Low dose radiation and childhood cancer, *J Clin Pathol* 45:378-381, 1992.
8. Bithell JF, Dutton SJ, Draper GJ, et al: Distribution of childhood leukaemias and non-Hodgkin's lymphomas near nuclear installations in England and Wales, *Br Med J* 309:501-505, 1994.
9. Waller LA, Turnbull BW, Gustafsson G, et al: Detection and assessment of clusters of disease: an application to nuclear power plant facilities and childhood leukaemia in Sweden, *Stat Med* 14:3-16, 1995.
10. Farwell J, Flannery JT: Cancer in relatives with central nervous system neoplasms, *N Engl J Med* 311:749-753, 1984.
11. Matsuo T: In vitro modulation of alkaline phosphatase activity in neutrophils from patients with chronic myelogenous leukemia by monocyte derived activity, *Blood* 67:492-497, 1986.
12. Heisterkamp N, Stephenson JR, Groffen J, et al: Localization of c-abl oncogene adjacent to a translocation breakpoint in chronic myelogenous leukemia, *Nature* 306:239-242, 1983.
13. Konoka JB, Watanabe SM, Singer J, et al: Cell lines and clinical isolates derived from Ph^1-positive chronic myelogenous leukemia patients express c-abl proteins with a common structural aberration, *Proc Natl Acad Sci* 82:1810-1814, 1985.

Suggested Readings

Henderson ES, Lister TA, editors: *Leukemia,* ed 5, Philadelphia, 1990, WB Saunders.

Pizzo PA, Poplack DG, editors: *Principles and practice of pediatric oncology,* ed 2, Philadelphia, 1993, JB Lippincott.

Pui CH: Childhood leukemias, *N Engl J Med* 332:1618-1630, 1995.

CHAPTER 51

Malignant Solid Tumors

•

Mark E. Weinblatt

Cancer, although a relatively uncommon disease in adolescents, is a leading cause of death among teenagers, surpassed only by accidents, suicide, and homicide. Despite increasing success in the treatment of this heterogeneous group of disorders, approximately 1400 individuals in the United States between the ages of 10 and 20 years die annually as a consequence of malignant disease. While the diagnosis of malignancy does not engender the same sense of hopelessness as it did in the past, the disease and its treatment burden an increasing number of survivors with enormous physical, emotional, and social costs during this already difficult time of life.

About 80% of newly diagnosed malignancies in adolescents are solid tumors. As shown in Figure 51-1, several common childhood tumors, particularly embryonal tumors (e.g., neuroblastoma and Wilms' tumor), are infrequently seen in adolescents, while the overwhelming preponderance of epithelial-derived carcinomas found in adults is also not manifest during the adolescent years. A noticeably significant transition in the incidence of many malignancies occurs during the teenage years (Fig. 51-2), with fewer cases of leukemia and brain tumors and an increased incidence of Hodgkin's disease and testicular and thyroid cancers. The frequency of several of these tumors peaks during the third decade of life before giving way to breast, colon, and lung carcinomas, which are common in adults. Although there is much speculation about the cause of the increased incidence of epithelial tumors in adults, the process behind this transition that begins in the adolescent years is not understood.

With the advent of more effective drug therapies, treatment of solid tumors has evolved considerably over the past few decades. Chemotherapy has effected a reduction in disfiguring and risky surgical procedures; a decrease in the need for and intensity of radiation therapy, with its potentially considerable long-term morbidity; and a significant improvement in survival for most teenagers diagnosed with a malignancy. Intensive chemotherapeutic regimens have been instrumental in shrinking inoperable tumors to a more manageable size, allowing easier surgical excision and reducing the need for a wide field of radiotherapy. Despite potentially serious adverse effects from these medications, their role in adjuvant therapy for destroying microscopic residua cannot be overemphasized. As a result of the complex interplay among the different treatment modalities and their considerable toxicities, careful coordination of each patient's therapy is of paramount importance and usually requires the experienced staff and well-equipped facilities of a cancer center. Just as important as antineoplastic therapy are the issues of supportive care, including the judicious use of antibiotics, transfusion therapy, fluids and electrolytes, and good nutrition. The demanding nature of the disease and its treatment also entails a great deal of emotional and social support for the patient and family.

NON-HODGKIN'S LYMPHOMA

Non-Hodgkin's lymphoma (NHL), which comprises a heterogeneous group of lymphoid malignancies, is one of the more common tumors encountered in teenagers, with an incidence of approximately seven cases per million in the U.S. population. The disease is more prevalent in adolescents than in children, with males affected three times more commonly than females (6:1 in B-cell lymphomas) and whites affected about twice as frequently as blacks.

Although the pathophysiologic mechanism involved in the origin of these tumors is unknown, speculation has focused on the immune system from which these tumors arise. The significantly higher risk of NHL in patients with immunodeficiency, both inherited and acquired, has increased speculation that lymphomas arise in the absence of appropriate regulatory controls in the body's immune system, particularly in patients with human immunodeficiency virus (HIV) infection and immunosuppressed transplant recipients. Most malignant cell lines contain some genetic abnormality (e.g., chromo-

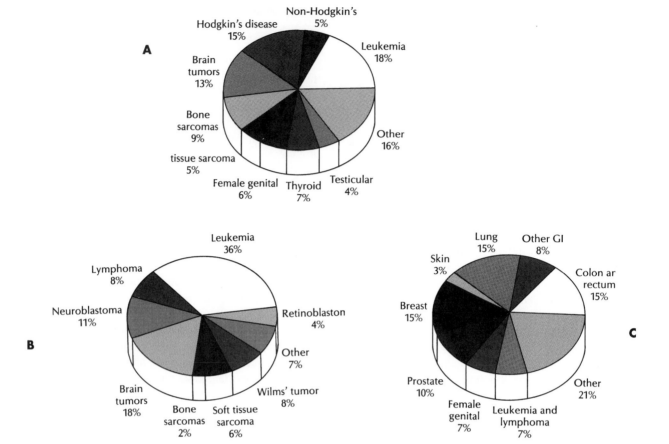

Fig. 51-1. Incidence of malignancy at different ages. **A,** Adolescent malignancies, ages 10 to 20 years. **B,** Childhood malignancies, age under 10 years. **C,** Adult malignancies, age over 20 years.

somal translocations, viral gene insertions, point mutations) that suggests another possible etiologic mechanism in the malignant transformation. The monoclonal nature of lymphomas, with all cells genetically identical to the malignant precursor, allows cytogenetic and immunophenotypic cell features to serve as markers for the disease and helps in gauging the patient's disease status during treatment and follow-up. The significant male preponderance might suggest some genetic protection associated with the X chromosome. Perhaps the strongest evidence for the genetic and molecular basis of NHL is found in Burkitt's lymphoma, a B-cell neoplasm with a characteristic translocation (t:8,14) that approximates the c-myc oncogene (the human homologue of an established oncogenic virus) on chromosome no. 8 to the DNA segment (14q32) responsible for production of immunoglobulin heavy chains. It has been determined that most chromosome breakpoints in NHL appear at sites of transformation-related genes or fragile sites.[1] The association of pseudolymphoma and NHL in patients treated with hydantoins, and the increased incidence of lymphoma in irradiated patients, might be mediated through damage to DNA, with inadequate repair and escape from

normal regulatory mechanisms. Finally, the role of infection in the interaction with the host DNA and the pathogenesis of NHL need further elucidation; there has been a well-established association with Burkitt's lymphoma and Epstein-Barr virus (EBV) infection (95% of patients in Africa, but only 20% in the United States) and an even stronger link between some T-cell lymphomas and the retrovirus, human T-cell leukemia virus type 1 (HTLV-1).

There are several distinct subtypes of adolescent NHL that present with characteristic features. Although most lymphomas are derived from T and B lymphocytes, only 34% of adolescent NHLs are lymphoblastic; the large cell (histiocytic) type accounts for 26%; undifferentiated (non-Burkitt's) lymphoma for 19%, Burkitt's lymphoma for 13%, and others for 8%. The immunologic expression of the tumor is frequently associated with the site of origin of the neoplasm, with B-cell tumors most commonly arising in the abdomen and T-cell tumors in the mediastinum. Seventy percent of patients with NHL have disseminated disease at presentation, with a tendency toward early involvement of extranodal sites. These tumors are among the fastest growing malignancies, with

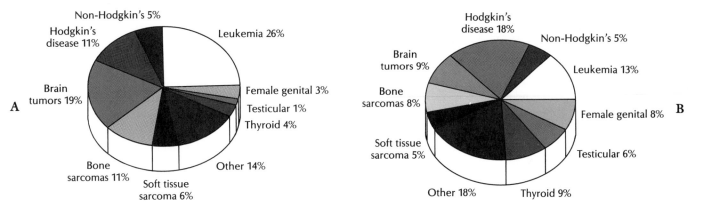

Fig. 51-2. Incidence of malignancies with transition during adolescent years. **A,** Ages 10 to 14 years. **B,** Ages 15 to 19 years.

a doubling time of 38 to 116 hours in Burkitt's lymphoma.

Lymphoblastic lymphoma, with typical L_1 cells (see Chapter 50, "Leukemia"), is often found in the mediastinum, and it nearly always possesses T-cell receptors. Patients complain of chest pain, dyspnea, or symptoms related to superior vena cava compression. Physical examination typically includes lymphadenopathy in the cervical, supraclavicular, and axillary area. Chest radiographs often reveal a pleural effusion in addition to the mediastinal mass. When a lymphoblastic NHL originates outside the mediastinum, the spectrum of immunologic expression is similar to that of lymphoblastic leukemia. The undifferentiated lymphomas most commonly originate in the abdomen, with pain or distention, emesis, gastrointestinal bleeding, or intussusception (with the tumor as the lead point). Origin in the jaw, frequent in endemic Burkitt's lymphoma in Africa, is rare in the United States, where the most common sites are the abdomen and the sinuses. The histiocytic subtypes are heterogeneous, with primary sites that include the gastrointestinal tract, the mediastinum, the neck, and other soft tissues.

The two most important sites of extranodal spread with important prognostic value are the central nervous system (CNS) and bone marrow. Central nervous system involvement includes meningeal, cranial nerve (especially VI and VII), or paraspinal infiltrations; these are most often sites of relapse and are uncommon at initial presentation. Burkitt's lymphoma in particular displays a propensity toward paraspinal encroachment with resultant paraplegia. Bone marrow involvement is common, particularly in the patient with lymphoblastic disease. The degree of involvement of the marrow will determine whether the patient is treated for lymphoma or leukemia (by convention, more than 25% of marrow involvement is considered leukemia).

Although several biochemical and hematologic abnormalities are suggestive of lymphoma in the patient with adenopathy (elevated erythrocyte sedimentation rate,

serum lactic dehydrogenase [LDH], and serum uric acid levels), diagnosis depends on examination of pathologic tissue from an involved lymph node. Obtaining a peripheral node with the patient under local anesthesia is usually preferable because of the inherent risks of general anesthesia in the patient with an anterior mediastinal mass and the surgical complications of laparotomy. Radiographic and radionuclide evaluation of the chest and abdomen is mandatory, with computed tomography (CT) and gallium scans the most helpful in delineating anatomic sites of disease. Serum electrolytes, uric acid level, liver function tests, bone marrow biopsies, and lumbar puncture all yield additional important information in the assessment of disease status. Enough tissue should be obtained for additional prognostic and diagnostic tests, including cells for karyotyping, immunophenotyping, and oncogene detection.

The prognosis for NHL rests primarily on the tumor burden at presentation. Localized disease of any subtype has a uniformly excellent outlook, whereas the more extensive the disease and the greater the number of involved sites, the more variable is the course and the poorer the outlook. The LDH level is a reflection of the tumor burden and has been used as a prognostic evaluator. Quantitation of interleukin-2 receptors is another promising prognostic marker.

In view of the excellent outlook for patients with localized disease, less aggressive therapy is indicated, and there is no role for radiation therapy in most instances. After surgery in most patients, very well tolerated chemotherapy is administered for only a few months, with generally minimal adverse effects and a cure rate greater than 90%.

Treatment for more advanced disease is considerably more demanding, with multiagent drug regimens tailored to the specific cell subtype. While initial surgical excision can substantially decrease the tumor burden by leaving fewer cells to be eliminated by other forms of treatment, this is usually not possible without significant morbidity and mortality. Because of the high growth fraction, tumor cells respond well to many drugs, and dramatic tumor responses can be obtained within days of instituting chemotherapy. Most drug protocols employ sequential intense pulsed cycles of multiple antineoplastic drugs given at brief intervals to prevent the emergence of resistant clones of cells. The best results for lymphoblastic NHL have been obtained from the LSA_2L_2 regimen, with a 75% to 80% long-term survival. Patients with undifferentiated and histiocytic lymphomas have a cure rate approaching 60% with a variety of cyclophosphamide- and doxorubicin-based regimens. Cure rates approaching 85% are being obtained for patients with Burkitt's lymphoma, using brief, very intense chemotherapy regimens. All patients with extensive disease receive prophylactic CNS therapy with some combination of intrathecal chemotherapy and CNS radiation. In most studies, radiotherapy to gross tumor sites has not been shown to increase overall survival, and because of additive toxicity it is reserved for emergency and other special situations (e.g., evolving paraplegia from a paraspinal mass or testicular disease).

A few complications must be resolved expeditiously to avoid emergency complications. Superior vena cava syndrome with plethora, headache, and swelling of the neck veins usually responds rapidly to chemotherapy without the need for surgical debulking or radiation. It is important to administer parenteral medications and all fluids through the veins of the lower extremities until the obstruction has been relieved, to avoid exacerbation of the syndrome. Before therapy is instituted in patients with bulky, extensive disease, correction of all biochemical abnormalities must be attempted. The acute tumor lysis syndrome that follows the destruction of rapidly proliferating cells can release large amounts of intracellular potassium and phosphates. Profound hyperkalemia, hyperuricemia, and hypocalcemia, aggravated by uric acid nephropathy and renal dysfunction, can result in a life-threatening situation. Prevention through vigorous hydration, administration of allopurinol, and judicious alkalinization of the urine is usually effective. Spinal cord compression should be treated with high-dose dexamethasone to reduce edema, along with chemotherapy and radiation (if needed), to prevent permanent neurologic deficits. Surgery plays less of a role in this situation.

Although most patients with NHL can be cured, the outlook for those with recurrent extensive disease has been dismal in the past, with only brief periods of partial remission before death. Promising results for cure in this patient population are now being achieved through the use of supralethal combinations of chemotherapy and radiation followed by rescue with allogeneic or autologous bone marrow or stem cell transplantation.

HODGKIN'S DISEASE

Hodgkin's disease (HD) differs from most other adolescent malignancies in its mode of spread, histologic appearance, diagnostic evaluation, and treatment. It is the only neoplasm in which the malignant cell (Reed-Sternberg) makes up a minimal portion of the tumor mass; it is the only malignancy in which successful treatment can consist exclusively of radiation; and it is the only cancer in which the less the radiographic evidence of involvement, the greater is the need for surgical diagnostic procedures to plan a therapeutic regimen.

The first of two age-incidence peaks in HD appears in adolescence, with the second after age 40. There is an equal male-to-female ratio, and the disease is more common in whites than in blacks. Although many patients with HD have a lifelong immune deficit, the malignancy is only seen with slightly higher incidence in patients with preexisting immunodeficiency diseases. There is some increased incidence of HD in patients with first-degree relatives who have HD, prompting speculation of a genetic predisposition. Reports of numerous clusters of the disease,[2] in addition to the frequent finding of high titers of EBV antibodies in many patients, have suggested a possible infectious etiology.

Most patients are diagnosed with disease restricted only to lymphoid tissue, prompting the hypothesis that the disease spreads initially along lymph vessels. However, this does not explain many findings, such as involvement of the spleen, which contains no afferent lymph vessels. Current theories suggest a multicentric appearance or even early hematologic metastases of a malignant cell line that grows preferentially in lymphoid tissue as a result of locally produced lymphokines. Regardless of the mechanism, this localization has allowed the cure of many patients by radiation therapy alone, with all sites of disease included in the field of radiation.

Most teenagers present with painless supraclavicular or cervical adenopathy and nodes of firm, rubbery consistency. Mediastinal involvement is common and is sometimes accompanied by superior vena cava compression, bronchial irritation and impingement with chronic cough, or pericardial effusion with some degree of tamponade. Splenomegaly is seen in more advanced disease, and the most common metastatic sites include liver, bone, bone marrow, and pulmonary parenchyma. About one third of patients have systemic (B) symptomatology, with fevers, night sweats, and more than 10% weight loss. Less common findings include pruritus with alcohol ingestion, immune thrombocytopenic purpura, and hemolytic anemia.

Diagnosis of HD is contingent on characteristic histologic findings, which include the presence of Reed-Sternberg cells. The four pathologic subtypes of HD are lymphocyte predominant, nodular sclerosis, mixed cellularity, and lymphocyte depleted. Nodular sclerosis is particularly common in adolescent girls. Inadequate node biopsy may reveal only reactive adenopathy, delaying the diagnosis until further pathologic evidence can be gathered on repeat biopsy, emphasizing the need for adequate tissue sampling. Additional diagnostic tests that help determine proper disease stage include CT or magnetic resonance imaging (MRI) scans of the chest and abdomen, gallium scan, LDH, sedimentation rate, and serum copper levels. Lymphangiography is less commonly performed at this time, although in experienced hands it is still a very useful tool for identifying abnormal abdominal nodes and following the progress of the disease during treatment.

Considerable controversy exists over the need for a staging laparotomy in many circumstances, in large part because of an increasing shift toward chemotherapy rather than radiation as the primary mode of treatment. If radiation is to be the sole therapy, accurate determination of the extent of disease is mandatory in order to include all sites in the radiation fields. If no gross disease is found through radiographic scans, laparotomy with extensive node sampling, splenectomy, and liver biopsy become necessary. However, for patients who will be receiving chemotherapy as part of the treatment, staging laparotomy is less important, since radiation is reserved for sites of bulky disease that are readily identified by radiographic means.

The prognosis for patients with HD has changed dramatically during the past few decades, with 80% to 85% overall cure rates currently achieved in most centers. These excellent results have made it difficult to establish one form of treatment as clearly superior to another, particularly for early-stage disease. The patient who has stage I or stage II disease with no systemic symptoms has more than a 90% disease-free survival with either radiation or chemotherapy. The older adolescent who has completed all growth is a better candidate for radiation treatment than the younger adolescent, who would be subject to radiation-induced growth retardation or scoliosis. Symptomatic patients with more advanced disease, with extensive involvement of both sides of the diaphragm (stage IIIB) or metastatic spread (stage IV), clearly do better with combination chemotherapy and radiation to sites of bulky disease. The patient with an intermediate prognosis (stages IIB and IIIA) often develops recurrent disease after radiation therapy alone, but the salvage rate with chemotherapy is high enough for many centers to continue to prefer radiation as first-line therapy for this group. It is particularly encouraging to note that most patients with metastatic disease are cured with currently available drug combinations. The most commonly used regimens are the original MOPP (nitrogen mustard, vincristine, prednisone, and procarbazine), ABVD (Adriamycin, bleomycin, vinblastine, and dacar-

bazine), or some combination of both. A treatment protocol gaining increased acceptance is a hybrid MOPP-ABV (or COPP-ABV) regimen that utilizes less anthracycline and alkylating medications. Even after previous chemotherapy treatment, patients with recurrent disease can be cured with either non–cross-reacting chemotherapeutic combinations or through stem cell or bone marrow transplantation as a rescue after supralethal doses of chemotherapy.

Controversy remains over therapeutic regimens because of the desirability of decreasing the amount of treatment and limiting the potential adverse effects.[3] Radiation can induce pneumonitis and pulmonary fibrosis, pericarditis (13%), thyroid dysfunction (more than 50% of patients have biochemical thyroid abnormalities), esophagitis with weight loss, secondary malignancies (sarcoma, lung, and breast carcinoma, NHL, melanoma, carcinoma of head and neck, and acute nonlymphoblastic leukemia), and gonadal dysfunction with sterility, as well as the aforementioned growth effects. An ongoing cooperative group study is currently assessing the need for consolidative radiation to sites of bulky disease in patients treated with chemotherapy. The risk of postsplenectomy sepsis also must be considered in the radiation-treated patient who has undergone staging laparotomy. Chemotherapy with MOPP has been associated with severe nausea and vomiting, myelosuppression, sterility (particularly in males), and secondary leukemia. ABVD is less likely to cause secondary malignancy or sterility, but concern for cardiac and pulmonary toxicity is greater, especially if adjunctive radiation is administered. The risk of secondary malignancy is greatest in the patient treated with MOPP and radiation, with a 6% to 10% incidence of a different neoplastic disease occurring within 10 years. Although results of therapy have been dramatic and the outlook is very promising, the considerable cost in long-term morbidity will ensure continuing debate over the best and least toxic treatment.

BRAIN TUMORS

Brain tumors are the most common malignant solid neoplasms diagnosed in adolescence. They are a diverse group of disorders whose signs and symptoms are related more to location than to histology. As a group these tumors are most difficult to treat because of their relatively slow growth rate, which results in less sensitivity to chemotherapy and radiation, late relapses many years after treatment, and the overall poor outcome.

The best-known predisposition to brain tumors is the presence of a neurocutaneous syndrome. Patients with neurofibromatosis are at significant risk of developing gliomas in any intracranial site (classically, attached to the optic pathway); tuberous sclerosis also has been associated with glial tumors. Previous radiation therapy to the head has been linked to meningioma and meningosarcoma. An increased risk of brain tumor also has been reported in children whose parents work with organic chemical compounds. Bizarre chromosomal aberrations, most commonly double minutes (extrachromosomal lengths of repeated DNA sequences), are common in high-grade gliomas, suggesting an alteration of DNA in patients with brain tumors.

The adolescent years mark a transition from the embryonal brain tumors of childhood to the glial malignancies of adults. Accompanying this shift is an increased incidence of supratentorial tumors, with a different constellation of presenting complaints. Several different pathologic classifications are currently in use, which adds confusion to any discussion of diagnosis and prognosis. Likewise, different emphasis is placed on histologic characteristics and special stains, which often makes treatment comparisons difficult.

Improvements in diagnostic tools, particularly the newer-generation CT and MRI scans, in addition to gauging treatment response, have enabled more precise objective measurements of tumors at diagnosis. Both types of scan yield important information regarding the extent of involvement, edema, shift of midline structures, and ventricular size. MRI often reveals earlier extensive infiltration because of the better delineation of normal tissue from neoplastic tissue and the ability to distinguish hemorrhage from calcification. As a result, MRI has become the preferred modality for many tumors, particularly infratentorial and brain stem lesions. Positron emission tomography can measure actual tissue metabolic activity and thus can differentiate recurrent or persistent disease from radionecrosis and scar tissue. Its use will expand as more experience with this modality is obtained. Radionuclide imaging, spinal fluid examination, electroencephalography, and angiography, which yield less useful information, are now used sparingly.

Supratentorial Astrocytoma

Supratentorial astrocytoma is the most common brain tumor diagnosed during the teenage years, with a 2 : 1 male-to-female incidence. The older the patient, the more likely it is that the tumor will be of a higher-grade malignancy. Most current systems of pathology grade these tumors according to cellularity, the presence or absence of mitotic figures and necrosis, the degree of cellular and nuclear pleomorphism, and the amount of distortion of normal brain architecture. Although often diffusely infiltrative, about 40% of low-grade tumors are cystic masses, which often can be completely excised and are associated with prolonged survival. The more aggressive, higher-grade anaplastic tumors, including glioblas-

toma multiforme, are histologically pleomorphic, with extensive necrosis and considerable mitotic activity. Such tumors are hypervascular and tend to distort normal surrounding structures. They usually have a poor outlook but have responded to aggressive chemotherapy/radiation regimens.

The duration of initial symptoms varies greatly, with more benign lesions characteristically exhibiting a longer prediagnostic prodrome. Signs and symptoms are a reflection of the site of the tumor rather than histologic grading, with the frequency of location corresponding to the amount of central white matter from which the tumor arises. Typical presenting findings include headaches, emesis, visual disturbances, and weakness. Seizures are more common in low-grade tumors (60%), whereas the incidence of elevated intracranial pressure and the pace of symptom progression are greater with more malignant masses because of the inability to compensate for the rapid growth and pronounced edema. Additional findings may include papilledema, cranial nerve palsies, and focal motor deficits.

Depending on the site and extent of tumor, gross total resection of the mass is commonly attempted, since the prognostic result is usually far superior to that of incisional biopsy. Ventriculoperitoneal shunting can be performed simultaneously to relieve obstructive hydrocephalus, if present. The less aggressive the histologic appearance, the greater is the need for surgical removal because of poor response to other treatment modalities; complete excision of a low-grade cystic astrocytoma is potentially curative, with at least 50% long-term survivors. Patients with high-grade tumors fare better if followed with combination chemotherapy and radiation rather than radiotherapy alone; studies from the 1980s yield a 45% versus 13% 5-year disease-free survival.[4] Unfortunately, late recurrences have been noted, and newer approaches are in great demand. More aggressive chemotherapy and the use of autologous bone marrow rescue have been shown to be of some benefit in relapsed patients, particularly those with glioblastoma, and are currently being used to treat newly diagnosed tumors.[5] Several novel radiotherapy approaches are currently under investigation. Hyperfractionation allows a higher total dose of radiation therapy with sparing of surrounding tissue. Brachytherapy, the application of radiation sources within or adjacent to the tumor, can now be performed safely using stereotactic neurosurgery: the stereotactic needle removes small pieces of tissue and leaves the small radioactive seeds behind. Radiosurgery using the γ-knife or linear accelerator has shown some promise, but these are designed for small, spherical metastatic lesions as opposed to the larger, irregularly shaped gliomas. Further refinements in the technology may ultimately be of benefit to these patients.

Primitive Neuroectodermal Tumor

Relatively common in younger adolescents, primitive neuroectodermal tumors (PNETs), termed *medulloblastomas* when found in the posterior fossa, often arise from the cerebellar vermis and extend into the brain stem and fourth ventricle, with resultant obstruction of spinal fluid and elevated intracranial pressure. The site of origin in adolescents is more commonly in the lateral cerebral hemispheres, with a short duration of symptoms that include headache, lethargy, emesis, and ataxia. Pathologic examination usually reveals sheets of anaplastic cells with pronounced mitotic activity. PNETs frequently spread to other CNS and systemic sites, including the spinal cord, bone, and bone marrow. Initial evaluation must include a thorough examination of the spinal cord (best done by a combination of spinal fluid analysis with cytology and MRI scan with gadolinium) to rule out often detected leptomeningeal spread; bone marrow aspiration and biopsy to rule out marrow infiltration; and bone scan to detect cortical involvement.

Better prognostic features in the newly diagnosed patient with PNET include small tumor volume, lack of involvement of adjacent structures, and absence of spinal or distant metastatic spread. Seeding to sites outside the CNS is apparently higher in patients with ventriculoperitoneal shunts, presumably as a result of seeding from the shunt catheter. Better surgical excision, including use of an operative microscope, the ultrasonic aspirator, and evoked-potential monitoring, has helped render more patients free of gross disease. Patients with this radiosensitive tumor also have shown a significant improvement in survival when craniospinal radiation is given in adequate doses. Patients with tumors that have had a poor prognosis have benefited substantially from simultaneous chemotherapy administration; survival in such cases is now about 80% 5 to 6 years after diagnosis, as a result of cisplatin-based regimens. Patients with recurrent disease have also benefited from high-dose chemotherapy followed by autologous marrow or stem cell rescue.

Brainstem Glioma

One of the CNS tumors with the poorest prognosis, brainstem gliomas deserve special mention because of their characteristic findings and the limitations of current treatment regimens. With about 70% arising in the pontomedullary region, these tumors often present with paresis of multiple cranial nerves (especially VI, VII, IX, X, and XI), with resultant visual abnormalities, dysarthria, and dysphagia. Additional symptoms may include ataxia, corticospinal tract dysfunction, and signs of elevated intracranial pressure. Brainstem tumors must be differentiated from arteriovenous malformations, in-

fections, and Leigh's disease (a rare, degenerative disease affecting the brain stem). Because of the inaccessibility of many of these tumors, the risks of biopsy, and the inaccuracy of tissue findings owing to tumor heterogeneity, diagnosis depends on radiographic studies, with MRI the most useful and accurate modality.

Although many tumors are histologically benign, survival is poor because of the location of the mass, with only a 20% to 30% survival rate at 5 years. Patients with dorsally exophytic tumors do best, with survival as high as 90%; such tumors can be excised and are more likely to be low grade. Cranial nerve dysfunction and hypodense intrinsic masses on CT scan are associated with a poorer outcome. Numerous experimental treatments for these patients, including very-high-dose, hyperfractionated radiation (>7000 cGy) and autologous bone marrow rescue after thiotepa-based preconditioning treatment, have not improved the outlook for this patient population.

Less Common Brain Tumors

Although less common than in younger children, cerebellar astrocytomas in adolescents are also predominantly cystic, low grade, and potentially curable through surgical excision alone. Complaints are generally of long duration and are often related to obstructive hydrocephalus (headache, papilledema, and emesis), gait abnormalities, nystagmus, dysmetria, and ataxia. Gross total excision with no further treatment results in prolonged survival in 75% of patients.

Craniopharyngiomas, which are rare, slow-growing, histologically benign tumors, arise in a dangerous location and exhibit a tendency toward destruction of hypophyseal structures. The hallmark of these tumors is an insidious onset of visual disturbances and endocrinopathies, a result of tumor encroachment on the optic nerve and hypothalamus. An excellent outcome is common, with treatment consisting of surgery, radiation to the tumor bed, and endocrine replacement as needed.

Germ-cell tumors peak in incidence in early adolescence, with germinoma the most common pathologic diagnosis and the pineal area the typical site. There is a male predominance in this type of tumor. Patients may present with visual field defects, vertical gaze paresis, diabetes insipidus, elevated intracranial pressure, hypothalamic/pituitary dysfunction, ataxia, and pyramidal tract signs. Metastases down the spine and to extraneural sites are common, which underscores the need for systemic therapy. After surgical excision, a combination of radiation and chemotherapy is administered if pathologic study confirms the presence of malignant tissue. Response to cisplatin-based therapy in germ cell tumors outside the CNS has led to its usage in pineal tumors also;

combination therapy has resulted in 60% to 85% disease-free survival at 5 years.

Primary intraspinal tumors, most of which are low-grade astrocytomas or ependymomas, grow slowly; contain large cysts; and characteristically produce localized or radicular pain, weakness, and gait and sphincter dysfunction. Some are associated with neurofibromatosis, and extensive involvement of a large segment of the cord is common. With current surgical advances, most patients can expect near-complete surgical excision with longer survival and less need for postoperative radiation. Radiotherapy is recommended after incomplete resection. Patients with low-grade tumors have a better than 70% disease-free survival at 5 years and 55% at 10 years. The outlook for high-grade malignancies remains dismal.

BONE TUMORS

Although rare in childhood, malignant bone tumors exhibit an incidence peak in adolescence, accounting for about 9% of teenage malignant disorders. Major advances in the treatment of these diseases during the past two decades have included significantly increased survival for nonmetastatic disease, innovative limb-sparing techniques, and overall superior quality of life in survivors.

Osteogenic Sarcoma

The most common malignant bone tumor, osteogenic sarcoma (OS), is found most frequently in older adolescents, with a higher incidence in males. The tumor has been well documented as appearing in anatomic sites and ages involving the most rapid bone growth. The most common primary sites are the metaphyses of the distal femur, proximal tibia, and proximal humerus. The age peak in teenagers corresponds to the adolescent growth spurt. Affected individuals are usually taller than average. This characteristic suggests a possible link between rapid bone growth and the etiology of OS. It is conceivable that rapidly proliferating normal bone cells are particularly susceptible to malignant transformation.[6] The inciting event might be radiation (approximately 3% of these tumors develop in sites of previous radiation), viruses (although there is evidence of viruses causing bone sarcomas in animals, no such association has been established in humans), or genetic predisposition. Inheritance clearly plays some role in patients with hereditary retinoblastoma, who have a risk of developing OS 500 to 2000 times greater than that of the average population; this risk is even higher if irradiation is administered. Although many patients present with a history of antecedent trauma, this is likely to be a serendipitous event that brings the mass to medical attention.

Presenting complaints are usually limited to the primary site of the tumor, with pain and swelling at the site and occasionally a pathologic fracture after minimal trauma. Duration of symptoms is usually related to the pathologic subtype; some slow-growing varieties are associated with a duration of years rather than months. Likewise, some tumors have an extensive soft tissue component rather than just bone involvement. Approximately 10% to 20% of patients have metastatic spread at presentation, with the lungs the most common site.

Diagnosis is confirmed through both typical radiographic appearance and pathologic characteristics. High-grade OS exhibits destruction of the normal bony trabecular pattern, lytic lesions with indistinct margins, periosteal elevation, and new bone formation (forming the classic Codman's triangle on x-ray film). Technetium bone scanning reveals "hot spots," areas of osteogenesis and bone destruction, which are helpful in locating other less obvious sites of disease. CT and MRI can delineate the extent of intramedullary and soft tissue involvement, information that is indispensable for potential limb-sparing procedures. CT scans of the chest are necessary to rule out pulmonary metastases. Both alkaline phosphatase and LDH are frequently elevated in patients with OS.

Biopsy is ultimately necessary to confirm the diagnosis, with adequate tissue sampling important because of tumor heterogeneity. The most common subtype, osteoblastic sarcoma, is usually high grade, with large, spindle-shaped malignant cells and abundant osteoid tissue present. Less common variants have differing presentations and prognoses. The rare telangiectatic sarcomas, which have a poorer outlook, are cystic and have little new bone formation. Paraosteal tumors are very slow growing, are typically located in the posterior distal femur, arise from the surface of the bone with no intramedullary invasion, and usually have a very good prognosis. Periosteal OS, which also arises from the surface of the bone, has a moderately good outlook. Generally, the more localized and smaller the mass, the more distal is the tumor, and the lower the alkaline phosphatase and LDH levels, the better is the prognosis.

Advances in chemotherapy have dramatically altered the outlook and therapeutic scheme for OS. Before the advent of effective systemic therapy, 80% of patients presenting with localized disease ultimately died of respiratory complications of pulmonary metastases, even after aggressive amputation procedures. The arrival of highly effective multiagent protocols, involving combinations of doxorubicin, vincristine, actinomycin D, cisplatin, supralethal doses of methotrexate with citrovorum rescue, and (more recently) ifosfamide, has effected cures in most patients with localized disease, while also offering some patients with few pulmonary metastases a chance of cure. The ability to control and shrink the primary tumor while preventing metastatic spread has given rise to a host of limb-sparing procedures that can be planned and customized during the first few months of therapy. More effective radiographic imaging also has enabled clearer delineation of the tumor margins, allowing less radical and less disfiguring surgical excision in addition to better follow-up. After the initial chemotherapy phase (which gives information regarding tumor sensitivity, response to medications, and prognosis), en bloc resection of the primary tumor with clear margins is performed, and the initial phase of limb replacement is begun. Generally, the more distal the lesion, the more amenable it is to limb salvage, whether by cadaveric implant (most successful for smaller lengths of bone), autologous bone transplant, or construction of a metal prosthetic device. Expandable steel or titanium implants are particularly effective in younger adolescents who have not yet completed growth or achieved full height. Thoracotomy should be attempted to remove accessible pulmonary metastases; in combination with chemotherapy, this procedure can be curative. Since OS is radioresistant, radiation therapy has a very limited role in the management of this type of tumor, offering palliative treatment of inoperable, symptomatic masses. An important component of care is early institution of physical therapy, rehabilitation, and psychological support to help the increasingly large number of survivors learn to use their altered limbs to the fullest and to enjoy a good quality of life.

Ewing's Sarcoma

The second most common malignant bone tumor, Ewing's sarcoma usually arises in the shaft of long bones rather than in the growth sites. It is very rare among blacks and Chinese and has no familial associations with or relation to previous radiation therapy. Unlike OS, which arises from primitive bone-producing mesenchymal cells, no definitive cell of origin has been established for this type of tumor. Most patients present with painful swelling of the involved bone. The most common primary sites are the upper or middle shaft of the femur and pelvis, with other lesions often noted in the tibia, fibula, scapula, humerus, and ribs. Patients with metastatic spread at diagnosis (most common sites are the lungs and other bones) present with fever, weight loss, and anorexia—signs often mistaken for osteomyelitis. Spinal metastases can cause back pain and neurologic dysfunction.

Radiographs usually reveal bone destruction and periosteal elevation, occasionally with an "onion skin" appearance. The intramedullary component of the tumor is normally extensive, and infiltration into surrounding soft tissue is common. Biopsy is necessary for definitive diagnosis, since the small round cell tumor can easily be confused with lymphoma, rhabdomyosarcoma, and neuroblastoma. The diagnosis is often one of exclusion. As with OS, CT, MRI, and bone scanning are helpful in delineating the extent of disease, and the LDH level is often elevated. Prognosis is better with more localized masses, distal primary sites, smaller tumors, absence of extraosseous soft tissue components, and low serum LDH levels.

Treatment for patients with radiosensitive Ewing's sarcoma consists of a combination of chemotherapy, surgery, and high-dose radiation therapy. Multiagent chemotherapy with vincristine, doxorubicin, cyclophosphamide, etoposide, and ifosfamide usually results in shrinkage of the primary tumor to a resectable size, enabling limb-sparing surgery. Tumors that respond poorly usually require amputation and high-dose radiation therapy for effective local control; adverse effects include fibrosis and contractures, osteopenia and fractures, and secondary malignancies. Disease-free survival ranges from 70% for distal lesions to 35% for metastatic disease.

SOFT-TISSUE SARCOMA

This group of heterogeneous tumors displays a broad array of histologic characteristics, primary sites, and prognostic implications. Although the variety of presentations and pathologic features is extensive, the treatment scheme is generally consistent.

Soft-tissue sarcomas have a slight male preponderance, and the incidence in whites is twice as great as in blacks. Reaching a peak in adolescence, the overall incidence of these malignancies declines during adulthood. Genetics probably plays some role in the etiology of sarcomas, many of these tumors being found in family cancer syndromes in association with glioblastomas and breast cancer. An increased incidence in patients with neurofibromatosis has also been noted. Sarcomas have appeared in sites of previous irradiation, and although oncogenic viruses and several noxious chemicals have been shown to cause sarcomas in several animal species, a clear-cut association in humans is lacking.

Because soft-tissue sarcomas arise from ubiquitous mesenchymal cells, primary masses are found in almost any anatomic site. While much controversy exists regarding many pathologic subtypes, the soft tissue sarcomas are divided into rhabdomyosarcoma (RMS) and non-RMS types. RMS, arising from embryonic skeletal muscle cells, accounts for approximately half of adolescent sarcomas. Diagnosis depends on the presence of typical cross-striations that imitate skeletal muscle and is further confirmed through immunocytochemical antibodies that stain muscle-specific proteins.[7] Pathologic categories of RMS include embryonal (most common), alveolar (resembling alveolar tissue in the lung, with rhabdomyoblasts in a glandlike arrangement), pleomorphic, undifferentiated, and extraosseous Ewing's sarcoma (also known as primitive neuroectodermal tumor). The undifferentiated and alveolar RMS types, having a poorer prognosis, are more common in adolescents than in children. There are many non-RMS sarcoma subtypes, most of which are found in the adult population but also appear with some regularity in adolescents. These include fibrosarcomas, neurogenic sarcoma, synovial sarcoma, malignant fibrous histiocytoma, malignant schwannoma, hemangiopericytoma, and liposarcoma.

Rhabdomyosarcomas most commonly arise from the head, neck, and genitourinary tract, but trunk and extremity sites are more common in adolescents than in children. Most of the head tumors involve the sinuses or the orbit, with symptoms including proptosis, ophthalmoplegia, and chronic nasal congestion with discharge. Meningeal extension can result in cranial nerve palsies or signs of elevated intracranial pressure. Orbital tumors often have a better outlook because of early diagnosis and lack of lymphatic spread; primary tumors in the sinuses, however, are often extensive at diagnosis, are incompletely resected, and are associated with a poorer survival. Primary bladder tumors are usually more localized, presenting with hematuria or urinary tract obstruction. Other genitourinary tumors are diagnosed after a mass has been discovered. One half of extremity tumors are alveolar; they usually cause a nontender swelling and frequently have spread via the lymphatics by the time of diagnosis. Likewise, primary tumors of the trunk and the intrathoracic and retroperitoneal areas are often very infiltrative, are difficult to eradicate, and have a high incidence of recurrence. All sarcomas have the potential to spread locally, by lymphatic drainage, and by hematogenous dissemination, with the most common metastatic sites being the lungs, bone, and bone marrow.

Although trauma is the most common nonmalignant etiologic consideration in the differential diagnosis, the continued painless enlargement of a nontender mass makes malignancy more likely. Other possible malignant disorders in the differential diagnosis include lymphoma, Ewing's sarcoma, and (rarely in adolescents) neuroblastoma. After biopsy confirmation, a complete evaluation of the disease status should include CT scans of the chest and primary site, bone scan, bone marrow, and lumbar puncture with head CT or MRI scan for parameningeal foci. Sonograms are particularly useful for following the progress of genitourinary primary tumors.

The prognosis for soft tissue sarcomas depends primarily on the extent of disease at diagnosis (the more localized, the better), the extent of initial surgical resection (the less residual disease, the better), primary site (trunk and extremity, poor outlook), and the pathologic subtype (alveolar pathology and anaplasia, poor outlook). Given these principles, treatment strategies have included fairly aggressive surgical excisions with wide margins to offer the best chance of cure. As more effective chemotherapeutic regimens have evolved, less disfiguring surgery, improved survival statistics, and better quality of life have become the rule. Intensive chemotherapy has enabled the complete removal of initially unresectable masses as well as the possibility of limb-sparing procedures for extremity masses. At the same time, radiation has been eliminated or sharply curtailed in several clinical situations, although it is still effective in improving disease-free survival when used in high doses early in the course of treatment for most patients. Chemotherapy protocols are still evolving, primarily under the direction of the Intergroup Rhabdomyosarcoma Studies, and currently use combinations of vincristine, actinomycin D, cyclophosphamide, doxorubicin, cisplatin, ifosfamide, etoposide, and decarbazine. Results range from a greater than 80% cure for patients with no gross residual disease after initial surgical excision to 60% for localized gross residual and 20% for metastatic disease. Nearly all patients showing no sign of recurrence 2 years after the end of therapy are cured.

Non-RMS types in adolescents are also more commonly noted in the extremities and the trunk. Many of these are slow growing, usually do not present with metastases at diagnosis, and have characteristic features. Neurogenic sarcomas (malignant schwannomas) are most often seen in patients with neurofibromatosis. Fibrosarcomas and synovial sarcomas are usually found in extremities. Surgery appears to be more important in the non-RMS types, in which the role of chemotherapy is still evolving. Disease-free survival in this group of tumors is comparable with that of adults with sarcomas, while approaching that of RMSs in teenage patients with localized disease. Because of the possibility of late recurrence, long-term follow-up is necessary before a patient can be pronounced cured.

TUMORS OF SEXUAL ORGANS

Although relatively rare in children, malignant gonadal tumors increase in incidence throughout the adolescent years. The overwhelming majority of testicular and ovarian tumors in adolescents are germ cell in origin. Many of these germ cells have no capability for further differentiation, as in germinomas (seminomas in males, dysgerminomas in females). Undifferentiated germ cells (embryonal carcinoma) have the potential to further differentiate along an embryonal course toward teratomas or an extraembryonal course toward yolk sac carcinoma (also known as endodermal sinus tumor).

Many of these masses are mixed and must be evaluated carefully before a therapeutic course is begun.

Testicular Malignancy

The incidence of testicular malignancy begins to increase after puberty, and by the third decade of life becomes a leading cause of cancer death. The only important predisposing condition is cryptorchidism, with affected patients having a 20 to 40 times greater risk of developing malignant degeneration than normal. Surgical correction at an early age significantly decreases the risk. Of patients with abdominal testicles, 5% to 10% will contract testicular malignancy.

Often mistaken for testicular torsion, hernia, hydrocele, or epididymitis, malignant tumors are the most common testicular masses of adolescence. Most patients present with a longer than 3-month history of painless scrotal swelling and discomfort. When the condition arises in high, undescended testicles, the physical examination is often remarkable for a large abdominal mass. Most patients have localized disease initially; others present with lymphatic spread to retroperitoneal nodes. However, only a few present with hematogenous metastases to the lungs, liver, or bone. Embryonal carcinoma is the most common malignant tumor.

Diagnostic work-up must include careful staging with radiographic evaluation of the retroperitoneum, chest, and bone. Human chorionic gonadotropin (hCG) and alpha-fetoprotein (AFP) levels are often elevated and are good markers for residual and recurrent disease.

Initial surgical treatment should include a radical orchiectomy with ligation of the spermatic cord to prevent tumor spillage. Ideally, a retroperitoneal node dissection should be performed to rule out lymphatic spread. After careful pathologic examination of all tissue, further treatment consists of chemotherapy for embryonal carcinoma and radiation for the more infrequent seminomas, which are highly radiosensitive. Effective chemotherapeutic regimens, including combinations of cisplatin, etoposide, ifosfamide, bleomycin, and vinblastine, have dramatically improved the outcome in patients with both localized and disseminated disease. Patients with localized disease have an 80% to 90% expected cure rate.

Other testicular tumors include hormone-producing masses, such as the Leydig cell and Sertoli cell tumors, which are endocrinologically active but rarely malignant. These masses are treated conservatively. Paratesticular malignancies, including RMSs and lymphomas, require aggressive combination therapy.

Ovarian Malignancy

The incidence of ovarian germ cell tumors increases during adolescence, but many older teenagers develop adult-type epithelial tumors, such as adenocarcinoma and undifferentiated carcinoma. Although the prognosis for these tumors is somewhat better than in adults, the initial extent of disease is the most crucial determinant of outcome.

Unlike testicular malignancies, ovarian tumors are usually more advanced at diagnosis because of the location and the longer time that elapses before they become clinically evident. Most patients present with abdominal pain, either with or without a palpable mass. The pain is sometimes severe and acute in onset, often heralding a torsion of the mass or rupture of its contents into the abdomen and pelvis. Some tumors, most notably embryonal carcinoma, are associated with amenorrhea, irregular vaginal bleeding, or false-positive pregnancy tests. Spread of tumor is often found on the surface of the bladder, pelvic organs, omentum, bowel, and liver. In addition to direct spread by contact, distal metastases to lung, bone, and liver are seen in advanced disease. Mixed tumor types occasionally have metastatic sites with only one component present, which makes it essential to obtain a biopsy sample of the primary tumor to plan proper treatment. Again, AFP and β-subunit hCG levels are frequently elevated and are helpful in following treatment progress.

Treatment varies greatly according to the pathologic diagnosis. The very common cystic teratomas are usually not highly malignant and require nothing more than excision and follow-up. Likewise, unilateral dysgerminomas do well with surgery alone. When recurrent or more extensive, these tumors are very sensitive to chemotherapy and radiation and generally have an excellent prognosis. Embryonal carcinomas cannot be treated with surgery alone. However, the prognosis with current chemotherapeutic regimens is very good. Finally, the outlook for the adult-type epithelial carcinomas depends on tumor staging; however, even patients with evidence of spread will respond to several antineoplastic agents (e.g., cyclophosphamide, 5-fluorouracil, methotrexate, cisplatin, and doxorubicin). As in males, Sertoli cell and granulosa cell tumors are rarely malignant.

Miscellaneous Female Malignancies

Females exposed to diethylstilbestrol (DES) in utero are at increased risk for development of clear cell adenocarcinoma of the vagina in the adolescent years. Appearing after menarche, this malignancy peaks at age 19 and then rapidly becomes less common. The mechanism of action remains unknown, although the consensus seems to be that this drug acts as a teratogen rather than a carcinogen. The tumors are often asymptomatic, although they sometimes cause vaginal bleeding. Patients at risk should undergo frequent examinations and cytologic sampling to diagnose the tumor at an early stage.

When tumors are discovered and found to be localized, surgery alone cures 90% of patients. Radiation is also effective treatment for early-stage disease.

Malignant breast masses are rare in adolescents, but the incidence begins to increase slightly in older teenagers. Masses, which are usually hard and painless, are nearly always found in proximity to the nipple. The most common malignancy, adenocarcinoma, is usually indolent and localized and carries an excellent prognosis. As with adults, the current trend is toward less disfiguring surgery and more adjuvant therapy with antineoplastic drugs.

MISCELLANEOUS ADOLESCENT MALIGNANCIES

Nasopharyngeal carcinoma is an uncommon tumor that shows increasing incidence during adolescence. Arising in the epithelial lining of the nasopharynx, undifferentiated carcinoma is the most common pathologic subtype in teenagers. Typical signs and symptoms include painless cervical adenopathy, nasal obstruction, sinusitis, epistaxis, chronic otitis, and headache. Extension to the base of the skull can cause multiple neurologic abnormalities, including cranial nerve involvement (present in 50% of affected patients), hoarseness, and dysphagia. Common metastatic sites include the lungs, liver, long bones, and vertebrae. This type of carcinoma has a strong association with EBV infection, most patients having elevated EBV antibody titers. After surgical diagnosis, the mainstay of therapy is high-dose radiotherapy (6000 to 7000 cGy) in combination with chemotherapy (cisplatin, 5-fluorouracil). The prognosis ranges from 80% survival for localized disease to 25% survival for tumors with invasion into surrounding bone or the CNS.

Hepatocellular carcinoma is the most common primary hepatic malignancy in adolescents. Predisposing conditions include long-standing hepatic inflammation, as seen in biliary cirrhosis, hereditary tyrosinemia, and hepatitis B infection. Patients treated with high doses of anabolic steroids for many years, such as children with Fanconi's anemia, have a significantly increased risk of developing hepatocellular carcinoma. Presenting symptoms include abdominal mass, distention, and pain; fever, weight loss, jaundice, and anorexia are also common. Occasional patients present with signs of acute abdomen, usually coinciding with rupture of the mass and internal bleeding. The tumor is extremely invasive, producing necrosis and hemorrhage. Seventy percent of patients have advanced, unresectable disease at presentation. Additional laboratory findings include thrombocytosis, elevated alkaline phosphatase level, other abnormal liver function test results, and, in 50% of patients, elevated AFP levels. Although a cure is very uncommon if the tumor has been incompletely resected, surgical excision is fraught with major complications, including exsanguinating hemorrhage, hypotension and shock, and biliary tract leakage with cholangitis. Recent success in shrinking hepatocellular tumors through aggressive chemotherapy (using cisplatin, 5-fluorouracil, doxorubicin, and etoposide) has enabled safer and more complete surgery with resultant increased survival. Liver transplantation followed by additional adjuvant chemotherapy has also yielded some degree of success in this patient population.

Renal cell carcinoma replaces Wilms' tumor as the most common primary renal tumor during the adolescent years. Although relatively rare, it is seen with increased frequency in patients with tuberous sclerosis and von Hippel-Lindau disease. Presenting complaints include abdominal pain and hematuria. The mass is often not palpable. Many patients have hypercalcemia and polycythemia as a result of increased secretion of erythropoietin. In advanced stages the tumor metastasizes to nodes, lungs, bone, and liver. When the tumor is completely resected with wide margins, the results are usually excellent and no further therapy is necessary. The value of chemotherapy and radiation has not been established in more advanced disease, but some dramatic responses have been obtained with interleukin-2, which can cause major life-threatening adverse effects.

Carcinoma of the colon is another uncommon malignancy in young patients. Predisposing conditions in adolescents include long-standing ulcerative colitis, polyposis coli, the family cancer syndrome, and possibly neurofibromatosis. Symptoms are usually subtle, with a change in bowel habit most commonly seen in the early stages. Most teenagers with colon carcinoma have more advanced disease at presentation than do adults, with spread to the regional lymph nodes or the liver. In adolescents, about half of these tumors are mucoid adenocarcinomas; they are frequently huge, containing large mucin pools. Localized disease can be treated successfully with surgical excision, with care taken to sample many regional nodes. Responses to therapy with 5-fluorouracil, citrovorum, and levamisole have offered some hope to patients with more extensive disease.

LONG-TERM PATIENT FOLLOW-UP

As survivors of childhood and adolescent malignancies increase in number, concern is being directed toward the quality of life and the potential long-term adverse effects of disease and treatment. Greater success in more advanced malignancy has come at the price of significantly more intense chemotherapy and/or radiation treatment, with the potential for debilitating and life-threatening complications appearing years after the completion of all treatment, as in some patients with HD. As a result, there has been an increasing trend toward reducing the amount of treatment without compromising survival. Some of these long-range concerns are summarized below.

1. *Reproductive capability.* Sterility has been associated with radiation therapy administered to the testicle or ovary after puberty. It is a significant complication in patients treated for stage III HD and sarcomas of the pelvis and lower abdomen. Some chemotherapeutic agents, most notably cyclophosphamide and nitrogen mustard, also affect gonadal tissue, depending on the number and size of doses. Many patients can recover some function, although decreased fertility is common even without sterility. In females, prophylactic treatment with oral contraceptives may offer some protection against the adverse effects of chemotherapy by suppressing the normal ovulatory cycle. Children of survivors of childhood cancer have not demonstrated any increase in congenital anomalies.

2. *Cardiac dysfunction.* Drug regimens that rely heavily on anthracyclines entail a greater risk of decreased cardiac contractility and outright cardiac failure. This effect is compounded by mediastinal radiation and high-dose cyclophosphamide. Particularly disturbing have been recent reports of a decline in cardiac function years after all therapy was discontinued. A recent trend has been toward continuous-infusion anthracycline therapy, which decreases cardiotoxicity significantly without sacrificing efficacy. Newer, less cardiotoxic anthracyclines are undergoing clinical trials.

3. *Pulmonary toxicity.* Radiation, methotrexate, bleomycin, and the nitrosureas all are associated with pulmonary fibrosis and restrictive lung disease. When these factors are superimposed on previous pulmonary parenchymal disease and pneumonitis, a cured patient may be left a pulmonary cripple, prone to frequent bouts of pneumonia and respiratory distress. Decreasing radiation doses and avoidance of other causes of pulmonary damage (e.g., high-concentration oxygen therapy in patients receiving bleomycin) may prevent this condition.

4. *Renal dysfunction.* The use of nephrotoxic chemotherapy (cisplatin and ifosfamide) has become more widespread as these agents have been shown to be efficacious in the treatment of many malignancies. Much of the kidney damage is irreversible, with interstitial nephritis, renal tubular acidosis, decreased renal filtration, and renal failure developing in some patients. Potentiating these deleterious effects are nephrotoxic antibiotics and radiation. Attempts to minimize renal damage by restricting nephrotoxic antibiotics and introducing less toxic chemotherapy (e.g., carboplatin replacing cisplatin) are being instituted.

5. *Orthopedic abnormalities.* Radical surgical excision of extremity tumors and high-dose radiation are associated with limb asymmetry and scoliosis. Additional problems with radiation-induced osteopenia and aseptic necrosis of the femoral heads can result in significant disability. Less disfiguring surgery has helped considerably. Early involvement of physical and occupational therapists—to evaluate the extent of disability, increase strength, provide adaptive equipment, teach new skills, and train the patient in the use of altered limbs—cannot be overemphasized. Simultaneously, comprehensive emotional and psychological support is necessary to achieve any degree of success.

6. *Secondary malignancies.* Whether a result of the original tumor or of an underlying genetic or immunologic predisposition, or a consequence of therapy, new malignancies are expected to be a major concern as patients age. Already a frequent event in patients with advanced HD or retinoblastoma, secondary malignancies pose a particular risk for a large number of patients who are undergoing treatment involving ionizing radiation, alkylating agents such as cyclophosphamide and nitrogen mustard, and other drugs such as etoposide. The substitution of less carcinogenic agents for these therapies might lessen the incidence of these devastating, poorly responsive tumors.

CANCER PREVENTION

The slow progress in treatment of adult malignancies has served to intensify the issues of cancer prevention. Since many of the most common malignancies have been linked to known carcinogenic entities, it is of paramount importance to begin education during the adolescent years, when many dangerous practices become ingrained.

Smoking tobacco is the most important cause of lung carcinoma and the leading cause of cancer death in males (also one that is increasing steadily in females). Continued strong educational efforts directed toward adolescents, who often develop the smoking habit in response to peer pressure and a perceived image of sophistication, are mandatory, particularly in younger adolescents who have not yet developed the habit.

Alcohol consumption, which is associated with carcinoma of the liver, pharynx, and esophagus, is another habit that begins in adolescence, often for the same reasons as does smoking. Because of the frequency of vehicular accidents, homicide, and other alcohol-related injuries, the risk of these behaviors warrants major education efforts in the adolescent age group.

Diet and its relationship to colon carcinoma presents an even more difficult challenge because adolescents develop a particular style of diet and eating over many years. Emphasis on lower fat and calories and increased fiber intake should be part of any educational program.

Patients at high risk for malignancy as a result of inheritance (e.g., retinoblastoma, family cancer syndromes), previous treatment with radiation, malignancies that carry increased risk of secondary neoplasms (e.g., HD), and exposure to carcinogenic agents (e.g., DES) should be aware of this risk and the early warning signs of possible malignancy. Frequent physical examinations and surveillance testing should become part of their routine. Good health habits for all adolescents also should include learning and applying self-examination techniques for malignancies of the breast and the testicles so that these curable tumors can be detected at an early stage.

References

1. Levine EG, Bloomfield CD: Cytogenetics of non-Hodgkin's lymphoma, *J Natl Cancer Inst* monogr 10:7-12, 1990.

2. Vianna NJ, Greenwald P, Davies JNP: Extended epidemic of Hodgkin's disease in high school students, *Lancet* 1:1209-1211, 1971.

3. Young RC, Bookman MA, Longo DL: Late complications of Hodg-kin's disease management, *J Natl Cancer Inst* monogr 10:55-60, 1990.

4. Sposto R, Ertel IJ, Jenkin RD, et al: The effectiveness of chemotherapy for treatment of high grade astrocytoma in children: results of a randomized study, *J Neurosurg* 7:165-177, 1989.

5. Finlay JL, August C, Packer R, et al: High-dose multi-agent chemotherapy followed by bone marrow "rescue" for malignant astrocytomas of childhood and adolescence, *J Neurooncol* 9:239-248, 1990.

6. Price C: Primary bone-forming tumours and their relationship to skeletal growth, *J Bone Joint Surg* 40:574-593, 1958.

7. Eusebi V, Ceccarelli C, Gorza L, et al: Immunocytochemistry of rhabdomyosarcoma: the use of four different markers, *Am J Surg Pathol* 10:293-299, 1986.

Suggested Readings

Pizzo PA, Poplack DG, editors: *Principles and practice of pediatric oncology,* ed 2, Philadelphia, 1993, JB Lippincott.

Pochedly C, editor: Cancer in children, *Hematol Clin North Am* 1:577-673, 1987.

Williams SF, Farah R, Golomb HM, editors: Hodgkin's disease, *Hematol Clin North Am* 3:187-343, 1989.

CHAPTER 52

Hemorrhage and Thrombosis

•

Mark E. Weinblatt

The hemostatic and fibrinolytic systems are part of an extremely complex interplay of proteins, blood cells, endothelial cells, electrolytes, and vascular structures that normally interact in a complementary fashion to maintain proper vascular integrity and blood flow. Although a delicate balance is normally maintained among these opposing forces, many factors can disrupt this equilibrium and cause either hemorrhage or thrombosis, depending on which system prevails.

The coagulation mechanism is usually set into motion in response to the traumatic exposure of subendothelial collagen. Platelet adhesion and aggregation at the site of injury normally occur, after which coagulation proteins interact until a meshwork of fibrin strands forms in and around the mass of platelets. Additional platelet aggregation and trapping of other cellular elements eventually result in formation of a plug to seal the ruptured blood vessels and damaged vascular lining and to begin the

process of repair. Finally, once the breach has been healed, the fibrinolytic system will dissolve the clot to allow the resumption of unimpeded blood flow.

Proper functioning of this process depends on adequate amounts of coagulation and fibrinolytic proteins, most of which are synthesized by the liver. Depletion or inhibition of any of the coagulation factors interrupts the smooth progression along the coagulation cascade to the final insoluble cross-linked fibrin strands. Similarly, a defect in any of the fibrinolytic components or coagulation inhibitors can lead to the pathologic deposition of fibrin, resulting in obstruction of blood flow and tissue ischemia. Finally, abnormal platelet activity or blood vessel wall reactivity can contribute to failure of normal hemostasis.

Virtually all patients with severe inherited hemostatic disorders are diagnosed early in life, long before the adolescent years. Therefore, a teenager who presents with a new onset of a significant hemorrhagic tendency most likely does not have a hereditary disorder. However, it is important for the clinician to have a basic understanding of many different hemostatic abnormalities, regardless of when diagnosed, since the adolescent may have special needs to be addressed in relation to permissible activities and long-term complications of recurrent internal hemorrhage.

DIFFERENTIAL DIAGNOSIS OF HEMORRHAGIC DISORDERS

A good history frequently yields important clues to the underlying cause of bleeding. The patient's family history of hemorrhagic tendency may uncover a previously undiagnosed hereditary disorder such as von Willebrand's disease, mild hemophilia, or platelet dysfunction. The bleeding pattern is another important part of the puzzle that can point to a particular hemostatic disorder. The patient who presents with hemarthrosis, delayed bleeding from superficial cuts and abrasions, and other deep tissue bleeding is very likely suffering from a coagulation disturbance rather than a platelet defect. On the other hand, petechial rashes, epistaxis, and immediate and prolonged bleeding from lacerations and dental extractions indicate abnormal behavior of the platelet-vascular interaction. Medication history is very important, since many relatively innocuous drugs, such as aspirin-containing compounds, can have profound effects on normal hemostasis.

As opposed to most other symptoms of disease, hemorrhage can be assigned to a category after a few simple blood screening tests have been obtained (Fig. 52-1). The platelet count can be easily ascertained with a simple complete blood count (CBC), while a bleeding time will reveal a defect in the platelet-endothelial interaction. The prothrombin time (PT) is an effective indicator of the health of the extrinsic and common pathways (particularly factor VII), while the partial thromboplastin time (PTT) can detect deficiencies of the intrinsic and common pathways (especially factors VIII, IX, XI, and XII). Subsequent, more specialized tests, including factor assays, platelet aggregation, and platelet morphology, can then be used to establish the diagnosis.

Classic Hemophilia

Classic hemophilia (factor VIII deficiency), a sex-linked, lifelong bleeding disorder limited almost exclusively to males, results from the production of a dysfunctional coagulation protein. With rare exceptions, patients with moderate or severe hemophilia are diagnosed early in childhood; only mildly affected patients (factor VIII:c levels between 5% and 20%) elude

diagnosis until their teenage years. Bleeding manifestations commonly sustained by teenagers include hemarthroses and intramuscular hematomas. As a result of patient education and prompt correction early in the course of bleeding episodes, the incidence of chronic hemarthroses with joint destruction has decreased dramatically, thus reducing a source of considerable debility. Head trauma is potentially the most serious type of injury in individuals with hemophilia, particularly in active adolescents who participate in sports. Gross hematuria is often a source of significant hemorrhage that may require red blood cell transfusions.

The diagnosis of mild hemophilia should be suspected in the male who reports protracted bleeding after dental procedures or prolonged epistaxis and who is found to have only an elevated PTT on initial screening. The family history is often positive for maternal male relatives who have had unusual bleeding manifestations, and definitive diagnosis is confirmed by finding a decreased factor VIII coagulant activity and a normal factor VIII antigen level.

Depending on the type of hemorrhage encountered, the treatment for nearly all bleeding episodes in moderately or severely affected patients entails infusion of reconstituted lyophilized factor VIII concentrate. This product, prepared from pooled plasma of thousands of donors, is usually very effective in raising the patient's factor level. In addition, with current manufacturing, purification, and cleansing processes, it is the safest product from the standpoint of infection transmission. Dosage varies according to the severity of hemorrhage, with 1 U/kg raising the factor level 2% in the factor VIII–deficient patient. Most patients with mild hemophilia A respond to intravenous infusions or intranasal administration of desmopressin (DDAVP), which induces release of factor VIII from endothelial cells and can triple the patient's circulating factor level. Administration of DDAVP is not as successful if done several times in a 24-hour period because of depletion of the storage sites. Another method of mitigating the amount of factor concentrate needed is simultaneous administration of antifibrinolytic agents (e.g., aminocaproic acid, tranexamic acid) that are effective in preventing rebleeding in mucous membranes. Prednisone is often of benefit in reducing the joint inflammation of recurrent acute hemarthroses, thus promoting quicker healing and fewer factor infusions.

Most adolescents with severe hemophilia are candidates for home infusion programs, in which family members, and ultimately the patients themselves, are taught how and when to infuse factor concentrate at home. The advantages of this program include prompt treatment of acute hemorrhagic episodes with as little disruption as possible in the patient's and family's schedule. This is particularly important for the adolescent, who can thereby achieve a greater sense of

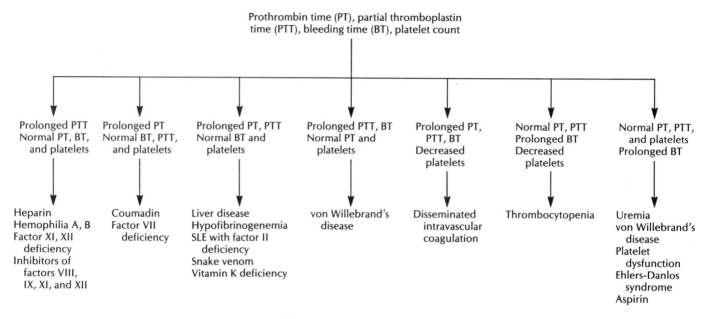

Fig. 52-1. Differential diagnosis of hemorrhagic disorders.

independence and responsibility. Prophylactic administration of factor concentrate can enable those with hemophilia to participate in more active sports. Physical activity and exercise help to strengthen muscles surrounding weakened joints, thus providing improved stability to the joint, allowing better handling of daily physical stress, and decreasing bleeding episodes. Although a good deal of trial and error is necessary for each teenager, activities such as swimming and golf are ideal for the patient with a bleeding disorder. Other sports, such as bowling, weightlifting, and bicycle riding, also provide opportunities for safe physical activities. As a rule, all contact sports should be avoided in patients with severe hemophilia.

An important complication of replacement therapy is infection. Although heat, detergent, and monoclonal antibody treatment of factor products have rendered current commercial concentrates almost virus free, most older adolescents with hemophilia presently have liver function abnormalities and hepatitis B surface antibody. A small percentage of patients are diagnosed as having chronic active hepatitis, with about 15% of patients showing biopsy evidence of cirrhosis.[1] Many adolescent patients also have human immunodeficiency virus (HIV) antibodies, a result of treatment with infected batches of factor concentrate prepared before widespread screening became available in 1985. Although some patients have progressed with development of typical AIDS-related complications and death, the majority are stable for many years, with only mild signs or symptoms (e.g., lymphadenopathy, chronic otitis, immune thrombocytopenic purpura [ITP]). The addition of widespread screening for hepatitis C, better methods of sterilizing products, and the

availability of factor products made by synthetic recombinant DNA techniques should further minimize the risk of infectious complications.

Another serious problem affecting the patient who has been treated with multiple infusions is that of inhibitors. Between 5% and 15% of individuals with hemophilia A develop antibodies against the factor VIII molecule because of frequent treatments and exposure to transfused proteins. Effective treatment for such patients includes prothrombin complex concentrates that bypass the factor VIII point in the coagulation cascade, porcine factor VIII concentrate, and high-dose factor VIII concentrates for selected hemorrhagic indications.

Miscellaneous Coagulation Deficiencies

Patients with factor IX deficiency generally display symptoms similar to those found in classic hemophilia. Again, patients with this sex-linked disorder who have a moderate or severe deficiency of the coagulation protein are likely to have been diagnosed earlier in childhood and will be familiar with the intricacies of hemorrhagic episodes and their treatment by the time they reach adolescence. Bleeding events are treated with factor IX concentrate, and patients usually require fewer infusions per bleed than those with classic hemophilia because of the longer half-life of the factor IX protein.

Deficiency of factor XI, also known as hemophilia C, is an autosomal recessive disorder primarily affecting Ashkenazi Jews. This deficiency is usually associated with milder hemorrhagic events, such as epistaxis, and delayed bleeding after surgery or dental procedures. Diagnosis is established with a prolonged PTT and low factor XI assay, and effective correction can be obtained with fresh frozen plasma.

Von Willebrand's disease is a heterogeneous group of disorders characterized by abnormal interaction between platelets and endothelial cells and reduced levels of factor VIII. There are many variants, and a hallmark of the disease is a fluctuation of platelet function and factor VIII levels over time in any given patient. The patient with classic von Willebrand's disease exhibits concomitantly low assays of factor VIII:c and VIII:ag, prolonged bleeding time, decreased ristocetin cofactor activity, and abnormal platelet aggregation in response to ristocetin stimulus. However, most variants of the disease involve only some of these abnormalities. Distinguishing subtypes in von Willebrand's disease is very important for therapeutic considerations. Classic von Willebrand's disease and several variants usually respond well to DDAVP administration, with a good correction of bleeding time and an elevation of ristocetin cofactor activity. In some subtypes, however, DDAVP is contraindicated because it can cause inappropriate platelet aggregation and thrombocytopenia (in type IIB). In other subtypes it is ineffective, and patients must be treated with cryoprecipitate infusion. Some responses have also been obtained in patients with von Willebrand's disease using Humate-P, an intermediate purity pasteurized factor VIII concentrate that possesses a nearly normal multimeric structure of the factor VIII molecule.

Any disease that severely affects the liver, the site of production of most coagulation proteins, can have pronounced effects on hemostasis. The liver-dependent proteins with the shortest half-life, particularly factor VII, are preferentially affected early in the course of hepatic dysfunction, resulting in a prolonged PT in most patients with acute hepatitis or liver failure. Other proteins, including factors II, V, X, and XIII, are also moderately reduced as a consequence of decreased synthesis, which can predispose the patient to severe bleeding. The patient with a severely cirrhotic liver typically has difficulty synthesizing most proteins and usually has abnormalities in most coagulation parameters, requiring frequent transfusions of fresh frozen plasma to replace all missing factors and to control bleeding.

Serious, often life-threatening bleeding complications are commonly encountered in the patient with disseminated intravascular coagulation (DIC). Both the coagulation and fibrinolytic systems are activated in this process, which can be triggered by many inciting events (Box 52-1) and may be associated with concurrent thrombosis and hemorrhage. Platelets and coagulation proteins are consumed and depleted in the process, with the overriding symptom complex dependent on which competing system is prevalent. Although platelet and plasma infusions are helpful in reducing hemorrhage, and plasma (as a source of antithrombin III) or antithrombin

---

BOX 52-1
Causes of Disseminated Intravascular Coagulation in Adolescents

Infections
  Sepsis
    Meningococcemia
    Gonococcus
    Staphylococcus
    Pseudomonas
    Klebsiella
    Pneumococcus
    Proteus
    Serratia
    Candida sepsis
    Aspergillus
  Malaria
  Rocky Mountain spotted fever
  Measles
  Cytomegalovirus
  Influenza
  Disseminated varicella/zoster
  Kala-azar
Severe asphyxia
Burns
Cyanotic cardiac disease
Acute promyelocytic leukemia
Sarcoma
Snake bite
Massive head injury
Massive trauma
Hemolytic transfusion reactions
Heat stroke
Retained dead fetus
Amniotic fluid embolus
Intrauterine infections
Abruptio placentae
Toxemia of pregnancy
Purpura fulminans
Hypothermia
Prolonged hypotension
Severe acidosis
Severe hepatic disease
Systemic vasculitis
Drowning

III concentrate may play a role in mitigating the consumption process, attention must be directed primarily toward eliminating the underlying cause.

Besides the specific coagulation antibodies that evolve in patients with hemophilia who are administered factor concentrates, acquired inhibitors may appear in patients with collagen vascular disease or even in those with no identifiable underlying disorder. Most of these natural anticoagulants are nonspecific, directed against several contact factors high in the intrinsic pathway, although on occasion they may be found to inhibit the activity of a particular factor. The presence of an inhibitor should be suspected after obtaining an isolated prolonged PTT that corrects poorly when mixed with normal plasma. Bleeding is rarely a problem in such patients if there is no associated factor deficiency. One particular type of antibody, the lupus anticoagulant, is often associated with thrombosis. In pregnant adolescents this antibody causes a significant number of spontaneous abortions and unexpected late intrauterine deaths as a result of placental thrombosis.[2]

Vitamin K deficiency is exceedingly uncommon in the healthy teenager, but it may be found in adolescents with cystic fibrosis, fat malabsorption, cholelithiasis, obstructive jaundice, or Crohn's disease or who have ingested warfarin compounds. Decreased activity of the vitamin K–dependent factors (II, VII, IX, and X) can result in prolongation of PT and PTT, with a range of hemorrhagic symptoms dependent on the severity of the deficiency. With administration of vitamin K, partial correction may be noted within 4 hours; if more rapid improvement is mandatory, fresh frozen plasma can be transfused.

Thrombocytopenia

Platelet defects, both quantitative and qualitative, cause characteristic bleeding, most often petechiae, ecchymoses, and epistaxis. The severity of bleeding in the patient with decreased platelets directly correlates with the degree of thrombocytopenia, with a serious risk of spontaneous internal hemorrhage when the platelet count is below 20,000/mm^3. The many causes of thrombocytopenia (Box 52-2) may be congenital or acquired. Although bone marrow examination will help to differentiate the pathophysiologic mechanism involved, a definitive diagnosis often requires careful analysis of the history, associated features, and other laboratory findings.

Immune thrombocytopenic purpura is the most common cause of low platelet count in the adolescent, with a behavior that is often different from that in children. Onset can be either abrupt or insidious, with the former more likely to be associated with acute ITP. The patient with a short history often reports an antecedent viral illness, the sudden appearance of petechiae and ecchymoses, and occasionally more serious gastrointestinal or urinary tract bleeding. Typically, the patient is in no distress, does not appear acutely or chronically ill, and, other than having hemorrhagic manifestations, is asymptomatic. Platelet counts are frequently under 20,000/mm^3, with normal hemoglobin levels and white blood cell counts, and bone marrow that shows a normal differential with increased megakaryocytes. Bleeding can begin during a viral infection, but more often hemorrhagic symptoms follow 1 to 2 weeks after the cessation of infectious symptoms. Nonspecific respiratory infections

are most commonly reported, although associations have been made with measles, rubella, varicella, Epstein-Barr virus, and HIV and after administration of live virus vaccines, particularly measles.[3,4] Immune complexes and antiplatelet antibodies have been detected in patients with ITP, and the spleen has been shown to be the most prominent site of platelet destruction, but the exact mechanism of destruction remains unclear.

Acute ITP is a generally benign illness that resolves within a few months in 80% to 90% of pediatric patients, regardless of age or therapy. Despite the severity of thrombocytopenia in most patients, only 2% to 4% of patients sustain serious hemorrhagic episodes, such as intracranial bleeding, and the mortality rate remains approximately 1%. A direct result of this excellent outcome is a lack of consensus about the best treatment or whether any treatment is indicated. The traditional use of prednisone remains prevalent in most centers, although high-dose intravenous gammaglobulin administered over 2 to 5 days also has proven efficacious, achieving a more rapid rise in platelet count in most patients. For the rare patient with an intracranial or another life-threatening hemorrhage, emergency splenectomy to remove the primary site of platelet destruction, along with platelet transfusion, corticosteroids, and/or gammaglobulin therapy, will result in the most rapid improvement in platelet counts.

Unlike children with ITP, adolescents exhibit a greater tendency toward chronicity. These patients are more likely to have insidious onset, platelet counts between 20,000 and 50,000/mm^3, and absence of any obvious viral prodrome. Females with this condition outnumber males by nearly 3 to 1, and more than 90% of patients have elevated levels of platelet-associated immunoglobulin. Many patients have underlying or associated diseases, including systemic lupus erythematosus, lymphoma, and HIV infection. Association with autoimmune hemolytic anemia (Evans' syndrome) and other autoantibody-mediated disorders usually warrants additional laboratory evaluation for autoimmunity, including Coombs' test, antinuclear antibody test, and anticardiolipin antibody measurement (often positive in patients with systemic lupus erythematosus). Although treatments for chronic ITP are similar to those for acute ITP, many more patients with chronic thrombocytopenia ultimately undergo elective splenectomy to alleviate the bleeding symptoms. Those patients who still exhibit a good response to prednisone or gammaglobulin and do not have an underlying illness are more likely to have sustained remission after surgery.[5] Long-term prednisone therapy plays less of a role in the management of chronic ITP because of adverse effects, and medical treatments currently in use include intermittent administration of gammaglobulin, danazol, vincristine, RhoGAM, and a variety of immunosuppressive medications.

BOX 52-2
Causes of Thrombocytopenia in Adolescents

DECREASED PRODUCTION
Aplastic anemia
Drug suppression
  Estrogen
  Chloramphenicol
  Alcohol
  Chemotherapy
  Thiazides
  Interferon
Leukemia
Sarcoma
Gaucher's disease
Myelofibrosis
Bernard-Soulier syndrome
May-Hegglin anomaly
Gray platelet syndrome
Radiation
Anorexia nervosa
Cyclic thrombocytopenia
Megaloblastic anemia
Severe iron deficiency
Paroxysmal nocturnal hemo-
  globinuria
Renal failure
Infection
  Tuberculosis
  Parvovirus
  Mumps
  Cytomegalovirus
  Dengue

SEQUESTRATION
Splenomegaly
Hypothermia
Liver disease
Cardiopulmonary
  bypass

INCREASED DESTRUCTION
Immune thrombocytopenic purpura
Drug-induced
  Heparin
  Valproic acid
  Phenytoin
  Penicillin
  Indomethacin
  Gold salts
  Heroin
  Sulfonamides
DIC
Massive transfusion
Collagen vascular disease
Infection
  Bacterial sepsis
  Malaria
  EBV infection
  HIV
  Rocky Mountain spotted fever
  Bacterial endocarditis
  Measles
  Measles vaccine
  Tuberculosis
Renal transplant rejection
Prosthetic heart valves
Indwelling catheters
Glomerulonephritis
Toxemia of pregnancy
Rheumatic heart disease
Hemolytic uremic syndrome
Thrombotic thrombocytopenic purpura
Burns
Fat embolism
Hemangiomas
Anaphylaxis

DIC, disseminated intravascular coagulation; *EBV,* Epstein-Barr virus.

Direct nonimmune platelet destruction may accompany a variety of serious medical disorders. Infections such as bacterial and fungal sepsis, toxic shock syndrome, Rocky Mountain spotted fever, and endocarditis often are associated with thrombocytopenia resulting from a combination of decreased platelet life span and production. Indwelling prosthetic devices (e.g., catheters, shunts, cardiac valves) and thermal injury in burn patients can directly injure platelets and enhance their removal from the circulation. Disorders associated with microangiopathic hemolysis, including hemolytic uremic syndrome, thrombotic thrombocytopenic purpura, and DIC, can cause profound thrombocytopenia and bleeding. Many drugs are associated with immune-mediated platelet destruction; the most commonly reported medications include quinidine, heparin, gold salts, and sulfonamide antibiotics. Resolution of thrombocytopenia in most of these disorders follows improvement in the underlying condition or cessation of medication use.

Decreased production of platelets also can be a consequence of infection or drug administration, but more often it is indicative of a primary disorder affecting the bone marrow. Pancytopenia is more common than isolated thrombocytopenia, and bone marrow examination is usually necessary to differentiate syndromes involving marrow failure from infiltrative processes. Inherited thrombocytopenias, such as the May-Hegglin anomaly and Bernard-Soulier syndrome, are rare and may be initially diagnosed at any age. Most of these disorders require platelet transfusions to control bleeding episodes.

In addition to specific therapy aimed at raising the platelet count in the thrombocytopenic patient, attention should be paid to minimizing any bleeding event. Patients with platelet counts above 75,000/mm^3 usually do not have any significant bruising, and restrictions should be limited to avoidance of contact sports and activities associated with risk of possible major trauma (e.g., climbing to heights). On the other hand, the patient with a platelet count below 30,000/mm^3 must be cautioned against most sports activities until the platelet count can be raised to safer levels. As a rule, patients with ITP bleed less than thrombocytopenic patients with a disorder of platelet production, owing in part to the large, very active circulating platelets that are produced in the healthy marrow. In any circumstance, care should be taken not to superimpose any additional hemostatic insult to the thrombocytopenic patients, such as the administration of medications that affect some component of hemostasis (e.g., aspirin and certain antihistamines).

Qualitative Platelet Disorders

Platelet dysfunction in the adolescent can be either acquired or congenital, can result from abnormalities in each phase of platelet function, and can produce a variable bleeding diathesis. Platelet adhesion, the initial response to exposure of subendothelial collagen, is abnormal in von Willebrand's disease and the autosomal recessive Bernard-Soulier syndrome. Von Willebrand's factor, a large multimeric glycoprotein synthesized by megakaryocytes and endothelial cells, is required for proper platelet adhesion. This protein is usually decreased in patients with von Willebrand's disease, whereas patients with Bernard-Soulier syndrome produce platelets that cannot interact with the factor. The bleeding time in both disorders is usually prolonged, and bleeding manifestations are similar to those in patients with thrombocytopenia. The rare patient with Bernard-Soulier syndrome will require platelet transfusions to halt bleeding related to the decreased number of platelets and their diminished function.

Inherited platelet aggregation dysfunction is seen in Glanzmann's thrombasthenia, which is usually diagnosed in childhood. This autosomal recessive disorder is a result of an abnormal or deficient glycoprotein of the platelet membrane that involves decreased binding sites of fibrinogen. Serious bleeding is treated with platelet transfusions. Another group of inherited platelet dysfunctions is seen in the storage pool disorders (gray platelet, Hermansky-Pudlak, and Chédiak-Higashi syndromes), all of which share a failure of normal granule secretion. These granules, which contain adenosine diphosphate, serotonin, and other materials, normally release their contents, which then migrate to the platelet surface and facilitate the generation of thrombin. Bleeding can be severe but often responds to DDAVP infusion or platelet transfusion.

Several acquired disorders can profoundly affect proper platelet functioning. Uremia can influence all phases of platelet function, possibly as a result of accumulation of materials such as guanidinosuccinic acid or phenolic acid. In addition to adhesion, aggregation, and secretory dysfunction, platelet procoagulant activity is routinely decreased. All these changes are reflected in a prolonged bleeding time. The defect often can be corrected by intensive dialysis, although both DDAVP and cryoprecipitate infusions have been effective in most patients.[6] Conjugated estrogens also have been used to shorten the bleeding time in patients with uremia. Patients who have undergone cardiopulmonary bypass may experience bleeding because of platelets that have been damaged by trauma or hypothermia and can no longer aggregate properly. When superimposed on thrombocytopenia (resulting from hemodilution, hepatic sequestration, and adherence to the bypass circuit) and heparinization, bleeding can be profuse. This aggregation dysfunction also can be improved with DDAVP, although at times platelet transfusions also are required.

Many drugs can interfere with normal platelet activity. The most common and well-known one is acetylsalicylic acid, which irreversibly inactivates cyclooxygenase, thus blocking normal platelet aggregation. Even small doses can result in some prolongation of the bleeding time in normal patients, with severe effects in patients with preexisting hemostatic defects (particularly von Willebrand's disease). These effects can last up to a week after ingestion. Other nonsteroidal antiinflammatory drugs, including indomethacin and ibuprofen, likewise inhibit cyclooxygenase, but the effect is reversible and the bleeding time normalizes within 24 hours. Finally, large doses of penicillins, especially carbenicillin, decrease aggregation and prolong bleeding time through an unknown mechanism in 50% to 75% of patients. Actual bleeding is uncommon and the effect is reversible.

Miscellaneous Purpuric Disorders

Henoch-Schönlein purpura produces characteristic hemorrhagic lesions on the buttocks and lower extremities. Often associated with fever, polyarthritis, colicky abdominal pain (occasionally with intussusception), and headache, the most serious complication of this disorder is renal dysfunction. The underlying pathologic dermatologic finding is aseptic vasculitis, and possible allergic or autoimmune mechanisms have been proposed. Although hematuria and melena may occur in 35% to 40% of patients, this bleeding is caused by vasculitic involvement of the kidney and bowel wall and not a generalized bleeding diathesis. Treatment with corticosteroids can alleviate joint and possibly renal complications, but it has demonstrated no effect on the hemorrhagic rash.

Purpura is a common feature of inherited connective tissue disorders, such as Ehlers-Danlos syndrome and pseudoxanthoma elasticum, with bleeding ranging from purpura and hematomas to life-threatening hemorrhage of the gastrointestinal or genitourinary tract. Hemostatic defects are usually a consequence of spontaneous rupture of friable blood vessels rather than any platelet-associated problems. Likewise, mechanical purpura associated with violent muscular activity results from ruptured blood vessels under increased intraluminal pressure. Factitious purpura, which may be a component of Munchausen's syndrome, usually presents with bizarre lesions and is seen most commonly in teenage girls. Suspicion of this disorder should be aroused by the unusual nature of the lesions (linear distribution, abrasions overlying bruises, and well-circumscribed areas of petechiae induced by suction) and the absence of abnormal hemostatic function.[7] Some teenage patients with severe emotional or psychiatric disturbances have self-administered anticoagulants to induce hemorrhage. It is important that such patients be tactfully confronted and expeditiously referred for psychiatric care.

THROMBOTIC DISORDERS

Thrombosis, the result of pathologic activation of hemostatic mechanisms, may be found in many diverse disorders. Any situation characterized by a hypercoagulable state, such as venous stasis, increased viscosity, and decreased blood flow, can lead to thrombus formation. Thrombotic disorders are not rare in adolescents, and early recognition of thrombophlebitis is mandatory to begin therapy and prevent clot propagation and pulmonary embolus.

In addition to conditions that increase blood viscosity (e.g., polycythemia, sickle cell disease, dehydration) and situations characterized by increased stasis (e.g., pregnancy, obesity, immobilization, heart failure, postoperative orthopedic surgery, cardiac surgery), many diseases are associated with increased risk of thrombophlebitis because of an altered balance between the fibrinolytic and coagulation processes. Studies of patients with diabetes mellitus, those with the nephrotic syndrome, and pregnant women have found higher levels of fibrinogen and factors V and VIII:c, and increased platelet aggregation. Therefore, all these patients are at risk for venous and arterial thrombosis. Inherited deficiencies of antithrombin III, protein C, and protein S—proteins that naturally inhibit the coagulation system—all are associated with recurrent deep vein thromboses in the teenage years. Acquired

deficiencies of these proteins can result from liver disease, DIC, and L-asparaginase therapy and can cause similar thrombotic complications. Indwelling central catheters, cardiac valves, and intracardiac patches provide thrombogenic surfaces, placing the patient at risk. Oral contraceptive use and smoking have been linked to an increased risk of venous and arterial thrombosis. Homocystinuria, an inherited disorder of homocysteine metabolism, is associated with demonstrable endothelial damage resembling classic atherosclerotic lesions. It is characterized by major thrombotic complications, including myocardial, cerebral, renal, and pulmonary infarctions. Inflammatory disorders, such as systemic lupus erythematosus, vasculitis, and Crohn's disease, are associated with a greater risk of thrombosis and embolism.

Early recognition and institution of therapy are critical in the management of thrombophlebitis. Suspicion of thrombosis should be aroused if a patient with any of the above conditions complains of pain and swelling in the lower extremities and has physical findings that include tenderness, increased warmth, and a typical "cord" on palpation. Doppler ultrasonography is very helpful in demonstrating blood flow patterns and obstruction in such patients. Sudden respiratory distress is an ominous finding of possible pulmonary embolus, which can have life-threatening implications.

Although the patient with superficial thrombosis can be managed conservatively with bed rest, hot compresses, and anti-inflammatory medications, anticoagulation with heparin remains the mainstay of therapy for deep vein thrombosis. More reliable heparin levels and fewer bleeding complications can be attained with continuous intravenous infusions rather than bolus infusions. After an initial loading dose of 75 to 100 U/kg, a continuous infusion of 10 to 25 U/kg/hr usually maintains the PTT in the desirable range of 1½ to 2 times normal. After improvement has been noted, oral warfarin therapy can be started, with an initial daily dose of 10 to 15 mg. Subsequent doses are aimed at keeping the PT in the same 1½ to 2 times normal range, or an international normalized ratio (INR) of 2 to 2½. The effects of heparin and warfarin can be easily neutralized with protamine and vitamin K, respectively, if bleeding complications arise. Patients with lifelong thrombotic disorders, such as protein C, protein S, or antithrombin III deficiencies, benefit from prophylactic heparin therapy. It is recommended that patients who have an indwelling cardiac prosthesis take a combination of anticoagulants and antiplatelet medications (aspirin or dipyridamole). The use of fibrinolytic therapy—with streptokinase, urokinase, and tissue plasminogen activator used to dissolve thrombi and emboli rapidly—has shown encouraging early results in dissolving coronary artery thromboses, massive pulmonary emboli, deep vein thromboses, and peripheral artery occlusion in adults. Fibrinolytic therapy may play a larger role in all age groups if success in controlling bleeding complications continues.

References

1. Aledort LM, Levine PH, Hilgartner M, et al: A study of liver biopsies and liver disease among hemophiliacs, *Blood* 66:367-372, 1985.
2. Gastineau DH, Kazmier FJ, Nichols WL, Bowie EJW: Lupus anticoagulant: an analysis of the clinical and laboratory features of 219 cases, *Am J Hematol* 19:265-275, 1985.
3. Oski FA, Naiman JL: Effect of live measles vaccine on the platelet count, *N Engl J Med* 275:352-356, 1966.
4. Nieminen U, Peltola H, Syrjala MT, et al: Acute thrombocytopenic purpura following measles, mumps, and rubella vaccinations. A report on 23 patients, *Acta Paediatr* 82:267-270, 1993.
5. Weinblatt ME, Ortega J: Steroid responsiveness as predictor of the outcome of splenectomy in children with chronic ITP, *Am J Dis Child* 136:1064-1066, 1982.
6. Mannucci PM: Desmopressin (DDAVP) for treatment of disorders of hemostasis, *Prog Hemost Thromb* 8:19-45, 1986.
7. Ratnoff CD: The psychogenic purpuras: a review of autoerythrocyte sensitization, autosensitization to DNA, "hysterical" and factitial bleeding, and the religious stigmata, *Semin Hematol* 17:192-213, 1980.

Suggested Readings

Colman RW, Hirsh J, Marder VJ, Salzman EW, editors: *Hemostasis and thrombosis. Basic principles and clinical practice,* ed 3, Philadelphia, 1994, JB Lippincott.

Colman RW, Rao AK, editors: Platelets in health and disease, *Hematol Clin North Am* 4:1-311, 1990.

Handin RI, Lux SE, Stossel TP: *Blood. Principles and practice of hematology,* Philadelphia, 1995, JB Lippincott.

Hilgartner MW, Pochedly C, editors: *Hemophilia in the child and adult,* ed 3, New York, 1989, Raven Press.

Loscalzo J, Schafer AI, editors: *Thrombosis and hemorrhage,* Oxford, 1994, Blackwell Scientific Publications.

Nathan DG, Oski FA: *Hematology of infancy and childhood,* ed 4, Philadelphia, 1993, WB Saunders.

Williams WJ, Beutler E, Erslev AJ, Lichtman MA: *Hematology,* ed 4, New York, 1990, McGraw-Hill.

CHAPTER 53

Lymphadenopathy and Splenomegaly

•

Mark E. Weinblatt

The lymph nodes and the spleen are integral parts of the lymphoid system that contain the largest accumulation of lymphocytes and cells of the reticuloendothelial system. These organs are at the vanguard of the body's defense system against foreign challenges and are responsible for generating appropriate immune responses to antigenic stimuli.

The lymphoid system grows rapidly in childhood, and palpable lymph nodes, particularly in the cervical and inguinal region, are nearly always found on routine physical examination. Palpable nodes begin to subside during the adolescent years until adulthood, when persistently enlarged nodes are unusual and often require investigation. The lymph nodes themselves are encapsulated structures—with well-defined, compact zones containing dense populations of lymphocytes—separated by bands of reticulum cells. The different internal lymph node regions vary and change with age, site, and immunologic or inflammatory stimuli. Enlargement can

result from proliferation of lymphocytes (or other resident cells) responding to outside stimuli, loss of normal control mechanisms (as in lymphomas), or invasion by cells normally foreign to the lymph node (storage cells, malignant cells, granulocytes).

The normal spleen is also composed of several distinct cellular components encased in a fibrous capsule. The outer white pulp contains dense collections of lymphocytes, plasma cells, and macrophages similar to those of the lymph node. The inner, larger red pulp is a spongy, highly vascular matrix through which blood flows. The splenic sinusoids are lined with endothelial cells covering a fenestrated basement membrane, all of which allows considerable flow and contact of blood components with the reticuloendothelial cells. Under normal conditions the spleen contains about 1% of the total blood circulation at any given time, including about one third to one half of the total blood platelets, and exhibits a much slower than expected blood transit time compared with other body

---

BOX 53-1
Differential Diagnosis of Lymphadenopathy

INFECTION
Bacterial
    "Strep" pharyngitis
    Regional pyogenic infections
    Cat-scratch disease
    Listeriosis
    Anthrax
    Bartonellosis
    Plague
    Diphtheria
    Rat-bite fever
    Leprosy
    Atypical mycobacteria
    Leptospirosis
Viral
    Upper respiratory infections
    Herpes zoster
    Dengue hemorrhagic fever
    Hepatitis
Fungal
    Sporotrichosis
    Coccidioidomycosis
    Tinea capitis
    Candidiasis
Miscellaneous
    Chlamydia

NEOPLASTIC DISEASES
Neuroblastoma
Rhabdomyosarcoma
Thyroid carcinoma
Nasopharyngeal carcinoma

RHEUMATIC DISEASES
Kawasaki's disease
Serum sickness
Scleroderma

MISCELLANEOUS
Adrenal insufficiency
Drug reactions: hydantoins, isoniazid, sulfasalazine, hydralazine, allopurinol
Seborrheic dermatitis
Sinus histiocytosis

---

sites. This arrangement allows for monitoring and filtering of blood, with both the necessary time and phagocytic cells available to complete the removal process. Damaged and senescent red blood cells (RBCs) are normally purged from the circulation during passage through the spleen. As evidenced by pathologic conditions that cause enlargement of the spleen, this hemodynamic status can be altered dramatically. Splenomegaly allows a larger volume of blood pooling, slowing of transit time, and increased cell trapping, resulting in the undesirable effect of a decrease in peripheral blood cells. The most extreme examples of this pathologic state are the splenic sequestration crisis in sickle cell disease and the severe pancytopenia of hypersplenism. As is true of lymph nodes, enlargement of the spleen can result from proliferation of intrinsic cells or infiltration of extrinsic cells. However, additional factors may be active in the pathogenesis of splenomegaly, including (1) abnormal hemodynamics of the splenic sinusoidal and portal circulation, (2) the spleen's role as a site of extramedullary hematopoiesis, and (3) the spleen's function as a preferential site for the deposition of lipid and other materials in storage disorders.

The spleen and the lymph nodes are often nonspecifically enlarged as a result of regional or generalized processes, including infection, inflammatory conditions, neoplasms, or storage diseases. As indicated in Boxes 53-1 to 53-3, the differential diagnosis of lymphadenopathy and/or splenomegaly is broad, and more specific direction must be provided prior to an extensive diagnostic evaluation. Since obtaining biopsy tissue for a pathologic examination is a painful, costly, and frequently nonproductive method of trying to ascertain the underlying problem, some general rules should be used to determine what features call for more invasive testing. An excellent algorithm for the work-up of lymphadenopathy can be found in a book by McMillan et al.[1]

The first question to be asked in evaluating the adolescent with lymphadenopathy is: What qualities make a lymph node a source of concern as a possible pathologic sign? Important criteria include the size of the node, with a measurement of more than 2 cm more likely to yield a pathologic diagnosis.[2] A history of a recent upper respiratory infection and a negative chest radiograph both would argue against the necessity of seeking an early tissue diagnosis.[2] The consistency of the node and its pattern of growth are helpful in the decision-making process. A node (or matted collection of nodes) having a rock-hard or firm, rubbery feel that is fixed and progressively enlarging is of greater concern than a node

---

BOX 53-2
Differential Diagnosis of Splenomegaly

HEMATOLOGIC DISORDERS
Sickle cell disease (SC and S-β-thalassemia double
    heterozygotes)
Thalassemia major
Other hemoglobinopathies (homozygous CC, EE)
Autoimmune hemolytic anemia
Thrombotic thrombocytopenic purpura
Erythropoietic protoporphyria
Splenic sequestration crisis*
Pyruvate kinase deficiency
Spherocytosis
Myelofibrosis
Myeloid metaplasia*
Chronic myelogenous leukemia*

LIVER DISEASE
Portal hypertension
Portal vein thrombosis
Budd-Chiari syndrome
Wilson's disease
Cirrhosis
Banti's syndrome (splenic venous obstruction)
Veno-occlusive disease

METABOLIC/STORAGE DISEASES
Gaucher's disease*
Niemann-Pick disease
Mucopolysaccharidoses (Hunter's and Hurler's)

INFECTION
Bacterial
    Sepsis
    Subacute bacterial endocarditis
    Salmonella
    Splenic abscess
Viral
    Colorado tick fever
    Hepatitis
Rickettsial
    Rocky Mountain spotted fever
    Typhus
Parasitic
    Malaria*
    Babesiosis
    Schistosomiasis
Miscellaneous infection
    Psittacosis
    Blastomycosis

MISCELLANEOUS
Felty's syndrome
Splenic hematoma
Splenic cyst (old infarcts, hematomas;
    echinococcal)
Hemangioma and lymphangioma
Mastocytosis
Chronic congestive heart failure
Rheumatic fever

*Often involves massive splenomegaly.

---

that is soft and mobile and has not changed in size over many months. Tender, firm lymph nodes, along with erythema of the overlying skin and fever, are more likely to be due to bacterial lymphadenitis, typically staphylococcal or streptococcal in origin. Location can be significant, with a supraclavicular site more worrisome than a cervical one, and inguinal nodes more often involved with a reactive process. Associated signs and symptoms also play a key role in judging the nature and gravity of the problem; for example, associated fever, weight loss, and pancytopenia would warrant an expeditious diagnostic work-up. These considerations confirm the important medical principle that nothing is as vital to a diagnostic evaluation as a thorough history and physical examination.

Although a palpable spleen is not necessarily enlarged, as is often the case in asthenic individuals or those with increased diaphragmatic excursion, this finding usually implies an increased size of 1.5 to 2.5 times normal, and efforts should be made to discover an underlying cause. However, an enlarged spleen has been found on routine examination in 3% of healthy college freshmen, with most of these organs returning to normal size on subsequent follow-up.[3] This example emphasizes the fact that isolated splenomegaly is not necessarily a significant finding and must always be placed in the context of the "company it keeps."

The degree of urgency involved in establishing a diagnosis varies, depending on the general condition of the patient, the rapidity of onset, and associated findings. Although increasing size of the spleen or lymph node is often a slow and painless process, the consequence of such enlargement sometimes can be profound. Lymphoid hypertrophy in Waldeyer's ring or in the mediastinum can cause life-threatening obstruction of the respiratory tree or the superior vena cava, necessitating emergency attention. Infiltration or hypertrophy of Peyer's patches in the terminal ileum, as seen in non-Hodgkin's lymphoma or mesenteric adenitis, is an important cause of intussusception. Acute splenomegaly places the patient at greater risk of rupture with resultant hypotension and shock, whereas a chronically enlarged spleen, causing hypersplenism and pancytopenia, may be associated with hemorrhagic or infectious complications involving sig-

---

BOX 53-3
Combined Lymphadenopathy and Splenomegaly

INFECTIONS
Bacterial
 Tuberculosis
 Tularemia
 Lyme disease
 Syphilis
 Brucellosis
Viral
 Infectious mononucleosis
 Cytomegalovirus
 Coxsackievirus
 Acquired immunodeficiency disease (AIDS)
 Adenovirus
 Rubella
 Measles
Rickettsial
 Q fever
 Scrub typhus
Parasitic
 Toxoplasmosis
 Kala-azar (leishmania)*
 Visceral larval migrans *(Toxocara)*
 Trypanosomiasis
Miscellaneous
 Lymphogranuloma venereum
 Mycoplasma
 Histoplasmosis
 Cryptococcosis

CONNECTIVE TISSUE DISORDERS
Systemic lupus erythematosis
Mixed connective tissue disease
Familial Mediterranean fever
Rheumatoid arthritis

HEMATOLOGIC DISORDERS
Leukemia/lymphoma
Chédiak-Higashi syndrome
Malignant histiocytosis
Histiocytosis syndromes
Chronic granulomatous disease

METABOLIC/ENDOCRINE DISORDERS
Hyperthyroidism
Hashimoto's thyroiditis
Cystic fibrosis

MISCELLANEOUS
Berylliosis
Splenic hamartoma
Behçet's disease
Sarcoid
Iodide treatment
IgA deficiency
Amyloidosis
Hemochromatosis

---

*Often involves massive splenomegaly.

nificant morbidity and mortality. Finally, lymphadenopathy and splenomegaly are two well-known signs of malignancy, and expeditious evaluation is often mandatory to allay the fears of an anxious, frightened adolescent and family. Since between 15% and 35% of cervical and supraclavicular node biopsies in patients in the 10- to 20-year age range show positive results for malignancy, this fear is well grounded.[1,4-8]

DIAGNOSTIC PARAMETERS

A routine blood count with examination of peripheral blood smear often discloses several clues that help narrow the differential diagnosis. The presence of atypical lymphocytes suggests a viral illness, whereas blast cells with cytopenia are the hallmark of acute leukemia. Abnormal erythrocyte shapes with reticulocytosis are expected in most hemolytic disorders associated with splenomegaly (e.g., sickle cell anemia, spherocytosis, pyruvate kinase deficiency, autoimmune hemolytic anemia), while liver disease is frequently associated with target cells and burr cells as well as macrocytosis. Finally,

the finding of erythrocyte inclusions, such as parasites, basophilic stippling, and Howell-Jolly bodies, or of lysosomal inclusions in granulocytes would expedite the diagnostic evaluation.

Additional blood screening tests are often very helpful in the work-up, with erythrocyte sedimentation rates, liver function tests, and serologic tests all providing more information about an underlying process, although not always a specific diagnosis. The adolescent with cervical adenopathy should receive antibody testing for tuberculosis and Epstein-Barr virus (EBV) performed to rule out two common causes of lymphadenopathy/splenomegaly. Very often, repeat serologic testing is necessary for some illnesses, particularly EBV infection and systemic lupus erythematosus, since definitive tests are commonly negative early in the course of the disease.

Although radiography rarely yields a definitive diagnosis, it can provide valuable information about the illness and its severity, as well as indicate the next logical step in the evaluation. A mediastinal mass found on chest radiography is strongly associated with granulomatous or malignant disease and strengthens the argument for an early biopsy. Ultrasonography of the abdomen can be used to detect cystic or nodular components in an enlarged spleen; provide accurate measurements; demonstrate intra-abdominal nodes; and clarify the arterial and venous circulation of the splenic, portal, and hepatic circulation. Radionuclide scanning, including the infusion of ^{51}Cr-labeled red blood cells, can define both splenic function and anatomy. Computed tomography (CT), magnetic resonance imaging, and occasionally angiography can provide the clearest picture of the anatomy, consistency, and extent of the problem, sometimes even disclosing the primary disorder. However, the final diagnosis of lymphadenopathy often is not made until an excisional biopsy is performed, after which definitive therapy can be considered. Tissue sampling is often necessary, but it is important to remember that more than 50% of biopsies of nodes show nonspecific hyperplasia. Therefore, many patients require a second biopsy several months later to establish a definitive diagnosis. This underscores the importance of carefully selecting the site and timing of the lymph node biopsy. It also serves to emphasize the need for an experienced pathologist who can help guide the surgeon during an operative procedure, to supply accurate and expeditious information regarding the initial tissue sampling. It is vital for the surgeon, in turn, to supply the pathologist with adequate tissue for the usual diagnostic stains, as well as for special stains required for confirmatory studies (including immunologic, histochemical, and cytogenetic analysis).

INFECTIOUS CAUSES

The most common infections associated with lymphadenopathy and/or splenomegaly in adolescents are EBV and other infectious mononucleosis–like illnesses. The classic picture in this group of infections includes fever, malaise, pharyngitis, lymphadenopathy, hepatosplenomegaly, and fatigue. The lymph nodes most commonly involved are the posterior cervical nodes, with epitrochlear enlargement a particularly consistent finding in EBV infection. Splenomegaly, although common, is rarely massive unless superimposed on a preexisting chronically enlarged spleen, as seen in hemolytic and storage disorders. However, the acute enlargement observed in infectious mononucleosis often causes left upper quadrant tenderness. Associated with infectious mononucleosis is a variety of possible hematologic abnormalities, including neutropenia; hemolytic anemia; thrombocytopenia; moderate pancytopenia; and atypical, sometimes very primitive-appearing lymphocytes on peripheral blood smear. These are usually immune-mediated and self-limited situations. While these complications are nearly always transient and cause only mild to moderate clinical problems, life-threatening aplastic anemia has followed EBV infection, with a permanent

marrow failure that is fatal without urgent medical intervention. Many of these hematologic findings may mimic leukemia and occasionally necessitate a bone marrow examination to clarify the diagnosis, particularly if the serologic tests for EBV are negative (as is often the case early in the course of the disease).

Although both cytomegalovirus and toxoplasmosis can cause symptoms similar to those of EBV infection, the degree of nodal and spleen enlargement is much less remarkable and hematologic abnormalities are less frequent. There should be a high index of suspicion for these two infectious disorders in the adolescent with infectious mononucleosis–like symptoms and negative serologic test results. Leptospirosis and brucellosis are two additional infections that primarily involve the cervical chain and have symptoms comparable with those of infectious mononucleosis; these should be considered in the differential diagnosis for teenagers who have been in contact with potential animal carriers of the causative organisms.

Given the large spectrum of infectious causes of lymphadenopathy and splenomegaly, it is helpful to consider the particular features of the lymph nodes and the spleen and any associated symptoms to give focus to the differential diagnosis. Important characteristics of lymphadenopathy include the location of the node, whether the adenopathy is localized or part of a generalized process, and the subsequent course of the involved node after the initial appearance. Likewise, the spleen may be very firm or very tender, and the size and changes on follow-up often provide the necessary clues to the diagnosis. Many of the following infectious processes have characteristic features that assist early diagnosis.

MEASLES. Now enjoying a recrudescence among adolescents, of whom at least 10% are not immune, measles can induce generalized adenopathy, with particular involvement of the anterior and posterior cervical chain. Mesenteric nodal enlargement can cause abdominal pain. The higher risk of pneumonitis and meningoencephalitis in adolescents makes this an important illness to prevent and identify early in its course. Teenagers may present with many classic features, including rash, cough, coryza, and conjunctivitis.

ADENOVIRUS. Adenovirus type 3, which is common in the adolescent age group, typically causes pharyngitis, conjunctivitis, and posterior cervical or submaxillary adenopathy that can persist for weeks. Type 7 is usually more virulent and associated with a toxic appearance, pneumonia, and splenomegaly.

LYMPHOGRANULOMA VENEREUM. A potential problem in the sexually active adolescent, this chlamydial infection causes a characteristic unilateral inguinal adenitis 1 to 4 weeks after the primary lesion appears. Firm and tender at first, the nodes become matted and fixed to the overlying skin, then turn erythematous and violaceous, and finally rupture to form a chronic sinus tract.

AIDS. AIDS is an increasing problem among adolescents who engage in high-risk sex, are intravenous drug abusers, or have hemophilia (as many as 80% of older hemophiliacs have antibodies to the HIV virus). Constitutional disorders such as weight loss and diarrhea, chronic lymphadenopathy, hepatosplenomegaly, and the appearance of opportunistic infections are classic findings in the infected patient. Complicating the chronic adenopathy that results from infection is the high incidence of B-cell lymphoma that develops in these patients.

RUBELLA. The rubella virus characteristically involves the retroauricular, posterior cervical, and postoccipital nodes, which show enlargement at least 24 hours before the appearance of a rash. Tender enlargement of these posterior nodes is usually more pronounced than in any other infection.

CAT-SCRATCH DISEASE. The hallmark of this gram-negative bacterial infection is regional lymphadenitis preceded by the bite or the scratch of a cat. Axillary and epitrochlear nodes are most commonly enlarged and tender, a sign that may last for weeks to months. Suppuration of the nodes occurs in 30% of patients, and lymph node biopsy typically shows tubercle-like granulomas and microabscesses.

MYCOPLASMA. This ubiquitous infection may present as tender cervical adenopathy or in a more generalized manner, with pneumonia and hilar adenopathy. Cold agglutinins are present in 75% of patients, inducing an immune hemolytic anemia and false extreme "macrocytosis" on Coulter counter blood counts (agglutinated cells are often recorded as giant erythrocytes, yielding mean corpuscular volume counts as high as 140) and markedly elevated erythrocyte sedimentation rates due to RBC agglutination at room temperature.

MYCOBACTERIAL INFECTIONS. Although tuberculosis most commonly affects superficial cervical, hilar, and supraclavicular nodes, the atypical mycobacterial organisms most often involve the submandibular and anterior cervical nodes, almost always unilaterally. These nodes usually suppurate, rupture, and form sinus tracts with chronic drainage. The diagnosis is confirmed by recovering the organism in excised granulomas.

TULAREMIA. The adenopathy of this bacterial infection, which is common in endemic rural areas, is pronounced and characteristic. After an abrupt onset of fever, chills, and malaise, most patients develop the ulceroglandular syndrome, evidencing ulceration of the nodes within 4 to 5 days. Typically, axillary and epitrochlear nodes are affected in rabbit-associated strains, with inguinal or femoral lesions noted in tick-borne *Francisella* infection.

MALARIA. Still an important worldwide health problem, malaria produces a characteristic symptom complex. Splenic involvement is important in the pathophysiology of hematologic abnormalities (e.g., leukopenia, anemia, thrombocytopenia), with the spleen serving as the site of both hemolysis and brisk erythrophagocytosis. The spleen may undergo infarction or rupture in acute attacks, and it becomes very large and hard after repeated episodes.

SCHISTOSOMIASIS. A serious problem in endemic regions in South America, the Far East, and the Middle East, schistosomiasis may present as a serum sickness–like syndrome with fever, chills, eosinophilia, lymphadenopathy, and hepatosplenomegaly. In its more chronic form, there is often no intestinal phase, and patients have hepatosplenomegaly, portal hypertension, ascites, and hematemesis at initial presentation.

NONINFECTIOUS CAUSES

Although fever and acute onset are less likely to be seen with noninfectious causes of lymphadenopathy and splenomegaly, unusual characteristic features of many of these disorders aid in establishing a rapid diagnosis. These disorders can be grouped into several broad categories: neoplastic diseases, storage diseases, portal hypertension, autoimmune disorders, and miscellaneous disorders.

Neoplastic Diseases

Frequently found through lymph node biopsy in adolescents, neoplastic disorders either can be primary (e.g., lymphomas) or can represent metastatic spread from other sites (e.g., sarcoma, carcinoma, and leukemia). These disorders are often suspected when they are associated with constitutional symptoms and other physical abnormalities; however, isolated adenopathy is sometimes the only presenting sign. A tissue diagnosis is always mandatory to establish a diagnosis before appropriate therapy is begun. Massively enlarged spleens are encountered in many patients with myeloproliferative disorders such as chronic myelogenous leukemia (see Chapter 50, "Leukemia").

Sinus histiocytosis is an uncommon disorder characterized by massive, painless lymphadenopathy and often confused with malignancy. This is a benign condition affecting only lymph nodes (nearly always cervical) that regresses spontaneously after a long course.[9]

Storage Diseases

Gaucher's disease, an autosomal recessive metabolic disorder seen primarily in Ashkenazi Jews, is caused by a deficiency of β-glucocerebrosidase and affects the monocyte/macrophage elements of the reticuloendothelial system. Glucocerebroside accumulates in senescent macrophages, which subsequently enlarge. These characteristic foamy cells are found in large numbers in the spleen, liver, bones, and skin. The adult form of Gaucher's disease, which may first appear in adolescence or may become more pronounced during the teenage years, is often manifested as massive splenomegaly, a consequence of involvement of the red pulp. Pancytopenia is common as the spleen continues to enlarge. Pathologic bone fractures, hepatomegaly, and aseptic necrosis of the femoral head are part of the syndrome. Although splenectomy cures pancytopenia in most patients, there is concern that deposition in other organs can accelerate after removal of the spleen. Enzyme replacement is effective in halting the progression of the disease in bones, liver, and marrow, occasionally helping to shrink an enlarged spleen also. Some patients have been cured by bone marrow transplantation, but this therapy is usually reserved for the very young child who develops significant complications of this illness.

Amyloidosis is a rare disorder characterized by extracellular deposition of a proteinaceous material throughout the body, with compression and destruction of involved tissue. In adolescents it most often appears in association with rheumatoid arthritis, Crohn's disease, and several different chronic infectious diseases (e.g., malaria). Infiltration of amyloid can result in massive hepatosplenomegaly; other sites of involvement include the kidneys, heart, tongue, and adrenal glands.

Portal Hypertension

A potential complication of many different pathologic conditions, portal hypertension can result from disturbances of blood flow of the splenic, portal, or hepatic vasculature. Underlying problems in teenagers include abdominal trauma, pancreatitis, hepatic vein thrombosis, Gaucher's disease, and inflammatory masses adjacent to the portal vein. Any of the many causes of cirrhosis, including Wilson's disease, chronic active hepatitis, α_1-antitrypsin deficiency, hemochromatosis, cystic fibrosis, venoocclusive disease, schistosomiasis, and biliary atresia, can result in enough intrahepatic scarring to distort the hepatic vasculature and increase vascular resistance. Increased vascular resistance also can be caused by hepatic fibrosis from abdominal radiotherapy for malignant disease (e.g., Wilms' tumor), and distorted hepatic regeneration after major liver resection (following hepatocellular carcinoma). Characterized by markedly increased splenic blood flow, splenomegaly will correlate with the rate of splenic arterial flow.[10] Increased splenic blood flow creates pressure on the portal outflow system; if vascular resistance is constrained by a rigid liver, collateral circulation forms, with bleeding esophageal varices and hemorrhoids. Complicating the anatomic abnormality, a hypersplenic hematologic picture evolves as the spleen enlarges, with

thrombocytopenia, neutropenia, shortened RBC life span, and reticulocytosis.

Autoimmune Disorders

Autoimmune disorders appear more commonly in teenagers, especially girls, than in younger children and may present with protean manifestations. In addition to splenic and nodal enlargement, complications of the joints, skin, kidneys, lungs, and gastrointestinal tract may cause considerable morbidity. Signs of inflammation are usually present, with elevated erythrocyte sedimentation rate and anemia of chronic inflammation. Lymph node biopsy is less likely to be helpful, and diagnosis is established by physical and serologic findings. For example, a characteristic facial "butterfly" rash or immune thrombocytopenic purpura in adolescent girls would make systemic lupus erythematosus a likely diagnosis, whereas predominant signs of arthritis with ancillary findings such as iridocyclitis are more typical of juvenile rheumatoid arthritis. Lymphadenopathy accompanied by urticaria, fever, and edema increases the suspicion of serum sickness.

Miscellaneous Disorders

Several hemoglobinopathies and other hemolytic disorders can result in substantial splenomegaly. Chronic hemolysis and extramedullary erythropoiesis in thalassemia major produce an enormous spleen, which usually necessitates removal to reduce transfusion requirements. Likewise, patients with S-β-thalassemia or SC sickle cell syndromes often have persistently enlarged spleens that have not infarcted and atrophied. Patients with severe pyruvate kinase deficiency, a hemolytic anemia caused by the most common enzyme disorder of the Embden-Meyerhof pathway, usually benefit from splenectomy, which can mitigate and occasionally eliminate the need for transfusion. Similarly, splenectomy is recommended for patients with hereditary spherocytosis to prevent biliary tract disease and aplastic crises. Splenomegaly is commonly found in autoimmune hemolytic anemia but is rarely massive.

Splenic cysts—with associated epigastric fullness, cough, shoulder pain, and left upper quadrant masses—can be either true cysts, as seen with dermoids, hemangioma, lymphangioma, and parasites (*Echinococcus* species), or false cysts occurring after hemorrhage, inflammation, or infarction. Ultrasonography or CT scanning readily demonstrate the lesions, although removal is usually necessary for diagnostic and therapeutic reasons.

Sarcoidosis is more prevalent in adolescents than in children and can mimic both infectious and malignant processes. The lung is the most commonly involved site, with nodules and prominent hilar and paratracheal adenopathy. Hepatic, ocular, and dermatologic abnormalities are common, in addition to frequently prominent peripheral lymphadenopathy.

Although several medications and other chemicals can result in nodal enlargement, a characteristic syndrome is associated with anticonvulsants, particularly phenytoin. This pseudolymphoma syndrome includes cervical, hilar, or generalized adenopathy; fever; hepatitis or hepatic necrosis; myositis; renal failure; nephrotic syndrome; and pancytopenia. Biopsy shows no obliteration of lymph node architecture or capsular invasion, and the syndrome slowly regresses when the medication is discontinued. A few patients with this syndrome have subsequently developed non-Hodgkin's lymphoma.

SPLENECTOMY

Persistent splenomegaly in an adolescent can become a source of considerable morbidity and often warrants excision. Destructive cytopenias, as seen in Gaucher's disease, spherocytosis, splenic sequestration, chronic immune thrombocytopenic purpura, and refractory autoimmune hemolytic anemia, usually benefit substantially from splenectomy. Transfusion requirements in several hematologic diseases can be lessened after splenectomy. Removal of the spleen, which is diagnostic and curative for many cysts and tumors, is still important for staging purposes in patients with early-stage Hodgkin's disease. In addition, extreme discomfort from massive spleen size and the risk of splenic rupture can be alleviated. Splenectomy is still necessary in most adolescents with a massive spleen before bone marrow transplantation, because the bone marrow graft can be sequestered in the enlarged spleen, with resultant engraftment failure. Although the risk of overwhelming sepsis from pneumococcus and *Haemophilus influenzae* organisms is much less of a concern in adolescents, who have antibody protection against most strains of these encapsulated bacteria, it is still advisable to administer Pneumovax and *H. influenzae*-B vaccines before surgery, and many patients considered to have a lifelong infection risk (e.g., Hodgkin's disease) should continue with prophylactic penicillin. There are many indications for surgery, and although the risks, morbidity, and complications of surgery have decreased, particularly with the advent of laparoscopic splenectomy, the risk of overwhelming sepsis must be weighed against the potential benefits conferred by surgery.

References

1. McMillan JA, Stockman JA, Oski FA: *The whole pediatrician catalog,* vol 3, Philadelphia, 1982, WB Saunders.
2. Slap GB, Brooks JSJ, Schwartz JS: When to perform biopsies of enlarged peripheral lymph nodes in young patients, *JAMA* 252:1321-1326, 1984.
3. McIntyre OR, Ebaugh FG: Palpable spleens in college freshmen, *Ann Intern Med* 66:301-306, 1967.
4. Lee YN, Terry R, Lukes RJ: Lymph node biopsy for diagnosis: a statistical study, *J Surg Oncol* 14:53-60, 1980.
5. Knight PJ, Mulne AF, Vassy LE: When is lymph node biopsy indicated in children with enlarged peripheral nodes?, *Pediatrics* 69:391-396, 1982.
6. Lake AM, Oski FA: Peripheral lymphadenopathy in childhood: ten year experience with excisional biopsy, *Am J Dis Child* 132:357-359, 1978.
7. Miller KB: Reactive lymphocyte disorders and lymphadenopathy. In Handin RI, Lux SE, Stossel TP, editors: *Blood: principles and practice of hematology,* Philadelphia, 1995, JB Lippincott; pp 661-674.
8. Miller D: Differential diagnosis of lymphadenopathy. In Miller DR, Baehner RL, editors: *Blood diseases of infancy and childhood,* ed 7, St. Louis, 1995, Mosby–Year Book; pp 745-749.
9. Rosai J, Dorfman RF: Sinus histiocytosis with massive lymphadenopathy: a pseudolymphomatous benign disorder, *Cancer* 30:1174-1188, 1972.
10. Witte CL, Witte MH, Renert W, et al: Splenic circulatory dynamics in congestive splenomegaly, *Gastroenterology* 67:498-505, 1974.

CHAPTER 54

Proteinuria and Hematuria

•

Marva M. Moxey-Mims and Edward J. Ruley

Proteinuria and hematuria are two of the more common urinary abnormalities seen in the practice of adolescent medicine. Isolated low-grade proteinuria and hematuria are relatively nonspecific findings and most often do not indicate serious renal disease; however, they demand thoughtful, cost-effective evaluation, which usually can be performed on an outpatient basis.

The American Academy of Pediatrics' Committee on Practice and Ambulatory Medicine recommends urine screening of asymptomatic children once during childhood and a "dipstick urinalysis for leukocytes for male and female adolescents."[1] The U.S. Preventive Services Task Force, the Canadian Task Force on the Periodic Health Examination, and the American Cancer Society have all advised against routine urine screening of asymptomatic individuals for proteinuria and hematuria, since efforts to detect serious and treatable disease in the otherwise well population are not cost effective.[2]

PROTEINURIA

Detection

Proteinuria usually is detected by testing a urine specimen with a bromphenol blue–impregnated dip-and-read strip that semiquantitatively indicates the concentration of protein by changing color. Very concentrated urine often gives a positive result in the low range (trace to 1+) even though the quantitated daily protein excretion is normal. False-positive results may occur with very alkaline urine (pH > 6.5). Occasionally, false-positive results occur with specimens contaminated with highly alkaline skin surface detergents (e.g., benzalkonium chloride), which are commonly used to cleanse the perineum for a clean-catch urine specimen. False-

negative results can occur in patients ingesting ascorbic acid.

Acid precipitation of protein, using sulfosalicylic acid, is another semiquantitative test of urinary protein. This test is very specific and is not affected by urine pH or ascorbic acid. The specimen is graded according to the amount of precipitate formed after the sulfosalicylic acid is added; results can range from negative (no precipitate) to 4+ (large amount of precipitate giving appearance of curdled milk). The acid precipitation test can be used to verify dipstick results; the disadvantage of this test is that it is much less convenient than the dipstick method.

The "gold standard" of urinary protein quantitation is chemical measurement of protein in a properly collected, timed urine specimen, most often a 24-hour specimen. The normal range of protein excretion is 150 to 200 mg/m^2/24 hr (this varies somewhat with the protein assay method used by the laboratory). Measurement of the urine protein/creatinine ratio in a random urine specimen also has been suggested as a way to assess quantitative proteinuria in lieu of a 24-hour collection.[3] A ratio of 0.2 or less is considered normal. Additionally, the formula

0.63 (urine protein/urine creatinine) = mg/m^2/day

has been shown to produce results that correlate well with 24-hour specimens in a variety of proteinuric diseases, within certain limitations.[4] Some investigators have suggested that the protein/creatinine ratio does not correlate with quantitative protein excretion as well in patients with interstitial nephritis, increasing renal insufficiency, or more severe proteinuria.[5] The urine protein/creatinine ratio test should not be used for patients in whom postural proteinuria is suspected, since it will produce erroneous results. However, the technique is an easier, more economical way to follow most patients with proteinuria.

Incidence

The incidence of proteinuria in any group depends on the definition of significant proteinuria, in terms of both degree and the number of specimens tested per individual. For example, when the children in one study were tested on their first visit to a neighborhood clinic, 6.3% were found to have a protein level of 1+ or higher by dipstick in a single void.[6] However, in a different study of children the prevalence was found to be only 0.45% for boys and 1.6% for girls when stricter criteria of 2+ or higher on two specimens was used.[7,8] Proteinuria is known to occur more often in adolescents than in children and is more common in girls than in boys in each age group. A variety of extrarenal factors can increase the apparent loss of protein in the urine, including posture, exercise, fever, and contamination by blood (as can occur during menstruation).[9] Investigating these factors in a patient with low-grade proteinuria will lower the reported incidence of pathologically significant proteinuria even more.

ETIOLOGY AND DIFFERENTIAL DIAGNOSIS. One clinical approach to the cause of proteinuria in a patient with a positive urinalysis result is presented in the algorithm in Figure 54-1. Although a carefully performed history, physical examination, and urinalysis are important in establishing the significance of the proteinuria, the key laboratory test is 24-hour urine collection in which each specimen is tested as it is voided. The instructions for the patient for this test are listed in Figure 54-2. The accuracy of the 24-hour collection can be determined by expressing the concentration of creatinine excreted in the urine in relation to the patient's weight (creatinine index). Normally, adolescents excrete 20 ± 3 mg of creatinine/kg/24 hr. Although there is some variation between individuals, the day-to-day creatinine excretion in one person is quite consistent. If the creatinine excretion is within the

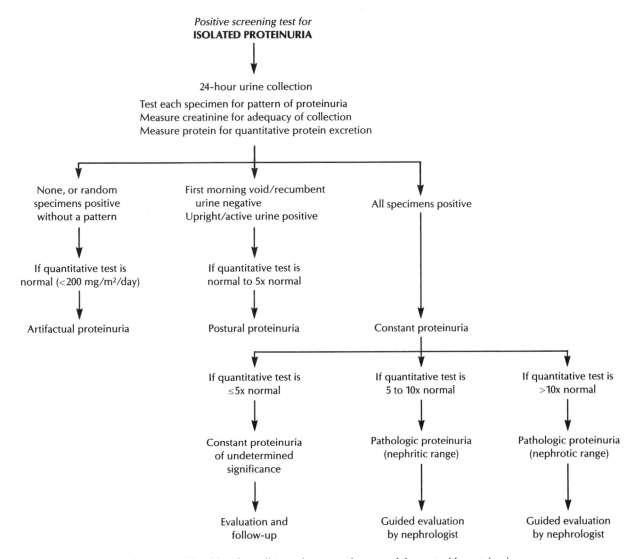

Fig. 54-1. Algorithm for a diagnostic approach to an adolescent with proteinuria.

PATIENT INSTRUCTIONS

24-HOUR URINE COLLECTION AND

POSTURAL PROTEIN TEST

This test involves the simultaneous collection of a 24-hour urine specimen (for quantitation of total urinary protein) and the testing of each individual urine specimen for protein. The amount of protein in each urination should be recorded along with the date, time of day, and the activities of the patient since the previous urination.

The specific instructions are as follows:

1) On the day the test begins, have the patient urinate immediately after rising (_____ a.m.), test for protein, record the results, and then **discard** the urine.

2) Test each subsequent urination, record the result and add the specimen to the 24-hour collection which should be kept refrigerated. A good intake of fluid is helpful throughout this test.

3) Sometime during the day have the patient exercise (bike riding, playing ball, etc.), so that there is a urine specimen to test after a period of vigorous activity. Test it, record the results, and add it to the collection as you did with the others.

4) During another time of day (evening is best) have the patient remain relatively quiet (doing home work, watching TV, etc.) so that there is a urine to test after a period of rest. Test it, and add to the collection.

5) On the next day, have the patient rise at the same time, urinate immediately, test for protein, record the results, and add to the 24-hour collection.

6) Bring this paper with the written urine test results, the unused urine protein test strips, and the 24-hour urine specimen to the Nephrology office. Bring the patient's hospital plate with you. The patient need not come to the office.

RESULTS

DATE	TIME	ACTIVITY	URINE PROTEIN

Fig. 54-2. Patient instructions for 24-hour urine collection and determination of the relationship of proteinuria to posture and activity.

BOX 54-1
Causes of Artifactual Proteinuria

Vulvovaginitis
   Infectious causes
      Bacteria (not related to sexually transmitted
         disease)
      Sexually transmitted diseases
      Fungi
   Contact irritation
   Foreign body
Urethritis/prostatitis
Contamination by menstrual blood

expected range, the clinician may presume that the urine was collected correctly and can proceed to assess the quantity and pattern of protein loss. The pattern of protein loss in relation to posture and activity will be evident from the diary kept by the patient. Since most 24-hour collections begin and end on rising, two "first morning voids" will be available with this test. As shown in Figure 54-1, patients can then be classified as having artifactual proteinuria, postural proteinuria, or constant proteinuria.

The more common causes of artifactual proteinuria are listed in Box 54-1. This type of proteinuria most often occurs in adolescent girls as a result of contamination of the urine specimen with a vaginal discharge, particularly when the patient has vulvovaginitis (vulvovaginitis can be caused by infection, contact irritation, or foreign bodies). Menstrual blood renders the color change on the dipstick uninterpretable, and its plasma and cellular proteins can produce a positive result on the acid precipitation test. Low-grade proteinuria that is not factitious but is nonrenal in origin occurs most often in adolescents of either sex who have urethritis and in boys with prostatitis. Sexually transmitted diseases should be strongly considered in these circumstances.

Artifactual nonrenal proteinuria is suggested by the clinical history and physical findings and by examining the centrifuged urinary sediment. Such symptoms as a vaginal discharge (often with a foul odor) and pruritus of the vulva frequently are present in a girl with vulvovaginitis; this possibility can be confirmed by direct visual examination of the vulva. The urinary sediment often contains many vaginal epithelial cells, bacteria, and leukocytes and considerable nonspecific debris suggesting contamination with vaginal secretions. The absence of true proteinuria can be confirmed by testing a urine specimen obtained by careful clean-catch technique or catheterization.

Adolescents with urethritis usually have such symptoms as dysuria, burning on urination, urinary urgency and frequency, and a urethral discharge. In these cases examination of a urine specimen obtained by catheterization will confirm the nonrenal origin of the proteinuria;

however, when the symptoms strongly suggest urethritis, a less traumatic approach may be to test the urine after treating the urethritis to determine whether the proteinuria has resolved. The urinary protein level in these patients usually is within the normal range despite positive test results from random specimens.

If artifactual proteinuria has been ruled out, the 24-hour urine collection and quantitation procedure then becomes the means by which the patient is further classified and further investigation is planned. As shown in Figure 54-1, a diagnosis of postural proteinuria can be made if the urinary protein level is insignificant (negative test result) or "trace" in the first morning specimen and highest in the specimens collected after more vigorous activity. The total quantitative urinary protein usually is within the normal range or low grade (i.e., less than five times normal for surface area; <1 g/m^2/24 hr). In addition, patients with postural proteinuria have no history of renal-related symptoms, a normal physical examination, and unremarkable urinary sediment.[10]

In contrast, some patients have a positive protein test result on *all* voidings; these patients are classified as having constant proteinuria. This category can be subdivided using the 24-hour quantitative urinary protein results. If the quantitated urinary protein is less than five times normal for the patient's size, the patient can be classified as having constant proteinuria of undetermined significance. Although the pattern of constant protein loss is disturbing, the amount lost is relatively low. In this group of patients, further evaluation must be individualized. In contrast, a diagnosis of nephritic-range proteinuria can be made if the quantitative urinary protein is five to 10 times normal for body surface area (1 to 5 g/m^2/24 hr). A diagnosis of nephrotic-range proteinuria is made if the urinary protein exceeds 10 times the normal for surface area (>5 g/m^2/24 hr). Although all the voidings will test positive for protein, it should be remembered that "all proteinuria is postural"; thus, the amount of protein may vary among specimens. Nonetheless, in patients with nephritic- or nephrotic-range proteinuria, it is unusual for a specimen to be protein free. In addition, the urinary sediment often is abnormal, showing granular, hyaline, or broad casts and/or concurrent hematuria. Constitutional symptoms such as headache, fatigue, and swelling, as well as physical examination findings of hypertension, edema, and other abnormalities, are more common in these patients.

Management

Proteinuria resolves in the adolescent with vulvovaginitis or urethritis after appropriate treatment. Patients who meet the criteria for postural proteinuria have a good prognosis.[10,11] The underlying reason for this functional problem is unclear, although studies suggest that hemodynamic changes in kidney perfusion may be the cause—either directly, by compression of the left renal vein between the superior mesenteric artery and the aorta, or indirectly, through stimulation of the renin-angiotensin system.[12] Whatever the cause, no intervention is necessary for postural proteinuria. However, it is important that these patients be reevaluated at least yearly by means of a history, physical examination, and repeat 24-hour urine collection. This will ensure that the diagnosis is correct and that the proteinuria is not a harbinger of a more serious renal condition. In most of these patients the proteinuria resolves with time.

For adolescents classified as having constant proteinuria of undetermined significance, the decision to investigate further must be individualized. If the patient has no hematuria, physical signs, or specific symptoms, the best course probably is regular follow-up and repeated evaluation of the degree of protein loss and kidney function. In many of these cases the proteinuria resolves without a definitive diagnosis being made. In others an increase in proteinuria, sometimes associated with the development of renal failure, necessitates more invasive evaluation. Individuals with nephritic- or nephrotic-range proteinuria need a comprehensive evaluation (often including renal biopsy), and their treatment should be based on a tissue diagnosis (See Chapter 56, "Nephritis and Nephrosis"). Consultation with a nephrologist is indicated in most of these cases.

In adolescents with a known chronic disease that can affect the kidney (e.g., systemic lupus erythematosus, diabetes mellitus, hypertension), urinary albumin excretion is a more sensitive measure of early renal involvement than total protein excretion.[13] Albuminuria can be detected before total protein excretion exceeds the normal range. In these cases, consultation with a nephrologist is indicated for further evaluation and management.

HEMATURIA

Hematuria can occur in a variety of clinical circumstances, ranging from grossly bloody urine to an unexpected chemical abnormality in the urine of an asymptomatic patient. It may be manifested as an isolated finding or occur in association with proteinuria and/or urinary sediment abnormalities. It may be either a finding of minor significance that does not require complicated, costly, or invasive testing or the harbinger of a more serious and progressive illness. The latter circumstance is more likely when hematuria occurs in association with other urinary, biochemical, or formed-element abnormalities.

Detection

The biochemical test for hematuria usually is performed with a dipstick that changes color in response to the peroxidase activity of hemoglobin and myoglobin. False-positive results may occur if the urine specimen is contaminated with oxidizing skin-cleaning agents (e.g., povidone-iodine) or surface cleaning agents (e.g., hypochlorite) or as a result of peroxidase activity of microbial origin. The dipstick does not differentiate hemoglobinuria from myoglobinuria or either of these two pigmenturias from hematuria. The dipstick also does not differentiate glomerular (renal parenchymal) bleeding from lower tract (urologic) bleeding.

Hemoglobinuria and myoglobinuria can only be differentiated by spectrophotometric analysis. Microscopic examination of the centrifuged urinary sediment can help differentiate hematuria from hemoglobinuria and myoglobinuria. The dipstick test for blood is positive in all of these conditions, but erythrocyturia is present only with hematuria. In hemoglobinuria and myoglobinuria the sediment usually shows reddish brown, finely granular casts of filtered pigment.

The type of formed elements in the sediment may help distinguish between upper tract bleeding and lower tract bleeding. With glomerular bleeding, the erythrocytes are dysmorphic; that is, they exhibit a wide range of morphologic abnormalities, including varying size, irregular outlines, and small blebs on their margins. Erythrocyte casts, originating in the glomerular tubules, usually are evident along with other granular and/or hyaline casts. With lower tract bleeding (i.e., from the ureters, bladder, or urethra), the erythrocytes usually are eumorphic; that is, they are uniform in size and shape, much like cells on a peripheral blood smear. Erythrocyte casts are absent.[14] Careful evaluation of the urinary sediment is the most important initial laboratory test for a patient with gross or microscopic hematuria.

Incidence

Grossly red urine has been reported as a symptom or sign in 1.4 patients for every 1000 consecutive emergency clinic visits.[15] Substances other than blood can give the urine a red color, including beets, vegetable dyes, blackberries, and drugs (e.g., phenytoin or phenothiazines).[16] When the urine of emergency clinic patients is tested by dipstick for blood or examined microscopically for erythrocytes, the incidence of gross hematuria falls to 1.3 patients per 1000 visits.

As with proteinuria, the incidence of microhematuria varies with the criteria. In an ambulatory setting the observed frequency of 4%, detected on a single random urinalysis, falls to 0.07% under a more stringent definition requiring positive test results from two urine specimens. Similar to the case in proteinuria, the incidence increases with age in both sexes and is higher in girls than in boys at each age.[17] The frequency of hematuria, either as an isolated finding or in association with proteinuria, is as high as 5.3%, as determined by hospital admission

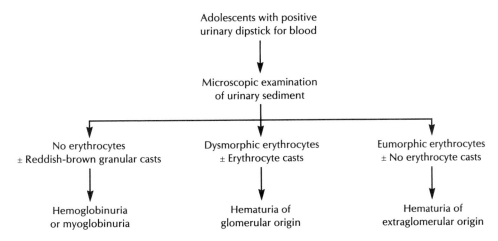

Fig. 54-3. Algorithm for a diagnostic approach to an adolescent with hematuria.

urinalysis in ill children. This figure falls to 2.2% if menstruating girls and children with fever are eliminated and the definition is made stricter by requiring two consecutive abnormal urinalyses.[18]

The incidence of abnormal degrees of erythrocyturia is even more vague. The average number of erythrocytes visible in each high-power field varies, principally depending on the amount of urine supernatant in which the sediment is resuspended and somewhat less on the time of centrifugation. It has been suggested that a finding of more than 10 erythrocytes per high-power field in two of three consecutive urine specimens should be considered abnormal.[18]

Etiology, Differential Diagnosis, and Management

It has been reported that in 56% of patients with gross hematuria the cause is readily apparent from the recent history, a physical examination, or a simple laboratory test such as a urine culture.[15] The most common diagnosis in this group (46%) is culture-proven urinary tract infection. Of the 44% of patients who have gross hematuria without a readily apparent cause, 53% will be suspected of having a urinary infection on the basis of the history and symptoms, even though the culture is negative. More serious diagnoses such as a tumor or acute glomerulonephritis are very uncommon in this unselected population, the two examples given accounting for less than 1% and 4% of cases, respectively.[15]

The diagnostic approach to microscopic hematuria is based on the clinical, patient, and family history; the physical examination; and the findings in the urinary sediment. An algorithm for the approach to these patients is given in Figure 54-3. With patients who have a positive result from the dipstick test for blood but no visible erythrocytes on microscopic examination of the urinary sediment, a working diagnosis of hemoglobinuria or myoglobinuria can be made. If the urine is grossly

---

BOX 54-2
Causes of Hemoglobinuria and Myoglobinuria

Hemoglobinuria
    Hemolytic anemia
    Sepsis/disseminated intravascular coagulation
    Mechanical erythrocyte damage
    Freshwater near-drowning
    Mismatched blood transfusions
Myoglobinuria
    Severe muscle injuries
    Myositis
    Rhabdomyolysis

---

discolored, it usually is the color of burgundy or rosé wine and clear. The differentiation of hemoglobinuria from myoglobinuria is suggested by the history and physical findings (e.g., pallor and icterus versus myositis and myalgia) and confirmed by spectrophotometric analysis of the urine. The causes of hemoglobinuria and myoglobinuria are listed in Box 54-2. Such illnesses are multisystemic in nature and have a variety of symptoms and signs that indicate the cause.

If the urinary sediment contains a large number of dysmorphic erythrocytes, as well as erythrocyte casts, a diagnosis of hematuria of glomerular origin is justified. With gross hematuria, the urine is usually brown or tea colored and looks opaque or cloudy. Some of the causes of hematuria of glomerular origin are listed in Box 54-3. A common and important cause is glomerulonephritis. In rare cases, patients with lifelong cystic or cystic-dysplastic malformations escape detection, only to manifest gross hematuria or microhematuria in adolescence. Acute tubular necrosis, sudden vascular catastrophes, and renal trauma are major events with multisystemic signs.

If most of the erythrocytes in the urinary sediment are eumorphic and no erythrocyte casts are evident, the

---

BOX 54-3
Causes of Hematuria
of Glomerular Origin

Glomerulonephritis
  Hereditary
  Acquired
Cystic and cystic/dysplastic malformations
Acute tubular necrosis
Acute arterial thrombosis or embolism
Renal vein thrombosis
Renal trauma

BOX 54-4
Causes of Hematuria
of Extraglomerular Origin

Infection
Trauma
Renal or urologic malformations
Nonspecific urologic bleeding
Hypercalciuria with or without calculi
Sickle cell hemoglobinopathy
Medications
Tumors

---

diagnosis of hematuria of extraglomerular origin can be made. The causes of this condition are listed in Box 54-4. Hematuria associated with urinary tract infection remains an important consideration in this working diagnosis. Trauma in general, but particularly trauma in a patient with an undiscovered renal malformation, can lead to extraglomerular bleeding. However, most patients have microhematuria as a result of minor bleeding of the urologic structures. This may be associated with exercise, fever, or other nonspecific events. With patients who have microhematuria, more invasive testing (e.g., cystoscopy, cystography) is almost never justified unless there is other strong evidence of a serious disease. Hypercalciuria with or without calculi can also be associated with microhematuria.[19,20] Normal calcium excretion varies by race and gender.[21] Urolithiasis as a specific cause of hematuria, as well as evaluation for hypercalciuria, is addressed below. Also, sickle cell trait or disease may be associated with gross or microscopic hematuria. Tumors rarely manifest with microhematuria as the only sign.

Whether gross or microscopic, hematuria is merely a sign of an underlying condition. As such, it generally does not require specific management. Rather, a thoughtful diagnostic plan to discover the underlying cause, followed by development of a specific treatment program, is the best course.

UROLITHIASIS

There are generally three circumstances predisposing to the development of nephrolithiasis: urinary tract infection; urinary tract obstruction; and metabolic disturbance, particularly hypercalciuria. The last-named can be seen in up to 60% of renal stone patients,[22] and 80% of all kidney stones contain calcium.[23] Other metabolic disturbances include hyperoxaluria, cystinuria, renal tubular acidosis, hyperuricosuria, and hypocitraturia. Urolithiasis is more common in males[24] and is less likely to occur in blacks in the United States than in other races,[24,25] likely because of difference in urinary calcium excretion.[21]

The clinical presentation of urolithiasis usually includes abdominal or flank pain (often colicky), nausea, and vomiting. Some patients may have localized tenderness along the flank. Microscopic hematuria is present in 100% of patients,[26] while gross hematuria occurs in 30% to 50%.[24] In some cases the stone(s) may even result in acute urinary tract obstruction and anuria.[27] Spontaneous passage of stones occurs in 30% to 40% of children and adolescents.[24]

A thorough history and physical examination and appropriate radiologic evaluation are key to establishing the diagnosis in these patients. Plain films will detect radiopaque stones such as calcium phosphate or calcium oxalate. Uric acid, xanthine, and cystine stones are usually radiolucent, while the radiopacity of infection stones (struvite) is variable. Renal ultrasonography is useful for identification of stones as well as for showing hydronephrosis or other structural renal anomalies. In the case of radiolucent stones within the urinary tract, intravenous urography is the test of choice for detection.

Once the diagnosis is established, the underlying cause should be sought, as more than half of all stone formers will experience recurrence.[28] Establishment of the etiology should lead to appropriate treatment and preventive measures. A urinalysis, particularly microscopic examination for crystals, is necessary. Calcium phosphate and calcium oxalate are the most common crystalline components of human stones.[29] Other crystals that might be visualized include magnesium-ammonium phosphate, cystine, and uric acid. Depending on the type of crystal, more specific evaluation can be pursued. A urine culture should be obtained, as recurrent urinary tract infection with urease-producing organisms is the underlying cause in 20% to 30% of children.[30] One must also keep in mind, however, that infection may be the consequence of urolithiasis, rather than its cause. Serum electrolytes can rule out renal tubular acidosis (evaluating for a normal anion gap, hyperchloremic, metabolic acidosis). The serum calcium level should be checked to look for hypercalciuria, and if found, to further evaluate for its etiology. Possibilities include hyperparathyroidism, hyperthyroidism, hyperadrenal corticoidism, vitamin D intoxication, sarcoidosis, malignancy, and immobilization. A check of BUN and creatinine levels will determine whether renal function is impaired.

It is important to determine urinary calcium excretion owing to the prevalence of hypercalciuria in this population. Hypercalciuria is defined as a spot calcium/creatinine ratio of >0.2 (mg/dl per mg/dl), or a 24-hour calcium excretion of >4 mg/kg/day. The spot ratio correlates well with 24-hour urinary calcium excretion in adults with hypercalciuria and urolithiasis.[31] If possible, urinary citrate excretion should also be checked, as low excretion rates of the inhibitor of stone formation have been shown to be a significant risk factor for nephrolithiasis.[22,32] If a stone is passed and retrieved, its chemical composition should be determined, as this is the most direct assessment of etiology.

Management of urolithiasis depends on the cause. The pain usually requires narcotic analgesia. If a urinary tract infection is present, it should be treated with appropriate antibiotics. Increased water intake should be encouraged, especially at night, to decrease urinary saturation with stone-forming elements. Extreme amounts of calcium supplementation should be eliminated. For hypercalciuria, thiazide diuretics reduce urinary calcium excretion.[33] For hypocitraturia, potassium citrate should be used; D-penicillamine and α-mercaptopropionylglycine should be considered for cystinuria.[34] If renal tubular acidosis is diagnosed, it should be treated with alkali therapy. Treatment of hyperoxaluria includes increased fluid intake and decreased dietary oxalate, as well as possible potassium citrate, thiazide diuretic, and orthophosphate. This should be done under the guidance of a nephrologist. Uric acid lithiasis is treated by maintenance of a high volume of alkaline urine. Allopurinol should be administered as appropriate for elevated serum uric acid levels. If obstruction develops, stone removal is necessary. A urologist should be consulted for extracorporeal shock-wave lithotripsy as a nonsurgical method for removal, or for open surgical removal as indicated.

BOX 54-5
Basic Evaluation for Nephrolithiasis

Urinalysis
Urine culture
Plain film/ultrasound/intravenous urogram
Serum electrolytes
Serum calcium
Parathyroid hormone level
Blood urea nitrogen/creatinine
Urinary calcium excretion
Urinary citrate excretion
Stone analysis

References

1. Committee on Practice and Ambulatory Medicine: Recommendations for preventive pediatric health care, *Pediatrics* 96:373, 1995.
2. Woolhandler S, Pels RJ, Bor DH, et al: Dipstick urinalysis screening of asymptomatic adults for urinary tract disorders. I. Hematuria and proteinuria, *JAMA* 262:1214, 1989.
3. Houser M: Assessment of proteinuria using random urine samples, *J Pediatr* 104:845, 1984.
4. Abitbol C, Zilleruelo G, Freundlich M, et al: Quantitation of proteinuria with urinary protein/creatinine ratios and random testing with dipsticks in nephrotic children, *J Pediatr* 116:243, 1990.
5. Teruel JL, Villafruela JJ, Naya MT, et al: Correlation between protein-to-creatinine ratio in a single urine sample and daily protein excretion, *Arch Intern Med* 149:467, 1989.
6. Gutgesell M: Practicality of screening urinalyses in asymptomatic children in a primary care setting, *Pediatrics* 62:103, 1978.
7. Silverberg DS: City-wide screening for urinary abnormalities in schoolboys, *Can Med Assoc J* 111:410, 1974.
8. Silverberg DS: City-wide screening for urinary abnormalities in schoolgirls, *Can Med Assoc J* 111:981, 1973.
9. Houser MT, Jahn MF, Kobayashi A, et al: Assessment of urinary protein excretion in the adolescent: effect of body position and exercise, *J Pediatr* 109:556, 1986.
10. Robinson RR: Isolated proteinuria in asymptomatic patients, *Kidney Int* 18:395, 1980.
11. Rytand DA, Spreiter S: Prognosis in postural proteinuria, *N Engl J Med* 305:618, 1981.
12. Vehaskari VM: Mechanism of orthostatic proteinuria, *Pediatr Nephrol* 4:328, 1990.
13. Shihabi ZK, Konen JC, O'Connor ML: Albuminuria vs urinary total protein for detecting chronic renal disorders, *Clin Chem* 37:621, 1991.
14. Stapleton FB: Morphology of urinary red blood cells: a simple guide in localizing the site of hematuria, *Pediatr Clin North Am* 34:561, 1987.
15. Ingelfinger JR, Davis AE, Grupe WE: Frequency and etiology of gross hematuria in a general pediatric setting, *Pediatrics* 59:546, 1977.
16. Koff SA: A practical approach to hematuria in children, *Am Fam Physician* 23:159, 1981.
17. Dodge WF, West EF, Smith EH, et al: Proteinuria and hematuria in schoolchildren: epidemiology and early natural history, *J Pediatr* 88:327, 1976.
18. Hermansen MC, Blodgett FM: Prospective evaluation of routine admission urinalysis, *Am J Dis Child* 135:126, 1981.
19. Stapleton FB, Roy S, Noe HN, et al: Hypercalciuria in children with hematuria, *N Engl J Med* 310:1345, 1984.
20. Heiliczer JD, Canonigo BB, Bishof NA, et al: Noncalculi urinary tract disorders secondary to idiopathic hypercalciuria in children, *Pediatr Clin North Am* 34:711, 1987.
21. Seifert-McLean CM, Cromer BA, Maosher G, et al: Urinary calcium excretion in healthy adolescents, *J Adolesc Health Care* 10:300, 1989.
22. Levy FL, Adams-Huet B, Pak CY: Ambulatory evaluation of nephrolithiasis: an update of a 1980 protocol, *Am J Med* 98:50, 1995.
23. Broadus AE, Thier SO: Metabolic basis of renal stone disease, *N Engl J Med* 300:839, 1979.
24. Gearhart JP, Herzberg GZ, Jeffs RD: Childhood urolithiasis. Experiences and advances, *Pediatrics* 87:445, 1991.
25. Stapleton FB, McKay CP, Noe HN: Urolithiasis in children: the role of hypercalciuria, *Pediatr Ann* 16:980, 1987.

26. Noronha RFX, Gregory JG, Duke JJ: Urolithiasis in children, *J Urol* 121:478, 1979.
27. Nicholson R, Hewitt I, Kam A: Ureteric sludge syndrome, *Arch Dis Child* 66:344, 1991.
28. Kreutzer ER, Folkert VW: Etiologic diagnosis of renal calculus disease. *Curr Opin Nephrol Hypertens* 2:949, 1993.
29. Khan SR, Glenton PA: Deposition of calcium phosphate and calcium oxalate crystals in the kidneys, *J Urol* 153:811, 1995.
30. Polinsky M, Kaiser BA, Baluarte HJ: Urolithiasis in childhood, *Pediatr Clin North Am* 34:683, 1987.

31. Matsushita K, Tanikawa K: Significance of calcium to creatinine concentration of a single-voided urine specimen in patients with hypercalciuric urolithiasis, *Tokai J Exp Clin Med* 12:167, 1987.
32. Cupisti A, Morelli E, Lupetti S, et al: Low urine citrate excretion as main risk factor for recurrent calcium oxalate nephrolithiasis in males, *Nephron* 61:73, 1992.
33. Yendt ER, Cohanim M: Prevention of calcium stones with thiazides, *Kidney Int* 13:397, 1978.
34. Pak CY: Etiology and treatment of urolithiasis, *Am J Kidney Dis* 18:624, 1991.

CHAPTER 55

Urinary Tract Infection

•

Marva M. Moxey-Mims and Edward J. Ruley

Urinary tract infections are among the most common infectious illnesses for which adolescents seek medical care. These infections pose a significant health problem because of their acute morbidity, their tendency to recur, their potential to damage kidney parenchyma, and the cost of diagnosis and treatment.

INCIDENCE

The exact incidence of urinary tract infection is unknown, since these infections can be asymptomatic or resolve without treatment. It is clear that the frequency of urinary tract infections increases with age throughout childhood, with a dramatic increase during adolescence that persists into adulthood. Girls have the highest incidence of symptomatic urinary infections at any age beyond 3 months, a gender-specific susceptibility attributed to the female's short urethra, which opens within the folds of the labia and is relatively close to the vagina and anus. It has been estimated that 10% to 20% of women will have at least one urinary infection and that 3% will have recurrent infections.[1]

In addition to age and gender, other factors that predispose adolescent girls to urinary infections include coitus, poor vulvar hygiene, pregnancy, and voluntary retention of urine.[2,3] Although some studies suggest that using a diaphragm for birth control is associated with a higher incidence of urinary infection,[4] others indicate that the method of contraception is not as important as the frequency of sexual intercourse.[5] Among adolescents, infection of the urinary system is less common in boys than in girls; however, certain complicating factors increase the incidence of urinary infection in both sexes and may predispose the patient to treatment failure, development of antibiotic-resistant organisms, or recurrent infections. These factors are listed in Box 55-1.

ETIOLOGY

Approximately 80% to 90% of urinary tract infections in young women are caused by *Escherichia coli*.[6,7] Other gram-negative organisms (e.g., *Proteus, Klebsiella, Enterobacter, Serratia,* and *Pseudomonas* spp.) are much less common. The coagulase-negative organism *Staphylococcus saprophyticus* has been reported to be an important pathogen in adolescents. Studies of college-age women found that *S. saprophyticus* accounted for 11% of urinary infections, making it the second most common infecting organism after *E. coli*.[7] *S. saprophyticus* infection is thought to be a sexually transmitted disease.

DIAGNOSIS

The problem of diagnosing urinary infections in adolescents has several dimensions, including (1) the occurrence of certain symptom patterns or clinical syndromes caused by urinary infection, (2) the use of specific laboratory tests to confirm the diagnosis, (3) the clinical dilemma of localizing the extent and site of the infection, and (4) the diagnosis of structural abnormalities and urolithiasis.

BOX 55-1
Complicating Factors
in Urinary Tract Infection

Indwelling urinary catheter
Recent urinary tract instrumentation
Recent use of antibiotics
Known urinary structural abnormality
Urolithiasis
Nosocomial infection
Pregnancy
Diabetes or other chronic debilitating condition

Syndromes of Infection

The common clinical syndromes caused by urinary tract infection include acute cystitis syndrome, urethritis, acute urethral syndrome, acute pyelonephritis, recurrent urinary infections, and asymptomatic bacteriuria.

Acute cystitis syndrome is characterized by the acute onset of symptoms of urinary outlet irritation, including dysuria (83%), urinary urgency (71%), and urinary frequency (43%), often associated with the voiding of small volumes or nocturia, or both.[7] Less common symptoms are tenderness over the flank or costovertebral angle (17%), fever (3%), and chills (4%). The physical examination usually reveals only suprapubic tenderness. The urine may be cloudy, malodorous, or frankly bloody.

Urethritis and acute urethral syndrome are manifested by symptoms of urinary outlet irritation, often similar to those of acute cystitis syndrome. The term *urethritis* is used for culture-proven bacterial urethral infections, whereas the term *acute urethral syndrome* is reserved for a patient of either sex who has bladder outlet symptoms but in whom the standard urinary culture is sterile. Boys usually have burning on urination, voiding hesitancy, and difficulty passing urine. Physical examination may reveal a milky or yellowish penile discharge. Microscopic examination of the urine usually reveals many leukocytes, and Gram's stain test of the urine sediment may demonstrate bacteria. Gram-negative intracellular diplococci, typical of *Neisseria gonorrhoeae,* are a common cause of urethritis in adolescent boys. The most common cause of acute urethral syndrome is *Chlamydia trachomatis,* although in girls mucosal irritation of the urethral os by chemical agents such as vaginal deodorants or douches may be a cause. It may be difficult to differentiate acute bacterial cystitis from acute urethral syndrome in girls. It has been suggested that because of its chlamydial origin, acute urethral syndrome is more often associated with a gradual onset and the symptoms are more chronic in nature, whereas suprapubic pain is less common. How-

ever, such a differentiation by symptoms can be very subtle, even in adults.[1]

Acute pyelonephritis syndrome is characterized by the relatively sudden onset of generalized signs of infection, including fever (often higher than 103°F [39.4°C]), shaking chills, nausea, vomiting, malaise, and pain in the flank or back. Symptoms of cystitis are often present but not always. The physical examination may reveal costovertebral angle and abdominal tenderness. The urine usually contains bacteria, leukocytes, and leukocyte casts.

Recurrent urinary infections can be a particular problem in some adolescent girls. The term *relapse* is used for the patient who has a recurrence of urinary infection with the same strain within 2 weeks of ending a course of antibiotic therapy. Relapse almost always results from incomplete eradication of a preceding infection. The term *reinfection* is used for a recurrent infection occurring at any time but caused by a different strain of bacteria than the previous infection.[8] Although the complicating factors listed in Box 55-1 should be considered in these situations, the urinary tract is normal in most women with recurrent urinary infections. In these individuals the recurrence occurs as a dysfunctional interaction between the host and the organism, allowing for chronic colonization of the vaginal mucosa. Under such circumstances, minor trauma or irritation (as occurs in coitus) can initiate an infection. Relapses of infection suggest one of the complicating factors, particularly structural abnormalities or urolithiasis.

Asymptomatic bacteriuria is the occurrence of at least two positive urine cultures in an individual who has no symptoms of urinary infection. In school-age girls the incidence ranges from 2% to 5%; in about half the positive culture will resolve spontaneously.[9] However, half of those with spontaneous clearing of the culture redevelop asymptomatic bacteriuria over the next year.

Laboratory Diagnosis of Infection

The laboratory diagnosis of urinary tract infection is based on the culture of 100,000 or more of an organism pathogenic for the urinary tract, as determined in a properly collected urinary specimen. A midstream urine specimen has been determined to be as good as one obtained by catheterization, provided that the proper collection technique and prompt processing are used.[10] Colony counts up to 100 in a properly collected and handled specimen can result from contamination with surface bacteria and are traditionally considered insignificant. It is currently recommended that colony counts from 100 to 100,000 be considered significant in girls or women who are symptomatic. As many as one third of adult women with acute lower urinary tract infection caused by *E. coli, S. saprophyticus,* or *Proteus* organisms have midstream colony counts in this range.[6] Although most bacterial pathogens grow very well on the commonly used urine culture media, optimal growth of *S. saprophyticus* requires blood agar media. Men or boys with symptoms of urethritis should have urethral swabs obtained for culture. *N. gonorrhoeae* is best isolated on a Thayer-Martin–type media or determined by the recently available DNA probes, whereas *C. trachomatis* can be detected by using monoclonal antibodies or DNA probes on smears made from urethral swabs.

Generally, urinalysis is not a good method to confirm a urinary tract infection. Although the presence of any bacteria in the Gram's stain of uncentrifuged, freshly voided urine suggests more than 100,000 organisms per milliliter, this technique is cumbersome and inconvenient and has value only as a screening test. Bacteriuria usually cannot be detected by this method in patients with urinary infections who have lower colony counts. Presumptive evidence of urinary tract infection is suggested by a positive result on a rapid-test to detect urinary leukocytes, bacteria, or their products. One study showed that a properly collected specimen processed within 10 minutes of collection by a certified technologist was actually very useful. Both sensitivity and negative predictive values were 100% when leukocyte esterase and nitrite tests were combined with microscopic examination for bacteria.[11] The nitrite test itself had a 100% specificity and positive predictive value.

Some authors suggest that patients with the signs and symptoms of urinary infection and no complicating factors can have treatment started without a urine culture, especially with a positive result on one of the rapid-tests or on microscopic examination of the unspun urine for bacteria. In contrast, urine culture and colony count are important pretreatment tests if the diagnosis of urinary infection is in question, if pyelonephritis is suspected, or if the patient has any of the complicating factors listed in Box 55-1.

Localization of Infection

An important consideration in any patient with a urinary tract infection is the extent of infection; that is, whether it involves only the lower urinary tract (cystitis and/or urethritis) or whether the upper tracts are also involved (pyelonephritis). Severity of constitutional symptoms has generally suggested more serious parenchymal infection. Renal cortical scintigraphy using technetium-99m-dimercaptosuccinic acid (DMSA) is considered the "gold standard" in detecting acute pyelonephritis, especially when there is clinical uncertainty.[12-14] In acute pyelonephritis, DMSA uptake is reduced in the infected areas of the kidney; in lower urinary infections, the kidneys are uninvolved and show normal uptake. Ultrasonography has very low sensitivity

and specificity for detecting acute pyelonephritis.[15,16] The DMSA renal scan has also been shown to be markedly superior to ultrasound for detecting residual renal scarring from previous kidney infections.[17,18]

Structural Abnormalities and Urolithiasis

Recurring urinary infections in adolescent girls or urinary bacterial infections in boys that are not part of the sexually transmitted disease group of organisms should motivate the clinician to investigate the integrity of the urinary tract. The initial screening test should be a sonogram of the kidneys, ureter, and bladder, followed by a renal scan. Intravenous urography is particularly valuable for the patient in whom urolithiasis is suspected. Isotope and contrast voiding cystourethrograms are indicated when there is evidence of ureteral dilation or if a kidney is small or misshapen, suggesting long-standing vesicoureteral reflux.

Constipation should also be ruled out as a contributing factor, as this may result in urine remaining in the bladder after voiding, and even upper tract dilation.[19]

DIFFERENTIAL DIAGNOSIS

In adolescent girls the condition that most commonly manifests itself similarly to lower urinary tract infection is vulvovaginitis. Girls with vulvovaginitis frequently have urinary symptoms, particularly dysuria.[20] Furthermore, dysuria is a relatively common symptom in mature women that can have a variety of causes. One study found that about 22% of otherwise normal adult women had this complaint over a 1-year period.[1] More than 75% of sexually active adolescent girls complain of dysuria at some time.[21] Some investigators have stated that approximately half of the young women with dysuria will be found to have a urinary infection,[22] but others have found that vaginitis is twice as likely as urinary infection to cause dysuria.[23] Some clinicians[24] have attempted to localize the cause of dysuria by having the patient classify the pain as external (pain as urine passes over the labia) or internal (pain deep inside the pelvis). However, use of this principle of differentiation has been disappointing in adolescents, because they are not as precise as adults in localizing the pain.[23]

Direct visual examination of the external genitalia and a careful pelvic examination are important initial steps in the differentiation. If a girl has pyuria, dysuria, or both and localizes the discomfort internally in the pelvis or cannot localize it, a tentative diagnosis of urinary infection should be made and a urine culture performed. In contrast, if the pain seems to be in the vulva, particularly if examination reveals a vaginal discharge or local irritation, the working diagnosis should be vulvovaginitis and a urine culture is less likely to be helpful.[17] Rather, cultures of the vaginal discharge should be taken.

Acute pyelonephritis may be difficult to distinguish from pelvic inflammatory disease, since fever, dysuria, abdominal pain, and direct and rebound tenderness may occur in either. Pelvic inflammatory disease is favored when a vaginal or cervical discharge is noted during the pelvic examination and pain occurs on movement of the cervix or direct palpation of the adnexa (see Chapter 140, "Sexually Transmitted Diseases").

TREATMENT

It is currently recommended that girls with symptoms of acute cystitis who have no complicating factors be treated with a single dose or short course (3 days) of oral antibiotics. Most such infections respond to these brief therapies, the cost of treatment and the incidence of side effects are significantly reduced, and the likelihood of compliance is increased.[6] The short-course (3-day) regimens have proved more effective than the single-dose regimens with no increase in side effects and only a modest increase in cost.[6,25] Trimethoprim and trimethoprim-sulfamethoxazole are the most commonly used antibiotics for these short-course programs and have proved very effective. Ampicillin and the more expensive oral β-lactam agents are less effective in that they are more often associated with treatment failures in the short-course regimens. Failure to respond to the single-dose regimen has been proposed as a screening test for either an upper tract infection or a lower tract infection associated with an unrecognized complicating factor.[26]

Cystitis in a patient with a complicating factor or any cystitis in a boy should be treated for at least 7 days. Urine culture and antibiotic sensitivities should be determined before the initiation of treatment. The acute urethral syndrome caused by *C. trachomatis* can be effectively treated with doxycycline.[27]

Treatment of pyelonephritis requires hospitalization for most patients. The degree of systemic symptoms in this parenchymal infection often necessitates intravenous antibiotics and other supportive care. Vomiting, a frequent finding with pyelonephritis, makes the oral route of antibiotics unreliable. In an adolescent with uncomplicated pyelonephritis, a single broad-spectrum intravenous antibiotic such as a third-generation cephalosporin or intravenous trimethoprim-sulfamethoxazole often suffices. Intravenous ampicillin alone is not a good choice, although ampicillin combined with an aminoglycoside is often effective. These patients can be changed to oral antibiotics when their condition has improved. The choice of an oral agent should be based on the results of the culture antibiotic sensitivity test. The duration of required

antibiotic treatment in pyelonephritis is undefined, although most recommend a 14-day course. A variant of renal scintigraphy, single photon emission computed tomography,[28] may also indicate the severity of the infection. In the future, a grading system may lead to more concrete recommendations for the type and duration of treatment. There have been reports of outpatient oral antibiotic treatment of "mild" pyelonephritis in adult women.[6,29]

Women and girls with recurrent urinary infections may benefit from low-dose, long-term antibiotic therapy. The trimethoprim-sulfamethoxazole combination, given as a single daily low dose, is often effective in preventing bacterial colonization of the vaginal mucosa. Changes in hygiene and behavior, such as voiding after coitus, may also reduce the recurrence of urinary infections.[3] Some have found that taking antibiotics prophylactically after coitus is very effective in preventing recurrent infection in susceptible individuals.[30]

In the past, many patients with asymptomatic bacteriuria were given antibiotics for fear they would develop a symptomatic infection. Although antibiotic treatment prolongs the period of sterile urine, it has no effect on the incidence of symptomatic urinary infections. It is currently recommended that asymptomatic bacteriuria in an otherwise healthy adolescent girl with no urinary tract abnormalities not be treated with antibiotics.[9] The exception to this may be the pregnant adolescent. The rate of progression of asymptomatic bacteriuria to overt cystitis or pyelonephritis during pregnancy may be as high as 40%, so it is recommended that this group be treated. Acute pyelonephritis in pregnancy is associated with premature delivery, intrauterine growth retardation, congenital anomalies, and even fetal demise.[31]

PROGNOSIS

The prognosis for urinary tract infection in adolescents is generally quite good. Recurrent lower tract infections are important primarily for their discomfort and minor morbidity. Uncomplicated acute pyelonephritis in adolescents rarely causes renal functional impairment or chronic renal disease.[32] However, in a kidney that is already compromised by scarring, pyelonephritis can result in a clinically significant reduction in function. Recurring urinary infections should prompt the physician to investigate the patient for an abnormality of urinary structure or urodynamics, or for urolithiasis. Repeated infections in these latter circumstances may be associated with renal parenchymal damage. The exact number of infections required to produce parenchymal damage is related to the extent and duration of renal parenchymal involvement. The interval between the onset of infection and onset of therapy has been shown to be of significance with regard to extension of kidney damage,[33] emphasizing the need for prompt diagnosis and treatment.

References

1. Sanford JP: Urinary tract symptoms and infections, *Annu Rev Med* 26:485, 1975.
2. Nicolle LE, Harding GKM, Preiksitis J, Ronald AR: The association of urinary tract infection with sexual intercourse, *J Infect Dis* 146:579, 1982.
3. Adatto K, Doebele KG, Galland L, Granowetter I: Behavioral factors and urinary tract infection, *JAMA* 241:2525, 1979.
4. Fihn SD, Latham RH, Roberts P, Running K, Stamm WE: Association between diaphragm use and urinary tract infection, *JAMA* 254:240, 1985.
5. Hsiao V: Relationship between urinary tract infection and contraceptive methods, *J Adolesc Health Care* 7:381, 1986.
6. Johnson JR, Stamm WE: Urinary tract infections in women: diagnosis and treatment, *Ann Intern Med* 111:906, 1989.
7. Latham RH, Running K, Stamm WE: Urinary tract infections in young adult women caused by *Staphylococcus saprophyticus,* *JAMA* 250:3063, 1983.
8. Nicolle LE, Ronald AR: Recurrent urinary infection in adult women: diagnosis and treatment, *Infect Dis Clin North Am* 1:793, 1987.
9. Zhanel GG, Harding GKM, Guay DRP: Asymptomatic bacteriuria: which patients should be treated?, *Arch Intern Med* 150:1389, 1990.
10. Walter FG, Knopp RK: Urine sampling in ambulatory women: midstream clean-catch versus catheterization, *Ann Emerg Med* 18:166, 1989.
11. Lohr JA, Portilla MG, Geuder TG, Dunn ML, Dudley SM: Making a presumptive diagnosis of urinary tract infection by using a urinalysis performed in an on-site laboratory, *J Pediatr* 122:22, 1993.
12. Tappin DM, Murphy AV, Mocan H, Shaw MR, Beattie TJ, McAllister TA, MacKenzie JR: A prospective study of children with first acute symptomatic *E. coli* urinary tract infection: early [99m]technetium dimercaptosuccinic acid scan appearances, *Acta Paediatr Scand* 78:923, 1989.
13. Majd M, Rushton HG, Jantausch B, Weidermann BL: Relationship among vesicoureteral reflux, P-fimbriated *Escherichia coli,* and acute pyelonephritis in children with febrile urinary tract infection, *J Pediatr* 119:578, 1991.
14. Benador D, Benador N, Sloman DO, Nusslé D, Mermillod B, Girardin E: Cortical scintigraphy in the evaluation of renal parenchymal changes in children with pyelonephritis, *J Pediatr* 124:17, 1994.
15. Bjorgvinsson E, Majd M, Eggli KD: Diagnosis of acute pyelonephritis in children: comparison of sonography and ^{99m}Tc DMSA scintigraphy, *Am J Roentgenol* 157:539, 1991.
16. Kass EJ, Fink-Bennett D, Cacciarelli AA, Balon H, Pavlock S: The sensitivity of renal scintigraphy and sonography in detecting nonobstructive acute pyelonephritis, *J Urol* 148:606, 1992.
17. Merrick MV, Uttley WS, Wild SR: The detection of pyelonephritic scarring in children by radioisotope imaging, *Br J Radiol* 53:544, 1980.
18. Rushton HG, Majd M, Jantausch B, Wiedermann BL, Belman AB: Renal scarring following reflux and nonreflux pyelonephritis in children: evaluation with [99m]technetium-dimercaptosuccinic acid scintigraphy, *J Urol* 147:1327, 1992.
19. Dohil R, Roberts E, Jones KV, Jenkins HR: Constipation and reversible urinary tract abnormalities, *Arch Dis Child* 70:56, 1994.
20. Krowchuk DP, Anglin TM, Lembo RM: Diagnostic efficacy of genitourinary symptoms and abnormal vaginal discharge for the recognition of lower genital tract infection in adolescent females, *Adolesc Pediatr Gynecol* 1:185, 1988.
21. Emans SJ, Goldstein DP: Vulvovaginal complaints in adolescents. In Emans SJ, Goldstein DP, editors: *Pediatric and adolescent gynecology,* ed 3, Boston, 1990, Little, Brown, p 334.
22. Leibovici L, Alpert G, Laor A, Kalter-Liebovici O, Danon YL: A clinical model for diagnosis of urinary tract infection in young women, *Arch Intern Med* 149:2049, 1989.
23. Demetriou E, Emans SJ, Masland RP: Dysuria in adolescent girls: urinary tract infection or vaginitis?, *Pediatrics* 70:299, 1982.
24. Komaroff AL, Pass TM, McCue JD, Cohen AB, Hendricks M, Friedland G: Management strategies for urinary and vaginal infections, *Arch Intern Med* 138:1069, 1978.
25. Norrby SR: Short-term treatment of uncomplicated lower urinary tract infections in women, *Rev Infect Dis* 12:458, 1990.
26. Sheehan G, Harding GKM, Ronald AR: Advances in the treatment of urinary tract infection, *Am J Med* 76:141, 1984.
27. Stamm WE, Running K, McKevitt M, Counts GW, Turck M, Holmes KK: Treatment of the acute urethral syndrome, *N Engl J Med* 304:956, 1981.
28. Kim SB, Yang WS, Ryu JS, Song JH, Moon DH, Cho KS, Park JS, Hong CD: Clinical value of DMSA planar and single photon emission computed tomography as an initial diagnostic tool in adult women with recurrent acute pyelonephritis, *Nephron* 67:274, 1994.
29. Safrin S, Siegel D, Black D: Pyelonephritis in adult women: inpatient versus outpatient therapy, *Am J Med* 85:793, 1988.
30. Stapleton A, Latham RH, Johnson C, Stamm WE: Postcoital antimicrobial prophylaxis for recurrent urinary tract infection, *JAMA* 264:703, 1990.
31. Lindheimer MD, Katz AI: The kidney and hypertension in pregnancy. In Brenner BM, Rector FC, editors: *The kidney,* ed 4, Philadelphia, 1991, WB Saunders, p 1567.
32. Kunin CM: Does kidney infection cause renal failure?, *Annu Rev Med* 36:165, 1985.
33. Jodal U, Winberg J: Management of children with unobstructed urinary tract infection, *Pediatr Nephrol* 1:647, 1987.

CHAPTER 56

Nephritis and Nephrosis

•

Marva M. Moxey-Mims and Edward J. Ruley

The terms *nephritis* and *nephrosis* represent very broad concepts based on the predominant clinical abnormalities in a particular patient. These concepts have a long history in the field of nephrology, originating from early attempts to construct clinicopathologic correlations for renal disease based on autopsy material. These concepts have undergone considerable revision and refinement as a result of increased use of percutaneous renal biopsy, improved techniques of tissue investigation, the development of theories of immune and nonimmune pathogenesis, and, more recently, the introduction of molecular techniques of investigation.[1]

The predominant clinical characteristics of nephritis are hematuria, hypertension, mild to moderate edema, and variable degrees of renal dysfunction. Proteinuria, hypoproteinemia, and hypercholesterolemia are less prominent. In contrast, the predominant clinical characteristics of nephrosis are massive proteinuria and hypoproteinemia, which produce generalized severe edema and hypercholesterolemia. Hematuria, hypertension, and renal failure are generally less common. However, it should be recognized that these distinctions are not exclusive and there can be overlap. For example, a patient with the nephritis of Henoch-Schönlein purpura, a condition that appears most commonly with nephritic manifestations, may occasionally appear with a fully manifested nephrotic syndrome. Traditionally, such combined features have been called *nephritic nephrosis* and have been associated with a worse prognosis.

NEPHRITIS

Nephritis has a variety of classifications, but a listing according to the acuity of onset has proved to be a practical concept. As seen in Box 56-1, nephritis can develop acutely or insidiously. Nephritis that develops acutely can be further subdivided into acute nephritic syndrome and the syndrome of nephritis with rapidly progressive renal failure. Acute nephritic syndrome most often has a sudden onset of gross hematuria, variable degrees of hypertension; and mild to moderate periorbital, suprapubic, or pretibial edema. Low-grade proteinuria and azotemia may be present but are not prominent. In contrast, the syndrome of nephritis with rapidly progressive renal failure has, as its name indicates, a prominent feature of relentless progression of renal failure associated with the features of acute nephritic syndrome. Some of the more common causes of acute nephritis, with and without rapidly progressive renal failure, are listed in Box 56-1.

The insidious presentation of nephritis can be subdivided into chronic nephritis syndrome and the syndrome of asymptomatic urinary abnormalities. The former is usually associated with vague constitutional symptoms that often result from chronic renal failure. The latter, by definition, has no symptoms and is most often discovered on a random screening urinalysis.

In addition to the acuity of onset, it is helpful to consider whether the predominant type of kidney dysfunction is glomerular or tubulointerstitial in each patient. Glomerular dysfunction usually involves oliguria with retention of fluid (manifested as decreased urine production, edema, and hypertension) and minerals (manifested as hyperkalemia). Tubulointerstitial dysfunction usually involves a sustained urinary output, making edema, hypertension, and hyperkalemia less likely. Azotemia occurs with both types of dysfunction. These functional considerations are useful in deciding on the most likely causes; postinfectious glomerulonephritis and the nephritis associated with multisystemic disorders predominantly demonstrate glomerular dysfunction, whereas drug- or toxin-induced nephritis and the hereditary forms of nephritis are usually characterized by tubulointerstitial dysfunction.

467

BOX 56-1
Clinical Syndromes of Nephritis

I. Acute onset
   A. Acute nephritic syndrome
      1. IgA/IgG nephropathy and Henoch-Schönlein purpura nephritis
      2. Postinfectious glomerulonephritis
         a. Poststreptococcal glomerulonephritis
         b. Postinfectious glomerulonephritis caused by other bacteria
         c. Postinfectious glomerulonephritis caused by viruses
      3. Membranoproliferative glomerulonephritis
      4. Acute interstitial nephritis
      5. Other
         a. Collagen vascular diseases
         b. Systemic vasculitis syndromes
   B. Rapidly progressive renal failure syndrome
      1. With glomerular crescents
         a. Postinfectious type
         b. Multisystem disorders
         c. Medications
         d. Idiopathic type
      2. Without glomerular crescents
         a. Acute tubular necrosis
         b. Acute interstitial nephritis
         c. Thrombotic microangiopathies
II. Insidious onset
   A. Chronic nephritis syndromes
      1. Glomerular in origin
      2. Tubulointerstitial in origin
   B. Syndromes of asymptomatic urinary abnormalities
      1. Thin basement membrane disease
      2. Hereditary nephritis

ACUTE NEPHRITIC SYNDROME

Several of the causes of acute nephritic syndrome are particularly common in adolescents and are discussed in more detail here.

Immunoglobulin A/Immunoglobulin G Nephropathy and Henoch-Schönlein Purpura Nephritis

INCIDENCE. IgA/IgG nephropathy is the most common primary glomerulonephritis in the world. It accounts for 10% of all primary glomerulonephritis in North America and 50% in Asia.[2,3] This geographic difference in occurrence may reflect styles of medical practice related to indications for biopsy that lead to differences in patient selection rather than differences in population susceptibility. Approximately 80% of cases occur be-

tween 16 and 35 years of age; the condition is unusual under the age of 10. Males are affected more than twice as often as females. This illness is very common in Native Americans and uncommon in blacks.[4]

ETIOLOGY. The cause and pathogenesis of IgA/IgG nephropathy are unknown. Pathologic and immunologic studies have suggested that it results from circulating immune complexes with the likelihood of alternate complement pathway activation. Although a specific antigen has not been identified, it has been suggested that this illness stems from the host's response to various dietary, infectious, or environmental antigens.[5] Genetic factors have also been suggested as playing a role, based on the occurrence of IgA/IgG nephropathy or the nephritis of Henoch-Schönlein purpura (or both) in the same family and the greater frequency of HLA-B-35, -B-12, and -DR-4, as well as the occurrence of the homozygous null C4 phenotype.

DIAGNOSIS. Although the clinical presentation of IgA/IgG nephropathy can vary considerably, the most common presentation is recurrent episodes of gross hematuria,[3,6] which most often occur within 24 to 48 hours of an upper respiratory infection. This "synpharyngetic" onset of gross hematuria differs from the delayed onset of hematuria following pharyngitis seen in poststreptococcal glomerulonephritis. Malaise, myalgia, vague back or loin pain, dysuria, and low-grade fever often accompany the episodes of gross hematuria. Hypertension is usually absent early in the course but may become a problem in patients with progressive kidney disease after several years. In some patients, reversible acute renal failure is associated with the episodes of gross hematuria. A few patients have episodes of gross hematuria after physical exertion or immunization.[6] Approximately 10% of patients have nephrotic syndrome when they seek treatment; in rare cases a patient has rapidly progressive renal failure.

There are no specific laboratory tests for IgA/IgG nephropathy. Examination of the urinary sediment reveals dysmorphic erythrocytes and erythrocyte casts. Microhematuria usually persists between episodes of gross hematuria. In most cases, proteinuria is mild to moderate. Serum C3 and C4 is usually normal. Approximately half of these patients have an elevated serum IgA, a finding that contributes little to establishing the diagnosis. Typically the diagnosis is made by renal biopsy. The usual findings with light microscopy are mesangial proliferation and expansion of the mesangial matrix. In more severe involvement, there may be glomerular crescent formation and glomerulosclerosis. Immunofluorescent examination reveals mesangial deposition of IgA and, to a lesser extent, IgA and C3. C1q and C4 are almost never present.

DIFFERENTIAL DIAGNOSIS. IgA/IgG nephropathy is considered the monosymptomatic variant of Henoch-Schönlein purpura glomerulonephritis.[7] The latter condition has the same urinary findings and an identical kidney biopsy appearance. However, the Henoch-Schönlein purpura syndrome also includes nonthrombocytopenic purpura, arthralgia, and/or abdominal pain, indicating more generalized vasculitis. Although IgA/IgG glomerular deposition is characteristically found in IgA/IgG nephritis, it is not limited to this syndrome. Similar deposition can be seen in patients with a variety of infections, neoplasms, or inflammatory diseases of the bowel.

MANAGEMENT. Currently, there is no specific therapy for IgA/IgG nephropathy, although corticosteroids have provided improvement for some patients with nephrotic manifestations.[5] In non-nephrotic patients the effect of corticosteroids (with or without cytotoxic drugs) has varied. In general, however, corticosteroids given early in the course of Henoch-Schönlein purpura do not appear to prevent the development of nephritis later on.[8] Control of hypertension and the metabolic derangements of renal failure are important and should be expected to deter the rate of progression of renal failure.

PROGNOSIS. Adolescents have a better prognosis than adults with this disease.[3,6] Approximately 20% to 30% of adolescents with IgA/IgG nephropathy progress to renal failure over 3 to 40 years. Most patients have symptom-free periods of varying duration between episodes of gross hematuria, although microhematuria is usually still present. An ultimately poor outcome has been associated with early onset of hypertension and persistent nephrotic-range proteinuria.[9] A finding of interstitial fibrosis on renal biopsy is also a poor prognostic sign. Pregnancy does not adversely affect the course of IgA/IgG nephropathy, and vice versa, provided that significant hypertension and renal failure are not present.

Poststreptococcal Glomerulonephritis

The prototype of an acute nephritic syndrome after an infection is poststreptococcal glomerulonephritis. However, postinfectious glomerulonephritis has been described after other bacterial infections (including pneumococcus, *Staphylococcus* spp., *Klebsiella* spp., gonococcus, and syphilis) and after viral infections (including measles, mumps, varicella, infectious mononucleosis, cytomegalovirus, hepatitis B, and coxsackievirus).[10]

INCIDENCE. The exact incidence of poststreptococcal glomerulonephritis is not known. The development of this renal complication of streptococcal infection depends on the presence of a nephritogenic strain of *Streptococcus* in a susceptible population, as well as on the interaction of host factors, many of which are incompletely understood. Poststreptococcal glomerulonephritis may occur as an epidemic of cases or only sporadically. Further complicating the determination of incidence is the fact that most episodes are subclinical, leading to underestimation of the number of affected individuals.[11] In some epidemics the clinical attack rate has been estimated at only 10% to 12%.[12]

ETIOLOGY. The causative agent is a group A, β-hemolytic streptococcus of certain subtypes. Type 12 is the most common, but at least 10 other types have been proved to be nephritogenic. Acute glomerulonephritis may follow either pharyngeal or skin infection.

DIAGNOSIS. Classically, acute nephritic syndrome caused by streptococcus begins after a latent period following the infection. In streptococcal pharyngitis the latent period may range from 6 to 21 days, with an average of 10 days. It is more difficult to determine the latent period in streptococcal impetigo. Clinically the patient usually has sudden onset of tea-colored or smoky urine and hypertension, although the occurrence and severity of this latter symptom varies. The hypertension is usually worse early in the nephritic episode. Hypertensive encephalopathy, manifested by irritability, altered states of consciousness, confusion, or seizures, can occur.[13] Occasionally, sudden onset of a grand mal convulsion is the presenting problem, with the hypertension detected subsequently, along with a urinalysis suggesting acute nephritis. Many patients have mild edema of the face, particularly in the periorbital regions. Less common signs are low-grade fever, petechiae, and flank or abdominal pain.

By laboratory investigation, hematuria is often evident grossly, and dysmorphic erythrocytes and erythrocyte casts are seen upon microscopic evaluation of the centrifuged urinary sediment. The urine-specific gravity is usually high, and low-grade proteinuria is common. Although the glomerular filtration rate usually is reduced, this may be evident only by a rise in blood urea; the blood creatine may be normal as a result of dilution from fluid retention. Mild dilutional hyponatremia, hypoproteinemia, and anemia may also be present. Hyperchloremia with mild hyperkalemia, as a manifestation of a type 4 renal tubular acidosis, is not uncommon.[14] Evidence of a streptococcal cause includes a positive culture and a rise in antibodies to streptococcal proteins. The antistreptolysin O titer rises over several weeks in 90% of patients with streptococcal pharyngitis, whereas antideoxyribonuclease B and antihyaluronidase become elevated in 90% of those with impetigo. One of the most important laboratory abnormalities supporting a poststreptococcal cause is the abnormality in serum complement values.[15] A variety of complement proteins have been studied, but the most readily available are C3 and C4. The former is reduced in 90% of cases early in the disease, whereas the latter is reduced 50% of the time. These values generally normalize with recovery, with the C3 reaching normal values by 8 weeks after the nephritic onset. In the typical patient with poststreptococcal glomerulonephritis, a renal biopsy is not usually necessary. It can be important in patients who have (1) no urine abnormalities,[16] (2) symptoms suggesting systemic diseases (see "Differential Diagnosis"), (3) normal complement levels, and (4) a C3 level that does not normalize within 8 weeks.

DIFFERENTIAL DIAGNOSIS. Poststreptococcal glomerulonephritis usually can be differentiated from the other causes of acute nephritis syndrome listed in Box 56-1 through the history, physical findings, and laboratory investigation. Some confusion is possible when acute nephritic syndrome begins without a latent period; that is, it coexists with a pharyngitis ("synpharyngetic"). Such patients should be suspected of having a preexisting renal disease (particularly IgA/IgG nephropathy) that has been exacerbated by the acute infection. Poststreptococcal glomerulonephritis must also be differentiated from other forms of hypocomplementemic glomerulonephritis that may appear to have an acute onset. These disorders include the nephritis of membranoproliferative glomerulonephritis, systemic lupus erythematosus, and chronic infection (e.g., hepatitis B, subacute bacterial endocarditis, and malaria). In membranoproliferative glomerulonephritis, C3 usually remains reduced even though the patient may clinically recover.[17] Systemic lupus erythematosus usually has other systemic manifestations of this collagen vascular disease, and C3 remains low also. In the nephritis of chronic infection, C3 usually returns to normal gradually, but the other physical manifestations suggest the correct diagnosis. Renal biopsy is indicated if these diagnoses are serious considerations.

MANAGEMENT. Antibiotic treatment of the patient and family contacts is indicated to prevent the spread of the nephritogenic streptococcus. Treatment of acute nephritic syndrome is symptomatic. Hypertension and fluid overload can be managed by restricting fluid and sodium and administering diuretic and antihypertensive medications. Bed rest is not indicated except as a precaution in patients with symptomatic hypertension. Neither corticosteroid nor cytotoxic therapy is needed.

PROGNOSIS. The prognosis for classic poststreptococcal glomerulonephritis in children is excellent, nearly all patients recovering completely without residual kidney damage.[18] It has been suggested that the long-term outcome is less predictable for adults who contract poststreptococcal glomerulonephritis. Although adolescents have not been studied as a specific group, they seem to have a prognosis similar to that for children. At all ages, the microhematuria may persist for several years without adversely affecting the prognosis.

Membranoproliferative Glomerulonephritis

Membranoproliferative glomerulonephritis, which is also called mesangiocapillary glomerulonephritis, is divided into at least three subtypes on the basis of the renal biopsy appearance.[19,20] Approximately 90% of patients with type 1 and 70% of those with type 2 are between 8 and 16 years of age. From 20% to 30% of patients (particularly those with type 2) have acute nephritic syndrome. The clinical characteristics cannot be differentiated from other causes of acute nephritic syndrome. However, a characteristic laboratory finding is reduced C3 that does not normalize after 8 weeks; this contrasts with the complement normalization seen in poststreptococcal glomerulonephritis. Failure of C3 to normalize within 8 weeks of onset is an indication for renal biopsy. Membranoproliferative glomerulonephritis can be diagnosed only by renal biopsy.

Acute Interstitial Nephritis

Adolescents with acute interstitial nephritis, particularly that caused by hypersensitivity reactions to antibiotics, can have acute nephritic syndrome.[21] These patients often have a rash, arthralgia, and low-grade fever in addition to hematuria. Laboratory investigation usually shows sterile pyuria, moderate proteinuria, azotemia, and peripheral eosinophilia. Salt wasting (increased fractional excretion of sodium) and an inability to conserve water (isosthenuria) as a result of the tubular damage intrinsic to this diagnosis are important differential findings.

Acute Nephritis Associated With Systemic Diseases

Other, less common causes of acute nephritic syndrome include collagen vascular diseases, such as systemic lupus erythematosus, and the systemic vasculitis syndromes, such as polyarteritis nodosa. Involvement of other organ systems and abnormalities in other laboratory tests suggest these diagnoses, although a renal biopsy may be necessary to be certain of the diagnosis.

RAPIDLY PROGRESSIVE RENAL FAILURE SYNDROMES

The characteristics of this presentation are an acute nephritis associated with oligoanuric renal failure that progresses rapidly to end-stage renal failure.

Most commonly, glomerular crescents are seen on renal biopsy. The crescentic glomerulopathies can be divided into four major categories (Box 56-1). The postinfectious causes include severe poststreptococcal glomerulonephritis and the glomerulonephritis of endocarditis, sepsis, or hepatitis B. A rapidly progressive presentation can be seen with various multisystemic disorders, including systemic lupus erythematosus, Henoch-Schönlein purpura, Goodpasture's syndrome, and the vasculitides.[22,23] In some instances, medications such as allopurinol or hydralazine have been implicated as the cause. When all other causes have been ruled out by clinical and laboratory findings, a diagnosis of idiopathic, rapidly progressive nephritis can be made. Less commonly, this type of presentation may be associated with conditions that are not associated with glomerular crescents, although the glomeruli may be abnormal on renal biopsy. Such causes include acute tubular necrosis, acute interstitial nephritis, and the thrombotic microangiopathies (including thrombotic thrombocytopenic purpura, hemolytic uremic syndrome, and disseminated intravascular coagulation).

Early involvement of a nephrologist in the diagnostic approach and clinical management of these cases is very important. Some of these disorders (e.g., Goodpasture's syndrome and systemic lupus erythematosus) have accepted therapies that often preserve renal function if they are implemented early. For others (e.g., acute interstitial nephritis and membranous glomerulopathy), therapy is controversial. Some causes are self-limited and reversible (e.g., poststreptococcal glomerulonephritis and acute tubular necrosis), although the patient may need comprehensive supportive care during the period of acute renal failure.

NEPHRITIC SYNDROMES WITH INSIDIOUS ONSET

Nephritis also may have an insidious onset. It may be associated with vague multisystemic complaints such as fatigue, gastrointestinal upset, or weight loss or may be entirely asymptomatic. In symptomatic patients it usually is discovered on a urinalysis performed as part of the general investigation of the nonspecific complaints, whereas in asymptomatic patients the urine abnormality usually is discovered during a health maintenance examination or sports physical examination. In these situations the hematuria discovered through laboratory tests is an unexpected clue to a renal problem. Further laboratory and radiologic evaluation are important in making a more specific diagnosis and determining the significance of the finding. The syndromes with an insidious onset are listed in Box 56-1.

The chronic nephritis syndromes are usually the ultimate result of a variety of renal insults that for some reason have escaped detection but over time have led to renal dysfunction. These insults may have been glomerular or tubulointerstitial in nature. Hematuria, proteinuria, and hypertension (usually mild to moderate) are typical clinical findings. The presence of azotemia reflects the advanced nature of renal damage. It is not unusual for a renal biopsy to be performed, but in late stages the renal damage is often so far advanced that the initiating processes cannot be identified. In these cases, therapy focuses on treating the complications of chronic renal failure.

One of the more common presentations is microhematuria in the asymptomatic adolescent (the stepwise

diagnostic approach to this problem is discussed in Chapter 54, "Proteinuria and Hematuria"). A renal biopsy is often necessary in patients who have persistent microhematuria with dysmorphic erythrocytes and erythrocyte casts. Diagnoses such as thin basement membrane disease,[24] familial nephritis,[25,26] and nonspecific focal glomerulonephritis can be made only by biopsy. Determining a tissue diagnosis allows the clinician to be more specific about the treatment possibilities and prognosis. The more widespread use of percutaneous renal biopsy and newer pathologic techniques have led to a more sophisticated classification and a better understanding of these conditions, which in the past were lumped into murky clinical diagnostic categories such as "benign familial hematuria" or "subacute nonprogressive glomerulonephritis." Consultation with a nephrologist usually is valuable in deciding on the sequence and extent of diagnostic tests.

NEPHROSIS

INCIDENCE

The incidence of nephrotic syndrome in adolescence is unknown, but it occurs less frequently in this age group than in younger children, where the peak occurrence is between 2 and 5 years of age.

ETIOLOGY

Nephrosis is more properly called nephrotic syndrome. As the term *syndrome* implies, it may occur in many different clinical circumstances and is a general pattern of renal response to many different insults. In most of these circumstances the exact cause is unknown. A pathologic classification of nephrotic syndrome based on renal biopsy is listed in Box 56-2. Serious forms of nephrotic syndrome occur more often in adolescents than in children. These types of nephrotic syndrome tend to resist treatment, are more likely to persist, and have a greater likelihood of progression to renal failure.

DIAGNOSIS

Classically, nephrotic syndrome consists of four components: (1) massive proteinuria (>3.5 g/1.73 m^2/day), (2) hypoproteinemia, (3) hypercholesterolemia, and (4) clinically detectable edema. The edema of nephrotic syndrome characteristically occurs in dependent areas, being more common in the face on rising in the morning and in the lower extremities at the end of the day. Ascites, if present, varies in degree. The patients with more severe

---

BOX 56-2
**Pathologic Classification and Common
Causes of Nephrotic Syndrome**

Minimal change disease
Focal segmental glomerulosclerosis
   Idiopathic
   Secondary to infection with HIV
   Secondary to vesicoureteral reflux
Membranoproliferative glomerulonephritis
   Idiopathic
   Associated with systemic lupus erythematosus
Membranous nephropathy
   Secondary to hepatitis B–antigen carrier state
   Associated with systemic lupus erythematosus
Focal proliferative glomerulonephritis
   IgA/IgG nephropathy
   Henoch-Schönlein purpura nephritis

---

ascites are the ones who usually have genital edema. Pleural effusions are seen in the more severely hypoproteinemic patients. Pericardial effusions are uncommon and should be investigated as resulting from other causes. Nephrotic syndrome without edema is called *biochemical nephrotic syndrome*.

Hematuria, hypertension, and azotemia occur more commonly in nephrotic syndrome in adolescents than in younger children.[27,28] The higher frequency reflects the more common severe diagnoses seen in this older age group.[28] In addition to the tests needed to confirm the diagnosis of nephrotic syndrome, laboratory investigation in adolescents should include measuring complement components, lupus serologies, and serologies for viral infections, particularly human immunodeficiency virus (HIV), hepatitis B, and herpesviruses. If the patient has a fever, blood and urine cultures should be performed. A percutaneous renal biopsy may be indicated in an adolescent with new onset of nephrotic syndrome because of the greater frequency of serious causes in this age group. However, an empiric trial of corticosteroid therapy may also be a reasonable approach.[29] An exact biopsy diagnosis also facilitates decisions regarding whether to treat, the choice of treatment, and the duration of therapy.

DIFFERENTIAL DIAGNOSIS

Although the clinical history, physical examination, and laboratory evaluation may give some clues to the cause and type of renal involvement in nephrotic syndrome in an adolescent, definitive diagnosis depends on the renal pathologic condition, as determined by renal biopsy. The pathologic classifications seen in adolescent nephrotic syndrome are listed in Box 56-2.

Minimal change disease, the steroid-responsive variety of nephrotic syndrome seen most commonly in infants and children (about 80%) is less common in adolescents (30%).[30] Clinical clues to its presence include the absence of organ involvement other than the kidney and the absence of hypertension, hematuria, and hypocomplementemia.

Focal segmental glomerulosclerosis is more common in adolescents than in younger children (18% versus 7%).[30] In this disease, hypertension and hematuria are commonly found whereas hypocomplementemia is absent. This pathologic finding is the most common kidney involvement seen with HIV and has been reported to be a late consequence of unrecognized vesicoureteral reflux.

Membranoproliferative glomerulonephritis is manifested with nephrotic syndrome in about 50% of patients.[31] Hypertension and hematuria are common, and the typical laboratory finding is reduced serum C3. This occurs most commonly in the type 2 variety of membranoproliferative glomerulonephritis. Membranoproliferative glomerulonephritis may also be seen as the renal manifestation of systemic lupus erythematosus. In about 12% of adolescent nephrotics the pathology consists of membranoproliferative glomerulonephritis.[30]

Membranous nephropathy can be seen in approximately 18% of adolescent nephrotics.[30] In adolescents it is often secondary to a carrier state for a virus, particularly hepatitis B. It can occur as a renal manifestation of systemic lupus erythematosus.

Finally, a minority of the focal proliferative diseases (e.g., IgA/IgG nephropathy or the nephritis of Henoch-Schönlein purpura) may be manifested as nephrotic syndrome. Nephritic manifestations are prominent in these circumstances.

MANAGEMENT

Symptomatic management of the edema in nephrotic syndrome should include limiting dietary salt and a prudent fluid intake for all patients. Diuretic therapy may be necessary if the edema interferes with the patient's daily activities. However, diuretics are usually only moderately effective in hypoproteinemic patients and they increase the risk of thrombotic complications. With very severe edema, intravenous administration of albumin is necessary, although it only temporarily reduces edema. The albumin should be administered on an inpatient basis, since it may exacerbate preexisting hypertension. Furthermore, recurrent administration may cause pulmonary edema. Diuretics and albumin should not be used merely for cosmetic purposes.

As mentioned earlier, specific treatment of nephrotic syndrome in the adolescent depends on the pathologic findings on biopsy. Some forms of nephrotic syndrome (e.g., minimal change disease or systemic lupus erythematosus) are treatable. In other types (e.g., membranoproliferative glomerulonephritis and focal glomerulosclerosis), treatment may be controversial.[32,33] Some types (e.g., membranous nephropathy secondary to viral diseases) have a tendency to resolve as the body adapts to the viral infection. In general, treatment of nephrotic syndrome is the subject of ongoing clinical trials; thus, the clinician should expect continual changes in the approach to the various diseases. Consultation with a nephrologist is important in developing any treatment program.

PROGNOSIS

The prognosis for these diseases varies according to their pathologic type and their potential responsiveness to therapy.[31] Some forms (e.g., focal segmental glomerulosclerosis and membranoproliferative glomerulonephritis) have a very high incidence of progression to chronic renal failure and end-stage renal disease. Once a patient has progressed to chronic renal failure, involvement of a nephrologist is mandatory if consultation has not been sought earlier. These patients have the potential to develop many problems of particular concern to adolescents, such as impaired growth (depending on the age of onset of the renal failure) and delayed sexual maturation. Recombinant human growth hormone is now available for clinical use and has generally shown good results when used in children with chronic renal failure.[34] The onset of puberty is often delayed in adolescents with chronic renal failure, with one study showing an average delay of 2 years.[35] In patients who have already entered puberty, reproductive function may be impaired; whether this is temporary or permanent seems to depend on the age of onset and duration of chronic renal failure before renal transplantation.[36,37] Some adults have recovered reproductive function after transplantation.[36] Numerous hormonal abnormalities have been implicated in the disorders of the reproductive system seen in chronic renal failure, including low dihydrotestosterone levels in males,[38] low estradiol levels in females,[37] and elevated luteinizing hormone and prolactin levels in both sexes.[39,40] These issues are best addressed in consultation with an endocrinologist, and many of the abnormalities appear to correct after transplantation. Despite decreased reproductive capacity, however, adolescents with chronic renal failure should still receive appropriate counseling on methods to prevent conception as well as sexually transmitted diseases.

References

1. Couser WG: Mechanisms of glomerular injury: an overview, *Semin Nephrol* 11:254, 1991.

2. Levy M, Berger J: Worldwide perspective of IgA nephropathy, *Am J Kidney Dis* 12:340, 1988.

3. Hogg RJ: IgA nephropathy: clinical features and natural history—a pediatric perspective, *Am J Kidney Dis* 12:358, 1988.

4. Jennette JC, Wall SD, Wilkman AS: Low incidence of IgA nephropathy in blacks, *Kidney Int* 28:944, 1985.

5. Clarkson AR, Woodroffe AJ, Aarons IA, et al: Therapeutic options in IgA nephropathy, *Am J Kidney Dis* 12:443, 1988.

6. D'Amico G: Clinical features and natural history in adults with IgA nephropathy, *Am J Kidney Dis* 12:353, 1988.

7. Waldo FB: Is Henoch-Schönlein purpura the systemic form of IgA nephropathy?, *Am J Kidney Dis* 12:373, 1988.

8. Saulsbury FT: Corticosteroid therapy does not prevent nephritis in Henoch-Schönlein purpura, *Pediatr Nephrol* 7:69, 1993.

9. Gallo GR, Katafuchi R, Neelakatappa K, et al: Prognostic pathologic markers in IgA nephropathy, *Am J Kidney Dis* 12:362, 1988.

10. Glassock RJ, Adler SG, Ward HJ, et al: Primary glomerular diseases. In Brenner BM, Rector FC, editors: *The kidney,* ed 4, Philadelphia, 1991, WB Saunders, p 1184.

11. Sagel I, Treser G, Ty A, et al: Occurrence and nature of glomerular lesions after group A streptococcal infections in children, *Ann Intern Med* 79:492, 1973.

12. Anthony BF, Kaplan EL, Wannamaker IW, et al: Attack rates of acute nephritis after type 49 streptococcal infections of the skin and respiratory tract, *J Clin Invest* 48:1697, 1969.

13. Yap H-K, Low P-S, Lee BW, et al: Factors influencing the development of hypertensive encephalopathy in acute glomerulonephritis, *Child Nephrol Urol* 9:147, 1989.

14. Don BR, Schambelan M: Hyperkalemia in acute glomerulonephritis due to transient hyporeninemic hypoaldosteronism, *Kidney Int* 38:1159, 1990.

15. Strife CF, McAdams AJ, McEnery PT, et al: Hypocomplementemic and normocomplementemic acute nephritis in children: a comparison with respect to etiology, clinical manifestations, and glomerular pathology, *J Pediatr* 84:29, 1974.

16. Albert MS, Leeming JM, Scaglione PR: Acute glomerulonephritis without abnormality of the urine, *J Pediatr* 68:525, 1966.

17. Northway JD, McAdams AJ, Forristal J, et al: A "silent" phase of hypocomplementemic persistent nephritis detectable by reduced serum β^{1C}-globulin levels, *J Pediatr* 74:28, 1969.

18. Clark G, White RHR, Glasgow EF, et al: Poststreptococcal glomerulonephritis in children: clinicopathological correlations and long-term prognosis, *Pediatr Nephrol* 2:381, 1988.

19. Donadio JV, Holley KE: Membranoproliferative glomerulonephritis, *Semin Nephrol* 2:214, 1982.

20. Jackson EC, McAdams J, Strife F, et al: Differences between membranoproliferative glomerulonephritis types I and III in clinical presentation, glomerular morphology, and complement perturbation, *Am J Kidney Dis* 9:115, 1987.

21. Ellis D, Fried WA, Yunis EJ, et al: Acute interstitial nephritis in children: a report of 13 cases and review of the literature, *Pediatrics* 17:862, 1981.

22. Southwest Pediatric Nephrology Study Group: A clinicopathologic study of crescentic glomerulonephritis in 50 children, *Kidney Int* 27:450, 1985.

23. Jennette JC, Falk RJ: Diagnosis and management of glomerulonephritis and vasculitis presenting as acute renal failure, *Med Clin North Am* 74:893, 1990.

24. Gauthier B, Trachtman H, Frank R, et al: Familial thin basement membrane nephropathy in children with asymptomatic microhematuria, *Nephron* 51:502, 1989.

25. Grunfeld J-P: The clinical spectrum of hereditary nephritis, *Kidney Int* 27:83, 1985.

26. Schroder CH, Bontemps CM, Assmann KJM, et al: Renal biopsy and family studies in 65 children with isolated hematuria, *Acta Paediatr Scand* 79:630, 1990.

27. International Study of Kidney Disease in Children: Nephrotic syndrome in children: prediction of histopathology from clinical and laboratory characteristics at time of diagnosis, *Kidney Int* 13:159, 1978.

28. Kher KK, Sweet M, Makker SP: Nephrotic syndrome in children, *Curr Probl Pediatr* 18:203, 1988.

29. Moxey-Mims MM, Stapleton FB, Feld LG: Applying decision analysis to management of adolescent idiopathic nephrotic syndrome, *Pediatr Nephrol* 8:660, 1994.

30. Hogg RJ, Silva FG, Berry PL, Wenz JE: Glomerular lesions in adolescents with gross hematuria or the nephrotic syndrome. Report of the Southwest Pediatric Nephrology Study Group, *Pediatr Nephrol* 7:27, 1993.

31. Chesney RW, Novello AC: Forms of nephrotic syndrome more likely to progress to renal impairment, *Pediatr Clin North Am* 34:609, 1987.

32. West CD: Idiopathic membranoproliferative glomerulonephritis in childhood, *Pediatr Nephrol* 6:96, 1992.

33. Tarshish P, Bernstein J, Tobin JN, Edelmann CM Jr: Treatment of mesangiocapillary glomerulonephritis with alternate-day prednisone. A report of the International Study of Kidney Disease in Children, *Pediatr Nephrol* 6:123, 1992.

34. Yadin O, Lippe B, Moulton L, et al: Five years' experience with recombinant human growth hormone (rhGH) treatment of children with chronic renal failure (CRF), *J Am Soc Nephrol* 3:291, 1992.

35. Schärer K: Study Group on Pubertal Development in Chronic Renal Failure. Growth and development of children with chronic renal failure, *Acta Paediatr Scand* 366(suppl):90, 1990.

36. Phadke A, MacKinnon K, Dossetor J: Male fertility in uremia: restoration by renal allografts, *Can Med Assoc J* 102:607, 1970.

37. Schärer K, Schaefer F, Trott M et al: Pubertal development in children with chronic renal failure. In Schärer K, editor: *Growth and endocrine changes in children and adolescents with chronic renal failure. Pediatric and adolescent endocrinology,* Basel, Switzerland, 1989, Karger; p 151.

38. Van Kammen E, Thijssen JHH, Schwarz F: Sex hormones in male patients with chronic renal failure. I. The production of testosterone and androstenedione, *Clin Endocrinol* 8:7, 1978.

39. Schaefer F, Seidel C, Mitchell R, et al: Cooperative Study Group on Pubertal Development in Chronic Renal Failure. Pulsatile immunoreactive and bioactive luteinizing hormone secretion in pubertal patients with chronic renal failure, *Pediatr Nephrol* 5:566, 1991.

40. Gomez F, de la Cueva R, Wauters J-P, et al: Endocrine abnormalities in patients undergoing long-term hemodialysis—the role of prolactin, *Am J Med* 68:522, 1980.

CHAPTER 57

Hypertension

•

Mary Ellen Turner

The adolescent with hypertension poses a challenging problem to the physician, in terms of both evaluation and treatment. To evaluate blood pressure in adolescent patients, one must be aware of the controversies surrounding the exact definition of hypertension and take into account contributing factors such as age, size, family history, and number of elevated readings. Identifying a hypertensive adolescent is important, since studies in adult patients have demonstrated a clear relationship between hypertension and the development of significant end-organ damage, in particular coronary heart disease, renal disease, and stroke.[1,2] There is now evidence that end-organ damage secondary to hypertension may begin in childhood or adolescence. Autopsy findings in children screened in the Bogalusa Heart Study have shown a significant correlation between systolic blood pressure and coronary artery fibrous plaques and fatty streaks.[3] In a study by Goldring et al,[4] high school students with persistent systolic/diastolic blood pressure elevations

1.65 standard deviations above the mean for age and sex showed evidence of cardiac hypertrophy on electrocardiography. In addition, the Bogalusa Heart Study showed that left ventricular wall thickness increases with increasing blood pressure.[5]

The implications of hypertension detected in childhood have become clear since the Muscatine Study revealed that patients with elevated systolic blood pressure as children had twice the risk of developing high blood pressure once they reached adulthood in comparison with the general population.[6] Thus, the public health implications of early detection and treatment of high blood pressure become very important.

Once hypertension has been identified in an adolescent patient, an individual treatment plan should be designed to ensure optimal compliance with a minimal disruption of life style. Although there are no definitive studies demonstrating that treatment of hypertension in childhood or adolescence reduces end-organ damage, studies

TABLE 57-1
Classification of Hypertension in Adolescent Age Group

Age Group (yr)	Significant (95th-99th percentile)	Severe (>99th percentile)
13-15	Systolic ≥136 mm Hg Diastolic ≥84 mm Hg	Systolic ≥144 mm Hg Diastolic ≥92 mm Hg
16-18	Systolic ≥142 mm Hg Diastolic ≥92 mm Hg	Systolic ≥150 mm Hg Diastolic ≥98 mm Hg

From Report of the Second Task Force on Blood Pressure Control in Children—1987, *Pediatrics* 79:1-25, 1987. Reproduced by permission of *Pediatrics.*

in adult populations have shown that successful reduction of blood pressure leads to diminished morbidity and mortality.[7-9]

DEFINITION

The Report of the Second Task Force on Blood Pressure Control in Children—1987 included revised distribution curves of blood pressure by age that also take into account height and weight.[10] In this report, normal blood pressure is defined as systolic and diastolic blood pressures less than the 90th percentile for age and sex; high normal blood pressure is considered average systolic and/or average diastolic blood pressure between the 90th and 95th percentiles for age and sex. Finally, hypertension is defined as average systolic and/or average diastolic blood pressures greater than or equal to the 95th percentile for age and sex with measurements obtained on at least three occasions (Table 57-1). It should be noted that the 95th percentile, the level that defines hypertension in adolescents, is lower than that given in earlier publications. Adolescents who have repeated blood pressure readings above the 95th percentile for age should be considered hypertensive and evaluated accordingly. One isolated high blood pressure reading should not be considered diagnostic, but it should suggest that further evaluation is necessary—initially as repeated measurements on subsequent visits over a specified time. Anyone with severe hypertension detected on an initial reading should be evaluated and treated promptly.

INCIDENCE AND PREVALENCE

The prevalence of hypertension reported from different parts of the world ranges from 1% to 20% of the adolescent population.[11] Reported prevalence may vary in the literature, depending on the ages of the subjects studied and the criteria used to define hypertension. In a study of 14,686 black and white American schoolchildren aged 10 to 15 years,[12] the incidence of "significant" hypertension, as defined by the revised blood pressure distributions of the Task Force on Blood Pressure Control in Children—1987, was approximately 1%. In a study of 17-year-old Israeli adolescents, the prevalence of systolic hypertension (defined in this study as >140 mm Hg) was 1.75% for males and 0.32% for females.[13] The prevalence of diastolic hypertension (>90 mm Hg) was 0.4% for males and 0.06% for females. Despite the low prevalence of hypertension in this age group, yearly measurement of blood pressure is indicated to identify those adolescents with real hypertension and to initiate appropriate intervention.

ETIOLOGY

It is now known that certain conditions that cause hypertension are statistically more common in particular age groups. In adolescents the most common causes of hypertension are primary hypertension and acquired renal parenchymal disease. The causes of secondary hypertension are listed in Box 57-1.

Primary Hypertension

Primary, or essential, hypertension is the leading cause of high blood pressure worldwide. Over the years, efforts have been directed toward finding the exact cause of this entity; however, no single cause has been identified. It is now thought that primary hypertension represents a heterogeneous disease with multifactorial causes.

In the adolescent population, over 50% of high blood pressure is due to essential hypertension. Patients with this type of hypertension usually have mild to moderate elevation in blood pressure and a strong family history of hypertension. Other characteristics of adolescents with this condition include excess weight in girls and increased height in boys, as well as a higher resting heart rate and a labile blood pressure pattern.[14]

Obesity has been associated with otherwise unexplained hypertension, and it is well known that weight reduction can be a successful treatment for many

---

BOX 57-1
Causes of Secondary
Hypertension in Adolescents

Renal parenchymal disease
  Glomerulonephritis
  Nephrotic syndrome
  Reflux nephropathy
  Chronic renal insufficiency
  Polycystic kidney disease
  Obstructive uropathy
  Trauma
Vascular and renovascular disease
  Renal artery stenosis
  Renal artery compression
  Coarctation of aorta
Endocrine disease
  Hyperthyroidism
  Pheochromocytoma
  Cushing's syndrome
  Primary hyperaldosteronism
  Hyperparathyroidism
Neurologic causes
  Increased intracranial pressure
  Head injury
  Posterior fossa lesions
Drugs/toxins
  Oral contraceptives
  Corticosteroids
  Sympathomimetics
  Amphetamines
  Methylphenidate
  Imipramine
  Lead
  Mercury

---

hypertensive patients. As the prevalence of childhood obesity increases, obesity-related hypertension has become more common in this age group.[15] The pathophysiology of this entity is not clear, although the results of one study suggest that salt sensitivity may play a role and that this sensitivity may be a result of the combined effects of hyperinsulinemia, hyperaldosteronism, and increased activity of the sympathetic nervous system, all of which are characteristic of obesity.[16]

Numerous investigators have attempted to identify specific physiologic or biochemical markers for essential hypertension. The role of electrolytes, specifically sodium, in primary hypertension has been researched extensively.[17] Although salt-sensitivity hypertension has been described in association with obesity, not all obese patients with hypertension are salt sensitive. Other electrolytes implicated in essential hypertension are potassium, magnesium, and calcium; however, none of these electrolytes is solely responsible for primary hypertension.[18,19] Other physiologic markers that have

been investigated include renin secretion, urinary kallikrein excretion, cellular sodium transport, and insulin levels. Again, none of these studies has been able to identify a reliable marker for essential hypertension in children, adolescents, or adults, suggesting that a variety of disease entities may be responsible for essential hypertension.[20-22]

Secondary Causes of Hypertension

Although primary hypertension may be more common in the adolescent population than in younger patients, secondary causes of elevated blood pressure should still be ruled out through history, physical examination, and (if necessary) diagnostic tests (especially in patients with severe hypertension). The list of secondary causes of hypertension is extensive. However, it is important to note that diseases of the kidney or the renal vasculature are the most common secondary causes of high blood pressure in the adolescent age group. Disorders affecting the renal parenchyma include acute or chronic glomerulonephritis, which may occur alone or in association with systemic diseases such as systemic lupus erythematosus, Henoch Schönlein purpura, and hemolytic uremic syndrome. The presence of a renal parenchymal disorder should become evident after history taking, physical examination, urinalysis, and serum creatinine determination. The diagnosis of anatomic renal disorders (e.g., reflux nephropathy, obstructive uropathy, congenital malformations of the kidney or urinary tract, cystic renal disease) requires additional imaging studies such as a renal sonogram or dimercaptosuccinic acid (DMSA) renal scan.

Renovascular hypertension, resulting from narrowing or obstruction of the renal artery or its branches, is usually more difficult to diagnose without resorting to invasive studies such as arteriography. Causes of this disorder in older children include fibromuscular dysplasia, neurofibromatosis, atherosclerosis secondary to inborn errors of lipid metabolism, arteritis, and extrinsic compression of the renal artery. Although some patients with renovascular hypertension may present with growth failure, abdominal bruit, hypokalemia, polydipsia, or enuresis, many patients are asymptomatic.

While plasma renin levels, Doppler ultrasonography, and captopril renal scanning may be useful screening tests for renovascular hypertension, renal arteriography remains the method of choice for determining the extent and location of arterial stenosis. This information is useful in guiding therapeutic decisions concerning medical versus surgical (angioplasty, nephrectomy) management.

Endocrine disorders are a relatively uncommon cause of hypertension in adolescents, yet it is important to keep these in mind. Increased systolic blood pressure and pulse pressure are characteristic of hyperthyroidism. Pheochromocytoma may have varying modes of presentation, ranging from malignant hypertension and encephalopathy to mild, labile, or sustained hypertension. Other symptoms include sweating, flushing, abdominal pain, and weight loss.

Hypertension also has been associated with various prescription and over-the-counter drugs such as cold medications containing ephedrine, corticosteroids, imipramine, and oral contraceptives. An adolescent girl should be asked specifically if she is taking birth control pills, since she may not consider them a medication or may be unwilling to offer such information.

EVALUATION

Once hypertension has been documented, an evaluation should proceed in a stepwise fashion beginning with a detailed medical history. In many cases the history may be the single most valuable diagnostic "test" in the hypertension work-up. Symptoms such as headache, palpitations, chest pain, rash, or gastrointestinal disturbances may suggest a possible cause for the elevated blood pressure. Specific questions concerning medications, especially stimulants and vasoconstrictors, should be asked. A detailed family history of primary or secondary hypertension also may help guide the evaluation of the adolescent with hypertension.

A thorough physical examination is important both for documenting any end-organ damage and for pinpointing possible causes of secondary hypertension. The evaluation of the hypertensive adolescent always should include four-extremity blood pressure measurements. Decreased lower extremity blood pressure suggests coarctation of the aorta. The presence of café au lait spots may suggest neurofibromatosis and point to an evaluation for renal artery stenosis or pheochromocytoma. Other physical signs associated with secondary hypertension include rash (vasculitis), goiter (hyperthyroidism), abdominal bruit (renal artery stenosis or arteriovenous malformation), and abdominal mass (polycystic kidneys, hydronephrosis, tumor). The finding of arteriolar nicking or narrowing on funduscopic examination would suggest that the patient's hypertension has been sustained and is of long standing.

The extent of further laboratory and radiographic evaluation of the adolescent with hypertension depends on the severity of blood pressure elevation and the findings from the history and the physical examination. Patients with mild elevation of blood pressure, a positive family history of essential hypertension, and other associated risk factors (e.g., obesity, labile blood pressure, high resting heart rate) are likely to have essential hypertension. In these cases, extensive diagnostic studies

---

BOX 57-2
Evaluation of Hypertension in Adolescents

History
Physical examination
Initial diagnostic studies
  Urinalysis
  Urine culture (if urinary tract infection
    suspected)
  BUN, creatinine, electrolytes
  Uric acid
  Cholesterol, triglycerides, lipid profile
  Echocardiogram*
Further diagnostic studies
  Renal ultrasonography
  Renal scanning with captopril
  Renal angiography with measurement of renal
    vein renins
  Digital subtraction angiography
  Abdominal CT
  Urine and plasma catecholamine levels
  Plasma renin
  Serum aldosterone

---

*Useful to determine end-organ damage and to establish baseline left ventricular mass before initiation of therapy.
BUN, blood urea nitrogen; *CT*, computed tomography.

---

are not indicated. Patients with severe hypertension or findings suggestive of secondary hypertension should undergo further studies to identify underlying disorders.

The Second Task Force on Blood Pressure Control in Children—1987[10] recommended a staged approach to the evaluation of hypertensive patients. The suggested stages of evaluation are listed in Box 57-2. The first stage is designed to detect renal disease, the presence of end-organ damage, and other cardiovascular risk factors. Diagnostic studies in the second stage of evaluation include abdominal ultrasonography, which can provide useful information concerning kidney size and the presence of any structural renal abnormality or tumor. Doppler ultrasonography of renal blood flow may be helpful in assessing renal artery flow; however, this technique has not replaced the arteriogram as the definitive test for renal artery stenosis.

The technetium-99m diethylenetriamine pentaacetic acid (DTPA) renal scan is a useful study for determining relative renal perfusion and glomerular filtration rate. When combined with administration of an angiotensin-converting enzyme (ACE) inhibitor, this study may reveal decreased renal perfusion in renal artery stenosis of a main renal artery.

In adolescents with severe hypertension and in whom a renal vascular lesion is suspected, detailed visualization of the renal vasculature and sampling of renal vein renin levels is indicated. Renal arteriography traditionally has been used to diagnose renal artery lesions, although digital subtraction angiography also has been used successfully in children. It has the advantages of a lower concentration of contrast material and less radiation exposure.[23]

When an endocrine cause of hypertension is suspected, the measurement of appropriate hormone levels (catecholamines, aldosterone) is indicated.

TREATMENT

Nonpharmacologic Therapy

Once the diagnosis of hypertension has been made in an adolescent patient, a therapeutic plan should be designed to foster compliance and adequate control of blood pressure and to minimize other cardiovascular risk factors. The Second Task Force on Blood Pressure Control in Children—1987[10] recommended that non-pharmacologic therapy, including weight reduction, physical conditioning, and dietary modification, be used as the first step in the treatment of hypertension in children. In many patients with mild hypertension, these measures may obviate the need for medication. However, for this type of therapy to succeed, changes in life style and diet are necessary for both patient and family.

For the obese adolescent with hypertension, weight reduction, although difficult, usually results in a lowering of blood pressure. This can be achieved by reducing caloric intake and increasing physical activity. Restriction of dietary sodium has been a mainstay of antihypertensive therapy for years, although recently its efficacy has been questioned. Reduction of sodium intake may decrease blood pressure in some patients, particularly those with salt-sensitive hypertension. The usual goal of dietary sodium restriction is to reduce sodium intake to 2.5 g/day. Education of the patient and parents concerning dietary salt reduction is key to the success of this intervention. The role of potassium in reducing blood pressure has been examined, and some studies suggest that increasing potassium intake may be beneficial in controlling blood pressure in some patients.[24] More studies are needed to confirm this; however, it is reasonable to suggest potassium-rich foods as a replacement for foods high in sodium.

Exercise has been recommended as an important adjunct to dietary management of hypertension. Aerobic exercise programs have been shown to lower blood pressure in hypertensive adolescents.[25] Static exercises, such as weight training or power lifting, remain controversial, since it has been shown that marked increases in blood pressure can occur with isometric exercise. However, other studies suggest that pure static or combined static and dynamic activity such as circuit training may produce a long-term antihypertensive effect.[26,27]

Patients with hypertension should not be restricted from participating in sports unless blood pressure elevation is severe and has not yet responded to therapy. Studies have failed to show that the elevation of blood pressure that occurs during strenuous exercise imposes a significant risk.[28]

Various relaxation techniques, including biofeedback, also have been shown to modestly reduce blood pressure in selected groups of adult patients, although there are no data on this effect for adolescents or children. Areas of stress in the patient's life should be addressed and appropriate support or counseling provided.

Adolescents with high blood pressure should be instructed to avoid or discontinue drugs that may contribute to blood pressure elevation, including oral contraceptives and sympathomimetic cold remedies. Elimination of other cardiovascular risk factors (e.g., cigarette smoking, alcohol consumption) also should be stressed.

Pharmacologic Therapy

Institution of pharmacologic intervention for management of hypertension in the adolescent is a major step that should be considered only when all nonpharmacologic measures have been tried and proved to be unsuccessful. The physician must weigh the possible risks and benefits of long-term medication use in this population of young patients. Antihypertensive drugs have potential side effects that can adversely affect serum electrolytes, glucose, and lipid metabolism as well as physical and cognitive performance.

The goal of pharmacologic management of hypertension in any age group should be used to attain maximal control of blood pressure with the minimal amount of medication. This approach should diminish side effects and ensure compliance. The Second Task Force on Blood Pressure Control in Children—1987[10] recommended a stepped-care approach to pharmacologic therapy that involves starting with a small dose of a single antihypertensive drug and then increasing the dose until blood pressure control is achieved or the maximal dose of the drug is reached. If adequate blood pressure control has not been achieved, a second drug can be either added or substituted. Traditionally, the medications used in this setting have been thiazide diuretics with the addition of an adrenergic blocking agent and then a vasodilator (Table 57-2). Although these drugs have proven effective, multiple daily doses or combinations of these medications may be necessary to control blood pressure. In addition, these medications may cause hypokalemia, hyperuricemia, and hypercholesterolemia. Recently, longer-acting preparations of these medications and new classes of

TABLE 57-2
Oral Antihypertensive Medications

	Dose	Doses per Day	Side Effects	Maximal Adult Dose
Diuretics				
Hydrochlorothiazide (HydroDiuril)	1-2 mg/kg	2	Hypokalemia	200 mg/day
Furosemide (Lasix)	0.5-2 mg/kg	1		600 mg/day
Spironolactone (Aldactone)	1-2 mg/kg	2	Hyperkalemia	200 mg/day
Triampterene (Dyrenium)	1-2 mg/kg	2		300 mg/day
Beta Blockers				
Propranolol (Inderal)	1-3 mg/kg	3	Bronchospasm	320-480 mg/day
Atenolol (Tenormin)	1-2 mg/kg	1	Increased triglyceride level	100 mg/day
Metoprolol (Lopressor)	1-4 mg/kg	2	Decreased cardiac output	450 mg/day
Vasodilators				
Hydralazine (Apresoline)	1-5 mg/kg	2-3	Tachycardia	200 mg/day
Minoxidil (Loniten)	0.1-1 mg/kg	2	Hirsutism, fluid retention	100 mg/day
Angiotensin-Converting Enzyme Inhibitors				
Captopril (Capoten)	25 mg	3	Neutropenia	450 mg/day
Enalapril (Vasotec)	5 mg	1-2	Proteinuria	40 mg/day
Lisinopril (Zestril)	10 mg	1	Rash	40 mg/day
Calcium Channel Blockers				
Nifedipine (Procardia)	0.25-0.5 mg/kg	3-4	Tachycardia	30 mg/dose
Nifedipine, long-acting (Procardia XL)	30 mg	1	Headache	120 mg/day
Verapamil (Calan)	40 mg	3	Constipation	360 mg/day
Verapamil, long-acting	120 mg	1		360 mg/day
Diltiazem (Cardizem)	30 mg	4		240 mg/day
Alpha-Blockers				
Prazosin (Minipress)	25-40 µg/kg	2-3	Syncope	20 mg/day
Central Adrenergic Inhibitors				
Clonidine (Catapres)	0.1 mg	2	Dry mouth	2.4 mg/day
Methyldopa (Aldomet)	10 mg/kg	2-4	Drowsiness	3 g/day

antihypertensive medications have been developed, and these have proven to be safe and in some cases more effective than traditional medications. They include ACE inhibitors and calcium channel blockers.

Angiotensin-convering enzyme inhibitors (e.g., captopril, enalapril, lisinopril) are especially effective in controlling hypertension secondary to renal vascular and parenchymal disease that is associated with high renin levels. The antihypertensive action of these agents is enhanced when used in conjunction with diuretics. These medications should not be used in patients with suspected bilateral renal artery stenosis, since acute renal failure

may result. Little has been reported on the use of these drugs for treatment of essential hypertension in the pediatric age group. In adults, captopril and enalapril have been used successfully to treat mild to moderate essential hypertension, usually in combination with a diuretic.[29]

Calcium channel blockers (e.g., nifedipine, verapamil, diltiazem) lower blood pressure by vasodilation. Nifedipine is the most potent arterial vasodilator and acts primarily on peripheral vessels. Verapamil and diltiazem, in addition to their vasodilatory effects, exert negative chronotropic and inotropic effects on the heart. Unlike hydralazine, these medications do not cause reflex tachycardia and in many cases can be used as a single agent to treat mild to moderate hypertension.

No matter which antihypertensive regimen is chosen, the adolescent with hypertension should be followed regularly to ensure compliance and adequate control of blood pressure. In addition, the patient should be monitored for physical and metabolic side effects of antihypertensive medications. Poor response may be caused by noncompliance, difficult dosage schedule, inadequate follow-up, or poorly tolerated side effects.

The Task Force on Blood Pressure Control in Children—1987[10] also recommends a "step-down" period in which an attempt is made at reducing or withdrawing medication after an extended period of blood pressure control. This may be possible, especially in cases in which nonpharmacologic therapy has been used maximally. However, the patient will continue to require close monitoring to determine whether hypertension will recur.

CONCLUSION

The adolescent with hypertension requires careful evaluation and an individualized treatment program with the goal of reducing blood pressure and other cardiovascular risk factors. A treatment program that includes patient education, reinforcement, and nonpharmacologic intervention should be instituted initially. If this approach fails, pharmacologic therapy should be added. The adolescent who is treated for hypertension should be followed closely and after a period an attempt should be made to decrease or withdraw medication.

References

1. Kannel WB, Wolf PA, Verter J, et al: Epidemiologic assessment of the role of blood pressure in stroke. The Framingham Study, *JAMA* 214:301, 1970.
2. Kannel WB, Castelli WP, McNamara PM, et al: Role of blood pressure in the development of congestive heart failure, *N Engl J Med* 287:781-787, 1972.
3. Newman WP, Fleedman DS, Voors AV, Gard PD, Srinivasan SR, Cresanta JL, Williamson JD, Webber LS, Berenson GC: Relation of serum lipoprotein levels and systolic blood pressure to early atherosclerosis. The Bogalusa Heart Study, *N Engl J Med* 314:138-144, 1986.
4. Goldring D, Hernandez A, Choi S, Lee JY, Londe S, Lindgreen FT, Burton RM: Blood pressure in a high school population. II. Clinical profile of the juvenile hypertensive, *J Pediatr* 95:298-305, 1979.
5. Burke GL, Arcila RA, Culpepper WS, Webber LS, Chiang YK, Berenson GS: Blood pressure and echocardiographic measures in children: the Bogalusa Heart Study, *Circulation* 75:106-114, 1987.
6. Lauer RM, Clarke WR: Childhood risk factors for high adult blood pressure: the Muscatine Study, *Pediatrics* 84:633-641, 1989.
7. Veterans Administration Cooperative Study Group on Antihypertensive Agents: Effect of treatment on morbidity and mortality: results in patients with diastolic blood pressures averaging 115 through 129 mm Hg, *JAMA* 202:1028-1034, 1967.
8. Veterans Administration Cooperative Study Group on Antihypertensive Agents: II. Results in patients with diastolic blood pressure averaging 90 through 114 mm Hg, *JAMA* 213:1143-1152, 1970.
9. Hypertension Detection and Follow-up Program Cooperative Group: The effect of treatment on mortality in "mild" hypertension. Results of the Hypertension Detection and Follow-up Program, *N Engl J Med* 307:976-980, 1982.
10. Report of the Second Task Force on Blood Pressure Control in Children—1987, *Pediatrics* 79:1-25, 1987.
11. Loggie JMH: Prevalence of hypertension and distribution of causes. In New MI, Levine LS, editors: *Juvenile hypertension,* New York, 1977, Raven Press.
12. Sinaiko AR, Gomez-Marin O, Prineas RJ: Prevalence of "significant" hypertension in junior high school-aged children: the Children and Adolescent Blood Pressure Program, *J Pediatr* 114:664-669, 1989.
13. Shohat M, Shohat T, Mimouni M, Nitzan M, Danan Y: Hypertension in Israeli adolescents: prevalence according to weight, sex and parental origin, *Am J Public Health* 79:582-585, 1989.
14. Falkner B, Kushner H, Onesti G, Angelakos E: Cardiovascular characteristics of adolescents who develop essential hypertension, *Hypertension* 3:251-258, 1981.
15. Gormaker SL, Dietz WH, Sobol AM, et al: Increasing pediatric obesity in the United States, *Am J Dis Child* 141:535-540, 1987.
16. Rocchini A, Key J, Bondie D, et al: The effect of weight loss on the sensitivity of blood pressure to sodium in obese adolescents, *N Engl J Med* 321:580-585, 1989.
17. Prineas RJ, Blackburn H: Clinical and epidemiologic relationship between electrolytes and hypertension. In Horan MJ, Blaustein MP, Dunbar JB, et al, editors: *NIH Workshop on Nutrition and Hypertension,* New York, 1985, Biomedical Information; pp 63-86.
18. Watson RL, Langford HG, Abernethy J, et al: Urinary electrolytes, body weight and blood pressure: pooled cross-sectional results among four groups of adolescent females, *Hypertension* 2:93-98, 1980.
19. Strazzulo P, Nunziata V, Cirrillo M, et al: Abnormalities of calcium metabolism in essential hypertension, *Clin Sci* 65:137-141, 1983.
20. Gruskin AB, Perlman SA, Baluarte HJ, et al: The utility of renin profiling in childhood hypertension, *Clin Exp Hypertens* 8:741-745, 1986.
21. Sinaiko AR, Glaser RJ, Gillem RF, et al: Urinary kallikrein excretion in children with high and low blood pressure, *J Pediatr* 100:938-940, 1982.
22. Ferranni E, Buzzigoli G, Bonadonna R, et al: Insulin resistance in essential hypertension, *N Engl J Med* 317:350-357, 1987.
23. Tonkin IL, Stapleton FB, Shane R: Digital subtraction angiography in the evaluation of renal vascular hypertension in children, *Pediatrics* 81:150-158, 1988.
24. Svetkey LP, Yarger WE, Feussner JR, et al: Double-blind placebo-controlled trial of potassium chloride in treatment of mild hypertension, *Hypertension* 9:444-450, 1987.
25. Hagberg JM, Goldring D, Ehsani AA, et al: Effect of exercise training on blood pressure hemodynamic features of hypertensive adolescents, *Am J Cardiol* 22:763-768, 1983.
26. Wiley RL, Dunn CL, Cox RH, Hueppchen NA, Scott MS: Isometric exercise training lowers resting blood pressure, *Med Sci Sports Exerc* 24:749-754, 1992.
27. Stewart KJ: Weight training in coronary artery disease and hypertension, *Prog Cardiovasc Dis* 25:159-168, 1992.
28. Wilson SL, Gaffney FA, Laird WP, et al: Body size composition and fitness in adolescents with elevated blood pressure, *Hypertension* 7:412-422, 1985.
29. Veterans Administration Cooperative Study Group on Antihypertensive Agents: Captopril. Evaluation of low doses, twice daily doses and the addition of diuretic for the treatment of mild to moderate hypertension, *Clin Sci* 63:443s, 1982.

CHAPTER 58

Systemic Lupus Erythematosus

•

Patricia L. Haber and Carol A. Smith

Systemic lupus erythematosus (SLE) is a syndrome characterized by chronic, episodic, multisystemic disease that results from a loss of immunologic tolerance. A hallmark of SLE is the presence of autoantibodies, particularly antinuclear antibodies (ANAs). Abnormalities of multiple facets of the immune system have been identified in SLE, but the underlying defects are not known.[1,2]

Systemic lupus erythematosus can affect virtually every organ system either simultaneously or sequentially. The onset may be either acute or insidious. While the entire range of manifestations can be seen in all age groups, there are some age-related variations in the frequency of different organ system involvement. For example, children have a higher incidence of severe renal disease and of pulmonary hemorrhage.[3]

In the past it was believed that the onset of SLE in childhood and adolescence was associated with a worse prognosis than onset in adulthood. More recently, it has been shown that the prognosis is dependent on the pattern of organ system involvement, and when this is taken into consideration survival rates are similar in children and adults.[4] As a consequence of the improved use of steroids and immunosuppressive agents, better management of problems such as hypertension, and the availability of dialysis and renal transplantation, survival in all age groups has improved substantially.[5]

EPIDEMIOLOGY

SLE predominantly affects young women. In most patients the onset of disease is between the ages of 15 and 25 years. The overall incidence is approximately 7 per 100,000; for patients under 15, the incidence is 0.6 per 100,000.[6,7] Although females predominate in all age groups, this tendency is most striking after menarche and before menopause. Adolescent girls are affected five times more frequently than boys; before puberty the ratio of girls to boys is about 3 : 1.[8] SLE is found worldwide, but susceptibility to the disease varies among different ethnic groups: African-Americans, Hispanics, and Asians are affected more commonly than Caucasians.

ETIOLOGY

The exact cause of SLE remains a mystery. Loss of immunologic tolerance could result from a variety of different defects. Indeed, abnormalities in multiple facets of the immune system have been identified in patients with SLE. These include polyclonal B-cell activation, specific autoantibody production, abnormal T-cell regulation, and aberrations in cytokine production and in the complement system.[1,2,9] The underlying defect, however, remains unclear.

Evidence strongly suggests that hereditary plays an important role. Multiple studies have identified an increased frequency of SLE in the relatives of patients with SLE. This is particularly true for patients presenting in childhood. In one pediatric series, 19 of 108 patients had affected first-degree relatives.[10] A 1992 study of twins reported a 24% concordance in monozygous twins versus 2% in dizygous twins.[11] HLA-specific associations with the disease are found for various ethnic groups. HLA-DR3 is increased in Caucasians with SLE and HLA-DR2 is increased in African-Americans, Chinese, and Japanese.[12] Hereditary deficiencies of almost all the components of the complement cascade have been associated with SLE-like disease.[13] Partial C4 deficiency seems to be a common risk factor for the development of SLE. In one report, complete C4A deficiency was present

TABLE 58-1
Causes of Drug-Induced Lupus Syndrome

Definite Association	Probable Association	Possible Association
Alpha-methyldopa	Beta blockers	p-aminobenzoic acid
Procainamide	Propylthiouracil	Estrogens
Isoniazid	Lithium	Gold salts
Hydralazine	Penicillamine	Penicillin
Chlorpromazine	Sulfasalazine	Griseofulvin
Quinidine	Captopril	Reserpine
	Phenytoin	Tetracycline
	Ethosuximide	
	Trimethadione	

Modified from Hess EV: Drug-related lupus (editorial), *N Engl J Med* 318:1460-1462, 1988.

in 10% to 15% of patients with SLE, and heterozygous C4A deficiency was found in 50% to 80%.[14]

Exogenous factors have also been implicated in the pathogenesis of SLE. Exposure to ultraviolet light may trigger or exacerbate the disease in some patients. The potential for a viral etiology is supported by studies that demonstrate an increased frequency of ANA positivity and lupus erythematosus (LE) cell phenomenon among laboratory technicians working with SLE sera.[15] Also, ingestion of certain drugs may cause a lupus-like syndrome (Table 58-1).[16]

Hormonal factors have been implicated in either the genesis or exacerbation of SLE. The disease can be aggravated by pregnancy, during the postpartum period, and by the use of oral contraceptives.[17]

CLINICAL MANIFESTATIONS

Although SLE can affect virtually every organ system, the most common presenting problems include fever, rashes, arthritis, and nephritis. Constitutional symptoms such as fatigue, myalgias, and weight loss are frequently present also.

SLE can cause several different cutaneous problems. The characteristic "butterfly" rash may appear as a malar erythema resembling a light rouge or as a follicular erythematous plaque over both cheeks and the bridge of the nose. Unlike seborrheic dermatitis, it spares the nasolabial folds. Vasculitic or discoid lesions can occur anywhere on the body and frequently result in scarring and atrophic changes. Alopecia is a common feature of SLE, and many patients experience either generalized thinning of the hair or patchy loss. Although the hair loss is disturbing, it is usually temporary, and regrowth generally occurs when the disease is under control.

Raynaud's phenomenon can result in scaling and paresthesias. In severe cases, digital ulcers and even gangrene may occur. Avoidance of cold exposure is important for patients with Raynaud's phenomenon.

Photosensitivity is another important problem for many SLE patients. Sunlight and ultraviolet light may cause skin eruptions but may also trigger or exacerbate other systemic manifestations. Although most patients are not overly photosensitive, it is prudent to limit sun exposure. The need to use sunscreen (SPF 26 or greater) and protective clothing should be stressed.

Arthritis and arthralgias occur in most patients with SLE. The arthritis is generally polyarticular, affecting large and small joints; it is rarely erosive, but deformities due to subluxation may result from capsular and ligamentous involvement. Patients with SLE are particularly susceptible to the development of avascular necrosis, and this always needs to be considered in patients with persistent hip or knee pain.

Pleurisy is the most common pulmonary manifestation. Other pulmonary problems include interstitial pneumonitis, which may mimic an infection, and pulmonary hemorrhage, which is a serious and often fatal complication of lupus lung involvement. Cardiac problems include pericarditis, which is common (although tamponade is rare), myocarditis, and a verrucous (Libman-Sacks) endocarditis. An increased risk of myocardial infarction exists in SLE owing to vasculitis and to premature atherosclerosis resulting from altered lipid metabolism caused either by the underlying disease or by corticosteroids used for treatment.

Abdominal pain is common during active disease. Nonspecific colitis, peritonitis, and malabsorption with diarrhea have been described. Acute pancreatitis may result from either corticosteroid therapy or the disease itself. Mesenteric arterial thrombosis is an ominous event that may lead to bowel necrosis and perforation; unfortunately, its symptoms may be masked by corticosteroid therapy. Mild hepatomegaly is frequent in children with SLE. Liver function test results may be abnormal, but jaundice is rare.

The hematopoietic system is frequently affected. Leukopenia, anemia (sometimes hemolytic), and thrombocytopenia are common. Lymphopenia is particularly diagnostic if malignancy and HIV infection are excluded. Splenomegaly is found in 25% and lymphadenopathy in 50% of children with SLE.

The "lupus anticoagulant" is a member of the group of antibodies currently referred to as antiphospholipid antibodies. Other antibodies in this group include anticardiolipin and the antibody responsible for the false-positive syphilis test seen in some SLE patients. The anticoagulation seen with the lupus anticoagulant is an in vitro phenomenon only. In fact, in vivo all the antiphospholipid antibodies are associated with an increased risk of thrombosis.[18] The mechanism for the hypercoagulability is still unclear, although multiple mechanisms have been proposed. Women with these antibodies also have an increased risk of miscarriage.[19]

Neuropsychiatric disease is a major cause of morbidity and mortality occurring in at least 20% to 35% of children with SLE. The range of manifestations is wide, including headaches (which may or may not be associated with other evidence of central nervous system [CNS] disease); a variety of psychiatric problems ranging from emotional lability to severe psychosis; chorea; seizures; strokes; and an organic brain syndrome characterized by disorientation, memory loss, and progressive intellectual deterioration.[20,21] It can be difficult to confirm a diagnosis of CNS lupus. A lumbar puncture is necessary to rule out infection or subarachnoid hemorrhage, but abnormalities of cerebrospinal fluid (CSF) protein, cell count, or glucose occur in less than 50% of patients with CNS disease. CSF complement determination is not clinically useful and serum levels are often normal. Detection of antineuronal antibodies may be useful.[22] Antiribosomal P antibodies seem to correlate with the presence of SLE-induced psychiatric disease.[23] Electroencephalography, computed tomography, and magnetic resonance imaging all carry a high frequency of abnormality in patients with SLE and are unlikely to help distinguish CNS disease unless localizing signs are present. Positron emission tomography and single photon emission computed tomography may be more useful.[24,25]

Lupus nephritis detectable by a kidney biopsy is present in virtually all patients with SLE. Clinically evident nephritis is present in about 75% of children. The earliest warning signs of renal involvement are proteinuria, microscopic hematuria, or hypocomplementemia. Development of nephrotic syndrome, red blood cell casts, white blood cells, white blood cell casts, and a decreasing creatinine clearance may be seen with more active disease. Since several different histopathologic subtypes have been identified, and these correlate to some extent with the prognosis and treatment, kidney biopsy is useful. Mesangial disease rarely progresses to cause significant problems. Focal proliferative disease also has a generally good prognosis. Diffuse proliferative disease carries a guarded prognosis and will progress to end-stage disease

if left untreated. Membranous glomerulonephritis is often associated with nephrotic syndrome and renal vein thrombosis and may show little response to therapy; however, for many patients it does not progress to end-stage renal disease. Diffuse proliferative glomerulonephritis is more common in children than in adults with SLE and contributes to the worse prognosis in pediatric SLE patients. Other features in the biopsy such as interstitial nephritis, glomerular sclerosis, and crescent formation may also contribute to the overall prognosis and likelihood of response to treatment.[26,27]

DIAGNOSIS

The diagnosis of SLE is based on both clinical findings and laboratory data. Table 58-2 shows the 1982 American Rheumatism Association criteria for the diagnosis of SLE, which were developed to ensure that most patients included in studies do indeed have SLE. The sensitivity and specificity of these criteria are each 96%.[28] However, not all patients with SLE fulfill these criteria, particularly early in the course of their disease. Patients with SLE have a variety of autoantibodies, but very few are specific for the disease. ANAs are detectable by immunofluorescence in virtually all children with SLE if HEp-2 cells are used as the substrate for the assay. However, the immunofluorescence ANA test lacks specificity, and positive tests can be seen in other rheumatic, chronic inflammatory, and infectious diseases; with tumors; after induction by certain medications; and in intravenous drug abuse. Also, approximately 5% of healthy adults have low-titer positive ANA tests.

Certain types of ANAs are more specific for SLE. Anti–double-stranded DNA antibodies are rarely present in any disease other than SLE. The same is true for antibodies to the extractable nuclear antigen (ENA) Sm. Antibodies to other ENAs such as RNP, SS-A(Ro), and SS-B(La), which are often found in SLE serum, are less diagnostic. Antibody to deoxyribonucleoprotein (anti-DNP) is responsible for the LE cell phenomenon. A positive LE cell test is strongly suggestive of SLE but not pathognomonic, and the low sensitivity of the LE cell test reduces its clinical utility.

Complement levels are useful both for diagnosis and as a measure of disease activity. Low or depleted complement suggest active SLE. C3 and C4 are consumed when the complement cascade is activated by immune complexes. CH50 should also be measured, because certain patients with SLE may have a hereditary complement component deficiency. A very low or absent CH50 level associated with a normal C3 suggests this possibility. Complement and anti-DNA levels are used as measures of disease activity. After treatment of the disease, they generally return to normal. However,

TABLE 58-2
Revised Criteria for Classification of Systemic Lupus Erythematosus

Criterion	Definition
Malar rash	Fixed erythema, flat or raised, over the malar eminences, tending to spare the nasolabial folds
Discoid rash	Erythematous raised patches with adherent keratotic scaling and follicular plugging; atrophic scarring may occur in older lesions
Photosensitivity	Skin rash as a result of unusual reaction to sunlight, by patient history or physician observation
Oral ulcers	Oral or nasopharyngeal ulceration, usually painless, observed by a physician
Arthritis	Nonerosive arthritis involving two or more peripheral joints, characterized by tenderness, swelling, or effusion
Serositis	Pleuritis—converting history of pleuritic pain or rub heard by a physician or evidence of pleural effusion *or* Pericarditis—documented by ECG or rub or evidence of pericardial effusion
Renal disorder	Persistent proteinuria >0.5 g per day or >3+ if quantitation not performed *or* Cellular casts—may be red cell, hemoglobin, granular, tubular, or mixed
Neurologic disorder	Seizures—in the absence of offending drugs or known metabolic derangements; e.g., uremia, ketoacidosis, or electrolyte imbalance *or* Psychosis—in the absence of offending drugs or known metabolic derangements; e.g., uremia, ketoacidosis, or electrolyte imbalance
Hematologic disorder	Hemolytic anemia—with reticulocytosis *or* Leukopenia—<4000/mm^3 total on two or more occasions *or* Lymphopenia—<1500/mm^3 on two or more occasions *or* Thrombocytopenia—<100,000/mm^3 in the absence of offending drugs
Immunologic disorder	Positive LE cell preparation *or* Anti-DNA: antibody to native DNA in abnormal titer *or* Anti-Sm: presence of antibody to Sm nuclear antigen *or* False-positive serologic test for syphilis known to be positive for at least 6 months and confirmed by *Treponema pallidum* immobilization or fluorescent treponemal antibody absorption test
Antinuclear antibody	An abnormal titer of antinuclear antibody by immunofluorescence or an equivalent assay at any point in time and in the absence of drugs known to be associated with "drug-induced lupus" syndrome

Four of 11 criteria provide a sensitivity of 96% and a specificity of 96%.
From Tan EM, Cohen AS, Fries JF, et al: The 1982 revised criteria for the classification of systemic lupus erythematosus, *Arthritis Rheum* 25:1271-1277, 1982.

occasional patients remain persistently hypocomplementemic or have elevated anti-DNA levels regardless of their clinical status.

PROGNOSIS AND TREATMENT

With careful medical management, many affected adolescents are currently able to continue a relatively normal life style. Certainly, life expectancy for this group has improved substantially. Thirty years ago the 5-year survival rate was only about 50%. By 1977 a study of 49 SLE patients under the age of 20 years showed an 86% 10-year survival rate for the entire group. However, in this same study survival was lower for patients with diffuse proliferative glomerulonephritis, who had a 5-year survival rate of 73%.[29] Currently the 5-year survival rate of patients with renal disease has improved substantially and is probably greater than 90%. Infection is now the leading cause of death followed by cerebritis, acute pancreatitis, pulmonary hemorrhage, and renal failure.[30]

Systemic corticosteroids remain the main treatment for active SLE, but other medications are used to minimize the dosage of systemic corticosteroids patients receive. Analgesics and nonsteroidal agents are the first choice for the treatment of arthralgias, arthritis, myalgias, and mild pleurisy and pericarditis. Antimalarials such as hydroxychloroquine have been used to treat certain rashes and may also be helpful for arthritis. Hydroxychloroquine is a generally well tolerated and safe medication, but occasional patients develop macular degeneration, so baseline and regular ophthalmologic examinations are necessary. Topical steroids are also useful for the treatment of certain rashes.

Systemic corticosteroids are generally required for major organ involvement such as in cerebritis, nephritis, and severe hematologic abnormalities. High doses are given initially and then tapered to the lowest dose required to control the disease. Most patients need daily doses, but alternate-day dosing has fewer side effects and may be used in certain patients. Immunosuppressive agents such as azathioprine and cyclophosphamide are added to the treatment regimen when steroids do not provide adequate control or as steroid-sparing agents to prevent excessive side effects. Several studies support the use of intravenous pulse cyclophosphamide for the treatment of diffuse proliferative glomerulonephritis. It may be more effective and less toxic than daily oral therapy and as such is now used for a variety of other severe disease manifestations.[31] The potentially severe side effects of immunosuppressive medications always need to be considered before they are administered. In addition to the frequent gastrointestinal discomfort during administration and alopecia, cyclophosphamide increases the risk of infection and the long-term development of malignancy. It is also associated with hemorrhagic cystitis and ovarian failure or azospermia.

Other forms of therapy, including intravenous gammaglobulin and danazol for the treatment of thrombocytopenia, dapsone for certain cutaneous problems, plasma exchange, and total lymphoid irradiation are discussed elsewhere.[32] Management of patients prone to thrombosis associated with antiphospholipid antibodies requires anticoagulants.

PREGNANCY

Adolescents are usually deeply concerned about attaining their goals of career accomplishment, marriage, and raising children. For women with SLE, active disease is often associated with menstrual irregularity. However, most women with SLE have normal fertility, and more than half of pregnancies in women with SLE conclude successfully. Pregnancy may cause a disease flare-up, particularly in patients with poorly controlled disease or

severe renal problems, but in well-controlled patients this is unlikely to occur.[33] Pregnant patients with SLE do have an increased risk of miscarriage that is largely the result of problems caused by antiphospholipid antibodies.[34]

Neonatal lupus syndrome results from the transmission of autoantibodies in utero. Certain problems such as rashes and thrombocytopenia are transient, but anti-SSA and anti-SSB antibodies are associated with cardiac disturbances, including congenital heart block, which is permanent.[35]

Corticosteroids are safe to use during pregnancy, but certain medications taken by patients with SLE, such as cyclophosphamide and methotrexate, are considered teratogenic. Patients on these medications should be cautioned to use birth control. Barrier methods are preferable. In the past, birth control pills have been associated with disease flare-ups, but it is not clear whether the newer very-low-estrogen pills or progesterone only medications have the same effect.

References

1. Elkon KB: Autoantibodies in systemic lupus erythematosus. In Klippel JH, Dieppe PA, editors: *Rheumatology,* Philadelphia, 1994, Mosby–Year Book.
2. Crow MK, Friedman SM: Systemic lupus erythematosus: cellular immunology. In Klippel JH, Dieppe PA, editors: *Rheumatology,* Philadelphia, 1994, Mosby–Year Book.
3. Miller RW, Salcedo JR, Fink RJ, et al: *J Pediatr* 108:576-579, 1986.
4. Lacks S, White P: Morbidity associated with childhood systemic lupus erythematosus, *J Rheumatol* 17:941-945, 1990.
5. Platt JL, Burke BA, Fish AJ, et al: Systemic lupus erythematosus in the first two decades of life, *Am J Kidney Dis* 2:212-222, 1982.
6. Nobrega FT, Ferguson RH, Kurland LT, et al: Lupus erythematosus, Rochester, Minnesota, 1950-65: a preliminary study. In Bennett PH, Wood PHN, editors: *Population studies of the rheumatic diseases,* International Congress Series, No. 148, New York, 1968, Excerpta Medica; p 259.
7. Siegel M, Lee ML: Epidemiology of SLE, *Semin Arthritis Rheum* 3:1-54, 1973.
8. Emery H: Clinical aspects of SLE in childhood, *Pediatr Clin North Am* 33:1177-1190, 1986.
9. Edberg JC, Salmon JE, Porges AJ, Kimberly RP: Systemic lupus erythematosus: immunopathology. In Klippel JH, Dieppe PA, editors: *Rheumatology,* Philadelphia, 1994, Mosby–Year Book.
10. Kosterking K et al: The clinical spectrum of SLE in childhood. III, *Arthritis Rheum* 20 (suppl 2):287-367, 1977.
11. Deapen D, Escalante A, Weinrib L, et al: A revised estimate of twin concordance in systemic lupus erythematosus, *Arthritis Rheum* 35:311-318, 1992.
12. Revielle J: The molecular genetics of systemic lupus erythematosus and Sjögren's syndrome, *Curr Opin Rheumatol* 4:644, 1992.
13. Liszewski MK, Kahl LE, Atkinson JP: The functional role of complement genes in systemic lupus erythematosus and Sjögren's syndrome, *Curr Opin Rheumatol* 1:347-352, 1989.
14. Atkinson JP: Complement deficiency: predisposing factor to autoimmune syndrome, *Am J Med* 85:45-57, 1988.
15. Carr RI, Hoffman AA, Harbeck RJ: Comparison of DNA binding in normal population, general hospital laboratory personnel and personnel from laboratories studying SLE, *J Rheumatol* 2:178-182, 1975.

16. Hess EV: Drug-related lupus (editorial), *N Engl J Med* 318:1460-1462, 1988.

17. Jungers P, Douglas M, Pelissier R, et al: Influence of oral contraceptive therapy on the activity of lupus erythematosus, *Arthritis Rheum* 25:618-623, 1982.

18. Appan S, Boley ML, Lin KE: Multiple thrombosis in SLE, *Arch Dis Child* 62:739-741, 1987.

19. Lockshin MD, Druzin ML, Qamar T: Prednisone does not prevent recurrent fetal death in women with anti-phospholipid antibody, *Am J Obstet Gynecol* 160:439-443, 1989.

20. Kaell AT, Shetty M, Lee BCP, Lochshin M: The diversity of neurologic events in systemic lupus erythematosus, *Arch Neurol* 43:273-276, 1988.

21. Denburg SD, Carbotte RM, Denburg JA: Cognitive impairment in systemic lupus erythematosus: a neuropsychological study of individual and group deficits, *J Clin Exp Neuropsychol* 9:323-329, 1987.

22. Long AA, Denbug SD, Carbotte RM, Sinai DP, Denburg JA: Serum lymphocytotoxic antibodies and neurocognitive function in systemic lupus erythematosus, *Ann Rheum Dis* 49:249-253, 1990.

23. Bonfa E, Golombek SJ, Kaufman LD, et al: Association between lupus psychosis and anti-ribosomal P protein antibodies, *N Engl J Med* 317:265-271, 1987.

24. Hirawa M, Nonaka C, Abe T, Io M: Positron emission tomography in systemic lupus erythematosus: relation of cerebral vasculitis to PET findings, *AJNR* 4:541-543, 1983.

25. Marienhagen J, Pirner K, Manger B, et al: Single-photon-emission computed tomography analysis of cerebral blood flow in the evaluation of central nervous system involvement in patients with systemic lupus erythematosus, *Arthritis Rheum* 36:1253-1262, 1993.

26. Nossent HC, et al: Contribution of renal biopsy data in predicting outcome in lupus nephritis. Analysis of 116 patients, *Arthritis Rheum* 33:970-977, 1990.

27. Baldwin DS, Gluck MC, Lowenstein J, et al: Lupus nephritis. Clinical course as related to morphologic forms and their transitions, *Am J Med* 62:12-30, 1977.

28. Tan EM, Cohen AS, Fries JR, et al: The 1982 revised criteria for the classification of SLE, *Arthritis Rheum* 25:1271-1277, 1982.

29. Fish AJ, et al: Systemic lupus erythematosus within the first two decades of life (review), *Am J Med* 62:99-117, 1977.

30. Abeles M, Yoman JD, Weinstein J, et al: SLE in the younger patient: survival studies, *J Rheumatol* 7:515-522, 1980.

31. McCune WJ, Golbus J, Zellis W, et al: Clinical and immunologic effects of monthly administration of intravenous cyclophosphamide in severe SLE, *N Engl J Med* 318:1423-1431, 1988.

32. Klippel JH: Systemic lupus erythematosus: management. In Klippel JH, Dieppe PA, editors: *Rheumatology,* Philadelphia, 1994, Mosby–Year Book.

33. Nossent HC, Swaak TJG: Systemic lupus erythematosus. VI. Analysis of the interrelationship with pregnancy, *J Rheumatol* 17:771-776, 1990.

34. Ramsey-Goldman R: Pregnancy in systemic lupus erythematosus, *Rheum Dis Clin North Am* 14:169-185, 1988.

35. Watson RM, et al: Neonatal lupus erythematosus: a clinical, serological and immunogenetic study with review of the literature, *Medicine* 63:362-378, 1984.

CHAPTER 59

Juvenile Rheumatoid Arthritis and Related Diseases

•

Patricia L. Haber and Carol A. Smith

Adolescents may experience chronic arthritis as a result of a variety of different diseases. Juvenile rheumatoid arthritis (JRA), beginning earlier in childhood, may persist into or through adolescence. In addition, certain diseases such as systemic lupus erythematosus (SLE), rheumatoid factor–positive JRA, and spondyloarthropathies often begin during adolescence. Box 59-1 contains a list of articular conditions that adolescents may experience. A discussion of SLE may be found in Chapter 58, "Systemic Lupus Erythematosus."

JUVENILE RHEUMATOID ARTHRITIS

JRA is one of the most crippling diseases of children, with incidence rates of 9 to 19 per 100,000 per year. According to some estimates the prevalence of JRA approaches 0.1%.[1,2] JRA is not one disease but rather is a group of partially overlapping joint syndromes that have their onset, by definition, before the age of 16 (Box 59-2). Although certain of these syndromes are relatively well defined, the diagnosis is primarily one of exclusion. The

---

BOX 59-1
Articular Syndromes in Adolescents

Juvenile rheumatoid arthritis
Rheumatoid arthritis
Systemic lupus erythematosus
Dermatomyositis/polymyositis
Spondyloarthropathies
    Ankylosing spondylitis
    Reiter's syndrome
    Arthritis of inflammatory bowel disease
    Psoriatic arthritis
Reactive arthritis
Rheumatic fever
Subacute bacterial endocarditis
Septic and infectious arthritis
Vasculitis
Neoplasms/malignancies
Sports and overuse injuries
Osteochondroses
Hemoglobinopathies
Hemophilias
Pigmented villonodular synovitis
Sarcoidosis
Angioimmunoblastic lymphadenopathy
Acquired immunodeficiencies
Reflex sympathetic dystrophy

BOX 59-2
Clinical Variants of Juvenile Rheumatoid Arthritis

SYSTEMIC
Most common age of onset 1 to 4; female/male ratio, 1:1; pattern of daily or twice-daily fever spikes and characteristic rash; other organ involvement; onset after age 16 is called "adult Still's disease"; antinuclear antibody (ANA) 10%, rheumatoid factor (RF) rare

PAUCIARTICULAR (1 TO 4 JOINTS INVOLVED)
One variant (early onset) usually presents before age 4; female/male ratio, 5:1; ANA 75%-85%, RF rare; asymptomatic uveitis is common
One variant (late onset) usually presents after age 7; female/male ratio, 1:4; ANA and RF rare; many eventually evolve into a spondyloarthropathy

POLYARTICULAR
May present throughout childhood, but peak is at 1 to 3 years; female/male ratio, 3:1; ANA 40%, RF 10% (increases with age); in older children it resembles adult disease with a tendency toward positive RF, chronicity, and progression

---

subsets of JRA are distinguished by the pattern of disease found during the first 6 months of illness. In approximately three fourths of cases the pattern remains constant. In the remainder, a change in "subset" occurs. The cause of the arthritis and the factors that predispose an individual to develop a certain subset remain unclear. However, it is suspected that environmental exposures such as infections, hormonal influences, and genetic factors all play roles.[3]

Certain of the JRA subsets occur predominantly in young children. For example, pauciarticular JRA, with a positive antinuclear antibody (ANA) and asymptomatic uveitis, rarely begins after early childhood. In contrast, polyarticular JRA, with a positive rheumatoid factor (RF), rarely occurs before puberty. This form of JRA is indistinguishable from adult rheumatoid arthritis (RA).

Since adolescents may be affected by all forms of JRA, each subset is discussed individually. For more complete descriptions, refer to Cassidy and Petty[4] and Jacobs.[5]

Systemic Juvenile Rheumatoid Arthritis

Systemic JRA is characterized by arthritis in association with fever as well as other evidence of systemic involvement such as lymphadenopathy, hepatosplenomegaly, pleuropericarditis, leukocytosis, thrombocytosis, and anemia. The fevers may be distinctive, with high spikes once or twice daily, returning to normal or subnormal between fever spikes. During the febrile period the patient may exhibit a characteristic rash that is an evanescent, macular, salmon-colored eruption found mostly on the trunk and proximal limbs. The arthritis may affect any number of joints and may appear in any joint, but wrists, elbows, and ankles are commonly involved. Although this form of JRA usually begins in early childhood, it may present at any age.

Laboratory findings are generally nonspecific. Rheumatoid factors are not present and only about 10% of patients have a positive ANA. Leukocytosis and thrombocytosis may be marked and the anemia may be severe. Other nonspecific evidence of inflammation such as increases in erythrocyte sedimentation rate, C-reactive protein, gammaglobulin, immune complexes and complement are also common findings.

As with all forms of JRA, the diagnosis of systemic JRA is one of exclusion, and other possible diagnoses such as infections, sarcoidosis, SLE, and malignancy need to be considered. The prognosis of patients with systemic-onset disease is generally good. Systemic symptoms usually decrease or totally resolve over time. For many patients the arthritis either totally resolves or remains fairly mild. However, a minority of patients may progress to have severely deforming arthritis. The persistence of systemic symptoms, particularly thrombocytosis, for more than 6 months has been shown to be associated with a high risk of severe progressive disease.[6]

Pauciarticular Juvenile Rheumatoid Arthritis

Pauciarticular arthritis is defined as arthritis in fewer than five joints. The most common form of pauciarticular JRA occurs primarily in girls, who have the onset of their disease at under 6 years of age. This subset of JRA has a high frequency of positive ANA and a 20% risk of chronic asymptomatic uveitis. Patients may have a moderately elevated erythrocyte sedimentation rate and a mild anemia, but fever and other evidence of systemic involvement are absent. The presence of fever should suggest another diagnosis. The antigenic specificity of the ANA has not been defined.

The outcome of patients with early-onset pauciarticular JRA is generally good. For most of these children the arthritis ultimately resolves and long-term disability is rare. However, these children (especially those with a positive ANA) require frequent ophthalmologic evaluations with slit-lamp examination to monitor for uveitis. The uveitis usually begins within several years of the onset of the arthritis, but occasional patients have had the onset of uveitis as late as 10 years after the onset of the arthritis, and the activity of the arthritis and the uveitis are unrelated.[7] In the past, many children with JRA who developed chronic uveitis became blind, but earlier identification and initiation of treatment seems to have improved the prognosis.[8]

Pauciarticular disease presenting in older children, particularly boys, is often the early manifestation of diseases such as ankylosing spondylitis, inflammatory bowel disease (IBD), and psoriasis. The most commonly involved joints are knees, ankles, and hips. Enthesitis (inflammation at the insertion of tendons or ligaments into bone) is common. Uveitis may also occur in these patients, but it is usually acute and symptomatic, unlike the uveitis found in early-onset pauciarticular JRA.

Genetic studies support the observations that the early-onset pauciarticular disease with chronic indolent uveitis and later-onset pauciarticular disease are distinct entities. Increased frequencies of HLA-DR5, DR8, and DPw2 are found in the early-onset patients. Patients with late-onset pauciarticular disease frequently carry the HLA-B27 gene.[9,10]

When patients present with arthritis in only one or two joints, particularly if it is of recent onset, joint aspiration is necessary to rule out problems such as infections or hemarthrosis. Synovial fluid cell count and protein and glucose determinations may be helpful but do not distinguish between infections and other inflammatory conditions such as JRA. Bone imaging studies are important to rule out conditions such as fractures,

osteomyelitis, and bone tumors. Early in the course of JRA, radiographic examinations are unlikely to show any bone changes except juxtaarticular osteopenia.[11]

Polyarticular Juvenile Rheumatoid Arthritis/Adult Rheumatoid Arthritis

Polyarticular JRA may begin early in childhood or during adolescence. At all ages, girls outnumber boys by approximately 3:1. The onset may be acute but is more often indolent. Mild systemic manifestations such as low-grade fever, lymphadenopathy, and mild pleural and pericardial effusions may be found. ANA may be present but is less common than in early-onset pauciarticular JRA. RF is present in some patients, most of whom have the onset of their disease in adolescence. JRA associated with a positive RF (seropositive) is more likely than seronegative JRA to have a chronic course persisting into adulthood. Seropositive JRA shares the clinical characteristics of classic adult RA. These patients are more likely to have symmetric disease with more small joint involvement, early onset of erosions, and extraarticular manifestations such as rheumatoid nodules, pericarditis, and rheumatoid vasculitis. Genetic studies show the same increased frequency of HLA-DR4 and -DR2 in seropositive JRA as in adult RA.[12]

Rheumatoid factor is not specific for RA or seropositive JRA. Rheumatoid factor may be found in chronic infections such as subacute bacterial endocarditis and tuberculosis as well as in other connective tissue diseases such as SLE, scleroderma, Sjögren's syndrome, and sarcoidosis. Since all of these disorders may present with joint symptoms, a careful history and special studies are necessary to exclude these diagnoses.

The prognosis is good for most polyarticular JRA patients, even those who are seropositive. Some seronegative patients have total resolution of the arthritis over time. This is unlikely for seropositive patients, but many will be able to continue a normal to somewhat modified life style without severe loss of function or serious joint deformities.

Treatment

The treatment of patients with JRA is directed toward improving patients' comfort and maximizing their functional status. Medications are used to reduce pain and decrease the inflammatory and immunologic responses that cause articular damage. The first line of therapy is generally nonsteroidal antiinflammatory medications (NSAIDs). For patients with poorly responsive disease, other medications are often required. Slow-acting antirheumatic drugs (SAARDs) such as gold salts, hydroxychloroquine, penicillamine, sulfasalazine, and methotrexate, as well as corticosteroids and immunosupressives, all play roles in the therapy of certain patients. These medications should be used only under the supervision of a rheumatologist. For patients with only one or two problem joints, intraarticular steroid injections may be useful.

In addition to drug therapy, patients benefit from a life style that permits regular rest and exercise. They should be encouraged to maintain the range of motion of their joints and the strength of their muscles by doing daily exercises. Participation of physical and occupational therapists in their care can be very important. The involvement of orthopedic surgeons may also be necessary. For children with severe arthritis of long duration, adolescence may be the time for joint replacement surgery. Growth abnormalities are common in all types of JRA. Localized growth problems are common in pauciarticular JRA and may result in leg length discrepancies that require special shoes or possible surgical intervention. Scoliosis may result from asymmetric spinal growth. Since JRA patients frequently have cervical spine disease, the stability of the cervical spine should be assessed before anesthesia is administered.

Attention to the educational needs of adolescents with arthritis is essential. Even those with severe arthritis can live very productive lives and every effort should be made to allow them to attend school regularly.

RELATED SYNDROMES

Spondyloarthropathies

The spondyloarthropathies are a group of interrelated arthropathies that have prominent involvement of spinal and sacroiliac joints. Enthesopathy, a painful low-grade inflammation at the sites of tendon insertions into bone or joint capsular surfaces, is also a characteristic finding in these diseases. Onset during adolescence is common. Many patients have a family history of similar problems, and all spondyloarthropathies are associated with an increased frequency of HLA-B27. This association is particularly strong in ankylosing spondylitis. Another distinguishing feature of this group of diseases is the strong male predominance. Table 59-1 outlines the overlapping features of the four major spondyloarthropathies.

Juvenile ankylosing spondylitis (JAS) is similar to the adult disease, except that radiographically evident changes (sacroiliac and spinal) are rarely noted at onset.[13] Common clinical findings include persistent or recurrent low back pain and stiffness not relieved by rest, thoracic pain and stiffness, limited lumbar spinal motion, and a history of acute iritis or conjunctivitis. These findings may occur with or without peripheral joint involvement and enthesopathy. The most common enthesopathy is at

the insertion of the Achilles tendon into the calcaneus, but virtually any site can be involved. The definitive diagnosis of ankylosing spondylitis cannot be made until sacroiliac changes are seen on radiographic examination. It is postulated that 8.6% of adults with ankylosing spondylitis had the onset of their disease in childhood, making the prevalence in children possibly as high as 0.08%, which is almost the same as that of JRA.[14] It is unclear how many adolescents with early signs and symptoms of possible ankylosing spondylitis actually develop significant spinal disease.[15-17]

Psoriatic arthopathy in young people commonly involves the peripheral joints alone, with reported figures of 17% to 47% developing sacroiliac changes and up to one third eventually having cervical spine manifestations. Skin disease may precede or follow the onset of the arthritis. The arthritis is typically asymmetric and may involve large or small joints. A family history, "sausage" digits, nailpitting, and skin lesions are helpful diagnostic clues, since the early arthritis may not be distinguishable from other spondyloarthropthies or from JRA.[18,19]

The arthropathies of IBD are those occurring before or during the course of regional enteritis or ulcerative colitis. Peripheral arthritis resembling that of pauciarticular JRA is the more common pattern, with sacroiliac and spinal problems occurring in somewhat fewer cases. The arthritis associated with IBD often responds to management that controls the gut inflammation.[20]

The Reiter's syndrome triad was initially described in a 16-year-old boy who developed arthritis, urethritis, and conjunctivitis after dysentery.[21] We now know that Reiter's syndrome may occur after *Salmonella, Shigella, Yersinia, Campylobacter,* and *Chlamydia* infections. It is considered to be a "reactive" arthritis since evidence of viable organisms in joint tissues is lacking. In addition to the Reiter's syndrome triad, mucocutaneous lesions such as balanitis, keratoderma blennorrhagicum (which may resemble psoriasis), and shallow oral ulcers may be seen. The course is usually self-limited, but in some cases it becomes episodic, and some patients may have chronic arthritis with significant sacroiliac and spine involvement.

"Reactive" arthritis often occurs without the other components of Reiter's syndrome. The term *reactive arthritis* is applied to apparently sterile joint inflammation occurring during or after infections with a variety of organisms, including those associated with Reiter's syndrome. Usually the course is self-limited, but occasionally there is evolution to another disease category.

Treatment of the spondyloarthropathies differs slightly from one syndrome to another. The arthritis, enthesitis, and spinal manifestations of ankylosing spondylitis and Reiter's syndrome are generally responsive to NSAIDs. Routine bending and chest expansion exercises are important to maintain flexibility.

TABLE 59-1
Overlapping Characteristics of the Spondyloarthropathies

	Enthesitis	Axial Arthritis	Peripheral Arthritis	B27 Positive	ANA Positive	RF Positive	Systemic Disease			
							Iritis	Skin	MM	GI
JAS	+++	+++	+++	+++	−	−	+	−	−	−
JPsA	+	++	+++	+	++	−	+	+++	−	−
IBD	+	++	+++	++	−	−	+	+	+	++++
RS	++	+	+++	+++	−	−	+	+	+	+++

JAS, juvenile ankylosing spondylitis; *JPsA,* juvenile psoriatic arthritis; *IBD,* inflammatory bowel disease; *RS,* Reiter's syndrome; *MM,* mucous membrane lesions; *GI,* gastrointestinal tract symptoms.
−, absent; +, <25%; ++, 25%-50%; +++, 50%-75%; ++++, 75% or more.
From Cassidy J, Petty R: *Textbook of pediatric rheumatology,* Philadelphia, 1995, WB Saunders, p 224.

Current evidence suggests that sulfasalazine may be useful in less responsive patients.[22] In IBD, sulfasalazine is useful in treating both the bowel and articular symptoms. Indeed, in IBD the joints are rarely active when the bowel disease is under control. Interestingly, inflammation is frequently seen in bowel biopsies of patients with spondyloarthropathies who do not have obvious evidence of IBD.[23] In Reiter's syndrome, antibiotics may be indicated if the offending organism is isolated from the bowel or genitourinary tract.

Psoriatic arthritis responds to medications similar to those used for JRA and RA. In particular, if NSAIDs are inadequate, gold and methotrexate have been useful.

Acute Rheumatic Fever

Discussion of the diagnosis and treatment of acute rheumatic fever (ARF) is found in Chapter 36, "Cardiac Infection and Inflammation: Rheumatic Fever, Endocarditis, and Myocarditis." The arthritis found in ARF is also a "reactive" arthritis, with group A streptococcus the initiating infection. Arthritis is the most common of the Jones criteria major manifestations. The arthritis is usually, but not always, a migratory polyarthritis and the pain is often very severe. Large and small joints can be affected, but the large joints of the lower extremity are the most commonly involved. Typically the arthritis shows a dramatic response to aspirin. The arthritis is nondeforming and rarely lasts more than several weeks for a single episode.

The Jones criteria (see Chapter 36) are not absolutely specific for ARF. Some patients with SLE and JRA may meet the criteria, since they may have fever and arthritis in association with elevated levels of antistreptolysin O. However, patients who fulfill the Jones criteria should receive prophylaxis to prevent potential cardiac complications until another diagnosis is made.

Treatment of patients with arthritis who show evidence of a preceding streptococcal infection but do not fulfill the Jones criteria is controversial. In some patients the arthritis may not be the result of a streptococcal infection, but in some it is. These patients with "poststreptococcal arthritis" may represent an incomplete form of ARF, but the clinical characteristics of certain patients are somewhat different. For example, the duration of the arthritis may be more prolonged. Although most of the patients with this disorder have a benign course, some may develop carditis.[24,25] Antistreptococcal prophylaxis is probably warranted.

Dermatomyositis/Polymyositis

During childhood and adolescence the prominent form of chronic inflammatory myositis is dermatomyositis. Idiopathic myositis in the absence of skin involvement (polymyositis) is very rare in adolescence. For dermatomyositis, the peak age of onset is between 10 and 14 years. Patients generally present with insidious onset of muscle weakness, fatigue, fever, and rash. For about three fourths of the patients, the rash is pathognomonic, including a violaceous hue over the upper eyelids (heliotrope) and symmetric, erythematous, shiny, atrophic plaques and papules over extensor surfaces (Gottron's papules). For other patients, the rash is less specific. Muscle involvement is generally proximal. Progressive muscle weakness is found in almost all patients; muscle tenderness may be present but is less common. Other evidence to support the diagnosis of dermatomyositis includes elevated serum levels of muscle enzymes, an electromyogram showing typical myopathic changes, and a muscle biopsy demonstrating inflammatory myositis. The biopsy in childhood dermatomyositis also usually shows evidence of vasculitis and vasculopathy, which is widespread and probably contributes to disease in other organs (gastrointestinal, joint, cardiac, lung) in some patients. As many as 10% of patients develop severe gastrointestinal ulceration.

When progressive muscle weakness occurs in conjunction with the typical rash, the diagnosis of dermatomyositis is straightforward. However, early in the course of the disease the rash may not be present and other etiologies for the myositis need to be considered. These include viral myositis, primary myopathies, and myositis accompanying other connective tissue diseases.

Treatment of dermatomyositis often requires the prolonged use of corticosteroids and perhaps other immunosuppressive medications also. Several reports of successful use of intravenous gammaglobulin have increased interest in this newer mode of therapy.[26] Early, vigorous treatment of the disease appears to be associated with the best outcome.

Vasculitis

Primary vasculitic disorders can be divided into several different groups.[27] The polyarteritis group is characterized by necrotizing vasculitis of small and medium muscular arteries. The arteritis is probably due to immune complex deposition. Hepatitis B surface antigen has been found in the immune complexes from many patients with polyarteritis nodosa, and other infections have also been associated with the disease.[28,29] The possibility of this disease should be considered in any patient with unexplained fever, weight loss, and an elevated erythrocyte sedimentation rate. Abdominal pain, arthritis, rash, and central nervous system problems are other common manifestations.

Leukocytoclastic vasculitis refers to conditions with a necrotizing vasculitis primarily affecting small vessels and postcapillary venules. Henoch-Schönlein purpura, hypersensitivity angiitis, and hypocomplementemic urticarial vasculitis fall into this category. The vasculitis found in connective tissue diseases such as SLE is also often of this type.

Wegener's granulomatosis is a granulomatous vasculitis that primarily affects the respiratory tract and kidneys. Antineutrophil cytoplasmic antibodies are strongly associated with this disorder. This is particularly true for C-ANCA, which reacts with proteinase 3.[30]

Giant cell arteritis predomintly affects large arteries. In young people the most common form is Takayasu's arteritis (pulseless disease), which usually involves the aorta and its major branches.

For a detailed discussion of these and other vasculitic syndromes, the reader is referred to Churg and Churg.[31]

Scleroderma

The most characteristic feature of scleroderma is thickening of the skin due to increased collagen deposition. The cause of this increased collagen deposition is uncertain, but hypotheses include a primary vasculopathy or an underlying disorder of fibroblasts.[32] Two broad categories of scleroderma have been defined: localized and systemic sclerosis. Localized scleroderma,

including morphea, linear scleroderma, and eosinophilic fasciitis, affects the skin and structures such as muscle and bone directly underlying the involved skin. Patients with systemic sclerosis may have multiple organ system involvement. Lungs, heart, gastrointestinal tract, and kidneys are commonly affected. Localized scleroderma is frequently a self-limited disease and rarely progresses to systemic sclerosis. Systemic sclerosis has a much worse prognosis, with reported 10-year survival rates of 35% to 90%.

Most patients with systemic sclerosis, and many with localized scleroderma, have positive tests for ANA. Raynaud's phenomenon occurs in more than 90% of patients with systemic sclerosis and may be the presenting problem. Approximately 60% of patients with new-onset Raynaud's phenomenon develop a connective tissue disease over the next 2 years. Individuals with positive ANA tests are at highest risk and need to be followed carefully.[33,34]

References

1. Laaksonen AL: A prognostic study of juvenile rheumatoid arthritis. Analysis of 544 cases, *Acta Paediatr Scand* 166 (suppl):1, 1966.
2. Gare BA, Fasth A, Andersson J, et al: Incidence and prevalence of juvenile chronic polyarthritis: a population survey, *Ann Rheum Dis* 46:277-281, 1987.
3. Lang BA, Shore A: A review of current concepts on the pathogenesis of juvenile rheumatoid arthritis, *J Rheumatol* 17 (S21):1-15, 1990.
4. Cassidy JT, Petty RE: *Textbook of pediatric rheumatology,* ed 3, Philadelphia, 1995, WB Saunders, pp 133-223.
5. Jacobs J: *Pediatric rheumatology for the practitioner,* New York, 1989, Springer Verlag, pp 179-273.
6. Schneider R, Lang BA, Reilly BJ, et al: Prognostic indicators of joint destruction in systemic-onset juvenile rheumatoid arthritis, *J Pediatr* 120:200-205, 1992.
7. Kanski JJ, Shun-Shin GA: Systemic uveitis syndromes in childhood: analysis of 340 cases, *Ophthalmology* 91:1247-1251, 1984.
8. Rosenberg AM: Uveitis associated with juvenile rheumatoid arthritis, *Semin Arthritis Rheum* 16:158-173, 1987.
9. Melin-Aldana H, Giannini EH, Glass DN: Immunogenetics of early onset pauciarticular juvenile rheumatoid arthritis, *J Rheumatol* 17 (S26):2-6, 1990.
10. Petty RE: HLA-B27 and rheumatic diseases of childhood, *J Rheumatol* 17(S26):7-10, 1990.
11. Pozanski AK: Radiological approaches to pediatric joint disease, *J Rheumatol* 19(S33):78-93, 1992.
12. Vehe RK, Begovitch AB, Nepom BS: HLA susceptibility genes in rheumatoid factor positive juvenile rheumatoid arthritis, *J Rheumatol* 17(S26):11-15, 1990.
13. Petty R: HLA-B27 and rheumatic disease of childhood, *J Rheumatol* 17(S26):7-11, 1990.
14. Bennet PH, Wood PHN: *Population studies of the rheumatic diseases,* International Congress Series, No. 148, New York, 1968, Excerpta Medica; p 456.
15. Olivieri I, Passero G: Longstanding isolated juvenile onset HLA-B27 associated peripheral enthesitis, *J Rheumatol* 19:164-165, 1991.
16. Burgos-Vargas R, Clarck P: Axial involvement in the seronegative enthesopathy and arthropathy syndrome and its progression to ankylosing spondylitis, *J Rheumatol* 16:192-197, 1989.

17. Van der Linden SM, Valkenburg HA, deJongh BM, et al: The risk of developing ankylosing spondylitis in HLA-B27 positive individuals. A comparison of relatives of spondylitis patients with the general population, *Arthritis Rheum* 27:241-249, 1984.

18. Lambert JR, Ansell BM, Stephenson E, et al: Psoriatic arthritis in childhood, *Clin Rheum Dis* 2:339-352, 1976.

19. Shore A, Ansell BM: Juvenile psoriatic arthritis—an analysis of 60 cases, *J Pediatr* 100:529-535, 1982.

20. Cassidy JT, Petty RE: *Textbook of pediatric rheumatology,* ed 3, Philadelphia, 1995, WB Saunders; pp 248-251.

21. Reiter H: Über eine bisher unerhannte spirochatenin Fektion *(Spirochaetosis arthritica), Dtsch Med Wochenschr* 42:1535, 1916.

22. McConkey B: Sulfasalazine and ankylosing spondylitis, *Br J Rheumatol* 29:2-5, 1990.

23. Mielants H, Veys EM, Goemaere S, et al: Gut inflammation in the spondyloarthropathies: clinical, radiological, biological and genetic features in relation to the type of histology: a prospective study, *J Rheumatol* 18:1542-1551, 1991.

24. Emery H, Wagner-Weiner L, Magilavy D: Resurgence of childhood post-streptococcal rheumatic syndromes, *Arthritis Rheum* 30:S80, 1987.

25. DeCunto CL, Giannini EH, Fink CW, et al: Prognosis of children with poststreptococcal reactive arthritis, *Pediatr Infect Dis J* 7:683-686, 1988.

26. Land BA, Laxer RM, Murphy G, et al: Treatment of dermatomyositis with intravenous gammaglobulin, *Am J Med* 91:169-172, 1991.

27. Jennette JC, Falk RJ, Andrassy K, et al: Nomenclature of systemic vasculitides: proposal of an international consensus conference, *Arthritis Rheum* 37:187-192, 1994.

28. Trepo CG, Zuckerman AR, Bird RC, et al: The role of circulating hepatitis B antigen/antibody immune complexes in the pathogenesis of vascular and hepatic manifestations in polyarteritis nodosa, *J Clin Pathol* 27:863-868, 1974.

29. Conn DL: Polyarteritis, *Rheum Dis Clin North Am* 16:341-362, 1990.

30. Van der Woude F, Rasmussen N, Lobatto S, et al: Autoantibodies against neutrophils and monocytes: tool for diagnosis and marker of disease activity in Wegener's granulomatosis, *Lancet* 1:425-429, 1985.

31. Churg A, Churg J, editors: *Systemic vasculitides,* New York, 1991, Ikagu-Shoin.

32. Yarom A, Levinson JE: Vasculopathy in scleroderma. In Hicks RV, editor: *Vasculopathies of childhood,* Littleton, MA, 1988, PSC Publishing.

33. Cardelli MB, Kleinsmith DM: Raynaud's phenomenon and disease, *Med Clin North Am* 73:1127-1146, 1989.

34. Gerbracht DD, Steen VD, Ziegler GL, Medsger TA Jr, Rodnan GP: Evolution of primary Raynaud's phenomenon (Raynaud's disease) to connective tissue disease, *Arthritis Rheum* 28:87-92, 1985.

Central Nervous System

CHAPTER 60

Headaches

•

Lawrence C. Newman and Shlomo Shinnar

Headaches are among the most common complaints in adolescents. By age 15 as many as 15% of teenagers will have recurrent headaches.[1] Chronic headaches constitute one of the most common reasons for referral to a pediatric neurology practice. Most headaches are not associated with intracranial structural lesions. Diagnosis can usually be made by careful history taking and physical examination, and laboratory investigations are rarely required. Most headaches can be managed with simple analgesics. For more severe cases, particularly of migraine, effective pharmacologic agents are available.

TYPES OF HEADACHE

Headaches may be classified as primary or secondary. The primary headache disorders (migraine, tension-type, and cluster headaches) represent illnesses in which the headache itself is the problem. In contrast, the term secondary headaches implies that headache is a manifestation of some underlying pathology such as a brain tumor, an infection, or some other systemic illness. Most headaches seen in clinical practice are primary, but headaches from secondary causes must always be excluded. An accurate diagnosis can usually be made on the basis of the history and physical examination.[2]

Harbingers of serious disease elicited during the headache history include

1. Headaches that are of sudden onset or described as "the worst headache ever"; these are suggestive of subarachnoid hemorrhage.
2. Progressively worsening headaches; these may be secondary to mass lesion.
3. Headaches that occur during exertion, straining, coughing, or during sexual activity; these may be a sign of posterior fossa masses or may be due to intracerebral hemorrhages.

4. Headaches associated with drowsiness, confusion, or memory disturbances; these may be a manifestation of either structural lesions or infections of the central nervous system.

Box 60-1 categorizes some common primary and secondary headache disorders.

PRIMARY HEADACHE DISORDERS

Migraine

Migraine headaches affect all age groups, although the clinical manifestations may differ. Children are less likely than adults to complain of severe headache and may therefore be less likely to have their headaches correctly diagnosed. There is an equal gender incidence before puberty, but in adolescents migraine occurs more frequently in girls. A first- or second-degree relative also has migraine in 70% to 80% of cases. Migraine headaches are typically unilateral, throbbing, and associated with nausea and vomiting. They occur at any time of day, last from 30 minutes to 2 or 3 days, and are often relieved by vomiting or sleep. Precipitating factors include stress, fatigue, exertion, head trauma, illness, and dietary factors.[3,4] In 1988 the International Headache Society (IHS) proposed new criteria for the diagnosis of migraine and other headaches.[5] Common migraine is now known as *migraine without aura,* and the term classical migraine has been replaced by *migraine with aura.* The IHS classification of migraine may be found in Box 60-2. The IHS criteria are quite restrictive and best reserved for research purposes. In clinical practice it is useful to divide migraine into four phases:

1. *Prodrome.* Many people with migraine experience premonitory symptoms that precede the aura or headache phase. These symptoms, which may

BOX 60-1
Headache Classification

PRIMARY
1. Migraine Headache
    Without aura
    With aura
        Typical aura
        Prolonged aura
        Familial hemiplegic
        Basilar[29]
    Ophthalmoplegic migraine
    Retinal migraine
    Childhood periodic syndromes that may
        be precursors to or associated with
        migraine[30-33]
        Benign paroxysmal vertigo of childhood
        Alternating hemiplegia of childhood
2. Cluster headache
    Episodic
    Chronic
    Chronic evolved from episodic
3. Tension-type headache
    Episodic
    Chronic

SECONDARY
    Mass lesions
        Tumors
        Hemorrhages
        Abscesses
    Infections
        Meningitis
    Metabolic
        Hypoxia
        Hypercapnia
        Hypoglycemia
    Posttraumatic
    Headaches associated with substances or their
        withdrawal
        Alcohol
        Monosodium glutamate
        Drug rebound
    Postlumbar puncture
    Pseudotumor cerebri
    Headaches due to disorders of cranium, neck,
        eyes, ears, nose, sinuses, teeth, mouth, or
        other facial or cranial structures

occur hours to days before the headache, occur in 30% to 80% of sufferers. Common prodromal symptoms include irritability, sluggishness, depression, excessive energy, increased yawning, impaired concentration, increased urination, fluid retention, hunger, food cravings, photophobia, phonophobia, and osmophobia.

2. *Aura.* Only 20% of migraine sufferers experience auras, and while their presence is not necessary to establish the diagnosis, many sufferers are misdiagnosed because of their absence. Auras are transient neurologic disturbances that last 5 to 60 minutes and then spontaneously resolve. They are believed to occur more commonly in adults than in children, although some studies have reported visual auras in up to 50% of childhood migraine sufferers.[1] The most common auras consist of visual disturbances such as scotomas, blurred vision, flashing lights, and hemianopsias. Other aura phenomena include paresthesias, hemiparesis, vertigo, aphasias, and visual hallucinations.

3. *Headache phase.* The headache is considered the hallmark of migraine. Typically, the pain is described as throbbing or pounding; is worsened with movement or exertion; and usually involves the temple, orbital, and frontal regions. Migraine headache tends to be hemicranial, although attacks demonstrate side-shift (i.e., they alternate sides during subsequent bouts). In children the headache may not be hemicranial; children complain of generalized or bifrontal headaches more frequently than of hemicranial pain. Hemicranial headaches occur in only 22% to 31% of childhood migraine.[1,6,7] Headaches may be associated with nausea, vomiting, photophobia, phonophobia, osmophobia, and tenderness of the scalp and pericranial muscles. During attacks, patients prefer to sleep or lie quietly in a dark room. Attacks last from 4 to 72 hours, although episodes tend to be shorter in children than in adults.

4. *Postdrome.* After the headache, many adolescents with migraines experience a period of decreased concentration, fatigue, and limited food tolerance for up to 24 hours.

Migraine with prolonged aura is the new IHS designation for complicated migraine.[4,5,8,9] These disorders consist of migraine with transient neurologic deficits or alterations in state of consciousness. In this subgroup of migraine, the aura symptoms last more than 60 minutes but less than 1 week. The deficits are presumably due to prolonged vasoconstriction and ischemia to the affected cerebral areas. The onset of the deficit usually precedes the headache. The symptoms are extremely diverse and depend on the vascular territory involved. The natural course of complex migraine is usually benign and most patients later go on to develop typical migraine. It is important to differentiate migraine syndromes from more serious intracranial pathology. In general, adolescents with complex migraine should be referred to a neurologist for evaluation. The more common complex migraine syndromes are listed in Box 60-1.

BOX 60-2
IHS Criteria for Migraine With and Without Aura

DIAGNOSTIC CRITERIA FOR MIGRAINE
WITHOUT AURA (COMMON MIGRAINE)
A. At least five attacks fulfilling B-D
B. Headache attack lasting 4-72 hours* (untreated or unsuccessfully treated)
C. Headache has at least two of the following characteristics:
   1. Unilateral location
   2. Pulsating quality
   3. Moderate or severe intensity (inhibits or prohibits daily activities)
   4. Aggravation by walking stairs or similar routine physical activity
D. During headache at least one of the following:
   1. Nausea and/or vomiting
   2. Photophobia and phonophobia
E. At least one of the following:
   1. History, physical and neurologic examinations not consistent with organic disease
   2. History and/or physical and/or neurologic examinations do suggest such disorder, but it is ruled out by appropriate investigations
   3. Such disorder is present, but migraine attacks do not occur for the first time in close temporal relation to the disorder

DIAGNOSTIC CRITERIA FOR MIGRAINE
WITH AURA (CLASSICAL MIGRAINE)
A. At least two attacks fulfilling B
B. At least three of the following four characteristics:
   1. One or more fully reversible aura symptoms indicating focal cerebral, cortical, and/or brain stem dysfunction
   2. At least one aura symptom develops gradually over more than 4 minutes, or two or more symptoms occur in succession
   3. No aura symptom lasts more than 60 minutes; if more than one aura symptom is present, the accepted duration is proportionally increased
   4. Headache follows an aura with a free interval of less than 60 minutes (it may also begin before or simultaneously with the aura)
C. At least one of the following:
   1. History, physical, and neurologic examinations not consistent with organic disease
   2. History and/or physical and/or neurologic examinations do suggest such disorder, but it is ruled out by appropriate investigations
   3. Such disorder is present, but migraine attacks do not occur for the first time in close temporal relation to the disorder

*In children under age 15, attacks may last 2-48 hours. If the patient falls asleep and wakes up without migraine, the duration of the attack is until the time of awakening.

From Headache Classification Committee of the International Headache Society: Classification and diagnostic criteria for headache disorders, cranial neuralgias, and facial pain, *Cephalalgia* 8(suppl 7):19-21, 1988.

Cluster Headache

Although cluster headache is sometimes included among the migraine syndromes, it is a distinct entity. Patients do not have a family history of migraine, nor do they progress to typical migraine. Cluster attacks are characterized by intense, nonthrobbing periorbital pain that may then generalize to the entire hemicranium. The headaches are often associated with unilateral conjunctival injection, ptosis lacrimation, and rhinorrhea ipsilateral to the headache. The attacks are brief, not preceded by an aura, last 15 to 180 minutes, and occur in groups of one headache every other day to eight attacks daily for a period of 6 to 12 weeks. The cluster of headaches is followed by prolonged periods of remission lasting months to years.[9] Cluster headaches are usually refractory to simple analgesic therapy and generally require treatment with preventive agents. Patients with cluster should be referred to a neurologist for treatment, as these

headaches tend to have a less favorable prognosis than migraine.[10]

Tension-Type Headache

Tension-type headaches are the most common form of headache in adolescents and adults. They were once called tension or muscle contraction headache, as they were believed to arise secondarily to increased contraction of the muscles of the head and neck. Recent evidence suggests this is not the case, and these headaches may in some way have pathophysiologic mechanisms similar to those of migraine. Tension-type headaches may be subdivided into episodic and chronic varieties. In chronic tension-type headache, sufferers report more than 15 headaches per month or more than 180 headache days per year.[5] Adolescents with these headaches typically describe a sensation of tightness or pressure in a bandlike distribution around the head. Physical examination may reveal tenderness or tightness of the muscles in the occipital scalp or posterior cervical region. These headaches are often quite frequent and may last all day if untreated. The episodic variety usually does not interrupt regular daily activities and often responds well to mild analgesics such as acetaminophen or ibuprofen. Tension-type headaches differ from migraine headaches by the absence of vomiting and associated autonomic symptoms and in the ability of patients to continue their daily activities during the attack.

SECONDARY HEADACHES

Posttraumatic Headaches

The existence of a posttraumatic headache is controversial, but in the authors' experience it is a real entity that occurs even when litigation is not an issue. The headaches are often self-limited and usually resolve after a few weeks. They can, however, persist for months to years even after relatively minor trauma. Other symptoms of the posttraumatic syndrome, such as sleep disturbances and behavior changes, are often present.[11] The headaches may be migraine or tension-type in character.

Headaches and Childhood Depression

A serious and often unrecognized cause of chronic headache is depression.[12] The patient usually complains of a dull, constant headache that may be generalized or localized to the occipital region. Other symptoms of depression can often be elicited, such as significant mood changes, withdrawal, increasingly poor school performance, school problems, sleep disturbances, aggressive behavior, lack of energy, weight loss, anorexia, and other somatic complaints. Appropriate treatment depends on recognition of the underlying depression. Headaches as a primary manifestation of depression are relatively uncommon and must be distinguished from tension-type or migraine headaches, whose frequency and severity are often increased by stress.[3]

Nonmigrainous Vascular Headaches

CONVULSIVE STATES. Headache may occur as a postictal symptom but is rarely the sole manifestation of a seizure.[13] On occasion, patients with nocturnal seizures may awaken afterward with a postictal vascular headache. Migraine and epilepsy are distinct syndromes that can usually be differentiated on clinical grounds.[2,14] Some cases of complex migraine that may involve altered states of consciousness and transient neurologic deficits may be difficult to distinguish from complex partial seizures.

TRACTION HEADACHE. As the name implies, a traction headache is caused by traction on the intracranial pain-sensitive structures. The traction may be exerted by a mass lesion such as a brain tumor, an abscess, or a subdural hematoma; by the weight of the brain after removal of cerebrospinal fluid by lumbar puncture; or by distortion of intracranial structures from increased intracranial pressure, as in hydrocephalus or pseudotumor cerebri. Although a relatively uncommon form of headache, it is often associated with serious intracranial pathology.

Although headache can be the first symptom of a brain tumor, brain tumors are an extremely rare cause of headache in adolescence. Several characteristics help to distinguish brain tumor headaches from more benign varieties. Headaches associated with brain tumors are usually chronic and progressive; present in the morning on first arising; and are exacerbated by changes in position, coughing, or a Valsalva maneuver. In a 1993 review, however, the classic triad of headache, sleep disturbance, and vomiting was present in only one third of patients with brain tumors.[15] Localization of the headache is also of limited value, because a mass lesion may cause distortion of distant pain-sensitive structures. Associated symptoms such as vomiting, diplopia, weakness, ataxia, and personality changes are usually present within a few weeks of the onset of headache.[16] The physical examination often reveals papilledema, nuchal rigidity, irritability, focal neurologic deficits such as a field cut, or a hemiparesis. As a general rule, the child with headaches of more than 6 months' duration who still has normal neurologic examination results is exceedingly unlikely to have a brain tumor.

PSEUDOTUMOR CEREBRI. This syndrome is characterized by the clinical manifestations of increased intracranial pressure in the absence of hydrocephalus or a mass lesion. It occurs most frequently in obese young women.[17] Headache is the most common presenting complaint and is frequently associated with nausea and vomiting. Visual symptoms such as diplopia are not uncommon and are usually present even between headaches. Imaging studies are typically normal. However, on examination papilledema is almost invariably present. Prompt treatment is necessary to prevent visual loss.

Headache Associated with Other Head or Neck Structures

Refractive errors and eye muscle imbalance are common but rarely cause frank headaches. Instead, they may cause dull pain localized to the periorbital or frontal area and clearly related to prolonged eye strain. Correction of the visual deficit will lead to prompt resolution of the headache. Headache from ear disease is usually associated with acute otitis externa, acute otitis media, or serous otitis media. The associated ear pain and the physical examination should make the diagnosis clear. Dental disease can also cause headache in association with severe local pain. However, in the absence of local pain, temporomandibular joint dysfunction is rarely a cause of headaches. Sinus disease can cause a chronic headache, with pain and tenderness to percussion over the forehead and maxillary regions. There is usually a history of chronic sinus disease or recurrent upper respiratory tract infection. Upon close inspection, most patients diagnosed with sinus headaches usually meet the criteria for migraine or tension-type headaches.

DIAGNOSIS

In most adolescents with headaches the diagnosis rests almost exclusively on the history. A detailed history should be obtained from both patient and parent, including information regarding the character of the headache, its frequency and severity, and associated symptoms. A change in the pattern of the headaches requires reevaluation. A detailed investigation of the triggering events and the events surrounding the first attack may provide a clue not only to the diagnosis but also to treatment. An aura may point to the diagnosis of migraine or temporal lobe seizures. Associated deficits between headaches, such as weakness, ataxia, personality change, and visual disturbances, should make one suspicious of a mass lesion. The type and number of medications used in the past is an indication of the perceived magnitude of the problem. Prolonged use of multiple medications should alert the physician to the potential of drug dependence or abuse. A therapeutic response to a previously used agent may be of diagnostic as well as therapeutic significance. At the end of the interview the physician should have a good idea as to the type of headache present.

Although usually normal in children and adults with headache, a complete general and neurologic examination is essential to rule out organic disease. In the general examination, blood pressure should be determined. Disturbances in growth parameters may indicate chronic disease or the presence of a pituitary tumor. Particular attention should be given to the structure of the head and neck.

In the neurologic examination, a thorough funduscopic examination, visual acuity, visual fields, and assessment of extraocular movements is essential. Abnormalities of other cranial nerve or cerebellar functions may indicate a posterior fossa mass. Gait disturbances and asymmetric motor findings also point to possible structural abnormalities. When a properly performed general and neurologic examination fails to reveal any significant abnormalities and the history is reassuring, the physician can

usually rule out an intracranial structural lesion and make a clinical diagnosis without laboratory testing.

In most adolescents with chronic headache, no laboratory studies are needed. When intracranial pathology is suspected, neurodiagnostic procedures are indicated. Both magnetic resonance imaging (MRI) and computed tomographic (CT) scanning of the head offer relatively safe, sensitive imaging for detecting a variety of structural lesions of the central nervous system, including brain tumors, hematomas, hydrocephalus, and hemorrhages. In the select group of adolescents in whom a mass lesion is suspected or a neurologic deficit is present even transiently, one of these imaging studies is mandatory. However, they are overutilized in the evaluation of patients with headache and are not indicated in the patient with no other symptom or sign of intracranial pathology. Imaging studies are often indicated in adolescents with complex migraine and in children in whom the headaches are consistently lateralized exclusively to one side. In general, MRI has become the imaging study of choice owing to its superior abilities to detect arteriovenous malformations and low-grade tumors and because it avoids the risks of intravenous contrast injection. Skull radiographs have been replaced by MRI and CT scans and no longer have a role in the evaluation of chronic headaches.

The electroencephalogram (EEG) is of minimal usefulness in the evaluation of headaches because of problems with both sensitivity and specificity. The EEG picture may be abnormal in many otherwise normal children with headache, particularly migraine. It may also be completely normal in adolescents with well-documented epilepsy. Even if the EEG is abnormal, the physician should always treat the patient and not the EEG. The EEG remains an important diagnostic test in children when the differential diagnosis includes both migraine and seizures.

TREATMENT

In treating recurrent headaches in adolescents, the emphasis should be placed on reassurance, removal of precipitating factors, and simple analgesics.

Nonpharmacologic Therapy

A large number of external and constitutional factors play a role in triggering and exacerbating both migraine and tension headaches in adolescents. Although these factors often cannot be completely eliminated, their identification and reduction will reduce the frequency and severity of the symptoms. Foremost among precipitating factors are the emotional stress of school, peer relations, and family tensions. In adolescents the stresses of maturation, puberty, and the struggle toward independence are additional factors. The irregular life style of many adolescents also contributes to their headaches, particularly in those with migraine. Fasting or missing meals, sleeping late, or lack of sleep have all been implicated in triggering headache attacks. Contrary to popular belief, dietary factors have not been conclusively implicated in studies of large numbers of people with migraines. However, in selected patients, when there is a clear history of headaches after the ingestion of specific foods, dietary manipulation may be beneficial. In adolescent girls, both migraine and tension headaches are often associated with menstruation, and oral contraceptives may exacerbate their headaches.

Biofeedback and relaxation techniques are relatively new nonpharmacologic tools that are achieving an increasingly accepted role in the management of chronic headaches. They are particularly effective in tension-type headaches but are also proving effective for migraine.[18,19] The safety of these techniques, and their avoidance of the potential pitfalls of drug dependency and abuse, make them very attractive for use in adolescents with chronic headaches of all causes. Biofeedback and relaxation techniques work best when provided in the context of a comprehensive stress management approach.

Pharmacologic Therapy

Pharmacologic therapies for headache are divided into three classes: abortive, symptomatic, and prophylactic agents. Abortive medications are taken at the onset of an attack to eliminate or shorten the duration of pain. Symptomatic medications are prescribed to treat the various accompanying symptoms, such as nausea, vomiting, or pain. These agents are also useful in treating an attack that has already begun (such as during sleep) in which abortive agents would be of no help. Prophylactic agents are used to prevent future attacks and are prescribed for patients who suffer three or more attacks monthly.

In many adolescents with chronic headaches, both migrainous and tension-type, therapy with a mild analgesic (e.g., acetaminophen or a nonsteroidal antiinflammatory agent) combined with rest in a quiet room will offer adequate relief. Drugs such as Fiorinal and its various congeners, which combine an analgesic with a short-acting barbiturate, should be used with restraint. They are effective in treating tension-type headaches, but not as useful for migraine. If used frequently, they may be habit forming and may induce rebound headaches. They are appropriate for the responsible adolescent with an occasional severe headache that is not frequent enough to warrant prophylactic therapy. They should also be used in conjunction with prophylactic agents, should headaches occur.

NONSTEROIDAL ANTIINFLAMMATORY AGENTS (NSAIDs). These agents are widely used to treat adult migraines, as they are potent analgesics. Double-blind studies in adults have found NSAIDs to be superior to placebo in the treatment of migraine. These agents have not been adequately evaluated in young children and adolescents.

In adolescents and adults, there is a wide variety of drugs to choose from; no one agent has proved superior, and treatment with this group may involve trial and error. If one drug is unsuccessful, switching to another may prove useful. Naproxen (750 mg at onset and 250 mg every hour if needed for a maximum of 1500 mg/day) has been shown to be beneficial. Other agents include naproxen sodium, ibuprofen, and ketoprofen. In an emergency department setting, ketorolac may be used intramuscularly: 60 mg IM at onset, 30 to 60 mg every 4 hours (maximal daily dose, 180 mg).

Isometheptene mucate (Midrin) is a useful abortive agent in adults as well as older children and adolescents. In children over age 8, the adult dosage is given: two capsules at headache onset and then one every hour as needed. The maximal daily dose is five capsules.

ERGOTAMINE COMPOUNDS. In adults with migraine, ergot compounds, usually given in combination with caffeine, were the mainstay of therapy in the past.[9] Because the medicine must be taken at the onset of symptoms, the patient must carry it at all times, including school and play, and be responsible for taking it. The usual dose is 1 to 2 mg orally at the onset of the aura and an additional 1 mg 30 to 60 minutes afterward if necessary, for a maximum of 12 mg/week. Ergotamine compounds are contraindicated in patients with complicated migraine, as they may theoretically prolong the ischemic phase. Ergotamine preparations should not be used in young children.

Intravenous dihydroergotamine (DHE) has been used to treat headaches in adults and adolescents. It has been successful for migraine attacks in patients as young as age 6 years.[20]

SUMATRIPTAN. The newest agent for migraine is sumatriptan (Imitrex), which is available as a subcutaneous injection or in tablet form. This drug is unique in that it treats the entire migraine complex (headache, nausea, vomiting, photophobia). Sumatriptan may be used in adults and adolescents. It is dosed subcutaneously as a 6-mg injection at headache onset, and may be repeated in 1 hour if needed (maximal daily dose, two injections). For patients with aura, the dose must be given after aura resolution to prevent the headache. Orally, sumatriptan is given as a 25- or 50-mg tablet at onset and repeated every 2 hours as needed (maximal daily dose, 300 mg).

Two randomized, double-blind, placebo-controlled studies of 50 mg and 100 mg oral sumatriptan in adolescents aged 11 to 18 with migraines have been conducted.[21] The drug was well tolerated, and adverse effects were similar to those in adults. Subcutaneous sumatriptan was evaluated in an open study of 50 consecutive children aged 6 to 18 years in a dose of 0.06 mg/kg.[22] The study reported 80% efficacy at 2 hours. Sumatriptan is contraindicated in patients with cardiac conditions and uncontrolled hypertension. Since it is a potent vasoconstrictor, it should not be used in patients with basilar or hemiplegic migraine or migraine with prolonged aura. Neither sumatriptan nor DHE is approved for the treatment of migraine in patients under 16 years of age.

Migraine Prophylaxis

In most adolescents with migraine, prophylactic therapy is neither necessary nor desirable. Given the choice of taking simple analgesics when the attack occurs or taking daily medications, all of which have potential side effects, most adolescents will either reject prophylactic therapy or become noncompliant after a short time. When prophylaxis is justified, several effective agents are available.

BETA BLOCKERS. Propranolol is an excellent agent for migraine prophylaxis and has been studied in both children and adults.[23,24] It is well tolerated by most adolescents. The most common side effects include nausea and easy fatigability on exertion. Since it is a beta blocker, it is contraindicated in patients with bronchial asthma, sinus bradycardia, and congestive heart failure. It is relatively contraindicated in patients with major affective disorders, because it can exacerbate them. Propranolol's effectiveness for the various types of migraine in all age groups, and the low incidence of side effects in children, make it a good choice for migraine prophylaxis. However, propranolol is only partially effective in tension-type headaches and rarely effective in cluster headaches. The starting dose in adolescents is 40 to 80 mg orally daily; this may need to be increased. Nadolol is also well tolerated and tends to produce fewer behavioral side effects.

TRICYCLIC ANTIDEPRESSANTS. Nortriptyline and amitriptyline are effective and well-tolerated agents in the prophylactic treatment of adult migraines, and chronic tension-type headaches. The headache prophylaxis effect is independent of the antidepressant activity.[25] We consider these agents the drugs of choice for adolescents with a combination of migraine and tension-type headaches, severe and frequent tension-type headaches, and posttraumatic headaches. The dosages of nortriptyline or amitriptyline for headaches are relatively small. They are well tolerated and relatively free of the disabling side effects associated with higher doses. In adolescents, a starting dose of 25 mg at bedtime (qhs) is often effective and can be increased if needed to 50 to 75 mg qhs.

Therapy must be instituted gradually, and a therapeutic effect may require several weeks. Other tricyclic antidepressants such as imipramine and doxepin may also be useful for these disorders.

CALCIUM CHANNEL BLOCKERS. Calcium channel blockers such as verapamil are effective in the prophylaxis of migraine headaches. They can be used in asthmatic children when beta blockers, such as propranolol, are contraindicated. We have found them to be poorly tolerated in young children, with a high incidence of gastrointestinal side effects, but relatively well tolerated in older adolescents, in whom they are often a first-line drug. These agents are the drug of choice in the treatment of basilar migraine, hemiplegic migraine, and migraine with prolonged auras.

Other Prophylactic Agents

Cyproheptadine (Periactin) is frequently prescribed as prophylactic therapy for childhood migraine although only one controlled trial has reported it to be efficacious.[23] The usual dose is 2 to 4 mg twice or three times daily. Side effects, including drowsiness, increased appetite, and weight gain, often limit the drugs' usefulness in treating adolescents.

Methysergide (Sansert) is an effective preventive agent in adult migraine and is used when other first-line agents fail. It has many side effects, including hallucinations, muscle cramping, and ischemic and gastrointestinal symptoms. Methysergide should be discontinued after every 6-month period for a 1-month "drug holiday" to prevent retroperitoneal fibrosis. The adult dose is 2 mg three or four times daily. This drug should not be used in children. Its use in adolescents should be limited to those with refractory headaches and given under the supervision of a neurologist.

PHENYTOIN. The anticonvulsant phenytoin is occasionally prescribed for children and adolescents with migraines, although studies supporting its efficacy are lacking.[25] Phenytoin may be given as 50 mg three times daily or 50 mg in the morning and 100 mg at bedtime for children up to age 12 years.[26] Adolescents usually require 200 to 300 mg. daily. A number of studies have demonstrated the usefulness of divalproex sodium as a migraine prophylactic agent for adults,[27,28] 500 to 3000 mg/day in divided doses. Owing to its potential toxicity, divalproex sodium should be reserved for patients with refractory headaches who have failed to respond to at least two first-line drugs. For more information on anticonvulsants and seizures, see Chapter 61, "Seizures."

Long-Term Management

Adolescents who are placed on prophylactic medication should generally also be treated with biofeedback and stress management techniques. Medications may be needed initially, but nonpharmacologic techniques alone may be sufficient at a later time or at least may reduce the need for chronic medications. Adolescents on long-term prophylactic treatment of migraine should make periodic attempts at medication withdrawal, as there is a high rate of spontaneous remission. A convenient time is after the end of the school year. Even if complete remission has not occurred, the symptoms may have improved sufficiently to warrant discontinuation of daily medication.

Since adolescents with chronic headaches may have them for many years, the potential for drug dependence in later life is high. One of the major problems faced in the treatment of adults with chronic headaches is trying to wean them from the veritable pharmacy of potent drugs that they are often taking. The physician caring for adolescents with headache will have a major influence on how they cope with headache and stress when they become adults. Emphasis on nonpharmacologic techniques and on prophylaxis of headaches rather than seeking acute pharmacologic relief for each symptom will help prevent some of the excesses commonly found in the treatment of chronic headaches.

References

1. Bille B: Migraine in school children, *Acta Paediatr Scand* 51(suppl 136):1-151, 1962.
2. Shinnar S, D'Souza BJ: The diagnosis and management of headaches in childhood, *Pediatr Clin North Am* 29:79-94, 1982.
3. Cooper PJ, Bowden HN, Camfield PR, Camfield CS: Anxiety and life events in childhood migraine, *Pediatrics* 79:999-1004, 1987.
4. Shinnar S: Headaches in children. In Kaufman DM, Solomon G, Pfeffer M, editors: *Pediatric neurology for psychiatrists,* Baltimore, 1991, William & Wilkins; pp 158-168.
5. Headache Classification Committee of the International Headache Society: Classification and diagnostic criteria for headache disorders, cranial neuralgias and facial pain, *Cephalalgia* 8(suppl 7): 1-96, 1988.
6. Congdon PJ, Forsythe WI: Migraine in childhood: a study of 300 children, *Dev Med Child Neurol* 21:209-216, 1979.
7. Prensky AL, Sommer D: Diagnosis and treatment of migraine in children, *Neurology* 29:506-510, 1979.
8. Barlow CF: *Headaches and migraine in childhood,* Clinics in Developmental Medicine No. 91, London, 1984, Spastics International Medical Publications.
9. Dalessio DJ, Silberstein SD: *Wolff's headache and other head pain,* ed 6, New York, 1993, Oxford University Press.
10. Maytal J, Lipton RB, Solomon S, Shinnar S: Childhood onset cluster headaches, *Headache* 32:275-279, 1992.
11. Levin HS, Eisenberg HM, Benton AL, editors: *Mild head injury,* New York, 1989, Oxford University Press.
12. Ling W, Oftedal G, Weinberg W: Depressive illness in childhood presenting as severe headache, *Am J Dis Child* 120:122-124, 1970.
13. Swaiman KF, Frank Y: Seizure headaches in children, *Dev Med Child Neurol* 20:580-585, 1978.
14. Andermann F, Lugaresi E, editors: *Migraine and epilepsy,* Boston, 1987, Butterworths.
15. Forsyth PA, Posner JB: Headaches in patients with brain tumors: a study of 111 patients, *Neurology* 43:1678-1683, 1993.
16. Honig PJ, Charney EB: Children with brain tumor headaches: distinguishing features, *Am J Dis Child* 136:121-124, 1982.
17. Weisberg LA, Chutorian AM: Pseudotumor cerebri of childhood, *Am J Dis Child* 131:1243-1248, 1977.
18. Adler CS, Adler SM: Biofeedback psychotherapy for the treatment of headaches: a 5-year follow-up, *Headache* 16:189-191, 1976.
19. Diamond S: Biofeedback and headache, *Headache* 19:180-184, 1979.
20. Silberstein SD: Twenty questions about headache in children and adolescents, *Neurology* 41:786-793, 1991.
21. Korsgaard AG: The tolerability, safety and efficacy of oral sumatriptan 50 mg and 100 mg for the acute treatment of migraine in adolescents, *Cephalalgia* 15(suppl 16):99, 1995.
22. Linder SL: Subcutaneous sumatriptan in the clinical setting: the first fifty consecutive patients with acute migraine in a paediatric neurology office practice, *Cephalalgia* 15(suppl 16):98, 1995.
23. Bille B, Ludvigsson J, Sanner G: Prophylaxis of migraine in children, *Headache* 17:61-63, 1977.
24. Ludvigsson J: Propranolol used in prophylaxis of migraine in children, *Acta Neurol Scand* 50:109-115, 1974.
25. Couch JR, Hassanein RS: Amitriptyline in migraine prophylaxis, *Arch Neurol* 36:695-699, 1979.
26. Millichap JC: Recurrent headaches in 100 children: electroencephalographic abnormalities and response to phenytoin (Dilantin), *Childs Brain* 4:95-105, 1978.
27. Hering R, Kuritzky A: Sodium valproate in the prophylactic treatment of migraine: a double-blind study vs. placebo, *Cephalalgia* 12:81-84, 1992.
28. Silberstein SD, Saper J, Mathew NT, et al: The safety and efficacy of divalproex sodium in the prophylaxis of migraine headache: a multicenter, double-blind, placebo-controlled trial, *Headache* 33: 264-265, 1993.
29. Lapkin ML, Golden GS: Basilar artery migraine: a review of 30 cases, *Am J Dis Child* 132:278-281, 1978.
30. Brown JK: Migraine and migraine equivalents in children, *Dev Med Child Neurol* 19:683-692, 1977.
31. Illingworth RS: *Common symptoms of disease in children,* ed 5, Oxford, 1975, Blackwell Scientific Publications; p 98.
32. Prensky AL: Migraine and migrainous variants in pediatric patients, *Pediatr Clin North Am* 23:461-471, 1979.
33. Vahlquist BO: Migraine in children, *Int Arch Allergy* 7:348-355, 1955.

CHAPTER 61

Seizures

•

Shlomo Shinnar

Epilepsy, one of the most common chronic neurologic disorders affecting adolescents, is defined as "recurrent seizures without immediate provocation."[1] Most cases of epilepsy begin in childhood and adolescence. The prevalence of epilepsy in the 10- to 19-year-old group has been conservatively estimated at 4.1 per 1000 population.[1-3] If one uses less strict criteria and includes single convulsions, prevalence rates as high as 20 to 30 per 1000 population have been reported.[2] Recent advances in the development of new antiepileptic drugs (AEDs) and improved understanding of their proper use have had a major impact on our ability to treat adolescents with epilepsy. Rational use of these drugs can result in complete control of seizures in many cases. Surgery is an increasingly available option for patients with intractable partial seizures. Recognition of psychosocial issues is also important, as many adolescents are hampered more by their fears than by their seizures. Proper management of the adolescent with epilepsy will help ensure a transition to life as an independent adult.[1]

CLASSIFICATION OF SEIZURES

A new internationally accepted classification of seizures has been adopted, replacing the often confusing older classification.[4] A simplified summary of the classification is shown in Table 61-1. The basic distinction in the new classification is between seizures with focal onset, which are referred to as partial seizures whether or not they generalize, and seizures that are generalized from the onset. The old "psychomotor" seizure is now referred to as a complex partial seizure, which is defined as a partial seizure with impaired consciousness. The new term recognizes that many complex partial seizures do not have motor phenomena. The new classification has a rational basis in terms of both common electrophysi-

ologic features of the various seizure types and the spectrum of drugs that are effective in their treatment.

EPILEPTIC SYNDROMES

The above is a classification of seizures, not of the epilepsies. The physician classifies a seizure on the basis of its clinical characteristics. An epileptic syndrome is defined on the basis of seizure types, characteristics of the electroencephalogram (EEG), age of onset, and other features. A full classification of epileptic syndromes is still being developed[3-6] and is outside the scope of this chapter. Selected epileptic syndromes with special relevance to adolescents are discussed below. Both primary generalized and partial epilepsies can have their onset in adolescence, but most adolescence-onset seizures are of partial origin. This is different from childhood-onset seizures, most of which are generalized. Almost three quarters of adolescents and adults with onset of seizures after age 15 years have a partial epilepsy.[1-3] This explains why neuroimaging studies, which are not usually necessary in children with a generalized tonic-clonic seizure, are routinely performed in adolescents with new onset of seizures.

Partial Epilepsies

Most adolescence-onset epilepsies are partial even if the patients present with what appears to be a generalized tonic-clonic seizure and a normal EEG picture. The temporal lobe is the most common site of onset for partial seizures, with the frontal lobe the next most common. Adolescence-onset partial seizures have the same clinical characteristics and prognosis as adult-onset epilepsy and represent part of the same spectrum.

One specific epileptic syndrome that should be mentioned is benign rolandic epilepsy, which is the best-described benign focal epilepsy of childhood.[3,5,6] It is thought to be an autosomal dominant disorder with

Supported in part by grant 1R01 NS26151 from the National Institute of Neurologic Disorders and Stroke.

501

TABLE 61-1
Classification of Seizures in Adolescents

Generalized	Partial
Absence	Simple partial
Atypical absence	Complex partial
Myoclonic	Partial with secondary generalization
Tonic	
Tonic-clonic	
Atonic	

Adapted from Commission on Classification and Terminology of the International League Against Epilepsy: Proposal for revised clinical and electroencephalographic classification of epileptic seizures, *Epilepsia* 22:489-501, 1981.

imperfect penetrance. Onset is between 4 and 10 years of age. Seizures tend to occur at night and can be generalized tonic-clonic or partial. When partial, they often involve the mouth and face. The EEG shows characteristic centrotemporal stereotyped spikes, with a horizontal dipole, that are often bilateral and increase with drowsiness and sleep. The seizures remit in early adolescence and the EEG abnormality generally disappears a few years later. Physicians caring for adolescents with this disorder must be aware that this epilepsy almost always remits in adolescence and that patients should be taken off medications at the appropriate time so they may enter adult life without medications. The other benign focal epilepsies of childhood are less well understood and have far more variable prognoses.[3,5,6]

Primary Generalized Epilepsies

Primary generalized epilepsies represent a spectrum of disorders with a presumed genetic basis. They all share the EEG marker of generalized spike and wave.[3,5,6] The most common are childhood absence, juvenile absence, and juvenile myoclonic epilepsy (JME). Childhood absence has a typical age of onset of 3 to 12 years, with a peak at 6 to 7 years of age. Affected children have multiple brief episodes of classic absences, usually easily provoked by hyperventilation. Most cases go into remission during adolescence with disappearance of both the seizures and the EEG trait.

Adolescents with a new onset of absence seizures more commonly have juvenile absence epilepsy, which has a typical age of onset of 8 to 17 years.[3,5,6] While the age of onset and clinical characteristics overlap with childhood absence, these children have somewhat fewer seizures. More importantly, however, they have a far worse prognosis in terms of eventually outgrowing the need for medications. As patients with juvenile absence get older, the absence seizures often disappear even if the EEG trait and the generalized tonic clonic seizures persist.

Juvenile myoclonic epilepsy is characterized by myoclonic jerks, which most often occur upon awakening.[3,5-7] Most patients have at least occasional generalized tonic-clonic seizures, which are what typically brings them to medical attention. The history of "morning jerks" must be specifically elicited, otherwise it is likely to be overlooked. Approximately 30% of patients with JME have absence seizures. The age of onset is in the second and third decades of life. Although most of these patients are well controlled on antiepileptic drugs, spontaneous remission of the underlying epileptic trait is rare.[6] The need for continued medications, as well as the underlying EEG abnormality, usually persists at least into the fifth decade of life. Relatives of patients with JME have an increased incidence of seizures, but the affected relatives do not necessarily have JME. Evidence suggests that the gene for JME may be located on chromosome 6.[7]

EVALUATION OF THE ADOLESCENT WITH NEW ONSET SEIZURES

All adolescents who present with an initial seizure require a comprehensive medical and neurologic evaluation. The evaluation should include a careful history, including potential precipitating factors and a description of the ictal event and postictal state, looking especially for any focal components. One must also ascertain that this is truly the first seizure, not merely the first convulsive event. Upon careful questioning, many adolescents who present with a first convulsion in fact have a history of nonconvulsive ictal events such as absence, myoclonic, or complex partial seizures. Indeed, in a prospective study of first seizures, approximately one third of children and adolescents who were referred with the diagnosis of a first seizure were found, upon careful history taking, to have had previous seizures.[8]

Laboratory studies in the emergency department should be performed with restraint.[3] Routine electrolyte and hematologic studies are rarely helpful in the afebrile patient. A lumbar puncture should be reserved for cases in which a central nervous system infection, such as encephalitis or meningitis, is suspected. In the afebrile patient with normal mental status and no focal deficits, a lumbar puncture is rarely indicated. In contrast, a toxicology screen is mandatory for all adolescents with a first seizure. Patients taking one of several popular drugs of abuse, most notably cocaine, can present with seizures after even occasional use. The author has seen a number of teenagers with recurrent seizures who experienced seizures each time they abused cocaine and never had any other seizures.

An EEG should be performed in all adolescents who present with new-onset seizures. The EEG is not only an important predictor of seizure recurrence but may also identify patients with those specific epileptic syndromes in which the long-term prognosis is known. If possible, an EEG in both the awake and sleep states should be performed. As most adolescence-onset seizures are of partial origin, a neuroimaging study is usually indicated, even in patients without obvious focal features. Magnetic resonance imaging (MRI) is the study of choice owing to its superior abilities to detect low-grade gliomas, vascular malformations, mesial temporal sclerosis, and heterotopias.[3] With current state-of-the-art neuroimaging, an increasing number of lesions are being detected. With the exception of patients known to have a primary generalized epilepsy, MRI should be considered for any adolescent who has long-standing epilepsy that is not in remission. In most cases, both the EEG and MRI can be performed electively.

PRINCIPLES OF ANTIEPILEPTIC DRUG THERAPY

The basic principle of AED therapy is to select the drug most likely to be effective for the individual patient's seizure type. The drug is then administered in a sufficient quantity to control seizures fully without undue toxicity. If the initial dose is inadequate, the drug is gradually increased until complete control of seizures is achieved or the patient experiences clinical toxicity. When several drugs with a similar spectrum of activity are available, one should select the drug with the least objectionable toxic effects for the given patient. When a patient has two or more seizure types, one should select, whenever possible, a single drug that will be effective against all the seizure types, rather than a different drug for each seizure type. Given the range of AEDs now available, initial therapy with a single agent is almost always possible.

Most adolescents with cryptogenic epilepsy can be controlled fully with a single drug. This is particularly true of primary generalized seizures. If the first drug is ineffective, a second drug is added and the dosage is gradually increased. If the second drug is effective, the physician should consider whether the original AED is still necessary. In principle, one should always try to use monotherapy because of its decreased toxicity, but some adolescents require treatment with more than one agent. If complete seizure control without toxicity is not achieved with two drugs, the patient should be referred to a neurologist specializing in epilepsy. Complete seizure control is attainable in only 70% to 80% of adolescents with epilepsy. However, since there is a major difference in quality of life between having complete control without toxicity and having an occasional seizure or toxic event, an attempt at complete control should be made in every adolescent. Also, adolescents with refractory epilepsy may be candidates for surgery, as discussed below.

Specific Antiepileptic Drugs

CARBAMAZEPINE. Carbamazepine was first introduced for the treatment of focal seizures, where, along with phenytoin, it is now considered by many to be the drug of choice. It is effective against both generalized tonic-clonic seizures and focal seizures. In most studies, its spectrum of activity is essentially identical to that of phenytoin. The Collaborative Study of New-Onset Seizures found carbamazepine and phenytoin to be equally effective. Both drugs were superior to phenobarbital and primidone.[9]

Initial rare reports of aplastic anemia associated with use of carbamazepine, and the possible need for frequent blood monitoring, created some concern about this drug. However, as increased experience with its use accumulates, many epileptologists are questioning the need for frequent hematologic monitoring, which now appears to have a purely medicolegal basis.[10] In using carbamazepine, one must start with a low dose and gradually titrate to a full maintenance dose. This is due to the unusual pharmacokinetic properties of the drug, which specifically autoinduces its own metabolism.

The relative lack of cosmetic and cognitive side effects, and its proven efficiency and safety, make carbamazepine a first-line drug for treating most adolescents, particularly girls, with generalized tonic-clonic or focal seizures. However, there are reports of spina bifida occurring in the offspring of women treated with carbamazepine.[11-13]

PHENYTOIN. Phenytoin is an effective AED for the treatment of both generalized tonic-clonic and focal seizures. Its advantages are that it is inexpensive and can often be given on a once-a-day schedule, which may improve compliance. It is also the only anticonvulsant for which a loading dose can be given with only minor side effects, making it most effective in cases in which a therapeutic level must be reached quickly. For this reason, phenytoin is the drug of choice in the emergency room setting and in situations in which short courses of therapy are indicated. In other settings, it should be considered a first-line drug along with carbamazepine. The major drawbacks of phenytoin are its chronic toxicities; these include gingival hyperplasia, coarsening of the facial features, and hirsutism, each of which can occur even with therapeutic doses. Although less severe and less frequent in adolescents than in younger children, these can still be a significant problem, particularly in young girls.

VALPROIC ACID. Valproic acid is very effective in the treatment of generalized seizures of all types, including general tonic-clonic, absence, myoclonic, and atonic seizures. It is also effective in the treatment of complex partial seizures. Its structure and clinical spectrum of activity are quite different from the AEDs discussed previously. Valproate is the drug of choice to treat (1) myoclonic and atonic seizures and photoconvulsive epilepsy, (2) patients with both absence and generalized tonic-clonic seizures, and (3) refractory absence seizures.[3,6] Some authors consider valproic acid the drug of choice for all primary generalized epilepsies.[6]

The major advantages of valproic acid are its broad spectrum of activity against all types of generalized seizures and its relative lack of cognitive side effects.[14] The disadvantages are its potential toxicities, the most common of which is nausea. Less common side effects include weight gain, alopecia (usually transient), tremor, and hyperammonemia. The last-named, which is often asymptomatic, may occur in the presence of otherwise normal liver function test results. The significance of this finding in the asymptomatic patient is unclear.

Of more concern is the occurrence of an idiosyncratic, fatal, hepatotoxicity, which has been reported in over 100 patients on valproic acid therapy to date.[15-17] At particular risk are children under 2 years of age who have neurologic handicaps and are on multiple drugs. However, this has also been reported in adolescents. Although the complication is rare in this age group (particularly in those on monotherapy), it is a major reason why, despite its efficacy, the American Academy of Pediatrics and many neurologists do not consider valproic acid the first-line drug for classic absence seizures.[17] Also of concern are reports of a high incidence of fetal malformations, including spina bifida, in infants born to women receiving valproic acid.[12,13,17,18]

PHENOBARBITAL AND PRIMIDONE. Phenobarbital is the oldest AED still in common use; it is effective against both generalized tonic clonic and partial seizures. Primidone, also a barbiturate, is metabolized to phenobarbital, but in addition has anticonvulsant properties of its own; it is primarily used to treat refractory partial seizures. The major drawbacks to these drugs are their cognitive and behavioral side effects and their sedative properties. In adolescents on barbiturates, one can demonstrate impaired cognitive function on formal neuropsychologic function, even in those who are "asymptomatic" with no obvious clinical complaints.[19,20] An increased incidence of depression and suicidal ideation has been reported in adolescents taking phenobarbital, particularly in those with a family history of major affective disorders.[21] In the prospective collaborative study of new-onset focal and generalized tonic-clonic seizures, both phenobarbital and primidone were less effective and less well tolerated than phenytoin or carbamazepine.[9] Additionally, since barbiturates are sedative hypnotics, they potentiate the sedative hypnotic effects of alcohol and other drugs. The physician must also remember that the half-life of phenobarbital in adolescents and adults is much longer than in children, which reduces the dosing requirements. In general, while phenobarbital remains a useful drug in selected cases, it is not usually the initial drug of choice in the management of adolescents with epilepsy.

ETHOSUXIMIDE. Ethosuximide remains the drug of choice for typical absence seizures.[3,17] However, classic petit mal epilepsy rarely has its onset in adolescence, and therefore, ethosuximide is rarely used in adolescents with new-onset seizures. However, it remains a valuable and relatively safe drug for selected patients.

CLONAZEPAM. Clonazepam is a benzodiazepine AED. It has a similar clinical spectrum to valproic acid, although it is usually not as effective. Clonazepam is rarely used as a first-line drug for any seizure type because of its sedative side effects. These side effects are also noted with the other recently introduced AEDs in the benzodiazepine class, such as lorazepam and nitrazepam.

New Antiepileptic Drugs

A number of new AEDs have been approved in the United States and Europe.[22] Although pediatric experience is limited, there is sufficient experience with adolescents to justify their use in selected patients. As with all new drugs that are first tried on intractable patients, the precise role of these drugs will be defined only after much more extensive experience in their use and when their efficacy and toxicity are understood more fully.

Among the new antiepileptic drugs, gabapentin, lamotrigine, and vigabatrin appear to be most promising for pediatric epilepsy. Felbamate, while an effective drug, is being used only for intractable cases owing to concerns about its hepatic and hematopoietic toxicity.

Gabapentin has been shown to be effective in adults with partial seizures.[22] The usual dose in adults is 900 to 1800 mg, although recent data suggest that higher doses are often needed. It is ineffective against absence seizures and may make them worse. Its main advantages are that it is not appreciably metabolized in humans and is excreted unchanged by the kidney. It does alter the levels of other AEDs or co-medications and does not induce the microsomal liver system. It should therefore not affect the metabolism and efficacy of oral contraceptives.

Lamotrigine has proved effective as add-on therapy in adults with both partial seizures and the Lennox-Gastaut syndrome. The most frequent side effects have been dizziness, diplopia, headache, somnolence, ataxia, asthenia, and rash. It should be used with caution when in combination with valproate.[22] The usual dose in adults is 300 to 500 mg in those not taking valproate, and 100 to 150 mg in those on valproate.

Vigabatrin has been approved and marketed in several European countries but is still investigational in the United States. It is effective for partial seizures of all types. Most common side effects include somnolence and behavioral disturbances.[22]

Therapeutic Dosage Range and Drug Monitoring

The ability to measure serum drug levels has led to a greater understanding of the pharmacokinetics of AEDs and has permitted correlations between serum levels and clinical efficacy and toxicity. While the availability of serum drug levels is important, it should be understood that the therapeutic range is a statistical concept based on studies of small populations of patients with epilepsy. Thus, many patients are fully controlled on a dose that produces a "subtherapeutic" level. Conversely, some adolescents may become toxic with serum levels in the therapeutic range. As a general rule, any adolescent patient on a single drug who is having no seizures and experiencing no clinical toxicity has a serum level that is therapeutic for that individual regardless of the numeric value. It should also be noted that the therapeutic range is calibrated for morning trough levels, whereas random levels obtained in the office or clinic are generally closer to peak levels. This is particularly important to consider when dealing with drugs such as valproate, which, because of their short serum half-life, have large differences between peak and trough levels.

With the above caveats, drug monitoring is a useful tool in the management of adolescents with epilepsy.[23] When initiating therapy, the concept of a therapeutic range enables one to choose a drug dosage that will usually result in full control without undue toxicity. If one achieves control of seizures with a given drug dosage, obtaining a baseline level is useful, particularly in the growing adolescent, in whom changes in metabolism and body weight over time may lead to significant changes in the serum drug level achieved by a given dose. Finally, serum drug levels are a useful, albeit imperfect, way of monitoring compliance, which is a major problem in adolescents. Compliance is a particularly difficult problem with AEDs, as they must be taken daily for years, often have unwanted side effects (hirsutism, sedation), and have a social stigma associated with their use. In addition, there are medicolegal issues that require the monitoring of compliance in the adolescent with epilepsy who wishes to drive.

The therapeutic range and average dose requirements for commonly used AEDs are shown in Table 61-2. The ranges listed are for adolescents and are the same as for adults. Unfortunately, for most drugs, there is no well-established dosage range for adolescents. Adolescence is a time of profound metabolic changes. The dosage requirements change throughout adolescence because of changes in body weight and composition as well as pharmacokinetic changes in the drug's half-life.

TABLE 61-2
Dosages of Commonly Used Antiepileptic Drugs in Adolescents

Drug	Dosage Range* (mg/day)	Therapeutic Range† (µg/ml)
Carbamazepine	600-1800	4-12
Ethosuximide	750-1500	40-100
Phenobarbital	90-180	10-30
Phenytoin	200-500	10-20
Primidone	500-1500	5-12
Phenobarbital (derived)	—	15-40
Valproic acid	1000-4000	40-150

*These dosage ranges are guidelines only for use in monotherapy. Individual patients may require more or less medication, depending on the severity of their seizure disorder, the individual metabolic rate and clearance of the drug, and the presence of clinical toxicity.
†Morning trough levels.

Drug Interactions

Several excellent monographs reviewing the drug interactions of AEDs are available.[24] A few general principles are worth noting. The most common drug interactions are due to competition for protein binding and induction of the hepatic microsomal enzyme system. The AEDs are all protein bound, some heavily so. The presence of another protein-bound drug will alter the protein-bound fraction of both drugs. This in turn affects the clearance, as well as the toxicity, both of which depend on the free fraction of the drugs. Antiepileptic drugs, particularly phenobarbital but also phenytoin and carbamazepine, induce the hepatic microsomal enzyme system. This induction causes increased biotransformation of all liver-metabolized drugs, including other AEDs, theophylline, steroids, and oral contraceptives. This last is of particular importance to the physician treating adolescents, as there have been several reports of failure of oral contraception in women also taking AEDs.[24-26] The interaction with theophylline is also important, because it is a drug with a very narrow therapeutic window that can be altered by initiating or stopping AED therapy.

EPILEPSY SURGERY

A major advance in the treatment of intractable epilepsy has been the increased availability of surgery for epilepsy.[3,27] Recent advances in our ability to localize the epileptic focus have made this procedure, which was sparingly used for more than 40 years, an increasingly utilized option in comprehensive epilepsy centers. There is some controversy regarding the use of epilepsy surgery in young children, as the long-term prognosis in this group is not well understood. In adolescents, however, the indications for epilepsy surgery are the same as for adults.

Candidates for epilepsy surgery must meet specific eligibility criteria, including the exclusion of nonepileptic events, failure to achieve control with optimal pharmacologic management, consistent localization of seizure onset to a single focus in a surgically accessible area that is not eloquent cortex and a high likelihood of substantial improvement in function or quality of life if seizure control is improved.

The protocol for evaluation of these surgical candidates requires recording, through videotape and EEG monitoring, of a sufficient number of seizures to localize electrographically the single source of origin. This is particularly important in patients who have more than one clinically distinguishable seizure type.

Initially, all patients receive an extensive outpatient evaluation, including an EEG, computed tomography (CT), MRI, and neuropsychological testing. These tests are designed to yield as much information as possible for the epileptologist. In patients previously followed in a community setting, an effort is made to manage their seizures with medications. Patients who are thought to be candidates for surgery after this initial screening then undergo prolonged video and EEG monitoring to record the precise location of the seizure onset site. To record a sufficient number of seizures, it is often necessary to reduce the antiepileptic medications. This then requires inpatient monitoring, as patients are at significant risk of having many or prolonged seizures. The monitoring data are then analyzed. If prolonged EEG monitoring (phase I) supports eligibility for surgery but does not adequately localize the focus, recording electrodes may be surgically placed by means of a craniotomy, either onto the surface of the brain or within it, using depth electrodes or a subdural grid (phase II). This allows more precise localization of the epileptic focus but requires an invasive procedure.

As part of the presurgical assessment, detailed neuropsychological evaluation is also required. This assists localization by defining specific areas of cognitive defect, as well as areas necessary for vital functions such as speech and memory. It also helps to assess patients' baseline level of functioning for comparison with their abilities after surgery and subsequent alterations in the pharmacologic regimen.

Patients who are deemed appropriate surgical candidates undergo focal resection. The ideal candidate is an adolescent or young adult who is otherwise neurologically normal and has normal intelligence, no motor deficits, and a single consistent EEG focus.[3,27] An abnormal MRI or CT scan with a focal abnormality in the same area is also a favorable prognostic sign, presumably because it increases the probability that the area being resected is in fact the site of origin of the seizures. The success rate in the best group is greater than 80%, success being defined as complete or almost complete seizure control with antiepileptic drugs. Excellent results are also achieved in patients with temporal lobe foci even when no mass lesions are present, particularly in the presence of mesial temporal sclerosis. Special coronal views with thin cuts are often needed to detect mesial temporal sclerosis, which can be missed on routine MRI. The field is rapidly evolving, with ever-improving neuroimaging modalities and EEG localization techniques. There are several comprehensive treatises on the subject.[3,27] At this time, surgery should be seriously considered for all adolescents with intractable partial seizures, particularly if they are otherwise neurologically normal and have a single EEG focus.

SINGLE SEIZURE

Prospective studies in recent years have shown that the risk of recurrence after a first unprovoked seizure in adolescents is 30% to 40%.[8,28-32] Risk factors for recurrence include a remote symptomatic etiology and an abnormal EEG result. However, even adolescents with positive risk factors have recurrence risks of 50% to 60%. Treatment with AEDs lowers the recurrence risk but does not alter the long-term prognosis.[31-33] For this reason, and because of the morbidity associated with drug therapy, many neurologists and pediatricians[8,28-33] now consider that therapy is usually not indicated for the adolescent with a first seizure. This is particularly true in females entering their childbearing years and in adolescents who are about to start driving. In both settings, waiting until at least a second seizure will avoid committing the youngster to long-term medications until it is certain that they are needed.

Whatever the decision, it must be made jointly by the physician and the family after careful discussion, including not only an assessment of the risks and benefits of treatment, but also a review of measures to be taken in the event of a recurrence. Even adolescents with good prognostic factors may experience a recurrence. Informed decision making will allow the adolescent and family to select the risks with which they are most comfortable. In my experience, when adolescents and families are informed of the risks of another seizure and its potential consequences, as well as the morbidity and consequences of antiepileptic drug therapy, they rarely opt to initiate or continue drug therapy after a single seizure.

PROGNOSIS OF SEIZURES

Studies based on data from tertiary care centers specializing in refractory epilepsy have shown a low rate of remission, but population-based studies show exactly the opposite.[3] The best available data on seizure remission come from longitudinal studies of the population of Rochester, Minnesota.[2,34] Within 6 years of the diagnosis of epilepsy, 42% of patients had been seizure free for 5 years either on or off medication. By 20 years, 70% had been seizure free for 5 years and 50% were seizure free off medications. The probability of attaining remission was highest in those with idiopathic epilepsy and onset of seizures before age 10. The probability of being at least 5 years seizure-free 10 years after diagnosis was 75% in those with onset of seizures before age 10, 68% in those with onset between 10 and 19 years of age, and only 63% in those with onset over 20 years of age.[34] The group with the worst outcome were those with neurologic dysfunction since birth. However, even these patients had a 46% probability of being seizure free for 5 years or more within 20 years of the onset of their epilepsy. Other studies report similar, although less detailed, results.[35,36] The favorable prognosis of a younger age of onset presumably reflects the capacity of the immature central nervous system to outgrow seizures as it matures.[37]

PUBERTY AND SEIZURES

A variety of disorders, both neurologic (epilepsy, migraine) and non-neurologic (asthma), tend to either remit or have their onset in adolescence. It would seem logical to conclude that, in addition to central nervous system development and maturation, systemic maturation may be an important variable in the onset and remission of seizures. Therefore, one would assume that neurologic factors associated with puberty most likely play a role. Nevertheless, at present, a definitive link between seizure onset and remission and puberty has not been shown.[3,34,37,38] In fact, a variety of epidemiologic studies, as well as studies on the remission of childhood seizures and on withdrawing antiepileptic drugs in children,[3,34,37-42] do not show a reproducible pattern that correlates with puberty. Studies of the long-term prognosis of seizures suggest that the probability of attaining remission is a function of the age of onset and the duration of the seizure disorder rather than showing a special role for puberty. However, studies of the relationship between puberty and seizure disorders have been less than satisfying owing to the inadequate definition of puberty. Few investigators have even used a Tanner score and none have used endocrine markers of puberty.

WITHDRAWING ANTIEPILEPTIC DRUGS

The available data suggest that adolescents who are seizure free on medication for 2 or more years have a very high likelihood of remaining in remission after medications are withdrawn.[32,36-41] The clinician must decide how long to maintain an adolescent on medications before attempting to discontinue them. This decision will be influenced by a variety of factors, including a given patient's probability of remaining seizure free after withdrawal and the potential risk of injury from a seizure recurrence, and the potential adverse effects of continued antiepileptic drug therapy.

Most adolescents who are seizure free on medications for at least 2 years will remain seizure free when medications are withdrawn. Many prospective and retrospective studies, involving over 4000 children and adolescents, have been conducted over the past 20 years and have been analyzed.[39,41,42] The overall results have been very similar.[32,39-43] Between 60% and 90% of children with epilepsy who have been seizure free for more than 2 years on medications remain seizure free when antiepileptic medications are withdrawn. Furthermore, most recurrences occur shortly after medication withdrawal, with almost half the relapses occurring within 6 months of medication withdrawal and 60% to 80% within 1 year.

Studies indicate no major differences between stopping after a 2-year seizure-free period and stopping after a 4-year period. Favorable risk factors for withdrawing medications include cryptogenic epilepsy, a normal picture before medications are discontinued, and an age of onset under 12 years.[32,39-43] Puberty has no effect on the success rate.[37-43] One should remember that the adolescent usually still lives in a relatively supervised environment. It is often far safer to attempt discontinuation of AEDs while adolescents are still living at home and before they start driving and/or become pregnant. The author and others[32,39-43] recommend attempting to discontinue AEDs in adolescents with reasonable risk factors as long as the patient and family understand the risks involved. The author is even more aggressive in trying to withdraw adolescent girls from antiepileptic drugs owing to the teratogenicity of the drugs and the need to determine whether they are necessary before pregnancy occurs.

When discontinuing AEDs, one must consider not only the half-life of the drug but also the potentially lower seizure threshold of the patient with epilepsy, even after a 2-year seizure-free interval. On the other hand, once the decision to withdraw medications has been made, there is no justification for tapering them over years. A 1994 randomized study found no difference in recurrence rates between children whose AEDs were tapered over 6 weeks and those tapered over 9 months.[43] The author generally tapers each drug over a 1- to 3-month period, depending on the dosage, the patient's serum level, and the type of medication.

EPILEPSY AND PREGNANCY

In treating a pregnant adolescent with seizures, the physician must try to maintain her in a seizure-free state while minimizing drug toxicity and the possible teratogenic effects on the fetus.[12,13] Pregnant women often require higher doses of their regular AEDs because of alterations of drug clearance (both volume of distribution and metabolism) in pregnancy. In addition, there is a much higher incidence of noncompliance, secondary to concerns about teratogenicity. Less commonly, the underlying seizure disorder is exacerbated by pregnancy. Several excellent reviews on the subject are available.[24,44]

Most of the teratogenic effects of AEDs occur in the first 6 to 8 weeks of gestation. Since adolescent pregnancies are often unplanned, this suggests that by the time the pregnancy is confirmed, these effects have generally already occurred. Therefore, it is usually too late to consider switching to other AEDs with lower teratogenicity. In general, major changes in the AED regimen during pregnancy are not recommended, because the risks of uncontrolled seizures during the changeover period that can cause damage to the fetus (owing to direct injury or metabolic factors such as maternal hypotension) outweigh the possible benefits to the mother and fetus.[12,13,23,43] In view of the high incidence of fetal malformations, including spina bifida, associated with the use of valproic acid, it has been recommended that pregnant women receiving this drug undergo prenatal diagnosis with amniocentesis and ultrasonography.[17,18] More recently, carbamazepine has also been linked with neural tube defects,[11] although the magnitude of the risk is not yet clear. Some authors have recommended supplementation with folic acid, 1 mg daily, for females of childbearing age on AEDs who are therefore at increased risk for neural tube defects in their offspring.[45] Other malformations, including nail hypoplasia, cleft lip and palate, ventriculoseptal defect, and (in severe cases) microcephaly, have been described with the use of phenytoin as well as phenobarbital and carbamazepine.[12,13,24,44]

SPORTS

In recent years, pediatricians and neurologists alike have recognized that with proper medical management, good seizure control, and proper supervision, adolescents with epilepsy may participate in most competitive sports. The American Academy of Pediatrics, in a major revision of its previous policy, has recommended that epilepsy per se should not be considered sufficient reason to exclude a child from contact sports, and that each case be evaluated on its own merits.[46] Certain activities, such as competitive underwater swimming, high diving, and rope climbing, in which the occurrence of a seizure could be unusually dangerous should be avoided. The new policy recognizes that sports and athletic activities are important

for the physical and emotional well-being of children and adolescents, and that undue limitations to "be on the safe side" do more harm than good.

DRIVING

Patients with epilepsy whose seizures are fully controlled on medications are legally allowed to drive in every state in the United States and in almost all developed countries. The precise reporting and certification requirements, as well as the required seizure-free period, vary tremendously among different jurisdictions. In the United States, specific information on the requirements in a jurisdiction can be obtained through the Epilepsy Foundation of America or through the local Epilepsy Society. Adolescents with epilepsy often view driving as an important issue. The ability to drive validates to them that they can indeed lead a relatively unrestricted life. I generally permit adolescents whose seizures are well controlled to drive as long as there is a reasonable expectation of compliance. However, accident rates in patients with epilepsy, particularly young males, are somewhat higher than in the general population.[47] It must be understood that driving is a privilege, not a constitutional right, and that, in return for the privilege, compliance with a medication regimen is expected. Since most adolescents who are seizure free for more than a year will remain so and become candidates for medication withdrawal, it is often reasonable to delay driving by a few years so that an attempt at medication withdrawal can be made first.

PSYCHOSOCIAL ADAPTATION

In treating the adolescent with epilepsy, the physician must recognize that controlling seizures with AEDs is not enough. Psychosocial problems in patients with epilepsy are frequent and often more debilitating than the seizures themselves.[3,48-50] It is not uncommon to see an adolescent with relatively mild, well-controlled epilepsy whose emotional development and growth have been severely hampered by the family's inability to deal with the fear of a seizure. The psychosocial problems noted in these patients are due to several factors, including the presence of chronic illness,[3,48-51] the patient's fears about epilepsy, and the social stigma associated with epilepsy.[3,48-51] Although only a few studies have investigated the specific psychosocial problems of adolescents,[3,50,51] these confirm the wide extent of such problems in adolescents with epilepsy. Additional studies are needed to evaluate the differences between psychosocial problems encountered in adolescents and adults, and to determine whether appropriate early interventions in adolescence may prevent some of the problems encountered in adult life.

References

1. Hauser WA, Annegers JF, Kurland LT: Incidence of epilepsy and unprovoked seizures in Rochester, Minnesota 1935 through 1984, *Epilepsia* 34:453-468, 1993.

2. Hauser WA, Hesdorffer DC: *Epilepsy: frequency, causes and consequences,* New York, 1990, Epilepsy Foundation of America–Demos Publications.

3. Shinnar S, Amir N, Branski D, editors: *Childhood seizures.* Basel, Switzerland, S Karger, 1995.

4. Commission on Classification and Terminology of the International League against Epilepsy: Proposal for revised clinical and electro-encephalographic classification of epileptic seizures, *Epilepsia* 22:489-501, 1981.

5. Roger J, Dreifuss FE, Martinez-Lage M, Munari C, Porter RJ, Seino M, Wolf P: Proposal for revised classification of epilepsies and epileptic syndromes, *Epilepsia* 30:389-399, 1989.

6. Roger J, Dravet C, Bureau M, Dreifuss FE, Wolf P, editors: *Epileptic syndromes in infancy, childhood and adolescence,* ed 2, London, 1992, John-Libbey Eurotext.

7. Greenberg DA, Durner M, Resor S, Rosenbaum D, Shinnar S: The genetics of idiopathic generalized epilepsies of adolescent onset: differences between juvenile myoclonic epilepsy and epilepsy with random grand mal and with awakening grand mal, *Neurology* 45:942-946, 1995.

8. Shinnar S, Berg AT, Moshe SL, Petix M, Maytal J, Kang H, Goldensohn ES, Hauser WA: Risk of seizure recurrence following a first unprovoked seizure in childhood: a prospective study, *Pediatrics* 85:1076-1085, 1990.

9. Mattson RH, Cramer JA, Collins JF, et al: Comparison of carbamazepine, phenobarbital, phenytoin, and primidone in partial and secondarily generalized tonic-clonic seizures, *N Engl J Med* 313:145-151, 1985.

10. Camfield CS, Camfield PR, Smith E, Tibbles JAR: Asymptomatic children with epilepsy: little benefit from screening for anticonvulsant-induced liver, blood and renal damage, *Neurology* 36:838-841, 1986.

11. Rosa FW: Spina bifida in infants of women treated with carbamazepine during pregnancy, *N Engl J Med* 324:674-677, 1991.

12. Committee on Drugs, American Academy of Pediatrics: Anticonvulsants and pregnancy, *Pediatrics* 63:331-333, 1979.

13. Commission on Genetics, Pregnancy and the Child, International League Against Epilepsy: Guidelines for the care of women of childbearing age with epilepsy, *Epilepsia* 34:588-589, 1993.

14. Vining EPG, Mellits ED, Dorsen MM, Cataldo MF, Quaskey SA, Speilberg SP, Freeman JM: Psychologic and behavioral effects of antiepileptic drugs in children: a double-blind comparison between phenobarbital and valproic acid, *Pediatrics* 80:165-174, 1987.

15. Dreifuss FE, Langer DH, Moline KA, Maxwell JE: Valproic acid hepatic fatalities. II. US experience since 1984, *Neurology* 39:201-207, 1989.

16. Scheffner D, St. Konig J, Rauterberg-Ruland I, Kochen W, Hoffman WJ, St. Unkelbach: Fatal liver failure in 16 children with valproate therapy, *Epilepsia* 29:530-542, 1988.

17. Committee on Drugs, American Academy of Pediatrics: Valproic acid: benefits and risks, *Pediatrics* 70:316-319, 1982.

18. Jager-Roman E, Deichl A, Jakob S, Hartmann AM, Koch S, Rating D, Steldinger R, Nau H, Helge H: Fetal growth, major malformations, and minor anomalies in infants born to women receiving valproic acid, *J Pediatr* 108:997-1004, 1986.

19. Masur DM, Shinnar S: The neuropsychology of childhood seizure disorders. In Segalowitz S, Rapin I, editors: *Handbook of neuropsychology,* vol 7, *Childhood neuropsychology,* Amsterdam, 1992, Elsevier; pp 457-470.

20. Committee on Drugs, American Academy of Pediatrics: Behavioral and cognitive effects of anticonvulsant therapy, *Pediatrics* 96:538-540, 1995.

21. Brent DA, Crumrine PK, Varma RR, Allan M, Allman C: Phenobarbital treatment and major depressive disorder in children with epilepsy, *Pediatrics* 80:909-917, 1987.

22. Wyllie E, editor: New developments in antiepileptic drug therapy, *Epilepsia* 36(suppl 2):S1-S118, 1995.

23. Commission on Antiepileptic Drugs, International League Against Epilepsy: Guidelines for therapeutic monitoring on antiepileptic drugs, *Epilepsia* 34:585-587, 1993.

24. Levy RH, Mattson RH, Meldrum BS, Dreifuss FE, Penry JK, editors: *Antiepileptic drugs,* ed 4, New York, 1995, Raven Press.

25. Janz D, Schmidt D: Antiepileptic drugs and failure of oral contraceptives, *Lancet* 1:1113, 1974.

26. Hempel E, Klinger W: Drug stimulated biotransformation of hormonal steroid contraceptives: clinical implications, *Drugs* 12:442-448, 1976.

27. Engel J Jr, editor: *Surgical treatment of the epilepsies,* ed 2, New York, 1993, Raven Press.

28. Hauser WA, Anderson VE, Loewenson RB, McRoberts SM: Seizure recurrence after a first unprovoked seizure, *N Engl J Med* 307:522-528, 1982.

29. Berg AT, Shinnar S: The risk of seizure recurrence following a first unprovoked seizure: a quantitative review, *Neurology* 41:965-972, 1991.

30. First Seizure Trial Group: Randomized clinical trial on the efficacy of antiepileptic drugs in reducing the risk of relapse after a first unprovoked tonic-clonic seizure, *Neurology* 43:478-483, 1993.

31. Musicco M, Beghi E, Solari A, First Seizure Trial Group: Effect of antiepileptic treatment initiated after the first unprovoked seizure on the long-term prognosis of epilepsy, *Neurology* 44(suppl 2):A337-338, 1994.

32. Shinnar S, O'Dell C: Treating childhood seizures: when and for how long. In Shinnar S, Amir N, Branski D, editors: *Childhood seizures.* Basel, Switzerland, 1995, S Karger; pp 100-110.

33. Shinnar S, Berg AT: Does antiepileptic drug therapy prevent the development of "chronic" epilepsy?, *Epilepsia* 37:701-708, 1996.

34. Annegers JF, Hauser WA, Elveback LR: Remission of seizures and relapse in patients with epilepsy, *Epilepsia* 20:729-737, 1979.

35. Brorson LO, Wranne L: Long term prognosis in childhood epilepsy: survival and seizure prognosis, *Epilepsia* 28:324-330, 1987.

36. Sofianov NG: Clinical evolution and prognosis of childhood epilepsies, *Epilepsia* 23:61-69, 1982.

37. Shinnar S, Moshe SL: Age specificity of seizure expression in genetic epilepsies. In Anderson VE, Hauser WA, Leppik IE, Noebels JL, Rich SS, editors: *Genetic strategies in epilepsy research,* New York, 1991, Raven Press; pp 69-85.

38. Diamantopoulos N, Crumrine PK: The effect of puberty on the course of epilepsy, *Arch Neurol* 43:873-876, 1986.

39. Gross-Tsur V, Shinnar S: Discontinuing antiepileptic drug therapy in patients with epilepsy. In Wyllie E, editor: *Treatment of epilepsy: principles and practice,* ed 2, Philadelphia, 1997, Lea & Febiger; pp 799-807.

40. Holowach-Thurston J, Thurston DL, Hixon BB, Keller AJ: Prognosis in childhood epilepsy: additional followup of 148 children 15 to 23 years after withdrawal of anticonvulsant therapy, *N Engl J Med* 306:831-836, 1982.

41. Shinnar S, Berg AT, Moshe SL, Kang H, O'Dell C, Alemany M, Goldensohn ES, Hauser WA: Discontinuing antiepileptic drugs in children with epilepsy: a prospective study, *Ann Neurol* 35:534-545, 1994.

42. Berg AT, Shinnar S: Relapse following discontinuation of antiepileptic drugs: a meta-analysis, *Neurology* 44:601-608, 1994.

43. Tennison M, Greenwood R, Lewis D, Thorn M: Discontinuing antiepileptic drugs in children with epilepsy: a comparison of a six-week and nine-month taper period, *N Engl J Med* 330:1407-1410, 1994.

44. Janz D, Dam M, Richens A, Bossi L, Helge H, Schmidt D, editors: *Epilepsy, pregnancy and the child,* New York, 1982, Raven Press.
45. Czeizel AE, Dudas I: Prevention of the first occurrence of neural-tube defects by periconceptual vitamin supplementation, *N Engl J Med* 327:1832-1835, 1992.
46. Committee on Children with Handicaps and Committee on Sports Medicine, American Academy of Pediatrics: Sports and the child with epilepsy, *Pediatrics* 72:884-885, 1983.
47. Hansotia P, Broste SK: The effect of epilepsy or diabetes mellitus on the risk of automobile accidents, *N Engl J Med* 324:22-26, 1991.
48. Dodrill CB, Breyer DN, Diamond MB, Dubinsky BL, Geary BB: Psychosocial problems among adults with epilepsy, *Epilepsia* 25:168-175, 1984.
49. Hoare P: Does illness foster dependency?: a study of epileptic and diabetic children, *Dev Med Child Neurol* 26:20-24, 1984.
50. Ziegler RG: Impairments of control and competence in epileptic children and their families, *Epilepsia* 22:339-346, 1981.
51. Westbrook LE, Silver EJ, Coupey SM, Shinnar S: Social characteristics of adolescents with idiopathic epilepsy: a comparison to chronically ill and non chronically ill peers, *J Epilepsy* 4:87-94, 1991.

CHAPTER 62

Motor Unit Disorders

•

Alfred J. Spiro

Motor unit disorders are those that affect the anterior horn cells of the spinal cord, various portions of the peripheral nerve, the myoneural junction, and/or the muscle cells. Although many of the more common disorders of the motor unit, such as infantile progressive spinal muscular atrophy and Duchenne's muscular dystrophy, are clinically apparent in infancy or childhood, several motor unit disorders characteristically become apparent or have their major impact on the patient and family during the adolescent years.

APPROACH TO THE PATIENT

The cardinal symptoms of a motor unit disorder are muscle weakness and/or sensory complaints such as numbness or tingling. Weakness may be manifested by difficulty in walking, running, rope climbing, and raising the arms above the head or a decrease in athletic abilities. To determine whether facial muscle weakness is present, for example, as in facioscapulohumeral muscular dystrophy, patients should be asked whether they can whistle normally or whether their eyelids are open during sleep. Appropriate questioning will reveal whether patients have been toe walkers in childhood, as in Becker's muscular dystrophy (BMD), or in juvenile progressive spinal muscular atrophy (JPSMA), or whether they trip easily while walking, which suggests weakness of the anterior tibialis muscles, as noted in peripheral neuropathies. Inquiries should be made about abnormal functional capacity of the hands, as seen in peripheral neuropathy or myotonic dystrophy: for example, by asking about difficulty in opening jars, using a screwdriver, or writing. Patients should be asked whether they have difficulty letting go of objects, a symptom common in myotonic dystrophy. Although it is occasionally difficult to ascertain when symptoms were originally noted, every effort should be made to obtain this information, since the duration of illness can be very important in establishing a definitive diagnosis. Old photographs or videotapes of the patient sometimes may provide useful information. Inquiries also should be made concerning the presence of muscle pain or pigmented urine. In addition, patients should be asked whether they have been paralyzed in the past, even for a brief period. They also should be questioned about easy fatigability, double vision, and dysphagia and about the variability of these symptoms, as observed in myasthenia gravis. Since many motor unit disorders are inherited, a careful genetic history should be undertaken. At times, examination of other family members for preclinical involvement is indicated.

Certain details of the physical examination should be stressed. These include assessment of gait, ability to walk on the heels and toes and to climb stairs, scoliosis, highly arched feet, increase in lumbar lordosis, and muscle enlargement or wasting; manual muscle testing; testing for deep tendon reflexes and sensory abnormalities and extraocular muscle weakness; and tests for shoulder, neck, and facial muscle weakness.

Genetic and other studies can be extremely helpful in arriving at a correct diagnosis when correlated to clinical data. Electromyography (EMG), performed with needle electrodes, records electrical activity from the muscle itself. Determination of nerve conduction velocities, both sensory and motor, is a test done with surface electrodes. The physician ordering these tests needs to remember that they are uncomfortable, sometimes painful, and expensive. For ancillary studies to be useful, they should be performed by a physician who has an understanding of the information sought. Serum muscle enzyme determinations, particularly creatine kinase (CK) levels, can be useful in searching for a primary muscular disorder. However, in some muscle disorders seen in adolescents, for example, facioscapulohumeral muscular dystrophy, the CK level may be normal. In selected instances a muscle biopsy can provide a definitive diagnosis, provided that appropriate morphologic, histochemical, biochemical, and other studies are performed.[1] A muscle biopsy should not be taken unless state-of-the-art studies can be obtained.

There are many clinics supported by the Muscular Dystrophy Association to which a patient with a motor unit disorder can be referred for diagnosis and multidisciplinary management.

ANTERIOR HORN CELL DISEASE

Since the virtual eradication of poliomyelitis, the most common disorder of anterior horn cells observed in adolescents is JPSMA, also known as Kugelberg-Welander disease.[2,3] This is a genetically determined disorder in which the primary lesion is degeneration of the anterior horn cells, resulting in wasting of the skeletal musculature. The inheritance pattern is generally autosomal recessive, but autosomal dominant types (in late-onset spinal muscular atrophy or, rarely, X-linked recessive forms) are known. The recessive form has been mapped to the long arm of chromosome 5, and prenatal diagnosis is possible in selected, informative families.[4]

The clinical characteristics of JPSMA include painless proximal and symmetric muscle weakness and atrophy, with manifestations more commonly in the legs than in the arms. Initial symptoms usually consist of difficulty in running, climbing stairs, or arising from a chair; toe walking, enlarged calves, and a waddling gait may be prominent. Intellectual function is generally normal, as are the muscles supplied by the cranial nerves. An increase in the normal lumbar lordosis may be apparent, and scoliosis and joint contractures may develop. Muscle fasciculations are present in only a few patients. Deep tendon reflexes are reduced or absent, and toe responses and sensations are normal. A mild irregular tremulousness of the outstretched hands may be apparent. JPSMA is usually very slowly progressive; however, in some patients it can lead to wheelchair status.

The diagnosis of JPSMA is established when the clinical picture is coupled with (1) normal serum muscle enzymes (although the CK level can be moderately elevated), (2) neuropathic EMG with normal nerve conduction velocities (although in some instances an element of myopathic dysfunction may be present), and (3) muscle biopsy indicating a predominantly denervating process.[1]

Similar patterns of weakness are observed in BMD, limb-girdle muscular dystrophy, and some metabolic muscle disorders, but these can usually be distinguished through the studies already noted.

Management is symptomatic, since there is no specific therapeutic agent that will alter the course of the disease. Physical therapy should be provided for the patient. A disorder that may be related to JPSMA has been termed "juvenile type of distal and segmental muscular atrophy of the upper extremities."[5] In this disorder, commonly seen in Japan but less commonly in the United States, the onset in approximately 90% of cases occurs in the age range from 18 to 22 years. Males are affected much more frequently than females. The distribution of muscular atrophy is initially limited to the hand and forearm. Deep tendon reflexes in the affected limb are hypoactive or absent, but no sensory abnormalities are noted. Rapid progression of the disease takes place during the initial 2 to 3 years after onset, with a slowly progressive course thereafter. No abnormal laboratory findings are noted, except for the results of EMG studies and structural changes on muscle biopsy that indicate neurogenic atrophy of the muscles. Although the cause of this disorder is unknown (and there does not seem to be a genetic pattern), the site of the lesion is thought to range from the fifth cervical to the first thoracic spinal segments, with intramedullary involvement. No specific therapeutic modality has been identified.

BRACHIAL PLEXUS AND PERIPHERAL NERVES

Brachial Plexus Neuropathy

Brachial plexus neuropathy[6] is observed in adolescents and adults. Although many patients with this disorder describe an antecedent illness (sometimes trivial) or injection, the pathogenesis of this disorder is unknown.

The major symptom of brachial plexus neuropathy is pain in one or both shoulders. This pain may be very severe and may last from hours to several weeks before it abates. Lessening or cessation of pain is accompanied or followed by varying degrees of weakness and atrophy of the arm muscles. Sensory loss is also extremely variable, but most patients do not exhibit weakness and/or sensory abnormalities of the entire arm, indicating incomplete or diffuse involvement of the brachial plexus. Electrodiagnostic studies may be helpful in substantiating the diagnosis of brachial plexus neuropathy.

Physical therapy, consisting of active exercise (when possible) and passive movement, should be prescribed, as well as measures to lessen pain. The prognosis for recovery is excellent, but full restitution of function may take place over a prolonged period.

Guillain-Barré Syndrome

Guillain-Barré syndrome (GBS)[7-9] has an incidence of 0.4 to 2 per 100,000 population. The incidence is moderately higher in females and somewhat lower in adolescents than in older individuals. Uncertainty still exists about the exact cause of the resultant polyradiculoneuropathy, but GBS is often associated with a preceding viral infection, and there is evidence for an autoimmune mechanism.

Characteristically, but not necessarily, GBS begins approximately 1 to 2 weeks after a viral infection or other illness, surgery, or inoculation. At that point in time the patient is usually afebrile. Symmetric weakness generally develops acutely or subacutely, and its degree may vary from very mild to severe, with paralysis of the facial, trunk, and bulbar muscles. The extraocular muscles also may become paralyzed; in fact, in some variants the disorder may begin with weakness of these muscles.

Areflexia is the rule in GBS, but sensory symptoms and signs are generally mild. Autonomic dysfunction, characterized by fluctuations in blood pressure and heart rate and postural hypotension, is common. Progression of weakness generally stops approximately 3 weeks after onset of the illness. Recovery usually begins a few weeks after the cessation of the progression. Although most patients recover fully, improvement may be delayed and may take place over several months. A few patients are left with some residual weakness and joint contractures.

Diagnosis can be made on the basis of the clinical pattern coupled with the results of cerebrospinal fluid (CSF) examination and electrodiagnostic studies. The CSF protein is usually increased after the first week of symptoms, and there are generally fewer than 10 mononuclear cells per cubic millimeter. Electrodiagnostic tests can provide diagnostic and prognostic information early in the disease. Possible infection with *Mycoplasma* spp., Epstein-Barr virus, and Lyme disease should be investigated. Other conditions, including poliomyelitis, paralysis resulting from a conversion reaction, botulism, toxic neuropathies (e.g., addictive glue sniffing), acute intermittent porphyria, tick paralysis, and hypokalemic periodic paralysis, occasionally may resemble GBS, but these possibilities can be readily excluded by appropriate studies. In addition, a GBS-like syndrome has been

described in adults with acquired immunodeficiency syndrome (AIDS).

During the first few weeks of GBS, management should take place in an intensive care unit with very careful monitoring of vital signs and respiratory function, since autonomic dysfunction and respiratory failure are important causes of complications and possible death in GBS. The immediate availability of respiratory assistance is mandatory. Intravenous administration of high doses of gamma globulin has been documented to shorten the course and lessen the severity of GBS; this should be begun as early as possible and may sometimes obviate the need for respiratory assistance.[9a] Physical therapy also should be begun early in the course of the disease to prevent joint contractures.

Peripheral Neuropathies

Peripheral neuropathies[10,11] are disorders of various causes—hereditary, toxic, traumatic, metabolic, idiopathic—that affect the function and/or structure of the peripheral nervous system. They occur in all age groups, and the manifestations can be recognized in adolescents. Sensory or motor symptoms may predominate but frequently coexist. The manifestations depend on the degree of involvement of large myelinated, small myelinated, or nonmyelinated fibers and on which portion of the peripheral nerve is involved. A peripheral neuropathy may occur with certain central nervous system (CNS) degenerative disorders in adolescents.

Symptoms include numbness, burning, or paresthesias (primarily in the hands or feet); insecurity of gait; and weakness in the fingers and/or dorsiflexors or plantiflexors of the feet. Weakness may be identified by functional muscle testing (e.g., by asking patients to walk on their heels or toes, which may be difficult or impossible) or by manual muscle testing. Sensation for pain, touch, or vibration may be reduced, and deep tendon reflexes, usually ankle jerks, are absent.

Electrodiagnostic studies are extremely useful for assessing patients in whom peripheral neuropathies are suspected. A demyelinating neuropathy results in a marked decrease in motor nerve conduction velocity. In neuropathies in which axonal degeneration is the primary pathologic alteration, there is either no change or only a minor decrease in nerve conduction velocity; however, there is EMG evidence of denervation. Sensory nerve action potentials also may be assessed in conventional electrodiagnostic studies, and these may be very useful in confirming the diagnosis of peripheral neuropathy.

Peripheral nerve trauma in adolescents is generally no different from trauma in other individuals. As in children and adults, there are certain vulnerabilities, such as injury to the radial nerve in the spiral groove, associated with fractures of the humerus, and trauma to the long thoracic nerve in backpackers, resulting in winging of the scapula. A problem encountered in adolescents who ride bicycles for long distances is compression neuropathy of the ulnar nerve at the wrist. This is related to riding with the hands in an extended position and the wrists pressing on the handlebars. This problem is found more commonly in the dominant hand. It is characterized by pain and tingling in the two ulnar fingers, with sensory abnormalities noted in the ulnar half of the ring finger; associated weakness of the muscles innervated by the ulnar nerve is sometimes also seen. A change in bicycle-riding habits usually results in alleviation of symptoms.

Diabetic peripheral neuropathy[12] is much less frequently a problem in adolescents than in adults. Manifestations include numbness and paresthesias, sometimes painful, of the toes and feet, and, to a lesser extent, the fingers and hands. Loss of pain, touch, and vibratory perception are found in a glove-stocking distribution; this sign is associated with depressed deep tendon reflexes, especially ankle jerks. Abnormalities can be documented by determinations of nerve conduction velocity. Rigorous control of the diabetes may delay the onset of peripheral neuropathy or lessen the severity when it exists. Relief of symptoms sometimes can be obtained with carbamazepine. Additional drugs such as imipramine, may be needed to provide symptomatic relief.

Uremic neuropathy may be observed in adolescents with chronic renal disease. Such patients develop a chronic, symmetric, and predominantly sensory neuropathy in which the major complaints are burning paresthesias, restless legs, and numbness spreading upward from the feet, and occasionally present in the hands. Motor problems, such as footdrop, also may be present. The severity of the involvement is not necessarily related to the degree of uremia. Nerve conduction velocity determinations can be used to substantiate the diagnosis. Renal dialysis may prevent the progression of the neuropathy or provide some degree of recovery when it exists. Renal transplantation, when indicated, also results in a good response.

Toxic neuropathy may be noted in adolescents who might be exposed to a wide variety of agents that potentially damage the peripheral nervous system. These include heavy metals, many industrial solvents and organic compounds, and nitrous oxide. In addition to the usual symptoms and signs of this disorder, toxic neuropathies are frequently associated with pain and weight loss. In any adolescent who has a peripheral neuropathy of unclear origin, a careful search for toxins should be undertaken.

Hereditary sensory motor neuropathies (HSMNs)[11] include several disorders in which various pathologic changes in peripheral nerves play a central role. HSMN type I, in which demyelination is the major alteration, and HSMN type II, in which axonal degeneration is the major

pathologic condition, are the most common. Both types may become clinically apparent in the adolescent years as motor and/or sensory problems, but it is often difficult to ascribe a date of onset because the symptoms are often insidious. HSMN disorders are often inherited in an autosomal dominant pattern, but individual differences in severity of symptoms occasionally make diagnosis in the parents or a sibling of the patient difficult when an affected relative is only subclinically involved. Elucidation of the hereditary pattern often necessitates careful neurologic and electrophysiologic studies of close relatives if possible.

Motor and sensory signs and symptoms are highly variable, but they generally involve the feet more than the hands. The initial complaints may be slowly evolving equinovarus deformity, generally symmetric, which may result in increasing tripping and difficulty in walking; this deformity also may be associated with increased fatigability after routine activities. The rate of progression is variable but is usually very slow. Wasting of the calf muscles may become apparent. Weakness of the hand muscles also can become a problem, as can wasting of the intrinsic muscles of the hands. Weakness, wasting, and difficulty in walking on the heels and/or toes usually can be detected at the time of examination. Sensory loss in a stocking or (less commonly) glove distribution, with diminished or absent ankle jerks, also may be noted at this time. Loss of vibratory perception is usually the most easily detected sensory abnormality. In some patients the ability to walk independently can be lost after many years.

The diagnosis can be confirmed by electrophysiologic studies, which also can be used to characterize the defect in the peripheral nerves as axonal or demyelinating. There is no specific medical treatment; however, physical therapy, prudent bracing with acceptable orthoses, and surgery, if needed, can be helpful. Genetic counseling should be provided; DNA studies can be useful in selected cases.

Chronic (or relapsing) inflammatory demyelinating polyradiculoneuropathy (CIDP)[13,14] can have its onset in adolescence, although it is more commonly observed in older individuals. The pathogenesis is not fully understood but is probably related to an abnormal immune response.

The onset of symptoms is subacute. Both proximal and distal symmetric muscle weakness, associated with sensory loss and diminished to absent deep tendon reflexes (especially ankle jerks), is the cardinal characteristic. Facial muscle weakness may also be present. A relapsing course is commonly observed.

Diagnosis is substantiated when the characteristic clinical pattern is coupled with slowed nerve conduction velocities, usually with conduction block; an elevated CSF protein level; and a nerve biopsy specimen with characteristic features. Most patients with CIDP respond to prednisone therapy. Initially, high single daily doses of prednisone are commonly used for 2 to 4 weeks. Subsequently, single-dose, alternate-day therapy can be given until clinical improvement is achieved. Some patients with CIDP require azathioprine; others respond very quickly to high-dose intravenous gamma globulin administration. After improvement, this therapy can be maintained, with doses given every few weeks if needed.

DISORDERS OF THE MYONEURAL JUNCTION

Myasthenia Gravis

Myasthenia gravis (MG),[15,16] an acquired autoimmune disorder affecting the myoneural junction, is not uncommon in adolescents. In this age group, MG is noted more frequently in females than in males.

The most common initial symptoms of MG are ptosis and/or diplopia because of selective vulnerability of the extraocular muscles. These symptoms may be variable in severity. They may not be present in the morning or if the patient is not fatigued, and therefore the diagnosis is sometimes missed. Spontaneous remission of symptoms may occur. Other clinically more severe forms of MG may occur; in these types, bulbar involvement with rapid development and progression of severe generalized weakness, and resultant ventilatory failure, are present. Because of muscle weakness, the patient may experience problems in speaking full sentences, chewing, and holding up the head. Deep tendon reflexes are characteristically preserved. No sensory abnormalities are noted.

Diagnosis can be established with edrophonium (Tensilon), an anticholinesterase drug that acts rapidly and briefly to provide prompt relief of myasthenic weakness. A test dose of 2 mg is given intravenously to determine whether the patient has any abnormal sensitivity to the drug or a beneficial response. If there are no untoward reactions, the edrophonium can be given in further small increments up to a total of 10 mg. After each dose, the response of the patient is determined by assessing changes in a specifically defined end point, such as the size of the palpebral fissue or the range of motility of the extraocular muscles.

Specialized electrodiagnostic studies are sometimes of great assistance in establishing the diagnosis. Antibodies against acetylcholine receptor sites, present in approximately 80% of patients with MG, also can be assessed as a definitive diagnostic measure. Since thymic enlargement or tumors are associated with MG, careful assessment of the thymus should be done with computed tomography or magnetic resonance imaging. Because of the association of dysthyroid states and MG, thyroid function should be assessed. In some cases of very mild

ocular MG, therapy may consist of eye-patching alone if diplopia is mild. Some patients experience spontaneous remission during the first 2 years of the disease. Most patients with ocular MG need anticholinesterase drugs, the most useful of which is pyridostigmine bromide (Mestinon), for relief of symptoms. The dosage needs to be titrated to the patient's activities and response. Single-dose, alternate-day administration of prednisone is frequently required in mildly to moderately severe generalized MG.

In adolescents with MG, thymectomy[17] may be indicated to provide long-term beneficial results, even if thymic enlargement is not demonstrated on imaging. The procedure can be done either through a sternal splitting operation or through a mediastinoscope. Each technique has its own advantages and disadvantages. Immunosuppression with azathioprine[18] can prove useful as therapy in some cases; although this drug is usually well tolerated, its effects may not be noted for several months after institution of treatment. When the patient experiences an acute exacerbation of severe or generalized weakness, plasmapheresis can be performed as part of the treatment. Administration of high doses of intravenous gamma globulin can be equally effective. In patients with MG in whom ventilatory failure is imminent, treatment in an intensive care unit is necessary, and intubation with respiratory assistance is frequently indicated.

Botulism

Botulism[19] is another disorder of the myoneural junction in which symptoms appear within hours after ingestion of contaminated food and often are manifested in several members of the same family. Diplopia and ptosis appear rapidly, with spreading of the paralysis to produce respiratory failure. Therefore, immediate respiratory support must be provided for the patient. There are no sensory abnormalities. Repetitive nerve stimulation demonstrates the defect of the myoneural junction. Bacterial testing may be used to confirm the diagnosis.

MYOPATHIES

Becker's Muscular Dystrophy

Becker's muscular dystrophy (BMD) and Duchenne's muscular dystrophy[20] (DMD) are X-linked recessive disorders of muscle, the major features of which are progressive muscular weakness and wasting.[20] The prevalence of DMD is about 3 in 100,000; that of BMD is approximately one tenth of that figure. The defective gene in both of these disorders has been isolated and is on the short arm of the X chromosome. Dystrophin, the protein product of the gene, has been identified; it is found to be absent in DMD and variably reduced or altered in BMD skeletal muscle.[21] There is a positive relationship between the amount of dystrophin present and the severity and onset of weakness. Since virtually all boys with DMD become wheelchair bound before the age of 12, they are all severely affected by adolescence. In contrast, patients with BMD generally become symptomatic at school age and frequently during adolescence or even adulthood.

Generally, painless weakness in BMD is noted initially in the proximal muscles of the legs, although a tendency to walk on the toes may be noted earlier, along with markedly enlarged calf muscles. Manifestations include difficulty with running, climbing stairs, and riding a bicycle, and a waddling gait. Weakness and wasting of the proximal arm muscles are seen later. Progression of weakness may be very slow, and patients with BMD may lead a relatively normal life for several decades. As in DMD, mental subnormality may coexist. The deep tendon reflexes are usually diminished or absent, with the exception of the ankle jerks, which are maintained indefinitely. No sensory abnormalities are present. Diagnosis of BMD is made when the characteristic clinical pattern is seen in association with very high serum levels of muscle enzymes, especially CK. Elevations of CK are noted at birth, long before weakness is clinically apparent. Results of EMG studies are consistent with a myopathy; muscle biopsy is characteristic, but quantitative or qualitative abnormalities of dystrophin can substantiate the diagnosis and aid in providing a prognosis.[22] About 65% of patients with BMD show a demonstrable lesion in DNA blood testing.

Differential diagnosis includes other syndromes in which limb-girdle weakness is present. Differentiation can be based on the changes noted in muscle biopsies, including studies of dystrophin. Elevated CK values can be observed in McLeod's syndrome, in which acanthocytes are seen; muscle weakness is absent.[23]

There is no specific medical management; however, appropriate physical therapy, including unlimited exercise, and genetic counseling should be provided. Daughters of affected patients are obligate carriers of the gene, but sons are uninvolved.

Limb-Girdle Muscular Dystrophy

Limb-girdle muscular dystrophy[24] represents a group of disorders of either autosomal recessive or autosomal dominant inheritance in which symptoms of proximal muscle weakness may begin at virtually any age, but commonly during the second decade of life and in adolescence. Proximal muscles in the legs are generally more involved than the proximal muscles of the arms, resulting in the gait difficulties that are usually the first symptoms. Weakness may be manifested by difficulty in climbing stairs or in running, and it can be documented by manual and functional testing. Deep tendon reflexes are usually reduced; however, the ankle jerks may be preserved. Sensory examination results are normal. Cardiac muscle involvement is exceptionally rare.

CK values are variable but generally elevated. EMG studies can be used to document the myopathic basis, and a muscle biopsy usually helps to delineate the myopathic nature of the disorder.

Treatment is symptomatic. In general, physical therapy should be aimed at preserving muscle function as long as possible and aborting joint contractures. The course of limb-girdle muscular dystrophy is extremely variable, but it may be severe enough to result in wheelchair status and/or dependence on a ventilator for respiration. Prenatal diagnosis is not yet possible.

Facioscapulohumeral Muscular Dystrophy

Facioscapulohumeral muscular dystrophy[25] is transmitted as an autosomal dominant trait. The onset may occur anytime from childhood until adulthood, but onset in adolescence is common. Facial musculature is involved initially, but there is a great potential for subsequent involvement of the shoulder-girdle musculature and of the leg muscles. Because of the limited involvement seen initially in this disorder, the patient may be described as being round-shouldered or having poor posture; diagnosis is made only when weakness is detected through manual muscle testing in the typical distribution. The diagnosis is substantiated when other members of the family are found to be similarly affected, even if muscle weakness is limited to the face and no other symptoms are present. A history of inability to whistle in the usual manner (with pursed lips), to blow up a balloon, or to puff up the cheeks frequently is noted. Winging of the scapulae is common. The CK values, although sometimes elevated, may be normal. Results of electrodiagnostic studies and muscle biopsies, when performed, may be extremely variable and should be correlated with the clinical findings.

Treatment of this type of muscular dystrophy is symptomatic, and physical therapy is aimed at preserving muscle function. Genetic counseling should be provided. The defective gene in facioscapulohumeral muscular dystrophy has been localized to chromosome 4; prenatal diagnosis will be available in the near future.

Myotonic Dystrophy

Myotonic dystrophy (MyD),[26,27] an autosomal dominant disorder with a prevalence of approximately 7 in 100,000 population, often has its symptomatic onset in adolescence or the school-age years. The gene responsible for MyD is located on the long arm of chromosome 19; an abnormal expansion of a trinucleotide repeat is present. Although myotonia, or difficulty in relaxing after muscular contraction, is the characteristic feature, MyD is a multisystemic disorder. It is often associated with distal muscle weakness and wasting, frontal baldness, presenile cataracts, cardiac conduction defects, testicular atrophy, and subnormal intelligence.

The clinical picture of MyD is extremely variable and the diagnosis is frequently overlooked. In some adolescents myotonia is recognized only when it is actively sought: for example, in mothers of "floppy babies" in whom infantile MyD is considered in the differential diagnosis. In other patients with mental retardation or hypernasality of speech, which are common features of MyD, the diagnosis is made only if percussion or reflex myotonia is sought specifically, since patients often do not complain of difficulty in relaxing muscles. Percussion myotonia is noted when the muscles of the thenar eminence are struck briskly with a reflex hammer; there is contraction of the muscle with markedly delayed relaxation. In reflex, or action, myotonia, the patient has difficulty opening the hand after grasping an object. Ptosis and an expressionless face are also very common signs. Wasting of the muscles of mastication and smallness of the sternocleidomastoid muscles are typical. Wasting and weakness of the distal muscles of the limbs, sometimes leading to footdrop, may be seen. Lenticular cataracts are frequently identified on slit-lamp examination in the adolescent age group.

Electrocardiographic (ECG) abnormalities are often observed. The course of MyD is very variable; in some cases there is a slow deterioration, usually over 15 to 20 years. There is an increased risk of complications during general anesthesia.

Diagnosis is verified by DNA testing. EMG findings are characteristic. Serum muscle enzyme levels are generally normal or only slightly elevated. There is usually no need for a muscle biopsy.

Treatment is symptomatic, but the patient should be provided with physical therapy and genetic counseling. However, because of the mental subnormalities so common in this disorder, these modes of therapy are not always useful. Prenatal diagnosis is readily available and extremely accurate. The judicious use of phenytoin or imipramine may be useful; however, as in other disorders in which mental subnormality is present, drugs should be administered with a great deal of caution.

Inflammatory Myopathies

Polymyositis and dermatomyositis,[28-30] both uncommon, occur in virtually all age groups, including adolescents. These disorders probably result from an alteration of normal immune mechanisms and are not genetically determined.

Onset of symptoms is generally subacute or subchronic, lasting over weeks or a few months, although rarely onset can be acute. Muscular weakness, generally proximal and more severe in the legs than in the arms, is the most common presenting complaint. Neck flexor muscles are very often weak, but extraocular and facial muscles are spared. Variably intense muscular pain is present infrequently in adolescence. Muscular atrophy or muscular enlargement, as seen in BMD or JPSMA, is not seen early in polymyositis or dermatomyositis. In dermatomyositis, skin manifestations are present in the periorbital and malar regions and on the extensor surfaces of the limbs; the skin over the metacarpophalangeal and interphalangeal joints also may be reddened. Arthralgias are present in about one quarter of patients. The course of the disease is variable: it may be limited, polycyclic, or continuous. Some patients may exhibit features of other connective tissue disorders.

Diagnosis can be established when the clinical pattern is correlated with appropriate biochemical, electrodiagnostic, and pathologic studies. Values of serum CK are generally elevated, but they may be normal in a few cases. Electrodiagnostic studies are very useful in verifying the diagnosis. These studies should be limited to one side of the body, to enable subsequent performance of a muscle biopsy in a muscle that has not been tested with a needle. A muscle biopsy, when done properly, can be diagnostic in that an inflammatory exudate and/or perifascicular atrophy is confirmatory. The erythrocyte sedimentation rate is abnormal in approximately one third of patients.

The differential diagnosis includes genetically determined or metabolic myopathies, anterior horn-cell disease, and sporadically occurring disorders; also included are acute viral myositis, "growing pains," conversion reactions, and toxic myopathies. In adolescents with an eating disorder, an ipecac (emetine)-induced myopathy can produce a pattern of muscle weakness similar to that seen in polymyositis. Careful analysis of the history in correlation with the clinical examination, negative genetic history, serum muscle enzyme values, results of electrodiagnostic tests, and muscle biopsy results generally serves to provide the correct diagnosis.

Prednisone is considered the preferential agent in the treatment of polymyositis or dermatomyositis. Treatment is usually begun with a daily, single morning high-dose regimen. After a period this may be switched to an alternate-date, single morning high-dose schedule to reduce the possibility of side effects. If patients do not experience a beneficial response after a reasonable period of prednisone therapy, or if they experience intolerable side effects, immunosuppressive agents (e.g., azathioprine, cyclosporine) may be added or substituted. High doses of intravenous gamma globulin have proved very effective. Physical therapy is generally part of the treatment plan.

With treatment the prognosis is generally good, although complications, which may be related to the disease itself or to the therapy, can be significant. These include severe respiratory involvement and dysphagia, gastrointestinal bleeding, subcutaneous calcifications,[31] recurrence, and death. The relationship of polymyositis or dermatomyositis with malignancy, as noted in older patients, does not exist in adolescents, with rare exceptions.

Miscellaneous Myopathies

Hypokalemic periodic paralysis,[32] a rare autosomal dominant disorder, frequently first appears in adolescence. This disorder is manifested by an acute quadriplegia with areflexia, most commonly occurring in the early morning hours. Results of an electrocardiogram may suggest hypokalemia, which is confirmed by a serum potassium determination. Treatment with potassium can overcome the paralysis, and diuretics can be used prophylactically to lessen the frequency and intensity of the attacks.

Carnitine palmityl transferase deficiency[33] may be manifested in adolescent males through sudden onset of severe weakness and myoglobinuria, frequently occurring after a fast. Respiratory difficulty is occasionally present during an attack. Serum muscle enzyme levels are elevated, and the diagnosis can be confirmed by specialized morphologic and biochemical studies of a muscle biopsy. In the presence of episodic myoglobinuria and weakness, other rare metabolic disorders of skeletal muscle that frequently have initial manifestations in adolescence, such as McArdle's disease (phosphorylase deficiency) and phosphofructokinase deficiency,[34] should be considered in the differential diagnosis.

Specialized studies of muscle biopsies can help to confirm the diagnosis in these disorders. Serum muscle enzyme levels, especially CK, are generally elevated in these myopathies and in myoadenylate deaminase deficiency of muscle, in which muscle pain and myoglobinuria may be present.

Intramuscular pentazocine (Talwin) or meperidine (Demerol) abuse in adolescents can result in induration and contracture of the muscles injected, with associated fibrosis. This effect may be severe and may produce a woodlike sensation to palpation of the muscles. Patients may complain of weakness, but diagnosis is frequently difficult because of their denial of drug abuse.

Ipecac abuse in adolescents with an eating disorder also can result in damage in both skeletal and cardiac muscles because of the toxic effect of emetine. This results in a generalized myopathy, with manifestations of proximal muscle weakness. Prognosis is guarded but generally good when the ipecac abuse is stopped.

In hyperthyroidism, *hyperthyroid myopathy*[35] may occur, frequently before the onset of symptoms of the underlying thyroid disorder. Proximal muscle weakness, which is the rule, is frequently associated with fatigability out of proportion to the degree of weakness. In addition, hyperthyroidism is occasionally associated with MG. The deep tendon reflexes are normal. EMG may be helpful in confirming the presence of an underlying myopathy, but the diagnosis is established on confirmation of the hyperthyroid state. Treatment of the underlying disorder is generally very successful.

Malignant hyperpyrexia,[36] which can be encountered in all age groups (including adolescents), is triggered by succinylcholine, halothane, and other anesthetic agents during the induction of anesthesia or shortly thereafter. The exact pathogenesis is unclear, but it is associated with a rapidly evolving metabolic acidosis with lacticemia, rapid rise in body temperature, muscle rigidity, hyperkalemia, extremely elevated CK levels, myoglobinuria, hypocalcemia, and other changes. Prompt termination of anesthesia and immediate administration of intravenous dantrolene, coupled with body cooling, rehydration, administration of sodium bicarbonate, and associated ventilatory assistance, have proved effective.

References

1. Dubowitz V: *Muscle biopsy: a practical approach,* ed 2, London, 1985, Bailliére Tindall.
2. Dubowitz V: *Muscle disorders in childhood,* Philadelphia, 1978, WB Saunders.
3. Gardner-Medwin D, Hudgson P, Walton JN: Benign spinal muscular atrophy arising in childhood and adolescence, *J Neurol Sci* 5:121, 1967.
4. Brzustowicz LM, Lehner T, Castilla LH, et al: Genetic mapping of chronic childhood-onset spinal muscular atrophy to chromosome 5q11.2-13.3, *Nature* 344:540, 1990.
5. Sobue I, Saito N, Iida M, Ando K: Juvenile type of distal and segmental muscular atrophy of upper extremities, *Ann Neurol* 3:429, 1978.
6. Beghi E, Kurland LT, Mulder DW, Nicolosi A: Brachial plexus neuropathy in the population of Rochester, Minnesota, 1970-1981, *Ann Neurol* 18:320, 1985.
7. McKhann GM: Guillain-Barré syndrome: clinical and therapeutic observations, *Ann Neurol* 27(suppl):S13, 1990.
8. Asbury AK, Cornblath DR: Assessment of current diagnostic criteria for Guillain-Barré syndrome, *Ann Neurol* 27(suppl):S21, 1990.
9. van der Meché FGA, van Doorn PA: Guillain-Barré syndrome and chronic inflammatory demyelinating polyneuropathy: immune mechanisms and update on current therapies, *Ann Neurol* 37(S1):S14-S31, 1995.
9a. Nicolaides P, Appleton RE: Immunoglobin therapy in Guillain-Barre syndrome in children, *Dev Med Child Neurol* 37:1110-1114, 1995.
10. Schaumburg HH, Berger AR, Thomas PK: *Disorders of peripheral nerves,* ed 2, Philadelphia, 1992, FA Davis.

11. Dyck PJ: *Peripheral neuropathy,* ed 3, Philadelphia, 1993, WB Saunders.

12. Dyck PJ: *Diabetic neuropathy,* Philadelphia, 1987, WB Saunders.

13. van Doorn PA, Vermeulen M, Brand A, et al: Intravenous immunoglobulin treatment in patients with chronic inflammatory demyelinating polyneuropathy: clinical and laboratory characteristics associated with improvement, *Arch Neurol* 48:217, 1991.

14. van der Meché FGA, Vermeulen M, Busch HFM: Chronic inflammatory demyelinating polyneuropathy: conduction failure before and during immunoglobulin or plasma therapy, *Brain* 112:1563, 1989.

15. Osserman KE, Genkins G: Studies in myasthenia gravis: review of a twenty-year experience in over 1200 patients, *Mt Sinai J Med* 38:497, 1971.

16. Lisak RP, editor: *Handbook of myasthenia gravis and myasthenic syndromes,* New York, 1994, Marcel Dekker.

17. Papatestas AE, Genkins G, Kornfeld P, et al: Effects of thymectomy in myasthenia gravis, *Ann Surg* 206:79, 1987.

18. Niakan E, Harati Y, Rolak YA: Immunosuppressive drug therapy in myasthenia gravis, *Arch Neurol* 43:155, 1986.

19. Lund BM: Foodborne disease due to *Bacillus* and *Clostridium* species, *Lancet* 336:982, 1990.

20. Bradley WG, Jones MZ, Mussini J-M, Fawcett PRW: Becker-type muscular dystrophy, *Muscle Nerve* 1:111, 1978.

21. Darras BT: Molecular genetics of Duchenne and Becker muscular dystrophy, *Pediatrics* 117:1, 1990.

22. Beggs AH, Kunkel LM: Improved diagnosis of Duchenne/Becker muscular dystrophy, *J Clin Invest* 85:613, 1990.

23. Swash M, Schwartz MS, Carter ND, et al: Benign X-linked myopathy with acanthocytes (McLeod syndrome): its relationship to X-linked muscular dystrophy, *Brain* 106:717, 1983.

24. Bradley WG: The limb-girdle syndromes. In Vinken PJ, Bruyn GW, Ringel SP, editors: *Diseases of muscle,* part 1. In Vinken PJ, Bruyn GW, editors: *Handbook of clinical neurology,* vol 40, Amsterdam, 1979, Elsevier/North-Holland Biomedical Press; pp 433-469.

25. Carroll JE: Facioscapulohumeral and scapuloperoneal syndromes. In Vinken PJ, Bruyn GW, Ringel SP, editors: *Diseases of muscle,* part 1. In Vinken PJ, Bruyn GW, editors: *Handbook of Clinical neurology,* vol 40, Amsterdam, 1979, Elsevier/North-Holland Biomedical Press; pp 415-431.

26. Harper PS: *Myotonic dystrophy,* ed 2, London, 1989, WB Saunders.

27. Jozefowicz RF, Griggs RC: Myotonic dystrophy, *Neurol Clin* 6:455, 1988.

28. Engel AG, Hohlfeld R, Banker BQ: Inflammatory myopathies. In Engel AG, Franzini-Armstrong C, editors: *Myology: basic and clinical,* ed 2, vol 2, New York, 1994, McGraw-Hill; pp 1335-1383.

29. Bohan A, Peter JB: Polymyositis and dermatomyositis (two parts), *N Engl J Med* 292:344, 403, 1975.

30. Bunch TW: Polymyositis: a case history approach to the differential diagnosis and treatment, *Mayo Clin Proc* 65:1480, 1990.

31. Randle HW, Sander HM, Howard K: Early diagnosis of calcinosis cutis in childhood dermatomyositis using computed tomography, *JAMA* 256:1137, 1986.

32. Riggs JE: The periodic paralyses, *Neurol Clin* 6:485, 1988.

33. Angelini C, Trevisan C, Isaya G, et al: Clinical varieties of carnitine and carnitine palmitoyl transferase deficiency, *Clin Biochem* 20:1, 1987.

34. Servidei S, DiMauro S: Disorders of glycogen metabolism of muscle, *Neurol Clin* 7:159, 1989.

35. Ruff RL: Endocrine myopathies. In Engel AG, Banker BQ, editors: *Myology,* New York, 1986, McGraw-Hill; p 1871.

36. Larew RE: Malignant hyperthermia: quick recognition and treatment to avoid death, *Postgrad Med* 85:117, 1989.

CHAPTER 63

Movement Disorders

•

Mitchell Steinschneider

Movement disorders are a diverse group of nervous system diseases characterized by involuntary movements impinging upon normal motor functions. These movements include: chorea, athetosis, dystonia, ballismus, tremors, tics, and myoclonus (Box 63-1). Rigidity, akathesia (increased movements), akinesia (paucity of movements), and bradykinesia (slowed movements) are related abnormalities. Except for tic disorders and movement abnormalities produced by drugs (especially neuroleptics), which are commonly seen in the adolescent population, involuntary movements caused by other genetic or acquired diseases range from infrequent to very rare. Once a movement disorder is identified that is not tic related or drug induced, however, a thorough investigation of all potential causes, including rare inborn errors of metabolism, must be performed.

BASAL GANGLIA ANATOMY AND PHYSIOLOGY

An appreciation of basal ganglia structure and function is helpful in understanding mechanisms underlying movement disorders. The basal ganglia make up a group of paired subcortical structures. The main input structure of the basal ganglia is the striatum, which is divided into

---

BOX 63-1
Definition of Movement Abnormalities

Chorea: rapid and nonrhythmic involuntary movements that flow from one to another

Athetosis: slow, writhing movements usually present with chorea (choreoathetosis)

Ballismus: violent movements of a limb

Dystonia: abnormal posturing of a body part

Tremor: oscillating movements of a body part

Tic: brief, stereotyped, and purposeless movements or vocalizations

Myoclonus: brief, shocklike muscle jerks

Rigidity: increased tone throughout a muscle group's range of motion

Akathesia: increased movements produced by a subjective feeling of restlessness

Akinesia (hypokinesia): decreased amount of movements

Bradykinesia: slowness of movements

---

two components called the caudate and the putamen. The principal remaining structures of the basal ganglia are the globus pallidus, substantia nigra, and subthalamus.

Intricate neuronal circuits connecting the basal ganglia, cerebral cortex, and thalamus are involved in the initiation and control of complex motor functions (Fig. 63-1).[1] The striatum receives massive excitatory input from the cerebral cortex. Different regions of cortex project to specific locations in the striatum, initiating complex loops of neuronal activity. One major loop begins with projections from the putamen to both the external and internal divisions of the globus pallidus. The external division projects to the subthalamus, which in turn sends its output back to both divisions of the globus pallidus. The internal division connects with the ventrolateral and ventroanterior nuclei of the thalamus, which completes the loop by projecting to multiple regions of frontal and motor cortex. The second major neuronal loop is initiated by caudate projections to the pars reticularis division of the substantia nigra, which in turn sends input back to the striatum by way of neurons in the pars compacta. Both circuits use an array of neurotransmitters for synaptic transmission. Glutamate serves as the principal excitatory neurotransmitter, while γ-aminobutyric acid (GABA) is the major inhibitory neurotransmitter. Outputs from the cortex, thalamus, and subthalamus are excitatory; striatal and globus pallidus outputs are inhibitory. Clinically significant pharmacologic manipulations affecting basal ganglia function involve compounds altering synaptic relations between the substantia nigra and striatum (*dotted box* in Fig. 63-1). Intrinsic striatal circuits use interneurons containing acetylcholine for synaptic transmission. The substantia nigra input to the striatum uses dopamine as its neurotransmitter, which has both excitatory and inhibitory effects on the caudate and putamen. The functional activity of acetylcholine and dopamine can be loosely thought of as being in antagonistic balance. For example, disorders that decrease substantia nigra function, epitomized by Parkinson's disease, can be treated by either increasing dopaminergic transmission (e.g., L-dopa) or decreasing striatal function

with anticholinergic compounds (e.g., diphenhydramine). Inversely, drugs that block dopaminergic transmission, such as the neuroleptic compound haloperidol, induce a parkinsonian state that can be countered by an anticholinergic agent. Disorders that decrease striatal function, exemplified by Huntington's disease, can be treated by restoring balance between the substantia nigra and striatum using neuroleptics. Drugs that affect GABAergic or glutamergic activities may also improve movement abnormalities.

DIAGNOSIS

Classification of abnormal movements is often difficult, yet is crucial for arriving at a correct diagnosis and instituting appropriate therapy. Detailed observation of the patient is needed to accurately describe the movements. Home videotapes may be invaluable in providing prolonged observation of the patient during daily activities. Consideration of the various diseases associated with a specific movement abnormality facilitates proper diagnosis. This chapter therefore groups these diseases according to the most prominent movement abnormality noted. Overlap of movement abnormalities is frequently observed in a given disease, making this grouping only a guideline for a patient's evaluation.

CHOREA, ATHETOSIS, AND BALLISMUS

Chorea consists of quick, nonrhythmic, and involuntary movements that are often incorporated into voluntary actions. This may give the appearance of a constant flow of motion, with one movement leading into another. Classic signs of chorea include the "milkmaid" sign, present when a "milking" action interferes with a patient's constant grip on the examiner's fingers. Athetosis is a slow, usually distal, writhing movement and is frequently associated with chorea (choreoathe-

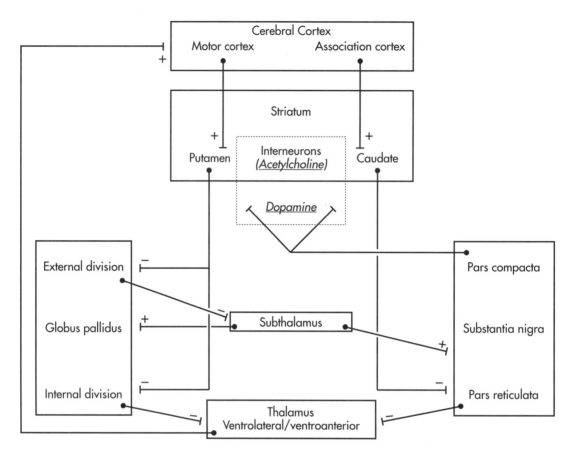

Fig. 63-1. Schematic representation of the major anatomical connections of the basal ganglia. The excitatory transmitter is glutamate and the inhibitory transmitter is α-aminobutyric acid (GABA). The basal ganglia is involved in complex loops of synaptic processing that begins with cortical input into the striatum (caudate and putamen), is followed by both serial and parallel excitatory and inhibitory connections intrinsic to the basal ganglia that finally modify thalamic activity, and ends with feedback from the thalamus back to the cortex. The most frequently used pharmacologic manipulations of these loops modify the activity of acetylcholine-containing interneurons in the striatum, and the dopaminergic pathway from the pars compacta division of the substantia nigra to the striatum *(dotted box)*.

tosis). Isolated athetosis is generally caused by perinatal injury (e.g., athetoid cerebral palsy caused by neonatal kernicterus or asphyxia). Ballismus is the violent flinging of a limb. It is usually unilateral in adults and is classically associated with a structural lesion of the contralateral subthalamus. In contrast, ballismus in children is most often an exaggerated form of chorea. Some selective causes that may produce choreoathetoid movements and their laboratory evaluation are listed in Box 63-2.

Genetic Disorders

HUNTINGTON'S DISEASE. Huntington's disease is a degenerative disorder characterized by progressive chorea, dementia, and psychiatric symptoms that usually begins in midadult life.[2-4] It is an autosomal dominant disorder with complete penetrance produced by an unusually long and unstable trinucleotide (CAG) repeat sequence on a gene residing on the short arm of chromosome 4. Repeat sequences longer than 37 are associated with the disease. There is an inverse relationship between the age of onset and the length of the trinucleotide repeat sequence. The neuropathologic hallmark of the disorder is degeneration of the caudate.

Juvenile Huntington's disease occurs in about 10% of patients, usually in the teenage years. These patients have the longest trinucleotide repeat sequences, and because the paternally derived DNA is more unstable, their disease is usually transmitted by the father. In contrast to the adult form of the disease, chorea is not a prominent symptom. Rigidity and rapidly progressive dementia are hallmarks of juvenile-onset disease. Psychiatric symptoms, seizures, gait abnormalities, tremor, and dysarthria are additional features of the disorder. Disease progression is more rapid than in the adult form, and death usually occurs within a decade.

Diagnosis is based on a family history of Huntington's disease, the patient's clinical constellation, and direct DNA testing that measures the length of the trinucleotide

---

BOX 63-2
Selective Causes of Choreoathetosis and Laboratory Analysis

Genetic causes
  Huntington's disease (rigidity in young patient)
  Fahr's disease
  Hallervorden-Spatz disease
  Paroxysmal dyskinesias (kinesigenic and nonkinesigenic)
  Wilson's disease
  Neuroacanthocytosis
Drugs
  Neuroleptics (acute and chronic)
  Stimulants
  Anticonvulsants
  Metaclopramide
  Antihistamines
  Lithium
  Birth control pills
Systemic causes
  Hyperthyroidism
  Systemic lupus erythematosus
  Sydenham's chorea
  Chorea gravidarum (consider systemic lupus erythematosus or Sydenham's chorea)

Hyperparathyroidism
Hypoparathyroidism (also pseudohypoparathyroidism and pseudopseudohypoparathyroidism)
Structural basal ganglia pathology

LABORATORY ANALYSIS (TEST: DISORDER)
Toxicology screen: drug ingestion
Ceruloplasmin/urinary copper excretion: Wilson's disease
EEG: rule out seizures for paroxysmal dyskinesias
MRI/CT scan of head: structural, metabolic, degenerative disorders
Erythrocyte sedimentation rate/antinuclear antibody level: systemic lupus erythematosus
Antistreptolysin O/anti-DNAse B titers: Sydenham's chorea
Serum calcium, phosphate, parathormone: parathyroid dysfunction
Thyroid function tests: hyperthyroidism
Blood acanthocytes: neuroacanthocytosis

Modified from Weiner WJ, Lang AE: *Movement disorders, a comprehensive survey,* Mt Kisco, NY, 1989, Futura.
CT, computed tomography; *EEG,* electroencephalography; *MRI,* magnetic resonance imaging.

---

repeat sequence. Neuroimaging studies classically reveal atrophy of the caudate nucleus, with additional cortical atrophy in patients with juvenile-onset disease. Therapy has been without lasting benefit and may exacerbate disabilities. For instance, neuroleptics can reduce chorea and some psychological symptoms, but parkinsonian and dementing symptoms may worsen. Drugs such as L-dopa (Sinemet) may improve rigidity yet exacerbate chorea and psychological difficulties. Counseling is necessary for at-risk presymptomatic family members, and is especially important with the advent of definitive DNA testing.[5]

CALCIFICATION OF THE BASAL GANGLIA (FAHR'S DISEASE). A number of movement disorders are characterized by calcifications within the basal ganglia. These diopathic familial disorders have been termed Fahr's disease, or bilateral symmetric striopallidodentate calcinosis, and tend to be inherited as autosomal dominant traits.[6-8] Calcifications may also be observed in the cerebellum, cerebral cortex, thalamus, and white matter. Onset of symptoms varies widely from early childhood through adulthood. Some patients have calcifications without clinical symptoms. Chorea, dystonia, dysarthria, and dysphagia are common. Diagnosis is made from the family history, clinical symptoms, radiographic findings, and exclusion of other disorders characterized by basal ganglia calcifications. Therapy beyond symptomatic

treatment, including Ca^{++} chelation, has been unsuccessful.

The rare occurrence of Fahr's disease mandates that more frequent causes of basal ganglia calcifications and dysfunction be excluded.[9] Abnormalities of Ca^{++} metabolism, including hyperparathyroidism, hypoparathyroidism, pseudohypoparathyroidism, and pseudopseudohypoparathyroidism, are all associated with basal ganglia calcifications. The latter two disorders are caused by the kidney's inability to respond to parathormone and are differentiated on the basis of serum Ca^{++} levels. They are congenital disorders with systemic signs that include short stature, rounded facies, and shortened fourth and fifth metacarpals. Tests to exclude disorders of Ca^{++} metabolism should include serum Ca^{++}, phosphate, and parathormone levels; slit-lamp examination for cataracts; and radiographic evaluation. Treatment of the endocrinologic imbalance can improve neurologic dysfunction. Other disorders with basal ganglia calcifications but not associated with Ca^{++} metabolism include tuberous sclerosis, AIDS, parainfectious processes, birth anoxia, carbon monoxide poisoning, and mitochondrial disease.

HALLERVORDEN-SPATZ DISEASE. Hallervorden-Spatz disease is a rare, progressively fatal, autosomal recessive disorder whose pathologic hallmark is massive iron deposition and degeneration within the globus pallidus and substantia nigra.[10-12] Onset is in childhood or adolescence with progressive choreoathetosis, dystonia, dysarthria, and rigidity. Dementia, seizures, spastic quadriparesis, and retinitis pigmentosa are frequent accompanying signs. Diagnosis is supported by characteristic, albeit nonspecific, magnetic resonance imaging (MRI) findings of decreased signal intensities in the globus pallidus, with a central area of increased signal on T2-weighted images ("eye-of-the-tiger" sign). Sea-blue histiocytes may be present in the bone marrow. Treatment is symptomatic. Iron chelating agents are not beneficial.

NEUROACANTHOCYTOSIS. Neuroacanthocytosis (choreoacanthocytosis) is a rare genetic disorder characterized by chorea, dystonia, tics, muscle weakness due to a myopathy, seizures, and behavioral changes.[2,13] Neuroimaging studies reveal bilateral atrophy of the caudate nucleus. Diagnosis rests on the demonstration of acanthocytes in peripheral blood smears. Incubation of the blood in saline or preparation in ethylenediaminetetraacetic acid (EDTA) for acanthocyte formation may be required in some patients.

HEREDITARY PAROXYSMAL DYSKINESIAS. Attacks of abnormal movements without altered consciousness or other evidence of seizure activity are the hallmarks of these disorders.[2,14,15] Paroxysmal kinesigenic choreoathetosis consists of brief episodes of chorea or dystonic posturing precipitated by sudden movements. Many attacks can occur in a single day. The movements can be focal or generalized and severe enough to precipitate falls. An aura may precede an attack. Paroxysms can occasionally be suppressed. Onset is in the first two decades of life, and the disorder tends to resolve over years. Neurologic examination results are normal. The disorder may be familial or sporadic. Anticonvulsants such as phenytoin or carbamazepine are useful in diminishing the attacks. Multiple sclerosis; head trauma; perinatal asphyxia; and abnormalities in glucose, electrolyte, and endocrinologic balance have also been associated with the disorder.

Paroxysmal dystonic choreoathetosis is a nonkinesigenic paroxysmal syndrome, usually of autosomal dominant inheritance, in which attacks either spontaneously occur or are precipitated by alcohol, coffee, tea, stress, or excitement.[2,16,17] Attacks generally begin in early childhood, are more prolonged than the kinesigenic variety, and occur less frequently. There is also more pronounced dystonic posturing instead of choreoathetosis. In contrast to the kinesigenic form, routine anticonvulsants are ineffective. Benzodiazepines offer the best relief.

Drug-Induced Chorea

Drugs are a frequent cause of chorea in adolescence.[9,18-20] Stimulants, cocaine, and metoclopramide are commonly cited offending agents. Acute dystonic reactions after the start of neuroleptic therapy occasionally include choreic components, especially of the face. Neuroleptics also acutely produce increased abnormal movements by inducing akathisia, a subjective feeling of restlessness. It is frequently mistaken for an increase in psychotic agitation, which might respond to increased medication, whereas the treatment of akathisia is a dose reduction. Oral contraceptives have also been an infrequent cause of chorea. Many of these women have had chorea from other etiologies in the past, especially Sydenham's chorea or systemic lupus erythmatosis (SLE), indicating that greater vigilance is required in these patients when they are placed on oral contraceptives. The chorea dissipates after withdrawal of the hormone. Other drugs rarely evoking chorea include tricyclic antidepressants, lithium, antihistamines, and benzodiazepines. Choreic movements may also be rarely precipitated by all the major anticonvulsant drugs.[21-25]

TARDIVE DYSKINESIA. Tardive dyskinesia is a choreic movement disorder caused by prolonged (>3 months) use of dopamine blocking agents such as neuroleptics.[26,27] Orofacial movements are the rule. Fine movements of the tongue are early signs, followed by an insidious progression of more pronounced tongue and other facial movements such as chewing, teeth clenching, and lip smacking. Other body motions such as "piano-playing" movements of the fingers, rocking, and pelvic thrusting may be seen. Movements are exacerbated by stress and abate with sleep. Increasing doses of the offending agent may mask symptoms. Tardive tics, dystonia, akathisia, and myoclonus also occur after prolonged neuroleptic therapy. While less common in young patients, children and adolescents are still at risk for developing tardive dyskinesia, especially with higher doses, more prolonged drug exposure, and neurologic dysfunction.[28,29] The risk in a 20-year-old is estimated at 10% after 2 years of neuroleptic exposure and 18% after 4 years of exposure.[30] A temporary tardive syndrome that occurs upon tapering neuroleptics, and lasts up to several months, is called withdrawal dyskinesia. Timely diagnosis rests upon careful serial observations of the patient, with special attention to tongue movements. This may be especially difficult in the psychotic patient whose behavior includes stereotypic movements. Therapy begins with discontinuation of the drug. Remission usually occurs in the young, although several years may be required. Benzodiazepines may be useful in selected patients, if only to decrease anxiety that might exacerbate the movements. Dopamine-depleting agents such as tetrabenazine or reserpine may help the most severely affected patients. Studies in recent years support the use of vitamin E for treating tardive dyskinesia.[31,32]

Systemic Disorders

Endocrine abnormalities. Chorea is an uncommon manifestation of hyperthyroidism.[33] Nevertheless, it is incumbent upon the physician to assess thyroid function in patients with chorea, because the abnormal movements resolve when the individual becomes euthyroid. Tremor is a much more common movement disorder associated with hyperthyroidism. Parathyroid dysfunction and electrolyte abnormalities may also elicit chorea.[2]

Systemic lupus erythematosus. Chorea is a well-described complication of SLE.[2,34,35] The diagnosis may be problematic because chorea can present as the initial manifestation of SLE, and characteristic laboratory findings may be absent at this time. Patients are often misdiagnosed as having Sydenham's chorea until additional evidence of SLE becomes apparent. Chorea as a manifestation of SLE is most common in adolescent women. The abnormal movements remit with steroid therapy, but relapses may occur. A role for antiphospholipid antibodies in the pathogenesis of chorea in patients with SLE and other disorders (e.g., primary antiphospholipid syndrome, cancer) has been postulated.[36,37] Strokes and other structural abnormalities of the basal ganglia must also be considered as a cause of chorea in these patients.

Sydenham's chorea. Sydenham's chorea is one of the major Jones criteria for the diagnosis of rheumatic fever, which remains a major health concern given its resurgence in many parts of the United States.[38-40] Diagnosis may be hampered by the frequent absence of other manifestations of rheumatic fever (e.g., carditis, arthritis, rash, subcutaneous nodules), a history of recent streptococcal pharyngitis in only one third of patients, and a prolonged 1- to 6-month latency of chorea after the pharyngitis. This latency often diminishes associated rises in streptococcal antibody titers. Correct diagnosis is needed, because one third of patients with Sydenham's chorea develop late-onset valvular disease of the heart if prophylactic antibiotic therapy is not instituted.

The cardinal signs of the disorder are chorea, emotional lability, and hypotonia. The chorea may be unilateral or generalized. Dysarthria and dystonic posturing may also be seen. The hypotonia may be severe, be associated with muscle weakness, and interfere with postural stability. Psychiatric symptoms include emotional lability, an organic confusional state, restlessness, diminished attention span, obsessive-compulsive behaviors, nightmares, and separation anxiety disorder. Gradual improvement of the chorea occurs over several months. Recurrences of the chorea may occur without other manifestations of rheumatic fever. Elaboration of antineuronal antibodies in response to streptococcal infection has been postulated as a cause of the chorea. MRI of the brain may demonstrate transient abnormalities in the basal ganglia, presumably reflecting a focal inflammatory response.[41] Elevations of antistreptococcal antibody titers are useful in supporting the diagnosis of Sydenham's chorea, but many patients have no associated titer increase. Elevations of acute-phase reactants are also unreliable indicators of disease. Thus, when the diagnosis is in doubt, caution dictates long-term prophylactic antibiotic therapy. One should also consider the diagnosis of SLE when no other rheumatic symptoms are present. Therapy for the chorea itself is usually not required. When the movements are severe enough to interfere with activities of daily living, treatment with benzodiazepines, neuroleptics, or valproate may be helpful.

Chorea gravidarum. Chorea is a rare complication of pregnancy. Its occurrence should precipitate an evaluation for an underlying cause, as many women with this disorder have SLE or a reactivation of Sydenham's chorea.[9,42,43]

Structural Basal Ganglia Pathology

Structural abnormalities of the basal ganglia can elicit choreoathetoid movements. Lesions produced by metabolic derangements (e.g., kernicterus, neonatal hypoxia) often evoke bilateral movements such as athetosis. In contrast, lesions such as mass lesions or strokes usually affect one hemisphere, eliciting unilateral movement abnormalities such as hemiballismus or hemichorea. A neuroimaging study should be undertaken to exclude these pathologic entities. Unilateral chorea may also be seen in Sydenham's chorea and SLE. Trauma, anoxia, status epilepticus, and complications of cardiac surgery have all been associated with the development of chorea.[44]

DYSTONIA

Dystonia is characterized by prolonged muscle spasms that position axial structures and limbs into abnormal postures. It is produced by simultaneous contractions of agonist and antagonist muscles. When the abnormal muscle activity is balanced, a dystonic posture results. Imbalance of the abnormal muscle activity elicits dystonic movements, which are often slow and repetitive. A classic dystonic posture is "spooning," a flexion of the wrists and hyperextension of the metacarpophalangeal joints best seen when the arms are extended. Dystonia is divided into four categories based on the extent of the abnormality. Focal dystonia involves only a single body part (e.g., torticollis). Progressively greater involvement is termed segmental, multifocal, or generalized dystonia. Hemidystonia involves an arm and leg on the same body side and warrants a search for a structural abnormality affecting the contralateral basal ganglia. The differential

---

BOX 63-3
Selective Causes of Dystonia

Genetic dystonia
  Idiopathic torsion dystonia
  Paroxysmal dyskinesia
  Wilson's disease
  Dopa-responsive dystonia
  Mitochondrial disease
  Hallervorden-Spatz disease
  Fahr's disease
Acquired dystonia
  Focal basal ganglia pathology (hemidystonia)
  Perinatal brain injury (athetoid cerebral palsy)
  Anoxia, carbon monoxide
  Postencephalitic
  Drugs
Psychiatric
Focal dystonia
  Isolated torticollis (structural lesions of cervical
  spine, spinal cord, base of brain or neck; hi-
  atal hernia; extraocular muscle dysfunction;
  idiopathic)

Modified from Weiner WJ, Lang AE: *Movement disorders, a comprehensive survey,* Mt Kisco, NY, 1989, Futura.

---

diagnosis of dystonia is extensive and summarized in Box 63-3. A brief description of important points in the evaluation and therapy of dystonia is given in Box 63-4.

Genetic Disorders

IDIOPATHIC TORSION DYSTONIA (DYSTONIA MUSCU-LORUM DEFORMANS). This fascinating disorder represents a genetically heterogeneous group of disorders characterized by dystonic postures and movements without other neurologic or intellectual abnormalities, without a medical history pointing to a cause for the dystonia, and without abnormal laboratory findings (e.g., normal copper metabolism, MRI). Most patients have an autosomal dominant pattern of inheritance with incomplete penetrance due to mutations of a gene on the long arm of chromosome 9.[45,46] There is a predilection for this disorder in Ashkenazi Jews. Different mutations of the chromosome 9 dystonia gene are responsible for the disorder in the Jewish and non-Jewish populations.

Clinically, torsion dystonia can be clinically segregated into two broad groups.[9,47] In the first group, onset is in childhood or adolescence. Dystonia usually begins in the legs or arms, tends to progress and generalize within a decade, and has the poorest prognosis for preserved motor function. Leg dystonia frequently begins as plantar flexion and inversion of the feet, producing gait disturbances. Occasionally, the gait abnormality is bizarre and difficult to characterize. Odd findings such as an improve-

---

BOX 63-4
Evaluation and Treatment of Dystonia

HISTORY
Acute onset: drug ingestion (especially neurolep-
  tics, if hyperthermia and rigidity, assume malig-
  nant neuroleptic syndrome)
Intermittent attacks: rule out seizures, hereditary
  paroxysmal dyskinesia, diurnal variation
  (dystonia-Parkinsonism syndrome)
Chronic dystonia
  Family history
  Perinatal history (hypoxia, kernicterus)
  Chronic exposure to neuroleptics: tardive dys-
  tonia
  Other neurologic, psychiatric, or hepatic symp-
  toms

PHYSICAL
Kayser-Fleischer rings: Wilson's disease (need slit-
  lamp examination)
Complete ophthalmologic examination: optic atro-
  phy suggests mitochondrial disease
Other neurologic signs: rule out idiopathic torsion
  dystonia
Hemidystonia: consider structural lesion
Parkinsonian signs (dopa-responsive dystonia)

LABORATORY ANALYSIS
Toxicology screen: acute dystonia
EEG: rule out seizures, especially for intermittent
  symptoms
MRI/CT of head: rule out mass lesion; bilateral le-
  sions common in metabolic or degenerative
  disease (low-density MRI lesions of basal gan-
  glia suggest Hallervorden-Spatz disease)
Ceruloplasmin: Wilson's disease
Urinary copper excretion: Wilson's disease
Serum lactate/pyruvate: mitochondrial disease
MRI/CT/radiography of cervical region: for iso-
  lated torticollis

THERAPY
Acute dystonia: parenteral diphenhydramine
Wilson's disease: penicillamine, trientine, zinc,
  ammonium tetrathiomolybdate
Paroxysmal dyskinesia: anticonvulsants, benzodi-
  azepines
Chronic dystonia: trihexiphenidyl (L-dopa
  [Sinemet] as initial trial therapy)

CT, computed tomography; *EEG,* electroencephalography; *MRI,* magnetic resonance imaging.

---

ment of gait with running or walking backward can be seen. As expected, psychiatric pathology is often the leading misdiagnosis, which is sometimes supported by unexplained remissions that may last for years. In the second group, onset is in adulthood and the condition is more often focal, usually presents with isolated hand and arm abnormalities (e.g., writer's cramp) or dystonia of the neck and trunk, has a lesser likelihood for progression, and a more favorable long-term prognosis.

Therapy is symptomatic.[48] Anticholinergics, such as trihexyphenidyl (Artane), at high doses ameliorate the dystonia in most young patients. Medication is well tolerated if started at a low dose and slowly increased. Central anticholinergic side effects may be troublesome and include memory dysfunction, personality change, and sleep alterations. Other useful drugs include benzodiazepines, carbamazepine, tetrabenazine, and neuroleptics. The use of dopaminergic agents is discussed under the next disorder. Local injections of botulinum toxin into selected dystonic muscles producing severe disability may be extremely beneficial.[49] A few patients may be candidates for surgical intervention at specialized centers.

DOPA-RESPONSIVE DYSTONIA. A subset of patients with childhood-onset dystonia have a syndrome incorporating parkinsonian features (rigidity, masked facies, tremor, postural instability, bradykinesia, and a stooped, shuffling gait).[50] This syndrome is a specific genetic disorder characterized by autosomal dominant transmission with incomplete penetrance. Some members of affected families may present in adult life with clinical parkinsonism without dystonia. Diurnal variation in symptoms is characteristic. The striking aspect of this dystonic syndrome is its responsiveness to antiparkinsonian drugs such as L-dopa. An abnormality in the synthesis of dopamine, or a deficiency in the connectivity of cells in the substantia nigra with the striatum, has been suggested as the pathophysiologic mechanism underlying this disorder.[51] Because it may not be possible to clinically differentiate idiopathic torsion dystonia from this syndrome at onset, a trial of a dopaminergic agent (e.g., L-dopa) is recommended for all cases of idiopathic childhood-onset dystonia.

WILSON'S DISEASE. Fatal when unrecognized, this rare but treatable autosomal recessive storage disorder must always be considered in younger individuals with a movement, psychiatric, or liver disorder of unexplained cause, or in relatives of patients with Wilson's disease. The genetic defect is located on the long arm of chromosome 13.[52-54] The gene codes for a copper-transporting ATPase enzyme with homology to a similar protein defective in X-linked Menkes' disease. Interestingly, both diseases reflect abnormal cellular transport of copper. In Wilson's disease, the apparent defect in transport impedes elimination of excess copper. Multiple genetic mutations have been identified and partially determine the wide phenotypic variability of Wilson's disease.

Extremely varied clinical manifestations are due to abnormal storage deposits of copper in the brain, liver, kidney, and cornea.[9,55-57] Onset is usually in the latter half of the first decade, during adolescence or early adulthood.

Patients are frequently misdiagnosed at clinical presentation by months to years, needlessly postponing life-saving therapy. Liver dysfunction tends to occur earlier than neurologic problems. In some, an acute hepatitis that resolves without permanent sequelae precedes neurologic dysfunction, indicating the need to question patients concerning previous liver abnormalities. Others suffer from chronic or fulminant forms of liver disease. The combination of hepatitis and hemolytic anemia is very suggestive of Wilson's disease. Neuropathologic degeneration within the brain is especially prominent in the basal ganglia, evoking the movement disorders characteristic of the disease. Additional lesions are noted in the subcortical white matter, cerebellum, thalamus, and brain stem. Neurologic problems usually begin with tremors, dystonia, dysarthria, incoordination, or gait ataxia. The classic tremor is a "wing beating" of the arms, although it is not present in most patients. Dysarthria is very common, is often accompanied by drooling, and may progress to total inability to speak (anarthria). When the condition is severe, dysphagia also occurs. Parkinsonian symptoms and chorea may also be seen, making Wilson's disease a potential cause of nearly all forms of movement disorders. Psychiatric presentations are almost as common as neurologic abnormalities. They range from mood disturbances and personality change to manic-depressive states and schizophrenia. Renal tubular dysfunction is another complication of Wilson's disease. The diagnosis of Wilson's disease is supported by diminished serum levels of the copper-containing protein ceruloplasmin, an increase in urinary copper excretion, and the presence of Kayser-Fleischer rings, which are greenish-brown deposits of copper around the limbus of the cornea. While Kayser-Fleischer rings are pathognomonic for neurologic involvement in Wilson's disease, they may either not be present or require slit-lamp examination by an experienced observer. Before the start of therapy, liver biopsy should be performed to demonstrate increased storage of copper.

Therapy consists of chelation for the lifetime of the patient.[58,59] Noncompliance, even after years of successful therapy, will result in clinical deterioration and death. Increased urinary excretion of copper can be used to monitor treatment effectiveness and patient compliance. Therapy should also be extended to include asymptomatic patients, because a chronic drug regimen can prevent the appearance of symptoms. High copper-containing foods (shellfish, liver, nuts, chocolate, mushrooms) should also be avoided. Classically, daily oral D-penicillamine has been used for chelation. Patients occasionally worsen after treatment onset, probably reflecting mobilization of copper stores. Unfortunately, some of these patients do not regain pretreatment functions. Penicillamine therapy may also precipitate side effects severe enough to at least temporarily halt therapy. These include nephrotic syndrome, proteinuria, bone marrow suppression, rash, fever, lymphadenopathy, and collagen disease–like reactions. Many of these can be treated by adding steroids to a reinitiated therapy. A pyridoxine-responsive anemia may also occur. If severe side effects persist, other chelating treatments such as trientine or zinc may be used. Ammonium tetrathiomolybdate has been advocated as an effective chelator that is safer than penicillamine.[60]

MITOCHONDRIAL DISEASE. Multiple different clinical syndromes caused by abnormalities of mitochondrial function have been associated with dystonia. One variety is characterized by childhood- or adolescent-onset dystonia associated with progressive, nonpainful visual loss.[61] The dystonia and visual loss may occur in the same patient or separately in different family members. The visual loss is associated with optic atrophy and is termed Leber's optic atrophy. Leigh's syndrome is another mitochondrial disorder that may manifest movement disorders, especially dystonia, as a prominent symptom.[62] Bilaterally symmetric abnormalities of the basal ganglia on neuroimaging studies are characteristic of these metabolic disorders.

Acquired Disorders

Any brain damage affecting the basal ganglia can produce dystonia.[9,63,64] Causes include space-occupying lesions such as tumors or vascular malformations, strokes, trauma, and encephalopathy. The latter may be from hypoxic, infectious, or metabolic insults (e.g., neonatal kernicterus). Space-occupying lesions and those resulting from trauma most commonly produce hemidystonia. Many of these disorders produce dystonia during the acute or subacute periods of the illness. However, encephalopathies and trauma can present with progressive dystonia years after the insult. The static encephalopathy causing adolescent-onset dystonia can occur from a distant neonatal event that left the patient with little or no neurologic deficits before the onset of dystonia.

Drug-Induced Dystonia

Dystonic reactions are a frequent complication of neuroleptic use in the early phase of therapy.[9,20] These acute dystonic reactions can involve any part of the body but most commonly affect muscles of the eyes, face, throat, and neck. Common reactions include torticollis, facial grimacing, tongue twisting, involuntary eye closure (blepharospasm), oculogyric crisis (forced eye deviation), and limb posturing. Therapy involves drug withdrawal and parenteral administration of an antihistamine such as diphenhydramine. When neuroleptic treatment must be continued, lowered doses or coadministration of an anticholinergic such as benztropine may be effective. Other medications producing an acute

dystonic reaction include metoclopramide and anticonvulsants. Prolonged use of neuroleptics may also produce a persistent dystonia that is a variant of tardive dyskinesia (tardive dystonia).

Neuroleptics produce two additional movement disorders of clinical significance.[20] The first is parkinsonism, and the drug-induced form may display all the classic disease features (akinesia, bradykinesia, shuffling gait with decreased arm swing, rigidity, tremor, postural instability, masklike facies). This effect is a result of the compounds' blockade of dopamine receptors and their interference with normal, dopamine-mediated synaptic transmission from the substantia nigra to the striatum. Dosage reduction or anticholinergic medications may be clinically beneficial. The second movement-related disorder is the neuroleptic malignant syndrome. The hallmarks of this potentially lethal complication (20% mortality rate) are hyperthermia, rigidity and akinesia, altered mental status, and autonomic instability. Seizures and other neurologic signs may develop. Leukocytosis and serum elevations of liver enzymes and creatine kinase from muscle may be seen. The latter indicates muscle damaged by the extreme contractions of rigidity. Rhabdomyolysis may precipitate renal failure. The disorder is an idiosyncratic response to neuroleptic therapy. Therapy includes dantrolene (a muscle relaxant) and bromocriptine (a dopamine agonist). Both drugs reduce the intense muscle contractions and therefore lessen hyperthermia, metabolic demands, and the risk of renal dysfunction. Neuroleptic malignant syndrome has been reported in adolescents, making its recognition incumbent upon caregivers in contact with children administered these drugs.[65]

Focal Dystonia

Focal dystonias are uncommon before adulthood and are usually the first manifestation of a more generalized dystonic process.[9] Of the four major locations for focal dystonia (face, neck, trunk, hand), torticollis in the neck is of the greatest importance in adolescence. A twisted neck may represent an isolated variant of idiopathic torsion dystonia. It can be successfully treated with intramuscular injections of botulinum toxin. Multiple structural lesions can also produce a contorted neck. Other important causes of neck tilt include cervical spine and spinal cord abnormalities, posterior fossa tumors, extraocular muscle palsies (especially from fourth cranial nerve dysfunction), local muscle trauma, and lymph node inflammation. Intermittent torticollis may rarely be associated with a hiatal hernia (Sandifer's syndrome), is exacerbated by eating, and is cured when the hernia is repaired.[66] Its onset is usually in the first decade, but patients may seek to medical attention while in their teens.

TREMOR

Tremor is an involuntary, rhythmic, and oscillating movement of a body part.[67,68] It should be characterized according to whether it occurs at rest, with maintenance of a posture, or with action. A normal, low-amplitude physiologic tremor can often be seen with the arms extended (postural tremor). It is accentuated by stress, exercise, fatigue, excitement, and several drugs (e.g., adrenergic agents, methylxanthines, caffeine, nicotine, steroids, lithium, tricyclic antidepressants, valproate). Fever, thyrotoxicosis, pheochromocytoma, hypoglycemia, Wilson's disease, heavy metal poisoning, and drug and alcohol withdrawal are other important causes of tremor. Tremor at rest suggests a parkinsonian state such as produced by neuroleptic use.

A common cause of action tremor is an autosomal dominant disorder termed essential tremor, which is a postural tremor that may be accentuated by movement. Its onset is often in adolescence and most frequently affects fine use of the hands, usually in the form of impaired handwriting. It is enhanced by fatigue or stress and relieved by even small amounts of alcohol. In contrast to the oscillations produced by cerebellar disease, the movements do not become worse at the end point (not dysmetric), and there are no other signs referable to cerebellar dysfunction. Abnormal signs other than tremor are not consistent with the diagnosis of essential tremor and should lead to a search for other causes. Hyperthyroidism should be excluded. Propranolol and the anticonvulsant drug primidone are usually effective in controlling tremor.

TICS/TOURETTE'S SYNDROME

Tics are brief, stereotyped, and purposeless movements or vocalizations. The most important tic disorder is Tourette's syndrome, which is characterized by an onset at under 21 years of age, multiple motor tics, vocal tics, and duration greater than 1 year.[69,70] Additional features include a waxing and waning variability in tic severity over time, a changing tic repertoire over time, and ability to temporarily suppress the tics. It differs from the more common transient tic disorder of childhood by the latter's shorter duration (less than 1 year), usual absence of vocal tics, and milder symptoms. Motor tics usually involve the head or neck. Repetitive eye blinking or deviations, facial grimacing, nose twitching, lip smacking, head jerks, and shoulder shrugs are frequently observed. Vocal tics usually begin after motor tics. Most frequent are throat clearing, grunting, sniffing, coughing, barking, and hissing. Echolalia may occur. Despite its notoriety, coprolalia is uncommonly seen. Temporary suppression of tics inevitably leads to increasingly unpleasant sensations that abate only with performance of a tic. The average age of onset for Tourette's syndrome is 7 years. The long-term prognosis is favorable, most patients having a marked decrease in tic severity by late adolescence. There is an almost 10:1 increase in Tourette's syndrome in boys compared with girls.[71] Prevalence estimates in school-age boys average about 0.1%.

Recent research on Tourette's syndrome has focused on the genetic features of the disorder and the frequent association with comorbid conditions, suggesting similar molecular mechanisms of pathogenesis. Both autosomal dominant and more complex patterns of inheritance involving multiple genes have been proposed.[72,73] The latter form of genetic expression is supported by the hypothesis that Tourette's syndrome represents the more severe end of a spectrum generated by multiple gene interactions modulating basal ganglia development.[74] Findings that the normal basal ganglia asymmetry (dominant hemisphere larger) is often absent in patients with Tourette's syndrome support these ideas.[75,76]

One of the most important conditions associated with Tourette's syndrome is obsessive-compulsive disorder.[77] Obsessions are recurrent and unwelcome thoughts, such as violent or sexual ideations, or feelings of severe self-doubt or of being contaminated, that interfere with daily living. Compulsions are repetitive and often ritualistic behaviors that are usually in response to obsessions. Repetitive handwashing, checking, and counting are several more common compulsions. It is estimated that about 50% of patients with Tourette's syndrome have obsessive-compulsive behaviors. Obsessive-compulsive disorder is common in first-degree relatives of patients with Tourette's syndrome. Women relatives are at greatest risk, suggesting that the molecular abnormality manifests as tics in boys and obsessive-compulsive disorder in girls.

Attention-deficit hyperactivity disorder (ADHD) is seen in up to one half of patients with Tourette's syndrome, may be clinically more disabling than the tics, and often antedates the onset of tics.[72] Concerns that stimulant treatment of ADHD may greatly exacerbate tics, or precipitate Tourette's syndrome in the genetically predisposed, generally appear exaggerated.[78] Tics may occur, or severity may increase, however, in some patients receiving stimulants for ADHD.[79] Conduct disorder may be a major problem in patients with Tourette's syndrome. Other comorbid conditions include learning disabilities, affective disorders, and sleep problems. An association with autism has also been suggested.[80]

Diagnosis of Tourette's syndrome is strictly by clinical criteria. Ancillary tests are not revealing. Psychological and social counseling are often sufficient therapy. Pharmacologic therapy must be based on the degree of patient distress and disability, weighed against the potential development of significant side effects.[78] Neuroleptics, such as haloperidol or pimozide, are the predominant drugs used in treatment and ameliorate symptoms in up to 80% of patients. Side effects of neuroleptics include those already discussed in this chapter, as well as sedation (worse with haloperidol), impaired cognitive performance, irritability, weight gain, anticholinergic signs, and gynecomastia or lactation. Prolongation of the QT interval on the electrocardiogram has been observed with pimozide use. Although statistically less efficacious in reducing tics, clonidine has the added benefits of a reduced side effect profile and the ability to improve hyperactivity.[78,81] In certain situations, stimulants may be necessary to treat the ADHD. Care is required to use the smallest effective stimulant dose and to monitor for exacerbation of tics. The tricyclic antidepressants nortryptyline and desipramine have proved to be effective agents for patients with both Tourette's syndrome and ADHD, although concern for cardiotoxicity has limited their clinical use.[82,83]

MYOCLONUS

Myoclonus consists of brief, shocklike muscle jerks that arise from the central nervous system.[84,85] The jerks may be regular or arrhythmic and may be due to brief lapses of muscle contractions (negative myoclonus) as in asterixis. They may be spontaneous or occur in response to a stimulus (reflex myoclonus) or a movement (action myoclonus). At times, it is difficult to differentiate myoclonus from other abnormal movements. Tics may also consist of brief muscle jerks but can be distinguished from myoclonus by their ability to be temporarily controlled, the presence of a conscious urge to perform the tic, and the usual more complex nature of the movement. Chorea is a constant flow of ever-changing movements in different muscle groups, whereas myoclonus repeats the same muscle jerks. Tremor is a sinusoidal movement, whereas myoclonus has a more discontinuous quality.

The causes of myoclonus range from normal events to lethal diseases (Box 63-5). Myoclonus can be classified into five broad categories: physiologic, essential, epileptic, symptomatic, and segmental. Examples of normal, physiologic myoclonus include hiccups; sleep jerks; and jerks brought out by anxiety, exercise, or fatigue. Essential myoclonus is characterized by movements without other neurologic deficits, onset before 20 years of age, a generally benign course, a normal electroencephalographic (EEG) picture, and an autosomal dominant or sporadic inheritance pattern. Segmental myoclonus refers to myoclonus restricted to a limited number of contiguous muscle groups and is caused by focal brainstem or spinal cord pathology. Epileptic causes are those pathologic processes in which seizures dominate the clinical picture. The most prominent epileptic cause of myoclonus in adolescents is primary generalized epilepsy, with juvenile

---

BOX 63-5
Selected Causes of Myoclonus

1. Physiologic: sleep jerks, anxiety-induced, exercise-induced, hiccups
2. Essential (no other abnormality): hereditary, sporadic
3. Epileptic (seizures are dominant symptom)
   a. Fragments of epilepsy: isolated epileptic jerks, epilepsia partialis continua, idiopathic, stimulus-sensitive myoclonus, photosensitive myoclonus, myoclonic absences in petit mal
   b. Childhood myoclonic seizures: juvenile myoclonic epilepsy
4. Symptomatic
   a. Progressive myoclonic epilepsies: mitochondrial diseases (MERRF), Unverricht-Lundborg disease (Baltic myoclonus), Lafora body disease, neuronal ceroid-lipofuscinosis, sialidosis, dentatorubral-pallidoluysian atrophy
   b. Spinocerebellar degeneration
   c. Wilson's disease
   d. Viral encephalopathies: SSPE, herpes simplex, postinfectious, arbovirus
   e. Metabolic: hepatic failure, renal failure, dialysis syndrome, electrolyte abnormalities, hypoglycemia, hypothyroidism, posthypoxic, multiple vitamin deficiencies, multiple drugs and intoxications[85]
   f. Paraneoplastic from occult neuroblastoma
5. Segmental: focal brain or spinal cord lesion (infectious and multiple structural etiologies)[84]

MERRF, myoclonus epilepsy with ragged red fibers; *SSPE*, subacute sclerosing panencephalitis.

---

myoclonic epilepsy especially common in this age group. The myoclonic jerks tend to be worse upon awakening from sleep in the morning. Seizures may also be present in symptomatic myoclonus, but the most prominent symptom is an encephalopathy that is usually progressive.

Important adolescent causes of symptomatic myoclonus are the progressive myoclonic epilepsies (PMEs). Six major types have been defined: mitochondrial diseases (MERRF [myoclonus epilepsy with ragged red fibers]), Unverricht-Lundborg disease (Baltic myoclonus), Lafora body disease, neuronal ceroid-lipofuscinosis, sialidosis (cherry-red spot myoclonus syndrome), and dentatorubral-pallidoluysian atrophy. Nonspecific findings for PME include generalized spike and wave discharges on EEG, epileptic photosensitivity, and giant somatosensory evoked potentials. PME may be difficult to differentiate at disease onset from more benign causes, such as juvenile myoclonic epilepsy. Evaluation of PME is outlined in Box 63-6. Symp-

---

BOX 63-6
Evaluation of Progressive Myoclonic Epilepsy

Mitochondrial disease (MERRF)[88-90]
 Genetics: maternal inheritance, point mutations
  in mitochondrial DNA
 Core features: onset before adulthood with
  myoclonus, ataxia, myopathy, tonic-clonic
  seizures
 Additional signs: dementia, sensorineural hearing loss, short stature, and other clinical features suggestive of mitochondrial disease
 Diagnosis: elevated lactate/pyruvate (CSF and
  serum), muscle biopsy yields ragged-red fibers, abnormal oxidative phosphorylation
  biochemistry, and mutations in mitochondrial DNA
Unverricht-Lundborg disease (Baltic myoclonus)[91,92]
 Genetics: autosomal recessive, chromosome 21
 Core features: onset between 6 and 16 years
  with myoclonus, tonic-clonic seizures
 Additional signs: ataxia (dementia not prominent)
 Diagnosis: clinical, genetic linkage analysis, no
  routine definitive tests
Lafora body disease[91]
 Genetics: autosomal recessive
 Core features: onset in teens with myoclonus,
  early and severe dementia
 Additional signs: occipital and tonic-clonic sei-
  zures
 Diagnosis: skin biopsy revealing Lafora inclusion
  bodies in eccrine sweat glands
Neuronal ceroid lipofuscinosis[93,94]
 Genetics: a group of different genetic diseases
  with variable-onset age and chromosomal
  defects, all autosomal recessive

Core features (juvenile form): visual loss with
  optic atrophy and macular degeneration
  (retinitis pigmentosa), seizures, dementia
 Additional signs: myoclonus, rigidity
 Diagnosis: abnormal electroretinogram, elevated
  urinary dolichols (lysosomal membrane component), specific inclusion body patterns on
  skin biopsy or in lymphocytes
Sialidosis (cherry red spot–myoclonus syndrome)[84,91]
 Genetics: autosomal recessive
 Core features: myoclonus, progressive visual
  loss
 Additional signs: tonic-clonic seizures, ataxia,
  peripheral neuropathy, lens opacities (dementia is absent)
 Diagnosis: retinal cherry red spot, increased urinary sialyloligosaccharides, deficiency of lysosomal enzyme alpha-N-acetylneuramini-
  dase in leukocytes or cultured skin fibroblasts
Dentatorubral-pallidoluysian atrophy[95]
 Genetics: autosomal dominant, abnormally long
  trinucleotide DNA repeat sequence, chromosome 12
 Core features: myoclonus, tonic-clonic seizures,
  dementia
 Additional signs: ataxia, choreoathetosis
 Diagnosis: DNA analysis

CSF, cerebrospinal fluid; *MERRF*, myoclonus epilepsy with ragged red fibers.

---

tomatic therapy is best accomplished with sodium valproate or benzodiazepines.

Viral infections, such as herpes virus and arbovirus, are another major cause of symptomatic myoclonus in the adolescent. The most important viral infection that classically produces myoclonus is the chronic brain infection with measles, subacute sclerosing panencephalitis (SSPE).[86] A mutation of the virus occurs that inhibits production of the measles M or matrix protein necessary for viral release from host cells. Cell-to-cell spread of the virus slowly occurs over time in the brain. SSPE has an incidence of 1 per million cases of measles infection and generally begins between 5 and 15 years of age. Four stages have been described. Dementia and behavioral signs begin in stage I. Stage II is the unique phase of the disease, dominated by new-onset myoclonus and a

worsening of the previous deficits. The EEG during this stage is almost pathognomonic, containing periodic epileptiform complexes associated with the myoclonus. The myoclonus and characteristic EEG changes disappear in the later two stages, which are dominated by progressive neurologic deterioration leading to a vegetative state and death. Besides the stage II EEG changes, diagnosis is confirmed by the presence of elevated CSF IgG levels, CSF oligoclonal bands, a high CSF measles antibody titer, and viral inclusion bodies (Cowdry bodies) in neurons and glia obtained from brain biopsy. These inclusion bodies contain viral nucleocapsids. Treatment is largely symptomatic, and most patients die 1 to 3 years after disease onset. Combined therapy with intraventricular α-interferon and oral inosiplex may retard disease progression.[87]

References

1. Afifi AK: Basal ganglia: functional anatomy and physiology. Part 1, *J Child Neurol* 9:249-260, 1994.

2. Feigin A, Kieburtz K, Shoulson I: Treatment of Huntington's disease and other choreic disorders. In Kurlan R, editor: *Treatment of movement disorders,* Philadelphia, 1995, JB Lippincott; pp 337-364.

3. Furtado S, Suchowersky O: Huntington's disease: recent advances in diagnosis and management, *Can J Neurol Sci* 22:5-12, 1995.

4. Gusella JF, MacDonald ME, Ambrose CM, Duyao MP: Molecular genetics of Huntington's disease, *Arch Neurol* 50:1157-1163, 1993.

5. International Huntington Association and the World Federation of Neurology Research Group on Huntington's Chorea Committee: Guidelines for the molecular genetics predictive test in Huntington's disease, *Neurology* 44:1533-1536, 1994.

6. Ellie E, Julien J, Ferrer X: Familial idiopathic striopallidodentate calcifications, *Neurology* 39:381-385, 1989.

7. Larsen TA, Dunn HG, Jan JE, Calne DB: Dystonia and calcification of the basal ganglia, *Neurology* 35:533-537, 1985.

8. Manyam BV, Bhatt MH, Moore WD, et al: Bilateral striopallidodentate calcinosis: cerebrospinal fluid, imaging, and electrophysiological studies, *Ann Neurol* 31:379-384, 1992.

9. Weiner WJ, Lang AE: *Movement disorders, a comprehensive survey,* Mt Kisco, NY, 1989, Futura.

10. Angelini L, Nardocci N, Rumi V, et al: Hallervorden-Spatz disease: clinical and MRI study of 11 cases diagnosed in life, *J Neurol* 239:417-425, 1992.

11. Savoiardo M, Halliday WC, Nardocci N, et al: Hallervorden-Spatz disease: MR and pathologic findings, *Am J Neuroradiol* 14:155-162, 1993.

12. Swaiman KF: Hallervorden-Spatz syndrome and brain iron metabolism, *Arch Neurol* 48:1285-1293, 1991.

13. Feinberg TE, Cianci CD, Morrow JS, et al: Diagnostic tests for choreoacanthocytosis, *Neurology* 41:1000-1006, 1991.

14. Kertesz A: Paroxysmal kinesigenic choreoathetosis: an entity within the paroxysmal choreoathetosis syndrome. Description of 10 cases, including 1 autopsied, *Neurology* 17:680-690, 1967.

15. Nardocci N, Lamperti E, Rumi V, Angelini L: Typical and atypical forms of paroxysmal choreoathetosis, *Dev Med Child Neurol* 31:670-674, 1989.

16. Kurlan R, Shoulson I: Familial paroxysmal dystonic choreoathetosis and response to alternate-day oxazepam therapy, *Ann Neurol* 13:456-457, 1983.

17. Lance JW: Familial paroxysmal dystonic choreoathetosis and its differentiation from related syndromes, *Ann Neurol* 2:285-293, 1977.

18. Daras M, Koppel BS, Atos-Radzion E: Cocaine-induced choreoathetoid movements ("crack dancing"), *Neurology* 44:751, 1994.

19. Klawans HL, Brandabur MM: Chorea in childhood, *Pediatr Ann* 22:41-50, 1993.

20. Miyasaki JM, Lang AE: Treatment of drug-induced movement disorders. In Kurlan R, editor: *Treatment of movement disorders,* Philadelphia, 1995, JB Lippincott; pp 429-474.

21. Bimpong-Buta K, Froescher W: Carbamazepine-induced choreoathetoid dyskinesias, *J Neurol Neurosurg Psychiatry* 45:560, 1982.

22. Ehyai A, Kilroy AW, Fenichel GM: Dyskinesia and akathesia induced by ethosuximide, *Am J Dis Child* 132:527-528, 1978.

23. Lancman ME, Asconape JJ, Penry JK: Choreiform movements associated with the use of valproate, *Arch Neurol* 51:702-704, 1994.

24. Nausieda PA, Koller WC, Klawans HL, Weiner WJ: Phenytoin and choreic movements, *N Engl J Med* 298:1093-1094, 1978.

25. Wiznitzer M, Younkin D: Phenobarbital-induced dyskinesia in a neurologically-impaired child, *Neurology* 34:1600-1601, 1984.

26. Casey DE: Neuroleptic-induced acute extrapyramidal syndromes and tardive dyskinesia, *Psychiatr Clin North Am* 16:589-610, 1993.

27. Rodnitzky RL, Keyser DL: Neurologic complications of drugs: tardive dyskinesias, neuroleptic syndrome, and cocaine-related syndromes, *Psychiatr Clin North Am* 15:491-510, 1992.

28. Gualtieri CT, Quade D, Hicks RE, et al: Tardive dyskinesia and other clinical consequences of neuroleptic treatment in children and adolescents, *Am J Psychiatry* 141:20-23, 1984.

29. Pourcher E, Baruch P, Bouchard RH, et al: Neuroleptic associated tardive dyskinesias in young people with psychoses, *Br J Psychiatry* 166:768-772, 1995.

30. Kane JM, Woerner M, Borenstein M, et al: Integrating incidence and prevalence of tardive dyskinesia, *Psychopharmacol Bull* 22:254-258, 1986.

31. Adler LA, Peselow E, Rotrosen J, et al: Vitamin E treatment of tardive dyskinesia, *Am J Psychiatry* 150:1405-1407, 1993.

32. Dabiri LM, Pasta D, Darby JK, et al: Effectiveness of vitamin E for treatment of long-term tardive dyskinesia, *Am J Psychiatry* 151:925-926, 1994.

33. Swanson JW, Kelly JJ Jr, McConahey WM: Neurologic aspects of thyroid dysfunction, *Mayo Clin Proc* 56:504-512, 1981.

34. Besbas N, Damargue I, Ozen S, et al: Association of antiphospholipid antibodies with systemic lupus erythematosus in a child presenting with chorea: a case report, *Eur J Pediatr* 153:891-893, 1994.

35. Herd JK, Medhi M, Uzendoski DM, Saldivar VA: Chorea associated with systemic lupus erythmatosus: report of two cases and review of the literature, *Pediatrics* 61:308-315, 1978.

36. Furie R, Ishikawa T, Dhawan V, Eidelberg D: Alternating hemichorea in primary antiphospholipid syndrome: evidence for contralateral striatal hypermetabolism, *Neurology* 44:2197-2199, 1994.

37. Schiff DE, Ortega JA: Chorea, eosinophilia, and lupus anticoagulant associated with acute lymphoblastic leukemia, *Pediatr Neurol* 8:466-468, 1992.

38. Aron AM, Freeman JM, Carter S: The natural history of Sydenham's chorea: review of the literature and long-term evaluation with emphasis on cardiac sequelae, *Am J Med* 38:83-95, 1965.

39. Janner D: Anxiety, insomnia and movement disorder in a fifteen-year-old Hispanic female, *Pediatr Infect Dis J* 14:82-85, 1995.

40. Swedo SE: Sydenham's chorea: a model for childhood autoimmune neuropsychiatric disorders, *JAMA* 272:1788-1791, 1994.

41. Heye N, Jergas M, Hötzinger H, et al: Sydenham chorea: clinical, EEG, MRI and SPECT findings in the early stage of the disease, *J Neurol* 240:121-123, 1993.

42. Agrawal BL, Foa RP: Collagen vascular disease appearing as chorea gravidarum, *Arch Neurol* 39:192-193, 1982.

43. Nausieda PA, Bieliauskas LS, Bacon LD, et al: Chronic dopaminergic sensitivity after Sydenham's chorea, *Neurology* 33:750-754, 1983.

44. Fowler WE, Kriel RL, Krach LE: Movement disorders after status epilepticus and other brain injuries, *Pediatr Neurol* 8:281-284, 1992.

45. Kramer PL, Heiman GA, Gasser T, et al: The DYT1 gene on 9q34 is responsible for most cases of early limb-onset idiopathic torsion dystonia in non-Jews, *Am J Hum Genet* 55:468-475, 1994.

46. Ozelius LJ, Kramer PL, de Leon D, et al: Strong allelic association between the torsion dystonia gene (DYT1) and loci on chromosome 9q34 in Ashkenazi Jews, *Am J Hum Genet* 50:619-628, 1992.

47. Stacy M, Jankovic J: Childhood dystonia, *Pediatr Ann* 22:53-58, 1993.

48. Greene P: Medical and surgical therapy of idiopathic torsion dystonia. In Kurlan R, editor: *Treatment of movement disorders,* Philadelphia, 1995, JB Lippincott; pp 153-181.

49. Brin MF, Jankovic J, Comella C, et al: Treatment of dystonia using botulinum toxin. In Kurlan R, editor: *Treatment of movement disorders,* Philadelphia, 1995, JB Lippincott; pp 183-246.

50. Nygaard TG, Marsden CD, Fahn S: Dopa-responsive dystonia: long-term treatment response and prognosis, *Neurology* 41:174-181, 1991.

51. Rajput AH, Gibb WRG, Zhong XH, et al: Dopa-responsive dystonia: pathological and biochemical observations in a case, *Ann Neurol* 35:396-402, 1994.

52. Bull PC, Thomas GR, Rommens JM, et al: The Wilson disease gene is a putative copper transporting P-type ATPase similar to the Menkes gene, *Nature Genet* 5:327-337, 1993.

53. Tanzi RE, Petrukhin K, Chernov I, et al: The Wilson disease gene is a copper transporting ATPase with homology to the Menkes disease gene, *Nature Genet* 5:344-350, 1993.

54. Thomas GR, Forbes JR, Roberts EA, et al: The Wilson disease gene: spectrum of mutations and their consequences, *Nature Genet* 9:210-217, 1995.

55. Oder W, Grimm G, Kollegger H, et al: Neurological and neuropsychiatric spectrum of Wilson's disease: a prospective study of 45 cases, *J Neurol* 238:281-287, 1991.

56. Starosta-Rubinstein S, Young AB, Kluin K, et al: Clinical assessment of 31 patients with Wilson's disease: correlations with structural changes on magnetic resonance imaging, *Arch Neurol* 44:365-370, 1987.

57. Walshe JM, Yealland M: Wilson's disease: the problem of delayed diagnosis, *J Neurol Neurosurg Psychiatry* 55:692-696, 1992.

58. Scheinberg IH, Jaffe ME, Sternlieb I: The use of trientine in preventing the effects of interrupting penicillamine therapy in Wilson's disease, *N Engl J Med* 317:209-213, 1987.

59. Starosta-Rubinstein S: Treatment of Wilson's disease. In Kurlan R, editor: *Treatment of movement disorders,* Philadelphia, 1995, JB Lippincott; pp 115-151.

60. Brewer GJ, Dick RD, Johnson V, et al: Treatment of Wilson's disease with ammonium tetrathiomolybdate: I. Initial therapy in 17 neurologically affected patients, *Arch Neurol* 51:545-554, 1994.

61. Novotny EJ Jr, Singh G, Wallace DC, et al: Leber's disease and dystonia: a mitochondrial disease, *Neurology* 36:1053-1060, 1986.

62. Macaya A, Munell F, Burke RE, DeVivo DC: Disorders of movement in Leigh syndrome, *Neuropediatrics* 24:60-67, 1993.

63. Lee MS, Rinne JO, Ceballos-Baumann A, et al: Dystonia after head trauma, *Neurology* 44:1374-1378, 1994.

64. Saint Hilaire M-H, Burke RE, Bressman SB, et al: Delayed-onset dystonia due to perinatal or early childhood asphyxia, *Neurology* 41:216-222, 1991.

65. Joshi PT, Capozzoli JA, Coyle JT: Neuroleptic malignant syndrome: life-threatening complication of neuroleptic treatment in adolescents with affective disorder, *Pediatrics* 87:235-239, 1991.

66. Kinsbourne M: Hiatus hernia with contortions of the neck, *Lancet* 1:1058-1061, 1964.

67. Franz DN: Tremor in childhood, *Pediatr Ann* 22:60-68, 1993.

68. Hallett M: Classification and treatment of tremor, *JAMA* 266:1115-1117, 1991.

69. Bruun RD, Budman CL: The natural history of Tourette syndrome, *Adv Neurol* 58:1-6, 1992.

70. The Tourette Syndrome Classification Study Group: Definitions and classifications of tic disorders, *Arch Neurol* 50:1013-1016, 1993.

71. Fallon T Jr, Schwab-Stone M: Methodology of epidemiological studies of tic disorders and comorbid psychopathology, *Adv Neurol* 58:43-53, 1992.

72. Comings DE: Tourette's syndrome: a behavioral spectrum disorder, *Adv Neurol* 65:293-303, 1995.

73. Eapen V, Pauls DL, Robertson MM: Evidence for autosomal dominant transmission in Tourette syndrome: United Kingdom Cohort Study, *Br J Psychiatry* 162:593-596, 1993.

74. Kurlan R: Hypothesis II: Tourette's syndrome is part of a clinical spectrum that includes normal brain development, *Arch Neurol* 51:1145-1150, 1994.

75. Peterson B, Riddle MA, Cohen DJ, et al: Reduced basal ganglia volumes in Tourette's syndrome using three-dimensional reconstruction techniques from magnetic resonance images, *Neurology* 43:941-949, 1993.

76. Singer HS, Reiss AL, Brown JE, et al: Volumetric MRI changes in basal ganglia of children with Tourette's syndrome, *Neurology* 43:950-956, 1993.

77. Como PG: Obsessive-compulsive disorder in Tourette's syndrome, *Adv Neurol* 65:281-291, 1995.

78. Kurlan R, Trinidad KS: Treatment of tics. In Kurlan R, editor: *Treatment of movement disorders,* Philadelphia, 1995, JB Lippincott; pp 365-406.

79. Lipkin PH, Goldstein IJ, Adesman AR: Tics and dyskinesias associated with stimulant treatment in attention-deficit hyperactivity disorder, *Arch Pediatr Adolesc Med* 148:859-861, 1994.

80. Comings DE, Comings BG: Clinical and genetic relationships between autism-pervasive developmental disorder and Tourette syndrome: a study of 19 cases, *Am J Med Genet* 39:180-191, 1991.

81. Steingard R, Biederman J, Spencer T, et al: Comparison of clinidine response in the treatment of attention-deficit hyperactivity disorder with and without comorbid tic disorders, *J Am Acad Child Adolesc Psychiatry* 32:350-353, 1993.

82. Singer HS, Brown J, Quaskey S, et al: The treatment of attention-deficit hyperactivity disorder in Tourette's syndrome: a double-blind placebo-controlled study with clonidine and desipramine, *Pediatrics* 95:74-81, 1995.

83. Spencer T, Biederman J, Wilens T: Tricyclic antidepressant treatment of children with ADHD and tic disorders, *J Am Acad Child Adolesc Psychiatry* 33:1203-1204, 1994.

84. Pappert EJ, Goetz CG: Treatment of myoclonus. In Kurlan R, editor: *Treatment of movement disorders,* Philadelphia, 1995, JB Lippincott; pp 247-336.

85. Pranzatelli MR: Myoclonic disorders, *Pediatr Ann* 22:33-37, 1993.

86. Dunn RA: Subacute sclerosing panencephalitis, *Pediatr Infect Dis J* 10:68-72, 1991.

87. Yalaz K, Anlar B, Oktem F, et al: Intraventricular interferon and oral inosiplex in the treatment of subacute sclerosing panencephalitis, *Neurology* 42:488-491, 1992.

88. DiMauro S, Bonilla E, Zeviani M, et al: Mitochondrial myopathies, *Ann Neurol* 17:521-528, 1985.

89. Graf WD, Sumi SM, Copass MK, et al: Phenotypic heterogeneity in families with myoclonus epilepsy and ragged-red fiber disease point mutation in mitochondrial DNA, *Ann Neurol* 33:640-645, 1993.

90. Hammans SR, Sweeney MG, Brockington M, et al: The mitochondrial DNA transfer RNA^{Lys}A→G$^{(8344)}$ mutation and the syndrome of myoclonus epilepsy with ragged red fibers (MERRF), *Brain* 116:617-632, 1993.

91. Berkovic SF, So NK, Andermann F: Progressive myoclonus epilepsies: clinical and neurophysiological diagnosis, *J Clin Neurophysiol* 8:261-274, 1991.

92. Cochius JI, Figlewicz DA, Kälviäinen R, et al: Unverricht-Lundborg disease: absence of nonallelic genetic heterogeneity, *Ann Neurol* 34:739-741, 1993.

93. Goebel HH: The neuronal ceroid-lipofuscinoses, *J Child Neurol* 10:424-437, 1995.

94. Nardocci N, Verga ML, Binelli S, et al: Neuronal ceroid-lipofuscinosis: a clinical and morphological study of 19 patients, *Am J Med Genet* 57:137-141, 1995.

95. Potter NT, Meyer MA, Zimmerman AW, et al: Molecular and clinical findings in a family with dentatorubral-pallidoluysian atrophy, *Ann Neurol* 37:273-277, 1995.

CHAPTER 64

Demyelinating Diseases

•

Mitchell Steinschneider

The hallmark of demyelinating diseases is myelin sheath disruption in the white matter, leading to an interruption of normal nervous impulses. Because white matter lesions can occur in any region of the central nervous system (CNS), signs and symptoms referable to these diseases vary widely. Cognitive, sensory, and motor functions may be affected to varying degrees, depending on the sites of the lesions. The ability to rapidly diagnose demyelinating diseases of the CNS has been greatly enhanced by magnetic resonance imaging (MRI), which easily demonstrates lesions within the white matter of the brain and spinal cord. Treatments that ameliorate symptoms can be given for most of the demyelinating disorders, so their accurate and rapid diagnosis is necessary. Infectious, parainfectious, metabolic, and idiopathic etiologies, the latter exemplified by multiple sclerosis (MS), are the main causes of CNS demyelination in the adolescent and are the topic of this chapter (Box 64-1). Other diseases of white matter that generally begin in early childhood, or those that may mimic MS in their presentations, are not discussed here and have been reviewed elsewhere.[1,2] As a group, demyelinating diseases are relatively common neurologic entities in adolescents, and a busy pediatric neurology practice or clinic can expect to see at least one new case per year.

INFECTIOUS CAUSES OF DEMYELINATION

CNS demyelination frequently results from infectious disorders, especially viral infections. Demyelination is usually caused by a parainfectious autoimmune response directed against white matter elements. In some instances, however, the demyelination is caused by a direct effect of the infectious agent. Retroviruses are important and increasingly more frequent causes of CNS demyelination. Human immunodeficiency virus (HIV) infection disrupts white matter in both the brain and spinal cord.[3,4] Spinal cord involvement is generally restricted to the cortico-

spinal tracts in children, in contrast to adults, who may have additional involvement of the posterior columns. The degree of white matter pathology in the brain is correlated with the degree of cerebral atrophy and ventricular enlargement, and associated with the severity of cognitive and behavioral dysfunction.[5,6] Progressive multifocal leukoencephalopathy, a lethal demyelinating disease caused by a papovavirus and seen in immunocompromised patients, has also been reported in children with HIV infection.[7] Tropical spastic paraparesis is a demyelinating disorder of the spinal cord's motor tracts caused by another retrovirus, human T-cell leukemia virus (HTLV-I). This disorder is endemic to tropical climates, and population mobility has increased its frequency in more temperate locations. While disease onset is generally in young adulthood, it has been diagnosed in children.[8] Diagnosis is made by demonstrating increased HTLV-I titers in serum and cerebrospinal fluid (CSF).

Demyelinating lesions of the brain are also a prominent manifestation of pediatric Lyme disease.[9-11] These lesions may be associated with a wide array of neurologic complications of Lyme disease, including Bell's palsy, aseptic meningitis, encephalitis, optic neuritis, pseudotumor cerebri, headache, and behavioral changes. There will be serologic evidence of Lyme disease in the CSF, and the white matter lesions resolve with antibiotic therapy. Thus, Lyme disease must be seriously considered in the differential diagnosis of demyelinating disease in endemic areas.

PARAINFECTIOUS CAUSES OF DEMYELINATION

Immunologic sequelae of infections are frequent causes of CNS demyelination. The disorder, called acute disseminated encephalomyelitis (ADEM), accounts for about 15% of cases of childhood-onset encephalitis.[12] Pathologically, ADEM is characterized by brain edema, vasculitis, perivascular inflammation, and demyelination.[13] ADEM may present fulminantly with more severe inflammation and hemorrhage. This form has been termed acute hemorrhagic leukoencephalitis.[14] Measles is the most common precipitating agent of ADEM worldwide, complicating 1 in 1000 cases.[15] *Mycoplasma pneumoniae* is another common precipitant of ADEM.[16-18] Other causes include a wide variety of viruses, other infectious agents, and immunizations; these are listed in Box 64-1.[19-23] It is often unclear whether the encephalitis is due to an immunologically mediated reaction or is a direct result of CNS invasion by the infectious agent.

Neurologic symptoms classically follow the systemic illness by several days to weeks.[20,24] For example, the onset of measles-induced ADEM generally occurs soon after the rash and fever have abated. Symptoms of ADEM vary widely, depending on the location of demyelination. Onset may begin with renewed fever, meningeal signs, acute mental status deterioration, seizures, and focal neurologic deficits. The CSF generally shows some abnormality with increased cells or protein, but this may be unimpressive. Increased CSF immunoglobulin (IgG)

and oligoclonal bands, indicative of an intrathecal immunologic response, may also be present. Neuroradiographic analysis with MRI usually demonstrates multiple asymmetric white matter lesions. Computed tomographic scans are less sensitive.

Diagnosis is based on the clinical picture, the history, and serologic evidence of a recent systemic illness. These criteria are supplemented by the CSF profile, by MRI findings, and occasionally by evoked potential studies when MRI is uninformative. ADEM may be confused with MS because their neurologic signs and CSF and radiographic findings overlap. They can usually be distinguished by the relationship of ADEM with a recent systemic illness and by the monophasic nature of ADEM, which contrasts with the multiple episodes of demyelination characteristic of MS. Large areas of demyelination that may include the cortex, as well as a relative paucity of periventricular and corpus callosal white matter lesions, are radiologic findings suggestive of ADEM and are infrequently observed in MS.[2] In general, however, there is no definitive test that distinguishes a first attack of MS from ADEM. ADEM is a serious disease: measles leukoencephalitis, for example, carries a 10% to 20% mortality rate and high neurologic morbidity. The outcome may be significantly better after ADEM due to other agents. Steroids are a standard treatment for ADEM and may induce significant neurologic improvement.[25] Therapy with intravenous IgG may also hasten recovery.[26]

MULTIPLE SCLEROSIS

The hallmarks of MS are multiple episodes of neurologic dysfunction produced by more than one demyelinating lesion in the CNS (dissemination in both space and time). The advent of sensitive laboratory studies such as MRI and evoked potentials has expanded the diagnostic criteria (Box 64-2).[27] While MS is generally a disease of young adults, 2% to 5% of cases begin in childhood, the majority in the teenage years.[28,29] Girls are more likely to be affected than boys by an average ratio of 2:1.[28-31] MS is a common disease, with a prevalence of about 0.5 in 1000 in northern latitudes that generally diminishes in lower latitudes.[2] Thus, although only a few new cases of MS occur in children, its high overall prevalence makes this a relatively common pediatric neurologic disorder. Its cause is unknown, although immunologic, environmental, genetic, and possibly infectious factors are involved. Pathologic lesions, termed plaques, are the foci of demyelination and have a predilection for periventricular and corpus callosal locations. Other common locations for plaques are the cerebellar hemispheres, brain stem, optic nerves, and spinal cord. Childhood cases of demyelination with characteristics identical to those of MS were in the past called Schilder's disease.[32]

Because demyelination can occur at any white matter site, the symptoms and signs of MS are protean.[28,29,33-35] Sensory disturbances, especially visual dysfunction, ataxia, and limb weakness, are common initial problems in childhood and are similar to those found in adults. The overall signs, symptoms, and pathologic mechanisms of MS are similar in children and adults, but focal seizures, headaches, altered mental status, and dementia occur more commonly in children. The initial presentation of MS in children may resemble ADEM and may begin with a febrile event associated with nausea and vomiting, headache, meningeal signs, altered mental status, and cerebral edema. The clinical course is characterized by periods of relapses and remissions in most patients. Initial remissions are usually associated with return to normal function, but further relapses tend to produce permanent residual deficits. More fulmanent and benign patterns of MS also occur. The clinical outcome of MS is variable and poorly predictable, with outcomes ranging from no long-term disabilities, to progressive acquisition of permanent deficits and loss of ambulation, to death.

Definitive diagnosis of MS rests on demonstrating multiple CNS lesions that produce acute episodes of CNS dysfunction separated in time. Ancillary tests are very useful in supporting the diagnosis of MS, with the caveat that these tests are nonspecific. MRI is the most sensitive test for confirming multiple lesions disseminated in space, many of which are asymptomatic. Evoked potentials may occasionally reveal lesions unseen on MRI.[36] The CSF cell count may show a mild mononuclear pleocytosis, and the protein content is usually elevated slightly. There is often an increase in CSF IgG levels and in the ratio of CSF IgG to total protein. CSF oligoclonal bands are found in most patients. Positive findings, while supportive of MS, are also found in many other chronic inflammatory and immunologic disorders affecting the CNS. Therefore, clinical judgment must always be the deciding factor in making the diagnosis, and other potential causes of the dysfunction must be excluded.

Management must be tailored to the individual patient. There is no cure for MS, but intensive research has led to multiple new therapies that can significantly ameliorate symptoms, reduce exacerbations of the disease, and retard its progression. The duration of acute exacerbations can be shortened by high-dose steroid therapy, although the overall clinical outcome is unaffected.[37] Newly approved interferon beta-1b, when subcutaneously injected every other day, significantly reduces the severity and frequency of acute exacerbations, as well as decreasing MRI abnormalities.[38] Copolymer 1, an experimental polypeptide compound that appears to be an immunologic modulator, also reduces the MS relapse rate and modestly reduces long-term deficits when subcutaneously injected on a daily basis.[39] Other immunologic therapies using methotrexate, cyclophosphamide, or cyclosporine may be of benefit in retarding the chronic progression of dysfunction in more seriously affected patients.[40-42] Adjunct therapies for the complications of MS are important features in the care of these patients.[43,44] For instance, medications are available to counter the effects of fatigue, dizziness, tremor, spasticity, muscle spasms, and urinary tract and bowel dysfunction.

Optic Neuritis

Optic neuritis is an inflammation of one or both optic nerves. Usually affecting young adults or children, it is manifested as a subacute loss of visual function often accompanied by local pain.[45-47] Onset often follows a prodromal viral illness. Associated symptoms and MRI findings may suggest that the optic neuritis is a component of ADEM. Recovery is usually excellent and occurs over several months. Although optic neuritis is usually an isolated demyelinating event caused by viral illnesses or Lyme disease, about 15% of children develop MS in the ensuing years. Whereas in the past low-dose corticosteroids were used to hasten recovery, later findings suggest that this regimen may increase the risk of developing recurrent optic neuritis without imparting any positive benefits.[48] In contrast, high-dose methylprednisolone (250 mg every 6 hours) for 3 days followed by low-dose prednisone (1 mg/kg/day) for 11 days and a rapid taper both hastened recovery of the optic neuritis and reduced the risk of later development of MS over the next 2 years.[49] These findings indicate that optic neuritis should either be treated with the more aggressive protocol or allowed to run its natural, generally favorable course.

Transverse Myelitis

Transverse myelitis is an inflammatory process of the spinal cord that has an acute or subacute onset and is usually the result of a parainfectious process similar to ADEM.[50,51] Signs and symptoms generally include back pain, leg weakness, diminished sensation below the thoracic level, and bowel and bladder dysfunction. Prognosis is guarded, and many patients are left with residual deficits. The association of optic neuritis and transverse myelitis is called Devic's disease. Many patients with transverse myelitis later develop MS.

METABOLIC CAUSES OF DEMYELINATION

Inborn errors of metabolism are an important cause of CNS demyelination or dysmyelination. Onset of disorders such as Krabbe's disease, metachromatic leukodystrophy, Pelizaeus-Merzbacher disease, mitochondrial disease, Canavan's disease, and Alexander's disease usually occurs in infancy or early childhood, and will not be discussed further here. The most important older childhood-onset demyelinating disease is adrenoleukodystrophy (ALD).

Adrenoleukodystrophy

ALD is an X-linked disorder with a male incidence of 1 in 20,000 to 50,000. It is associated with serum elevations and impaired beta-oxidation within peroxisomes of very-long-chain fatty acids (VLCFAs)—saturated fatty acids with carbon chain lengths of 24 to 30.[52] The genetic defect mutates a membrane protein involved in the transport into the peroxisome of the enzyme ligoceroyl-CoA ligase, which catalyzes the formation of the CoA derivative of the VLCFA required

for beta-oxidation.[53,54] There are multiple phenotypic expressions of the disorder even within the same kindred, implicating factors other than mutation of the X-linked gene in determining the disease state.

Classic ALD is characterized by a severe white matter demyelination that is most prominent in the parietooccipital region. Onset generally begins at 6 to 7 years of age, although adolescent-onset ALD occurs in 4% to 10% of patients with this phenotype.[55,56] Initial neurologic symptoms usually include behavioral problems that may resemble attention-deficit disorder with hyperactivity. Seizures occur in about 30% of patients. Dementia, hearing and visual loss, and visual and motor disturbances are also common symptoms. Adrenocortical insufficiency (Addison's disease) occurs in about 25% of patients and may be the only clinical manifestation of ALD; laboratory evidence of abnormal adrenal function is present in many others. The disease is slowly progressive, leading to a vegetative state and subsequent death within several years after onset of symptoms.

Adrenomyeloneuropathy (AMN) is another common phenotypic expression of the disorder (28% to 43%) and generally has an onset in the third decade, although onset occurs before 20 years of age in 10% to 20% of patients. It is characterized by neurologic dysfunction of the spinal cord and peripheral nerves, leading to a progressive spastic paraparesis and sphincter dysfunction. Both adrenal gland and cerebral dysfunction can also occur. Older women who are heterozygotes may also develop symptoms of AMN.

Diagnosis is based on the clinical constellation of neurologic and adrenal abnormalities and confirmed by demonstration of elevated serum levels of VLCFAs supplemented by genetic analysis. Prenatal diagnosis is available. Adrenal function should be evaluated, and if abnormal treated with steroid replacement. MRI of the head reveals demyelination with a predilection for posterior head regions in ALD. Dietary treatment that reduces serum levels of VLCFAs, combining restricted intake with supplementation of shorter-chain fatty acids that cause a reduction in endogenous synthesis, has been disappointing in reversing or retarding the rate of disease progression in symptomatic patients.[57-59] However, it may be useful in delaying disease onset in presymptomatic children.[55] Thrombocytopenia and leukopenia are common side effects of dietary therapy. Bone marrow transplantation may be the treatment of choice for patients with early neurologic involvement.[55,60]

CONCLUSIONS

Adolescent demyelinating diseases of the CNS are produced by a limited number of disease classes. Infections of the CNS, ADEM, MS, and ALD are the most prominent causes of demyelination. Confusion may arise

BOX 64-3
Laboratory Evaluation
of Demyelinating Disorders

MRI/CT scan of head (MRI is the most sensitive laboratory indicator of demyelinating lesions)

MRI of spinal cord (if spinal cord disease is suspected)

Evoked potentials (visual, auditory brain stem, somatosensory; often indicated only if MRI is not informative)

CSF (IgG, oligoclonal bands; consider specific serologic tests [e.g., Lyme titers], routine studies)

Serologic studies (see Box 64-1 for list of infectious agents)

Vasculitic/rheumatologic studies

Very-long-chain fatty acids (for adrenoleukodystrophy; consider other metabolic studies if all tests not informative)

CSF, cerebrospinal fluid; *CT,* computed tomography; *IgG,* immunoglobulin; *MRI,* magnetic resonance imaging.

in differentiating these disorders from other diseases that may also produce white matter lesions, such as vasculitic syndromes and a long list of other genetic and metabolic abnormalities.[1,2,61] (Box 64-3 lists laboratory tests that may assist in the diagnosis of demyelinating diseases.) Prompt diagnosis may lead to early, and more effective therapy. Progress in therapies requires that physicians stay abreast of new treatment developments, possibly referring patients to centers conducting clinical trials.

References

1. Natowicz MR, Bejjani B: Genetic disorders that masquerade as multiple sclerosis, *Am J Med Genet* 49:149-169, 1994.
2. Poser CM: The epidemiology of multiple sclerosis: a general overview, *Ann Neurol* 36(suppl 2):S180-S193, 1994.
3. Belman AL: AIDS and pediatric neurology, *Neurol Clin* 8:571-604, 1990.
4. Belman AL: Central nervous system involvement in pediatric HIV-1 infection, *Int Pediatr* 7:126-135, 1992.
5. Brouwers P, DeCarli C, Civitello L, et al: Correlation between computed tomographic brain scan abnormalities and neuropsychological function in children with symptomatic human immunodeficiency virus disease, *Arch Neurol* 52:39-44, 1995.
6. DeCarli C, Civitello LA, Brouwers P, Pizzo PA: The prevalence of computed tomographic abnormalities of the cerebrum in 100 consecutive children symptomatic with the human immune deficiency virus, *Ann Neurol* 34:198-205, 1993.
7. Vandersteenhoven JJ, Dbaibo G, Boyko OB, et al: Progressive multifocal leukoencephalopathy in pediatric acquired immunodeficiency syndrome, *Pediatr Infect Dis J* 11:232-237, 1992.
8. Yoshida Y, Sakamoto Y, Yoshimine A, et al: Three cases of juvenile onset HTLV-1–associated myelopathy with pseudohypoparathyroidism, *J Neurol Sci* 118:145-149, 1993.
9. Belman AL, Coyle PK, Roque C, Cantos E: MRI findings in children infected by *Borrelia burgdorferi, Pediatr Neurol* 8:428-431, 1992.
10. Belman AL, Iyer M, Coyle PK, Dattwyler R: Neurologic manifestations in children with North American Lyme disease, *Neurology* 43:2609-2614, 1993.
11. Bingham PM, Galetta SL, Atheya B, Sladky J: Neurologic manifestations in children with Lyme disease, *Pediatrics* 96:1053-1056, 1995.
12. Hart MN, Earle KM: Haemorrhagic and perivenous encephalitis: a clinical-pathological review of 38 cases, *J Neurol Neurosurg Psychiatry* 38:585-591, 1975.
13. Reik L: Immune-mediated central nervous system disorders in childhood viral infections, *Semin Neurol* 2:106-114, 1982.
14. Byers RK: Acute hemorrhagic leukoencephalitis: report of three cases and review of the literature, *Pediatrics* 56:727-735, 1975.
15. Johnson RT, Griffin DE, Hirsch RL, et al: Measles encephalomyelitis—clinical and immunological studies, *N Engl J Med* 310:137-141, 1984.
16. Fernandez CV, Bortolussi R, Gordon K, et al: *Mycoplasma pneumoniae* infection associated with central nervous system complications, *J Child Neurol* 8:27-31, 1993.
17. Fisher RS, Clark AW, Wolinsky JS, et al: Postinfectious leukoencephalitis complicating *Mycoplasma pneumoniae* infection, *Arch Neurol* 40:109-113, 1983.
18. Nara T, Matoba M, Numaguchi S, Ito F, Maekawa K: Postinfectious leukoencephalopathy as a complication of *Mycoplasma pneumoniae* infection, *Pediatr Neurol* 3:171-173, 1987.
19. Fujii Y, Kuriyama M, Konishi Y, Sudo M: MRI and SPECT in influenzal encephalitis, *Pediatr Neurol* 8:133-136, 1992.
20. Kesselring J, Miller DH, Robb SA, et al: Acute disseminated encephalomyelitis: MRI findings and the distinction from multiple sclerosis, *Brain* 113:291-302, 1990.
21. Munn R, Farrell K, Cimolai N: Acute encephalomyelitis: extending the neurological manifestations of acute rheumatic fever?, *Neuropediatrics* 23:196-198, 1992.
22. North K, de Silva L, Procopis P: Brain-stem encephalitis caused by Epstein-Barr virus, *J Child Neurol* 8:40-42, 1993.
23. Rantala H, Uhari M: Occurrence of childhood encephalitis: a population-based study, *Pediatr Infect Dis J* 8:426-430, 1989.
24. Johnson RT: The pathogenesis of acute viral encephalitis and postinfectious encephalomyelitis, *J Infect Dis* 155:359-364, 1987.
25. Pasternak JF, De Vivo DC, Prensky AL: Steroid-responsive encephalomyelitis in childhood, *Neurology* 30:481-486, 1980.
26. Kleiman M, Brunquell P: Acute disseminated encephalomyelitis: response to intravenous immunoglobulin?, *J Child Neurol* 10:481-483, 1995.
27. Poser CM, Paty DW, Scheinberg L, et al: New diagnostic criteria for multiple sclerosis: guidelines for research protocols, *Ann Neurol* 13:227-231, 1983.
28. Duquette P, Murray TJ, Pleines J, et al: Multiple sclerosis in childhood: clinical profile in 125 patients, *J Pediatr* 111:359-363, 1987.
29. Sindern E, Haas J, Stark E, Wurster U: Early onset MS under the age of 16: clinical and paraclinical features, *Acta Neurol Scand* 86:280-284, 1992.
30. Gall JC, Hayles AB, Siekert RG, Keith HM: Multiple sclerosis in children: a clinical study of 40 cases with onset in childhood, *Pediatrics* 21:703-709, 1958.
31. Hanefeld F, Bauer HJ, Christen HJ, et al: Multiple sclerosis in childhood: report of 15 cases, *Brain Dev* 13:410-416, 1991.
32. Poser CM, Goutieres F, Carpentier MA, Aicardi J: Schilder's myelinoclastic diffuse sclerosis, *Pediatrics* 77:107-112, 1986.
33. Bye AME, Kendall B, Wilson J: Multiple sclerosis in childhood: a new look, *Dev Med Child Neurol* 27:215-222, 1985.
34. Cole GF, Stuart CA: A long perspective on childhood multiple sclerosis, *Dev Med Child Neurol* 37:661-666, 1995.
35. Guilhoto LMFF, Osório CAM, Machado LR, et al: Pediatric multiple sclerosis: report of 14 cases, *Brain Dev* 17:9-12, 1995.

36. Giesser BS, Kurtzberg D, Vaughan HG Jr, et al: Trimodal evoked potentials compared with magnetic resonance imaging in the diagnosis of multiple sclerosis, *Arch Neurol* 44:281-284, 1987.

37. Thompson AJ, Kennard C, Swash M, et al: Relative efficacy of intravenous methylprednisolone and ACTH in the treatment of acute relapse in MS, *Neurology* 39:969-971, 1989.

38. IFNB Multiple Sclerosis Study Group: Interferon beta-1b is effective in relapsing-remitting multiple sclerosis, *Neurology* 43:655-661, 1993.

39. Johnson KP, Brooks BR, Cohen JA, et al: Copolymer 1 reduces relapse rate and improves disability in relapsing-remitting multiple sclerosis: results of a phase III multicenter, double-blind placebo-controlled trial, *Neurology* 45:1268-1276, 1995.

40. Goodkin DE, Rudick RA, Medendorp SV, et al: Low-dose (7.5 mg) oral methotrexate reduces the rate of progression in chronic progressive multiple sclerosis, *Ann Neurol* 37:30-40, 1995.

41. Multiple Sclerosis Study Group: Efficacy and toxicity of cyclosporine in chronic progressive multiple sclerosis: a randomized, double-blinded, placebo-controlled clinical trial, *Ann Neurol* 27:591-605, 1990.

42. Weiner HL, Mackin GA, Orav EJ, et al: Intermittent cyclophosphamide pulse therapy in progressive multiple sclerosis: final report of the Northeast Cooperative Multiple Sclerosis Treatment Group, *Neurology* 43:910-918, 1993.

43. Schapiro RT: Symptom management in multiple sclerosis, *Ann Neurol* 36(suppl):S123-S129, 1994.

44. Weiner HL, Hohol MJ, Khoury SJ, et al: Therapy for multiple sclerosis, *Neurol Clin* 13:173-196, 1995.

45. Kriss A, Francis DA, Cuendet F, et al: Recovery after optic neuritis in childhood, *J Neurol Neurosurg Psychiatry* 51:1253-1258, 1988.

46. McDonald WI, Barnes D: The ocular manifestations of multiple sclerosis. 1. Abnormalities of the afferent visual system, *J Neurol Neurosurg Psychiatry* 55:747-752, 1992.

47. Sedwick LA: Optic neuritis, *Neurol Clin* 9:97-114, 1991.

48. Beck RW, Cleary PA, Anderson MA, et al: A randomized, controlled trial of corticosteroids in the treatment of acute optic neuritis, *N Engl J Med* 326:581-588, 1992.

49. Beck RW, Cleary PA, Trobe JD, et al: The effect of corticosteroids for acute optic neuritis on the subsequent development of multiple sclerosis, *N Engl J Med* 329:1764-1769, 1993.

50. Dunne K, Hopkins IJ, Shield LK: Acute transverse myelopathy in childhood, *Dev Med Child Neurol* 28:198-204, 1986.

51. Jeffrey DR, Mandler RN, Davis LE: Transverse myelitis. Retrospective analysis of 33 cases, with differentiation of cases associated with multiple sclerosis and parainfectious events, *Arch Neurol* 50:532-535, 1993.

52. Naidu S, Moser HW: Peroxisomal disorders, *Neurol Clin* 12:727-739, 1994.

53. Mosser J, Douar AM, Sarde CO, et al: Putative X-linked adrenoleukodystrophy gene shares unexpected homology with ABC transporters, *Nature* 361:726-730, 1993.

54. Ligtenberg MJL, Kemp S, Sarde CO, et al: Spectrum of mutations in the gene encoding the adrenoleukodystrophy protein, *Am J Hum Genet* 56:44-50, 1995.

55. Moser HW: Clinical and therapeutic aspects of adrenoleukodystrophy and adrenomyeloneuropathy, *J Neuropathol Exp Neurol* 54:740-745, 1995.

56. van Geel BM, Assies J, Weverling GJ, et al: Predominance of the adrenomyeloneuropathy phenotype of X-linked adrenoleukodystrophy in the Netherlands: a survey of 30 kindreds, *Neurology* 44:2343-2346, 1994.

57. Aubourg P, Adamsbaum C, Lavallard-Rousseau MC, et al: A two-year trial of oleic and erucic acids ("Lorenzo's oil") as treatment for adrenomyeloneuropathy, *N Engl J Med* 329:745-752, 1993.

58. Korenke GC, Hunneman DH, Kohler J, et al: Glyceroltrioleate/ glyceroltrierucate therapy in 16 patients with X-linked adrenoleukodystrophy/adrenomyeloneuropathy: effect on clinical, biochemical and neurophysiological parameters, *Eur J Pediatr* 154:64-70, 1995.

59. Poulos A, Gibson R, Sharp P, et al: Very long chain fatty acids in X-linked adrenoleukodystrophy brain after treatment with Lorenzo's oil, *Ann Neurol* 36:741-746, 1994.

60. Aubourg P, Blanche S, Jambaque I, et al: Reversal of early neurologic and neuroradiologic manifestations of X-linked adrenoleukodystrophy by bone marrow transplantation, *N Engl J Med* 322:1860-1866, 1990.

61. Kissel JT: Neurologic manifestations of vasculitis, *Neurol Clin* 7:655-673, 1989.

CHAPTER 65

Immunizations and Related Infectious Diseases

•

Victor Israele and Philip A. Brunell

Adolescents are traditionally the orphans of immunization practice, because the recommended pediatric immunization schedules have tended to emphasize infants and school-age children. However, the adolescent population is susceptible to a variety of diseases that are preventable by immunization. Present-day adolescents have been raised in an era when many new vaccines have been introduced and often administered inconsistently. Many may have escaped natural infection, may not have been immunized, may have received less than optimal vaccines, or may have received adequate vaccine at an age when passively acquired maternal antibodies could interfere with immunization (e.g., live measles vaccine before 12 months of age).

In this chapter, immunizations recommended for adolescents are reviewed. These include measles, mumps, rubella, tetanus, diphtheria, poliomyelitis, varicella, and hepatitis B (Table 65-1). Brief descriptions of the manifestations of these illnesses in adolescents are included, along with the rationale for current immunization recommendations.

The indications for immunizations in special circumstances, such as pregnant adolescents, immunocompromised adolescents, adolescents with occupational exposure, and immigrant adolescents, are also reviewed. Also included are the new vaccines that were licensed in 1995 (varicella and hepatitis A) and their recommended uses in adolescents.

DISEASES REQUIRING IMMUNIZATION

Measles

ETIOLOGY. The measles virus is a member of the family Paramyxoviridae and the genus *Morbillivirus;* only one antigenic type exists. Measles virions are pleomorphic particles with an average diameter of 150 nm. Virions consist of an outer lipoprotein envelope covered with short surface projections. This envelope also contains specific proteins associated with the hemagglutination, hemolytic, and membrane fusion properties of the measles virus. These proteins play an important role in pathogenesis. A helical nucleocapsid composed of protein and a single-stranded RNA genome is enclosed within the envelope. Humans are the natural host for the measles virus, although primates also may be infected.

EPIDEMIOLOGY. Before the measles vaccine became available in 1963, more than 400,000 measles cases and approximately 500 deaths from measles were reported each year in the United States. The licensure of measles vaccine in 1963 and its subsequent widespread use resulted in a 95% reduction in the number of reported cases by 1968. A record low of 1497 cases was reported in 1983, a greater than 99% reduction from the years preceding vaccine availability. In 1989, however, over 18,000 cases were reported. Increases in the incidence rates of measles were seen in all age groups, but two groups were most affected: preschool-age children (most of whom were unvaccinated) and those 15 to 19 years of age. Accordingly, the routine measles vaccination schedule was modified.

Outbreaks in persons over 19 years of age are rare, with few reported cases, but such outbreaks continue to occur on college campuses, perhaps because of student mobility, which facilitates measles transmission. Most cases on college campuses have occurred in those who were previously immunized. These cases have raised concerns about issues of primary vaccine failure and waning immunity. The total number of measles cases reported in 1995 were 309, which is the lowest number ever recorded in the United States. In 1994, 963 measles

TABLE 65-1
Routine Immunizations for Adolescents

Vaccine	No Proof of Primary Immunization	Proof of Primary Immunization
Measles	Two doses (MMR)	One dose at 11 to 12 yr (MMR)
Mumps	One dose (MMR)	MMR is administered to provide
Rubella	One dose (MMR)	second measles dose
Poliovirus	<18 yr, OPV, three doses	
	>18 yr, IPV, three doses	
Tetanus-diphtheria	Three doses	One dose every 10 yr

cases were reported, the second lowest. The reduction in reported measles cases may reflect cyclic changes in measles cases, as well as increases in vaccination coverage among preschool children and increased use of a second dose of measles vaccine among school and college-age persons.

TRANSMISSION AND PATHOGENESIS. The measles virus is labile to temperature, light, acidity, dryness, and certain enzymes. Measles is spread by respiratory droplets and by aerosol created by coughing and sneezing. The peak incidence of infection is during winter and spring. It is one of the most highly transmissible of the infectious diseases. Within family settings, nearly 100% of susceptible individuals become infected when exposed to a measles case. Infectiousness is maximal during the late prodromal phase (3 to 5 days before the rash). Respiratory isolation for a 7-day period is recommended.

The incubation period from exposure to onset of the first symptom (i.e., fever) is about 10 days, and the average interval from fever to appearance of the rash is 3 to 4 days.

The primary portal of entry and the site for virus replication is the respiratory tract epithelium of the nasopharynx. An early primary viremia leads to infection of the reticuloendothelial system, including tonsils, lymph nodes, spleen, and lungs. A secondary viremia, caused by release of virus from the infected reticuloendothelial cells, occurs 5 to 7 days after the initiation of infection, heralding the onset of clinical symptoms.

CLINICAL MANIFESTATIONS. Measles is a systemic infection. The clinical manifestations of uncomplicated illness consist of a prodromal phase of fever, malaise, and anorexia, followed by signs and symptoms of upper respiratory tract infection, including cough, coryza, and conjunctivitis. Koplik's spots, pathognomonic of measles, are bluish-gray spots on a red base that are seen most frequently on the buccal mucosa opposite the second molars from 2 days before to 2 days after the onset of rash.

The rash classically begins near the hairline on the neck and spreads rapidly to involve the face and upper trunk. Over 2 to 3 days, the rash extends to the distal extremities to include the palms and soles. The rash is erythematous and maculopapular. As the disease progresses, the rash becomes confluent, mainly on the face and neck, and generally lasts 5 to 7 days. In adults the rash tends to be more confluent and violaceous and may be slightly raised. During convalescence, the rash fades rapidly and may cause a brownish epidermal desquamation in cases in which the rash was extensive.

Two to 3 days after the onset of the rash, the fever peaks and then rapidly diminishes by lysis. The course of uncomplicated measles lasts 7 to 10 days, but a dry cough may persist for several weeks.

COMMON COMPLICATIONS. The most common complications of measles involve the respiratory tract and central nervous system (CNS). The disease is often complicated by ear infections and pneumonia in 5% to 15% and 1% to 6% of cases, respectively. Pneumonia is the most common cause of death. This may be due either to secondary bacterial infection or to the measles virus directly infecting the lung parenchyma and producing a giant cell pneumonia.

Measles encephalitis is an acute inflammatory reaction in the CNS that is temporally associated with measles infections. It complicates approximately 1 in 1000 cases of measles. CNS symptoms in such cases generally appear 2 to 7 days after the onset of the rash. Of cases of measles encephalitis, 10% to 15% are fatal, and 25% of survivors have permanent neurologic sequelae such as mental retardation, personality disorders, deafness, hemiplegia, or seizures.

Subacute sclerosing panencephalitis (SSPE) is a chronic degenerative neurologic disease that may begin insidiously several years after an attack of measles. Approximately 1 in every 100,000 patients develops this entity, apparently the cause of a persistent infection with a defective measles-like virus. An insidious onset of intellectual deterioration, myoclonic seizures, dystonia, and extrapyramidal and cranial nerve abnormalities precedes the appearance of cortical blindness, decerebrate posturing, coma, and death in patients with SSPE. Fortunately, the measles vaccine has dramatically decreased the occurrence of SSPE.

OTHER COMPLICATIONS. Less frequent complications of measles include laryngotracheobronchitis, diarrhea, emesis, myopericarditis, hepatitis, and thrombocytopenic purpura.

Measles in patients with congenital or acquired immunodeficiencies can be especially severe, with shedding of measles virus from the respiratory tract for prolonged periods and increased mortality from giant cell pneumonia, which can occur before or up to a year after the rash. A chronic, fatal encephalitis resembling SSPE has been reported in persons with cellular immune deficiencies.

Malnourished children, especially in developing countries, have also been reported to develop severe measles with a higher likelihood of a poor outcome. This may be caused by a poor cell-mediated immune response secondary to the effects of malnutrition.

MEASLES IN PREGNANCY. Measles in pregnancy may be associated with increased maternal morbidity but does not cause congenital anomalies. However, measles has been associated with spontaneous abortion, premature delivery, and low birthweight. Perinatally acquired measles can cause severe disease in the newborn, leading to a mortality rate as high as 15%.

MODIFIED MEASLES. Modified measles is a milder form of measles occurring in children or adults who acquire the infection in the presence of antibodies, such as young infants who have received maternal antibodies passively, or individuals who have received immunoglobulins parenterally. The incubation period is longer, and symptoms are similar to those seen in typical measles but milder. At times the infection may be subclinical.

ATYPICAL MEASLES. Atypical measles has been described in persons who received killed measles vaccine in the past or who received killed vaccine and live attenuated vaccine in the same schedule and were subsequently exposed to wild measles virus. The killed vaccine was available in the United States from 1963 to 1967. Thus, although cases of atypical measles were seen in adolescents in the 1970s and 1980s, all present cases now occur in young adults.

Atypical measles is believed to be caused, in part, by the failure of the killed vaccine to induce antibody to the measles virus F protein. After the usual incubation period, a 2- to 3-day prodromal phase begins and includes high fevers, dry cough, pleuritic chest pain, and myalgias. Koplik's spots are not seen.

The rash in atypical measles begins on the extremities, involves the palms and soles, and spreads centrally to the trunk. It may be maculopapular, urticarial, hemorrhagic, or vesicular. Many patients develop peripheral edema. Involvement of the lower respiratory tract is common, including interstitial pneumonitis and pleural effusions. Some have reported pulmonary disease in the absence of rash.

Infrequent findings include hepatitis and peripheral neuropathy. The diagnosis is clinical but is usually associated with extremely high measles antibody titers, which may be absent at the onset of the rash. The measles virus has not been recovered from patients with atypical measles, suggesting that such patients are not contagious. Recovery occurs within 4 to 7 days.

DIAGNOSIS. The presence of cough, conjunctivitis, coryza, Koplik's spots, and the characteristic rash, associated with an epidemiologic history of exposure, is sufficient to make a clinical diagnosis.

Measles virus can best be isolated in tissue culture from respiratory tract secretions, before or occasionally shortly after the onset of rash. However, virus isolation is technically difficult and usually not available. Viral isolation can be useful in immunosuppressed patients, in whom antibody responses may be minimal. In some cases, measles virus antigen has been demonstrated by fluorescent antibody techniques in cells collected from nasopharyngeal secretions or urinary sediments. The diagnosis is usually confirmed by a serologic response to the virus. A fourfold or greater increase in specific measles antibody titers in acute and convalescent sera collected 1 to 3 weeks apart is considered diagnostic for measles. The presence of specific immunoglobulin M (IgM) antibodies in a single specimen is evidence of primary measles infection. The IgM assay, however, is technically difficult. In a properly performed assay, antibodies are usually detectable from shortly after the onset of rash until 3 to 4 weeks later. The antibody capture enzyme immunoassay is the optimal assay in current use.

MEASLES VACCINE. Moraten, the live measles virus vaccine most widely used in the United States, is prepared in chick embryo cells from the Edmondston B strain. A combined measles-mumps-rubella vaccine (MMR), licensed in 1971, which contains the Moraten strain, is the preferred method of measles vaccine administration. The reconstituted vaccine should be protected from light, kept at 2° to 8° C, and used within 8 hours of reconstitution. Measles vaccine causes a subclinical or mild noncommunicable infection, inducing both humoral and cellular immunity. Because of the difficulty of measuring the latter, a response to the vaccination is determined by measuring measles antibody titers. Antibody titers induced by vaccination are lower than those following natural infection. An initial rise of IgM antibodies is followed by a rise in IgG antibodies. The IgG antibody titers decrease with time but are believed to persist throughout life. One unconfirmed report has documented measles occurring in 5% of persons who were known to seroconvert after vaccination; these individuals were all low seroconverters.

Since 1980, vaccine-induced serum conversion has occurred in over 98% of susceptible children who were vaccinated at 15 months of age. Before this time, immunization was less effective; this phenomenon may be related to the addition of an improved stabilizer to the vaccine in 1979.

Most vaccine failures are unexplained. Higher attack rates have been found among infants vaccinated at under 12 months of age, compared with older infants; this may reflect neutralization of vaccine virus by persistent maternal antibodies that interfere with the immune response.

ROUTINE VACCINATION. Until recently, the recommended age for immunization in the United States was 15 months. In 1989, because of the persistence of measles outbreaks in highly vaccinated populations, it was recommended by both the Committee on Infectious Diseases of the American Academy of Pediatrics (AAP) and the Advisory Committee on Immunization Practices (ACIP) of the Centers for Disease Control (CDC) that routine immunization be changed from one dose to a routine two-dose schedule. In usual circumstances, the first dose should be given as the MMR vaccine at 12 to 15 months of age.

The ACIP prefers the second dose of MMR at school entry (4 to 6 years of age), whereas the AAP recommends that the second dose be given at entry to middle school or junior high school (11 to 12 years of age). Revaccination at 11 or 12 years of age, as recommended by the AAP, is designed to achieve a more rapid impact on the current adolescent population but is more difficult to implement in the public sector. It also is postulated that revaccination in early adolescence might boost waning immunity more immediately before the high-risk period of increased measles exposure at 15 to 19 years of age.

Other candidates for the two-dose regimen include persons entering college or starting employment in medical facilities who do not have (1) documented evidence of two doses of live attenuated measles vaccine, (2) physician-diagnosed measles, (3) laboratory evidence of measles immunity, or (4) a birthday before 1957.

Measles vaccination also is recommended for outbreak control. Any person without documentation of having received two doses of measles vaccine after the first birthday or evidence of measles immunity (previous physician diagnosis or laboratory evidence of immunity) should be vaccinated during an outbreak. There is no contraindication to vaccination of persons born before 1957 if they are susceptible.

Care should be taken that persons traveling abroad should be immune to measles. Immunization of persons born in or after 1957, who have not been vaccinated with two doses of measles vaccine, or who do not have other evidence of measles immunity is crucial. This recommendation includes travel to western Europe as well as to other areas.

Measles vaccine can be given for 3 days after exposure. This has proved reasonably successful in preventing the disease.

PASSIVE IMMUNIZATION. Immune globulin, 0.25 ml/kg, with a maximal dose of 15 ml, should be given to those who are unprotected. Those who are immunocompromised should receive 0.5 ml/kg, with a maximal dose of 15 ml. This dose should be given as soon as possible after exposure; it is believed to have some effect for up to 6 days.

PRECAUTIONS AND CONTRAINDICATIONS. Although the measles vaccine virus has not been shown to cross the placenta and infect the fetus, the live measles vaccine should not be given during pregnancy, and women should be advised to not become pregnant for at least 3 months after vaccination. In adolescents it is prudent to be sure that sexually active females are using an appropriate method of birth control before measles immunization is undertaken.

Minor illnesses, such as mild upper respiratory tract infections, are not a contraindication to measles vaccination. Persons with moderate to severe febrile illnesses can be vaccinated. Vaccination of persons who have received immunoglobulins or whole blood products should be postponed for a 3-month period to avoid interference with seroconversion.

Other persons who are immunocompromised should not receive the vaccine. However, because severe measles has been reported in symptomatic persons with human immunodeficiency virus (HIV) infection, measles vaccine is recommended for this group.

Persons with known anaphylactic reactions to neomycin should not receive the vaccine. Individuals with egg allergies, even those with severe hypersensitivity, may be immunized in the usual manner.

Mumps

Mumps is an acute generalized viral infection characterized by nonsuppurative swelling of the salivary glands. It occurs primarily in school-age children and adolescents and is usually self-limited.

ETIOLOGY. The mumps virus is a *Paramyxovirus* related to the parainfluenza viruses. Mumps virus is polymorphic, with a diameter ranging from 90 to 300 mm. The helical nucleocapsid contains a single negative-strand RNA and is surrounded by an envelope consisting of three layers. The external layer presents two glycoproteins, one with hemagglutination and neuraminidase functions and the other with cell fusion activity. Only one serotype of mumps virus is known.

EPIDEMIOLOGY. Mumps is endemic throughout the world and in the United States. Before the live attenuated mumps vaccine was licensed for use in 1967, mumps was a disease of children and young adults, with a peak incidence between 5 and 9 years of age. In recent years, the highest incidence has been observed among teenagers.

After licensure of the vaccine, the number of reported mumps cases decreased from 152,000 in 1968 to 2982 cases in 1985. A relative resurgence of mumps was observed in 1986 (7790 cases) and 1987 (12,848 cases), with a decrease to 5712 in 1989.

The disease occurs throughout the year, peaking in late winter and early spring. Epidemics have been reported in high schools, colleges, and military and occupational settings.

Males and females have the same attack rates, and almost all adults have evidence of mumps-neutralizing antibodies. Humans are the only known natural host. The disease, which is considered slightly less contagious than measles and chickenpox, provides lifelong immunity; no carrier state is known to exist. The period of communicability is usually 1 to 2 days but may be as long as 7 days before the onset of parotid swelling. Patients are considered to be contagious until the parotid swelling disappears, but no more than 7 days after its onset.

CLINICAL MANIFESTATIONS. The incubation period for mumps is usually 16 to 18 days, but cases may occur 12 to 25 days after exposure. The route of transmission is through infected droplets containing live virus, derived from respiratory tract secretions. Subclinical infection occurs in 30% of patients.

A prodromal phase, including low-grade fever, anorexia, malaise, myalgia, and headaches, is followed by swelling of the parotid glands that may be unilateral (25%) or bilateral (75%). The enlarged parotid gland obscures the angle of the mandible, making it possible to differentiate the condition from cervical lymphadenopathy, which does not hide this anatomic point. The pain caused by the swollen parotid glands may be described as an earache. The swelling progresses for 2 to 3 days and thereafter regresses. Reddening and swelling of Stensen's ducts may be present, as may trismus. Swelling of the submaxillary and sublingual salivary glands is seen in up to 10% of patients, but these glands are rarely enlarged in the absence of parotid involvement. Clinical mumps infection can also occur without demonstrable parotitis.

Mumps causes more severe infections in older children, adolescents, and adults. Epididymoorchitis is the most common nonsalivary manifestation in adult males. It is age related, with the highest attack rate in those 15 to 29 years of age, and it occurs in 20% to 38% of postpubertal boys. Unilateral testicular involvement is most common; this can lead to atrophy of the involved testis in one third to one half of cases. Impotence is not a sequelae and sterility is rare. The onset is abrupt, usually after the onset of parotitis, with a high temperature and vomiting. Marked swelling, warmth, and pain of the testes occur, along with erythema of the scrotum. The fever resolves in 5 to 7 days, but the tenderness can persist for 2 weeks or longer. Testicular malignancy after mumps orchitis leading to atrophy has been reported.

Postpubertal females develop mastitis in 15% of cases. Oophoritis with fever, nausea, vomiting, and lower abdominal pain occurs in 5% of cases. Mumps can cause aseptic meningitis and encephalitis with or without the presence of parotid swelling. Before vaccination, mumps was the most common cause of aseptic meningitis and viral encephalitis in the winter and spring. The mumps virus is remarkably neurotropic, causing cerebrospinal pleocytosis in 50% of patients in the absence of clinical symptoms. Neurologic involvement is three times more common in males than in females; adults are at increased risk for mumps meningoencephalitis.

Typically, the meningitis is mild with headaches, vomiting, and nuchal rigidity. Typical spinal fluid abnormalities include mononuclear pleocystosis, normal to mildly elevated protein levels, and normal to low glucose levels. Early in the infection, polymorphonuclear cell predominance can be detected in 25% of patients. When decreased glucose levels are present, the differential diagnosis should include bacterial meningitis. In cases with lymphocyte predominance, fungal and tuberculous etiologies should be considered. Mumps meningitis is benign, leading to full recovery without sequelae in a 3- to 10-day period. In contrast, mumps encephalitis may be associated with seizures, cranial nerve palsies, paralysis, hydrocephalus, and aphasia, leading to permanent sequelae and a mortality rate of 1%. Encephalitis may be observed soon after the onset of parotitis and is a much rarer complication than meningitis.

Other neurologic syndromes associated with mumps include nerve deafness, cerebellar ataxia, facial palsy, Guillain-Barré syndrome, polyneuritis, and transverse myelitis. Other uncommon complications include arthritis, pancreatitis, thyroiditis, myocarditis, nephritis, and thrombocytopenia.

Mumps infection during the first trimester of pregnancy has been associated with increased fetal mortality. Mumps infection during gestation does not cause congenital anomalies.

Immunocompromised people who acquire mumps have not been reported to develop unusual manifestations, although the duration of symptoms and viral shedding may be prolonged.

DIAGNOSIS. In most instances the diagnosis of mumps is made by the history of exposure and the presence of parotid swelling accompanied by mild to moderate constitutional symptoms. When parotitis is absent or other extraordinary manifestations are present, a variety of laboratory diagnostic aids are available.

The virus is present in the saliva for approximately 5 to 9 days, both before and after the onset of parotitis. It also can be isolated from the saliva of asymptomatic patients and from the cerebrospinal fluid (CSF), urine, and (rarely) blood. The mumps virus can be isolated in many tissue culture cell lines, such as monkey kidney cells, chick embryo fibroblast cells, human embryonic kidney, HEP-2, and HeLa cells. The virus causes giant cell formation and syncytia. If no cytopathic effect is observed, mumps virus can be detected by hemadsorption or by fluorescence microscopy.

In serologic testing a fourfold rise between acute and convalescent sera by complement fixation or hemagglutination inhibition can confirm the diagnosis. Virus neutralization and the enzyme-linked immunosorbent assay (ELISA) are used to test for susceptibility. The skin test should not be used for this purpose, as it is very inaccurate.

MUMPS VACCINE. A live attenuated mumps vaccine, derived from the Jeryl Lynn strain, was licensed in 1967. It is stored in lyophilized form and rehydrated just before use. Clinical trials have determined that the seroconversion rate after one subcutaneous dose of mumps vaccine is 93% to 97%. Epidemiologic and serologic data indicate the persistence of immunity. When mumps vaccine is combined with rubella and measles vaccines, similar conversion rates are noted.

RECOMMENDATIONS FOR VACCINE USE. The ACIP has recommended that mumps vaccine be given to all susceptible children, adolescents, and adults, unless vaccination is contraindicated. Persons who did not receive the mumps live attenuated vaccine after the first year of life and do not have either laboratory evidence of mumps or physician-diagnosed mumps should be considered susceptible and should be vaccinated.

Mumps vaccine can be given effectively after the disappearance of passively transferred maternal antibodies, which usually is considered to have occurred by the first birthday. Ordinarily, mumps vaccine is given between 12 and 15 months of age as part of the MMR vaccine. Most states now require evidence of immunity to mumps (vaccine antibody tests or physician-diagnosed infection) for school admittance.

For practical purposes, adults born before 1957 are considered immune to mumps. Since persons who have received the mumps vaccine or had mumps disease are not at increased risk for adverse reactions to the live attenuated mumps vaccine, it is not necessary to ascertain immune status before administering the vaccine. It is preferable to administer the MMR vaccine when reimmunizing adolescents or school-age children against measles.

The mumps vaccine has not been shown to prevent infection if administered after exposure has occurred, but it may prevent infection if exposure occurs subsequently. The simultaneous administration of other vaccines, such as those for diphtheria and tetanus or poliomyelitis, does not interfere with the immunogenicity of the mumps vaccine.

Mumps vaccine is safe and has few side effects. Mild parotitis and fever are rare. No causal association has been reported between vaccine administration and CNS involvement such as seizures, deafness, or encephalitis.

Pregnant women or women who plan to become pregnant within 3 months should not receive mumps vaccine. Immunocompromised patients and persons with severe febrile illnesses should not receive the vaccine. Asymptomatic HIV-infected children should receive the MMR vaccine at 15 months of age. Because the vaccine is prepared in chick embryo and contains traces of neomycin, it should not be given to persons with a history of anaphylactic reactions to neomycin or eggs.

Passive protection with intravenous immune globulin or hyperimmune mumps immunoglobulin is not efficacious in preventing or ameliorating mumps or its complications. Vaccine should not be given within 2 weeks before or 3 months after administration of immunoglobulins.

Rubella

Rubella is an acute exanthematous viral infection characterized by rash, fever, and lymphadenopathy. In childhood it is generally an inconsequential disease, but when it occurs during pregnancy the fetus is at significant risk for severe damage and resultant birth defects.

ETIOLOGY. Rubella virus is a member of the *Rubivirus* genus of the Togaviridae family. It is spherical and moderately large (60 to 80 mm in diameter), containing single-strand infectious RNA, an icosahedral capsid, and a lipoprotein envelope. There is a hemagglutinin in the outer envelope, two distinct complement-fixing antigens, and two precipitating antigens designated "theta" and "iota."

EPIDEMIOLOGY. Rubella has a worldwide distribution. Before the advent of rubella vaccine in 1969, children 5 to 9 years of age had the highest attack rate. By contrast, the highest incidence of reported cases in more recent years are in the 15- to 19-year-old age group.

Before the licensure of rubella vaccine, periodic increases in cases occurred at 6- to 9-year intervals, with major epidemics at 10- to 30-year intervals. Since 1964, no large national outbreaks of rubella have been reported, although localized epidemics have occurred, especially in unimmunized older children and young adults. Rubella peaks in late winter and early spring in temperate climates.

Humans are the only source of infection. The virus is transmitted through direct or droplet contact from nasopharyngeal secretions. Although considered very contagious, rubella is not quite as contagious as measles.

Primary replication begins in the respiratory tract epithelium and in local lymphoid tissue. A viremic stage leads to widespread viral dissemination. Viremia ends with the appearance of the rash and development of neutralizing antibodies. The period of maximal transmissibility appears to be a few days before and after the onset of rash. Prolonged respiratory shedding of virus, up to 21 days after onset of the rash, has been documented. The incubation period for postnatal rubella ranges from 14 to 21 days and is usually 16 to 18 days.

CLINICAL MANIFESTATIONS. Rubella is usually a mild disease characterized by an erythematous maculo-papular rash, postauricular and suboccipital lymphade-nopathy, and low-grade fever. Adolescents and adults frequently report a prodrome consisting of headaches, malaise, and anorexia. Transient polyarthralgia and polyarthritis are frequent in rubella, particularly in young women. Encephalitis and thrombocytopenic purpura are less common.

The most important consequence of rubella in the adolescent occurs if infection is acquired during pregnancy, causing congenital infection in the fetus. The infection can result in miscarriage, stillbirth, or the congenital rubella syndrome. The major manifestations of congenital rubella syndrome include the classic triad of cataracts, heart defects (pulmonary artery stenosis, patent ductus arteriosus), and deafness. Intrauterine growth retardation, other ocular defects (micro-ophthalmia, ret-initis, cloudy cornea, glaucoma), psychomotor behavior, and psychiatric disorders also occur. Neonatal findings of rash, hepatosplenomegaly, hyperbilirubinemia, hepatitis, pneumonitis, myocarditis, bone lucencies, encephalitis, hemolytic anemia, and thrombocytopenia are common.

The risk of anatomic defects because of maternal rubella varies from 60% to 100% in the first 11 weeks of gestation and declines as gestation progresses. Beyond the twentieth week, little risk exists.

LABORATORY DIAGNOSIS. The laboratory diagnosis of rubella can be made by viral culture or appropriate serologic tests. Since viral isolation from nose and throat swabs, blood, urine, CSF, or other body fluids is technically difficult, the laboratory diagnosis of rubella is most often made by serologic testing.

Acute rubella infection may be diagnosed either by the demonstration of specific IgM in one serum sample, or by a fourfold or greater increase in IgG rubella antibody titer in an acute serum specimen obtained as soon as possible and a convalescent serum specimen obtained 2 to 3 weeks later. Both sera should be evaluated by the same test. ELISA, latex agglutination, fluorescent immunoassays, hemagglutination-inhibition, and hemolysis in gels are the most commonly used tests. Suceptibility testing is generally performed by ELISA or agglutination.

RUBELLA VACCINE. In 1969, three live attenuated vaccines were licensed for use in the United States: HPV-77 (duck embryo), HPV-77 (dog kidney), and Cendehill (rabbit kidney). Since 1979 the only licensed rubella vaccine is the RA-27/3, which is grown in human diploid cell cultures and contains no penicillin. Serum antibody is induced in almost all vaccinees and vaccine-induced immunity probably is lifelong. Rubella vaccine may cause viremia and excretion of virus in nasopharyn-geal secretions for 2 to 3 weeks after vaccination, but no person-to-person spread of the virus subsequent to vaccination has been a problem.

Rubella vaccine can be combined with measles and mumps vaccines and administered as MMR and can be simultaneously administered with DTP, oral polio, inac-tivated polio, *Haemophilus influenzae* b conjugate, hepa-titis A or B, or varicella vaccines. The dose is 0.5 ml of reconstituted vaccine administered subcutaneously.

Indications. Rubella vaccine is recommended for all adolescents unless there is proof of immunity or the vaccine is contraindicated. Proof of immunization re-quires documentation of rubella vaccination on or after the first birthday or serologic evidence of rubella immunity. Confirmation of clinical rubella is not accept-able, since the clinical syndrome is often misdiagnosed. Special emphasis should be given to vaccination of nonpregnant, susceptible adolescent females, premari-tally or postpartum. Sexually active adolescents should be informed about the theoretical risk of infection of the fetus if they are pregnant or become pregnant within 3 months of vaccine administration. Premarital serologic tests for rubella immunity are useful in identifying susceptible women in need of immunization. Testing during pregnancy should be routine and the vaccine should be administered to susceptible women in the immediate postpartum period. Routine serologic testing of adolescents has become less important in recent years, since larger numbers of teenagers receive a second dose of MMR during their adolescent years.

College students, day care personnel, military per-sonnel, and healthcare personnel should have evidence of rubella immunity. Persons without evidence of rubella immunity who travel abroad should be vaccinated against rubella, since this disease is endemic in many countries.

Side effects and adverse reactions. Side effects are usually mild. Low-grade fevers, rash, and lymphadenop-athy can occur. Arthralgias and transient arthritis are more commonly reported in postpubertal females and may develop in 2.5% of adults. Arthritis occurs 13 to 19 days after immunization, lasting 1 to 11 days, whereas arthralgia occurs 10 to 25 days after rubella vaccine and lasts 1 to 9 days. The joints of the fingers, wrists, and knees generally are affected. There are no cases of persistent arthritis or arthralgias.

Precautions and contraindications. Pregnant women should not receive rubella vaccine. If a pregnant woman is vaccinated or if a woman becomes preg-nant within 3 months after immunization, she should be counseled about the potential risks for the fetus. In more than 500 susceptible pregnant women who have been immunized with the RA-27/3 and have been reported by the CDC, not a single case of congenital rubella syndrome has resulted from those vaccinations. Termination of pregnancy for this indication has therefore become uncommon.

Patients with congenital or acquired immunodeficiency diseases should not receive rubella vaccine because replication of the vaccine viruses can be enhanced. Vaccine should be withheld for 3 months after cessation of immunosuppressive therapy to enable the immune response to be effective. The exception to this rule occurs in symptomatic HIV-infected patients, who should be vaccinated against measles with MMR, because measles can be severe in these children.

Since rubella vaccine is produced in human diploid cell cultures, a history of anaphylaxis to egg ingestion is not a contraindication to monovalent rubella vaccine. As mumps and measles vaccines are produced in chick-derived tissue culture, caution is advised in the use of MMR in these patients. Upper respiratory tract infections are not a contraindication to rubella vaccination.

The rubella vaccine should be given at least 14 days before administration of immune globulin or deferred for 6 weeks, but preferably 3 months, after administration, because passively acquired antibodies may interfere with the response to the vaccine. Previous administration of blood products or Anti-Rh⁰(D) immunoglobulin does not interfere with the immune response and is not a contraindication to postpartum vaccination.

Diphtheria and Tetanus

The occurrence of diphtheria and tetanus in the United States has decreased markedly because of the high level of appropriate immunization among children. Since the mid-1980s, only one to five cases of diphtheria and 50 to 100 cases of tetanus have been reported yearly to the CDC. Most of the cases of tetanus have been in older persons. It is essential to have a tetanus-diphtheria immunization every 10 years to maintain immunity. A dose is routinely given at age 14 to 16 years and every 10 years thereafter; this follows the DTP shot given before school entry at age 5. Pertussis immunization is not given beyond age 7 or 8 owing to the greater severity of vaccination complications in older children and adolescents.

GUIDELINES FOR IMMUNIZATION. Diphtheria and tetanus toxoids are prepared by formaldehyde treatment of the respective toxins. The combined tetanus and diphtheria toxoids, absorbed, for adult use (Td), containing not more than 2 flocculating units (Lf) of diphtheria toxoid per dose, are a fraction of the amount used in infant and child immunization. This decreases the reactivity of Td and thus is the preparation of choice for the immunization of adolescents. The route of administration is intramuscular.

Primary immunization. If adolescents have not previously received a primary series, a series of three doses of Td should be given intramuscularly, the second dose 4 to 8 weeks after the first, and the third dose 6 to

12 months after the second. If interruption or delay of the scheduled doses occur, the series need not be restarted, regardless of the time elapsed between doses. Two doses of Td produce protective antibody titers to tetanus in 100% and to diphtheria in 94% of vaccinees. A third dose produces protective titers in 100% of vaccinees against diphtheria.

Side effects and adverse reactions. The most common side effect is a local reaction at the injection site. Fever and other systemic reactions are uncommon.

The Td vaccination should ordinarily be deferred until the second trimester in pregnancy to minimize any theoretical risk of teratogenecity.

Tetanus prophylaxis in wound management. Wound cleaning, debridement if needed, and immunization are important in the management of wounds. The need for tetanus toxoid (active immunization) and tetanus immune globulin (TIG) (passive immunization) depends on the wound and the immunization status of the patient.

A complete series of primary immunizations with tetanus toxoid provides protection for 10 years. Therefore, booster injections need be given only every 10 years. If the wound is clean, a booster injection should be administered only if the last tetanus shot was given more than 10 years before. In heavily contaminated or tetanus-prone wounds (e.g., those contaminated with feces or dirt, puncture wounds, avulsions, frostbite, burns, crushing wounds), a booster is appropriate if the patient has not received a tetanus toxoid within the preceding 5 years.

In patients with unknown or incomplete tetanus vaccination and in whom the wound is other than a clean, minor wound, the Td vaccination should be administered with TIG. The TIG dose is 250 units intramuscularly. Separate syringes and separate sites should be used. Td is the preferred preparation to be used in adolescents for wound management because it also enhances diphtheria protection.

Poliomyelitis

Poliomyelitis is an acute neurologic disease caused by three distinct antigenic serotypes of polioviruses, which are enteroviruses belonging to the family of Picornaviridae. Humans are the only natural reservoir for polioviruses. Since the introduction of inactivated polio vaccine in 1955 and an oral polio vaccine in 1962, the number of cases has dropped dramatically. In the United States, five to 15 cases of paralytic poliomyelitis were reported yearly to the CDC in the 1980s, all of which were due to vaccine. A massive effort to immunize all children in the Western hemisphere greatly reduced the number of cases, so that the World Health Organization declared that poliomyelitis had been eradicated in that hemisphere.

Polioviruses replicate in the nasopharynx, the gastrointestinal tract, and adjacent lymphoid tissue. Inapparent infection, which can be recognized only by the recovery of virus or by a rise in antibody titers, occurs in about 95% of infections. Fever, headaches, sore throat, anorexia, vomiting, and myalgias, which are indistinguishable from any other viral illness and last about 48 hours, occur in 4% to 8% of poliomyelitis infections.

Nonparalytic poliomyelitis occurs in about 1% of patients, with the development of aseptic meningitis. The signs and symptoms include stiffness of the neck and back, vomiting, headaches, and high fever.

Polioviruses can cause extensive necrosis of the neurons in the gray matter of the brain and spinal cord, resulting in paralytic poliomyelitis in 0.1% of all poliovirus infections. A biphasic course is seen in one third of infected children; this includes a preparalytic phase, which consists of the symptoms observed in those with abortive and nonparalytic poliomyelitis. The first symptom of the paralytic phase is usually muscle pain, lasting for 1 or 2 days, followed by a flaccid paralysis that is asymmetric in distribution. The paralysis usually progresses for a few days and stops when the patient becomes afebrile. Sensory loss is rare.

Bulbar poliomyelitis involves the cranial nerves with respiratory and vasomotor effects. Polioencephalitis is uncommon, in contrast to spinal paralytic poliomyelitis. The occurrence of spastic paralysis reflects involvement of the upper motor neurons. The complications of paralytic poliomyelitis include respiratory failure, aspiration pneumonia, pulmonary edema, pulmonary embolism, myocarditis, gastrointestinal hemorrhage, ileus, and gastric dilation.

VACCINES. Two poliovirus vaccines are used in the United States: the oral polio vaccine (OPV) and the enhanced-potency inactivated polio vaccine (IPV-Ep).

Developed by Albert Sabin in 1960, OPV is a live attenuated vaccine containing the three poliovirus types. It is highly immunogenic, generating specific antibodies in 97% to 100% of vaccinees to all three types after three doses. The mucosal and systemic immunity that results is believed to be enduring. Virus excretion, which may result in secondary spread, occurs for weeks after vaccination. Vaccine-associated cases of poliomyelitis, which are rare, occur once in every half million first doses and are less common with subsequent doses. Vaccinees and their contacts are both at risk.

OPV should not be given to immunocompromised individuals or their contacts because of the much higher incidence (10,000 times greater) of poliovaccine-related complications observed in this population. OPV can be administered at the same time as other vaccines.

Killed polio vaccine (IPV), which was developed by Jonas Salk and licensed in 1955, has been replaced by IPV-Ep developed by A.L. Van Wezel. The extent of mucosal immunity produced is uncertain but is less than that with OPV. No viral excretion or secondary spread

follows the vaccine administration, and no cases of vaccine-associated poliomyelitis have been reported. These vaccines are the choice for immunodeficient patients and their contacts. There has been extensive experience with this type of vaccine in European countries, where it has been used exclusively and with great success. IPV-Ep can be administered simultaneously with other vaccines. No serious side effects have been reported. Because the vaccine contains traces of streptomycin and neomycin, persons with anaphylactic reactions to these antibiotics should not receive the inactivated vaccine.

IMMUNIZATION RECOMMENDATIONS. In 1997 the ACIP changed its poliomyelitis vaccine recommendations. Adolescents aged 11 to 21 years who did not receive the primary series should receive the first two doses of IPV-Ep 2 months apart. In adolescents under the age of 18 years, the completion of the primary series is attained by administering two doses of OPV 12 to 18 months and 4 to 6 years after the first two IPV-Ep doses. In adolescents over 18 years of age, IPV-Ep is the recommended vaccine to be administered. IPV-Ep is also recommended for immunocompromised adolescents and their contacts. IPV-Ep is preferred to OPV for the latter group because paralysis after OPV, although rare, is more common in adults. Other acceptable schedules, recommended by the ACIP, the American Academy of Pediatrics, and the American Academy of Family Practice include the use of four consecutive IPV-Ep doses at 0, 2, and 12 to 18 months and at 4 to 6 years, or four consecutive doses of OPV at 2, 4, and 6 to 18 months and at 4 to 6 years, when the adolescent is less than 18 years of age.

Persons traveling for the first time to areas where wild poliovirus is prevalent should complete a primary series of polio vaccine or should receive a booster dose of either OPV or IPV, regardless of the vaccine used previously, if they have completed the series. IPV-Ep is recommended for persons over 18 years, but OPV can be given if there is insufficient time to complete a series of IPV-Ep. If less than 4 weeks are available, a single dose of OPV is recommended, with remaining doses given at the appropriate intervals.

Unimmunized pregnant women should receive primary vaccination against poliomyelitis only when the risk of exposure is high, such as in foreign travel to areas where wild poliovirus is epidemic or endemic. A sequential schedule has recently been implemented in which two doses of OPV are followed by two doses of IPV-Ep. For unimmunized adolescents through secondary school age (generally up to 18 years of age) the primary sequential series of IPV and OPV consists of four doses. The first two doses, given 2 months apart, consist of IPV followed 12 months and again 4 to 6 years after the second dose with two OPV doses.

Varicella

Varicella-zoster virus (VZV) causes two diseases, varicella (chickenpox), which is the primary infection, and zoster (shingles), caused by the reactivation of latent VZV. In the United States, varicella occurs predominantly in children under 10 years of age. Approximately 10% of adolescents and adults remain susceptible.

Chickenpox presents with a rash, low-grade fever, and malaise. A sentinel lesion in the trunk can be present 1 to 3 days before the appearance of the rash. For the most part, chickenpox is a benign disease in immunocompetent children with temperatures ranging from 100° to 103° F of only 3 to 4 days' duration. Constitutional symptoms include malaise pruritus, anorexia, and restlessness. The skin lesions consist of maculopapules, vesicles, and scabs in varying stages of evolution. They appear on the trunk and face and rapidly spread centripetally to involve other areas of the body, including mucosal surfaces. Successive crops of lesions appear over 3 to 5 days; the crusts fall off within 1 to 2 weeks, generally leaving no scars.

Compared with children, adolescents and adults are at an increased risk for a prolonged course and visceral dissemination, most commonly pneumonitis, encephalitis, and hepatitis. Pregnant and immunocompromised adolescents are also likely to develop a disease with increased severity. The mortality rate in adults is 25 times greater than in children.

Herpes zoster, or shingles, is seen in 15% of individuals after they have had chickenpox. It is characterized by a unilateral vesicular eruption with a dermatomal distribution. The thoracic and lumbar dermatomes are most commonly involved. It can also involve the fifth nerve, and if keratitis is present, a sight-threatening condition may occur.

The onset of disease is preceded by pain within the dermatome; 48 to 72 hours later, macropapular lesions on an erythematous base develop, rapidly evolving into a vesicular rash. The vesicles may coalesce, forming bullous lesions. In the normal host the total duration of the rash is 10 to 15 days. The most significant clinical manifestations include acute neuritis and, later, postherpetic neuralgia. Extracutaneous manifestations involve the CNS, as manifested by meningoencephalitis.

Healthy adolescents with varicella may benefit from administration of 800 mg acyclovir by mouth 5 times a day, begun within 24 hours of onset of disease, for 5 to 7 days. Early therapy with oral acyclovir has been found to decrease the time to cutaneous healing, decrease the duration of fever, and lessen symptoms. Oral acyclovir has not been observed to be associated with fetal malformations when given during pregnancy. If varicella becomes progressive or complications develop, intravenous acyclovir, 10 to 15 mg/kg every 8 hours, should be administered rather than the oral drug.

Immunocompromised adolescents or healthy adolescents with visceral dissemination, such as in varicella pneumonitis, should receive intravenous acyclovir, 5 to 10 mg/kg every 8 hours. Susceptible immunocompromised and pregnant adolescents are candidates to receive varicella zoster immunoglobulin (VZIG), when exposed to VZV. VZIG modifies primary VZV infections and should be given as soon as possible, but no more than 96 hours, after exposure. VZIG is given by intramuscular injection. Each vial contains 125 units. The dosage is one vial every 10 kilograms of body weight to a maximal dose of 625 units (5 vials).

Varicella vaccine. Varicella vaccine (VARIVAX) was licensed for use in the United States in March 1995. It is a live attenuated virus vaccine prepared from the Oka strain of VZV. This vaccine has been used in Europe and Japan for several years. Since 1989, more than 2 million doses have been given and serious side effects have been rare.

Immunogenicity. Seroconversion rates of 79% to 82% after one dose and 94% after two doses have been reported in adolescents over 12 years of age and in adults. Antibodies to VZV have been detected as late as 10 years after immunization in more than 95% of vaccinees, taking into consideration that wild VZV had continued to be present, which could have served as a natural booster of vaccine-associated antibodies.

Efficacy. In studies of VARIVAX to date, approximately 70% of adults who have seroconverted after vaccination are completely protected after household exposure to VZV. The remaining 30% have developed an attenuated disease characterized by fewer than 100 lesions, many of them papular with little or no systemic signs or symptoms.

Vaccine safety. Within 1 month of vaccination, approximately 8% of adolescents and adults develop a mild maculopapular or varicelliform rash consisting of two to five lesions. Transient pain and tenderness or redness at the site of injection occurs in 25% to 35% of adolescent and adult vaccinees; a temperature of 100.4° F or more is observed in 10% of vaccinees. Upper respiratory tract symptoms, headache, and fatigue are associated with immunization in less than 1% of healthy vaccinees.

In studies in the United States, more than 1500 adolescents and adults received Varivax vaccine and only one case of zoster was reported after 11 to 13 years of follow-up; this case was shown to be caused by a wild strain of virus.

Recommendations for vaccine use. A single dose of vaccine should be given to persons who have not reached their thirteenth birthday, have not been immunized previously, and have no history of varicella infection. Older individuals should be given two 0.5-ml doses subcutaneously, the second dose 4 to 8 weeks after the first. The vaccine is lyophilized and must be stored frozen. When reconstituted as recommended, the vaccine must be used within 30 minutes; vaccine not used within that time should be discarded. It is desirable to immunize college students and persons working with children, traveling abroad, in the military, and in institutions. The immunity of healthcare workers should be ensured.

CONTRAINDICATIONS AND PRECAUTIONS

Immunocompromised patients. Varicella vaccine should not be given routinely to immunocompromised adolescents, such as those with congenital immunodeficiencies, blood dyscrasias, leukemia, lymphoma, HIV infection; those receiving immunosuppressive therapy for malignancies; and those receiving high doses of systemic steroids (2 mg/kg/day or more of prednisone or its equivalent or 20 mg/day or more for at least 1 month).

Adolescents with acute lymphocytic leukemia who have been in remission for at least 1 year and have more than 700 lymphocytes/ml and a platelet count over 100,000/ml are eligible to receive the varicella vaccine through a research protocol.

Pregnancy. As the effects of vaccine virus on fetuses are unknown, pregnant adolescents should not be vaccinated. Nonpregnant adolescents who receive varicella vaccine should defer pregnancy for at least 1 month after receiving each dose.

Others. Allergy to neomycin, manifested by an anaphylactoid reaction, is a contraindication to the administration of varicella vaccine; the administration of salylates within 6 weeks after varicella vaccination is not recommended owing to the association among Reye's syndrome, natural varicella, and salicylates. If immunoglobulin has been administered, varicella vaccination should be delayed for at least 3 months because of its potential interference with antibody responses. Moderate to severe acute disorders are also a reason to defer varicella vaccination. There is a very small risk of spread of vaccine virus to contacts, and its use in households with immunodeficient, HIV-seropositive, or pregnant females in the household should be considered with this in mind.

SPECIAL SITUATIONS REQUIRING IMMUNIZATIONS

Influenza Vaccine

Children over 12 years of age can receive either inactivated whole influenza virus vaccine or split-virus vaccine. Both vaccines contain two type A viral strains and one type B. Vaccine strains are changed to reflect those that are expected to circulate the following winter. Of vaccinated individuals, 70% to 80% develop protective hemagglutination-inhibition antibody titers and protection against illness. Immunocompromised individuals develop lower postvaccination antibody titers, which may

not protect as well but offer substantial protection against lower respiratory tract infection or death.

SIDE EFFECTS AND ADVERSE REACTIONS. The most frequent side effect is soreness at the vaccination site for up to 2 days. Reactions are few and generally mild. Infrequent reactions (fever, malaise, myalgia, and other systemic symptoms) occur most often in persons without previous exposure to influenza infection or vaccine. Because influenza virus vaccines are produced in embryonated eggs, individuals with anaphylactic reactions to eggs should not receive an inactivated influenza vaccine. Patients who have egg allergies and medical conditions requiring influenza vaccination may receive it with appropriate skin testing and, if needed, desensitization. Persons with acute febrile illness should not be vaccinated until their symptoms have resolved.

TARGET GROUPS FOR SPECIAL VACCINATION PROGRAMS. The ACIP recommends targeting specific groups of patients for influenza vaccination. As appropriate to the adolescent age group, these include the following three categories.

Groups at increased risk for influenza-related complications. These include (1) adolescents with chronic disorders of the pulmonary or cardiovascular systems, including cystic fibrosis and asthma; (2) adolescents who have required regular medical follow-up or hospitalization during the preceding year because of chronic metabolic diseases (including diabetes mellitus), renal dysfunction, hemoglobinopathies, or immunosuppression (including immunosuppression caused by medications); and (3) adolescents who are receiving long-term aspirin therapy and are therefore at risk of developing Reye's syndrome after influenza.

Groups that can transmit influenza to high-risk persons. These include (1) adolescents working in hospital or outpatient care settings who are in contact with high-risk persons in all age groups, including infants; and (2) adolescents employed in nursing homes or chronic care facilities who have contact with patients or residents and those who provide home care to high-risk persons (e.g., volunteer workers) or live in households with high-risk persons (e.g., elderly grandparents).

Other groups. These include (1) students or other persons in institutional settings (schools and colleges), who may be considered for vaccination to minimize the disruption of routine activities during outbreaks; (2) pregnant women with other medical conditions; (3) adolescents infected with HIV; and (4) adolescents who are planning foreign travel.

DOSE. Adolescents should receive one 0.5-ml dose of whole or split-virus influenza vaccine intramuscularly in the deltoid area. Annual vaccination is necessary because immunity declines after 1 year. The vaccine is generally administered in the fall, before the influenza season.

High-risk adolescents may receive the influenza vaccine at the same time as the MMR, pneumococcal, and polio vaccines. The vaccines should be administered at different sites.

Hepatitis A Virus

In the United States the hepatitis A virus causes an estimated 75,000 to 125,000 cases of acute hepatitis each year, resulting in approximately 100 deaths per year. The virus is spread by the fecal-oral route, including spread via water and food contaminated by feces. The mean incubation period is 28 days, with a range of 2 to 7 weeks. A persistent carrier state or chronic hepatitis is not caused by this virus. Subclinical infection is more common in children than in adolescents. The most common risk factors include personal contact with a person who has active hepatitis, employment in or attendance at a day care center, intravenous drug use, recent international travel, and association with a suspected food- or water-borne outbreak. Approximately 40% of individuals with hepatitis A have no known risk factor.

HEPATITIS A VACCINE. The hepatitis A vaccine (Havrix) was licensed in 1995. It is a killed, formalin-inactivated whole virus vaccine prepared in human diploid cells. In 1996, a new vaccine with similar characteristics was licensed (Vaqta).

IMMUNOGENICITY. Both Havrix and Vaqta have been shown to be highly immunogenic. The adult dose for Havrix (1440 ELISA units) is four times (360 ELISA units) the dose used for children and adolescents under 18 years of age, whereas the adult dose (50 units) for Vaqta is double the dose used in children and adolescents.

When children and adolescents up to age 17 years have been vaccinated with 360 ELISA units of Havrix at 0, 1, and 6 months, more than 95% and 99%, respectively, responded after each of the first two doses. The antibody titers after the second and third doses reached 300 and 4000 mIU/ml, respectively. Eighty percent to 90% of adults responded with protective antibody levels to a single 1440 ELISA unit dose of vaccine after 15 days, while more than 96% responded after 30 days. With a booster dose at 6 months, essentially 100% of vaccinees had high levels of protective antibodies.

Adults receiving serum immune globulin concurrent with the first dose of vaccine had the same seroconversion rates, but their antibody titers increased to only half of the values of adults who received the vaccine alone.

Efficacy. Two large prospective pediatric randomized trials have shown the efficacy of these two vaccines.

The Havrix vaccine was found to be 94% effective after administration of two doses in preventing clinical hepatitis, when 40,119 children were randomized to receive either hepatitis A or hepatitis B vaccine.

The Vaqta vaccine was shown to be 100% effective when over 1000 children were randomized to receive either the Vaqta vaccine or placebo. No cases of hepatitis were seen from 21 days after immunization.

Protective efficacy data in adults have not been published. There are also no published data regarding the use of hepatitis A vaccine in pregnant women or immunocompromised persons, including those with HIV infection.

Safety. These hepatitis A vaccines have proved very safe and no serious side effects have been reported. Of more than 1000 children who received Havrix, 75% showed no side effects, 15% developed soreness at the injection site, and 3% developed temperatures of 37.5° C or more. When Vaqta vaccine was tested in more than 500 children in one study, less than 13% developed local reactions and less than 9% had a temperature of 37.8° C or higher.

RECOMMENDATIONS FOR VACCINATION. Pre-exposure immunization with hepatitis A vaccine is recommended for adolescents in the following groups:

1. Travelers to endemic areas
2. Military personnel
3. Homosexual males
4. Patients with chronic liver disease
5. Native Americans and Pacific Islanders
6. Laboratory workers who handle live hepatitis A virus

Adolescents up to 18 years of age should receive three 360 ELISA unit doses of the Havrix at 0, 1, and 6 to 12 months or two 25 unit doses of the Vaqta vaccine at 0 and 6 months. Adolescents over 18 should receive two 1440 ELISA unit doses at 0 and 6 to 12 months or two 50 unit doses 6 months apart of the Havrix and Vaqta vaccines, respectively.

Hepatitis B Virus

Among the estimated 300,000 persons infected with hepatitis B virus (HBV) yearly, 25% develop jaundice, more than 10,000 patients require hospitalization, and approximately 250 die of fulminant disease. There are 750,000 to 1 million infectious carriers in the United States, 25% of whom develop chronic active hepatitis, which can lead to cirrhosis and primary hepatocellular carcinoma. Approximately 4000 persons die annually from HBV-related cirrhosis, and more than 800 die from HBV-related liver cancers.

HEPATITIS B VIRUS VACCINES. Two types of hepatitis B vaccines are licensed for use in the United States. A plasma-derived vaccine from chronic hepatitis B surface antigen (HB_sAg) carriers consists of noninfectious 22-mm HB_sAg particles that are inactivated and alum adsorbed. The antigen is separated from human plasma by a combination of ultracentrifugation and biochemical procedures. These procedures render all known viruses inactive, including HIV. Its use is restricted to immunocompromised persons, hemodialysis patients, and individuals with yeast allergy. This vaccine is no longer produced in the United States. A recombinant hepatitis B vaccine has been developed through genetic engineering using the yeast *Saccharomyces cerevisiae* into which a plasmid containing the gene for the HB_sAg has been inserted. The purified HB_sAg particles are obtained by lysing the yeast cells and separating the particles from yeast components by biochemical and biophysical techniques. HB_sAg protein constitutes more than 95% of the vaccine content.

A plasma-derived hepatitis B vaccine (Heptavax-B) and two recombinant vaccines (Recombivax HB and Engerix-B), when administered in the recommended dose, have comparable immunogenicity (>95% after three intramuscular doses in healthy adolescents) and efficacy (80% to 90% in preventing infection or clinical hepatitis). The antibody response in patients receiving hemodialysis ranges from 60% to 70%, in those with HIV infection from 50% to 70%, and in those with diabetes from 70% to 80%. Complete protection is defined by anti-HB_s levels of 10 mIU (international standard units) or more when tested by radioimmunoassay.

Vaccine use. Primary vaccination of adolescents and adults includes three intramuscular doses of vaccine. The first two doses should be given 1 month apart and the third dose 5 months after the second. A schedule of four doses at 0, 1, 2, and 6 months has been approved for postexposure prophylaxis or for more rapid induction of immunity. Hepatitis B vaccine in adolescents should be given only in the deltoid muscle. Administration in the buttocks has been found to be less immunogenic.

Healthy adolescents should receive 20 µg in 1 ml, 5 µg in 0.5 ml, and 20 µg in 1 ml of Heptavax-B, Recombivax HB, and Engerix-B, respectively. Heptavax-B vaccine in a dose of 40 µg in 2 ml (i.e., two 1-ml doses at different sites); Recombivax HB, 40 µg in 1 ml; and Engerix-B, 40 µg in 2 ml is recommended when using a four-dose schedule at 0, 1, 2, and 6 months for patients undergoing hemodialysis or for other immunosuppressed patients.

Serologic screening to detect susceptible persons before vaccination may or may not be cost effective, depending on the cost of vaccination, the cost of testing for susceptibility, and the estimated risk of previous infection. Testing for immunity after vaccination is not recommended routinely. Booster doses are not recommended at the present time in healthy adolescents. For hemodialysis patients, yearly anti-HB_s testing and booster doses to maintain anti-HB_s above 10 mIU/ml has been recommended.

Side effects and adverse reactions. The vaccine is well tolerated. The most common adverse reaction has been local soreness at the injection site. Less common local reactions include erythema, swelling, warmth, or induration, which usually subsides within 48 hours. Transient low-grade fever, malaise, fatigue, vomiting, dizziness, myalgias, and arthralgias have been rare.

Postvaccination surveillance has shown a borderline significant association between Guillain-Barré syndrome and receipt of the first plasma-derived vaccine dose. The estimated attributable risk is 0.5 cases per 100,000 vaccines. No information regarding the risk is available for the recombinant hepatitis B vaccines. Plasma-derived vaccines have proved extremely safe in regard to potential transmission of infectious viral agents, including HIV.

Groups recommended for pre-exposure hepatitis B vaccination. In October 1994 the ACIP approved recommendations expanding the vaccination strategy to eliminate HBV transmission in the United States. These include vaccination of *all* 11- to 12-year-old children who have not previously received HBV vaccine and a general recommendation that adolescents should be immunized against HBV infection. Special efforts should be made to vaccinate adolescents at high risk for HBV, such as

Homosexual males

Users of illicit injectable drugs

Patients with clotting disorders

Populations with high rates of HBV infection: Alaskan natives, Pacific Islanders, immigrants from HBV-endemic areas

Household and sexual contacts of HBV carriers

Clients and staff of institutions for the developmentally disabled

Hemodialysis patients

Healthcare and public safety workers who are exposed to human blood

Sexually active heterosexual adolescents and adults with more than one sexual partner in the past 6 months or other sexually transmitted diseases

Adoptees from countries where HBV infection is endemic and members of households with adoptees who are HB_sAG positive

Inmates of long-term correctional facilities

International travelers to endemic HBV areas who plan to reside for more than 6 months and have close contact with the local population, or short-term travelers who are likely to have contact with blood or sexual contact

Postexposure prophylaxis for hepatitis B. The recommendations for hepatitis B prophylaxis after percutaneous or permucosal exposure are shown in Table 65-2.

Sexual exposure to hepatitis B. Susceptible sexual partners of persons with acute HBV infection or hepatitis B carriers should receive a single dose of hepatitis B immunoglobulin (0.06 ml/kg intramuscularly) within 14 days of the last sexual contact and should begin the hepatitis B vaccine series with a 1-ml dose intramuscularly. Then, either the three-dose series should be completed, or the individual should be tested for HB_sAg; if results are positive, the series should be completed.

TABLE 65-2
Hepatitis B Recommendations

Exposed Person	Treatment When Source Is Found to Be:		
	HB$_s$Ag Positive	HB$_s$Ag Negative	Source Not Tested or Unknown
Unvaccinated	HBIG × 1 and initiate HB vaccine	Initiate HB vaccine	Initiate HB vaccine
Previously vaccinated			
Known responder	Test exposed for anti-HB$_s$: 1. If adequate,* no treatment 2. If inadequate, HB vaccine booster dose	No treatment	No treatment
Known nonresponder	HBIG × 2 or HBIG × 1 plus one dose HB vaccine	No treatment	If known high-risk source, may treat as if source were HB$_s$Ag positive
Response unknown	Test exposed for anti-HB$_s$: 1. If inadequate,* HBIG × 1 plus HB vaccine booster dose 2. If adequate, no treatment	No treatment	Test exposed person for anti-HB$_s$: 1. If inadequate,* HB vaccine booster dose 2. If adequate, no treatment

From Centers for Disease Control and Prevention. Hepatitis B virus: a comprehensive strategy for eliminating transmission in the United States through universal childhood vaccination: recommendations of the Immunization Practices Advisory Committee (ACIP), *MMWR* 40(RR-13):22, 1991.
HBIG, hepatitis B immune globulin; *HB$_s$Ag*, hepatitis B surface antigen.
*Adequate anti-HB$_s$ is ~10 sample ratio units by radioimmunoassay or positive by electroimmunoassay.

IMMUNIZATION IN PREGNANCY

Adolescents of childbearing age ideally should be immune to poliomyelitis, measles, mumps, rubella, tetanus, diphtheria, hepatitis B, and varicella. Pregnant women are immunologically competent and generate adequate serologic responses to live attenuated vaccines, inactivated vaccines, and toxoids. In general, live attenuated vaccines are contraindicated in pregnancy because of their ability and potential to cause placental and fetal infection; the exceptions to this rule are polio and yellow fever virus vaccines, which may be administered if the risk of exposure is high. Inactivated vaccines and toxoids such as rabies, poliomyelitis, cholera, plague, typhoid fever, influenza, diphtheria, tetanus, and pertussis can be administered if indicated. Table 65-3 contains the recommendations for active and passive immunizations in pregnancy.

OCCUPATIONAL EXPOSURES

College Students

College students, particularly those living in dormitories, are at increased risk for certain infectious diseases, as are military recruits. Outbreaks of measles, rubella, and meningococcal disease have been reported on college campuses. Universal immunization against measles and rubella is recommended unless documented immunization, laboratory proof of seropositivity, or a documented measles diagnosis made by a physician is available. Also, all students should be vaccinated against tetanus, diphtheria, hepatitis B, and varicella, as mentioned. Influenza vaccination should be encouraged. Meningococcal vaccination should be considered as an adjunctive measure to chemoprophylaxis with antibiotics if a meningococcal disease outbreak is recognized on a college campus. Many states have passed legislation mandating immunization against certain diseases as a condition of college attendance.

Healthcare Personnel

Healthcare personnel, including adolescent volunteers with patient care contact, are at increased risk of acquiring certain preventable infectious diseases. Persons working in hospitals, nursing homes, laboratories, blood banks, clinics, physician offices, prisons, and schools are included in this category.

All healthcare workers should be immune to measles, mumps, rubella, poliomyelitis, tetanus-diphtheria, hepatitis B, and varicella. An annual influenza vaccination is strongly recommended to reduce morbidity among healthcare personnel and the likelihood of transmission of influenza to patients.

Pneumococcal vaccine is indicated for persons who have underlying heart or lung disease or asplenia. To

TABLE 65-3
Immunizations in Pregnancy

Disease	Vaccine	Active Immunization: Indications and Schedule	Passive Immunization: Agent and Schedule
Measles	Live attenuated virus	Contraindicated (to be given post partum to susceptible women)	Pooled immune globulin 0.25 ml/kg up to 15 ml must be given within 6 days of exposure
Mumps	Live attenuated virus	Contraindicated (to be given post partum to susceptible women)	Not indicated
Rubella	Live attenuated virus	Contraindicated (to be given post partum to susceptible women)	Not indicated
Poliomyelitis	Live virus	Not routine. Indicated when risk of exposure is high, such as travel to endemic area or during epidemics. If time allows: IPV, three doses q 1-2 mos. If less than 4 wk available: OPV, two doses q 6-8 wk. If primary series has been completed, single booster dose is recommended.	Not indicated
Yellow fever	Live virus	Travel to high-risk areas. One dose given subcutaneously.	Not indicated
Influenza	Inactivated virus, whole or split vaccine	Pregnant women at high risk because of cardiovascular, pulmonary, and chronic diseases (diabetes, chronic severe anemia, immunodeficiency states). Administer in early fall. Primary series: two doses, 6-8 wk apart; booster: one dose.	Not indicated
Rabies	Inactivated virus	Indications are same for nonpregnant women. Pre-exposure prophylaxis to veterinarians, animal handlers, field personnel, hunters, or people visiting or living in countries where rabies is prevalent. (See text for doses.)	Human rabies immune globulin is used for prophylaxis after exposure to rabies in previously unimmunized individual. Rabies immune globulin should be given as soon as possible after exposure; 20 IU/kg are given, 50% locally and 50% intramuscularly.
Cholera	Killed bacteria	Primary immunization consists of two 0.5-ml intramuscular doses given 4 wk apart. A booster dose of 0.5 ml should be given at 6-mo interval while danger of infection exists. Given to meet international travel requirements or during epidemics. Efficacy is 50%. Protection lasts 6 mo.	Not indicated
Typhoid fever	Typhoid Vi (ViCPS) polysaccharide	Typhoid vaccine is indicated for travelers to endemic areas. One 0.5-ml intramuscular dose constitutes primary series. Similar efficacy with other typhoid vaccines.	Not indicated
Plague	Killed bacteria	Plague vaccine is indicated for laboratory and field personnel working with *Yersinia pestis* or enzootic or epidemic plague and for exposed individuals. The primary series consist of three intramuscular doses: first, 1 ml; 4 wk later, 0.2 ml; 5 mo later, 0.2 ml.	Not indicated
Meningococcus	Polysaccharide group A, C, Y, W135	Indicated in control of outbreaks in closed or semiclosed populations, such as college, military, or epidemic disease and high-risk patients with terminal complement component deficiencies or asplenia. Single intramuscular injection provides protection in more than 90% of recipients.	Not indicated

Continued.

TABLE 65-3
Immunizations in Pregnancy—cont'd

Disease	Vaccine	Active Immunization: Indications and Schedule	Passive Immunization: Agent and Schedule
Pneumococcus	Polysaccharide with 23 serotypes	Indication as for influenza vaccine and patients with asplenia. One 0.5-ml intramuscular injection constitutes required immunization.	Not indicated
Tetanus-diphtheria	Toxoid	Lack of primary series or no booster in 10 yr. Primary series, three intramuscular doses at 1-mo intervals. Booster, 0.5 ml q 10 yr.	Tetanus postexposure prophylaxis with hyperimmune globulin should be administered as indicated in text.
Hepatitis B	Plasma-derived or recombinant vaccines	Indications are same as for nonpregnant individuals. (Refer to hepatitis B section.)	Hepatitis B immune globulin should be used after parenteral exposure or direct mucous membrane contact at dose of 0.06 ml/kg intramuscularly. Vaccines should be delayed for 2 mo after immune globulins are administered.
Hepatitis A	Inactivated virus	Not indicated owing to lack of data	Recommended for household contacts, other contacts with similar intensity, and travelers to epidemic areas. Also indicated in certain situations where member of household attends day care. Immune serum globulins, 0.02 ml/kg, should be given as soon as possible after exposure.
Varicella	Live attenuated virus	Contraindicated	Varicella-zoster immune globulin modifies infection. Susceptible pregnant woman after significant exposure to varicella may receive varicella zoster immune globulin at dose of 125 U/10 kg with maximal dose of 625 U intramuscularly as soon as possible after exposure.
Japanese encephalitis	Inactivated virus	Vaccine should be offered to pregnant women spending >30 days in endemic areas during transmission season, especially in travel in rural areas. Primary series: 3 1.0-ml subcutaneous doses at days 1, 7, and 30. 91% efficacious.	Not indicated

OPV, oral polio vaccine; *IPV,* inactivated polio vaccine.

ascertain immune status and vaccine schedules, refer to the sections on specific diseases in this chapter.

IMMUNOCOMPROMISED INDIVIDUALS

HIV Infection

The ACIP recommends that adolescents with HIV infection should receive Td, *Haemophilus influenzae* type B polysaccharide conjugate, pneumococcal, and inactivated influenza vaccines. IPV should be given in place of OPV. MMR vaccine is recommended in all but the most severely ill individuals, because of reports of severe measles and even deaths in symptomatic individuals infected with HIV. People infected with HIV and involved in high-risk behavior for acquiring hepatitis B infection (male homosexuals and intravenous drug users) should also receive active immunization with HBV. Bacillus Calmette-Guérin (BCG) is contraindicated in people infected with HIV.

Malignancies

Adolescents receiving immunosuppressive therapy for a malignancy should not receive live attenuated vaccine because of the risk of serious adverse effects. Viral vaccines should be administered no less than 3 months after all immunosuppressive therapy has been discontinued. Adolescents with acute lymphocytic leukemia in remission for more than 1 year may receive the live attenuated varicella vaccine through a research protocol.

Inactivated vaccines are not a risk to immunocompromised patients. If possible, these vaccines should be administered before the initiation of chemotherapy, radiotherapy, and splenectomy because of the reduced efficacy observed when vaccines are given with concurrent immunosuppressive therapy.

Many people with malignant diseases are at increased risk for invasive pneumococcal, *H. influenzae* type B, and influenza disease, and for hepatitis B infection from multiple exposures to blood products, and should be vaccinated against these pathogens. Patients recovering from bone marrow transplantation should be considered unimmunized and should be revaccinated with inactivated vaccines, including IPV. Transplant recipients receiving immunosuppressive therapy need to be vaccinated with pneumococcal, influenza, and hepatitis B vaccines.

Asplenia

Individuals with functional or anatomic asplenia, including those with sickle cell disease, have an increased risk of fulminant bacteremia caused by *Streptococcus pneumoniae, Neisseria meningitidis,* and *H. influenzae* type B, each of which carries a high mortality rate.

The polyvalent pneumococcal vaccine is recommended for all asplenic patients over 2 years of age in a single 0.5-ml intramuscular or subcutaneous injection. Protective antibody titers appear in 85% of patients. Many experts recommend revaccination every 2 to 5 years and continuous penicillin prophylaxis in addition to vaccination. Meningococcal vaccine also should be given to these individuals. This vaccine contains four group-specific antigenic capsular polysaccharides (A, C, Y, and W-135). Unfortunately, approximately 50% of meningococcal disease in the United States is caused by group B, which is not covered by the present vaccine. The vaccine consists of 50 μg each of the purified capsular polysaccharides, administered subcutaneously as a single 0.5-ml dose. Antibody responses in patients who have undergone splenectomy for either trauma or nonlymphoid tumors is comparable with that achieved in normal individuals; however, asplenic individuals who have received previous chemotherapy or radiation respond poorly. The duration of antibody response to the meningococcal vaccine in asplenic individuals is currently unknown.

Although little information is currently available concerning the efficacy of vaccination and the duration of antibody response in asplenic individuals, it is reasonable to immunize these patients with the *H. influenzae* type B

polysaccharide conjugate vaccine in a single 0.5-ml intramuscular dose.

No known contraindications exist to simultaneous administration of pneumococcal and meningococcal vaccines together with *H. influenzae* type B vaccine in separate syringes at different sites.

Chronic Diseases

Adolescents with chronic disease (cardiorespiratory, allergic, hematologic, metabolic, collagen vascular, and renal disorders) may be more susceptible to complications of influenza and pneumococcal infection and should be immunized with influenza and pneumococcal vaccines. Hepatitis B vaccine is also recommended for adolescents undergoing hemodialysis because of their frequent exposure to blood products.

Congenital Immunodeficiency Disorders

Live virus vaccines of all types, as well as BCG, are contraindicated in adolescents with congenital disorders of immune function. Inactivated vaccines (e.g., IPV) are preferable and should be administered. Individuals with deficiencies in antibody synthesis may not respond to vaccination; these individuals need to receive monthly doses of intravenous immune globulin, which provides passive protection against many infectious diseases.

Adolescents with selective IgA deficiency can be vaccinated with influenza and pneumococcal vaccines; however, they should not receive intravenous immune globulin, because this preparation contains insufficient amounts of IgA for replacement but enough to cause sensitization and lead to anaphylactic reactions if subsequent blood transfusions are administered.

Immigrants

Comprehensive medical evaluation of adolescent immigrants usually is performed before emigration from their home country. Immigrant adolescents who arrive in the United States illegally undergo no specific screening examination, and their preventive health care may be delayed or completely omitted.

The adolescent immigrant should have documentation of the required immunizations with which every adolescent should comply: measles, mumps, rubella, poliovirus, tetanus, diphtheria, and varicella. Testing for hepatitis B, including tests for HB_sAg, anti-HB_c, and anti-HB_s, will determine the need for hepatitis B vaccination. HIV testing by ELISA may be desirable in some instances. If HIV positivity is determined, expanded vaccination with pneumococcal and inactivated influenza vaccines, along with a switch from OPV to IPV, is recommended.

A Mantoux tuberculin skin test with a *Candida* antigen test for anergy, is important to rule out tuberculosis in view of the high prevalence of this disease in developing countries. Immigrants from countries in which BCG is used routinely may test positive, but these adolescents should be treated no differently from those who have not received previous BCG vaccination (see Chapter 68, "Tuberculosis").

POSTEXPOSURE IMMUNIZATION

Rabies

Pre-exposure immunization with the human diploid cell vaccine (HDCV) consists of three 1-ml doses intramuscularly in the deltoid area, one each on days 0, 7, and 28. Vaccination is recommended for groups at high risk for rabies infection, such as people working with animals (including veterinary students) and hunters exposed to potentially rabid dogs, cats, raccoons, foxes, skunks, or bats. Civilians and military personnel living or visiting countries where rabies is endemic also should be vaccinated.

Most rabies exposures come from unanticipated animal contact from a bite, a scratch, or mucosal contamination. The decision to provide specific antirabies treatment after contact depends on the type of exposure, species of animal, circumstances of the accident, and geographic location.

Postexposure treatment should begin with an immediate and thorough cleansing of all wounds with soap and water. Persons not previously immunized should receive rabies immune globulin, 20 IU/kg of body weight, half at the bite site and the rest intramuscularly; and five 1-ml doses of HDCV on days 0, 3, 7, 14, and 28. For persons previously immunized, two 1-ml doses of HDCV on days 0 and 3 should suffice. Rabies immune globulin should not be administered.

Local reactions such as pain, erythema, swelling, or itching at the injection site are reported in 25% of recipients of rabies vaccine. Mild systemic symptoms such as headache, nausea, abdominal pain, muscle aches, and dizziness are reported in approximately 20% of recipients.

Immune complex–type reactions (type III hypersensitivity reactions), appearing as a generalized pruritic rash or urticaria with or without arthralgia, arthritis, angioedema, nausea, vomiting, fever, and malaise, are seen in about 6% of patients receiving booster doses as part of a pre-exposure immunization regimen. Guillain-Barré syndrome has been reported rarely after vaccination, resolving without sequelae in 12 weeks. No deaths have been reported.

Hepatitis A

Immune globulin is recommended for postexposure prophylaxis in close household and sexual contacts of persons with hepatitis A, staff and household contacts of diapered children attending day care centers in which hepatitis A transmission is occurring, and food handlers with hepatitis A. A single 0.02-ml/kg dose of immune globulin should be administered as soon as possible, up to 2 weeks after exposure.

Pertussis

Although whole cell vaccine is highly reactive in adults, this is not the case with the acellular vaccines. Thus, these vaccines may find a role either in exposures or for routine immunization of adolescents (e.g., as dTaP). Exposed adolescents should receive erythromycin orally for 2 weeks.

Suggested Readings

American Academy of Pediatrics: *Report of the Committee on Infectious Diseases,* ed 23, Elk Grove Village, IL, 1994, American Academy of Pediatrics.

American College of Obstetricians and Gynecologists: Technical Bulletin no. 64. Washington DC, 1982, The College.

American College of Physicians Task Force on Adult Immunization and Infectious Diseases: *Guide for adult immunization,* Philadelphia, 1994, American College of Physicians.

Centers for Disease Control and Prevention: General recommendations on immunization, *MMWR* 40/No RR-1, 1994.

Centers for Disease Control and Prevention: *Health information for international travel,* Atlanta, 1994, US Department of Health and Human Services. Public Health Service.

Feigin RD, Cherry JD: *Textbook of pediatric infectious diseases,* ed 3, Philadelphia, 1992, WB Saunders.

Infectious Disease Clinics of North America, vol 4, nos. 1 and 2, Philadelphia, 1990, WB Saunders.

Mandell GL, Gordon Douglas R Jr, Bennet JE, editors: *Principles and practice of infectious diseases,* ed 4, New York, 1995, Churchill Livingstone.

Pediatric Clinics of North America, vol 37, no. 3, Philadelphia, 1990, WB Saunders.

Centers for Disease Control: Recommendations of the Advisory Committee on Immunization Practices, The American Academy of Pediatrics, The American Academy of Family Physicians, and The American Medical Association: Immunization of adolescents, 45(13):1996. Printed by the Massachusetts Medical Society Publishers of The New England Journal of Medicine.

American Academy of Pediatrics Committee on Infectious Diseases: Recommendations for the use of live attenuated varicella vaccine, *Pediatrics* 95:791-796, 1995.

Gardner P, Eickhoff T, Poland GA, et al: Adult immunizations, *Ann Intern Med* 124:35-40, 1996.

CHAPTER 66

Infectious Mononucleosis and Epstein-Barr Virus Infections

•

Nathaniel A. Brown

The Epstein-Barr virus (EBV) was discovered in 1964, when particles with typical herpesvirus morphologic characteristics were observed in electron micrographs of cultured Burkitt's lymphoma cells. Extensive seroepidemiologic and virologic studies during the 1960s and 1970s unexpectedly revealed that EBV infection was ubiquitous and was not limited to patients with Burkitt's lymphoma. These studies suggested that, on a worldwide basis, most persons become persistently infected with EBV by young adulthood. The discovery that EBV is the principal cause of infectious mononucleosis (IM) was serendipity. A technician in an EBV research laboratory was noted to have developed antibodies to EBV antigens when she developed mononucleosis. With this clue, further serologic studies established that EBV infection is the major cause of the mononucleosis syndrome.

Since the initial discovery, much has been learned about the pathogenesis of IM, which is now established as the most common illness recognizably associated with acute primary (initial) EBV infection. However, the universality of EBV infection continues to confound the study of the clinical consequences of persistent (chronic) EBV infection. For any group of patients with a clinical syndrome putatively related to "reactivated" chronic EBV infection, a high prevalence of EBV antibody, indicating EBV infection, generally can be found in groups of control subjects. Thus, specialized virologic, immunopathologic, and molecular biologic procedures are needed to implicate reactivated EBV infection in disease causation. Hence, the clinical consequences of chronic EBV infection remain incompletely understood. At present, it is thought that persistent EBV infection in normal subjects is generally without clinical consequences. This indeed appears to be the case for most adults, just as most adults silently carry other herpesviruses, such as herpes simplex virus, herpesvirus-6, herpesvirus-7, cytomegalovirus, and varicella-zoster virus.

Adolescent primary care is the clinical setting in which symptomatic EBV infection is most frequently encoun-

tered, usually in the form of acute IM or its complications. This chapter reviews the biologic and clinical aspects of EBV infection, with the aim of providing a knowledge base for sound clinical decisions regarding EBV infections as they are encountered in the practice of adolescent medicine. Because IM is a common and debilitating condition in adolescents, and because the complications of EBV infection are sometimes serious, it is important for clinicians to have a good working knowledge of EBV infection, including its epidemiology, pathogenesis, clinical manifestations, treatment, and prognosis.

EPIDEMIOLOGY

The EBV has been called the most prevalent viral infection of man, although the recently described human herpesvirus 6 (HHV-6) may infect human populations even more widely. In all worldwide populations studied to date, it appears that at least 90% to 95% of individuals are infected with EBV by the age of 30 years. However, there are large geographic differences in the age-related incidence of primary EBV infection in the first three decades of life. In some countries or locales, virtually 100% of individuals become infected with EBV by the age of 3 to 6 years. In contrast, in socioeconomically advanced countries, including the United States, primary EBV infection is still most common in early childhood. However, an appreciable number of initial EBV infections do not occur until the second or third decades of life, presumably because of different patterns of interpersonal contact and differences in hygiene. The age-related prevalence of EBV antibody varies among different cultural and socioeconomic groups, but overall it appears that about 50% of U.S. individuals are infected with EBV by the age of 10 years. Thus, by the high school and college years, about 30% to 40% of U.S. adolescents remain EBV seronegative and are potentially susceptible to primary EBV infection. Numerous studies have shown that EBV-related IM develops only in these seronegative (or susceptible) individuals. As would be expected, then, IM is rare in countries or among socioeconomic groups in which primary EBV infection occurs universally in early childhood. This is the case for many developing countries in Africa, Asia, and Central and South America. IM is more frequently observed in North America, Europe, and Australia.

BIOLOGY

Electron microscopic studies established that EBV has the ultrastructural features common to herpesviruses. EBV virions are enveloped particles measuring approximately 150 to 200 nm in diameter. Inside the lipoprotein envelope is a spherical (icosahedral) nucleocapsid 110 nm in size. A proteinaceous capsid shell encloses the linear, double-stranded DNA genome of the virus. The EBV genome contains more than 170,000 nucleotide base pairs (170 Kb). Rapid progress is being made regarding the molecular genetics of EBV and expression of the viral genome inside infected cells. The viral genome potentially encodes more than 80 proteins, but full expression of the genome occurs only in cells that support the entire viral replicative cycle. Such cells are said to be lytically infected, and it is thought that this state of viral replication is eventually fatal to the cell. An alternative state of the EBV genome inside cells involves restricted expression of the viral genome (i.e., expression of about 10 gene loci). Such cells are said to be latently infected. All herpesviruses share this ability to persist inside some cells as latent genomes with limited viral gene expression. It is this property that results in lifelong carriage of these viruses in various tissues of the body after the initial (primary) infection.

The predominant tissue tropisms of EBV are for B lymphocytes and certain epithelial cells—for example, in salivary glands, the oropharynx, and perhaps the mucous membranes of the genitourinary tract. Recent evidence suggests that lymphoid precursor cells or rare T lymphocytes may also occasionally become infected with EBV. In attaching to cells, EBV parasitizes a receptor for the third component of the complement cascade, the C3d receptor (CR2, or CD21). This cell surface moiety appears to be distributed mostly on mature B lymphocytes and certain epithelial cells. Although the distribution of the C3d receptor appears to be the major determinant of EBV tissue tropism, there may be other cell surface molecules that can serve as EBV receptors for some cell types.

After attachment, the enveloped viral particle undergoes pinocytosis into the cytoplasm, where the viral envelope and capsid shell are removed, and the viral genome enters the cell nucleus. Then, a critical event occurs. The two ends of the linear viral DNA genome become covalently joined, resulting in a circularized extrachromosomal DNA plasmid (episome), which is stable and has self-replicative capabilities inside the cell nucleus. This circularized viral episome persists inside cells even when the viral replicative cycle is effectively inhibited, for example, by currently available antiviral drugs. Thus, drugs that inhibit the viral replicative cycle can be virustatic but are not virucidal, since no means have yet been discovered to "cure" cells of their intranuclear herpesvirus episomes.

After circularization, the EBV genome is amplified in copy-number, so that a typical latently infected cell contains two to 60 intranuclear copies of the circularized EBV episome. Cellular gene products, interacting with specific EBV gene loci and with EBV "early" gene products, appear to be critical to the subsequent pattern of expression of the virus in infected cells. In salivary gland and perhaps oropharyngeal tissue, it appears that a pattern of chronic semipermissive viral infection is established, resulting in relatively heavy virus shedding in saliva for several months after initial infection, followed by lifelong low-level shedding of virus in the oropharyngeal secretions of most individuals. In the B lymphocytes of most persons, the most common state is viral latency, with rare B cells sporadically entering the viral replicative cycle. In vitro, EBV has the interesting property of growth-transforming ("immortalizing") the B lymphocytes of humans and several primate species, resulting in the ability to propagate such cells indefinitely in tissue culture. It is thought that this property of growth transformation of cells in vitro may be related to the association of EBV with several neoplasias in vivo.

The primary sites of somatic persistence of EBV are still controversial. It was previously thought that somatic persistence derived mainly from chronic semipermissive infection of the salivary glands. However, recent studies of patients who underwent bone marrow transplantation and who received cyclophosphamide for lymphoid ablation before transplantation suggest that lymphocytes may be the most important somatic compartment for EBV latency and persistence. After lymphoid ablation, the transplant patients appeared to lose evidence of infection with their previous EBV strain, and some subsequently became infected with new EBV strains.

CLINICAL ASPECTS AND PATHOGENESIS OF EPSTEIN-BARR VIRUS–RELATED DISEASES

Initial Infection

Infection with EBV is usually acquired through oropharyngeal exposure to the oral secretions of an

EBV-infected family member or other social contact: hence, the traditional reference to IM as "the kissing disease." However, it is likely that contact with virus-contaminated secretions on shared drinking vessels and eating utensils, and other forms of nonsexual family contact, play important roles in EBV transmission. After entry of the virus into the oropharynx, EBV infection becomes established in the salivary glands, where a chronic semipermissive infection occurs, apparently for life. Secondary infection of lymphocytes and the lymphoid organs occurs either by way of a viremia originating in the salivary glands or by direct infection of lymphocytes as they traffic through oropharyngeal and salivary gland tissues.

Silent Primary Infection

In most young children and in one half to two thirds of adolescents and adults, the initial (primary) infection with EBV does not result in appreciable clinical illness. Such infections are said to be silent or subclinical, yet they are important because they make up the preponderance of EBV infections worldwide. Silently infected individuals remain persistently infected with EBV; they apparently develop a full immunologic response and are thought to be protected against clinically significant reinfections with EBV later in life.

Infectious Mononucleosis

Individuals who remain EBV seronegative into their teenage years or beyond are most susceptible to the clinical consequences of EBV infection. After contracting primary EBV infection, about 30% to 50% of adolescents develop the clinical symptoms and signs of the mononucleosis syndrome. A tetrad of findings makes up the classic syndrome of IM: fever, tonsillopharyngitis, lymphadenopathy, and an absolute lymphocytosis with many circulating "atypical" lymphocytes. Frequently, the classic tetrad is preceded by a prodrome of malaise, fatigue, and headache, with or without low-grade fever, usually lasting 1 to 5 days. In patients having typical IM, initial findings on physical examination usually include tonsillopharyngitis, with or without exudate, and bilateral anterior and posterior cervical lymphadenopathy. The lymphadenopathy is sometimes generalized and usually becomes maximal in the second or third week of illness. Within the first 3 weeks of illness, splenomegaly is noted in about 50% to 60% of patients and hepatomegaly in 10% to 25%. Many patients develop enanthema consisting of petechiae on the soft palate. A maculopapular or morbilliform rash appears in 5% to 10% of patients. Clinically evident jaundice is found in 5% to 10%. Chemosis and facial puffiness are evident in some patients. Rarer physical findings include signs of arthritis,

severe skin rashes (e.g., erythema multiforme, Stevens-Johnson syndrome), and signs referable to complications involving major organ systems (e.g., blood dyscrasias, pneumonia, cardiac or renal manifestations). The severity of the discomforts of IM can sometimes result in markedly decreased oral intake and subsequent dehydration. A concurrent group A streptococcal pharyngitis is noted in approximately 5% to 20% of patients. The manifestations of acute IM are summarized in Box 66-1. The incubation period from the time of initial oropharyngeal infection until the development of IM is about 4 to 7 weeks.

BOX 66-1
Manifestations of Infectious Mononucleosis

CLINICAL SYMPTOMS AND SIGNS
Prodrome (1 to 5 days)
  Fatigue, malaise, headache
  Fever (usually low grade)
Acute illness
  Usually present:
    Fatigue, malaise, headache
    Fever (low to moderate, usually <39.5°C
      [<104°F])
    Sore throat/tonsillopharyngitis
    Anterior and posterior cervical lymphadenopathy
  Often present:
    Diffuse lymphadenopathy
    Organomegaly (splenomegaly in 50%, hepatomegaly in 10%-25%)
    Enanthema (petechiae on soft palate)
  Sometimes present:
    Chemosis/periorbital edema
    Rash (maculopapular, morbilliform)
    Jaundice
    Interstitial pneumonia
    Organ system complications

LABORATORY FEATURES
Complete blood count
  Absolute lymphocytosis (>50% lymphocytes on differential)
  Increased "atypical" lymphocytes (>5%)
Serologic tests
  Heterophil antibodies (Paul-Bunnell type)
  EBV-specific antibody pattern consistent with primary infection
Other tests
  Mildly elevated serum aminotransferases (ALT, AST)
  Occasional hyperbilirubinemia

ALT, alanine aminotransferase; *AST,* aspartate aminotransferase.

Because of the low availability of susceptible seronegative persons and the long incubation period for the clinical illness, EBV-associated IM is generally observed not as an epidemic illness but as a sporadic endemic illness. "Epidemics" of IM-like illnesses are usually not caused by EBV but rather are the result of other viral causes of illnesses having some features of the mononucleosis syndrome, including adenoviruses, influenza A and B viruses, and parainfluenza viruses. Also, illnesses clinically resembling IM can be observed with cytomegalovirus infection, in HHV-6 infection, in primary infection with the human immunodeficiency virus (HIV), in acute toxoplasmosis, or in infections with hepatitis A or rubella viruses. Overall, EBV causes 80% to 90% of cases of bona fide mononucleosis syndromes, and it is the only cause of mononucleosis in which Paul-Bunnell–type heterophil antibodies develop. Thus, the other potential microbial agents should be considered, as appropriate, in heterophil-negative cases of IM-like illness, although it is important to be aware that EBV is also the most common cause of heterophil-negative mononucleosis.

The pathogenesis of IM has been likened to a self-limited lymphoma. In individuals experiencing the first week of acute IM, a mild increase in total B lymphocytes is noted, and about 0.1% to 20% of circulating B cells are infected with EBV. A protean cellular and humoral immune reaction occurs in response to this viral invasion of the lymphoid compartment, involving brisk responses by natural-killer mononuclear cells and cytotoxic/suppressor T lymphocytes and antibody responses to multiple EBV antigens. It is thought that the strong immune response is responsible for the characteristic lymphadenopathy, organomegaly, and other clinical manifestations of IM. The net effect of this massive immune response is a rapid reduction in the number of circulating EBV-infected cells. Within several weeks after the acute stage of IM, the number of circulating EBV-infected B lymphocytes is reduced to about 1 per million lymphocytes. This small proportion of EBV-infected cells remains in the blood of most persons for life, although it may increase again under conditions of debilitation or immunodeficiency.

Excretion of infectious EBV in saliva becomes maximal shortly after the onset of acute IM and can persist at high levels for more than 6 to 12 months. It was previously thought that salivary shedding of EBV was observable in only 10% to 20% of healthy, EBV-seropositive persons. However, more sensitive techniques have revealed that virtually all EBV-seropositive individuals shed virus in the oropharynx, probably for life. This observation and the epidemiologic data summarized above suggest that most adults in the world shed EBV continuously in their throats, generally in low amounts. Therefore, silently infected older family members are the likely source of most infections in children, through interpersonal contact within families.

One study indicated that, in most persons undergoing acute IM related to primary EBV infection, there is also serologic evidence suggesting marked reactivation of a preexisting HHV-6 infection. Thus, it is possible that some of the clinical features or some of the occasional complications of IM result from reactivated HHV-6 infection in conjunction with primary EBV infection. However, the pathogenetic role of HHV-6 reactivation in patients with IM remains to be elucidated.

Atypical Clinical Syndromes and Complications

Patients undergoing primary EBV infection sometimes manifest unusual clinical features, which may represent the presenting syndrome or may occur in conjunction with the clinical signs of IM. In individual reports, EBV infection has been associated with dysfunction of nearly every organ system. Overall, it appears that the complications of EBV infection are associated with several dozen deaths yearly in the United States. The most common serious complications involve blood dyscrasias or neurologic syndromes. EBV infection also has been associated with hemolytic anemia, aplastic anemia, hemophagocytic syndromes, transient pancytopenia, isolated leukopenia or thrombocytopenia, and red cell aplasia. Marrow hypoplasia and the hemophagocytic syndrome often occur in conjunction with a moderate or severe degree of hepatitis. Serious neurologic consequences of EBV infection have included parainfectious encephalitis, Alice in Wonderland syndrome, Guillain-Barré syndrome, cerebellar ataxia, transverse myelitis, Bell's palsy, and peripheral neuropathy. Splenic rupture occurs occasionally but appears to be rarer than previously thought. Other serious complications include severe hepatitis, cardiac dysfunction, renal disease (both nephritis and nephrosis have been reported), and pancreatitis. Polyarticular or pauciarticular arthritis occurs occasionally but is generally not serious by itself. Interstitial pneumonia occurs in as many as 5% of patients with IM but is often inapparent and not usually clinically serious.

The pathogenesis of most of the rare complications of EBV infection appears to involve disordered immunologic responses to EBV, but the pathogenetic details of these disorders are difficult to establish because of their rarity, the need for specialized research studies, and the difficulty of providing corollary results in appropriate controls.

Severe Chronic Infection

Several reports have described rare patients who appear to suffer from chronic symptomatic EBV infection with severe manifestations. The clinical descriptions vary somewhat, but such patients typically have recurrent episodes of moderate to high fever, intermittent blood dyscrasias (e.g., leukopenia, anemia, thrombocytopenia), intermittent organomegaly and hepatitis, putative autoimmune phenomena (e.g., arthritis or uveitis), and episodes of interstitial pneumonia. Some patients have died, usually of intercurrent bacterial sepsis or pneumonia. In some patients the disease appears to be familial, but sporadic cases also have been noted. Such patients are rare, and they are distinguished by very high antibody titers to EBV-replicative antigens and the typically impaired antibody response to the EBV nuclear antigen complex.

Associated Tumors

Although not commonly encountered in primary adolescent care settings in the United States, various neoplastic processes are associated with EBV infection, and clinicians should be aware of these. In particular, the endemic form of Burkitt's lymphoma and undifferentiated nasopharyngeal carcinoma represent monoclonal, neoplastic expansions of EBV-infected cells. EBV is also associated with B lymphomas and B-lymphoproliferative disorders in immunodeficient or immunosuppressed hosts, which appear to result from unchecked proliferation of EBV-transformed B cells. Recent evidence also suggests that EBV may somehow be involved in 50% or more of cases of Hodgkin's disease, and EBV has been implicated in parotid carcinomas, primary central nervous system lymphoma (especially in AIDS patients), and certain lymphoepithelial lesions.

Other Associated Disorders

EBV appears to be the cause of oral hairy leukoplakia, a condition involving whitish, mosslike epithelial lesions on the margins of the tongue and the buccal mucosa. This condition is found only in immunodeficient hosts, especially as a component of the AIDS-related complex. The presence of oral hairy leukoplakia in an adolescent or adult should alert the clinician to the possibility that the patient has progressive immune deficiency related to HIV infection. Oral hairy leukoplakia has also been noted in organ transplant patients and in patients with other forms of immune deficiency.

Chronic Fatigue Syndrome

EBV infection was previously implicated in a symptom complex that was initially called chronic EBV infection or chronic mononucleosis but is now most commonly known as the chronic fatigue syndrome (CFS) (see Chapter 107, "Chronic Fatigue Syndrome"). The clinical signs of this disorder are vague and are not generally agreed, although case definitions have been proposed for the purpose of epidemiologic studies.

Fundamentally, CFS is a symptom complex in which the dominant complaint is life style dysfunction due to severe and intractable fatigue of more than 6 months' duration. Other symptoms, especially cognitive dysfunction, and mild physical signs also can be part of the CFS syndrome. The symptom complex, which may have multiple causes, may be temporally associated with any of a number of physical or psychiatric stresses. Recent controlled studies suggest that EBV is probably not a major cause of CFS, although occasional CFS patients may have experienced recent mononucleosis or a subclinical primary EBV infection. The latter group of patients can be detected by testing for heterophil antibodies and assessment of the EBV-specific antibody profile. However, at this time such serologic tests are not indicated for most patients with the CFS syndrome, since EBV involvement is generally unlikely and because antiviral therapy has been found to lack benefit in a controlled trial involving patients with CFS.

LABORATORY DIAGNOSIS

In patients with the typical clinical signs of IM, two laboratory tests are useful to establish the diagnosis of EBV-related IM: a complete blood count (with leukocyte differential) and a test for heterophil antibodies.

Complete Blood Count

The complete blood count typically shows an elevated total leukocyte count, usually in the range of 10,000 to 18,000 white blood cells per cubic millimeter, with an absolute lymphocytosis (> 50% lymphocytes) and with an increased number of atypical lymphocytes, usually more than 5%. The lymphocytosis is often maximal in the second or third week of illness. Platelet counts may be mildly depressed in the first week of illness, or they may become elevated as a component of an acute-phase reaction. Similarly, neutrophil counts are sometimes mildly decreased in the first 1 or 2 weeks, or they may be elevated as part of an acute-phase response.

Heterophil Antibody Testing

Heterophil antibodies are immunoglobulin M (IgM) antibodies that agglutinate erythrocytes of several animal species, including sheep, oxen, and horses. It has been known for more than 50 years that heterophil agglutinins develop during acute IM, and heterophil antibody testing remains the single most useful means of confirming a diagnosis of IM. A number of tests for heterophil antibodies are commercially available. Since the mid-1980s, most laboratories have preferred to use tests based on the agglutination of horse red blood cells (RBCs) on glass slides (e.g., Mono-Spot, Mono-Test, Mono-Diff).

Horse RBCs are a more sensitive indicator substrate than sheep RBCs, which were used formerly. However, with either RBC indicator system it is important to first absorb the sera with guinea pig kidney extract and erythrocyte stromal material to ensure specific detection of IM-related (Paul-Bunnell–type) heterophil antibodies. When such absorption is not done, the agglutination assays with horse or sheep RBCs can give a high false-positive rate because of the presence in most persons of two other types of heterophil agglutinins, Forssman and serum sickness–type antibodies. Also, with the use of the sensitive horse RBC-based heterophil assays, it is important to remember that such tests remain positive for prolonged periods after acute IM; for example, 75% of patients maintain a heterophil agglutinin titer of 1:40 or greater for at least 12 months, although there is generally a quantitative decline within the first 2 to 4 months after onset of illness.

Epstein-Barr Virus–Specific Serologic Tests

For unknown reasons, heterophil agglutinins are often absent in very young children with mononucleosis syndromes, especially in those under 5 years of age. After age 8 to 10 years, however, most subjects (80% to 90%) with EBV-related mononucleosis have a positive heterophil test result. Only about 50% are positive in the first week of illness, and repeated (weekly) testing during the first 3 to 4 weeks of illness may be needed to detect the development of heterophil antibodies. When a patient has typical features of IM and exhibits a positive heterophil antibody test, it is neither necessary nor desirable to perform EBV-specific serologic testing, since interpretation of the latter can be problematic and the results are sometimes equivocal. However, when results of the heterophil antibody test are negative, it may be desirable to perform EBV-specific serologic testing to detect evidence of recent primary EBV infection. Such testing is desirable if the differential diagnosis is difficult, the patient is seriously ill, and accurate prognostication is required.

The pattern of the usual serologic response to EBV antigens is illustrated in Figure 66-1. An individual who is not infected with EBV will be seronegative in all assays, including tests for IgG antibody to the EBV viral capsid antigen (VCA) complex, which is used as the initial screening test in most laboratories. Individuals who have experienced recent primary infection will develop IgM and IgG antibodies to the EBV viral capsid antigens, along with antibodies to the early antigen (EA) complex. Appreciable levels of antibody to the EBV nuclear antigen (EBNA) complex are usually lacking in the first 1 to 2 months of illness, but they develop subsequently in most persons. Thus, the cardinal serologic evidence of recent primary EBV infection is a

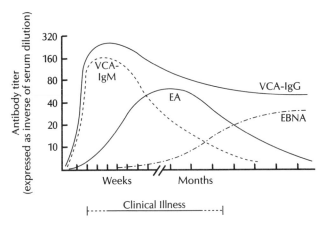

Fig. 66-1. Typical human serologic response to Epstein-Barr virus infection. At clinical presentation (usually 4 to 7 weeks after exposure), anti–viral capsid antigen (anti-*VCA*) response may consist of *IgM* and *IgG* antibodies, anti–early antigen (anti-*EA*) response is often present, and anti–EBV nuclear antigen (anti-EBNA) is commonly negative. IgM anti-VCA response usually subsides within 2 to 4 months, and anti-EA response usually disappears within 2 to 6 months. Chronically infected, asymptomatic persons maintain measurable IgG anti-VCA and anti-EBNA titers for life. (Modified from Andiman WA, McCarthy P, Markowitz R, et al: Clinical, virologic, and serologic evidence of Epstein-Barr virus infection in association with childhood pneumonia, *J Pediatr* 99:880-886, 1981.)

positive IgG anti-VCA test and a negative anti-EBNA test. Positive results in the assays for IgM anti-VCA antibodies and IgG anti-EA antibodies can be supportive of the interpretation of recent primary EBV infection, but such results are absent in as many as 40% to 50% of cases, depending on the timing of the clinical presentation and the assay methods used for testing. In most persons, IgM anti-VCA antibodies become undetectable within 1 to 3 months, and anti-EA antibodies decline to undetectable levels within 2 to 6 months after initial infection. The serologic pattern of chronic ("normal") EBV infection thus consists of positive tests for IgG anti-VCA and anti-EBNA antibodies. Also, in as many as 10% to 30% of apparently normal individuals, anti-EA antibodies remain detectable in low titer (generally <1:40) in tests using immunofluorescence. The various interpretations of EBV serologic tests are summarized in Box 66-2. As noted earlier, cases of the rare syndrome of severe chronic EBV infection can be confirmed by adjunctive use of EBV serologic tests. Such patients usually develop very high titers of antibody to EBV-replicative antigens—for example, titers more than 1:5000 for IgG anti-VCA antibody and titers more than 1:640 for IgG anti-EA antibodies, when these tests are done by immunofluorescence. These results are often found in conjunction with absent or low levels of anti-EBNA antibody, resulting from a diminished response to the chief antigenic component of the EBNA complex.

*Normal titer ranges vary among different laboratories. Abnormal titers should be judged according to specific laboratory normal values. The clinical significance of a "reactivated" pattern is unclear.
VCA, viral capsid antigen; *EBNA,* EBV nuclear antigen; *EA,* early antigen.

Other Laboratory Tests

Other tests are sometimes indicated in assessing patients with acute EBV infections. Up to 80% of patients exhibit mild elevations of serum hepatocellular enzyme levels. Serum aspartate and alanine aminotransferase levels generally remain below 200 IU/ml, but more severe hepatitis is observed occasionally. Thus, patients with significant hepatomegaly or jaundice should be evaluated with serial tests of liver function. In such patients it is also advisable to perform serial complete blood counts with leukocyte differentials and platelet counts, since a severe hepatitis picture often precedes EBV-related marrow hypoplasia or hemophagocytic syndromes. Other biochemical tests, such as of serum electrolytes and renal function, should be performed according to clinical indications and the need for parenteral fluid support. Throat cultures to rule out concurrent group A streptococcal pharyngitis should be performed liberally in patients with IM, especially in those with evidence of severe pharyngitis or exudate.

Specialized tests are indicated for patients in whom complications are evident. For example, hemolytic anemia develops in some patients and is usually due to anti-I antibodies, which can be detected in laboratory tests.

Patients with complications of major organ systems should be assessed by relevant techniques (electrocardiograms, cardiac ultrasonography, chest radiography, computed tomography or magnetic resonance imaging, lumbar puncture) as appropriate. Patients with severe IM often develop diffuse organ enlargement, which is sometimes noted on radiographs or body scans. By itself, moderate organ enlargement is not a bad prognostic marker and tends to resolve spontaneously. In general, however, significant organ system dysfunctions require hospitalization and a full evaluation, including subspecialty consultations.

TREATMENT AND PROGNOSIS

Antiviral Therapy

To date, antiviral therapy has not been shown to be consistently beneficial in acute IM or in other forms of EBV infection, except for oral hairy leukoplakia. In several studies, treatment of patients who have acute IM with high-dose intravenous or oral acyclovir has been shown to reduce pharyngeal excretion of EBV. However, the treatment had minimal impact on clinical manifestations, probably because (1) IM is essentially an immunologically mediated disease that is well established within the usual 4- to 7-week incubation period before clinical recognition and treatment, (2) acyclovir has no impact on the resolution of this immunologic reaction, and (3) the inciting EBV viremia is typically already abating at the time of the clinical presentation. Thus, there is no current evidence that patients with typical acute IM should be treated with acyclovir or another antiviral agent. However, in patients with serious complications (especially those requiring adjunctive steroid therapy) or in immunocompromised patients with early lymphoproliferative disease, most specialists empirically use antiviral therapy in conjunction with other supportive care. If acyclovir is used in patients with severe complications, maximal dosage should be administered (30 mg/kg/day intravenously, divided every 8 hours, or 1500 mg/m^2/day intravenously, divided every 8 hours). Therapy should continue for a minimum of 10 days. It has been noted in several reports that acyclovir in high oral doses also has been found to be effective for the treatment and suppression of hairy leukoplakia in AIDS patients. Other antivirals, such as ganciclovir, also have in vitro activity against EBV, but these agents have undergone minimal clinical evaluation.

Supportive Therapy

Acetaminophen or aspirin and adequate fluid intake are the mainstays of supportive therapy. Corticosteroids are used by some physicians for the management of uncomplicated acute IM, but controlled data supporting this practice are lacking, and the potential for exacerbating EBV replication and its consequences cannot be readily dismissed. Thus, most infectious disease specialists reserve steroid use for evidence of complications, especially hematologic or neurologic complications, in which steroid use is also empiric but the risk-benefit consideration may be more advantageous. One exception is the hemophagocytic syndrome, in which some reports suggest that steroids may be contraindicated. Some clinicians also use steroids when evidence of coarse-sounding "tonsillar breathing" develops. However, it is usually the upper poles of the tonsils that are enlarged in acute IM; enlargement of the lower poles that leads to true respiratory obstruction is unusual.

As with other debilitating conditions, patients with acute IM require clinical evaluation and serial follow-up to ensure that adequate hydration and nutrition are maintained and to detect complications as soon as possible. In typical IM cases, patients should be assessed at least weekly during the first 3 weeks, then subsequently as needed. It is customary to encourage rest during the early phase of acute IM. Patients are usually advised not to take part in contact sports, bicycling, skating, and other activities that might result in abdominal trauma until they are feeling better and organomegaly is no longer evident (thus limiting the risk of rupture of a tensely enlarged spleen through trauma). However, a risk of spontaneous splenic rupture remains. The overall risk of splenic rupture appears small, probably less than 1 in 1000 cases of IM. Patients and parents should be advised to seek medical help immediately when signs of possible complications develop. In most cases of acute IM, substantial resolution of clinical signs and symptoms occurs within 2 to 4 weeks. However, lymphadenopathy, organomegaly, or both sometimes remain appreciable for 3 to 4 months. Despite substantial resolution of the signs of illness, patients with IM have a notorious propensity for experiencing protracted fatigue, which may persist for several months. In extreme cases, fatigue may not resolve for 1 to 2 years. In the absence of complications or other underlying conditions, patients should be encouraged to resume normal activities as tolerated, in conjunction with an adequate diet and an appropriate exercise regimen.

Although acute IM is distressing and often debilitating to the patient, it requires only simple management considerations and is generally benign in eventual outcome in the normal host. Conscientious follow-up will provide early detection of most complications, allow supportive care, and usually result in eventual spontaneous recovery. On the other hand, immunocompromised patients, or patients with advanced stages of serious complications, have a potentially life-threatening condition that may require hospitalization and multidisciplinary subspecialty management.

Suggested Readings

Bailey RE: Diagnosis and treatment of infectious mononucleosis, *Am Fam Physician* 49:879-888, 1994.

Brown N: The Epstein-Barr virus: infectious mononucleosis, B-lymphoproliferative disorders. In Feigin RD, Cherry JD, editors: *Textbook of pediatric infectious diseases,* ed. 2, Philadelphia, 1987, WB Saunders, pp 1566-1577.

Connelly KP, DeWitt LD: Neurologic complications of infectious mononucleosis, *Pediatr Neurol* 10:181-184, 1994.

Epstein MA, Achong BG, Barr YM: Virus particles in cultured lymphoblasts from Burkitt's lymphoma, *Lancet* 1:702-703, 1964.

Miller G: The Epstein-Barr virus: biology, pathogenesis, and medical aspects. In Fields B, Knipe DM, editors: *Virology,* ed. 2, New York, 1990, Raven Press, pp 1921-1958.

Miller G, Grogan E, Rowe D, Rooney C, Heston L, Eastman R, Andiman W, Niederman J, Lenoir G, Henle W, Sullivan J, Schooley R, Vossen J, Straus S, Issekutz T: Selective lack of antibody to a component of EBV nuclear antigen in patients with chronic active Epstein-Barr virus infection, *J Infect Dis* 156:26-34, 1987.

Niederman JC, McCollum RW, Henle G, Henle W: Infectious mononucleosis: clinical manifestations in relation to EB virus antibodies, *JAMA* 203:205-209, 1968.

Schlossberg D, editor: *Infectious mononucleosis,* ed. 2, New York, 1989, Springer-Verlag.

Sullivan JL: Epstein-Barr virus and lymphoproliferative disorders, *Semin Hematol* 25:269-279, 1988.

CHAPTER 67

HIV Infection and AIDS

•

Donna Futterman, Neal Hoffman, and Karen Hein

The 1990s mark the second decade of the acquired immunodeficiency syndrome (AIDS) pandemic, and adolescents and young adults represent a dynamic and expanding proportion of those newly infected. Human immunodeficiency virus (HIV) infection and AIDS have already had a profound medical and social impact on adolescents. Since 1988, AIDS has been the sixth leading cause of death among youth in the United States aged 15 to 24 years.[1] Of the nation's 548,102 cases through June 1996, 19% are young people aged 20 to 29 years.[2] Because there is an average 10-year latency period from HIV infection (acquisition of the virus) to the development of AIDS, many of these individuals were infected while still teenagers.[3] The National Cancer Institute estimates that 25% of the people with HIV in the United States were infected before age 22.[4] The World Health Organization has estimated that 50% of the 12 to 14 million people with HIV in the world were infected before age 25 years.[5]

AIDS and HIV infection pose a particular threat to adolescents, because the same behaviors that can expose them to HIV infection are often at the intersection of risk-taking behaviors and normative developmental tasks of adolescence. Those who provide medical services for adolescents are faced with the challenge of incorporating AIDS prevention programs, screening for HIV, and direct medical care for HIV-infected youth into already existing adolescent services.[6] Elements of this care are discussed in this chapter, along with the epidemiology of AIDS and HIV infection among adolescents.

EPIDEMIOLOGY: HIV TRANSMISSION

AIDS Cases

National reporting of AIDS cases to the Centers for Disease Control and Prevention (CDC) includes two age groups for adolescents: 13 to 19 years and 20 to 24 years.[2] This age breakdown complicates an understanding of the epidemic among adolescents who are 13 to 21 years of

age. Through June 1996, there were 2574 reported cases of AIDS among 13- to 19-year-olds and 19,997 reported cases among 20- to 24-year-olds. Adolescents aged 13 to 21 years represent approximately 1% of the total AIDS caseload. Approximately half of adolescents aged 13 to 19 years and 90% of adolescents and young adults aged 20 to 24 years with AIDS were infected through sexual exposure or intravenous drug use.

Exposure categories vary by gender according to age group. Adolescents with AIDS are primarily male (66% of 13- to 19-year-olds and 75% of 20- to 24-year-olds), but the male-to-female ratio is lower among 13- to 19-year-old adolescents (2:1) than among adults (7:1). Among youths 13 to 19 years old, receipt of blood products accounted for 41% of male cases and male-to-male sex for 32%, while male-to-female sexual contact accounted for 52% of female cases. Among 20- to 24-year-olds with AIDS, sex with males accounted for 63% of transmission in males, while heterosexual exposure again accounted for 55% of transmission in females. In contrast, perinatal transmission accounts for almost 90% of AIDS cases among children younger than 13 years; the remaining cases are associated with the receipt of infected blood products.

Ethnic and racial minorities are disproportionately represented. African-Americans and Hispanics represent 61% of 13- to 24-year-old AIDS cases, although they are only 27% of the U.S. population in this age group. Adolescents with AIDS have been reported from at least 45 states, Puerto Rico, and the District of Columbia, but most (54%) have been reported from five states (Florida, New York, California, Texas, New Jersey) and Puerto Rico.[7]

HIV Seroprevalence

Focusing solely on the number of AIDS cases provides a substantial underestimation of the scope of the epidemic among adolescents, given the average 10-year period from infection to the development of advanced HIV disease or AIDS. Therefore, a description of youths with

AIDS must include data on HIV infection and behaviors that put adolescents at risk for HIV infection.

Although it is not known how many adolescents in the United States are infected with HIV, small-scale seroprevalence studies have been useful in estimating the extent of the epidemic and in providing portraits of certain at-risk subpopulations. Since 1985, all applicants to the U.S. military have been tested for HIV antibodies. Up to December 1992, among youth 17 to 19 years of age (n = 2,053,708), a seroprevalence of 0.03% was noted, increasing to 0.14% among applicants aged 20 to 24 years (n = 1,077,106).[7] The Job Corps, a federal training and employment program for socioeconomically disadvantaged youths, began screening entrants in 1987. They reported an overall seroprevalence of 0.3% among 269,956 youths aged 16 to 21 years, with a significant increase among female students from 0.21% in 1988 to 0.42% in 1992. The highest HIV seropositivity rates were seen among older students from the south and northeast and among African-Americans.[8] Since the military does not enlist people who acknowledge their homosexuality, and neither the military nor the Job Corps admits known intravenous drug users, these data do not accurately represent HIV seroprevalence among youths at highest risk for HIV infection.

A shelter serving runaway and homeless youths aged 16 to 20 years in New York City reported a seroprevalence rate of 5.4% up to 1989.[9] Among adolescents under 20 years of age seen at sexually transmitted disease (STD) clinics in Baltimore, a 2.2% seroprevalence rate was reported.[10] Substantial increases in HIV seroprevalence were reported in a Washington, DC clinic for 13- to 21-year-olds rising from 0.4% in 1987 to 1.9% in 1992.[11] Data from New York City studies of newborn blood tested for HIV (which indicates maternal HIV antibody serostatus) noted an HIV prevalence of 0.58% among mothers under 20 years of age and a ninefold increase in HIV seroprevalence in mothers aged 14 to 24 years.[12]

Behavioral Risk Factors

Although there is a wide range of rates of HIV infection among adolescents studied to date, the data show the continued presence and growth of this epidemic among youths, most particularly those with specific behavioral risk factors.[13] It is during adolescence that many teenagers begin to explore their sexuality and engage in behaviors that put them at risk for HIV infection. Most adolescents (80% of males and 70% of females) have initial sexual intercourse by age 20.[14] In the 1993 National Youth Risk Behavior Survey of high school students, only 53% of currently sexually active youths reported that they or their partners had used condoms during their last sexual intercourse.[15] These behaviors put adolescents at risk for STDs, unwanted

pregnancy, and drug addiction, all of which may affect HIV transmission rates and the progression of HIV disease.

Despite the fact that condoms are the only form of protection against both pregnancy and STDs, including HIV, widely varying rates of condom use are reported by sexually experienced youths. In a national survey of adolescent males in 1988, 58% of 17- to 19-year-olds reported condom use at last intercourse, but these rates were significantly lower among males who had five or more sexual partners, had paid for sex, or had used drugs intravenously.[16] In a survey conducted among middle-class urban adolescents at a health clinic in 1985 to 1986, only 2% of females and 8% of males reported using condoms every time they had intercourse.[17] In another survey of urban minority adolescent females at a health clinic, 26% reported engaging in anal intercourse, but condoms were used in only one third of these encounters.[18]

Sexually Transmitted Diseases and Biologic Susceptibility

HIV is a sexually transmitted pathogen, and the dynamics of its transmission reflect both host (behavioral and physiologic susceptibility) and viral factors.[19] HIV acquisition during adolescence may be facilitated by incomplete development of the female genital tract. In the United States, menarche begins at an average age of 12.5 to 13 years, and it is followed by anovulatory cycles for a period of several months to years. The lack of progesterone that accompanies the anovulatory cycles during this time may create a more permeable cervical mucus that allows sperm and infectious agents in semen to ascend more easily into the upper genital tract. Early puberty is also characterized by ectopy of the uterine cervix (i.e., extension of endocervical columnar cells onto the vaginal surface of the cervix). This single layer of columnar cells is more susceptible to gonorrheal infection and may be more susceptible to HIV infection than the multilayer squamous epithelial cells that replace them as puberty proceeds. These physical factors may influence the rate of transmission of HIV infection among adolescents. Infection with other STDs, particularly genitoulcerative infections such as syphilis, herpes, and chancroid, facilitates transmission of HIV. Acquisition of an STD also may serve as a marker for sexual behaviors that are associated with the spread of HIV.[20,21]

Homosexuality and Bisexuality

Male adolescents who have unprotected intercourse with other males are at particular risk for HIV infection, given the high prevalence of HIV infection among gay and bisexual adult men. Studies of 18- to 24-year-old males who had sex with males in San Francisco (1992-1993) and New York (1990-1991) demonstrated an HIV seroprevalence of 4.8% and 9%, respectively.[22,23] Surveys estimate that 17% to 35% of young males have had same-sex experiences to orgasm,[24] yet behavior is not the same as a gay or bisexual identity. Societal and familial prejudices against homosexuality often interfere with gay youths' ability to build an integrated gay identity or "come out" to themselves and others. The prevention of open socialization with gay peers increases the pressure on gay adolescents to explore their sexuality in secretive and sometimes unsafe ways.[25] Despite an abundance of safe-sex messages aimed at the gay community, the gay adolescent who is just "coming out" frequently does not have access to these messages or does not yet identify with the gay community, and therefore ignores them. Gay male and lesbian adolescents also frequently engage in heterosexual sex to hide their homosexuality from themselves and others,[26] which also can result in potential exposure to HIV infection.

Sexual Abuse

Sexual abuse poses yet another risk for HIV transmission. Of reported sexual abuse cases, 17% to 30% of the victims are in the adolescent age group.[27] In addition to direct risk from an HIV-infected abuser, sexual abuse puts adolescents at risk by increasing the likelihood of future high-risk behavior and by interfering with self-esteem and the ability of youths to negotiate safer sex with future partners. Adolescents who have been sexually abused have a lower age of initiation into both intercourse and the use of alcohol and illicit drugs.[28] A study examining adult risk behaviors that were associated with HIV infection reported a fourfold increase in prostitution ("survival sex," see below) among females and an eightfold increase among males who had been sexually abused during childhood.[29] For these reasons, providers and ethicists published a paper in 1994 calling for increased attention to HIV risk and follow-up care for sexual assault survivors.[30]

Survival Sex

Adolescents who engage in "survival sex," or the exchange of sex for money, drugs, food, or shelter, are at particularly high risk for HIV infection (see Chapter 101, "Prostitution and Pornography"). An estimated 900,000 youth engage in some form of survival sex or "sex work," and two thirds of these are female with an average age of 15. These youths often engage in unprotected intercourse with many high-risk partners.[31] There is some overlap between teen sex workers and the estimated 1 million teenagers who run away from home each year. There are approximately 250,000 homeless teenagers, many of whom engage in high-risk sexual behavior in exchange

for food, shelter, protection, or companionship in order to survive on the streets.[1]

Substance Use

The link between injection drug use, needle sharing, and HIV infection was established within the first year of the reported AIDS epidemic. Injectable drug use continues to be described as the sole risk activity by 10% of U.S. adolescents with AIDS.[2] A variety of drugs are injected, including heroin, cocaine, amphetamines, hormones, and anabolic steroids, although the percentage of adolescents who are self-administering these drugs intravenously and engaging in needle-sharing practices is unknown. An analysis of anabolic steroid use from the 1992 CDC National Youth Risk Behavior Survey found that 4% of males and 1% of females reported anabolic steroid use, injection drug use being the highest predictor of steroid use.[32] Reports of needle sharing by 25% of teenage steroid users, and a higher proportion of shared steroid vials, highlight their ongoing risk for HIV infection.[33]

The use of crack cocaine also appears to be closely associated with risk-related sexual behaviors and increased rates of STDs. Crack is a smokable form of cocaine that is inexpensive and rapidly addictive; it is also a sexual stimulant and disinhibitor that can increase sexual arousal while impairing judgment and self-control. Because crack is so highly addictive, its use has become associated with the exchange of sex for crack or for money to purchase crack.[34] In addition, many adolescents are using other substances (e.g., alcohol, marijuana, "designer drugs") that can impair their judgment and increase the likelihood of engaging in risk-related sexual behaviors and drug use. Use of these substances before or during intercourse can impair adolescents' ability to practice safe sex.

Hemophilia and Blood Transfusions

Males with hemophilia who received HIV-infected clotting factors before 1985 have a prevalence of HIV infection paralleling the severity of their clotting disorder; of those with severe hemophilia, approximately 75% are infected with HIV compared with 25% of those with mild hemophilia.[35] Although hemophilia accounts for only 1% of adult cases of AIDS, this is a much more significant risk factor in adolescents aged 13 to 21 years. Adolescents infected by way of blood products, from one-time transfusions or from chronic illnesses that require multiple transfusions, also may engage in high-risk sexual behaviors (e.g., intercourse without condoms) that can cause the transmission of HIV. A study of adolescents who have hemophilia demonstrated that, despite a good knowledge base about safe sex, only one of nine males who were having sexual intercourse used condoms consistently.[36]

Perinatally Infected Adolescents

As knowledge has grown concerning the natural history of HIV infection in children, and as more effective treatments have been developed, more children who were perinatally infected with HIV have reached adolescence. An Italian multicenter study reported that 50% of surviving children had reached 9 years of age.[37] A U.S. case series described 42 perinatally-infected adolescents who were older than 9 years (mean age 11.3 years, range 9 to 16 years). One quarter of the youths remained asymptomatic, while 57% had developed AIDS.[38] The full impact of HIV infection on the physiologic, psychological, and sexual development of these youths remains to be described, yet multisystemic illness, growth failure, delayed puberty, issues surrounding disclosure of illness, and maternal death from AIDS have already been noted.

HIV TESTING AND COUNSELING

As the benefits of treatment for HIV infection have been demonstrated, early identification of HIV infection has become more important. Although risk-related activities can identify some of the adolescents who should be offered HIV counseling with voluntary consent for testing, studies have shown that traditional "risk assessment" misses a significant portion of HIV-infected adolescents.[39,40] There are currently few regulations or laws specifically related to adolescents and HIV testing.[41] Thus far, laws governing testing vary from state to state and have focused on adults. Before the HIV epidemic, adolescents in most states had the right to consent to confidential treatment of STDs without parental notification or consent. However, in all states they did not have the same right with regard to certain contraceptive services and abortion. Debates over the right of minors to provide consent for confidential testing, issues of parent and sexual partner notification, and persistence of discrimination against those who are HIV positive highlight some of the social and ethical complexities in testing adolescents for HIV.[42] However, with advances in medical treatments for persons infected with HIV, the standard of care has become to offer HIV counseling and testing as a routine part of care. In 1995 the CDC began recommending that all pregnant women be routinely offered HIV counseling and testing, the first group to be targeted.[43] The challenge for adolescent providers is to balance the need to develop and implement a simple, provider- and patient-friendly, adolescent-specific HIV counseling and voluntary testing protocol, yet ensure that it remains developmentally appropriate for youth.

Consensus recommendations for principles governing HIV counseling for adolescents were published in 1988 and are summarized in Box 67-1.[44] Elements of adolescent-appropriate HIV counseling and testing are summarized in Box 67-2.

BOX 67-1
Consensus Principles for HIV Testing in Adolescents

HIV testing should be voluntary

Pretest and post-test counseling must be offered and be developmentally and culturally appropriate

Adolescents capable of giving informed consent should be allowed to consent to HIV testing, preferably with a family member or other responsible adult who can provide emotional support during the testing process

Testing should not be coercive or mandatory as a prerequisite for admission to programs

Confidentiality should be ensured, with special care taken in settings such as foster care, residential institutions, and detention facilities

Adolescents should be assured access to all appropriate care and research protocols

---

BOX 67-2
Elements of HIV Counseling and Testing in Adolescents

Assess reasons for HIV testing, including adolescents' knowledge about HIV transmission and their actual risk behaviors

Provide information about the benefits of early diagnosis and medical intervention

Explain confidentiality and clarify who will have access to test results

Identify a support adult for the testing process and establish a plan for emotional support during the waiting process

Assess potential reactions to a positive or negative result

Assess plans for partner or family notification of positive results

Communicate information about risk-reduction strategies and skills

Determine the risks and benefits of HIV testing at this time for the youth and formalize a decision to have or defer an HIV test

Obtain written informed consent in accordance with local laws and the ability of the youth to consent

Give the HIV test result in person

Provide appropriate health, mental health, and social service referrals

MEDICAL MANAGEMENT

Comprehensive guides to the medical and psychosocial management of HIV-infected adolescents[45] and those with early HIV infection[46] are available. Elements of this care are summarized below.

Risk Assessment

A complete history of sexual behavior and drug use should be obtained from all adolescents to assess the risk for infection and to develop an understanding of the adolescent's actual behaviors. Individualized risk reduction plans are based on this information. Boxes 67-3 and 67-4 highlight areas that should be assessed.

Classification and Natural History

Medical management of an adolescent infected with HIV begins with a staging evaluation that helps to determine the susceptibility to opportunistic infections and the appropriate course of treatment. This assessment includes characterization of the patient as asymptomatic (including persistent generalized lymphadenopathy), symptomatic with HIV-related symptoms, or having AIDS. The CDC 1993 classification system for adolescent and adult HIV infection[47] is presented in Tables 67-1 and 67-2. This classification system added three clinical conditions (pulmonary tuberculosis, recurrent pneumonia, and invasive cervical cancer) and a laboratory marker of severe immunodeficiency (CD4 + T-lymphocyte count $< 200/mm^3$) to the case definition of AIDS. Since the criteria used for this surveillance system were not developed specifically for adolescents, they may need to be modified as the natural history of HIV infection in adolescents becomes better understood.

In contrast to the adult male and female population and children, the natural history of HIV infection in adolescents has not yet been systematically studied. The year 1995 marked the first effort by the National Institutes of Health to assess disease progression and spectrum of disease among HIV-infected teenagers in a multisite cooperative study by the Adolescent Medicine HIV/AIDS Research Network. The impact of puberty on HIV progression and conversely the impact of HIV on pubertal growth and development, as well as other clinical and basic science questions, is addressed in this multisite study. In the meantime, clinical care for youths infected with HIV is based on the assumption that their course will more likely follow that of adults than that of perinatally infected children, since most youths were infected after their immune systems had developed.

Several studies published in 1995 altered the understanding of HIV pathogenesis, demonstrating that HIV multiplies at a very high rate from the earliest stages of

---

BOX 67-3
Elements of Sexual Risk History

1. At what age did you begin sexual intercourse (oral, vaginal, or anal) and how old was your partner?
2. Do you have sex with men, women, or both?
3. Do you consider yourself heterosexual, homosexual, or bisexual?
4. Have you ever had the following sexual experiences (if so, how often and with how many partners): oral, vaginal, or anal intercourse; receptive or insertive? What percentage of the time were condoms used? Describe those experiences in the past month.
5. Describe the number of sexual partners you have had, their ages, and if any of them had known risk factors for HIV infection.
6. Have you ever had an STD? (Name all of them, describe symptoms, ask for treatment history.)
7. What forms of birth control have you used? Describe. Have you done anything to try to prevent STDs? What?
8. Have you ever been pregnant, had a baby, had an abortion or miscarriage?
9. Have you used drugs or alcohol before or during sex?
10. Have you ever had sex in exchange for food, money, drugs, or a place to sleep or live?
11. Has anyone ever forced you to do something sexually that you did not want to do?
12. Do you have any questions or concerns about your current sexual experiences?
13. What are you doing to protect yourself and your sex partners from being infected with HIV?
14. What do you know about safe and safer sex? How do you feel about changing your sexual behaviors to prevent HIV infection? What sexual behaviors will you miss? How does your partner feel about safe sex?
15. Do you think condoms can prevent the spread of HIV and STDs? If so, what makes it hard for you to use condoms? Did you use a condom the last time you had intercourse? Why or why not?

From Futterman DC, Hein K: Medical management of adolescents. In Pizzo P, Wilfert C, editors: *Pediatric AIDS: the challenge of HIV infection in infants, children and adolescents*, Baltimore, 1990, Williams & Wilkins; pp 757-772. Copyright © 1990, Williams & Wilkins.
STDs, sexually transmitted diseases.

---

infection. Viral replication at a rate of 1 billion viruses per day gradually overwhelms the body's ability to keep up with production of new CD4 lymphocytes.[48,49] Thus, it appears that clinical latency does not equal viral latency, but rather there is a constant high-volume production

BOX 67-4
Elements of Drug Use History

1. Do you, your friends, or your sexual partners ever use any of the following: alcohol, marijuana, crack, cocaine, heroin, amphetamines, hallucinogens (LSD, PCP), barbiturates, sedatives, steroids? Are you using them in combinations? How?
2. For each drug describe age of first use, frequency of use in past month, average daily use, and ways used (pills, snorted, smoked, injected).
3. In what settings do you use drugs: alone, with friends or lovers, at parties, where you buy the drugs (crack houses, shooting galleries)?
4. For those who have injected drugs, describe needle use: sharing frequency, with whom, use of works in shooting galleries, cleaning practices.
5. For those who smoke crack, describe frequency of use, percentage of use in crack houses, frequency of sex in crack houses, and types of sex.
6. How do you get money to obtain drugs?
7. Have you ever had sex in exchange for drugs?
8. Have you ever had a medical problem (i.e., visited a doctor or hospital) or tried to hurt or kill yourself in relation to drug use?
9. Have you ever been in trouble with the law, your family, school, or a job in relation to drugs?
10. Do you think you are addicted to or have a problem with drugs?
11. Have you ever tried to "get off" drugs? What treatment programs have you tried? How else have you tried?

From Futterman DC, Hein K: Medical management of adolescents. In Pizzo P, Wilfert C, editors: *Pediatric AIDS: the challenge of HIV infection in infants, children and adolescents,* Baltimore, 1990, Williams & Wilkins; pp 757-772. Copyright © 1990, Williams & Wilkins.

of HIV. Over time, as the infected person's CD4 + T lymphocytes decline, they become susceptible to the symptoms and opportunistic infections that characterize HIV disease and AIDS. There is therefore a strong possibility that clinical strategies will shift and emphasize early treatment with antiretroviral agents rather than the current policy of waiting until the CD4 count declines.

Medical History

A medical history should include an assessment of previous illnesses or medical treatments that may be HIV related. Evidence of the acute HIV seroconversion illness

should be sought, because this information can help to date the acquisition of HIV. Symptoms, which are frequently similar to those of a mononucleosis-like syndrome, include fever, malaise, lymphadenopathy, and variable involvement of multiple organ systems.[50] A medical history for late-presenting, congenitally infected adolescents should include a history of their parents' drug use, risk behaviors, and medical illnesses.

Other elements of a medical history include (1) history of sexual behavior and drug use; (2) previous illnesses, especially STDs, recurrent pneumonia, or tuberculosis, which may reactivate in the presence of HIV infection or during adolescence; (3) hospitalizations; (4) menstrual history; (5) use of contraception in females and males; (6) history of sources of medical care; (7) history of blood transfusions or receipt of blood products; (8) immunizations; (9) medications; (10) allergies, especially to medications; (11) family history (medical and psychiatric); and (12) diet history. A psychiatric history should include assessment of past or present functioning, depression, anxiety, psychosis, hospitalizations, medications, and suicidal thoughts or attempts. A social history should include the current living situation (with family, with friends, alone, in an institution, or homeless), school and work status, and (importantly) social supports (including who knows about the adolescent's HIV status).

Review of Systems

An HIV-oriented review of systems should include general assessment of fatigue, weight loss or failure to gain weight during the growth spurt, anorexia, nausea, prolonged or high fevers, night sweats, lymph node enlargement, and any skin lesions or rashes. The head, eyes, ears, nose, and throat (HEENT) review should include a notation of any visual or hearing changes, sinusitis, dysphagia, thrush, gum disease, tooth decay, or oral ulcers. Persistent cough or shortness of breath should be ascertained. Questions should be asked regarding diarrhea, abdominal pain or masses, and anal pain or discharge. Similarly, penile or vaginal discharge and herpes, yeast, or other persistent infections should be noted, along with any complaints of pelvic pain. A neuromuscular review should seek evidence of weakness, myalgia, or abnormal pain or sensations. A neuropsychiatric review should focus on evidence of personality changes, dementia, depression, anxiety, or headaches. For some of these complaints, it may be difficult to distinguish those effects caused by HIV from those associated with less severe illnesses or with chronic use of illicit drugs.

Physical Examination

Because adolescence is characterized by dynamic changes in somatic growth and cognitive function,

TABLE 67-1
Centers for Disease Control and Prevention HIV Classification/AIDS Surveillance Case Definition for Adolescents and Adults

Category A

One or more of the conditions listed opposite

Asymptomatic HIV infection
Persistent generalized lymphadenopathy
Acute (primary) HIV infection with accompanying illness or history of acute HIV infection

Category B

Symptomatic conditions that are attributed to HIV infection or indicative of a defect in cell-mediated immunity or are considered by physicians to have a clinical course or management that is complicated by HIV infection

Bacillary angiomatosis
Bacterial enocarditis, meningitis, or sepsis
Candidiasis, oropharyngeal
Candidiasis, vulvovaginal: persistent, frequent, poorly responsive to therapy
Cervical dysplasia, severe
Constitutional symptoms, such as fever (>38.5° C) or diarrhea lasting more than 1 month
Hairy leukoplakia, oral
Herpes zoster involving at least two distinct episodes or more than one dermatome
Idiopathic thrombocytopenic purpura
Listeriosis
Nocardiosis
Peripheral neuropathy

Category C

Conditions strongly associated with severe immunodeficiency

Bacterial pneumonia, recurrent
Candidiasis of bronchi, trachea, or lungs
Candidiasis, esophageal
Cervical cancer, invasive
Coccidiodomycosis, disseminated or extrapulmonary
Cryptosporidiosis, chronic intestinal (duration >1 month)
Cytomegalovirus disease (other than liver, spleen, or nodes)
Cytomegalovirus retinitis (loss of vision)
HIV encephalopathy
Herpes simplex: chronic ulcer(s) (duration >1 month); or bronchitis, pneumonitis, or esophagitis
Histoplasmosis, disseminated or extrapulmonary
Isosporiasis, chronic intestinal (duration >1 month)
Kaposi's sarcoma
Lymphoma, Burkitt's (or equivalent term)
Lymphoma, immunoblastic (or equivalent term)
Lymphoma, primary in brain
Mycobacterium avium complex, disseminated or extrapulmonary
Mycobacterium, other species or unidentified species, disseminated or extrapulmonary
Pneumocystis carinii pneumonia
Progressive multifocal leukoencephalopathy
Pulmonary tuberculosis
Salmonella septicemia, recurrent
Toxoplasmosis of brain

---

assessment should include the notation of failure to progress as well as actual regression.[51] A complete physical examination is performed, with special attention to vital signs and growth assessment, including weight and height velocity. During the second decade of life, weight is expected to double and height should increase by 15% to 20%. Failure to gain weight or to increase height at the expected rate during puberty may be significant. Normal ranges of pulse rate and blood pressure increase during adolescence. Nutritional status should be noted. Adolescence is a time when skin problems such as acne first appear, but many other

TABLE 67-2
Centers for Disease Control Classification System for HIV Infection (1993)

	Clinical Categories		
CD4+ T cell	**A** Asymptomatic, Acute (Primary) HIV or PGL	**B** Symptomatic, Not (A) or (C) Conditions	**C** AIDS-Indicator Conditions
1. ≥500/μl	A1	B1	C1
2. 200-499/μl	A2	B2	C2
3. <200/μl AIDS-indicator T-cell count	A3	B3	C3

PGL, persistent generalized lymphadenopathy.

common dermatologic disorders are seen with HIV infection and may signal the progression of disease.[52]

The lymph nodes should be examined and any lymphadenopathy fully described (location, number, size, consistency, persistence). Adenopathy can be a sign of benign intercurrent illness; if confined to the inguinal area, it may be associated with sexually transmitted infections or lower extremity trauma. Axillary adenopathy in the absence of upper extremity trauma is rarely seen in conditions other than HIV infection. Adolescence is a stage when lymphoid tissue normally begins to regress, but regression of adenopathy also may be seen in advanced AIDS.

A HEENT examination should include assessment of visual acuity, a funduscopic examination, and a thorough oral examination. Early oral *Candida* infection (thrush) can present as an erythematous, denuded patch on the mucous membrane rather than the more typical white plaques. Gum disease, ulcers (apthous or herpetic), and dental caries are frequently seen. The lungs and heart should be examined. An abdominal examination should focus on the presence of masses or hepatosplenomegaly.

The genitalia should be assessed and the sexual maturity staging of Tanner and Whitehouse, describing the development of secondary sexual characteristics, noted.[51] A yearly or twice-yearly pelvic examination with appropriate laboratory tests and inspection for vaginal *Candida* infection should be performed for females who have had sexual intercourse, those who have unexplained pelvic pain, or those over age 19. A rectal inspection is also needed for both females and males.

The neurologic examination should include a mental status assessment. It is not currently known how HIV infection affects cognitive development in the adolescent. Assessment of the adolescent's ability to generalize or to think abstractly is important so that age-appropriate explanations can be given to the patient. Neuropsychological testing should also be performed if neurologic involvement is suspected.

Laboratory Assessment

Laboratory assessment must take into account adolescent-specific normal values when these are available and when they differ from those of other age groups. Markers have been identified that are useful in assessing HIV disease stage and predicting progression, and these may be used to guide therapy; however, normal values during puberty have not been established. The most useful markers to date have been the lymphocyte cells, particularly the helper, or CD4 + T lymphocyte, the decline of which remains the best marker of disease stage and susceptibility to opportunistic infections.[53,54] However the CD4 count is not as reliable a predictor of response to medications; that is, an improvement in the number of CD4 cells does not always correlate with increased survival or delayed disease progression.[55] A CD4 count of less than 500/mm^3 is an indication of immune dysfunction; a CD4 count of less than 200/mm^3 is classified as AIDS, indicating susceptibility to opportunistic infections. One program that handled HIV-infected adolescents reported that almost 50% of the patients had CD4 values of less than 500/mm^3 at presentation to the clinic.[56] Measurement of CD4 cell counts and percentages should be performed as a baseline and at 3- to 6-month intervals.

In 1996, it was first demonstrated that the amount of virus (as measured by viral load testing of HIV RNA in the blood) was the strongest predictor of the course and duration of HIV diseases and that lowering viral load improves clinical outcome.[55] Measures of viral load have been licensed by the Food and Drug Administration and are available for clinical use (including when to initiate or change antiretroviral treatments).

A complete blood count (CBC) is necessary to assess the presence of anemia, lymphopenia, and neutropenia or thrombocytopenia. An elevated erythrocyte sedimentation rate is common with HIV. A chemistry panel, including evaluation of renal and liver function, is advisable. HIV renal involvement may be accompanied by increased blood urea nitrogen, creatinine, or potassium levels or by a decreased serum bicarbonate level. Albumin is decreased in the presence of chronic malnutrition, diarrhea, or malabsorption, whereas an elevated total protein level is generally noted with an increased immunoglobulin fraction. Increased liver enzymes may denote liver involvement. An elevated alkaline phosphatase level can be seen during the adolescent growth spurt but is typically higher with disseminated *Mycobacterium avium* complex. An elevated lactic dehydrogenase level may signal lymphoma or pulmonary disease, especially *Pneumocystis carinii* pneumonia.

All adolescents having intercourse should be screened for sexually transmitted pathogens, since asymptomatic infections are possible. The work-up of a patient for STDs includes serologic testing for syphilis and hepatitis B, gonorrheal and herpes cultures, a test for *Chlamydia* (immunofluorescent slide test or culture), a Gram's stain to detect inflammation or *Candida* organisms in males and females or to detect gonorrhea in males, potassium hydroxide (KOH) prep for *Candida* organisms, and a "wet prep" for *Trichomonas* and for the clue cells seen with bacterial vaginosis. HIV infection has been associated with a rapid progression of cervical neoplasia,[57] indicating the need for cervical cytologic examination via (Papanicolaou smear) every 6 to 12 months in females who are infected with HIV and are sexually experienced.[58] The utility of anal cytology in screening for human papillomavirus and neoplasia in youths engaging in anal intercourse remains to be determined.[59]

A tuberculin skin test (PPD) with anergy panel (Merieux multitest or *Candida,* mumps, and tetanus antigen) should be performed to assess the presence of tuberculosis infection and cell-mediated immunity. A baseline chest radiograph should be obtained in those who are anergic to check for tuberculosis and in patients with a history of pulmonary disease. Baseline titers for toxoplasmosis should be obtained, because this infection can reactivate in HIV-positive adolescents with immune dysfunction.[60] Serologic assessment of immunity to rubella should be performed routinely in adolescent females.

Immunization

Although there is sometimes a decreased antibody response to immunizations in immunocompromised patients, the following immunizations are recommended for patients infected with HIV.[61] Adolescents should be given Pneumovax and a yearly influenza vaccine.[62] They should also receive the vaccinations appropriate for their age, such as Td (tetanus and diphtheria) and MMR (measles, mumps, and rubella).[63,64] Hepatitis B vaccine should be given to all HIV-positive adolescents who are not immune. Varicella vaccine is not approved for adolescents with HIV infection but is recommended for nonimmune household contacts to minimize exposure risk.

Treatment for HIV Infection

ADOLESCENTS AND MEDICATIONS. Until 1989, virtually all the antiretroviral medications used in the treatment of HIV were developed in clinical trials among children or adults. Although adolescents have been included in clinical trials since 1989, most adolescent enrollees have been either males with hemophilia or pregnant women in perinatal trials. In 1992, seven clinical trial sites were funded to focus specifically on adolescents. In addition to issues of access and consent to participate in trials, care must still be taken to include adolescent-specific normal values when evaluating medications and outcomes. The dose, dose interval, toxicity, and effectiveness of various medications differ among neonates, children, adolescents, adults, and elderly persons (see Chapter 16, "Pharmacologic Considerations"). During the adolescent years, there are gender-related changes in body composition. Proportional differences include greater increases in body fat among adolescent females and bone and muscle mass among adolescent males. These differences in body habitus alter drug distribution and have a direct effect on drug dose. Changes in drug metabolism during adolescence affect drug half-life and therefore the dosing interval.[65] Age-related differences in response to medications have already been demonstrated. For example, prophylaxis against *P. carinii* pneumonia (PCP) is recommended for patients infected with HIV who have CD4 counts of less than 200/mm^3.[66] Young children have had fewer adverse reactions to trimethoprim-sulfamethoxazole than adults.[67,68] The rates of adverse reactions in adolescents are currently unknown. Adolescents in Tanner stages 1 and 2 should receive pediatric dose schedules; those in Tanner stages 4 and 5 should receive adult dose schedules, regardless of their chronologic age. Further studies are needed to determine appropriate dose schedules for adolescents in Tanner stage 3.[69]

ANTIRETROVIRAL THERAPY. 1996 ushered in a new era of treatment for persons infected with HIV with the development and licensing of a powerful new class of anti-HIV medicines (protease inhibitors), which in combination with other antiretroviral medicines, are highly effective in improving both the duration and quality of life for those who are infected.[70-76]

Current suggestions of viral load monitoring include two baseline tests (to establish a reliable starting point) and then repeat testing every 3 months and/or within 3 to 4 weeks of a change in treatment. The goal of antiretroviral treatment is to reduce the viral load to undetectable by the most up-to-date test system. The most recent Consensus Recommendations[70] for treatment initiation are listed in Table 67-3.

Combination Therapy

Combination therapy (the use of at least two antiretroviral medicines) is now the standard of care because this is the most effective way to lower viral load and help prevent viral resistance to medications. Combinations must be designed for each individual and take into account: current disease status, prior antiretroviral medication use, other current medications/drug interactions, side effects, and dosing schedules. As knowledge is increasing at a rapid pace and new medications are rapidly being approved by the Food and Drug Administration, providers must seek the latest publications/consensus panels for current treatment recommendations regarding combination therapies. Medications as of January 1997 are summarized in Table 67-4.

In 1994 a clinical trial (ACTG 076) in pregnant women and their offspring demonstrated efficacy in reducing perinatal HIV transmission to their babies from 25% to 8% when ZDV was used during three stages: orally by the mother from the 14th to 34th week of gestation to delivery, intravenously to the mother during delivery, and orally by the baby for the first 6 weeks of life.[77] Since the study was not designed to ascertain which stage of medication was most useful, the Public Health Service now recommends this complete regimen for all pregnant women who are HIV positive.[78] This positive clinical finding helped form the basis for the CDC recommendation that all pregnant women should know their HIV status.[43] Of note, 25% of the original trial participants were mothers under the age of 21.

OPPORTUNISTIC INFECTION PROPHYLAXIS. Some of the most exciting improvements in HIV treatment have been in the area of prevention (primary and secondary) and treatment of opportunistic infections. This treatment strategy has been referred to as MOPP (multiple opportunistic pathogen prophylaxis). In 1995 the CDC released new guidelines for the prevention of opportunistic infections[79] that call for prophylaxis against PCP when the patient has had PCP, if the CD4 cell count is below 200/mm^3, if the patient has developed oral thrush, or there is a 2-week history of unexplained fever. The first-line agent remains trimethoprim/sulfamethoxazole (TMP/SMX), but if an allergic reaction develops, desensitization should be attempted; if that fails, dapsone is now the recommended alternative. TMP/SMX also provides recommended prophylaxis for patients who have antibodies to *Toxoplasma gondii* and CD4 counts of less than 100/mm^3, but pyrimethamine must be added if dapsone is used.

Prophylaxis against *Mycobacterium avium* complex with rifabutin, clarithromycin, or azithromycin is recommended when the CD4 count is less than 75/mm^3. Prophylaxis for exposure to *Mycobacterium tuberculosis* with isoniazid or rifampin is also recommended for patients who have a positive PPD test or have been exposed to tuberculosis. Prophylaxis against fungal infections (*Candida, Cryptococcus, Histoplasma,* and *Coccidioides*) with fluconazole can also be considered for patients with CD4 count less than 50/mm^3, as can prophylaxis against cytomegalovirus (CMV) retinitis with oral ganciclovir for patients who are CMV antibody positive in this CD4 cell range.

Patient Adherence

Adherence to medical regimens is a challenge for all age groups, with unique issues for adolescents centering on their developmental stage and life circumstances (see Chapter 17, "Compliance with Health Recommendations"). For adolescents with HIV, coming to medical providers and taking antiviral medications is an unwanted reminder of their potentially fatal disease. Many adolescents have difficulty understanding the concept of disease latency and asymptomatic infection. Concrete thought processes, expressed as "I feel and look good—how can I be sick?," may be combined with developmental self-perceptions of immortality and invincibility to inten-

TABLE 67-3
Consensus Recommendations for Treatment Initiation

Status	Recommendation
Symptomatic HIV Disease	Therapy recommended for all patients
Asymptomatic, CD4 <500/mm^3	Therapy recommended (some would defer therapy if CD4 350 to 500/mm^3 and viral load <10,000 copies/ml)
Asymptomatic, CD4 >500/mm^3	Therapy recommended for patients viral load >30,000 to 50,000 or rapidly declining CD4
	Therapy should be considered if viral load >5,000 to 10,000 copies/ml

Carpenter C, Fischl M, Hammer S, et al for the International AIDS Society USA: *JAMA* 276:146-154, 1996.

TABLE 67-4
Antiretroviral Medications

Medication (generic/ *brand* name, FDA approval date)	Dosage	Side effects/considerations
Nucleoside Analogues		
Zidovudine (AZT/ZDV) *Retrovir (1986)*	200 mg (2 capsules) every 8 hours	Anemia, granulocytopenia, headache, malaise.
Didanosine (ddI) *Videx (1991)*	200 mg (2 tabs) every 12 hours	Pancreatitis, neuropathy, diarrhea, rash. Take on empty stomach.
Zalcitabine (ddC) *HIVID (1992)*	0.75 mg (1 pill) every 8 hours	Pancreatitis, neuropathy, mouth ulcers.
Stavudine (d4t) *Zerit (1992)*	40 mg (1 capsule) every 12 hours	Neuropathy.
Lamivudine (3TC) *Epivir (1995)*	150 mg (1 tablet) every 12 hours	Anemia, headache, malaise, nausea.
Protease Inhibitors		
Saquinavir *Invirase (1995)*	600 mg (3 capsules) every 8 hours	Nausea, diarrhea, headache. Must take with food.
Indinavir *Crixivan (1996)*	800 mg (2 capsules every 8 hours)	Nausea, vomiting, diarrhea, kidney stones, rash. Must take on empty stomach, drink lots of water.
Ritonavir *Norvir (1996)*	600 mg (6 capsules) every 12 hours	Bitter taste, nausea, vomiting, diarrhea, tingling around mouth. Refrigerate; take with food.
Nonnucleoside Reverse Transcriptase Inhibitors		
Nevirapine *Viramune (1996)*	200 mg (1 tablet) every 12 hours	Rash, fever, nausea, headache.

sify denial. These factors may decrease compliance with complicated medical regimens.

There is a documented decrease in compliance in all age groups when chronic therapies and complex regimens are used.[80] Adolescents should be assisted in developing plans to integrate medications into their daily lives, and obstacles to this should be anticipated and discussed. Most adolescents do not respond to abstract notions of efficacy such as good health or longevity; they are frequently more responsive to reaching concrete goals that they have helped to set. Bolstering the patient's social supports (e.g., family, friends, agencies) is another strategy for encouraging compliance and serving the many needs of adolescents infected with HIV.

For the subset of disenfranchised teenagers who are infected with HIV (e.g., those who are homeless, prostitutes, or drug addicts), compliance with medication schedules is often a much lower priority than securing food and a place to sleep. For these, money to purchase medications and literally having a place to keep their medicines are important factors in the compliance equation. A particular challenge is posed by homeless youth who are infected with tuberculosis, and directly observed therapy programs are crucial for the prolonged treatment required.[60]

Psychological Issues

Adolescents may have a wide range of psychological reactions to being informed they are infected with HIV. These reactions include fear, depression, and anxiety and are often an appropriate response to the loss of a healthy future. For many, a positive test result represents a death sentence. However, a review of adolescents found no increase in suicide attempts and a minimal increase in suicidal ideation after discovery of their HIV-positive status,[81] findings similar to those reported in adults.[82]

Many youths fear the potential loss of support from family, friends, and present and future sexual partners. Providers can help youths solve problems regarding when and to whom to disclose their infection. Particularly among females, there is often a focus on their perceived inability to have children. Most feel ambivalent about wanting a child, yet not wanting to pass on their infection.

Some teenagers report a loss of interest in sexual expression. Others become empowered by strictly adhering to safe sex (or safer sex) guidelines or finding another partner who is HIV positive with whom to have safe sex. Still others, in anger or denial of HIV infection, engage in unprotected intercourse. A nonjudgmental response can help adolescents voice their concerns and communicate honestly about their actual behaviors; this then serves as the basis for risk-reduction strategies. Linkage of youths who are HIV positive to opportunities for peer support is important. Providers must also help youths address such issues as choosing a healthcare proxy and preparing a living will in which they make choices about care in the terminal phase of their illness.

PREVENTION

Limiting the further spread of HIV infection among adolescents is an urgent priority that requires the development and dissemination of effective prevention programs. Some of the key principles of prevention have been termed the "correlates of immunity" and include "sound policies promoting HIV risk reduction; access to health and social services, condoms, needles and syringes; interventions shown to motivate behavioral change; organizations capable of reaching those at risk; and development and diffusion of technologies to interrupt the spread of the virus."[83]

Adolescents must be addressed in their homes, schools, and communities before they begin to engage in risk-related activities. Because family members may be reluctant or may not have the skills or knowledge to discuss sex and drug use, it is important to achieve access to resources that can help families begin a dialogue.[84] Excellent curricula are available for school-based education programs; however, there have often been difficulties in implementing these curricula on a local level.[85] There have been significant debates over whether the education message should be a "moralistic" one, urging sexual abstinence, or a "realistic" one, encouraging risk reduction.[86] All adolescents, regardless of their risk, should be provided with information about HIV transmission and programs that can help them understand and modify risk-related behaviors.

During adolescence, peer identification is a major factor in the young person's move from total dependence on family to independent functioning. This identification has provided the basis for many innovative HIV-oriented peer education programs. Interventions for prevention and risk reduction should include three components: (1) HIV/AIDS education; (2) discussion of safer sex, including a condom demonstration; and (3) exercises that will help adolescents develop decision making, assertiveness, and communication skills. For adolescents who are infected with HIV or at high risk for infection, the interventions should also be directed toward the information obtained during an individualized risk assessment.

Basic information about HIV infection should include a discussion about the differences between AIDS and HIV infection and between high- and low-risk behaviors. Adolescents need to learn that they can protect themselves either by abstaining from or delaying sexual intercourse, or by practicing safer sex by using condoms during sexual intercourse. The risks of unprotected (i.e., without a condom) vaginal, anal, and oral intercourse should be explained and these activities discouraged.

For adolescents at a critical stage in the development of their sexual identity, sex should not be equated with possible death. The full range of options for expressing intimacy and sensuality should be presented. Differentiation between risk-related intercourse and risk-free "outercourse" may be useful. "Outercourse" can be defined as sensual touching on the outside of the body, including kissing, massage, and masturbation. The challenge is to help adolescents learn how to explore their feelings and sexuality in ways that are safe and healthy. This is particularly important for gay and lesbian youths, who face many obstacles in developing a positive identity.

Latex condoms with nonoxynol 9 spermicide, but not animal skin condoms or polyurethane female condoms, are effective in reducing the risk of HIV transmission through sexual intercourse. Most adolescents have not had the opportunity to talk about condoms or to learn how to use them properly. Survey data indicate that adolescents are more likely to use condoms if they perceive them as enjoyable, view themselves as able to get a sexual partner to use condoms, and believe that they can effectively negotiate condom use with a sexual partner. Demonstrating proper condom use and letting adolescents practice on a penis model or their fingers can desensitize the issue and enable adolescents to use condoms correctly. Role-play exercises also can be used to help adolescents develop decision making, assertiveness, and communication skills. With these skills, adolescents can successfully negotiate risk reduction and condom use with a sexual partner and resist peer pressure to use drugs and engage in unprotected intercourse.[87]

CONCLUSION

HIV infection clearly exists in the adolescent population. The time for primary prevention alone has passed. By 1994, the worldwide incidence of 1.6 million new AIDS cases surpassed the cumulative number of cases in the 1980s. The greatest impact of this epidemic is yet to come. The extent of HIV infection among U.S. adolescents is unknown, but many subgroups of adolescents across the United States are infected. Advances in understanding of HIV-related illnesses have highlighted the importance of early intervention to forestall many of the complications of this disease. Those caring for teenagers should play a key role in providing services to meet their preventive and medical needs as this epidemic progresses.

References

1. Novello A: *Report of the Secretary's Work Group on Pediatric HIV Infection and Disease,* Washington, DC, 1988, Department of Health and Human Services.
2. Centers for Disease Control and Prevention: HIV/AIDS Surveillance Report 8:1-33, 1996.
3. Brookmeyer R: Reconstruction and future trends of the AIDS epidemic in the United States, *Science* 253:37-42, 1991.
4. Rosenberg P, Biggar R, Goedert J (letter): Declining age at HIV infection in the United States, *N Engl J Med* 330:789, 1994.
5. Goldsmith M: Invisible epidemic now becoming visible as HIV/AIDS pandemic reaches adolescents, *JAMA* 270:16-19, 1993.
6. Hein K. AIDS in adolescence: exploring the challenge, *J Adolesc Health Care* 10(suppl):10-35, 1991.
7. Lindgren ML, Hanson C, Miller K, Byers R, Onorato I: Epidemiology of human immunodeficiency virus infection in adolescents, United States, *Pediatr Infect Dis J* 113:525-535, 1994.
8. Conway G, Epstein M, Hayman C, et al: Trends in HIV prevalence among disadvantaged youth: survey results from a national job training program, 1988 through 1992, *JAMA* 269:2887-2889, 1993.
9. Stricof R, Kennedy J, Nattell T, Weisfuse I, Novick L: HIV seroprevalence in a facility for runaway and homeless adolescents, *Am J Public Health* 81(s):50-53, 1991.
10. Quinn T: Evolution of the HIV epidemic among patients attending STD clinics, *J Infect Dis* 165:541-544, 1992.
11. D'Angelo L, Getson P, Brasseux C, et al: The increasing prevalence of HIV infection in urban adolescents: a five year study. Abstracts of the Annual Society for Adolescent Medicine Meeting, *J Adolesc Health* 14:46, 1993.
12. Novick L, Glebatis D, Stricof R, MacCubbin P, Lessner L, Berns D: Newborn seroprevalence study: methods and results, *Am J Public Health* 81(s):15-21, 1991.
13. National Research Council: In Miller HG, Turner GF, Moses LE, editors: *AIDS: the second decade,* Washington, DC, 1991, National Academy Press; pp 147-252.
14. U.S. National Research Council Panel on Adolescent Pregnancy and Child Bearing: In Hayes CD, editor: *Risking the future: adolescent sexuality, pregnancy and child bearing,* Washington, DC, 1987, National Academy Press; pp 33-74, 95-121.
15. Centers for Disease Control and Prevention: Youth risk behavior surveillance—U.S 1993, *MMWR* 44:1-55, 1995.
16. Sonenstein FL, Pleck JH, Ku LC: Sexual activity, condom use and AIDS awareness among adolescent males, *Fam Plann Perspect* 21:152-158, 1989.
17. Kegeles SM, Adler NE, Irwin CE: Sexually active adolescents and condoms: changes over one year in knowledge, attitudes and use, *Am J Public Health* 78:460-461, 1988.
18. Jaffe L, Seehaus M, Wagner C, Leadbeater B: Anal intercourse and knowledge of AIDS among minority-group adolescents, *J Pediatr* 112:1005-1007, 1988.
19. Holmberg SD, Horsburgh CR, Ward JW, Jaffe HW: Biological factors in the sexual transmission of human immunodeficiency virus, *J Infect Dis* 160:116-125, 1989.
20. Simonsen JN, Cameron DW, Gakinya MN, et al: Human immunodeficiency virus infection among men with sexually transmitted diseases: experience from a center in Africa, *N Engl J Med* 319:274-278, 1988.
21. Hook EW: Syphilis and HIV infection, *J Infect Dis* 160:530-534, 1989.
22. Osmond D, Page K, Wiley J, et al: HIV infection in homosexual and bisexual men 18-29 years of age: The San Francisco Young Men's Health Study, *Am J Public Health* 84:1933-1937, 1994.
23. Dean L, Meyer I: HIV prevalence and sexual behavior in a cohort of NY City gay men (aged 18-24), *J Acquir Immune Defic Syndr* 8:208-211, 1995.
24. Remafedi G: Preventing the sexual transmission of AIDS during adolescence, *J Adolesc Health Care* 9:136-143, 1988.
25. Martin AD: Learning to hide: the socialization of the gay adolescent, *Ann Am Soc Adolesc Psychiatry* 10:52-65, 1982.
26. Paroski PA: Health care delivery and the concerns of gay and lesbian adolescents, *J Adolesc Health Care* 8:188-192, 1987.
27. Hampton RL, Newberger EH: Child abuse incidence and reporting by hospitals: significance of severity, class and race, *Am J Public Health* 75:55-60, 1985.
28. Harrison PA, Hoffman NG, Edwall GE: Differential drug use patterns among sexually abused adolescent girls in treatment for chemical dependency, *Int J Addict* 24:499-514, 1989.
29. Zierler S, Feingold L, Laufer D, Velentgas P, Kantrowitz-Gordon I, Mayer K: Adult survivors of childhood sexual abuse and subsequent risk of HIV infection, *Am J Public Health* 81:572-575, 1991.
30. Gostin L, Lazzarini J, Alexander D, et al: HIV testing, counseling and prophylaxis after sexual assault, *JAMA* 271:1436-1444, 1994.
31. Sanders JM: Guidelines to health care providers of the sexually active adolescent. In: Schinazi RF, Nahmias AJ, editors: *AIDS in children, adolescents and heterosexual adults,* New York, 1988, Elsevier, pp 350-351.
32. DuRant R, Escobedo L, Heath G: Anabolic steroid use, strength training and multiple drug use among adolescents in the U.S., *Pediatrics* 96:23-28, 1995.
33. DuRant R, Rickert V, Ashworth, Newman C, Slavens G: Use of multiple drugs among adolescents who use anabolic steroids, *N Engl J Med* 328:922-926, 1993.
34. Fullilove R, Fullilove M, Bowser B, Gross S: Risk of sexually transmitted disease among black adolescent crack users in Oakland and San Francisco, California, *JAMA* 11163:851-855, 1990.
35. Goedert JJ, Kessler CM, Aledort LM: A prospective study of human immunodeficiency virus type 1 infection and the development of AIDS in subjects with hemophilia, *N Engl J Med* 321:1141-1148, 1989.
36. Overby KJ, Lo B, Litt IF: Knowledge and concerns about acquired immune-deficiency syndrome and their relationship to behavior among adolescents with hemophilia, *Pediatrics* 83:204-210, 1989.
37. Tovo P, DeMartion M, Gabiano C, et al: Prognostic factors in survival in children with perinatal HIV infection, *Lancet* 339:1249-1253, 1992.
38. Grubman S, Gross E, Lerner-Weiss N, et al: Older children and adolescents living with perinatally acquired HIV infection, *Pediatrics* 95:657-663, 1995.
39. Hein K, Dell R, Futterman D, Rotheram MJ, Shaffer N: Comparison of HIV+ and HIV− adolescents: risk factors and psychosocial determinants, *Pediatrics* 95:96-104, 1995.
40. D'Angelo L, Getson P, Luban N, Gayle H: HIV infection in urban adolescents: can we predict who is at risk?, *Pediatrics* 88:982-985, 1991.
41. English A: Expanding access to HIV services for adolescents: legal and ethical issues. In DiClemente R, editor: *Adolescents and AIDS: a generation in jeopardy,* Newbury Park, CA, 1992, Sage; pp 262-283.
42. Hein K: Mandatory HIV testing for youth: a lose-lose proposition, *JAMA* 266:2430-2431, 1991.
43. Centers for Disease Control and Prevention: U.S. Public Health Service recommendations for HIV counseling and voluntary testing for pregnant women, *MMWR* 44:1-15, 1995.

44. English A (editor) and the AIDS Testing and Epidemiology for Youth Workgroup: *J Adolesc Health Care* 10(suppl): 52-57, 1989.

45. Kunins H, Hein K, Futterman D, Tapley E, Elliot A: Guide to Adolescent HIV/AIDS program development, *J Adolesc Health* 14(s):1-140, 1993.

46. El-Sadr W, Oleske J, Agins B, et al: *Evaluation and management of early HIV infection: clinical practice guidelines,* USDHHS, AHCPR publication No. 94-0572, 1994.

47. Centers for Disease Control and Prevention: Revised adult and adolescent HIV classification system and expanded surveillance case definition for severe HIV disease (AIDS), *MMWR* 11-23, 1992.

48. Ho D, Neumann A, Perelson A, Chen W, Leonard J, Markowitz M: Rapid turnover of plasma virions and CD4 lymphocytes in HIV-1 infection, *Nature* 373:123-126, 1995.

49. Coffin J: HIV population dynamics in vivo: implications for genetic variation, pathogenesis and therapy, *Science* 267:483-489, 1995.

50. Tindall B, Imrie A, Donovan B, Penny R, Cooper D: Primary HIV infection. In Sande M, Volberding P, editors: *The medical management of AIDS,* ed 3, Philadelphia, 1992, WB Saunders; pp 67-86.

51. Tanner JM: *Growth at adolescence,* ed 2, London, 1962, Blackwell Scientific.

52. Goodman DS, Teplitz ED, Wishner A, et al: Prevalence of cutaneous disease in patients with AIDS or AIDS-related complex, *J Am Acad Dermatol* 17:210-220, 1987.

53. Masur H, Ognibene FP, Yarchoan RY, et al: CD4 counts as predictors of opportunistic pneumonias in HIV infection, *Ann Intern Med* 111:223-231, 1989.

54. Fahey JL, Taylor JMG, Detels R, et al: The prognostic value of cellular and serologic markers in infection with human immunodeficiency virus type 1, *N Engl J Med* 322:166-172, 1990.

55. Saag M, Holodniy M, Kuritzkes D, et al: HIV viral load in clinical practice, *Nat Med* 2:625-629, 1996.

56. Futterman D, Hein K, Reuben N, Dell R, Shaffer N: HIV-infected adolescents: the first 50 patients in a NYC program, *Pediatrics* 91:730-735, 1993.

57. Vermund S, Kelley K, Klein R, et al: High risk of human papilloma virus infection cervical squamous intraepithelial lesions among women with symptomatic HIV infection, *Am J Obstet Gynecol* 165:392-400, 1991.

58. Minkoff H, DeHovitz J: Care of women with the human immunodeficiency virus, *JAMA* 88:2253-2258, 1991.

59. Palefsky J, Gonzales J, Greenblatt R, et al: Anal intraepithelial neoplasia and anal papilloma virus infection among immunosuppressed homosexual males with group IV HIV disease, *JAMA* 263:2911-2916, 1990.

60. Hoffman N, Kelly C, Futterman D: TB infection in HIV+ adolescents: a NYC cohort, *Pediatrics* 97:198-203, 1996.

61. Centers for Disease Control and Prevention: Recommendations of the Advisory Committee on Immunization Practices: use of vaccines and immune globulins in persons with altered immunocompetence, *MMWR* 42:1-18, 1993.

62. Centers for Disease Control: Recommendations of the Immunization Practices Advisory Committee: immunization of children with human immunodeficiency virus, *MMWR* 37:181-183, 1988.

63. Peter G, editor: *Immunization in special clinical circumstances: adolescents and college populations. Report of the Committee on Infectious Diseases,* ed 21, Elk Grove Village, IL, 1988, American Academy of Pediatrics.

64. Centers for Disease Control: Measles prevention: recommendations of the Immunization Practices Advisory Committee, *MMWR* 38:1-18, 1989.

65. Hein K: The use of therapeutics in adolescence, *J Adolesc Health Care* 8:8-35, 1987.

66. Centers for Disease Control: Guidelines for prophylaxis against PCP for persons infected with HIV, *MMWR* 38 (suppl 5):1-9, 1989.

67. McSherry G, Wright M, Oleske J, Connor E: *Frequency of severe adverse reactions to TMP-SMX and pentamidine among children with HIV infection,* Presented at the 28th Interscience Conference on Antimicrobial Agents and Chemotherapy, 1988.

68. Gordon FM, Simon GL, Wofsy CB, et al: Adverse reactions to trimethoprim-sulfamethoxazole in patients with AIDS, *Ann Intern Med* 100:495-499, 1989.

69. El-Sadr W, Oleske J, Agins B, et al: *Evaluation and management of early HIV infection: AHCPR Publication No. 94-0572,* Rockville, Md., 1994, U.S. Department of Health and Human Services.

70. Carpenter C, Fischl M, Hammer S, et al for the International AIDS Society USA: Consensus statement: antiretroviral therapy for HIV infection in 1996, *JAMA* 276:146-154, 1996.

71. Deeks S, Smith M, Holodniy M, Kahn J: HIV-1 protease inhibitors: a review for clinicians, *JAMA* 277:145-153, 1997.

72. Mellors J, Kingsley L, Rinaldo C, et al: Quantitation of HIV-1 RNA in plasma predicts outcome after seroconversion, *Ann Intern Med* 122:573-579, 1995.

73. Ho D: Time to hit HIV, early and hard, *N Engl J Med* 333:450-451, 1995.

74. O'Brien W, Hartigan P, Martin D, et al: Changes in plasma HIV-1 RNA and CD4+ cells per cubic millimeter, *N Engl J Med* 334:425-431, 1996.

75. Katzenstein D, Hammer S, Hughes M, et al: The relation of virologic and immunologic markers to clinical outcomes after nucleoside therapy in HIV-infected with 200 to 500 CD4 cells per cubic millimeter, *N Engl J Med* 334:1091-1098, 1996.

76. Hammer S, Katzenstein D, Hughes M, et al: A trial comparing nucleoside monotherapy with combination therapy in HIV-infected adults with CD4 cell counts from 200 to 500 per cubic millimeter, *N Engl J Med* 335:1081-1090, 1996.

77. Connor E, Sperling R, Gelber R, et al: Reduction of maternal-infant transmission of HIV with zidovudine treatment. *N Engl J Med* 331:1173-1180, 1994.

78. Centers for Disease Control and Prevention: Recommendations for the use of zidovudine to reduce perinatal transmission of HIV, *MMWR* 43:1-20, 1994.

79. Centers for Disease Control and Prevention: USPHS/IDSA guidelines for the prevention of opportunistic infections in persons infected with HIV: a summary, *MMWR* 44:1-34, 1995.

80. Litt IF, Cuskey WR: Compliance with medical regimens during adolescence, *Pediatr Clin North Am* 27:3-15, 1980.

81. Futterman D, Hein K, Kipke M: *HIV+ adolescents: HIV testing experiences and changes in risk-related sexual and drug use behaviors,* Presented at the 6th International Conference on AIDS, San Francisco, 1990.

82. Perry S, Jacobsberg L, Fishman B: Suicidal ideation and HIV testing, *JAMA* 263:679-682, 1990.

83. Stryker J, Coates T, DeCarlo P, et al: Prevention of HIV infection: looking back, looking ahead, *JAMA* 273:1143-1148, 1995.

84. Hein K, DiGeronimo T: *AIDS: trading facts for fears: a guide for young people,* New York, 1995, Consumer Reports Books.

85. Kirby D, Short L, Collins J, et al: School-based programs to reduce sexual risk behaviors: a review of effectiveness, *Public Health Rep* 109:339-360, 1994.

86. National Research Council: In Turner CF, Miller HG, Moses LE, editors: *AIDS: sexual behavior and intravenous drug use,* Washington, DC, 1989, National Academy Press; pp 372-401.

87. Kipke MD, Futterman DC, Hein K: HIV infection and AIDS during adolescence, *Pediatr Clin North Am* 74:1149-1167, 1990.

CHAPTER 68

Tuberculosis

•

Marguerite M. Mayers

Tuberculosis is a potentially fatal communicable disease with significant morbidity. It has been present since antiquity and remains a worldwide problem even though it is both preventable and curable. Its incidence in the general U.S. population increased between 1985 and 1992 for several reasons: an influx of new cases from foreign-born immigrants, the resurgence of tuberculosis in communities infected with human immunodeficiency virus (HIV), and the spread of tuberculosis in group settings such as prisons, hospitals, and shelters.[1] This increase occurred at a time when public health programs were inadequately supported.

Since 1993, the number of new cases of active tuberculosis has decreased with the systematic identification, containment, and treatment of infected individuals and their contacts through an increased public health commitment. Nevertheless, the number of new cases is still higher than that documented in 1985.[2]

ETIOLOGY

The genus *Mycobacterium* is characterized by the ability of the bacteria to absorb a carbol-fuchsin stain (Ziehl-Neelsen) when heated and then to resist decolorization by acid alcohol: hence, the name *acid-fast bacilli.* The organisms grow slowly, replicating every 16 to 20 hours, and thrive at pH 7.4 with a PO_2 between 100 and 140 mm Hg. They exist with different degrees of metabolic activity within cavities, in granulomas filled with caseating material, and within macrophages. *M. tuberculosis* is the most common cause of tuberculosis in the United States. *M. bovis* was previously an important etiologic agent of tuberculosis, both in man and in cattle, but universal pasteurization of milk in the United States and the destruction of infected herds of cows in the early part of the twentieth century have eliminated this species as an important pathogen. Atypical mycobacteria, including *M. scrofulaceum, M. kansasii, M. marinum, M. fortuitum,* and *M. chelonei,* can cause disease in man, but these species are more likely to produce only a mild or subclinical infection. Clinically apparent infections include lymphadenitis and cutaneous manifestations. *M. avium-intracellulare* complex represents the two atypical species of *Mycobacterium* that have become significant pathogens, affecting patients infected with HIV and indicating the dysfunction of their immune systems. Atypical mycobacteria, however, because they share some antigens with *M. tuberculosis,* may cause false-positive reactions in adolescents being skin tested for evidence of *M. tuberculosis* infection.

PATHOPHYSIOLOGY

Tubercle bacilli usually enter through the respiratory tract, although infection can be acquired via the skin or the gastrointestinal tract. The infection spreads from the initial focus in the lung by way of lymphatics to the regional lymph nodes and then proceeds hematogenously to other sites throughout the body. Air-droplet nuclei containing *M. tuberculosis* are inhaled and infection begins in the alveoli, usually in the lower lobes of the lung. The bacilli are phagocytized by alveolar macrophages, which either kill the bacilli or are themselves killed. The killed macrophages then lyse and release proteolytic enzymes and viable organisms, attracting blood monocytes (macrophages) to the site of infection. These recruited monocytes phagocytize the bacilli, carry the viable organisms to the regional lymph nodes, and enter the circulation, spreading infection preferentially to highly vascular organs. The target organs include the lungs, liver, bone marrow, spleen, kidneys, adrenals, central nervous system (CNS), bones, and joints. This dissemination usually occurs silently and is unchecked, with clusters of epithelioid cells called *tubercles* being formed. With the activation of macrophages by the T-helper cells, there is enhancement of phagocytosis and destruction of the tubercle bacilli instead of containment. This cell-mediated immune response usually occurs 6 weeks to 3 months after the initiation of the primary infection. The host immune response halts the spread of infection, eliminates many of the bacilli, and contains the remainder of the disseminated organisms in a dormant state. If incomplete cell autolysis occurs, central caseation of these tubercules develops. If a cell-mediated response does not occur because of immunosuppression or overwhelming disease, the progression of untreated disease may be fatal.

CLINICAL MANIFESTATIONS

Primary disease is the most common type of tuberculosis seen in adolescents. Most adolescents remain completely asymptomatic throughout their primary infection and its bacillemia, and total containment of the bacilli by the host occurs. These dormant foci of infection, however, represent a lifelong source for endogenous reactivation of disease. Age, immunosuppression, and malnutrition are factors in reactivation. During adolescence, those individuals infected in childhood may experience reactivation because the teenager, a relatively recent converter, undergoes a period of metabolic stress during accelerated growth. Pregnancy creates a negative nitrogen balance and is a time of increased risk for complications both in newly infected individuals and in those with reactivation disease. Clinical manifestations of tuberculosis in the minority of individuals (< 5%) who are symptomatic are usually nonspecific. The adolescent may present with fever, anorexia, malaise, weight loss, or night sweats. In some instances, symptoms may be specifically referable to the organ system involved. However, symptoms also may be subtle, and therefore the clinician must suspect an organic basis for a variety of complaints, including headache, vague abdominal pain, and chronic fatigue.

Primary pulmonary disease initially manifests as a nonproductive cough. Partial containment of the bacilli may result in a symptomatic progressive primary process with pleural effusion. This typically occurs within the first year after acquisition of tuberculosis, peaking at 4 months. A productive cough with hemoptysis and chest pain may be seen with reactivation or advanced disease. Chest pain and/or respiratory distress may accompany this presentation.

Miliary disease usually presents with the nonspecific signs and symptoms that characterize symptomatic primary disease, but these manifestations are unrelenting and progressive. The name *miliary* comes from the presence of fine nodular lesions ("millet seeds") found on chest radiograph examination. These lesions are uniformly and diffusely distributed throughout the lung fields. Central nervous system disease has a varied presentation. Tuberculous meningitis presents insidiously with fever, headache, and vomiting followed by signs of increased intracranial pressure and focal neurologic signs.

There are changes in mental status with stupor, seizures, coma, and death ultimately occurring in untreated individuals after several weeks of progressive illness. Tuberculomas frequently present as mass lesions with signs and symptoms of increased intracranial pressure or focal neurologic signs.

Tuberculous adenitis and bone, peritoneal, renal, and genitourinary tuberculosis may involve pain and/or swelling or other symptoms referable to the organ system involved.

DIAGNOSIS

The intradermal Mantoux test is the most reliable noninvasive diagnostic test for tuberculosis. The most sensitive and specific results are obtained when 0.1 ml of 5 tuberculin units of purified protein derivative (5 TU PPD) is injected intracutaneously on the volar forearm, forming a 6- to 10-mm wheal at the site of injection. At 48 to 72 hours the area should be inspected and the diameter of induration measured transversely to the long axis of the forearm. A positive reaction, indicating infection with *M. tuberculosis* either now or at some time in the past, is defined as induration of more than 10 mm. Populations infected with HIV or adolescents who are immunosuppressed are considered positive for tuberculosis if the induration is more than 5 mm. Similarly, contacts of recent converters, those individuals with active disease, or those who have chest x-ray film evidence suggestive of old tuberculosis are also considered positive with 5 mm or more of induration. Previous exposure with atypical mycobacteria may produce a reaction between 5 and 10 mm of induration. A negative reaction may occur in recently infected adolescents who have not yet had time to develop cell-mediated immunity. If this situation is suspected, the adolescent should be retested in 3 months and advised to seek medical care in the interim for any suspicious clinical illness. Anergy, a negative test when a patient is truly infected, may be seen in those overwhelmed by disease or immunocompromised for any reason.

Repeated testing of uninfected individuals does not sensitize them to tuberculin. However, when it is suspected that delayed hypersensitivity to tuberculin may have waned over the years, a second skin test should be performed in 1 to 2 weeks in an attempt to boost the size of the induration. This second reaction then becomes the baseline against which all subsequent tests are measured. A positive reaction is defined as an increase in size of the induration of more than 6 mm over the baseline. Multiple puncture tests, which use old tuberculin or PPD as an antigen, are sensitive but not specific and do not enable the observer to quantitate the response to the administered antigen. Positive reactions should be verified by intradermal placement of 5 TU PPD.

A chest x-ray examination must be performed to assess the presence of active pulmonary disease in any adolescent with a positive 5 TU PPD test. The x-ray film may show an infiltrate and hilar adenopathy in a Ghon complex or reveal an infiltrate alone. A snowstorm or millet seed appearance may indicate miliary tuberculosis. A pleural effusion may indicate progressive primary disease. Calcifications of hilar lymph nodes represent old healed disease. Apical abnormalities or a cavity suggests reactivation. A negative chest radiograph examination indicates a low inoculum of organisms or healed disease within the respiratory tract. The radiograph examination may be negative in as many as half of the individuals with extrapulmonary tuberculosis, even though the pathophysiology of the infection indicates that almost all tuberculosis is acquired through the respiratory tract.

An attempt should always be made to obtain an organism for culture and sensitivity either before the initiation of therapy or, in the event of life-threatening disease, concurrently with the start of therapy. Once specimens have been obtained for culture, empiric therapy should be started, because cultures processed by standard methods can require 3 to 10 weeks to show growth. Sensitivity tests for various antituberculous chemotherapeutic agents are performed on the organism grown from a subculture of the original specimen, not by direct plating, and these results may not be available for weeks to months. Current technology, however, epitomized by the BACTEC method, which is both automated and radiometric, uses a culture media with a carbon-labeled substrate specific for *Mycobacterium* organisms, and under optimal conditions may give a positive culture in as little as 2 weeks, and drug sensitivities in 3 weeks.[3]

All body fluids obtained should be examined by Ziehl-Neelsen staining for acid-fast bacilli, or should be stained with auramine O and examined by blue-light fluoroscopy. Pathologic specimens also should be stained for the presence of tubercle bacilli.

Sputum may be obtained by expectoration. In the cooperative adolescent, it may also be induced by nebulized normal saline and postural drainage with the assistance of a respiratory therapist. In the patient without a productive cough, morning gastric aspirates of at least 50 ml of fluid have a 10% yield for organisms, but the discomfort involved with placement of the nasogastric tube may be unacceptable to the adolescent patient, in whom bronchoscopy is better tolerated. Bronchial lavage through the bronchoscope usually yields a sufficient specimen for culture and pathologic examination. The bronchorrhea that frequently occurs after bronchoscopy is even more valuable for laboratory examination. Morning urine cultures, even in a patient with sterile pyuria, have a very low yield but are an adjunct examination acceptable to the adolescent. In tuberculous meningitis the cerebrospinal fluid (CSF) classically shows pleocy-tosis with lymphocytes predominating, a low glucose level, and a high protein level. The cellular reaction present in the CSF represents a serous response to organisms contained by the host defenses within the tubercule. Stains and cultures of the fluid are positive only when tubercules on the meninges rupture into the cerebrospinal space. Blood cultures for mycobacteria should be obtained if miliary tuberculosis is suspected.

Enzyme-linked immunosorbent assay (ELISA) serology, gas chromatography, DNA probes, and polymerase chain reaction (PCR) amplification are now commercially available techniques that augment but have not replaced the standard methods of identification and drug sensitivity testing of the mycobacteria.[3]

Liver and bone marrow biopsies show caseating granulomas on pathologic examination in 60% and 30%, respectively, of patients with pulmonary tuberculosis. Biopsy is indicated in adolescents when the diagnosis is obscure, and it is obtained both to confirm tuberculosis and to rule out other pathologic conditions.

Radiographs may show destruction of the bones and joints affected by tuberculosis. A radiograph examination of the spine, in an untreated patient with advanced disease, may show destruction of two adjacent vertebral bodies with anterior collapse and loss of intervening disk space. This classic finding correlates clinically with a prominent posterior kyphosis or gibbous deformity of the spine.

Computed tomography may demonstrate the basilar meningitis and hydrocephalus characteristic of tuberculous meningitis, or it may reveal single or multiple calcified intracranial tuberculomas. This type of imaging is also a useful noninvasive procedure for delineating the extent of the infection in other affected systems.

DIFFERENTIAL DIAGNOSIS

Pulmonary and extrapulmonary disease must be differentiated from bacterial, viral, and fungal infections, and from sarcoidosis and neoplasms. The diagnosis is made from the clinical presentation, history and physical examination, laboratory tests, pathologic examination, and culture and sensitivity results. Occasionally, tuberculosis and other processes may exist concurrently, and in such cases each disease must be appropriately treated.

TREATMENT

When active tuberculosis is suspected or diagnosed, the patient should be hospitalized for culture, initiation of antituberculous therapy, and some evidence of effective control of the disease process. The adolescent and family should be educated concerning the disease and its implications for future health. An assessment should be made of the probable compliance of both patient and family. In addition, the family and close social and school contacts of the adolescent should be screened for tuberculin positivity and active disease. The index case should be sought from among these contacts. While the adolescent is still hospitalized, outpatient follow-up should be arranged to ensure compliance with medication regimens, and a mechanism should be developed to notify the provider if the patient does not comply with treatment.

Current chemotherapy is based on the following four principles:

1. In vivo, the tuberculous bacilli exist in three different sites: the caseating lesion, the macrophage, and the cavity. Each site has its own metabolic milieu, contains a characteristic number of organisms, and places unique demands on the chemotherapeutic agents available. Primary disease has relatively few slow-growing organisms that multiply in the acidic pH of the macrophage and in the neutral pH of caseating granuloma. In cavities the bacilli exist in a metabolically more active state and at a neutral-to-alkaline pH.

2. There are spontaneously occurring drug-resistant mutations in every population when the bacterial density is equal to or greater than 10^6 organisms. Individuals with a positive PPD and a negative chest x-ray examination have between 10^3 and 10^4 organisms. When an infiltrate is seen on chest x-ray film, between 10^5 and 10^7 organisms are usually found. In cavities, 10^7 to 10^8 organisms are found. The number of organisms present, as suggested by the clinical picture, mandates the number of chemotherapeutic agents to be used to prevent the selection of drug-resistant organisms.

3. Bactericidal drugs are more effective in totally eliminating the mycobacteria and are active in a shorter time than are bacteriostatic agents.

4. Primary or selected drug resistance is found in geographic areas and in populations with endemic disease where widespread antituberculous drug therapy has been used. Such areas include Southeast Asia, South America, Central America, Africa, and the Caribbean. Resistant organisms are also commonly seen in reactivation disease in patients with a history of previous chemotherapy, and in primary disease in individuals whose source of infection is someone with a resistant organism.

The chemotherapeutic agents that have been widely studied and are in general use are listed in Table 68-1. Bactericidal drugs kill the mycobacteria even in the presence of host immune dysfunction, while bacteriostatic agents contain the bacilli but depend substantially on the integrity of host immunity to completely eradicate disease. Of the bactericidal drugs, isoniazid (INH) is most

effective in cavities, although it has some activity at other sites. Rifampin (RIF) is the most active agent at all sites, especially against the intermittently multiplying organisms in caseating lesions. Streptomycin (SM), the first antituberculous agent to be developed, is effective against extracellular organisms only. Pyrazinamide (PZA) is active only in acid environments, and so its principal effect is on the macrophage, especially during the first few months of treatment. The bacteriostatic agents listed in Table 68-1 are those commonly included in regimens in which drug resistance is suspected or documented. Given the effectiveness of the new bactericidal drugs, and on the basis of many clinical studies obtained throughout the world, the American Thoracic Society recommends intensive short-course therapy in the adult patient, which is as effective as and less expensive than older regimens.[4] Multiple bactericidal drugs are used initially for 2 months, followed by at least two drugs of known sensitivity for 4 to 7 more months. There is a strong emphasis on patient compliance, with direct administration of medication by healthcare workers two or three times a week if necessary. With these regimens, because of early and rapid sterilization of all or most disseminated bacilli, a bacteriologic cure can be achieved even if the patient does not complete the full course of therapy. In the *1994 Red Book,* the Committee on Infectious Disease of the American Academy of Pediatrics recommends as standard these same short, intensive treatments for children and adolescents with tuberculosis.[5] Short-course therapy is that which is administered for 9 months, whereas intensive short-course therapy may be completed in 6 months. Supervised therapy, also called directly observed therapy (DOT), is defined as that administered by a healthcare worker. Such therapy may be intermittent, with drugs being given only two or three times a week. Regimens that contain mainly the bacteriostatic drugs, either because of multiple drug resistance or because of patient intolerance of the bactericidal agents, must be continued for up to 18 to 24 months, usually on a daily treatment schedule.

RECOMMENDATIONS FOR SPECIFIC CLINICAL SITUATIONS

Pulmonary Tuberculosis

Intensive short-course therapy is now the standard recommendation for pulmonary disease, including hilar adenopathy, in which sensitive organisms are documented or strongly suspected. The following basic therapeutic regimens are suggested if there is less than 4% of primary INH resistance in the community:

1. Daily INH, RIF, and PZA for 2 months, followed by INH and RIF either daily or twice a week with

TABLE 68-1
Antituberculous Agents

| | Dosage | | | |
	Daily	Twice Weekly	Route	Side Effects
Bactericidal Drugs				
Isoniazid (INH)*	10-15 mg/kg (300 mg max)	20-40 mg/kg (900 mg max)	Oral/IM (IV avail.)	Hepatitis Peripheral neuropathy Hypersensitivity
Rifampin (RIF)†	10-20 mg/kg (600 mg max)	10-20 mg (600 mg max)	Oral/IV	Hepatitis Thrombocytopenia Flulike reaction
Streptomycin (SM)	20-40 mg/kg (1 g max)	20-40 mg/kg (1 g max)	IM	Ototoxicity Nephrotoxicity Dermatitis
Pyrazinamide (PZA)	20-40 mg/kg (2.5 g max)	40-50 mg/kg (2.5 g max)	Oral	Hepatotoxicity Increased uric acid Arthralgia Skin rash
Bacteriostatic Drugs				
Ethambutol (EMB)‡	15-25 mg/kg (2.5 g max)	50 mg/kg	Oral	Optic neuritis Visual acuity Color vision GI hypersensitivity
Para-aminosalicylic acid (PASA)	200 mg/kg TID (12 g max)		Oral	GI intolerance Hepatotoxicity Hypersensitivity
Ethionamide (ETH)	10-20 mg/kg (1 g max)		Oral	GI intolerance Hepatitis

*Add 10 mg pyridoxine for each 100 mg INH in patients whose diets are deficient of pyridoxine.
†Give ½ hr before meals or 3 hr afterward; urine, tears, saliva become red; may interfere with the action of oral contraceptives, stain contact lenses, and accelerate clearance of drugs metabolized by the liver.
‡Use higher dose if INH resistance is suspected, and decrease to 15 mg/kg after 2 months.
GI, gastrointestinal; *IM,* intramuscular; *IV,* intravenous; *TID,* three times daily (daily dose is given in three divided doses).

supervision for 4 months, for a total of 6 months of therapy.

2. Daily INH and RIF for 9 months.
3. Daily INH and RIF for 1 month, followed by INH and RIF twice a week with supervision for 8 months, for a total of 9 months of therapy.

Extrapulmonary Tuberculosis

Miliary disease, meningitis, and bone or joint tuberculosis generally require more intensive and prolonged treatment. In these presentations the disease may be life-threatening and the number of organisms infecting the patient may be greater than those seen in pulmonary disease. The therapeutic regimens recommended consist of daily INH, RIF, PZA, and SM for 2 months, followed by INH and RIF either daily or twice a week under supervision, for 10 months.

When CNS tuberculosis is being treated, it is imperative to use those agents that cross the blood-brain barrier and achieve therapeutic concentrations in the CSF. Although INH and PZA both cross the meninges, RIF and SM achieve therapeutic levels in the CSF only when meningeal irritation is present.

Other forms of extrapulmonary disease, including cervical lymphadenopathy, may be treated according to the regimen used for pulmonary tuberculosis.

Multiple Drug-Resistant Tuberculosis

If the incidence of primary INH resistance in the community exceeds 4%, initial therapy should include four drugs until an organism has been cultured and its sensitivity pattern has been determined. The initial regimens recommended include the following[6]:

1. Daily INH, RIF, PZA, and ETH or SM.
2. Daily INH, RIF, PZA, and ETH or SM for 2 weeks followed by these same drugs given under direct supervision, twice a week.
3. INH, RIF, PZA, and ETH or SM administered

under direct supervision, three times a week. If the bacillus isolated is in fact sensitive to INH and RIF, intensive short-course therapy can be resumed. If resistant organisms are found, the number of drugs and the duration of therapy depend on how many effective bactericidal drugs can be included in the regimen. The greater number of available bactericidal drugs that can be used, the shorter is the course of therapy. Therapy can be stopped 6 months after negative cultures are obtained.

For multiple drug-resistant strains of tuberculosis (MDR-TB), in which the mycobacteria are resistant to both INH and RIF and frequently to other first-line drugs also, the bacteriostatic agents listed in Table 68-1 may need to be included in the patient's regimen. If only bacteriostatic drugs can be used, 18 months or more of therapy may be necessary. Other potentially useful drugs for the patient with MDR-TB include cycloserine, kanamycin, and capreomycin. The use of these drugs is limited, however, because they are toxic to bone marrow and kidney. In addition, there are other drugs that may be effective but have not had widespread use in the treatment of tuberculosis. These drugs include amikacin and the quinolones ciprofloxacin and ofloxacin, all of which have been found to be both bactericidal in vitro and effective in many of the clinical situations in which they have been used.

Adjuvant Therapy

Surgical biopsy may be indicated for diagnosis and culture. Surgical incision and drainage is indicated when large collections of pus are life-threatening or effectively impeding the action of the chemotherapeutic agents.

Corticosteroids have been used to decrease intracranial pressure in meningitis, inflammation in pericarditis, and respiratory obstruction caused by large hilar adenopathy. These agents must be used in conjunction with the appropriate antituberculous drug therapy.

ISOLATION AND INFECTION CONTROL

Primary pulmonary tuberculosis without a productive cough is rarely contagious. Thus, a teenager need not be isolated in the hospital or at home but may return to school and normal activities as soon as he or she feels capable of resuming them. However, family members and close contacts should be tested.

Adolescents with a productive cough and smear-positive sputum must be placed on respiratory isolation until an examination of the sputum is negative for acid-fast bacilli and the cough has diminished. This clinical picture is usually seen with reactivation pulmonary disease and requires respiratory isolation for about

2 weeks after the initiation of therapy. The teenager should be instructed to wear a mask if coughing frequently, and to dispose properly of all expectorated material.

Unless there is drainage from an infected lymph node or skeletal site, extrapulmonary tuberculosis does not require isolation. When there is drainage of infected material, the site should be covered, and gloves should be used when dressings are changed. If renal infection is suspected, urine should be considered as potentially infectious material and not splashed in the bathroom or left standing in open containers.

OUTPATIENT MANAGEMENT

The goal of hospitalization for the adolescent with tuberculosis, after specimens are taken for culture and sensitivity and drug therapy is initiated, is to return the patient to the family, school, and social milieu quickly and in a state of optimal health. To this end, discharge planning should begin on admission with an assessment of the ability of the adolescent to take and complete the prescribed medications. Whenever possible, DOT should be arranged for the adolescent to ensure maximal compliance.

A dietary history should be obtained. Adolescents who have diets deficient in meat and milk risk peripheral neuropathy while taking INH. Pregnant and lactating teenagers are at similar risk. The addition of pyridoxine (vitamin B_6) is required for such patients.

Baseline liver function tests should be obtained in adolescents suspected of having preexisting liver disease because of a history of hepatitis, drug use, or alcohol abuse. In all other patients, liver function may be presumed to be normal and checked only for clinical indications. The potential side effects of the medication prescribed should be discussed with the adolescent. Chemical hepatitis is the most serious of potential side effects. It is seen in patients receiving INH and/or RIF, usually when these drugs are being administered in high doses, and frequently in patients in whom there is preexisting liver disease. The individual complains of anorexia, malaise, and abdominal pain and the liver function tests are found to be elevated, more than three times baseline. When these drugs are discontinued, liver function usually returns to normal. In life-threatening disease or in the treatment of MDR-TB, some experts have cautiously reinstituted these drugs at lower dosages.

During the course of therapy, cultures of the body fluids that were initially positive should be repeated until negative specimens are obtained, indicating a sterilization of the body site. Positive radiographic and scan results should also be followed until there is improvement or resolution of the abnormal process.

The cost of therapy to the patient is substantial, but the cost to society of allowing individuals with active tuberculosis to remain untreated is even greater, considering the deleterious effect on the individual and the spread of infection to others. Some costs, such as the hospitalization and diagnostic tests, the physician's fees, and the cost of the chemotherapeutic agents, can be measured. Table 68-2 shows the estimated monthly cost of the most commonly prescribed antituberculous drugs. Fixed-combination drugs have been recommended, both to improve compliance by reducing the number of pills to be taken at one time and to prevent the emergence of resistant organisms by the patient's self-modification of the drug regimen. The physician should ascertain who is financially responsible for payment of the adolescent's medical bills to ensure that an expensive but necessary course of therapy is not prescribed to a teenager who will be unable to afford it. Social service and public health agencies should be involved if there is no obvious third-party insurance or responsible parent to pay for the prescribed medications and medical monitoring.

SCREENING

Current recommendations for routine tuberculin screening in the pediatric population include testing at 12 to 15 months, at school entry (4 to 6 years), and in adolescence.[5]

High-risk populations are targeted for annual screening. These include minority teenagers (blacks, Hispanics, Asians, Native Americans), those living in urban areas, those from low socioeconomic backgrounds, and those who are or whose parents are emigrants from high-risk areas (Africa, Asia, South America, Central America, the Caribbean, and the Middle East). Incarcerated youth, the homeless, and those living in shelters are also populations at risk. Teenagers from these groups are more likely to be exposed to tuberculosis in these settings and are more likely to ignore any symptoms of medical illness. In all teenagers, however, the physician should have a high index of suspicion for tuberculosis.

CHEMOPROPHYLAXIS

Chemoprophylaxis with isoniazid, 10 mg/kg/day up to 300 mg/day for 9 months, is recommended by the American Academy of Pediatrics[5] for all children and adolescents with a positive tuberculin skin test and a negative chest radiograph examination. This approach is designed to reduce subsequent reactivation of dormant foci of tubercule bacilli, a lifelong risk in the untreated person. Epidemiologic studies have shown that 6 months of INH therapy is associated with a 65% disease reduction, which increases to 75% after 1 year of therapy. Modifications of this recommendation that are also acceptable include either 6 to 12 months of continuous therapy or 9 months of twice-weekly therapy. If the index case is found to be infected with INH-resistant organisms, rifampin, 10 mg/kg/day (up to 600 mg), may be added to INH therapy, or it may be used alone if it is suspected that the entire population of tuberculous bacilli is INH resistant. For contacts of patients infected with MDR-TB,

---

TABLE 68-2
Estimated Monthly Cost of Therapy

Drug	Daily Dosage*	Cost of a 30-Day Supply	
		HHC†	AWP‡
Isoniazid (INH):			
100-mg, 300-mg tablets	300 mg	$ 1	$ 2
50 mg/5 ml syrup			
Rifampin (RIF):			
150-mg, 300-mg capsules	600 mg	$ 24	$127
Pyrazinamide (PZA):			
500-mg tablets	1 g	$ 42	$ 65
Ethambutol (EMB):			
400-mg tablets	800 mg	$ 43	$100
RIF (300 mg)/INH (150 mg)§	2 capsules	$ 36	$146
RIF (120 mg)/INH (50 mg)/PZA (300 mg)	5 capsules	$113	$270

*Frequently prescribed adolescent/adult dose.
†Cost to New York City HHC (Health & Hospitals Corporation) pharmacy, July 1995, based on contract and volume purchases.
‡Average wholesale price, New York City, December 1996 (excluding pharmacist's overhead costs).
§Fixed-combination drugs.

observation alone in the asymptomatic, immunocompetent individual has been suggested, because there is no tested drug regimen. However, for individuals with a high risk of developing active tuberculosis (i.e., the HIV infected), PZA and ETH, or PZA and a quinolone, have been recommended as chemoprophylaxis.[7]

SPECIAL SITUATIONS

Compliance

Compliance is the most significant factor affecting the successful outcome of treatment of tuberculosis in adolescents. Adolescents may not take their medications and may miss their appointments. This type of behavior leads to increased morbidity and mortality in the individual patient and affects the ecology of the disease in general, since drug-resistant organisms may be selected and disseminated throughout the population. Supervised twice-weekly therapy, visiting nurse referrals, and social service support may help with this problem. Adolescents should be seen monthly for assessment of their disease status and their compliance with medication regimens.

Interruption of therapy raises many questions. How long was the interruption? At what stage of the disease and the therapy did the interruption occur? What was the adolescent's clinical condition—findings on radiograph and potential inoculum of tubercle bacilli? If the teenager stopped therapy early in the course, he or she is presumed to still have predominantly sensitive organisms and may simply resume therapy. If the disruption of chemotherapy occurred very late in the course, a cure may have already been achieved, especially if the interval from the cessation of therapy to the present has been long and the patient has remained asymptomatic. Of most concern is an interruption that occurs substantially into the course of therapy, at which time most sensitive organisms may have been eliminated, a long interval has passed, and the adolescent is again clinically symptomatic. In such a situation, resistant organisms must be suspected and therapy modified until repeat cultures and sensitivities are obtained.

Pregnancy

Pregnant teenagers who are tuberculin positive are at increased risk for reactivation. Diagnostic tests and drug therapy are dictated by the clinical presentation of the patient. If a positive tuberculin reaction is found but there is no clinical suspicion of any active disease, the chest x-ray examination and chemoprophylaxis can be postponed until after delivery to protect the developing fetus from any possible harm of radiation or drugs. However, if there is evidence of active disease, an appropriate

evaluation is obtained (including x-ray examinations and a lumbar puncture if indicated) and therapy is initiated to treat the state of the disease found. In either case the adolescent's family and contacts should also be screened for active disease in preparation for the discharge of a newborn into the household.

HIV Infection

HIV infection presents a dual risk to the teenager. First, populations in which HIV is present have a higher incidence of tuberculosis, and therefore acquisition of the disease is more likely. Second, those who are HIV infected may have more difficulty in being cured of tuberculosis. Some experts recommend that all patients with tuberculosis be tested for HIV.[8] In HIV-infected patients, 5 mm of induration is considered a positive Mantoux test indicative of tuberculosis, although anergy may render the tuberculin skin test unreactive and the clinical presentation of disease may be subtle because of immunosuppression. Extrapulmonary tuberculosis is more common and should be strongly suspected in the adolescent with HIV infection. All clinical material obtained from the patient should be examined pathologically and cultured for tuberculosis. If the diagnosis of *M. tuberculosis* is made, initial therapy should include at least four drugs until sensitivities are available. Therapy should be continued for at least 9 months, or for at least 6 months after three negative cultures have been documented. A positive PPD without evidence of disease in an HIV-infected individual should mandate chemoprophylaxis for 1 year.

Immunosuppressive drugs or medications, such as steroids or cancer chemotherapy, used in the treatment of chronic illness or the underlying disease itself can be factors in increasing the risk of reactivation of tuberculosis in the teenager.

Bacille Calmette-Guérin

The bacille Calmette-Guérin (BCG) vaccine frequently presents the physician caring for teenagers with a diagnostic dilemma. Many teenagers from Third World countries where tuberculosis is endemic and epidemic have been given BCG at birth, at school entry, or in refugee camps. Without documentation of BCG negativity before vaccination or documentation of conversion to tuberculin positivity after vaccination, all PPD tests that produce induration of 10 mm or greater should be considered positive for *M. tuberculosis*. A chest x-ray examination should be obtained and treatment initiated. In some circumstances however, when the adolescent originates from a country with a low rate of endemic tuberculosis, has documentation of recent BCG administration, a negative chest x-ray examination, and a PPD between 10 and 15 mm of induration, the provider may elect to consider the PPD reaction only as proof of BCG-induced immunity and not prescribe chemoprophylaxis. The PPD should then be repeated in 1 year. However, most patients in this category usually are given chemoprophylaxis because of probable exposure to *M. tuberculosis*. A PPD of 15 mm or greater induration is always considered evidence of *M. tuberculosis* infection.

PROGNOSIS

With current therapy available in the United States, tuberculosis should involve minimal morbidity and mortality in adolescents and in the population as a whole, provided that it is diagnosed in the early stages and therapy is appropriate in intensity and duration.

References

1. Centers for Disease Control: A strategic plan for the elimination of tuberculosis in the United States, *MMWR* 38(suppl S-3), 1989.
2. Centers for Disease Control: Tuberculosis morbidity—United States, 1994, *MMWR* 44:387-395, 1995.
3. Witebsky FG, Conville PS: The laboratory diagnosis of mycobacterial disease, *Infect Dis Clin North Am* 7:359-376, 1993.
4. American Thoracic Society: Treatment of tuberculosis and tuberculosis infection in adults and children, *Am J Respir Crit Care Med* 149:1359-1374, 1994.
5. American Academy of Pediatrics: Tuberculosis. In *Report of the Committee on Infectious Disease,* ed 23, Elk Grove Village, IL, 1994, American Academy of Pediatrics; pp 480-500.
6. Centers for Disease Control: Initial therapy for tuberculosis in the era of multidrug resistance. Recommendations of the Advisory Council for the Elimination of Tuberculosis, *MMWR* 42(RR-7):1-8, 1993.
7. Centers for Disease Control: Management of persons exposed to multidrug-resistant tuberculosis, *MMWR* 41:59-71, 1992.
8. Centers for Disease Control: Tuberculosis and human immunodeficiency virus infection: recommendations of the Advisory Committee for the Elimination of Tuberculosis (ACET), *MMWR* 38:236-238, 243-250, 1989.

Suggested Readings

American Thoracic Society: Diagnostic standards and classification of tuberculosis, *Am Rev Respir Dis* 142:725-735, 1990.

Centers for Disease Control: Screening for tuberculosis and tuberculosis infection in high risk populations; and The use of preventive therapy for tuberculosis infection in the United States: Recommendations of the Advisory Committee for the Elimination of Tuberculosis, *MMWR* 39(RR-8):1-12, 1990.

Huebner RE, Schein MF, Bass JB: The tuberculin skin test, *Clin Infect Dis* 17:968-975, 1993.

Schluger NW, Rom WN: Current approaches to the diagnosis of active pulmonary tuberculosis, *Am J Respir Crit Care Med* 149:264-267, 1994.

Starke JR, Correa AG: Management of mycobacterial infection and disease, *Pediatr Infect Dis J* 14:455-470, 1995.

CHAPTER 69

Lyme Disease

•

Leonard R. Krilov

Lyme disease was initially described from investigations of a cluster of cases of oligoarticular arthritis reported from Old Lyme, Connecticut in 1975.[1] Subsequent evaluations have shown Lyme disease to be a multisystem disorder affecting the skin, heart, nervous system, and joints that is caused by the spirochete *Borrelia burgdorferi.*[2] The spectrum of clinical manifestations continues to expand, and reported cases of Lyme disease in the United States have increased almost twenty-fold from 1982 (497 cases) to 1994 (13,083 and 1995 (11,603).[3] The disease is particularly common in the adolescent age group, with the highest incidence reported in individuals under 20 years of age.[4,5] Cases appear to be evenly distributed between the 10- to 19-year-old age group and the under-10 age group.

EPIDEMIOLOGY

The geographical and seasonal clustering of Lyme disease cases suggested an infectious, arthropod-borne vector for this disease. Most cases occur in summer and early autumn, with clustering of cases in wooded and sparsely populated areas. This is consistent with the location and life cycle of ticks, whose nymphal stage matures at this time of year. In 1982, Burgdorfer et al isolated a spirochete, now named *Borrelia burgdorferi,* from *Ixodes scapularis* (previously *I. dammini*) ticks (deer ticks).[2,6] The organism was subsequently recovered from patients with Lyme disease, and specific host immune responses to the organism were identified.[7]

In the northern United States, *I. scapularis* is the major vector of transmission. Elsewhere, other members of the *Ixodes* genus can transmit the spirochete: *Ixodes pacificus* on the U.S. west coast and *Ixodes ricinus* in Europe. In experimental situations, the ticks generally need to remain attached for at least 24 hours before *B. burgdorferi* transmission occurs.[8] These ticks are small, 1 to 4 mm in diameter (about the size of a nail head or pencil point). Therefore, they may not be readily apparent, and the person with Lyme disease may not recall a tick bite at any time before the development of clinical signs and symptoms. Mosquitoes, deer flies, and other species of ticks (*Amblyomma americanum, Dermacentor variabilis*) can harbor the spirochete, but their role in Lyme disease transmission is less certain.[9] One report documented fly transmission of Lyme disease.[10]

Lyme disease is currently the most common arthropod-borne disease reported to the Centers for Disease Control and Prevention.[3] Cases occur in areas where *Ixodes* ticks are found, and the frequency of disease in a given area depends on the presence of ticks and the degree of parasitism of the ticks. In the United States three sectors of the country account for over 90% of reported cases: coastal areas of the northeast (up to 80% of cases); Minnesota and Wisconsin; and parts of California and Nevada. The disease has been reported from all 50 states, although in seven (Alaska, Arizona, Hawaii, Montana, Nebraska, New Mexico, Wyoming) indigenous cases have not been identified. The disease is also widely distributed in Europe and has been found in Australia. In areas with a high incidence of Lyme disease, infection rates for ticks with *B. burgdorferi* are quite high. Up to 35% of ticks in Connecticut[11] and 60% of ticks in Shelter Island, New York[6] carry the Lyme disease spirochete.

Lyme disease has been reported in all age groups and without a clear-cut dominance in either sex. Several studies suggest an age-specific variation in the incidence of the disease, with the highest rate observed in individuals under 20 years of age. In New York state, almost half of the 600 cases of Lyme disease reported from 1983 to 1988 occurred in individuals under 20 years of age (278 of 600), and those were evenly distributed between 10- to 19-year-olds and children under age 10.[5] Again, nationally, in 1995 the highest proportion of cases occurred among 0-14 year olds (2760 [24%]).[3] Petersen et al,[4] in their analysis of 1149 infected individuals from

Connecticut, reported the highest Lyme disease incidence in children 5 to 14 years of age. The reasons for the increased incidence in this age group are unknown. Possibilities include (1) increased tick exposure because children and adolescents are more likely to go into wooded areas and off trails, (2) increased susceptibility to *B. burgdorferi* infection and/or increased likelihood of developing symptoms after infection, (3) a higher likelihood of disease being reported in these patients, and (4) decreased attention to self-observation for and removal of ticks after potential exposures.

In addition to age-specific differences in the incidence of Lyme disease, individuals under 20 years of age are also more likely to present with arthritis alone as their first manifestation of the disease than are persons 20 years of age or older. One third or more of children and adolescents (ages 1 to 19 years) reported as having Lyme disease did not have erythema migrans (EM).[12,13] In comparison, it has been noted that adults have EM in up to 80% of cases.

CLINICAL MANIFESTATIONS

The clinical manifestations of Lyme disease have been divided into three stages (Table 69-1). Although conceptually useful to an understanding of the manifestations of Lyme disease, any of the findings can occur in isolation. Furthermore, the protean manifestations of disease within a given organ system have led to this disease being referred to as the "latest great imitator."[14]

Stage I

The earliest and most distinctive aspect of Lyme disease is erythema migrans or erythema chronicum migrans. EM begins as an erythematous macule or papule at the site of the infected tick bite. It first appears 3 to 32 days after exposure. The lesion expands over days to weeks, reaching a median diameter of 16 cm (range, 3 to 68 cm). Central clearing accompanying the outward expansion is characteristic (Fig. 69-1), although some lesions may exhibit diffuse erythema, vesication, or ulceration. The rash most commonly occurs on exposed areas of the skin, especially the lower extremities and trunk. Biopsy of the periphery of the skin lesion may reveal *B. burgdorferi* organisms on Warthin-Starry stain, and cultivation of the spirochete is possible, although not routinely available. Up to 50% of patients develop multiple smaller secondary EM lesions in close proximity to the original lesion. Only about one third of individuals with documented Lyme disease recall a tick bite, and up to 40% or more (especially children and adolescents) do not give a history of EM or recall a rash consistent with EM. Systemic manifestations are frequently reported in

TABLE 69-1
Clinical Manifestations of Lyme Disease

Time of Occurrence After Tick Bite	Skin	Nervous System
Stage I: Local infection (3-32 days)	Erythema migrans	Nonspecific: headaches, musculoskeletal pain
Stage II: Disseminated, recurrent infection (4-6 wk)	Erythema migrans	Aseptic meningitis Cranial nerve palsies Peripheral radiculoneuritis Other (see discussion)
Stage III: Persistent infection (4-6 wk to months or years)	Acrodermatitis chronica atrophicans	Chronic encephalitis; subtle mental disorders; chronic polyneuritis

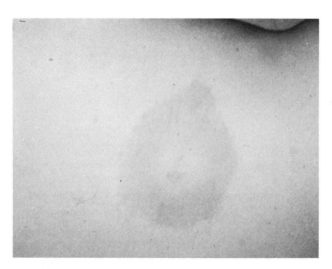

Fig. 69-1. Typical lesion of erythema migrans. Note large size and peripheral erythema with central clearing and papule at center.

patients with EM. In summer months a flulike illness with headaches, malaise, lethargy, fever, stiff neck, myalgias, arthralgias, and diffuse adenopathy occurring in an endemic area raises the specter of Lyme disease. Given the nonspecific nature of these findings, they have not been systematically associated with Lyme disease in the absence of EM. Without treatment, the rash and other symptoms of stage I Lyme disease persist for up to 3 to 4 weeks and then gradually resolve. Skin lesions can recur for up to 1 year from the initial presentation. As many as 20% of untreated patients develop stage II disease with significant neurologic and/or cardiac abnormalities. More than 50% of patients who are not treated develop the intermittent episodes of arthritis lasting weeks to months that are characteristic of stage III Lyme disease.[15]

Stage II

The clinical manifestations of stage II Lyme disease typically occur 4 to 6 weeks after the initial onset of symptoms and reflect hematogenous dissemination of the infection. The heart, nervous system, and skin are most commonly affected.[16] About half of the patients with stage II disease develop recurrent skin lesions resembling EM, but these lesions tend to be smaller and migrate less.[7]

The most common cardiac manifestation of Lyme disease is atrioventricular block, which can range from first-degree to complete heart block.[17-19] Evidence of myocarditis also may be seen on an electrocardiogram or echocardiogram. Less than 10% of patients with Lyme disease develop cardiac abnormalities, and those that do occur generally remain for a brief period (less than 1 week), even in the absence of therapy. Most patients with cardiac abnormalities also display other evidence of Lyme disease.

The characteristic neurologic findings in Lyme disease are the triad of aseptic meningitis, cranial nerve palsies, and peripheral radiculoneuropathy.[20] However, they may not all be observed in a given patient. Nervous system involvement, which occurs in 10% to 20% of patients with Lyme disease, can occur weeks to months after tick exposure. The most common manifestation is aseptic meningitis, which involves severe headache and mild stiff neck. This effect may be intermittent and last for days to weeks. Cerebrospinal fluid analysis reveals a lymphocytic pleocytosis with up to 100 cells, normal glucose level, and normal to mildly elevated protein level. Subtle findings of encephalitis, such as poor concentration, memory loss, somnolence, emotional lability, and behavioral changes, are also frequently seen.[21,22] Isolated seventh cranial nerve palsy, unilateral or bilateral, may be the only nervous system manifestation of Lyme disease, or it may occur in association with aseptic meningitis. Other cranial nerve palsies occur less frequently. Motor and/or sensory nerves also may be affected. Less common neurologic syndromes reported in association with Lyme disease include transverse myelitis,[23] Guillain-Barré syndrome,[24] pseudotumor cerebri,[25] and cerebellar ataxia.[20]

Joints	Heart	Other
		Flulike syndrome; regional lymphadenopathy Severe malaise and fatigue
Migratory arthralgias; brief bouts of arthritis	Atrioventricular block, myocarditis	
Prolonged and/or recurrent attacks of arthritis		Fatigue

Stage III

Stage III is the chronic phase of Lyme disease. It is characterized by recurrent intermittent episodes of monoarticular, oligoarticular, or migratory polyarthritis, which can last from weeks to months and which generally develop weeks to many months after the EM is noted. The large joints, especially the knees, are most commonly involved. Typically, the involved joints are swollen, warm, and painful but not red; morning stiffness is generally not described.[15] The first episode usually lasts about 1 week. Recurrent episodes may occur frequently, with intervals of weeks to years between attacks. As noted earlier, arthritis frequently occurs in the absence of a history of EM, especially in children and adolescents. Thus, Lyme disease needs to be considered in the differential diagnosis of juvenile rheumatoid arthritis. An association has been made between chronic Lyme arthritis and particular class II major histocompatibility genes, suggesting that host susceptibility factors are necessary for the development of this form of Lyme disease that does not respond to antibiotics.[26] Chronic, or stage III, neurologic involvement also has been described months to years after the initial infection. These findings include neuropsychiatric symptoms, focal encephalitis, and severe incapacitating fatigue.[27,28]

LABORATORY DIAGNOSIS

The specific diagnosis of Lyme disease is currently dependent on detection of host antibody response to *B. burgdorferi*. This is most commonly accomplished by enzyme-linked immunosorbent assay (ELISA) or immunofluorescent antibody staining (IFA) techniques. There are a number of commercially available reagents and kits for these purposes. Unfortunately, the best antigen of the organism to use in detecting host antibody response is not defined, and great variability has been reported among laboratories and commercial kits in evaluating patient specimens.[29] Low levels of antibody and specific IgM responses are not reliably detected by these assays. Early in the course of Lyme disease, antibody responses to the organism may not be detectable by standard assays. Less than 50% of patients with stage I Lyme disease have positive titers by currently available methods.[30] Thus, recognition of EM should prompt treatment regardless of the serologic status of the patient. Furthermore, early antibiotic therapy may abort the antibody response. Patients in this situation with persistent symptoms have been documented to have T-lymphocyte responses to *B. burgdorferi*.[31] False-positive results for Lyme serology have been reported in individuals with syphilis, Rocky Mountain spotted fever, other spirochetal infections (including oral treponemes), leptospirosis, autoimmune diseases, and (rarely) infectious mononucleosis.[32] In addition to false-positive results, patients may have asymptomatic *B. burgdorferi* infections.[33] If such patients have symptoms caused by another condition, these may be erroneously attributed to Lyme disease if serologic specimens are obtained.

The usefulness of serologic testing for Lyme disease is limited by the issues described, and therefore results need to be interpreted in the context of the clinical presentation of the patient. The incidence and prevalence in a given area also have a bearing on the interpretation of the results. For example, if the specificity is 98% (2% false positive) and the incidence of true disease is 25%, for every 1000 patients evaluated, 250 will have the disease and 20 will be falsely positive. Furthermore, the sensitivity and specificity of commercially available Lyme disease tests are much lower than this (26% to 57% sensitivity and 12% to 60% specificity in one review[12]), giving the tests a very poor predictive value. If the likelihood of disease is 0.1%, as is the case presently on Long Island, New York, then for every 1000 sera tested at random, there will be one true positive along with 20 false positives. Thus, for proper interpretation of results, it is crucial to reserve the test for patients with symptoms strongly suggestive of Lyme disease. Unfortunately, the vagueries of the clinical findings match the difficulties in interpreting the laboratory results.

Additional methods of detecting *B. burgdorferi* infection that are less readily available may offer assistance in difficult cases. Western blot detection of antibody responses to *B. burgdorferi* appears to offer more sensitive and specific results.[34] A national consensus panel has recommended uniform criteria for interpretation of such immunoblots and advises their use to confirm a positive or equivocal ELISA or IFA test.[35] These criteria require the presence of at least five of the 10 most frequent IgG bands after the first week's infection (18, 21, 28, 30, 39, 41, 45, 58, 66, and 93 kD). Early in the course of disease, two or more of the most common IgM bands (18, 21, 28, 37, 41, 45, 58, and 93 kD) are required to be interpreted as positive. An IgM blot is considered a valid assay only in the first 4 weeks of illness. Immunologic staining for the organism may be useful when pathologic specimens are available for study (e.g., synovial biopsy). Other methodologies, including polymerase chain reaction and antigen detection (instead of antibody) response to the organism, are under investigation as possible modalities for improving the diagnostic capabilities for Lyme disease.

Additional difficulties are encountered in the diagnosis of central nervous system (CNS) disease. Intrathecal production of antibody to *B. burgdorferi,* evaluated by comparing the CNS level of antibody with the serum level, may be useful in determining active CNS infection.[36]

DIFFERENTIAL DIAGNOSIS

The classic picture of EM should make the diagnosis of Lyme disease straightforward. If it is absent (as is frequently the case in adolescents), unrecognized, or atypical, the differential diagnosis will vary with the patient's presentation. With migratory arthralgias or arthritis, it may be necessary to differentiate Lyme disease from acute rheumatic fever. In Lyme disease there should be no evidence of antecedent streptococcal infection or the development of valvular heart disease. The arthritis of Lyme disease needs to be differentiated from rheumatoid arthritis, Reiter's syndrome, gonococcal arthritis, reactive or postinfectious arthritis, and psoriatic arthritis.[16] A particular problem noted in adolescents is the increasing number who present with vague symptoms of headache, musculoskeletal pain, and fatigue. Differentiating Lyme disease from chronic fatigue syndrome or an infectious mononucleosis syndrome in such patients can be extremely difficult. Typically, individuals with these complaints as part of Lyme disease have shown more objective findings of the disease.[7] In view of these observations and the poor predictive value of current available Lyme serology tests, caution should be used in obtaining and interpreting Lyme disease tests in patients with only nonspecific manifestations of the disease.

TREATMENT

Even before the cause of Lyme disease was known, antibiotic therapy with oral penicillin or tetracycline was shown to hasten the resolution of the EM rash and associated stage I symptoms.[37] Subsequent in vitro and clinical studies have confirmed the utility of these agents in the treatment of Lyme disease. Parenteral therapy with high-dose penicillin[38] or ceftriaxone[39] has proved useful in patients with arthritis or neurologic disease. Controversies still exist regarding the optimal therapeutic regimen and duration of treatment at various stages of the disease. A suggested treatment schedule is offered in Table 69-2. Patients with EM should be treated regardless of serologic status, since up to 50% of patients at this early stage of disease may not yet have detectable antibodies to the organism. Even with appropriate therapy, many patients have minor degrees of headache, musculoskeletal pain, and fatigue after treatment. Treatment failures have been reported at all stages of Lyme disease. Despite this observation, there are no data to suggest a benefit from prolonged treatment regimens with oral and/or intravenous antibiotic regimens beyond the durations listed in Table 69-2. Correlation of treatment response with age has not been reported.

PREVENTION

Prevention of Lyme disease depends on avoidance of potentially infectious ticks. This can be accomplished by wearing long pants, a long-sleeved shirt, and high socks and shoes if going into tick-infested areas. Insect repellants such as diethyltoluamide (DEET) for skin and permethrin for clothing also may be of value. Since tick attachment for at least 24 to 48 hours appears necessary for *B. burgdorferi* transmission, careful daily examination for ticks should be made when in an endemic area. If a tick is found, it should be removed carefully by pulling straight out with a forceps or gloved hand. Using a twisting motion or applying an agent to kill the tick prior to removal should be avoided, because these maneuvers may lead to injecting organisms into the involved skin.[40] At present, there is not sufficient evidence for recommending prophylactic antibiotic therapy following a tick bite.[41] A potential vaccine for prophylaxis of Lyme disease is in early clinical trials.[42]

TABLE 69-2
Treatment Recommendations for Lyme Disease

	Regimen
Stage I	Doxycycline,* 100 mg PO bid (or tetracycline,* 250 mg PO qid) *or* Amoxicillin, 500 mg PO bid *or* Cefuroxime axetil, 500 mg PO bid *or* Newer macrolide (clarithromycin, 500 mg bid; azithromycin, 500 mg PO day 1; 250 mg days 2-5) *Duration:* 10-30 days (except 5 days for azithromycin)†
Stage II	
A. Recurrent skin lesions	Ceftriaxone 2 g IV qd for 14-28 days (alternative penicillin G, 20 million units IV qd for 30 days)
Carditis with first-degree atrioventricular block (PR interval >0.3 sec)	Penicillin-allergic patient: doxycycline, 100 mg PO bid for 30 days
Isolated Bell's palsy (unilateral or bilateral)	Oral Rx as for stage I may be sufficient
B. Generalized neurologic disease	IV Rx as above
Stage III	IV Rx as above

*Individuals 8-10 years of age or older.
†Exact duration dictated by clinical response.

References

1. Steere AC, Malawista SE, Snydman DR, et al: Lyme arthritis: an epidemic of oligoarticular arthritis in children and adults in three Connecticut communities, *Arthritis Rheum* 10:7-17, 1977.
2. Steere AC, Grodnicki RL, Kornblatt AN, et al: The spirochetal etiology of Lyme disease, *N Engl J Med* 308:733-740, 1983.
3. Centers for Disease Control: Lyme disease—United States, 1995, *MMWR* 45:481-484, 1996.
4. Petersen LR, Sween AH, Checko PJ, et al: Epidemiological and clinical features of 1,149 persons with Lyme disease identified by laboratory-based surveillance in Connecticut, *Yale J Biol Med* 62:253-262, 1989.
5. Epidemiology Notes: Lyme disease, *Newsletter of the New York State Department of Health* 3(3):1-2, 1988.
6. Burgdorfer W, Barbour AG, Hayes SF, et al: Lyme disease—a tick-borne spirochetosis? *Science* 216:1317-1319, 1982.
7. Steere AC: Lyme disease, *N Engl J Med* 321:586-596, 1989.
8. Piesman J, Mather N, Sinsky RJ, Spielman A: Duration of tick attachment and *Borrelia burgdorferi* transmission, *J Clin Microbiol* 25:557-558, 1987.
9. Magnarelli LA, Anderson JF, Barbour AG: The etiology agents of Lyme disease in deer flies, horse flies and mosquitoes, *J Infect Dis* 154:355-358, 1986.
10. Luger SW: Lyme disease transmitted by a biting fly, *N Engl J Med* 322:1752, 1990.
11. Magnarelli LA, Anderson JF: Ticks and biting insects infected with the etiologic agent of Lyme disease, *Borrelia burgdorferi, J Clin Microbiol* 26:1482-1486, 1988.
12. Shapiro ED: Lyme disease in children, *Am J Med* 98(suppl 4A):69S-73S, 1995.
13. Reed AM, Pachman LM: Lyme disease in children and adolescents, *Compr Ther* 15:31-36, 1988.
14. Stechenberg BW: Lyme disease: the latest great imitator, *Pediatr Infect Dis J* 7:402-409, 1988.
15. Steere AC, Schoen RT, Taylor E: The clinical evolution of Lyme arthritis, *Ann Intern Med* 107:725-731, 1987.
16. Steere AC, Bartenhagen LH, Craft JE, et al: The early clinical manifestations of Lyme disease, *Ann Intern Med* 99:76-82, 1983.
17. Steere AC, Batsford WP, Weinberg M, et al: Lyme carditis: cardiac abnormalities of Lyme disease, *Ann Intern Med* 93:8-16, 1983.
18. Olson LJ, Okafor EC, Clements IP: Cardiac involvement in Lyme disease: manifestations and management, *Mayo Clin Proc* 61:745-749, 1986.
19. McAlister HF, Klementowicz PT, Andrews C, et al: Lyme carditis: an important cause of reversible heart block, *Ann Intern Med* 110:339-345, 1989.
20. Reik L, Steere AC, Bartenhagen NH, et al: Neurologic abnormalities of Lyme disease, *Medicine* 58:281-294, 1979.
21. Finkel MF: Lyme disease and its neurological complications, *Arch Neurol* 45:99-104, 1988.
22. Reik L Jr, Burgdorfer W, Donaldson JO: Neurologic abnormalities in Lyme disease without erythema chronicum migrans, *Am J Med* 81:73-78, 1986.
23. Rousseau JJ, Lust C, Zangerpe PF, Rigaignon G: Acute transverse myelitis as presenting neurological feature of Lyme disease, *Lancet* 2:1222-1223, 1986.
24. Sherman AB, Nelson S, Barclay P: Demyelinating neuropathy accompanying Lyme disease, *Neurology* 32:1302-1305, 1982.
25. Raucher HS, Kaufman DM, Goldfarb J, et al: Pseudotumor cerebri and Lyme disease: a new association, *J Pediatr* 107:931-933, 1985.
26. Steere AC, Dwyer E, Winchester R: Association of chronic Lyme arthritis with HLA-DR4 and HLA-DR2 alleles, *N Engl J Med* 323:219-223, 1990.

27. Broderick JP, Sandok BA, Mertz LE: Focal encephalitis in a young woman 6 years after the onset of Lyme disease: tertiary Lyme disease?, *Mayo Clin Proc* 62:313-316, 1987.

28. Wokke JHJ, Van Gijn J, Elderson A, Stanek G: Chronic forms of *Borrelia burgdorferi* infection of the nervous system, *Neurology* 37:1031-1034, 1987.

29. Hedberg CW, Osterholm MT, MacDonald KL, White KL: An interlaboratory study of antibody to *Borrelia burgdorferi, J Infect Dis* 155:1325-1327, 1987.

30. Shrestha M, Gradzicki RL, Steere AC: Diagnosing early Lyme disease, *Am J Med* 78:235-240, 1985.

31. Dattwyler RJ, Volkman DJ, Luft BJ, et al: Seronegative Lyme disease, *N Engl J Med* 319:1441-1446, 1988.

32. Duffy J, Mertz LE, Wobig GH, Katzmann JA: Diagnosing Lyme disease: the contribution of serologic testing, *Mayo Clin Proc* 63:1116-1121, 1988.

33. Steere AC, Taylor E, Wilson ML, Levine JF, Spielman A: Longitudinal assessment of the clinical and epidemiological features of Lyme disease in a defined population, *J Infect Dis* 154:295-300, 1986.

34. Dresser F, Whalen JA, Reinhardt BN, Steere AC: Western blotting in the serodiagnosis of Lyme disease, *Clin Infect Dis* 167:392-400, 1993.

35. Centers for Disease Control: Recommendations for test performance and interpretation from the second national conference on serologic diagnosis of Lyme disease, *MMWR* 44:590-591, 1995.

36. Halperin JJ, Luft BJ, Anand AK, et al: Lyme neuroborreliosis: central nervous system manifestations, *Neurology* 39:753-759, 1989.

37. Steere AC, Malawista SE, Newman JH, et al: Antibiotic therapy in Lyme disease, *Ann Intern Med* 93:1-8, 1980.

38. Steere AC, Pachner AR, Malawista SF: Neurologic abnormalities of Lyme disease: successful treatment with high-dose intravenous penicillin, *Ann Intern Med* 99:762-772, 1983.

39. Dattwyler RJ, Halperin JJ, Volkman DJ, Luft BJ: Treatment of late Lyme borreliosis—randomized comparison of ceftriaxone and penicillin, *Lancet* 1:1191-1194, 1988.

40. Needham GR: Evaluation of five popular methods of tick removal, *Pediatrics* 75:997-1002, 1985.

41. Costello CM, Steere AC, Pinkerton RE, Feder HM Jr: A prospective study of tick bites in an endemic area for Lyme disease, *J Infect Dis* 159:136-139, 1989.

42. Keller D, Koster FT, Marks DH, Hosbach P, Erdile LF, Mays JP: Safety and immunogenicity of a recombinant outer surface protein A Lyme vaccine, *JAMA* 271:1764-1768, 1994.

Suggested Readings

Burgdorfer W, Barbour AG, Hayes SF, et al: Lyme disease—tick-borne spirochetosis: *Science* 216:1317-1319, 1982.
> *Original paper describing the organism now known to be the causative agent of Lyme disease.*

Shapiro ED: Lyme disease in children, *Am J Med* 98(suppl 4A): 69S-73S, 1995.
> *Largest series in pediatric patients, including adolescents, with Lyme disease.*

Hedberg CW, Osterholm MT, MacDonald KL, White KL: An interlaboratory study of antibody to *Borrelia burgdorferi, J Infect Dis* 155:1325-1327, 1987.
> *Highlights some of the pitfalls in serodiagnosis of Lyme disease.*

Steere AC: Lyme disease, *N Engl J Med* 321:586-696, 1989.
> *Excellent review of all issues related to Lyme disease.*

Steere AC, Malawista SE, Snydman DR, et al: Lyme arthritis: an epidemic of oligoarticular arthritis in children and adults in three Connecticut communities, *Arthritis Rheum* 10:7-17, 1977.
> *Classic article describing investigation in Lyme, Connecticut, leading to unraveling of the mystery of this disease.*

CHAPTER 70

Toxic Shock Syndrome

•

Elizabeth Rose

Toxic shock syndrome is a systemic illness characterized by high fever, hypotension, rash, and desquamation. It was first described by Todd et al in 1978.[1] It gained widespread notoriety in the scientific and medical community as well as the lay press and public in 1980 when many healthy menstruating adolescent females who used tampons became very ill and several died. The syndrome is caused by absorption of an enterotoxin produced by a noninvasive phage group I *Staphylococcus aureus* that may be cultured from a variety of body sites.[2]

In several studies, a particular toxin, TSST-1 (toxic shock syndrome toxin 1), alone or with other toxins, was isolated in more than 90% of patients diagnosed with toxic shock.[3,4]

Although most commonly seen in menstruating females who use tampons, toxic shock syndrome has been associated with many other medical and surgical nonmenstrual conditions and circumstances, including the postpartum period, use of contraceptive sponges and diaphragms, wounds, osteomyelitis, orthopedic procedures, sinusitis and nasal packings, burns, influenza, pneumonia, and cellulitis.

EPIDEMIOLOGY

The overall U.S. incidence of toxic shock syndrome is low at 0.53 per 100,000. There have been only about 2600 reported cases in the United States and fewer than 1000 reported cases in Britain. Cases have also been reported in other European countries, Japan, Australia, New Zealand, Israel, Canada, and South Africa.

It is important for epidemiologic purposes to divide the disease into two clinical entities: menstrual toxic shock and nonmenstrual toxic shock. The latter affects men and women equally, with age ranges from newborn to elderly with a mean of approximately 30. The mortality rate is slightly higher than that of menstrual toxic shock syndrome at 9% to 12%, particularly in cases associated with pneumonia and burns and isolation of enterotoxin B. Menstrual toxic shock has been shown to have an increased incidence of 1.52 per 100,000 in 15- to 19-year-old females that is out of proportion to the number of teenagers using tampons.[5,6] In addition, there is a higher incidence in whites than in nonwhites that is not in proportion to the racial distribution of the U.S. population. The mortality rate in menstrual toxic shock varies between 2% and 4%.

Several theories have been advanced to explain the increased incidence of toxic shock syndromes in certain populations. These include lack of antibodies to specific toxins, perhaps caused by some mild immune deficiency; nonhygienic tampon use; overuse of superabsorbent tampons; and use of nonintroducer tampons.

A study in Northern California revealed that the incidence of the disease in 15- to 44-year-old women began increasing in about 1977 when tampon formulations began to change to make them more absorbent.[7] In 1980 one particular brand that had been associated with toxic shock syndrome was removed from the market, with a reduction of incidence that was also not statistically significant. In 1985, tampons containing polyacrylate rayon (a superabsorbent material) were removed from the market, and another reduction in incidence was noted that was also not statistically significant.

CLINICAL PRESENTATION, DIAGNOSTIC CRITERIA, AND DIFFERENTIAL DIAGNOSIS

A previously well patient classically presents with headaches, high fever, malaise, vomiting, diarrhea, myalgia, rash, abdominal pain, and/or syncope. Typically, menses will have begun up to 5 days before the onset of illness.

Physical examination reveals a high fever, tachycardia, and tachypnea with orthostatic hypotension. There is also likely to be a widespread symmetric blanching macular rash, a strawberry tongue, abdominal tenderness, and tenderness of the extremities. A pelvic examination may reveal tender external genitalia, erythematous vaginal mucosa, and a malodorous cervical discharge.

No single laboratory test is diagnostic for toxic shock syndrome. Consistent hematologic findings might include an elevated white blood cell count with a left shift, thrombocytopenia, a mild normochromic normocytic anemia, and possibly elevated prothrombin time and partial thromboplastin time. Chemistries may reveal hypocalcemia, elevated blood urea nitrogen and creatinine, elevated transaminases, and bilirubin. Typically blood, urine, and cerebrospinal fluid cultures are all negative. Vaginal, cervical, or wound cultures grow *S. aureus*. In 1982 the Centers for Disease Control published a strict case definition of toxic shock syndrome to provide unified criteria for subsequent studies (See Box 70-1).[8] The differential diagnosis includes Kawasaki's disease, scarlet fever, staphylococcal scalded skin syndrome, Stevens-Johnson syndrome, bacteremia with shock, meningococcemia, acute rheumatic fever, Rocky Mountain spotted fever, measles, leptospirosis, and Reye's syndrome.

TREATMENT

The most important aspect of treatment involves rapid fluid replacement to correct hypotension with the utilization of large volumes of colloid or crystalloid. Most patients need intravenous calcium chloride as part of their fluid replacement to correct hypocalcemia. Patients who do not respond to fluid replacement may need vasopressors.

If a tampon is in place, it should be removed, as should infected packs and sutures, to eliminate the source of preformed toxin. Wounds, abrasions, and surgical sites should be irrigated. To prevent additional toxin from being produced, a staph-sensitive, beta-lactamase-resistant antibiotic should be administered.

The remainder of possible treatments depend on the course of the individual patient. Patients who develop renal failure may need dialysis; those who develop adult

---

BOX 70-1
Diagnostic Criteria for Toxic Shock Syndrome

MAJOR CRITERIA (ALL FOUR MUST BE PRESENT)
Temperature ≥38.5° C for <14 days
Diffuse macular erythroderma (without discrete lesions)
Convalescent desquamation
Hypotension (any one)
   Systolic or diastolic blood pressure less than fifth percentile for age.
   Orthostatic hypotension
      Syncope
      ≥30 mm Hg fall in systolic blood pressure
      ≥20 mm Hg fall in diastolic blood pressure

MINOR CRITERIA (AT LEAST THREE MUST BE PRESENT)
Mucous membrane hyperemia (any one)
   Conjunctival
   Pharyngeal
   Strawberry tongue
Cardiopulmonary (any one)
   Diffuse pulmonary infiltrates on chest radiograph
   Cardiothoracic ratio >50% on chest radiograph
   Gallop rhythm (two listeners)
   Cardiac index >2.2 L/min/m²
   Arterial oxygen tension <75% normal with arterial carbon dioxide tension <40
Renal (any one)
   Serum
      Blood urea nitrogen ≥1.5 upper limit of normal for age

Creatinine ≥1.5 upper limit of normal for age
Urinalysis (in absence of urinary tract infection)
   ≥5 white blood cells/high-power field
   ≥1 red blood cells/high-power field
   ≥2+ protein
Hematologic (any one)
   Platelets <100,000/mm³
   Neutrophils >10,000/mm³
   Nonsegmented neutrophils >1000/mm³
Hepatic (any one)
   Total bilirubin >1.5 upper limit of normal for age
   Serum transaminase >1.5 upper limit of normal for age
Gastrointestinal: history or observation of water-loss stools or vomiting
Central nervous system: change in level of consciousness not associated with fever or hypotension

EXCLUSIONARY CRITERIA (MUST BE NEGATIVE IF OBTAINED)
Blood culture not growing pathogen other than *Staphylococcus aureus*
Viral cultures negative
Serologic titers negative (e.g., group A streptococcus *Leptospira* rickettsia)
Absence of other definitive diagnosis (e.g., drug reaction, autoimmune disorder)

---

respiratory distress syndrome may require ventilatory assistance; and those who develop disseminated intravascular coagulapathy may need fresh frozen plasma and other blood products.

There is evidence, albeit not conclusive, that steroid treatment may decrease the number of days that patients are hemodynamically unstable.[9] For this stabilization to be effective, the steroids must be given within 48 hours of the onset of the illness. There is no evidence, however, that intravenous steroids will change the ultimate mortality rate of the illness.

PREVENTION

There is up to a 28% risk of recurrence in patients who have had toxic shock syndrome, and this risk is highest in the first or second month after the initial illness. One method of prevention of recurrence is proper antistaphylococcal antibiotics during the initial illness and cessation of tampon use during the four to six subsequent periods.

Other methods of preventing toxic shock syndrome include proper education on menstrual hygiene to include all prepubertal girls. Such education should not forbid tampons but rather instruct young females to use less absorbent tampons whenever possible and to change them frequently.

References

1. Todd J, Fishaut M, Kapral F: Toxic shock syndrome associated with phage group I staphylococci, *Lancet* 2:1116-1118, 1978.
2. Davis JP, Chesney PJ, Wand PJ, et al: Toxic shock syndrome: epidemiologic features, recurrence, risk factors, and prevention, *N Engl J Med* 303:1429-1435, 1980.
3. Crass BA, Borgdoll MS: Toxin involvement in toxic shock syndrome, *J Infect Dis* 153(3):918-926, 1986.
4. Marples RR, Weneke AA: Enterotoxins and toxic shock syndrome toxin-1 in nonenteric staphylococcal disease, *Epidemiol Infect* 110:477-488, 1993.
5. Markowitz LE, Hightower AW, Broome CV, et al: Toxic shock syndrome: evaluation of a National Surveillance Data using a hospital discharge survey, *JAMA* 258:75-78, 1987.

6. Gaventa S, Reingold AL, et al: Active surveillance for toxic shock syndrome in the United States, 1986, *Rev Infect Dis* II:528-534, 1989.

7. Petitti DB, Reingold AL: Recent trends in the incidence of toxic shock syndrome in northern culture, *Am J Public Health* 8:1209-1211, 1991.

8. Reingold AL, Hargrett NT, Shands KN, et al: Toxic shock syndrome surveillance in the United States, 1980-1981, *Ann Intern Med* 96:875-880, 1982.

9. Todd JK, Ressman M, et al: Corticosteroid therapy for patients with toxic shock syndrome, *JAMA* 252:24, 1984.

CHAPTER 71

Parasitic Infections

•

Murray Wittner

Parasitic infections are encountered in all age groups from the newborn to the geriatric. However, in this chapter only those parasitic diseases particularly pertinent to, although not exclusive of, adolescence are considered. Therefore, and perhaps arbitrarily, protozoan infections such as toxoplasmosis, giardiasis, cryptosporidiosis, and dientamoebiasis and helminthic infections such as ocular toxocariasis, enterobiasis, and cysticercosis will be emphasized.

Although parasitic infections are frequently associated with eosinophilia, there is a wide range of nonparasitic causes of this condition such as allergy, skin disorders, collagen vascular diseases, gastrointestinal disease, and neoplastic and hereditary disorders. Nevertheless, most clinicians relate eosinophilia to parasitic infections.

Eosinophils usually represent 3% to 6% of the peripheral granulocyte population. It is important, however, to determine the absolute eosinophil count when evaluating what appears to be an increase in circulating eosinophils, since the relative or percentage increase in eosinophils can lead to erroneous conclusions. Thus, an individual with a 9% eosinophilia and a total white cell count of less than 4000/mm^3 would not have eosinphilia, since there are usually 350 to 400 eosinophils/mm^3 in the peripheral circulation. Furthermore, it is important to recognize that the number of eosinphils are influenced by many patient factors such as circulating levels of corticosteroids, epinepherine, and estrogens; and that eosinophil counts tend to peak around midnight and are at their nadir at noon. In addition, the degree of eosinophilia can fluctuate widely from day to day.

The eosinophilia associated with various allergies such as hay fever, asthma, and eczema is generally mild, whereas high levels may be seen as a result of a drug reaction and especially in aspirin-sensitive asthma. In general, protozoan infections such as malaria, amebiasis, and giardiasis are not associated with eosinophilia, although exceptions have been reported, notably in toxoplasmosis, isosporiasis, and dientamebiasis.

Undoubtedly, helminthic infections are the most important causes of parasite-related eosinophilia. It is likely that the extent of tissue invasion is associated with the level of eosinophila. Thus, worms that inhabit the bowel lumen usually provoke little or no eosinophilia (ascaris and various tapeworms), whereas larvae migrating in tissue such as hookworm and ascaris, filaria, schistosomula, and trichinella stimulate very high eosinophilia as related to their invasion of host tissues.

TOXOPLASMOSIS

Toxoplasmosis is an infection of birds, humans, and other mammals with the protozoan *Toxoplasma gondii,* an obligate intracellular parasite.

Etiology

Toxoplasma are coccidian parasites whose definitive hosts are cats and other felines. In nonfelines, *Toxoplasma* exhibits two extraintestinal forms: the trophozoite or proliferative form (tachyzoite) and the tissue cyst (bradyzoite). A third form, the oocyst, is found only in felines in which an enteroepithelial cycle takes place and is passed in the feces in an immature noninfective stage. Depending on temperature, oocysts become infective in 1 to 5 days. Nonfeline mammals and birds ingest infective oocysts, with resultant widespread infection of host tissues by intracellular reproduction of trophozoites (tachyzoites); eventually, transition to bradyzoites occurs in which the organisms accumulate in tissue cysts. The latter may be present for years or for the life of the host. After human ingestion of tissue cysts in rare or uncooked meat, bradyzoites are released and transform to tachyzoites; they reside briefly in the intestinal epithelium before they disseminate throughout the body and reproduce in many cell types. Thus, infection can be acquired by ingesting infective oocysts from the soil or cat litter, by ingesting tissue cysts in rare or raw meat, or by congenital transmission during acute infection during pregnancy.

The *T. gondii* trophozoite in peritoneal exudate or tissue culture is crescentic, measuring 4 to 7 μm by 2 to 4 μm. Masses of organisms seen within parasitophorous vacuoles of host cells superficially resemble *Leishmania* or *Histoplasma* organisms. The organisms multiply rapidly and may so distend the cell that it bursts. The released trophozoites can then invade other cells, or be phagocytosed and subsequently destroyed. The intracellular proliferative forms can be found in almost every type of tissue cell.

Tissue cysts vary in size and contain from a few to thousands of organisms. They are frequently found in the brain, heart, and skeletal muscle. *Toxoplasma* can be transmitted experimentally by feeding tissue cysts or oocysts to numerous mammals and birds, and large numbers of naturally infected animals have been found, including dogs, rodents, chickens, pigeons, and ducks.

Epidemiology

Congenital or transplacental transmission of toxoplasmosis generally takes place only if the primary infection occurs during pregnancy. Nevertheless, evidence suggests that the disease is transmitted to the offspring in fewer than half the instances of maternal toxoplasmosis acquired during pregnancy and that, when transmitted, the infection is often subclinical. The severity of fetal disease is associated with the trimester when maternal infection occurs; thus, maternal toxoplasmosis acquired in the first trimester is associated with more severe fetal disease but with fewer instances of fetal acquisition, whereas maternal infection acquired late in pregnancy is associated with mild to inapparent disease but more frequent transmission to the offspring. The suggestion that toxoplasmosis gives rise to habitual abortion is not settled. Transmission of postnatal or acquired toxoplasmosis to humans by carnivorism has been established by several observations, most notably in France, where raw or rare meat is traditionally eaten, and in the United States, when a group of Cornell University medical students acquired the infection after eating rare hamburger. Inadequately cooked meats (e.g.,

lamb, beef, pork) frequently contain the infective tissue cysts. There have been recent reports of *Toxoplasma* transmitted to immunosuppressed hosts after organ transplantation or whole blood or leukocyte transfusion. Individuals with acquired immunodeficiency syndrome (AIDS) frequently develop severe toxoplasmosis. The disease usually involves the central nervous system (CNS) and is often fatal. Experimental studies have shown that *Toxoplasma* could be transmitted in milk; however, transmission during breast feeding in humans has not been confirmed.

The incidence of infection increases with age, but the rate of increase differs, depending on the population, its eating habits, and the locality studied. Areas in which moisture and warmth favor viability of *Toxoplasma* oocysts demonstrate the highest prevalence of *Toxoplasma* antibodies. In the United States, the yearly antibody acquisition rate is 0.5% to 1%; the rate for children is lower than for adults. The U.S. prevalence rates are similar for males and females, and there seems to be greater prevalence in regions at lower altitudes. The prevalence of positive *Toxoplasma* titers ($\geq 1:32$) in women of childbearing age for various areas of the United States has been reported to be 38%. The incidence of congenital toxoplasmosis has been estimated conservatively to be about 1.3 per 1000 live births in New York City and Birmingham, Alabama.

Pathology

Pathologic lesions may affect multiple organs and tissues. In congenital toxoplasmosis the CNS is always affected, and neurologic and ocular lesions are generally more common than in acquired disease. In congenital toxoplasmosis, focal disseminated areas of necrosis and miliary granulomatous inflammation are found, especially in the periventricular and periaqueductal tissues. Many yellow soft areas are seen in the cortex, basal ganglia, medulla, and leptomeninges. Calcification, microcephalus, and hydrocephalus are common sequelae. *Toxoplasma* cysts may persist for years without provoking cellular reaction. Pulmonary involvement usually consists of parasitized alveolar cells in areas of interstitial pneumonia. Proliferation of organisms in the myocardium, hepatic parenchyma, spleen, and adrenal glands is commonly associated with focal necrosis.

The lymphadenitis of acute acquired toxoplasmosis is morphologically distinct, showing reactive follicular hyperplasia with focal necrosis and karyorrhexis. The principal inflammatory ocular lesions are in the retina and choroid, although secondary changes involve the iris and lens. The exudative process heals by fibrosis, and the degree of impairment depends on the location and extent of involvement. Free organisms or cysts are often found in retinal lesions.

Clinical Manifestations

Serologic evidence strongly suggests that most human and animal infections are asymptomatic. Acute maternal infection acquired immediately before or during pregnancy may cause fetal infection. The disease may be immediately apparent at birth, presenting as a mild to severe neonatal infection that may be fatal, or may have a delayed onset of varied severity sometime during the first month of life. The onset of symptoms may be later in life, often presenting as chorioretinitis (Plate 1) or a seizure disorder; more likely, however, congenital toxoplasmosis may be an inapparent infection of little consequence. The factors that determine this spectrum are only partially known but are believed to be related to host immunity, the virulence of the infecting strain, and the size of the inoculum.

The implications of clinically inapparent neonatal infections have only recently come under careful study. In a few patients the disease was progressive with marked developmental retardation, but in most only subtle abnormalities of CNS function, such as significantly lower IQ and retarded development of gross and/or fine motor functions, were noted. Inapparent congenital toxoplasmosis may ultimately present later in life as chorioretinitis. Furthermore, most studies suggest that most *Toxoplasma* chorioretinitis infections are the result of congenital infection and that only a very small number are attributable to acquired disease.

Acquired toxoplasmosis is usually asymptomatic, although the acute acquired form can be a fulminating disease with an erythematous rash, fever, malaise, myositis, dyspnea, acute myocarditis, and encephalitis. The outcome can be fatal, but this form of toxoplasmosis is rare. The most common clinical presentation of acquired infection is a relatively asymptomatic localized lymphadenopathy syndrome. The lymphadenitis may wax and wane for months and finally resolve spontaneously. Lymphadenopathy associated with an infectious mononucleosis–like picture is common. These patients often exhibit malaise, fever, and localized to generalized lymphadenopathy. Circulating atypical lymphocytes may be seen. Cervical nodes are frequently involved, although lymphadenopathy can be generalized. Within several weeks to months, spontaneous resolution is to be expected, although in a minority of patients the symptoms may continue for an inordinate period and prompt therapeutic intervention. Undoubtedly, chorioretinitis can result from acquired disease, but it is usually the result of congenital infection.

In the immunocompromised host, toxoplasmosis can sometimes be fulminant or even fatal. This is presumably the result of reactivation of a latent tissue infection. Encephalitis is reported in the vast majority and is an important complication in AIDS patients.

Diagnosis

Toxoplasmosis can be extremely difficult to diagnose, especially in neonates. Examining the cerebrospinal fluid (CSF) or, better yet, the ventricular fluid in newborns can be suggestive if there is a marked rise in CSF protein and a pleocytosis. Eosinophilia has been described in neonatal disease.

The IgM fluorescent antibody test (IgM-IFA) measures the early rise of IgM, presumably during the acute stage of infection, and precedes the appearance of IgG antibodies. In the neonate, IgM antibodies suggest infant origin and therefore infection, because these antibodies do not cross the placenta as do IgG antibodies. In acquired infection, a simple positive IFA or enzyme-linked immunosorbent assay (ELISA) titer signifies only that the patient has the infection, not whether it is active or latent. Therefore, rising titers in serum taken 3 weeks apart and tested together or seroconversion should be obtained before concluding that a patient has acute disease. Inasmuch as titers might have stabilized before the first serum sample was obtained, the IgM-IFA or IgM-ELISA test should also be performed. Currently, any patient with an IFA of 1:1000 or more and a positive IgM-IFA or IgM-ELISA titer must be presumed to have active toxoplasmosis until it is proved otherwise. Thus, because very high titers may persist for a year or more, only the findings of a single high IgM or rising titers in other tests establish the diagnosis of acute infection.

In a recent study of congenital toxoplasmosis, the diagnosis was established using several criteria such as the presence of *Toxoplasma*-specific IgM in neonatal serum and/or CSF, or the presence of *Toxoplasma*-specific IgM and/or an acute pattern in the differential aggluttination test in maternal serum. Several studies have shown that *Toxoplasma*-specific IgA and IgE can be found in the serum of congenitally infected infants as well as in children with retinochoroiditis. Detection of IgM and IgA in fetal blood obtained by chordocentesis is currently being performed at specialized centers. The polymerase chain reaction (PCR), using primers to detect the multiple copy gene B1, including amniocentesis and chorionic villus biopsy, has been used to detect *Toxoplasma* DNA in a variety of body fluids and tissues.

The diagnosis of *Toxoplasma* chorioretinitis is often difficult to establish by serologic methods. Antibody titers are often low (1:2 or 1:8) even during clinically active disease, and one must presume that the patient has toxoplasmosis if the clinical picture is consistent. A more specific procedure for diagnosing ocular toxoplasmosis is direct serologic testing of aqueous humor.

Diagnosis of toxoplasmosis in patients with AIDS is problematic, as AIDS patients with active *Toxoplasma* encephalitis may have low antibody titers. Computed tomography (CT) is useful, but fungal or mycobacterial infections as well as intracerebral lymphomas or progressive multifocal leukoencephalopathy must also be considered. Brain biopsy performed with immunoperoxidase staining is often the only way to arrive at a definitive diagnosis; however, sampling errors occur with this technique. Presumptive therapy is given if the serologic results are positive and the CT scan suggestive but biopsy cannot be obtained. A therapeutic trial may also be justified in the presence of CNS symptoms even with a normal CT scan.

Treatment

Chemotherapy is based on the experimental evidence that pyrimethamine (Daraprim) and sulfonamide have marked synergistic activity against *Toxoplasma* organisms. The evaluation of therapy in infants and adults has been difficult, however, because few controlled studies have been done and the outcome of untreated infection is highly variable. Moreover, because congenital toxoplasmosis is associated with such severe long-term morbidity as well as mortality, few clinicians are willing to withhold therapy for diagnosed disease. Therapy probably does not entirely eliminate infection. Tissue cysts, especially in the CNS, may be sufficiently sequestered to be unaffected by chemotherapy. A recent study on the early therapeutic intervention for congenital toxoplasmosis in infants and children clearly demonstrated that most children with severe CNS involvement at birth developed normally, whereas delay in diagnosis and therapy was associated with irreversible damage.

Pyrimethamine and sulfonamides remain the mainstay of therapy for congenital and acquired toxoplasmosis. Treatment is recommended in the following circumstances: (1) infants with clinical or subclinical infection, (2) healthy newborns in whom the disease has not been established but whose mothers definitely acquired the infection during pregnancy, (3) healthy newborns of mothers with high antibody titers but with unknown date of infection, (4) active ocular infection, (5) reactivation of toxoplasmosis in the immunosuppressed host, and (6) clinically persistent active acquired infection. Treatment should be provided for 1 year. Adults receive an initial loading dose of 75 mg pyrimethamine once then 25 mg/day for 3 to 4 weeks. Pyrimethamine, a potent folic acid antagonist, may cause reversible bone marrow depression, thrombocytopenia, leukopenia, and anemia. Therefore, peripheral blood cell and platelet determinations should be made several times a week during therapy. Folinic acid, 10 to 25 mg/day, is usually given to prevent bone marrow suppression.

Several studies indicate that treatment of acquired infections during pregnancy significantly diminishes the incidence and severity of congenital infection. Of some concern, however, is the known teratogenicity of pyrimethamine in rodents.

Spiramycin, a macrolide only available from the manufacturer in the United States, seems to reduce the number of congenital infections, and toxicity does not seem to be a problem with this antibiotic. It is given orally, 50 mg/kg twice a day for 30 to 45 days. Once it has been established that fetal transmission has occurred, and in view of the seriousness of congenital disease, it is reasonable to use pyrimethamine and sulfadiazine together with folinic acid in the second and third trimesters when organogenesis has been completed. Spiramycin apparently can be used as soon as the diagnosis is established. Clindamycin has been reported to be effective in treating ocular as well as systemic toxoplasmosis. Its role in the therapy for this disease remains to be evaluated.

Therapy is usually unnecessary for individuals with *Toxoplasma* lymphadenopathy because it is usually short-lived and self-limited. Occasionally, however, an individual may have persistent and debilitating symptoms; some authors advocate therapy with a course of pyrimethamine and sulfadiazine as described above.

Treatment of AIDS patients for CNS toxoplasmosis is often complicated by allergies to sulfonamide or leukopenia caused by pyrimethamine. Both of these complications are more common in AIDS patients because there is no clear end point to therapy. In sulfonamide-intolerant patients, pyrimethamine alone at doses of 75 to 100 mg daily together with folinic acid has been used. Some authorities add clindamycin to the regimen. No clear prophylactic regimen to prevent toxoplasmosis in AIDS patients has been established. However, to prevent relapse subsequent to primary therapy, all AIDS patients should receive life-long secondary prophylaxis. Various regimens have been suggested.

Daily prophylaxis with pyrimethamine and sulfadiazine with folinic acid is associated with the lowest relapse rate. Recent studies have shown that in patients maintained on high-dose pyrimethamine alone the relapse rates were very low.

Prognosis

Congenital toxoplasmosis may have short- and long-term prognostic implications. In severely affected infants the outcome may be disastrous. The outcome in children with inapparent infection is uncertain. The possibility of mental and developmental retardation is just beginning to be appreciated. Chorioretinitis in later life is an important long-term complication. The risk of ocular disease appears to increase with age, at least during early life. Reactivation during immunosuppressive therapy in later life is also an ever-present hazard. Rehabilitation of handicapped children may improve the prognosis. Importantly, as described above, early diagnosis and treatment dramatically improves the clinical outcome.

Prevention

Several simple measures may prevent toxoplasmosis. Ingestion of raw and rare meats should be avoided; infected meat or eggs can be made safe by thoroughly heating to at least 60°C. Individuals who handle raw meat should wash their hands carefully. It has been shown that smoking, curing in brine, and freezing at −40°C for 9 days will kill the bradyzoites in pork; a typical home freezer is not a certain method of killing the cysts, however.

Because cats, an important source of oocysts, defecate in loose soil and sand, children must be protected from these sites. Cat litter should not be handled by vulnerable pregnant women unless they wear disposable gloves. Young domestic cats that are fed raw meat that is often contaminated may be an important source of human infection. The handling of this raw meat by pet owners has been suggested as a more important source of infection than oocyst discharge by cats. Household cats that are not permitted to roam and are fed only dry, canned, or cooked food have little opportunity to become infected. Nevertheless, their feces should be discarded every day before the oocysts have had a chance to sporulate (1 to 5 days) and become infective. Cat feces should be buried or flushed down a toilet.

GIARDIA LAMBLIA

Giardia lamblia is a flagellated protozoan that is a major cause of parasitic diarrhea worldwide and is said to infect approximately 4% of the U.S. population. Between 1972 and 1982, 60 separate outbreaks affecting over 20,000 people were reported. Transmission usually occurs by drinking contaminated water, but food-borne and person-to-person transmission are now documented with increasing frequency.

Giardiasis may afflict anyone but is more frequent among certain groups such as campers, tourists, skiers, gay men, residents of institutions such as homes and hospitals for the retarded, day care centers, patients with immunodeficiencies (e.g., dysgammaglobulinemia, low serum IgA, and low mucosal IgA), and those with a decreased or absent gastric acidity. From 20% to 50% of children under the age of 3 years in day care centers and 20% of gay men may be asymptomatic cyst passers.

Clinical Disease

Clinical symptoms usually begin 9 to 14 days after ingestion of cysts and consist of flatulence, abdominal pain, tenderness to palpation, midepigastric distress, watery diarrhea, and weight loss. Fever and bloody stools are not associated with this infection and should raise the possibility of another diagnosis. A chronic infection with persistent, soft, grumatous stools is often seen. This may be associated with lactose intolerance and flatulence, which may or may not resolve promptly with appropriate therapy.

The presence of the parasite in the small intestine can be associated with a variety of histologic changes ranging from normal to minimal cellular infiltrates in the lamina propria, reduction in the height and number of villi, loss of the brush borders, cell damage, and an increase in epithelial cell mitosis. Malabsorption occurs to some degree in over 50% of patients with giardiasis. The most frequently malabsorbed materials include fats, lactose, vitamin B_{12}, and D-xylose.

Diagnosis

Diagnosis of a *Giardia* infection is usually made by stool examination. It has been reported that by means of direct smears and formalin-ether concentration, 76% of infected persons were detected with the first specimen, 90% with two specimens, and 97.6% with three. Trophozoites (Plate 2) can be found in diarrheic stools, while cysts are encountered in formed or semiformed stools. A concentration technique should be employed to enhance the chances of finding the cysts. Trophozoites must be found on direct examination, however, as they do not survive concentration techniques. It seems reasonable to conclude that if the parasite cannot be found after four or five stool examinations, alternative diagnostic techniques may be needed. The use of a weighted duodenal gelatin capsule containing 140 cm of 3-ply nylon string (Enterotest) or duodenal aspiration also may be effective in recovering the organism. Purgatives have not proved useful in increasing the number of positive stools.

Immunity, both humoral and cellular, is thought to play an important role in host defenses against this parasite. In this regard, a number of reports have documented specific anti-*Giardia* IgG antibodies in symptomatic patients using the indirect fluorescent antibody (IFA) and enzyme-linked immunoabsorbent assay (ELISA) techniques, utilizing whole trophozoites as antigens. ELISA and monoclonal antibody antigen detection techniques are available to enhance the detection of *Giardia* in the stool and may be used as valuable adjuncts in the diagnosis of giardiasis.

Treatment

Therapy for giardiasis should be provided for all individuals, including asymptomatic cyst passers. Metronidazole, 250 mg three times a day for 5 days, is usually effective for this infection. Furazolidone is less effective than metronidazole but is available as a suspension for young children.

CRYPTOSPORIDIOSIS

Cryptosporidiosis is now acknowledged as an important cause of diarrhea in man. Recognition of its ubiquitous and nearly worldwide presence began to emerge contemporaneously with the AIDS epidemic, as almost all individuals infected with *Cryptosporidium* also had AIDS. Currently, it is evident that *Cryptosporidium* infects gastrointestinal tract, biliary tract, and respiratory epithelium in man and other animals, causing self-limited diarrhea in the immunocompetent and severe and sometimes fatal diarrhea in the immunocompromised.

The mature oocysts of *C. parvum* are infectious when passed in the feces and are about 4 to 5 μm in diameter. In humans, when ingested with contaminated water or food, oocysts sporulate and the escaped sporozoites invade enterocytes. The organism resides in a parasitophorous vacuole close to the microvillous border of the host cell where the developmental cycle takes place. In man the prepatent period has been reported to be 5 to 21 days; oocyst shedding may extend for many weeks and occasionally for months. Since oocysts are fully infectious when shed, hospitalized patients with cryptosporidiosis should be isolated and stool precautions strictly observed.

Epidemiology

Fully sporulated oocysts resist adverse environmental conditions and can survive for long periods if stored moist and cold. The usual water purification procedures (chlorination and ozonation) are ineffective in sterilizing *Cryptosporidium* oocysts, and oocysts are 30 times more resistant to ozone and 14 times more resistant to chlorine than cysts of *Giardia*.

As in giardiasis, waterborne transmission of cryptosporidiosis has been well documented as an important route of infection in the United States and United Kingdom. Runoff of waste and surface water into the local water supply has been suggested as an important source of this contamination in the massive Milwaukee, Wisconsin, outbreak. It is now believed that person-to-person spread occurs much more frequently than was previously acknowledged. This has been especially evident in the many day-care–center and nosocomial outbreaks. Zoonotic reservoirs of transmission of *Cryptosporidium* such as farm animals (calves), rodents, puppies, and kittens are no longer thought to be as important. Interestingly, *Cryptosporidium* is now being recognized as one of the many causes of traveler's diarrhea.

Clinical Disease

Cryptosporidiosis, whether in immunocompetent or immunocompromised patients, is characterized by profuse, almost cholera-like watery diarrhea. It is unusual to find red or white cells in the stools, although mucus may be present occasionally. Cramping abdominal pain, nausea, and vomiting may sometimes be present, and low-grade fever (<39°C) occasionally is seen. Peripheral eosinophilia or leukocytosis is not characteristic. Intestinal malabsorption and lactose intolerance is frequently present, especially in AIDS patients, who become so markedly wasted and unable to feed that they may need total parenteral nutrition (TPN).

Generally, immunocompetent patients have a self-limited infection that usually lasts from several days to 2 weeks, although occasionally it persists for 3 to 5 weeks. In these patients, and especially in malnourished children, oral and parenteral dehydration therapy may become necessary; in immunocompromised patients, diarrhea can be relentless and profuse with fluid loss of up to 17 L/day. The severity and extent of the symptoms appear to depend on the level of immunodepression. It has been reported that in malnourished children the diarrheal episode can be significantly prolonged.

Biliary tract disease due to direct invasion of the common bile duct is not uncommon in AIDS patients. The presenting symptoms are similar to non–HIV-1–infected persons and include right upper quadrant pain, fever, vomiting, and a cholestatic biochemical profile as well as jaundice. Acalculous cholecystitis and cholangitis can be a secondary disorder concomitant with *C. parvum* infection. The wall of the gallbladder and common duct may be thickened, and when papillary stenosis occurs, dilation may be seen distally.

Cryptosporidium has been found in the sputum, in bronchoalveolar lavage fluid within alveolar macrophages, and in the bronchial epithelium. Most patients have been severely immunodepressed children with other pulmonary infections. It is unclear whether *Cryptosporidium* is an important cause of respiratory tract disease in these patients.

Diagnosis

Many techniques have been advocated for the diagnosis of *Cryptosporidium* infection. Concentration methods are usually employed to detect small numbers of oocysts. Stools are usually submitted in sodium acetate–acetic acid–formalin (SAF), and formalin-ether is used for concentration. A modified acid-fast stain is then used to visualize the oocysts (Plate 3). Currently, a mixed monoclonal immunofluorescence method is used to detect small numbers of oocysts. When biliary tract infection is suspected and oocysts cannot be found in the stool, endoscopic retrograde cholangiography (ERCP) may be especially helpful in obtaining bile as well as tissue for diagnosis. *Cryptosporidium* must be differentiated from cyclospora (see next section).

Treatment

Immunocompetent individuals with cryptosporidial diarrhea may receive oral or intravenous hydration. They may frequently respond to nonspecific antidiarrheal agents such as loperamide (Imodium), diphenoxylate (Lomotil), tincture of camphorated opium, or bismuth subsalicylate (Pepto-Bismol). Generally, symptoms abate within a few days to weeks with full recovery.

Unfortunately, the treatment of cryptosporidiosis in immunodepressed patients can be an extremely vexing problem that responds to few treatment modalities. Sometimes the diarrhea can be moderated with nonspecific antidiarrheal agents, but often it cannot. In patients in whom diarrhea has been relentless and of large volume and who have not responded to any other therapy, the somatostatin-like agent octreotide has been used with some success, but the response has been unpredictable.

The development of specific therapy has been hampered by the lack of suitable in vitro and in vivo models in which to test candidate compounds. Nevertheless, large numbers of anticoccidial agents and other antiprotozoan chemotherapeutic compounds have been tried with little success. Some patients have responded to paromomycin, 25 to 35 mg/kg for 14 to 21 days. However, they usually relapse and antibiotic therapy must be reinstituted. Limited experience with azithromycin has been promising. In some patients the infection is eradicated entirely; in others the frequency and volume of diarrhea are markedly diminished. Treatment is initiated with 1250 mg daily for 2 weeks and then continued with 500 mg daily. Stools are monitored regularly to ascertain whether the infection has been eliminated.

CYCLOSPORIASIS

Recently, several diarrheal outbreaks in AIDS patients, as well as in travelers, were reported from Nepal and Chicago, Illinois, and were ascribed to a *Cyanobacteria*-like body (CLB) or "blue-green alga." These organisms were subsequently shown to be not algae but a coccidian parasite closely related to *Cryptosporidium,* termed *Cyclospora* spp. For diagnostic purposes, cyclosporan oocysts measure 8 to 10 μm, whereas *Cryptosporidium* organisms are 4 to 5 μm. They are also acid-fast stain reactive and will autofluoresce under ultraviolet light. Therefore, it is essential to measure the oocysts carefully to differentiate between these two organisms. *Cyclospora* organisms cause a clinical syndrome similar to *Crypto-*

sporidium infection, although it tends to wax and wane over a period of several weeks before remitting. In AIDS patients it is not self-limited, biliary tract disease may occur, and these patients must be maintained on drug therapy indefinitely. In immunocompetent patients, successful treatment has been achieved with trimethoprim/sulfamethoxazole, 160 mg/800 mg twice daily for 7 days.

ISOSPORIASIS

Isosporiasis was a relatively uncommon diarrheal disease of man until the AIDS epidemic uncovered large numbers of patients with this disease. It is caused by the apicomplexan coccidian protozoan parasite *Isospora belli,* which is found in enterocytes of the proximal small intestine. Like *Cryptosporidium, Isospora* may cause a life-threatening diarrheal state in patients with AIDS, and self-limited disease in immunocompetent patients.

Infection follows ingestion of mature oocysts. After ingestion, the liberated sporozoites invade enterocytes, primarily in the proximal portion of the small bowel, and become trophozoites. Asexual multiplication (schizogony) occurs and a sexual cycle soon intervenes (sporogony) in which ooysts are produced. These are passed with the feces, and maturation is subsequently attained in approximately 2 to 3 days, depending on the environmental temperature. Infection follows ingestion of the mature oocysts in contaminated food or water.

Pathology and Clinical Disease

In experimental studies in volunteers, focal to widespread mucosal changes occurred that varied from severe flattened villi to mild nonspecific alterations and increased inflammatory cells in the lamina propria. The severity of the histopathologic changes appeared to correlate with the severity of the symptoms.

The onset of symptoms occurs about 1 week after ingestion of oocysts, the principal symptoms being profuse watery diarrhea, abdominal cramping, foul-smelling gas, loss of appetite, and low-grade fever. Peripheral mild eosinophila and Charcot-Leyden crystals are often found in the stool.

The clinical presentation is reminiscent of giardiasis or cryptosporidiosis. In AIDS patients, diarrhea as well as the other symptoms may persist indefinitely; in immunocompetent patients, the clinical episode gradually diminishes over 2 to 3 weeks. Oocyst shedding may persist many weeks after the patient returns to normal.

Treatment

In most patients, therapy with trimethoprim (160 mg) and sulfamethoxazole (800 mg) (TMP/SMX) four times a day for 10 days followed by TMP/SMX twice a day for 21 days is usually curative. Generally the symptoms respond in the first week of administration. However, in immunosuppressed patients there is a high rate of recurrence shortly after therapy is discontinued. Daily pyrimethamine (25 mg) and folinic acid (5 to 10 mg) prophylaxis has prevented recurrence in patients with AIDS. If sulfa drug intolerance or sensitivity is present, high-dose pyrimethamine, 75 mg four times a day together with folinic acid, 10 to 25 mg daily, has also been effective. Prophylaxis for these patients is necessary and they are continued on 25 mg pyrimethamine daily together with 5 to 10 mg folinic acid. Isolated reports that metronidazole, quinacrine, furazolidone, roxithromycin, and other macrolides may be effective therapy for isosporiasis have not been substantiated.

DIENTAMOEBIASIS

Dientamoeba fragilis is a protozoan parasite of the human colon that has been associated with diarrheal disease. This organism belongs to the class Mastigophora (flagellates) and in the ameboid stage is quite small, averaging 6 to 12 μm in diameter. This organism is often overlooked by inexperienced laboratory personnel because of its small size.

It has been postulated that *Dientamoeba* is transmitted with the egg of the pinworm *Enterobius vermicularis*. In a recent report, *D. fragilis* and pinworm infection were found together about nine times more frequently than would be expected on the basis of random distribution of these parasites. Attempts to culture *D. fragilis* from pinworm eggs or larvae, however, were always unsuccessful.

D. fragilis has been found in most parts of the world, the incidence varying widely from about 1% to 20% in some countries. Surveys of inmates in mental institutions and Native Americans from Arizona have shown a very high incidence of 19% to 47%; in New York City the incidence is about 4%.

Patients may have frank diarrhea or soft, mushy, or normally formed stools. They may complain of mild to severe abdominal pain, perianal pruritus, abdominal distention, and flatulence. Frank red blood in the stools is unusual. The organisms are not known to invade the colonic mucosa. Some authors have reported low-grade eosinophilia with this infection. Many individuals harbor this protozoan and have no complaints. The diagnosis depends on finding the parasite in a stool specimen that has been properly collected and promptly examined.

Adults should be treated with iodoquinol, 650 mg three times a day for 20 days; children should receive 40 mg/kg/day in three divided doses for 20 days. Alternatively, adults may be given tetracycline, 500 mg four times a day for 10 days, and children over 8 years of age 10 mg/kg four times a day for 10 days (maximum of 2 g).

ENTEROBIASIS

Enterobiasis is caused by the nematode pinworm *Enterobius vermicularis*. The adult worms inhabit the cecum, appendix, and adjacent areas of the ileum and ascending colon, although immature worms have been seen in the rectosigmoid. The gravid female detaches from the cecal mucosa and migrates distally, usually passing out of the anus onto the perianal and perineal skin, leaving a trail of eggs on the surface of the skin. In about 5% of patients, eggs are deposited in the bowel and may be found in feces. Migration out of the anus most often commences around 10 or 11 PM and continues until midnight.

Epidemiology

Enterobiasis is ubiquitous and unrelated to poor sanitary facilities or tropical climates. In the United States, infection rates in young schoolchildren vary from 10% to 45%. Infection in families is common. Young girls have pinworm more frequently than do boys of the same age, and whites are infected more often than blacks. It is not unusual to find this infection in young adolescents and occasionally in adults, especially young mothers.

Reinfection is by hand-to-mouth transmission, such as by scratching the contaminated anal area and subsequently ingesting the eggs. Nail biters or those who habitually put their fingers in their mouths are difficult to treat successfully. Inhaling and ingesting freshly deposited eggs in a room is also a common means of infection. There is no good evidence that retrograde infection occurs. For unknown reasons, some individuals seem to be predisposed or vulnerable to reinfection. In modern communities the "pinworm season" usually begins in October, peaks during the winter months, and declines in late spring.

Clinical Manifestations

Serious pathologic lesions are rarely caused by pinworms. Perianal and perineal pruritus are the most common complaints. Pruritus may provoke such severe scratching that local bleeding, secondary pyogenic infection, and lichenification may result. Whether pinworms are a primary cause of appendicitis remains unsettled. Some authors believe that pinworm infection may cause irritability and nervousness in children, and that perineal itching in young girls may lead to vaginitis and masturbation. Pinworms have occasionally been found in the fallopian tubes, peritoneal cavity, or spleen, where they have served as a nidus of symptomatic granulomatous inflammation.

Diagnosis

Nocturnal perianal pruritus strongly suggests pinworm infection. Small, creamy-white worms are often found if the perianal region is examined when the patient is awakened or disturbed by itching. Ova are not often seen in the stools, and the Scotch tape swab technique (National Institutes of Health swab) is the diagnostic method of choice. One swab on three to five consecutive mornings before getting out of bed is usually sufficient to detect the eggs.

Treatment

Treatment of pinworm infection is simple and effective. Since infection is often present in several members of a household, each family member should be examined, or the entire family should be treated simultaneously; otherwise, reinfection often occurs. Patient and parents alike should be instructed about the nature of pinworm infection and about the usual widespread dissemination of the ova throughout the household. Initially, bed sheets, underwear, and night clothes should be washed, and the household should be vacuum-cleaned and damp-mopped to reduce the number of ova. This vigorous program need not be undertaken more than once or twice as a means of reducing the opportunity for reinfection.

Mebendazole (Vermox), 100 mg (1 tablet) once, chewed thoroughly, is all that is necessary. Pyrantel pamoate, 11 mg/kg (maximum, 1 g) is equally effective. In each instance, therapy should be repeated after 2 to 3 weeks to ensure an almost 100% cure. All household members are usually treated simultaneously.

Prevention

Fingernails should be cut short and hands washed frequently. Infected persons should sleep alone and wear tight-fitting night clothes to discourage direct finger contact with the perianal region as well as dissemination onto bed linens and to the remainder of the household. Bedclothes, linens, and underclothes of those infected should be handled carefully and not shaken, to avoid dispersing ova into the air, and should be laundered daily for several days. It is almost impossible, however, to control dust-borne infective eggs.

TOXOCARIASIS (VISCERAL LARVA MIGRANS)

Visceral larva migrans (VLM) is caused by one of several species of parasitic helminth larvae of lower vertebrates that ordinarily cannot complete their life cycle in man. These larvae may wander through extraintestinal viscera, cause tissue necrosis, and provoke marked eosinophilic granulomatous inflammatory lesions.

Etiology and Epidemiology

The clinical syndrome of VLM is often caused by larvae of the common dog and perhaps cat ascarids, *Toxocara canis,* and *T. cati.* The disease is universal.

Adult worms living in the dog's small intestine deposit ova together with the dog's feces. If ova are swallowed by young dogs, second-stage larvae hatch in the small intestine, penetrate the intestinal wall, migrate to the lungs, ascend the bronchi and trachea, and are swallowed; they finally reach the small intestine, where they mature. In older dogs, larvae may undergo somatic migration and encyst in the tissues; encystment occurs more often in bitches, and the encysted larvae serve as the source of perinatal infection in puppies. Thus, in late pregnancy encysted larvae are activated, penetrate the uterus, and invade the developing fetus. Eggs can be found in the puppy's feces by about 21 days post partum. The infection can also be transmitted to newborn pups via the colostrum.

In humans, most infections have been reported in children 1 to 4 years of age with a history of pica, especially geophagia. Moreover, because young children are most likely to play carelessly with puppies and have little awareness of personal hygiene, they are especially at risk. After ingestion of the embryonated egg, the second-stage larva emerges in the small intestine, penetrates the intestinal wall, and initiates a somatic migration that may last for many weeks or months. Ingestion of *T. canis* ova by older children and young adolescents in whom pica (e.g., geophagia) is uncommon may cause ocular larva migrans (OLM) (Plate 4). The eye is invaded in this syndrome, which in the past was misdiagnosed as retinoblastoma.

Recent seroepidemiologic surveys have shown surprisingly high prevalence rates for *Toxocara* antibodies in children and adolescents. Moreover, the VLM syndrome has now become recognized in adults and older adolescents, causing mild to severe pulmonary symptoms. These studies suggest widespread subclinical infection in the United States, but they do not address the long-term consequences of this infection, such as late-onset seizures.

Pathology

The liver is most often involved in toxocariasis where eosinophilic granulomas can be found. These lesions also can be found in the lung, kidney, lymph node, eyes, brain, heart, and skeletal muscle.

Clinical Disease

The clinical presentations can vary from clinically silent eosinophilia to fever, hepatomegaly, hyperglobulinemia, and marked eosinophilia. Some children have pulmonary symptoms, signs of myocarditis, or CNS disease. Undoubtedly, the most dramatic symptoms are those involving the retina in OLM. In patients with OLM, the immune response as measured by antibody titers is often low or sometimes absent.

Diagnosis

The diagnosis is usually made on clinical grounds. Close association with a dog or cat is common; with VLM a history of pica is frequently elicited, but not with OLM. A biopsy can be helpful, particularly if it can be done by direct observation and if larvae are found. A persistently elevated eosinophil count, markedly elevated anti-A or anti-B isohemagglutinin antibody titers in patients who are not blood type AB, a moderate to high increase in IgG, and an elevated erythrocyte sedimentation rate all help to confirm the diagnosis. A specific and sensitive ELISA test is available; a titer of 1:16 or more is diagnostic and is associated with elevated serum IgM and IgG but not IgA. Patients with VLM usually have elevated ELISA titers (1:1024), but those with ocular manifestations alone may have low or absent titers.

Treatment

Because most VLM infections resolve spontaneously, it is difficult to evaluate therapy. Symptomatic VLM appears to respond to oral diethylcarbamazine, 6 mg/kg/day in three doses for about 7 to 10 days. It may be necessary to initiate treatment at 1 mg/kg and gradually increase the dose because of an allergic response to dying parasites. Albendazole, 100 to 200 mg twice daily for 5 days, has also been used successfully. In ocular disease, local and/or systemic steroids are usually advocated together with the specific agent.

Prevention

Since puppies and kittens are usually infected, they should be dewormed as soon as possible. Dogs often roll in contaminated feces, and their fur may carry the infective ova for a short period. Children should be protected from young dogs and cats. Although older dogs may carry the intestinal infection, they generally develop immunity. Bitches that have recently given birth to a litter may have an intestinal infection for a number of weeks before immunity intervenes. All dogs and cats should be dewormed periodically.

CYSTICERCOSIS

Human cysticercosis is the infection by the larval stage of the pork tapeworm *Taenia solium,* which is acquired by ingestion of *T. solium* eggs. The CNS and subcutaneous and intermuscular tissues are the most frequent infected sites.

Epidemiology

In underdeveloped countries, contamination of food, water, or hands with *T. solium* eggs from human feces is the primary source of infection. Most U.S. cases are found in immigrants from endemic areas.

In a review of 162 U.S. cases of neurocysticercosis (NCC), more than 95% of patients traveled to or came from endemic areas. In a recent survey from Los Angeles, immigrants accounted for most cases of cysticercosis. Travel-associated and autochthonous cases have accounted for 6.5% and 7.2%, respectively. None of the individuals had ever left the United States or had a history of eating raw pork. More recently, four cases were diagnosed in an orthodox Jewish U.S. community. The most likely sources of infection were believed to be women who had recently emigrated from Latin America and worked in patients' homes. The recent dramatic increase in the diagnosis of NCC is most likely accounted for by the introduction of CT and magnetic resonance imaging (MRI) and by advances in the immunologic diagnosis.

Clinical Disease

NCC, the most important of the clinical manifestations of cysticercosis, has been classified into parenchymal and extraparenchymal types. The latter, which is less common, is often subdivided into intraventricular, subarachnoid, and spinal NCC. Clinical presentation and pathogenesis vary depending on whether the cysts are active (living) or inactive (dead), the host's immune response, the number of cysts present, and the location of the cysts.

In the active type of disease, cysts may be solitary or multiple and located in several regions of the CNS. The most frequent site, however, is the subarachnoid space, causing arachnoiditis with detectable changes in the CSF. In about half of these cases, obstructive hydrocephalus is evident and is caused by occlusion of the foramina of Luschka and/or Magendie. In many cases, parenchymal cysts may be found. It is now recognized that when live cysts degenerate either as a result of the host's immune mechanisms or through chemotherapy, an inflammatory reaction may ensue that can cause severe symptoms. When these cysts are adjacent to or in contact with the subarachnoid space, there are protein, glucose, and cellular changes in the CSF. Cerebral edema may be present, associated with an increase in intracranial pressure.

Other less common findings include vasculitis associated with infarction; intraventricular cysts causing ependymitis and hydrocephalus; and spinal cysts, producing spinal cord compression or radicular syndromes. Racemose cysts are large, lobulated cysts without a scolex; these are usually found in the ventricular system and in the subarachnoid space. Although it is the least common form, it is often the most serious; it may be found rarely in the cerebral parenchyma.

More than 50% of cases of NCC are inactive at presentation. They are usually calcified and histologically are associated with granulomatous inflammation. This is thought to indicate previously destroyed cysts. It is not uncommon to have inactive and active forms of NCC coexisting in the same patient. Frequently, these calcified lesions are incidental findings at autopsy, CT, or MRI scan in otherwise asymptomatic or epileptic patients. Another form of NCC associated with inactive cysts is hydrocephalus, which is the result of meningeal fibrosis following the inflammatory response to cyst death. In these cases, cranial nerve involvement is common.

The clinical incubation period is unknown. However, a study of British troops stationed in India suggested a median of 3.5 years. Clinical manifestations of NCC are varied, with almost any neurologic and psychiatric syndrome attributable to this infection. With both inactive and active lesions localized in the parenchyma, focal seizures are the most common clinical manifestation. In urban U.S. settings, late-onset seizures in Hispanic immigrants are often the presenting complaint of NCC, although chronic severe headaches are also a frequent presenting complaint. Focal neurologic deficits are frequent and varied. Pyramidal tract signs are the most common, followed by signs of brainstem dysfunction, cerebellar ataxia, involuntary movements, and sensory deficits. Intellectual deterioration is also common. A particularly severe form of NCC is cysticercotic encephalitis, in which there are multiple cysts associated with an intense inflammatory reaction. These patients may have signs and symptoms of increased intracranial pressure, mental disturbances, diminution of visual acuity, and generalized seizures. Encephalitis is more frequent in children and young adolescents, in whom cerebral edema is a common accompaniment. Hydrocephalus is less frequent in children than in adults in this form of the disease. In a retrospective study of U.S. children it was found that most cases presented with inflammatory cysts diagnosed by CT.

Diagnosis

The widespread use of CT scanning was an important advance in the diagnosis of NCC; MRI is indicated where CT is not conclusive. These imaging methods, as well as new modalities in immunodiagnosis, have made possible the presumptive diagnosis of NCC. Brain biopsy should be limited to difficult diagnostic problems, especially when malignancy is a likely possibility and when other noninvasive diagnostic tools have been exhausted. Soft tissue radiographic studies should be performed to look for small curvilinear calcifications. If these are found, biopsy can be helpful for the diagnosis, as is the removal and reexamination of a palpable subcutaneous nodule.

Until recently, ELISA has been the diagnostic procedure most frequently used to detect *Cysticercus* antibodies in both serum and CSF. However, these tests used crude or partially purified antigens that may cross-react with other helminth antibodies, especially *Echinococcus* organisms. The sensitivity of these tests depend on the antigen preparation and the type of disease. Frequently, sensitivity was as low as 44%, especially in patients with few or calcified parenchymal cysts. Comparison with the recently introduced enzyme-linked immunoelectrotransfer blot (Western blot) in NCC has shown nearly 100% sensitivity, while ELISA had 74% sensitivity. In NCC the sensitivity of the immunoblot was shown to decline when individuals had fewer than two parenchymal cysts.

Lumbar puncture is contraindicated in cases with intracranial pressure. The CSF may be normal on examination. However, frequently, active cases are associated with elevated protein, hypoglycorrhachia, and a lymphocytic pleocytosis with occasional eosinophiles.

Treatment

Patients may require hospitalization during the initial phase of therapy. Treatment of NCC varies according to the stage of the disease, the number and location of the cysts, and the clinical manifestations. When viable cysts are present in the parenchyma, therapy with albendazole is indicated; the daily dose is 15 mg/kg (usually 800 mg/day) in divided doses. The duration of treatment has varied; the usual length is 28 days, but some clinicians have administered therapy for several months, and some Mexican investigators have recommended periods as short as 8 days. A ventriculoperitoneal shunt is often required to relieve intracranial pressure as a result of subarachnoid NCC hydrocephalus. When active arachnoiditis is present, anticysticercal drugs are also useful. Clumps of cysticerci in the subarachnoid space are usually treated by surgical extirpation. The presence of intraventricular cysts requires surgical resection. These may be of the racemose type, for which the anticysticercal drugs may not always be effective.

Most cases of spinal NCC are treated by surgery, although medical treatment may be beneficial. In mixed forms, a combination of treatment, both medical and surgical, is used.

Anticonvulsive treatment should be maintained when epilepsy is present before initiating anticysticercal drug therapy. CT scans are recommended 3 to 6 months after specific treatment and are a more valuable parameter of cyst viability than serology for evaluating treatment.

In 3% to 7% of cases the eye is involved and the diagnosis is made by funduscopic examination. Imaging techniques such as ultrasonography may be helpful. Cysticerci float freely in the eye and are found in the anterior and vitreous chambers. They may also adhere to subretinal tissues. Subretinal cysts are associated with vasculitis and retinal edema. In the vitreous they are associated with chorioretinitis and retinal detachment. Rarely, cysts may be found in the eyelid and lacrimal glands. Antiparasitic therapy should be avoided and surgery is usually indicated.

Prevention

The prevention and control of cysticercosis has been especially difficult, since an improvement in sanitation and personal hygiene in the poor areas of the world does not occur unless living standards are elevated. Screening of household contacts to detect positive tapeworm cases may be done by inquiring whether these large tapeworm proglottids have been seen in the stool. While it is unusual to find intestinal infection in patients with NCC, contacts of such patients are more frequently positive. Stool examinations may not be reliable and serology is often unavailable in endemic areas. Even where these studies are possible, the presence of intestinal tapeworm does not often result in a positive serologic test. The identification of contacts is important in controlling cysticercosis; they should be treated with praziquantel. Food handlers from endemic areas should also be considered for empiric praziquantel therapy.

Suggested Readings

Toxoplasmosis

Brooks RG, McCabe RE, Remington JS: Role of serology in the diagnosis of toxoplasmic lymphadenopathy, *Rev Infect Dis* 9:775-782, 1987.

Daffos F, Forestier F, Capella-Pavlvsky M, et al: Prenatal management of 746 pregnancies at risk of congenital toxoplasmosis, *N Engl J Med* 318:271, 1988.

Dannemann BR, Vaughn WC, Thulliez P, et al: The differential agglutination test for diagnosis of recently acquired infection with *Toxoplasma gondii*, *J Clin Microbiol* 28:1928-1933, 1990.

Desmonts G, Couvreur J: Congenital toxoplasmosis. A prospective study of 378 pregnancies, *N Engl J Med* 290:1110, 1974.

Dorfman RF, Remington JS: Value of lymph node biopsy in the diagnosis of acute acquired toxoplasmosis, *N Engl J Med* 289:878, 1973.

Frenkel JK: Toxoplasmosis: parasite life cycle, pathology and immunology of toxoplasmosis. In Hammond DM, Long P, editors: *The coccidia:* Eimeria, Toxoplasma, Isopora, *and related genera,* Baltimore, 1973, University Park Press; p 225-241.

McCabe RE, Brooks RG, Dorfman RF, Remington JS: Clinical spectrum in 107 cases of toxoplasmic lymphadenopathy, *Rev Infect Dis* 9:754-774, 1987.

McCauley J, Boyer KM, Patel D, et al: Early and longitudinal evaluations of treated infants and children and untreated historical patients with congenital toxoplasmosis. The Chicago Collaborative Treatment Trial, *Clin Infect Dis* 18:38-72, 1994.

Remington JS, Araujo FG, Desmonts G: Recognition of different *Toxoplasma* antigens by IgM and IgG antibodies in mothers and their congenitally infected newborns, *J Infect Dis* 162:270-273, 1985.

Remington V, Desmonts G: Toxoplasmosis. In Remington JS, Klein JO, editors: *Infectious diseases of the fetus and newborn infant,* ed 4, Philadelphia, 1995, WB Saunders.

Ruskin J, Remington J: Toxoplasmosis in the compromised host, *Ann Intern Med* 84:193, 1976.

Weiss LM, Harris C, Berger M, Tanowitz HB, Wittner M: Pyrimethamine concentrations in serum and cerebrospinal fluid during treatment of acute *Toxoplasma* encephalitis in patients with AIDS, *J Infect Dis* 157:580-583, 1988.

Wilson CB, Remington JS, Stagno S, Reynolds DW: Development of adverse sequelae in children born with subclinical congenital *Toxoplasma* infection, *Pediatrics* 66:767, 1980.

Wong S-Y, Remington JS: Toxoplasmosis in the setting of AIDS. In Broder S, Merigan TC, Bolognesi D, editors: *Textbook of AIDS medicine,* Baltimore, 1994, Williams & Wilkins.

Cryptosporidiosis

Crawford FG, Vermund SH: Human cryptosporidiosis, *Crit Rev Microbiol* 16:113-159, 1988.

Current WL, Garcia LS: Cryptosporidiosis, *Clin Microbiol Rev* 4:325-358, 1991.

Dehovitz JA, Pape JW, Boncy M, Johnson WD Jr: Clinical manifestations and therapy of *Isospora belli* infection in patients with the acquired immunodeficiency syndrome, *N Engl J Med* 315:87-90.

Kreinik G, Burstein O, Landor M, Bernstein L, Weiss LM, Wittner M: Successful treatment of intractable cryptosporidial diarrhea with intravenous octreotide (Sandostatin), a somatostatin analogue, *AIDS* 6:765-767, 1991.

Centers for Disease Control: Outbreaks of diarrheal illness associated with *Cyanobacteria* (blue-green algae)–like bodies—Chicago and Nepal, 1989 and 1990, *MMWR* 40:325, 1991.

Sifuentes-Osinio J, Porras-Cortes G, Bendell RP, et al: *Cyclospora cayetanensis* infection in patients with and without AIDS: biliary disease as another clinical manifestation, *Clin Infect Dis* 21:1092-1097, 1995.

Weiss LM, Perlman D, Sherman J, Tanowitz HB, Wittner M: *Isospora belli* infection: treatment with pyrimethamine, *Ann Intern Med* 109:474, 1988.

Dientamoebiasis

Millet V, Spencer MJ, Chapin M, et al: *Dientamoeba fragilis:* a protozoan parasite in adult members of a semicommunal group, *Dig Dis Sci* 28:335, 1983.

Schein R, Gelb A: Colitis due to *Dientamoeba fragilis, Am J Gastroenterol* 78:634, 1983.

Yang J, Scholten T: *Dientamoeba fragilis:* a review with notes on its epidemiology, pathogenicity, mode of transmission, and diagnosis, *Am J Trop Med Hyg* 26:16, 1977.

Cysticercosis

Diaz JF, Verastegul M, Gilman RH, et al: Immunodiagnosis of human cysticercosis *(Taenia solium)*: a field comparison of an antibody-enzyme-linked immunosorbent assay (ELISA), an antigen-ELISA and an enzyme-linked immunoelectrotransfer blot (EITB) assay in Peru, *Am J Trop Med Hyg* 46:610, 1992.

Schantz PM, Moore AC, Munoz J, et al: Neurocysticercosis in an Orthodox Jewish community in New York City, *N Engl J Med* 327:692, 1992.

Carpio A, Santillán F, León P, et al: Is the course of neurocysticercosis modified by treatment with anthelminthic agents?, *Arch Intern Med* 155:1982-1988, 1995.

CHAPTER 72

Dermatologic Problems

•

Amy S. Paller, Elizabeth A. Abel, and Ilona J. Frieden

To many physicians and patients, adolescent dermatology is virtually synonymous with acne. Acne *is* a common skin problem during adolescence, and any physician seeing adolescents should have a good understanding of its pathogenesis and treatment. However, many other skin disorders are seen during adolescence. Some of these have their onset during adolescence; others are modified in their course at this time. Some of these dermatologic disorders are directly related to the profound changes in hormonal production occurring during adolescence, whereas others are either indirectly related or unrelated to hormonal changes. Although this chapter cannot be a comprehensive review of all these disorders, the diagnosis and management of some of the more common disorders are discussed, and some of the less common ones that a physician caring for adolescent patients may encounter are noted.

One important aspect of skin disease, especially chronic skin disease such as acne, psoriasis, or atopic dermatitis, is its impact on the psychological well-being of the affected individual. Both clinical observations and projective psychological testing have demonstrated anxiety, depression, and lowered self-esteem in patients with chronic skin disease. In severe cases, withdrawal from social interactions may be seen. During adolescence, self-concept and body image are especially important for normal psychological development. A relatively minor problem, such as dandruff, may seem trivial to the physician but may be extremely embarrassing to the adolescent patient. Conversely, patients with mild, non-scarring acne may not be interested in treatment since many of their peers have the same problem. The psychological impact of any skin disorder should be assessed before therapy is planned. Finally, the physician seeing adolescent patients has a good opportunity

to practice preventive medicine by counseling them about the harmful effects of ultraviolet irradiation from sunlight. Many adolescent patients may accept this information more readily if they understand that premature aging and wrinkling of the skin and skin cancer are the sequelae of long-term sun exposure. They should be encouraged to wear protective clothing or to use a sunscreen appropriate for their skin pigmentation type; for example, fair-skinned individuals should be advised to use a preparation with a sun protection factor (SPF) of at least 15.

ACNE

Acne is the most common skin disorder seen during adolescence, and 40% of children develop early lesions of acne between the ages of 8 and 10 years. Eventually, 85% of adolescents develop some degree of acne, but the spectrum of severity is broad.

Acne is a treatable disease. In the past, when treatment was less effective, many physicians and parents advised teenagers with acne that they would outgrow their disease, and no treatment other than over-the-counter soaps and astringents was given. Unfortunately, emotional and physical scarring from acne is not rare. For this reason, adolescents with any significant degree of acne, and especially those with scarring, should be given the option of treatment. This includes patients who do not specifically seek treatment for acne but are in the office for other concerns. Many adolescents do not ask about treatment of acne, even when it concerns them, because of embarrassment or the misapprehension that there is no effective treatment. Many also believe that they are to blame for their acne because of dietary indiscretions or lack of frequent face washing, both of which are of dubious significance as causes of acne.

Management of acne requires a basic understanding of its pathogenesis. The earliest changes leading to acne occur when the pilosebaceous unit begins to enlarge and produce sebum. This often occurs 1 to 2 years before the onset of puberty, probably secondary to adrenal androgenic stimulation. This sebaceous gland activation apparently cannot take place without the sebaceous gland converting circulating testosterone to dihydrotestosterone by way of the enzyme 5α-reductase. The higher circulating testosterone levels in males probably contribute to the increased incidence and severity of acne in that group. As the sebaceous gland hypertrophies, sebum becomes measurable at the skin surface. Sebum consists of a mixture of triglycerides, squalene, wax esters, and sterol esters. Most patients with acne produce increased amounts of sebum, noted clinically as an oily complexion. Not all patients with acne have elevated sebum excretion, and it alone does not fully explain the pathogenesis of acne. However, the face, back, and chest (the main sites of acne) are the areas with the highest concentration of pilosebaceous glands.

The initial clinical sign of acne is the comedo, a papule created when the follicular opening to the pilosebaceous gland becomes plugged. This pore plugging is caused by abnormal keratinization of the epithelial lining of the follicular orifice. Rather than emptying the more superficial epithelial cells from the orifice in an orderly process, the follicle retains them and creates a keratinous plug to the follicular opening. When the plug is retained with a widely dilated follicular opening, it appears as an open comedo, or "blackhead." The darkened tip of an open comedo is not caused by dirt; it results from compaction and oxidation of keratinous material as well as from melanin pigment. Open comedones rarely lead to inflammatory papules or pustules because the follicular contents can move more readily to the skin surface. When a plug occurs with a small follicular orifice, a closed comedo, or "whitehead," is formed. Closed comedones are the precursors of inflammatory lesions because their contents are more likely to rupture into the surrounding dermis and cause inflammation. The depth of rupture determines whether the lesion will appear as a pustule, papule, or nodule.

The anaerobic bacterium *Propionibacterium acnes* appears to play an important role in the pathogenesis of acne. *P. acnes* is capable of releasing lipolytic enzymes that convert the triglycerides in sebum into irritating fatty acids and glycerol. Although comedones can form in the absence of *P. acnes,* the bacteria may promote comedo genesis and follicular rupture. They also may promote chemotaxis by activation of the classic or alternate complement pathways. Indirect evidence of the importance of bacteria comes from the therapeutic efficacy of using antibiotics that are active against *P. acnes.* The dramatic effect of a synthetic vitamin A derivative, isotretinoin (Accutane), in the absence of antibiotics suggests that the altered keratinization and excessive sebum production may be of primary importance in the pathogenesis and that the bacterial effects are secondary.

Diet does not appear to play a significant role in the etiology of acne. A double-blind study in which volunteers were fed huge quantities of chocolate refuted the myth that chocolate exacerbates acne. Dietary iodides and fatty foods also have been discounted as etiologic agents. Stress may cause flares of acne, but the exact mechanism of this effect is not known. In some cases mechanical factors, such as frequent touching of the face during times of stress, may cause increased numbers of inflammatory lesions. In addition, many female patients note a worsening of acne at the beginning of the menstrual cycle, presumably because of hormonal alterations.

There are six types of acne lesions: comedones, papules, pustules, nodules, cysts, and scars. Individual patients may have one predominant type of lesion or a mixture of many. Early in adolescence, comedones tend to predominate, regardless of the eventual pattern. For many adolescents, acne begins on the midface with later involvement of the jawline, neck, chest, and back. Assessment of the type of acne lesions, sites of involvement, and degree of severity should be made in all patients before therapy is begun.

Treatment Approaches

The treatment of acne requires flexibility in using different therapeutic modalities to achieve both a clinical response and patient satisfaction. One crucial factor is to make the patient understand that virtually no therapy will produce a significant response before 4 to 6 weeks. Without this understanding, the patient will become discouraged and label the therapy a failure before it has a chance to work. Another important point of education is to explain that many topical medications can be irritating. To minimize this effect, these medications should never be applied shortly after washing and they should be introduced gradually. For example, tretinoin (Retin-A) may be applied every second or third day for a week, and then the frequency of application can be slowly increased to nightly applications. If significant irritation occurs, the frequency of application should be decreased or the strength of medication lowered as tolerated. Patients should be instructed to apply the medications to the entire areas in which acne occurs, not just to individual pimples. Topical medications should not be applied simultaneously, since they may inactivate one another.

Several acne medications, including oral tetracycline and topical tretinoin, cause enhanced photosensitivity.

Therefore, patients need to be warned that they may sunburn more easily while undergoing therapy. Cleansing of the affected areas, although emphasized in the past, is probably of minor importance because the surface oils are not the cause but a symptom of acne. Too frequent washing, especially with harsh or gritty soaps, should be avoided because the combined irritancy with topical medications may make therapy less effective. A mild soap, such as Neutrogena Acne Soap or Purpose, may be used. Acne scrubs, containing gritty materials, and rough sponges may be useful in some patients, but they also can be irritating and are generally discouraged.

Commonly Used Agents

Benzoyl peroxide has been used widely as a topical agent in acne therapy since the 1960s. It acts as a keratolytic agent and suppresses the growth of *P. acnes.* This agent comes in a number of formulations, including creams, lotions, and gels. The gels seem to have a better ability to penetrate into the pilosebaceous glands and may be somewhat more effective. Water-based gels (e.g., Desquam-X, Benzac W, Persa-Gel W, Panoxyl AQ) may be slightly less irritating than the alcohol- or acetone-based gels (e.g., Persa-Gel, Benzac, and PanOxyl). Benzoyl peroxide is available in concentrations of 2.5%, 4%, 5%, 8%, and 10%; as a 5% or 10% wash; and as a soap bar. The wash and soap formulations may be useful for large areas, such as the back, or in patients who cannot remember to use the topical medications regularly.

Vitamin A acid (a component of tretinoin) is effective in decreasing comedo formation and in loosening already existing comedones. It acts by altering keratinization and reversing the epidermal cell cohesiveness that causes the comedones to form. Some patients may experience a flare of inflammatory lesions when first using this agent. Patients with fair complexions or sensitive skin should begin by using Retin-A 0.025% cream every second to third day; those with more oily skin may tolerate the 0.05% cream or the 0.01% gel. When tolerance has been established, the strength may be increased as needed to the 0.1% cream or the 0.025% gel, applied nightly.

Topical Antibiotics

Commercially available topical antibiotics include preparations of erythromycin, clindamycin, and meclo-cycline. Many trials have confirmed the efficacy of these medications, but no one of these has been shown conclusively to be superior. Nevertheless, many practitioners have the clinical impression that clindamycin is somewhat more effective than the other agents. The risk of pseudomembranous colitis from this or other topical antibiotics appears to be extremely low, but patients using these medications should be cautioned to

seek medical attention if severe diarrhea develops, since rare cases have been reported. Meclocycline sulfosalicylate (Meclan) is the only topical antibiotic formulated in a cream base. It may be useful in patients who have very sensitive skin, such as those with concurrent atopic dermatitis. The other topical antibiotics come in liquid, gel form or lotion, or as medicated swabs (pledgettes) and are applied twice daily. A combination gel of benzoyl peroxide and erythromycin (Benzamycin) may improve patient compliance, but its disadvantage is that it must be refrigerated.

The traditional peeling agents such as sulfur, resorcinol, and salicylic acid may have a beneficial effect and can be bought over the counter. Since these agents can be irritating, they are often avoided in patients with significant acne so that more effective preparations can be employed without additional irritation.

Oral Antibiotics

Tetracycline, erythromycin, minocycline, doxycycline, clindamycin, and trimethoprim/sulfamethoxazole have all been used orally with some success in the treatment of acne. Tetracycline and erythromycin are used most commonly. The dosages of these medications are adjusted according to the severity of disease. As a group, their most common side effects are the production of candidal vulvovaginitis and gastrointestinal upset. Patients with severe acne who are undergoing long-term, high-dose antibiotic therapy may develop a gram-negative folliculitis, which usually appears as clustered follicular pustules around the nose. *Enterobacter* or *Klebsiella* organisms may often be cultured from these lesions. Treatment consists of the use of isotretinoin or high-dose oral antibiotics (usually ampicillin).

Tetracycline is extremely useful in treating inflammatory acne. Beginning doses are usually 1 to 1.5 g/day divided two to three times daily. An attempt should be made to taper the dose once control has been achieved. Patients should be instructed to take the medication 1 hour before or 2 hours after meals. Tetracycline should be used with caution in sexually active female adolescents, as it is contraindicated during pregnancy. It has been suggested that tetracycline itself might decrease the effectiveness of oral contraceptive pills. The actual risk of contraceptive failure while the patient is taking tetracycline is not known, but in view of the lack of many case reports, it is probably low.

Rarer side effects of tetracycline include fixed drug eruption, phototoxicity (including separation of the nail from its plate, or photoonycholysis), and a rise in blood urea nitrogen. Yellow staining of the brain in patients undergoing long-term therapy with tetracycline for treatment of acne has been found incidentally at autopsy without associated neurologic signs or symptoms.

Erythromycin is administered in dosages from 0.5 g to 2 g/day, depending on severity. The main toxic effect is gastrointestinal. Nausea and diarrhea are fairly common, but these effects may be reduced by using enteric-coated erythromycin, such as E-Mycin 333-mg tablets.

Minocycline is a semisynthetic derivative of tetracycline and can be extremely effective in cases in which tetracycline or erythromycin has failed. It is usually reserved for more severe cases, however, because of its side effects and great cost. Minocycline rarely causes dizziness and vertigo and may cause photosensitivity. If used chronically, it may increase skin pigmentation. Rare instances of tooth discoloration have been reported recently. Dosage ranges from 50 to 200 mg every day.

Doxycycline is also very effective, given in dosages from 50 to 200 mg each day. It is less expensive than minocycline but causes more photosensitivity than either tetracycline or minocycline.

Isotretinoin

Isotretinoin is a synthetic vitamin A derivative that represents a major advance in the therapy for severe inflammatory acne (see Plate 5). Its use in dosages of 1 mg/kg/day for 4 to 5 months seems to give long-lasting remissions (up to several years) in many patients. Some patients (less than 30%) require a second course of therapy. Improvement is often noted to continue even after use of the drug is stopped. Isotretinoin should be administered only to patients with severe cystic acne that has been recalcitrant to other systemic therapy, including appropriate courses of antibiotics.

The major side effect of isotretinoin is its teratogenicity, and effective contraception *must* be used during treatment. Reported congenital anomalies include hypoplastic external ears, ocular and central nervous system (CNS) abnormalities, congenital heart disease, and thymic aplasia. In female patients, pregnancy testing must be performed before initiating therapy and monthly thereafter. The drug is begun on day 2 or 3 of the menstrual cycle. Pregnancy should be avoided for 1 month after discontinuation of the drug. Isotretinoin is not mutagenic and has no known adverse effects on spermatogenesis or sperm motility.

The drug has many additional side effects. Commonly reported toxicities include cheilitis (90%); dry skin, especially on the face (80%); conjunctivitis (60%); dry mouth (30%); and pruritus (25%). Fasting triglyceride levels, complete blood count, calcium level, alkaline phosphatase level, and liver function tests should be obtained initially at 2 weeks and followed monthly thereafter during therapy. Elevated triglycerides have been reported in up to 25% of patients and tend to occur early in therapy. Decreasing the dose of isotretinoin and restricting fats may help to reduce triglyceride levels.

Musculoskeletal discomfort occurs in 16% of patients, particularly in athletic male adolescents. The creatine kinase level may be elevated, and if this persists, therapy may need to be discontinued.

Estrogen Therapy

Estrogen therapy in the form of oral contraceptives is rarely used as primary therapy but may benefit some female adolescents with acne. Certain oral contraceptives, including Ortho-Cept, Orthocycline, and Desogen, can be particularly helpful either as a therapy or as an adjunct to other therapies.

Antiandrogens

Spironolactone (200 mg/day) and cyproterone acetate, systemic antiandrogens, control inflammatory acne lesions but produce side effects, particularly breast tenderness and menstrual irregularity.

Acne Surgery

Acne surgery consists of the mechanical removal of comedones and the draining of cysts. It can be very useful in hastening the resolution of inflammatory lesions and in preventing the development of new comedones when used in conjunction with antiacne therapy. Acne surgery should be performed with clean, proper equipment by a trained practitioner. Patients should be cautioned not to attempt to perform such surgery on themselves. The use of tretinoin may ameliorate the response to acne surgery.

Intralesional Corticosteroids

Intralesional corticosteroids are extremely useful in treating cystic and nodular acne. Triamcinolone, 2.5 to 5 mg/ml, is injected into lesions, with up to 0.1 ml used per lesion. The injection must be directed into the center of the lesion. If the injection is too superficial, cutaneous atrophy (usually reversible) may occur. Patients should be warned of this potential complication. Hypopigmentation also may occur after injection.

Ultraviolet Light

Ultraviolet light probably does not significantly improve acne, although the tan it produces may conceal acne activity. Known side effects of skin aging and carcinogenesis probably outweigh any benefit it might offer.

Treatment of Scars

Superficial scarring may be treated with chemical peels, such as those in which trichloroacetic acid is used.

Deeper scars may require dermabrasion, in which the epidermis and upper dermis are removed to the level of scarring. Side effects may include erythema, milia, pigmentary alterations, and hypertrophic scarring. Synthetic collagens may be injected into deep scars to smooth the skin, but the effect is not permanent. Intralesional corticosteroids may be injected into keloidal acne scars.

DERMATITIS

Dyshidrotic Eczema

Dyshidrotic eczema is characterized by recurrent crops of vesicles and eczematous patches on the palms, soles, and lateral aspects of the fingers. Although relatively rare in early childhood, this disorder is more common during adolescence. Occasionally, it is a manifestation of atopic dermatitis, but it can be seen in nonatopic individuals. Stress seems to play an important role in flares of dyshidrotic eczema. The role of excessive sweating is controversial. Some patients have hyperhidrosis, but others sweat normally. Itching and burning can cause significant discomfort. Treatment consists of the application of potent topical steroids such as fluocinonide (Lidex) or betamethasone valerate 0.1% (Valisone) in cream or ointment form. For severe cases, class I steroids such as Temovate, Diprolene, or Ultravade may be used for up to 2 weeks. Occasionally the use of systemic corticosteroids is necessary during a severe exacerbation. The differential diagnosis includes contact dermatitis and inflammatory tinea infection of the feet.

Seborrheic Dermatitis

Seborrheic dermatitis is a very common disorder that frequently begins during adolescence. It is characterized by scales (frequently greasy) as well as erythema and pruritus in areas of the body having a high concentration of sebaceous glands (scalp, central face, eyebrows and eyelashes, postauricular areas, central chest). Less commonly, it can involve intertriginous areas. The pathogenesis of this disorder is unknown, although overgrowth of *Pityrosporum* yeast has been implicated. Mild scaling of the scalp (dandruff) is a normal variant. In seborrheic dermatitis the scales on the scalp are thicker and frequently inflammation is also present. The differential diagnosis includes psoriasis (plaques are usually thicker and more discrete but may be localized to the scalp), tinea capitis (especially that caused by *Trichophyton tonsurans),* and contact dermatitis.

Treatment of seborrheic dermatitis consists of frequent shampooing with antiseborrheic shampoos. These are usually over-the-counter preparations that contain sulfur, salicylic acid, zinc pyrithione, selenium sulfide, and/or tar. Shampooing should be done every day or every other day, and the shampoo should be left on the scalp for at least 5 minutes before rinsing. For severe scalp erythema and pruritus, topical corticosteroid solutions (e.g., Valisone, Fluonid, or Synalar solutions) can be very useful when applied once or twice a day. In recalcitrant cases, topical ketoconazole cream may be used as an adjunct, or ketoconazole in the form of a shampoo, twice weekly.

Seborrheic dermatitis on the face should be treated with hydrocortisone cream, 1% to 2.5% two to three times daily. In other areas of the body, hydrocortisone or slightly more potent corticosteroid creams may be used. The condition waxes and wanes in severity, and treatment should take place when the dermatitis is present. The application of ketoconazole cream once a day may add to the treatment effect.

Atopic Dermatitis

Atopic dermatitis, a very common skin disorder seen in up to 10% of children, may persist into adolescence. The onset frequently occurs before 2 years of age, and the disease usually improves during adolescence. A few patients may have a flare of disease activity during adolescence; others may continue to have about the same degree of activity.

The pathophysiologic basis of atopic dermatitis is incompletely understood. The predisposition is usually inherited and found in families with other "atopic" diseases such as asthma and hay fever. Atopic dermatitis involves immunologic abnormalities, such as elevated IgE level and increased rates of sensitization to common contact allergens and response to intradermal skin tests. Other parameters of cell-mediated immunity have been reported to be abnormal, including decreased numbers of some T-lymphocyte subsets.

In general, the skin of patients with atopic dermatitis is different from that of other individuals in the following respects:

1. Increased tendency toward dryness
2. Lowered threshold for pruritus from minor irritants such as soaps, wool, or polyester
3. Tendency toward lichenification and production of a rash when the skin is rubbed or scratched
4. Frequent colonization with *Staphylococcus aureus* and increased risk of *S. aureus* impetigo and severe herpes simplex infections

Many cases of atopic dermatitis resolve after early childhood, but those that persist into adolescence often have a somewhat different distribution and morphology. More often, patches are hyperpigmented and lichenified rather than red and acutely eczematous. Lesions may be more nummular (round) and circumscribed. Although the antecubital and popliteal fossae are still frequently involved, the face (especially eyelids), neck, shoulders, lower legs, and hands are often affected. Fingertips and the lateral area of the fingers are frequently involved; cutlike fissures are common (see Plate 6). The condition of some patients with atopic dermatitis will clear completely except for recurrent bouts of hand eczema, sometimes with vesiculation of the interdigital surfaces (dyshidrotic eczema). Unilateral or bilateral nipple dermatitis is occasionally seen in adolescent females (see Plate 7).

Keratosis pilaris, a follicular hyperkeratosis found most commonly on the outer upper arms and anterior thighs, is a frequent finding in patients with atopic dermatitis. The condition is rarely symptomatic and its onset usually occurs before adolescence, but it may first come to medical attention during adolescence, since the small red bumps and follicular hyperkeratosis may be cosmetically bothersome. The application of ammonia lactate 12% lotion may improve the condition because of its keratolytic effect.

The management of atopic dermatitis involves both the prevention of precipitating factors and treatment of the existing dermatitis. The skin must be kept well lubricated, and exposure to skin irritants, such as hot water and harsh soaps, must be avoided. Bathing or showering should be done with lukewarm water and a mild soap (e.g., Dove). Regular lubrication with bland emollients (e.g., Eucerin or Moisturel cream) is extremely important, especially after bathing. If sweating and sweat retention are problematic, less occlusive lubricants (e.g., Cetaphil, Shepard's Lotion, or Nutraderm) may be applied. Most patients with atopic dermatitis can tolerate strenuous physical activity, but excessive sweating may occur, necessitating restriction of vigorous exercise. Work requiring frequent use of water or irritating chemicals may cause atopic dermatitis to flare. Thus, career counseling is extremely important for adolescents with chronic atopic dermatitis. These individuals should avoid occupations such as beautician, food handler, and dishwasher and certain jobs in nursing and medicine that would require frequent hand washing or exposure to irritating chemicals.

Topical corticosteroids are the mainstay of atopic dermatitis therapy. Atopic dermatitis that is recalcitrant to topical corticosteroid therapy can be treated with ultraviolet light and tar preparations. Systemic corticosteroids occasionally may be needed in a severe flare, but their use should be avoided on a regular basis because of the long-term side effects. Patients who are flaring badly and those who have denuded skin with excoriations (even without obvious crusting and oozing from impetiginization) should receive a course of oral antistaphylococcal antibiotics.

Contact Dermatitis

Allergic contact dermatitis is more common in adolescents than in younger children, probably because of the increased opportunity for allergic sensitization over time. This type of contact dermatitis must be distinguished from irritant contact dermatitis, a common form that is caused by chemically irritating substances, such as soaps, detergents, acids, and alkalis, and is not immunologically mediated.

Common allergic sensitizers in the adolescent age group include the *Rhus* antigen (poison ivy, oak, and sumac), nickel, and ingredients in cosmetics, including a variety of sensitizing chemicals. The acute phase of both allergic contact dermatitis and irritant contact dermatitis may appear as an eczematous eruption, with erythematous papules and edema; if severe, vesicles and bullae will also be noted. The distribution of lesions is often a clue to the cause. In *Rhus* dermatitis, linear lesions are frequently present (see Plate 8). Nickel dermatitis usually occurs at sites where jewelry is worn, such as the earlobe, neck, and wrist (see Plate 9). Erythema and oozing at the site of pierced ears is often attributed to "infection" but is almost always the result of nickel allergy, unless the ears have been very recently pierced. The wearing of surgical stainless steel posts or wires usually alleviates this problem. Nickel allergy also can occur around the waistline from studded jeans or belt buckles. Dermatitis associated with cosmetics frequently involves the eyelids, even if the make-up is not directly applied to the lids themselves. Nail polish, for example, may cause eyelid dermatitis instead of paronychial changes because of the transfer of allergen to the thinner, more susceptible skin of the eyelids.

Subacute contact dermatitis is characterized by erythema, crusting, scaling, and some lichenification. Chronic contact dermatitis involves little erythema, but the skin is usually lichenified and scaly and sometimes becomes fissured. The diagnosis of allergic contact dermatitis can be confirmed by patch testing for suspected common allergens. The patch test kits used are designed to specifically differentiate irritant reactions from true allergic reactions. Such testing is particularly important in cases of chronic or recurrent contact dermatitis, especially those that are occupation related. In these cases, avoidance of the allergen is usually the only effective means of resolving the dermatitis.

Severe acute contact dermatitis, such as a generalized *Rhus* dermatitis, should be treated with 40 to 60 mg/day of prednisone, gradually tapered over 2 to 3 weeks. In addition, soothing compresses with colloidal oatmeal (Aveeno) can be used. Itching can be controlled with oral antihistamines such as diphenhydramine or hydroxyzine. In less severe cases of contact dermatitis, moderate- to high-potency topical steroids can be applied three or four times a day. Antipruritic lotions (e.g., Sarna, PrameGel, calamine) may be helpful.

SKIN DISORDERS OF PREGNANCY

Many skin changes may be noted during pregnancy. The most common of these are striae (stretch marks), which develop in 90% of pregnant women. These are pink to purple atrophic bands, commonly seen on the abdomen, breast, and thighs. They may occur in nonpregnant adolescents during a growth spurt. The tendency to form striae is often familial. With time, the color of these marks usually fades and they become less apparent; however, they do not disappear completely. No treatment is effective, nor is there an effective means of preventing this problem.

Other physiologic changes during pregnancy include increased pigmentation of the areolae, linea alba, and genitalia. Nevi and freckles also may darken. Many pregnant women develop increased body hair, which usually decreases several months after delivery. The development of vascular lesions (angiomas) on the face or upper chest is also very common. Acne may improve or worsen during pregnancy. Mild acne can be left untreated, but moderate cases can be treated safely with topical antibiotics such as erythromycin solution.

Several rashes specific to pregnancy also may occur. Pruritic urticarial papules and plaques of pregnancy (PUPPPs), seen in the last trimester of pregnancy, consist of pruritic erythematous papules and plaques that frequently begin in the abdominal striae during the third trimester (see Plate 10). The eruption may generalize. There is no increased incidence of fetal difficulties, and the rash clears spontaneously after delivery. Treatment is limited to symptomatic relief of pruritus.

Itching during pregnancy without skin rash (pruritus gravidarum) is usually caused by mild cholestatic hepatitis. This commonly begins in the third trimester. Excoriations may be present. The diagnosis is confirmed by elevated levels of alkaline phosphatase and/or bilirubin. Treatment is routinely symptomatic; in more severe cases, oral cholestyramine is administered.

ECCRINE AND APOCRINE DISORDERS

Hyperhidrosis (excessive sweating) and bromhidrosis (foul-smelling sweat) are relatively common complaints in adolescence and can cause anxiety and embarrassment. Sweat comes from two sources. Eccrine glands are located anywhere on the skin, with the highest concentration on the forehead, palms, and soles; these function throughout childhood and adolescence. In contrast, apocrine glands are quiescent during childhood, but in adolescence they become active under hormonal influence. Apocrine glands are located in the axillae, perineal area, and areolae of the breasts. When sweat reaches the surface of the skin, it is sterile and odorless, but bacterial action on the sweat and stratum corneum can produce a rather potent odor. This is found most commonly in the axillae and on the soles of the feet.

Hyperhidrosis can be treated with regular application of aluminum chloride to the affected area. A 20% aluminum chloride solution (Drysol) can be applied with plastic wrap occlusion nightly until decreased sweating is achieved; this is followed by intermittent application as needed. If irritation occurs, 7.5% aluminum chloride (Xerac AC) is usually well tolerated. Bromhidrosis also may respond to this treatment, particularly if an antibacterial soap (e.g., Dial or Hibiclens) is used. Dusting powders such as Zeasorb can be used on the feet to absorb excessive sweat.

Miliaria (heat rash) is a common skin condition. In adolescents it is seen most frequently with intense physical exertion, particularly when heavy protective padding or garments are worn, such as in school athletics. The lesions consist of multiple discrete erythematous papules and papulovesicles that can be asymptomatic or highly pruritic. They are caused by plugging of the eccrine ducts. When plugging occurs, the proximal duct ruptures and the extravasated sweat induces an inflammatory response. Because the duct always empties away from hair follicles, miliaria is never follicular in location, which helps to distinguish it from folliculitis. Management consists of preventing the hot, humid conditions from occurring, for example, by wearing lighter clothing and avoiding excessive exertion. Bland shake lotions, such as calamine, may be of limited benefit.

Hidradenitis suppurativa is a chronic inflammatory disease of the apocrine sweat glands. It is seen more frequently in females and blacks. The onset is usually during adolescence. Although the exact pathogenesis is not understood, the disease is believed to be caused by plugging of the apocrine duct, with consequent dilation and bacterial superinfection in a manner reminiscent of acne. There is a higher than expected incidence of hidradenitis in patients with cystic acne. Obesity and tropical climates are aggravating factors. Antiperspirants do not appear to cause hidradenitis suppurativa but may exacerbate it.

Lesions first appear as tender, flesh-colored nodules; they then enlarge into abscesses that drain and scar (see Plate 11). The lesions may form fistulous tracts to the skin and to contiguous abscesses. The sites of predilection are the axillae, buttocks, perianal area, and inguinal areas, reflecting the high concentration of apocrine glands in these sites. When they first appear, the lesions are frequently mistaken for furuncles, especially since *S.*

PARASITIC INFECTIONS

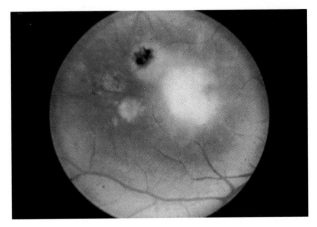

PLATE 1

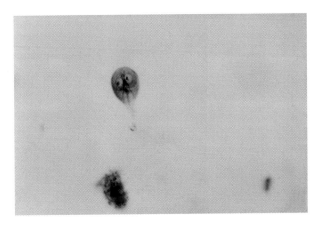

PLATE 2

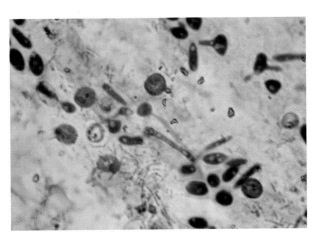

PLATE 3

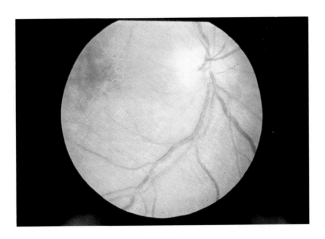

PLATE 4

PLATE 1   Toxoplasma chorioretinitis—old and new lesions (Courtesy of Dr. Herman Zaiman, Mercy Hospital, Valley City, N.D.).

PLATE 2   *Giardia lamblia* trophozoite showing the characteristic double nucleus and terminal axostyle. The 4 pairs of flagella are not evident.

PLATE 3   Oocysts of cryptosporidium showing their characteristically acid-fast staining.

PLATE 4   Ocular larva migrans—early invasion of the retina by *Toxocara canis* larva.

DERMATOLOGIC PROBLEMS

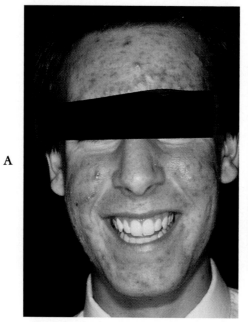
A

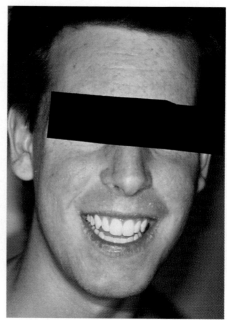
B

PLATE 5

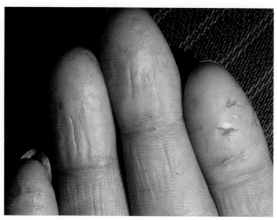

PLATE 6

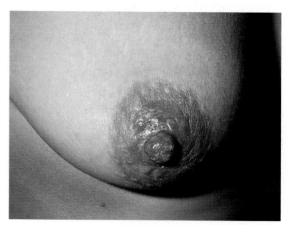

PLATE 7

PLATE 5   Severe inflammatory acne before (**A**) and following (**B**) treatment with isotretinoin. (From Acne in the pediatric population. The Child's Doctor 7:2, 1990. Copyright © 1990 The Children's Memorial Hospital, Chicago, Ill. Reprinted with permission.)

PLATE 6   Atopic dermatitis.

PLATE 7   Atopic dermatitis with nipple involvement.

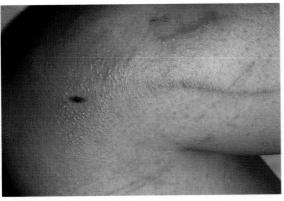

PLATE 8

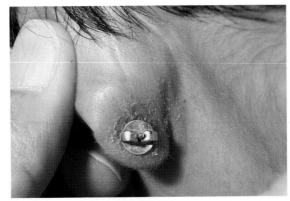

PLATE 9

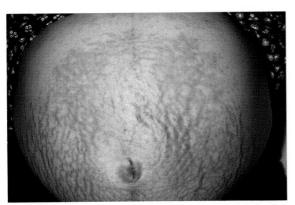

PLATE 10

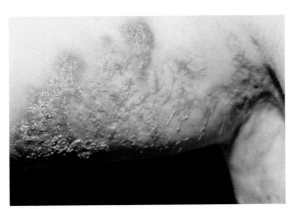

PLATE 11

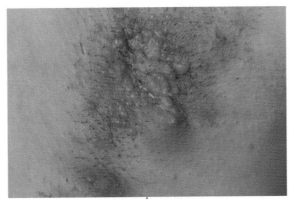

PLATE 12

PLATE 8   Poison oak. Linear streaks from contact with branches or leaves are common. Black resin in central area is uncommon, usually seen with large dose of inoculum.

PLATE 9   Nickel dermatitis.

PLATE 10   Pruritic urticarial papules and plaques of pregnancy.

PLATE 11   Hidradenitis suppurativa resulting in cysts, sinus tracts, and scarring in axilla. (Courtesy Leonard Winograd Memorial Slide Collection, Department of Dermatology, Stanford University Medical Center, Stanford, Calif.)

PLATE 12   Fox-Fordyce disease (apocrine miliaria). (Courtesy Leonard Winograd Memorial Slide Collection, Department of Dermatology, Stanford University Medical Center, Stanford, Calif.)

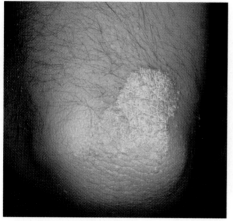

PLATE 13

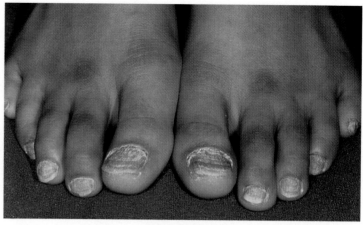

PLATE 14

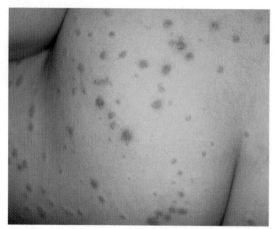

PLATE 15

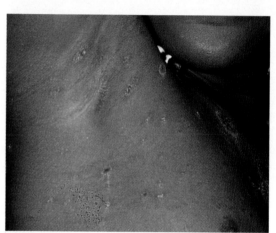

PLATE 16

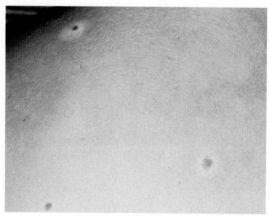

PLATE 17

PLATE 13 Psoriasis with well-circumscribed, thick plaque of scale overlying erythematous area of elbow.

PLATE 14 Psoriasis with pitting, discoloration, and onycholysis of toenails.

PLATE 15 Guttate psoriasis.

PLATE 16 Pityriasis rosea.

PLATE 17 Halo nevi. (Courtesy Leonard Winograd Memorial Slide Collection, Department of Dermatology, Stanford University Medical Center, Stanford, Calif.)

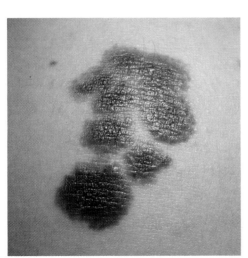

PLATE 18

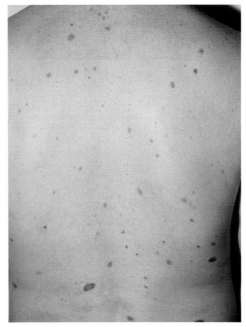

PLATE 19

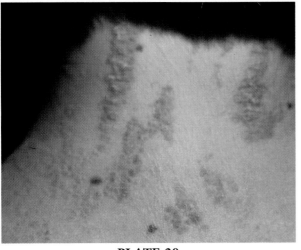

PLATE 20

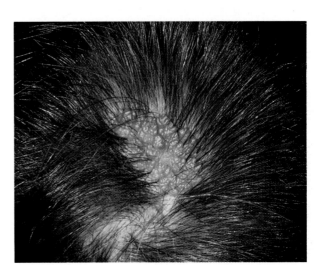

PLATE 21

PLATE 18   Large congenital melanocytic nevi.
PLATE 19   Dysplastic nevi.
PLATE 20   Epidermal nevi.
PLATE 21   Nevus sebaceus.

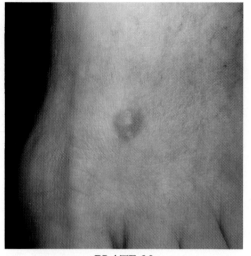

PLATE 22

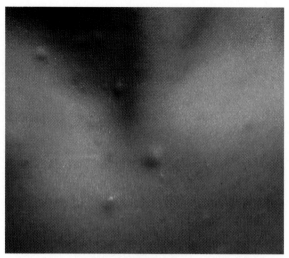

PLATE 23

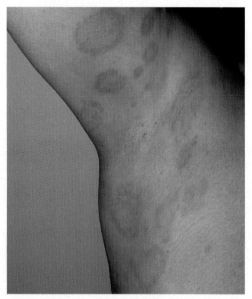

PLATE 24

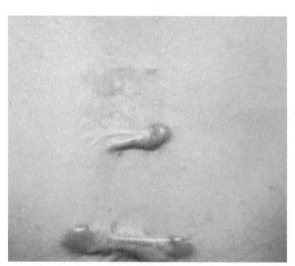

PLATE 25

PLATE 22   Dermatofibroma.
PLATE 23   Steatocystoma multiplex.
PLATE 24   Granuloma annulare.
PLATE 25   Postacne keloids.

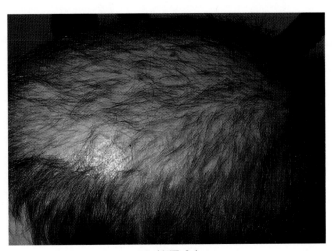

PLATE 26

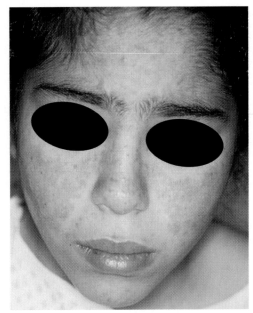

PLATE 27

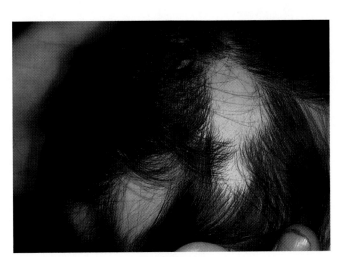

PLATE 28

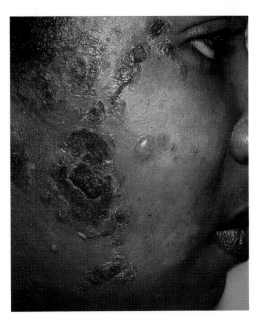

PLATE 29

PLATE 26 Trichotillomania.

PLATE 27 Malar flush ("butterfly" rash) of systemic lupus erythematosus with violaceous erythema and mild scaling in sun-exposed area.

PLATE 28 Alopecia areata.

PLATE 29 Extensive bullous impetigo.

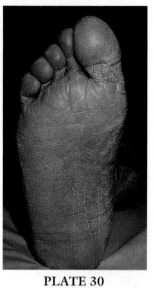

PLATE 30

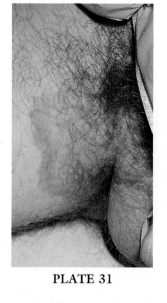

PLATE 31

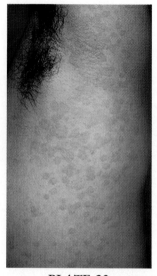

PLATE 32

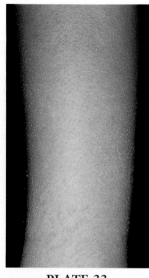

PLATE 33

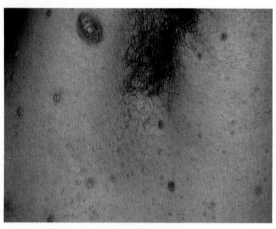

PLATE 34

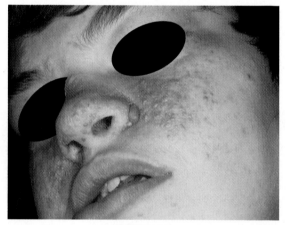

PLATE 35

PLATE 30 Tinea pedis with extensive scaling on plantar foot. This "moccasin form" is usually caused by *Trichophyton rubrum*. (From Frieden IJ. Tinea infections in adolescents. In Shapiro SC, Strasburger VC, Greydanus DE, eds. Adolescent Dermatology, vol 2, no 1, p 336. State of the Art Reviews. Adolescent Medicine. Philadelphia: Hanley & Belfus, 1990. Reprinted with permission.)

PLATE 31 Tinea cruris.

PLATE 32 Tinea versicolor with hyperpigmentation. (From Frieden IJ. Tinea infections in adolescents. In Shapiro SC, Strasburger VC, Greydanus DE, eds. Adolescent Dermatology, vol 2, no 1, p 338. State of the Art Reviews. Adolescent Medicine. Philadelphia: Hanley & Belfus, 1990. Reprinted with permission.)

PLATE 33 Ichthyosis vulgaris.

PLATE 34 Neurofibromatosis with axillary freckling and neurofibromas.

PLATE 35 Tuberous sclerosis.

aureus organisms sometimes can be cultured from the pus. The presence of multiple such lesions (noted by history or examination) or their occurrence in more than one area should help to confirm the diagnosis. The spectrum of disease severity is wide. Some patients have only an occasional lesion; others have a chronic, unremitting, painful, scarring process. Rarely, this severe form has been associated with fever, arthralgia, and anemia.

Treatment is notoriously difficult. In mild cases, oral antibiotics such as tetracycline, 1 to 2 g/day for several weeks, may be helpful. Useful adjunctive measures include cleansing with an antibacterial soap such as Hibiclens and use of topical antibiotics such as Cleocin. Intralesional triamcinolone injections may help to resolve the nodules. In severe cases in which scarring has occurred, surgery for removal of the apocrine glands may be the treatment of choice, especially in the axillae. Isotretinoin has been effective in some patients.

Fox-Fordyce disease (apocrine miliaria) is a relatively rare condition seen almost exclusively in women, with onset in adolescence or early adulthood. It consists of tiny, round follicular papules in the apocrine-bearing areas, particularly the axillae and areolae (see Plate 12). The major symptom is intense pruritus. The condition appears to be a form of superficial obstruction of the apocrine duct, with consequent sweat retention similar to the "prickly heat" seen in eccrine sweat retention. Hair growth and sweating are decreased or absent in the affected areas. Treatment is difficult, but most effective is administration of oral contraceptives. Topical corticosteroids may be of limited benefit in the disorder.

PAPULOSQUAMOUS DISORDERS

Psoriasis

Psoriasis is a common dermatologic disorder affecting 1% to 3% of the population. Significantly, in approximately 25% of those with psoriasis, the onset of disease occurs between the ages of 10 and 20 years. The pathogenesis of psoriasis has not been completely elucidated. Epidermal hyperproliferation and increased cell turnover of the epidermis are involved. The rapid turnover results in incomplete differentiation and leads to the accumulation of scale noted clinically. The exact factors leading to this hyperplasia and high rate of cell division are not precisely understood, but they may relate to immunologic factors, abnormal metabolism of inflammatory mediators, and abnormalities in the regulation of cell turnover.

Psoriasis is characterized by sharply circumscribed, scaly, erythematous plaques. Common sites of involvement are the scalp, elbows, knees, gluteal cleft, genitalia, and lumbosacral area, but any area of the skin can be affected (see Plate 13). Typical lesions have a silvery, micaceous scale, which may leave pinpoint bleeding when removed ("Auspitz's sign"). Scale may be less prominent on the genitalia and in intertriginous areas, owing to increased heat and moisture. Pruritus is variable but can be severe. Psoriasis has a tendency to occur in sites of local skin trauma (Koebner's phenomenon), a fact that is important in management of the disease. Well-circumscribed plaques in the scalp with adherent asbestos-like scale and minimal disease elsewhere are common findings in adolescents with psoriasis. The differential diagnosis includes eczema, tinea capitis, and seborrheic dermatitis.

Nail changes may be helpful in confirming the diagnosis of psoriasis (see Plate 14). Pitting is characteristic but nonspecific; patients without psoriasis occasionally develop a pit from trauma. Nailpitting may also be seen in other childhood disorders, particularly eczema and alopecia areata. Onycholysis (loosening of the distal nail from the nail bed) is probably the most common nail abnormality in psoriasis. Discoloration, nail grooving, and accumulation of subungual debris also may occur, mimicking onychomycosis.

Variant forms of psoriasis may be noted during adolescence. Psoriasis confined to intertriginous areas and the umbilicus is known as "inverse psoriasis." Guttate psoriasis (see Plate 15) first appears as the sudden onset of multiple small lesions, 2 to 10 mm in size, usually with truncal predominance. It frequently follows an upper respiratory infection, such as streptococcal pharyngitis. Antibiotics are indicated if streptococcal infection has been documented. Many cases of guttate psoriasis clear readily with treatment, but some evolve into more persistent disease.

Pustular psoriasis is rare in adolescence; the condition is difficult to treat, and its generalized form can be life-threatening. Erythrodermic psoriasis, which is also rare in adolescents, requires prompt medical attention. Psoriatic arthritis, although uncommon, can occur in adolescents with psoriasis. It most commonly presents as a seronegative polyarthritis involving both large and small joints.

Psoriasis is a disease characterized by remissions and exacerbations. Treatment depends on the extent and severity of disease. One important aspect of care is prevention. As mentioned previously, skin injury frequently causes new psoriatic lesions to develop. This may not be as important in patients with stable, limited disease, but patients with more labile disease should be very careful when shaving their legs, since small cuts frequently lead to psoriatic plaques on healing. Work with irritating or caustic substances can cause recalcitrant psoriasis of the palms. Adolescents who participate in sports may develop psoriasis at sites of frictional trauma, and therefore good padding is advisable.

Treatment of the scalp is similar to that of seborrheic dermatitis. In addition to steroid solutions, tar shampoos are extremely useful. If scalp involvement is severe, a tar oil or a mixture of phenol and saline in oil (Baker's P&S) can be used nightly and washed out in the morning.

Plaques on the body may respond to medium- to high-potency corticosteroids, but they may require the addition of either a keratolytic agent (e.g., Keralyt [6% salicylic acid]), or a tar, Lac-Hydrin lotion (12% ammonium lactate), cream, gel, or oil (e.g., Fototar, AquaTar, PsoriGel, Estar gel, or T-Derm), which can be applied once or twice a day. Other topical treatments include tar baths and the use of topical anthralin—a synthetic compound related to chrysarobin that produces the side effects of irritancy and red-brown staining of the skin. Most patients with psoriasis find that their skin improves when they are exposed to sunlight. Such exposure should be encouraged but with the caution that burning is unnecessary and, in fact, may result in exacerbation of psoriasis by way of Koebner's phenomenon. The observation that sunlight improves the condition has been incorporated into a treatment that combines ultraviolet B light and tar on a daily basis—the so-called Goeckerman regimen. This regimen should be undertaken only with the close supervision of a dermatologist.

Systemic therapies are reserved for patients with more severe generalized disease. Psoralen, a drug that produces a phototoxic effect, combined with ultraviolet A light (PUVA) is an effective treatment for psoriasis, but its long-term side effects include an increased risk of squamous cell carcinoma of the skin. There is a long-term risk of cataracts in patients who do not take precautions to shield the eyes from ultraviolet A light. This treatment probably should not be used in adolescents, except in the most recalcitrant cases for only a limited course of therapy. Weekly administration of methotrexate in low doses is effective in the treatment of psoriasis, but it can cause liver damage (with long-term use) and hematologic abnormalities. This agent should be used only when all other therapies have been exhausted and must be appropriately monitored by tests of hematologic and hepatic function. Etretinate and isotretinoin, synthetic vitamin A derivatives, are beneficial in some severe cases of psoriasis, particularly the erythrodermic and pustular forms, but retinoid treatment has many potential side effects and should be reserved for recalcitrant cases. Etretinate, a known teratogen, is generally contraindicated in women of childbearing potential because of its prolonged half-life.

Pityriasis Rosea

Pityriasis rosea is a benign, self-limited disorder that frequently develops in adolescents. The annual incidence rate is approximately 170 per 100,000 person years. The average age of onset is 22 years, with approximately 27% of cases occurring between ages 10 and 20 years. The cause of pityriasis rosea is not known, although a viral etiology is suspected.

Many patients have a "herald patch," a single oval, scaly plaque that precedes the eruption by 5 to 10 days. Subsequently, there is an eruption of oval papulosquamous lesions distributed on the trunk, neck, and extremities (see Plate 16). Occasionally, the lesions also occur on the face, especially the preauricular area. The distal extremities tend to be relatively spared, and the palms and soles are rarely involved. A variable degree of pruritus is present, but patients usually have no concomitant systemic complaints.

The lesions of pityriasis rosea follow the skin lines of cleavage, leading to the "fir tree" distribution on the chest and back. The outer axilla is a particularly useful place to look, since it is a common site of involvement and the lines of cleavage are particularly distinctive in this area. Another helpful hint is the presence of a collarette of scale. Although classic lesions are oval-pink with a fine collarette of scale, pityriasis rosea can be eczematous, hemorrhagic, annular, or diffusely papular. The diagnosis is made from a constellation of findings: history of onset, morphology, distribution, and lack of other etiologic agents. Skin biopsy findings tend to be nonspecific. The differential diagnosis includes secondary syphilis, a drug eruption, papular eczema, and guttate psoriasis. The disease remits spontaneously, usually in 4 to 6 weeks, but it may persist for a few months; it rarely recurs. Treatment is supportive and consists of emollients, topical corticosteroids in eczematous and pruritic cases, and oral antihistamines for severe itching.

Mucha-Habermann disease (pityriasis lichenoides et varioliformis acuta) is an unusual disorder with a peak incidence during childhood. It consists of crops of papules, vesicles, and occasionally necrotic (varioliform) lesions that crust over and gradually resolve, at times leaving pitted scarring. Lesions are most frequently seen on the extremities and trunk, but any area can be affected. The crops of vesicular lesions, crusting, and scarring are reminiscent of "chronic chickenpox," but a viral cause has never been proved. Diagnosis is made by biopsy, which reveals a lymphocytic vasculitis. The disease is limited to the skin.

Treatment may be unsuccessful, but many cases respond to oral tetracycline or erythromycin. Ultraviolet light, in the form of either natural sunlight or artificial ultraviolet irradiation, is often helpful. Longer-wave ultraviolet light (UVA) with oral psoralen may be efficacious but should be used only for a limited time because of its long-term side effects, including the potential for skin cancer.

Pityriasis lichenoides chronica may appear de novo or may represent the evolution of the more acute Mucha-

Habermann disease into a chronic phase. Scaly papules are present, but pustules, vesicles, and necrotic lesions are absent in this form. When resolution occurs, extensive pigmentary changes may persist, particularly in dark-skinned persons. Individual lesions tend to resolve gradually and the eruption can continue for many years. Treatment is similar to that for Mucha-Habermann disease. No systemic abnormalities are found and the later development of lymphoreticular malignancy has rarely been reported.

Lichen planus is most common in adults over the age of 30 but can be seen during adolescence. The cause is unknown. The primary lesions are small, violaceous, flat-topped papules found most frequently on the flexural surfaces of the arms and legs and on the genitalia. On close inspection, delicate white lines (Wickham's striae) may be seen on the surface of the papules. The cutaneous lesions tend to be very pruritic and often leave intense hyperpigmentation on resolution. Mucous membrane lesions are found in up to 70% of patients; they consist of tiny white papules that form lacelike patterns on the buccal mucosa. Occasionally, patients also demonstrate nail dystrophy.

The diagnosis usually can be made clinically, but a biopsy may be necessary to confirm the diagnosis. In most patients the condition clears spontaneously after approximately 1 year of recurrent bouts of lesions. Local symptomatic treatment with topical or intralesional steroids may be beneficial. Antihistamines, such as hydroxyzine, may help for pruritus. Short courses of systemic steroids may be required for severe cases. Mucous membrane lesions usually require no treatment unless they are symptomatic.

PIGMENTED NEVI, NODULES, AND PAPULES

Pigmented nevus cell nevi continue to appear frequently during adolescence. They usually appear as flat, darkly pigmented junctional nevi. Over decades, they slowly progress to benign, elevated, compound, or intradermal nevi. Halo nevi, also called leukoderma acquisition centrifugum, appear commonly as junctional or compound nevi surrounded by a zone of depigmentation. The central nevus eventually may disappear by means of an autoimmune mechanism. Lesions develop more commonly in adolescents than in older adults, and they may be associated with a personal or family history of vitiligo (see Plate 17).

Changes in already existing nevi, such as enlarging size and darkening of pigmentation, also occur. With a heightened public awareness of melanoma, many patients and parents may become concerned about a change in one or more moles. Although melanoma is rare in adoles-

cence, it does occur. Situations of particular concern are changes in congenital nevi (see Plate 18) and changes in nevi of a patient with a family history of melanoma or with atypical nevi. In these situations the patient should be referred to a dermatologist for further evaluation. In addition, the physician should become familiar with the early signs of malignant melanoma, such as disproportionately rapid growth, focal increase or loss of pigment, irregularity of contour, bleeding, ulceration, itching, and inflammation. If there is any question of an abnormality, or if parental or patient anxiety is high, a referral should be made to a dermatologist for evaluation.

The dysplastic nevus syndrome is characterized by multiple nevi that tend to be larger than normal nevi (>6 mm), to be irregular in outline and color, and to have an irregular surface (see Plate 19). The nevi are found most frequently on the trunk and upper extremities, but they are also seen on the buttocks, groin, and scalp. This disorder may be inherited as an autosomal dominant condition (B-K mole syndrome or familial dysplastic nevus syndrome) or may occur sporadically. Patients with dysplastic nevi have an increased risk of the development of melanoma, and the dysplastic nevi themselves may transform into melanoma. The prognosis for melanomas arising in dysplastic nevi is slightly better than for other melanomas, but extremely close follow-up with a dermatologist is necessary to watch for further changes in other dysplastic nevi.

Epidermal nevi are hamartomas of the epidermis that either are present at birth or develop shortly thereafter. During adolescence, epidermal nevi frequently become more verrucous and elevated (see Plate 20). Occasionally they extend to previously normal-appearing skin.

Epidermal nevi vary in color from light to dark brown. They may consist of a few small, warty-looking papules or may be extensive, with large plaques or linear arrays of lesions. Particularly during adolescence, they may become macerated and develop an odor from bacterial overgrowth. Pruritus is variable and can be bothersome to some patients. Unfortunately, excision is the only definitive treatment when problems occur. Malignant degeneration is rare. Epidermal nevi may be associated with skeletal, CNS, and other systemic abnormalities, but these abnormalities are generally recognized before adolescence. The cause of epidermal nevi is unknown, but one type has recently been shown to result from gene mosaicism for a mutation for a keratin gene.

Nevus sebaceus of Jadassohn is present at birth and represents a hamartomatous collection of sebaceous glands. In the newborn period these lesions are generally flat, well-circumscribed, hairless plaques. They are usually on the scalp or face. During adolescence, the sebaceous glands within the nevi hypertrophy and the nevi become more elevated, often with a verrucous surface (see Plate 21). Approximately 10% to 20% of these nevi develop secondary neoplastic changes. These include basal cell carcinoma and syringocystadenoma papilliferum. For this reason full-thickness excision of these lesions is usually recommended.

Dermatofibromas are benign dermal lesions that are more common in adolescents than in young children. They are among the most common benign skin tumors in adults. Dermatofibromas are firm nodules, usually measuring from 1 to 4 mm in size, and often have a hyperpigmented, slightly scaly surface (see Plate 22). The tumor is embedded within the dermis and moves freely over subcutaneous fat. The most common location is on the legs, but dermatofibromas may be seen on other parts of the body. They are usually solitary and appear de novo or after trauma to the skin (e.g., from an insect bite). The diagnosis can be established either by the typical clinical appearance or through biopsy. No treatment is necessary, but if removal is desired for cosmetic reasons, complete excision is necessary to avoid recurrence.

Epidermal inclusion cysts can occur at any age but are frequently seen during adolescence in association with acne. Many people refer to these cysts as "sebaceous cysts," but this term is inaccurate since the cyst lining is epidermal in origin and the contents of the cyst are keratin, not sebum. True sebaceous cysts occur in steatocystoma multiplex, an autosomal dominantly inherited condition in which multiple cysts containing an oily material appear on the trunk and extremities. Cysts can occur in areas of acne or trauma, or they may form de novo. Initially, they are cystic nodules with normal skin overlying them. Sometimes a small follicular punctum is visible, connecting the center of the cyst to the surface of the skin. Cyst size may vary from a few millimeters to several centimeters.

If cysts rupture, keratin is released into the dermis and an inflammatory foreign body reaction may be elicited. At this time the cysts are tender, warm, red, and filled with purulent material. Because of this, they are frequently mistaken for bacterial abscesses and treated with antibiotics. Cultures are either sterile or show the presence of *Staphylococcus epidermidis*.

Treatment should consist of expression of the contents of the cyst with as small an incision as possible and intralesional corticosteroid injection with 0.1 to 0.3 ml triamcinolone acetonide, 5 to 10 mg/ml. With this treatment, there is usually prompt resolution of acute inflammation. Some cysts resolve after they become inflamed; others persist and may be surgically excised when inflammation subsides. Cysts that have not been previously ruptured may be left alone or excised, depending on the size and patient preference.

Steatocystoma multiplex is a relatively rare condition characterized by the appearance of multiple 2- to 4-mm cystic nodules, primarily on the chest, with occasional involvement of the face, arms, and thighs (see Plate 23).

The onset is usually during adolescence. The disorder is inherited in an autosomal dominant manner. Initial lesions are usually thought to be epidermal cysts, but the appearance of multiple lesions and the characteristic skin histopathology help to confirm the diagnosis. There is no effective treatment, although individual lesions that are bothersome may be excised.

Granuloma annulare is a relatively common skin disorder of unknown cause, often occurring in adolescence. Typical lesions of this disease appear as smooth plaques or coalescing papules with little or no epidermal involvement (see Plate 24). They have an accentuated border and a clearing center; hence, the term *annulare*. The lesions vary in size from a few millimeters to several centimeters. They may be flesh-colored, pink, dull-red, or violaceous. Characteristic locations include the dorsal aspects of the hands, feet, elbows, and knees, but lesions may be found elsewhere. When granuloma annulare is located in the subcutaneous tissue of the skin, it may be mistaken for a rheumatoid nodule, which it closely resembles histologically. Unlike rheumatoid nodules associated with rheumatoid arthritis, granuloma annulare has no associated systemic symptoms. The differential diagnosis includes sarcoidosis, lichen planus, and sometimes erythema multiforme. On first glance it may be confused with tinea corporis because of its annular configuration, but tinea corporis shows scaling, whereas granuloma annulare does not.

Diagnosis of granuloma annulare can be made clinically or by skin biopsy. In most cases the lesions involute spontaneously within 2 years, but in some patients lesions persist for many years. Treatment is not necessary unless the lesions are pruritic or cosmetically disturbing to the patient. High-potency steroids under occlusion or intralesional triamcinolone acetonide may hasten the resolution of lesions.

Keloids are scars in which fibroblasts produce excessive collagen. They are fairly common, especially in darkly pigmented individuals, and the tendency toward keloids is often inherited. They can begin at any site of injury and occasionally appear without known previous trauma. Acne scars and sites of ear piercing are frequent locations in adolescents. Although keloids are cosmetically distressing, they do not tend to become malignant. They should be differentiated from hypertrophic scars, which are seen within the first 6 months of injury, stay within the boundaries of the existing area of trauma, and tend to flatten with time. In contrast, keloids extend beyond the original area of trauma and do not resolve spontaneously (see Plate 25). They are usually pink and firm and may be tender or pruritic.

Treatment usually involves administration of intralesional triamcinolone acetonide, 10 to 40 mg/ml, repeated every month for several months until flattening has been achieved. Reinjection at a later time is sometimes necessary. Cryotherapy coupled with intralesional steroids and reexcision with injections are alternative therapies. Reexcision, however, often results in regrowth and enlargement of the keloid.

Syringomas are benign tumors of eccrine origin. They are seen predominantly in female patients, and the onset is frequently during adolescence. The lesions are usually multiple, firm, skin-colored to yellowish papules 1 to 3 mm in size. Several papules may merge to form small plaques. The lesions are most commonly found on the lower eyelids, but they may be on the face, neck, and chest. The diagnosis can be made clinically or by the characteristic skin histopathology. Treatment is unnecessary except for cosmetic reasons. Electrodesiccation, excision, and cryotherapy have been used as treatment.

PSYCHODERMATOSES

Psychological factors can influence the course of many common skin diseases, including atopic dermatitis, acne, psoriasis, seborrheic dermatitis, and dyshidrotic eczema. Another group of skin diseases are actually caused by the secondary manipulation of skin, hair, or nails, usually as a response to psychological factors. These diseases often have their onset during adolescence.

The two most common forms of this behavior during adolescence are the manipulation of acne lesions and nail biting. Although the squeezing of pimples is an extremely common response to acne, excessive manipulation of acne can result in scarring and worsening of the condition. The best management of this problem is effective acne therapy to decrease the number of comedones and inflammatory lesions. A minority of patients, however, engage in this activity to an extreme degree by either digging deeply into their skin or by creating lesions where none exist. This is probably more common in young women ("acne excoriée de jeune fille"), but it also can occur in men. This situation should be suspected in patients with numerous scabbed areas but only a few inflammatory lesions. Occasionally the lesions can be quite deep and disfiguring. Excessive or deep manipulation of acne lesions should prompt a psychiatric evaluation.

Trichotillomania is a disorder in which hair is compulsively pulled out or broken (see Plate 26). The scalp is the most commonly affected site, but occasionally the eyebrows, eyelashes, and even the pubic hair may be involved. Trichotillomania is not a rare disorder during adolescence, and it is more common in female than in male teenagers. Extensive areas of scalp hair may be pulled out and the patient may be nearly bald; typically, a fringe of frontal hair is left intact. In some cases, smaller circular or linear patches may be present. Close inspection of the scalp usually reveals short broken hairs, often with focal areas of hemorrhage or excoriations. Some patients with trichotillomania are unaware or deny that they are pulling out their hair, making the diagnosis more difficult. The differential diagnosis includes tinea capitis (excluded by KOH examination and fungal culture of short broken hairs), damage from improper use of chemicals applied to the hair (permanents or hair dyes), and alopecia areata, in which the affected patch is generally devoid of hair and rarely shows the stubbled appearance of trichotillomania. If the diagnosis is in doubt, a scalp biopsy demonstrating empty hair follicles, perifollicular hemorrhage, and increased numbers of catagen hairs usually helps to differentiate these disorders.

During adolescence, trichotillomania is often a subconscious response to stressful events, and the condition resolves when the stress becomes less intense. Like nail biting, it does not necessarily denote severe psychopathology. Nevertheless, it can be a distressing habit; if persistent, it may indicate more severe psychological problems such as an obsessive-compulsive disorder or even psychosis. Management may be difficult, but confronting the patient with the problem, along with supportive counseling or behavioral therapy, may be helpful. The tricyclic antidepressant drug clomipramine also has proved helpful.

Neurotic excoriations can be seen in areas of acne but also occur elsewhere on the body, including sites with no previous skin disease. These superficial excoriations or deeper ulcerations usually are found on the face or arms and have a characteristic linear pattern. In factitial dermatitis the patient may use external agents, such as acids, alkalis, or cigarettes, to produce injury to the skin. Patients with delusions of parasitosis are convinced that their skin (and sometimes other body parts) are infested with bugs. Similar ideation may be caused by the ingestion of certain drugs, particularly cocaine. All three conditions—neurotic excoriations, factitial dermatitis, and delusions of parasitosis—are associated with significant psychopathology and are difficult to treat. Psychiatric consultation is advised.

IMMUNE-MEDIATED DISORDERS

Lupus erythematosus, although rare in early childhood, is seen with increasing frequency during adolescence. It is more common in female patients, especially blacks. Both the degree and the type of skin involvement vary widely. The most common skin lesion is the discoid lesion, characterized by sharply marginated, violaceous, scaly plaques with telangiectasias, atrophy, and pigmentary changes. Discoid lesions are most commonly seen on the face and scalp but may occur on the extremities and trunk. Most patients with discoid lupus skin lesions show no evidence of systemic lupus erythematosus, but a few patients later develop manifestations of systemic disease. As a result, monitoring for clinical or serologic changes is important. Scarring alopecia is another manifestation of lupus erythematosus that may be seen in both cutaneous and systemic types.

Additional cutaneous manifestations of lupus noted in patients with systemic disease include (1) fixed urticarial plaques often seen on sun-exposed areas; (2) frontal hair breakage or generalized thinning of the hair; (3) livedo reticularis, a mottled blue discoloration, especially of the lower extremities; (4) a malar flush ("butterfly" rash), which is not specific for lupus erythematosus (see Plate 27); (5) vasculitis, with or without ulceration; (6) telangiectasias, especially palmar or periungual; (7) mucosal inflammation, hemorrhage, or ulcerations; (8) bullae; and (9) Raynaud's phenomenon (vasospasm of digital arterioles in response to cold).

The diagnosis of cutaneous lupus can be confirmed by skin biopsy, with both conventional light microscopy and immunofluorescent staining for the deposition of immunoglobulins at the dermal-epidermal junction. In systemic lupus, clinically normal skin as well as involved skin may show a granular deposition of immunoglobulins and complement at this junction. The serologic evaluation of patients with cutaneous lupus should include antinuclear antibody, serum complements, anti–double-stranded DNA, anti-Ro and anti-La antibodies, sedimentation rate, and a complete blood count with differential and platelet count. If indicated, other tests should be ordered for a complete review of systems and physical examination. Treatment of active skin disease depends on the severity of involvement. Localized disease may be treated with high-potency topical or intralesional steroids. The scarring alopecia of lupus should be treated promptly, since it may respond to therapy and prevent permanent hair loss. More severe cutaneous disease may require the administration of oral antimalarial agents such as hydroxychloroquine. Systemic disease often requires systemic corticosteroids or other immunosuppressive agents.

Scleroderma is uncommon during adolescence. When it does occur, it is usually limited to localized areas of the skin, a form referred to as *morphea*. The trunk and proximal extremities are most often affected. In *linear morphea* the sclerosis involves one extremity or one side of the face. This form is rare, but when it does occur it frequently begins in late childhood or early adolescence. The muscle, fat, and bone in the affected area also may become sclerotic, causing a significant cosmetic deformity. In both localized and linear morphea, the skin is firm and bound-down, with ill-defined sclerotic plaques. The plaques may be depigmented centrally with a violaceous halo peripherally, and they often become more pigmented as the lesion ages. The diagnosis can be confirmed by skin

biopsy. Laboratory evaluation sometimes demonstrates a positive rheumatoid factor, ANA, or positive anti–single-stranded DNA antibodies, particularly in the linear form. There is no effective treatment, but physical therapy may help to preserve limb function in the linear form.

Henoch-Schönlein purpura is a vasculitis seen most commonly in school-age children and adolescents. It appears to be a hypersensitivity reaction, often to a recent viral or bacterial infection, and results in localized or widespread vascular damage. The skin disease is characterized by crops of nonblanching papules and urticarial plaques that become hemorrhagic. Other features include abdominal pain, melena, arthritis, and nephritis. Hepatosplenomegaly, scrotal swelling, CNS effects, and pulmonary involvement are unusual manifestations. Most patients recover without therapy. The prognosis is slightly poorer, however, for older children because of the higher incidence of renal involvement. The value of corticosteroid therapy remains controversial. Other causes of vasculitis in adolescence are rare but include drug reactions, systemic lupus erythematosus, and sepsis (including gonococcal).

Erythema nodosum is a septal panniculitis characterized by erythematous, tender nodules, usually in the pretibial areas. It is thought to be a hypersensitivity reaction with a variety of possible underlying etiologies. Among these are recent streptococcal or other respiratory infection, sarcoidosis, tuberculosis, deep fungal infections, drug reactions (including birth control pills), pregnancy, and inflammatory bowel disease. The cause often remains obscure, and extensive laboratory work-up is probably unnecessary unless the condition recurs frequently.

The lesions are often symmetric and become bruise-like in appearance after a few days. New lesions may appear for up to several weeks, and rarely the condition becomes chronic. Fever, malaise, and arthralgia may be associated signs. The diagnosis usually can be made on clinical grounds, but histologic confirmation may be helpful in atypical cases. If known, the underlying cause should be treated. Otherwise, treatment includes bed rest, leg elevation, and administration of salicylates or other nonsteroidal antiinflammatory agents.

Alopecia areata is one of the most common causes of hair loss in adolescents. Round, well-circumscribed patches of alopecia develop within days of onset (see Plate 28). The underlying scalp appears normal and is usually completely devoid of hair. The hair at the margin of the alopecia tends to pull out easily during active disease. Localized loss of hair in the beard area is sometimes seen. Occasionally, the alopecia may be more diffuse, with complete loss of scalp, eyebrow, eyelash, or body hair. Nail dystrophy is seen in 10% of patients. Rarely, thyroiditis or other autoimmune disease is present.

The diagnosis is usually made clinically, although a scalp biopsy may be helpful if the pattern is atypical. Trichotillomania, with broken hairs of different lengths and irregular patches, and tinea capitis, usually with scalp scaling, must be distinguished. The prognosis is better in adolescence than in early childhood. In mild disease, with one or a few patches, 95% of patients experience regrowth within a year. More extensive involvement portends a much poorer prognosis. About 30% of patients experience recurrent hair loss. It is difficult to assess therapy in view of spontaneous regrowth. Potent topical steroids or intralesional steroid injections appear to accelerate regrowth but probably do not influence the overall prognosis.

Other treatment regimens include anthralin therapy, topical minoxidil, PUVA therapy, and contact sensitization. Supportive counseling, either individually or through alopecia areata support groups, is extremely important in cases of extensive hair loss. In such cases, the patient should also be given information about manufacturers of high-quality wigs.

CUTANEOUS INFECTIONS

Several cutaneous infections caused by bacteria, fungi, and viruses are common during adolescence; these include impetigo, bacterial folliculitis, tinea versicolor, tinea pedis, tinea cruris, and warts. Sexually transmitted diseases of the skin, such as molluscum and human papillomavirus, are discussed in Chapter 140, "Sexually Transmitted Diseases."

Impetigo is a superficial skin infection, usually caused by *S. aureus* or group A streptococcus. The most frequent sites of involvement in adolescents are the face, neck, and extremities. Lesions may be bullous (see Plate 29) or crusted. The bullous-type lesions are usually caused by *S. aureus,* phage group II. Crustaceous lesions are characterized by honey-colored crusts on an erythematous base; most result from *S. aureus* but some are caused by group A streptococcus. Associated adenopathy of regional lymph nodes and fever are occasionally seen.

Small, very localized areas of impetigo can be treated with topical antibiotics (e.g., bacitracin or mupirocin) applied three times a day. More extensive areas should be treated with either cephalexin (250 mg three times a day), dicloxacillin (250 mg four times a day), or if the patient is penicillin allergic, erythromycin (250 mg four times a day for 7 to 10 days). Heavily crusted areas may be soaked with an aluminum acetate solution (Burow's solution) to cleanse the area of accumulated debris.

Bacterial folliculitis is usually caused by infection with *S. aureus*. Erythema and tiny pustules are seen at the orifices of hair follicles. Lesions are most commonly on the scalp and the extremities but may be seen on the face,

especially in the beard area in male patients, and on the legs in women who shave their legs. Mild localized folliculitis often resolves through topical therapy with mupirocin. Extensive or recurrent folliculitis may be treated with oral erythromycin or dicloxacillin as well as with the regular use of antibacterial soaps (e.g., Hibiclens or pHisoDerm). Recurrent bacterial folliculitis should prompt an evaluation of other family members, including nasal cultures to determine whether one or more is a nasal carrier of *S. aureus*. Oral rifampin or intranasal mupirocin given in conjunction with oral dicloxacillin may help in clearing the nasal carriage of *S. aureus*.

Folliculitis in the beard area should be differentiated from pseudofolliculitis barbae, a noninfectious inflammatory process. Folliculitis is seen most commonly in blacks or individuals with kinky hair. It is due to shaved hairs that become ingrown, eliciting a foreign body reaction in the skin. Management is difficult unless shaving is avoided entirely.

During adolescence, *Candida albicans* is a common cause of intertrigo, involving either the inguinal folds, the axillae, or the inframammary area in large-breasted females. Involved skin, which is intensely erythematous, is characterized by scaling and by papules and pustules at the periphery (satellite lesions). A KOH preparation that demonstrates spores and pseudohyphae may help confirm the diagnosis, although false-negative results may occur. Treatment consists of topical application of anticandidal cream, such as nystatin, miconazole, or clotrimazole cream, used two to three times daily.

Dermatophyte infections are superficial skin, hair, and nail infections caused by a group of fungi dermatophytes. Although many body sites may be affected, the feet (tinea pedis), inguinal folds (tinea cruris), and toenails (tinea unguium) are the most common sites during adolescence. Fungal hair infection (tinea capitis) was once rare after the age of 10 years but is becoming more common.

Tinea pedis commonly causes toe-web scaling, but it may cause diffuse scaling and hyperkeratosis of the soles of the feet as well as erythema and vesiculation (see Plate 30). Tinea cruris causes scaling in the crural folds with a discrete accentuated border and often with central clearing (see Plate 31). In male patients the scrotum is usually spared. Tinea capitis may cause patchy hair loss with broken hairs, or it can be associated with a diffuse, seborrheic dermatitis–like scaling with little evidence of hair loss.

The diagnosis of tinea may be established with a KOH wet mount of scale, demonstrating hyphae. In tinea of the skin, branching hyphae are present, whereas in tinea capitis, arthrospores are seen either within or surrounding the hairs. All suspected nail or hair infections should be cultured on Sabouraud's agar or Mycosel growth medium to confirm the diagnosis, since prolonged oral antifungal therapy is required for treatment of tinea capitis.

The treatment of localized tinea infections of the skin consists of application of topical antifungal agents such as clotrimazole, miconazole, or econazole. More extensive lesions, recalcitrant conditions, tinea capitis, and tinea unguium require treatment with oral griseofulvin, 250 to 500 mg twice daily, or new antifungal agents, such as itraconazole. The duration of therapy depends on the site being treated. Toenail infections usually require 12 to 18 months of treatment with griseofulvin and tend to recur after therapy is stopped. Treatment of toenail infections with itraconazole, 200 to 400 mg good for 1 week of each month for 4 to 6 months, is also effective. Itraconazole is retained in the nail for months after termination of administration. Adjunctive therapy for tinea pedis involves minimizing exposure of the feet to warmth or moisture. This is accomplished by avoiding nylon socks or occlusive footwear, by using absorbent powder (e.g., Zeasorb or Desenex), and, if necessary, by using antiperspirants (e.g., Drysol) to minimize hyperhidrosis.

Tinea versicolor, an extremely common disorder in adolescents, is caused by the overgrowth of a saprophytic yeast, *Pityrosporum orbiculare* (see Plate 32). Lesions are most common on the trunk and upper extremities, but they may occur virtually anywhere, including the face and lower extremities. The lesions may be mildly erythematous and hyperpigmented or hypopigmented, but they are rarely symptomatic, although mild pruritus may be present. The infection frequently worsens in warm weather.

The diagnosis can be made easily on clinical grounds and confirmed by KOH wet mounts that show clusters of spores and thick, short mycelia. Because the *Pityrosporum* organism is a normal skin inhabitant, its complete eradication cannot be achieved. The most effective means of controlling the overgrowth without excessive cost is to use either selenium sulfide lotion, 2.5%, or a zinc pyrithione lotion, commonly found in dandruff shampoos (e.g., Danex or DHS Zinc). The medication is applied for 2 to 12 hours two to three times a week for the first month of therapy, then decreased in frequency to prevent recurrence. Alternative treatments include topical miconazole and clotrimazole, but these are more costly and no more effective. Oral ketoconazole, taken as 400 mg in a single dose, is often effective but may need to be repeated if the eruption recurs.

Warts are a very common skin infection of adolescents. The hands are the most common site, but infection of the plantar surface of the feet (plantar warts) is also common. Common warts, if untreated, usually disappear spontaneously within 2 years, but in addition to possible symptoms of pain or bleeding, most adolescents are self-conscious about their appearance and want them removed.

Since no specific antiviral therapy for common warts has been developed, virtually all treatments are nonspecific, causing localized irritation, damage to the stratum corneum and epidermis (where the infection occurs), or production of a subepidermal blister in an attempt to remove the wart or to enhance immunologic reaction to it. Cryotherapy with liquid nitrogen, a common and effective treatment, is particularly well suited to one or two warts on the hand, since the pain involved is tolerable and the response is usually rapid. Multiple hand warts or plantar warts are more practically treated with keratolytics containing salicyclic or lactic acid (e.g., DuoFilm, Occlusal, Mediplast). The preparations in plasters or patches are particularly helpful for plantar warts; those in a liquid form are best for hand warts. Treatment may require weeks to months for resolution of the warts, and occasionally warts persist or spread despite these treatments. In such cases, referral to a dermatologist is advised. A 2- to 3-month course of cimetidine, 30 to 40 mg/kg/day, has been found to clear warts in some patients, presumably because of its immunomodulatory effects.

GENODERMATOSES

A number of dermatologic conditions are hereditary. Although some of these conditions are rare, the physician seeing adolescents should have some familiarity with the genodermatoses that have their onset during adolescence. Other conditions may be present during childhood, but their course is modified during adolescence.

The ichthyoses are a group of scaling disorders of varying genetic patterns, etiologies, and clinical features. The most common of these is ichthyosis vulgaris an autosomal dominant disorder found in approximately 1 in 500 persons. It is characterized by generalized fine scaling, especially on the lower extremities (see Plate 33) and hyperlinear palms and soles, but sparing of the flexural creases. The condition tends to improve during adolescence. Atopic diseases, such as eczema, hay fever, and asthma, may be associated with this disorder.

X-linked ichthyosis, which occurs less commonly, is caused by an absence of a sulfatase enzyme. It is inherited in an X-linked recessive manner. This form of ichthyosis is characterized by large brown scales involving all areas, including the face and flexural creases, but sparing the palms and soles. It frequently worsens during adolescence.

Patients with lamellar ichthyosis usually have severe scaling of the skin, including flexural creases, palms, and soles. Ectropion is almost always present and can result in keratitis. The condition tends to remain stable during adolescence. It is an autosomal recessive disorder that may result from mutations in the gene that codes for transglutaminase I, an enzyme necessary for normal maturation of skin.

Epidermolytic hyperkeratosis is a form of ichthyosis characterized by small, verrucous, and hyperkeratotic scales that are most prominent on the extensor surfaces and in flexural and intertriginous areas. The palms and soles are often hyperkeratotic. Superficial blistering is associated and secondary bacterial infections are common. The condition tends to remain stable but can worsen during adolescence. It is an autosomal dominant condition that occurs owing to mutations in keratin 1 or 10 genes.

The ichthyoses are all improved somewhat by topical emollients and keratolytic agents, including lactic and salicylic acids, topical retinoic acid, and urea. Treatment of the more severe ichthyoses is difficult. Retinoids such as isotretinoin and etretinate are often useful in high doses, but their use can lead to adverse side effects, including abnormalities of bone growth, so they are not generally recommended for an adolescent.

Darier's disease (keratosis follicularis) is an autosomal dominant disorder that usually has its onset during late childhood or adolescence. It is characterized by skin-colored papules that quickly become darker and covered with a greasy scale, and may coalesce into plaques. The eruption is generally symmetric and most commonly occurs in the seborrheic distribution—on the midface, behind the ears, in the scalp, and on the anterior chest. Punctate keratoses or pits are commonly seen on the palms and soles. The condition flares in warm weather. Pruritus is often severe and secondary bacterial infections may occur. The diagnosis is made by characteristic findings on skin biopsy. Treatment may be difficult and many modalities, including keratolytics, topical corticosteroids, and tar preparations, have been used. Systemic retinoids also may be helpful for patients with Darier's disease but are not recommended for adolescents.

Familial benign chronic pemphigus (Hailey-Hailey disease) is usually first seen in the late teens or early twenties. It is inherited in an autosomal dominant fashion, with incomplete penetrance. In 70% of affected individuals there is a positive family history. The primary lesions are grouped blisters that quickly rupture and leave an eroded base covered with crust, resembling impetigo. The border of the lesions is often serpiginous. Sites of predilection are the neck, axillae, groin, and flexural surfaces. The diagnosis is established by skin biopsy of an affected area. As in Darier's disease, lesions worsen during the summer and with exposure to ultraviolet light. The disease tends to run a chronic course with exacerbations and spontaneous improvement. Although no treatment is universally effective, systemic and topical antibiotics may be helpful. In severe cases, excision with grafting of affected areas may produce long-term improvement.

Epidermolysis bullosa refers to a group of hereditary blistering diseases that have different hereditary patterns, different levels of cleavage in the skin, and varied clinical manifestations. Although a complete review of these conditions is not possible here, several points should be emphasized. Blistering in scarring forms of epidermolysis bullosa appears early in life. These types may be inherited in either an autosomal dominant or recessive manner and result from collagen VII gene mutations. Squamous cell and basal cell carcinomas of the skin have been reported in these conditions, often during the adolescent years. The nonscarring forms usually are first seen early in life and tend to improve with age. The exception is Weber-Cockayne syndrome in which recurrent blisters appear after trauma and are usually limited to the hands and feet. This is an autosomal dominant condition often first manifested during adolescence and due to mutations in keratins 5 or 14.

Oculocutaneous albinism is a heterogeneous group of disorders manifested by congenital depigmentation of hair, skin, and eyes. The extent of eye pigmentation, photophobia, and nystagmus depends on the type of albinism. The major cutaneous problem for albinos during adolescence is the high incidence of actinic damage to the skin, which may result in actinic keratoses, basal cell and squamous cell carcinomas, and melanomas. Patients should be instructed to avoid sunlight and to wear sunscreen and protective clothing when outdoors. The most severe forms of albinism occur with mutations in tyrosinase, a key enzyme for pigment synthesis.

Neurofibromatosis has an incidence of at least 1 in 3000 individuals. There are several types of neurofibromatosis, with NF-1 (von Recklinghausen's disease) the most common (see Chapter 73, "Congenital and Genetic Disorders"). NF-1 is inherited as an autosomal dominant disorder with variable expressivity, and spontaneous mutations account for 50% of cases. The characteristic skin lesions include café au lait spots, cutaneous and plexiform neurofibromas, and axillary freckling. Although café au lait spots are present in childhood and usually during infancy, during puberty the intensity and number of pigmentary lesions markedly increases and cutaneous neurofibromas first appear in large numbers (see Plate 34).

The café au lait spot is a homogeneously pale-brown patch found anywhere on the body, but usually not on the face. These spots may not be present at birth but usually appear by 5 years of age. The diagnosis of NF-1 can be suspected in prepubertal adolescents without neurofibromas when there are five or more café au lait spots measuring 1.5 cm in diameter. Freckling of the axillae, which is present in 20% of patients, is pathognomonic of NF-1. Freckling also may be generalized or concentrated in other intertriginous sites.

Cutaneous neurofibromas may vary in size from small, soft papules to large, pendulous tumors that are extremely disfiguring. Neurofibromas characteristically invaginate through the ring of surrounding skin when pushed lightly with the finger ("buttonholing"). When neurofibromas are subcutaneous and run along the course of nerves, especially trigeminal or upper cervical nerves, these are called plexiform neurofibromas. The skin overlying plexiform neurofibromas is often hyperpigmented and thickened, and the borders of pigmentation are concordant with the borders of the neurofibromas. The neurofibromas tend to be destructive because of their size and they may undergo malignant transformation, usually when the patient is over age 40. In addition to cutaneous manifestations, a diagnostic feature that is present in 94% of affected adolescents is the iris hamartoma (Lisch nodule), which may be detectable only by slit-lamp examination.

The severity of cutaneous involvement is completely unrelated to the extent of other organ involvement. Up to 50% of patients have skeletal defects, especially kyphoscoliosis. Neurologic disease occurs in up to 40% of affected patients, especially optic gliomas, learning disabilities, and speech disorders. Adolescents with neurofibromatosis have an increased risk of malignancy, because the gene mutation of NF-1 affects a tumor suppressor gene. In addition, affected teenagers may develop pulmonary fibrosis and vascular stenosis. There is no treatment for neurofibromas except excision. Facial lesions have been removed by dermabrasion with good results. Genetic and psychological counseling for the affected adolescent are imperative.

Tuberous sclerosis is an uncommon neurocutaneous disorder that has an autosomal dominant pattern of inheritance with irregular penetrance. In 50% to 70% of cases the disorder arises from new mutations. There are a variety of pathognomonic cutaneous changes, some of which may not be present until adolescence.

The "hypopigmented macule" (often ash leaf in shape), which is the earliest marker of the disorder, tends to appear at birth or shortly thereafter in about 90% of patients. This hypopigmented macule may be more easily identified with a Wood's lamp. The macule varies in size and is often oval with smooth margins, but also may be dermatomal or resemble a thumbprint or confetti. The hypopigmented patches persist throughout life. The trunk is the most common site. Fibrous forehead plaques occur in 25% of patients and are often present at birth.

Adenoma sebaceum consists of angiofibromas usually first seen between the ages of 2 and 5 years, but they may not appear until puberty. These small, red-yellow, waxy papules tend to be symmetric and are most commonly found on the medial cheeks and midface (see Plate 35). Shagreen patches are connective tissue hamartomas that tend to develop during childhood. These yellowish to flesh-colored thick plaques are usually in the lumbosacral area. Periungual and subungual fibromas, as well as gingival fibromas, appear at puberty in 50% of patients.

They are firm, skin-colored digitate growths. Other common noncutaneous features of tuberous sclerosis include mental retardation, seizures (especially myoclonic), retinal gliomas, renal angiomyolipomas and cysts, cardiac rhabdomyomas, and cerebral cortical calcification. As in NF-1, at least one of the gene mutations that causes tuberous sclerosis involves a tumor suppressor gene. Once again, genetic counseling of affected adolescents is important.

In the basal cell nevus syndrome basal cell carcinomas appear between puberty and the middle thirties and are usually found on sun-exposed areas of the body. Associated cutaneous findings are milia, cysts, and palmar and plantar pits. Associated systemic features may include a typical facies, cystic lesions, skeletal abnormalities, and medulloblastomas and other neoplasms. Since the disorder is progressive, frequent inspection for the tumors and their removal is important.

Cowden's disease, also known as multiple hamartoma syndrome, includes multiple facial trichilemmomas that may resemble facial warts, adenoma sebaceum, or the lesions of Darier's disease. Other cutaneous findings are keratoses on the hands and feet and oral mucosal fibromas. The disorder is most significant for the later development of malignancies, especially carcinomas of the breast and thyroid.

Multiple trichoepitheliomas, which may appear on the face, scalp, and trunk, are commonly noted during the second decade. These firm, skin-colored papules are especially prominent on the scalp and trunk and are occasionally mistaken for basal cell carcinomas. In general, multiple trichoepitheliomas are not associated with any systemic abnormalities.

The mucosal neuroma syndrome (multiple endocrine neoplasia type III) is characterized by neuromas at multiple sites—for example, lips, tongue, eyes, and gastrointestinal tract. The neuromas may be congenital or may be noted during the first years of life. Intestinal ganglioneuromas, a marfanoid habitus, and later development of medullary carcinoma of the thyroid and pheochromocytoma are associated findings. Early recognition of the disorder and its malignant potential is important, since patients often die from malignancy during early childhood. Elevated levels of serum calcitonin provide the earliest evidence of thyroid cancer.

CORTICOSTEROIDS

Topical glucocorticosteroids are probably the most commonly prescribed medications for pruritic and inflammatory dermatoses such as contact dermatitis, atopic eczema, and insect bite reactions. In psoriasis, these agents produce an antimitotic effect and serve to mediate inflammation. Most topical steroids are applied twice daily. Some of the new preparations are designed for once-daily application.

Topical steroids are available in a variety of forms, including creams, ointments, solutions, and gels, for ideal application to various body sites. For example, an ointment preparation would be cosmetically unacceptable for scalp application, whereas a solution is less greasy and easier to apply to the scalp. Ointments are more lubricating and occlusive but are less aesthetically appealing because of their greasiness. Creams, which are generally more cosmetically acceptable, may be irritating and drying to some patients. Steroid preparations with emollient bases (e.g., Synemol or Lidex-E) are a compromise between creams and ointments. The key to finding the proper form of preparation involves determining patient preference for a particular skin site, with the option of switching to another form if a problem arises.

Topical steroids are classified according to their potency, which is based on the vasoconstriction assay. Examples of topical steroids in six different categories—ranging from low, medium, or high potency to the newer superpotent preparations—are listed in Table 72-1. It is important to point out to the patient that the percentage strength does not indicate potency; the chemical formulation determines the potency. For example, 0.05% fluocinonide is much stronger than 1% hydrocortisone. Most of the high-potency steroids are fluorinated. Low-potency steroids should be used on the face and skinfolds, where absorption is enhanced. Prolonged use of high-potency steroids, particularly under occlusion, may result in side effects such as cutaneous atrophy and striae, prominent superficial vessels known as telangiectasias, acneiform eruptions such as rosacea, and perioral dermatitis. Repeated use of high-potency steroids on extensive skin areas, especially with occlusion, can suppress the hypothalamic-pituitary-adrenal axis. This suppression also can occur with even limited use of the newer superpotent steroids. For this reason, high-potency steroids are best prescribed for no more than a 2-week course, followed by a rest period. Chronic use of steroids in the periorbital areas is associated with a risk of cataract formation. Therefore, for dermatitis around the eyes, the lowest-strength steroids are used for a limited time. Ophthalmologic consultation should be obtained for any patient requiring chronic therapy.

Another caution to be noted with the use of topical steroids involves the treatment of the inflammatory component of a disorder without eliminating the primary cause. For example, steroid treatment of an eczematous dermatophyte infection may temporarily help the pruritus but will not clear the tinea infection. The clinical appearance may be altered, resulting in a "tinea incognito" that is difficult to diagnose. Similarly, steroid treatment of a scabies infestation controls only the

TABLE 72-1
Classification of Topical Corticosteroids According to Potency*

Drug	Generic Name
I: Super Potency	
Diprolene 0.05%	Betamethasone dipropionate optimized vehicle
Psorcon 0.05%	Diflorasone diacetate
Temovate 0.05%	Clobetasol propionate
II-III: High Potency	
Alphatrex 0.05%	Betamethasone dipropionate
Aristocort HP 0.5%	Triamcinolone acetonide
Cyclocort 0.1%	Amcinonide
Diprosone 0.05%	Betamethasone dipropionate
Florone 0.05%	Diflorasone diacetate
Halog 0.1%	Halcinonide
Kenalog 0.05%	Triamcinolone acetonide
Lidex 0.05%	Fluocinonide
Maxiflor 0.05%	Diflorasone diacetate
Maxivate 0.05%	Betamethasone dipropionate
Topicort 0.25%	Desoximetasone
IV-V: Medium Potency	
Aristocort 0.1%	Triamcinolone acetonide
Betatrex 0.05%	Betamethasone valerate
Cordran 0.05%	Flurandrenolide
Kenalog 0.1%	Triamcinolone acetonide
Synalar 0.025%	Fluocinolone acetonide
Synalar-HP 0.2%	Fluocinolone acetonide
Topicort LP 0.05%	Desoximetasone
Valisone 0.1%	Betamethasone valerate
VI-VII: Low Potency†	
Aclovate 0.05%	Alclometasone dipropionate
DesOwen 0.05%	Desonide
Locoid 0.1%	Hydrocortisone butyrate
Tridesilon 0.05%	Desonide
Westcort 0.2%	Hydrocortisone valerate
VIII: Lowest Potency	
Any brand hydrocortisone	Hydrocortisone

*In general, ointment preparations are more potent than equivalent cream preparations in categories II-III and VI-VII.
†All drugs listed in this group are nonfluorinated products.

secondary symptoms and may actually exacerbate the infestation.

Careful clinical assessment with appropriate diagnostic evaluation must be performed before topical steroids are prescribed. When used appropriately, topical steroids are extremely useful for their antiinflammatory effect, either alone or as an adjunct to other therapies.

Suggested Readings

General

Berger TG, Elias PM, Wintroub BU: *Manual of therapy for skin diseases,* New York, 1990, Churchill Livingstone.

An excellent, concise, current manual that discusses initial therapy, alternative modalities, and pitfalls of therapy.

Shapiro SC, Straburger VC, Greydanus DE, editors: *Adolescent dermatology. Adolescent medicine: state of the art reviews,* Philadelphia, 1990, Hanley & Belfus.
   A recent multiauthored review of most facets of adolescent dermatology, including acne, infections and infestations, and foot and scalp disorders. The chapter on "Diagnosis and management of disorders of the scalp and hair in adolescents" (S. Hurwitz) is noteworthy.

Acne

Bergfeld WF, Odom RB, editors: New perspectives on acne, *J Am Acad Dermatol* 32:S1, 1995.

Leyden JJ: Retinoids and acne, *J Am Acad Dermatol* 19:164, 1988.

Pochi PE, Ceilley RI, Coskey RJ, et al: Guidelines for prescribing isotretinoin (Accutane) in the treatment of female acne patients of childbearing potential, *J Am Acad Dermatol* 19:920, 1988.

Dermatitis

Fisher AA: *Contact dermatitis,* ed. 3, Philadelphia, 1986, Lea & Febiger.

Hanifin JM: Atopic dermatitis in infants and children, *Pediatr Clin North Am* 38:763, 1991.

Skin Disorders of Pregnancy

Hanno R, Saleeby ER, Krull EA: Pruritic eruptions of pregnancy, *Dermatol Clin* 1:553, 1983.

Wong RC, Ellis CN: Physiologic skin changes in pregnancy, *J Am Acad Dermatol* 10:929, 1984.

Winton GB: Skin diseases aggravated by pregnancy, *J Am Acad Dermatol* 20:1, 1989.

Eccrine and Apocrine Disorders

Dicken CH, Powell ST, Spear KL: Evaluation of isotretinoin treatment of hidradenitis suppurativa, *J Am Acad Dermatol* 11:500, 1984.

Sato K, Kang WH, Saga K, Sato KT: Biology of sweat glands and their disorders. II. Disorders of sweat gland function, *J Am Acad Dermatol* 20:713, 1989.

Thomas R, Barnhill D, Bibro M, Hoskins W: Hidradenitis suppurativa: a case presentation and review of the literature, *Obstet Gynecol* 66:592, 1985.

Papulosquamous

Bleicher PA, Dover JS, Arndt KA: Lichenoid dermatoses and related disorders. I. Lichen planus and lichenoid drug-induced eruptions, *J Am Acad Dermatol* 22:288, 1990.

Nanda A, Kaur S, Kaur I, Kumar B: Childhood psoriasis: an epidemiologic survey of 112 patients, *Pediatr Dermatol* 9:19, 1990.

Pigmented Nevi, Nodules, and Papules

Abel EA, Farber EM: Benign cutaneous tumors. In Rubenstein E, Federman DD, editors: *Scientific American medicine,* vol 2, Sect 2, *Dermatology,* New York, 1995, Scientific American, Chapter 11; pp 1-12.

Mehregan AH, Mehregan DA: Malignant melanoma in childhood, *Cancer* 71:4096, 1993.

National Institute of Health Consensus Conference: Precursors to malignant melanoma, *JAMA* 251:1864, 1984.

Rigel DS, Rivers JK, Kopf AW, et al: Dysplastic nevi: markers for increased risk for melanoma, *Cancer* 63:386, 1989.

Slade J, Marghoof AA, Salopek TG, et al: Atypical mole syndrome: risk factor for cutaneous malignant melanoma and implications for management, *J Am Acad Dermatol* 32:479, 1995.

Williams ML, Sagebiel RW: Melanoma risk factors and atypical moles, *West J Med* 160:343, 1994.

Psychodermatoses

Koblenzer CS: Compulsive habits and obsessional concerns as they relate to the skin. In *Psychocutaneous disease,* New York, 1987, Grune & Stratton, p 143.

Koo JYM: Psychodermatology, *Curr Probl Dermatol* (in press).

Siegel RK: Cocaine hallucinations, *Am J Psychiatry* 135:309, 1978.

Swedo SE, Leonard HL, Rapoport JL, et al: A double-blind comparison of clomipramine and desipramine in the treatment of trichotillomania (hair-pulling), *N Engl J Med* 321:497, 1989.

Immune-Mediated Disorders

Paller AS: Juvenile dermatomyositis and overlap syndromes, *Adv Dermatol* 10:309, 1995.

Singsen BH: Scleroderma in childhood, *Pediatr Clin North Am* 33:1119, 1986.

Watson R: Cutaneous lesions in systemic lupus erythematosus, *Med Clin North Am* 73:1091, 1989.

Cutaneous Infections

Frieden IJ: Tinea infections in adolescents. In Shapiro SC, Straburger VC, Greydanus DE, editors: *Adolescent dermatology. Adolescent medicine: state of the art reviews,* Philadelphia, 1990, Hanley & Belfus, p 333.

Gellis SE: Warts and their management in adolescents. In Shapiro SC, Straburger VC, Greydanus DE, editors: *Adolescent dermatology. Adolescent medicine: state of the art reviews,* Philadelphia, 1990, Hanley & Belfus, p 345.

Prose NS, Mayer FE: Bacterial skin infections in adolescents. In Shapiro SC, Straburger VC, Greydanus DE, editors: *Adolescent dermatology. Adolescent medicine: state of the art reviews,* Philadelphia, 1990, Hanley & Belfus, p 325.

Genodermatoses

Alper JC: *Genetic disorders of the skin,* St. Louis, 1991, Mosby-Year Book.

Fine J-D, Bauer EA, Briggaman RA, et al: Revised clinical and laboratory criteria for subtypes of inherited epidermolysis bullosa, *J Am Acad Dermatol* 24:119, 1991.

Riccardi VM: Neurofibromatosis: past, present and future, *N Engl J Med* 324:1283, 1991.

Shwayder T, Ott F: All about ichthyosis, *Pediatr Clin North Am* 38:835, 1992.

Worobec-Victor SM, Shanker DB, Bene-Bain MA, Solomon LM: Genodermatoses. In Schachner LA, Hansen RC, editors: *Pediatric dermatology,* New York, 1988, Churchill Livingstone.

Zvulonov A, Esterly NB: Neurocutaneous syndromes associated with pigmentary skin lesions, *J Am Acad Dermatol* 32:915, 1995.

Corticosteroids

Cornell RC, Stoughton RB: The use of topical steroids in psoriasis, *Dermatol Clin* 2:397, 1984.

Goa KL: Clinical pharmacology and pharmacokinetic properties of topically applied corticosteroids, *Drugs* 36:51, 1988.

Stoughton RB: Topical corticosteroids in psoriasis. In Roenigk HH Jr, editor: *Psoriasis,* New York, 1985, Marcel Dekker.

Tan PL, Burnett GL, Flowers FP, Araujo OE: Current topical corticosteroid preparations, *J Am Acad Dermatol* 14:79, 1986.

SECTION 12

Genetic Disorders

CHAPTER 73

Congenital and Genetic Disorders

•

Robert W. Marion and Marcie B. Schneider

In recent years the field of medical genetics has undergone a revolution. Because of changes in prevailing ethical views and improved and more aggressive medical and surgical care delivered during infancy and childhood, increasing numbers of children born with congenital malformations and genetic syndromes are living longer. They are "aging out" of the pediatric population and appearing in increasing numbers in the waiting rooms of physicians who provide care to adolescents and young adults. Better, more sophisticated diagnostic techniques, such as fluorescent in situ hybridization (FISH), prophase chromosome banding, and recombinant DNA technology, have allowed earlier diagnosis of inherited and chromosomal disorders and have led to intervention at a younger age and the elucidation of the natural history of a number of these disorders from infancy into adulthood. Because of these facts, it has become increasingly important for professionals caring for adolescents to have a working knowledge of genetic disorders so that correct, sensitive counseling can be offered and medical problems such as hypothyroidism, in individuals with Down syndrome, can be anticipated and treated in an early stage.

Care providers generally encounter a patient with or at risk for a genetic disorder in one of three ways. First, and most common, is the situation in which a diagnosis has already been established and the adolescent comes for assessment or management of a specific complaint. Most children with congenital or genetic disorders will have had their conditions diagnosed well before entering adolescence. Between 3% and 8% of all U.S. newborns are found, during early life, to be affected with one or more congenital malformations, which are abnormalities in morphogenesis that interfere with normal form or function. Although some of these individuals die in infancy, most survive, often requiring sophisticated medical and surgical treatment throughout their lives. Although this group represents only a small percentage of adolescents, they are often overrepresented in adolescent clinics and inpatient services; it is estimated that individuals with congenital or genetic disorders account for between 20% and 35% of all inpatient pediatric admissions.[1]

The second situation in which a knowledge of genetic disorders is important occurs when an individual whose condition has not been previously diagnosed seeks evaluation. Confirmation of the diagnosis of disorders such as Prader-Willi syndrome, Turner syndrome in females, or Klinefelter syndrome in males must await the development of characteristic phenotypic changes that may become apparent only around or after puberty. Therefore, it is essential that those caring for adolescents, in addition to knowing about the management of these conditions, be able to recognize the signs and symptoms, so that the diagnosis will not be missed.

Finally, because they may be providing care for young women during pregnancy, it is important for clinicians to have knowledge of techniques for prenatal diagnosis of genetic disorders, such as amniocentesis and chorionic villus sampling, and to know when to refer pregnant women for appropriate testing. Also, an understanding of teratogenesis is important in order to know what should be done to monitor the pregnant woman whose embryo or fetus has been exposed to a potential teratogen.

This chapter offers a simple approach to the adolescent affected with, or at risk for, genetic disorders. After a review of the categories of genetic diseases and standard prenatal diagnostic techniques, the natural history of specific disorders will be discussed and guidelines regarding management of these disorders offered.

GENETIC DISORDERS

CATEGORIES OF GENETIC DISORDERS

When evaluating a patient with an apparent syndrome, the clinical geneticist attempts to classify the disorder into one of four categories: (1) chromosomal abnormalities, (2) single gene mutations, (3) multifactorially inherited disorders, and (4) teratogenically induced syndromes.

Chromosomal abnormalities account for approximately 7% of all congenital anomalies in the newborn period. Although individuals with some of the more common chromosomal disorders, such as trisomies 13 and 18, may be unlikely to survive infancy, patients with other aberrations, such as Down, Turner, and Klinefelter syndromes, most often do survive to adulthood.

Single gene mutations, which account for approximately 7.5% of all congenital malformations and illustrate mendelian inheritance patterns, include four major subcategories. In autosomal dominant inheritance, a single copy of an abnormal gene is sufficient to cause symptoms. As such, these disorders are usually passed vertically, from parent to child, and each child of an affected parent has a 50% chance of also being affected. In autosomal recessive inheritance, two copies of an abnormal gene are necessary to produce symptoms. Thus, parents who carry one copy of the abnormal gene are usually themselves healthy, and each child born to such carrier parents has a 25% chance of being affected. X-linked recessive inheritance is marked by male preponderance of affected individuals. In this form of inheritance, an abnormal gene causing disease is carried on the X chromosome. Females, who have two copies of the X chromosome, do not usually manifest symptoms; males who carry the abnormal gene, however, because of their hemizygous state, suffer the full consequences of the disorder. Thus, male offspring of a woman known to be carrying an X-linked recessive trait have a 50% chance of being affected. Female children of such women are not at risk but have a 50% chance of being a carrier, like their mother. Finally, in X-linked dominant inheritance, a single dose of an abnormal gene that is carried on the X chromosome is sufficient to cause symptoms. In X-linked dominant inheritance, males and females are affected in equal numbers, but male-to-male transmission, a hallmark of autosomal dominant inheritance, does not occur.

In multifactorial inheritance, abnormalities result from an interplay of many factors, both genetic and environmental. This form of inheritance accounts for 20% of all congenital malformations, including such common conditions as meningomyelocele and nonsyndromic cleft lip and palate, as well as a great number of diseases of later life, such as atherosclerotic heart disease and some forms of cancer.

Teratogen-induced disorders, such as fetal alcohol syndrome, result from the adverse effects of drugs, chemicals, and other environmental agents on the developing embryo and fetus. Teratogens account for approximately 7% of all congenital malformations.

Over half of all congenital disorders do not fit into any of these four categories. Presumably, as more information about the human genome becomes available, these disorders will ultimately be classified into the known categories.

PRENATAL DIAGNOSIS OF GENETIC DISORDERS

It is essential that those providing care for pregnant adolescent women have an understanding of prenatal diagnostic techniques so that appropriate referrals can be made. Some women affected with congenital disorders, such as meningomyelocele, are themselves at increased risk for having a child with a similar condition. Others, like those who have had multiple spontaneous abortions of unknown cause or who have a brother with muscular dystrophy, may, by virtue of their medical or family history, be at increased risk for having a child with a specific problem. Finally, some women are exposed to drugs or chemicals, such as *cis*-retinoic acid (Accutane), that are known teratogens during early embryogenesis. All of these women should be offered the opportunity to have their pregnancy monitored for specific anomalies; all deserve sensitive, accurate risk counseling, performed either by their primary care provider or by a genetic counselor.

Prenatal diagnosis originated in the 1960s with the first midtrimester amniocentesis performed for detection of fetal chromosomal abnormalities. Since that time, the field has blossomed and other diagnostic modalities, including ultrasonography, chorionic villus sampling, and percutaneous umbilical blood sampling, have been developed. As a result of these new techniques, a greater number of congenital anomalies can now be safely detected at a relatively early stage of pregnancy.[2]

Maternal Serum Biochemical Screening

During pregnancy, alpha-fetoprotein (AFP), a normal component of fetal serum, "leaks" in low concentration into the amniotic fluid and subsequently into the maternal blood. When defects exist in the fetal skin, such as occurs in meningomyelocele, excess leakage of AFP into the maternal serum occurs. AFP screening is thus useful as an indicator of fetal neural tube defects and other malformations.

In 1984 an association between low levels of AFP and chromosomal trisomies, such as Down syndrome, was reported. Although the cause of the lowered AFP level has not been adequately explained, this association has led to the use of AFP as a screening test for chromosomal disorders. Subsequently, levels of two other biochemical markers, unconjugated estriols (uE) and human chorionic gonadotropin (hCG), have been found to be useful additions to the AFP screen. Using all three of these tests, commonly referred to as the triple screen, coupled with information regarding maternal age and underlying medical conditions, a risk profile for a fetal chromosomal abnormality can be developed for every pregnancy.

Maternal serum biochemical testing is ideally performed between 15 and 18 weeks of gestation. Because it is used only as a screening test, an abnormal triple screen must be followed up with further testing (amniocentesis and/or ultrasonography). In most cases, abnormal levels of AFP, uE, and hCG are not associated with any fetal abnormality; similarly, a normal result does not completely rule out the possibility that a defect will be found in the newborn. However, because of both the low risk and the low cost of testing, maternal serum biochemical screening is a valuable initial step in the evaluation of women at risk for having a child with a neural tube defect or chromosomal abnormality.

Ultrasonography

Currently the most commonly used form of indirect fetal imaging, ultrasonography uses sound waves generated by a transducer that "bounce off" the uterine contents, producing an echogenic "picture" of the fetus and uterine contents. At levels used for diagnosis, ultrasonography does not have any harmful effect on the fetus. Commonly used for assessment of fetal age, evaluation of gestational bleeding, and evaluation of intrauterine growth retardation, ultrasonography can also be helpful in the diagnosis of a growing number of structural congenital malformations and as an adjunct to other forms of prenatal diagnosis (e.g., amniocentesis, AFP screening, and chorionic villus sampling).

At present, most women receiving prenatal care in the United States have at least one ultrasonographic examination during pregnancy. The examination is relatively inexpensive and can be performed at any time, but for the detection of fetal malformations it is best done after 16 weeks of gestation.

Amniocentesis

Amniocentesis currently forms the cornerstone of prenatal diagnosis. When used for detection of fetal genetic disorders, it usually is performed between 14 and 18 weeks of gestation. The procedure is carried out under ultrasonographic guidance to assess fetal age, rule out gross structural anomalies, and choose a suitable site for placement of the needle. After a site has been chosen and the area cleaned with an antiseptic solution, a needle is inserted through the abdominal and uterine walls and into the amniotic sac. Approximately 30 ml of amniotic fluid is aspirated, and aliquots of this fluid are placed in a culture medium (to allow growth of fetal cells so that chromosomal or DNA analysis can be performed) and are also used to determine the AFP level. If the latter is significantly elevated, a study of acetylcholinesterase, a specific marker for neural tube defects, is also performed.

The principal use of amniocentesis today is for detection of chromosomal abnormalities in women at increased risk for having a child with one of these anomalies. As such, the applicability of amniocentesis in adolescent women is limited to those who have a family history of a chromosomal aberration in a first-degree relative (e.g., a sibling or child), or who have had an abnormal triple screen. In addition to detection of chromosomal abnormalities, however, amniocentesis is used when the fetus is at increased risk for (1) neural tube defects (e.g., when the mother or a first-degree relative has meningomyelocele, or when the fetus has been exposed to teratogens known to cause such defects); (2) specific X-linked disorders (e.g., when the mother carries the gene for Duchenne muscular dystrophy or hemophilia); (3) inborn errors of metabolism in which an enzyme defect (e.g., Tay-Sachs disease) or an abnormal metabolite (e.g., congenital erythropoietic porphyria) can be detected; or (4) any single gene defect that can be diagnosed through analysis of DNA (e.g., cystic fibrosis).

The risk incurred from amniocentesis is usually cited as 1 in 300, believed to be the frequency with which fetal loss, either through introduction of infection or from other complications, is actually caused by the procedure. The reliability of information obtained through amniocentesis is extremely high; incorrect information, caused by sampling and growing maternal cells rather than those from the fetus, failure of growth of the cells in culture, or laboratory error, occurs much less than 1% of the time.

After detection of an abnormality through amniocentesis, two options are available. The pregnant woman may choose to continue the pregnancy, knowing that her baby will be affected with a specific disorder, or she can choose to terminate it. By the time the diagnosis is relayed to the woman, the pregnancy is relatively far advanced, often between weeks 18 and 21, and the abortion techniques available are psychologically and medically more complicated than those performed during the first trimester. As a result of these problems, prenatal diagnosis through chorionic villus sampling has been developed.

Chorionic Villus Sampling

This modality has been developed in response to the need for a safe, accurate test that will provide information about anomalous pregnancies during the first trimester. The technique employs sampling of the chorionic villi, structures derived from fetal mesenchymal tissue that eventually form the cytotrophoblast and the placenta.

Removing a small number of villi is relatively easily accomplished between 8 and 11 weeks of gestation. The cells of the villi, embryonic in origin, are actively dividing, and analysis of the karyotype and isolation of DNA can be rapidly performed. As a result, these investigations can be completed within a week after the procedure, allowing detection of chromosomal defects and single-gene mutations within the first trimester, a marked advantage over amniocentesis.

At present, chorionic villus sampling is performed through a transcervical or transabdominal approach. The procedure is preceded by ultrasonographic examination to assess fetal viability. Data concerning the risks for transcervical chorionic villus sampling indicate that the fetal loss rate is only 0.8%, suggesting that it is a safe and effective technique for the early prenatal diagnosis of cytogenetic abnormalities, but that it entails a slightly higher risk of procedure failures and of fetal loss than does amniocentesis. Also, as in amniocentesis, analysis of cells obtained from chorionic villus sampling is not always guaranteed. Cells may fail to grow in the culture, and occasionally inadvertent inclusion of maternal cells may occur. In chorionic villus sampling, however, an additional problem has occasionally been seen, that of chromosomal mosaicism; experience has shown that detection of an abnormal karyotype during chorionic villus sampling does not always reflect an underlying fetal anomaly. Some aberrations, such as tetraploidy, trisomy 16, and monosomy X, may be found in direct chorionic villus preparations but not in the embryonic tissue.

Chorionic villus sampling is useful for diagnosing many of the same conditions as detected by amniocentesis, such as chromosomal anomalies, certain inborn errors of metabolism, and single-gene mutations in which DNA defects are known. Detection of neural tube defects through AFP determination cannot be accomplished by chorionic villus sampling, however.

Percutaneous Umbilical Blood Sampling

Occasionally, rapid and accurate assessment of a fetus's karyotype is necessary in the second and third trimesters of pregnancy. Chorionic villus sampling is not possible at this stage, and diagnosis through amniocentesis may require more time than is available. In these instances, direct sampling of fetal blood and culturing of lymphocytes is an appropriate technique. In this procedure a catheter equipped with a small needle and a syringe allows sampling of a small aliquot of blood from an umbilical cord vessel, which can be used for appropriate testing.

The applicability of percutaneous umbilical blood sampling is limited to those instances in which an immediate obstetric or neonatal decision must be made. For instance, percutaneous umbilical blood sampling can be helpful when significant intrauterine growth retardation is found or in a fetus noted to have congenital malformations on routine ultrasonography.

APPROACH TO THE ADOLESCENT

CHROMOSOMAL DISORDERS

Down Syndrome

As more infants and children with Down syndrome survive to adolescence and adulthood, a clearer picture of the disorder's natural history has emerged. Down syndrome, which occurs in 1 in 700 newborns, is caused by an extra copy of chromosome 21 in every cell of the body. Full trisomy 21, caused by nondisjunction, is present in over 94% of affected individuals; the remaining cases are due to chromosomal translocation (in 3.3%) and mosaicism (in 2.4%).

MEDICAL PROBLEMS. The management of adolescents with Down syndrome must reflect current knowledge of the medical problems that occur in patients with this disorder.

Central nervous system. Every individual with Down syndrome has some degree of developmental disability, ranging from mild (low normal or borderline range) to profound retardation. Most patients fall in the mild to moderately retarded range, with IQs in the 50s. Because of the developmental delay, few adolescents or adults with Down syndrome are able to live independently; most live with their families or in supervised group homes, and hold jobs in sheltered settings.

Young adults with Down syndrome are at increased risk for developing presenile dementia. This condition, which rarely begins before the age of 20 but is seen with some frequency during the third decade of life, resembles Alzheimer disease both clinically and pathologically. This association is interesting in that a cluster of genes believed to play a role in the pathogenesis of Alzheimer disease has been mapped to the distal portion of the long arm of chromosome 21 (21q11.2-q21), a region that also is important in producing some of the phenotypic features of Down syndrome.

Craniofacial features. The facial phenotype, a hallmark of Down syndrome in infancy, becomes less striking with advancing age, so that by adolescence many features may be lacking. With age the nasal bridge becomes more prominent and the epicanthal folds may vanish. Dental disease is common in older patients because of a predilection for infections and poor oral hygiene. Therefore, regular dental follow-up is essential in the management of these patients.

Controversy has developed over the issue of performing facial plastic surgery in people with Down syndrome in an effort to mask some of the dysmorphic features. Requests for such surgery often come from parents who are disturbed by their child's "stigmatized" appearance. Because subjecting a child or young adult to surgery for his or her parents' sake seems inappropriate, it is our opinion that such procedures should be offered only when patients themselves request them; thus, these operations would be reserved for higher-functioning individuals.

Cardiovascular system. Between 33% and 50% of newborns with Down syndrome have congenital heart disease, most commonly because of endocardial cushion defects, including especially atrioventricular canals, and ventricular or atrial septal defects. Since most of these anomalies are now repaired surgically, the cardiovascular complications in adolescents and adults with Down syndrome do not differ from those in older patients who have survived congenital cardiac disorders.

Endocrinologic features. Abnormalities of thyroid function are common in young adults with Down syndrome. By the age of 18, 20% have hypothyroidism and 3% have hyperthyroidism. These figures increase through adult life. In nearly all cases the thyroid disease represents an autoimmune defect. Pathologically, the thyroid tissue resembles that seen in Hashimoto thyroiditis. Since the number affected increases with age, it is essential that thyroid function testing be performed frequently in all adolescents and adults with Down syndrome.

Obesity is another significant problem in young adults with Down syndrome. In some cases a marked increase in weight may herald the onset of hypothyroidism. Often, however, no thyroid dysfunction can be uncovered. In these individuals, weight gain is caused by a combination of complicated factors, including a sedentary life style and excessive caloric intake. In addition, early in life, behavior modification techniques that involve food as a reward are often used in children with Down syndrome. This clearly can contribute to the later obesity and make it more difficult to use other types of rewards in adolescence. It is essential that the care provider aid these families by helping them devise appropriate, nutritious diets; encouraging increased physical activity; and using rewards other than food in behavior modification efforts.

Sexual development in the adolescent with Down syndrome is usually less complete than normal. Females are fertile, however, and there have been many reports of affected women bearing children. As expected, the incidence of trisomy 21 in progeny of women with Down syndrome is markedly increased over the general population. Birth control counseling is indicated but is made difficult by the developmental disability that occurs with Down syndrome, a fact that makes barrier methods of birth control unreliable. Methods of birth control applicable in women with Down syndrome therefore are limited to medroxyprogesterone (Depo-Provera), levonorgestrel (Norplant), and birth control pills. The issue of birth control raises a major ethical concern: Who should make the decision regarding use of birth control in women with Down syndrome? The answer to this complex question is beyond the scope of this chapter.

There have been no proven cases of paternity in men with Down syndrome. Although testicular histology appears to be normal, the semen produced by affected men contains no viable sperm. This may be due to a postmeiotic maturational defect or to some other as yet unidentified endocrinologic abnormality.

Skeletal system. Adult height is significantly shorter than that seen in the general population; mean height is 154 cm for males and 144 cm for females. Growth hormone has been found to be normal in these patients.

Atlantoaxial instability, related to an increased distance between the first and second cervical vertebrae, occurs in 15% of individuals with Down syndrome and is believed to predispose them to spinal cord compression. It has been recommended that lateral radiographs of the cervical spine in full flexion, extension, and neutral positions be performed in children with Down syndrome, and that participation in contact sports be restricted if the atlantoaxial distance is greater than 4.5 mm. It has further been recommended that these radiographs be repeated again at least once on completion of puberty. In adults in whom atlantoaxial instability was present in childhood, osteoarthritis of the cervical spine has been reported. Therefore, radiographs of the spine should be taken in adolescents and young adults complaining of neck pain. Individuals with abnormalities should be referred to appropriate specialists.

Eyes and ears. Strabismus, common in childhood, continues to be a problem in adults with Down syndrome. Conductive hearing loss, related to recurrent otitis media in childhood, is significantly increased in the adult population.

Hematologic features. Individuals with Down syndrome have a markedly higher risk for developing leukemia during their lives compared with the general population. Other forms of cancer are believed to be more common, but there are no figures available to support this. The reason for this predilection is not certain but probably relates to errors in basic cellular regulatory mechanisms caused by the chromosomal aneuploidy that exists in these individuals.

CLINICAL MANAGEMENT. The management of adolescents with Down syndrome must be geared toward the

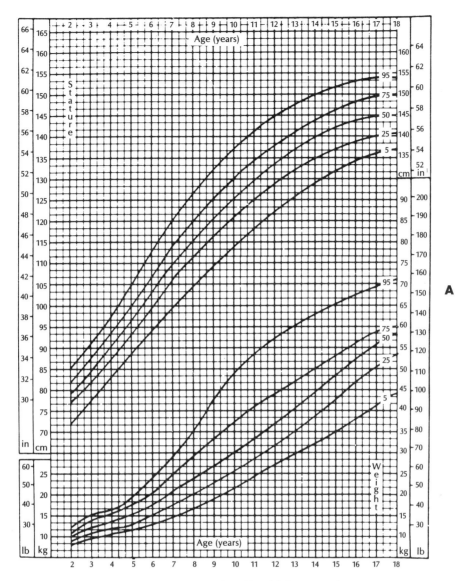

A

Fig. 73-1. A, Growth chart for girls with Down syndrome.

Continued.

medical problems just noted.[3] The first visit should include the following:

1. Full history and physical examination, with height and weight plotted on the Down syndrome growth curve (Fig. 73-1, *A* and *B*).
2. Hearing and vision testing, with referral if abnormalities are found.
3. Blood work to include a complete blood count and thyroid function tests.
4. Lateral radiographs of the neck in neutral, flexion, and extension positions, to rule out atlantoaxial instability. These radiographs should be performed during childhood, during adolescence, and after age 30.

5. Check of school placement to confirm that it is appropriate.
6. Confirmation that vocational and long-term living arrangement planning is ongoing.
7. Reinforcement of genetic counseling for the family and the beginning of birth control counseling, if the patient is female.

For subsequent visits:

1. Continue to plot height and weight.
2. Annually check thyroid function, and perform ophthalmologic examination to rule out keratoconus and cataracts.
3. If obesity is present, help with dietary advice and behavioral modification.

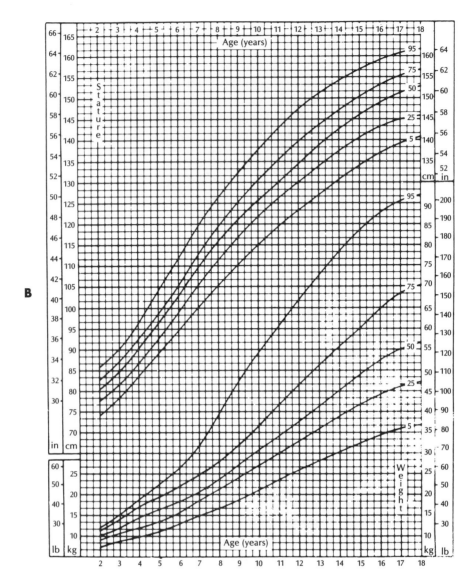

Fig. 73-1, cont'd. B, Growth chart for boys with Down syndrome. (From Cronk C, Crocker A, Püeschel S: Growth charts for children with Down syndrome: 1 month to 18 years of age, *Pediatrics* 81:102-110, 1988. Reprinted with permission of *Pediatrics.*)

Turner Syndrome

Although Turner's description of seven adolescent and adult women with short stature, "sexual infantilism," webbed neck, and cubitus valgus appeared in 1938, the chromosomal basis of the syndrome was not discovered until 1959, when a single copy of an X chromosome was found in the cells of a girl with clinical Turner syndrome. Since that time, it has been learned that the phenotype of Turner syndrome, which occurs in 0.4 per 1000 live-born females, represents the mildest expression of the 45,X genotype: over 95% of 45,X conceptuses are lost during early gestation. Furthermore, 40% of females with clinical Turner syndrome have karyotypes other than 45,X, including partial monosomy X caused by structural anomalies of the X chromosome (in 20%) and monosomy

X mosaicism (in 20%). This observation suggests that such aberrations may produce a milder phenotype. Studies of women with deletions of portions of the X chromosome have produced a "phenotypic map," short stature being associated with monosomy of the short arm of the chromosome (Xp−) and failure of sexual development associated with deletions of the long arm (Xq−).

MEDICAL PROBLEMS. Clinically, Turner syndrome is variable. The classic neonatal features, including lymphedema of the extremities, redundant skinfolds, and webbing of the neck, occur in less than 25% of affected girls. The diagnosis is more commonly made later in childhood or adolescence, during an evaluation for either growth failure, delayed thelarche or puberty, or primary amenorrhea. Because many affected girls are diagnosed after infancy, it is essential that the clinician not only understand the natural history of Turner syndrome, but be able to recognize the clinical features of the disorder so that appropriate chromosomal testing can be performed.[4]

Endocrinologic features. Three major endocrinologic problems occur commonly in women with Turner syndrome: (1) hypogonadism, (2) growth failure, and (3) Hashimoto thyroiditis, as well as other forms of autoimmune endocrinopathies. Careful evaluation of each of these is vital in the management of patients with Turner syndrome. Ovarian dysgenesis, with hypoplasia to absence of germinal elements, occurs in over 90% of women with a 45,X karyotype and less commonly in women with Turner syndrome who have other X chromosome anomalies. This pathologic finding, resulting in ovarian failure and lack of estrogen production at adolescence, leads to failure of development of the clinical signs of puberty.

It is stressed that in women with Turner syndrome the timing and extent of ovarian failure varies. Approximately 10% of patients have sufficient estrogen production to enter thelarche spontaneously. A smaller percentage may initiate menarche, but the continuation of regular menses throughout adolescence is rare. Finally, there are multiple reports of successful conceptions and pregnancies in women with both 45,X and variant karyotypes, but they account for far less than 1% of all affected females.

The second major endocrinologic problem in women with Turner syndrome is growth failure. Short stature, the cause of which is as yet unidentified, is the single most common clinical finding, occurring in 100% of females with 45,X karyotypes and 95% of those with structural variants or mosaicism. Children with Turner syndrome tend to deviate progressively from the normal height percentages until 14 years of age when, because of delayed closure of the epiphyses, growth approaches more closely the normal percentile chart. Adult stature, not usually reached until the early 20s, ranges from 142 to 147 cm. The growth chart for females with Turner syndrome is reproduced in Figure 73-2.

The final group of endocrinologic disorders occurring commonly in Turner syndrome are autoimmune endocrinopathies, Hashimoto thyroiditis being the most frequent. Although thyroid autoantibodies are found in 30% to 50% of women with Turner syndrome, only 10% manifest clinical hypothyroidism. In addition to Hashimoto disease, other autoimmune phenomena, including Graves' disease, Addison disease, vitiligo, and type 2 diabetes mellitus, may be seen. The clinical approach and management of these endocrinologic problems are covered in the chapters on endocrinology (Chapters 23 to 28).

Cardiovascular problems. Cardiovascular anomalies occur in approximately 30% of girls with Turner syndrome. The major malformations, in descending order of frequency, include bicuspid aortic valve, coarctation of the aorta, mitral valve prolapse, and dissecting aortic aneurysm resulting from median cystic necrosis. Although some of these anomalies may be diagnosed in infancy or childhood, others, such as mitral valve prolapse, may not be detected until adolescence or adulthood. Therefore, it is essential that every woman with Turner syndrome undergo a cardiac evaluation at some time during childhood or adolescence.

Renal features. Abnormalities of the kidneys have been found in 25% to 70% of women with Turner syndrome. Most anomalies, including horseshoe and pelvic kidneys and partial or complete duplication of the collecting system, can remain clinically silent. Occasionally, however, urinary tract obstruction may occur and result in hydroureter, hydronephrosis, and recurrent infections. Because of the high frequency of anomalies, a renal ultrasound examination should be performed as part of the initial evaluation of affected females.

Skeletal system. A large number of skeletal anomalies have been reported in females with Turner syndrome, including disproportionately short legs, leading to an increased upper- to lower-segment ratio; a "shieldlike" chest; hypoplasia of the cervical vertebrae; short fourth and fifth metacarpals; and genu valgum. These features, although helpful in establishing the diagnosis, do not cause medical problems. Nevertheless, they should be sought whenever the diagnosis of Turner syndrome is being considered.

Neurodevelopmental problems. Although most women with Turner syndrome have normal intelligence, their performance on tests of mathematical ability, visual-motor coordination, and spatial-temporal processing may be below average. However, with appropriate remedial assistance and counseling, individuals with Turner syndrome can succeed, often attending college and graduate school.

CLINICAL MANAGEMENT. When, because of the presence of one or more of the clinical features, a diagnosis of Turner syndrome is suspected in an adolescent female, chromosomal studies should be performed immediately. For diagnostic purposes, karyotype analysis should always be carried out on lymphocytes cultured from peripheral blood. Analysis of Barr bodies, obtained from smears of buccal mucosa, is unreliable and should never be used for primary confirmation of the diagnosis.

The informing interview after cytogenetic confirmation of the diagnosis must be conducted in a respectful and sensitive manner. The diagnosis, unsuspected by the adolescent and her parents, often comes as a blow. Virtually assured that she will be infertile, with no possibility of bearing children without advanced technological assistance, and learning that she will be strikingly shorter than most of her friends, the adolescent may react angrily or violently to the care provider delivering the news. In some instances, it may prove valuable for the information to

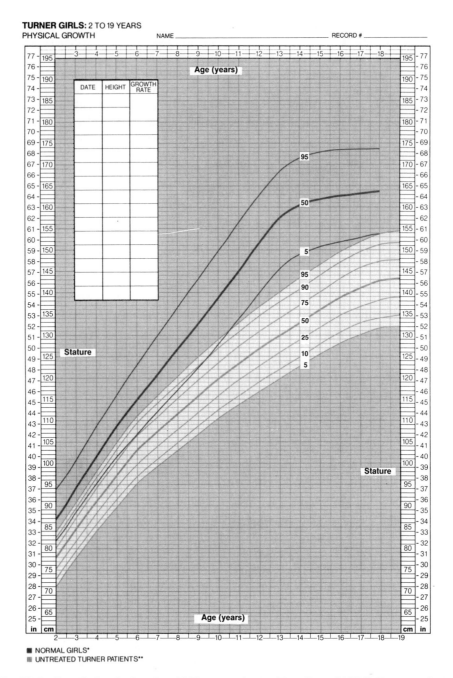

TURNER GIRLS: 2 TO 19 YEARS
PHYSICAL GROWTH

■ NORMAL GIRLS*
▨ UNTREATED TURNER PATIENTS**

Fig. 73-2. Growth chart for females with Turner syndrome. (From Rosenfeld RG: *Turner syndrome: a guide for physicians,* Copyright Turner's Syndrome Society of the United States, Wayzata, Minn.)

come from the geneticist, who may not be involved in providing ongoing medical care. On the other hand, hearing the news from the primary care provider, who has been offering care and support for the patient and her family, may soften the blow. The decision should be made by the primary care provider on a case-by-case basis.

After the informing interview, a comprehensive work-up should be performed in all patients and generally includes the following:

1. *Endocrinologic evaluation.* First, thyroid function and growth hormone secretion should be tested.

More specific testing for the other associated endocrinologic abnormalities that occur in Turner syndrome should be performed only if the patient is symptomatic.

2. *Renal evaluation.* Because of the association of urinary tract anomalies, a renal ultrasound examination and voiding cystourethrography should be performed.

3. *Cardiovascular evaluation.* As previously stated, cardiovascular anomalies occur in 30% of females with Turner syndrome, and some may not be

detected until adulthood. A full evaluation, including chest radiography, electrocardiography, and echocardiography, should be performed in all patients in whom Turner syndrome has been confirmed.

4. *Other.* Radiographic examination of the skeletal system should be considered in any woman who has symptoms such as bone or joint pain. Special consideration is given to other anomalies, as mentioned previously. In addition, hearing loss, both sensorineural and conductive, occurs in affected women. For this reason, an audiographic evaluation should be performed.

After completion of this evaluation, the adolescent should be monitored on a routine basis. Because the diagnosis may lead to a great deal of emotional distress, it may be propitious for the primary caretaker to see the patient at least once a month to reinforce the counseling and to check on the patient and her family's understanding and acceptance of the diagnosis. In addition to helping support the patient through these emotionally difficult times, it will also allow the primary caretaker, by checking on the woman's compliance with subspecialty appointments and medications, to coordinate and monitor the patient's medical progress.

The use of growth hormone to increase the adult height of women with Turner syndrome has been advocated by many endocrinologists in recent years. Also, estrogen replacement therapy, to produce secondary sexual characteristics, has been very helpful in normalizing the lives of many women with Turner syndrome. For these reasons, a good rapport and long-term follow-up with an endocrinologist is essential in the management of women with Turner syndrome.

In recent years, advances in in vitro fertilization techniques have been instrumental in helping some women with Turner syndrome to bear children. In these cases, eggs obtained from a donor and fertilized in vitro have been implanted in those women who have been hormonally primed. This breakthrough offers a significant hope to young women with this disorder who previously had no possibility of bearing children.

Klinefelter Syndrome

In the first half of the twentieth century, Klinefelter first described males with gynecomastia, testicular atrophy with azoospermia but without atrophy of Leydig's cells, and increased excretion of follicle-stimulating hormone, although it was not until 1959 that a 47,XXY karyotype was demonstrated. Since virtually none of the clinical findings are expressed in infancy and childhood, nearly all cases of Klinefelter syndrome are diagnosed in adolescence.[5] Because of this and because of its relatively high frequency (1 to 2 per 1000 males), it is essential that

the adolescent care provider be able to recognize the phenotype of Klinefelter syndrome and respond appropriately.

MEDICAL PROBLEMS

Endocrinologic problems. Commonly, gynecomastia is the initial sign of Klinefelter syndrome, a finding that occurs in one third of affected patients. The breast enlargement, which may be present by 12 years of age, is of moderate volume and is not associated with hyperpigmentation; although it may be strikingly asymmetric at the outset, symmetry is present by adulthood.

Gynecomastia also occurs commonly in males who do not have Klinefelter syndrome during early to middle adolescence. This syndrome should be suspected only when additional phenotypic features (listed below) are present or when the gynecomastia persists into later adolescence.

Testicular atrophy, the only constant feature, is usually the second sign noted. The testes are small, measuring less than 5 cc, and are soft to the touch; this is in sharp contrast to the apparent normal development of the penis and the relatively normal pubertal development. Although puberty is usually normal, clinical manifestations related to the testicular dysfunction include the absence of beard and body hair, a high-pitched voice, a decreased libido, and lack of muscular development.

Histologically, at puberty, the seminiferous tubules are sclerotic and atrophic, containing almost nothing but Sertoli cells. Although elements of germinal maturation are present, mature sperm are almost never seen.

Skeletal problems. The typical Klinefelter syndrome phenotype includes a tall, long-limbed, and somewhat eunuchoid body habitus, but these features are extremely variable. The absence of the typical skeletal pattern in a male with small testes and normal pubertal development should not impede the evaluation process.

Neurodevelopmental problems. Although most men with Klinefelter syndrome have normal intelligence, the incidences of psychiatric disturbances and developmental delay are higher than in the general population. The literature is replete with reports of men with Klinefelter syndrome who have immature emotional development. However, the frequency of this finding in the Klinefelter syndrome population is not known.

CLINICAL MANAGEMENT.

The initial management of patients suspected of having Klinefelter syndrome is similar to that of those with Turner syndrome. Chromosome analysis of peripheral blood lymphocytes should be performed in any male in whom microorchia is found during adolescence. Again, analysis of buccal mucosal cells for the presence of Barr bodies is unreliable and should never be used to confirm this diagnosis. As in Turner syndrome, the professional informing the patient and his family of the diagnosis must be sensitive and respectful. Once the diagnosis is explained, the patient must begin to deal with its consequences, most importantly the infertility that is virtually always a feature. After the informing interview, frequent visits to the primary care provider should be encouraged to assess and reinforce acceptance of the diagnosis and compliance with the medical regimen. After confirmation of the diagnosis, testosterone production should be evaluated and testosterone replacement therapy offered.

Prader-Willi Syndrome

Although Prader-Willi syndrome is not a commonly encountered disorder, it is important for the practitioner caring for adolescents to recognize its features because, as in Klinefelter syndrome and Turner syndrome, this diagnosis is often made during adolescence. Prader-Willi syndrome has been classified here as a chromosomal disorder because, during the past two decades, evidence has pointed to the fact that a small deletion of the long arm of chromosome 15 (del 15q11-13) is associated with the phenotype in most cases. For this reason, for purposes of diagnosis and genetic counseling of both the patient and other family members, a FISH study, with a probe specific for this region of chromosome 15, should be performed in every individual in whom the diagnosis of Prader-Willi syndrome is being considered.

MEDICAL PROBLEMS. The clinical features of Prader-Willi syndrome are variable and change as the affected individual grows older. In infancy the hallmark of the disorder is hypotonia, with failure to thrive because of the inability to suck and swallow. During early childhood, the hypotonia resolves and the course is marked by the development of an unusual eating pattern: affected individuals develop a seemingly insatiable appetite, often eating anything that is available to them. As a result, pica is a common feature. Obtaining food becomes a major activity for these children, and affected individuals have been known to steal or beg for food on the streets and eat garbage. As a result of the insatiability of the appetite, obesity usually is present by 3 or 4 years of age and becomes progressively more striking. In the older child, adolescent, and young adult, this obesity leads to serious, ongoing medical problems such as type 2 diabetes mellitus and coronary artery disease.

Developmental delay is usually not severe in adolescence. Adolescents typically have outgoing, cheerful personalities. Because of their loquaciousness, the examiner may conclude that these patients can function at a level higher than that indicated by schoolwork or IQ tests. However, behavioral problems, such as stubbornness and rage-type outbursts (frequently centered around issues of obtaining food), tend to be common in adolescence and young adulthood.

Hypogonadotropic hypogonadism is an important feature of Prader-Willi syndrome. In males, this may be manifested early in life by the finding of micropenis and cryptorchidism. In females, however, the hypogonadism may become apparent only when the changes of puberty or menarche do not occur at an appropriate age. It is for this reason, especially in females with Prader-Willi syndrome, that the diagnosis may first be considered by the adolescent care provider.

CLINICAL MANAGEMENT. As mentioned above, when the diagnosis of Prader-Willi syndrome is suspected, a sample of blood for FISH studies should be obtained. As in Turner and Klinefelter syndrome, counseling of the adolescent and his or her family must be sensitive and respectful. Because of the developmental problems in the affected individual, more time than might be expected may have to be allotted before the information is clearly understood. Therapy for the adolescent with Prader-Willi syndrome must be aimed at three major problems: weight reduction and control, treatment of hypogonadism, and management of the behavioral and psychological sequelae of the disorder.[6]

Weight reduction and control. Because weight gain is directly caused by the eating disorder that occurs in Prader-Willi syndrome, weight control must be attempted through correction of the eating disorder. This is not a simple task. By the time their child is an adolescent, most parents of children with Prader-Willi syndrome have placed a padlock on their refrigerators and cabinets. This is rarely successful. Because of their compulsive need for food, the patients usually solve this dilemma quickly by obtaining food from a neighbor's kitchen or through some other source. In fact, the only method that has enjoyed any success in controlling the food intake is behavior modification. Surgical intervention to reduce stomach capacity should be avoided. Surgery fails to get at the cause of the problem, and thus such procedures are rarely, if ever, successful.

In addition to trying to reduce the weight and control the eating compulsion, the care provider must be vigilant for signs of obesity-related disease. Periodic testing for glycosuria, with appropriate follow-up of glycohemoglobin and serum cholesterol levels, must be done.

Treatment of hypogonadism. Because these patients have hypogonadotropic hypogonadism and are therefore deficient in either estrogen or testosterone, they may never spontaneously enter puberty. As a result, replacement therapy should be attempted during adolescence.

Management of behavioral and psychological sequelae. Dealing with the psychologic aspects of Prader-Willi syndrome often goes hand in hand with management of the compulsive eating disorder. As a result, the clinician supervising the patient's behavior modification should also address this issue.

SINGLE GENE MUTATIONS

Disorders caused by a single gene mutation demonstrate one of four mendelian inheritance patterns: autosomal dominant and recessive patterns and X-linked dominant and recessive patterns. Because few disorders result from X-linked dominant inheritance, this discussion includes only entities falling into the other three categories.

AUTOSOMAL DOMINANTLY INHERITED DISORDERS

Marfan Syndrome

Although Antoine Marfan's description of a patient with long, spidery fingers and other skeletal abnormalities appeared in 1896, the underlying cause of Marfan syndrome has only recently been elucidated. Since the features of the disease, involving the skeletal, ophthalmologic, and cardiovascular systems, are related to the fact that aberrations in connective tissue lead to the pathologic findings, research efforts focused on the composition of the extracellular matrix. Within the last decade, two breakthroughs have occurred in Marfan syndrome research: (1) demonstration of abnormalities in the myofibrillar array in the connective tissue of some Marfan syndrome patients, coupled with a defect in the production of fibrillin, a major constituent of these myofibrils; and (2) linkage of at least one gene responsible for Marfan syndrome to the long arm of chromosome 15. These findings will undoubtedly lead, in the near future, to an understanding of the molecular pathogenesis of Marfan syndrome and the potential for treatment. At present, however, the diagnosis can be made only on the basis of phenotypic features, and only symptomatic treatment can be offered.[7] Marfan syndrome is an autosomal dominantly inherited disorder; thus, each offspring of an affected individual has a 50% chance of also being affected. Although it might be expected that one of the parents of an affected individual would be similarly affected, the fact is that in most cases no such history is available. This phenomenon is explainable in one of two ways: either, because of variability of expression of the gene, the features are so subtle in the affected parent that a diagnosis has not been made; or the disorder may have arisen as the result of a spontaneous mutation in the affected individual. Before it is concluded that the latter is the case, it is essential that both parents be examined carefully for features of the disorder.

MEDICAL PROBLEMS

Skeletal problems. Perhaps the best known of the abnormalities that occur in Marfan syndrome are those of the skeletal system: dolichostenomelia (a tall, thin body habitus) with distal lengthening of the extremities (on examination, the upper- to lower-segment ratio is often greater than 2 standard deviations below the mean, and the arm span is greater than the height); and arachnodactyly, with long, "spidery" fingers and excessive and disproportionately long hand measurements. Additional manifestations include progressive scoliosis and lumbar lordosis, joint laxity, and abnormalities of the sternum, most commonly pectus excavatum.

Cardiovascular problems. Weakness in the wall of the aorta (caused by a deficiency or absence of the protein fibrillin) leads to the most dramatic and life-threatening of the clinical features of Marfan syndrome: aneurysmal dilation of the ascending aorta with dissection. The natural history of this catastrophic event is now well known. Individuals with Marfan syndrome show progressive dilation of the aortic root, often beginning in infancy, frequently accompanied by aortic regurgitation. Eventually, the wall weakens and dissection occurs. Prior to recently developed therapies, which are detailed below, the average age at death in individuals affected with Marfan syndrome was approximately 45. Dilation and dissection of other parts of the aorta (the thoracic and abdominal segments), as well as of other vessels (the pulmonary artery and the ductus arteriosus), have also been known to occur.

Ophthalmologic problems. Subluxation of the lens (ectopia lentis) caused by a defect in the lens' suspensory ligament, is a common feature of Marfan syndrome. The subluxation often occurs in an upward and outward direction. In addition, myopia is nearly constant, and the sclerae often have a bluish tinge.

DIAGNOSIS. The initial step in managing the patient with Marfan syndrome is to confirm the diagnosis. Marfan syndrome is often diagnosed in childhood, but it is not unusual for patients to reach puberty without the diagnosis having been made. Because molecular diagnostic techniques are not yet widely available, the diagnosis of Marfan syndrome must still be based on phenotype and family history. In our experience, the diagnosis should be made only in individuals who demonstrate two or more of the following: (1) involvement of the cardiovascular system, including aortic root dilation or aortic valve insufficiency; (2) skeletal manifestations, including dolichostenomelia, with an aberrant upper- to lower-segment ratio, abnormally long total hand and foot lengths, and evidence of pectus excavatum or carinatum; (3) ophthalmologic abnormalities (ectopia lentis and/or "high" myopia); and (4) a history of Marfan syndrome, diagnosed by these criteria, in a first-degree relative. Thus, an individual with only a dolichostenomelic body habitus does not have Marfan syndrome.

CLINICAL MANAGEMENT

Cardiovascular system. In recent years, many "marfanologists" have advocated the long-term use of beta-adrenergic blocking drugs, such as propranolol and atenolol, in the treatment of all patients with Marfan syndrome. Theoretically, the decrease in cardiac preload induced by these medications serves to decrease the pressure with which cardiac output reaches the proximal aorta, thus cutting down on the "wear and tear" affecting this vulnerable vessel.

In addition, echocardiograms are performed at least every 6 months to monitor the size of the aortic root. Because the risk of dissection increases significantly in individuals whose aortic root diameter exceeds 6 cm, replacement of the ascending aorta with a composite graft (replacing the aorta and valve) is performed electively in such patients.

The need for a decrease in physical activity and for the daily taking of medication represents a marked change in life style for many patients with Marfan syndrome.

Ophthalmologic management. Careful ophthalmologic follow-up is a necessity because of the risk of blindness, from either untreated ectopia lentis or vitreoretinal degeneration (secondary to high myopia).

Skeletal system. Orthopedic care must be directed toward two complications: the progressive scoliosis, which may be treatable with bracing but often requires surgery; and pectus excavatum, which can be a confounding factor in the cardiac surgery described earlier and may lead to respiratory compromise. For these reasons, orthopedic surgery is not unusual in patients with Marfan syndrome, and close follow-up is necessary.

Genetic counseling. The risk of Marfan syndrome occurring in each child born to an affected individual is 50%. Because molecular diagnostic techniques are not yet commonly available, a definitive prenatal diagnosis cannot usually be offered. Although some infants with Marfan syndrome are symptomatic and the diagnosis has been reported by ultrasonographic demonstration of disproportionately long arms and legs in some fetuses, this has generally been unreliable. Therefore, affected adults must currently make a decision about reproduction based only on risk estimates.

In addition, in some women with Marfan syndrome, pregnancy has accelerated aortic dilation, leading to dissection during the third trimester. However, most affected women remain relatively stable throughout the pregnancy. Because the risk of pregnancy may be considerable and affected teenagers may be sexually active, the issue of family planning needs to be addressed early in adolescence. Furthermore, birth control pills are not contraindicated in this disorder; they can be safely prescribed for women with Marfan syndrome, even those in whom cardiovascular disease has been diagnosed.

Psychologic concerns.. Marfan syndrome is a disorder that is often first diagnosed during adolescence. Suddenly, the "normal" adolescent must come to grips with the fact that he or she is not "perfect"; in addition, the teenager must begin taking cardiac medications, limit physical activity, and face difficult reproductive decisions. Because of the risk of aortic dissection, compliance with the medical regimen may be crucial. Thus, the primary caretaker must encourage compliance, facilitate understanding and acceptance of the disorder, and monitor the psychosocial development of these adolescents.

Neurofibromatosis

In recent years a great deal of progress has been made in the delineation of the neurofibromatoses.[8] Table 73-1 outlines the eight currently accepted types of neurofibromatosis (NF) and lists the chromosomal map position of NF-1 and NF-2. This discussion will be limited to these two most important forms of NF.

NEUROFIBROMATOSIS-1. Formerly called von Recklinghausen disease, NF-1 is an autosomal dominantly inherited condition that occurs in 1 in 4000 people. The disease, characterized by a large number of seemingly unrelated clinical findings, is caused by a gene defect that has been mapped to the long arm of chromosome 17. This discovery will, in the near future, permit a better

TABLE 73-1
Neurofibromatoses

NF-Type	Alternate Name	Chromosome Localization
NF-1	von Recklinghausen disease	17q11.2
NF-2	Central or bilateral acoustic neurofibromatosis	22q11.21-q13.1
NF-3	Mixed type (features of neurofibromatosis I and II)	
NF-4	Variant neurofibromatosis	
NF-5	Segmental neurofibromatosis	
NF-6	Multiple café au lait spots	
NF-7	Late-onset neurofibromatosis	
NF-NOS	Not otherwise specified (features do not fit other types)	

understanding of the pathogenesis of NF-1, as well as allowing more precise prenatal and postnatal diagnoses.

The clinical features of NF-1, summarized in Box 73-1, include café au lait spots (pigmented nevi 5 mm or more in diameter that increase in number throughout childhood), axillary or inguinal freckling (clusters of small, 1- to 3-mm macules, similar in color to café au lait spots), and neurofibromas (benign tumors of the Schwann cells and fibroblasts that can arise virtually anywhere and, because of their presence, cause a large variety of complications). Rarely present in the newborn, neurofibromas gradually increase in number and size through life. During puberty, they may grow rapidly or become apparent for the first time. Optic gliomas (neurofibromas of the optic nerve, which have the potential to cause blindness), Lisch nodules (melanocytic hamartomas of the iris, identifiable through slit-lamp examination, which cause no symptoms but are a unique, pathognomonic hallmark of NF-1), skeletal defects (including scoliosis, a serious problem in adolescents with NF-1), and sphenoid wing dysplasia are other cardinal features of NF-1. In addition to these features, growth (the average height in adolescents with NF-1 is at the 33rd percentile on the normal growth curve), development (attention deficit hyperactivity disorder, learning disabilities, and, less commonly, mental retardation), neurologic function (headaches, seizures), and emotional status are often affected by NF-1. Finally, individuals with NF-1 are at increased risk for the development of many types of malignancies, including soft tissue sarcomas and astrocytomas.

Clinical management. As in Marfan syndrome, the initial step in managing the adolescent with NF-1 is to confirm the diagnosis. The individual in whom NF-1 is suspected must have at least two of the seven features listed in Box 73-1. Thus, a patient with multiple café au lait spots and no other symptoms, signs, or family history does not have NF-1 and is not at risk for any of the other disorders that occur in this disease.

Over 90% of patients with NF-1 have nothing more than café au lait spots, axillary and/or inguinal freckling, Lisch nodules, and subcutaneous neurofibromas. For this reason, the care provider should help the patient maintain a positive attitude while providing careful surveillance for signs of more serious symptoms. In 10% of affected individuals, more severe complications occur. Once the diagnosis of NF-1 has been confirmed, possible courses of action include surgery, surveillance, and genetic counseling.

Surgery. In most cases, surgery to remove subcutaneous neurofibromas is inappropriate or unnecessary and should be discouraged. The reasons for this include medical factors (tumor regrowth is likely) and psychologic factors (the patient must come to grips with the fact that removal of all neurofibromas would be impossible in most cases). With this in mind, there are several clear indications for removal of neurofibromas: (1) when the size becomes excessive, (2) when pain becomes significant, (3) when the tumor causes disfigurement, and (4) when a tumor interferes with normal function.

Surveillance. The care provider must maintain a constant search to identify any of the serious complications that may accompany NF-1. At the time the diagnosis is made, we recommend initial magnetic resonance imaging (MRI) of the head and orbits (to search for hamartomas in the basal ganglia, common concomitants to NF-1 that in most cases are associated with no symptoms), yearly ophthalmologic examinations (to evaluate the development of optic gliomas), and vision and hearing tests every 6 to 12 months. Any complaint made by the patient should be seriously evaluated. Because of the increased risk of malignancy in NF-1 patients, some authors have recommended a regular series of radiographic studies such as a periodic skeletal survey, along with computed tomographic scans of the brain, orbits, cervical and thoracic spine, abdomen, and pelvis. In our opinion, these tests should not be routinely performed unless appropriate symptoms occur.

Genetic counseling. Because the gene for NF-1 has been identified, direct prenatal diagnosis, through amniocentesis or chorionic villus sampling, is currently available. Since each child born to an affected individual has a 50% chance of being affected, such testing should be offered. However, because of the marked variability of clinical features in NF-1, the decision concerning abortion of an affected fetus will undoubtedly be a difficult and troubling one.

BOX 73-1
NF-1: Major Diagnostic Criteria

Two or more of the following features must be present to confirm a diagnosis of NF-1:

1. Café au lait spots:
   Prepubertal: five or more of at least 0.5 cm in diameter
   Postpubertal: six or more of at least 1.5 cm in diameter
2. Axillary or inguinal freckling
3. Neurofibromas: two or more of any type or one plexiform
4. Optic glioma (neurofibromas of the optic nerve)
5. Lisch nodules (melanotic hamartomas of the iris)
6. Skeletal defects: include scoliosis, pseudarthrosis, and sphenoid wing dysplasia
7. Family history of first-degree relative with NF-1, diagnosed by these criteria

Neurofibromatosis-2. Although characterized by skin hyperpigmentation and neurofibromas, NF-2 presents a markedly different clinical picture from that of NF-1. The hallmark of NF-2, the presence of bilateral acoustic neuromas and other central nervous system (CNS) tumors, is a serious, life-threatening complication. After confirmation of this diagnosis, all efforts must be focused on identifying small neuromas at a point at which they can be surgically removed and function can be preserved.

Like NF-1, NF-2 has an autosomal dominant inheritance pattern, but it is genetically distinct, the gene responsible having been mapped to the long arm of chromosome 22. The position of this gene is adjacent to a gene responsible for familial meningiomas, and these CNS tumors also occur commonly in individuals with NF-2.

Clinical management. Clinically, the adolescent with NF-2 generally has fewer café au lait spots than does the patient with NF-1. Because there is a good deal of overlap between these two entities, management of NF-2 parallels that of NF-1, except for the addition of surveillance MRI scans to determine the presence of CNS tumors. Since early detection of acoustic neuromas is the only method of preventing deafness, we recommend that MRI be performed at least once a year in these patients.

Achondroplasia

The most common bone dysplasia in humans, achondroplasia is a condition that affects 1 in 10,000 newborns. A disorder of endochondral bone, it causes rhizomelic ("root of the limb") shortening of the extremities, as well as many other clinical signs and symptoms.[9] Achondroplasia is an autosomal dominantly inherited condition, with 80% presumably arising secondarily to spontaneous mutations. Recently, the gene responsible for the condition was mapped to the short arm of chromosome 4. Further studies have shown that achondroplasia is due to a mutation in the gene that codes for fibroblast growth factor receptor type 3, a protein important in early bone development. This breakthrough has opened the door to allow early prenatal diagnosis in fetuses of affected parents.

Medical problems

Orthopedic problems. The most striking feature in individuals with achondroplasia is the disproportionate shortening of stature. The mean adult height (131.5 cm in males, 123.4 cm in females) renders affected individuals immediately obvious and carries with it the potential for significant psychologic and orthopedic dysfunction. The growth chart for individuals with achondroplasia is shown in Figure 73-3.

In adolescence, knee pain becomes a common complaint. Associated with obesity and progressive genu varum (related to unequal growth of the tibia and fibula), the pain is caused by strain on the lateral collateral ligaments and is difficult to treat. In addition, spinal disorders are common orthopedic problems in young adults with achondroplasia, occurring in 70%. Exaggerated lumbar lordosis is seen first, and spinal stenosis is common later in life, leading to a spectrum of problems. If spinal surgery is indicated in these individuals, the use of instrumentation, such as rods, should be avoided, because these devices have been known to leave the patient with permanent neurologic sequelae.

Neurologic problems. Complaints referrable to neurologic dysfunction occur in 70% of young adults with achondroplasia. Early in life, hydrocephalus and other problems related to dysplasia of the cranial base and upper cervical spine may occur. Later, spinal deformities causing nerve root compression may lead to diverse symptoms (central apnea, paraplegia, claudication, numbness).

Respiratory problems. Hypoventilation and apnea, caused by cord compression, can occur at any age. It has also been our experience that obstructive apnea, resulting from a combination of factors, including an acute cranial base angle and obesity, may become a significant problem in early adolescence. Changes in school performance, daytime somnolence, and alterations in sleeping patterns should lead to a careful evaluation of the airway in such patients.

Obstetrics/family planning. Both males and females with achondroplasia have normal genitalia and endocrine functioning. Pregnancies are not significantly different from those of unaffected women during the first two trimesters. However, because of a markedly increased risk of stillborn infants when delivered vaginally (because of abnormalities in the size and shape of the pelvis), elective cesarean section is indicated in women with achondroplasia.

Like children with neurofibromatosis and Marfan syndrome, children born to men or women with achondroplasia have a 50% chance of also being affected. However, as a result of involvement with social organizations such as Little People of America, patients with achondroplasia frequently meet and mate with other affected individuals. In such matings, although each offspring still has a 50% chance of having heterozygous achondroplasia, there is a 25% risk that the child will inherit both abnormal genes and have homozygous achondroplasia, an almost universally lethal disorder. Because of this and the need for cesarean section, the decision to bear children is a significant one.

As noted above, because of the recent discovery that achondroplasia is caused by a mutation in the fibroblast growth factor receptor type 3 gene, prenatal diagnosis through amniocentesis or chorionic villus sampling is now available to many affected individuals. This is

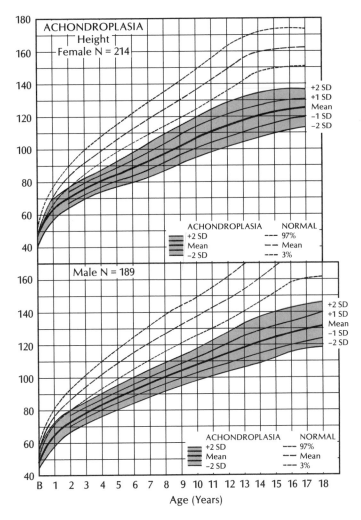

Fig. 73-3. Growth charts for children with achondroplasia. (From Jones KL: *Smith's recognizable patterns of human malformations,* ed 4, Philadelphia, 1988, WB Saunders; p 298.)

especially important in matings between individuals with achondroplasia, because the diagnosis of the homozygous condition can be accomplished.

Psychosocial problems. Nearly all people with achondroplasia have normal intelligence. Because of the short, disproportionate size of adolescents with achondroplasia, many in society react to them with curiosity, surprise, fear, and concern. Affected adolescents, faced with the frequent disruptions of their lives caused by people's reactions, adopt one of four defense mechanisms: (1) withdrawal and isolation (a combination that may contribute to obesity); (2) denial (a defense that is likely to last for only a short time); (3) accepting the role of "mascot" (which leads to poor body image and serious psychologic problems); and (4) finally, realizing the effect their size has on other people and helping society cope with their abnormality by learning methods of putting people at ease. According to Little People of America, the last-named is the most effective and healthy mechanism.

School and employment present special problems for people with achondroplasia. At school, special tools, such as a step stool at the toilet and a second set of books so that heavy books need not be carried, may be necessary. Traditionally, people with achondroplasia have been forced to find work in the entertainment field and have often had a difficult time finding white-collar jobs.

Finally, because of the rarity of achondroplasia and other bone dysplasias, it is not uncommon for affected adolescents never to have seen another person with achondroplasia. As a result, organizations such as Little People of America and the Human Growth Foundation have served an important role in the social development of young adults with achondroplasia. Through local functions and annual national conventions, people with achondroplasia have an opportunity to meet others with bone dysplasias. In addition, these groups deal with such day-to-day problems as the inability to buy life or health insurance, the need to purchase appropriate clothing, and discrimination in the workplace.

CLINICAL MANAGEMENT. The diagnosis of achondroplasia is always made in infancy or early childhood. By the time of adolescence, the psychologic and physical effects of achondroplasia have already been felt.

Growth. At present, no consistently effective treatment is available for the disproportionate short stature that occurs in achondroplasia. Growth hormone therapy currently has little place in the management of these patients. Leg-lengthening procedures, performed surgically, have been successful in some cases; however, these procedures take an extremely long time, require a great deal of dedication and compliance on the part of both patient and family, are expensive, and are fraught with complications. These procedures should therefore be offered only to highly motivated individuals on whom the shortened stature is having the most serious effects.

Orthopedic surgery. Surgery to repair the genu varum is important and should be performed in early adolescence. Surgical correction of the spinal malalignment may be needed later in life. For these reasons, it is important that patients with achondroplasia be monitored by an orthopedist.

Respiratory management. As noted previously, there is a significant risk for the development of obstructive apnea. The care provider must be ever-vigilant for symptoms and signs of airway obstruction. If such symptoms are evident, the practitioner should (1) conduct a sleep study to confirm the presence of apnea, (2) evaluate the airways (through endoscopy) to find any causes of obstruction, and (3) select a treatment aimed at specific causes (some patients may require continuous positive airway pressure, others a tracheostomy).

Genetic counseling. Careful counseling is imperative in adolescence. Patients need to know their risks of having an affected child, as well as the risk of having an unaffected child (which may prove more of a burden). As already discussed, prenatal diagnosis through amniocentesis or chorionic villus sampling is possible. Ultrasonographic and radiologic prenatal diagnosis can also be accomplished.

AUTOSOMAL RECESSIVELY INHERITED DISORDERS

The two most common autosomal recessively inherited disorders, sickle cell disease and cystic fibrosis, are discussed in depth in Chapters 49 and 42, respectively. This section focuses only on genetic counseling.

Sickle Cell Anemia

More information about the molecular genetics of sickle cell anemia is known than about nearly any other genetic disorder. All clinical signs and symptoms in this disease are caused by a single base change in the gene coding for the beta-globin chain, which has been mapped to the short arm of chromosome 11. This minute change, leading to a substitution of the amino acid valine for glutamine at the sixth position from the protein's amino terminal end, affects the conformation of the hemoglobin molecule and leads to its sickled shape when oxygen saturation is low.

Because so much of the molecular genetics of sickle cell anemia are known, definitive prenatal diagnosis, through either amniocentesis or chorionic villus sampling, is possible. However, only women at risk of having an affected child should be referred. Therefore, one of the following criteria should be met: (1) both parents have previously had a child with sickle cell anemia, either together or separately; (2) both parents have been tested and found to be heterozygotes (have the sickle cell trait); or (3) one parent has had a child with sickle cell anemia and the other has tested positive. Each child born to a couple in which any of these criteria have been fulfilled has a 25% chance of having sickle cell anemia and a 50% chance of inheriting the sickle cell trait. Children born to couples in which one parent is affected with sickle cell anemia and the other has a trait each have a 50% chance of being affected with the disease. If both parents are affected, all offspring will have sickle cell anemia.

In counseling couples who fulfill these criteria, it is important to emphasize that sickle cell anemia is clinically variable; some affected individuals are chronically ill and others only mildly symptomatic. The decision to undergo prenatal diagnosis and then to continue or interrupt the pregnancy must be made by the couple.

Cystic Fibrosis

A massive research effort has been aimed at attempting to understand the molecular basis of cystic fibrosis, and the mystery has now been unraveled. Through a procedure known as "reverse genetics," in which a candidate protein is synthesized from a region of DNA known to be abnormal in affected patients, the gene responsible for cystic fibrosis has been mapped to the long arm of chromosome 7 (7q31.3-q32), and a protein, found to be deficient in affected individuals, has been synthesized. These exciting breakthroughs, as in sickle cell anemia, have permitted the development of prenatal diagnosis through amniocentesis and chorionic villus sampling.

The criteria for referral for prenatal diagnosis of cystic fibrosis are similar to those for sickle cell anemia. Although women with cystic fibrosis are fertile and can bear children, there has been no documented case of a man with cystic fibrosis fathering a child.

X-LINKED RECESSIVELY INHERITED DISORDERS

The two most common disorders in this group are Duchenne muscular dystrophy and hemophilia. Again, both have been covered in Chapters 62 "Motor Unit Disorders" and 52 "Hemorrhage and Thrombosis," respectively. As a result, only the genetics of these disorders will be discussed here.

Duchenne Muscular Dystrophy

Although Duchenne muscular dystrophy (DMD) has long been known to be linked to the X chromosome, characterization of the gene responsible for this disorder was accomplished only in the 1980s. By means of reverse genetics, the protein dystrophin has been identified as the component of muscle cells that is deficient in men with this and some other forms of muscular dystrophy. The characterization of dystrophin has led to major advances in both the diagnosis and potential treatment of DMD.

Since Duchenne muscular dystrophy shows an X-linked recessive inheritance pattern, the overwhelming majority of affected patients are male, and the disorder occurs in 1 in 3500 boys. Mothers and sisters of affected males may or may not be carriers of the abnormal gene. In the past, counseling was offered on the basis of statistical probabilities: the chances that a first-degree female relative of a male affected with Duchenne muscular dystrophy carried the abnormal gene depended on the number of other affected males in the family and the level of creatine kinase in the woman's blood. Furthermore, in women believed to be carriers, fetal sex determination was the only possible method of prenatal diagnosis. Because of the identification of the actual gene defect responsible for Duchenne muscular dystrophy, however, counseling with certainty can now be offered after testing of affected relatives. In addition, once a female has been identified as a carrier, direct prenatal diagnosis can now be offered through amniocentesis or chorionic villus sampling.

Because of the inheritance pattern, those men with Duchenne muscular dystrophy who reproduce cannot have children who are affected. Rather, all daughters born to such men will be obligate carriers, whereas sons, having received their father's Y chromosome, will be completely free of disease. Because of the risk of carrier status in first-degree female relatives of men with Duchenne muscular dystrophy, all such women should be offered definitive testing. Since such testing should ideally be performed before childbearing has begun, much of this testing will take place in adolescence.

Hemophilia

Appropriate genetic counseling in hemophilia is nearly identical to that for Duchenne muscular dystrophy.

Similarly, the gene responsible for producing the clotting factors deficient in both hemophilia A and B, as well as for some of the other inherited bleeding diatheses, has been characterized, and direct DNA diagnosis is possible. As in Duchenne muscular dystrophy, children of males affected with hemophilia cannot be themselves affected; however, daughters will all be carriers and should be offered prenatal diagnosis. First-degree relatives of affected males (i.e., mothers and sisters) should routinely be offered the opportunity to be tested and, if found to be carriers, be referred for prenatal diagnosis by either chorionic villus sampling or amniocentesis.

MULTIFACTORIALLY INHERITED DISORDERS

Multifactorially inherited traits result from a combination of many factors, both genetic and nongenetic, each of which makes a significant contribution to the overall picture. These disorders tend to cluster in families, but the inheritance does not conform to simple mendelian patterns. Approximately 20% of all congenital malformations are multifactorially inherited; included in this group are neural tube defects, congenital heart disease, nonsyndromic cleft lip and palate, and hypospadias. In addition, many diseases of adult life, such as type 1 diabetes mellitus, alcoholism, alcoholism, atherosclerotic heart disease, and some forms of cancer, are determined by the interplay between genetic background and environmental exposures. One of the multifactorially inherited disorders faced commonly by those providing care to adolescents, meningomyelocele, is discussed in this section.

MENINGOMYELOCELE

Present in 1 in 1000 newborns in the United States, meningomyelocele is the most commonly occurring physically disabling birth defect in humans.[10] Thanks to the development of the ventricular shunt for the treatment of hydrocephalus and aggressive surgical management, children with meningomyelocele now routinely survive into adulthood and lead productive lives. Because of the need for close, ongoing medical attention, it is imperative that the care provider understand the medical problems associated with this disorder.

In meningomyelocele, because of a failure of closure of the neural tube during early fetal life, a defect of the spinal cord occurs, leading to disruption of the distal nervous system. Depending on the level of the spinal lesion, the child may be born with a spectrum of medical problems, including (1) paraplegia of the lower extremities; (2) multiple orthopedic anomalies of the legs, including clubfeet, contractures of the knees, and dislocation of the hips; and (3) neurogenic bladder. In addition, obstructive hydrocephalus, caused by Arnold-Chiari malformation, occurs in 90% of affected individuals, necessitating the placement of a ventricular shunt.

CLINICAL MANAGEMENT. Because of the complex and chronic medical problems, adolescents with meningomyelocele should be managed by a team consisting of (1) a neurosurgeon, who manages care of the ventricular shunt, if shunting is necessary; (2) a urologist, who manages the patient's neurogenic bladder and, through a program of clean intermittent catheterization, treatment with prophylactic antibiotics, and frequent radiographic surveillance, attempts to prevent recurrent urinary tract infections, vesiculoureteral reflux, and the development of chronic renal failure; (3) an orthopedic surgeon, who may surgically repair congenital defects of the lower extremities and spine in an attempt to allow the patient to become as ambulatory as possible; and (4) a physiatrist, who, through a coordinated plan with the orthopedic surgeon, prescribes therapy and braces to allow ambulatory stability.

The primary care provider must take an active role in patient management. In addition to providing routine healthcare maintenance, the primary care physician should ensure that the adolescent with meningomyelocele is in an appropriate school setting (children with meningomyelocele are at increased risk for learning disabilities and mental retardation); that his or her vision (strabismus and astigmatism are more common) and hearing are normal; and that psychiatric services, if indicated, are available. Perhaps the most important contribution of the primary caretaker is to coordinate subspecialty services; encourage compliance, especially with self-catheterization, in which noncompliance may affect renal function; and attend to the teenager's psychosocial development, including sexual activity, counseling regarding reproduction, the risk of bearing a child affected with meningomyelocele, and prenatal diagnostic options.

Although most women with meningomyelocele have normal gynecologic functioning, the majority of affected men are infertile. Taken as a group, approximately 50% of these men are unable to maintain an erection; of those who can do so, some cannot reach orgasm and others have retrograde ejaculation. As a result, only 10% to 25% of men with meningomyelocele can father children. Generally, the higher the spinal lesion, the less likely the patient is to be fertile, but each case must be evaluated on an individual basis.

Recently, it has been noted that, with advancing age, most individuals with meningomyelocele develop an allergy to latex. Sudden death, due to anaphylaxis, has occurred and, because of the frequency of the allergy and the suddenness with which it can manifest itself, we have chosen to label all patients with meningomyelocele latex allergic. In general, avoidance of latex has not interfered with routine medical management, but it has created a problem in the area of family planning. Because latex condoms are the only effective barrier against the spread of the human immunodeficiency virus (HIV), these have become an important component in the fight against the spread of AIDS. Men with meningomyelocele should avoid the use of latex condoms, as should partners of women who have meningomyelocele.

Each child born to a parent affected with meningomyelocele has a 2% to 4% chance of also being affected. Although this represents a twenty- to fortyfold increase in risk over the general population, the odds are still dramatically against recurrence in a patient's progeny. However, since the risk is present, prenatal diagnosis is indicated in such pregnancies; all women who have meningomyelocele, or whose partner is affected, should be offered counseling and testing.

Epidemiologic studies have shown that the risk of recurrence of neural tube defects can be reduced by as much as 70% through the use of periconceptual folic acid supplementation. To be effective, supplementation must begin 2 to 3 months before conception. Currently, the U.S. Department of Health recommends that all women of childbearing age receive 0.4 mg of folic acid per day. The dose suggested for individuals who have a first-degree relative with meningomyelocele is 4 mg per day.

Meningomyelocele and other neural tube defects can be detected through the measurement of AFP and, if this is elevated, acetylcholinesterase in the amniotic fluid, and sonography. These diagnostic tests should be offered to women whose fetuses are at risk for these conditions.

ENVIRONMENTALLY INDUCED CONGENITAL MALFORMATION SYNDROMES

A "teratogen" is defined as any chemical or environmental agent that has the potential to damage embryonic tissue primordia, ultimately resulting in one or more congenital malformation. Since the early 1960s, when it became apparent that the drug thalidomide, a tranquilizer often prescribed during pregnancy, caused phocomelia and a series of other life-threatening congenital malformations, information has been collected for a large series of drugs and chemical agents that, when administered during pregnancy, appear to induce birth defects. Today, teratogens are responsible for approximately 6.5% of all malformations recognized in the newborn period.

There are three major reasons why those providing care to adolescents need to understand teratogenesis. First, within the patient population being served, some individuals are bound to be affected with such entities as fetal alcohol and congenital rubella syndromes. To provide optimal care to such individuals, the care provider must understand the natural history of these disorders. Second, because of the growing number of women who become pregnant during adolescence, the care provider should question the patient about use of such agents as crack cocaine, alcohol, and other teratogenic agents. Finally, the care provider, in treating the pregnant adolescent, may wish to prescribe drugs, such as *cis*-retinoic acid, hydantoin, or tetracycline, all of which have been implicated in causing birth defects. For these reasons, the concepts of when and how teratogens cause their adverse effects, the work-up after a teratogen exposure, and the natural history of some resulting syndromes will be covered in this section.

Teratogenesis

Before specific teratogenic agents are discussed, three concepts need elucidation. First, teratogens often have different effects when administered at different periods during gestation. The three important periods during fetal life are (1) the preimplantation phase, from conception until 10 days after conception, when implantation is completed; (2) the organogenic phase, from implantation to approximately 8 weeks after conception, when formation of all major organ systems has been completed; and (3) the fetal phase, from 9 weeks after conception until birth. When a teratogen is administered during the preimplantation phase, either it will cause such severe damage to the blastocyst that the conceptus will be lost and a spontaneous abortion will occur (at a time when the woman may be completely unaware that she is pregnant), or no harmful effects will occur and normal implantation will take place. This latter phase has been referred to as the safe period; although this is technically inaccurate, it is understood that if pregnancy does ensue, no significant harm has been done to the embryo. The same teratogen administered during the organogenic phase may cause serious harm to many developing structures, but if it is administered after the completion of organogenesis, it is possible that no harmful effects will occur. Alcohol, described later in greater detail, provides a good example of this phenomenon. If a woman drinks alcohol heavily during the preimplantation phase and then stops, any surviving offspring will be unharmed; if she drinks in the organogenic phase, her child may be affected with the fetal alcohol syndrome; if she abstains from alcohol until the second trimester of pregnancy, her infant will appear morphologically normal but is at risk for serious developmental abnormalities. Alcohol is therefore considered both a structural (capable of causing congenital malformations) and a behavioral (capable of inducing behavioral alterations) teratogen.

A second important concept of teratogenesis is that of tissue specificity. Some agents known to be teratogenic exert harmful effects on only one or two tissue types. The antibiotic tetracycline is a good example; it is harmful only to developing bone and teeth. If it is administered during the early first trimester, before this tissue has begun to develop, no harmful effects will result. If it is administered later, in the second and third trimester, tooth defects (hypoplasia of enamel) and diminished growth of long bones may result.

A third concept that should be understood is that of facilitation. In the context of teratogenesis, facilitation refers to the enhancement or alteration of an agent's effect by the presence of a second agent or factor. For example, the anticonvulsant hydantoin causes different effects on the embryo and fetus when the mother who uses the drug is free of seizures than it does when seizures occur. Therefore, facilitation may have a confounding effect on epidemiologic analysis and majy affect the type of counseling offered to the mother.

Teratogens

MATERNAL FACTORS
Maternal infections. Table 73-2 lists some of the more common infectious agents that produce harmful effects and the consequences of infection on the conceptus. The effect of each of these infectious agents on the developing embryo or fetus is related to the timing of infection. Generally, the earlier the infection, the more devastating are the effects.

Noninfectious maternal illness. The fetus is sensitive to a number of maternal metabolic disturbances. In most cases, strict control of the underlying metabolic abnormality in the mother will serve to protect the fetus.

Diabetes mellitus. Infants of diabetic mothers are at significantly greater risk for congenital malformation than are infants whose mothers do not have diabetes. It is estimated that approximately 10% of these infants have an abnormality in form or function that is detectable in the neonatal period.[11] Malformations that occur more commonly in this group include the caudal regression sequence (a severe defect in the development of the posterior blastema, in which absence of the sacrum, defects of the lower limb, imperforate anus, and abnormalities of the genitourinary tract combine); and the VACTERL association (association of *v*ertebral anomalies, *a*nal stenosis, *c*ardiac anomalies, *tr*acheo-*e*sophageal fistula, and *r*enal and *l*imb malformations). The presence and severity of anomalies appear to be directly related to the degree of glycemic control during the first trimester of pregnancy.

In addition to these congenital malformations, infants of diabetic mothers are at greater risk for nonmalformation-related disorders at the time of birth. Macrosomia, cardiomyopathy, hypoglycemia, polycythemia, and hyperbilirubinemia are all known neonatal sequelae of gestational diabetes.

TABLE 73-2
Selected Infectious Teratogens

| Agent | Central Nervous System | Congenital Malformations | | | |
		Eye	Ear	Heart	Other
Rubella virus	MR, microcephaly	Cataract, glaucoma, other	Deafness	VSD, ASD, PDA	Growth deficiency, bone dysplasia, other
Cytomegalovirus	Microcephaly, calcifications, MR	Microphthalmia, blindness	Deafness		Miscarriage
Taxoplasma gondii	Microcephaly, calcifications, MR	Microphthalmia, chorioretinitis			Miscarriage
Herpes simplex virus	Microcephaly, MR	Microphthalmia, retinal dysplasia			
Varicella	Microcephaly, MR	Cataracts, microphthalmia			Limb deficiency, cicatricial skin lesions
Human immunodeficiency virus	Microcephaly, calcifications, MR	Prominent eyes, blue sclerae			Characteristic facies, immunodeficiency

ASD, atrial septal defect; *MR*, mental retardation; *PDA*, patent ductus arteriosus; *VSD*, ventricular septal defect.

Maternal phenylketonuria. Through the use of neonatal screening and the institution of special diets low in phenylalanine, phenylketonuria (an inborn error of metabolism caused by a deficiency of phenylalanine hydroxylase) has become a relatively innocuous disease since the 1960s. The tendency in the past has been to limit intake of phenylalanine in affected individuals until late childhood, when liberalization of the diet has occurred. However, Mabry et al, in 1966, were the first to note that offspring of women with phenylketonuria are at significant risk for mental retardation, microcephaly, and congenital heart disease.[12] In the late 1980s, suggestions were made that women in the childbearing years be returned to a low phenylalanine diet; it has been shown that, if this diet is instituted before the start of pregnancy, the fetus is at little or no increased risk for these anomalies.

DRUGS AND CHEMICALS AS TERATOGENS. This category of teratogenic agents has special significance because, to some extent, their use by pregnant women is determined by the physician, whose prescription and advice can cause these agents to be used or avoided. Therefore, it is essential for the physician to have a clear understanding of drugs and chemicals that can cause birth defects.

Nonprescription drugs. Alcohol, cocaine, marijuana, and heroin are all nonprescription drugs with teratogenic potential. Also considered as part of this group are caffeine and nicotine, but these agents are believed to have no teratogenic potential.

Fetal alcohol syndrome. In 1973, Jones et al[13] described a recognizable pattern of malformations in infants born to chronic alcoholic women. Features of fetal alcohol syndrome include prenatal and postnatal growth deficiency; microcephaly with developmental delay; various skeletal defects, such as radioulnar synostosis and atlantoaxial instability; cardiac anomalies, including ventricular and atrial septal defects; and a characteristic facial appearance, including short palpebral fissures, ptosis, a hypoplastic malar region, a flat philtrum, and a thin upper vermilion border of the lip. The full-blown syndrome occurs in 3 to 5 per 1000 newborns, making fetal alcohol syndrome the most common teratogenic syndrome encountered in humans.[14] Medical problems that occur in the adolescent with fetal alcohol syndrome include growth retardation, serious developmental defects and mental retardation, and seizure disorders. Adolescents and adults with fetal alcohol syndrome are fertile; if affected women refrain from drinking alcohol during their pregnancies, their offspring are at no increased risk for congenital defects.

Cocaine embryopathy. Over the past few years, use of cocaine and crack has reached epidemic proportions in inner-city areas. A spectrum of anomalies has been observed in some offspring of women using these substances. Malformations, including intracranial hemorrhages leading to developmental disabilities and microcephaly, intestinal atresias, limb reduction defects, and striking urinary tract anomalies such as the prune-belly syndrome, have been reported.[15] The cause of these anomalies appears to be related to vascular disruption. Thus, the vasoconstrictive effects of the drug occurring at critical times of gestation lead to this pattern of anomalies.

Although this pattern of malformations has been seen repeatedly in infants of cocaine-using women, the overall incidence of congenital malformations in this group of infants does not exceed the 3% expected in all populations. This suggests that some exposed embryos and fetuses are lost as spontaneous abortions, and that cocaine effects can be seen in only a small minority of exposed conceptuses who survive to term.

More troubling is the recent evidence that offspring of women who used cocaine during pregnancy are at significant risk for the development of behavioral and psychologic disturbances during childhood and later in life. Although the pathogenetic mechanism yet for this association has not yet been firmly established, it appears that these neurodevelopmental aberrations are direct sequelae of exposure to cocaine during gestation, and thus represent behavioral teratogenic effects.

Prescription drugs. Thalidomide was the first prescription drug known to cause malformations. The effects of two other drugs are described below.

Accutane embryopathy. A vitamin A congener, *cis*-retinoic acid is an effective agent in the treatment of cystic acne, which is common in adolescence. In the early 1980s, this drug, marketed in the United States as Accutane, was also found to be a potent teratogen. Up to 70% of the fetuses exposed to Accutane during the first trimester were found to be abnormal. Some of the pregnancies ended in spontaneous abortion. Others resulted in the birth of a child with what has become known as Accutane embryopathy, a pattern of anomalies including severe craniofacial disorders (abnormalities of the skull, ears, eyes, nose, and palate), cardiac defects, and DiGeorge syndrome (hypoparathyroidism and T-cell deficiency). Because of the clear cause-and-effect relationship, *cis*-retinoic acid, as well as all other vitamin A congeners, should never be prescribed, recommended, or used during pregnancy.[16]

Hydantoin. Convincing epidemiologic evidence of an association between the anticonvulsant hydantoin and congenital anomalies was provided by Fedrick.[17] In 1975, Hanson and Smith described a recognizable pattern of malformations in offspring of women using hydantoin to control seizures during pregnancy. Features of the fetal hydantoin syndrome include a characteristic facies (ocular hypertelorism, a broad depressed nasal bridge, low-set ears with abnormal pinnae, cleft lip and palate); occasional mild mental retardation; and hypoplasia of the distal phalanges of the fingers and toes, with tiny or absent nails, a striking characteristic of the disorder.[18] In recent years, the pathogenetic mechanism responsible for the malformations has been described. The risk of the syndrome is low; less than 10% of exposed embryos prove to have features of the disorder. Therefore, recommended counseling at this time is as follows: if a woman is already pregnant and taking hydantoin, she

should continue taking the medication; if she is not pregnant, she should be switched to an anticonvulsant that has not been shown to be teratogenic.

ENVIRONMENTAL AGENTS AS TERATOGENS. This category of teratogens represents a group apart from those mentioned previously because, in contrast to prescription and street drugs, exposure to chemicals and agents in the environment is not easily controllable. One agent and some "nonagents" are described here.

Radiation. From the experience in the Japanese cities of Hiroshima and Nagasaki at the conclusion of World War II, it became clear that radiation exposure during fetal life can have lethal or devastating consequences. In addition to a significantly higher rate of spontaneous abortion, pregnant women exposed to high doses of radiation from the atomic bomb explosions (i.e., those close to "ground zero") gave birth to a higher number of children with microcephaly, mental retardation, and skeletal malformations. However, the dose of radiation needed to induce these defects is greater than 5 rad and probably closer to 25 rad. The radiation dose used in diagnostic radiology is extremely low, with most exposure in the range of a few millirad. The literature offers no good evidence that a single (or even multiple) chest radiograph, upper gastrointestinal tract series, or other commonly performed radiologic study can harm the developing fetus.

Nonteratogenic environmental agents. Contrary to some media reports, there is no convincing evidence that exposure to video display terminals, electromagnetic fields, or caffeine causes malformations. Finally, although the active inhalation of cigarette smoke can cause a decrease in birthweight, there is no evidence that the smoking of cigarettes induces malformations in exposed fetuses.

EVALUATION OF EMBRYO/FETUS WITH POTENTIAL TERATOGEN EXPOSURE. Women who have been exposed to potential teratogens often seek advice from their physician. To serve the best interests of both mother and baby, a careful evaluation must be carried out, as follows:

1. Obtain a complete history of the agent, including the dates, type, and length of exposure. The woman should bring any information about the agent (e.g., package insert, label information) in her possession.

2. Obtain a complete history of the pregnancy, including last menstrual period, last normal menstrual period before the last menstrual period (to ascertain the length of the menstrual cycle), date when the pregnancy test became positive, and any symptoms of pregnancy noted. It is essential to make sure that the putative exposure actually occurred during the pregnancy and after the "safe period," as defined earlier, before proceeding with the evaluation.

3. Perform a literature search to investigate previously reported teratogenic effects of the agent. Because it does not give sufficiently helpful or specific information, the *Physicians' Desk Reference* should never be used for purposes of teratogen counseling. Rather, use appropriate on-line computer services and textbooks,[19,20] or refer to specific articles that cite large retrospective or prospective studies.

4. Armed with the information obtained from the literature, counsel the woman regarding the risks. She may then opt to terminate the pregnancy. If she decides to continue the pregnancy, proceed to the next step.

5. Plan an evaluation, using prenatal diagnostic modalities (see earlier discussion), looking for anomalies previously reported after agent exposure.

6. Provide the information necessary so that an intelligent decision can be made about the pregnancy, and support the woman in any decision she has made.

References

1. Hall JG, Powers EK, McIlvaine RT, Ean VH: The frequency and financial burden of genetic disorders in a pediatric hospital, *Am J Med Genet* 1:417, 1978.

2. Evans MI: *Reproductive risks and prenatal diagnosis,* East Norwalk, CT, 1991, Appleton & Lange.

3. Down syndrome preventive medicine check list: *Down Syndrome Papers and Abstracts for Professionals* 12:2, 1989.

4. Rosenfeld RG: *Turner syndrome: a guide for physicians,* Los Angeles, CA, 1989, Mason Medical Communications; pp 1-23.

5. Caldwell PD, Smith DW: The XXY syndrome in childhood: detection and treatment, *J Pediatr* 80:250, 1972.

6. Butler MG, Meaney FJ, Palmer CG: Clinical and cytogenetic survey of 39 individuals with Prader-Labhert-Willi syndrome, *Am J Med Genet* 23:793, 1986.

7. Pyeritz RE: The Marfan syndrome, *Am Fam Physician* 34:83, 1986.

8. Riccardi VE, Eichner JE: *Neurofibromatosis: phenotype, natural history, and pathogenesis,* Baltimore, 1986, Johns Hopkins University Press.

9. Jones KL: *Smith's recognizable patterns of human malformations,* ed. 4, Philadelphia, 1988, WB Saunders, p 298.

10. Marion RW, Chambers P, Schendel LF: Myelomeningocele. In Johnson RT, editor: *Current therapy in neurologic disease—3,* St Louis, 1990, Mosby–Year Book; p 85.

11. Merlob P, Reisner SH: Fetal effects from maternal diabetes. In Buyse ML, editor: *Birth defects encyclopedia,* Cambridge, MA, 1990, Blackwell Scientific Publications; p 700.

12. Mabry CC, Denniston JC, Coldwell JG: Mental retardation in children of phenylketonuric mothers, *N Engl J Med* 275:1331, 1966.

13. Jones KL, Smith DW, Ulleland CN, Streissguth AP: Pattern of malformations in offspring of chronic alcoholic women, *Lancet* 1:1267, 1973.

14. Jones KL: Fetal alcohol syndrome, *Pediatr Rev* 8:122, 1986.

15. Bingol N, Fuchs M, Diaz V, et al: Teratogenicity of cocaine in humans, *Pediatrics* 110:93, 1987.

16. Lammer EJ, Chen DT, Hoar RM, et al: Retinoic acid embryopathy, *N Engl J Med* 313:837, 1985.

17. Fedrick J: Epilepsy and pregnancy: a report from the Oxford Record linkage study, *Br Med J* 2:442, 1973.

18. Hanson JW, Buehler BA: Fetal hydantoin syndrome: current status, *J Pediatr* 101:816, 1982.

19. Shepard TH: *Catalog of teratogenic agents,* ed 6, Baltimore, 1989, Johns Hopkins University Press.

20. Briggs GG, Freeman RK, Yaffe SJ: *Drugs in pregnancy and lactation,* ed 2, Baltimore, 1986, Williams & Wilkins.

SECTION 13

Allergic Disorders

CHAPTER 74

Allergic Disorders

•

Paula Thomas Ardron and Robert Henry Schwartz

Twenty-five percent of the U.S. population has at least one allergic disorder, such as asthma, allergic rhinitis, or atopic dermatitis. Diseases of allergic origin account for one out of every nine visits to a physician. Asthma alone costs the U.S. economy more than 6 billion dollars per year. Chronic rhinitis affects 20% of the population and each year accounts for a loss of 3 million work days and 2 million school days, and a medical cost of $500 million.

Allergic disorders are mediated by different types of immunologic and inflammatory mechanisms. Atopy, the most common type, requires a genetic predisposition to develop immunoglobulin E (IgE) antibodies, an initial sensitizing exposure to an allergen, and a repeat exposure that triggers the release of acute and longer-lasting inflammatory mediators. Allergens that affect the respiratory and gastrointestinal tracts are proteins derived from organic substances such as house dust, pollens, mold spores, animal danders, and foods. They often cause not only allergic rhinoconjunctivitis and asthma, but also urticaria and anaphylaxis. Other common sensitizers include medications, venoms from stinging insects, synthetic compounds such as latex, and metals such as nickel. Despite common perceptions, chocolate, household detergents, and tobacco rarely cause allergic reactions; they elicit adverse reactions by other nonimmunologic mechanisms (chemical, irritant, toxic).

Immunogenic proteins (allergens, antigens) that penetrate the mucosal barriers of the respiratory and gastrointestinal tracts or skin are captured by antigen-presenting cells (macrophage, dendritic cell, Langerhans cell, B cell). The allergens are then processed for presentation to CD4 ("cluster of differentiation") and TH2 lymphocytes (type 2 helper T cells). In susceptible individuals, through class II proteins of the major histocompatibility complex (HLA-DP, HLA-DQ, HLA-DR), TH2 cells recognize the antigen as foreign and secrete cytokines (lymphokines). Cytokine IL-4 (interleukin-4) induces B-cell proliferation, a switch from IgG (immunoglobulin G) and IgM to IgE antibody (specific IgE) production, and mast cell activation. Specific IgE binds to high-affinity Fc receptors (FcεRI) on mast cells. Upon second exposure, allergens bridge the specific IgE on mast cells, inducing degranulation and immediate (within minutes) release of preformed mediators (histamine, tryptase, chymase, cathepsin G). Later (hours to days), newly formed spasmogenic, vasoactive, and chemotactic mediators (leukotrienes and prostaglandins) and other proinflammatory cytokines are released from mast cells and other inflammatory cells. GM-CSF (granulocyte-macrophage colony-stimulating factor) and the cytokines IL-3, IL-4, and IL-5 promote eosinophil growth, migration, and activation. Thus, the TH2 lymphocyte, the B cell, IgE, the mast cell, and the eosinophil are central to the development of acute and chronic allergic reactions. This chapter reviews the clinical manifestations of allergic reactions occurring in disorders of the airway, skin, and eyes, and also other allergic disorders (anaphylaxis, stinging insect allergy, food allergy, drug allergy) that may affect the adolescent.

DISORDERS OF THE AIRWAY

Rhinitis

EPIDEMIOLOGY AND PATHOPHYSIOLOGY. Chronic rhinitis is not a trivial illness. It affects 20% of the population and accounts for 2% of all physician office visits. Approximately 50% of those with chronic rhinitis have nonallergic disease. The incidence of allergic rhinitis, the most common form of atopy, peaks during childhood and adolescence.

The nose protects the trachea and lower airways by warming and humidifying inhaled air and by filtering inert pollutants, aeroallergens, and microorganisms. Turbulent airflow, created by three turbinates, aids in deposition of these particles on the mucosal surface. The beating cilia of pseudostratified columnar epithelial cells transport particles trapped in mucus to the pharynx. Airflow obstruction can result from an anatomic deformity, mucosal swelling, or the physical barrier caused by thick nasal secretions. Sneezing is the result of local irritation of nerve endings and central reflexes.

Studies using nasal provocation tests have clarified the roles of chemical mediators in the nasal mucosa. Histamine produces pruritus. Serotonin induces sneezing and rhinorrhea without congestion. Leukotrienes, kinins, and prostaglandin D_2 cause congestion and rhinorrhea.

Inhaled allergens induce immunologic degranulation of sensitized mast cells, and physical stimuli, such as cold air, may cause nonimmunologic degranulation of mast cells and basophils. Both mechanisms release the preformed chemical mediators that can cause acute rhinitis. The late-phase allergic reaction results pathologically in inflammation with eosinophils. The clinical counterpart is chronic rhinitis.

DIAGNOSTIC CONSIDERATIONS. Seasonal allergic rhinitis and/or conjunctivitis (hay fever, rose fever, pollenosis) is manifested by nasal congestion, repetitive sneezing, clear rhinorrhea, and ocular tearing. Patients describe intense nasal, ocular, and sometimes palatal itching. These symptoms are often associated with fatigue that may be aggravated by the side effects of medication. The family history is often positive for atopic disease. Nasal congestion associated with headaches, purulent postnasal discharge, and halitosis suggests infectious rhinosinusitis. Seasonal symptoms result from sensitivities to tree pollens in the spring, grass pollens in the early summer, or weed pollens and mold spores in the late summer and fall.

Perennial allergic rhinitis symptoms may be due to dust mites, indoor animal danders, or indoor molds. Environmental irritants such as tobacco smoke, air pollution, perfumes, or ammonia can aggravate both seasonal and perennial rhinitis.

Vasomotor rhinitis is manifested by symptoms that are provoked by exercise, emotional upset, changes in temperature, the ingestion of spicy foods or alcohol, or exposure to bright sunlight or perfumes. This condition is thought to be neurally mediated but the exact mechanism has not been ascertained; it is not mediated by IgE. The most effective form of treatment is avoidance of the provoking events.

Acute rhinitis is triggered by viral upper respiratory tract infections with rhinovirus, adenovirus, or respiratory syncytial virus. Symptoms may include fever. The rhinorrhea is often clear and the disease process is self-limited.

If symptoms last longer than 2 weeks and/or a purulent discharge is present, bacterial rhinosinusitis should be suspected. Some patients present with symptoms and signs of allergic rhinitis, including sneezing, watery rhinorrhea, and nasal pruritus associated with nasal eosinophilia, but still have negative skin tests. These patients fit into a subset of perennial rhinitis called the nonallergic rhinitis with eosinophilia syndrome (NARES). A triad of symptoms consisting of rhinitis, nasal polyps, and asthma, called Samter's syndrome, is associated with an allergy to aspirin and other nonsteroidal antiinflammatory drugs. Several other prescribed medications can cause nonallergic rhinitis, including antihypertensives (such as reserpine) and oral contraceptives containing estrogen. An adolescent who has a history of allergic rhinitis should be encouraged, when appropriate, to use the injectable or implanted forms of progestin for birth control, because rhinitis is not an associated side effect of these. Rhinitis is also associated with pregnancy and usually resolves after delivery. Chronic rhinitis may be a symptom of hypothyroidism or diabetes.

PHYSICAL EXAMINATION. Infraorbital cyanosis ("shiners") may be evident in the physical examination of patients with allergic rhinitis. This bluish hue under the eyes occurs in both allergic and nonallergic forms of chronic rhinosinusitis and is the result of vascular engorgement of nasal sinusoids and venous stasis of cutaneous blood flow around the eyes. A transverse nasal crease at the distal end of the nasal bridge is pathognomonic of persistent nasal itching and a strong indication that inhalant allergy exists. Patients with allergic rhinitis have a pale bluish appearance to the nasal mucosa along with a clear nasal discharge. Those with infectious nonallergic rhinitis have a reddish hue that may be associated with either clear or purulent nasal discharge. An effusion behind the tympanic membrane denotes eustachian tube dysfunction frequently associated with chronic rhinitis. Cobblestoning, a follicular collection of lymphoid tissue in the posterior pharynx, results from the constant irritation of postnasal mucus. Further examination may reveal other associated conditions. Hyposmia or anosmia suggests the presence of nasal polyposis. A barrel chest is a result of chronic air trapping and asthma. Dry, scaly, lichenified patches of skin distributed over the flexor surfaces of the extremities signal the presence of chronic atopic dermatitis.

ALLERGY TESTING. Microscopic examination of stained (Wright's or Hansel's stain) specimens of nasal mucus (nasal smears) can help to distinguish nonallergic from allergic forms of rhinitis. A predominance of neutrophils suggests bacterial infection. Eosinophilia (>10% of cells) usually indicates an allergic etiology, but it is also seen in the uncommon NARES. Epicutaneous skin tests (prick or puncture techniques) using commonly inhaled allergens or in vitro immunoassays (radioallergosorbent test [RAST], enzyme-linked immunosorbent assay [ELISA]) identify specific IgE and help to confirm the sensitization suggested by the patient's history. Skin tests are more sensitive and less expensive than in vitro tests. In vitro immunoassays are used when skin testing cannot be done because the patient has extensive dermatitis or severe dermatographism or must remain on antihistamine or tricyclic antidepressant drugs. Decongestants and glucocorticosteroid medications do not inhibit immediate IgE-mediated wheal and flare skin test reactions.

MANAGEMENT

Nonpharmacologic. After the cause of allergic rhinitis has been identified by the history alone or by history and appropriate testing, avoidance measures should be discussed. Avoidance of outdoor allergens such as pollens and mold spores is difficult. Hiking and camping trips can be planned during nonpollen seasons. Driving with the car windows closed during allergy seasons is helpful. Keeping windows in the house closed and cooling the house with an air-conditioning system will reduce indoor exposure to outdoor pollens. The amount of pollen deposited on the hair and skin and transferred to bedding can be reduced by taking showers in the evening during the pollen season. Avoidance of indoor allergens may be a difficult task, especially when there is significant sensitization to cats and dogs. Cockroaches, a source of major indoor allergens, are found especially in multiple family dwellings in the inner cities. Aeroallergens (the fecal pellets) derived from house dust mites (*Dermatophagoides farinii* and *pteronyssinus*) are powerful inducers of allergic responses in children and adults. If sensitization has been shown to exist, measures to reduce exposure to mite allergens should be taken when managing patients with allergic rhinitis and asthma (Box 74-1).

BOX 74-1
House Dust Mite Control Measures

ESSENTIAL
1. Encase the mattress in an airtight cover
2. Either encase the pillow or wash weekly
3. Wash the bedding in 130° F water weekly
4. Avoid sleeping or lying on upholstered furniture
5. Remove carpets that are laid on concrete

DESIRABLE
1. Reduce indoor humidity to less than 50%
2. Remove carpets from bedroom
3. Use chemical agents to kill mites or alter their antigens

Pharmacologic. Antihistamines are effective first-line choices for the treatment of allergic rhinitis because they work quickly and relieve the sneezing, itching, and rhinorrhea. However, they are not very effective for the treatment of nasal congestion. Sedation is the most common side effect of the classic antihistamines but it is less likely to occur with the newer nonsedating antihistamines such as loratadine and astemizole, which do not readily cross the blood-brain barrier. Oral decongestants (alpha-adrenergic sympathomimetic amines) relieve nasal congestion by constricting blood vessels, decreasing blood flow to the nasal mucosa, and reducing nasal mucosal edema. Their most common side effects are irritability, insomnia, tremor, tachycardia, and increased blood pressure. Topical decongestants also are effective. However, repetitive use of alpha-adrenergic topical nasal sprays for more than 7 days can lead to rhinitis medicamentosa manifested by chronic rebound nasal obstruction and dependency. Since these medications are available without a prescription, parents may not be aware that their children are taking them. Adolescents may not regard them as medications and need to be specifically asked about use. The nasal mucosa will appear beefy red with punctate regions of bleeding. Similar findings occur among adolescents who use other forms of vasoconstrictors, such as cocaine.

Topical intranasal antiinflammatory drugs, such as cromolyn sodium and glucocorticoids, are safe and effective medications for the treatment and prevention of allergic rhinitis. Cromolyn sodium stabilizes mast cells, preventing degranulation. It works best when initiated before the patient's allergy season begins or before episodic exposures. It has virtually no adverse side effects. Compliance with its prescription may be a problem because it is most effective when used frequently (four times a day) and its onset of action is slow. Topical glucocorticosteroids are safe because, in the dose and concentrations used, they act locally and are not significantly absorbed. Their antiinflammatory action begins at the level of gene expression in the nucleus, which is why there is a delay between administration and the onset of clinical activity. The vasoconstrictive and antipruritic actions are more immediate. Preparations containing beclomethasone, budesonide, dexamethsone, flunisolide, fluticasone, and triamcinolone are now available in the United States. For the treatment of chronic allergic rhinitis, topical glucocorticosteroids are more effective than antihistamines, decongestants, and cromolyn. The most common side effects are local nasal irritation, burning, and sneezing, which occur in about 10% of patients. Bloody nasal discharge is seen in about 2% of patients, and septal perforations can occur with long-term use. Nasal overgrowth with *Candida* organisms is uncommon. A major advantage for the adolescent patient is the once or twice daily dosing regimen now possible with the newer antihistamines, topical and oral decongestants, topical glucocorticosteroids, and cromolyn sodium.

Immunologic. Specific-allergen immunotherapy is a form of treatment based on an individual's specific sensitivities. It involves weekly to monthly subcutaneous injections of allergen extracts of pollens, mold spores, dust mites, epidermoids, and Hymenoptera venoms. Immunotherapy is effective for patients who find it impossible to avoid allergens or for whom pharmacotherapy has failed (Box 74-2). Immunologic changes that occur during immunotherapy include an increase in serum allergen-specific IgG antibody levels, and an initial increase followed by a significant decrease in serum allergen-specific IgE levels. IgA and IgG antibody concentrations increase in nasal secretions. There is also a reduction in the late-phase allergic inflammatory response and a decrease in the number of eosinophils in nasal secretions. Clinical improvement occurs over 1 to 2 years. Therapy should be continued for 1 to 2 years after all symptoms have resolved; if a patient shows no sign of improvement after 2 years of treatment, immunotherapy should be stopped. The duration of immunotherapy need not exceed 5 years and it should be carried out only under the supervision of a physician trained in its use. The most common side effects are local reactions at the site of the injection. Infrequently, patients develop systemic reactions, including urticaria, bronchospasm, or hypotension. If these reactions occur, they usually happen during the initial build-up phase, during a symptomatic pollen season, or when freshly prepared injection material is first used. Life-threatening anaphylactic reactions can occur if an excessively high dose or the wrong extract is given, or if the dose is inadvertently administered intravenously. Since these reactions usually occur within 30 minutes after the injection is given, patients should remain in the physician's office for at least this time. The busy adolescent patient may be reluctant to do this.

BOX 74-2
When to Consider Immunotherapy

1. A specific allergic trigger is identified
2. Environmental control is ineffective (allergic rhinitis, allergic asthma)
3. Avoidance is not possible (e.g., occupational exposure)
4. Pharmacologic therapy fails to control asthmatic and/or allergic rhinitis symptoms
5. Patients or families do not or cannot administer medication or carry out adequate environmental control
6. The patient has experienced a life-threatening anaphylactic reaction to an insect sting

---

Sinusitis

ANATOMIC AND PATHOPHYSIOLOGIC CONSIDERATIONS. The paranasal sinuses include the maxillary, ethmoidal, frontal, and sphenoidal sinuses. The maxillary sinuses are present at 10 weeks' gestation; the ethmoid, sphenoid, and frontal sinuses are present at 3 to 5 months' gestation. Radiographically, the maxillary and ethmoid sinuses appear during infancy, the frontal sinuses are evident between the ages of 3 and 7 years, and the sphenoid sinuses come into view around the age of 9 years. Each sinus drains through an opening, or ostium, on the lateral aspect of the nasal cavity. The anterior and middle ethmoidal, the maxillary, and the frontal sinuses drain into a common area (osteomeatal complex [OMC]) and then into the middle meatus, located between the middle and inferior turbinates. The posterior ethmoidal sinuses and the sphenoidal sinus drain into the spheno-ethmoidal recess (SER) and then into the superior meatus. The opening to the nasolacrimal duct is below the inferior turbinate.

The epithelial surface of the sinuses functions as a mucociliary apparatus and facilitates drainage by propelling foreign particles and microorganisms trapped in a mucus blanket toward the ostia. Obstruction of the OMC or SER and patency of the ostia are the most important factors in the development of sinusitis. The most common cause of ostial obstruction is edema from inflammation associated with a viral upper respiratory infection. The allergic reaction can act similarly. Mucus movement will be impaired if cilia are dysfunctional (dysmotile cilia syndrome) or if secretions become viscous because of infection or dehydration. Nasal polyps, nasal tumors, and anatomic abnormalities (deviated nasal septum) can also contribute to obstruction.

Sinusitis is classified by the duration of symptoms: acute (less than 30 days), subacute (3 weeks to 2 months), and chronic (more than 2 to 3 months). The most frequent pathogens found in acute and chronic sinusitis are *Streptococcus pneumoniae, Haemophilus influenzae,* and *Moraxella catarrhalis.* Chronic sinusitis, in young otherwise healthy adolescents and in patients with hypogammaglobulinemia and antibody deficiency syndromes, is often caused by the same organisms. When chronic sinusitis in adolescents and adults does not respond to conventional antibiotics, infections with *Staphylococcus aureus* and with anaerobic organisms *(Bacteroides fragilis)* should be suspected. Patients with cystic fibrosis commonly have *Pseudomonas aeruginosa* as the etiologic pathogen.

DIAGNOSIS AND PHYSICAL EXAMINATION. Acute sinusitis should be suspected in patients whose symptoms fail to resolve after a viral upper respiratory tract infection. Patients present with cough, turbid or yellow to green nasal discharge and pharyngeal drainage, headache (frontal, between the eyes, vertex, retroorbital, bitemporal), fever, chills, facial pain (maxillary, dental), and discomfort worsened by bending. Physical examination reveals purulent nasal discharge, erythema of the nasal mucosa, and evidence of edema.

Chronic sinusitis presents with similar symptoms of purulent nasal discharge, sore throat, malaise, and halitosis. Pain or systemic symptoms are often not present. Because secretions pool in the posterior pharynx, complications involving chronic coughing or wheezing may also be present. On physical examination, direct sinus tenderness may or may not be present. Posterior pharyngeal lymphoid hyperplasia (cobblestoning) may be evident. The nasal mucosa will appear edematous and erythematous. A fungal infection should be suspected if a thick, peanut butter–like discharge is seen. Complications of sinusitis include orbital or periorbital cellulitis, epidural or dural abscesses, osteomyelitis, mucoceles, and pyoceles. Sinusitis can both complicate and intensify bronchial asthma.

DIAGNOSTIC TESTS. Nasal smears show sheets of polymorphonuclear neutrophils and bacteria. Nasal cultures reflect bacteria in the anterior nares and do not give an adequate picture of the organisms found in the sinuses. Antral puncture aspirates are considered the gold standard, but these can be obtained only by a skilled otolaryngologist and should be reserved for refractory cases.

Radiographic studies include the Waters view, displaying the maxillary sinuses; the Caldwell view, revealing the ethmoid and frontal sinuses; and the lateral view, showing the sphenoid sinuses. Radiographic evidence of sinusitis includes the presence of air-fluid levels, opacification, and mucosal thickening. Coronal computed tomography (CT) is the gold standard for diagnosing sinusitis, but it should not yet be considered a routine procedure because of its high cost.

MANAGEMENT: MEDICAL, ALLERGIC, AND SURGICAL. Medical therapy for acute sinusitis includes topical (oxymetazoline hydrochloride) and/or oral decongestants (pseudoephedrine, phenylpropanolamine) for their vasoconstricting effect, allowing the sinuses to drain. Limiting the use of topical decongestants such as oxymetazoline hydrochloride to 3 to 4 days usually is adequate and prevents the addictive results of rhinitis medicamentosa. Topical or oral steroids can assist in decreasing the nasal mucosal edema due to inflammation, thus augmenting the effects of nasal decongestants. Antibiotics such as amoxicillin, sulfatrimethoprim, erythromycin, and first-generation cephalosporins serve as good first-line drugs, but treatment failures are becoming more common because beta-lactamase–producing organisms are on the rise and often are resistant to these medications. Antibiotics effective against these pathogens include clavulanic acid in combination with amoxicillin, and azithromycin

or clarithromycin. To ensure eradication of the offending organism, the duration of therapy should be 2 to 3 weeks for acute sinusitis and 4 to 6 weeks for chronic sinusitis. Guaifenesin, a mucoevacuant, can help to thin tenacious nasal mucus and enhance response to therapy. Systemic glucocorticosteroids may need to be used cautiously if nasal polyps are present. Management of fungal sinusitis includes debridement and use of antifungal agents. The allergic form of sinusitis caused by colonization of the sinuses with organisms like *Aspergillus* responds to debridement and systemic steroids. *Pseudomonas* infections can be treated with ciprofloxacin.

Referral to an allergist should be considered if perennial or seasonal allergies are present in individuals with recurrent or chronic sinusitis. Those who have specific allergies identified by history and skin testing can be taught avoidance measures. Further medical management can be implemented and immunotherapy considered.

Referral to an otolaryngologist should be considered for patients who fail medical management or who show evidence of anatomic abnormalities contributing to obstruction, such as nasal septal deviation, spurs, and polyps. Functional endoscopic sinus surgery (FESS) is a contemporary form of sinus surgery that enlarges the OMC or SER regions and relieves anatomic and inflammatory obstruction associated with unremitting chronic sinusitis.

Chronic Cough

Along with phagocytosis by alveolar macrophages, mucociliary clearance, lymphatic drainage, and the gag reflex, cough removes abnormal secretions and foreign substances from the respiratory tract. Chronic cough is the principal reason for 16 million office visits in the United States, or 2.5% of total office visits per year. In the adolescent patient the most common causes of chronic cough include asthma and sinusitis. Other conditions associated with exacerbations of asthma that may be manifested by cough include allergic bronchopulmonary aspergillosis, exercise-induced bronchospasm, certain drug and food additive idiosyncrasies, gastroesophageal reflux, and pregnancy.

The term *asthma* is derived from the Greek word for panting or breathlessness. Pathophysiologically, it is characterized by airway inflammation (eosinophilic bronchitis), obstruction of airflow (bronchospasm, edema, mucus), and hyperresponsiveness of the airway to a variety of stimuli (exercise, cold air, methacholine, histamine). A detailed discussion of the pathophysiology of asthma may be found in Chapter 41. Many specialists believe that cough occurring as a cough-variant of asthma is a more common symptom and sign of asthma than is wheezing. Since allergy is the primary event in 90% of children with asthma over the age of 3 years and under the age of 16 years, and in 70% of people with asthma under the age of 30 years, it should be considered in the etiology of cough. Asthma should be suspected in patients who have a family history of atopy, whose cough exacerbations are seasonal, who have a history of other atopic diseases (e.g., allergic rhinitis or atopic dermatitis), or who have eosinophils in the sputum. Nedocromil sodium by inhalation has been shown to be effective in the management of the allergic asthmatic cough. Other drugs used in the treatment of asthma (inhaled beta agonists, inhaled glucocorticosteroids, theophylline) can also be tried.

Allergic bronchopulmonary aspergillosis is a complication of asthma characterized by cough and wheezing, production of brown chunky sputum, blood and sputum eosinophilia, elevated serum levels of IgE, and large positive immediate wheal and flare reactions to allergenic extracts of *Aspergillus fumigatus.* Chest radiographs reveal fleeting acute infiltrates and evidence of chronic proximal bronchiectasis. Treatment consists of an oral glucocorticosteroid and an inhaled bronchodilator.

Exercise-induced asthma and cough occur in 70% of adolescent asthma patients. Symptoms begin 5 to 10 minutes after the initiation of strenuous prolonged exercise; in some patients, symptoms begin after exercise is completed. This form of asthma can be prevented by warm-up exercises and by using cromolyn sodium, nedocromil sodium, or a beta$_2$-adrenergic agonist 15 to 20 minutes before exercise. Patients with exercise-induced asthma perform better when breathing warm humidified air. Activities such as swimming or short-distance running are excellent alternatives to endurance sports.

Idiosyncratic reactions to drugs such as aspirin and other NSAIDs occur in a small subset of patients who develop rhinorrhea and bronchospasm or urticaria and angioedema. Aspirin-sensitive asthma should be suspected in patients who have nasal polyposis, chronic sinusitis, and eosinophilia. Management consists of aggressive treatment of the rhinitis and polyposis, as well as strict avoidance of aspirin, NSAIDs, and tartrazine (a yellow food dye). Recently developed lipoxygenase inhibitors and leukotriene receptor antagonists may become the treatments of choice because they inhibit the production and action of leukotrienes in these patients who have an aberration of arachidonic acid metabolism. Sulfites, bisulfites, and metabisulfites are chemicals used as food preservatives to prevent nonenzymatic browning and inhibit the growth of microorganisms. When ingested, these agents liberate sulfur dioxide in the mouth and stomach. Subsequent inhalation of sulfur dioxide results in bronchospasm. Lastly, chronic cough is a frequent side effect of angiotensin-converting enzyme (ACE) inhibitor drugs used in the treatment of hypertension.

Although a cough is an unusual manifestation of pregnancy, it can be a stressful symptom for the pregnant adolescent with asthma. The severity of asthma during pregnancy can be predicted by the number of exacerbations the patient has during the first trimester. One third get better, one third stay the same, and one third get worse. During this time, patients experience an increase in tidal volume and up to a 50% increase in minute ventilation. These changes are thought to be due to circulating progesterone.

Psychogenic cough presents as a dry, honking cough that is most pronounced during the daytime. Patients are typically able to sleep through the night without coughing. Patients with gastroesophageal reflux present with symptoms of heartburn after meals that increase while bending over or lying down. Gastroesophageal reflux should be suspected in patients with nighttime exacerbations of their cough.

Patients suspected of having an allergic cough or cough-variant of asthma can be evaluated by skin testing with commonly inhaled aeroallergens and by pulmonary function testing. Airflow obstruction can be identified by a reduction in FEV$_1$ (forced expiratory volume in 1 second). A measurement 20% below the value predicted for age, sex, height, and race is significant. A 15% or more improvement in this expiratory flow parameter, after the use of an inhaled bronchodilator, is considered significant.

ANAPHYLAXIS

Anaphylaxis results from the release of bioactive mediators that exert damaging effects on target organs. It can affect a single organ system or crescendo into a concerted response involving multiple organ systems. The manifestations of anaphylaxis are of sudden onset and specific to each organ system. The cutaneous response results in urticaria and angioedema; the respiratory response in bronchospasm and laryngospasm; the gastrointestinal response in nausea, vomiting, and diarrhea; the cardiovascular response in tachycardia, arrhythmias, hypotension, and shock; and the central nervous system (CNS) response in incontinence and a feeling of impending doom.

IgE-mediated anaphylaxis occurs in both atopic and nonatopic individuals. Atopic patients are not at increased risk for this form of anaphylaxis unless they are receiving immunotherapy. Other sensitizing agents that can cause this form of anaphylaxis include drugs, especially beta-lactam antibiotics (penicillins); foods (peanuts, tree nuts, egg white, shell fish, fish, milk); certain food additives (sulfites); and Hymenoptera venom (Box 74-3).

Immune complex–mediated anaphylaxis can occur after exposure to blood or its products. Immune complexes activate the classic pathway of the complement cascade. This mechanism can be operative in some IgA-deficient patients who have IgG antibodies to IgA and are treated with intravenous immunoglobulin (IVIG). If the IVIG contains IgA, immune complexes are formed, complement is activated, and bioactive mediators are released, resulting in urticaria, bronchospasm, and hypotension.

Abnormalities in arachidonic acid metabolism explain the anaphylactic reactions to aspirin and other NSAIDs that sometimes occur. The mechanism is thought to be an inhibition of the cyclooxygenase pathway by NSAIDs and augmentation of the lipoxygenase pathway with the generation of leukotrienes.

Anaphylactoid reactions mimic anaphylactic reactions but are caused by nonimmunologic degranulation of mast cells and basophils, resulting in the release of histamine and other mediators. Precipitating agents in this group include morphine, codeine, curare, plasma expanders, aminoglycosides, and radiocontrast media.

Exercise-induced anaphylaxis is a syndrome with symptoms similar to anaphylaxis caused by IgE-dependent mechanisms. It is increasingly recognized to occur in some young adults with interest in physical fitness activities such as jogging, bicycling, racquet sports, soccer, skiing, and aerobic exercise. Clinical features include early symptoms of diffuse warmth, pruritus, and erythema followed by urticaria and angioedema most prominent on the face, palms, and soles. The cutaneous manifestations last from 30 minutes to 4 hours. Vascular collapse and loss of consciousness, as well as choking, stridor, colic, nausea, and vomiting, are common. Most episodes resolve in 2 hours, but a disabling headache may persist for as long as 72 hours. In contrast to cholinergic urticaria, patients do not develop symptoms after a hot bath or shower, with febrile episodes, or with anxiety or stress. However, elevated serum histamine levels occur in both conditions. Since exercise alone does not reproduce attacks, additional factors have been implicated. These include exercise on warm, humid days; antecedent ingestion of alcohol; aspirin ingestion; and eating of certain foods such as shellfish, celery, cabbage, peach, wheat, and chicken. Management is identical to that of anaphylaxis of any cause. It is essential to avoid precipitating and associated factors, stop exercise at the earliest symptom, carry a syringe with epinephrine, wear a medical identification bracelet, and exercise with an informed companion.

Treatment of anaphylaxis should begin immediately. Once an open airway is secured, breathing is established, and supplemental oxygen is in place, the circulatory system can be stabilized by using injections of epinephrine, intravenous fluids, and other vasopressors as needed. Antihistamines block histamine receptors; H_1 blockers affect the respiratory mucosa and skin, and H_2 blockers exert their effect on the stabilization of the vascular bed. Nebulized albuterol reverses bronchospasm, and nebulized epinephrine decreases upper airway edema. Glucocorticosteroids should be used, because anaphylaxis can be biphasic and even lethal during the second phase. They decrease the intensity of the late-phase reaction by reducing further release of inflammatory mediators.

Patients who have life-threatening anaphylaxis should be admitted to the hospital for treatment and observation. Upon discharge, they should be given an emergency plan, including instructions for the use of an epinephrine syringe (EpiPen, ANA kit). They should be counseled to avoid the circumstances that have initiated the event and to wear a medical alert bracelet.

HYMENOPTERA REACTIONS (INSECT STINGS)

Stinging insects are members of the order Hymenoptera, which is divided into two groups: vespids and apids. Vespids are yellow jackets, wasps, and hornets. Yellow jackets are more likely to sting because their nests are found in the ground or on walls and are frequently disturbed by lawn mowing, gardening, or other outdoor activities. Their attraction to food compels them to be the uninvited guests to picnics and barbecues. Their stinging apparatus, consisting of a venom sac connected to a stinger, can deliver multiple stings to their victim. Apids are honeybees and bumblebees. Honeybees are the most common stinging insects in this group. They generally are docile and sting only when provoked. Because their stinging apparatus contains many barbs, they can sting only once. Injection causes evisceration of their organs, resulting in their death. Fire ants are nonwinged Hymenoptera found in the southeastern and south central United States. They bite their victims and then inflict a series of stings in a circular pattern as they rotate around the bite site. Patients develop sterile pustules within 24 hours of the sting.

Typical reactions to stings consist of localized pain, swelling, and erythema. Treatment with analgesics and cold compresses results in rapid resolution. Large local reactions typically peak 48 hours after the sting and slowly resolve over 7 days. The reaction is often associated with fatigue and nausea. Treatment with analgesics and an antihistamine is often sufficient, but in patients who have severe local swelling, corticosteroids are beneficial. Subsequent reactions in these patients present similarly but with a less than 5% risk of anaphylaxis. The risk of generalized anaphylactic reactions secondary to an insect sting is highest in those under age 20 years. Symptoms usually begin within 10 to 20 minutes of the sting. The risk of anaphylaxis with subsequent stings is 50% to 60%.

Anaphylaxis from insect stings can be prevented by minimizing exposure to the insect, having available and using appropriate medication (liquid diphenhydramine and an epinephrine syringe), and receiving venom immunotherapy. Protective measures include the wearing of shoes, pants, and long-sleeve shirts when outside. Cosmetics, hair sprays, perfumes, and brightly colored clothing attract Hymenoptera, so their use should be avoided.

Venom immunotherapy should be considered by any patient who has had a generalized anaphylactic reaction to an insect sting. Children with only cutaneous reactions need not be given this therapy, since subsequent reactions will usually be limited to the skin. Adolescents 16 years of age or older have been shown to benefit from venom immunotherapy, which significantly reduces their risks of life-threatening respiratory and cardiovascular reactions. Patients should be skin-prick tested to detect specific IgE to one or more purified Hymenoptera venoms. RASTs are a less specific and more expensive alternative to skin tests. The duration of venom immunotherapy is 3 to 5 years. It is considered successful in those patients whose repeat skin tests are negative. Once therapy is completed, the subsequent risk of anaphylaxis plummets to as low as 2%.

DISORDERS DUE TO FOOD ALLERGY

The real prevalence of food allergies is 1% to 2% in the adult population and 6% in young children, but the perceived prevalence may be as high as 33%. The discrepancy is due to improper terminology used by both the lay public and "informed" health professionals. Adverse reactions to foods can be divided into two categories: IgE-mediated allergic reactions and non–IgE-mediated intolerance reactions that result from abnormal physiologic responses that are not immunologic in nature (toxic, pharmacologic, metabolic, or idiosyncratic).

The gastrointestinal mucosa serves as a barrier to more than 98% of ingested antigens. Factors that prevent absorption of these intact antigens include enzymatic digestion, increased stomach acidity, the presence of other food in the gut, and the local immune IgA system. Despite these defenses, a minute amount of an intact antigen can breach this barrier. Typically, these intact antigens are unable to cause adverse reactions because of the body's ability to develop tolerance to them. Food antigens are presented to TH2 lymphocytes. If they are perceived as foreign, cytokines are released, B lymphocytes are activated, specific IgE antibodies are produced, and mast cells are sensitized. When the same food antigens bind to membrane IgE on basophils and mast cells, a cascade of bioactive amines, including histamine, are released. These mediators induce immediate hypersensitivity, resulting in the signs and symptoms of anaphylaxis.

Clinically, local gastrointestinal reactions include cramping, bloating, vomiting, and diarrhea that can be self-limited or protracted. Systemic reactions result from the spread of food antigens throughout the body by way of the bloodstream and lymphatics, causing urticaria and angioedema, laryngeal stridor, bronchospasm, rhinorrhea, nasal congestion, and oral or pharyngeal pruritus. In adolescents and adults, severe life-threatening reactions are most often associated with the ingestion of peanuts, tree nuts, fish, and shellfish. Reactions to milk, egg, and wheat rarely occur in adolescence.

Allergic eosinophilic gastroenteritis is an eosinophilic inflammatory late-phase allergic reaction occurring in the mucosal, muscular, and/or serosal layers of the stomach or small intestine. These three locations represent the three variants of the disease. All of them are characterized by a peripheral eosinophilia and absence of vasculitis. Infiltration of the muscular wall with eosinophils leads to thickening and rigidity and to signs of obstruction. When it involves the serosal layer, ascites with eosinophils is predominant. Patients present with postprandial nausea, vomiting, diarrhea, and abdominal pain. There is weight loss in adults and failure to thrive in infants. A gastrointestinal biopsy in the mucosal type shows eosinophilic infiltrates in the lamina propria and loss of intestinal villi, explaining the other clinical features of malabsorption, gastrointestinal blood loss, and protein-losing enteropathy. Elevated serum IgE levels and multiple positive immediate skin test reactions or RASTs to food antigens are found almost exclusively in the mucosal variant type. Many of these patients have other atopic diseases such as asthma or allergic rhinitis. The mucosal variant type is thought to be IgE mediated. Elimination of suspected foods from the diet for 6 to 12 weeks may help to resolve symptoms. However, long-term treatment with systemic glucocorticosteroids is often required. Ketotifen, a new H_1 receptor blocker, has shown some promise in controlling symptoms.

Oral allergy syndrome symptoms begin within 5 to 30 minutes of ingestion of certain foods, most commonly fruits or vegetables. Oral tingling, burning, and pruritus occur with or without oral mucosal blebs, angioedema, throat tightness, hoarseness, and facial flushing. These symptoms can be a prelude to systemic anaphylaxis. Ragweed-sensitive adolescents frequently experience these symptoms when eating melons or bananas.

Atopic dermatitis is the "itch that rashes." Food allergies can exacerbate the condition by releasing histamine and causing cutaneous erythema and pruritus. The foods involved most commonly include eggs, milk, peanuts, soy, fish, and wheat. Elimination of these foods may help the skin to return to its normal state.

Dermatitis herpetiformis is a non–IgE-mediated reaction consisting of a chronic, intensely pruritic, burning or stinging, papulovesicular rash that is distributed symmetrically over the extensor surfaces of the extremities (elbows and knees) and can involve the buttocks. It is associated with an asymptomatic gluten-sensitive enteropathy in 75% to 90% of patients. Diagnosis depends on finding granular immunofluorescent IgA deposits at the dermal-epidermal junction of normal-appearing and lesional skin. Treatment with sulfones ameliorates skin symptoms, and strict elimination of gluten from the diet may normalize intestinal findings.

Diagnosis

Epicutaneous skin tests for reactions to specific foods are sensitive but not specific. False-positive reactions for certain foods may be as high as 60% to 65%, but the false-negative rate is very low. Therefore, the negative predictive value is high for IgE-mediated allergic reactions to foods. Negative skin test results occur, of course, in intolerance reactions. RAST testing should be done in patients who have extensive skin disease, in those who have significant dermatographism, and in those who might have life-threatening reactions to minute amounts of food antigens used in skin testing.

Double-blind, placebo-controlled food challenge (DBPCFC) is the gold standard for proving an adverse reaction to food. Food is administered with the patient in a fasting state at a dose unlikely to cause a reaction. The dose is doubled every 15 to 60 minutes until an objective reaction is observed or a dose equivalent to 10 g is administered. If the DBPCFC is negative, an open challenge should be done to rule out the rare chance of a false-negative reaction. The DBPCFCs and open challenges can be performed in an office, clinic, or hospital. However, they should be carried out only by trained personnel who have access to emergency equipment suitable for treating systemic anaphylaxis.

Management

Avoidance of the offending food is the only currently proved preventive therapy for food allergies. Patients must be instructed to read labels carefully, looking specifically for hidden allergens. Diets must be constructed properly so that complications resulting from malnutrition do not occur. With allergen avoidance of 1 to 2 years' duration, one third of children will lose their clinical reactivity to milk, egg, and fruit. Older patients who have allergies to tree nuts, fish, peanuts, shellfish, or fish rarely lose their clinical reactivity. Celiac disease, caused by gluten sensitivity, requires a lifelong avoidance of gluten.

Instructions should be given on the use of a syringe containing epinephrine, which the patient should carry at all times with liquid diphenhydramine. If administration of these drugs is required, the patient should be evaluated and observed by medical personnel so that if late-phase reactions occur, they can be treated.

DISORDERS DUE TO DRUG ALLERGY

Drug reactions occur in 1 to 2 million Americans each year. Adverse drug reactions are primarily caused by antibiotics, aspirin and other nonsteroidal antiinflammatories, and CNS depressants. The most common manifestation is the eruption of a skin rash.

Drugs given in frequent, intermittent courses are more likely to cause IgE-mediated reactions than those given for prolonged periods without interruption. The route of drug administration also influences the risk of sensitization; oral administration carries the lowest risk of sensitization, followed by intravenous, intradermal, and topical routes.

Drugs and their metabolites can function as haptens, simple low-molecular-weight chemicals capable of combining with body proteins (carriers) and being recognized by the immune system. An example is the beta-lactam ring of penicillin that conjugates to body proteins through the penicilloyl moiety, the major metabolite (determinant) of penicillin. Upon repeat exposure, hapten-protein conjugates bind to specific IgE on sensitized mast cells, leading to their degranulation. The release of vasoactive, chemotactic, and bronchospastic mediators affects multiple organ systems, resulting in symptoms ranging from pruritus and urticaria to bronchospasm, laryngeal edema, anaphylactic shock, and death.

A maculopapular or morbilliform eruption is the most common allergic reaction to drugs. It occurs in 40% of college students treated with ampicillin or amoxicillin for sore throats associated with infectious mononucleosis. A pruritic or nonpruritic rash typically has a symmetric distribution that begins on the extremities and spares the palms and soles. Drugs causing this form of reaction include beta-lactams, sulfonamides, and anticonvulsants.

Erythema multiforme is characterized by urticaria, angioedema, and the classic target skin rash. It can progress to Stevens-Johnson syndrome, one of the febrile mucocutaneous syndromes. These patients develop fever and vesicular bullous lesions involving at least two or more mucosal surfaces. Toxic epidermal necrolysis is another of the more severe forms of the febrile mucocutaneous syndromes resulting in full-thickness sloughing of the epidermis. The mortality rate is low for erythema multiforme but increases to 30% with toxic epidermal necrolysis. Drugs most often implicated in these reactions include trimethoprim/sulfamethoxazole, phenytoin, beta-lactams, aspirin, and NSAIDs.

Serum sickness is an allergic reaction due to the formation of both specific IgE and IgG. IgE sensitizes mast cells and is responsible for urticaria and angioedema. In antigen excess, IgG forms soluble complexes with the antigen, and these antigen-antibody complexes circulate, become deposited in tissues, and activate the complement system cascade locally. Patients present with fever, malaise, urticaria, and arthralgia 1 to 3 weeks after receiving the offending agent. The classic skin rash involves erythema with a serpiginous border along the side of the palms and soles. Serum sickness is self-limited and resolution occurs with clearing of the circulating immune complexes. Antihistamines and oral glucocorticosteroids provide symptomatic relief. Drugs that commonly cause serum sickness include beta-lactam antibiotics, sulfonamides, and equine thymocyte globulin.

IgE-mediated skin tests are available for beta-lactam antibiotics, heterologous antiserum, and vaccines containing egg proteins. In vitro antigen-specific skin tests are available but are generally less sensitive than skin testing. In evaluating serum sickness–like reactions, specific IgG antibody levels in conjunction with immune complex assays and complement levels (decrease in C3, C4, and CH50) can be used to confirm the diagnosis and establish its cause.

Management of drug reactions requires stopping the suspected agent, treating clinical symptoms, and (if necessary) identifying an adequate substitute for the drug implicated. If the drug causing the reaction is necessary for treatment in spite of the allergy, acute desensitization should be considered. This is another reason to consult an allergist. Drug rechallenge is contraindicated in patients who have had drug-associated febrile mucocutaneous syndromes.

DISORDERS OF THE SKIN

Langerhans cells in the skin phagocytose antigens, process them and present them to TH2 cells that release cytokines that stimulate B cells to produce specific IgE antibodies. The cross-linking of membranous IgE by antigen causes degranulation of mast cells, resulting in the release of mediators like histamine, prostaglandin D_2, leukotrienes, and platelet-activating factor, all resulting in an increased vascular permeability, inflammatory cell infiltration, and dermal edema.

Urticaria and Angioedema

IgE-mediated urticaria typically results from the ingestion of or parenteral exposure to an antigen such as food, medication, or an insect sting. A food allergy is the most common cause of urticaria, followed by medication allergy to penicillin or sulfonamides.

Complement-mediated urticaria occurs when antigen-antibody complexes activate the complement cascade. Patients receiving intravenous immunoglobulin or other blood products are at risk for this form of urticaria. This mechanism is also responsible for urticaria and angioedema in patients with vasculitis and serum sickness.

Hereditary angioedema has an autosomal dominant pattern of inheritance with variable penetrance. This genetic defect has two forms. Type I results in low levels of C1 esterase inhibitor (C1 INH) protein and its activity. Type II has normal levels of the inhibitor protein, but the protein is dysfunctional. C1 INH deficiency may also be acquired. There are also two types. Type I, found in B-cell lymphoproliferative disorders, is due to massive consumption of C1 by antiidiotypic immune complexes. In Type II, not associated with underlying disease, anti-C1 INH inactivates inhibitor function. Patients present with recurrent, self-limited attacks of nonpitting angioedema involving tissues of the skin and gastrointestinal and respiratory tracts. Local trauma frequently triggers attacks. Death can occur from airway obstruction. C4 levels are depressed between attacks and are undetectable during attacks; C2 levels are normal between attacks but reduced during attacks. Anabolic steroids stimulate hepatic production of normal C1 INH and can be used to prevent attacks. Fresh frozen plasma and purified C1 INH can be used to treat life-threatening attacks.

Chronic urticaria (lasting more than 6 weeks) can have many different causes, including chronic infections (e.g., dental abscesses, sinusitis), systemic vasculitis, autoimmune disease, physical stimuli (e.g., solar urticaria, ultraviolet light exposure, cholinergic and heat urticaria, cold urticaria, vibration, dermatographism), food and food additives (e.g., preservatives, colorings), and over-the-counter medications. However, an etiology is found in only 5% to 10% of patients, the remainder having what is called chronic idiopathic urticaria. The laboratory evaluation includes a complete blood count, sedimentation rate, antinuclear antibodies, CH50, urinalysis with urine culture, chest radiograph, and thyroid-stimulating hormone testing. Treatment is with H_1 and H_2 antihistamines and sympathomimetics. Corticosteroids should be avoided if possible.

Atopic Dermatitis

Atopic dermatitis is characterized by a pruritic rash with a classic morphologic pattern and distribution. Acute lesions are erythematous, edematous, and vesicular, but chronic lesions are dry and scaly with evidence of lichenification. In adolescents the distribution includes the neck, hands, feet, and flexor surfaces. IgE-mediated hypersensitivity should be suspected in patients having a family history of atopic disease, an elevated IgE level, or a history of allergens that exacerbate the dermatitis.

Emollients applied to the skin after bathing maintain hydration. Topical corticosteroids are effective in treating acute flares. High-potency creams can be used for the first 7 to 10 days but should be decreased to low- to mid-potency creams for longer periods to avoid local cutaneous atrophy. High-potency corticosteroids should not be used around the eyes or on the eyelids because of the risk of developing glaucoma or cataract formation. Antihistamines offer relief of pruritus and are especially beneficial at night. Antibiotics may be required to treat staphylococcal or streptococcal superinfections.

Allergic Contact Dermatitis

Allergic contact dermatitis is a form of delayed hypersensitivity (stimulation of TH1 CD8 cells) commonly encountered in occupational settings. Common etiologies include sensitization to topical medications (neomycin), soaps, metals (nickel), rubbers (latex), cosmetics, fragrances, and plants (rhus dermatitis [poison ivy]).

Acute contact dermatitis presents within 1 or 2 days after reexposure to a sensitizing agent as pruritic, macrovesicular lesions progressing to a weeping dermatitis. The subacute form presents with erythema and dyshidrotic vesicles. Chronic forms appear as cracked, scaly, lichenified lesions.

A detailed history of the type of jewelry worn or cosmetics used and of the patient's outdoor exposures, hobbies, and occupational exposures gives the best clues to possible etiologies. Patch testing, done by a dermatologist, is helpful in confirming the diagnosis or when the cause remains elusive.

Treatment of allergic contact dermatitis includes identification and avoidance of the offending sensitizer, and the use of emollients to decrease dryness and reduce itching. Topical steroids are beneficial in reducing the inflammatory reaction. A short course (7 to 10 days) of high-potency topical steroids with a tapering dose of low- to mid-potency preparations over 2 to 3 weeks is effective. Antihistamines reduce the discomfort from itching. For severe contact dermatitis, such as extensive poison ivy, a tapering dose of oral prednisone over 14 to 21 days is recommended. Shorter courses may result in a flare-up of the dermatitis. Attempts at desensitization by oral administration or injection have not been generally effective.

DISORDERS OF THE EYE

Pathophysiology

The eyelids protect the eye from environmental insults. The conjunctiva is highly vascular and the stroma beneath its epithelium is composed of loose connective tissue and blood vessels. Mast cells are found throughout the conjunctival stroma and are highly concentrated in the limbal region, the junction between the cornea and the sclera. Immunoglobulin-producing plasma cells are found in the lacrimal gland, and tears in allergic patients often elevate IgE levels.

The eye has many protective mechanisms in the cornea, conjunctiva, tears, and lids. The lids protect the eyes from trauma and foreign bodies through the blink mechanism. They also contain many glands that secrete tears containing antimicrobial substances such as lysozyme, lactoferrin, and immunoglobulin. IgA is the major immunoglobulin found in tears. The conjunctiva normally has a satin smooth appearance and contains many inflammatory cells. When the conjunctiva is exposed to an irritant, it responds by forming papillae, which are nonspecific collections of lymphocytes adherent to the tarsal plate or the limbus. This reaction is seen commonly in viral, bacterial, and allergic conjunctivitis. Large collections of these lymphocytes (follicles) can be found in conjunctivitis due to *Chlamydia,* adenovirus, or herpesvirus. A brilliant red appearance of the conjunctiva suggests a bacterial infection; a pink, milky appearance due to obscured blood flow because of conjunctival edema suggests allergies. The cornea is considered a "privileged" site because of the paucity of blood vessels in this region. A general discussion of conjunctivitis may be found in Chapter 145, "Ophthalmology." When exposed to environmental irritants, it responds by forming small, punctate defects in its surface, called epithelial keratitis, which is found most commonly in response to drug allergy or toxicity due to ocular medications such as neomycin, atropine, and thimersol and certain topical anesthetics such as tertracaine. Trantas' dots are white deposits composed of eosinophils found at the limbus in patients who have atopic dermatitis or vernal conjunctivitis.

An ocular allergy should be suspected if there is a history of recurrent episodes, a strong history of systemic allergy, and a family history of atopy. Determining whether the patient uses over-the-counter medications such as artificial tears, contact lens solutions, vasoconstrictors, or cosmetics helps rule out the presence of contact allergic dermatoconjunctivitis or conjunctivitis medicamentosa.

The hallmark of allergic conjunctivitis is itching, which can be intense and may last for days. The ocular discharge typically is "stringy." Most airborne allergens cause bilateral irritation. Contactant allergic reactions can be unilateral, but a lacrimal duct obstruction, a retained foreign body, or drug-induced disease should also be considered.

Diagnostic Considerations

Allergic rhinoconjunctivitis (also known as hay fever or rose fever) is usually seasonal. Recurrent inflammation of the conjunctiva occurs in response to exposure to airborne allergens such as tree, grass, and weed pollens; mold spores; or animal danders. Patients complain of itching, burning, and tearing. Antihistamine eyedrops such as antazoline or pheniramine combined with a topical vasoconstrictor such as naphazoline hydrochloride provide rapid relief for mild disease. A 4% cromolyn ophthalmic solution used regularly before and during the pollen season is effective in controlling mild to moderate

symptoms. Corticosteroids are very effective for allergic conjunctivitis. Because this condition may be chronic and ocular glucocorticoids increase the risk of herpetic keratoconjunctivitis, they should be used only in extreme situations.

Atopic keratoconjunctivitis is found in individuals with severe chronic atopic dermatitis. The skin of the eyelid becomes erythematous with exudative lesions. These patients are at risk for blepharitis secondary to *S. aureus* infection. The conjunctiva shows hyperemia, filamentous discharge, and chemosis. Giant papillary hypertrophy may be present on the palpebral conjunctiva, with Trantas' dots at the limbus. Patients complain of photophobia and tearing and are at risk for scarring, vascularization, or keratoconus (a cone-shaped ectasia) of the cornea. A 4% cromolyn solution has been used with some success. The eyelid lesions should be treated in the same way as other areas that have atopic dermatitis, although fluorinated steroids should never be used near the eyes. Hydrocortisone in concentrations of 0.25% to 0.5% is safe to use on the eyelid but should not touch the eye. Keratoconus can be successfully treated with the use of contact lenses or, in severe cases, corneal transplants.

Vernal keratoconjunctivitis begins in the prepubertal years, has a male predominance, and is more common in warm climates. Patients with this disease often have a history of atopic disease such as hay fever, asthma, or atopic dermatitis. Vernal keratoconjunctivitis is a recurrent, bilateral, seasonal condition typically occurring in the spring and summer. Patients present with photophobia, tearing, and severe itching. The hallmark of vernal keratoconjunctivitis is the presence of giant papillae on the conjunctiva of the upper palpebral surface. Trantas' dots are visible at the limbus. Corneal ulcers and plaques can be found in severe cases. This is typically a self-limited disease that lasts no longer than 10 years. Cromolyn has been used successfully in its treatment, but most cases require systemic or topical steroids.

Giant papillary conjunctivitis is seen in patients who wear contact lenses and is thought to be due to an allergic reaction to the contacts or the chemicals used to clean them. Some believe it to be due to repetitive trauma of the palpebral surface against the lens surface. It is treated easily by stopping the use of contacts. If this is not possible, frequent cleaning with enzyme solutions to prevent build-up of deposits is recommended. Another alternative consists of disposable contacts so that a new lens can be used each week.

Conjunctivitis medicamentosa is due to excessive use of ophthalmic medications. It is a delayed hypersensitivity reaction that can involve the eyelids, conjunctiva, or cornea. Patients may present acutely with eczema consisting of vesicular lesions and hyperemia of the conjunctiva with a mucopurulent discharge. Clues to the diagnosis of contact allergic dermatoconjunctivitis in-

BOX 74-4
When to Consult an Allergist

1. Signs and symptoms are atypical and diagnosis is uncertain
2. The patient has life-threatening allergic, anaphylactic, or asthmatic episodes
3. Other clinical conditions complicate asthma:
   Chronic rhinitis
   Sinusitis
   Allergic bronchopulmonary aspergillosis (ABPA)
   Hypogammaglobulinemia or antibody deficiency
   Gastroesophageal reflux (GER)
   Nasal polyposis and/or aspirin sensitivity
   Pregnancy
4. Additional diagnostic testing is indicated to delineate and manage allergic triggers
5. The patient does not respond to standard therapy or does not achieve therapy goals
6. The patient needs comprehensive education and self-management instruction
7. The patient may benefit from allergen immunotherapy
8. The patient needs desensitization to a drug or other biologic agent

clude a history of cosmetic application or drug use, the most common offenders being phenylephrine, aminoglycosides (e.g., neomycin, idoxuridine), and atropine and its derivatives.

SUMMARY

Allergic disorders are common in the adolescent patient and can involve many different organ systems. Primary care physicians can manage most of these atopic conditions. An allergist should be consulted when signs and symptoms escape diagnosis, when special diagnostic tests are required, when a patient has a serious complication of an allergic condition, or when standard forms of medical treatment fail (Box 74-4). Immunotherapy, although not indicated for every patient, should be considered part of the medical management of certain allergic disorders (see Box 74-2).

Suggested Readings

Bierman CW, Pearlman DS, Shapiro GG, Busse WW, editors: *Allergy, asthma, and immunology from infancy to adulthood,* ed 3, Philadelphia, 1996, WB Saunders.

deShazo RD, Smith DL, editors: *JAMA primer on allergic and immunologic diseases,* ed 3, New York, 1992, Marion Merrell Dow.

Holinger LD, Saunders AD: Chronic cough in infants and children: an update, *Laryngoscope* 101:596-605, 1991.

Jackson WB: Differentiating conjunctivitis of diverse origins, *Surv Ophthalmol* 38:91-104, 1993.

Lawler GJ Jr, Fischer TJ, Adelman DC, editors: *Manual of allergy and immunology,* ed 3, Boston, 1995, Little, Brown.

Lichtenstein LM, Fauci AS, editors: *Current therapy in allergy, immunology, and rheumatology,* ed 4, St. Louis, 1992, Mosby–Year Book.

Mabry RL: Rhinitis of pregnancy, *South Med J* 79:965-971, 1986.

Middleton E Jr, Reed CE, Ellis EF, Adkinson NF, Yunginger JW, Busse WW, editors: *Allergy: principles and practice,* ed 4, St. Louis, 1993, Mosby–Year Book.

Naglerio RM: Allergic rhinitis, *N Engl J Med* 325:860-869, 1991.

Nguyen KL, Corbett ML, Garcia DP, Eberly SM, Massey EN, Le HT, Shearer LT, Karibo JM, Pence HL: Chronic sinusitis among pediatric patients with chronic respiratory complaints, *J Allergy Clin Immunol* 92:824-830, 1993.

Reisman RE: Insect stings, *N Engl J Med* 331:523-527, 1994.

Rice DH: Indications for endoscopic sinus surgery, *Ear Nose Throat J* 73:461-466, 1994.

Stites DP, Terr AI, Parslow TG, editors: *Basic & clinical immunology,* ed 8, Norwalk, CT, 1994, Appleton & Lange.

Ten RM, Klein JS, Frigas E: Laboratory medicine and pathology: allergy skin testing, *Mayo Clin Proc* 70:783-784, 1995.

SECTION 14

Selected Medical Emergencies

CHAPTER 75

Overdose

•

Edward E. Conway, Jr

An overdose may result from environmental, occupational, or unintentional exposure to a toxic agent; a therapeutic drug error (incorrect dose or route of administration, administration to the wrong patient, or administration of the wrong substance); or unintentional misuse of a toxic agent when the exposure was unplanned or not foreseen by the patient. Drugs may also be intentionally misused or abused. Such intentional acts were responsible for over 600 reported deaths in the United States in 1993.[1] A total of 1.7 million exposures were reported to the American Association of Poison Control Centers in 1993, and even this large number underestimates the true incidence of poisoning. Poisoning accounts for approximately 7% of all emergency department visits and also contributes to suicide, which is the second leading cause of death in adolescent patients.[2]

Patients are classified according to symptoms as *minor* (minimally bothersome and resolving rapidly with no residual disability), *moderate* (signs or symptoms that are more pronounced and prolonged and usually require some type of treatment), and *major* (signs and symptoms that are life threatening or result in significant residual disability or disfigurement). In 49% of 13- to 19-year-olds who sought emergency care, there was either no effect or a minor effect; 8% had a moderate effect; and 1% had a major effect, with 61 deaths reported.[1] The duration of the moderate and major effects ranged between 8 and 72 hours.[1] Approximately 50% of patients received decontamination therapy, which included dilution/irrigation, activated charcoal, cathartic, ipecac syrup, multidose activated charcoal (MDA), other emetics, and whole bowel irrigation. Substances associated with the largest number of deaths included analgesics, antidepressants, stimulants, sedative/hypnotics/antipsychotics, cardiovascular drugs, alcohols, gases and fumes, chemicals, asthma therapies, hydrocarbons, and cleaning substances.[1]

Approximately 5% of patients who are poisoned require admission to a hospital, although specific antidotes were administered in only 1.3% of the reported cases.[1] The approach to the poisoned patient should consist of initial resuscitation and stabilization, diagnosis, nonspecific therapy, specific therapy for the toxin, and aggressive supportive care.

TOXIDROMES

In light of the large number of pharmacologic substances that may be ingested, it is best to approach the poisoned patient by using what has been termed *toxidromes*.[3] Toxidromes are groups of related signs and symptoms seen after the ingestion of certain classes of pharmacologic substances. The best-described include sympathomimetic, cholinergic, anticholinergic, and opiate/sedative/ethanol syndromes.

Presenting signs of the sympathomimetic toxidrome include changes in mental status (hyperactivity, delusions, paranoia), tachycardia, hypertension, hyperpyrexia, diaphoresis, mydriasis, and hyperreflexia. Seizures and dysrhythmias may also occur, and hypotension is a late finding. Agents associated with this syndrome include cocaine, amphetamines, methamphetamine, phencyclidine, lysergic acid diethylamide (LSD), theophylline, caffeine, phenylpropanolamine, and beta$_2$ agonists.

Presenting signs of the anticholinergic toxidrome include changes in mental status (delirium and hallucinations), tachycardia, dry flushed skin, mydriasis, myoclonus, hyperthermia, urgency and urinary retention, decreased bowel sounds, respiratory failure, seizures, and dysrhythmias. The symptoms are the opposite of those seen in cholinergic poisoning and are best remembered by the paraphrase from *Alice in Wonderland:* "mad as a hatter, blind as a bat, red as a beet, hot as a hare, and dry as a bone." Agents commonly associated with this syndrome include antihistamines, atropine, scopolamine, amantadine, antipsychotic medications, antidepressants, antispasmodics (belladonna alkaloids), mydriatics, mushrooms, and jimsonweed.

The cholinergic toxidrome presents with central nervous system (CNS) changes (confusion, depressed CNS), weakness, salivation, lacrimation, urinary and fecal incontinence, gastrointestinal cramping, emesis, diaphoresis, muscle fasciculations, miosis, bradycardia, and seizures. The symptoms can be remembered by the mnemonic SLUDGE (*s*alivation, *l*acrimation, *u*rination, *d*efecation, *g*astrointestinal upset, and *e*mesis). Agents associated with this syndrome include organophosphate and carbamate insecticides, acetylcholine, tobacco, physostigmine, edrophonium, and some mushrooms.

Presenting signs of the opiate/sedative/ethanol toxidrome include CNS depression, hypoventilation, hypotension, hypothermia, miosis, hyporeflexia, bradycardia, and decreased bowel sounds. Seizures may occur after some narcotic overdoses. Agents commonly associated with this syndrome include narcotics, barbiturates, benzodiazepines, ethanol, clonidine, chloral hydrate, and methaqualone.

MANAGEMENT

The management of the patient who presents with an overdose begins with immediate assessment of the ABCs: airway, breathing, and circulation. Examination of the presenting vital signs and their continuous monitoring is essential. An intravenous line should be placed and an immediate determination of serum glucose performed. Patients who are hypoglycemic (serum glucose <50 mg/dl) should receive an immediate bolus of 50% dextrose, but if hypoglycemia is suspected, therapy should not be withheld while a confirmatory laboratory value is awaited. Arterial blood gas, blood samples for serum electrolytes, urea nitrogen, and creatinine levels should be obtained. These results may be used to calculate the anion gap (serum sodium − bicarbonate + chloride); a normal anion gap is between 12 and 16. The mnemonic MUDPILES will indicate the causes of an elevated gap and perhaps suggest which toxin was ingested: (*m*ethanol, *u*remia, *d*iabetic ketoacidosis, *p*araldehyde, *i*ron, *i*soniazid, *l*actic acidosis [any toxin that may cause hypoxia or hypotension], *e*thylene glycol, and *s*alicylates). A pregnancy test should be considered in female patients, and a complete blood cell count obtained. The decision to use electrocardiography or chest radiography should be guided by the history and physical examination; routine use of these tests has a very low yield. Other therapeutic

interventions should include oxygen administration and a trial of naloxone. Specific antidotes are summarized in Table 75-1.[4]

As noted above, after stabilization of the ABCs, the patient's vital signs and level of consciousness should be monitored. The Glasgow Coma Scale (described in Chapter 80, "Altered States of Consciousness") is helpful; patients with a score of less than 8 are considered comatose. The cause of the coma must be quickly determined. The mnemonic AEIOU THIPS may prove helpful and even suggest a toxic agent (*a*lcohol, *e*ncephalopathy, *e*ndocrinopathy, *e*lectrolytes, *i*ngestions, *o*piates, *u*remia, *t*rauma, *h*yper/hypothermia, *h*yper/hypotension, *h*ypoglycemia, *i*nfection, *p*sychogenic, *s*tructural lesions, *s*eizures, *s*yncope).

Hypotension may be seen after the ingestion of many agents, but it usually results from nonspecific autonomic dysfunction, which produces venous pooling. Patients should receive a fluid challenge (20 ml/kg) with a crystalloid solution (lactated Ringer's solution or 0.9% sodium chloride). Tachycardia may also represent the body's attempt to compensate for the venous pooling. Bradycardia may result from the ingestion of parasympathomimetic agents, cholinesterase inhibitors, beta blockers, cardiac glycosides, or antidysrhythmics. Hyperthermia may be seen after the ingestion of sympathomimetic compounds and must be recognized early and treated aggressively. Hypothermia may be seen after the ingestion of CNS depressants such as ethanol, barbiturates, benzodiazepines, and narcotics. Many substances may cause seizures, either directly or indirectly, by causing metabolic derangements.

In many patients who present after an ingestion, a history may not be available. The selection of urine and serum toxicology studies should be guided by the history and physical examination. Studies have shown that physicians are not very accurate in identifying the toxin ingested.[5] The important question is whether a drug screen or level will alter the patient's management. Serum levels usually correlate poorly with the clinical condition. Quantitative levels to be obtained in all patients include those of acetaminophen and salicylate. Other levels to consider include those of iron, theophylline, anticonvulsants, and carbon monoxide, as these will guide patient management.

Nonspecific therapy involves measures to slow the absorption or remove the offending agent, such as emesis, gastric lavage, catharsis, whole bowel irrigation, and the administration of activated charcoal. Many publications in recent years have reassessed the management of the overdosed patient.[6-8] Emesis induced by administration of syrup of ipecac may be useful for the first hour after an ingestion, but a definite benefit has not been adequately demonstrated. Emesis should never be induced in a patient with a depressed sensorium or absent gag reflex.

TABLE 75-1
Antidotes

Toxin	Antidote	Dose and Comments*
Opiates	Naloxone	Starting dose 2 mg. More may be needed for doses of some synthetic narcotics; less may be used in addicts to avoid precipitating withdrawal symptoms.
Methanol, ethylene glycol	Ethanol	Loading dose 10 ml of 10% per kg body weight. Titrate to a blood ethanol level of 22 mmol/L (100 mg/dl).
Anticholinergic agents	Physostigmine	1-2 mg intravenously over 5 min. Use only for severe delirium. May be useful to treat seizures or tachydysrhythmias, but strong clinical evidence is lacking.
Organophosphate or carbamate insecticides	Atropine	Test dose 2 mg intravenously. Repeat in larger increments until drying of pulmonary secretions occurs.
Isoniazid	Pyridoxine	Give in gram-per-gram equivalent doses to what was ingested. If amount ingested is unknown, start with 5 g intravenously. An overdose of pyridoxine may cause neuropathy.
Beta blockers	Glucagon	Starting dose 5-10 mg intravenously. Titrate to response (normalization of vital signs). Maintenance dose of 2-10 mg/hr may be used.
Tricyclic antidepressants	Bicarbonate	1-2 mmol/kg intravenously for substantial cardiac conduction delay or ventricular dysrhythmias. Titrate to response and arterial pH.
Digitalis, glycosides	Digoxin-specific antibody fragments	Equimolar to ingestion: the number of milligrams of digoxin ingested divided by 0.6 is the number of vials required. If amount ingested is unknown and patient has life-threatening dysrhythmias, give 10-20 vials intravenously. If serum digoxin concentration is known, the number of vials to administer is concentration in ng/ml × 5.6 × weight in kg divided by 600.
Benzodiazepines	Flumazenil	0.2 mg over 30 sec. If no response after 30 sec, give 0.3 mg over 30 sec. If no response after 30 sec, give 0.5 mg over 30 sec at 1-min intervals up to a total dose of 3 mg. Should not be given if patient shows signs of serious overdose from coingestion of tricyclic antidepressants or was taking benzodiazepines for control of seizures.
Calcium channel blockers, hydrofluoric acid fluorides	Calcium	1 g calcium chloride given over 5 min by intravenous infusion with continuous cardiac monitoring. May be repeated often in life-threatening situations, but serum calcium level should be monitored after third dose.

From Kulig K: Initial management of ingestions of toxic substances, *N Engl J Med* 326:1677-1681, 1992.
*Doses are for adults.

Gastric lavage may be performed using 2 to 3 ml/kg of isotonic 0.9% saline at either body or room temperature, instilled and removed by way of an orogastric or nasogastric tube. With gastric lavage, there is a risk of aspiration and the patient may require elective intubation. Cathartics are used to limit drug absorption and speed up gastrointestinal transit time. They are generally given in conjunction with activated charcoal.

Whole bowel irrigation is a relatively new method of decontamination that involves the administration of polyethylene glycol electrolyte lavage solution (Go-Lytely) by way of an orogastric or nasogastric tube. It has proved useful for iron and lead overdose; as therapy for swallowed batteries, lithium, and sustained-release products; and to cleanse the bowel of "body packers and stuffers" who ingest condoms filled with cocaine.[9]

Administration of activated charcoal is the mainstay of decontamination therapy. Activated charcoal has a large surface area and allows for the adsorption of many toxic substances. It is thought to work through gastrointestinal dialysis. It serves as an adsorbent sink in the gastrointestinal tract by both interrupting enterohepatic circulation and adsorbing drugs that enter the gut by active secretion. Drugs that are not protein bound pass by simple diffusion across the gastrointestinal cell membranes and into the gut lumen, where a diffusion gradient ensues, causing more drug to complex with the activated charcoal.[10] The only contraindication to the use of activated charcoal is an ileus or mechanical bowel obstruction. Although activated charcoal is relatively nontoxic to the lungs, aspiration of swallowed charcoal introduces stomach acid and oral bacteria into the lungs. The standard adult dose is 100 g, administered either orally or via an orogastric or nasogastric tube. It may also be administered as a continuous nasogastric drip.[11] A cathartic (sorbitol) should be administered at least twice daily to patients receiving multiple doses of charcoal, to prevent bezoar formation. Patients who have ingested substances that have a low volume of distribution, low plasma protein binding, biliary or gastric secretion, or the formation of active recirculating (enterohepatic) metabolites are candidates for the use of repetitive doses of activated charcoal. Multiple doses of activated charcoal have been shown to be useful after the ingestion of carbamazepine, tricyclic antidepressants, dapsone, digitoxin, disopyramide, nadolol, phenobarbital, phenytoin, and theophylline.[10]

Most acutely poisoned patients who arrive at the hospital are not critically ill. They are assessed in the emergency department and either treated and released or admitted to the hospital for further therapeutic interventions or observation. Criteria for high-risk patients to be admitted to the intensive care unit include the need for intubation, unresponsiveness to verbal stimuli, seizures, $PaCO_2$ >45 mm Hg, systolic blood pressure <80 mm Hg, and any irregular cardiac rhythm.[12]

Thousands of over-the-counter medications are available for relief from pain, symptoms of the common cold, allergies, dysmenorrhea, nausea, insomnia, and minor gastrointestinal complaints. These medications are usually presumed to be safe because they are available without a prescription.[13] They may contain acetaminophen, salicylates, antihistamines, dextromethorphan, ephedrine, pseudoephedrine, phenylpropanolamine, or phenylephrine. Any of these substances taken in large enough doses may be toxic. Other potential toxins include vitamins (A, D, C, B_6), nutritional supplements such as zinc and L-tryptophan, nonprescription herbal preparations, and other toxic traditional remedies.

The patient who presents after an unknown ingestion represents a challenge to the physician. Rapid stabilization and assessment of the ABCs is all that is required in most instances of ingestion. Careful assessment and reassessment of the vital signs, a thorough history and physical examination, and selective use of laboratory studies will produce an excellent outcome in most poisoned adolescents.

References

1. Litovitz TL, Clark LR, Soloway RA: 1993 Annual Report of the American Association of Poison Control Centers Toxic Exposure Surveillance System, *Am J Emerg Med* 12:546-584, 1994.
2. Hoffman RS, Goldfrank LR: The impact of drug abuse and addiction on society, *Emerg Med Clin North Am* 8:467-480, 1990.
3. Mofenson HC, Greensher J: The unknown poison, *Pediatrics* 336, 1974.
4. Kulig K: Initial management of ingestions of toxic substances, *N Engl J Med* 326:1677-1681, 1992.
5. Krenzelok EP: Toxicological screens: their role in the diagnosis and management of acute poisoning emergencies, *Clin Tox Forum* 2:1-5, 1990.
6. Fine JS, Goldfrank LR: Update in medical toxicology, *Pediatr Clin North Am* 39:1031-1051, 1992.
7. Perrone J, Hoffman R, Goldfrank LR: Special considerations in gastrointestinal decontamination, *Emerg Med Clin North Am* 12:285-299, 1994.
8. Phillips S, Gomez H, Brent J: Pediatric gastrointestinal decontamination in acute toxin ingestion, *J Clin Pharmacol* 33:497-507, 1993.
9. Kirshenbaum LA, Matthews SC, Sitar DS, et al: Whole-bowel irrigation versus activated charcoal in sorbitol for the ingestion of modified release preparations, *Clin Pharmacol Ther* 46:264-271, 1989.
10. Lee DC, Roberts JR: Use of oral charcoal in medical toxicology, *Contemp Management Crit Care* 1:43-57, 1991.
11. Ohning BL, Reed MD, Blummer JL: Continuous nasogastric administration of activated charcoal for the treatment of theophylline intoxication, *Pediatr Pharmacol* 5:241, 1986.
12. Brett A, Rothschild N, Gray R, et al: Predicting the clinical course in intentional drug overdose, *Arch Intern Med* 147:133-137, 1987.
13. Cetaruk EW, Aaron CK: Hazards of nonprescription medications, *Emerg Med Clin North Am* 12:483-507, 1994.

CHAPTER 76

Pneumothorax

•

Deborah M. Lopez and Edward E. Conway, Jr

Pneumothorax (PTX) is the accumulation of air in the intrapleural cavity resulting from rupture of the pulmonary parenchyma and visceral pleura. Spontaneous (PTX) is an uncommon condition with an incidence of 5 to 10 per 100,000 in the general population and a male-to-female ratio of approximately 6:1. The highest incidence of spontaneous PTX is in the 16- to 24-year-old age group. Most pneumothoraces in the pediatric population result from trauma; mechanical ventilation; and pulmonary conditions such as asthma, cystic fibrosis, and Marfan's syndrome. PTX may be either primary or secondary. Primary PTX occurs in healthy individuals without any predisposing medical condition; secondary PTX is associated with underlying pulmonary disease.

During normal breathing, the pressure in the pleural space is negative in comparison with alveolar pressure. The elastic recoil of the lungs creates a pressure gradient between the alveoli and pleural space. Pleural pressure in a spontaneously breathing person is negative with respect to the atmospheric pressure. Pneumothoraces develop when a communication is created between the alveolus or other intrapulmonary air space and the pleural space, or when a communication develops through the chest wall between the atmosphere and the pleural space. In either case, air enters the pleural space until there is equalization of pressure or the communication is closed. When a critical volume of air is introduced into the pleural space, an increase in pleural pressure occurs. The resultant decreases in vital capacity (VC being the maximal amount of air that can be exhaled after a maximal inspiration) and PaO_2 are frequently well tolerated by patients without underlying pulmonary pathology but can be life threatening for patients with compromised lung function. The increased work of breathing that results from a decrease in VC produces respiratory insufficiency with consequent hypoxemia and respiratory acidosis. The resultant hypoxia appears to be caused by ventilation-perfusion mismatch (areas of the lung that are ventilated but poorly perfused or well perfused but poorly ventilated), alveolar hypoventilation, and anatomic shunts. These changes are reversible after evacuation of the pleural air.

PRIMARY SPONTANEOUS PNEUMOTHORAX

Primary PTX is predominantly a disease of young adult males with an asthenic body habitus and a history of smoking.[1] The median age of primary PTX is 16.7 years and the male-to-female ratio is 2:1.[2] The most common cause of primary PTX is rupture of a subpleural bleb or bulla.[3,4] A study of chest computed tomography (CT) of 20 patients revealed various types of emphysematous lesions located predominantly in the apical fields.[5]

Symptoms are most often mild and consist of dyspnea and chest pain on the side of the pneumothorax. Primary PTX frequently develops when the patient is at rest, contrary to the popular belief that there is an association with strenuous physical activity.[6] Physical examination may reveal loss of tactile fremitus, hyperresonance to percussion, and decreased breath sounds. Tension pneumothorax should be suspected if the patient has severe acute dyspnea, cyanosis, and/or a tracheal shift.

The usual radiographic finding in a patient with a PTX is the demonstration of a distinct visceral pleural line with the absence of lung markings in the periphery (Fig. 76-1). Chest radiographs taken during expiration or in a lateral decubitus view with the side of the suspected pneumothorax superior may accentuate a small pneumothorax not apparent on routine chest radiographs.

Pneumothoraces that are less than 20% in a healthy adolescent may not require any treatment to reexpand the lung. It has been estimated that the rate of air reabsorption in the pleural space is 1.25% per 24 hours; therefore, it can take up to 2 weeks for a 20% pneumothorax to resolve. Because of the risk of developing a trapped lung as a result of fibrotic peels being laid down on the visceral pleura, pneumothoraces that have not resolved within 2 weeks should be evacuated with either tube thoracostomy or percutaneous aspiration. Patients given 100% oxygen by face mask absorb pleural air approximately four times faster than those who do not receive 100% oxygen. The nitrogen gradient between the alveoli and pleural air enhances absorption.[7] Pneumothoraces that are greater than 25%, are increasing in size, are causing clinical deterioration, or involve a significant pleural effusion should be evacuated. Pneumothoraces can be evacuated with simple percutaneous aspiration and then monitored by serial chest radiography. If resolution does not occur, tube thoracotomy should be considered. Evacuation of a PTX by way of percutaneous aspiration, tube thoracotomy with underwater suction, pleurodesis, open thoracostomy with apical bullectomy, or thoracoscopy and video-assisted thoracic surgery (VATS) should be individualized.

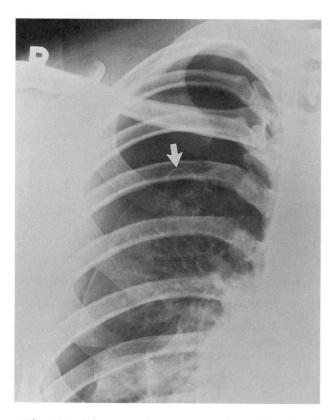

Fig. 76-1. Primary spontaneous pneumothorax. The visceral pleural line is clearly demonstrated together with the lateral avascular space. There is pleural bleb at the apex of the lung *(arrow)*, a common finding. Such blebs are usually not detectable when the lung reexpands. (From Armstrong P, Wilson AG, Dee P, Hensell DM: *Imaging of diseases of the chest,* ed 2, St. Louis, MO, 1995, Mosby–Year Book, p 696.)

SECONDARY SPONTANEOUS PNEUMOTHORAX

The incidence of secondary PTX is similar to that of primary PTX. An estimated 7500 new cases per year are diagnosed in the general population, with males affected three times more commonly than females. Clinically, multiple disorders are associated with secondary PTX (Box 76-1). Currently, the entity most commonly associated with secondary PTX is seen in patients infected with the human immunodeficiency virus and underlying *Pneumocystis carinii* pneumonia.[8,9]

Secondary PTX is a more serious condition because underlying pulmonary function is already compromised. Interpretation of the physical examination is difficult in patients with suspected secondary PTX because they may have underlying hyperexpanded lungs, decreased tactile fremitus, hyperresonance to percussion, and distant breath sounds. Secondary PTX should be suspected when an adolescent with an underlying pulmonary disorder experiences severe acute dyspnea, tachypnea, chest pain, or cyanosis.

Once the diagnosis of a secondary PTX is considered, chest radiography should be performed. Its interpretation in patients with underlying lung disease may be difficult. Pneumothoraces as small as 5% to 10% in this population can produce severe symptoms. If the distinction between a pneumothorax and a bulla cannot be made, a CT scan should be obtained.

The main objective in treating patients with secondary PTX is to decrease the possibility of a recurrence. Therapy is usually more aggressive than for primary PTX because of an increased risk of pulmonary deterioration and death.

Virtually all patients with underlying pulmonary pathology require tube thoracostomy. Deterioration in respiratory status necessitating mechanical ventilation

---

BOX 76-1
Diseases Associated with Secondary Spontaneous Pneumothorax

Asthma
Cystic fibrosis
Tuberculosis
Atypical mycobacteria
Drug abuse
Congenital cystic lung disease
Pulmonary embolism
Collagen vascular disease
Marfan's syndrome
Ehlers-Danlos syndrome
Cutis laxa (generalized elastolysis)

will require immediate insertion of a chest tube because of the possible continued enlargement of the pneumothorax or of the development of a tension pneumothorax. Tube thoracostomy is less effective at reinflating the lung in secondary PTX than in primary PTX. The median time for lung reexpansion in secondary PTX is 5 days, and patients often require multiple, prolonged use of chest tubes. Once the lung has reexpanded, it is recommended that agents such as minocycline can be instilled into the pleural space to decrease the incidence of recurrence.[10] These agents produce pleuritis, with resultant adhesions between the visceral and parietal pleurae. Surgical intervention should be considered in patients whose lungs remain unexpanded for more than 5 days or if an air leak persists for several days after pleurodesis.

Pneumothorax is a well-recognized complication of both inhalational and intravenous drug abuse. Drugs used for inhalation include cocaine, marijuana, nitrous oxide, and amphetamine.[11] Pneumothorax following inhalation of these agents is related to a prolonged Valsalva maneuver or other vigorous inhalation maneuvers performed by users of these substances to enhance the effects of the drug. During the Valsalva maneuver, the alveoli are overdistended and the vessels that they contact are devoid of blood. The pressure gradient created between the alveolus and the vessel leads to rupture of the alveolar wall into the perivascular adventitia, which may in turn lead to formation of a pneumothorax.

Primary PTX is a relatively uncommon occurrence seen most frequently in tall, thin adolescent males with a history of smoking. Secondary PTX is associated with underlying lung pathology or drug abuse. Treatment should be individualized, ranging from observation to serial chest radiographs and, in some cases, surgical intervention. The major complication associated with PTX is the development of a tension pneumothorax, which should be recognized and treated promptly and aggressively.

References

1. Deslauriers J, Beaulieu M, Desprese J, et al: Transaxillary pleurectomy for treatment of spontaneous pneumothorax, *Ann Thorac Surg* 30:569-574, 1980.
2. Poenaru D, Yazbeck S, Murphy S: Primary spontaneous pneumothorax in children, *J Pediatr Surg* 29:1183-1185, 1994.
3. Kjaergaard H: Spontaneous pneumothorax in the apparently healthy, *Acta Med Scand* 43(suppl):1-159, 1932.
4. Brock RC: Recurrent and chronic spontaneous pneumothorax, *Thorax,* 3:88-111, 1948.
5. Lesur O, Delorme N, Fromaget JM, Bernadac P, Polu JM: Computed tomography in the etiologic assessment of idiopathic spontaneous pneumothorax, *Chest* 98:341-347, 1990.
6. Bense L, Wiman LG, Hedenstierna G: Onset of symptoms in spontaneous pneumothorax: correlations to physical activity, *Eur J Respir Dis* 71:181-186, 1987.
7. Chadha TS, Cohn MA: Non-invasive treatment of pneumothorax with oxygen inhalation, *Respiration* 44:147-152, 1983.
8. Byrnes T, Brevig J, Yeoh C: Pneumothorax in patients with acquired immunodeficiency syndrome, *J Thorac Cardiovasc Surg* 98:546-550, 1989.
9. Sepkowitz KA, Telzak EE, Golds JW, et al: Pneumothorax in AIDS, *Ann Intern Med* 114:455-459, 1991.
10. Tanaka F, Itoh M, Esaki H, Isobe J, Ueno Y, Inoue R: Secondary spontaneous pneumothorax, *Ann Thorac Surg* 55:372-376, 1993.
11. Seaman M: Barotrauma related to inhalation drug abuse, *J Emerg Med* 8:141-149, 1990.

CHAPTER 77

Pulmonary Embolus

•

Diana King and Edward E. Conway, Jr

EPIDEMIOLOGY

Although the epidemiology of pulmonary embolism (PE) has been studied extensively in adults, there are very few data concerning its occurrence in pediatric patients. There has been a decrease in the incidence and case-fatality rate among adults as a result of anticoagulant use, but PE continues to be a common, often fatal event. Pulmonary embolism is diagnosed in 120,000 adult patients in the United States each year and contributes to death in one quarter of these patients.[1] The incidence and case fatality of PE in children and adolescents are not known. Most published pediatric series are based on autopsy records. This method underestimates the true incidence in younger patients, whose healthier cardiopulmonary systems rarely succumb to PE. In one study, pulmonary emboli were found in 4.2% of 1098 autopsied children and were the direct cause of death in fewer than one third (n = 36).[2]

A retrospective review of 24,250 adolescent patients over a 15-year period identified pulmonary embolism in only 19 cases. The diagnosis was confirmed by pulmonary angiography, radionuclide scanning, or autopsy. PE was the direct cause of death in only one of these patients. The diagnosis was delayed in many of these patients because of a low index of suspicion.[3]

PRESENTATION

Pleuritic pain is the most common symptom of PE, followed by dyspnea, cough, and hemoptysis. Other associated findings include lower extremity deep vein thrombosis (DVT), tachypnea, and fever. Abnormal breath sounds and a prominent pulmonic component of the second heart sound may be noted.[3]

In over 50% of young adults 18 to 40 years of age with documented PE, there is no evidence of cardiopulmonary abnormality or DVT on physical examination.[4] Therefore, if a clinical suspicion of PE exists, diagnostic tests should be pursued, even if the patient "looks well."

DIAGNOSIS

Clinical suspicion of PE is the crucial step in making a diagnosis. Risk factors and physical findings consistent with PE should prompt an investigation. Underlying conditions associated with the risk of PE are summarized in Box 77-1.

Hypoxemia (PaO_2 < 80 mm Hg) is a frequent laboratory finding. A widened alveolar-arterial gradient (>20 mm Hg) may also be noted. Chest radiography should be performed to exclude other processes, such as pneumothorax; results are abnormal in 50% of adolescents with PE,[3] most commonly revealing atelectasis or parenchymal abnormalities. Electrocardiography should be performed to exclude such entities as pericarditis or myocardial infarction. Sinus rhythm is the most frequent finding, but nonspecific ST-segment or T-wave abnormalities are common.[5] A low quantitative plasma D-dimer level can help to exclude the presence of a pulmonary embolus. A level less than 500 ng/ml (normal range, <500 ng/ml) has a negative predictive value of 97%.[6]

The initial diagnostic test, following those noted above, should be a ventilation/perfusion (V/Q) scan. The perfusion portion consists of an intravenous injection of technetium-labeled albumin that is distributed into the

---

BOX 77-1
Risk Factors for Pulmonary Embolism

Central venous catheters
Immobility
Congenital heart disease
Ventriculoatrial shunt
Lower extremity trauma
Abdominal trauma
Neoplasm
Oral contraceptives
Elective abortion
Infection
Collagen vascular disease
Intravenous drug abuse
Colitis
Dehydration
Obesity
Renal transplant
Recent surgery
Hypercoagulable state

Data from Buck et al.[2] and Bernstein et al.[3]
Adapted from Bernstein D, Coupey S, Schonberg SK: Pulmonary embolism in adolescents, *Am J Dis Child* 140:667-671, 1986. With permission of the American Medical Association.

---

pulmonary circulation. If any perfusion defect is found, a ventilation scan should be performed. [133]Xenon gas is inhaled and its distribution recorded with a gamma camera. The perfusion scan is then compared with the ventilation scan to identify areas of mismatch. The degree of perfusion defect is then categorized as high probability (that a pulmonary embolus is present), intermediate probability, low probability, or normal.[7] A normal V/Q scan makes the possibility of PE unlikely. A low-probability scan combined with clinical assessment of low likelihood yields a 96% negative predictive value. A positive predictive value of 96% is obtained when a high-probability scan is combined with a high level of clinical suspicion.[8]

If the V/Q scan is nondiagnostic (intermediate or low probability), venous studies of the lower extremities may be helpful in deciding further management. Proximal DVTs (femoral, iliac, or inferior vena cava) carry a higher embolic risk than distal thromboses.[9] Impedance plethysmography and duplex ultrasonography are two noninvasive techniques to evaluate venous flow. Both methods are better at detecting proximal than distal thrombi. In the presence of thrombosis, there will be decreased impedance to flow, revealed by plethysmography. This technique detects proximal thrombi in symptomatic patients with 92% sensitivity and 95% specificity. The sensitivity is poor (22%) in asymptomatic patients. Duplex scanning is real-time B-mode ultrasonography coupled with Doppler flow detection imaging, which visualizes blood flow in any vessel. This

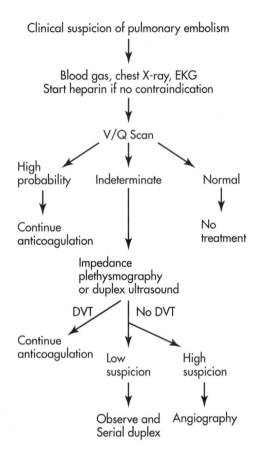

Clinical suspicion of pulmonary embolism

Blood gas, chest X-ray, EKG
Start heparin if no contraindication

V/Q Scan

High probability → Continue anticoagulation

Indeterminate → Impedance plethysmography or duplex ultrasound

Normal → No treatment

DVT → Continue anticoagulation

No DVT →
Low suspicion → Observe and Serial duplex
High suspicion → Angiography

V/Q, ventilation/perfusion; DVT, deep-vein thrombosis

Fig. 77-1. Diagnostic algorithm for pulmonary embolus.

method has 97% sensitivity and 97% specificity for detecting proximal thrombi in symptomatic patients. In asymptomatic patients, the sensitivity is only 59%.[10]

The gold standard for diagnosing PE is angiography. This is an invasive technique that requires special equipment and personnel and should be reserved for cases in which the diagnosis by V/Q scan is indeterminate and a high level of clinical suspicion exists. Figure 77-1 summarizes the approach to the patient with suspected PE.

PATHOPHYSIOLOGY

Thrombosis can occur when any component of Virchow's triad is present: stasis of blood flow, injury to the vessel wall, or a hypercoagulable state. Primary and secondary hypercoagulable states are risk factors for PE. Antithrombin III, protein C, and protein S deficiencies should be considered in a patient with recurrent thromboembolic disease, particularly if there is a family history of thrombosis. Acquired deficiencies of these proteins may occur with disseminated intravascular coagulation,

liver disease, nephrotic syndrome, acute respiratory distress syndrome, or pregnancy or after surgery or L-asparaginase chemotherapy. Low protein S levels have been noted in patients infected with the human immunodeficiency virus.[11]

After a PE, right heart failure may develop as a result of acute pulmonary hypertension. The degree of obstruction produced by the embolus is proportional to the severity of the pulmonary hypertension. Alveolar dead space increases as lung units continue to be ventilated and are not perfused because the embolus obstructs blood flow through the pulmonary artery. Hypoxemia and an increased alveolar-arterial oxygen gradient commonly occur as a result of V/Q mismatch, intracardiac shunt, reflex bronchoconstriction, atelectasis, or lung infarction. Proprioceptors that respond to stretch and irritation contribute to the hyperventilation seen in many patients with PE. Loss of pulmonary surfactant distal to the vascular occlusion results in atelectasis and edema. This makes the lungs less compliant. Obstruction of smaller pulmonary arteries and hemorrhage into the airways can result in infarction if the extravasated blood is not cleared.[12]

TREATMENT

Heparin should be administered as soon as there is clinical suspicion of PE. An intravenous bolus of 50 units/kg should be given, followed by a constant intravenous infusion at 10 to 25 units/kg/hr. Absolute contraindications to its administration include active or potential internal or central nervous system (CNS) bleeding, and a cerebrovascular accident within 2 months.[7] Heparin activates antithrombin III, which inhibits thrombin, preventing propagation of a thrombus.[11] Heparin should be administered intravenously for 5 days and the dose adjusted to maintain an activated partial thromboplastin time (PTT) of 1.5 to 2 times the control. Long-term anticoagulation with warfarin should be initiated 1 to 2 days after heparin administration so that there is an overlap of 4 to 5 days. Studies have shown low-molecular-weight heparin to be as effective as and possibly safer (fewer major bleeding events) than conventional heparin.[13] The duration of oral anticoagulant therapy should be 6 months in order to prevent recurrences effectively. The international normalized ratio (INR) of 2.0 to 2.8 is targeted for anticoagulation.[14] When anticoagulation is contraindicated, an inferior vena caval filter should be considered.[7]

Angiographically proved PE or emboli diagnosed by high-probability V/Q scan with a high clinical suspicion can be treated with thrombolytic therapy. Three regimens currently available include streptokinase, urokinase, and recombinant tissue–type plasminogen. The major complication of thrombolytic therapy is bleeding; therefore, recent or active CNS hemorrhage is a contraindication to thrombolysis.[15] Surgical embolectomy is rarely necessary now that thrombolytic agents are in use.[7]

PREVENTION

Heparin prophylaxis with small subcutaneous doses (5000 units two to three times a day) is recommended in patients at moderate risk for thromboembolic disease. Graduated-compression stockings and intermittent external pneumatic compression are alternatives in patients who have undergone neurosurgery and in whom heparin is contraindicated.[10]

CONCLUSION

Pulmonary embolism is rarely suspected in children and adolescents. The presenting signs and symptoms may be subtle, so the physician's index of suspicion must be high to make this frequently elusive diagnosis. Early consideration of PE and initiation of anticoagulant therapy can be lifesaving.

References

1. Gillum RF: Pulmonary embolism and thrombophlebitis in the United States, 1970-1985, *Am Heart J* 114:1262-1264, 1987.
2. Buck JR, Connors RG, Coon WW, Weintraub WH, Wesley JR, Coran AG: Pulmonary embolism in children, *J Pediatr Surg* 16:385-391, 1981.
3. Bernstein D, Coupey S, Schonberg SK: Pulmonary embolism in adolescents, *Am J Dis Child* 140:667-671, 1986.
4. Green RM, Meyer TJ, Dunn M, Glassroth J: Pulmonary embolism in younger adults, *Chest* 101:1507-1511, 1992.
5. Stein PD, Terrin ML, Hales CA, et al: Clinical laboratory, roentgenographic, and electrocardiographic findings in patients with acute pulmonary embolism and no pre-existing cardiac or pulmonary disease, *Chest* 100:598-603, 1991.
6. Goldhaber SZ, Simons GR, Elliott CG, et al: Quantitative D-dimer levels among patients undergoing pulmonary angiography for suspected pulmonary embolism, *JAMA* 270:2819-2822, 1993.
7. Evans DA, Wilmott RW: Pulmonary embolism in children, *Pediatr Clin North Am* 41:569-584, 1994.
8. Quinn DA, Thompson T, Terrin ML, et al: Value of the ventilation/perfusion scan in acute pulmonary embolism, *JAMA* 263:2753-2759, 1990.
9. Monreal M, Ruiz J, Olazabal A, Arias A, Roca J: Deep vein thrombosis and the risk of pulmonary embolism, *Chest* 102:677-681, 1992.
10. Weinmann EE, Salzman EW: Deep-vein thrombosis, *N Engl J Med* 331:1630-1640, 1994.
11. Nachman RL, Silverstein R: Hypercoagulable states, *Ann Intern Med* 119:819-827, 1993.
12. Elliott CG: Pulmonary physiology during pulmonary embolism, *Chest* 101(suppl):163S-171S, 1992.
13. Hull RD, Raskob GE, Pinco GF, et al: Subcutaneous low-molecular-weight heparin compared with continuous intravenous heparin in the treatment of proximal vein thrombosis, *N Engl J Med* 326:975-982, 1992.
14. Schulman S, Rhedin A-S, Lindmarker P, et al: A comparison of six weeks with six months of oral anticoagulant therapy after a first episode of venous thromboembolism, *N Engl J Med* 332:1661-1665, 1995.
15. Goldhaber SZ: Contemporary pulmonary embolism thrombolysis, *Chest* 107(suppl):45S-51S, 1995.

CHAPTER 78

Hyperthermia

•

Lewis P. Singer and Edward E. Conway, Jr

Body temperature is closely controlled by a balance between heat production generated by normal metabolism and heat dissipation from the skin and lungs. This complex thermoregulation is governed by a thermostat located in the preoptic nucleus of the anterior hypothalamus.[1] *Fever* is defined as an elevation of body temperature due to the resetting of this thermostat by circulating pyrogenic cytokines. *Hyperthermia* (temperature >40°C), in contrast, occurs when the normal thermoregulatory mechanisms are overwhelmed by excessive heat production, decreased heat dissipation, or extreme environmental heat and humidity. During hyperthermia the hypothalamic set point is normal, but autonomic mechanisms are unable to dissipate sufficient heat.[1] Common etiologies of hyperthermia are summarized in Box 78-1.

Normally, a rise in body temperature causes cutaneous vasodilation and sweating, both mediated by the autonomic nervous system. Vasodilation causes heat loss by convection, while perspiration promotes heat loss by evaporation. In cold environments the hypothalamus maintains body heat by vasoconstriction and diminished sweating. Body heat can be produced by increased skeletal muscle activity, ranging from barely perceptible increased muscle tone to overt shivering.[1]

CLASSIC HEATSTROKE AND EXERTIONAL HEATSTROKE

Classic heatstroke occurs during heat waves in the summer months. Over 5000 deaths in the United States were attributed to excessive heat between 1979 and 1991.[2] Adolescents at particular risk for heat-related deaths include the obese, those physically active in hot environments who fail to rest or drink sufficient liquids, and those unable to obtain adequate fluid intake or avoid excessive heat. The major mechanism of this disorder is diminished heat dissipation.[1] Heat may be the primary cause of death or it may worsen a preexisting disease state (cardiac or pulmonary problems).

People are at increased risk for environmentally induced hyperthermia until they become acclimatized to high temperatures. Acclimatization, which requires 10 to 14 days, is initially characterized by increased plasma volume with subsequent augmented stroke volume and decreased heart rate.[2] This is accomplished by increased secretion of aldosterone, resulting in renal sodium absorption with increased potassium loss in the urine and decreased salt loss in sweat. With maximal acclimatization, sweat volume increases up to two to three times normal.[3] Access to air conditioning clearly reduces the risk, so that heat-related hyperthermia is a more common condition in lower socioeconomic groups. Fans are not protective when ambient temperatures are over 32°C.[4]

Exertional heatstroke occurs during strenuous activity in hot, humid weather, usually by healthy individuals such as athletes (football and rugby players, marathoners), military recruits, and workers in heavy industries (steel workers). Lack of acclimatization and cardiovascular conditioning, dehydration, and heavy clothing place these individuals at additional risk. The pathophysiology of exertional heatstroke is excessive heat production when heat dissipation is limited. Although elevated levels of pyrogenic cytokines have been reported in some patients, it is not clear whether these cytokines are part of the pathophysiology or just a response to the heatstroke. Patients who survive exertional heatstroke have normal skeletal muscle, unlike those who have anesthesia-related hyperthermia.[1]

Both classic and exertional heatstroke have similar clinical presentations that include sudden onset of hyperthermia with body temperature greater than 40.5°C; altered mental status characterized by confusion, convulsions, delirium, or coma; hypotension; tachycardia; tachypnea; and hot and dry skin in classic heatstroke or moist skin in exertional heat stroke. Vomiting and diarrhea commonly occur. Heat exhaustion is a less severe form of exertional heatstroke in which the patient's temperature is approximately 40°C and mental status remains normal. The major differential consideration is

BOX 78-1
Causes of Hyperthermia

DISORDERS OF EXCESSIVE HEAT PRODUCTION
Exertional hyperthermia
Exertional heatstroke*
Malignant hyperthermia
Neuroleptic malignant syndrome*
Lethal catatonia
Thyrotoxicosis
Pheochromocytoma
Salicylate intoxication
Cocaine or amphetamines
Delirium tremens
Status epilepticus
Generalized tetanus
Hemorrhagic shock and encephalopathy

DISORDERS OF DIMINISHED HEAT DISSIPATION
Classic heatstroke*
Extensive occlusive dressings
Dehydration
Autonomic dysfunction
Anticholinergics
Neuroleptic malignant syndrome*

DISORDERS OF HYPOTHALAMIC FUNCTION
Neuroleptic malignant syndrome*
Stroke
Encephalitis
Sarcoidosis and granulomatous infections
Trauma
Hemorrhagic shock and encephalopathy*

Reprinted with permission of *The New England Journal of Medicine.*
From Simon HB: Hyperthermia, *N Engl J Med* 329:483-487, 1993,
Massachusetts Medical Society.
*Mixed etiology.

sepsis, especially in patients with underlying chronic disease.

Management

Heatstroke is a medical emergency that requires rapid recognition and aggressive care. In the prehospital setting, patients' clothing should be removed and they should be fanned and bathed in cool water or covered with ice packs. In the hospital, patients should be rapidly cooled to 38.5°C with ice packs and cool intravenous fluids. Aggressive cardiovascular and respiratory support should be initiated. Close monitoring and correction of metabolic disturbances are essential. Even with aggressive therapy, death from arrhythmias, shock, myocardial ischemia, renal failure, and neurologic dysfunction is possible. The best therapy is prevention. Effective measures include reducing physical activity, drinking additional liquids, and increasing the amount of time spent in air-conditioned environments.[1]

Malignant Hyperthermia

Malignant hyperthermia (MH) may affect normally healthy individuals during and immediately after general anesthesia. Findings in MH include muscle rigidity; severe rhabdomyolysis; myoglobinuria; and a hypermetabolic state, including hypoxia, hypercapnia, and both metabolic and respiratory acidosis. Ventricular arrhythmias are caused by hyperkalemia from rhabdomyolysis. Body temperature may be elevated, often exceeding 42°C. Renal failure, hepatic failure, disseminated intravascular coagulopathy, and neurologic damage may occur.[5] MH develops in susceptible individuals a few minutes to many hours after exposure to halothane, other volatile anesthetics, or a depolarizing muscle relaxant such as succinylcholine. It may also recur hours after successful therapy. The incidence is 1 in 15,000 in children and 1 in 40,000 in adults receiving general anesthesia. Presentation includes sudden generalized muscle rigidity, cardiac arrest, immediate hyperkalemia, rhabdomyolysis, and myoglobinuria. Patients with underlying neuromuscular disease such as Duchenne muscular dystrophy may be at increased risk.[5] Individuals with a positive family history should be referred for a muscle biopsy rather than risk the emergence of this syndrome at the time of an emergency intervention.

When MH occurs, all triggering anesthetics must be discontinued and the patient should be hyperventilated with 100% oxygen. Intravenous dantrolene, a muscle relaxant that works by inhibiting the movement of calcium into the cell, is the primary therapy. Intravenous fluids and infusions of sodium bicarbonate may be needed to treat metabolic acidosis and hypovolemia. Insulin and glucose may be necessary to treat hyperkalemia. Surface cooling, and iced saline lavage of the stomach, bladder, or rectum, may be required to treat the hyperthermia. Mannitol and furosemide are administered to maintain adequate urinary output.[5] MH-susceptible patients should be informed of the disorder. Referral to the Malignant Hyperthermia Association may be useful for education and family support.[5]

Neuroleptic Malignant Syndrome

Neuroleptic malignant syndrome (NMS) is a rare form of drug-induced hyperthermia initiated by butyrophenones (haloperidol) and piperazines (chlorpromazine, fluphenazine) neuroleptic drugs. The reported incidence varies from 0.1% to 5.5%.[6] It is more common in young adults. NMS usually occurs within 10 days of initiating neuroleptic therapy, with a range of 1 to 44 days.[6] Early signs and symptoms include changes in mental status, tachycardia, tachypnea, hypertension, dysarthria or dysphagia, diaphoresis, sialorrhea, fever, rigidity, myoclonus, other extrapyramidal signs, and unexplained elevation of the serum creatine kinase (CK). These signs do not necessarily suggest that the patient will develop NMS. However, hyperthermia and profound muscle rigidity are invariable features of NMS. Sinus tachycardia and respiratory distress may progress to respiratory arrest.[7] Elevated CK, aldolase, and myoglobinuria are frequently present.

Once neuroleptic therapy is discontinued, NMS is a self-limited disorder. Prompt recognition and supportive therapy, as outlined for MH, are the mainstays of treatment.[7]

Drug-Related Hyperthermic States

Various drugs can cause hyperthermia. Cocaine, amphetamines, methamphetamines (ecstasy), phencyclidine (angel dust), and neuroleptics undermine thermoregulation. Use or misuse of these drugs is frequently associated with hyperthermia-related deaths.[2] Medications with anticholinergic effects (antihistamines, tricyclic antidepressants, benztropine) diminish sweating and impair heat loss.[3] Salicylate ingestions may cause excessive heat production as the salicylate uncouples oxidative phosphorylation in mitochondria.[1] Alcohol consumption leads to dehydration and is also associated with hyperthermia.[3]

Hyperthermia is an emergency requiring prompt recognition and therapy. Any underlying condition must be treated while cardiovascular and metabolic support is given. In contrast to those with fever, patients with hyperthermia will not benefit from centrally acting antipyretic medication.[1] Physical cooling is the appropriate method for lowering body temperature. Dantrolene is indicated in MH and may well be useful in heatstroke. Despite rapid recognition and therapy, hyperthermia may still be fatal.

References

1. Simon HB: Hyperthermia, *N Engl J Med* 329:483-487, 1993.
2. Heat-related deaths—Philadelphia and the United States 1993-1994, *MMWR* 43:453-455, 1994.
3. Delaney KA, Vassallo SU, Goldfrank LR: Thermoregulatory principles. In Goldfrank LR, editor: *Toxicologic emergencies*, ed 5, Norwalk, CT, 1994, Appleton & Lange; pp 159-170.
4. Kilbourne EM, Choi K, Jones TS, et al: Risk factors for heatstroke—a case control study, *JAMA* 247:3332-3336, 1982.
5. Kaus SJ, Rockoff MA: Malignant hyperthermia, *Pediatr Clin North Am* 41:221-237, 1994.
6. Naganuma H, Fujii I: Incidence and risk factors in neuroleptic malignant syndrome, *Acta Psychiatr Scand* 90:424-426, 1994.
7. Caroff SN, Mann SC, Campbell EC: Hyperthermia and neuroleptic malignant syndrome, *Anesthesiol Clin North Am* 12:491-512, 1994.

CHAPTER 79

Shock

•

Anthony L. Palomba and Edward E. Conway, Jr

Shock is a physiologic disturbance characterized by tissue perfusion that is inadequate to meet the body's metabolic demands for oxygen and nutrients. It may occur with normal blood pressure, elevated blood pressure, or hypotension. The most common causes of shock in adolescent patients include trauma (hemorrhage), sepsis, anaphylaxis, respiratory failure, and drug ingestion.

Shock is the failure of tissue oxygenation that may ultimately cause cellular dysfunction and death. Tissue oxygenation is the product of cardiac output and arterial oxygen content. Cardiac output is the product of ventricular stroke volume (milliliters of blood per beat) and

heart rate (number of beats per minute). Arterial oxygen content depends on the saturation of hemoglobin, and in healthy adolescents with a hemoglobin concentration of 13 to 15 g/dl, arterial blood carries 16 to 20 ml/dl of oxygen.

Tissues extract oxygen at different rates at different times according to their metabolic needs. As the delivery of oxygen decreases, a critical point is reached where the cells no longer receive an adequate oxygen supply and therefore cannot carry out oxidative phosphorylation. In the absence of sufficient oxygen, cells then rely on anaerobic mechanisms of adenosine triphosphate production, which is much less efficient and results in an increased production of lactic acid. Eventually, cell energy levels and pH fall, resulting in an inability to carry out essential functions necessary for survival. The subsequent dysfunction and breakdown of the cell and its mitochondrial membranes leads to a cascade of secondary events resulting ultimately in cell death and organ insufficiency.[1] Early recognition of the signs of shock followed by the institution of timely and aggressive resuscitative measures is of paramount importance for a successful outcome.

ETIOLOGY AND CLASSIFICATION

Identification of disturbances of the major components of the perfusion system allows for a physiologic classification of shock. These include (1) blood—the oxygen- and nutrient-carrying fluid; (2) heart—the pump that moves the blood to and from the lungs and out to (3) the peripheral vasculature, which includes the arteries, veins, and microcirculation.

Hypovolemic shock is precipitated by an absolute or relative decrease in effective circulating blood volume. Etiologies include traumatic hemorrhage, gastrointestinal bleeding, obstetric hemorrhage, excessive fluid and electrolyte losses as seen in diabetic ketoacidosis and diarrheal dehydration, and the loss of protein-rich fluids as occurs in major burns and peritonitis.[2]

In cardiogenic shock the major disturbance results from the heart's failure as a pump. It is the least common cause of shock in the pediatric age group but can accompany various forms of congenital or acquired heart disease. Examples include myocarditis, rheumatic fever, dilated cardiomyopathies, valvular heart disease, subacute/acute bacterial endocarditis, tachydysrhythmias, bradydysrhythmias, and pump failure after cardiac surgery or anoxic-ischemic injury.

Mechanical obstruction to right or left ventricular filling or outflow is termed obstructive shock. Cardiac tamponade and tension pneumothorax are two rapidly reversible causes of obstructive shock. Cardiac tamponade occurs when blood, fluid (usually an inflammatory exudate), or air fills the pericardial space. A rare but poorly recognized cause of obstructive shock is massive pulmonary embolism, which can be rapidly fatal.

Distributive shock states are characterized by severe alterations in peripheral vascular tone. There is vasodilation and maldistribution of microcirculatory flow secondary to loss of autoregulation. Severe arteriovenous shunting of blood away from capillary beds, and capillary leak syndrome, which produces a loss of intravascular volume into the interstitial space, also occur. Causes include sepsis, anaphylaxis, drug intoxication, and spinal cord injury.

PATHOPHYSIOLOGY AND CLINICAL RECOGNITION

Hypovolemic shock triggers a number of early compensatory adjustments in response to the decrease in organ perfusion. The decrease in central venous pressure and cardiac filling results in an increase in antidiuretic hormone release from the pituitary. On the arterial side of the circulation, baroceptors and chemoreceptors sense an inadequate pressure and flow, which produces a marked increase in sympathetic nervous system tone. There is an increased release of norepinephrine and epinephrine (from the adrenal) into the circulation. A decrease in renal perfusion activates the renin-angiotensin system, and local changes in the microcirculation promote movement of fluid from the interstitium into the capillaries. The result is an attempt to restore or maintain blood volume by retaining water and salt through translocation of extracellular fluid into the intravascular space at the capillary level. The increase in circulating catecholamines provides for an early increase in heart rate and contractility, as well as centralization of blood volume via venoconstriction and maintenance of systemic blood pressure via arterial vasoconstriction. Circulation to the more vital organs (brain, heart, lungs) is maintained at the expense of the periphery (skin, muscle, and splanchnic beds, including the kidneys).

These changes result in the clinical signs of early compensated hypovolemic shock. Patients are tachycardiac with cool mottled extremities that demonstrate a decrease in capillary refill. Peripheral pulses are diminished in amplitude, and blood pressure is often normal, with a narrowed pulse pressure. Urinary output is diminished and maximally concentrated. Neurologic status is usually normal, although mild impairment may be manifested as lethargy or irritability.

A continued loss of blood or ineffective therapy can lead to later decompensation as microperfusion in the vital organs becomes more and more inadequate. The heart will eventually fail as a pump. Pulmonary and renal function will deteriorate rapidly. There will be progressive neurologic deterioration, including impairment of those autonomic centers providing for neurohumoral support of the circulation and breathing. Metabolic acidosis becomes severe and intractable. Mortality is high in late decompensated shock.

In cardiogenic shock, the same attempt at compensation is triggered by the decrease in stroke volume of the right and left ventricles. However, unlike the situation in hypovolemic shock, these adjustments may worsen the situation. The increase in pressure and volume in the ventricle mediated by sodium and water retention will cause increased distention, leading to subendocardial ischemia and an increase in wall tension. The increase in peripheral vascular resistance will further increase the afterload on a failing myocardium and increase its oxygen demands. Pulmonary edema will worsen gas exchange, and oxygen saturation will fall.

The clinical findings are similar to those described in patients with hypovolemic shock but with some differences. The cardiopulmonary examination frequently reveals signs of pulmonary congestion and heart failure. Murmurs, gallops, irregular rate and rhythm, neck vein distention, hepatomegaly, and peripheral edema are additional clues to the diagnosis. Central venous pressure will be high rather than low as in hypovolemia. Progression to a decompensated state may be rapid. Patients with tamponade demonstrate muffled or distant heart sounds, neck vein distention, and hepatomegaly but do not have signs of pulmonary congestion.

Septic and anaphylactic shock typify the pathophysiologic profile of distributive shock. The offending agent triggers the production and release of bioactive mediators into the circulation.[3,4] These mediators initiate a number of secondary events that lead to a systemic inflammatory response. It is characterized by fever, generalized vasodilation, venous pooling, capillary endothelial leak, accumulation of leukocytes and platelets in the microcirculation, and arteriovenous shunting of blood away from tissue capillary beds. Septic shock is more common and may carry a mortality rate as high as 60%.[3] The offending agents are usually substances produced by or actual components of the infecting agent.[5] Lipopolysaccharide from gram-negative bacteria and toxic shock toxins produced by *Staphlococcus* and *Streptococcus* infection are examples.[6] They stimulate the production of cytokines such as tumor necrosis factor and interleukin-1 by macrophages. These cytokines then initiate the production of a myriad of substances that mediate the inflammatory response and alter cellular metabolism.[7]

Clinically, most of these patients present with an early hyperdynamic or "warm shock" phase. They are febrile and the skin is plethoric and warm to touch. Peripheral pulses are easily felt and blood pressure may be normal, with a low diastolic component and a widened pulse pressure. Patients are tachypneic and urinary output may be preserved early on. If the condition is left unrecognized and untreated, there is a progressive decrease in cardiac output, and clinical findings are similar to those described for hypovolemic and cariogenic shock.

Regardless of the cause of shock, a state of late decompensation may be reached as microperfusion becomes more marginal, cellular function deteriorates, and cell energy production mechanisms are irreversibly damaged. There is progressive and severe dysfunction of the brain, heart, kidneys, and lungs. Metabolic acidosis is intractable and profound.

TREATMENT

The key to a successful outcome for a patient in shock is the early institution of aggressive measures titrated to the clinical goal of restoration of tissue perfusion and oxygenation.[8,9]

The more common causes of shock result in either an absolute (hypovolemic) or relative (distributive shock) hypovolemia. Patients with septic shock have considerable loss of fluid through capillaries leaking into the interstitium.[7] The hallmark of therapy becomes the timely restoration of an effective circulating blood volume by rapid intravenous (or intraosseous) administration of an appropriate solution. Isotonic crystalloids such as Ringer's lactate, 0.9% sodium chloride, and isotonic colloids such as 5% albumin and 6% hetastarch (pectin-derived polymer) are the more commonly used and readily available solutions.[10] There is no one best solution to administer, so the selection is a matter of individual preference and availability. Crystalloids are less expensive and must be given in larger volumes (at least two to three times that of a colloid solution), as they readily equilibrate into the interstitial space. The larger albumin and hetastarch molecules are more impermeable to the capillary membrane and stay in the intravascular compartment longer. In patients suffering from hemorrhagic shock, blood and blood products become the fluid of choice for resuscitation as soon as they become available. Ideally, the large volumes administered should be titrated to clinical and physiologic end points to provide adequate resuscitation and minimize complications such as pulmonary edema. Rapid bolus administration of 20 ml/kg of crystalloid or 10 ml/kg of colloid is followed by an assessment for an improvement in heart rate, blood pressure, capillary refill, strength of peripheral pulses, and urinary output. If little or no improvement is noted, a second bolus is administered.

Hypothermia, acidosis, hypocalcemia, anemia, and hypoglycemia produce a marked depression of cardiovascular function, and their presence must be determined and treated to ensure successful resuscitation. Patients in shock should be intubated early in the course of their resuscitation to ensure ventilation and the delivery of a high concentration of oxygen to the lungs while decreasing the oxygen demand of breathing.

Not all patients in shock respond to early volume replacement. Placement of intra-arterial, central venous, and Foley catheters provides additional physiologic data for further titration of volume infusion and institution of pharmacologic support of the circulation. Low central venous pressure requires additional volume infusion; high central venous pressure indicates the need for inotropic support. Patients in advanced stages of shock with multiple organ system involvement may require placement of a pulmonary artery catheter for a more detailed evaluation of their physiologic disturbances in oxygen supply and demand.[11]

Inotropic agents improve cardiac performance by increasing myocardial contractility. The most widely used and efficacious agents are dopamine, dobutamine, norepinephrine, epinephrine, and isoproterenol. They differ in their actions on heart rate (chronotropic properties) and peripheral vascular tone.[12] They are administered as a continuous intravenous infusion, with doses titrated to clinical and physiologic end points. Their onset of action is within minutes and they have an extremely short half-life (minutes).

Dobutamine is a semisynthetic derivative of isoproterenol and a beta-receptor stimulator. It increases cardiac contractility with little or no increase in heart rate. Its action on the peripheral vasculature is to vasodilate peripheral and pulmonary arterioles. The usual dosage range is 5 to 15µg/kg/min.

Dopamine is a naturally occurring catechol precursor of norepinephrine. Its cardiovascular effects are dose dependent, making it a good drug for initiation of inotropic support. Low doses (0.5 to 2 µg/kg/min) vasodilate the splanchnic and renal vascular beds. It is often used in combination with other inotropes to improve renal blood flow and urinary output. Doses of 2 to 12 µg/kg/min provide mostly beta-receptor stimulation, which increases both heart rate and contractility. Doses greater than 15 µg/kg/min cause increasing degrees of vasoconstriction and an increase in blood pressure.

Norepinephrine is the major catechol neurotransmitter of the sympathetic nervous system. It has potent vasoconstrictor and inotropic effects in the dosage range of 0.1 to 1 µg/kg/min. It is particularly useful in restoring peripheral vascular tone, blood pressure, and tissue perfusion in early septic shock during the hyperdynamic "warm shock" phase.

Epinephrine has potent vasoconstrictor, chronotropic, and inotropic effects. It is used in a dosage range of 0.1 to 1 µg/kg/min in combination with other inotropes for patients in severe shock states. It is the drug of choice for support of the circulation in anaphylactic shock. Its potent metabolic effects may cause hyperglycemia and lactic acidosis.

Isoproterenol has a very narrow spectrum of use. It is a potent chronotropic agent and is best used in situations in which bradycardia is a major contributor to low cardiac output. The usual dose is 0.1 to 1 µg/kg/min.

It must be emphasized that the various etiologies and stages of shock effect significant alterations in drug metabolism and response, making it necessary to titrate the dose against clinical effect.

Once perfusion is reestablished and the patient is adequately resuscitated, a definitive diagnosis can be pursued. Appropriate cultures should be obtained from and antibiotics administered to patients in septic shock. Victims of shock should be transferred to an intensive care setting where the technology and expertise exists for definitive physiologic monitoring and management of the disturbances that can occur after reperfusion.[13]

In summary, shock is the pathophysiologic state of perfusion that is inadequate to meet the body's metabolic demands for oxygen and nutrients. All forms of shock share oxygenation failure, which produces cell dysfunction and death. Clinically, shock manifests as tachypnea, tachycardia, weak pulses, acrocyanosis, altered level of consciousness, and low or no urinary output. It may occur with normal, elevated, or decreased blood pressure. Early recognition and aggressive fluid resuscitation are the keys to an improved outcome.

References

1. Perkin RM, Levin DL: Shock in the pediatric patient. Part I, *J Pediatr* 101:163-169, 1982.
2. Hayashi R: Obstetric hemorrhage and hypovolemic shock. In Clarke SL, Colton DB, GDV Hankins GDV, Phelan JP, editors: *Critical care obstetrics* Boston, 1991, Blackwell Scientific; pp 199-211.
3. Saez-Lloreno X, MaCracken GH Jr: Sepsis syndrome and septic shock in pediatrics: current concepts of terminology, pathophysiology, and management, *J Pediatr* 123:497-508, 1993.
4. Bochner BS, Lichtensein LM: Anaphylaxis, *N Engl J Med* 324:1785-1790, 1991.
5. Wiles JB, Cerra FS, Siegel JH, et al: The systemic response: does the organism matter?, *Crit Care Med* 8:55-57, 1990.
6. Givner LB, Abramson JS, Wasilauskas B: Apparent increase in the incidence of invasive group A beta-hemolytic streptococcal disease in children, *J Pediatr* 118:341-346, 1991.
7. Parillo J: Pathogenic mechanisms of septic shock, *N Engl J Med* 328:1471-1477, 1993.
8. Perkin RM, Levin DL: Shock in the pediatric patient. Part II, *J Pediatr* 101:319-332, 1982.
9. Carcillo JA, Davis AL, Zaritzky A: Role of early fluid resuscitation in pediatric septic shock, *JAMA* 266:1242-1245, 1991.
10. Imn A, Carlson RW: Fluid resuscitation in circulatory shock, *Crit Care Clin* 9:313-333, 1993.
11. Katz RW, Pollack MM, Weibley RE: Pulmonary artery catheterization in pediatric intensive care, *Adv Pediatr* 30:169-190, 1983.
12. Perkin RM, Anas NG: Nonsurgical contractility manipulation of the failing circulation, *Clin Crit Care Med* 10:229-256, 1986.
13. Carden DL, Smith KJ, Zimmerman BJ, et al: Reperfusion injury following circulatory collapse: the role of reactive oxygen metabolites, *J Crit Care* 4:294-307, 1989.

CHAPTER 80

Altered States of Consciousness

•

Edward E. Conway, Jr

Consciousness is maintained by the interaction of both cerebral cortices and the reticulating activating system (RAS) located within the brain stem. Coma is caused by extensive damage to both cortices or to the RAS. Normal consciousness requires the interaction of neurons at the cellular level with specific central nervous system (CNS) structures at the gross anatomic level.[1] CNS function may be disrupted either at the cellular level (hypoglycemia, hypoxia, electrolyte abnormalities) or at a more gross anatomic level.[1] A change in the level of consciousness may be caused either by a diffuse toxic/metabolic state (approximately 80% of coma cases) or by structural damage to the CNS.

COMA

Coma is defined as the absence of awareness of one's self and one's environment.[2] It is a state of unarousable unresponsiveness in which the patient lies without spontaneous movement with eyes closed. The patient may respond to noxious stimuli by purposeful withdrawal but cannot localize with discrete movements. There is a range of alterations in mental status, including lethargy, confusion, delirium, obtundation, and stupor. Lethargy is a state in which one is easily distracted and misjudges sensory perceptions but retains the ability to communicate. Delirium is characterized by disorientation, fear, irritability, and visual hallucinations. Obtundation is a state of mental blunting with a decreased interest in the environment. Stupor is a state of deep sleep from which the patient can be aroused for short periods only by vigorous and repeated stimuli.

Coma is best assessed and described using the Glasgow Coma Scale (GCS) (Table 80-1).[3] A fully alert patient is given a score of 15, whereas a score below 8 indicates coma. The scale is easily applied and repro-

duced. The ability to speak is a cortical function, eyelid opening is a brain stem function, and the motor responses require both the cortical and brain stem pathways to be intact. The GCS therefore allows assessment of the integrity of the cortex and its interconnections on the basis of a simple clinical examination.

Coma should always be considered a neurologic emergency. The major goal in evaluating and treating the patient is to prevent further CNS injury. The initial assessment should consist of the ABCs: airway, breathing, and circulation. The physician must identify conditions that are rapidly correctable (hypoxemia, hypotension, hypoglycemia) and be able to identify a deteriorating CNS status. After the ABC assessment, it should be immediately determined whether there are any signs of increased intracranial pressure (ICP) or if the patient is at risk for cerebral herniation. These include vomiting, headache, a decrease in GCS score, papilledema (a late finding), hypertension, bradycardia, apneustic breathing, posturing, and unilateral dilation of a pupil. If there is a suggestion of increased ICP, the patient should be hyperventilated, administration of 1 g/kg of mannitol considered, and a prompt neurosurgical consultation obtained.

One must carefully assess for focal neurologic signs that may suggest a structural CNS lesion. After the initial stabilization of the patient, history taking and a careful physical examination must be performed. The history may have to be obtained from emergency personnel, bystanders, or someone other than the patient. Specific items to evaluate in the history include chronic underlying diseases (pulmonary, renal, hepatic, immunodeficiency), ingestion of any drugs or substances (including over-the-counter medications), trauma, seizures, previous episodes, thyroid disease, metabolic disease (diabetic ketoacidosis [DKA]), malignancy, psychosocial history, and possible exposure to any environmental toxins (carbon

TABLE 80-1
Glasgow Coma Scale

Test	Finding	Score
Eye opening	Spontaneously	4
	Response to voice	3
	Response to pain	2
	No response	1
Verbal response	Oriented and appropriate	5
	Disoriented conversation	4
	Inappropriate words	3
	Incomprehensible sounds	2
	No response	1
Motor response	Obeys commands	6
	Localizes pain	5
	Flexion withdrawal	4
	Decorticate posturing	3
	Decerebrate posturing	2
	No response	1
	Maximal total score	15

monoxide). The time course of the change in mental status and focal findings may also suggest an etiology.

The physical examination includes evaluation of the vital signs: heart rate, blood pressure (either hyper- or hypotension), respiratory pattern (often abnormal in patients in coma), and temperature (hyper- or hypothermia). Each of these is a possible cause of coma. The patient should be examined for signs of trauma and the scalp palpated for possible hematomas or the presence of a ventriculoperitoneal shunt. The neck should be stabilized until a C-spine fracture can be safely excluded. Nuchal rigidity may not be present in the deeply comatose patient. Examination of the pupils may suggest a possible cause of the coma. In toxic/metabolic coma the pupils are small but react symmetrically, whereas there may be dilation or asymmetry in patients with a CNS lesion. A funduscopic examination should evaluate signs of papilledema or absent venous pulsations suggesting an increase in ICP.

A detailed neurologic examination begins with assessment of the GCS score. An important clue to a structural CNS lesion is focality on the neurologic examination. Respiratory patterns should be observed. The position, posture, and spontaneous movements of the patient should be noted. Decorticate positioning (flexor posturing of the upper extremities) is usually associated with a CNS injury above the midbrain, whereas decerebrate positioning (extensor posturing) is associated with damage to the midbrain or diencephalon. These postures may be produced by a variety of lesions in many different locations and do not of themselves suggest the location of the lesion. Babinski's sign (an extensor upgoing toe) may be present bilaterally when consciousness is depressed

from any cause, but a unilateral upgoing toe is a good indicator of a CNS structural lesion.[4]

The choice of laboratory studies should be guided by the history. All patients must undergo an immediate determination of serum glucose levels and arterial blood gases to ascertain their acid-base status. Serum electrolytes to be evaluated include sodium, calcium, bicarbonate, urea nitrogen, and creatinine. If the history and physical examination suggest an infectious cause, appropriate cultures should be obtained along with a complete blood count. A spinal tap should be performed unless contraindicated. Serum and urine toxicologies should be guided by the most likely substance ingested, keeping in mind the possibility of administering an antidote. The decision to perform head computed tomography (CT) will be guided by the patient's presentation and physical examination.

The differential diagnosis of coma is extensive. The mnemonic AEIOU THIPS can help to classify the causes of coma (Box 80-1). A major consideration is whether the coma is the result of a correctable toxic/metabolic etiology (ingestion or electrolyte abnormality) or of a structural lesion (CNS hemorrhage, trauma, or tumor).

Infection

Most infections of the CNS are life-threatening and there must be a high index of suspicion. Fever, photophobia, headache, vomiting, and a change in mental status suggest CNS infection. Kernig's and Brudzinski's signs may be absent in patients in deep coma. Cerebrospinal fluid (CSF) studies should be performed in all patients

---

BOX 80-1
Etiologies of Coma

A Alcohol/abuse/anoxia
E Encephalopathy/endocrinopathy/electrolytes
I Ingestions/insulin
O Opiates
U Uremia
T Trauma
H Hypo/hypertension/hyper/hypothermia/hypo-
    glycemia
I Infection
P Psychogenic
S Structural lesions/seizures/syncope

---

with symptoms suggesting CNS infection; however, in patients with papilledema or focal neurologic findings a head CT scan should be performed to rule out a mass lesion. An opening pressure should be determined and CSF obtained for cell counts, chemistries (glucose and protein), and bacterial and viral cultures. Cryptococcal antigen determination should be performed in all immunocompromised patients.

Antibiotics should be started empirically, and the major bacterial organisms to consider in adult meningitis are *Streptococcus pneumoniae* and *Neisseria meningitidis*. Complications associated with meningitis that may lead to coma include seizures, subdural effusions, subdural empyema, cerebral abscess, cerebral venous infarcts, the syndrome of inappropriate antidiuretic hormone (SIADH) (hyponatremia), and both communicating and obstructive hydrocephalus.[5]

Encephalitis

Encephalitis is an unusual complication of common viral infections. These usually involve the meninges, as in aseptic meningitis, or cause a mild clinical syndrome of meningoencephalitis.[6] They present with the acute onset of fever; headache; altered mental status; disorientation; behavioral and speech disturbances; and neurologic signs, sometimes focal, but generally diffuse, such as hemiparesis or seizures.[6] There is no evidence of bacteria, fungi, spirochetes, or parasites in the CSF, but there is usually a mild elevation in the cell count, usually lymphocytes, with normal chemistries. The differential diagnosis includes parameningeal infections and carcinomatous meningitis.

The most common viral cause of sporadic acute focal encephalitis is herpes simplex. In the absence of therapy, mortality exceeds 70%, and only about 2.5% of persons affected regain normal function.[6] There is an associated classic electroencephalographic picture called PLEDs

(periodic lateralized epileptiform discharges) that shows periodic focal spikes from the temporal area where the virus localizes. Treatment should be instituted with acyclovir as soon as a herpes infection is suspected.

Lastly, patients with AIDS may present with chronic encephalitis. The virus itself may cause damage to deep cortical structures, and these patients may have unusual opportunistic infections of the CNS. Unusual primary and secondary malignancies have also been noted.[7]

Ingestions/Alcohol/Opiates/Abuse

Drugs that are commonly ingested and lead to changes in mental status and coma include barbiturates, opiates, psychedelics, amphetamines, cocaine, ethanol, atropine, tricyclic antidepressants, phenothiazines, methaqualone, benzodiazepines, anticonvulsants, and antihistamines. Some agents have a direct effect on the CNS (barbiturates, opiates, ethanol, benzodiazepines). Others induce seizures or other physiologic changes that produce a coma (hyper/hypotension, hyperthermia). Drug withdrawal (opioids and benzodiazepines) produces neurologic findings including confusion, hallucinations, myoclonus, seizures, hyperthermia, and pupillary constriction.

The initial assessment of adolescents with a change in mental status may begin in the field. Such patients are usually administered dextrose (discussed below), thiamine, and a trial of naloxone, a narcotic antagonist. The routine empiric naloxone dose is intravenous administration of 0.8 to 2.0 mg. It may also be administered endotracheally, intramuscularly, or subcutaneously or injected intralingually.[8] The half-life of naloxone is 40 to 90 minutes, a much shorter time course than that of the opioid being reversed. A continuous infusion should be considered if the initial dose is successful. Naloxone should be administered to patients with a respiratory rate less than 12 breaths per minute, those with pinpoint pupils, and those with circumstantial evidence of opioid abuse (drug paraphernalia, needle tracks, bystander corroboration).[8] Flumazenil, a new benzodiazepine antagonist, has been administered to patients with multiple drug ingestions, but its use has precipitated seizures in patients who have ingested both tricyclic antidepressants and benzodiazepines. It is a reversal agent that should be viewed with great caution in pediatric patients.[9,10]

Metabolic/Electrolyte/Endocrine Abnormalities

Metabolic etiologies of coma most commonly include hypoglycemia and hypoxia. Both globally disrupt neuronal function at the cellular level and produce a change in consciousness. Hypoglycemia is defined as a blood concentration less than 50 mg/dl in an adult patient; a glucose determination should be one of the first investigations in a comatose patient. If it is not possible to obtain an immediate serum glucose level, 50 ml of D50W should be administered intravenously.

Hypoglycemia has three important effects on the CNS: (1) it invokes a stress response, (2) it causes cerebral blood-flow disturbances, and (3) it alters cerebral metabolism, ultimately leading to permanent neurologic damage.[11] Common causes include fasting, liver and renal disease, excess insulin, glucocorticoid deficiency, sepsis, malnutrition, heart failure, and drugs (oral hypoglycemics, ethanol, salicylates, propranolol).

The effects of hypoxia are different for different cell types, but brain cells can be permanently damaged after only 4 to 6 minutes of hypoxia.[12] Neuronal dysfunction is caused by the development of cellular acidosis, generation of free radicals, an increase in the concentration of metabolic products, and degradation of membrane phospholipids. CNS anoxia is most commonly seen after cardiopulmonary arrest. In the United States, there are over 1000 cardiac arrests daily; 80% of persons successfully resuscitated are unconscious at 1 hour, and 39% of victims never regain consciousness.[13]

Extremes of temperature may cause neuronal dysfunction. Hyperthermia is directly toxic to neurons and it produces renal and hepatic failure that contribute to neuronal dysfunction. Electrolyte abnormalities that cause a change in consciousness include hyponatremia, hypercalcemia, hypermagnesemia, and hypernatremia. Extreme changes in serum osmolarity (seen in DKA, diabetes insipidus, and SIADH) also contribute to cellular dysfunction. Toxic metabolites may accumulate in patients with renal and hepatic failure and cause neuronal depression. Endocrinopathies that produce a change in mental status include DKA, hypo- or hyperthyroidism, and adrenal disease. Extremes of acid-base disturbance produce cellular neuronal dysfunction.

Structural Processes

Structural processes cause focal disruption or destruction of either the cerebral cortices or the RAS. CNS lesions may be subdivided as occurring in either the supra- or subtentorial regions. Trauma resulting in an epidural, subdural, or intracerebral hematoma or diffuse cerebral swelling is the leading cause of supratentorial lesions. Cerebrovascular accidents (in sickle cell disease and systemic lupus erythematosus patients), venous thrombosis, subdural empyema, or intracerebral tumor may also produce supratentorial lesions. These lesions may produce focal destruction in one hemisphere, which in turn may cause cerebral swelling or pressure on the other hemisphere or on the brain stem and, ultimately, coma.

Subtentorial (posterior fossa) lesions result from tumors, trauma, and primary hemorrhage into the brain stem. These directly affect the RAS and thus depress consciousness.

Subarachnoid hemorrhage (SAH), although a focal lesion, may cause global dysfunction because the blood released is transported by way of the CSF to the entire CNS. Approximately one third of patients with SAH present in a comatose state. The most common causes are a ruptured aneurysm or an arteriovenous malformation.

Trauma

Head injury accounts for almost 25,000 deaths per year in pediatric patients. Younger patients with severe head injury (GCS score of <8) have better outcomes than adults and approximately one half the mortality rate. Alcohol and drugs play an increased role in head injury in adolescent patients. Recovery from severe head injury depends on the severity of injury, rapid initiation of medical treatment, and rehabilitation. A concussion is a head injury associated with a transient loss of consciousness, but patients may also exhibit confusion and disorientation.

Seizures/Psychiatric Syndromes

Patients may present in a postictal state after a protracted seizure that may not have been witnessed. Several psychiatric syndromes are associated with a depressed mental state, including "locked-in syndrome," akinetic mutism, psychogenic unresponsiveness, conversion disorder, and catatonia. These syndromes are not life-threatening but must be differentiated from other potentially reversible causes of coma.

The patient who presents in a comatose state represents a true diagnostic dilemma for the physician. The goal of therapy is to prevent further CNS injury and to stabilize the patient quickly. Rapid identification and reversal of toxic or metabolic causes of coma may be lifesaving. Once the patient is hemodynamically stable, one may then consider the AEIOU THIPS approach to elucidate the cause of the coma.

References

1. Peterson J: Coma. In Rosen P, editor: *Emergency medicine: concepts and clinical practice*, St. Louis, 1993, Mosby–Year Book; pp 1728-1751.

2. Plum F, Posner JB: *The diagnosis of stupor and coma*, ed 3, Philadelphia, 1980, FA Davis; pp 1-86.

3. Teasdale G, Jennett: Assessment of coma and impaired consciousness, *Lancet* 2:81-84, 1974.

4. DeMyer W: Examination of the patient who has a disorder of consciousness. In DeMyer W, editor: *Technique of the neurologic examination*, New York, 1980, McGraw-Hill.

5. Kornelisse RF, de Groot E, Neijens HJ: Bacterial meningitis:

mechanisms of disease and therapy, *Eur J Pediatr* 154:85-96, 1995.

6. Whitley RJ: Viral encephalitis, *N Engl J Med* 323:242-250, 1990.

7. Levy RM, Berger JR: Neurologic critical care in patients with human immunodeficiency virus infection, *Crit Care Clin* 9:49-72, 1993.

8. Doyon S, Roberts JR: Reappraisal of the "coma cocktail," *Emerg Med Clin North Am* 12:301-316, 1994.

9. Sugarman JM, Paul RI: Flumazenil: a review, *Pediatr Emerg Care* 10:37-43, 1994.

10. Winkler E, Almog S, Kriger D, et al: Use of flumazenil in the diagnosis and treatment of patients with coma of unknown etiology, *Crit Care Med* 21:538-542, 1993.

11. Sieber FE, Traystman RJ: Special issues: glucose and the brain, *Crit Care Med* 20:104-114, 1992.

12. Guiterrez G: Cellular energy metabolism during hypoxia, *Crit Care Med* 19:619-626, 1991.

13. Shewmon DA, De Giorgio CM: Early prognosis in anoxic coma: reliability and rationale, *Neurol Clin* 7:823-843, 1989.

PART THREE

Psychosocial Issues

CHAPTER 81

Communication Between Parent and Adolescent

•

Arthur L. Robin

Adolescents often complain that they are misunderstood, unduly restricted, and unfairly treated by their parents. Parents often complain that their adolescents either fail to communicate or communicate their feelings in a hostile manner. How should the practitioner in adolescent health care decide when a family has significant communication problems, and what should the practitioner do about these problems? What types of anticipatory guidance can the physician give to the family to prevent parents and adolescents from developing significant communication problems? To answer these questions, we must understand the "chemistry" of parent-adolescent communication. The "atoms" or "molecules" of family communication consist of specific skills in expressing messages, receiving messages, and solving interpersonal problems. In addition, expectations and beliefs about family life greatly influence communication skills.

Table 81-1 summarizes common negative and positive communication skills and is designed for family use. Effective communicators clearly and concisely express their feelings and attitudes without accusations, put-downs, ridicule, or sarcasm. They accept responsibility for their actions. Good communicators listen attentively, maintaining eye contact and a receptive posture, and watch for signs of the listener's understanding of their comments. They acknowledge the speaker's points to clarify their understanding. When interpersonal disagreements arise, the effective communicator engages in a mutual problem-solving process, as follows:

1. Define the problem by pinpointing situations and actions that create a conflict.
2. Generate a variety of alternative solutions creatively and without premature criticism or evaluation.
3. Evaluate the solutions, considering the benefits and risks and the impact of the solutions on themselves and others.
4. Negotiate a mutually acceptable compromise.
5. Plan the details necessary to implement the solutions.

Early to middle adolescence is a time when individuals separate from parents and assume personal responsibility for their own behavior. As a normal part of the individuation process, the young adolescent will argue and disobey parental rules. The manner in which parents react to these rebellious acts helps shape the adolescent's resultant sense of personal efficacy. It is easy for parents to react by feeling threatened and restricting the teenager's freedom. Such reactions inevitably evoke reciprocal negative adolescent reactions, which may take the form of defensiveness, further rebelliousness, evasiveness, or withdrawal. Before long, a repetitive pattern of accusatory/defensive communication and coercion/disobedience pervades the parent-adolescent relationship, leading to clinically significant conflict.

Rigid, perfectionist expectations and malicious accusations also elicit an angry response. Parents who are infuriated because the adolescent did not live up to their expectations, however unreasonable, will be unable to have a rational discussion of the important issues in the parent-child relationship. For example, parents may believe that if they give an adolescent too much freedom, the adolescent will ruin his or her life ("If I let her stay out late, she will become pregnant, an alcoholic, or a drug addict."). They may demand complete obedience and perfection from the adolescent and interpret normal rebelliousness as misbehavior that is maliciously and purposely designed to aggravate the

TABLE 81-1
Negative Communication within Families

Check if Your Family Does This:	**More Positive Way to Do It:**
____ Call each other names	Express anger without hurt
____ Put each other down	"I" statements: "I am upset that . . ."
____ Interrupt each other	Take turns and keep it short
____ Criticize all the time	Point out the good and the bad
____ Get defensive when attacked	Listen, then calmly disagree
____ Give a lecture	Tell it straight and short
____ Use big words	Stick to simple words
____ Dredge up the past	Stick to the present
____ Talk in a sarcastic tone	Talk in a normal tone
____ Get off the topic	Stick to the topic
____ Think the worst	Keep an open mind
____ Command, order	Ask nicely
____ Look away from the speaker	Look at the speaker
____ Slouch	Sit up attentively
____ Give the silent treatment	Say it if you feel it
____ Deny you did it	Take responsibility for your actions
____ Nag about small mistakes	Overlook small things

parent ("He should obey my order to be home by midnight. His failure to do so is a sign of serious disrespect, done on purpose to get me mad."). Adolescents may also adhere to extreme beliefs. They often have a keen sense of injustice or unfairness, believing that it is their birthright to be completely autonomous and that parental restrictions are intrinsically unfair, purposely designed to ruin their teenage years ("Why can't I stay out as late as Sally? Her parents really understand teenagers. You just want to make me lose all my friends."). Such extreme beliefs are associated with clinically significant distress and disruptive behavior disorders.[1]

ASSESSMENT

The best way for the practitioner to assess parent-adolescent communication and beliefs is through a combination of clinical interviews, direct observations, and standardized self-report questionnaires. The following two-step screening procedure is recommended:[2]

1. At regular intervals when adolescents come to the office for routine medical care, the practitioner should provide brief, well-validated screening questionnaires designed to establish possible significant parent-adolescent relationship problems.
2. When scores on the screening questionnaires are high compared with normative data, the practitioner should set aside approximately 30 minutes for a family-functioning check-up.

The Conflict Behavior Questionnaire (CBQ)[3] is one example of such a screening tool. It is a 20-item true/false questionnaire that assesses communication, problem solving, and general dissatisfaction with a relationship and takes about 5 minutes to complete. The number of items endorsed in a negative direction make up the total score; adolescents without significant clinical distress endorse an average of two items; those with clinical distress endorse an average of eight items. The Issues Checklist (IC),[3] another useful tool, is a list of 44 issues, such as chores, curfew, and homework, about which parents and adolescents commonly disagree. The respondent indicates the frequency of disagreements and the associated anger-intensity level for each issue during the previous few weeks. Parents and adolescents complete these measuring tools independently. We have found the CBQ and the IC to be reliable, valid questionnaires in our research with families.[3]

During the family-functioning check-up, it is best to interview the adolescent and parents together, since the goal is to assess their interaction. When feasible, it is a good idea to invite both parents to participate, since the practitioner can then observe the widest variety of parent-child and spouse interactions. Confidentiality is not a major problem because the goal is to gather information about interactions, not about inner feelings and secrets. It should be explained to the participants that the purpose of the interview is to learn how the family members get along with each other. The parents should be asked to reassure the adolescent that there will be no negative repercussions for speaking freely during the interview. The interview is begun with broad questions about the parent-child relationship, and later moves to pointed questions. Several illustrations of typical questions follow:

- In general, how well do you get along?
- In the past 2 weeks, how many arguments have you had? Pick a recent argument. Give me a "blow by blow" description of what happened.
- What topics do you disagree about? How much anger is involved in each of these disagreements?
- What gets you mad about the way your parent/child talks/communicates with you?
- When you have a disagreement about something such as chores, curfew, or homework, how do you work it out?
- *(To parents)* If you give your teenager more freedom, what do you think will happen? How much obedience do you expect from your teenager?
- *(To teenager)* How unfair are your parents' rules compared with the rules at your friends' houses? How much freedom should someone your age be given?

While conducting this inquiry, the practitioner should be alert for any negative communication patterns (Table 81-1). The interchange should be interrupted if an argument breaks out or if clear-cut instances of negative communication occur. The practitioner needs to label the negative behaviors, inquire about their impact on the family members, and investigate the extent to which similar responses occur at home. To maintain rapport with both the parents and the adolescent, the practitioner must resist the temptation to take sides with one or the other and remain a neutral mediator available to all.

On the basis of the interview and the self-report questionnaires, the practitioner can decide on the overall level of negative communication, specific negative communication patterns, and unreasonable beliefs and plan an appropriate course of intervention.

INTERVENTION

The practitioner can promote positive communication between parents and adolescents by (1) teaching positive communication skills during office visits, (2) encouraging home practice of problem-solving skills learned during an office visit, and (3) giving anticipatory guidance concerning possible communication problems before their actual occurrence.

Teaching Communication Skills

If assessment reveals that a family is experiencing significant parent-adolescent conflict and engaging in many negative communication skills, a short-term skill-oriented intervention may be very helpful. The average family beginning to experience unpleasant conflict with a young adolescent needs four to six 1-hour training sessions to acquire basic positive communication and problem-solving skills. The expert in adolescent health care can undertake such training and would need to refer to a mental health specialist only in complicated cases.

First, the practitioner conducts a didactic review of the communication assessment shown in Table 81-1 to increase the family's awareness of specific negative communication patterns. Family members are asked to indicate how often each negative response occurred within the past few days.

Second, the practitioner teaches the family general guidelines for having a positive conversation: (1) be a good listener by looking at the speaker, waiting for a good time to respond, and indicating understanding even when you disagree; (2) make your own points in concise, nonaccusatory language, being specific and constructive; and (3) take turns at speaking and listening without interruptions.

Third, the practitioner instructs the family in ways to correct the specific negative communication habits identified during the didactic review. For example, consider a mother who lectures her son in an accusatory, critical manner: "You should really stop being irresponsible about your pigsty of a room. You are old enough to clean it up without my nagging. Who's going to hire a slob anyway? And what wife would put up with a slob for a husband?" The practitioner might discuss with the mother the negative impact of her communication, suggesting a more positive alternative: "I am very upset about the big mess in your room. I want to help you find a way to keep it clean without my nagging. I'm worried about your future because you are not learning to take care of your things."

The family members then would be required to rehearse the positive communication skills in the office. They might be asked to conduct a brief conversation about the day's events, and the practitioner would point out instances of negative communication. Each negative response would be corrected through feedback, instructions, demonstrations of more positive responses, and requests to rehearse the positive responses.

Encouraging Problem-Solving Skills

After one or two training sessions devoted to communication, the practitioner might begin to teach problem-solving skills. As a general introduction, the practitioner should point out that (1) adolescence is a time for children to grow up, become independent, and learn to make their own decisions; (2) parents inevitably will lose power if they simply try to dictate to adolescents; and (3) therefore, whenever possible, disagreements should be resolved through mutual problem solving that involves input from the adolescent. Outlines of problem-solving steps (Box

81-1) can be distributed. The practitioner then serves as a mediator, guiding the family to discuss a problem using the problem-solving steps. Each step is explained to the family; each family member is given a chance to perform the step, with coaching and feedback from the practitioner, who functions as a stage director in a play.

Normally, a topic of mild to moderate intensity is appropriate for this first problem-solving discussion. It is important for the practitioner to maintain neutrality, not siding with any one family member, and to keep the family on task, interrupting when irrelevant comments are made and redirecting the family members to the steps of problem solving. By the end of 30 to 40 minutes, the family can usually reach an agreement to implement a particular solution. The practitioner sends them home to do so and has them report back at the next session. If the family members verify that the solution worked, a new problem is discussed. If not, the original problem is renegotiated. Family members also are encouraged to practice problem-solving and communication skills at home. The practitioner can ask the family to schedule a regular meeting time to practice the steps of problem solving or new communication skills. Specific "homework" assignments often are given, with instructions to audiotape the discussions for review by the practitioner.

Anticipatory Guidance and Effectiveness

Many of the points discussed in this chapter about positive communication skills, mutual problem solving, and reasonable expectations can be converted into anticipatory guidance rather than being reserved for use during a crisis. When parents bring their preadolescent for routine medical check-ups, the practitioner should prepare them for the onset of puberty by emphasizing the following points:

1. A certain amount of rebelliousness and moodiness is normal and most prevalent during the first year after the onset of puberty.
2. Adolescents cannot establish their own identity without some overt rejection of parental values and beliefs.
3. Mothers are more likely than fathers to be the targets of early adolescent rebellion.
4. Overreacting to the first signs of rebellion by becoming more restrictive is inappropriate; instead, parents need to move slowly toward a democratic approach to problem solving as children enter adolescence.
5. Maintenance of open, positive parent-child communication is very important.

During medical office visits with 12- to 14-year-old adolescents, the practitioner should distribute handouts, such as those presented in Table 81-1 and Box 81-1, and

---

BOX 81-1
Problem-Solving Outline for Families

I. Define the problem
   A. Tell the others what they do that bothers you and why
   B. Start your definitions with an "I"; be short, clear, and don't accuse
   C. Ask the other to paraphrase your definition to see whether you got your point across
   D. If they understood you, go on; if not, repeat your definition

II. Generate a variety of alternative solutions
   A. Take turns listing solutions
   B. Follow three rules:
      1. List as many ideas as possible
      2. Don't evaluate ideas
      3. Be creative; anything goes
   C. One person writes down ideas to keep track of them

III. Evaluate the ideas and decide upon the best one
   A. Take turns saying whether you like each idea and what would happen if you followed it
   B. Vote "Yes" or "No" for each idea and record your vote in writing next to the idea
   C. Look for ideas voted "Yes" by everyone
   D. Select one of these ideas or combine several
   E. If none were voted "Yes" by everyone, negotiate a compromise
      1. Select an idea voted "Yes" by one parent and the adolescent
      2. List as many possible compromises as you can
      3. Evaluate the compromises as you did the original ideas
      4. Try to reach an agreement

IV. Plan to implement the selected solution
   A. Decide who will do what, where, how, and when
   B. Decide who will monitor compliance with the solution
   C. Decide upon the consequences for compliance or noncompliance
      1. Penalties for noncompliance
      2. Rewards for compliance

---

give brief advice about how to identify and correct negative communication and ineffective problem solving. Requests to comment on specific issues such as curfew, chores, and homework might be handled by helping the family understand how the adolescent's striving toward independence underlies the specific disagreements, and by explaining that they need to learn the process of mutual problem solving to find the solutions that will best meet their needs. The practitioner cannot give the family the best solutions but can help them learn the problem-solving process.

The effectiveness of problem-solving communication training interventions for reducing parent-adolescent conflict has been demonstrated in a series of outcome studies comparing it with no-treatment controls and alternative forms of treatment.[3] This research indicates that such interventions help reduce parent-teenager conflict in up to 75% of the families with mild to moderately severe problems. Such interventions also have been tested and found to be effective for reducing family conflict in adolescents with attention deficit hyperactivity disorders[4] and eating disorders.[5]

CONCLUSION

The practitioner who understands that parents and teenagers need knowledge and skills to negotiate the process of adolescent individuation can be extremely helpful to patients through both anticipatory guidance and intervention. Skill training in family communication and problem solving can be done within a primary care pediatric and/or adolescent medicine setting. Cognitive restructuring of unreasonable attitudes and beliefs is more difficult to achieve without specialized psychologic training and often may require referral to a specialist. Practitioners who wish to conduct the type of family interventions outlined here might sharpen their skills by attending workshops or by reading selected references.[3] Such workshops are typically sponsored by organizations such as the Association for the Advancement of Behavior Therapy, the Society for Adolescent Medicine, and the Society for Developmental and Behavioral Pediatrics.*

References

1. Vincent-Roehling P, Robin AL: Development and validation of the Family Beliefs Inventory: a measure of unrealistic beliefs among parents and adolescents, *J Consult Clin Psychol* 54:693-697, 1986.
2. Schubiner H, Robin AL: Screening adolescents for depression and parent-teenager conflict in an ambulatory medical setting: a preliminary investigation, *Pediatrics* 85:813-818, 1985.
3. Robin AL, Foster SL: *Negotiating parent-adolescent conflict: a behavioral family systems approach,* New York, 1989, Guilford Press.
4. Robin AL: Guiding the adolescent with ADHD, New York, 1997, Guilford Press.
5. Robin AL, Siegel PT, Moye A: Family versus individual therapy for anorexia: impact on family conflict, *Int J Eat Disord* 17:313-322, 1995.

*Association for the Advancement of Behavior Therapy, 15 West 36th St., New York, NY 10018.
Society for Adolescent Medicine, 1916 NW Copper Oaks Circle, Blue Springs, MO 64015-8300.
Society for Developmental and Behavioral Pediatrics, 19 Station Lane, Philadelphia, PA 19118-2939.

CHAPTER 82

Anticipatory Guidance for Parents

•

Morris Green

In a time of physical, biologic, psychologic, cognitive, and social transition, the goals of anticipatory guidance for parents of preadolescents may be viewed as prospective adaptation to and mastery of these pervasive changes. Anticipatory guidance is an effort to make parents aware of and prepared for the developmental changes—physical, social, psychologic, and behavioral—that lie ahead. The desired outcome is a healthy, well-functioning young adult and a happy family. Although helping children, adolescents, and families adapt and cope has been a traditional part of clinical practice, enhancement of their adaptation to the various stressors of today's society is a more recent development.

In an overly simplistic manner, adolescence has often been viewed as either a highly problematic period or a time of robust health. Although these perceptions may apply to some individuals, most adolescents demonstrate a spectrum of strengths, potentialities, vulnerabilities, and problems.

The rapidity of recent social changes and the current causes of adolescent morbidity and mortality mandate increased attention by the primary care physician to prospective parental adaptation before the teenage years. Many parents welcome such anticipatory advice, particularly when the approach is a constructive and optimistic one that values the continuing contribution of the parents.

Although it is useful for the primary care physician to meet with the parents of a preadolescent alone, parent group sessions offer special advantages. Such meetings not only save time but also facilitate a broad range of questions and a sharing of concerns, and foster a resolve to strengthen community resources. Handouts and a reading list also may be distributed at these meetings. In addition, these occasions may be used to advise the parents of the physician's approach of seeing the adolescent alone, without a parent always present. If the parents are willing to pay for such visits without violating their youngster's wish and right to confidentiality, the physician and parents may work out an arrangement in which the physician will see the youngster at his or her own request.

Mastery of the changes and transitions of adolescence is greatly enhanced by growth-promoting strengths in the family, the child, and the community (including the school). When such strengths are present in abundance, identified vulnerabilities or risks are contained, and problems such as a chronic illness or disability are appropriately managed. In such circumstances the adolescent can be expected to do very well. Anticipatory guidance that is sufficiently detailed to achieve optimal effectiveness requires a careful assessment of strengths and vulnerabilities of child and family, as well as problems. This can be done most efficiently with a computerized screening instrument if such is available. A highly developed computer program can permit the printout of an individual health plan for each preadolescent and family. Such a document provides reinforcement of strengths and offers suggestions for appropriate interventions.

GOALS FOR PROSPECTIVE ADAPTATION

Each set of parents needs to identify their personal goals for their preadolescent; become knowledgeable about the developmental characteristics, potential problems, and strengths of adolescents; have the opportunity to discuss their personal concerns with the primary care physician; and approach the adolescent years with a sense of confidence and efficacy.

The goals that parents envision differ from family to family, depending on cultural heritage, socioeconomic status, educational background, and personal histories. However, certain developmental targets for the adolescent are shared by most parents. These include the establishment of a developmentally appropriate level of independence and autonomy; attainment of self-responsibility for health, schoolwork, and decisions;

development of a clear identity and high self-esteem; acquisition of good health behaviors; avoidance of habits that are self-injurious; ability to deal with peer pressures; achievement of comfortable relationships with peers of both sexes; and mastery of the developmental, social, psychologic, educational, and vocational challenges of adolescence.

KNOWING WHAT TO EXPECT

An awareness of the range of normal adolescent behaviors is an important aspect of anticipatory guidance for adolescence. Typical factors include the extensive influence of peers, who largely set the behavioral standards; a change in communication patterns between the adolescent and the parents; the occurrence of sudden challenges to parental authority; conflicts over issues of indepen-dence; an unwillingness to participate in some family activities; moodiness; risk-taking behaviors; and sexuality.

Although communication is a complex issue during adolescence (see Chapter 81, "Communication between Parent and Adolescent"), some common myths should be refuted as part of anticipatory guidance. These include the popular beliefs that parents communicate better with the adolescent than is actually the case; that the adolescent actually hears and understands what the parents are saying; that adolescents are not hesitant to ask questions; and that adolescents know what parents are thinking, feeling, or expecting without being told explicitly.

BEHAVIORS THAT MERIT CONCERN

Although the range of normal adolescent behavior is very wide, parents should be advised that certain

---

BOX 82-1
Strengths of Parents

Maintenance of comfortable communication with the adolescent, with channels kept open but periods of poor communication and transient estrangement anticipated

Respect for adolescent's privacy: bedroom, telephone, mail

Establishment of fair rules, based on reasonable and realistic expectations, to be followed at home, with minor episodes of noncompliance anticipated

Establishment of reasonable consequences if these expectations are not met

Provision of ethical and behavioral role models

Maintenance of an unconditional positive regard for and trust in the adolescent

Encouragement, praise, and support for the adolescent's evolving independence and friendships, activities, and achievements

Presence at athletic events, musical recitals, theatrical performances, and other public activities in which the adolescent participates

Spending time with the adolescent

Showing affection for the adolescent

Provision of adult supervision when the parents are not at home

Avoidance of laughing at the adolescent's frustrations or trivializing his or her worries

Avoidance of seeming to be indifferent, overly critical, nagging, distant, or derogatory

Being available at times of failure and excessive stress

Appreciation of the importance of family warmth, cohesion, support, communication, and mutuality in the life of the adolescent

---

BOX 82-2
Strengths of Adolescent

Positive role models

Good health habits

Physical fitness, endurance, and vigor

Self-confidence, sense of pride in accomplishments, strong sense of personal competence

Self-responsibility for health and schoolwork

Supportive social network, ability to mobilize social support

Social skills and one or more close friends

Ability to ask for help with comfort

Ability to enjoy life

Ability to express feelings

Close interaction with peers of both sexes

Ability to form trusting relationships

Sense of belonging to a valued group

Ability to persist in achieving goals

High self-esteem, constructive assessment of personal capacities

Achievements, successes, special interests or talents

Recognition of efforts and achievements by parents and other significant persons

Opportunities for mastery of new challenges; access to educational, vocational, and social opportunities

Expectation of personal success

Belief that he or she knows what to do and can do it

Set of moral and ethical values

behaviors warrant a call or visit to the physician. These include indications of low self-esteem, a decline in school performance, poor social skills and lack of close friends, antisocial behaviors, unusual anxiety, and depressive behavior.

STRENGTHS OF PARENTS AND PREADOLESCENT

The content of anticipatory guidance should underline the crucial role of protective factors within the family and the strengths of the preadolescent in ensuring an adaptive rather than a maladaptive outcome to adolescence. Box 82-1 shows a list of strengths of the parents or family that provide an optimal environment for growth, development, and mastery. Box 82-2 offers a similar list of strengths of the preadolescent or adolescent. These checklists afford opportunities for self-assessment and family assessment with the dual goal of maintaining current strengths and identifying targets for further development (perhaps in consultation with the physician). Likewise, an assessment of vulnerabilities, such as those listed in Box 82-3, helps to ensure that appropriate preventive strategies or therapeutic interventions are used.

Anticipatory guidance that builds on present and potential strengths offers parents a prospectus of the adolescent years based on a positive rather than a deficit model—one to which parents can make major contributions.

BOX 82-3
Vulnerabilities of Adolescent

Lack of social skills, friendships, and good peer relationships
Lack of a sense of self-efficacy
Multiple or cluster of stressors, especially losses or discontinuities
Feeling that one's potential cannot be fulfilled
View of the world as unpredictable
Lack of social support, social isolation
Low socioeconomic status, poverty
Absence of a feeling of being loved and valued by parents
Long-term illness or handicap
Childhood depression
Low self-esteem
Learned helplessness
Belief that nothing he or she does matters
Family discord and violence
Lack of communication within family
Parental psychiatric illness
Attendance at substandard schools

Suggested Readings

Elster AR, Kuznets NJ: *American Medical Association guidelines for adolescent preventive services (GAPS): recommendations and rationale,* Baltimore, 1994, Williams & Wilkins.

Green M, editor: *Bright futures: guidelines for health supervision of infants, children, and adolescents,* Arlington, VA, 1994, National Center for Education in Maternal and Child Health.

CHAPTER 83

Allowances, Household Chores, and Curfews

•

Doris R. Pastore

Allowances, household chores, and curfews are often matters of conflict between parents and teenagers. Pediatricians have a unique opportunity to guide parents in the use of a developmental focus as they plan, execute, and enforce these aspects of home life.

ALLOWANCES

Many parents want their adolescent to be "financially mature" but do not know how to offer financial guidance. The idea of using the adolescent's allowance as an educational tool is not widely recognized by parents. However, the allowance is an ideal instrument for teaching skills of budgeting, purchasing, decision making, and goal setting, which are necessary for fiscal soundness.[1]

National surveys indicate that approximately half of all teenagers receive allowances, with the highest prevalence among junior high students.[1] White and minority students, in one study, were equally likely to have received allowances, although white students started receiving theirs earlier and had more in savings.[2]

Money—and the right to manage it—is a symbol of power and thus is central to the struggle for independence that occurs during adolescence.[3] The significance of allowances lies more in the characteristics of their arrangement as opposed to the actual receipt of money. It is not uncommon for parents to attempt to control their adolescent through the manipulation of money, for example, by dispersing funds for some items and not others.

Many households use the "envelope method" for their own budgeting, and this approach can be suggested to the teenager. Budget categories, such as "save," "clothes," "gifts," and "fun," can be set up for an adolescent to monitor his or her own cash flow. The exact amount an adolescent can or should spend per month is a matter of family and individual priorities and objectives. In general, an allowance should be consistent with the overall life style of the family. The 1994 Rand Youth Poll indicated monthly income and expenditures for teenagers surveyed. Teenagers aged 13 to 15 reported an average weekly allowance of $16.70 with additional earnings of $16.20 for males, and a weekly allowance of $20.10 with additional earnings of $18.80 for females. Teenagers aged 16 to 19 reported a weekly allowance of $30.75 plus earnings of $46.45 for males, and an allowance of $33.75 with earnings of $51.55 for females.[4] Types of expenditures traditionally differ by age and sex; females spend more on clothing and personal grooming, and older teenagers spend more on auto and entertainment costs. However, contrary to the gender differences noted in the Rand Youth Poll, another study found no such gender difference as reported by students.[5]

Some financial advisors who are familiar with household money management suggest that by the early teenage years allowances be given monthly, rather than weekly, to encourage the adolescent to take responsibility for the money.[1] This also allows the adolescent the freedom of decision making as well as the freedom to fail in budgeting.

Parents need to acknowledge that all family members have financial needs, and that therefore teenagers should receive allowances because they are a part of the family. Parents also need to recognize that all family members should assume a portion of the responsibility for living in the household by having chores to perform. These two factors should be completely independent of each other. Chores may be divided into two categories: expected and optional. The understanding could be established that performing optional chores would entitle the adolescent to additional monetary compensation.

An allowance should have an explicit and firm basis. It should not be based on the performance of chores, withheld for disciplinary reasons, or used to influence behavior. The amount should not constantly vary once it has been agreed on and set. This firm structure allows the adolescent a sense of ownership and fosters positive motivation for independent money management. Teenager-directed goal setting (for example, saving money to buy a car) teaches the value of both long- and short-term goals, an important aspect of economic maturity. It is also useful for adolescents to learn the mechanics of balancing and maintaining a checkbook before moving away from home. Only 17% of teens have checking accounts, and most of these are 18- to 19-year-olds often preparing for college life. Planning for college provides a convenient opportunity for parents to review budgeting, saving, and investing.[2]

Although some teenagers may appear to be sophisticated in the area of finance, many make the mistake of viewing credit cards as another form of currency and do not understand that these are more correctly likened to a loan. Some financial advisors recommend only the use of secured credit cards where teenagers may make deposits into a savings account and then charge up to the amount in that account.[2]

Parents often cannot remember to give the allowance on time, which can be a source of continual frustration to the teenager and the family. To avoid this problem, parents should view this transaction as being as important as any other bill and choose a particular day of the month that this "bill" is due.

Adolescents often report getting far less allowance than their peers. If this situation is found to be true, a reevaluation of the budget may be in order. In some families, no limits are set on spending and adolescents may be allowed access to unlimited credit card use. In such cases the issue is one not only of money but of different family values.

Parents may have difficulty in accepting the spending choices that their adolescents make. However, it is important for parents to realize that choices that are different are not inherently wrong. In fact, it would be surprising if parents and adolescents—individuals from two such different age groups—spent their money in similar ways. In addition, there is the need to tolerate, along with their teenager, the consequences that may follow. Most important, parental love should not be conditionally based on the adolescent choosing the parent-approved options.

HOUSEHOLD CHORES

A common complaint of parents, and a source of great tension, is that their adolescent does not act responsibly about household chores. A study by Cogle and Tasker reported that 88% of children aged 6 to 17 years perform at least one chore, and that time spent on chores averages 3.5 hours per week.[6] Parents tend to believe that an adolescent who fails to complete assigned chores will be unable to meet life's responsibilities, particularly in the business world. Such parental concern frequently be-

comes more intense as the teenager approaches the senior year of high school. This is a time when society expects greater responsibility of the adolescent, whether the individual plans to enter college or the workforce.

It is helpful to divide household chores for the adolescent into two categories: (1) those that reflect the distribution of responsibility among everyone living within the home and (2) those that are optional for the teenager and result in cash compensation. Motivation based on guilt or pure bribery may get the job done, but it never teaches a true sense of responsibility.

The pediatrician can be helpful in explaining to parents the context within which the adolescent is functioning. When younger, the child may have taken great pleasure in completing household chores. However, as an adolescent, the individual is now concerned, even preoccupied, with new social interactions. Every new social experience consumes the adolescent, requiring serious planning and thought. As is developmentally appropriate, the adolescent's view of the "future" may extend only to next Saturday night. Therefore, household chores assume a low priority and may be repeatedly forgotten, much to the dismay of the parents. Further, compliance with parental demands interferes with the very autonomy and independence the teenager is seeking. Thus, chores may become the battlefield for parents and teenagers in their attempt to define a new parent-child relationship.

It is often desirable to set a contractual type of agreement for chores.[7] The pediatrician is in a position to mediate such an agreement, which ideally involves the adolescent and both parents. The "contract," which should be stated explicitly or put in written form, lists the teenager's household responsibilities and the consequences of not fulfilling them. The consequences, which need to be reasonable and enforceable, should be applied automatically if chores are not done as agreed. The responsibilities of the parents are (1) not to nag and (2) not to add chores that were not part of the original agreement. The pediatrician should follow up on such a mediated contract in 2 to 4 weeks to assess the successes and failures of the contract and the possibility to negotiate changes.

Studies show that older female adolescents who usually were assigned tasks within the home and involved family needs had a greater sense of motivation than male adolescents who were assigned tasks outside the home and were often isolating.[8] A study of 152 single and dual income families indicated that adolescent males had highest scores on perceived competence when their parents, especially the fathers, had positive attitudes about males performing "traditional" female chores such as cooking and cleaning dishes.[9]

The adolescent, when treated as a responsible and reasonable person, is more apt to act like one. If parents take the first step toward reasonable interaction, they communicate an understanding of the adolescent's age of development and become role models for the teenager's behavior. If parents constantly nag their teenager about a chore that they themselves will eventually complete, no behavior change should be expected. Last, parents should choose those areas of household responsibility that are of most concern to them and ignore issues that are relatively inconsequential.

CURFEWS

Another aspect of family life that often becomes an area of parent-teenager conflict is the setting of curfews. At adolescence, parents commonly are confronted with a teenager who expects adult-level autonomy. The goal of parenting thus changes from protecting the child to helping the teenager achieve independence without undue risk. Ideally, parents should take pride in their adolescent's increasing autonomy, but if they expect their teenager to need continual direct supervision, however subtle this expectation may be, such an attitude may become a self-fulfilling prophecy. When parents set rules and values, they give teenagers a framework to establish their own values.[10]

With adolescents, it is especially important to incorporate a democratic process in setting up family rules. The parent who tyrannically wins every single battle risks losing the war.[8] The goal is for both the parents and the adolescent to discuss guidelines for weeknight and weekend curfews and then negotiate an agreement. Discussion that excludes the adolescent should be discouraged. In fact, watching parents resolve their differences by compromise is a useful process for the teenager. Parents often have difficulty realizing that their child is growing up, and they may be quite pleased to discover that their offspring can be a reasonable young adult. Ultimately, however, the parents' wishes must prevail, especially for the younger adolescent, but it is better for the outcome to be influenced by the adolescent's arguments and desires. In one study of the relationship of drug use to involvement in home life and other activities, teenagers with later or no weekend and weeknight curfews reported greater drug use.[11]

If adolescents realize that they will not be able to meet a curfew, a telephone call home is sufficient and acceptable to most parents. However, the consequences of infractions should be known to the adolescent ahead of time, and the "punishment should fit the crime." For example, confinement to home for one weekend night might be appropriate punishment for staying out 2 hours past curfew. However, "grounding" the adolescent for 1 month in a moment of anger amounts to overkill, and parents typically relent on such harsh punishments, making future consequences more a threat than a reality.

ROLE OF THE PEDIATRICIAN

During adolescence the pediatrician, as an objective outside observer, has the opportunity to facilitate the establishment of intrafamily communication techniques. Problem solving that involves effective communication should include the following steps: (1) defining the problem, (2) "brainstorming" to create a variety of solutions, (3) evaluating the impact of solutions on both parents and adolescents, (4) negotiating a compromise beginning with the alternative that appealed to both parties, (5) planning implementation steps, and (6) reviewing the effect of the solution (see Chapter 81, "Communication Between Parent and Adolescent"). A study of 139 adolescents and the influence of parenting style indicated that authoritative parents who were highly demanding of *and* highly responsive to their teenager were remarkably successful in generating competence and deterring problem behavior at all developmental stages.[12] In this study, authoritarian (demanding but *not* responsive), permissive, and rejecting-neglecting parenting styles were unable to foster the secure attachments of adolescents to their parents that would enable teenagers to pursue personal emancipation and individuation simultaneously, and to assert the social values they share with their parents.

Parents may have unspoken fears that are projected onto their adolescent and are manifested as conflicts over allowances, household chores, and curfews. Curfews and other restrictions, such as use of the family car, may be justified as necessary to allow time for homework. Although the need for homework time represents a good reason for the restriction, the real reason typically is to limit exposure to drugs and sex. The pediatrician may significantly improve parent-teenager communication when conflicts arise by bringing the real issues out for discussion, frequently allaying parental fears and thereby promoting adolescent autonomy. Parents often have misconceptions about teenage behavior in general and unwarranted fears about their own teenager. Thus, the pediatrician may have a dual role: education and family counseling.

References

1. Blue R: *Money matters for parents and their kids,* Nashville, TN, 1988, Thomas Nelson.
2. Bodnar J: *Kiplinger's money-smart kids,* Washington, DC, 1993, Kiplinger Books.
3. Miller J, Yung S: The role of allowances in adolescent socialization, *Youth Society* 22:137-159, 1990.
4. *Rand Youth Poll* (news release), New York, 1994, Youth Research Institute.
5. Peters J: Gender socialization of adolescents in the home: research and discussion, *Adolescence* 29:913-934, 1994.
6. Cogle FL, Tasker GE: Children and housework, *Family Relat* 21:395-399, 1982.

7. Bauman L, Riche R: *The nine most troublesome teenage problems and how to solve them,* New York, 1986, Ballantine Books.

8. Duckett E, Raffaelli M, Richards M: "Taking care": maintaining the self and the home in early adolescence, *J Youth Adolesc* 18:549-565, 1989.

9. Crouter AC, McHale S, Bartko WT: Gender as an organizing feature in parent-child relationships, *J Soc Issues* 49:161-174, 1993.

10. Elkind D: *Parenting your teenager,* New York, 1993, First Ballantine Books.

11. Buckhalt J, Halpin G, Noel R, Meadows M: Relationship of drug use to involvement in school, home, and community activities: results of a large survey of adolescents, *Psychol Rep* 70:139-146, 1992.

12. Baumrind D: The influence of parenting style on adolescent competence and substance use, *J Early Adolesc* 11:56-95, 1991.

CHAPTER 84

Divorce

•

Robert E. Emery

Divorce rates increased dramatically from the 1960s into the early 1980s, but since that time divorce rates have stabilized—at a very high level. The commonly cited statistic about divorce is accurate: approximately half of all children born to married parents will experience their parents' divorce. However, this statistic masks some important influences on children's family living circumstances and the prevalence of divorce, including the frequency of nonmarital childbirth, ethnic differences, remarriage and the influence of marital history on the likelihood of divorce, and the differing rates of divorce experienced by children according to their age and sex.

The number of children born to unmarried parents has increased together with divorce rates over recent decades, but unlike divorce, nonmarital childbirth is still rising, particularly among whites. Currently, about one quarter of American children are born outside of marriage. Teenage childbirth contributes significantly to birth out of wedlock, but an increasing number of adult couples are cohabiting not only before marriage but also after they have a child or children together. Many cohabiting couples eventually marry, but divorce rates are higher, not lower, among couples who cohabited before marriage.[1]

Both divorce and especially nonmarital childbirth are more common among African-Americans than in other major American ethnic groups. Over 60% of black children currently are born outside of marriage in contrast to about 20% of white children. Of those children born to married parents, 40% of whites will experience a divorce, as will nearly three quarters of African-American chil-

dren. Statistics for Latino and Asian children are less certain than for blacks and whites, in part because large numbers of Latinos and Asians have immigrated to the United States only in recent years. Nevertheless, estimates consistently indicate that divorce and nonmarital childbirth rates are higher among Latinos than among white Americans, but lower among Latinos than among African-Americans. Asian-Americans have the lowest rates of divorce and childbirth outside of marriage.

Many children experience the remarriage of one or both of their parents after divorce. Currently, nearly 15% of children live with a stepparent and one biologic parent, more commonly the mother, and an unknown but significant number of children live with a divorced or never married biologic parent and the parent's cohabiting partner. Contrary to some impressions, remarriage does not recreate the two-parent family but is a second transition that presents new and often difficult challenges for children. Second marriages also are more likely to lead to divorce than are first marriages, as about 60% of remarriages end in divorce. As a result, many children experience not one but two or more divorces during their childhood. In fact, a second divorce is more likely if one of the partners brings children to the marriage.

Fewer couples today stay together "for the children's sake" and about 60% of all divorces involve children. Still, the presence of children does influence the likelihood of divorce. As noted, a remarriage is more likely to end in divorce when there already are children. In other circumstances, children serve as something of a deterrent to divorce, at least when they are of preschool age. Controlling for the length of marriage, parents with preschoolers are about half as likely to divorce as are childless couples, while the likelihood of divorce is nearly equal for childless couples and couples with school-aged children. Because most divorces occur early in marriage, however, young children are considerably more likely to experience a parental divorce than are older children. About half of all children who experience divorce are aged 5 years or younger when their parents separate.[2] Finally, it is of some interest to note that divorce is slightly less likely in families with a boy than in those with all girls.

SHOULD PARENTS STAY TOGETHER FOR THE CHILDREN'S SAKE?

There is no doubt that, on average, divorce creates substantial emotional and practical challenges for children. The potential problems caused by divorce include not only mental health concerns but also many practical problems. For example, financial pressures can mean that children may have to move out of their primary family residence; change schools; lose contact with familiar peers; or cope with increased parental employment, increased time in childcare, more time alone at home, and their parents' worrying and arguing about money. Children are better off in a happy, well-functioning two-parent family than in a divorced family. Unfortunately, many marriages are unhappy and many families are not well functioning. Thus, parents frequently are faced with the choice of divorce as opposed to staying together "for the children's sake."

Whether parents should stay together is a question that individual pediatricians cannot answer in their clinical practices. Different pediatricians surely have different values, religious beliefs, and personal experiences in regard to marriage, divorce, and childrearing, and some may choose to identify and share their personal positions. Nevertheless, the question of whether to stay together ultimately must be addressed by each unhappily married adult. Pediatricians can empathize with the struggles divorce poses for parents, however, and can provide parents with information that bears on their personal decision.

Perhaps the foremost advice a pediatrician can offer is an objection to the very question of whether parents should stay together—or divorce—for the children's sake. This question places an inappropriate and unfair burden for adult decisions onto a child or children. For example, the author has worked with a number of young people whose parents stayed together for their sake, and then announced their sacrifice and their intention to divorce shortly after a high school or college graduation.

The parents apparently took pride in their fortitude but failed to understand that their children still were distressed by the divorce, even as young adults, and now the young people also felt responsible for their parents' unspoken misery during marriage. The point of the example, and the reason to reject the "children's sake" question, is that adults need to accept responsibility for their own choices about their marriage or divorce rather than shifting the burden onto the children, even if only by implication.

CONSEQUENCES OF DIVORCE FOR CHILDREN

Of course, parents who are considering divorce legitimately want information about the potential consequences of divorce for their children, and the pediatrician also can be of help here. Although the massive popular literature on divorce invariably highlights its negative emotional consequences for children, the weight of research indicates that most children successfully cope with divorce.[3] Extensive research indicates that, in the long run, most children from divorced families function no less well than do children whose parents are married in terms of their emotional adjustment. Given the number of emotional, relationship, and practical stressors that accompany divorce, the evidence of children's eventual, positive adjustment to divorce is testimony to the resilience of children in overcoming adversity.[4]

The resilience perspective offers an optimistic and scientifically accurate perspective on children's long-term emotional adjustment to divorce, but this characterization of research evidence must be tempered by several cautions. Children are resilient but not invulnerable. Successful coping is the most common long-term outcome for children, but in the short term most children, including most adolescents, are very distressed by divorce. Coping with divorce can involve an extended process of adjustment, one that may be akin to grief for many parents and at least some adolescents. Unlike bereavement, however, the process of grieving over a divorce is complicated by family changes that continue to unfold after a marital separation or legal divorce. Central complications include the ongoing possibility of reconciliation, continued parental conflict, custody battles, changes in children's living arrangements, lost contact with one parent, remarriage, and relocation.

Divorce and the Adolescent

Teenagers may express their distress with the upheaval of divorce by becoming sad, angry, embarrassed, or frightened for their parents and themselves. Some adolescents turn away from one or both of their parents and seek refuge in relationships with peers, or perhaps with a teacher or a friend's parents. Other teenagers are drawn into what may seem to be a very close relationship with one parent, who treats the adolescent like a peer or confidant.

A parental divorce also can challenge adolescents' views of themselves and their relationships. Some of the identity issues that the adolescent faces are relatively minor, such as feeling embarrassed or stigmatized by the divorce or coming to terms with what it means to be a "child of divorce." Some concerns are more profound or lasting, however, such as worries about one's own ability to love and to maintain a romance.

Concerns about their own ongoing or future love relationships are common among children from divorced families, and the risk of divorce increases 25% to 50% among adults whose own parents divorced. There are practical explanations for the increased risk, however, such as the greater acceptance of divorce as a solution to an unhappy marriage. In fact, many normal worries about relationships are compounded unnecessarily by the perceived stigma of divorce. There is a tendency among teenagers and parents to interpret everything they do through the filter of divorce.

The pediatrician can help parents and adolescents by "normalizing" the process of adjustment to divorce, that is, by pointing out that the teenager's negative reactions are expected, normal, and probably adaptive in the long run. When children show distress in the days, weeks, and months following a marital separation, parents should not rush them to "health" by attempting to allay every emotion, and probably should not rush them to a psychotherapist either. At the opposite extreme, emotionally overwhelmed parents must offer their teenagers some support and some space for experiencing and expressing their distress. Parents may have to ask an adolescent to assume more practical chores around the house. However, teenagers should not be put in the role of becoming a substitute spouse, friend, or therapist who puts the needs of a distraught parent before his or her own developmentally appropriate needs and reactions. Shortly after a marital separation, the goals for parents are to allow their children some time to adjust to the situation, while working toward establishing supportive, clear, and consistent relationships in the postdivorce family—relationships that are as similar as possible to predivorce family relationships. The goals for teenagers are to recognize and express their feelings (to some one, not necessarily to a therapist or to a pediatrician), to offer a reasonable degree of help to other family members, and (most of all) to be a teenager—to continue to have fun with friends, to work hard in school, and to gain independence responsibly. Divorce clearly entails many difficult changes in emotions, relationships, living circumstances, and family economics. Despite the distress,

however, teenagers survive divorce, and most thrive in a family that is different but a family nevertheless.

The Disturbed Adolescent and Predictors of Risk

Although most children eventually bounce back from the many stressors posed by divorce, it also is true that a significant number do not cope successfully with divorce in either the short or long run. Children from divorced families are two to three times as likely to be referred to mental health professionals as children whose parents are married.[5] Divorce also is associated with a number of emotional problems among children and adolescents, including disruptive behavior disorders, depression, lower academic achievement, school dropout, precocious sexuality, and eventually an increased likelihood that their own marriage will end in divorce.[2,6] These problems are found among only a minority of children from divorced families, but divorce is nevertheless a risk factor for emotional troubles among children.

Social science research has identified several factors that impede children's and adolescents' adjustment to divorce, as well as a number of conditions that apparently do not predict outcome. A child's age at the time of divorce has little relation to long-term outcome. There is no "right" or "wrong" age, including adolescence, for children to experience their parents' divorce. However, children of different ages clearly do require more or less elaborate explanations about the reasons for a divorce and are likely to demonstrate their emotional distress in a manner consistent with their age.

Boys and girls also may differ in how they express their negative feelings about divorce and its associated disruptions in family life. Boys tend to externalize emotions in response to stress, becoming angry, aggressive, and disobedient. On the other hand, girls often internalize their reactions to negative life events and become worried, sad, or overly responsible in caring for others. However, divorce is not easier or harder for either boys or girls, and gender differences in children's long-term adjustment to divorce appear to be minimal.

In general, the characteristics of children or adolescents predict little about risk or resilience in the face of divorce. What is much more important is the manner in which parents manage the divorce process and establish family relationships after divorce. In this regard, the pediatrician can tell parents that the consequences of divorce for their children depend largely on the parents' actions during and after the marital separation. Parents do not give up control over their children's development with the decision to divorce. Rather, their children's adjustment will depend on how well both parents are able to (1) minimize their own conflicts and avoid placing the children in the middle of their disputes, (2) continue to demonstrate warmth and affection to their children, (3) continue to monitor and discipline the children appropriately, (4) cope with and rebound from their own emotional struggles, (5) provide social and economic stability for their children, and (6) manage further family transitions, especially remarriage.

PARENTAL CONFLICT

One of the strongest predictors of risk for psychologic problems among children from divorced—and married—families is exposure to and involvement in conflict between their parents. In fact, evidence demonstrates that many of the psychologic problems found among children after divorce actually begin *before* the marital separation while they are living in the conflict-ridden two-parent family.[7] Thus, many of the emotional difficulties found in children appear to be consequences of parental conflict and related family dysfunction, not consequences of divorce itself.

The central role of conflict also has been highlighted by some provocative, but still tentative, evidence. A 1995 study found that children fared *better* after a divorce if their parents showed a high degree of conflict during marriage, yet fared *worse* after divorce if marital conflict was contained during marriage.[8] This study points to the destructive role of parental conflict inside marriage, and it indicates that divorce can be a relief from the stress of conflict. However, the evidence also implies that divorce may *not* be the better alternative when parents are able to accept their marital unhappiness and shield their feelings from the children.

Of course, one purpose of a marital separation is to end the conflict stemming from an unhappy marriage, but one of the ironies of divorce is that conflict between spouses who remain parents may not end once they separate. Unfortunately for children, parental conflict not only can become more intense after a marital separation, but also can become focused on the children who are the link between the former spouses. Thus, children too often are witnesses to their parents' angry fights, are told inappropriate details about the other parent's transgressions and shortcomings, are told to carry inappropriate messages back and forth between parents, are not allowed to bring personal items one parent bought for them to the other parent's household, are urged to take sides in parental disputes, or are the subject of protracted and venomous custody battles supposedly designed to serve the "child's best interests."[9]

Pediatricians can help divorced families by pointing out to parents that their conflicts have destructive effects on their children. The advice to contain conflict is more likely to be followed if it is given early in the divorce process before the disputes become entrenched or legal battles are waged. If possible, it is also best to offer advice to *both* parents in an even-handed manner. Such an approach may not only help to keep children out of the middle of parental disputes, but also help to prevent the pediatrician from becoming caught in the parents' crossfire. At this time, the pediatrician may also want to tell both parents about policies concerning each parent's access to medical records, obtaining parental consent, and similar matters.

At the same time that cooperation is encouraged, it is essential to be realistic and to acknowledge parents' painful feelings about divorce. Parents can be given permission to feel hurt and angry but still be urged to keep their children out of their disputes. To allow adolescents to have a relationship with the "other" parent, each parent needs to recognize that the child's perspective differs from his or her own. A father or a mother may be a horrible partner in the eyes of the former spouse, but that person remains a parent from the adolescent's perspective. In short, divorced parents must disentangle their ongoing roles as parents from their former roles as spouses.

When conflict is entrenched, a referral for therapy or mediation is in order. One or both feuding parents may benefit from individual psychotherapy, or they may benefit from seeing a skilled therapist together. If the disputes involve legal issues, the pediatrician should consider a referral to a divorce mediator, who will help parents to negotiate cooperatively outside the legal system. When there is no hope of alleviating the parents' fighting, referral of an adolescent for individual therapy may be appropriate, but the clinician should take great care not to label the teenager as the problem.

PARENT-CHILD RELATIONSHIPS

Research indicates that children's relationships with nonresidential, and especially residential, parents can be vital to their adjustment to divorce and to their continuing development. The quality of these parent-child relationships needs to be considered on two levels. The first involves the transition in parent-child relationships that all divorced families face. Children confront a transition not only in their parents' relationship but also in their own relationships with each of their parents. The second level concerns the quality of the new relationship that eventually is formed. Parent-child relationships may be better than, worse than, or just different from what existed before the divorce.

Residential Parents

Although some children live with their fathers (10% to 15%) and joint physical custody is not uncommon (perhaps 5% of divorced families), most children live primarily with their mothers after divorce. An important point of comparison—and contention—often raised about father- and mother-residence families is the relative adjustment of boys and girls. Some past research found that children who lived with their same-sex parents were better adjusted than children who lived with their opposite-sex parents. This conclusion has been strongly questioned by more recent evidence, however, as there appear to be few if any differences in the adjustment of children living with mothers or fathers regardless of the child's gender.

Residential parent-child relationships are frequently strained during the first years after the divorce. Parenting concerns focus on the general areas of affectional relationships, discipline, and household management. Residential mothers and fathers typically must leap different hurdles, with each having greater difficulties assuming the roles traditionally fulfilled by the opposite-sex partner. Thus, discipline is a more common problem for residential mothers, whereas affection and household management more frequently pose problems for residential fathers.

Researchers have found that the parenting of residential mothers is more negative, more inconsistent, and less affectionate than that of married mothers. Overloaded with their own emotional turmoil or with the tasks of managing children and finances alone, many single mothers simply have fewer resources to devote to parenting. For the adolescent whose parents have divorced recently, this may mean that he or she encounters less patience and more anger, less predictability, and less affection from a mother whose support previously may have been taken for granted. Adolescents whose parents have divorced recently also may find fewer or less consistent limits on their behavior. Ineffective discipline undermines appropriate parental control, and it also disrupts the sense of security that teenagers derive from parental limit setting.[5]

Teenagers whose parents were divorced many years earlier are likely to have completed the transition in their relationships with their residential parents. Discipline becomes more consistent as time passes after a divorce, but teenagers from divorced families still may have somewhat less strict rules than their peers. The same adolescents also may have more duties at home, perhaps including responsibilities for caring for younger siblings, because of the added demands of managing a single-parent household.

Nonresidential Parents

In contrast to residential parenting, the changes involved in children's relationships with their nonresidential parents are much more dramatic, both during the divorce transition and afterward. In fact, the small amount of contact between children and their nonresidential

fathers is startling. The amount of contact diminishes as time passes after a divorce, and it is complicated by changes such as remarriage or geographic relocation. According to a national study, over 25% of children from divorced families had not seen their fathers in a year, and less than 20% saw their fathers as often as once a week.[10] Other evidence indicates that nonresidential mothers maintain somewhat more frequent contact with children.

In the short term, both children and nonresidential parents must cope with the difficulties of defining a "visiting" relationship. These include adjusting to contact based on schedule, the tension or disruption of pickups and dropoffs, and learning to feel at home in a new residence. In the long run, research indicates that the interaction between visiting fathers and their children is often more social than parental in nature. Nonresidential fathers who infrequently see their children emphasize "fun" and have laxer rules and lower expectations for their children's conduct than do married fathers. When contact is rare, children have to cope with the sense of rejection, or unrealistically positive fantasies, felt toward a parent they hardly know.

Unlike residential parent-child relationships, children's relationships with their nonresidential parents have *not* been strongly linked to difficulties or enhancements in their psychologic functioning. Nevertheless, children often regard nonresidential parents as important figures in their life, even when relationships are distant. Moreover, interest in nonresidential parents may increase during adolescence, and some teenagers wish to change residence as a result. In addition, older adolescents often want to explore or rekindle lost relationships with their nonresidential parents, particularly as they grapple with issues of autonomy and identity.

Joint Custody

Some parents and professionals continue to be confused about the meaning of joint custody. In *joint legal custody,* legal authority for the children is shared, but the children spend considerably more time living with one parent. In *joint physical custody,* children spend approximately equal amounts of time with each parent. Joint legal custody is far more common, but questions about joint physical custody are more likely to be asked of the pediatrician.

Several findings about joint custody are worth noting. First, numerous studies suggest that children can function well even under complex joint physical custody arrangements; thus, joint custody should not be rejected out of hand. Second, the potential benefits of joint custody for children are not so great that the option should be strongly pushed on unwilling parents. Third, joint custody seems to be both the best and the worst parenting arrangement for children from divorced families. When parents can integrate their lives and cooperate in childrearing, children living in joint custody arrangements are the best adjusted. When joint custody is a way for contentious parents to "divide the child," however, the repeated exposure to conflict outweighs the benefits of a relationship with both parents, and joint custody is the worst alternative.[11] The custody label is far less important to children's adjustment than is the quality of postdivorce family relationships.

Understanding is one valuable service that pediatricians can offer to single parents. The parent who has primary responsibility for rearing the children may feel overwhelmed and exhausted. The parent who no longer lives with the children may feel powerless and alone. Often, an adult's personal struggles with divorce are so great that a pediatrician should suggest that the parent seek individual counseling. In all cases, parents will be more ready to follow the pediatrician's advice on parenting when their own struggles are recognized.

Exactly what parenting advice the pediatrician should offer varies, because different divorced parents develop different problems with their children. Common topics include urging parents to be very consistent in their schedules for sharing time with the children; work toward consistency in rules and discipline between households (including communicating about the children's medication and medical treatments); discipline their children appropriately despite the parents' guilt or uncertainty following divorce; and stop practices indicative of a parent's emotional dependence, such as sleeping with older children or confiding in them inappropriately. The pediatrician can also emphasize that the best outcome is for children to have good relationships with *both* parents after divorce. When hostility between parents is intense, however, it is more important for the teenager to be kept out of parental conflicts, even if this means having less contact with one parent.

Many parents find comfort from having the opportunity to voice their concerns and from hearing that things will get better as time passes. Referrals for psychotherapy are appropriate when relationship troubles are severe or prolonged. Family therapy is the most appropriate recommendation, because it may include one or all of the children together with one, or perhaps even both, of the parents. Teenagers and parents also may benefit from individual therapy, especially when the chances of relationship change are remote, or when the individual's anger or depression seems out of proportion to the family's relationship difficulties.

FAMILY FINANCES

Divorce causes financial strains for all but the wealthiest families, because it is more expensive to live in two households than in one. Economic research indicates that costs rise by 10% to 25% after divorce, but because income does not rise, a family's standard of living falls. Evidence also makes it clear that women and children suffer most of the economic hardships. The standard of living of divorced women and children falls about 20%, and it remains below predivorce levels (except after remarriage). In contrast, the standard of living of married couples—and divorced men—increases over time. Income transfers from men to women, namely, child support and spousal support, often are too small, are not paid regularly or at all, and in any case cannot fully make up for the disparities because of the increased expenses.

The pediatrician can do little about the financial problems of divorced families, but recognition of a parent's struggles can help. For example, parents may not follow medical advice because they cannot afford the care. They may be too embarrassed to admit this to the pediatrician, however, especially if money was not a concern previously. Medical insurance for the children also can be a major financial issue, as many women and children are insured through their husband's employment. Children (and spouse) still should be covered after a separation, but the pediatrician can forewarn parents to address medical coverage for the children in their legal agreements.

DATING AND REMARRIAGE

Sooner or later, divorced parents begin to form new romantic lives. As a rule, later is better than sooner, because dating and remarriage present their own complications. Dating should be acknowledged but (at least in the early stages) should generally take place apart from the family. Discretion is the key to sexual relationships. As a romantic relationship becomes more serious and likely to last, the new partner can be introduced to the child or adolescent gradually.

Even when a romance leads to remarriage (or committed cohabitation), the relationship between stepparents and children should be allowed to develop slowly over time. In general, it is easier for stepparents eventually to become more close and more firm with stepchildren than it is to become more distant or more lenient. Thus, the biologic parent does well to remain as the principal disciplinarian, since the stepparent gradually develops a more friendlike relationship with the teenager. Once warmth and credibility are established, the stepparent can assume more of a disciplinary role. It may take considerable time for both warmth and discipline to develop, if they develop at all, as the children, a former spouse, or even the remarried parent may view stepparents as rivals or intruders in the family.[12]

One important piece of advice about remarriage is that it will involve a new set of family transitions. The parent who is getting remarried is presumably happy about the event, but the children may have a different perspective. Children and the stepparent need time to adjust to one another, especially if they have not had much time to develop a relationship previously. Even if children have a relationship with the new stepparent, the symbolism of marriage may make a change in their eyes or in the eyes of the stepparent. Often, the change is positive, but a teenager may also view the remarriage as a final confirmation of the divorce or as an intrusion on family life. A biologic parent or stepparent also may mistakenly view the remarriage as a symbol of the stepparent's readiness to assume full parental authority, or may perhaps even change custody because they are now a "real" family. Conflicts with the children's other biologic parent may develop because of real or perceived threats to their parenting role or because of rekindled jealousies. Basic advice that is critical to remarriage is to go slow and expect some difficulties.

PEDIATRICIAN'S RESOURCES

The busy pediatrician can offer some psychologic advice directly to parents and adolescents, but educational videos, self-help books, and a list of local referral sources are helpful and time-saving additions to this service. A list of referral sources can be compiled from telephone calls to local psychologists, psychiatrists, social workers, and family courts. A few favorites among self-help books are listed below.

References

1. Cherlin AJ: *Marriage, divorce, remarriage,* ed 2, Cambridge, MA, 1992, Harvard Univ. Press.
2. Emery RE: *Marriage, divorce, and children's adjustment,* ed 2, Beverly Hills, Sage.
3. Amato PR, Keith B: Parental divorce and the well-being of children: a meta-analysis, *Psychol Bull* 110:26-46, 1991.
4. Emery RE, Forehand R: Parental divorce and children's well-being: a focus on resilience. In Haggerty RJ, Sherrod L, Garmezy N, Rutter M, editors: *Risk and resilience in children,* London, 1994, Cambridge University Press; pp. 64-99.
5. Hetherington EM: Coping with family transitions: winners, losers, and survivors, *Child Dev* 60:1-14, 1989.
6. Zill N, Morrison DR, Coiro MJ: Long-term effects of parental divorce on parent-child relationships, adjustment, and achievement in young adulthood, *J Fam Psychol* 7:91-103, 1993.
7. Cherlin AJ, Furstenberg FF, Chase-Lansdale PL, Kiernan KE, Robins PK, Morrison DR, Teitler JO: Longitudinal studies of effects of divorce on children in Great Britain and the United States, *Science* 252:1386-1389, 1991.
8. Amato PR, Loomis LS, Booth A: Parental divorce, marital conflict, and offspring well-being during early adulthood, *Social Forces* 73:895-915, 1995.
9. Emery RE: *Renegotiating family relationships: divorce, child custody, and mediation,* New York, 1994, Guilford Press.
10. Seltzer JA: Relationships between fathers and children who live apart: the father's role after separation, *J Marriage Family* 53:79-101, 1991.
11. Maccoby EE, Mnookin RH: *Dividing the child: social and legal dilemmas of custody,* Cambridge, MA, 1992, Harvard Univ. Press.
12. Hetherington EM, Clingempeel WG: Coping with marital transitions. *Monogr Soc Res Child Dev* (serial no. 227) 57:1-229, 1992.

Resources for Families

Ricci I: *Mom's house, dad's house,* New York, 1982, Macmillan.

Trafford A: *Crazy times: surviving divorce,* New York, 1984, Bantam.

Visher E, Visher J: *Stepfamilies,* New York, 1982, Doubleday.

CHAPTER 85

Adolescents with Gay or Lesbian Parents

•

Melanie A. Gold and Ellen C. Perrin

The traditional structure of two married parents with a working father, a homemaker mother, and one or more siblings no longer describes the majority of North American adolescents' home environments. According to the 1990 U.S. Census, only 37% of U.S. families consist of a once married, two-parent couple with children.[1] Adolescents may live in a variety of other family environments. They may live with a single father or mother, with a parent and stepparent, with a relative of the extended family or foster parent, or with a blended family composed of a parent and new spouse and step- or half-siblings. Adolescents can flourish in various family environments as long as these include adequate nurturance and guidance for optimal development.

One family environment for an adolescent is with a gay father and/or a lesbian mother, either with or without the parent's same-sex partner. Current estimates suggest that there are up to 5 million lesbian mothers, 3 million gay fathers, and 6 to 14 million people who have at least one gay or lesbian parent in the United States. These figures probably underestimate the true total, because many gay and lesbian parents are reluctant to reveal their sexual orientation.

Most of today's adolescents with gay or lesbian parents were conceived at a time when their parents were involved in a heterosexual relationship before recognizing or acknowledging their homosexuality. These parents may continue to live with their heterosexual spouse and children, may divorce their spouse and live as single parents, or may form stable relationships with a gay or lesbian partner. They may have full or joint custody or regular visitation with their children. Currently, as gay men and lesbian women choose increasingly to "come out" in their youth, growing numbers are becoming parents in the context of an ongoing homosexual relationship by adoption or insemination techniques. This new pattern will yield a generation of adolescents whose parents are gay or lesbian, but whose family lives are unmarred by the disruption involved in parents' "coming out" or parental divorce.

RESEARCH ON ADOLESCENTS WITH HOMOSEXUAL PARENTS

Most studies on gay or lesbian parenting have focused on younger children rather than adolescents and have been limited by small sample sizes, nonrandom subject selection, a narrow range of demographic variables, and lack of long-term follow-up. The majority of studies are not double-blind. They have focused on demonstrating the absence of pathology rather than elucidating patterns of resilience. In a review of the literature, Patterson[2] described twelve studies that, when combined, include more than 300 offspring of gay or lesbian parents. The studies' sample sizes ranged from 12 to 56 children whose parents were gay or lesbian, and equal numbers of children with heterosexual parents. No differences were found in personality characteristics, locus of control, moral maturity, intelligence, or the incidence of psychiatric disturbance or behavioral problems, nor in the development of sexual or gender identity or gender role behavior. In those studies that differentiated adolescents in their samples, equal proportions of adolescents in both groups report homosexual attraction or behavior.

Little research specifically focuses on the impact of gay or lesbian parenting on the developmental processes of adolescence. In one study the self-esteem of 18 adolescent children of lesbian divorced mothers was compared with that of a similar-sized sample of adolescent children of heterosexual divorced mothers.[3] Self-esteem was assessed using the Coopersmith Self-esteem Inventory and interviews with mothers and adolescents. No statistically significant differences were found. The same study found that children of mothers who were currently living with a male or female lover or had remarried reported higher self-esteem than adolescents whose mothers did not have a stable live-in relationship, irrespective of their mother's sexual orientation. Consistent with the known relationship between critical attitudes toward a parent and poor self-esteem, adolescents whose mothers were lesbians with low self-esteem were more likely to have a negative view of their mother's homosexuality than those with lesbian mothers with high self-esteem.

In the only published longitudinal study of adults raised as children in lesbian families, 25 young adults with lesbian mothers were compared with 21 adults of heterosexual single mothers on characteristics such as family and peer relationships, sexual orientation, and psychologic adjustment.[4] Individual interviews revealed that young adults who had been raised in lesbian households reported their relationship with their mother's partner to be significantly more positive than that reported by those raised by a heterosexual mother and her male partner. There were no significant differences in the reported quality of their current relationship with their mother(s) and/or father. No differences were reported in the memories of their feelings during adolescence about their mothers' relationships, but young adults raised by lesbian mothers were currently more positive about their mother's unconventional relationships than were those young adults raised by single heterosexual mothers. Young adults with lesbian mothers, especially males, recalled more frequently having been teased about being gay or lesbian themselves. Young adults from a lesbian family background were more likely to have considered or to have engaged in a same-gender sexual relationship. The two groups did not differ significantly in reported anxiety or depression. Overall the investigators concluded that children of lesbian mothers functioned well during adolescence and did not seem to experience long-term detrimental effects. A 1995 study of 76 adolescents in San Francisco who had lesbian mothers found their self-esteem to be equivalent to that of the normative sample, and even improved in the presence of strong learned coping skills.[5]

Adolescents growing up with gay fathers have been studied less extensively than those with lesbian mothers. However, Bailey et al[6] report the largest study to date on the sexual orientation of 82 sons of 55 gay or bisexual men recruited from advertisements in gay publications. Both fathers and their sons were surveyed by questionnaire and personal interview about the son's sexual orientation, and 91% (68/75) of the sons who could be rated reported themselves to be heterosexual. Sexual orientation was not correlated with the amount of time that the sons had lived with their fathers. This study reinforces the view that child custody decisions should be made irrespective of parents' sexual orientation.

ADVOCACY

There is no evidence to suggest an obstacle to the healthy development of an adolescent with gay or lesbian parents. Nevertheless, because of the extent of homopho-

bia, these adolescents may be faced with criticism and stigmatization that thus may be hurtful and isolating, and may affect their self-esteem. Healthcare providers have an opportunity, which some may consider a responsibility, to play an active role in helping to change social attitudes and restrictive legal codes that are damaging to gay and lesbian parents and their children. Healthcare providers may choose to be available as consultants to gay or lesbian support groups, participating in parent-teacher association meetings and various community programs.

ISSUES IN PROVIDING ADOLESCENT CARE

Early adolescence is the time when children of gay or lesbian parents are most likely to feel stigmatized and isolated because their family is perceived as nontraditional or "different." Furthermore, adolescence may be accompanied by anger and rebellion on the part of young people toward their parents. Like all adolescents, those whose parents are gay or lesbian may express reluctance to participate in family activities and may concentrate instead on peer relationships, be preoccupied with their physical development, and experience conflicts related to independence and autonomy. Healthcare providers can help adolescents and their gay or lesbian parents understand and cope with these issues by listening sympathetically and nonjudgmentally, and by providing information about community and national support groups for adolescents of gay and lesbian parents. Healthcare providers also can provide a bibliography of books for adolescents and parents and a list of local and national resource groups. They can help parents to anticipate and understand possible increasing ambivalence, or even anger, from their adolescent toward the parents' sexual orientation despite previous acceptance and support.

Adolescents who have gay or lesbian parents, like adolescents in heterosexual families, may explore and experiment in both homosexual and heterosexual relationships (see Chapter 99, "Sexual Orientation and Gender Identity"). The data suggest that adolescents who have gay or lesbian parents are no more inclined toward either sexual orientation than are adolescents of heterosexual parents. Healthcare providers and parents should make themselves available for open discussions about sexuality, and also offer support for whatever intrinsic sexual orientation the adolescent may express and guide him or her to do so safely.

Healthcare providers should convey their support of all forms of caring families, being careful not to assume that all adolescents are heterosexual, or have parents who are heterosexual. Healthcare providers who care for adolescents whose parents are gay or lesbian should communicate trust and respect; be sensitive and aware of the special needs, expectations, and concerns of these parents; and focus on the families' strengths and resources as they pertain to the adolescents' care and development. They should be wary of giving unconscious signals of negative feelings toward homosexuality, which can interfere with a supportive and helpful role. Those providers who cannot reconcile their personal beliefs with their professional obligation to provide supportive, understanding, and respectful care to gay and lesbian-headed families should refer these families to a provider who *can* meet these needs.

Discussion of nontraditional family structures can be facilitated by evidence of the healthcare provider's acceptance of diverse families. Questions on standardized office intake forms using gender-neutral terms such as "parent" or "family member" instead of mother/father; pictures of diverse families in the waiting room; and brochures, books, and magazines that acknowledge same-sex parents communicate the provider's availability to assist *all* families in their parenting challenges. Such office modifications create an environment in which adolescents also can feel at ease in discussing issues relating to their own sexual identity and behavior. Healthcare providers can create and implement a policy against lesbian and gay slurs, jokes, and putdowns in the office that might be hurtful or offensive to patients, parents, and staff.[7]

Gay or lesbian parents may choose not to identify their sexual orientation to their healthcare provider despite the latter's efforts to create a safe and inclusive environment. They may worry that latent homophobia or bias in professional and nonprofessional staff may jeopardize the care their adolescents receive, or that the healthcare provider will not honor their confidentiality, particularly if the parents are concerned about legal challenges to their custody rights. Adolescents with gay or lesbian parents also may choose not to share their parents' sexual orientation with their provider because they too may worry about the impact this may have on their relationship with their provider. Adolescents also may believe their parents' life style to be separate from and unrelated to their own life style, and may thus omit to inform the provider of the family environment.

When healthcare providers are aware of the family structure, they should openly discuss issues of confidentiality with parents and their adolescent(s), such as whom have parents told and from whom do they wish to withhold disclosure of their family structure (e.g., school officials, hospital and office personnel), and honor that request when it is not to the detriment of the adolescent's care. It is also important to point out to the parents, as well as to the adolescent, the importance of legal consent to care. In the frequent circumstance that only one of a same-sex couple is legally recognized as an adolescent's

parent, the healthcare provider should clarify how responsibility for medical decisions and consent for treatment for the adolescent will be shared. In the event of serious illness, injury, death, or voluntary separation of the legal parent, a prior written agreement giving the other parent power of attorney in making medical decisions for the adolescent is necessary. Healthcare providers should discuss consent for medical care and clarify in writing any power of attorney granting the nonbiologic/nonadoptive parent the right to make medical decisions. Box 85-1 shows an example of a consent to medical care.

Physicians and other healthcare providers are an important resource for many families as their children become adolescents and then adults. They have an important role to play in initiating and supporting community advocacy and in providing sensitive and accessible health care to families of every imaginable structure and constellation, including those in which one

---

BOX 85-1
Authorization to Medical, Surgical, or Dental Examination of a Minor

I, _____ , being the parent with legal custody of my son/daughter _____ , born on the _____ day of the month of _____ , in the year of _____ , hereby authorize _____ , into whose care my son/daughter has been entrusted, to consent to any examination, immunization, medication, x-ray, laboratory test, anesthetic, medical or surgical diagnosis, or treatment and hospital care to be rendered to my son/daughter _____ under the general or special supervision and upon the advice of a physician or surgeon licensed to practice medicine in any state of the United States, or to consent to an x-ray, examination, anesthetic, dental or surgical diagnosis, or treatment and hospital care to be rendered to my son/daughter _____ by a dentist licensed to practice dentistry in any state in the United States.

This authorization is valid from the _____ day of the month of _____ , in the year of _____ , to the _____ day of the month of , in the year _____ .

Dated: _____ Signature: _____
                                    Parent with legal custody

Dated: _____ Signature: _____
                                    Guardian to consent to care

Notarization _____

Adapted from Curry H, Clifford D, Leonard R: *A legal guide for lesbian and gay couples,* ed 7, Berkeley, CA, 1993, Nolo Press.

or both adults is/are gay or lesbian. They can be especially helpful to adolescents who may be grappling with the stigma associated with their parents' sexual orientation. Physicians and other healthcare providers can demonstrate their support by using gender-neutral language in reference to the adolescent's parents, by posting bulletin boards in their offices about resources for children of similar family constellations, and by serving as a resource for schools or extracurricular groups interested in learning about family diversity.

References

1. U.S. Bureau of the Census Current Population Report: Series P20, No. 486, 467, Statistical Abstract of the U.S.: 1992, ed 112, Washington, DC, 1992.
2. Patterson CJ: Children of lesbian and gay parents, *Child Dev* 63:1025-1042, 1992.
3. Huggins SL: A comparative study of self-esteem of adolescent children of divorced lesbian mothers and divorced heterosexual mothers. In Bozett F, editor: *Homosexuality and the family,* New York, 1989, Harrington Park Press; pp 123-135.
4. Tasker F, Golombok S: Adults raised as children in lesbian families, *Am J Orthopsychiatry* 65:203-215, 1995.
5. Gershon TD, Tschann JM, Jemerin JM: The effect of stigmatization on the adolescent children of lesbian mothers (poster abstract), *Arch Pediatr Adolesc Med* 149:49, 1995.
6. Bailey JM, Bobrows D, Wolfe M, Mikach S: Sexual orientation of adult sons of gay fathers, *Dev Psychol* 31:124-129, 1995.
7. Perrin EC, Kulkin H: Pediatric care for children whose parents are gay or lesbian, *Pediatrics* 97:629-635, 1996.
8. Curry H, Clifford D, Leonard R: *A legal guide for lesbian and gay couples,* ed 7, Berkeley, CA, 1993, Nolo Press.

Recommended Reading

Gold MA, et al: Children of gay or lesbian parents, *Pediatr Rev* 15:354-358, 1994.

Martin A: *The lesbian and gay parenting handbook: creating and raising our families,* New York, 1993, Harper Collins.

Support Groups

Children of Lesbians and Gays Everywhere (COLAGE), 2023 North Clark, Box 121, Chicago, IL 60657.

Gay and Lesbian Parents Coalition International (GLPCI), PO Box 50360, Washington, DC 20004. Telephone: (202) 583-8029.

These national organizations can assist in locating local support and a network of information in communities. They also provide an extensive reference list of books, articles, and videos for a nominal fee.

CHAPTER 86

Mourning

•

Morris A. Wessel

All physicians will have among their adolescent patients some who experience the death of a parent, grandparent, sibling, other relative, adult friend, or peer. The extent of a physician's involvement with a patient who is suffering a significant loss depends on that professional's confidence in his or her ability to cope with the bereaved individual's distress and conviction as to how worthwhile it is to assume this task.

Adolescence is a transitional phase in human development when individuals vacillate between moments of extreme independence, setting off with determination to make their way in the world, and moments, particularly evident during times of stress, when they regress to a less mature level, seeking parental care, sympathy, and advice. Even during moments of intense independence, adolescents normally have the comforting option of returning to an earlier phase and being taken care of by their parents. These alternating ways of relating to adults are important considerations when an adolescent experiences the death of a parent. Because of the fragmented parental situation, the option of returning to the earlier relationship is no longer possible.

Mourning the loss of a parent in adolescence is unique because the young individual, even while being emancipated from family and home, depends on the parents to be available as needed. After the death of a parent, adolescents are likely to deny the loss, often acting as if nothing has happened. Indeed, a visit to the home or a phone call often evokes a response such as "We're all fine" or "No one is sick here." Yet, despite the appearance of living in a normal manner, there are usually indications that the family members are struggling to adapt to the loss. Bereaved adolescents tend to long incessantly for and dream of the deceased. They often have difficulty sleeping; experience hallucinations ("I thought I saw my father coming up the road"); and suffer somatic symptoms such as nausea, abdominal discomfort, diarrhea, headaches, and weight loss. They commonly report an overwhelming loneliness and difficulty in focusing on school or social activities. Similar symptoms occur with the death of a relative, close friend, or teacher or even a public hero such as President John F. Kennedy.

ROLE OF PRIMARY CARE PHYSICIAN

Any call from a bereaved child or adolescent concerning somatic symptoms merits a careful examination and discussion of the findings. If there is no evidence of specific disease, the physician should clearly state this and mention that the symptoms are well known to be manifestations of the bereavement process. This visit relieves the adolescent of fears that he or she has a serious illness or is "going crazy." The examination and the sharing of concerns with the physician with whom there is a long-standing trusting relationship is reassuring.

However, one must take into consideration the fact that the stress associated with the loss of a loved one may be associated with the onset or recurrence of a significant illness, such as malabsorption syndrome, regional ileitis, colitis, peptic ulcer, cardiac arrhythmia, asthma, or arthritis.

If it is important to reach out to adolescents who suffer a significant loss, how do physicians learn of a tragic event among their patients? Physicians can state at the initial visit that they wish to be available in the event of an unusual family crisis. Many parents and adolescents phone their physician when a death occurs in the family. Also, in small- and moderate-sized communities, a newspaper account of the death of an individual in a family is readily available to the primary physician.

In caring for a critically ill child, adolescent, or adult, the primary physician may be acquainted with the family. Although colleagues with specialized skills may assume the care of the patient during critical phases, a primary physician's long-standing relationship offers the opportunity to support the patient and members of the family during this crisis.

Parents and siblings of the patient appreciate the continual interest of their primary physician when the illness is critical or a death is anticipated. Visits to the home, hospital, or hospice or (if distance makes this impossible)

frequent phone calls are usually welcome. A comment such as "Please call me if there is a major change . . . I want to know about it" offers tremendous support to siblings and other family members. A personal contact when a death occurs, either at the hospital or at home, or a phone call or hand-written condolence note to the parents and each of the siblings is well worth the effort.

Many parents also appreciate contact from the physician 3 or 4 months following a death, when there is an attempt to resolve the acute grief reaction. A physician cannot prevent the pain and anguish of the death, because the loss is real and devastating. However, the physician's genuine interest and concern are reassuring and supportive even though the physical and psychologic discomfort associated with bereavement may continue for many months or years.

ROLE OF PHYSICIAN IN SCHOOL

A physician serving as a medical advisor or health director at a local high school, preparatory school, or college has an important role when a student dies. This event, whether due to illness, drug overdose, accident, or suicide, is not a private matter. High school and college students, as they mature and separate from their parents and home setting, develop intense and meaningful relationships with other students. The death of a schoolmate is a significant stress for the students since it represents the loss of a friend. It also reminds them of their own vulnerability. They may say "It could have been me."

A physician can serve administrators, faculty, and students at this tragic moment. A meeting with the staff offers the opportunity to consider their feelings about the student's death. It also provides time to anticipate the reactions of the students as they grapple with the loss of their schoolmate.

Students who attend preparatory school or college are in the process of relinquishing their intimate family setting and developing new and intense alliances with schoolmates and faculty members. Students may express their feelings quite openly by saying "What's the use? You're here now but may be gone tomorrow." A physician's attentive interest is comforting to students as they struggle to accept their loss.

Small group meetings, such as a class, dormitory unit, athletic team, or other activity group, chaired by a physician, nurse, administrator, social worker, counselor, or teacher, offer the opportunity for discussion of feelings of grief.

Students often feel isolated and confused when one of their fellow students dies. They are relieved when their classmates also report feelings of alienation, malaise, lethargy, anorexia, loneliness, and difficulty in concentrating on educational or social activities. Such discussions are essential because parents and school personnel often urge students to "forget it," "snap out of it," or "stop thinking about it." Yet this advice is impossible to follow and not appropriate. Bereavement is a healthy human response to a significant loss.

The suggestion that a physician's role is "to cure sometimes, to relieve often, to comfort always" is as true now as when stated by Dr. Edward Trudeau, a pioneer in the treatment of tuberculosis, many decades ago. This theme serves as a guideline for physicians who serve adolescents when they suffer the loss of a beloved family member, friend, or classmate.

Suggested Readings

Parkes CM: *Bereavement: studies of grief in adult life,* New York, 1979, International University Press.
> *A classic description of the natural history of grief in adults that applies equally well to adolescents.*

Podell C: Adolescent mourning: the sudden death of a peer, *Clin Soc Work* 17:64, 1989.
> *A beautiful presentation of how social workers counseled students and faculty when five children were burned to death in a fire while visiting an amusement park.*

Sahler OJZ: *The child and death,* St. Louis, 1978, Mosby–Year Book.
> *A presentation of a 1977 symposium held at the University of Rochester Medical Center that deals with the needs of children and adolescents and also those of caregivers.*

Schonfeld DJ: Crisis intervention for bereavement support: a model of intervention in the children's school, *Clin Pediatr* 28:27, 1989.
> *Describes how the author, as a pediatric consultant, served staff and students in a school when the death of a child occurred.*

Wolfenstein M, Kliman G, editors: *Children and the death of a president. Multidisciplinary studies,* New York, 1965, Doubleday.
> *Offers detailed presentations by 13 professionals who reported how children reacted to the death of President John F. Kennedy. Includes a wealth of information about childhood bereavement presented in vivid and poignant terms.*

CHAPTER 87

Family Illness

•

Murray M. Kappelman

Adolescents view their personal world as a dynamically changing environment that is influenced by their own developmental coping methods—the hyperbolic nature of viewing everyday events, the sense of time being constricted and immediate, and the struggles with development of personal identity. Illness within the family, similar to divorce or death, disrupts the equilibrium of that tenuous world, necessitating a course correction at a time when the developmental voyage is fraught with unknown and fearful turbulence under unexceptional conditions. The adolescent takes for granted the organization of the family and the way the particular family operates, according to previous experience. This framework provides a state of equilibrium that helps to balance the effects of unsettling developmental forces of the adolescent years. Family illness is a threat to the family's organization because it is a threat to its equilibrium, the steady state that has been achieved to guarantee the continuity necessary for the growth of each family member and the family as a whole. To state it simply, there is a disruption in the "family machinery."[1]

RESPONSIBILITY

One of the major problems for the adolescent is the illness of one or both parents during the teenage years. There are a number of developmentally normal reactions that, if magnified more than normally expected within the pattern of everyday family living, can result in significant problems for the adolescent and potentially for the family unit as a whole. One reaction is a heightened sense of responsibility felt by the adolescent when confronted by the illness of a parent. There are two aspects to this problem. The first is the issue of responsibility and blame. Because adolescence is a period of rebellion, withdrawal, and self-actualization, an aura of chaos and anger often exists between the parental authority figures and the adolescent over both major and minor issues of daily living. This struggle for authority and autonomy can suddenly can become counterproductive for the adolescent when a parent becomes seriously ill, causing the adolescent to wonder and worry about how much the heightened tension contributed to the parent's illness and potential recovery. It is important for the healthcare providers of both the adolescent and the parent to make clear to the adolescent the nature and cause of the parent's illness, thereby absolving the adolescent of all blame, whether the illness is physical or emotional in origin.

Another area of responsibility deals with the adolescent's natural developmental tendency to become a rescuer. The feeling often grows within the adolescent that not only should he or she attempt to work to make the parent well and whole again but also that many of the duties and jobs previously undertaken by the parent now are the adolescent's specific responsibility. Asen[1] noted that the redistribution of function and power within the family with an ill parent requires adaptation within that family and that some families are better at making a healthy adaptation than others. It is clearly not healthy to expect a 15-year-old male to assume the full burden of the activities and responsibilities assigned to his unexpectedly ill 37-year-old father (even if he heroically offers or attempts to do so). The analogy with the teenage female with an ill mother (or father) is clear.

VULNERABILITY

The next issue faced by the adolescent coping with an ill parent is the sense of vulnerability of self and family. Vulnerability comes in two distinctly different forms. One aspect of vulnerability is the decreased degree of resiliency to other external and internal negative forces associated with daily living. Sargent[2] noted that children of mentally ill parents are often vulnerable, partly because they may not be receiving adequate nurturing and partly because they feel stigmatized by their parents' disabilities. Winicott[3] noted that this parental problem can leave the child desperate to establish supportive, nurturing ties to others (often in inappropriate ways) or feeling emotionally destitute with no hope of connection. He claimed that children may develop a "false self" in defense against a disturbed family environment. An interesting comment by Winicott is that adolescents may experience rage, dread, and dislike in the face of the psychic loss of the parent just at the time when the external world is anticipating compassion from the teen-

ager. This suggests that the natural developmental stage of adolescent withdrawal from adults (parents) is accentuated by parental illness at the time when the teenager is feeling most vulnerable to the outside world because of his or her inability to approach the parent during times of need. This only increases the adolescent's sense of vulnerability. The healthcare provider must be sensitive to this heightened vulnerability and needs to assist the adolescent in locating alternative sources of support within family, friends, or community.

There is another side to the issue of vulnerability. Adolescents may relate the illness, particularly if it is emotional, to themselves and begin to ponder the question: "Will I get it?" The question may not be asked explicitly, but often it is lurking in the recesses of the troubled adolescent's mind. It is the healthcare professional's responsibility to answer that question honestly and clearly, a response that is likely to provide strong reassurance for the adolescent. The concomitant vulnerability issue for the teenager may be the confrontation with the proximity of death for the first time. The vulnerability of the parent to death often causes adolescents to reflect on their own vulnerability to illness and death. Some of the teenager's anxiety associated with a parent's sickness therefore, can be of a very personal, internalized, self-centered nature.

REBELLION

Another adolescent developmental landmark that may be disturbed by the illness of a parent is that of rebellion. It is developmentally normal for a teenager to withdraw from the authority and strong personal impact of parents in order to find self, self-actualize, and eventually return to the family unit to present self as a fully realized and personally accepted individual. This can be a long and arduous journey that begins at any age during the teenage years or may be inappropriately delayed until a later age. The "pulling back" of the adolescent often takes the form of rebellious behavior, covert or overt. With an ill parent, many adolescents resist the turmoil and confrontation engendered by the developmentally normal rebellion and defer maturation as the solution to dealing with the parent's illness. Occasionally this temporary deferral of developmental passaging may be appropriate for short crisis periods, but prolonged delays can lead to emotional and social maladaptation. It becomes necessary to counsel the family and the teenager that the young person needs to be allowed the necessary new autonomy and conflict of thought and action between self and parents to a healthy degree, especially when the adolescent is faced with a parent who has a long-term chronic illness.

LOSS

A very serious phenomenon for adolescents to handle during the teenage years is loss. All individuals have difficulty adapting to loss, but teenagers—with developmental issues of hyperbole, time-perspective problems, and struggles with formation of personal identity—find the issue of loss at times not only paralyzing but sometimes cause for thoughts of withdrawal and self-harm. There are three areas of loss that are faced by the adolescent and must be understood by the health professional who wants to counsel the young person and family intelligently. The first is feared loss of an ill parent to death. The second is the loss of both parents at a crucial time in adolescent development secondary to the refocused energies of the adults in the family relative to coping with the parent's illness. The third is the loss of the expected stable daily family dynamics that create the necessary equilibrium for the adolescent, whose personal physical and emotional life can be legitimately chaotic and seemingly out of control. As stated by a 14-year-old in a book written by his mother and him about the mother's bouts with breast cancer, "One day, normal will come back into our house."[4]

There is a fourth loss that should be elucidated and discussed by the healthcare provider with the family. Not only is there potential loss of emotional family support for the teenager during this period, but there is also potentially loss of financial support at a time when many adolescents face future educational plans that require family fiscal help. For example, the answer to the question "Will there be enough money for me to go to college?" needs to be addressed openly and honestly, and alternative fiscal coping mechanisms need to be initiated by the well parent and the adolescent together.

HELPLESSNESS

When a parent becomes ill, the teenager suddenly experiences an accentuated sense of helplessness. All too often, the healthcare professional, in collusion with the other parent, "spares" the children the details of the illness and the treatment. This only heightens the extreme anxiety experienced by a teenager when a parent becomes ill, as described by Power.[5] Teenagers have a heightened sense of rescuing; knowing may not enable them to do more, but it will help them put into perspective what they can do and why other things are not their responsibility or within the realm of possibility for them.

As already noted, the loss of structure within everyday life creates a nightmarish vacuum for teenagers who have not yet established sufficient personal skills, adaptation techniques, and "roots" within the family and community

to "make it on their own." Attempts by the healthcare professional to assist families to reframe the family structure in a healthy, practical manner during the parental illness, no matter how long, may permit adolescents to regroup their resources and move forward in the developmental trip through the teenage years.

It is imperative that the healthcare professional bear in mind the impact on the adolescent when he or she is faced with the illness of a single parent. There is no authority cushion to fall back on, no guarantee of fiscal or emotional support, and no reassurance that someone is in control to reframe and maintain the family unit. No time should be lost by the healthcare professional in assisting both an ill single parent and the adolescent in locating all possible alternative sources of assistance within and outside the family. Social agencies should be considered for appropriate crisis or long-term support, even when members of the extended family live within the immediate vicinity. In a situation involving an ill single-parent, attempts at helpful intervention always should have as a first priority maintaining the teenager within his or her usual environment as physically close to the ill single parent as possible.

ILLNESS OF SIBLING

Illness of a sibling must be considered in regard to the impact that such an event may have on the adolescent. Gayton et al[6] postulated that 14- to 18-year-old siblings and patients with cystic fibrosis appeared to be functioning within normal limits in terms of personality functioning. Another example of normal function was the lack of any evidence of negative psychologic impact on sibling development when brothers or sisters had cystic fibrosis. On the other hand, Adams and Deveau[7] believe that the stress of having a sibling with cancer may distort the ability of adolescent siblings to cope, thus making them vulnerable to emotional turmoil and disruption of social and family relationships.[8] This disparity suggests that the impact on the adolescent relative to sibling illness may be related to the nature of, longevity of, and outlook for the disease process.

It should be stated clearly, however, that no matter whether the outcome of the sibling illness is positive or negative, there are vital areas of the teenager's development and adaptation to daily living that will be significantly affected by the serious illness of a sibling.

BLAME, GUILT, AND FEAR

Two closely allied areas of concern for the adolescent when a sibling is significantly ill are those of blame and guilt. It has been noted that siblings are distressed by the visibility of the illness and their tendency to identify with it.[7] Some siblings even feel guilty about being healthy. As siblings grow older toward and within the teenage years, their distress is manifested by their own physical symptoms, their seeking of affection, and their complaints about disorganized family routines.[8] Cairns et al[9] indicated that siblings aged 6 to 16 have significant levels of anxiety and fear for their own health. There is a very real fear of contagion that adolescents fantasize about when dealing with the illness of a sibling. As with the illness of parents, adolescents must be reassured, whenever possible, that their past behavior has not in any way precipitated or prolonged their sibling's illness; that their good health is an asset to the sibling and family rather than a shame; and that they are not susceptible to the illness unless there are genetic reasons, when counseling might be indicated.

LACK OF INVOLVEMENT

Another key problem that is dealt with best by caregivers is the adolescent's sense of total lack of involvement in the caring process for the ill sibling, whether hospitalized or at home. This sense of inadequacy, both personally and viewed as a parental assessment of the adolescent's worth, reinforces the impotence and magnifies the mystery surrounding the future of the sibling's illness (and therefore that of the family as a whole). It is essential to involve the adolescent from the very beginning in any family illness—from the time of diagnosis through the various stages of acute and chronic treatment, whether the ill person is a parent, a sibling, or a grandparent close to the teenager.

Loss becomes a real issue with sibling illness. Along with the sense of loss from the adolescent perspective is an additional one when a sibling becomes significantly ill—that of loss of parental involvement. The mobilization of parental emotional, physical, and fiscal resources to come to the immediate aid of the ill sibling all too often leaves the adolescent sibling bereft of the support systems so desperately needed at this stage of development. As with divorce, loss of parental involvement is probably most serious in relation to a pathologic outcome during the turbulent adolescent years. Despite the usual outspoken and acting-out nature of many normal adolescents going through the detachment/reattachment phases of the teenage years, Rosen[10] notes that most adults, when they had ill siblings as adolescents, shared their feelings with no one and felt isolated and neglected. Caregivers to the ill child must always remember that there are other children in the family. They need not only to program their involvement in the care process but also to assist the parents in finding the time to maintain the supportive

parent-child relationship expected and needed by each child. Adams and Deveau[7] concluded that if an open, honest, and trusting relationship is established with all family members early in a child's illness, adolescent siblings will not be overlooked, their vulnerability will be lessened, and serious sequelae can be prevented.

UNRESOLVED ANGER

Adolescents have great difficulty in dealing with the feeling that they are entrapped in a situation over which they have no control. This can lead to hostility that is either internally or externally directed. When a sibling is ill, the adolescent has the normal rescue fantasies, but he or she is helpless to do more than support, care, and watch the illness "win over whatever we do." This leads to the phenomenon seen with parents, but even more so with siblings, of unresolved anger at the illness that leads to diffuse displaced hostility that affects other important educational and social and family areas of the teenager's life. Spinetta[11] noted that sibling anger begins to surface most clearly during remissions of cancer in siblings. This is probably because the diffuse anger is lost in the turmoil of the acute phase but does not abate when the sibling seems better. The anger persists because parental involvement does not lessen, treatments continue without reassurance of a "cure," and (most important) the family is more able to become aware of the angry vibrations being sent out by the teenage sibling. These often are misinterpreted as self-centered reactions; it is the family's healthcare provider who can assist them in defining the true cause of, and solutions to, the hostile behavior of this adolescent. As stated by Adams and Deveau,[7] distancing may be mistaken for rejection.

ABSENCE OF PEER

When a sibling has a prolonged serious illness, it is vital to remember that, in the family constellation, it is not uncommon for the adolescent to feel the real absence of a peer whether the sibling was a close friend, a rival, or a figure to support or from whom to receive support. Loss of a different type again occurs; it is more peer related, is more personal on an intimate basis, and disturbs the balance of the adolescent's daily social dynamics, which are usually tenuous without the added stress. It is important to enable the adolescent to interact with the sick sibling as often as is appropriate and to attempt to allow that interaction to be a normal, age-relevant activity. This advice can be offered by the healthcare professional at the time when the ill sibling is able to participate in this role.

ROLE OF HEALTHCARE PROFESSIONAL

Power[5] listed several ways in which the healthcare professional can assist the adolescent in coping with chronic illness of the parent. This expert advice applies equally well to the case of the adolescent with an ill sibling:

1. If deterioration is anticipated, assist the young person to come to terms with this fact.
2. Help the young person master the threat of loss. Reestablish contact if distancing has become the coping mechanism.
3. Clarify the genetic aspects and minimize the contagion, if appropriate.
4. Act as teacher, activator of family discussions (family meetings), and interpreter of family dynamics and address the reactions of all family members.
5. As appropriate, assist the adolescent to find self-help groups that deal with family illness and/or loss.

Many positive actions can be undertaken by the healthcare professional, from the moment of diagnosis and throughout therapy and maintenance, in assisting the adolescent to adapt to the unsettling issue of significant illness in a family member. To be ready to intervene appropriately, it is necessary for the caregiver to understand the dynamics of what is causing the actions of the teenagers—in other words, to recognize the true message behind the behavioral signal. The teenager's needs should be an integral part of every treatment plan for each family with a member who has been diagnosed as having a prolonged or serious illness.

References

1. Asen K: Illness and the family, *J R Soc Med* 8(suppl)78:21-25, 1985.
2. Sargent KL: Helping children cope with parental mental illness through use of children's literature, *Child Welfare* 64:617-628, 1985.
3. Winicott DW: *The family and individual development,* New York, 1965, Basic Books.
4. *The Sunpapers,* August 12, 1990, Section H, pp 1, 6.
5. Power PL: Adolescent reaction to parental neurological illness: coping and intervention strategies, *Pediatr Soc Work* 3:45-52, 1984.
6. Gayton WF, Friedman S, Tavormina J, et al: Children with cystic fibrosis: psychological test findings of patients, siblings, and patients, *Pediatrics* 59:888-894, 1977.
7. Adams DW, Deveau EJ: When a brother or sister is dying of cancer: the vulnerability of the adolescent sibling, *Death Studies* 11:279-295, 1987.
8. Sourkes B: Siblings of the pediatric cancer patient. In Kellerman J, editor: *Psychological aspects of childhood cancer,* Springfield, IL, 1981, Charles C Thomas; p 56.
9. Cairns NU, Clark GM, Smith SD, et al: Adaptation of siblings to childhood malignancy, *J Pediatr* 95:484-487, 1979.
10. Rosen H: *Unspoken grief,* Lexington, MA, 1986, DC Health; p 16.
11. Spinetta JJ: The siblings of the child with cancer. In Spinetta JJ, Deasy-Spinetta P, editors: *Living with childhood cancer,* St. Louis, 1981, Mosby–Year Book; p 137.

CHAPTER 88

The Adopted Adolescent

•

Edward L. Schor

Adopted children face unique challenges during adolescence. As they move toward adult relationships and responsibilities, they must realign ties, both real and imagined, with two families—the family in which they were raised and their family of origin. Adopted children approach the tasks of adolescence in the context of ambiguity of origin and recapitulation of previous loss.

ADOPTION STATISTICS

In the United States, accurate data about adoptions and adoptees are limited by the absence of a national registry. The adoption of adolescents by nonrelatives is a rare event; estimates place the figure at about 5% of the roughly 51,000 annual nonrelative adoptions. Not even such rough estimates are available for the approximately 53,000 annual adoptions by relatives, although the proportion of adolescents is likely higher. Since a federal agency is involved in the adoption of foreign-born children, it is known that children above 10 years of age constitute about 5% of the nearly 10,000 foreign-born children adopted annually in the United States.

About 2% of U.S. children live in families with adoptive parents, neither of whom is biologically related to the child. Early in the 1980s, almost 9% of children lived in homes with a stepparent and a biologic parent, usually their mother. It appears that stepparent adoption constitutes a large proportion of recent adoptions and reflects the large number of children involved in divorce proceedings (see Chapter 84, "Divorce"). About 1.7% of children live with a grandparent or other relative. In total, nearly 13% of U.S. children have been adopted.

BACKGROUND

Present-day knowledge and understanding of many aspects of the adoption process have been hampered by the social stigma and secrecy that have often characterized adoption in the past. Women who completed an unwanted or out-of-wedlock pregnancy sought confidentiality in the relinquishment and placement of their child. For adoptive parents, their inability to conceive a child created much personal anguish and led to the emotional, often tedious pursuit of an adoptable child. Face-to-face contact between adoptive and biologic parents was discouraged, and identifying information was not shared or made available to either set of parents. Children often were told very little about their adoption, and some reached adulthood without discovering that they were adopted. The secrecy that enshrouded the adoption process has prevented the research studies necessary to describe the consequences of adoption. As a result, there are few population-based studies or even case-controlled studies from which to draw valid and generalizable conclusions about adoption.

Historically, for social and legal reasons, adoption usually has involved a public or a private adoption agency. However, changes in the availability of adoptable children, in the stigma associated with out-of-wedlock pregnancies, in the public airing of topics such as infertility and adoption, in the increased rates of divorce and remarriage, and in other personal and social factors that accompany adoption, have led to changes in the process of adoption. One evident change is a decrease in agency adoptions and a corresponding increase in private adoptions handled through attorneys. Private adoptions now constitute nearly one third of all domestic adoptions by nonrelatives. Families involved in private adoptions may incur considerable expenses, and con-

sequently such adoptions are more frequently initiated by affluent parents.

Until recent years, agency adoptions were synonymous with "closed" adoptions, that is, adoptions in which neither party, the biologic parents nor the adoptive parents and their adopted child, knew or had access to identifying information about each other. Since the mid-1970s decades, adopted persons, usually adults and older adolescents, have spearheaded a movement to allow access to previously confidential adoption records. Although there has been much consequent public debate and legislative activity, most adoption records remain "closed." However, in most states, adult adopted persons and their biologic parents can meet each other, typically through a mutual-consent adoption registry or through an intermediary system known as "search and consent." Adoption records remain confidential in all but a few states. Despite the continuing legal veil of secrecy and confidentiality, as the proportion of private adoptions has increased, so too has the number of biologic parents and adoptive parents who know each other. Even adoption agencies are finding that biologic mothers want to meet the prospective adoptive parents of the child they are relinquishing. Thus, recent adoptions, in contrast to adoptions of the past, can be distinguished by their degree of "openness": that is, the information and familiarity that members of the "adoption triad" (biologic parents, adoptive parents, and the adoptee) often have of one another. The consequent familiarity adoptees have with their biologic families has great meaning for the adopted adolescents, who are in the process of developing mature concepts of themselves.

Apart from adoptions by relatives, most U.S. children who are adopted during adolescence are those who have been in the foster care system for a great portion of their lives. They commonly enter foster care primarily because their parents were unwilling or unable to care for them, and it is likely that they experienced varying degrees of physical or sexual abuse and neglect. These children may have lived in a stable foster home for the greater part of their lives, and their adoption by their foster parent is a recognition of the attachment that has developed between them. Alternatively, these children may have foster parents whose age and increasing disability has impaired their ability to continue providing care for them and led to their placement in an adoptive home. For such children, this is at least the second relinquishment of them by "parents." More often than not, these adolescents have lived in multiple foster homes. As teenagers, they have left these homes because their foster parents were unable to cope with their sometimes typical, sometimes exaggerated, adolescent behavior. The alternatives for such adolescents are limited, and most spend their remaining dependent years in group homes.

Finally, the foster care system provides services for

children with a variety of chronic emotional and physical problems, since finding an adoptive family for such children is often a difficult and lengthy process. Thus, the experiences of children adopted from foster care are greatly variable. Time is not on the side of adoptable children in foster care: they often wait years for the social service and judiciary systems to meet their needs. About 40% of children in foster care who are awaiting adoption are more than 11 years old, and the median age of children in foster care is between 11 and 12 years.

THE ADOPTION EXPERIENCE

Few generalizations can be made about how children fare in adoption or how adopted children will traverse adolescence. Children adopted in infancy from biologic parents, children adopted from the foster care system, and children adopted by a relative or a stepparent have strikingly different life experiences. However, for all members of the adoption triad adoption is a lifelong condition that colors many aspects of their lives.

Successful Adoption

Successful adoption of an adolescent should begin with full and open discussions between a professional and the adoptive family about the social and personal history and special needs of the child. Similarly, the adolescent should be fully informed about the adoptive family and the reasons for their wishing to adopt. Both parents need to be committed to the adoption, and their biologic children need to approve of their parents' plans. The adoptive family must be prepared for and be able to deal with their own and the adoptee's ambivalence and even negative feelings. The adoptive parents should be able to postpone their own needs for intimacy and emotional gratification. Adoptive parents should not act with the intention of changing the child; rather, they need to accept the child and negotiate from that starting point. Families who are able to seek and accept support and help from outside the family, particularly those who participate in planned professional postadoptive services, are more likely to succeed with adoption.

Disrupted Adoption

A failed adoption can be of great consequence to both the adolescent and the adoptive parents, jeopardizing future adoptions and damaging self-esteem. Children who are adopted during adolescence are at special risk for disruption, with failure rates of 10% to 24% reported. Many factors work against successful adoption. Adolescents who are adopted from foster care are likely to have had multiple foster care placements, inconsistent parent-

ing, and a history of abuse. They also may have been separated from their siblings. In addition, most of the adolescents in disrupted adoptions have some special problem, such as a chronic medical condition, a developmental disability, or an emotional or behavioral disorder. Homes in which biologic children of the adoptive parents are present, and with whom the adopted adolescent feels a sense of competition, are also at greater risk for unsuccessful adoption. Transracial adoptions seem not to be at special risk for disruption.

Often preexisting factors within the adoptive family contribute to or are responsible for a failed or a strained adoption. Sometimes the adoptive parents' commitment to the adoption is not sufficiently strong to see them through the difficulties of forming a lasting relationship with someone else's child, especially when their resolve is tested by difficult adolescent behavior. Marital problems between the adoptive parents or among previous spouses also can interfere with adoption. Other stresses within the household, such as financial problems, physical illness, or change in household composition, can prevent successful incorporation of an adopted child. Sometimes the adolescent's motivation to be adopted, or his or her ability to be emotionally close to others, is insufficient for the adoption to succeed. Physicians caring for adopted adolescents need to be aware of all these factors in order to anticipate difficulties and to intervene appropriately.

OUTCOMES OF ADOPTION

Emotional Outcomes

Adopted adolescents may have been adopted as infants or young children, as stepchildren to their biologic parent's new spouse, or through the foster-care system. Generalizations about their development and adjustment to life must acknowledge not only their shared adoptive status but also their very different life experiences—hence, the seeming paradox that although adopted children generally adjust to life about as successfully as nonadopted children, adoptees are almost uniformly overrepresented in mental health clinics and psychiatric practices and hospitals.

There are a number of explanations for this apparent discrepancy. First, the life experiences of adopted children differs in fundamental ways from those of other children. During adolescence, these differences modify the usual developmental tasks and may be manifested in the behavior of adopted children. Second, seeking therapy may be a healthy response by an adoptive family. Because of adoptive parents' sensitivity to putative signs of emotional distress, they may misread normal adolescent behavior as abnormal. This may contribute to adoptees being referred to social and psychiatric services with about twice the frequency of the general population. Finally, as an adopted adolescent, the previous foster child often has experienced abuse and neglect during childhood, has suffered from a lack of stability within relationships, and has excessive burdens of chronic health conditions, and thus is at increased risk for emotional disturbances.

Currently, in the absence of substantial evidence based on research, it is prudent to recognize adoptees' increased risk for poor adjustment during adolescence, but to tailor predictions and interventions to the individual circumstance of each adolescent. Emotional disturbances in adolescent adoptees are rarely a result of the simple fact of being adopted. More likely, such disturbances reflect the child's preadoptive life experiences or the ongoing relationship between the child and the adoptive parents.

Social and Educational Outcomes

Parents who place their children for adoption do so in the hope and expectation that their child will have a better life than they are able to provide. Children who are removed from their parents' custody by the courts are also placed in the homes of other families to offer them better care and a more secure future than their parents are expected to be able to provide. In general, adoption does succeed in advancing the socioeconomic status of the children. As a group, adopted children have IQ scores and scholastic attainment equal to that of the general population and substantially better than might be expected on the basis of their background. This outcome seems to be related to the fact that their adoptive parents are better educated, of higher socioeconomic status, older, and more settled than average. In addition, there are usually fewer children in adoptive families, so the child receives more individualized attention and a larger share of the family's resources than in other families.

Tasks of Adolescence

The tasks of adolescence, of course, are not discrete challenges but a developmental continuum for both the adoptee and the adoptive parents. The success of this stage depends most on the previous establishment of an open and respectful communication between parents and adolescent, one in which feelings can be acknowledged and explored freely. Much has been written about telling children that they are adopted. In the narrow sense, the process of "telling" is not an issue for those children who are adopted at an older age. However, "telling" is not a discrete event but rather an ongoing dialogue that goes beyond informing the child of his or her adoptive status. It includes discussing the circumstances surrounding the adoption, and the feelings that were and continue to be

attached to adopting and being adopted. How these topics are initially presented reflects the adoptive parents' comfort with discussing sensitive issues and can set the stage for future communication on this and other subjects.

It is important that adoptive parents acknowledge the differences between adoptive and biologic parenthood. They should regard their child's life experiences and concerns as different from theirs, and from those of other children, and speak freely about adoption. "Telling," and then sharing relevant information about the child's background, should be done in the form of developmentally appropriate answers to the child's questions. All children have a need to know about their background and roots. Adolescent adoptees are likely to have a special interest in their biologic parents' level of education, work, and abilities and in what sort of people they are. In late adolescence, as they contemplate their own procreative potential, adopted adolescents may develop a special interest in the medical and social histories of their biologic parents.

All adolescents develop their individual identities apart from their families, while simultaneously building on their experiences within those families. Adopted adolescents have additional real and fantasized experiences within another family, their family of origin. To varying degrees, adopted children feel the loss of a relationship with an emotionally, if not materially, significant person. Thus, while learning about themselves and separating from their family, they also must separate from another family about whom they may know very little. In one sense, along with the loss of their birth parents, adopted children lose their ties to an ethnic, cultural, social, and perhaps religious heritage. The lack of knowledge about their roots makes separating from their family of origin more difficult, and adopted adolescents are quite naturally anxious to learn more about these families.

Developmentally, adopted adolescents must know something of their past in order to see their future as a rational synthesis of experience. The struggle to achieve this unity, in spite of a real break in continuity, may take the form of exaggerated fantasies, disruption and testing of the adoptive family, and a search for information about the biologic family. Since adoption is created out of the loss of a biologic family, one unique task for adopted adolescents is to grieve and accept that loss, and the implicit rejection that it implies.

Adopted adolescents' experience within their adoptive family should reinforce a sense of permanence and belonging. A successful adoption then will have laid a firm groundwork for the adolescent task of individuation. Adoptees who use their status as a weapon or a threat to test family unity and commitment will *not* succeed unless that family relationship is unstable.

Adopted adolescents are unlikely to have a peer group

of other adoptees. Their adoptive parents are similarly lacking role models. Nonetheless, most adoptees and their families accomplish the social transitions of adolescence without unusual difficulty. Adopted adolescents are not unique in having trouble with their parents or with peer acceptance, or in having doubts about their abilities. Some may have excessive difficulty with the normal tasks of social development and may display adjustment, conduct, oppositional, and antisocial disorders. Some may deny their adoptive status, or alternatively wear it as a badge for all to see. Dating can be affected if fears of intimacy and rejection are excessive, if there is fear of establishing an incestuous relationship with an unknown biologic relative, or if the adolescent is seen by the adoptive parents as a symbol of their own infertility. However, despite these potential problems, adopted adolescents need not experience any excessive difficulty with adolescent development, and they have been found in some instances to function better than other adolescents.

ROLE OF THE PHYSICIAN

The issues involved in adoption take new, but predictable, forms during adolescence. Physicians can be most helpful to the adolescent and the adoptive parents by assisting with the identification and management of the underlying adoption-related concerns that are accentuated during this developmental stage, and differentiating them from problems with other sources. Caution should be exercised so that the adoption does not become the focus of other conflicts or unresolved issues within the family, such as marital tension between the parents. During adolescence, adoptees can developmentally be expected to have increased interest and concern regarding their adoptive status. Adolescent adopted children often become more vocal about their interest in their biologic parents. Adoptive parents who have difficulty communicating with their adolescents about this subject are likely to find their relationship with them strained.

Failure to resolve disputes and conflicts can cause adolescents and adults to feel alienated from one another, and this situation creates anxiety and consternation on both sides. Those who feel secure and able to discuss their concerns with one another will cope more easily with the stresses this period places on both the adolescent and the family.

Adolescents, particularly adopted ones, need sources of support outside their immediate family. Physicians or other professionals working with adopted adolescents can offer a safe, supportive, and structured professional relationship in which to explore questions about the adolescent's personal and biologic origins. Most of these questions are merely normal adolescent concerns, perhaps exaggerated by being adopted. Some adolescents' distress may reflect a continuing need to mourn real or perceived past losses, and to integrate those experiences into an emerging adult identity. Counseling about this grief should be provided.

The health care of adolescents usually includes the goal of facilitating family dialogue by providing information, interpreting, or actually mediating between the adolescent and parents. In some families the adopted adolescent may correctly anticipate that discussion of his or her normal, adoption-related developmental issues may be too emotionally charged and threatening for the adoptive parents to face. In such cases the physician should provide an opportunity for the adolescent to explore his or her own concerns, while guiding the family into appropriate counseling and postadoptive services. Normal adolescent development cannot take place when important issues remain taboo topics within the family or when the parents and adolescent feel insecure with one another. Physicians caring for adopted adolescents need to assess the degree of comfort within the family concerning the adoption; they should anticipate whether adolescence is likely to accentuate normal family developmental issues unduly; they should be able to recognize when adoptive status is causing dysfunctional behavior on the part of the adolescent and family; and they should ensure that both the adolescent and the adoptive family have access to the appropriate resources to deal effectively with their concerns.

Suggested Readings

Adoption factbook, Washington, DC, 1989, National Committee for Adoption.

Berry M, Barth RP: A disrupted adoptive placement of adolescents, *Child Welfare* 69:209, 1990.

Bourguignon J-P, Watson KW: *After adoption: a manual for professionals working with adoptive families,* Springfield, IL, 1987, Illinois Department of Children and Family Services.

Brodzinsky DM, Schechter DE, Braff AM, Singer LM: Psychological and academic adjustment in adopted children, *J Consult Clin Psychol* 52:582, 1984.

Committee on Adolescence: *Normal adolescence: its dynamics and impact,* 1968, Group for Advancement of Psychiatry.

Marquis KS, Detweiler RA: Does adopted mean different? An attributional analysis, *J Pers Soc Psychol* 48:1054, 1985.

The future of children. Adoption, Los Altos, CA, 1993, David and Lucile Packard Foundation.

Wolff S: The fate of the adopted child, *Arch Dis Child* 49:165, 1974.

CHAPTER 89

Out-of-Home Living Arrangements

•

Edward L. Schor and Elizabeth Goodman

Most children in the United States live with both of their biologic parents, although 27% live with a single parent or in a household with a biologic parent and a stepparent (14.9%). There remain a large number of children who live out of their family home for a variety of reasons. Some of these children require out-of-home care because their parents are physically or emotionally absent. Others have parents who are unable or unwilling to care for them because the child's needs outweigh the parents' physical, emotional, social, or financial resources. This latter group includes youths with emotional and sociobehavioral problems, often arising from experiences within their families or communities, that require intensive professional services apart from their families. There is also a small group of adolescents whose families choose to have them live away from home, for example, in a boarding school, in order to offer them more opportunities for personal, social, and academic growth than are available in their own community. Finally, a significant number of adolescents are homeless and without shelter or support from their families or community.

The child welfare system is charged with supporting and thus preserving the biologic family as the most desirable intervention for troubled families with children. A number of programs of intensive family support have been developed to preserve families and enhance parents' ability to care for their children. However, these programs are limited in size and number and serve only a small proportion of eligible families. Most families, especially those with adolescents, continue to rely on out-of-home care for dependent youths.

Most of adolescents living out of home have been placed in structured alternative living arrangements. Except for preparatory schools, most of the placements have been arranged by public child welfare or juvenile justice agencies. These agencies strive to select residential settings that provide a therapeutic milieu. These settings form a placement continuum that ranges from individual, family foster homes at one end to residential centers and psychiatric hospitals at the other, with group homes somewhere in between. In theory, the choice of placement should be based on the needs and experiences of the youth. In practice, placement decisions frequently are dictated by the availability and cost of a room or a bed. In addition, placements are commonly viewed hierarchically, and residential care is often used as a placement of last resort rather than as one of a number of options that provide for appropriate care and services to the adolescent.

The explanations of why youths require out-of-home care differ according to whether the reason is thought to be the environment in which the child has been reared (e.g., family and community) or is intrinsic to the adolescent. Most adolescent children in out-of-home care have been physically abused, sexually abused, or neglected. Some of the reasons cited to justify placement are that (1) the parents are unable to control a child's behavior, (2) the child is severely emotionally disturbed and in need of care, (3) an adolescent girl is pregnant, (4) the teenager is substance abusing, or (5) the adolescent has run away from home or been denied access to the family home.

Out-of-home placement should be considered a temporary solution whenever possible. Each teenager's care should be guided by an individualized treatment plan, with long-range goals of reunification with the family, other permanent placement, or emancipation. Good treatment plans begin with an accurate assessment of the adolescent's needs and capabilities—educational, developmental, behavioral, and emotional. A variety of factors including, the age of the adolescent, his or her own strengths, the integrity and functioning of the family, and the availability of community resources, determine whether an adolescent once placed in out-of-home care will ever return to live with the family. These same factors are also central to the success of a placement in helping adolescents attain their potential to function in society.

Adolescence is, by definition, a process of separation from the family and the progressive development of independence and individuation. By focusing too closely on the adolescent's acute needs and finding a safe haven, some programs have disregarded or de-emphasized the ongoing role and influence of the adolescent's family. Families play important roles both as antecedent to the adolescent's current status and as possible supports during the youth's placement and after discharge. Physical separation from the family, often abruptly instituted, is a common occurrence in out-of-home care for adolescents. Although placement decisions are well intended and carefully considered, placement invariably disrupts the emancipation process and disturbs important relationships with peers and families. Good residential care is in many ways a type of family support that provides family-centered care. Many programs espouse a family systems approach to therapy, and maintaining the integrity of the family is a goal of the treatment they provide.

Therapy in the milieu of a residential program also provides some aspects of a substitute family that might be called childrearing if it occurred at home. An important difference is that good out-of-home care protects adolescents from having to meet their care provider's expectations of intimacy. Children and adolescents who have experienced early developmental disruptions, especially of attachments, can have much difficulty settling into new, residential environments. Thus, good programs provide a lot of structure, clear expectations, and emotional and social support.

Foster and residential care are often not a solution but only part of a continuum of care that involves the family and the youth's community. Support services to provide for the adolescent's needs must continue after discharge from the facility or home. Ideally, the overall goal should be to release healthier children to the care of healthier families.

TYPES OF SETTINGS OF OUT-OF-HOME CARE

Foster Home Care

Family foster care is the most frequently used form of out-of-home care. Adolescents usually enter foster care during a crisis such as newly discovered sexual abuse or being thrown out of their home. After a brief stay in an emergency shelter home or facility, and after a preliminary investigation of the family's circumstances, one option is for the child to be placed in a foster home. In general, foster parents are individuals who have applied to open their home to dependent children and youths. They receive a modest monthly stipend and usually a clothing allowance. Most foster parents are raising or have raised their own children. The training that foster parents receive before accepting a child and during the placement is usually minimal and not sufficient to enable them to provide the type of therapeutic care many of these youths need. Almost all adolescents in foster care are eligible for publicly funded health care. However, access to these services may be limited, and the quality of care available may not be sufficient to meet the youths' medical and mental health service needs.

Compared with children in most group care facilities, adolescents in foster family homes find themselves in environments that are more child oriented. Since foster homes are private homes, the space available to an individual adolescent may be limited, but his or her opportunity to be integrated into the local community is greater. Perhaps the greatest advantage to the adolescent in a foster family home is the personalized care that is possible in such a setting. Despite its poverty of resources and professional services, foster home care can be beneficial for adolescents, especially in such areas as school attendance and academic performance.

When adolescents stay in foster care for an extended period, the 18-year age limitation for foster services creates a forced transition to independent living and a serious problem for most of these youths. Unless their foster parents adopt the adolescent, a rare event for a recently placed youth, or voluntarily and without public assistance allow the emancipated adolescent to remain in their home, many of these youths risk homelessness or at least an insecure living situation. The lack of structured preparation for emancipation is a serious problem within the foster care system.

Group Homes and Residential Communities

Individual foster homes are limited in the number of children and youths they can house. In addition to foster homes, adolescents reside in a wide variety of settings that range from community-based group homes with a small number of youths to comprehensive, self-enclosed residential communities. These facilities all have salaried staff who must comply with state licensure requirements that may not apply to volunteer foster parents. Otherwise, there is enormous variability among these settings. Out-of-home care facilities may be run by public agencies, by not-for-profit entities, or by proprietary companies. Staff may be professionally trained or marginally supervised. While some placements are voluntary, most adolescents are placed by the child welfare system or by the juvenile justice system through an order of the courts. The underlying philosophies of care can span a spectrum from militaristic, boot camp regimentation to empathetic, permissive sensitivity groups. In some cases, treatment plans may be intuitive and poorly articulated; in others, they may be based on substantiated research and extensive professional experience. Because of the large number of variables involved in placement and out-of-home care, good evaluation and comparative research is limited.

A number of long-standing problems are common among group care facilities. First, staff salaries are low and benefits poor. Consequently, staff may have little professional training, and staff turnover is high. Quality of care can suffer accordingly. Structured relationships with professional providers of health, mental health or social services may be absent or tenuous, causing there to be little or no supervision and consultative support available to the staff. Mechanisms to ensure communication among caregivers within the group home may be lacking. Similarly, there may be poor communication with the adolescent's family or with professionals working with them outside the facility. There are circumstances in which essential services such as appropriate individual therapy or family counseling may not be provided.

ADOLESCENTS' RESPONSE TO PLACEMENT IN FOSTER OR RESIDENTIAL CARE

Placement in out-of-home care, although sometimes clinically indicated, is a distortion of the usual developmental process of emancipation and can foster maladaptive behavior. Especially during the early phases of out-of-home placement, adolescents in residential care may manifest behavior that is predictable but maladaptive. In ways that are similar to the regressive behavior of highly stressed young children, some adolescents revert to behavior more appropriate of a preadolescent. In both foster home and group care settings, staff often report a "honeymoon" period during which the recently placed adolescent is superficially cooperative and compliant. This behavior is not genuine, and the pseudoconformity and false adaptation provide the adolescent with time to assess the new environment and caretakers. The honeymoon period often is followed by a period of testing during which rebellious, aggressive, or provocative behavior is apparent. Because of their preplacement life experiences within their family, which may have been compounded by multiple placements in the foster care system, adolescents in group care are likely to have difficulty developing emotional attachment with adults. Thus, early measures of success should not rest on interventions that depend on forming bonds with adult caretakers. In addition, teenagers may view removal from their family as a punishment instead of a therapeutic intervention. This response should be openly discussed with the young person by a professional, and the beneficial and nonpunitive aspects of placement should be emphasized early in the placement.

ELEMENTS OF GOOD-QUALITY RESIDENTIAL CARE FOR ADOLESCENTS

Residential care for adolescents is more likely to be successful if (1) the placement matches the youth's needs—clinically, culturally, socially, and personally; (2) the treatment program is based on clearly articulated concepts, and its objectives are well communicated to the adolescent, the family, and the staff; and (3) the adolescent remains in one facility until ready to be reunited with his or her family, adopted or emancipated. The characteristics of good-quality residential care are essentially the same whether the facility is a juvenile detention center, a group or foster home, or a psychiatric hospital.

The physical characteristics of a residential environment should be designed to support the developmental needs of the adolescent. The facility should be attractive and appropriate to adolescents and should include access to television, music, and telephones. It should be well maintained and afford a reasonable degree of privacy. The total number of adolescents in one group should be limited, and the staff-to-adolescent ratio should be sufficiently small to provide adequate supervision and treatment.

Most of the elements of good-quality residential care are the same as those of good parenting. Adolescents in care need to be involved in the major decisions that affect their lives, and to have some personal choice over things such as clothing, food, and recreation. They need to have reliable, consistent, and explicit behavioral limits and expectations. Caregivers should provide abundant emotional support, including the opportunity to safely express anger, fear, and anxiety that is related to placement. Rules will be tested and broken, and expectations of desirable attitudes and behaviors will not be fully met. These circumstances offer opportunities for building and reinforcing respectful and trusting relationships between adolescents and caregivers. Good programs also offer opportunities for adolescents to develop healthy peer relationships and to develop or maintain constructive relationships with their families. Finally, adolescents and their families should be provided with a written list of patients' rights, including rights to privacy and confidentiality, the right to refuse medication and treatment, the prohibition of physical restriction and restraint, and access to legal counsel.

OTHER OUT-OF-HOME LIVING SITUATIONS

Boarding Schools

Attendance at boarding schools usually involves a choice in which the adolescent and family actively participate in the decision to leave home. Boarding schools were first established in the United States in the 1700s. Today, there are approximately 280 boarding schools in North America with nearly 36,000 students in attendance. They can be roughly grouped into three types: (1) schools focusing on academics, (2) schools focusing on special learning needs, and (3) reform or behavior modification schools. The first type includes schools geared to students who have demonstrated high levels of academic achievement, schools for students who require academic motivation to achieve their potential, and schools structured to give students who have failed academically elsewhere another chance. Some specialized schools focus on developing skills for a particular trade, whereas others are designed to serve students with special academic needs due to a learning disability.

The boarding school environment allows students to obtain a comprehensive educational experience in addition to intensive socialization. The low student-to-teacher ratio promotes student-faculty interaction both inside and outside the classroom. Many faculty live on campus, often residing in the student dormitories to function "in loco parentis." School styles and policies vary in this regard, and families should take these styles into consideration when selecting schools. Separation of the adolescent from the family is one of the facets of boarding school existence that can be both beneficial and difficult for the teenager. Families should be aware that the admission selection process gives both students and school staff an opportunity to assess whether a particular school meets the academic and social needs of the individual adolescent. Tuition fees can be quite high, and although most schools have scholarship programs, cost may be prohibitive for many families.

Role of the Healthcare Provider in the Decision to Attend Boarding School

Like other forms of out-of-home care, attendance at a boarding school should never be used as a punishment or threat. Such schools may serve adolescents whose current academic environments are unable to meet their needs or (rarely) those whose family are in crisis and for whom the structured environment of the boarding school may be a temporary haven. Healthcare providers should be aware of the strengths and limitations of the boarding school environment. They should be prepared to help families determine an adolescent's readiness for attendance at such a school. Boarding schools may be particularly helpful when the healthcare provider believes the adolescent may benefit from the neutral environment and that the family may benefit from the separation. Providers should be aware, however, that not all schools have staff trained to deal with dysfunctional families.

The most common reasons for which students at boarding schools seek medical attention are gastritis, first aid, headaches, and fatigue. Immunizations must be up to date and students should be screened for tuberculosis before attendance. Because of the close living quarters in the dormitories, many boarding schools recommend yearly influenza vaccination for all students. Healthcare providers for students attending boarding schools should also keep in mind that, although the environment is structured and supervised, teenagers will continue to engage in risky behaviors. Providers should discuss tobacco product use, drug and alcohol use, and sexual behaviors with all adolescents in boarding school or those about to begin attending. They should be prepared to provide information, preventive services, and (if needed) therapeutic options.

Homeless Youths

Many adolescents are homeless and have no structured living arrangement. Estimates of the number of homeless adolescents in the United States range between 1.3 million and over 2 million annually. Despite these large numbers, homeless youths are among the most understudied of the homeless population. Male and female adolescents are equally represented among the homeless. Most of these come from families in which the parents were divorced or were never married. The Society for Adolescent Medicine has suggested a four-part typology for runaway and homeless youth in the United States. First are *situational runaways,* who make up the largest group, and are teenagers who run away from home for a day or two, most often after a disagreement with parents. Second are *runaways,* who leave home for long periods mostly because of serious problems at home such as abuse, neglect, or conflicts surrounding sexual orientation. Third are *throwaways,* many of whom have been in and out of foster care and have left home because their parents have asked them to leave, have abandoned them, or have subjected them to profound levels of abuse or neglect. Fourth are *systems youth,* who may not have had family contact for a while and were unable to tolerate their current living situation whether it was foster care or residential placement. Whatever the cause of their homelessness, most of these adolescents stay within a

50-mile radius of their family or original living situation; those youths who travel longer distances tend to gravitate toward larger urban areas.

Health Consequences of Homelessness

Previous experiences often encourage homeless adolescents to be mistrustful of adults and systems of care. Homeless youths have serious health needs. They are more likely than their nonhomeless peers to experience depression; suicidal ideation and attempts; alcohol and drug abuse; sexually transmitted diseases (STDs); and hosts of other medical illnesses, including peptic ulcer disease, pharyngitis, sinusitis, tonsillitis, bronchitis, allergies/asthma, upper respiratory infections, pediculosis, and trauma. To provide for their basic needs such as food, clothing, and shelter, up to one quarter of homeless youths may engage in prostitution, otherwise known as "survival sex." Their high rate of sexual activity, low rates of condom use, and high rates of injection drug use put these adolescents at increased risk for HIV infection. These risks are compounded for homosexual or bisexual adolescents or those struggling with sexual identity issues. For physical, monetary, or emotional reasons, homeless adolescents often have limited access to health care. Healthcare providers should maintain an open-minded, nonjudgmental attitude and be sure to include in the social history they obtain whether their adolescent patients are currently homeless or have been in the past. If currently homeless, adolescents should be referred to social services so that safe housing can be arranged and the cause of homelessness explored further with them. Referral for mental health and other specialized services may also be necessary.

Suggested Readings

Child developmental issues: risk factors for abused and neglected children and implications for quality shelter care, Sacramento, CA, 1989, The Children's Research Institute of California.

Colton M: Dimensions of foster and residential care practice, *J Child Psychol Psychiatry* 29:589-600, 1988.

Deisher RW, Rogers WM: The medical care of street youth, *J Adolesc Health* 12:500-503, 1991.

Farrow JA, et al: Health and health needs of homeless and runaway youth: a position paper of the Society for Adolescent Medicine, *J Adolesc Health* 13:717-726, 1992.

Johnson RL: Drug abuse, *Pediatr Rev* 16:197-199, 1995.

Robertson JD: Homeless youth: an overview of the recent literature. In Kryder-Coe JH, Salamon LM, Molnar JM, editors: *Homeless children and youth: a new American dilemma,* New Brunswick, NJ, 1991, Transaction Publishers, pp 33-68.

Stricof RL, et al: HIV seroprevalence in a facility for runaway and homeless adolescents, *Am J Public Health* 81(suppl):50-53, 1991.

Weisman ML: When parents are not in the best interests of the child, *Atlantic Monthly,* July 1994.

CHAPTER 90

Physical Abuse

•

Murray A. Straus and Desmond K. Runyan

The term *physical abuse* usually evokes images of battered babies. The research evidence, however, suggests that physical abuse of adolescents occurs at least as frequently as abuse of infants and toddlers. However, it comes to the attention of child protection services less often because adolescents are less fragile than young children and therefore less likely to require emergency medical care. Nevertheless, physical abuse of adolescents poses serious health risks, especially mental health risks. If healthcare providers are aware of the extent and seriousness of the problem, primary prevention and treatment is facilitated.

DIFFERENTIATING PHYSICAL ABUSE FROM CORPORAL PUNISHMENT

Parents in every state of the United States are permitted to use corporal punishment on minor children in their care. The permission is usually in the form of an exemption from the crime of physical assault. These exemptions give parents the right to use "reasonable force" for purposes of discipline and control. However, the specific acts considered to be reasonable force are not identified by the law. Thus, the boundary between "reasonable force" and "physical abuse" is left to the judgment of the law enforcement and judicial systems. The definition of physical abuse has therefore reflected informal cultural norms concerning what exceeds reasonable force. Perhaps the most important criterion embedded in these cultural norms concerns injury. Essentially,

parents are permitted to use any degree of force that does not result in an injury or does not involve an extremely high risk of injury. This includes hitting a child with traditionally approved objects such as belts and wooden paddles.

There is an inherent tension between the criterion of injury that defines abuse on the basis of infliction of injury and the criterion of abuse as constituting acts that entail a high risk of injury, such as kicking and punching an adolescent, even though in most cases no injury occurs. This is in contrast to physical assault of adults and sexual abuse of children, both defined on the basis of whether the act occurred rather than whether it resulted in an injury. From 1960 to 1970, every state passed legislation to define, prevent, and treat child abuse. The definitional aspect of this legislation, however, changed little. These statutes make the presence of injury the primary criterion but allow for determination of abuse on the basis of a high risk of injury. This may seem to expand the definition to include severe assaults by parents that do not result in an injury, but in practice it is rare for physical abuse to be confirmed unless it results in injury that requires medical attention and treatment. In fact, this is the law in nearly half the states, because their statutes specify that only "serious injury" is reportable abuse.[1] Moreover, this legislation had the ironic effect of reinforcing the right of parents to hit children by declaring that it was not intended to prohibit corporal punishment. Thus, the criminal justice system, the child protective system, and informal cultural norms are in agreement that if an assault by a parent results in an injury that requires medical care, it is physical abuse, but if no injury results, it is simply bad parenting but not child abuse in the legal sense. This principle was illustrated by a New Hampshire Supreme Court ruling that a mother who was hitting her child with a leather belt had not committed physical abuse because the child did not suffer an injury that required medical care.[2] Although the child abuse leg-

This paper is part of a research program on family violence at the Family Research Laboratory, University of New Hampshire, Durham, NH 03824. A publications list will be sent on request. It is a pleasure to express appreciation to Nancy Asdigian for assistance with the literature review and statistical analysis. The work has been supported by grants from several organizations, including National Institute of Mental Health grants T32MH15161.

islation did not clarify the boundary between corporal punishment and physical abuse, it may have laid the basis for long-term change in what is accepted as corporal punishment and what is considered abusive.

CORPORAL PUNISHMENT OF ADOLESCENTS AS A FORM OF ABUSE

There are important reasons to include corporal punishment in a consideration of physical abuse of adolescents. One reason is the evidence that most cases of physical abuse occur when corporal punishment escalates out of control.[3,4] In addition, as shown below, ordinary corporal punishment of adolescents is associated with an increased risk of many serious social and psychologic problems.

Although the law continues to give parents the right to hit adolescents, the cultural norms are changing. Today, even pediatricians who advocate corporal punishment as a mode of discipline say it should be limited to early childhood.[5] Thus, there are grounds for regarding any hitting of adolescents as physical abuse. Using that criterion, the fact that 52% of American parents use corporal punishment on children aged 13 and 14[6] can be taken to mean that over 50% of early adolescents are victims of physical abuse by parents.

PREVALENCE STUDIES

Two main types of data have been used to compute rates of physical abuse of adolescents: reports of abuse to state child protection agencies and interviews with parents in household epidemiologic surveys.

Reports to Child Protection Agencies

CHILD PROTECTIVE SERVICES. The most widely used rates are based on reports to state child protective service (CPS) agencies under the mandatory reporting acts (called CPS data from here on). The statistics on age in the 1994 report[7] show the highest rate of confirmed reports for infants (16 per thousand children). The rate decreases slightly with age and is about 25% lower for children aged 12 to 14 years (12 per thousand). Thereafter the rate decreases more rapidly to about 11 per thousand at ages 15 to 17 years. However, these rates include neglect and sexual abuse as well as physical abuse. About one fourth of all confirmed cases are for physical abuse. If this proportion also applies to adolescents, it means a rate of physical abuse of about 3 per thousand children aged 12 to 14 years, and about 2.3 per thousand children aged 15 to 17 years.

The CPS data measure treatments or other interventions in the form of someone reporting and a subsequent investigation. Since many cases are unknown and there is therefore, no report or investigation, the CPS data underestimate the prevalence of abuse. Moreover, as pointed out earlier, the older the child, the lower are the chances of an attack resulting in injury and thus of being reported and confirmed. Consequently, the decrease with age in the CPS rate may reflect age differences in reporting rather than a lesser underlying prevalence.

NATIONAL INCIDENCE STUDIES. Another source of data for estimating physical abuse of adolescents is the National Incidence Studies (NIS) conducted in 1980 and 1986.[8,9] The NIS interviewed a variety of human service professionals in a national sample of 29 counties. The respondents were asked for information on all instances of children who had suffered demonstrable harm from maltreatment in the previous 12 months. The NIS data include only cases known to service providers. Consequently, the NIS data, like the CPS data, result in a measure that is closer to an intervention rate than to a prevalence rate. A key difference, however, is that the service providers were asked about all cases, regardless of whether they had been reported to CPS. The inclusion of cases that were not officially reported probably explains why the 1986 NIS rate (6 per thousand for children aged 12 to 17 years[10]) is almost 2.5 times higher than the estimate from CPS reports. The NIS findings on adolescents also differ from the CPS rates in demonstrating a greater prevalence of physical abuse of adolescents than that of younger children. This, too, could be the result of including cases that are known but not officially reported because these did not involve an injury that required medical attention.

Household Epidemiologic Surveys

NATIONAL FAMILY VIOLENCE SURVEYS. These surveys (NFVS), conducted in 1975, 1985, and 1992,[11,12] interviewed one parent from each household in large and nationally representative samples. The NFVS measured physical abuse by means of the Conflict Tactics Scales (CTS).[13,14] The CTS ask parents about how often they engaged in each of a list of acts during the previous 12 months when they had trouble with a randomly selected child. These acts are used to compute four scales: nonviolent discipline (e.g., explaining), psychologic aggression (e.g., calling the child a name), corporal punishment (e.g., slapping or spanking), and physical abuse (e.g., kicking or punching).

The physical abuse rate for children aged 12 to 17 years in the NFVS was about 25 per thousand in all three surveys, which is ten times greater than the CPS rate and four times greater than the NIS rate. Moreover, these are lower bound estimates because it can be assumed that some of the parents interviewed did not disclose instances of abuse. In addition, only one parent was interviewed in each household. If the rate of 25 per thousand applies to the 24 million U.S. adolescents, it means that a minimum of 600,000 adolescents were severely assaulted by one of their parents during the survey year. Fortunately, this does not mean 600,000 adolescents required medical care, because the NFVS measured severe assaults in terms of parents, not injuries. Typical severe assault of an adolescent does not always result in an injury that comes to medical attention.

SURVEY OF ADOLESCENTS. Beginning in 1990, the Youth Risk Behavior Surveys (YRBS), survey of adolescents in grades 9 to 12, have been sponsored by the Centers for Disease Control and Prevention. The 1993 Oregon survey included three questions about physical abuse. The survey asked whether the person had ever been physically abused (hit, kicked, or struck with an object) when not involved in a fight. It also asked when was the last time this occurred and whether the adolescent tried to talk with someone about it.[15] This survey was administered to 3211 students in 25 high schools in Oregon, using a stratified cluster design. A total of 32% of the adolescents reported that they had ever been abused. For some the abuse was quite recent, 3.7% reported having been abused in the past week, and 16.3% reported that the most recent occurrence was in the last year. This rate is dramatically higher than that reported by the other sources.

Subsequent Trends

Reports of abuse to child protective services increased steadily since these data began to be compiled in 1976. The 1988 NIS also found a substantially higher rate than the first NIS found in 1980. Child maltreatment rates based on CPS and NIS reports roughly doubled from 1980 to 1990. However, for adolescents the rates were the same in all three NFVS. These seemingly contradictory trends are consistent if it is recognized that the CPS and NIS data measure interventions to treat and prevent child abuse, and that the focus of these interventions has been on infants and young children. To the extent that these interventions are effective, it should result in a decrease in the incidence rates for young children, but not for adolescents, and that is exactly what the NFVS have found. This should not be taken to mean that treatment and prevention efforts are the only, or even the main, reason for the decrease in the prevalence of physical abuse found by the NFVS. Many other changes in American society also served to lower the risk of child maltreatment, including a decrease in the prevalence of

alcoholism, later marriage, more equalitarian marriages, and fewer children per couple. These have probably outweighed other changes that increase the risk of child abuse, such as a growing underclass, the crack cocaine epidemic, and a greater proportion of children in one-parent households.

CLINICAL CHARACTERISTICS

Adolescents versus Younger Children

Three of the four sources of data on the prevalence of physical abuse permit comparison by age. The three studies provide conflicting data over whether the rate of physical abuse of adolescents differs from that for younger children. The CPS report data indicate less abuse of adolescents, the NIS data indicate more abuse of adolescents than of younger children, and the NFVS found about equal rates for all age groups. The higher rate for younger children in the CPS reports probably occurs because younger children are more likely to be injured and thus to be confirmed as cases of physical abuse. Similarly, the equal rates of abuse of adolescents and younger children in the NFVS may occur because those surveys counted severe assaults such as kicking or punching a child as abuse, regardless of whether an injury occurred.

Adolescent and Family Characteristics

Analyses of the NFVS show that more boys than girls are physically abused, and that the difference becomes greater as children age. Adolescent boys are physically abused twice as often as girls. The rates of abuse by mothers and fathers also change as children grow older. Although among infants the rate of abuse by mothers is about five times greater than that by fathers, the rate of physical abuse of adolescents by fathers is about double that by mothers.

A similar reversal of differences between white and minority children occurs with age. Among infants and toddlers, the rate for minority children in the NFVS was half again greater than for white children, but among adolescents it was half again greater for whites.

In contrast to the NFVS, data from the YRBS for high school girls reported a higher rate of physical abuse for the past year than for boys (17.6% vs. 14.8%). However, the definition used in the YRBS did not specify that the perpetrator be a parent. Dating violence or other unprovoked hitting may have been included by the girls. There were no differences in reports of physical abuse by high school students in terms of race of urban versus rural origin in the YRBS in Oregon.

ETIOLOGY OF ADOLESCENT ABUSE

Onset During Adolescence

Little is known about the extent to which abuse of adolescents begins during the adolescent years as opposed to cases that are a continuation of a long-standing pattern. This information could be helpful in determining prevention and treatment, because the dynamics of adolescent-onset abuse might be different from those of early-onset abuse. Libbey and Bybee[1] found that in nearly half their 24 cases abuse began in adolescence, and that these cases were less often characterized by major disorganization and parental inadequacy than early-onset cases. This is consistent with the report of Moran and Eckenrode,[16] who found that adolescent onset is associated with a lower risk of psychologic injury to the child. It is also consistent with the theory that much adolescent abuse occurs as a response by previously nonabusive parents to delinquency and rebelliousness emerging during adolescence. If this is correct, treatment and primary prevention of such cases must include work with the adolescent as well as the parents.

Etiologic Theories

Libbey and Bybee[1] argue that understanding abuse of adolescents requires considering not only the characteristics of the parents but also the characteristics of the child, and the social circumstances of the family such as stress, poverty, and social isolation. They identify theories that emphasize one or the other of these three types of etiologic factors, starting with what might be called "developmental vulnerability" theories. These theories postulate that the developmental tasks of separation and control during adolescence make the adolescent vulnerable. What they perceive to be the typical case involves parents who have not previously abused but who, in responding to adolescent misbehavior may tend to "go too far."

A second theoretical approach involves parental "inadequacy theories." Researchers who advocate this perspective focus on characteristics of the parents that put them at risk of abusing an adolescent, such as psychopathology, alcoholism, disorganized and dysfunctional family patterns, and rigid and controlling discipline.

The third theoretical approach is "sociologic." These theories focus on socially generated stresses such as social isolation, unemployment, and poverty.

As useful as it is to identify the predominant focus of these three theories, Libbey and Bybee emphasize that "all of these models include the relation parent + child + crises = abuse." In addition, although they do not identify it as a theory, these authors put forward what can be called an escalation from corporal punishment theory.[3,4] They

report that 22 of the 24 most recent abusive incidents were immediately preceded by "typical adolescent-parent conflicts." They also found that most of the abusing parents believed they were disciplining the youth.

PSYCHOSOCIAL HEALTH RISKS ASSOCIATED WITH PHYSICAL ABUSE

Physically abused adolescents experience a greater risk of a wide variety of psychosocial and behavioral problems than other adolescents. The YRBS found a strong association between a history of abuse and a variety of serious outcomes. When adolescents who were physically abused were compared with those who were not, the odds for a poor self-image were 1.6; the odds for having seriously considered suicide in the past year, 2.1; the odds for alcohol, cigarettes, and marijuana use, all approximately 1.7; and the odds for more than three sex partners in a lifetime and for involvement in a pregnancy, 1.9. Aggressive behaviors in physically abused adolescents were also increased. The odds of fighting in the previous year were increased to 2.2 and the odds for carrying a weapon in the past 30 days were 1.9. These findings are all consistent with previously reported associations.[15]

As mentioned previously, in addition to physical abuse, over half of American adolescents experience less severe assaults by parents in the form of corporal punishment, such as a slap in the face.[6,17] This widely occurring practice is associated with an increased risk of such problems as depression, delinquency, and impaired school performance in the adolescent.[18]

PREVENTION AND TREATMENT

Primary Prevention

Because over 90% of parents spank and slap toddlers, and just over 50% use corporal punishment on adolescents, it is likely that most abuse of adolescents represents an escalation of a pattern that began with slapping the hand of an infant. This suggests that the most important step for primary prevention of adolescent abuse is the same as the most important primary prevention step to prevent physical abuse of young children: total avoidance of corporal punishment as a means of discipline.[4] A prevention approach that begins with avoiding corporal punishment of toddlers is also likely to apply to parents who gradually reduce the amount of corporal punishment as the child grows older. About 40% stop by the time the child is 10 or 11 years old.[18] For these parents, the onset of adolescence, with attendant difficulties in monitoring and directing the child's behavior, can lead some to revert to corporal punishment. During adolescence, a slap in the face for "mouthing off" or staying out late carries a greater risk of escalation into physical abuse because the adolescent may retaliate verbally or physically. The furious parent may use physical force in retaliation.

Treatment

Treatment and secondary prevention is more difficult because it often involves addressing the combination of an entrenched pattern of harsh but inconsistent discipline, including corporal punishment, and the acting out of rebellious youth.[19,20] The combination manifests itself as a vicious circle of coercion, abuse, and acting out. To end this pattern, parents can be helped (1) to understand that corporal punishment, especially at this age, is counterproductive; and (2) to learn and practice more effective disciplinary methods.

Mandatory reporting laws require the reporting of abuse of adolescents to child protective service agencies in all 50 states. The process of recognizing and reporting adolescent abuse can serve to begin a discussion directed at helping the family and the adolescent. Treatment begins at the point of recognition of the problem through the responses of the observing professional. It may first be necessary to deal with concerns related to making the mandatory report. Protective service agency involvement connotes both treatment and punishment. In most states the protective service agency must share all confirmed reports with police authorities. However, child protective service agencies have a mandate to protect the child and preserve the family. The risk of foster home placement and/or criminal prosecution is low. Adolescents whose physical abuse is substantiated by protective service agencies are less likely to be put into foster care than either adolescents associated with sexual abuse allegations or younger children.[21] This may result from the increased difficulty in finding placements for adolescents, or from a perception by CPS workers that physical abuse of adolescents is less serious.

Successful treatment of adolescent abuse is likely to involve multiple agencies and disciplines working with families. In addition to working with parents, treatment may involve agencies that deal with the adolescent's behaviors. The schools, courts, police, and protective service agencies all play an important role in supporting the adolescent and the family engaged in treatment. Treatment must be directed at the child and parents as individuals and at the family unit. The behaviors and responses of abusing parents and their children have developed over a long time. Consequently, treatment is not likely to be brief.[22]

The more effective treatments are based on the discipline already practiced by almost all parents, but not consistently enough. These include providing clear standards and expectations, recognizing and praising good behavior, and the sparing use of nonviolent punishments.[23] The behavior of the acting-out or rebellious youth must also be addressed. Just as parents need to understand that corporal punishment is counterproductive and dangerous, adolescents should recognize that the defiance and delinquency are also counterproductive. The methods of resolving conflicts with peers being taught in school-based violence prevention programs are also effective in preventing conflicts with parents. Mediation is an element of these programs that is applicable to parent-child conflict. In some states such as New Hampshire, parent-child mediation is currently the largest single category of cases among members of the mediators association.

Adolescents experience a very high rate of severe physical violence by parents. In addition, just over half of early teenagers experience less dangerous forms of violence by parents, such as a slap. Although the less serious violence rarely results in a physical injury requiring treatment, it puts the child at an increased risk of serious social and psychologic problems resulting in reduced school performance, violence, delinquency, and depression.[18,24] Efforts to prevent and treat abuse for all children under age 18 are explicit national goals for the year 2000.[25] Adolescents must be included as beneficiaries in this national enterprise.

References

1. Libbey P, Bybee R: The physical abuse of adolescents, *J Soc Issues,* 35:101-126, 1979.
2. NH vs Johnson. No. 90-533 (Supreme Court, Hillsborough. June 25, 1992). 1992;.
3. Kadushin A, Martin JA: *Child abuse: an interactional event,* New York, 1981, Columbia University Press.
4. Straus MA, Yodanis CL: Physical abuse. In Straus MA, editor: *Beating the devil out of them: corporal punishment,* San Francisco, 1994, Jossey-Bass/Lexington Books, pp 81-97.
5. Trumbull DA, Ravenel D, Larson D: Letter to editor: corporal punishment, *Pediatrics* 96:792-793, 1995.
6. Straus MA, Donnelly DA: Hitting adolescents. In Straus M, editor: *Beating the devil out of them: corporal punishment in American families.* San Francisco, 1994, Lexington/Jossey-Bass, pp 35-48.
7. National Center on Child Abuse and Neglect: *Child maltreatment 1993: reports from the states to the National Center on Child Abuse and Neglect,* Washington, DC, 1995, U.S. Government Printing Office.
8. National Center on Child Abuse and Neglect: *Study findings: National Study of Incidence and Severity of Child Abuse and Neglect,* Washington, DC, 1981, Department of Health and Human Services.
9. National Center on Child Abuse and Neglect: *Study findings: Study of National Incidence and Prevalence of Child Abuse and Neglect,* Washington, DC, 1988, Department of Health and Human Services.
10. Sedlak AJ: *Supplementary analyses of data on the national incidence of child abuse and neglect,* 1991, National Clearinghouse on Child Abuse and Neglect.
11. Straus MA, Gelles RJ: *Physical violence in American families: risk factors and adaptations to violence in 8,145 families,* New Brunswick, NJ, 1990, Transaction Publishers.

12. Straus MA, Kaufman Kantor G: *Trends in physical abuse by parents from 1975 to 1992: a comparison of three national surveys.* In Annual Meeting of the American Society of Criminology, Boston, MA, 1995.

13. Straus MA, Hamby SL: Measuring physical and psychological maltreatment of children with the Conflict Tactics Scales. In Kaufman Kanto G, Jasinski JL, editors: *Out of the darkness: contemporary perspectives on family violence,* Thousand Oaks, Calif., 1997, Sage.

14. Straus MA, Hamby SL, Finkelhor D, Moore DW, Runyan D: Identification of child maltreatment with the Parent-Child Conflict Tactics Scale (CTSPC): development and psychometric data for a national sample of American parents, *Child Abuse Negl* (in press).

15. Nelson D, Higginson G, Grant-Worley J: Physical abuse among high school students, *Arch Pediatr Adolesc Med* 149:1254-1258, 1995.

16. Moran P, Eckenrode J: Protective personality characteristics among adolescent victims of maltreatment, *Child Abuse Negl* 16:743-754, 1992.

17. Straus MA, Donnelly DA: Corporal punishment of adolescents by American parents, *Youth Society* 24:419-442, 1993.

18. Straus MA: *Beating the devil out of them: corporal punishment in American families,* San Francisco, 1994, Jossey-Bass/Lexington Books.

19. Patterson G: *Parents and adolescents: living together: Part 1: The basics,* Eugene, OR, 1987, Castalia Publishing.

20. Forgatch M, Patterson G: *Parents and adolescents: living together: Part 2: Family problem solving,* Eugene, OR, 1989, Castalia Publishing.

21. Runyan D, Trost D, Loda F: The determinants of foster care for the maltreated child, *Am J Public Health* 71:706-711, 1981.

22. Kaplan S: Adolescent abuse, *Womens Health Issues* 4:65-67, 1994.

23. Burke RV, Herron RW: *Common sense parenting: a practical approach from Boys Town,* Boys Town, NE, 1992, Boys Town Press.

24. Durant RH, Getts A, Cadenhead C, Emans SJ, Woods ER: Exposure to violence and vicitimization and depression, hopelessness, and purpose of life among adolescents living in and around public housing, *J Dev Behav Pediatr* 16:233-237, 1995.

25. Public Health Service: *Healthy people 2000: national health disease prevention objectives,* 1991, U.S. Department of Health and Human Services.

CHAPTER 91

Peer Relationships

•

Gary W. Ladd and Jennifer T. Parkhurst

Adolescents' peer relationships are an important resource for individual and interpersonal growth. It is within this context that they search for a sense of identity and self-worth. Moreover, through participation in peer relationships, most adolescents learn important lessons about interpersonal trust, intimacy, and commitment. Yet adolescents' peer relationships are also the stage on which many traumas and difficulties are acted out, often to the dismay of both family members and helping professionals.

Efforts to understand or evaluate adolescents' peer relationships, especially if the aim is to identify potential risks and resources for their health and development, require careful consideration of several key focal points, including adolescents' social history, personal characteristics, search for autonomy, social competence, and peer relationships.

SOCIAL HISTORY

It is often helpful to begin the assessment by examining the history of the adolescent's peer relationships during childhood. This focus can be summarized in the following question: What were the adolescent's previous peer relationships like, and how might they have contributed to the current situation? Interpersonal and peer relationship problems, especially serious ones, may have their roots in childhood.[1] For example, antisocial tendencies, such as the display of aggression and violent behavior, often emerge during childhood and remain stable over time. Rejection or alienation from peers is also a relatively stable characteristic during childhood and adolescence. Not surprisingly, it is strongly related to the display of antisocial and deviant forms of behavior in the peer group. Moreover, both antisocial behavior and peer rejection in childhood are among the best predictors of adjustment difficulties in adolescence and early adulthood, including mental health problems, school truancy and failure, and delinquency.[2]

PERSONAL CHARACTERISTICS

A second question to consider is: What personal characteristics may affect the ease or difficulty with which adolescents negotiate peer relations? Physical maturation and its timing appear to create both benefits and risks for the young adolescent.[3] Teenagers who mature early are often popular with their peers. However, the social risks associated with early maturation can be substantial for both males and females. Adolescents who appear more mature than is typical for their age are more likely to be drawn into family conflicts and relationships with older peers. Moreover, in the context of older peers, adolescents are expected to conform to more advanced norms and pressures. Those adolescents who mature early are likely to feel greater pressure at a young age to engage in sexual relationships, experiment with alcohol and drugs, and defy parental authority. Early-maturing males may be at greater risk for family conflict and rebellious behavior, especially with their mothers.[4] Early-maturing females may encounter higher risks because they are often pursued by older males and, as a result, tend to experience higher levels of parental restriction and punishment. Also, females who mature early, unlike their male counterparts, tend to develop more internalizing disorders, such as lower levels of self-esteem.

BECOMING A SEPARATE, INDEPENDENT PERSON

Parents' concerns about their adolescent's choice of friends and activities with peers are the problems presented to physicians and counselors in many cases. Family conflicts in these areas may be skirmishes in larger battles over the adolescent's attempts at self-determination. Where this is true, a third question to be addressed is: What avenues are available to the adolescent to establish autonomy while satisfying his or her needs for connectedness with others?

To establish a sense of autonomy, and ultimately a separate (or at least a seemingly self-established) identity, many adolescents choose to distance themselves from family members and family activities and to challenge parental authority and regulations. One result is often less closeness between the adolescent and other family members.[5] Instead, needs for connectedness with others are often met through relationships with peers. Time-use studies show that, by the early to middle teens, most adolescents spend more waking hours with peers than with parents or siblings.[6] Because peer norms are often at odds with family values, peer group pressures compete directly with parental demands for many teenagers, creating internal conflict for them and often overt conflict with family members.

About 15% to 20% of families in the United States experience severe and persistent parent-adolescent conflict, and an additional 15% to 20% must cope with occasional or sporadic crises.[7] Both parents and adolescents may contribute to the severity of conflicts. Parents may fail to adjust their expectations to permit some forms of autonomy seeking by their adolescent child and to include him or her in decision making. This may inadvertently promote rebelliousness and stronger ties with peers. Adolescents may contribute to these conflicts by choosing dysfunctional ways to achieve independence from the family, and by associating with a peer group that supports antisocial behavior.

Escalating cycles of conflict between parents and adolescents often emerge when parents respond to rebellious behavior and negative peer group involvement by tightening their controls. Such action may precipitate more extreme forms of behavior or a total disregard for parental sanctions. Conflicts also tend to be exacerbated by other issues or problems in the family, such as divorce, midlife crises, unemployment, and poverty.[8] In such cases, relief from the conflict may require attention to the family's basic needs.

Tensions are often eased when parents allow adolescents means to gain independence, to participate in making decisions, and to form an identity that is not totally defined by the parents. There is also less conflict when one or both parents are able to maintain an emotional tie with their adolescent. It is important for parents to nurture such ties by empathizing with the adolescent's needs and increasing their connection with him or her in areas of common interest. In some cases, professional assistance in the form of counseling or family therapy may be needed.

ONGOING PEER RELATIONSHIPS

Research suggests that membership in peer groups and friendship plays an important role in adolescent health and development. However, the specific contributions of each form of relationship differ, and it is also important to consider the quality of the relationships that adolescents develop with peers. For diagnostic purposes, a fourth focal point can be summarized with the question: What kinds of peer relationships has the adolescent developed or failed to develop?

Adolescent peer groups are seldom homogeneous and tend to fragment into a number of crowds, each possessing a separate identity or social reputation.[9] Adolescents are very aware of these crowds and often invent names to describe them (e.g., nerds, jocks, druggies, dirts). Moreover, individuals begin to define themselves and others by their membership in particular crowds.

Crowds affect their members in various ways. The internal dynamics of peer groups lead to various forms of social organization, including status hierarchies. Group members may develop more or less status, depending on the degree to which they possess characteristics valued by the group, such as toughness, attractiveness, or humor. Adolescents who become members of "popular" groups or achieve higher status within a group tend to feel greater self-esteem.

Crowds also establish their own sets of norms for behavior and expect members to conform to these. Typically, the pressure adolescents feel to conform stems from their fear of censure or rejection by the group. Conformity pressures are strongest during early adolescence. Although peer pressure is implicated in various forms of adolescent deviance (e.g., substance abuse, sexual promiscuity, delinquency, and criminality), conformity demands often support activities that are consistent with parental and societal values (e.g., school achievement, sports). Thus, the conformity pressures exerted by a given crowd may work for or against adult values.

Adolescents differ in their susceptibility to peer pressures. Adolescents who have low self-esteem and lack friendships tend to be more susceptible; those who have many close ties and sources of support appear to be less vulnerable to peer pressure.[10] Parents are an important part of this network and can help to offset negative peer pressures if they are able to maintain a close emotional relationship with the adolescent.

Friendships, unlike crowds, are dyadic in nature and represent a voluntary rather than an imposed form of relationship. Children and adolescents derive considerable support from their friendships, which help to buffer stress and promote coping in many types of life situations.[11] Both same-sex and opposite-sex friendships become an important source of closeness and companionship for adolescents, especially during high school and early college years. By late adolescence, teenagers rely less on peer groups and more on friendships to meet their needs for support and identity. This shift helps to explain why peer conformity pressures decline throughout high school.

Children and adolescents who lack friendships or who are rejected by peer groups appear to be vulnerable to loneliness, depression, and interpersonal anxiety.[12] Although most adolescents are lonely at one time or another, 15% to 20% of U.S adolescents suffer from severe and persistent loneliness and social alienation.[13] These and other forms of social dissatisfaction are often cited as a basis for the rising rates of adolescent suicide.

Reactions to severe loneliness vary. Adolescents who attribute social difficulties to external causes, or perceive that they have little control over their lives, may blame others and react against their social situations. These adolescents may be more likely to perpetuate antisocial acts, run away from home, use drugs, or drop out of school. Adolescents who blame themselves for their social difficulties may be at greater risk for depression, anxiety, and suicide.

SOCIAL COMPETENCE

To be socially competent means that one's social presentation and behavior is of a kind that others will approve. Adolescents' social competence in the area of peer relations is reflected in their acceptance and prestige among their peers. Another diagnostic question to be asked, then, is: Is this adolescent's self-presentation and behavior of a kind that will gain him or her adequate liking and standing among peers? Those adolescents who are most popular with their peers tend to be those who avoid deviant behaviors; whose grooming, dress, and manners conform to widely accepted norms; who are perceived to be friendly, cooperative, kind, supportive, and trustworthy; and who have a good sense of humor and widely shared interests and values. While they stick up for themselves, they do not engage in disruptive or hurtful behaviors or provoke fights, and, although often leaders, they are not "stuck up." These characteristics overlap with, yet also differ from, those characteristics associated with *perceived* popularity. Being perceived as popular by peers is not the same as actually being popular. Those adolescents who are perceived to be popular tend to

be those with greatest social dominance and prestige. Prestige and perceived popularity are more strongly associated than is actual popularity with being self-assured and outgoing, being able to hold one's own in conflicts, being a leader, excelling at sports (among boys), being attractive and fashionable (among girls), holding a position of importance at school (e.g., team member, cheerleader), and obtaining membership in a high-status peer group.[14] Perceived popularity is less strongly associated than is actual popularity with being nice; indeed, those perceived to be most popular are often seen as aggressive and "stuck up."[15]

Two behavioral styles have been identified as maladaptive because they contribute to rejection and/or lack of social standing among young adolescents.[16] A pattern of aggressive and disruptive behavior, especially if accompanied by a lack of positive qualities, often leads to dislike and rejection. However, aggressive adolescents are often perceived as more popular than they actually are, often have little awareness of the extent of their actual rejection, and (even if rejected) often experience relatively little loneliness. A second pattern of behavior consisting of oversensitivity, timidity, unassertiveness, undue submissiveness, and withdrawal from social interaction is associated with rejection, low social dominance, and low perceived popularity. Extreme shyness and social withdrawal can put young adolescents at risk for being misperceived as unfriendly and "stuck up," while undue submissiveness appears to put them at risk for being bullied. Rejected adolescents with this behavioral style are commonly aware of their poor acceptance, often worry about being teased and pushed around, and for both reasons frequently experience extreme levels of loneliness. They are also often characterized by particular vulnerability to feelings of shame and depression and other internalizing problems.

Peer rejection, especially when it begins during childhood and continues into adolescence, may be a source of many other problems and may itself contribute to social incompetence, maintaining a self-defeating cycle that, once established, may be difficult to modify. Adolescents often react to rejection by either withdrawing from peers or acting out against their rejection in aggressive and disruptive ways. Children who are rejected over long periods often develop debilitating self-perceptions. Moreover, prolonged rejection may remove children and adolescents from important learning experiences in the peer group, and erode their social skills and interpersonal confidence.

TEASING AND VICTIMIZATION

Another question that should be asked is: How well does the adolescent handle teasing, and to what extent is the adolescent either the victim or the perpetrator of bullying?

Young adolescents care a great deal about their acceptance and influence among peers. They also have much greater capacities for introspection and for understanding and predicting others' feelings, motives, and reactions than do children. These characteristics make them more self-conscious and vulnerable to embarrassment, humiliation, and shame and simultaneously more adept at inducing such reactions in their peers. Combined with a strong value placed (especially during early adolescence) on maintaining poise and on controlling the expression of negative and tender feelings, these attributes contribute to a great deal of teasing among adolescents. Teasing ranges from friendly teasing that is meant to convey affection indirectly or to communicate criticism without producing hurt feelings, to cruel teasing that is clearly designed to cause humiliation, either in order to induce pain or in order to establish dominance.

It is an important social task of early adolescence to develop the abilities to distinguish between friendly and hostile teasing, to respond to teasing appropriately, to direct teasing away from hostile exchanges toward more friendly ones, and to keep one's own teasing within appropriate bounds. Research suggests that those adolescents fare best socially who can take friendly teasing and respond to it in kind; who react to less friendly teasing with spunk, poise, and humor; and who do not engage in excessive or cruel teasing of others.

Hurtful teasing is only one of several forms of bullying that can be observed among adolescents, especially young adolescents. Besides ridiculing peers, calling them names, and making verbal threats against them, adolescents may subject peers to physical attack or intimidation, ostracize them, spread damaging rumors, play cruel jokes, put peers in humiliating social situations, or engage in sexual harassment.

Adolescents are more likely to be victimized if they are widely rejected and if they are oversensitive and easy to push around. The last type of problem may be contributed to by physical slightness and ineptness, and also by an unassertive behavioral style. Studies of children and adolescents indicate that being subjected to persistent bullying can produce immediate loneliness, depression, and negative attitudes toward school. Longitudinal studies of bullied young adolescents have also shown that being victimized by peers can lead to a lasting drop in self-esteem and to increased vulnerability to depression in adulthood.[17]

Adolescents are more likely to bully others if their parents have been unaffectionate and harsh in their dealings with them or have permitted their children to be cruel. Bullies tend to have high self-esteem, which they support through their domination of others. While bullying peers is socially maladaptive, and may be a precursor

of similar behavior in adult relationships, bullies tend to have an entourage of hangers-on whose reactions encourage them to behave as they do. Bullying is a problem that can be addressed through the establishment by schools of effective antibullying programs.[18]

In summary, during adolescence, the peer culture serves as one of the most important contexts for psychological growth and development. The adolescent's peer relationships take many forms and serve many functions, some of which may pose both risks and resources for health and development. It is important for professionals who wish to understand and effect change in the social lives of adolescents to assess their social history, the interface between their physical and social maturation, their strategies for resolving autonomy needs, their social competence, and their friendship and peer-group relations.

References

1. Ladd GW: Friendship patterns and peer status during early and middle childhood, *J Dev Behav Pediatr* 9:229-238, 1988.
2. Parker J, Asher SR: Peer acceptance and later interpersonal adjustment: are low accepted children at risk?, *Psychol Bull* 102:357-389, 1987.
3. Simmons RG, Burgeson R, Carlton-Ford S, Blyth DA: The impact of cumulative change in early adolescence, *Child Dev* 58:1220-1234, 1987.
4. Steinberg L: Impact of puberty on family relations: effects of pubertal status and pubertal timing, *Dev Psychol* 23:451-460, 1987.
5. Steinberg L: Reciprocal relation between parent-child distance and pubertal maturation, *Dev Psychol* 24:122-128, 1988.
6. Csikszentmihalyi M, Larson R: *Being adolescent,* New York, 1984, Basic Books.
7. Montemayor R: Family variation in parent-adolescent storm and stress, *J Adolesc Res* 1:15-31, 1986.
8. Silverberg SB, Steinberg L: Adolescent autonomy, parent-adolescent conflict, and parental well-being, *J Youth Adolesc* 16:293-312, 1987.
9. Brown BB: The role of peer groups in adolescents' adjustment to secondary school. In Berndt TJ, Ladd GW, editors: *Peer relationships in child development,* New York, 1989, John Wiley, pp 188-215.
10. Delgato-Gaitan C: Adolescent peer influence and differential school performance, *J Adolesc Res* 1:449-462, 1986.
11. Berndt TJ: The features and effects of friendship in early adolescence, *Child Dev* 53:1447-1460, 1983.
12. Asher SR, Parkhurst JT, Hymel S, Williams GA: Peer rejection and loneliness in childhood. In Asher SR, Coie JD, editors: *Peer rejection in childhood,* New York, 1990, Cambridge University Press, pp 253-273.
13. Brennan T: Loneliness in adolescence. In Peplau LA, Perlman D, editors: *Loneliness: a sourcebook of current theory, research and therapy,* New York, 1982, John Wiley; pp 269-290.
14. Weisfeld GE, Block SA, Ivers JW: Possible determinants of social dominance among adolescent goals, *J Genet Psychol* 144:115-129, 1984.
15. Eder D: The cycle of popularity: interpersonal relations among female adolescents, *Sociol Educ* 15:154-165, 1985.
16. Parkhurst JT, Asher SR: Peer rejection in middle school: subgroup differences in behavior, loneliness, and interpersonal concerns, *Dev Psychol* 28:231-241, 1992.
17. Olweus D: Victimization by peers: antecedents and long-term

outcomes. In Rubin KH, Asendorpf JB, editors: *Social withdrawal, inhibition, and shyness in childhood,* Hillsdale, NJ, 1993, Lawrence Erlbaum Associates.

18. Olweus D: *Aggression in the schools: bullies and whipping boys,* New York, 1978, John Wiley.

Suggested Readings

Berndt TJ, Ladd GW: *Peer relationships in child development,* New York, 1989, John Wiley.

Reviews of research by prominent investigators on the contributions of friendships and peer relations to child and adolescent development; topics include relationship processes, family and school contexts, and intervention strategies.

Kupersmidt JB, Coie JD, Dodge KA: The role of poor peer relationships in the development of disorder. In Asher SR, Coie JD, editors: *Peer rejection in childhood,* New York, 1990, Cambridge University Press; pp 253-273.

An excellent review of research on the linkages between problematic childhood peer relations and adjustment problems during adolescence and adulthood.

Parke RD, Ladd GW: *Family-peer relations: modes of linkage,* Hillsdale, NJ, 1992, Lawrence Erlbaum Associates.

Reviews of research on family factors that influence the development of children's and adolescents' competence in peer relations; topics include parenting styles, discipline, divorce, abuse/maltreatment, and parental psychopathology.

Simmons RG, Blyth DA: *Moving into adolescence: the impact of pubertal change and school context,* Hawthorne, NY, 1987, Aldine de Gruyer.

A review of research and findings from impressive longitudinal studies on pubertal growth and psychosocial development during adolescence.

CHAPTER 92

The Media

•

Victor C. Strasburger

Children have more need of models than of critics.
        Joseph Joubert

Children have never been very good at listening to elders, but they have never failed to imitate them.
        James Baldwin

After parents and peers, the media probably constitute the single greatest influence on adolescents today. The media present "idealized" versions of parents and peers to teenagers—role models discussing everything from sex and alcohol to food and careers. The media's role as a powerful teacher, shaping attitudes and influencing behavior, is known as the *cultivation effect.* For example, it is well known that heavy viewers of television tend to believe that the television world is "real" and that people in everyday life should behave accordingly. The cultivation effect has an even more significant impact when adult society refuses to permit widespread dissemination of information, such as sex education in the schools, and the media must fill an important gap as a source of information, however inaccurate it sometimes may be.

Teenagers spend more time watching television and listening to the radio than they do performing any other activity except sleeping. By the time today's children reach age 70, they will have spent 7 to 10 years of their lives watching television. Thus, the media also exert a *displacement effect:* because so much time is spent watching television, other, less passive activities (e.g., reading, sports, hobbies) are shortchanged.

Aside from the displacement effect, the media are neither intrinsically good nor bad. They can teach pro-social ideas just as easily and effectively as antisocial ones. Unfortunately, the United States has the least socially responsible media in the Western world, and American society pays the price with high rates of pregnancy, suicide, violence, and alcohol abuse among teenagers.

TYPES OF MEDIA

Television

Of all the media, television ranks as the most important influence on youth because of its accessibility and its effectiveness as a "teacher." On average, young people aged 5 to 17 years spend more time in front of the television set (15,000 to 18,000 hours) during those 13 years than they do in formal classroom instruction (12,000 hours). Although younger children watch more television, teenagers spend 21 to 23 hours a week watching television. With the advent of cable, video-cassette recorders, videogames, and Music Television (MTV), this figure may be an underestimate. In one survey, two thirds of teenagers had a television set in their room, and over half of 15- to 16-year-olds had seen the most popular R-rated movies. Another survey found that teenagers with access to MTV viewed an average of 1 to 2 hours a day.

Radio

Although radio does not offer the compelling visual aspect of television, it also can be a major influence on adolescents. Radio frequently is used as a back-ground accompaniment for doing homework, driving, or visiting with friends. Since teenagers spend an average of 3.7 hours on weekdays and 6.4 hours on weekend days listening to the radio, this medium could represent one of the most important and underutilized methods of transmitting positive health messages to teenagers.

Movies

Adolescents spend only 10% to 15% as much time watching movies as they spend viewing television. In addition, since movies are frequently viewed with friends, the process of socialization may temper whatever unhealthy effects are associated with this medium. Nevertheless, contemporary movies contain seven times as many sexual acts or references as prime-time television does; these movies also depict violence and hard drug use much more openly. In particular, the "slice 'em and dice 'em" genre of slasher movies can desensitize young males to violence against women.

Print

Few data exist concerning adolescents' taste in magazines. One 1993 survey found that *Seventeen, Sports Illustrated, Teen, Time, Ebony, Young Miss, Jet, Newsweek,* and *Vogue* accounted for more than half of all reported reading. Adolescents who read sports or music magazines were more likely to report engaging in risky behaviors.

Print media continue to exploit female sexuality in unhealthy ways. For example, sex is used without regard to the product advertised but rather to simply gain the

---

BOX 92-1
Examples of Inappropriate Use of Sexuality in Print Advertising

"LIGHT MY LUCKY" (THE AMERICAN TOBACCO COMPANY)
An attractive young woman in a bathing suit is shown sitting on a beach, her hand holding an unlighted cigarette over her shoulder. She pouts at the camera, and the caption reads, "Light my Lucky." Similar ad shows an attractive young man in an identical pose.

"THE JOCKEY FASHION STATEMENT IS BOLD" (JOCKEY INTERNATIONAL, INC.)
Jim Palmer, ex-star pitcher for the Baltimore Orioles hands on hips, gazes at the camera with nothing on except a smile and a pair of Jockey briefs.

"CALVIN KLEIN FRAGRANCE FOR MEN" (CALVIN KLEIN, INC.)
A young stud, naked to the waist, is shown in bed, passionately embracing a recumbent (dressed) female.

"HOW A WOMAN RESPONDS TO SAX" (RICHARDSON-VICKS, INC.)
A young man and woman are shown in three separate frames: meeting, touching, then passionately kissing. Underneath them is pictured a bottle of Saxon after-shave lotion. The copy reads: "Even if it's the first time, most women love Sax. Of course, you can't base a relationship on Sax. But it can make a difference. Discover the Joy of Sax."

From Strasburger VC: Adolescent sexuality and the media, *Pediatr Clin North Am* 36:747-774, 1989.
Note: All the above companies were contacted and asked for permission to reproduce the above-described ads, and all refused.

---

reader's attention (Box 92-1). In addition, although cigarette advertising is no longer permitted on television, cigarettes are the second most widely advertised product in print and on billboards (autos are first), producing an expenditure of over $6 billion a year. Beer and alcohol are also advertised heavily.

Pornography remains a highly controversial topic. Although virtually no research exists on pornography with regard to adolescents under college age, current research seems to indicate that pornography that is explicit but nonviolent carries little risk. However, studies have shown that the combination of violence and pornography may desensitize males to rape and make them more callous toward females.

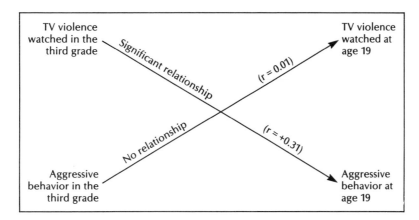

Fig. 92-1. Does TV violence watched in the third grade correlate with aggressive behavior at age 19? Results of a 10-year longitudinal study. (From Lefkowitz MM, Eron LD, Walder LO, Huesmann LR: Television violence and child aggression: a follow-up study. In Comstock GA, Rubinstein EA, editors: *Television and social behavior,* vol 3. *Television and adolescent aggressiveness,* Washington, DC, 1972, U.S. Government Printing Office; p 49.)

This classic study is ongoing and these boys have been followed through age 40 years. See Eron LD: Media violence, Pediatr Ann 24:84-87, 1995.

EFFECTS OF MEDIA

If parents could package psychological influences to administer in regular doses to their children, I doubt that many would deliberately select Western gunslingers, hopped-up psychopaths, deranged sadists, slap-stick buffoons and the like, unless they entertained rather peculiar ambitions for their growing offspring. Yet such examples of behavior are delivered in quantity, with no direct charge, to millions of households daily.

Albert Bandura

Television Violence and Aggressive Behavior

American television is the most violent in the world, with teenagers viewing approximately 200,000 murders, rapes, assaults, and armed robberies—vicariously—by the time they reach adulthood. The United States also has a preoccupation with guns, as demonstrated on such prime-time shows as *America's Most Wanted* and *Cops.* Weapons appear an average of 9 times per hour in prime-time programming. Guns are often involved in teenage homicides and suicides, the second and third leading causes of death (auto accidents are first); the United States leads the Western world in both handgun availability and handgun deaths. The *concentration* of violence on American television has not changed significantly since the early 1980s despite strong concerns by parents and public health organizations.

The connection between media violence and aggressive behavior in children and adolescents is the most thoroughly researched (and convincing) in all the communications literature. Over 1000 studies and reviews attest that exposure to heavy doses of television violence can increase the likelihood of aggressive or antisocial behavior. Longitudinal studies over 20 years have established such links (Fig. 92-1). The messages implicit on television are that violence is an acceptable solution to complex problems and that violence is justified if the "good guy" must resort to it. Abundant research documents the fact that aggressive behavior is learned early and that, once learned, it is resistant to modification.

Sex and Sexuality

American teenagers seem to have inherited the worst of all possible worlds regarding their exposure to messages about sex: Movies, music, radio and TV tell them that sex is romantic, exciting, titillating: premarital sex and cohabitation are visible ways of life among adults they see and hear about . . . . Yet, at the same time, young people get the message good girls should say no. Almost nothing they see or hear about sex informs them about contraception or the importance of avoiding pregnancy.

1985 Guttmacher Report

Television has become the leading sex educator in American society. Why? First, only a minority of parents discuss sexual matters in detail with their children. Second, only an estimated 10% to 30% of schools offer comprehensive sex education; even then, the courses

TABLE 92-1
Television and Birth Control

(n = 1250 adults)	Yes (%)	No (%)
Should characters on TV shows be shown using birth control?	59	34
Is contraception too controversial to be mentioned on TV shows?	32	64
Are you in favor of advertising birth control on TV?	60	37
Would birth control advertising:		
encourage teenagers to have sex?	42	52
encourage teenagers to use contraceptives?	82	14

Modified from Harris L, et al: *Attitudes about television, sex and contraception advertising,* New York, 1987, Planned Parenthood Federation of America.

often do not begin until after many teenagers have begun having sexual intercourse. Consequently, the media fill in the blanks. However, the "education" is inadequate. Content analyses of television programs reveal that American teenagers view over 14,000 sexual references, innuendoes, and jokes a year, yet fewer than 175 of these deal with birth control, sexually transmitted disease, or abstinence. Birth control advertisements remain banned from national television, despite the fact that most American adults favor them (Table 92-1). Although the subject of AIDS loosened up the network censors slightly in the 1990s, the mention of birth control as a means of preventing pregnancy, rather than as a means of preventing AIDS, is still strongly discouraged. Soap operas, which are extremely popular with teenage girls, have always been the worst offenders. In the "soaps," sex is frequently portrayed as being impersonal and exploitative, birth control is rarely mentioned, and sex between unmarried partners is 24 times more common than sex between spouses.

These examples are reflected in the realities of teenage pregnancy. The 1985 Guttmacher Report demonstrated that the United States has the highest teenage pregnancy rate in the Western world, despite the fact that American teenagers are no more sexually active than European or Canadian teenagers. Many studies document the media's importance as a source of information for teenagers about sex. Unfortunately, at present, young people are getting more unhealthy than healthy information from the media. When sex is used to sell everything from cars to shampoo, and when human sexuality is displayed irresponsibly, children and adolescents derive cues about adult behavior. Compounding this situation is the television networks' refusal to air birth control advertising, which has led many observers to accuse the networks (and American society) of a hypocrisy that is tragic in terms of pregnancy, sexual abuse, and sexually transmitted infections among teenagers.

Alcohol and Alcohol Advertising

You don't see dead teenagers on the highway because of corn chips.
Jay Leno (when asked why he does commercials for Doritos corn chips but refuses to do beer ads)

Slogans that teach young people to "Say no" to drugs or sex have a nice ring to them. But they are as effective in prevention of adolescent pregnancy and drug abuse as the saying "Have a nice day" is in preventing clinical depression.
Michael Carrera

A major paradox exists in American television: why are birth control ads forbidden, when they could be used to prevent untold numbers of teenage pregnancies and sexually transmitted diseases, yet beer and wine ads are encouraged, when alcohol is the leading drug threat to teenagers' lives? Beer and wine manufacturers spend over $1 billion a year on advertising. That is far too high a price tag for "influencing brand choice," which is what advertisers claim their commercials are limited to doing. In Sweden, where such ads were banned in the mid-1970s, per capita consumption of alcohol has decreased 20%. In America, per capita consumption has increased 50% since 1960. One 1988 survey of Washington, DC, 8- to 12-year-olds found that they could identify more alcoholic beverages (by brand name) than American Presidents.

Much attention and energy has been focused on cocaine and marijuana and "Just Say No" counteradvertising (Fig. 92-2). Such ads are extremely clever and well done, yet they fail to address the most significant drug in America today—alcohol. On the other hand, beer ads give many unhealthy messages to teenagers: drinking beer is fun, sexy, and likely to make you more popular and has no negative repercussions. In addition, for every "Know

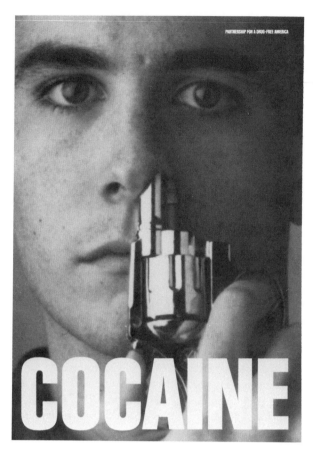

Fig. 92-2. Example of counteradvertising in the media. (Courtesy of Partnership for a Drug-Free America.)

When to Say When" public service announcement teenagers see, they are exposed to 25 to 50 beer and wine ads. This amounts to a total of 1000 to 2000 ads per year that are seen by the average teenager.

In television programming, the portrayal of alcohol use has changed considerably in the past 15 years. The funny, falling-down drunk is now rarely seen on television. In contrast, the dangers of drinking and driving are being dramatized through the efforts of organizations such as the Harvard Alcohol Project. Such changes illustrate that responsible network programmers and Hollywood producers can offer wholesome programs that give healthy messages about such topics as alcohol, cigarettes, and other drugs.

Suicide

It's not enough to say that Shakespeare and Marlowe were violent and civilization still survived. Technology has brought a new amplification into play. Never before has so much violence been shown so graphically to so many.
Joseph Morgenstern

The media may contribute to adolescent suicide in two ways: by glamorizing guns and by modeling adult behavior. Several studies have documented that the presence of a gun in the household is one of the most significant risk factors in teenage suicide. Also, studies have demonstrated a link between television programming or news reports about suicide and a subsequent increase in teenage suicide rates. Such studies point to the risk of imitative behavior in certain susceptible teenagers.

Anorexia Nervosa and Obesity

Television presents viewers with two sets of conflicting messages. One suggests that we eat in ways almost guaranteed to make us fat; the other suggests that we strive to remain slim.
Lois Kaufman

With the incidence of anorexia nervosa as high as 1 in 200 middle-class females, the role of the media is undergoing increasing scrutiny. Studies show that television characters usually are portrayed as happy in the presence of food. However, food is rarely used to satisfy hunger; rather, it is used as a means of bribing others or facilitating social interactions. Like other media, television has an obsession with thin people: of all television characters, 88% are thin or average in body build, and obese people are rarely portrayed positively.

Along with aggressive behavior, obesity is an area in which television's influence achieves the level of cause and effect rather than being simply contributory. The numbers of hours spent watching television is a strong predictor of adolescent obesity, with the prevalence increasing 2% for each hour of television viewed above the norm. This may result from the passiveness of television viewing, the excess of poor nutritional products being advertised, or the unhealthy nutritional practices being depicted in prime-time programming.

Influence of Rock Music and Music Videos

*Sounds like an animal panting to the beat
Groan in the pleasure zone, gasping from the heat.
Gut wrenching frenzy that destroys every joint.
I'm gonna force you at gun point
To eat me alive . . . . squealing in passion
as the rod steel injects.*
"Eat Me Alive" by Judas Priest *in* Defenders of the Faith *(Columbia Records), 2 million copies sold*

Rock music has always been provocative, antiestablishment, and offensive to many adults. This simply means that rock music, as a badge of adolescence, is doing its job properly. Although violent or sexually suggestive lyrics serve no useful purpose, no adverse behavioral effects from them have been shown either. In fact, efforts to label record albums and publicize lyrics on record jackets may actually be counterproductive. Research indicates that only 30% of teenagers know the lyrics to their favorite songs and that comprehension of lyrics is age dependent. Even so, nearly half of college students mistakenly believed that Bruce Springsteen's hit, "Born in the USA" was a song of patriotism, not alienation. Perhaps the only significant behavioral finding has been that heavy metal music, which lies at the outer limits of rock 'n' roll, may serve as a useful marker for depressed or disturbed adolescents.

Music videos are more akin to television. These videos may focus on either performance (the band playing) or concept (telling a story). Content analyses show that 75% of concept videos contain sexually suggestive material, 56% contain violence, and the violence shown often is directed against women. Although only a handful of behavioral studies exist, one does show that viewing violent videos may desensitize young people to violence. Another study found that music videos are self-reinforcing and produce a magnified effect; if viewers hear a song after having seen the video version, they "flash back" to the visual imagery in the video. *MTV* estimates that it now reaches the majority of U.S. teenagers. Therefore, *MTV* and music videos represent an extremely compelling medium that could be used to transmit positive, rather than negative, health messages.

ROLE OF THE PRACTITIONER

The media are neither good nor bad, but they are powerful teachers of children and adolescents. At the present time the media transmit more unhealthy messages (e.g., about sex, violence, and alcohol) than pro-social messages (e.g., about racial harmony, good nutrition, respect for women). However, this situation can be changed by counseling parents and teenagers about the effects of media and by encouraging practitioners to become politically active to create more positive programming.

Counseling

Practitioners who treat young children should advise parents to limit television time to no more than 1 to 2 hours a day and to monitor what shows are selected. Although teenagers deserve greater freedom in deciding what programs to watch, they also should be advised to curtail their TV watching. Discussing teenagers' cultural milieu also demonstrates a certain respect for

them as individuals and may help to make rapport easier. In particular, practitioners should elicit a "television history" when treating teenagers who are obese, aggressive, or suicidal or having school or learning difficulties. For example, obese teenagers who are watching 5 hours of television a day should have their hours cut sharply. Teenagers with academic difficulties who come home from school and turn on the television in their room should be advised that homework comes first.

Research

Health professionals need to familiarize themselves with television research, even though most of it is published in journals that may be unfamiliar to them. Furthermore, they need to avoid the intellectual trap of minimizing the importance of the media simply because the literature is complex, it does not contain straightforward "bench research," and there is no "smoking gun" in much of the work to date. Television is such a ubiquitous medium that studying its effects can be a real "mission impossible." Nevertheless, researchers have produced a considerable body of knowledge about the effects of the media.

School Programs

Much research attests to the power of the specialized school programs to cut dramatically the use of cigarettes, alcohol, and marijuana among teenagers. Unfortunately, such programs are time consuming, costly, and more complex than simple "Jusy Say No" sloganeering. Media literacy programs could well have similar effects on aggressive behavior and early sexual intercourse, and a wide variety of programs are now available.

Political Advocacy

The United States has the poorest quality programming in the Western world. Despite the efforts of Congress (the Telecommunications Act of 1996) and the Federal Communications Commission, networks have shown little interest in producing educational programming for children and adolescents. The recent addition of network ratings is not likely to have a major impact, because virtually all shows are rated PG. Banning beer and wine advertisements, encouraging birth control advertising, and the responsible portrayal of human sexuality (Box 92-2), and eliminating gratuitous violence and gunplay would have far-reaching effects that could benefit the health and welfare of America's children and teenagers. Health professionals should be on the frontlines of such efforts.

BOX 92-2
Guide to Responsible Sexual Content in Media

- Recognize sex as a healthy and natural part of life
- Parent and child conversations about sex are important and healthy and should be encouraged
- Demonstrate that not only the young, unmarried, and beautiful have sexual relationship
- Not all affection and touching must culminate in sex
- Portray couples having sexual relationships with feelings of affection, love, and respect for one another
- Consequences of unprotected sex should be discussed or shown
- Miscarriage should not be used as a dramatic convenience for resolving an unwanted pregnancy
- Use of contraceptives should be indicated as a normal part of a sexual relationship
- Avoid associating violence with sex or love
- Rape should be depicted as a crime of violence, not of passion
- The ability to say "no" should be recognized and respected

From Strasburger VC: *Adolescents and the media: medical and psychological impact,* Thousand Oaks, CA, 1995, Sage. Modified from Haffner DW, Kelly M: Adolescent sexuality in the media, SIECUS Report, March-April, 1987, pp 9-11.

Suggested Readings

For a comprehensive overview of the field

Dietz WH, Strasburger VC: *Children, adolescents, and television, Curr Probl Pediatr* 21:8-31, 1991.

Huston AC, Donnerstein E, Fairchild H, et al: *Big world, small screen: the role of television in American Society,* Lincoln, NE, 1992, University of Nebraska Press.

Liebert RM, Sprafkin J: *The early window—effects of television on children and youth,* ed 3, New York, 1988, Pergamon Press.

Strasburger VC, Comstock GC, editors: Adolescents and the media, *Adolesc Med: State of Art Rev* 4:479-657, 1993.

Strasburger VC: *Adolescents and the media: medical and psychological impact,* Thousand Oaks, CA, 1995, Sage.

Strasburger VC, editor: Children, adolescents, and the media, *Pediatr Ann* 24:73-108, 1995.

Specific topics

Sex and Sexuality

Brown JD, Greenberg BS, Buerkel-Rothfuss NL: Mass media, sex, and sexuality, *Adolesc Med: State of Art Rev* 4:511-525, 1993.

Greenberg BS, Brown JD, Buerkel-Rothfuss NL: *Media, sex, and the adolescent,* Cresskill, NJ, 1992, Hampton Press.

Strasburger VC: Adolescent sexuality and the media, *Curr Opin Pediatr* 4:594-598, 1992.

Drugs

Atkin CK: Effects of media alcohol messages on adolescent audiences, *Adolesc Med: State of Art Rev* 4:527-542, 1993.

Strasburger VC: Adolescents, drugs and the media, *Adolesc Med: State of Art Rev* 4:391-416, 1993.

Rock 'n' Roll Music/Music Videos

Brown EF, Hendee WR: Adolescents and their music: insights into the health of adolescents, *JAMA* 262:1659-1663, 1989.

Strasburger VC, Hendren RO: Rock music and music videos, *Pediatr Ann* 24:97-103, 1995.

Violence

Committee on Communications, American Academy of Pediatrics: Media violence (policy statement), *Pediatr* 95:949-951, 1995.

Comstock GC, Strasburger VC: Media violence: Q & A, *Adolesc Med: State of Art Rev* 4:495-509, 1993.

Eron LD: Media violence, *Pediatr Ann* 24:84-87, 1995.

Mediascope Inc: *National Television Violence Study,* Studio City, Calif, 1996, Mediascope.

Suicide

Shaffer D, Garland A, Gould M, et al: Preventing teenage suicide: a critical review, *J Am Acad Child Psychiatry* 27:675-687, 1988.

Movies

Jowett G, Linton JM: *Movies as mass communication,* ed 2, Newbury Park, CA, 1989, Sage.

CHAPTER 93

The Military and the Adolescent

•

David E. Suttle

This chapter is not solely for the practitioner wearing a military uniform or working as a government employee. The provider caring for adolescents, no matter what the practice setting, can reasonably expect to care for adolescents associated with the military. Not all medical care for military families is provided in the services' own hospitals and clinics. These patients have an insurance program (acronym CHAMPUS) that allows them to seek outpatient care from providers of their own choosing on a cost-sharing basis and without previous organizational approval.

Practicing in an area that is not situated in close proximity to a military installation is not exemptive. Many military families move close to their extended families during times of parental separations owing to remote assignments for the service member. Knowing that their insurance continues gives them a sense of security and no hesitancy about seeking health care for their children.

The military, like large corporations attempting to control the spiraling cost of health care, is rapidly implementing its own managed care program called TriCare (for the three military services). There will continue to be a need for nonmilitary care providers because of the approximately 3 million children, including adolescents, eligible for military health care. The total number of military officers on active duty is capped by Congress for each service. Thus, healthcare providers must compete with other branches such as Infantry officers and pilots for positions. As the services become smaller over the next few years, this competition will become even greater, but the population served medically will not decrease at the same rate. The percentage of married service members approaches 60%. This fact, together with larger losses among the younger (and therefore unmarried) service members, will result in continued needs for medical care to family members that uniformed healthcare providers alone will not be able to meet.

DEMOGRAPHICS

The implementation of the all-volunteer military force in the mid-1970s resulted in many significant changes in the demographics of its members. While actual percentages of various groups do not follow exactly the percentages within our society, virtually all races, ethnicities, religions, and genders are represented. The socioeconomic strata found in society is mirrored in the military. The degree of poverty is not as severe, and homelessness is not an issue, but young married enlisted members and their children may well find themselves eligible for food stamps and other Federal assistance programs such as Women, Infants, and Children (WIC).

Ambulatory services are free in military facilities, and inpatient services require payment of a small administrative fee only, less than $20 a day. Therefore, families at the lower end of the military socioeconomic spectrum resemble families insured by Medicaid in both their health status and utilization patterns.[1]

In addition to men and women in the services who have adolescent family members, the services themselves contain many adolescents. Service members aged 17 to 21 years make up 24.5% of all males and 24.4% of all females in the services. To ensure that the new all-volunteer system was successful, Congress enacted laws providing new entitlements and benefits, including increased pay. As the number of volunteers steadily increased, the selectivity of the services also increased, to the point that it is extremely difficult to join the military without a high school diploma. Coupling this with the services' programs for college assistance benefits and skills training makes it easy to understand that the adolescent military service member of today mirrors his or her civilian counterpart in being aggressively goal oriented.

MILITARY BRATS

The term "military brat" is fairly universal. To military people it is usually an affectionate term, most often used in response to the question, "Where are you from?" The answer will be something like, "Oh, I'm a military brat, so nowhere in particular," or "I've lived all over." Most accounts say that the origin of this term stems from the belief that the children of military families were often poorly behaved and not prone to adequate socialization. The frequent moves, stereotypical strong family discipline, and frequently absent father figure were all given as developmental reasons for this behavior. However, solid data have never validated these hypotheses. In fact, studies in this population, although limited in number, have shown just the opposite—that children of military families develop similarly to the rest of the population, but with particular strengths in socialization, ability to adapt to change, independence, and feelings of worth.[2]

This is not to say that there are no problems. The military has long recognized that life for its members and families involve unique stresses. Many of these are no longer unique in that society has incorporated them into its own definition of normality, and thus military adolescents are not viewed as different among their peer groups. Mobility and the loss of the support of the extended family is as common to IBM as it is to the Navy. Frequent, long absences from home of either parent occur in the diplomatic corps as well as the Army. An even risk of death occurs among police and firefighters.

However, the military family remains unique in having to deal with all, or at least most, of these stresses at one time, and this is not limited only to times of war. Training for war and standing in the face of an aggressor to deter conflict ("peace-keeping" missions) are often just as risky as war itself. The family dynamics used in coping with stress are a major factor influencing the development of the adolescent. As with their civilian counterparts, families that are overtly or borderline dysfunctional have adolescents who have difficulty coping. Parents who approach stress as positive events and as providing learning opportunities will greatly assist the adolescent in negotiating the dilemma successfully.[3]

Notwithstanding the above, families in the military move, on average, every 2.9 years, compared with 5.8 years for their civilian counterparts. Every military installation in the world with families has packets of resource material available on schools, recreational facilities, and living accommodations for all the other installations in the world. The practitioner needs to understand that there is a potential for healthy adjustment to these stresses. A history of healthy family dynamics should provide reassurance that hidden problems do not exist. The practitioner can easily gain clues to any problems the adolescent may be experiencing by including open-ended statements about how exciting, interesting, or rewarding living in a foreign country must be, along with any problems that might arise. The response can be revealing and often lead to fertile areas for further exploration and assistance.

The transition to a largely married armed force and the services' concerted efforts to reduce the stresses for family members have resulted in a markedly different environment from even 10 years ago. Many of the stereotypes concerning military fathers and families come from earlier life styles. Movies, television scripts, and books, while telling the truth as the authors remember it, should not influence the care provider into assuming that all adolescents of military families are living through similar experiences. Each adolescent should be evaluated and treated individually. The rigid, authoritarian disciplinarian like that described in Mary Wertch's 1991 autobiography[4] portraying a father who runs his family as he runs a boot camp still does exist, although rarely. If found, the adolescents of these families will usually welcome the open, accepting provider.

Practitioners caring for all adolescents, and this military population in particular, would do well to ponder the writings of Ostrov and Offer[5] on loneliness in this age group. These authors differentiate among being alone, loneliness, and depression and discuss the usefulness of the first two on normal development during adolescence. While loneliness is not unique to adolescents, the intensity of feelings associated with it probably is. Practitioners can have a major positive impact by helping the parents to understand that this intensity is far greater than they themselves would feel in similar situations, and suggesting alternative coping mechanisms for the family. Loneliness is thought to be the major underlying factor in the adolescent's difficulties surrounding geographic moves. Properly handled, the adolescent can mature into an adult who is comfortable with being alone, is not being forced into superficial relationships to avoid it, and is not experiencing feelings of inadequacy because of it.

One positive consequence of our society's recent acceptance of increased responsibility on the part of fathers in rearing their children has been the creation of more quality family time for parents frequently absent from home. Studies of military families show them to be generally much more involved in family activities during free time than their nonmilitary contemporaries. The resultant emotional support adolescents can receive is probably the reason for the strengths found in military adolescents. Problems the practitioner will have in assisting the adolescent in attaining emancipation will most likely be similar to those seen in cultures with strong family ties.

Care providers should also review the recommendations of Fisher et al.[6] The needs of adolescents in military families mirror those described in that study. Adolescent services in military facilities are more oriented toward primary care than is usually the case in the civilian sector, and youths use them for treatment of acute infectious processes, injuries, and other health issues more readily. Once adolescents perceive the staff as truly interested in them as individuals, future visits for health questions and emotional disturbances will be assured. Providers in settings not specifically established for adolescents need to realize that the latter may be receiving fragmented care, or not receiving care for all that is bothering them. Therefore, it is wise in this setting to probe a little deeper to identify areas of concern.

THE UNIFORMED ADOLESCENT

The 154,000 adolescents in uniform require medical care no different from that of other adolescents engaged in strenuous activity. Field training exercise, physical training, and working on heavy equipment produce injuries and overuse syndromes similar to those seen in college athletic programs. Living in close quarters with people from various geographic locations results in a variety of infectious diseases. The autoimmune and collagen vascular diseases, malignancies, and other conditions seen late in adolescence also occur, albeit infrequently.

The care provider new to treating adolescents in uniform must always be cognizant of the aura of maturity their patients will display. The regimentation that is the daily life within the military often produces a facade of maturity greater than that the adolescent has actually reached. The author's experience at the U.S. Military Academy at West Point and in caring for service members with acute illness confirms this. However, behind the closed examination room door, the intuitive interview techniques required for any adolescent the provider wishes to assist psychosocially, as well as physically, will produce a provider-patient relationship as rewarding for the former as it is for the latter. Adolescents respond to empathy with forthright answers about their struggles for emancipation in such a regimented environment and are proud of their accomplishments.

Since the lowest age for military entry is 17 years, the concept of, and problems associated with, "babies having babies" are not irrelevant. Practitioners providing well-baby services to military families must remember that there will often be two or three young, psychologically developing patients in the room: the baby, the mother, and the father. An adolescent orientation is often of use in determining why earlier advice is not being followed by the family or why priorities in certain families are set the way they are. Parents will accept responsibility for their children's health and safety only after they have accepted the same for themselves.

The adolescent in uniform, like all adolescents, is attempting to successfully accomplish the goals of emancipation and establishment of self-identity. The stresses unique to the military *family* mentioned earlier do not apply to single adolescents in uniform, for the military itself has become their immediate family and peer group combined. The frequent moves, strong discipline, and risk of potential imminent danger are indeed stresses, but the service member has volunteered for them, and these factors therefore contain less negative developmental significance.

The healthcare provider concerned with this group will most likely be in uniform also or hired by the particular military service as a civilian employee. However, providers who cared for these adolescents before their entry into the military may see them again as patients when they return on vacation and illness occurs. Other providers may see them in emergency rooms. Even though these patients now wear a uniform, they remain adolescents in varying stages of development, and as such require the same type of care as any other adolescent.

References

1. Newacheck PW: Improving access to health services for adolescents from economically disadvantaged families, *Pediatrics* 84:1056-1063, 1989.
2. Watanabe HK: A survey of adolescent military family members' self-image, *J Youth Adolesc* 14:99-107, 1985.
3. Levai M, Kaplan S, Ackerman R, Hammock M: The effect of father absence on the psychiatric hospitalization of navy children, *Mil Med* 160:104-106, 1995.
4. Wertsch ME: *Military brats: legacy of childhood inside the fortress,* 1991, Crown/Harmony.
5. Ostrov E, Offer D: Loneliness and the adolescent, *Adolesc Psychiatry* 34-36, 1978.
6. Fisher M, Marks A, Treiller K: Meeting the health care needs of suburban youth: review of a clinical service, *Pediatrics* 80:8-13, 1988.

CHAPTER 94

Affluence

•

Elizabeth M. Alderman and William A. Shine

Most people would agree that it is more desirable to be wealthy than to live in poverty. According to the 1990 United States Census, there are over 1 million families with earned annual income of $100,000 or greater.[1] This represents 5.8% of American households, up from 3.7% in 1979.[2] Wealth also may be measured by other valuable assets such as property, investments, and inheritance. The behavior of affluent youth has recently undergone scrutiny in the lay press such as *New York Times* and *Forbes.* Coles, in his book *Privileged Ones: Children in Crisis,* describes significant developmental and emotional problems in affluent children and adolescents, despite their resources.[3] However, scientific literature describing adolescents of affluence remains scant.

This chapter discusses the unique developmental issues affluent adolescents face as they grow toward adulthood against the backdrop of high economic and social status. These adolescents may develop a sense of entitlement, as well as problems seen commonly in the wealthy, such as social isolation and unrealistic expectations of high academic achievement. Not surprisingly, as with their less affluent counterparts, wealthy adolescents may be involved in delinquency and substance abuse.

DEVELOPMENTAL AND FAMILY ISSUES

Entitlement is the emotional expression of the class-bound prerogatives of money and power.[3] The beneficial aspect of entitlement includes the fact that wealthy teenagers have the money and time to serve on local charities and participate in political activities and committees, in many of which their parents also participate. In the worst form, narcissistic entitlement describes a spoiled adolescent who is self-centered, takes being rich for granted, and thinks he or she can use the privileged class and money to control any situation.[3] These adolescents feel that they and their families are shielded from harm because of their wealth.

A sense of entitlement brings with it the inflated sense of self-worth experienced by some adolescents in affluent families.[4] They are so intent on fulfilling their own needs that there may be no sensitivity to the needs of others.

The "silver spoon syndrome" also has been described in wealthy adolescents.[5] Its roots are in the emotional deprivation affluent adolescents experience owing to the absence of parents who have a multitude of social, recreational, and professional commitments. This deprivation results in little time for parental nurturance of the child and few family-centered interactions.[6] Adolescents with the "silver spoon syndrome" have low self-esteem and a need to display a facade of confidence, when in reality they are insecure. Because these adolescents often feel superfluous, they may become depressed or may "act out" in the form of substance abuse or delinquency.

In some wealthy families, parents deluge the adolescent with gifts, such as a new car or a trip to Europe, to allay their feelings of guilt for not spending much time with the teenager. These adolescents may not be able to delay gratification and may believe that their parent's money will pave their way in life. Adolescents whose needs are immediately gratified learn little about independence. They cannot develop a sense of achievement and are unable to deal effectively with frustration.[7]

In the book *Kids Who Have Too Much,* Miner describes the "rich kids syndrome" in which adolescents have too many material goods, too much freedom, too much independence, and little advice at home.[8] The increased independence these adolescents have may be a result of deficient discipline from their parents. The combination of independence and the impression that money and idle time are unlimited may lead to risk-taking behaviors, such as premature sexual activity and drug and alcohol use.

Affluent adolescents may rely on employed housekeepers and chauffeurs, instead of doing chores on their own.[4] They have an excessive dependency on others and cannot take care of themselves, even as adults. Many of these adolescents may be raised by caretakers, and their closest confidantes may be family employees such as housekeepers, governesses, or nannies.[9] Because these caretakers are often viewed as the primary loving adult in his or her life, a constant turnover of caretakers may be painful to the adolescent.[6]

EDUCATION

School is a significant life experience for all adolescents. Affluent adolescents generally attend culturally and cognitively partitioned schools or school programs, suburban public schools, or urban private schools. Their ego ideal is developed in a culture that places an extraordinary emphasis on individual achievement.[10] Wealthy families of these adolescents belong to a subgroup that has increasingly focused on the primacy of academic success over all other aspects of life.

Students who are academically talented and affluent have unlimited choices. When their parents consider a school, its climate, enrollment diversity, location, degree of specialization, and range of programs are all considerations. However, the overarching criterion for school choice is the emphasis on gaining admission to a competitive college. Acceptance at a "noncompetitive" college has, regrettably, become a mark of academic failure.

If parental expectations are congruent with the child's or adolescent's ability, it is likely that the adolescent will exhibit competence and control over his or her school environment. If expectations and ability differ, and the adolescent is goaded or seduced into accepting unrealistic academic or vocational goals, the variance between actual self and ideal self often results in turmoil.

For affluent children of average or below-average academic abilities, attending a school driven by "meritocratic principles" can be a tragic experience. Their learning problems increase their vulnerability to emotionally handicapping conditions that make academic success more problematic, and threaten their mental health. By seventh grade, a series of academic failures has, for most such children, set an enduring negative perception of their cognitive ability.[11] Because such individuals' actual self varies widely from their ideal self, these vulnerable adolescents are at risk for engaging in "acting-out" behavior.

Even more damaging, highly successful parents of academically average or below-average adolescents may have a lesser opinion of their children's social competence than do the adolescents themselves.[12] A child who consistently fails to meet family expectations perceives a loss of familial respect that often results in estrangement.

Schools where most affluent adolescents are educated are usually characterized by a high degree of parental involvement. According to the National Education Longitudinal Study (NELS) of eighth graders, more than 60% of affluent parents had contacted their child's school to discuss either academic programs or performance.[13] For the adolescent, this involvement is a mixed blessing. Adolescents' need for privacy becomes more important as it relates to the task of developing their individual personality. The triangular tension that exists among child, parent, and school is altered when parental control of the school is so dominant that the teachers and school authorities lack the credibility of an independent voice. The teacher then becomes an extension of the parent, whose view of the child's capabilities and needs is not always normatively informed.

DELINQUENCY

Many theories exist as to why affluent youth participate in delinquent activities. One theory is that delinquency is a means to sabotage parents and their "affluent values."[14] The youth culture theory describes delinquency as a way for the adolescent to escape the boredom of a life style of affluence. Another perspective is the socialization theory—the permissive environment of the wealthy leads to self-indulgence and poor self-control.[15]

It is difficult to ascertain the extent to which affluent youths participate in delinquent activity. Criminal activity is usually discussed in the context of poverty. However, police and court records may be skewed toward lower socioeconomic classes because adolescents with financial resources may be "slapped on the wrist" for minor offenses or may be able to employ attorneys who are able to negotiate a sentence of community service rather than incarceration.[16] Self-report studies of adolescents have circumvented this bias; thus, there is a growing recognition that delinquency is not limited to the poor.

A study of suburban youth in the 1970s by Richards et al. reported a relatively high degree of minor forms of delinquency such as shoplifting, stealing school property, vandalism, cheating on a test, or stealing from another student.[17] In fact, the *New York Times* has written about gangs in Westchester County, an affluent suburb of New York City.[18] These gang members were from middle class and upper middle class families and caused problems at school, shopping malls, and movie theaters. Gang members had been involved in shootings, automobile theft, and minor assaults on fellow students at school.

SUBSTANCE ABUSE

Alcohol and substance use are major causes of morbidity and mortality in all adolescents regardless of socioeconomic status. It has been hypothesized that drugs are used by affluent youth to combat the perceived meaninglessness of their lives and social isolation. Drug abuse is influenced by peer and sibling use and may be a result of anger at parents.[17] Elkind described the use of alcohol in affluent youth as a reflection of the affluence of American society in which teenagers have enough disposable income and time to buy alcohol and illicit drugs.[19]

The Washington Regional Alcohol Program reports that alcohol is the most commonly used substance for affluent teenagers in the suburbs of Washington, DC.[20] The average age of first alcohol use was 14 years, and over half of the teenagers surveyed by the Program had engaged in binging and drinking more than five drinks at one time.

The 1993 Monitoring the Future Study of American High School Students used parental education in describing family socioeconomic status, as adolescents are more likely to have this information than to know their parents' income.[21] The study found that for drugs such as marijuana, inhalants, and LSD there is a positive correlation between use by high school seniors and higher parental education. Cocaine, which had been thought to be a drug of choice for the rich, was not found to be used more by affluent students than by other students.

Using private school attendance as a marker for affluence, a national high school study found that seniors attending private high schools were more likely to drink alcohol (76% vs. 64%) and smoke cigarettes (22% vs. 18%) than those in public school. Additionally, more private school students than public school students (62% vs. 56%) reported illicit drug use during their lifetime.[22]

CONCLUSION

All adolescents are influenced by their social context. For some, affluence has a major impact on their lives. Too many choices, loss of intimacy, adjusting to a wide range of surrogates, and precocious success and anxiety are some of the major forces flowing from the affluent life style. For most adolescents these forces are manageable, and for persons outside the situation they often appear trivial. For troubled adolescents, however, these forces are often insurmountable obstacles that turn entitlement into despair.

It is important for the practitioner working with affluent adolescents and their families, as with all patients and their families, to inquire about supervision and activities after school, parental-child interactions, current behavior such as possible sexual activity, illicit drug use, delinquent activity, and school progress. Parental expectations and aspirations for their child should also be determined in order to judge whether they are congruent with the child's abilities. It is often difficult for physicians to address these issues in families that are very similar to their own. Nevertheless, there is growing evidence that affluent adolescents and their families are not exempt from typical adolescent concerns and indeed carry the potential for unique behavioral problems.

References

1. Bureau of Census: Money income of households, families and persons in the U.S., 1991, Series P-60, No. 180.
2. Hacker A: Who they are, *New York Times Magazine;* Nov 19:70-71, 1995.
3. Coles R: *Privileged ones: children in crisis,* vol V, Boston, 1977, Atlantic-Little, Brown.
4. Hausner L: *Children of paradise, successful parenting for prosperous families,* Los Angeles, 1990, Jeremy Tarcher.
5. LeBeau, J: The "silver spoon syndrome" in the super rich: the pathologic link of affluence and narcissism in family systems, *Am J Psychother* 21:425-436, 1988.
6. Wise PH, Schor L: The neighborhood—poverty, affluence and violence. In Levine MD, Carey WB, Crocker AC, editors: *Developmental-behavioral pediatrics,* ed 2, Philadelphia, 1992, WB Saunders; pp 160-170.
7. Wixen BN: *Children of the rich,* New York, 1973, Crown.
8. Miner RE, Proctor W: *Kids who have too much,* Nashville, TN, 1987, Thomas Nelson.
9. Warner SL: Psychoanalytic understanding and treatment of the very rich, *J Am Acad Psychoanal* 19:578-594, 1991.
10. Beiberg E: Adolescence, sense of self, and narcissistic vulnerability, *Bull Menninger Clin* 52:211-228, 1988.
11. Sandler AD, Levine MD: Learning and attention deficit disorders. In Friedman SB, Fisher M, Schonberg SK, editors: *Comprehensive adolescent health care,* St. Louis, 1992, Quality Medical Publishing.
12. Casey R, et al: Impaired emotional health in children with mild reading disability, *J Dev Behav Pediatr* 13:256-260, 1992.
13. National Center for Education Statistics: *A profile of parents of 8th graders—National Education and Longitudinal Study (NELS) of 1988,* Washington, DC, 1992, U.S. Dept. of Education, Office of Educational Research and Improvement, U.S. Government Printing Office.
14. Elkind D: Middle class delinquency, *Ment Hyg* 51:80-84, 1967.
15. Hagen J: Juvenile justice and delinquency in the life course, Criminal Justice Research Bulletin 7(1), 1992.
16. Rutter M, Giller H: *Juvenile delinquency—trends and perspectives,* New York, 1992, Guilford Press.
17. Richards P, Berk R, Forster B: *Crime as play: delinquency in a middle class suburb,* Cambridge, MA, 1979, Ballinger Publishing.
18. Henneberger M: Gang membership grows in middle-class suburbs, New York Times, July 24, 1993.
19. Elkind D: *All grown up and no place to go—teenagers in crisis,* Reading, Mass, 1984, Addison-Wesley.
20. Milk L, Jaffe H: Saturday night in the suburbs, Washingtonian 28:78-82, 1993.
21. O'Malley PM, Johnston LD, Bachman JG: Adolescent substance use: epidemiology and implications for public policy, *Pediatr Clin North Am* 42:241-260, 1995.
22. O'Malley PM, Bachman JG, Johnston LD: Student drug use in America: differences among high schools, 1986-1987, Monitoring the Future, Ann Arbor, Mich., 1987, Occasional Paper Series.

CHAPTER 95

Poverty

•

Gloria Johnson-Powell

With its social, educational, health, and economic ramifications, poverty is the greatest and most severely handicapping condition of childhood and adolescence.[1] Therefore, a thorough understanding of the complex mechanisms of poverty and its persistent nature is a prerequisite to any viable solutions for preventing its continuation and devastating effects on youth.

According to Wilber,[2] poverty can be viewed as a consequence of the interaction between resources and their mobilization. As such, it is part of the life cycle and an integral element in the social processes that take place over time. Therefore, it is crucial, as emphasized by Gronberg et al,[3] to examine how society creates, maintains, and selects the victims of poverty.

Bane and Ellwood[4] offered an explanation of why children are poor and gave a definition of poverty that includes its historical, demographic, and economic dimensions. These authors note that in the 1960s the federal government's poverty standard was originally determined by calculating how much a family of four needed for a minimum amount of food. Low-income families, it was estimated, spent one third of their income on food. Therefore, the minimum amount of food needed to sustain a family was multiplied by three. Families having incomes below the level thus calculated were considered poor.

A universal poverty line has many limitations, the most important of which is the variation in cost of living from one region to another. A second important point is that only cash income is included in the determination of the poverty line; no other economic factors, such as home-grown crops or barter transactions, are considered. Therefore, the poverty line is basically an arbitrary standard applied to annual income alone.

Several other important concepts need to be considered in the definition of poverty[4]: (1) the poverty line may convey a more serious, continuing condition; (2) the poverty line does not convey the vast differences among poor families; (3) the poverty line does not address the serious problem of *persistent* poverty; (4) regional cost-of-living indexes are not reliable; and (5) the exact definition of "income" is still debatable.

Many scholars argue that poverty is relative rather than absolute and that it ought to be defined in relation to the median income in the population.[5,6] Others argue that a cutoff level does not give an accurate picture of the severity of poverty and the vast differences in family income that occur below the poverty level. Grienstein[7] defined the "poverty gap," or the total dollar amount by which the incomes of the poorest fall below the poverty level. He noted that in 1986 the poverty gap was $49.2 billion, representing an increase of more than 50% from 1977. The definition of the poverty gap illustrates the following significant trends: (1) decreasing rates of poverty until the early 1970s, (2) increases through the early 1980s, (3) more stability in the late 1980s, and (4) an increase in income inequality from 1976 to 1986.[8]

By 1992, the child poverty rate was 21.9% and included 14.6 million children.[9] By 1993 the federal poverty line was $11,890 per year for a family of three, yet the annual salary at a minimum wage of $4.25 was $8840 (Fig. 95-1). By 1994, the poverty line for a family of four was $15,441.[26] Between 1975 and 1994, the percentage of children living in extreme poverty or in a family with an income less than one half the poverty line increased with $7,570 for a family of four in 1994.

An examination of the patterns and prevalence of childhood poverty over 15 years indicates that much childhood poverty is short-lived and most of the data fail to measure the persistence of poverty across an individual's childhood.

Duncan and Rodgers[10] used data from the Panel Study of Income Dynamics, which began in 1968 with children under the age of 4 years and examined the family economic conditions of their childhood for 15 years. They found that many more children come into contact with poverty than experience persistent poverty.[4] One third of all children experienced poverty for at least 1 year and one child in 20 experienced poverty over 10 years or more.

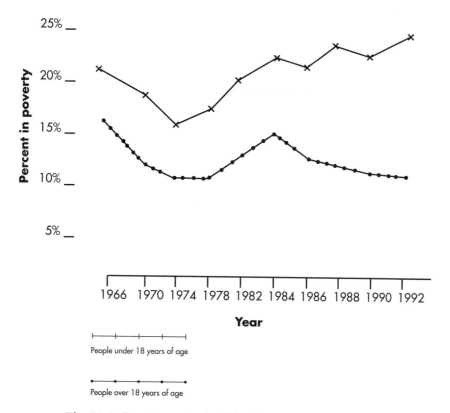

Fig. 95-1. Poverty rates in the United States from 1965 to 1992.

WHY ARE SO MANY CHILDREN POOR?

In 1991, 14.3 million children were living in poverty, and by 1992 the number increased to 14.6 million, the largest number since 1965.[11] The younger the child, the higher was the prevalence of poverty: for example, 25% of all children under 6 years of age and 27% of all children 3 years old and younger lived in poverty in 1992. In 1992, more children were living in extreme poverty, defined as an annual income of less than $5593 for a family of three, than in any year since 1975.[12] In fact, the U.S. poverty rate was higher in the late 1980s than in 1980. Between 1949 and 1959, poverty rates for all ethnic groups fell about 20%.[8] Poverty rates have been rising since the early 1970s, and by the mid 1980s the childhood poverty rate had risen about 1% every 4 years. Between 1975 and 1993, the proportion of children at or below the poverty line increased by 47 percent (U.S.D.H.H.S., 1996). In 1995, 20.8% of children under age 18 lived in poverty and represented 40% of all the poor people and 25% of the total population of the United States[13] (Table 95-1).

The increase in childhood poverty has been caused by an accumulation of several factors[8]: (1) a sluggish macroeconomic environment resulting in a decrease in the distribution of income, (2) a greater inequality in the distribution of income, (3) an increase in female heads of

household, (4) fixed wages for young workers, and (5) a decline in the labor force involvement of men, especially minority men. Indeed, an increasingly unequal income distribution resulted in more childhood poverty in 1986, with families in the top fifth receiving a 27% higher income in 1986 than in 1970.[8,11]

Any discussion of poverty in childhood is incomplete without noting the fact that the incidence of poverty among female-headed families continues to be 7 to 8 times that among married couples.[4] Family structure changes from 1970 to 1980 are considered a major factor producing higher rates of childhood poverty along with income inequality. Those two factors, together, with the recessions in the mid-1970s and early 1980s, also added to the changes in the prevalence of child poverty. In 1992, among children in female-headed households with no other adult, 54%, or 14.8 million children, were poor.[9] Although this is a factor in the increase of poverty in childhood, many children in two-parent families live in poverty.

Figures alone do not present a complete picture of children in poverty. Glasgow[12] referred to the ethnic and racial nature of the "underclass." It seems that class, not caste, has become a prevailing theme in American social demography.[12] In 1989 Wilson[13] analyzed the origin and nature of this class phenomenon and its growing conse-

TABLE 95-1
Proportion of Children Under Age 18 Living Below Selected Poverty Thresholds by Age and Race/Hispanic Origin, 1975 to 1994

	1975	1980	1985	1990	1991	1992	1993	1994
Under 50% of Poverty								
Related Children Under 18	5	7	8	8	9	10	10	—
White	4	5	6	6	6	6	6	—
Black	14	17	22	22	25	27	26	—
Hispanic	—	—	—	14	14	15	14	—
Under 100% of Poverty								
Related Children Under 18	17	18	20	20	21	22	22	21
White	13	13	16	15	16	17	17	—
Black	41	42	43	44	46	46	46	—
Hispanic	33	33	40	38	40	39	40	—
Under 150% of Poverty								
Related Children Under 18	30	29	32	31	32	33	33	—
White	24	24	26	25	26	27	27	—
Black	60	57	59	57	60	60	61	—
Hispanic	—	—	—	55	58	58	60	—
Under 200% of Poverty								
Related Children Under 18	43	42	43	42	43	44	44	—
White	38	37	38	37	38	38	38	—
Black	73	70	71	68	70	71	72	—
Hispanic	—	—	—	69	72	70	72	—

Note: The poverty level is based on money income and does not include noncash benefits, such as food stamps. Poverty thresholds reflect family size and composition and are adjusted each year using the annual average Consumer Price Index (CPI) level. The average poverty threshold for a family of four was $13,924 in 1991 and $10,989 in 1985. The levels shown here are derived from the ratio of the family's income to the family's poverty threshold. For example, a child living under 125% of poverty is from a family with income above their poverty threshold but below 125% of their poverty threshold. If the family's poverty threshold was $10,000, under 125% of poverty would mean their income was between $10,000 and $12,500. Related children include biologic children, stepchildren, and adopted children of the householder and all other children in the household related to the householder (or reference person) by blood, marriage, or adoption.
Sources: Rates for 1975, 1980, and 1985 were calculated by Child Trends, Inc. based on data from the U.S. Bureau of the Census, Series P-60, No. 106, Table 7; No. 133, Table 4. Rates for 1990 through 1993 are from the U.S. Bureau of the Census, Series P-60, No. 175, No. 185, No. 188, and revised data for 1992 provided by the U.S. Bureau of the Census, Poverty Branch. Data for 1994 from unpublished tables supplied by the U.S. Bureau of the Census.

quences. Most social policy commentators concur that there is a "poverty problem" in the United States and that the large numbers of poor people represent a disproportionate number of youths. Many also agree that there have been two significant evolving processes.[3,4,7,8] First, by 1974 children had displaced the elderly as the poorest age group in the nation. Second, in 1959 the child poverty rate was 25%, whereas that for the elderly was 35.2%. However, by 1979 the poverty rate for children was increasing rapidly and approached 26.9%, but the elderly poverty rate continued to decline.

These extraordinary phenomena can be explained by the major disparities existing between the benefit programs provided for the elderly and those for children.[4] Data from 1970 to 1984 show that the Old Age and Survivors Insurance increased by 54%, but the mean Aid to Families with Dependent Children (AFDC) decreased by 34%. Indeed, since the mid-1980s or earlier the Social Security Old Age, Survivors, and Disability Insurance (OASDI) payments to children and their parents was greater than the AFDC benefits: the OASDI payments reached $10.5 billion, 40% more than the amount for the AFDC.

Clearly, no matter how child poverty is defined, there is consensus that it does exist, that it has increased over the past decade or longer, and that this increase is greater than most Americans have realized or cared to realize. Poverty rates for U.S. children have exceeded those for children in Canada, Germany, Norway, Sweden, and the United Kingdom.[8] At present, it is not clear whether similar calculations have been made in other Western countries.

Since most U.S. youths under 18 years of age live in families, it is important to understand the different family structures and life styles; the quality of family relationships; and the stresses faced by parents, adolescents, and communities. An examination of the family structure of poor adolescents has revealed an increase over more than a decade in the number of youths who are poor and residing in households with a female as its head. Bane and Ellwood[4] confirmed that for a decade the yearly increases in poverty among youths reflect increases in the number of poor children in two-parent families, leading to a persistent long-term increase in poor children in two-parent homes. Three major forces have shaped family poverty: (1) the persistent incremental increase, over almost two decades, of children in single-parent families; (2) a persistent and high poverty rate among children in single-parent homes; and (3) a constantly changing rate of poverty for children in two-parent homes. A review of the data on family structure and poverty shows the following changes: (1) between 1959 and 1969 the decrease in poverty was the result of less poverty for two-parent families; (2) from 1969 to 1979 the increase in poverty rates was caused by persistent incremental changes in family structure; and (3) from 1979 to 1987 the increase of poverty among two-parent families was responsible for 50% of the increase in poverty—with the change in the family structure accounting for 25% and the increase in poverty for families with a female as its head accounting for about 25%.[11]

Although the prevailing view is that most poor adolescents come from households with a female as its head, that view is not accurate for all poor adolescents in the United States. It is a stereotypical view of poor youths—one on which many subsequent judgments are made. In reality, there are many two-parent families in which both parents work, but they are still unable to support a family.

Most Americans think of urban ghettos when poverty is mentioned. However, the rates of poverty in rural America are as high as that in central cities.[6] The poor in rural areas are more often married and have a working head of the family. The rural poor are less often nonwhite, less often have children, receive fewer welfare benefits, and more often live in states that do not provide AFDC for two-parent families.

The average child growing up in a middle-class family is more likely to complete high school or college and to enjoy a higher-paying and higher-status job than a child raised in a poor family. Indeed, the income and assets of the family throughout childhood matters a great deal in shaping the life chances of children, because "the advantages provided by higher incomes are presumed to persist even after accounting for the effects of other characteristics associated with more affluent families."[8]

Growing up very poor throughout one's entire childhood compounds the difficulties an adolescent encounters. Such an adolescent is less likely to finish high school and even less likely to go on to college. In fact, there are approximately 20 million youths between 16 and 24 years of age who are not likely to go to college and are finding it difficult to cope with the economic changes and pressures they face. Adolescents who grow up in poverty are more likely to fall into the following categories, which present additional problems: (1) high school dropouts with lower income; (2) more working youths with continuously decreasing earning power, and more of them reporting no earnings; (3) less than 50% of these youths earning only enough to support a family of three above the poverty level.

Adolescents who grow up in one of the census tracts of 100 U.S. cities that comprise the underclass are at high risk for school failure, alcohol and substance abuse, teenage pregnancy, and juvenile delinquency. Such youngsters typically have never had a childhood free from want, homelessness, and fear. For them, the common theme of life is not just drugs, guns, and violence, but daily survival, despair, and death.[14,16]

THE PERSISTENCE OF POVERTY

There is a marked distinction between those who are poor and those who are part of the underclass, in both degree and persistence of poverty. It is the deprivation characterizing the underclass that is the focus of growing national concern. By definition, the underclass typically includes minority-group people living in the poorest areas of large cities; this group represents the poorest census tracts in the 100 largest cities.[5,11-13] In these areas the poverty rates exceed 40%, but it should be emphasized that less than 9% of all poor children live in such areas.[4] Consequently, if the underclass is defined as including only the *persistently* poor, the following groups would be represented: (1) large numbers of African-Americans or Hispanics, (2) a disproportionate number of families headed by unmarried mothers, (3) fewer of the working poor or the near-poor, and (4) most of the poor who live outside the major urban ghettos.[12]

Duncan and Rodgers[10] found that persistent poverty is far from insignificant, that 4.8% of all children are exposed to poverty for at least two thirds of their childhood, and that some children are poor for 5 to 9 of the 15 years. The study also highlighted the racial differences: for example, less than one in seven African-American children live comfortably above the poverty line, more than one quarter are poor for at least 10 of the 15 years, and African-Americans account for about 90% of the children who are poor during at least 10 out of the 15 years. Most surprisingly, the data showed that the expected prevalence of poverty among African-American children living in continuously two-parent families is about as high as the prevalence of poverty for white children who spend their entire childhood in single-parent families. It was concluded by the researchers that family structure differences between white and black families are not the major reason for the differences between the amounts of poverty experienced by the two groups. Disability of the household head and rural location are the most powerful factors associated with African-American child poverty.[15,16] Educational attainment of the household head has only modest effects on the prevalence of childhood poverty, especially for African-Americans.

Poverty among children in households with a single female as its head has been considered the most important contributor to the persistently high rate of poverty among children and the alarmingly high rate of poverty among these families. Indeed, from many accounts it has been estimated that 50% or more of all children born in the United States will spend some time in a single-parent home.[4] Careful scrutiny of the data on poverty among families with a single female as head reveals that 60% of absent fathers contribute no child support or alimony, compared with 91% of married fathers, who contribute a minimum of $5000.[5,7,9] The poverty rate for children in single-parent families is about 50%. More recently, particular attention has been given to the fact that the percentage of custodial mothers who were due child support awards and received the full amount was only 26%.[9] The complex social and economic factors involved result in a cycle of single parents who either work all the time or collect welfare. However, welfare benefits are not high enough to keep families out of poverty.

There is consensus that the growing proportion of children born to unmarried mothers in minority communities represents the greatest concern associated with the very high and persistent rates of poverty among single females who are the heads of households. For a young, unmarried (or never married) mother to escape from poverty and welfare, she must be able to find a job that pays twice the minimum wage and keep that job. To keep a job, such a mother needs to have adequate child care benefits and good medical benefits, since such mothers are least likely to receive child support. In the face of many obstacles, such families live in poverty while collecting welfare benefits for a long time. Without adequate financial and psychosocial support to meet their roles as parents and providers, they often lack the resources to meet the needs of their adolescent children. Although all adolescents have difficult rites of passage to face in this society, these difficulties are compounded for adolescents who are poor. Such difficulties are even more severe if the youths are part of a household in the underclass. The situation is extremely bleak if such a household is made up of minority-group members and the adolescent is male, particularly an African-American male.[17]

THE CONSEQUENCES OF POVERTY FOR SOCIAL AND EMOTIONAL HEALTH

There are about 28 million adolescents in the United States.[16] The inner city youth population of all ethnic and cultural groups is about 8.5 million for youth between 10 and 17 years of age and represents 30% of the total adolescent population.[16] By the year 2000, nonwhite and Spanish-speaking youths under 18 years old are expected to represent 30% of the youth population, and by the year 2020, 38%.[17] Inner city youth of all ethnic/racial and cultural backgrounds have a poverty rate of 47.5%, which is 30% more than the poverty rate for white youths in general.[8] However, all poor youths share the same consequences of high-risk and socially maladaptive behavior problems that often continue into maladaptive adult life styles, thus continuing the cycle of poverty or persistent poverty. Indeed, the issues of poverty and an impoverished environment place all adolescents in similar psychosocial crisis, and these adolescents are at risk for failure to complete adolescent tasks.[17] Although the family is an important influence in the psychosocial development of adolescents, the community—and, most important, the social context in which the community exists—and the peer group are vital factors. Equally important is how adolescents think that the world perceives them and how they perceive the world—not only the immediate world of their families and communities, but also the world on a national, international, and global level.[17-19]

The path to healthy psychosocial development is often fraught with a bewildering array of freedoms and choices, as well as ambiguous responsibilities that may be conflicting and confusing to many adolescents. Most adolescents are able to use resources available to them and negotiate the demands and challenges of adolescent task development, but for many there are obstacles encountered in attaining their goals because such resources are tenuous or unavailable.[8] For adolescents with compromised cognitive and social skills, in addition to being poor, their lack of appropriate social skills acquisition and their compromised cognitive and academic skills make it difficult for them to negotiate parent and other authority relationships, forge and commit to lasting peer relationships, and develop a separate and autonomous self[17] (see Chapter 8, "Psychosocial Development"). Also, the explicit and implicit messages received from social violence, illegal drug trafficking, and substandard economic conditions profoundly influence the adolescent's personal code of ethics and value system, or enhances attitudes and values that lead to maladaptive behaviors and the consequences that such high-risk behavior brings. Additionally, reviews of extensive data on child health indicate that poor physical health is intrinsically linked to academic failure and maladaptive social behaviors.[20-22]

THE EFFECTS OF POVERTY ON HEALTH CARE AND HEALTH STATUS

The Medicaid program is financed by federal and state governments and provides medical care to those who are receiving AFDC or who are eligible for the Supplemental Security Income program. Medicaid programs vary from state to state, depending on whether a state extends coverage to the medically needy and other groups such as the aged, blind, and disabled. In 1993, 49% of Medicaid recipients were children and youths 21 years of age or under, but children and youths accounted for only 16% of expenditures.[23] Eighteen percent of Medicaid recipients were treated under the early and periodic screening program, with an average cost per child of $143, which accounted for less than 1% of Medicaid expenditures.

The extent to which those with incomes below the poverty line are covered by Medicaid varies greatly from state to state. The variability in Medicaid eligibility is due in large part to each state's eligibility levels for AFDC. States that have higher income ceilings for welfare programs and/or extend eligibility to families with unemployed male heads are more likely to have larger proportions of their poverty population covered by Medicaid. From 1991 to 1993 the ratio of Medicaid recipients to persons below the poverty level ranged from 48 per 100 in Nevada to 117 per 100 in New York (U.S.D.H.H.S., 1995). During the same period, ten states had the highest ratios of Medicaid recipients to persons below the poverty level, which meant 93 or more per 100. Four of the top ten were located (1) in the New England area—Vermont, Massachusetts, and Connecticut; (2) in the Pacific area—Alaska, Washington, and Hawaii; (3) in the Midwest area—Ohio, Nebraska, and Iowa; and (4) in the South Atlantic area—Delaware. Those ten states with the lowest ratios of Medicaid recipients to persons below the poverty level or less than 65.8 per 100 were located in the South and in the mountain states. The average payments per Medicaid recipients in 1993 had more than a twelvefold variation among the states, with a low of $524 in Arizona to a high of $6402 in New York.[23] The ten states with the highest average Medicaid payments per recipient were those in the Northeast, as well as Minnesota, North Dakota, Indiana, and Maryland. The District of Columbia is also included in this group.

In the early 1980s, children under 5 years of age and young adults 15 to 44 years of age were more likely than other groups to be uninsured. It is estimated that between 1980 and 1993 the percentage of persons 15 to 44 years of age without health insurance increased more than 50%. Within that same period, the percentage of persons who were uninsured increased for all age groups except those under 5 years of age, for whom the expansions in the Medicaid program resulted in a decline from 18% in 1984 to 14% in 1993.[23]

It has been well documented that problems in accessing the healthcare system lead to lower healthcare utilization and poorer health outcomes.[24,25] This is particularly true for poor persons and other disadvantaged groups. *Health United States 1994* documents the socioeconomic and racial disparities in healthcare utilization (U.S.D.H.H.S., 1994). Among children with good to excellent health status, nonpoor children had close to 30% more physician contacts than poor or near-poor children. For children with fair or poor health status, there are significant differences in physician utilization by family income. From 1991 to 1993, in children with fair or poor health status, nonpoor children had 28% to 31% more physician contacts than poor or near-poor children.

Poor children are more likely to become ill and have more serious illnesses because of increased environmental exposures, poor housing, hazardous neighborhoods, poor nutrition, and inadequate preventive care.[24,25] The higher rates of more serious problems and the increased death rates from diseases at all childhood ages are a result of poor access to medical care. Low income is responsible for much if not most of the disadvantages found among children in racial minority groups. Indeed, the relative frequency of health problems in low income children and youth is significantly higher than that of other youth living in families with adequate and high income levels.

CONCLUSION

Child poverty has been increasing rapidly since the 1970s and continued through the 1980s and now into the 1990s. The increase in the prevalence of poverty by the mid-1980s was due primarily to several factors: (1) an increase in the prevalence of single-parent families, (2) a sluggish labor market, and (3) declining benefit levels in transfer programs. Although the greatest numbers of children who are poor are 6 years of age and under, persistent childhood poverty is not insignificant. The racial differences among children who remain in poverty for a significant number of years are striking. African-Americans accounted for nearly 90% of the children who were poor for at least 10 out of 15 years.[8] Many Hispanics and immigrants do not fare much better.

With already overburdened budgets and demands for funds from many sources, there will be few state or federal monies for new programs in the near future. Therefore, to prevent the colossal waste of our greatest future natural resource—our youth—we will need to create bold strategies for their survival. It is imperative to monitor monies earmarked for youth and to rechannel those resources in an efficacious and cost-effective manner. Restructuring of bureaucratic agencies and development of cost-sharing strategies may be a means of providing money to create needed programs.

References

1. Powell R, Johnson-Powell G: Poverty as the most disabling condition of childhood. In Johnson-Powell G, Yamamoto J, Romero A, Morales A, editors: *The psychosocial development of minority group children,* New York, 1983, Brunner/Mazel.
2. Wilber GL: Determinants of poverty. In Wilber GL, editor: *Anticipating the poverties of the poor,* Monograph No. 1, Lexington, KY, 1971, University of Kentucky Social Welfare Research Institute.
3. Gronberg K, Street D, Suttles GD: *Poverty and social change,* Chicago, 1978, University of Chicago Press.
4. Bane MJ, Ellwood DT: One fifth of the nation's children: why are they poor?, *Science* 245:1047-1053, 1989.
5. Danziger SH, Haveman RH, Plotnick RD: Antipoverty policy: effects on the poor and the non-poor. In Danziger SH, Weinberg DH, editors: *Fighting poverty: what works and what doesn't,* Cambridge, MA, 1986, Harvard University Press; pp 50-77.
6. Huston AC: Children in poverty: developmental and policy issues. In Huston AC, editor: *Children in poverty,* New York, 1994, Cambridge University Press.
7. Grienstein R: Children and families in poverty: the struggle to survive. Testimony at the hearing before the Select Committee on Children, Youth, and Families, U.S. House of Representatives, Washington, DC, February 25, 1988.
8. Duncan GJ: The economic environment of childhood. In Huston AC, editor: *Children in poverty,* New York, 1994, Cambridge University Press.
9. Children's Defense Fund: *The state of America's children: yearbook 1994,* Washington, DC, 1994, Children's Defense Fund.
10. Duncan GJ, Rodgers W: Longitudinal aspects of childhood poverty, *J Marriage Family* 50:1007-1021, 1988.
11. Danziger S, Gottschalk P: How have families been faring? Discussion paper presented at the Institute for Research on Poverty, University of Wisconsin, Madison, WI.
12. Glasgow DG: *The black underclass: poverty, unemployment, and entrapment of ghetto youth,* San Francisco, 1980, Jossey-Bass.
13. Wilson WJ: *The declining significance of race: blacks and changing American institutions,* Chicago, 1989, University of Chicago Press.
14. Wilson WJ, Neckerson K: Poverty and family structure: the widening gap between evidence and public policy issues. In Danziger S, Weinberg PH, editors: *Fighting poverty: what works and what doesn't,* Cambridge, MA, 1986, Harvard University Press.
15. Jensen L: Rural-urban difference in the utilization and ameliorative effects of welfare programs, *Policy Studies Rev* 7:782-794, 1988.
16. U.S. Bureau of the Census, Money, Income, Income of Households, Families and Persons in the United States, 1987: *Current population reports,* Series P-20, No. 162, Washington, DC, 1989, U.S. Government Printing Office.
17. Palmer-Castor J: The grey girls: America's youthful shadows. Doctoral dissertation. The Heller Graduate School for Advance Study in Social Welfare, Waltham, Mass., 1993, Brandeis University.
18. Johnson-Powell G: Urban anger: take back the streets, *Harvard Med Alum Bull,* Winter 1990-1991, pp 7-12.
19. Johnson-Powell G: Academic self-concept and achievement of Afro-American children. In Berry GL, Asamen JK, editors: *Black students and academic achievement,* Newberry Park, CA, 1989, Sage.
20. National Research Council: *Adolescents in high risk settings,* Washington, DC, 1993, National Academy Press.
21. Dryfoos J: *Adolescents at risk: prevalence and prevention,* New York, 1990, Oxford University Press.
22. Schorr L, Schorr D: *Within our reach: breaking the cycle of disadvantage,* New York, 1988, Doubleday.
23. National Center for Health Statistics, 1995: *Health, United States, 1995,* Hyattsville, MD, Public Health Service.
24. Klerman LV: *Alive and well?: a research and policy review of health programs for poor young children,* New York, 1991, National Center for Children in Poverty, Columbia School of Public Health.
25. Klerman LV: The health of poor children. In Huston AC, editor: *Children in poverty,* New York, 1994, Cambridge University Press.
26. U.S. Department of Health and Human Services: Trends in the well-being of America's children and youth: 1996, Washington, D.C., 1996, Office of the Assistant Secretary for Planning and Evaluation.

CHAPTER 96

Cults

•

Margaret Thaler Singer

The spread of cults began in the late 1960s, but it was not until the tragic mass suicide/murder of 913 U.S. citizens in Guyana in 1978 that people began to focus on the tremendous influence that cult leaders can have over their followers.[1,2] Since that time, countless families in the United States and elsewhere have had to cope with the problems that arise when a member of the family becomes involved with a cult.

The first wave of cults that sprang up in the United States tended to recruit 18- to 25-year-olds. Most of these were religious cults. Soon the variety of cults increased and the age range of those recruited widened.[3] Families sought assistance from health professionals, clergy, and educators about how to cope with the cult issue.

TYPES OF CULTS

Because the first wave in the late 1960s and early 1970s tended to be religious cults, some people mistakenly think that all cults are religious in nature. However, there are political cults; psychologic cults; communal living groups that become cults; flying saucer cults; women's separatist cults; and diet, health, philosophical, and Satanic cults—to name a few. In recent years, some attention has been paid to the smaller individualized, or one-on-one, cults.[4]

PUBLIC CONCERN ABOUT CULTS

Public concern has focused on the recruitment activities; apparent personality changes reported to result from membership; and general public awareness of reported child abuse, deaths, bizarre crimes, and acts of terrorism associated with cults.[5] In addition, parents are concerned about the "lost years" youths have spent in some of these groups. As with any organization, each cult must be evaluated on its own conduct. Cults vary from relatively benign groups to ones whose records are replete with illegalities, including murder. As each group is considered individually, the focus must be on its conduct and

behavior, not its beliefs. The First Amendment protects belief absolutely, but it leaves the behavior of all citizens and groups open to public review and the requirements of law. Cults have been studied from theological, social, psychologic, and legal standpoints.[6] However, one of the sagest overviews has been by a physician who analyzed cults from a public health standpoint.[7]

CULT MEMBERS

Requests to physicians and others for consultation are not limited to the need to know what to do about teenagers and young adults who have joined cults. Currently, when one spouse leaves a cult but has children and a marital partner still in the group, that individual may seek legal, medical, and psychologic consultation about his or her rights in regard to the children. Grandparents also may have concerns about the welfare of their grandchildren when they are being reared in cults. Finally, adult children often seek help about what to do when their parents are recruited by cults. Because of the breadth and complexity of issues involved in discussing cults, the focus here will be on youth participation.

PERVASIVENESS OF CULTS

It is estimated that in the past two decades 20 million people in the United States have been involved with one or another of the reportedly 5000 cults and cultlike groups in the country. These groups range in size from ones composed of a dozen or fewer members to large international groups claiming membership in the millions.[3,4]

MYTHS ABOUT WHO JOINS CULTS

Many people mistakenly think that youths who join cults are psychologic misfits, products of bad or broken families, or seekers of the very cult they joined. These myths have not been validated by research and they appear to be related to the common tendency to blame victims. This attitude allows many people to avoid serious thought about cults—how they form and operate and their impact on individuals, families, and society—by simply blaming those who join cults or their families as being inadequate or having pathologic problems. In turn, many parents believe that they must be at fault in some way when their offspring joins a cult. Such self-blame often causes them to fail to seek help. However, families in this situation need assistance from people and agencies knowledgeable about how cults operate in a general way; in particular, they need information about the specific group the family member has joined. Ex-members of many of these groups, parent support groups, and professionals often can provide information, reading materials, and assistance. (See Resources listed at the end of this chapter.)

Research indicates that approximately two thirds of the young adults who have joined cults come from normal-functioning families and demonstrate age-appropriate behavior when they enter the cult. Of the remaining third, about 6% had major psychologic difficulties before joining the cult. The rest of those with problems had diagnosable depression related to a personal loss (e.g., death in the family, failure to gain entry to the college of choice, broken romance) or were struggling with age-related sexual or career dilemmas.

Other myths include the idea that people freely choose to get involved in a cult and that they are happy and content. Studies indicate that most cults apply organized, intense tactics of influence to induce people to join. Furthermore, there is often widespread deception involved in recruitment. At best, the new recruit is not fully informed about what membership will entail. Cult apologists tend to present "seeker" theories and ignore the active recruiting efforts of cults.

After joining a cult, new members are exposed to concentrated social and psychologic influence techniques designed to change their demeanor, behavior, and expressed attitudes to conform to those that will benefit the group's goals. The welfare and life plans of the members are rarely a consideration. Most cults apply what researchers have termed "coordinated programs of coercive influence and behavior control."[8] Other terms, such as "thought reform," "coercive persuasion," and "brainwashing," have been used to describe the variety of social and psychologic techniques used to induce substantial changes in belief or opinion. These organized influence programs are often effective in eliciting compliance. An obvious goal in most cults is to teach the members to avoid expressing criticism and negative feelings so that the public and potential new members see only positive signs and enthusiasm for the group. Divergence from this pattern can result in ostracism,

social pressure to conform, and a loss of status in the group.

Former members commonly reveal that they were looking only for companionship and the chance to do something to benefit themselves and mankind. They often say that they were not looking for the particular cult they joined and were not intending to belong to the cult for a lifetime. Instead, they were actively and/or deceptively pressured to join, soon found themselves enmeshed in the group, were slowly cut off from their past and their families, and became totally dependent on the group.

POTENTIAL CULT MEMBERS

It appears that almost anyone, at a vulnerable period in his or her life, is a potential cult recruit. Research shows that no "type" is prone to join cults, nor is membership linked to a previous psychopathologic condition. Rather, anyone who is at a vulnerable period in life (e.g., period of transition, time of loss, period of loneliness) is open to persuasion and influence. Although vulnerability is transient, if a cult recruiter appears and adeptly and insistently applies simple lures and influence procedures during these periods, the individual can be easily influenced. Mild to moderate depression is the most frequently noted cause of vulnerability to cult lures. When a youth is depressed because of a recent disappointment, loss, or failure, a cult recruiter's offering of a group that will accept the person unconditionally and provide a supposedly positive, simplistic way to improve oneself and a means of helping mankind is more likely to appeal to the young person than it would at other times.

STRESS FACTORS

Another kind of vulnerability evolves when youths begin to feel overwhelmed by the multitude and complexities of the choices they need to make in the late teenage and early adult years. In addition to those personal decisions that must be addressed, many adolescents are attempting to come to grips with their overall values, beliefs, and purposes. The sheer number of choices an adolescent needs to make, the ambiguity of life at this age, the complexity of the world, and the amount of conflict associated with many aspects of daily life can be overwhelming. Many former cult members report that certain classes that they took in late high school and early college contributed greatly to their bewilderment. They commonly describe classes, teachers, and experiences that they felt had destabilized their views of the world. As a result, they felt a need to find affiliation and some simple ways to make life work. They literally felt "at sea" about so many things and were frightened by the complexity of how to make seemingly endless decisions. They felt lost and alone. Without intending to make such a choice, they found themselves swept along into a group that offered simple and "guaranteed" paths to follow. Sometimes the young person had been handed an invitation or a brochure on the street or on campus, approached in the dorm to attend a social meeting, and in a short time induced to join a type of cult.

Other appeals are found in free lectures on campus about the supposedly scientifically based benefits of meditation, which soon lead to joining a cult. Other youths are directly approached and asked to attend a particular event that would appeal to many in their age group. One large cult has a rock band that tours the country and serves as an attraction in malls and large assembly areas. Members of the cult personally approach and invite young persons to their local headquarters. Other teenagers are recruited into a cult while they are traveling at home or abroad. Thus, being in a transitional state, whether psychologic or physical, increases openness to persuasion and influence.

TRUST, GULLIBILITY, AND PERSUADABILITY

Cults are seeking friendly, obedient, altruistic, and malleable people, because such individuals are easy to persuade and control. Cults do not want to deal with recalcitrant, disobedient, self-centered youths. Such individuals are simply too difficult to mold into highly controlled, tightly disciplined organizations that use guilt and social pressure as their main methods of control.

Tough, insolent, self-centered, or street-smart youths are difficult to change easily. They do not trust others and do not simply go along with the requests or offerings of others. Such youths have been "burned" enough by life and do not politely trust people who try to influence them. Therefore, they are not compliance prone. They are wary of offers of instant companionship, group living, seemingly altruistic work, and a sense of security. Such youths are likely to have been lied to and to have experienced or carried out street hustles or con jobs. They sense from experience that people who approach them with offerings have a double agenda—the surface one and a hidden agenda. Trusting individuals and those from protected backgrounds are more likely simply to respond without sufficient critical thinking about what is behind the offerings and claims made by others.

Some of the large cults have handbooks that describe types of individuals to enlist and how to set up recruiting encounters. Cult members are trained in persuasive methods for approaching potential new members. Some cults assign members to recruit on junior high and senior high school grounds, in college dormitories, and outside counseling offices. The cult's program is sold by calculated persuasion procedures. The recruitment practices used belie the myth that people freely join the cult.

To lure people, one large cult offers free personality tests as a means of learning to communicate better. No one ever attains an acceptable score on the test. Instead, each person is told that he or she is in dire need of help that only this particular organization can provide, and that without such help the individual's psychologic stability will deteriorate. At this point of entry the youthful "buyer" is unaware that he or she is joining a religion. Other groups are more open about their core contents but do not provide sufficient information about what the "bottom line" will be. Most people who join cults have little real knowledge of what will eventually happen to them. It is rare for a new member to exercise fully informed consent. The individual is usually making an emotionally based acquiescence to organized persuasion tactics.

ENTRY INTO CULT GROUPS

With cults, individuals are gradually exposed to a series of lectures, events, and experiences that, one step at a time, cut them off from their past. They come to accept the idea that their family and their past have been "bad." They are led to think that to survive and to help the world, they must give their life to the cult leader, who has some special knowledge, facts, talents, and mission in life.

New members are changed so gradually that they do not notice. Eventually, however, they no longer call or write to their family and friends. They may drop out of school, or school may be relegated to such a low priority that eventually it becomes impossible to keep up with schoolwork because the cult activities occupy so much time.

THOUGHT MANIPULATION

In growing up, it is almost impossible to avoid having mixed feelings about one's parents. Even the most beloved mothers and fathers have had encounters with offspring that leave memorable feelings of anger, and parents have some habits or peculiarities that can be aggravating. Cults play upon such normal ambivalences.

For example, one large cult has its members adopt vegetarianism, the wearing of light-colored clothing, and chanting. Soon new members are indoctrinated to regard their parents as "flesh-eating parents who wear ungodly clothing" (red, yellow, and black colors) and who "intellectualize" and are not "enlightened." New cult members soon cut off ties with the flesh-eaters, wear light-colored clothes; avoid reflective, critical thinking about the group ("intellectualizing"); and occupy their minds with almost continuous internal chanting.

SIBLINGS OF CULT MEMBERS

The brothers and sisters of cult members are rarely discussed, yet they should be kept in mind when a physician or other consultant works with a family. Often the siblings are involved in a replay of the prodigal son story. The brothers and sisters want to say to the parents, "Why don't you pay attention to me? Why is all the emotion and time being focused on the person in the cult?" Often the siblings are angry and disappointed in the cult member. Usually they are unaware of the deceptions commonly associated with cult recruitment, the marked social and psychologic pressure brought to bear on members while they are in the cult, and the fears the cult member is inbued with about leaving the group. The siblings recall childhood memories of disappointments and anger toward the individual and inwardly dwell on the injustice that appears to be transpiring. They are in school, working, helping the family, and yet the parents focus almost solely on having lost a child to a cult. If parents can be counseled to understand the hidden resentments often harbored by siblings about the unequal attention the missing cultist receives, much good can be achieved.

CULTS, MARRIAGE, AND DIVORCE

Some cults arrange marriages between members, often for immigration purposes or to maintain tight control of members by the leader, who may pair partners. When children have been born and one partner leaves the cult and the other remains, the issue of group custody arises. Many legal cases are being noted in which the parent who has left the cult seeks legal assistance to secure visitation and custody rights to gain some control over the education, health, and care of the child or children still in the cult. Physicians are often consulted in such cases and need to have firm knowledge about the practices of the cults, because some groups have printed "answers" that the cult parent provides to outsiders to make cult practices appear different from what they actually are.

CULTS AS INTERNATIONAL PHENOMENA

In the past two decades, the growth of cults and their effects on youth, family life, and certain economic and political areas have come to public attention. However, only in recent years, because of cult-related tragedies in the United States, Canada, Switzerland, and Japan, have citizens become cognizant of the cults' impact on our society.[9] Some cults have grown so large and wealthy that their land holdings affect local tax rates because of the sizable amount of cult property that is excluded from taxes.

RESOURCE INFORMATION

Until a few years ago, health professionals, clergy, educators, and families had few places or people to turn to for consultation about dealing with cult issues. Currently, numerous cult veterans and organizations are available to provide consultation and aid to the practitioner and family.[4,6,10] (See the resources listed at the end of this chapter). The American Family Foundation publishes the *Cultic Studies Journal* and other material about cults, and also serves as a referral and information service for former members, families, and professionals in all fields who might be concerned about the cult issue. This agency can put callers in touch with local resource people across the nation and provide referral sources in Canada, England, France, Germany, Spain, and Sweden. reFOCUS (Recovering Former Cultists Support) also can provide information and referrals to local resources. Families, health professionals, and others also can find individuals in their own localities who can be of assistance and help with information about cults, cult processes, and working with families who have members in cults.

References

1. Wooden K: *The children of Jonestown,* New York, 1981, McGraw-Hill.
2. Reiterman T, Jacobs J: *Raven: the untold story of the Rev. Jim Jones and his people,* New York, 1982, E.P. Dutton.
3. Singer MT, with Lalich J: *Cults in our midst: the hidden menace in our everyday lives,* San Francisco, 1995, Jossey-Bass.
4. Tobias ML, Lalich J: *Captive hearts, captive minds: freedom and recovery from cults and abusive relationships,* Alameda, CA, 1994, Hunter House.
5. Ofshe R, Singer MT: Attacks on peripheral versus central elements of self and the impact of thought reforming techniques, *Cult Stud J* 3:3-24, 1986.
6. Langone MD, editor: *Recovery from cults: help for victims of psychological and spiritual abuse,* New York, 1993, Norton.
7. West LJ: Persuasive techniques in contemporary cults. In Galanter M, editor: *Cults and new religious movements,* Washington, DC, 1989, American Psychiatric Press; pp 165-192.
8. Singer MT, Ofshe R: Thought reform programs and the production of psychiatric casualties, *Psychiatr Ann* 20:188-193, 1990.
9. Singer MT, Lalich J: The social meaning of Aum Shinri Kyo, *The Cult Observer* 12(7), 1995.
10. Giambalvo C: *Exit counseling: a family intervention,* ed 2, Bonita Springs, FL, 1995, American Family Foundation.

CHAPTER 97

Cross-Cultural Views of Adolescence

•

Alice Schlegel

It is commonly believed that adolescence as a *social* stage is a product of the industrial age. However, evidence from across the world indicates that the behavior of young people and the way they are treated differentiate them from both children and adults. The need for an adolescent stage is clear in societies that demand a lengthy period of schooling or apprenticeship, but it is not so obvious in tribal societies. Nevertheless, in the Standard Cross-Cultural Sample, a representative worldwide sample of 186 preindustrial societies ranging from foraging bands to traditional states, this stage is reported to be present in every case for boys and also for girls (with one possible exception). The information presented in this chapter comes from a study that used that sample, with supplementation from historical and contemporary accounts of adolescent life.[1]

PARAMETERS OF ADOLESCENCE

Members of both sexes most commonly enter the stage of adolescence at the approximate time of puberty. In a study that also used the standard sample, ceremonies marking the transition from childhood to adolescence were reported as present in 36% of societies for boys and in 46% of societies for girls.[2] One aspect of adolescent initiation ceremonies is preparation for adult gender roles. These ceremonies occur most often in tribal societies, in which gender is likely to be the single most salient feature of social identity. Ritual recognition may be limited to one sphere of activity. Such is the case for the contemporary Jewish bar mitzvah, in which a boy is given adult religious responsibilities but is not moved into full social adulthood.

In most societies, marriage marks the end of adolescence and the beginning of adulthood. Adolescence is usually longer for boys than for girls, probably because a boy must prove his competence before parents are willing to release their daughter to him. Girls are likely to be married young, particularly when parents stand to benefit materially from a daughter's marriage by receiving goods or labor from their son-in-law. The factors that precipitate or delay marriage usually determine the length of the adolescent stage. Although an Eskimo boy married and entered adulthood at about age 20, his sister usually did so shortly after menarche, at about age 14 or 15.

When marriage is delayed beyond the late teens, there is generally a social stage intervening between adolescence and adulthood. It is useful to distinguish this youth stage and not to see it as merely a prolongation of adolescence.[3] Our contemporary youth stage, which extends from the end of high school to marriage or serious employment, is not new. Europe and America have a long history of a youth stage, since delayed marriage (in the middle or late twenties) for both sexes was common before the Industrial Revolution.[4,5]

ADOLESCENCE ACROSS CULTURES

Parents and Family

A major task for adolescents in Western society is preparing themselves for independence. However, such preparation is unnecessary when children remain in the household of parents (or parents-in-law). A struggle for autonomy is not a major problem in such cases, since control over one's own activities and those of others is achieved gradually as parents age and adult children grow into the roles of heads of the household.

This does not imply that conflict or antagonism never arises. Adolescent children can resent parental authority, especially when their own goals are thwarted. For example, an African cattle-keeper may prefer to use his animals for bride wealth to acquire another wife for himself rather than one for his son, or a peasant family might deny education to a bright and motivated child and insist that he or she remain at home to work on the family farm. Nevertheless, there is little evidence in the sample of much overt conflict, possibly because in most preindustrial societies adolescent children are too dependent on family resources for their future well-being to risk alienating their parents through rude or rebellious behavior.

As measured for this sample, parent-child relationships differ somewhat between the sexes. Although conflict between parents and children is low in most societies, it tends to be somewhat higher between fathers and children, particularly sons, than between mothers and children. Children are also more subordinate to fathers than to mothers and more intimate with mothers than with fathers.

Parent-child relationships are not simply a function of contact, because the highest level of contact is between mother and daughter and then between father and son, mother and son, and father and daughter, in that order. Therefore, separation of the sexes exists to some degree even within the home. In modern societies, in which fathers usually work away from home, the contact between father and son is greatly reduced. In this sample, fathers and sons generally work together, except when adolescent boys have specialized occupational roles such as herding animals.

Peers and Community

The children's play group assumes greater importance when it is transformed into the peer group of adolescents. Peers in most societies in the sample associate during leisure hours. Unlike Western adolescents, who spend most of their waking hours with peers in school, boys in other societies are together for most of their waking hours in only a few cases. (There are no societies in the sample in which girls spend most of their waking hours with peers.)

Peer groups exist for both sexes, but boys' groups are likely to be larger and more formally organized than are girls' groups. Girls often see their friends in the company of mothers and other older women, whereas boys are more likely to associate with one another away from adult supervision or interaction.

Interacting with adults other than kin is usually done in groups of same-sex peers. In many places, such as in Japanese villages, the adolescent boys' group is held responsible for certain aspects of community welfare, in this case keeping the paths to the village shrine cleared. Organizing events in community festivities or religious rituals was a prominent feature of adolescent life in early modern Europe and persists into the present in parts of eastern and southern Europe. Adolescents may often be called on to do the social "dirty work" of the community by punishing deviant behavior of adults through mockery and harassment or by chasing away undesirables, all with the approval of adults. Examples include the Mbuti pygmies of Africa, European peasants, and the boys of Chinatowns in the United States.

Social Deviance

Every society has its occasional deviant, but only a minority of societies in the sample are like modern societies in that antisocial behavior is expected from some adolescents, usually boys. Since there were too few cases of such expectations for girls to permit testing, the following discussion applies only to boys.

The most common forms of antisocial behavior are violence and theft, although destruction of property and sexual misbehavior also occur. Violence takes the form of fighting, which rarely results in death or serious injury. Theft is commonly small-scale. Although adults publicly deplore antisocial behavior, there is evidence of some ambivalence about it; for example, such behavior may be used against a hated or envied neighbor or his child; or it may be secretly admired as a sign of masculine daring, as among the Gros Ventre Indians of the North American Great Plains.

Boys are more likely to behave in antisocial ways in societies in which they have less contact with men (not necessarily their fathers) and more contact with peers. They are also likely to commit antisocial acts when men also often do so. Childhood socialization also plays a role; for example, reliance on certain child-socialization techniques such as lecturing or rewarding good behavior appears to be ineffective in teaching children the restraint of impulses.

There is no evidence that antisocial behavior in these preindustrial societies arises out of antagonism toward, or alienation from, the family or the community. It appears to be a response to impulses and is usually directed toward other adolescents. For example, in societies in which some boys are expected to steal, there is likely to be little emphasis on productive work, yet an important technique for socializing children in these societies is to reward them with gifts. Thus, boys are taught to prize material possessions without learning to work for them. Theft is an obvious way of gratifying an acquisitive impulse, not a protest against family or society.

Although boys' peer groups may encourage or at least allow for antisocial behavior, the available evidence for girls suggests that their peer groups tend to promote conformity.

Sexuality

For most societies in the sample, premarital virginity is not expected for either sex. However, sexuality is prohibited in those societies (or social classes) in which the choice of a son-in-law is a critical issue for the social status of the girl's family.[6] These societies tend to be the more complex ones in which dowry or indirect dowry is given to the new couple, or elaborate gifts are exchanged between the families of the bride and groom. When girls' adolescence is short and girls marry within a few years after menarche, the premarital pregnancy rate is low because of widespread adolescent subfecundity.

A few societies, such as the Muria tribe of India, promote sexual behavior through the use of adolescent houses, dormitories in which boys and girls frolic and sleep together after the day's chores are done. In other cases, parents pretend ignorance of their children's sexual adventures. Peers in these kinds of societies usually pressure one another to spread their sexual "favors" among the adolescents of the community rather than to pair off, recognizing that the solidarity of the peer group is threatened by exclusive romantic attachments.

Homosexual acts are tolerated in some societies as an expression of youthful experimentation or as a substitute for relations with the opposite sex. This does not appear to lead to an adult preference for homosexuality.

Development of Self

In preindustrial societies, adolescence is often a time of pressure for both sexes not only to exhibit competence but also to excel, since one's future spouse, in-laws, social connections, and activities are determined to some extent by how one succeeds as an adolescent. Memories are long in small communities, and one rarely has the opportunity to start over elsewhere. Data on adolescence have been compared with data on childhood for the same sample to determine the pattern of development.[7] Measures of socialization for character traits leading to compliance (responsibility, obedience, sexual restraint) show an increase from early to late childhood and from late childhood to adolescence, whereas the measures of socialization for traits leading to assertion (achievement, aggressiveness, competitiveness, self-reliance) show a decrease from late childhood to adolescence. This shift in socialization comes at a time when adolescents are straining against the bonds of childhood discipline, and what is tolerated in the child may be disapproved of or even punished in the adolescent. Although there is pressure on both sexes for compliance, it is somewhat stronger for girls than for boys. This gender difference should not be exaggerated, however, because societies that emphasize certain traits for one sex are likely to do so for the other.

The inculcation of character traits varies according to features of the social setting. The form of the household is one such feature; for example, boys exhibit significantly lower levels of aggressiveness in societies with the stem-family (three-generation) household, and girls exhibit significantly higher levels of aggressiveness in societies with the nuclear-family household. The peer group is another such feature; boys' higher level of aggressiveness is significantly related to increased contact with peers and increased competitiveness within the peer groups.

Gender Differences

The greatest gender difference in the organization of adolescent life lies in relations with adults and peers. Girls remain embedded in their families more than do boys; conversely, boys are extruded more than girls. Boys' peer groups play a larger role in their lives than do girls' groups in theirs. Girls are more often in the company of women than boys are in the company of men. This sex difference seems to arise before adolescence and is intensified at that stage. Such different settings have profound consequences for behavior and personality features.

Mixed age groups are hierarchical, whereas peer groups are egalitarian. There is less of a disjuncture between the social settings of childhood and adolescence for girls than for boys, which may ease the transition from childhood for girls. Age-stratified structures tend to inhibit competition for status within the group, whereas egalitarian structures promote it. Thus, in their peer groups boys learn to compete. However, they also learn to cooperate in organizing action, since boys' peer groups tend to have more goal-oriented activities, such as team sports or community activities, than do girls' groups, which are more likely to be engaged in conversation or unstructured play.

Although all groups pressure members toward conformity to the norms of the group, the senior members in mixed age groups enforce conformity to community norms. This may help to account for the lesser social deviance exhibited by girls in general. It is also likely that in their closer relations with mothers and other women, girls learn to "read" the actions of the adults in order to judge a situation and the appropriate responses to it, and they learn to influence rather than to dominate. Thus, they commonly acquire a style of interaction that is less assertive and less competitive than the style that boys learn in their peer groups.

The findings on the inculcation of aggressiveness and other character traits support this gender difference. Although both sexes respond to various features of the family, boys more than girls respond to features of the peer group in that peer-group variables show more correlations with other variables for boys than they do for girls.

MODERN ADOLESCENTS

The greatest difference in the activities of modern adolescents in comparison with adolescents in preindustrial societies is the amount of time spent with adults and peers. In most preindustrial societies adolescents spend most of their waking hours with adults of the same sex, even when they spend their free time, or the entire night in the case of adolescent dormitories, with age mates. Adolescents in such societies are working alongside adults, except for some herding societies (in which boys may herd together) or some hunting societies (in which boys may hunt together or alone). These adults are usually family members, although a boy or girl may be an apprentice to a recognized craftsman and spend considerable time working with that person.

Schooling makes the difference. Mass education is a product of industrialization, and it is increasingly widespread in formerly tribal societies.[8] In earlier times, schooling as we know it was limited to the elite or to very young children, or it was of a religious nature and occupied only a few hours a week. Universal education puts all adolescents in contact with peers for much of the day. Often, the after-school and weekend jobs that adolescents have also put them in contact with other adolescents rather than with adults.

Findings from the cross-cultural study indicate that antisocial behavior of boys is related to lesser contact with men (not necessarily their fathers), organized peer groups that have names, and a high level of competition among peers. Competitiveness and a low degree of cooperation and trust are associated with violence (fighting). Thus, without ameliorating influences such as frequent contact with fathers or other male mentors, a certain proportion of adolescent boys in modern societies can be expected to misbehave. Given the rise of the female-headed household and the diminishing importance of community structures that bring boys into interaction with men (e.g., religious organizations), it is possible that adolescent misbehavior will increase. (If the mentors are themselves delinquent, however, boys will be socialized for delinquency.)

A close bond between mother and daughter may insulate the adolescent girl, more than the boy, from adverse peer or neighborhood influences. On the negative side, the girl may not find her affiliative needs satisfied as much from peers as boys do, and a rupture in the family ties may affect her more severely. Teenage girls in the United States seem to show more signs of emotional distress than do boys.[9] Decreasing the girl's contact with women, and thus reducing her emotional support, may make her vulnerable to feeling lonely and directionless.

The study of adolescence in preindustrial societies lends support to the widespread recognition that young people need contact with trusted adults to be successful during this stage of their lives. In preindustrial societies these adults are likely to be of the same sex as the child. The need for close ties with same-sex adults also may be true for modern societies, although that cannot be inferred from the data available. It is not necessary that the adults be parents or family members. Both the nature and the amount of contact may be important features. Since antisocial behavior is associated with competitiveness, noncompetitive activities (e.g., building a structure, organizing an event) appear to be more conducive to compliance than are competitive games or sports.

Sexuality is another area that is often viewed as troublesome, especially when disease or inappropriate pregnancy result. However, in most societies adolescents take a rather light-hearted attitude toward sexual activity, and that seems to be the approach that adolescents in the United States are taking. Socialization for responsible sexuality is needed to keep pace with the changing mores of our teenage children.

Young people can be helped to achieve a successful adolescence by being in settings that include a high ratio of concerned adults to adolescents. The three-generation family has such a ratio, but this family form seems unlikely to develop in the contemporary world, where the single-parent household is becoming a widespread "normal" alternative. Schools are not and cannot be such settings. It is time, perhaps, to rethink education to include apprenticeships or other practical arrangements for bringing adolescents and adults together.

References

1. Schlegel A, Barry H III: *Adolescence: an anthropological inquiry,* New York, 1991, The Free Press.
2. Schlegel A, Barry H III: The evolutionary significance of adolescent initiation ceremonies, *Am Ethnologist* 7:696, 1980.
3. Keniston K: *Youth in dissent: the rise of a new opposition,* New York, 1971, Harcourt Brace Jovanovich.
4. Stone L: *The family, sex and marriage in England, 1500-1800,* New York, 1977, Harper & Row.
5. Kett JF: *Rites of passage: adolescence in America, 1790 to the present,* New York, 1977, Basic Books.
6. Schlegel A: Status, property, and the value on virginity, *Am Ethnologist* 18:719, 1991.
7. Barry H III, Josephson L, Lauer E, Marshall C: Traits inculcated in childhood: cross-cultural codes 5. In Barry H III, Schlegel A, editors: *Cross-cultural samples and codes,* Pittsburgh, 1980, University of Pittsburgh Press; p 237.
8. Schlegel A, guest editor: Special issue on adolescence, *Ethos 23,* no. 1, 1995.
9. Offer D, Sabshin M: Adolescence: empirical perspectives. In Offer D, Sabshin M, editors: *Normality and the life cycle,* New York, 1984, Basic Books; p 76.

CHAPTER 98

Sexual Dysfunction

•

Alwyn T. Cohall and Theresa M. Exner

It is a tribute to the resilient adolescent spirit that, despite our society's failure to promote healthy sexual development, most young people survive their sexual exploits during adolescence and go on to become sexually adjusted adults. However, for a variety of reasons, some adolescents may have difficulty achieving satisfactory sexual functioning. Left unattended, these early difficulties may become firmly entrenched by adulthood.

ADOLESCENT PSYCHOSEXUAL DEVELOPMENT

There are several developmental tasks that adolescents must complete on the pathway toward adulthood, such as emancipation from parents, development of abstract reasoning, achievement of moral identity, development of plans for the future, and the means for making those plans come true. Just as important are the tasks of psychosexual development.

Sarrel and Sarrel[1] posited that, to become a "sexually healthy" adult, several "mini-tasks" must be completed. These include (1) the development of a positive gender-specific body image that is relatively free from distortion, (2) acceptance of oneself as a sexual person, (3) resolution of gender identity conflicts and sexual orientation, (4) the ability to make personally and socially responsible sexual decisions, and (5) a gradually increasing ability to experience eroticism as one aspect of interpersonal intimacy.

Failure to master these tasks completely may impair sexual functioning. There are many rapids to negotiate in navigating the waters of psychosexual development; relatively few adolescents approach their first sexual experiences with a knowledge and acceptance of their capacity for sexual expression. Early sexual exploration is typically covert and rushed. Mixed parental, peer, religious, and cultural messages can foster confusion and guilt; combine these with sexual ignorance, identity concerns, relationship issues, and performance demands, and the situation is ripe for the development of sexual problems.

Scattered case reports and studies[2-6] provide some insight into adolescent sexual complaints, but it is not possible to determine the true incidence or prevalence of sexual dysfunction among sexually active adolescents since there have been no population-based studies in this age group. In the absence of such data, we must guardedly use extant adolescent studies in conjunction with those involving adults to estimate the dimensions of the problems affecting adolescents. Before briefly describing the DSM IV[7] psychosexual dysfunctions, it is important to frame the discussion within the context of the sexual response cycle.

THE HUMAN SEXUAL RESPONSE

In their pioneer 1966 volume, Masters and Johnson[8] provided the first clear description of the physiology of the human sexual response. Their findings were based on observations of 694 men and women aged 18 to 89 during more than 7000 cycles of sexual response. Table 98-1 presents a summary of each phase of the cycle.

During the response cycle, complementary physiologic changes occur in both sexes. There is a noted increase in heart rate, blood pressure, genital vasocongestion, muscle tension, breathing rate, and skin flush. Orgasmic contractions occur at the same 0.8-second interval for both men and women. The only substantial sex differences identified by Masters and Johnson concern ejaculation (women do not ejaculate) and

TABLE 98-1
The Sexual Response Cycle

	Desire	Arousal	Orgasm	Resolution
Subjective Recognition	Cognitive perception	Female: Vaginal lubrication Male: Erection	Female: Genital throbbing Male: Emission, ejaculation	Relaxation Detumescence in male
Primary Physiologic Process	Hormonal?	Genital vasocongestion	Muscular contraction	

multiple orgasm (men do not experience multiple orgasm). A critical contribution has been Masters and Johnson's debunking of the vaginal orgasm myth: that *all* orgasms are the result—directly or indirectly—of clitoral stimulation.

Kaplan[9] conceptually simplified Masters and Johnson's model and speaks in terms of a biphasic model of sexual response. She states that the sexual response consists of two distinct and relatively independent components: (1) a general vasocongestive reaction (arousal), which is controlled by the parasympathetic system; and (2) reflexive clonic muscular contractions (orgasm), which are controlled by the sympathetic system. Since the two components are controlled by different parts of the central nervous system, one can be inhibited or impaired while the other functions normally.

CONCEPTUALIZING SEXUAL PROBLEMS

Before specific dysfunctions and possible etiologic factors are discussed, a general framework for evaluating sexual difficulties is in order. When conceptualizing problems of sexual functioning, it is useful to distinguish between lifelong and acquired dysfunctions. In the former case, the individual has never experienced a period of normal functioning; in the latter, a period of adequate functioning occurred before the sexual dysfunction developed. Typically, lifelong dysfunctions are the most intransigent, the exception being inhibited female orgasm, where it is often easier to treat preorgasmic women. Prognosis is better for problems that are situational (occurring only in limited contexts) than for those that are generalized. Finally, it is useful to distinguish between etiologic factors that are medical, psychologic, or both. Combined factors are at play when (1) psychologic factors have a role in onset, severity, exacerbation, or maintenance of the dysfunction; and (2) a general medical condition or substance use (including medication side

---

BOX 98-1
Problem Dimensions Checklist

1. Has the problem always existed?
2. Does it exist in all situations? With all partners? During all sexual activities? During masturbation?
3. Are there health or organic problems that may be playing a role? Are any medications being taken by the patient?
4. Are there serious psychologic problems? Depression? Anxiety? Substance abuse?
5. Are there environmental problems that are interfering with functioning and/or will interfere with working on the problem?
6. Are there relationship problems within the couple?
7. Is there more than one sexual problem?

---

effects) is contributory but not sufficient to account for the dysfunction. Box 98-1 presents brief questions useful for clarifying these dimensions. The more questions that can be answered affirmatively, the more difficult is the probable course of treatment.

SEXUAL DYSFUNCTION

How common are sexual dysfunctions? The DSM IV acknowledged that the prevalence of sexual dysfunctions is not known. Data from a representative U.S. probability sample, which provides rates of specific self-reported sexual "problems" lasting several months or more in the previous year, show that difficulties with functioning, at least in a milder form, are not rare.[10] The dysfunctions most likely to be encountered in clinical practice are summarized in Table 98-2, along with available prevalence information.

TABLE 98-2
Definition and Estimated Prevalence of Selected Psychosexual Dysfunctions

Dysfunction	Response Cycle Phase	Definition	Prevalence
Hypoactive sexual desire	Desire	Persistent or recurrently deficient (or absent) sexual fantasies and desire for sexual activity	Absence of all desire present in 1% to 3% of married men and women and in 15% to 20% of single heterosexual women[11] Among those 18-24 years of age, 13.6% of men and 32% of women report problems with lack of interest in sex[10]
Female sexual arousal disorder	Arousal	A recurrent and persistent condition in which there is a partial or complete failure to attain or maintain lubrication/swelling until completion of intercourse	Dysfunction rates in women cannot be estimated Among women 18-24 years of age, 19.3% report problems with lubrication[9]
Male sexual arousal disorder	Arousal	A recurrent and persistent condition in which there is a partial or complete failure to attain or maintain an erection until completion of intercourse	In men under age 60, rates of erectile failure (of varying severity) range from 10% to 20%[11] Among men 18-24 years of age, 5.6% report inability to keep an erection[10]
Male orgasmic disorder	Orgasm	A recurrent or persistent delay or absence of ejaculation following a normal sexual excitement phase judged by the clinician to be adequate in focus, intensity, and duration	Kinsey reported a base rate of 15/10,000[12] In less severe forms, it may be present in about 5% of the population[11] Among men 18-24 years of age, 4.6% report problems with ability to orgasm[10]
Female orgasmic disorder	Orgasm	A recurrent or persistent delay or absence of orgasm following a normal sexual excitement phase judged by the clinician to be adequate in focus, intensity, and duration (*Note:* A fairly large subset of women can experience orgasm during noncoital stimulation but not during vaginal intercourse in the absence of direct clitoral stimulation)	Among white, middle-class married women surveyed, 15% reported total inability to reach orgasm; 46% reported difficulty in achieving orgasm[13] Among sexually active adolescent girls surveyed, 25% reported never achieving orgasm, 33% were "unsure," and 42% had experienced orgasm[6] Among women 18-24 years of age, 26% report problems with ability to orgasm[10]
Premature ejaculation	Orgasm	The recurrent inability to exert reasonable control over orgasm and ejaculation during sexual activity	Prevalence of this disorder is 22% to 35%[11] Among men 18-24 years of age, 26.6% report climaxing too early[10] Kinsey suggests that ejaculation occurs within 2 minutes of intromission for three quarters of American men[13]
Dyspareunia	—	Pain during intercourse	Among those 18-24 years of age, 5.7% of men and 21.5% of women report pain during sex[10]
Vaginismus	—	A condition that involves involuntary contraction of the pelvic musculature and the vaginal introitus	Rates cannot be estimated

ETIOLOGIES

From their review of the literature, Spector and Boyle[14] provided a useful framework for conceptualizing the cause of sexual dysfunction. Although there is some overlap, the causes fall broadly into four categories: physical, psychosocial, practical, and sexual.

Physical Causes

Search for the cause of sexual dysfunction should always address possible organic factors. The likelihood of organic contributions tends to vary with the specific disorder. In males, physiologic factors are rarely implicated as a reason for premature ejaculation. Organicity is more likely to come into play when erectile difficulties are discovered,[15] although psychologic impotence is the usual reason for erectile dysfunction among adolescent males.[5] In general, conditions associated with low levels of circulating testosterone—or more precisely, its active metabolite dihydrotestosterone—may cause problems with erection, since testosterone is essential for the achievement of adequate erectile function (Table 98-3). Conditions associated with increased levels of prolactin may similarly be problematic, since prolactin interferes with the bioactivity of testosterone.[16]

Vascular occlusion or diversion of blood supply to the pelvic organs can also result in erectile problems[17] and probably to lubrication and swelling difficulties in females. Similarly, conditions resulting in sensory neuropathy may decrease genital sensation and feedback. Autonomic neuropathy may prevent adequate maintenance of the venous constriction needed to keep the corpora cavernosa engorged. It may also impair arousal in females. Infections of the prostate gland in males (usually secondary to gonorrhea or *Chlamydia* infection) also may be implicated in erectile dysfunction and premature ejaculation.[3]

In females, local irritation secondary to vaginal infections may contribute to the development of vaginismus. Abnormalities, endometriosis, or infections involving the cervix, uterus, or fallopian tubes may cause discomfort or pain during intercourse. Vaginismus may then develop as a protective measure in cases involving these internal genital tract abnormalities[9] (Table 98-3).

There are rarely any organic causes for lifelong or acquired orgasmic phase disorder or for lifelong excitement-phase dysfunctions, but acquired excitement-phase dysfunctions may be caused by many factors. The recent development of a systemic medical illness may leave the patient temporarily enervated and unable to participate fully in sexual relations. Dyspareunia may cause the patient to suppress the desire to have sex. Invasive surgical procedures and concomitant scarring can affect an adolescent's sense of attractiveness and body integrity, which subsequently can have an impact on sexual feelings.[5]

Medication that affects the parasympathetic or sympathetic systems may interfere with arousal or orgasm responses, presumably in both sexes, although there has been little research on such effects in females.[9] Table 98-3 presents a more complete review of organic causes.

Psychosocial Causes

SEX-NEGATIVE ATTITUDES. Children who grow up in sex-negative, morally repressive environments are likely to experience guilt and anxiety about their bodies, their sexual thoughts, their sexual feelings, and (ultimately) their sexual behavior. Those who learn that sex is "dirty" carry a burden that may impede the natural and mature expression of sexual feelings. Evidence indicates that individuals with high levels of "sex guilt" have less knowledge about sex, less frequently use condoms and other contraception, and find it more difficult to communicate about sex.[18] Sex guilt also has been specifically implicated in the development of sexual dysfunction.[19]

Against this backdrop, we should also mention the effect that HIV and AIDS have had on the sexual functioning of many adolescents and young adults. Concern, bordering on preoccupation, about acquisition of the virus has led some young people to shun having sex because they are afraid. The task for the clinician is to arm adolescents with the tools they need to make responsible, healthy sexual choices that are sex positive, not sex phobic, and are based on a mature assessment of their goals and needs.

TRAUMA. Prevalence studies of child molestation indicate that 6% to 62% of females and 3% to 31% of males have been sexually abused as children.[20] In addition, adolescent girls are twice as likely to be victimized by rape than are older women. Many survivors of sexual abuse and rape experience both immediate and long-term disturbances in sexual functioning. The most common sexual dysfunctions involve response-inhibiting reactions (fear of sex, and desire and arousal dysfunctions).[21]

It is critical that issues of abuse be evaluated in a gentle, supportive manner; the patient may be further traumatized by a physician who either overtly or covertly suggests that the adolescent initiated or invited the abuse.

SOCIAL FACTORS. Adolescents face conflicting and confusing sexual messages from society at large. Although there are prominent campaigns that exhort teens to "Just Say No!" to sex, there are omnipresent signals that beckon "Just Do It!"

The mass media exploits sex to sell everything from cars to chewing gum to compact discs. Too frequently, media portrayals of sexuality are stereotyped, idealized, and unrealistic, thereby creating standards that are

TABLE 98-3
Physical Causes of Sexual Dysfunction

	Disorder/Cause	Possible Effect on Functioning
Cardiovascular	Aortic coarctation; internal iliac/pudendal artery stenosis; thrombosis of arteries or veins of penis	Impairment of erection in men
Metabolic	Sickle cell disease; chronic cardiac, pulmonary, renal, and hepatic disorders; autoimmune diseases; cancer; anemia	May decrease libido and impair arousal response in men and women
Endocrine	Addison's disease; hypoprolactinemia; hypothyroidism; hypogonadism; Cushing's disease; Klinefelter's syndrome; acromegaly; diabetes mellitus	May decrease libido and impair arousal response in men and women
Systemic infections	Infectious mononucleosis; hepatitis	May decrease libido and impair arousal response in men and women
Local genital disease	Penile trauma, priapism, chordee, phimosis, hypospadias; bilateral orchitis due to mumps; balanitis	May decrease libido and impair arousal in men
	Urethritis; prostatitis; urethral pathology	Impaired arousal, premature ejaculation
	Vulval and vaginal pathology; endometriosis; PID, prolapse of uterus; ovarian and uterine cysts and tumors	Dyspareunia and consequent decrease in libido; vaginismus—orgasm may be unaffected
	Neisseria gonorrhoeae; Chlamydia trachomatis	Decreased libido, impaired arousal in men and women
Neurologic	Spinal cord injury; peripheral neuropathy (metabolic drug induced); epilepsy; cardiovascular accident; head injury; spina bifida; cerebral palsy; muscular dystrophy; MS; syringomyelia	May affect arousal and/or orgasm response in men and women
	Surgery or trauma of sacral or lumbar cord, cauda equina, pelvic sympathetic nerves	May cause increase or decrease in libido and changes in sexual behavior in men and women
Medication/drugs	Sedatives (narcotics, tranquilizers, alcohol)	May impair arousal and orgasm
	Stimulants (amphetamines, cocaine)	In acute doses, increased libido
	Antidepressants (fluoxetine [Prozac], imipramine [Tofranil])	May increase libido, impair orgasm
	Antipsychotics (haloperidol [Haldol])	May decrease libido, impair arousal
	Antihypertensives (propanonol, hydrochlorothiazide)	May impair arousal
	Chemotherapeutic agents (cisplatinum)	May decrease libido
	Hormonal contraceptive agents (oral contraceptives, Depo-Provera, Norplant)	May decrease libido, vaginal lubrication

Derived from references 2 and 8, adapted for adolescents. See Kaplan[9] for more comprehensive coverage.
PID, pelvic inflammatory disease; *MS,* multiple sclerosis.

impossible for "normal" people to reach.[22] It is important to help teenagers reexamine skewed standards against which their sexuality is measured.

RELATIONSHIP PROBLEMS. Problematic sexual relationships are often characterized by poor communication. As a consequence, sexual activity is frequently based on unverified assumptions of the other person's sexual attitudes, preferences, and tastes. Helping teenagers improve verbal and nonverbal sexual communication skills can go a long way toward improving sexual functioning.

When couples engage in fixed "sexual scripts," sex can become routine.[19,23] Rigid seducer-seducee roles may limit a fuller experience of sexuality. The stereotypic male role of stud and "sexual expert" can lead to performance anxiety, and the female partner may not learn to take fuller responsibility for and delight in her own pleasure.

PSYCHIATRIC CONDITIONS. Depression and anxiety have long been linked to difficulties in sexual functioning.[9,24,25] At times, it may be difficult to assess whether depression or anxiety is primarily or secondarily implicated in the development of sexual dysfunction (usually loss of desire, failure of arousal, or premature ejaculation).

Adolescents (and adults) may use sex to cope with nonsexual problems (e.g., anger, jealousy, boredom, stress).[25] This becomes problematic, first, because the conflict or force driving the sexual experience is not dealt with effectively. Second, since the pleasure inherent in the sexual experience becomes diffused as these other feelings compete for the adolescent's attention, satisfaction with sex is blunted. Failure to cope appropriately with underlying psychologic disturbances may ultimately result in sexual dysfunction as these problems overwhelm the adolescent's problem-solving ability.

Alcohol and drugs, like sex, can temporarily distance the adolescent from environmental and intrapsychic problems. Additionally, many adolescents believe that mood-altering substances may have aphrodisiacal properties. However, the psychologically disinhibiting effects of small amounts of alcohol yield to erectile and lubrication deficits as the quantity of alcohol builds up in the body. While many cocaine and crack users report an initially elevated sex drive and level of sexual stamina, these reported effects diminish over time as the quest for the drug overrides all other concerns.

Studies also indicate that individuals with eating disorders may have disturbances in sexual functioning.[27] Obesity itself is not a deterrent to a satisfactory sex life, but for some, excessive weight can be an obstacle. Concerns about body image, hygiene, and size of genitalia may affect sexual expression. On the other end of the scale, individuals with anorexia nervosa frequently eschew sex altogether, reporting low desire and strongly negative feelings about sexuality.

Practical Causes

Despite the prevailing wisdom that adolescents are "know-it-alls" when it comes to sex, clinical experience indicates that they harbor many misconceptions about sex. Adolescent girls often have no idea what an orgasm is; both female and male teenagers have often never even heard of the clitoris; and many young men inculcated with "knowledge of the street" develop deep feelings of insecurity after hearing the long-distance exploits of peers who can "stay hard for hours" when, according to Kinsey, three fourths of American men ejaculate within 2 minutes of intromission. Often the clinician will discover that providing basic sexual information and normalizing an

adolescent's experience can substantially reduce concerns and enhance sexual functioning.

Just as ignorance can precipitate sexual anxiety, so too can the fact that many adolescents have sex in places not conducive to relaxed sexual activity, which is the case for many. Trying to have sex while watching the clock or listening for a parent's key in the lock can exacerbate feelings of anxiety.

Sexual Causes

When couples vary in preferences for specific sexual practices or in preferred sexual frequency, difficulties may arise. In a different vein, many sexual problems stem directly from stimulation that lacks adequate focus, intensity, or duration (e.g., rushed foreplay, stimulation of the breasts but not the genitals). Unresolved issues of gender identity or of sexual orientation also can interfere with sexual functioning. It is fairly common for multiple sexual problems to coexist. Low desire may develop on the wings of erectile failure; an individual who has difficulty with orgasm may also experience problems with arousal.

ASSESSMENT ISSUES

Adolescents rarely present at a clinician's office with a chief complaint of sexual dysfunction. In our experience, many adolescents (and adults) feel uncomfortable talking about sexual issues and tend not to volunteer information that is not specifically elicited. Patients often won't ask if you don't, even if it is a side effect of treatment. Burnap and Golden[28] demonstrated that the frequency of sexual problems encountered in a physician's practice was directly related to his or her comfort with the topic of sexuality. In their study, 66% of physicians who routinely took sexual histories identified sexual problems in at least 50% of their patients, while 75% who did not actively inquire about sexual issues said that less than 10% of their patients had sexual difficulties. Taking the time to ask about sexual questions or problems can have large payoffs for the patient. Such assessment should be incorporated into routine history taking, during physical or reproductive care examinations, when medications that may affect functioning have been prescribed, before and after any surgical procedures that may affect body image or sexual functioning, and during the routine evaluation of any mental health condition. Screening questions that can be incorporated into a basic history questionnaire or can be used in a clinical interview appear in Box 98-2.

The ease the physician models in discussing sex will help to set the pace for the adolescent. Assurances of confidentiality and acknowledgment of potential client (and clinician) discomfort, while validating the impor-

BOX 98-2
The Adolescent Sexual Functioning and Satisfaction Questionnaire

Note to health providers: This instrument may be appended to any other database forms currently used to obtain information from patients. Alternatively, it may be used by itself. The questionnaire is not intended to be comprehensive; rather, it is best used as an "ice breaker." Responses to questions should be verified by the interviewer. Elaboration of positive responses should be explored.

Note to clients: By now you are probably used to filling out a lot of papers when you come to the clinic. Well, we have one more for you! As you know, we ask a lot of questions about your health, your feelings, your family, and your friends. Some of these questions are kind of personal. We don't mean to be nosy; we're just trying to find out as much as we can about you, so that we can better help you take care of your health and your future. This questionnaire in front of you asks about your feelings or experiences in your sexual relationships. Sometimes, we get so busy asking you about everything else, we forget to ask you about this important topic. Also, sometimes young people may be a little shy about asking their health providers for help. So please take a few minutes and fill out this survey. When you finish, we can talk about anything you had concerns about in the survey. As with everything else, your answers are private and confidential—they are just between us. There are no right or wrong answers. Relax! This is not a test! Ready? OK—here we go. . . .

1. Have you ever been in a sexual relationship with anyone? Y N

2. Are you involved in a sexual relationship with someone now? Y N

3. Are your sexual partner/s male, female, or both? (circle one)

    (a) male only   (b) female only   (c) both

4. How satisfied are you with your sexual relationship/s? (circle one)

    (a) it's usually great   (b) it's usually ok   (c) it's usually boring

    (d) other _____

5. How satisfied do you think your partner/s have been in your sexual relationship/s? (circle one)

    (a) they think it's been great   (b) they think it's been ok

    (c) they think it's been boring   (d) I don't know

    (e) other _____

6. Do you ever experience any unwanted pain or discomfort during sex? Y N

7. Have you ever had any difficulties in talking with your partner/s about:
    where to have sex Y N
    when to have sex Y N
    how often to have sex Y N
    using protection during sex Y N
    what feels good during sex Y N
    what feels painful during sex Y N

8. Are you having any sexual difficulties or concerns? Y N

    If No: Please skip to QUESTION 22, *for both males and females*

    If Yes: Please answer the following questions:

9. Do you feel that it is sometimes difficult to 'get in the mood' for sex? Y N

For males only:

10. Do you sometimes have difficulty in having an erection (getting hard)? Y N

11. Do you sometimes have difficulty in keeping an erection (staying hard)? Y N

12. Does wearing a condom affect your ability to get hard or stay hard? Y N

13. Do you ever have difficulty in putting your penis into your partner's vagina or rectum? Y N

14. During sex, do you sometimes ejaculate ("cum") before you or your partner is ready (satisfied)? Y N

    14a. If this is a problem or concern for you, how long do you think it takes from the time you

       start to have sex to the time you ejaculate? _____

15. Does it ever take you a longer time to ejaculate ("cum") than you (or your partner) would like? Y N

Continued

BOX 98-2
The Adolescent Sexual Functioning and Satisfaction Questionnaire—cont'd

For females only:

16. Do you sometimes have difficulty in becoming lubricated (getting wet)?   Y   N

17. Do you sometimes experience discomfort when your partner touches your vagina or puts
    anything inside the vagina?   Y   N

18. Do you sometimes experience discomfort when your partner touches your rectum or puts
    anything inside the rectum?   Y   N

19. Do you sometimes experience discomfort during sex, when your partner is thrusting
    (pumping)?   Y   N

20. Do you know what an orgasm is?   Y   N
    In your own words, please describe what an orgasm is:
    _____

21. Do you ever have difficulty in reaching an orgasm?   Y   N

For both males and females:

22. Have you had any sexual experiences that were disturbing to you, or that you felt you had to
    keep secret?   Y   N
    If so, please describe below: _____
    _____
    _____

23. Have concerns about AIDS affected your sexual relationships or how you feel about sex?   Y   N
    If so, please describe below: _____
    _____
    _____

24. Would you like to talk to someone today about any of the questions you have answered in this
    survey?   Y   N

---

tance of the discussion, are important initial steps in the evaluation. As with many sensitive topics, once these concerns are broached, the adolescent often feels a tremendous sense of relief at finding someone to talk to about them. It is important to keep the tone conversational. When talking to adolescents about sex, check to make sure that the terms used are clearly understood. We recommend using formal vocabulary, and then inviting the adolescent to let you know what terms are most comfortable for him or her.

When an assessment of sexual dysfunctions is performed, it is useful to go from the general (e.g., attitudes about sexuality and toward the same and the opposite sex, current activity, satisfaction with sex life) to the more specific (e.g., sexual practices, arousal, orgasm). It is important to explore each phase of functioning that occurs during partner sex and/or masturbation. For many adolescents, anxiety and ignorance are the major contributors to sexual problems, and simple information or reassurance often can resolve the problem. One should not pathologize when minor concerns are reported that are not especially problematic—if it's not broken, don't fix it. Normalization of sexual difficulties and concerns can frequently do much by itself to ameliorate the problem.

During the discussion, if the existence of a problem is disclosed by an adolescent, information should be obtained on its parameters: onset, duration, and situational/generalized dimensions. In addition, it is important to attend to the adequacy of stimulation and to other contextual factors. The clinician should be clear about determining whether the dysfunction is lifelong or acquired. Client characteristics such as health, cultural and religious background, history of sexual abuse, expectations, relationship factors, sexual orientation, and life style need to be taken into account. An exploration of what the client (and partner) believe about causal factors can often provide important diagnostic information.

In many cases, if an organic cause for the dysfunction is identified, it may be remediable through medical treatment. In the case of drugs, discontinuation or switching to an alternative medication may be enough to reverse the situation. It must be remembered that sexual problems can have both organic *and* psychogenic causes. Some problems may be out of the clinician's depth, some not. Addressing psychosocial issues may be far more complex, and in this regard the clinician may want to enlist the aid of a trained sex therapist. A list of certified sex therapists practicing in the area can be obtained from the American Society of Sex Educators, Counselors, and Therapists (ASSECT).

CASE EXAMPLES

To provide a flavor for the types of dysfunctions most likely to be encountered, two case studies are provided.

J.T. is an 18-year-old college freshman who presented for evaluation of headaches. In reviewing the various stressors in his life, he related that one principal area of concern was the fact that his girlfriend was due to visit him from Boston at the end of the month. Their first sexual encounter (which was also J.T.'s first), 6 weeks previously, had been a "disaster." J.T. related being so "excited" that the entire episode was over in less than a minute. Despite his girlfriend's understanding statement, J.T. felt embarrassed and inadequate. Treatment issues focused on decreasing J.T.'s performance anxiety. He was also instructed in the squeeze masturbatory technique[29] to learn how to better control his responses to sensations.

Mary, a 16-year-old high school sophomore, presented at the clinic for a routine examination required by her school for all athletes. During the examination, she reported feeling "down" about her relationship with her boyfriend, but could not point to any real problems. In reviewing their sexual relationship, Mary disclosed that she had never had an orgasm. She felt that this must mean either that something was wrong with the relationship or that she was "frigid." Education about the female sexual response cycle, clarification of the misconception that "love equals orgasm," and normalization of her lack of orgasm constituted the first treatment step. Mary was given an assignment to familiarize herself with and explore her genitals, and initial concerns were discussed. Using Barbach's book *For Yourself: the Fulfillment of Female Sexuality*[30] as an aid, Mary was instructed in self-pleasuring techniques. Mary's partner was invited to join her on a subsequent visit to address both parties' feelings and concerns, and to learn sexual communication and sensate focus techniques that could facilitate her becoming orgasmic with him.

CONCLUSION

Adolescent medicine practitioners are the front-line forces in addressing the physical, psychologic, and psychosexual problems of young adults. By incorporating an assessment of sexual functioning into the standard examination, the practitioner can play a crucial role not only in providing basic sexual information, but also in fostering the development of healthy, satisfying sexual expression. In addition, early identification and referral of those young people who need further counseling and treatment may prove beneficial in reducing future sexual morbidity.

References

1. Sarrel LJ, Sarrel P: *Sexual unfolding,* Boston, 1979, Little, Brown.
2. Farrow JA: An approach to the management of sexual dysfunction in the adolescent male, *J Adolesc Health Care* 6:397-400, 1985.
3. Johnson RL, Stanford P: Sexual dysfunctions in adolescent males with prostatic enlargement, *J Curr Adolesc Med* 2:31-35, 1980.
4. Miller GD, Cirone J: Sexual dysfunction in college sexuality course attenders and course treatment benefits, *J Am Coll Health Assoc* 27:107-108, 1978.
5. Greydanus DE, Demarest MS, Sears JM: Sexual dysfunctions in adolescents, *Semin Adolesc Med* 1:177-187, 1985.
6. Haas A: *Teenage sexuality: a survey of teenage sexual behavior,* New York, 1979, Macmillan.
7. American Psychiatric Association: *Diagnostic and statistical manual of mental disorders (DSM-IV),* ed 4, Washington, DC, 1994, American Psychiatric Association; p 495.
8. Masters WH, Johnson VS: *Human sexual response,* Boston, 1966, Little, Brown.
9. Kaplan HS: *The new sex therapy,* New York, 1974, Brunner-Mazel.
10. Lauman EO, Gagnon JH, Michael RT, Michaels S: *The social organization of sexuality: sexual practices in the United States,* Chicago, 1994, University of Chicago Press.
11. Nathan SG: The epidemiology of DSM III psychosexual dysfunctions, *J Mar Sex Ther* 12:267-281, 1986.
12. Kinsey AC, Pomeroy WB, Martin CE: *Sexual behavior in the human male,* Philadelphia, 1948, WB Saunders.
13. Frank E, Anderson C, Rubenstein D: Frequency of sexual dysfunction in "normal" couples, *N Engl J Med* 229:111-115, 1978.
14. Spector KR, Boyle M: The prevalence and perceived etiology of male sexual problems in a nonclinical sample, *Br J Med Psychol* 59:351-358, 1986.
15. Krauss D: The physiologic basis of male sexual dysfunction, *Hosp Pract* 2:193-222, 1983.
16. Frank S, Jacobs HS, Martin N, Narbarro JD: Hyperprolactinaemia and impotence, *Clin Endocrinol* 8:277-287, 1978.
17. Jevitch MJ: Vascular noninvasive diagnostic techniques. In Krone RJ, Sirosky MB, Goldstein I, editors: *Male sexual dysfunction,* Boston, 1983, Little, Brown.
18. Mosher DL: The meaning and measurement of guilt. In Izard CE, editor: *Emotions in personality and psychopathology,* New York, 1979, Plenum Press.
19. LoPiccolo L, Nowinski JK: Sex therapy. In Frank C et al, editors: *Handbook of medical psychology and behavioral medicine,* Philadelphia, 1981, Grune & Stratton.
20. Finkelhor D: *Sourcebook on child sexual abuse,* Beverley Hills, CA, 1986, Sage.
21. Becker JV, Skinner L, Abel G, Axelrod R, Cichon J: Level of postassault sexual functioning in rape and incest victims, *Arch Sex Res* 15:37-49, 1986.
22. Strasburger VC: Normal adolescent sexuality, *Semin Adolesc Med* 1:101-115, 1985.
23. Mosher DL: Three dimensions of depth of involvement in human sexual response, *J Sex Res* 16:1-42, 1980.
24. Nowinski J: *Becoming satisfied: a man's guide to sexual fulfillment,* Englewood Cliffs, NJ, 1980, Prentice-Hall.
25. Beck AT: *Depression,* Philadelphia, 1967, University of Pennsylvania Press.
26. Hajcak F, Garwood P: Quick-fix sex: pseudosexuality in adolescents, *Adol* 23:755-760, 1988.
27. Renshaw DC: Sex and eating disorders, *Med Asp Hum Sex* 24:69-77, 1990.
28. Burnap DW, Golden JS: Sexual problems in medical practice, *J Med Educ* 42:673-680, 1967.
29. Semans JH: Premature ejaculation: a new approach, *South Med J* 49:353-358, 1956.
30. Barbach LG: *For yourself: the fulfillment of female sexuality,* New York, 1975, Doubleday.

CHAPTER 99

Sexual Orientation and Gender Identity

•

Robert James Bidwell

Until the recent past, issues of adolescent sexual orientation and gender identity were only briefly discussed in the medical literature. Adolescent homosexuality, for example, was ignored or seen either as a passing phase or indicative of a deeper pathologic condition leading to adult homosexuality. The phenomenon of adolescent transgenderism (transsexualism) was even less recognized. In the past 25 years, however, it has become increasingly clear that a significant number of adolescents are dealing with issues of sexual orientation and gender identity. Many homosexual adolescents traverse the adolescent years with minimal outward signs of scarring, yet the experience of growing up gay, lesbian, bisexual, or transgender in our society can be especially difficult. A study suggests that gay and lesbian adolescents may be three to five times more likely to attempt suicide than other teenagers.[1] This statistic is not surprising in a society that often classifies those who are gay, lesbian, or transgender as sick, sinful, or dangerous. It was not until 1973 that the American Psychiatric Association removed homosexuality from its list of mental disorders.[2] More recently, the American Academy of Pediatrics formally recognized the existence of adolescent homosexuality and acknowledged the responsibility of health providers to address the needs of homosexual youths.[3] Unfortunately, transgendered teenagers for the most part remain ignored.

THEORETICAL CONSIDERATIONS

Much research has been done on the nature and origins of human sexuality. The variability of populations studied and the terminology and methods employed make conclusions difficult.[4] Nevertheless, it is clear that sexuality is a complex concept composed of several interrelated elements. An individual's genetic sex usually directs the development of anatomic sex in a predictable manner. It also may direct another element of sexuality— core gender identity—that is, that deepest psychic sense of being either male or female. Transgendered individuals, for example, although genetically and anatomically male or female, feel as if they are "trapped" in the body of the opposite sex because their core gender does not match their genetic and anatomic sex. Another element of sexuality is gender role: the agreement between an individual's interests, dress, and mannerisms and society's expectations related to male and female roles. For example, a 12-year-old boy who cross-dresses (dresses as a girl) might be considered as having a female gender role in respect to that particular behavior. Finally, sexual orientation generally refers to a persistent pattern of sexual partner preference (homosexual, heterosexual, or bisexual). Lesbian and gay adolescents necessarily differ from their heterosexual peers only in this last aspect of sexuality.

Theories attempting to explain origins of human sexuality tend toward either a biologic or an environmental viewpoint.[4] Some have suggested that an interplay of "nature" and "nurture" is involved in the unfolding of an individual's sexuality. It is generally believed that an individual's sexual orientation and gender identity are established by early childhood. There is some debate, however, as to how immutable gender identity might be. For example, whereas some have claimed that it is very difficult to change the acquired gender identity of children "misassigned" to the opposite sex because of ambiguous genitalia, others have claimed some success in this area. There also has been controversy concerning the origins of transgenderism, with some research implicating parental influences and other studies suggesting biologic factors.

Similar controversy typifies inquiry into the origins and nature of sexual orientation.[5] There is as yet no generally accepted evidence that supports either a single biologic or a single environmental explanation for sexual orientation. Among biologic theories are those that suggest a genetic predisposition toward homosexuality or heterosexuality. Both family and twin studies provide supportive evidence yet do not rule out social or environmental influences.[6,7] The influence of hormones on sexual orientation also has been examined. There is no consistent evidence that homosexual adults differ from heterosexual adults in their levels of sex hormones. More recent inquiry has examined the possible prenatal influence of sex hormones on sexual orientation.[8] Results have been intriguing but inconclusive. There have also been several reports of differences in the brains between homosexual and heterosexual individuals that have not yet been replicated in other studies.[5]

Several theories have examined the development of sexual orientation in psychoanalytic or sociologic terms. Psychoanalytic theories often find significance in the preoedipal or oedipal relationships between parents and child (e.g., a close-binding mother and a cold, weak, hostile father). They often imply that a homosexual orientation develops when the normal process of individuation has gone awry. Sociologic theories, on the other hand, tend to view homosexuality as a learned behavior. According to the labeling theory, for example, a child who is either an effeminate male or a masculine female may be labeled as homosexual on the basis of his or her gender-atypical behavior or mannerisms. The child in turn accepts this label as a real description of who he or she is, and thus eventually becomes homosexual in fact. According to the conditioning theory, an individual is born as a tabula rasa, with no predisposition toward heterosexuality or homosexuality. Through circumstance, an individual has experiences that are either homosexual or heterosexual, and if these experiences are pleasurable, the individual is reinforced in that particular orientation, seeking out further experiences.

In 1981, Bell et al[9] published their study of more than 1500 homosexual and heterosexual men and women. The study sought to determine which, if any, of the prevailing psychoanalytic and sociologic theories were plausible. In-depth interviews failed to support either set of theories. Gay men and lesbians were remarkably similar to their heterosexual peers in terms of family and sociologic background. The researchers concluded that although they were not able to test the various biologic explanations for homosexuality, these were the only theories that were consistent with their data.

PREVALENCE

There are no certain data regarding the prevalence of homosexual feelings and behaviors during adolescence. The same is true of transgenderism, although it appears to be much less common than homosexuality. Adolescence is a time of sexual exploration and experimentation. Therefore, sexual activity, whether heterosexual or homosexual, does not necessarily reflect either present or future sexual orientation. Yet it is sexual behavior, and more often male sexual behavior, that is best described in the literature. Kinsey's work in the 1930s and 1940s revolutionized thought about human sexuality.[10,11] In addition to demonstrating that exclusive heterosexuality and exclusive homosexuality were merely opposite end points on a continuum of human sexual behaviors, Kinsey discovered that homosexuality was far from a rare phenomenon. Among his subjects, 13% of women and 37% of men had had at least one homosexual experience leading to orgasm, and 10% of males had been more or less exclusively homosexual for at least 3 years. In 1973, Sorenson's report[12] on adolescent sexuality stated that of his sample of adolescents, 17% of boys and 6% of girls between the ages of 16 and 19 years had had at least one homosexual experience. In a 1989 large-scale survey of adolescent homosexual behavior in Minnesota, among 18-year-old high school students, 3.2% of males and 2.1% of females acknowledged homosexual activity.[13] In a review of the literature on the prevalence of homosexual behavior in the adult population, Diamond reported that 5% to 6% of males and 2% to 3% of females regularly engage in, or have since adolescence at least once engaged in, homosexual activity.[14]

Less is known about the incidence of homosexual attraction and self-definition as gay or lesbian during adolescence. The Minnesota study cited above found that homosexual attractions were acknowledged by 5% of male twelfth graders and 8.5% of female eleventh graders. Whereas only 1% of students described themselves as mostly or completely homosexual, more than 10% said they were unsure of their sexual orientation.[13]

It is generally accepted that the roots of sexual orientation are established before puberty.[15] Troiden[16] proposed a four-stage theoretical model describing homosexual identity acquisition from childhood through adulthood. The first stage, *sensitization,* occurs before puberty when a child does not see homosexuality as personally relevant, but later attaches meanings to childhood experiences that relate to his or her homosexuality. In a number of studies, for example, homosexual adults describe feelings of marginality or of being different during their childhood years. In the second stage, *identity confusion,* these adolescents begin to see that their feelings or behaviors could be interpreted as homosexual. This realization can lead to significant turmoil as these adolescents attempt to reconcile all they believe and know about themselves with an attribute that has extremely negative connotations. Some adolescents suppress or deny their feelings, while others begin the slow process of self-acceptance. The third stage, *identity assumption,* occurs when the gay or lesbian identity is acknowledged, accepted, and explored, often surreptitiously. The final stage, *commitment,* occurs when gays and lesbians see their orientation as both natural and healthy, form healthy same-sex relationships, and acknowledge their identity honestly and openly.

Many homosexual adults report awareness of homosexual attractions in early adolescence, sometimes even in childhood.[15] The average age of first awareness of homosexual attraction is 13 years for boys and 14 to 16 years for girls. These attractions, however, are not acted upon by most teenagers until at least 2 years after first awareness. The average age of self-identification as homosexual is 19 to 21 years old for males and 21 to 23 years old for females. There are some teenagers, however, who recognize and accept their gay or lesbian orientation at a much younger age. Remafedi[17] provided evidence that the assumption of gay identity during adolescence is made neither casually nor arbitrarily and that self-identification as gay remains stable over time. Unfortunately, the process of identity acquisition for lesbian teenagers, rural homosexual youth, and homosexual youth of color is less well understood than that for white gay urban males.

In short, although many teenagers may not label themselves as gay or lesbian until their later adolescent years, almost all gay and lesbian adults recall adolescence as a time of confusion and distress related to homosexual feelings and behaviors. Failure of professionals in the past to recognize this turmoil has resulted in significant physical and psychologic harm to gay and lesbian teenagers, their families, and their friends.

HOMOSEXUALITY AND LESBIAN/GAY IDENTITY

The Experience

Most lesbian and gay youths are ordinary adolescents from ordinary families faced with the same developmental tasks as other teenagers. However, they are also faced with the challenge of growing up in a society that is often unaccepting of their sexual orientation.[5,18,19] Unlike most other minorities, gay and lesbian teenagers grow up in profound isolation. They often believe they are the only teenagers in their school who have homosexual feelings. Although they may have close friends with whom they share personal concerns, knowledge of their homosexuality or of the possibility of being gay or lesbian is often considered too horrible to tell anyone, whether friend, relative, or counselor. To protect their "awful secret," they distance themselves emotionally and socially from those who would otherwise be closest to them. They live in constant fear of being found out. They, like their heterosexual peers, have almost no access to supportive information about homosexuality and gay or lesbian identity. Instead, they hear and accept the myths and stereotypes about homosexuality that, though disproved, continue in the public mind and are often voiced by those whom they love and respect. Gay and lesbian immigrant

youths and youths of color may be especially isolated.

The experience of growing up as a gay or lesbian adolescent is fraught with real and immediate dangers.[20] Those teenagers whose sexual orientations are discovered or who choose to "come out" (reveal their sexual identity to others) may be rejected by their families, friends, and churches. Often they are both emotionally and physically abused. It is not uncommon for these teenagers to run away or be forced from their homes. Many find the ridicule and harrassment at school intolerable and drop out. Some turn to street life, supporting themselves through prostitution, dealing drugs, and participating in other illegal activities. Many engage in serious substance abuse and are vulnerable to sexually transmitted diseases, pregnancy, and sexual exploitation. For males, especially, sexual activity may involve multiple anonymous encounters, not through choice but because there are no socially approved outlets for safe sexual exploration. For street youths whose main concern is day-to-day existence, safer sex practices are seldom employed. Those teenagers who have come out must also face the realities of discrimination in employment and housing. Those who enter the juvenile justice and social service systems often encounter institutional ignorance, disapproval, and abuse. These systems may minimize or be fearful of addressing issues of sexual orientation. Sometimes they adopt a "blame the victim" stance, in which gay adolescents are seen as provoking the abusive situations in which they find themselves.

Most gay and lesbian adolescents, however, reveal their sexual orientation to no one. A primary preoccupation is learning to hide a very important part of who they are as human beings. Some adolescents do this through denial of the feelings they may be experiencing. Others are acutely aware of their sexual orientation but channel their energies into other areas such as athletics, academics, or hobbies. These teenagers may be heterosexually or homosexually active or, perhaps most commonly, not sexually active at all. They often avoid the usual social rituals and sexual experimentation of adolescence. If homosexual activity does occur, it often takes place anonymously and with deep feelings of guilt. An unfortunate consequence of isolation is that many lesbian and gay adolescents begin to see their futures as somehow circumscribed by their sexual orientation. Educational, career, and family goals are often readjusted in light of what they see as society's imposed limitations on homosexual individuals. Declining school performance, school truancy and dropout, substance abuse, parent-teenager conflict, social withdrawal, runaway behavior, and a variety of acting-out and self-destructive behaviors often accompany the anger and despair of these alienated adolescents. Unfortunately, many turn to suicide. The 1989 Report of the Secretary's Task Force on Youth Suicide[1] stated that most suicide attempts among homosexuals occur during their adolescence, and that an estimated 30% of completed adolescent suicides are among teenagers dealing with issues of sexual orientation.

Medical Concerns

The medical needs and concerns of gay and lesbian adolescents are similar to those of heterosexual teenagers, especially since teenagers of any sexual orientation may be heterosexually or homosexually active. Some concerns, such as substance abuse, are common to any group of alienated youths. Nevertheless, certain medical issues are especially important in working with gay or lesbian adolescents. Not the least of these is the fact that denial and fear make homosexual youths less likely to seek medical care or admit to homosexual behaviors. In addition, these adolescents are less likely to have received preventive health education specific to their sexual orientation.

LESBIAN ISSUES. Studies have shown that lesbians who are exclusively homosexual are less likely than other groups to have sexually transmitted diseases (STDs). However, there are reports of vaginitis due to *Gardnerella vaginalis, Candida* organisms, and *Trichomonas* organisms in lesbians without a history of heterosexual or bisexual contact. Some adolescent lesbians are heterosexually or bisexually active. This interaction and possible sexual abuse may place them at risk for STDs or pregnancy. Careful and nonjudgmental history taking will help guide appropriate physical examination, laboratory evaluation, and counseling. Lesbians face the same risks of breast and pelvic malignancies as other women. All lesbian teenagers should be instructed in breast self-examination and undergo yearly pelvic examinations for evidence of infection, pregnancy, and malignancy. Serologic testing for syphilis should be performed if there is a history of bisexual or heterosexual activity. Rubella immune status should be determined and the patient immunized if susceptible.

Contraception and safer sex practices should be discussed with all adolescent patients. Like other female patients, lesbian teenagers may experience dysmenorrhea and other menstrual problems. They also may be concerned about sexual functioning, including anorgasmia or partner incompatibility related to sexual practices and frequency. Lesbians are becoming increasingly interested in parenting issues, including artificial insemination, child custody, and advice on parenting. Since gay men are often chosen by lesbians as sperm donors, the risk of possible human immunodeficiency virus (HIV) transmission should be assessed. The health professional should be able to address these issues or to refer the individual to supportive resources.

GAY MALE ISSUES. Sexually active gay male teenagers are at high risk for the traumatic and infectious complications stemming from homosexual activity.[4,21] Few, if any, sexual behaviors are the exclusive domain of homosexual youths. Gay male youths may be at increased risk, however, because they are often forced by societal norms to engage in these practices with anonymous partners and without the information they need to protect themselves medically. As a whole, adult gay males appear to have a higher incidence of gonorrhea, syphilis, hepatitis B, enteric pathogens, and HIV infection than the general population. It is uncertain to what extent the nature of sexual behaviors and the incidence of STDs among gay teenagers differs from that of adult gay populations.

Because of the frequent unreliability of the medical history, a screening physical examination of all male teenagers should include a careful examination of the skin, lymph nodes, oropharynx, abdomen, genitals, and anorectal region. Homosexually active youths should be screened regularly with gonorrhea cultures of the pharynx, urethra, and rectum; *Chlamydia* cultures of the urethra and rectum; and syphilis serologic testing. Testing for hepatitis B and HIV should also be performed. Additional laboratory evaluation is determined by the specific historical and physical findings. The traumatic sequelae of male homosexual activity may include hemorrhoids, anorectal fissures and tears, rectal foreign bodies and allergic proctitis, fecal incontinence, penile edema, and inhaled nitrite burns. Most of these problems are secondary to anal intercourse, which may or may not be part of a gay male teenager's sexual repertoire. The most common infectious conditions among homosexual men are urethritis, anogenital dermatologic conditions, oropharyngeal conditions, gastrointestinal disease, hepatitis, and AIDS.

Urethritis. Gonorrhea and *Chlamydia* organisms are the most common agents responsible for urethritis in homosexual men. Some carriers may be asymptomatic. Urethral, pharyngeal, and rectal gonorrhea cultures and urethral and rectal *Chlamydia* cultures should be obtained. Urethral and rectal Gram's stains should be obtained in symptomatic patients. The treatment for urethritis is the same as in heterosexual men.

Anogenital dermatologic conditions. Pediculosis pubis, scabies, tinea cruris, and molluscum contagiosum are dermatologic conditions that are diagnosed and treated as in the heterosexual population. Penile, anal, and rectal condylomata acuminata (venereal warts) are also frequently present. Ulcerative lesions generally represent primary syphilis, chancroid, or herpes simplex. Although usually painless, the chancre of primary syphilis, if in the rectal area, may be painful and may have an atypical appearance. Because the chancre may be painless and/or hidden, a teenager may be unconcerned or unaware of a primary syphilitic infection. These disease characteristics also lead to frequent underdiagnosis of syphilis by practitioners. Uncommon in the United States, chancroid (caused by infection by *Haemophilus ducreyi*) presents as painful penile ulcers with regional lymphadenopathy progressing to suppuration. Herpes simplex may occur on the penis and in the anorectal region. Herpetic lesions are painful and begin as multiple blisters that proceed to painful, punched-out ulcers with shaggy erythematous borders. The lesions may be accompanied by fever, difficult defecation and urination, sacral paresthesias, and regional lymphadenopathy. Diagnosis and treatment of the above conditions in homosexual males are the same as in heterosexual individuals.

Oropharyngeal conditions. Gonorrhea, syphilitic chancres, herpes simplex, condylomata acuminata, and molluscum contagiosum can be found in the oropharynx of homosexual men. *Chlamydia* infection may also be present but is of uncertain pathogenicity. Gonorrhea may present as an exudative pharyngitis, but asymptomatic infection is common, which emphasizes the importance of obtaining cultures for gonorrhea from the pharynx, urethra, and rectum in all symptomatic or asymptomatic sexually active gay men. Sexual partners also should be treated. Kaposi's sarcoma and infection with *Candida* organisms, both associated with AIDS, may also be present in the oropharynx of homosexual men. Diagnosis and treatment is the same as for heterosexual individuals.

Gastrointestinal disease. Sexually transmitted gastrointestinal infections can occur in any patient who engages in anal intercourse and oropenile or oroanal contact. Gonorrhea, *Chlamydia* (both lymphogranuloma venereum and nonlymphogranuloma strains), herpes simplex, primary syphilis, and human papillomavirus can cause proctitis with rectal pain and discharge, tenesmus, constipation, and fever. Proctitis may be severe enough to resemble Crohn's disease. Rectal gonorrhea may often be asymptomatic, however. Proctocolitis may present as abdominal pain, bloody diarrhea, and fever. Causative agents include *Shigella* spp., *Salmonella* spp., *Campylobacter* spp., *Yersinia* spp., and *Entamoeba histolytica*. Enteritis with symptoms of abdominal pain, diarrhea, bloating, and nausea is most frequently due to *Giardia lamblia*. HIV infection can result in a number of other opportunistic infections of the gastrointestinal tract, including those caused by *Isospora, Cryptosporidium,* and *Candida* species. Finally, anal pruritus may indicate pinworms. A teenager with symptoms of proctitis should undergo proctoscopy. Cultures should be obtained for evidence of gonorrhea and *Chlamydia* infection, and serologic testing for syphilis should be performed. Symptoms of proctocolitis and enteritis should prompt the performance of stool cultures and ova and parasite examination for the above enteric pathogens. The treatment regimen depends on the pathogens found.

Hepatitis. Homosexual males are at high risk for hepatitis A, B, and C. All male and female adolescents, regardless of sexual activity, should be tested for hepatitis B immunity (hepatitis B surface antigen [HB^{s}Ag] and antibody to hepatitis B core antigen [anti-HB^c]). If the patient is found to be susceptible (negative HB^{s}Ag or anti-HB^c), a three-dose series of hepatitis B vaccine should be given.

Cytomegalovirus infection may or may not present with acute hepatitis. More often it either is asymptomatic or presents as a mononucleosis-like illness. The incidence of cytomegalovirus infection is high among very sexually active homosexual males. Epstein-Barr virus serologic testing or a Monospot testing should be a part of the evaluation of any teenager with hepatitis or mononucleosis-like illness.

AIDS. Homosexually active gay youths are at very high risk for HIV exposure. At the present time, many adolescents with a diagnosis of AIDS have a history of homosexual activity. HIV infection may present in many ways, making initial diagnosis difficult if the health practitioner has not taken a careful history related to substance use, sexual behaviors, and sexual orientation. During the physical examination, the practitioner should be especially alert for skin lesions, lymphadenopathy, oropharyngeal lesions, and signs of anogenital infection that might indicate homosexual activity. Because of the recommended treatment of some asymptomatic HIV-positive individuals with zidovudine (AZT) or multiple-drug regimens, HIV-antibody testing should be recommended to all homosexually active teenagers. Testing should be accompanied by informed consent, careful protection of confidentiality, and comprehensive counseling before and after testing.

Interview and Counseling Issues

THE INTERVIEW. Health professionals work with lesbian and gay teenagers in a variety of contexts. Most of these teenagers do not identify themselves as gay or lesbian and present with the same medical and psychosocial concerns as other teenagers. Occasionally, teenagers are brought by their parents or referred by schools or youth-service agencies for evaluation of acting-out behaviors together with homosexual behaviors or sexual orientation concerns. A few teenagers seek counseling on their own. Working with issues of sexual orientation requires time, patience, assurance of confidentiality, and an accepting and caring demeanor on the part of the health professional. If he or she cannot provide these factors, referral should be made to an appropriate counselor.

The content of the initial interview varies with the individual teenager and the nature of the presenting complaint. Usually, sexual issues are explored over a series of visits as trust and rapport grow. It is important that the practitioner not presume heterosexual or homosexual orientation in any adolescent. Questions related to both homosexual activity and gay or lesbian identity should be a part of all well-teenager visits, as well as any visits suggestive of underlying psychosocial concerns such as recurrent abdominal pain, declining school performance, or depression. Adolescents should be informed at the beginning of the interview that some very personal questions will be asked, that these questions are asked of all patients, and that honest and open answers will help in providing them with the appropriate medical care.

Questions about homosexual activity and sexual orientation can be raised in a number of ways, usually in the context of a broader psychosocial history. It is helpful to move from less threatening to more sensitive areas of inquiry. One might begin, for example, by asking, "Have you ever dated or are you now dating anyone?" This can be followed by questions such as "Have you ever had sex with another person?" "Do you usually have sex with girls (women) or with boys (men)?" "Some of the teenage boys (girls) I see in my clinic have had sex with or been attracted to other boys or men (girls or women). I'm wondering if this is something you've ever done or been concerned about." If a teenager acknowledges such activity or concerns, the practitioner may continue the discussion and address pertinent issues. If a teenager denies homosexual activity or orientation, the practitioner should add, "This may or may not ever be a part of your life or the life of a friend or relative, but you should know that it is now believed that being gay (lesbian) is quite common and natural. If you ever would like to talk more about this, you should feel free to come and see me." Most gay and lesbian adolescents will not admit to homosexual feelings or behaviors at a first visit. This final message, however, lets them know that they are all right, that they are not alone, and that there is someone to whom they can talk when they are ready to do so.

A comprehensive sexual and psychosocial history should be taken of all adolescents (Box 99-1). A careful sexual history will determine a teenager's risks for infection, pregnancy, and abuse and guide the practitioner's counseling. In the psychosocial history, one should determine why a teenager thinks he or she might be gay or lesbian. A teenage boy, for example, may fear that a single homosexual experience means that he is gay. He should be told that although he may or may not be gay, his sexual orientation is not determined by a single or even a series of homosexual experiences. At the same time, he should not be told that his behaviors are "just a phase," since he may in fact be gay. It is also important to determine what being gay or lesbian means to teenagers. Is homosexuality seen as sinful, for example, or is it seen as somehow defining in stereotypic terms who they are or must become? The extent of a teenager's isolation should be determined. Has the teenager had any access to information on sexual orientation or known of any other gay or lesbian teenagers or adults? Has he or she had any friend or counselor to turn to for support? The possibility of verbal, physical, and sexual harrassment at home, in school, and among peers should also be

---

BOX 99-1
Medical History

Sexuality
  Activity: practices, partners, places
  Condom/contraceptive use
  Signs/symptoms of STDs/HIV
  History of pregnancy
  Sexual abuse/sexual offense
  Exchange of sex for money, drugs, shelter
Substance use
Other psychosocial issues
  Knowledge/beliefs about homosexuality, gay/
    lesbian identity
  Degree of acceptance/uncertainty/concern
  Isolation from/access to resources
  Awareness/acceptance of family, peers, com-
    munity
  Violence/harassment
  School attendance/performance
  Runaway history
  Depression/suicidal ideation
  Decision-making skills (sex, drugs)
  Experience with juvenile justice, social service
    systems

---

addressed. The possibility of involvement with drugs, runaway behavior, and the exchange of sex for money, drugs, or shelter should be explored as well. It is important to remember that many teenagers, although acutely aware of their homosexual feelings and perhaps sexually active, may lack the insight, vocabulary, or perspective to discuss these issues as might an adult.

COUNSELING. The role of the counselor working with adolescents is to facilitate their healthy physical, sexual, and emotional development.[22] This is done by providing them with information, positive role models, supportive resources, and anticipatory guidance. It is not the role of the primary care practitioner to "make a diagnosis" of heterosexuality or homosexuality. Only the adolescent can come to this conclusion. The practitioner can, however, resolve much of an adolescent's confusion by providing information about the nature and origins of sexual orientation and dispelling myths or stereotypes that the patient may believe about homosexuality. The practitioner should convey the single most important message for any teenager: no matter who you are, whether straight or gay or somewhere in between, you are all right. Lesbian and gay teenagers should understand that their orientation is normal and healthy, that it is not a choice, that there are millions of young people like them, and that their adult lives can be as personally and professionally fulfilling as those of heterosexual adults. Some teenagers struggling with a gay or lesbian identity will resist these messages. It is important to remember that self-understanding and self-acceptance is an evolutionary process. The teenager must be allowed time to contemplate, to explore, and to accept who he or she might be.

It is helpful to provide the teenager with a variety of supportive resources. Several books for gay and lesbian teenagers are listed in the Suggested Readings at the end of this chapter. Many communities have gay and lesbian teenager support groups in which these youths can meet one another in a safe and supportive environment. There are counselors in many communities who are able to counsel lesbian and gay teenagers in an accepting manner. One should not refer a gay or lesbian teenager, even one who is distressed by his or her emerging identity, to a therapist who claims an ability to change sexual orientation. Such therapy is generally believed to be ineffective, unethical, and dangerous.

Anticipatory guidance for all adolescents should include information on safer sex practices that is specifically targeted to their present and future needs. Safer sex guidelines include avoiding unprotected anal intercourse and the exchange of blood, semen, and vaginal fluid; limiting the number of sexual partners; refraining from anonymous sex; using condoms or other barrier methods; and exploring alternative ways of sharing intimacy. Gay and lesbian teenagers should understand that they can lead healthy and enjoyable sexual lives even in the age of AIDS and should be given permission to begin the safe exploration of their sexuality. They should be encouraged, too, to have regular medical checkups with a health provider who is accepting of their sexual orientation. The counselor also can help provide the skills necessary for healthy decision making related to sex, drugs, and other risky behaviors. For example, it is not very helpful to be told how to obtain and use condoms if one is unable to insist on their use in a sexual encounter.

Gay and lesbian teenagers also should receive guidance in how to survive and thrive in a society that is often nonaccepting.[23] Rejection, discrimination, and violence are very real dangers for gay and lesbian youths, yet these issues can often be confronted in ways that enhance self-esteem. Many gay and lesbian people avoid challenging these injustices owing to their own internalized homophobia, thinking that they must conform to society's expectations. The counselor should empower the teenager to challenge unjust treatment in a judicious manner.

Coming-out issues, that is, when and how to tell parents and friends about one's sexual orientation, also should be explored. Only the teenager can decide when to come out. The practitioner can help the teenager weigh the consequences of coming out or "staying in the closet." Coming out should not be used as a weapon by the adolescent in an argument with parents. There are also significant risks in coming out to a parent before a teenager has attained financial independence. Nevertheless, coming out should be supported as an eventual goal.

Family Issues

The parents and siblings of lesbian and gay youths experience a mix of confusion, pain, fear, guilt, anger, and loss.[24] Even in families that are otherwise healthy and intact, the revelation of a teenager's gay or lesbian identity often leads to disapproval, rejection, or a search for an immediate "cure." Parents often believe the negative myths and stereotypes related to homosexuality and may feel overwhelming guilt for having caused their teenager's orientation. They may not know where to turn for information or support, often fearing rejection or disapproval by relatives, friends, and counselors. They mourn the loss of all they had hoped for in their child and also fear for his or her well-being in a disapproving society. Siblings, too, often react negatively. Many are fearful of what a gay or lesbian sibling implies about their own sexuality. They fear the loss of friends and are angry at the perceived loss of family as they had known it. Anger sometimes translates into violence and almost always into a distancing or outright rejection. The experience of watching one's family in turmoil may be especially painful for another sibling who may also be coming to terms with a gay or lesbian identity.

When such families are counseled, it is important to listen carefully to their expressed fears, anger, and guilt. One should determine what homosexuality and a gay or lesbian identity mean to each of the family members. The health practitioner should respect the reality and sincerity of the family's pain and, through regular contact, allow them as much time as they need to assimilate the information and resources provided. Gay and lesbian teenagers are often frustrated by the inability of parents to accept their homosexuality immediately and unconditionally. While acknowledging their impatience, the practitioner should also gently help them understand that acceptance takes time.

The provider should help the family understand that they are not alone, that they have done nothing wrong, and that (as hard as it may be for them to accept or believe) there is nothing unhealthy or unnatural in their adolescent's sexual orientation. They must be advised that now, more than ever, their daughter or son needs their love and support. They must also be told of the very real and serious dangers inherent in family disapproval or rejection, such as substance abuse, runaway behavior, and suicide. Many families seek professional help to change their teenager's sexual orientation. The practitioner should be understanding of these requests but must clearly point out that therapies aimed at changing sexual orientation are of dubious effectiveness and may be dangerous. However, referral to a supportive counselor for family therapy may be helpful.

Parents should also be introduced to books written for the families of gay and lesbian youths (see Suggested Readings). They should be made aware of community resources, such as supportive religious counselors and local chapters of Parents, Families and Friends of Lesbians and Gays,* which hold monthly support groups and publish informational literature for parents.

TRANSGENDERISM

Among the most isolated of adolescents are those coming to terms with a transgendered (transsexual) identity. Transgendered individuals are those who, while biologically male or (less frequently) female, emotionally and psychologically are of the opposite gender. They describe themselves as feeling "trapped" in the body of the opposite sex. Transgenderism may appear in early childhood and is usually well established by puberty, manifested not only in cross-dressing but in the mannerisms, vocal inflections, and interests of the opposite sex. Unlike some individuals who engage in transvestitism, the transgendered person often displays these characteristics with an easy and unexaggerated naturalness. Most transgenders are heterosexual, choosing sexual partners of the opposite sex relative to their core gender identity. There are some gay or lesbian adolescents who in their early teenage years express a desire to be of the opposite sex. This wish is perhaps due to their lack of knowledge about the nature of sexual orientation or perhaps represents a desire to be "normal" (i.e., "If I were a woman, it would be all right to love another man."). This situation should not be confused with transgenderism.

Despite the *Diagnostic and Statistical Manual of Mental Disorders* (fourth edition) classification of transgenderism as a "gender identity disorder," it is harmful to treat transgendered adolescents as disordered individuals.[2] The goal in working with transgendered teenagers is not to "cure" but rather to provide counseling, information, and anticipatory guidance. The medical physician and psychiatrist should work with the adolescent to establish a plan that will help the teenager achieve his or her life goals. For some transgendered teenagers, this plan will include eventual sex-reassignment surgery as an adult. During adolescence, the transgendered teenager will need psychologic evaluation to determine how ready he or she is for the first steps in gender reassignment. For the young male transgendered, the appearance of secondary sexual characteristics, such as beard growth and deepening voice, may be especially disturbing. When determined to be psychologically ready, the teenager may begin experimental living in the gender of reassignment, including cross-dressing and name change. If this transition is successful, hormonal therapy may be started in the later teenage years after completion of the growth

spurt. A typical regimen for transgendered males consists of Premarin, 1.25 to 2.5 mg per day.[25] The physician should be aware that adolescents may increase their estrogen dosage above recommended amounts to maximize physical changes. The possible complications of estrogen therapy include thromboembolism, cardiovascular effects with smoking, hepatic adenoma leading to hemorrhage, and hypertension. Patients should be examined at least every 6 months for hypertension, liver changes, and changing sexual characteristics. Expected changes include breast growth, more rounded body contour, testicular atrophy, voice change, decreased body hair, and decreased erections and libido. Transgendered females undergo a similar course of masculinizing hormonal treatment. It is not unusual for some teenagers to go in and out of their assumed gender of reassignment. This ambivalence should be expected and tolerated. The cost of estrogen therapy may also result in inconsistent compliance. Since sex-change surgery is not an option during adolescence, hormonal therapy and ongoing counseling may be literally lifesaving for many transgendered teenagers. The high suicide rate among transgendered teenagers may be due in part to their seeing no hope in finding a supportive physician willing to help them work out a therapeutic plan.

TRANSVESTITISM

Transvestitism is a gender-role paraphilia referring to the practice of wearing clothes generally ascribed to the opposite sex, primarily for erotic satisfaction. This behavior is usually a male phenomenon and may first appear before puberty. Most adult transvestites are heterosexual males. However, in childhood and adolescence, cross-dressing may occur as an early expression of homosexuality, transgenderism, or transvestitism. The small minority of gay adolescents who cross-dress usually do so for nonerotic reasons. Some may believe that this is the social script they must follow to express their sexual orientation. Others may cross-dress as a means to attract other males, as a form of protection, or as an expression of defiance. Those gay adolescents who cross-dress often abandon this behavior in adulthood.

During counseling, it is important to define the significance of cross-dressing for the teenager and to help him learn skills to cope with the negative reactions he may receive from family, peers, and society. If a youth seems to be cross-dressing more out of defiance than as an expression of individuality, one might point out that while defiance may feel satisfying in the short run, it may be self-defeating if the result is dropping out of school, physical violence, frequent institutionalization, and serial foster home placements. Nevertheless, it is often easier

---

*PFLAG, 1101 14th Street NW Suite 1030, Washington, DC 20005.

for cross-dressing adolescents to work with the health professional than with nonaccepting agencies and institutions.

ADVOCACY

Because gay, lesbian, bisexual, and transgendered youths are unable to advocate for themselves, it is important that youth-serving professionals speak out on the experience and needs of these teenagers. In the past, many potential advocates have not spoken out because they feared losing their jobs or having their own sexual orientation questioned. Recently, however, several communities have developed innovative projects to begin to address the needs of these adolescents. These projects include school- and community-based counseling programs, in-service training programs for youth workers, gay and lesbian teenage hotlines, support groups, theater projects, job training programs, and community-sponsored recreation events. Although these programs have sometimes been met with disapproval, more often there has been a community openness to learning more about these teenagers and how their needs might be met. Advocacy, to be effective, must come from within each community. It is driven by the recognition that these teenagers exist in every community and that their lives are endangered by a failure to address their needs.

References

1. U.S. Department of Health and Human Services: *Report of the Secretary's Task Force on Youth Suicide,* Washington, DC, 1989, DHHS Pub. No. (ADM) 89-1623.
2. American Psychiatric Association: *Diagnostic and statistical manual of mental disorders,* ed 4, Washington, DC, 1994, American Psychiatric Association.
3. American Academy of Pediatrics Committee on Adolescence: Homosexuality and adolescence, *Pediatrics* 92:631-634, 1993.
4. Rowlett JD, Greydanus DE: Homosexuality in adolescence, *Adolesc Med State of Art Rev* 5:509-525, 1994.
5. Friedman RC, Downey JI: Homosexuality, *N Engl J Med* 331:923-930, 1994.
6. Pillard RC, Weinrich JD: Evidence of familial nature of male homosexuality, *Arch Gen Psychiatry* 43:808, 1986.
7. Heston LL, Shields J: Homosexuality in twins: a family study and a registry study, *Arch Gen Psychiatry* 18:149-160, 1968.
8. Gladue BA, Green R, Hellman RE: Neuroendocrine response to estrogen and sexual orientation, *Science* 225:1496-1499, 1984.
9. Bell AP, Weinberg MS, Hammersmith SK: *Sexual preference: its development in men and women,* Bloomington, 1981, Indiana University Press.
10. Kinsey A, Pomeroy W, Martin C: *Sexual behavior in the human male,* Philadelphia, 1948, WB Saunders.
11. Kinsey A, Pomeroy W, Martin C, Gebbard P: *Sexual behavior in the human female,* Philadelphia, 1953, WB Saunders.
12. Sorenson RC: *Adolescent sexuality in contemporary America: personal values and sexual behavior ages 13 to 19,* New York, 1973, World Publishing.
13. Blum R: *The state of adolescent health in Minnesota,* Minneapolis, 1989, Adolescent Health Database Project.
14. Diamond M: Homosexuality and bisexuality in different populations, *Arch Sex Behav* 22:291-309, 1993.
15. Remafedi GJ: Homosexual youth: a challenge to contemporary society, *JAMA* 258:222-225, 1987.
16. Troiden RR: Homosexual identity development, *J Adolesc Health Care* 9: 105-113, 1988.
17. Remafedi GJ: Male homosexuality: the adolescent's perspective, *Pediatrics* 79:326-330, 1987.
18. Hetrick ES, Martin AD: Developmental issues and their resolution for gay and lesbian adolescents, *J Homosex* 14:25-44, 1987.
19. Sturdevant MS, Remafedi G: Special needs of homosexual youth, *Adolesc Med State of Art Rev* 3:359-371, 1992.
20. Remafedi GJ: Adolescent homosexuality: psychosocial and medical implications, *Pediatrics* 79:331-337, 1987.
21. Remafedi GJ: Sexually transmitted diseases in homosexual youth, *Adolesc Med State of Art Rev* 1:565-581, 1990.
22. Martin AD: Learning to hide: the socialization of the gay adolescent. In Feinstein SC, Looney JG, Schwartzberg AZ, Sorosky AD, editors: *Adolescent psychiatry,* Chicago, 1982, University of Chicago Press; p 52.
23. Remafedi GJ: The healthy sexual development of gay and lesbian adolescents, *SIECUS Rep* 17:7-8, 1989.
24. Borhek MV: Helping gay and lesbian adolescents and their families, *J Adolesc Health Care* 9:123-128, 1988.
25. Cooper MA: Hormone treatment clinic for transsexuals, *Hawaii Med J* 43:5, 1984.

Suggested Readings

Bell R: *Changing bodies, changing lives: a book for teens on sex and relationships,* New York, 1988, Random House.
> *A supportive section on homosexuality makes this an excellent book for all teenagers, including those with concerns about being lesbian or gay.*

Garden N: *Annie on my mind,* New York, 1982, Farrar Straus Giroux.
> *A supportive teenage novel of two girls who fall in love.*

Griffin CW, Wirth MJ, Wirth AG: *Beyond acceptance: parents of lesbians and gays talk about their experiences,* Englewood Cliffs, NJ, 1986, Prentice-Hall.
> *An informative and supportive book for parents on homosexuality and being gay or lesbian.*

Rench JE: *Understanding sexual identity: a book for gay teens and their friends,* Minneapolis, 1990, Lerner Publications.
> *A clear and straightforward discussion of what it means to be gay or lesbian.*

Snyder A, Pelletier L: *The truth about Alex,* New York, 1981, New American Library.
> *A teenage novel about a gay teenager and his straight friend that provides both hope and an honest look at the prejudice facing them.*

Whitlock K: *Bridges of respect: creating support for lesbian and gay youth,* Philadelphia, 1989, American Friends Service Committee.
> *A resource book for professionals working with adolescents, including a list of organizations working with gay and lesbian adolescents.*

CHAPTER 100

Sexual Abuse

•

Kent P. Hymel and Richard D. Krugman

Physicians frequently are asked to evaluate adolescents for current or past sexual abuse. Sexual abuse is defined as the engaging of the child or adolescent in sexual activities that the child does not understand, to which the child cannot give informed consent, and that violate the social or legal taboos of society. This broad definition includes all forms of sexual misuse, including exhibitionism; voyeurism; all forms of oral, genital, or anal contact; fondling; pornography; and the engaging of a child or adolescent in prostitution.

Normal sexual activity should occur between developmentally equal individuals, should be consensual, and should be engaged in without coercion. In contrast, sexual abuse exists when sexual activity occurs between individuals who are disparate in terms of age and level of development, when there is a lack of consent, and/or when coercion is involved. The element of coercion often involves secrecy in which the victim is warned that if the abuse is disclosed, there will be dire consequences.

INCIDENCE

In a 1977 address to the American Academy of Pediatrics, C. Henry Kempe, MD, described the sexual abuse of children as "a hidden pediatric problem." Two decades later, the problem is anything but hidden. In 1976, 6000 reports of sexual abuse of children were tabulated by the American Humane Association. By 1986, this number had increased to 132,000. In 1994, reports of suspected sexual abuse accounted for approximately 11% of the 3.1 million reports nationally of all forms of abuse and neglect.[1] In our own experience, it appears that reports of adolescent sexual abuse or assault are handled within emergency services or law enforcement agencies and are less frequently reported to social services as child sexual abuse. Estimates of adolescent sexual abuse derived from social service agencies may therefore be flawed.

Characteristics associated with greater risks of sexual abuse include female gender, preadolescence or early adolescence, having a stepfather, living without a natural parent, having an impaired mother, poor parenting, and witnessing of family conflict.[2] By the time adolescents reach college age, approximately one in five girls and one in ten boys will have experienced some form of sexual abuse. Thus, sexual abuse is a significant problem for adolescents in that a number of them are victims at some point in their lives.

PRESENTATION

Adolescents who may have been sexually abused usually come to the attention of the practitioner primarily in one of three ways. They may present with behavioral changes, genital-rectal or medical complaints, or a specific disclosure of developmentally inappropriate sexual contact.

Behavioral Changes

None of the behaviors listed in Box 100-1 are diagnostic of sexual abuse. Sexualized play, excessive masturbation, promiscuity and prostitution, and perpetration of sexual abuse to others are more specific than the rest. It is critical that physicians not treat behavioral symptoms with "behavior modification" without first attempting to understand the underlying cause, which may be intra- or extrafamilial abuse or neglect.

Among the most worrisome outcomes for the sexually abused adolescent is the transition from victim to victimizer. Warning signs for adolescent perpetration are listed in Box 100-2. Most adolescent perpetrators are male, although it is possible that as more is learned about sexual abuse, more adolescent female perpetrators will also be identified. An adolescent perpetrator's victims may be either male or female. Studies have shown that many adolescents who sexually abuse children have been sexually abused themselves, and a significant proportion are sexually abused outside their own families.

BOX 100-1
Presentations of Sexual Abuse

Behavioral changes
    Sleep disturbances (e.g., nightmares, night
       terrors)
    Appetite disturbances (e.g., anorexia, bulimia)
    Neurotic or conduct disorders
    Phobias, avoidance behavior
    Withdrawal, depression
    Guilt
    Temper tantrums, aggressive behavior
    Excessive masturbation
    Runaway behavior
    Suicidal behavior
    Hysterical or conversion reactions
    School problems
    Promiscuity/prostitution
    Substance abuse
    Perpetration of sexual abuse to others
    Sexualized play
Medical symptoms
    Abdominal pain
    Genital, urethral, or rectal trauma
    Sexually transmitted diseases
    Recurrent urinary tract infections
    Enuresis
    Encopresis
    Pregnancy
Direct statements
    Partial or complete disclosure of inappropriate
       sexual contact

BOX 100-2
**Warning Signs of Adolescent
Perpetration**

"Red flags"
    Compulsive masturbation (especially chronic or
       public)
    Degradation/humiliation of self or others with
       sexual themes
    Attempting to expose others' genitals
    Chronic preoccupation with sexually aggressive
       pornography
    Sexually explicit conversation with significantly
       younger children
    Touching genitals without permission (e.g.,
       grabbing, goosing)
    Sexually explicit threats (verbal or written)
"Illegal behaviors" (defined by law)
    Obscene phone calls, voyeurism, exhibitionism,
       frottage
    Sexual contact with someone of significant age
       difference (child sexual abuse)
    Forced sexual contact (sexual assault)
    Forced penetration (rape)
    Sexual contact with animals (bestiality)
    Genital injury to others

Adapted from Ryan G, Blum J, Christopher D, et al: *Understanding and responding to the sexual behavior of children: trainer's manual,* Denver, CO, 1993, Kempe National Center.

Medical Symptoms

The medical presentations listed in Box 100-1 are also nonspecific for sexual contact, with the exception of gonorrhea, syphilis, and pregnancy. Genital, urethral, or rectal trauma or teenage pregnancy are all highly associated with previous sexual abuse. Abdominal pain, recurrent urinary tract infections, enuresis, encopresis, school problems, and substance abuse are also potential presentations for an adolescent who has been sexually abused.

Direct Statements

Partial disclosures of sexual victimization by adolescents may involve a generalized statement such as "There's a lot of raping and molesting going on in our school." Such statements are often attempts to "test the waters," since children who have been sexually abused are often coerced into keeping the molestation a secret. They may gauge the practitioner's response to see whether the abuser was correct in telling them that disclosure would prompt a negative and punitive response. If early warnings are responded to in this manner, the child or adolescent may not disclose more information.

More direct statements about sexual abuse may occur under any circumstance. These are often spontaneous or in response to a question. Occasionally, they are disclosed in anger. Not all direct statements of sexual abuse are reliable. Fictitious reports do exist, but studies have shown that these tend to be the minority. Although it is false to state that "children never lie," all direct statements about sexual abuse should be taken seriously, be reported to the appropriate investigatory agencies, and result in a multidisciplinary investigation.

In the course of normal adolescent health care, a physician may recognize that the sexually active relationship of a young adolescent with her or his significantly older partner constitutes statutory rape. Although legal definitions vary, many states define statutory rape as sexual contact when the victim is under 15 years of age and the "perpetrator" is at least 4 years older. Many adolescents define these relationships with their older partners as entirely normal. Data on teen pregnancy published in 1993 revealed that adult men over 20 years of age fathered over one half of infants born to school-age girls (11 to 18 years of age) in California during 1990.[4] Although intervention by law enforcement or social services is less likely than in cases of sexual abuse involving children, physicians caring for adolescents are legally required to report illegal statutory relationships as sexual abuse.

DIAGNOSIS

The diagnosis of sexual abuse generally requires a multidisciplinary approach. Cases involve physicians, law enforcement agencies, social services, mental health facilities, civil and criminal courts, and educational institutions. When the presenting complaint is not overtly one of sexual abuse, the diagnosis may depend on the physician's index of suspicion and willingness to consider sexual abuse as a possibility in the differential diagnosis.

History

The history is usually the most critical component of the diagnostic evaluation. Because of the secrecy that may be enforced by the perpetrator, the physician must open the discussion and give the adolescent the opportunity to disclose information about sexual abuse if it has occurred. For example, the practitioner might begin with the following statement: "There are lots of reasons why kids your age have nightmares or fears or exhibit runaway behavior. In some cases, it is because someone has sexually abused them. Is that a possibility with you?" The history of sexual abuse must be elicited through supportive, nonaccusatory, and nonleading questioning. When open-ended questioning is complete, more specific questions should be asked for clarification. It is vital to record the interview in maximum detail in the medical record.

Physical Examination

There are many reasons why the genital and rectal examinations in adolescents who have been sexually abused are often entirely normal or reveal only nonspecific findings. Vaginal vestibular tissues are elastic, are well vascularized, and usually heal rapidly. Early pubertal estrogen effects increase hymenal elasticity, hymenal redundancy, and physiologic vaginal secretions. Longitudinal studies of sexually abused prepubertal children reveal that hymenal defects become less visible after puberty.[5] Because of the possibility (or in the older adolescent, probability) of developmentally appropriate sexual activity, physical examination findings are less often specific. Ideally, a genital and rectal examination should be performed routinely (with consent) during adolescent health maintenance examinations. The clear documentation of an adolescent with a normal hymen at a routine check-up may become important in the evaluation of a later case of sexual abuse or sexual assault.

After acute sexual assault, physical findings may include bruising, hymenal or rectal tears, bite marks, pinch marks, and other trauma. The American Academy of Pediatrics has published guidelines on the evaluation of the acutely sexually assaulted adolescent.[6] We have seen instances in which adolescent boys and girls who have been acutely sexually assaulted displayed hysterical conversion reactions and underwent many days of neurologic work-up before physicians considered the possibility of sexual abuse or performed an adequate physical examination (including rectal examination).

In the chronically sexually abused female, abnormalities considered specific for penetrating sexual abuse are limited to the posterior genital structures. There may be hymenal defects, scarring, or narrowing posteriorly as well as anal scars. In males, there may be evidence of genital injury or rectal scarring or trauma.

Laboratory Evaluation

Medical evaluation of the acutely sexually assaulted adolescent requires skill, sensitivity, and patience. Forensic tests provided in the "rape kit" must be performed as soon as possible after the abuse. If these tests are performed more than 72 hours from when the incident occurred, the results are usually unrewarding and inconclusive. Evaluation for sexually transmitted diseases (STDs) should be accomplished acutely and repeated in 2 weeks. Serologic testing for syphilis, human immunodeficiency virus, and hepatitis B should be repeated at 12 weeks after the assault to exclude acquired infection more definitively. Finally, pregnancy and STD "prophylaxis" should also be considered. (See Chapter 102 for a complete discussion of sexual assault.)

The presence of STDs in adolescents may be of diagnostic importance, and victims of chronic sexual abuse should be screened for these. Contact tracing and history taking should address the possibility that a "sexually active" adolescent may be sexually active with an older sibling, parent, stepparent, or other relative. (See Chapter 140 for a complete discussion of STDs.)

MANAGEMENT

If child sexual abuse is suspected, a report to the mandated child protective services and/or law enforcement agency is required. The 50 states vary somewhat with respect to reporting requirements. Generally, adolescents below the age of 16 to 18 years who are suspected to be victims of sexual abuse should be reported.

Appropriate follow-up should be obtained. All sexually abused children and adolescents should be evaluated by a competent mental health professional. Most will need treatment. If other siblings or friends are involved, they also should be evaluated.

PROGNOSIS

The prognosis for sexually abused adolescents is not known. Retrospective studies have revealed that adolescents with a history of sexual abuse are at increased risk for behavioral/emotional problems, running away, substance abuse, suicide attempts, bulimia, sexual dysfunction, borderline personality disorder, multiple personality disorder, STDs, menstrual disorders, and pregnancy.[7] In addition, in abusive and neglectful parents there is a high rate of previous sexual abuse during their own childhood or adolescence. These data do not mean that every abused adolescent will grow up to be an abusive parent (two out of three probably will not), but the risk for these individuals is substantially higher than for adolescents in the general population who have not been abused.

If any perpetration behavior in an adolescent is recognized, there should be immediate intervention. Most studies of adult sexual offenders have indicated that the deviant behavior begins in adolescence or much earlier. Thus, efforts to interrupt a potentially escalating pattern of sexually offending behavior by treating identified adolescent offenders could prevent future cases of sexual abuse and assault. Specialized, offense-specific treatment needs to involve a combination of behavioral and insight therapy, which is instituted most commonly (and most effectively) in group settings. There are relatively few published studies on the outcomes of treatment of adolescent offenders. A much longer treatment regimen is necessary for violent offenders, who must be treated in a closed setting. It is probably prudent to suggest that sexual offending behaviors in adolescents can be controlled in some instances but not cured, and long-term follow-up is required for the protection of both the adolescent and any potential victims in the community.

References

1. Wiese D, Daro D: *Current trends in child abuse reporting and fatalities: the results of the 1994 fifty state survey,* Chicago, Ill., 1995, National Center on Child Abuse Prevention Research.
2. Finkelhor D: Epidemiological factors in the clinical identification of child sexual abuse, *Child Abuse Negl* 17:67-70, 1993.
3. Ryan G, Blum J, Christopher D, et al: *Understanding and responding to the sexual behavior of children: trainer's manual,* Denver, CO, 1993, Kempe National Center.
4. Males M: Schoolage pregnancy: why hasn't prevention worked?, *J Sch Health* 63:429-432, 1993.
5. McCann J, Voris J, Simon M: Genital injuries resulting from sexual abuse: a longitudinal study, *Pediatrics* 89:307-317, 1992.
6. American Academy of Pediatrics Committee on Adolescence: Sexual assault and the adolescent, *Pediatrics* 94:761-765, 1994.
7. Jenny C: Sexual abuse in adolescents, *Curr Opin Pediatr* 3:575-579, 1991.

Suggested Reading

Hymel KP, Jenny C: Child sexual abuse, *Pediatr Rev* 17:236-250, 1996.

CHAPTER 101

Prostitution and Pornography

•

William M. Rogers II and Robert W. Deisher

Although there is growing awareness of the extent and sequelae of adolescent homelessness, it is less commonly recognized that prostitution represents an important, indeed principal means of survival for youths who are extensively involved in street life.[1] The term *survival sex* is often used in this context to distinguish the sexual exploitation of street-involved adolescents from the stereotypic exchange of sex for money between (typically heterosexual) adults. Male and female street youths of all ages can become involved in "hustling" through a variety of circumstances, often in exchange for shelter, food, or drugs instead of money.

Clearly, this phenomenon is not a common adolescent experience, but neither is it entirely negligible. Although the epidemiology of adolescent homelessness is fraught with methodologic difficulties, it is estimated that there are between 1 and 2 million runaways each year and that, at any given time, 100,000 to 300,000 youths are living permanently on the street.[2] The forces that propel these adolescents into street life are the very factors that favor their entrance into prostitution: early and coercive sexual experiences at home; histories of unsatisfactory foster home placement and institutional care; delinquency and incarceration; depression and poor self-esteem; and family histories of sustained substance abuse. This profile of profound psychosocial jeopardy all but guarantees that homeless adolescents will experience the exploitive exigencies of street life with grim familiarity. Indeed, many have migrated into street life precisely because it represents an improvement over life at home.[3]

Even so, most of those who become involved in survival sex do so without having ever considered it before coming to the streets. However, without education, work experience, or vocational skills, their prospects for legitimate employment are limited and uninviting.

Other aspects of their lives are equally detrimental. At a critical stage in their development, they are not in school and lack positive role models. They are active on the street at night, asleep during the day, frequently incapacitated by their use of alcohol and drugs, and almost entirely deprived of the age-appropriate experiences that are necessary for success in the conventional world.

FEMALE ADOLESCENT PROSTITUTION

In urban areas, runaway female teenagers often fall prey to predatory male taskmasters in the sex industry ("pimps"). These individuals actively maintain surveillance for new arrivals in their territory and contrive to establish ostensibly protective relationships with them. It is not uncommon for young women to become involved with pimps within 2 days of their arrival on the street. Given their backgrounds of emotional deprivation, it is not surprising that these girls are inclined to construe the solicitous attentions of pimps as serious romantic overtures. However, any pretense of romance is soon replaced by the demand to produce income, and either by force or sometimes by mutual agreement, these girls are introduced to prostitution. Drugs, the alternative currency of street life, are frequently an important feature of the bond that connects young women with their pimps. Indeed, pimps may actively cultivate drug dependency in the young women who work for them as a means of maintaining control.

Pregnancy

Many homeless girls who are involved in prostitution become pregnant. Their age, chaotic life styles, and unsettled backgrounds render them uniquely ill prepared for parenthood, yet they actively seek this outcome. Many of them sincerely believe that having a child will provide them with a source of love. Thus, even though their knowledge of birth control may be limited, these pregnancies are often not accidental and would not be prevented by improved access to contraceptive technology. Also, these girls are not often willing to consider adoption or abortion once they become pregnant.

In a study conducted at the University of Washington,[4] 19 of 62 infants born to adolescent prostitutes in the Seattle area were taken from their mothers at the time of birth by local child protective services. Of the 40 infants who were initially released to the custody of their mothers, 15 were known to have been taken from their mothers within the first 18 months of life as a result of abuse or neglect, perpetuating a seemingly ineluctable cycle of intergenerational misfortune. Longitudinal studies of this population are very difficult; these 18-month follow-up data thus represent conservative estimates of the long-term risk for termination of maternal custody among adolescent prostitutes.

Heavy maternal drug use, particularly cocaine, frequently complicates the pregnancies of these girls, with uncertain ramifications for the cognitive and behavioral development of their offspring.[5] In addition, most of these young women continue to engage in prostitution and substance abuse while raising their children. Their itinerant, disorderly life styles and efforts to avoid child protection agencies and other authorities complicate the task of providing even basic care for them and their infants.

MALE ADOLESCENT PROSTITUTION

Although young women who are homeless often find that they have few options for survival other than prostitution, adolescent males on the street frequently seek recourse in a variety of petty crimes and drug dealing. Nevertheless, up to 60% of chronically homeless young men have been found to have depended on survival sex.[6] First noted in the medical literature in 1969,[7] the epidemiology of adolescent male prostitution remains obscure. The transience of all street populations, in combination with the natural reticence of young males to discuss their experience in prostitution, complicates the task of achieving even a replicable cross-sectional view of this phenomenon. However, reports suggest that the proportion of homeless youths who are engaged in prostitution has declined since this phenomenon was first described.[8]

For many male runaways, their first contacts on the street are other adolescent males involved in prostitution. These early, formative social experiences among peers with similar unfortunate backgrounds and impaired self-esteem render prostitution less frightening and foreign as a means of livelihood. The prospect of easy money in a setting that encourages survival by picaresque, delinquent activities provides additional incentive for participation in the established folkways of street life, particularly among young males who are developmentally inclined to seek validation through group identity. Amplified within the crucible of street life, the risks associated with these normal developmental processes are profound, but, typically, they are overshadowed by momentary needs and impulses. Full awareness of the perils of prostitution may not emerge until these young men enter their third decade, long after significant physical and psychic harm has been sustained.

There are two distinct groups of adolescent male prostitutes: those self-identified as heterosexual and those self-identified as homosexual. Approximately 30% to 40% of males engaged in prostitution have a homosexual or bisexual identity, although a substantial number indicate some uncertainty about their sexual orientation.[3] Those who are self-identified as homosexual are most likely to be homeless because of family and peer rejection. Even in the harsh context of street life, they view contact with other gay-identified individuals (both peers and customers) as preferable to a life of isolation and stigmatization at home. Gandy and Deisher,[6] in a study of the rehabilitation of young male prostitutes, found that those who are self-identified as homosexual have a better prognosis for leaving prostitution and seeking educational or vocational opportunities than those who are self-identified as heterosexual. Heterosexually identified males are more likely to use prostitution encounters as opportunities to commit crimes (e.g., robbing their customers).

It is uncommon for adolescent male prostitutes to have pimps. They are less likely to feel endangered by their customers and are also better able to defend themselves. Some of these young men cultivate ongoing "sugar daddy" relationships with customers, an arrangement that affords greater safety than street hustling. Rarely do these situations evolve into sustained relationships that provide young males with secure niches outside of street life.

Youthfulness is an especially important attribute among young male prostitutes. Many women can remain active in prostitution until middle age, but few young men can continue in street hustling beyond the age of 20. Those who are not physically scarred by the vicissitudes of street life may be able to work in the escort or pornography industries for a few additional years, but they are obviously ill prepared to enter the mainstream job market when their perceived desirability in these underworld arenas finally expires. Frequently, drug involvement, alcoholism, and crime dominate their futures.[9] Necessity, maturity, rehabilitation, fortuity, and opportunity are all likely to influence the exit of these young men from street life and prostitution, but the significance and interaction of these factors have not been elucidated.

PORNOGRAPHY

The recent explosive growth of the video industry has augmented the already substantial role of adolescents in the production of pornographic material. Young people are often recruited into this work as a result of prostitution encounters. This employment is usually brief in duration and frequently entails substantial risk of further degradation through drug abuse and violence. Although pornographic material depicting minors is unlawful, many adolescents conceal their true ages to secure money or drugs. As a result, they may become involved in the production of pornography at a very young age. It is uncommon for medical or social service personnel to be aware of this activity, even among adolescents who are known to be involved in prostitution.

PROSTITUTION AND SEXUALLY TRANSMITTED DISEASE

The prevalence of sexually transmitted disease (STD) is high among homeless adolescents.[10] Although frequently the targets of "safe sex" campaigns by public health agencies, they are uniquely vulnerable to circumstances conducive to the transmission of STDs. These adolescents' use of condoms is sporadic; they sometimes use them with customers but rarely with their peers. Their developmental status, haphazard housing, lack of adult supervision, and extensive involvement with psychoactive substances together with other psychosocial risks combine to make routine STD surveillance critical in this population. Unfortunately, even in the large urban areas where these services are available to them, they may be unwilling to seek appropriate diagnostic and preventive services. This may be due to perceived inability to pay for services or aversion to conventional sources of health care. Free clinical facilities established specifically for these adolescents (and located near the areas that they frequent) have been successful in providing STD-related services.[11]

The elevated prevalence of conventional STDs among this population raises particular concern regarding their risk for infection with the human immunodeficiency virus (HIV). A 1994 survey of five sites providing services to runaway youths found seroprevalence rates ranging from

0% to 7.3%.[12] Given their frequent high-risk contacts with concentrated reservoirs of HIV seroprevalence (injection drug users, adult male homosexuals, and heterosexuals with unprotected multiple sexual partners), it is surprising that the seroprevalence rates detected among homeless adolescents are so low. Chapter 67 contains an in-depth discussion of HIV infection and AIDS. Risk behaviors of street youths warrant specifically targeted interventions.[13] Social isolation and depression may be factors in their poor response to conventional interventions.[14,15] Although customers of adolescents who engage in prostitution are virtually impossible to study, there is some anecdotal evidence to suggest that increased AIDS awareness among customers has resulted in decreased patronage of adolescent prostitutes.

ROLE OF THE PHYSICIAN

Most adolescent prostitutes receive their medical care in free clinics, emergency rooms, and detention centers. They are generally wary of mainstream medical providers, whom they perceive, often correctly, as condescending and disapproving. For this reason, they may be hesitant to discuss the very circumstances and concerns that affect their health most directly, such as homelessness, poverty, STDs, pregnancy, previous physical and sexual abuse, confusion about sexual orientation, the effects of chronic use of psychoactive substances, depression, and suicidal impulses. Contacts with medical providers may represent rare opportunities to influence these young people favorably, and so it is particularly important for interviews to be conducted in an objective, nonjudgmental manner.

Information about living arrangements, sexual behavior, and social support should be routinely gathered. It is a mistake to assume that adolescents' knowledge of the physical and psychologic aspects of sexuality is commensurate with their levels of activity. Condoms should be available in every clinical setting in which these young people are regularly served.

Interviews and physical examinations should not overlook developmental issues and other core indicators of health that define the care of mainstream adolescents. Although this discussion has focused on the exceptional and extreme conditions that characterize prostituting adolescents, it is also true that they benefit from attention to acne, weight control, and other minor medical problems that may have been neglected for years for lack of care. Given the chaotic conditions that have often prevailed in the families of origin, serious congenital disorders often go unrecognized.[11]

Treatments should be as simple as possible. It is often futile to issue a prescription for medication, since money and adult supervision are typically unavailable. When possible, medications and medical supplies should be dispensed directly to these patients at the time of their evaluations. Their compliance with follow-up recommendations is erratic and they often discontinue prescribed treatments prematurely; thus, single-dose regimens of antibiotics, particularly for STDs, are warranted. Single dose treatment regimens for STDs are described in Chapter 140. Continuity of care is often a frustrating goal for these patients and their healthcare providers owing to their mobility and their distrust of adults. However, with appropriate allowance for the exigencies of street life, empathetic providers can sometimes establish enduring bonds with these youths that favorably influence their development.

References

1. Weisberg DK: *Children of the night; a study of adolescent prostitutes,* Lexington, MA, 1987, D.C. Heath, p 114.
2. Data from the National Network of Runaway and Youth Services, cited in U.S. General Accounting Office: *AIDS education: programs for out-of-school youth slowly evolving,* HRD-90-111, May 1990, p 2.
3. James J, Meyerding J: Early sexual experience as a factor in prostitution, *Arch Sex Behav* 7:31-42, 1978.
4. Deisher RW, Farrow JA, Hope K, et al: The pregnant adolescent prostitute, *Am J Dis Child* 143:1162-1165, 1989.
5. Fulroth R, Phillips B, Durand DJ: Perinatal outcome of infants exposed to cocaine and/or heroin in utero, *Am J Dis Child* 143:905-910, 1989.
6. Gandy P, Deisher R: Young male prostitutes: the physician's role in social rehabilitation, *JAMA* 212:1661-1666, 1970.
7. Deisher R, Eisner V, Sulzbacker S: The young male prostitute, *Pediatrics* 43:936-941, 1969.
8. Manzon L, Rosario M, Rekart ML: HIV seroprevalence among street involved Canadians in Vancouver, *AIDS Educ Prevent* 4(suppl):86-89, 1992.
9. Farrow JA, Deisher R: A practical guide to the office assessment of adolescent substance abuse, *Pediatr Ann* 15:675-684, 1986.
10. Luna GC, Rotheram-Borus MJ: Street youth and the AIDS pandemic, *AIDS Educ Prevent* 4(suppl):1-13, 1992.
11. Deisher RW, Rogers WM: The medical care of street youth, *J Adolesc Health* 12:500-503, 1991.
12. Allen DM, Lehman JS, Green TA, et al: HIV infection among homeless adults and runaway youth, United States, 1989-1992, *AIDS* 8:1593-1598, 1994.
13. Sugerman ST, Hergenroeder AC, Chacko MR, et al: Acquired immunodeficiency syndrome and adolescents; knowledge, attitudes, and behaviors of runaway and homeless youths, *Am J Dis Child* 145:431-436, 1991.
14. Federal Centre for AIDS, National Health Research and Development Program: *Street youth and AIDS,* Ottawa, Canada, 1989, Health and Welfare Canada.
15. Governor's AIDS Advisory Committee; Subcommittee on Out-of-Home Adolescents, HIV Infection and AIDS: *Out of home adolescents, HIV infection and AIDS,* Olympia, WA, 1989, State of Washington Department of Health.

CHAPTER 102

Sexual Assault

•

Suzanne P. Starling and Richard D. Krugman

Acute sexual assault is a term used to describe sexual activity performed against the will of the victim. In the case of adolescent sexual assault, medical practitioners are often the first to be notified. This contact may be in an office or emergency room. Proper procedures and examination techniques should be used to ensure the comfort and safety of the patient.

Adolescents are the targets of assault more frequently than are adult women. Nearly 700,000 women are raped each year in the United States; 61% of these are teenagers.[1] Victimization rates peak at the 16- to 19-year age range.[2] Studies have found that as many as 12% of boys and 18% of girls experience unwanted sexual activity before the age of 16.[3] Although males can be sexually assaulted, adolescent boys rarely present acutely for examination.

EPIDEMIOLOGY AND RISK FACTORS

The epidemiology of adolescent sexual assault differs from that of adults. Assailants are known to the adolescent victim in 87% of the cases; 57% are acquaintance or date rapes. Over half the assaults start as a voluntary social interaction, with nearly half of the victims willingly going to the home or car of the assailant.[2,4,5] In 1988, Jenny found that most adolescent assaults occur between 10 PM and 4 AM and are likely to be alcohol related.[5]

Date rape is more common in this age group. In 1989, Koval found that 17% to 52% of college students and 12% to 27% of high school students had experienced violence in dating.[6] Date rape is more likely to involve verbal coercion and alcohol, whereas stranger assault more typically involves weapons and has an increased level of violence and trauma.[3,7] For this reason, date rape may cause less physical trauma to the victim.[4,5]

MANAGING THE ADOLESCENT ASSAULT VICTIM

History of the Assault

Adolescents are often brought to medical attention by a parent or friend several hours to days after an assault, although some adolescents may not disclose that they have been assaulted for months or years. At first presentation, many teenagers may not have contacted law enforcement authorities. A detailed history of the event is required to determine whether an assault has occurred and to delineate the extensiveness of the assault. Although wording varies among jurisdictions, mandatory reporting laws exist throughout the United States. If a history of sexual assault is obtained from the adolescent or caretaker, the case should be reported to the proper law enforcement agency. State laws may dictate the need to contact social services if the case was an intrafamilial assault. Chapter 100 discusses sexual abuse in detail.

The history taking should include details such as the place and time of the assault, and specific sexual activities. Physical complaints and behavioral changes should be elicited from both the patient and the parent in separate interviews. Adolescents frequently minimize their symptoms, and a careful history from a parent may help to further delineate both physical and behavioral changes. A complete medical history, including medications such as oral contraceptive pills (OCPs) and chronic illnesses, is important. Social history is also pertinent in many cases. See Box 102-1 for a sample sexual assault protocol.

Carefully document all physical and historical data in a thoughtful and legible fashion. These cases are often prosecuted months to years after the examination has taken place, and a complete record will assist the examiner should legal testimony be required.

Medical Examination

The medical examination of assault should always include a thorough general physical examination. Vital signs such as blood pressure and pulse can help in the evaluation of stress level. Weight and any history of weight loss are also important. Pay special attention to the skin, looking for evidence of abrasions or lacerations, especially on the hands and forearms. Examine the mouth for evidence of trauma to the tongue and buccal mucosa.

The genital examination should be documented with a detailed descriptions of all structures, using correct terminology. Specifically describe the areas of trauma that may be present. Look for trauma to the hymen, particularly posteriorly. A moist cotton swab can facilitate separation of the hymenal leaflets in the estrogenized hymen. Complete or partial acute transections of the hymen indicate recent trauma. Examine the posterior fourchette and fossa navicularis for trauma, as these areas frequently are injured in acute assault. Abrasions, lacerations, and bruising are common in this area after assault. Internal speculum examinations are indicated for postpubertal adolescents. Describe any areas of trauma to the walls of the vagina or the cervix. Describe the buttocks and anus with the same detail. Look carefully for damage to the anal rugae, using gentle traction. Photocolposcopy

---

BOX 102-1
Acute Sexual Assault Protocol for Adolescents

I. Identifying information
  A. Patient name, date of birth, address, parent's names
  B. Alleged perpetrator's name, age, address (if known)
II. History of present event (obtain separate histories from patient and parent/caretaker)
  A. Description of event: sexual acts, exact place and time
  B. Physical complaints: discharge, bleeding, pain
  C. Other injuries sustained in event: cuts, bruises, fractures
  D. Behavioral complaints: nightmares, anorexia
III. Medical history
  A. Previous illnesses: include medications (esp. oral contraceptive pills), surgeries, previous STDs
  B. Onset of menarche and last menstruation
  C. Allergies and immunizations
  D. History of previous assaults
IV. Social history
  A. Names/relationships of people in patient's home
  B. Educational level, including any developmental delay or special classes
  C. Support of friends and family members (obtain separate histories from patient and family/friends)
V. Physical examination
  A. Thorough general examination including vitals, height, and weight
  B. Special attention to skin, mucous membranes, hair
VI. Genital examination
  A. Tanner stage of breasts and genitals
  B. Indicate examination position and use of any instrumentation
  C. Describe labia majora and minora, urethra, clitoris, periurethral and perihymenal tissue
  D. Describe hymen: configuration, margins, evidence of trauma
  E. Describe posterior fourchette and fossa navicularis
  F. Internal speculum examination to describe injury to vaginal walls and cervix, physical evidence of STDs
  G. Collection of specimens for STDs
  H. Forensic kit (see text for details)
  I. Photographs: colposcopy or 35 mm
VII. Anal examination
  A. Indicate examination position and any instrumentation
  B. Describe buttocks and surrounding skin
  C. Document anal tone, tags, tears, fissures, or other evidence of trauma
  D. Photographs: colposcopy or 35 mm
VIII. STD testing and prophylaxis (see Table 102-1)
  IX. Pregnancy prophylaxis
  A. 2 tablets 50 µg ethinylestradiol/0.5 mg norgestrel (Ovral) within 72 hours of assault
  B. 2 tablets 12 hours after first dose
  C. Consider antiemetic prior to both doses
X. Follow-up
  A. 7-14 days for repeat STD testing
  B. 12 weeks for repeat serum syphilis test, HIV, hepatitis B antibodies
  C. Mental health counseling for patient and family members

Adapted from The Child Advocacy and Protection Team, The Children's Hospital, Denver, CO.
STDs, sexually transmitted diseases.

is helpful in delineating microtrauma to the external anogenital area and in obtaining photographs for legal purposes, but is not mandatory.

Absence of trauma to the genitals in acute assault should not deter a full investigation of the case. There are many reasons for lack of trauma in these cases. Full penetration of the vulva by the perpetrator may not have been achieved. Even in cases of complete penetration, there may not be physical signs. The hymenal and vaginal structures of the adolescent are elastic in nature and can stretch without extensive damage to the structures. This is particularly true if the patient has experienced intercourse before the time of the assault. In this case, signs of healed transections of the hymen may be present, which should not be confused with the acute findings of the assault.

Forensic Evaluation

Forensic or "rape kits" are often necessary to obtain physical evidence that may be used in a court of law. They are only used if the examination takes place within 72 hours of the assault. These tests are more likely to yield useful information if the victim is still in her original clothing and has not bathed, although adequate samples can be retrieved in other cases. This evidence collection is time consuming and can be stressful to the patient. Careful explanation of the need for the tests often results in better patient compliance, but the patient does have the right to refuse any or all portions of the testing. Collection of this evidence for legal purposes must be weighed against the patient's mental status and ability to complete the examination.

The specimen collection protocol varies from state to state. It involves gathering vaginal swabs from genital and extragenital sites to look for the presence of sperm and biochemical evidence. The victim's clothing is collected. Hair samples from the head and genitals are collected to compare with samples from the scene. Bite marks and areas of dried semen are swabbed for the presence of genetic markers that may aid in identification of the perpetrator. Skin can be scanned with a Wood's lamp to illuminate areas of dried semen. The blood type of the victim is also tested.

The forensic kit becomes legal evidence in the assault case and must be handled with care. Strict chain of evidence applies, and all parties involved in the handling should sign the kit. The evidence is ultimately delivered to law enforcement for processing.

Laboratory Evaluation (Table 102-1)

In postpubertal females, sexually transmitted disease (STD) cultures should be obtained from the endocervical canal as well as any extragenital site indicated by the history. Positive cultures for gonorrhea should be confirmed by two different laboratory methods. Only cell culture for *Chlamydia* infection should be used, since the antigen detection tests for *Chlamydia* have lower sensitivity and specificity than culture and are not approved for use on nongenital sites.[8] Examine a normal saline preparation for evidence of motile sperm and trichomonads. A 10% potassium hydroxide preparation that exudes the odor of amines is suggestive of bacterial vaginosis. Culture for *Trichomonas vaginalis* is indicated.

TABLE 102-1
Laboratory Evaluation and STD Prophylaxis in Acute Sexual Assault

STD	Diagnostic Test/Site	Prophylaxis*
Neisseria gonorrhoeae	Culture of cervix, mouth, anus	Ceftriaxone, 125 mg IM in 1 dose, or cefixime, 400 mg PO in 1 dose†
Chlamydia trachomatis	Culture (not antigen testing) of cervix, anus, mouth	Doxycycline, 100 mg PO bid for 7 days, or azithromycin, 1 g PO in 1 dose†
Trichomonas vaginalis	Culture and wet mount of vaginal swabs	Metronidazole, 2 g PO in one dose
Bacterial vaginosis	Wet mount of vaginal swabs	Metronidazole, 2 g PO in one dose
Syphilis	Serum syphilis testing	None recommended
HIV	Serum antibody	None recommended‡
Hepatitis B	Serum antibody	Consider vaccination if nonimmune

*Adapted from Centers For Disease Control and Prevention: 1993 sexually transmitted diseases treatment guidelines, *MMWR* 42:97-99, 1993.

†Alternate regimens suggested for treatment are not specifically recommended for prophylaxis by the CDC, but are often used in clinical practice as prophylaxis secondary to their ease of administration or lack of invasiveness. See CDC guidelines for specific recommendations.

‡Recommendations are subject to change. For known or suspected HIV contact where prophylaxis is requested, consult an antiretroviral expert.

If STD prophylaxis is given and the original cultures are negative, no follow-up cultures are needed.[8] However, if medications were not given or the original cultures were positive, cultures should be repeated in 7 to 14 days.

Blood samples should be drawn for the evaluation of syphilis, and hepatitis B antibody. Some centers also test for HIV initially. Because of their longer incubation periods, repeat specimens are also drawn at a 12-week follow-up visit. Blood or urine samples for pregnancy are also indicated.

TREATMENT

STD Prophylaxis (Table 102-1)

In cases of sexual assault with genital contact of any orifice, STD cultures should be obtained. Prophylaxis can be offered in cases of known or suspected STD in the assailant, unknown assailants, patient or parental concerns, and suspected lack of follow-up.

Pregnancy Prophylaxis

Often the patient and family members are particularly concerned about the possibility of pregnancy. After appropriate counseling and a negative pregnancy test, prophylaxis can be offered. Two tablets of 50 µg ethinylestradiol/0.5 mg norgestrel (Ovral) should be given within 72 (preferably within 12 to 24) hours of the assault. Two additional tablets are taken 12 hours after the first dose. With this method, the rate of pregnancy after assault is approximately 2%.[10] The pills work by promoting luteal phase dysfunction, out-of-phase endometrial development, and disordered tubal transport of the ovum. Because they may cause excessive nausea, antiemetics prior to both doses are recommended. Follow-up serum or urine pregnancy testing should be done 2 weeks after the assault to ensure the effectiveness of the treatment.

PSYCHOLOGIC SEQUELAE AND TREATMENT

Adult victims of rape often report the signs and symptoms of rape trauma syndrome.[11] These include complaints of pain, headache, amenorrhea, insomnia, and nightmares; psychologic reactions of fear, anger, depression, and heightened startle response; and a change in interpersonal reactions, including fears of intimacy; sexual dysfunction; and distrust of men. While adolescents often experience many of these symptoms, they also have concerns unique to themselves. Many experience feelings of shame, self-blame, and guilt. They may fear

for their lives or experience irrational fears of bodily harm such as undetected internal injuries, inability to have children, or disfigured genitals.[11]

Anger at the assailants is expressed less commonly by adolescents. This can be in sharp contrast to their parents, who often demand investigation and prosecution of the perpetrators against their children's wishes. If the adolescent refuses, the parents may blame the child for the assault. Teenagers often report increased communication problems with their parents after the assault.[11]

Posttraumatic stress disorder (PTSD) is a concern for both adult and adolescent rape victims. It is defined as symptoms lasting longer than 1 month in the following categories: (1) intrusive re-experience of the event, (2) avoidance of previously pleasurable experiences, (3) persistent avoidance of stimuli related to the trauma, and (4) persistent autonomic symptoms of anxiety. PTSD can last for many months, affecting the adolescent's daily functioning. Its incidence is higher in the case of stranger assaults and assaults involving the use of physical force or weapons, and in cases in which injuries were sustained.[12]

Some experts advocate crisis intervention and intense individual and group therapy for the rape victim.[13] Mann believes that teenagers respond less well to individual therapy than do adults.[11] He feels that the psychologic outcome in most adolescents depends greatly on the support of their families. He recommends separate interviews for the parents and patients, with attention paid to each person's particular concerns.[11] Active inquiry regarding the patient's fears, and assisting the parent to understand these issues, can be pivotal.

PREVENTION

Prevention of adolescent sexual assault hinges on prevention of the activities often associated with it. Alcohol consumption, late night hours, and poor date choices often increase risk. Other suggestions, such as planning a first date for a public place, not entering a car without checking the backseat for intruders, and using a "buddy" system when walking or shopping, can be offered to adolescents during routine health maintenance examinations. Renshaw suggests that adequate sexual education of children may help prevent assault in later years by giving the adolescent the basis for understanding healthy relationships.[13] Medical professionals can help prevent adolescent sexual assault through education offered in routine health maintenance examinations.

References

1. American Academy of Pediatrics, Committee on Adolescence: Sexual assault and the adolescent, *Pediatrics* 94:761-765, 1994.

2. Koss MP, Gidycz CA, Wisniewski N: The scope of rape: incidence and prevalence of sexual aggression and victimization in a national sample of higher education students, *J Consult Clin Psychol* 55:162-170, 1987.

3. Erickson PI, Rapkin AJ: Unwanted sexual experiences among middle and high school youth, *J Adolesc Health* 12:319-325, 1991.

4. Peipert JK, Domagalski LR: Epidemiology of adolescent sexual assault, *Obstet Gynecol* 84:867-871, 1994.

5. Jenny C: Adolescent risk-taking behavior and the occurrence of sexual assault, *Am J Dis Child* 142:770-772, 1988.

6. Koval JE: Violence in dating relationships, *J Pediatr Health Care* 3:298-304, 1989.

7. Bownes I, O'Gorman E, Sayers A: Rape—a comparison of stranger and acquaintance assaults, *Med Sci Law* 31:102-109, 1991.

8. Schwarcz SK, Whittington WL: Sexual assault and sexually transmitted diseases: detection and management in adults and children, *Rev Infect Dis* 12:s682-s689, 1990.

9. Centers for Disease Control and Prevention: 1993 sexually transmitted diseases treatment guidelines, *MMWR* 42:97-99, 1993.

10. Hatcher RA, Trussell J, Stewart F, et al, editors: *Contraceptive technology,* ed 16, New York, 1994, Irvington.

11. Mann BM: Self reported stressors of adolescent rape victims, *J Adolesc Health Care* 2:29-33, 1981.

12. Bownes IT, O'Gorman EC, Sayers A: Assault characteristics and post traumatic stress disorder in rape victims, *Acta Psychiatr Scand* 83:27-30, 1991.

13. Renshaw DC: Treatment of sexual exploitation: rape and incest, *Psychiatr Clin North Am* 12:257-277, 1989.

Suggested Reading

Heger A, Emans SJ: *Evaluation of the sexually abused child: a medical textbook and photographic atlas,* New York, 1992, Oxford University Press.

CHAPTER 103

Enuresis

•

Michael W. Cohen

Enuresis is defined as involuntary discharge of urine, although the term is often used to refer to wetting during nighttime sleep (nocturnal enuresis). Daytime wetting is termed diurnal enuresis or incontinence. Primary enuresis is present when a child has never achieved consistent dryness. Secondary or relapse enuresis refers to a condition in which wetting occurs after a period of dryness that lasts at least 3 to 6 months.

The symptom of enuresis may cause enormous stress and anxiety for the adolescent patient. It is an embarrassing symptom that often affects the progression of normal development. Enuresis can adversely affect adolescents' social confidence and their ability to develop a positive self-concept. The "secret" may be held with great vigilance, often at substantial emotional expense. The desire to be emancipated does not allow youths to share their worries and anxieties with their parents. Their friends may not understand how the enuretic symptoms could persist into adolescence. Adolescents may mistakenly assume that there is a relationship between bladder adequacy and sexual functioning that can limit their formation of a sexual identity. They may, in fact, be too embarrassed to seek medical attention, thus allowing unnecessary perpetuation of the symptoms.

Primary nocturnal enuresis exists in approximately 15% of all 5-year-olds, 8% of 8-year-olds, and 3% of 12-year-olds. Symptoms of enuresis that persist beyond 15 years of age are more common than generally appreciated. The incidence has been reported as 2% in one longitudinal study and as 1.2% among military draftees (Fig. 103-1). Further, it has been estimated that 1% of 20-year-olds are enuretic.

At age 12 years and beyond, more than 50% of cases of enuresis are of the secondary type. Statistics indicate a 15% annual spontaneous cure in youngsters beyond age 5 or 6 years. As enuresis persists into young adulthood, diurnal symptoms are more common, with over 50% of adults reporting associated frequency, urgency, or urge incontinence. Lower socioeconomic groups, families with lower educational levels, and institutionalized populations have a higher reported prevalence of enuresis. In general, bedwetting is more common in boys, although daytime frequency and wetting tend to be more common in girls. At age 12 years the boy-to-girl ratio of incidence is 4.5:1.

Hereditary factors contribute to enuresis. It is estimated that when both parents have had enuresis, approximately 75% of children will be enuretic. If only one parent has had enuresis, about 40% to 45% of children will have enuresis. If neither parent has had enuresis, only 15% of the children will be affected. Support for the hereditary and genetic nature of primary nocturnal enuresis was provided by a genetic study that, through multipoint analysis, localized the genetic marker on chromosome 13.

ETIOLOGY

Developmental Delay

Enuresis must be considered a symptom with multiple causes. Although definite proof is lacking, many believe that a maturational delay in adequate neuromuscular bladder control is the major cause in most cases of enuresis occurring at all ages. This view is supported by (1) the primary nature of most instances of enuresis, (2) the common familial pattern, (3) the common history of frequency of voiding and urgency, (4) cystometric studies that indicate the presence of a small functional bladder capacity in enuretic children despite an anatomically normal-appearing bladder, and (5) the high incidence of

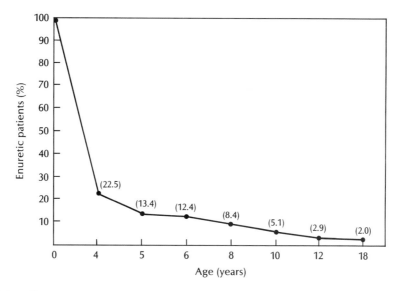

Fig. 103-1. Frequency of enuresis at selected ages. (From Garfinkel BD: The elimination disorders. In Garfinkel BD, Carlson GA, Weller EB, editors: *Psychiatric disorders in children and adolescents,* Philadelphia, 1990, WB Saunders; p 328.)

spontaneous remission or developmental maturation. It is unclear which variables are most influential in allowing the spontaneous resolution of bedwetting resulting from maturational advancement. Environmental factors, such as the emotional response of others, the family context in which the condition occurs, the child's general developmental status, and the original efficacy of toilet training all predict resolution potential. Adolescents with resolved developmentally based primary enuresis may have relapses during periods of stress.

Sleep Disorder

Investigations of sleep in enuretic children have evolved along with technologic advances. Early studies described nocturnal enuresis as a "disorder of arousal," with the voiding episodes beginning in the deepest stages of sleep, from which patients lightened their sleep but were unable to wake completely. More recently, researchers have concluded that nocturnal enuresis is independent of sleep stage and is not specifically related to the depth of sleep. Enuretic episodes have been noted throughout the night on a random basis, with wetting occurring in each stage of sleep and in proportion to the amount of time spent in that stage. However, the most advanced sleep research indicates that there may be a subset of youngsters with enuresis who have accentuated "delta" waves during sleep and who wet only during this phase.

Psychologic Factors

The psychologic contributions to the development and persistence of enuresis have received much attention.

According to the results of behavioral questionnaires, interviews, and observations, older youngsters with enuresis have somewhat more behavioral and school-related problems than younger children. Most studies have shown a low-order association with passive-aggressive behavior, mild depression, and inability to resolve high levels of anxiety. Fergusson and Horwood, in a New Zealand study,[1] have reported that for children whose primary or secondary enuresis persisted beyond age 10 years, there was a small but detectable increase in the risk of conduct problems, attention deficit behaviors, and anxiety/withdrawal in early adolescence. They point out that much of the apparent increase in behavioral disturbances occurs because the age of cessation of bedwetting is correlated with a series of factors (gender, social maturity, childhood IQ, family social background, family stress, and parental conflict) that are also associated with an increase in rates of adolescent behavior problems.

Psychoanalysts have viewed the symptom of enuresis as an expression of a child's wish to return to an immature stage of development that was more comfortable and less demanding than the present one. This viewpoint is particularly strong when primary enuresis persists beyond a reasonable time and when secondary enuresis occurs during a time of personal or family stress. However, it is difficult to discern the exact psychologic status of youngsters with enuresis because the profile of those who seek medical attention may differ from that of the population of enuretic children who do not. Enuresis in conjunction with behavioral and school-related problems may precipitate a visit to the physician, whereas an isolated symptom may not. Overall, studies do not support the conclusion that psychopathology is a *significant* cause of enuresis for most individuals at any age.

Organic Factors

Recent studies of adolescents have focused on the role of polyuria and diuresis in nocturnal enuresis.[2] The patients studied were urodynamically normal. They had a sleep diuresis that exceeded their daytime bladder capacity by up to several hundred percent. In contrast to the normal nighttime increase in antidiuretic hormone (ADH) (arginine vasopressin), constant serum levels were noted in these patients at night. It is also speculated that some enuretic individuals have an impaired renal sensitivity to this hormone. Enuresis for this group of patients appears then to be related to polyuria, either secondary to a lack of circadian rhythm or to a relative renal insensitivity to ADH secretion. This information is consistent with parental reports of multiple nighttime wetting episodes and an apparent excessive urinary output in their enuretic children. Because of the expense and cumbersome nature of defining this possible cause of enuresis, no data are available to determine the incidence of enuresis from this cause at any particular age, nor is it clinically feasible to prove this cause in any specific patient.

Other organic explanations for enuresis have focused primarily on the genitourinary tract and nervous system. Obstructive lesions of the distal outflow tract, such as posterior urethral valves, have received particular attention both as a cause of urinary tract infection and as an independent cause of enuresis. Also, recurrent urinary tract infection or a history of previous infection may be causal factors. Studies have reported significant improvement in enuresis with the use of antibiotics, particularly in girls with bacteriuria. Urinary tract infection should be strongly considered when there is secondary-onset enuresis in an adolescent female, particularly if it is associated with dysuria. Most patients who have urologic causes of enuresis will have been diagnosed before their teenage years.

Nervous system dysfunction may be associated with enuresis either through lumbosacral disorders that affect bladder innervation or as a symptom of global retardation. Diabetes mellitus, diabetes insipidus, sickle cell anemia, sickle cell trait, food allergies, and ingestion of foods or medications with diuretic actions all have been implicated as infrequent causes of enuresis.

DIURNAL INCONTINENCE IN FEMALES

Urethrovaginal reflux of urine may lead to postmicturition leakage of urine. Girls with this problem are often obese and have an anterior displacement of the posterior labial frenulum. Giggle incontinence is the sudden, completely involuntary emptying of the bladder with laughter. This symptom, which is relatively uncommon, occurs primarily in otherwise fully continent females and may be noted at any age. Urgency incontinence results in wetting secondary to intense bladder spasm due to detrusor instability. Those affected often have a lifelong history of urinary urgency and frequency.

EVALUATION

For most adolescents, enuresis is a highly sensitive topic, even with a physician. However, a thorough assessment will reflect that all potential causes and treatments are being considered and thus reassure the patient and the family. Interviews should be conducted separately with the adolescent and the parents. The primary or secondary nature of the symptom and a family history provide an important perspective. Management techniques previously used by the family as attempts to control the symptom should be explored. The youth's perception of the family's involvement may reflect issues that have actually perpetuated the symptom. The effect of the symptom on the adolescent's age-appropriate activities should be elicited. The limitation of social interaction with peers may reveal that the symptom is having a detrimental effect on the child's social adaptation and self-esteem. Inquiry regarding youngsters' sexual activity may provide an entree into their perception of their sexual and genital normality. An associated medical symptom, such as encopresis, may reflect an underlying cause of nervous system dysfunction or a psychologic basis.

Possible relevant psychosocial experiences that should be explored include (1) marital and family discord, (2) physical and sexual abuse, (3) separations and removal from the home, (4) episodes of depression, (5) the impact of new siblings, (6) bereavement and loss, (7) developmental delays and learning disabilities, (8) disruptive behavioral disorders, (9) separation anxiety disorder symptoms, and (10) ineffective toilet-training practices.

A full physical examination is mandatory to discover any potential organic causes of enuresis. Renal disease may be reflected in poor growth or elevated blood pressure. Examination of the genitalia should include observation of the youngster during micturition if this is comfortable for both clinician and patient. The strength of the urinary stream, the inability to interrupt voiding, or the presence of dysuria or dribbling may reflect urinary tract abnormalities. If the age of the patient or wish for privacy precludes such observations, the interview should be used to elicit the patient's self-observation. The neurologic examination should focus on peripheral reflexes and the evaluation of perineal sensation and anal sphincter tone, in addition to observation of gait and visual inspection of the lower back for evidence of sacral dimpling or cutaneous anomalies suggestive of a spinal abnormality.

Rushton[3] divided the evaluation recommendations into "complicated" and "uncomplicated" enuresis. Youngsters with nocturnal enuresis, a normal physical examination, and negative urinalysis and urine culture have uncomplicated enuresis, even though they may have associated mild daytime urinary frequency or urgency. These children often have a family history of enuresis and require no further evaluation. In contrast, patients who have an abnormal physical examination, a positive urinalysis or urine culture, or a history of significant voiding dysfunction have complicated enuresis and require further evaluation. This evaluation may include a pelvic sonogram initially and then consideration of intravenous pyelography, voiding cystourethrography, cystoscopy, cystometric studies, or referral for a urologic consultation as indicated (Fig. 103-2).

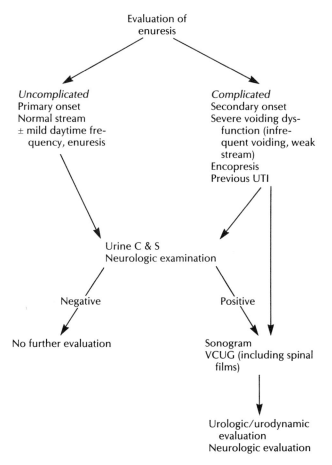

Fig. 103-2. Flow chart for evaluation of uncomplicated and complicated enuresis. *C & S,* culture and sensitivity testing; *UTI,* urinary tract infection; *VCUG,* voiding cystourethrogram. (From Rushton HB: Nocturnal enuresis: epidemiology, evaluation and currently available treatment options, *J Pediatr* 114 (suppl):691, 1989.)

MANAGEMENT

Principles

After a thorough evaluation, the clinician should provide a thoughtful definitive response. The anxious adolescent will not have the patience or tolerance for a delay in decision making. Supporting evidence for any diagnostic consideration should be shared with the patient. If further diagnostic tests are required, the exact nature of the studies and their specific purpose should be explained. A list of therapeutic options and the anticipated response should be discussed with the teenager, along with a timetable for decision making. Both the patient's and the family's attitudes regarding previous therapeutic efforts must be considered. If a previously unsuccessful therapy is to be recommended, a positive attitude must be engendered by emphasizing the child's current older age. The adolescent's active involvement will promote a sense of control and help ensure a return for subsequent visits and compliance with a treatment regimen.

Support for the adolescent's psychologic needs must be an integral aspect of all treatment plans. This may simply involve encouragement for participation in the treatment program, which may extend over time and include periods of relapse. At times, more intense psychologic counseling may be required for the patient and perhaps for the family, depending on the etiologic role of psychologic factors and the impact the enuresis is having on the family and the adolescent. The importance of these services to the treatment outcome must be emphasized to the family. Psychologic support services can best be accomplished in the primary care setting, unless the magnitude of the problem requires referral to a specific mental health resource. A mental health professional who understands the developmental nature of adolescence and the intrafamily dynamics of adolescent-parent relationships is essential for success.

Conditioning

An enuresis conditioning instrument involves a moisture-activated sensor connected to an alarm that provides auditory stimulation to wake the patient or parent at initiation of wetting. The new auditory sources of stimulation are contained in a wristwatch or small pin-type battery-powered alarm. Because the temporal relationship between the wetting episode and the alarm is critical for effective conditioning, a refined instrument with adequate sensitivity is required. Controlled studies have yielded cure rates between 60% and 85%. Since many enuretics are deep sleepers, they may not respond to the alarm and awaken. If they do not wake, parents should wake them during the initial stage of treatment. Before falling asleep in the evening, the adolescent should listen to the alarm several times as a means of training for awakening to the familiar sound. In addition, he or she can use imagery before sleep, mentally practicing awakening to the sound of the alarm. Permanent responders require an average of 2 months of therapy.

A 20% to 40% relapse rate is reported in all studies of conditioning with enuresis. A learning-model explanation of the conditioning approach should be emphasized to the patient. Effective learning requires practice. Relapses often can be explained by inadequate time allowed for learning, with more practice required for a "cure." A second course of treatment usually results in more permanent dryness. Gradual tapering of the use of the conditioning device after dryness has been achieved for 3 months may reduce the relapse risk. Tapering can be begun with use of the device every other night, then every third and every fourth night. Encouragement should be given to the adolescent when independent dryness is accomplished on the non-alarm nights. If relapse occurs during tapering, the schedule should revert to the previously successful routine (every other night or every third night), and that schedule should be maintained for a few weeks before further tapering is attempted. After full dryness at every fourth night for approximately 1 month, use of the conditioning device can be discontinued. Outcome studies have supported the relative long-term superiority of conditioning compared with pharmacologic interventions.

Self-Hypnosis

Self-hypnosis has been demonstrated to be effective for primary nocturnal enuresis. The enuretic episode is viewed as a "habit disorder" that allows the wetting episode without the youth's awakening. Youths are taught the technique of self-induced relaxation to be practiced before sleep. During this trance state, they tell themselves that they will wake up when they experience a need to void, thus allowing a dry bed and comfortable feelings on awakening in the morning. This comfort can be associated with a visual image of some warm, tranquil, enjoyable experience in the youngster's memory to enhance the desirability of the feeling of a dry bed. Significant improvement and cure rates (80%) have been reported after only a few training visits.[4] The benefits of other treatments may be enhanced by adopting this approach; for example, imagining the sound of the conditioning alarm before sleep with the goal of awakening more rapidly during the night. Practicing imagery before sleep may assist waking with a full bladder, or imagining the alarm sound may improve awakening to the sound.

Pharmacologic Treatment

Drugs such as sedatives, stimulants, and sympathomimetic agents have not proved beneficial in the treatment of enuresis. Oxybutynin, an anticholinergic agent often prescribed for enuresis, is not significantly better than a placebo, for noctural enuresis.

Tricyclic antidepressants, particularly imipramine, have been used extensively to treat enuresis and have achieved a short-term success rate of 40% to 45% but with a relatively high relapse rate. Desipramine has been used with comparable success. The exact beneficial mechanisms of action for both drugs are unknown. Detrusor muscle relaxation, an antidepressant effect, and an alteration in sleep patterns have been proposed as the mechanisms but are unlikely as full explanations. Imipramine is generally given 30 minutes to 1 hour before bedtime, with no proven advantage noted in administering multiple daily doses. The initial dose of imipramine is 25 mg for children under 12 years and 50 mg for older children or adolescents. The maximal recommended dose is 75 mg at bedtime. Although many youngsters experience improvement with imipramine during the first week of treatment, the drug should be continued for no less than 4 to 6 weeks before nonresponsiveness is concluded. The dose may be increased with the youngster self-monitoring his or her bedwetting by maintaining a calendar of successes and failures. Direct follow-up contact with the teenager is imperative to provide the necessary encouragement. Once a successful therapeutic response has been achieved, the teenager should be maintained on the medication for approximately 3 months of total dryness. At the end of this period, a gradual tapering and discontinuation of the drug will decrease the likelihood of relapse. Tapering can begin with a lowering of the dose followed by administration every other night and every third night over a period of 4 to 6 weeks. Although one study has shown a correlation between clinical success and imipramine levels, monitoring of serum levels is not necessary on a routine basis unless there is concern regarding toxicity.

It is important to note that imipramine has been shown to increase the resting pulse by 10 beats per minute or more and to have the potential for causing an increase in diastolic blood pressure. Nervousness, sleep disorders, lethargy, and mild gastrointestinal disturbances may occur, but these effects usually disappear with a reduction in dose. Constipation, convulsions, anxiety, and syncope have been reported infrequently. Abrupt discontinuation of the medication after prolonged treatment can lead to withdrawal symptoms of nausea, headache, and malaise. Increased incidence of dental caries has been reported with the use of tricyclic antidepressants. Overdose can lead to a triad of coma, convulsions, and cardiac conduction disturbances that can be fatal. Deaths have been reported in preadolescents whose "magical" thinking led them to increase their intake of medication to the level of overdose in an attempt to solve their enuresis permanently. Owing to the inherent risks associated with the use of imipramine, this drug should be reserved for use in adolescents whose condition is refractory to other approaches.

Desmopressin, the synthetic analog of vasopressin or ADH, has been in use for more than 12 years. This agent is used intranasally at bedtime as a substitute for the apparent lack of circadian increase in ADH at night in some children with nocturnal polyuria. Oral treatment with desmopressin tablets has yielded comparable results. The starting dosage is 20 µg, with the dosage increased by 10 µg on a weekly basis to a maximum of 40 µg. If 20 µg seems adequate, 10 µg should be tried. A literature review of articles published from 1966 to 1992 indicated that desmopressin is effective in reducing the number of wet nights but that only about one quarter of subjects studied become completely dry.[5] The best response is seen in children over the age of 10 years with nocturnal polyuria whose urine osmolality was 1000 mOsm/kg *after* desmopressin therapy, and those who have a positive family history of enuresis. The relapse rate may be as high as 80%, either immediately or up to 3 months after discontinuation of treatment. Prolonged use may be necessary for many responders and is viewed as being well tolerated, safe, and appropriate for adults, such as a military population.

When after 3 to 6 months of treatment sustained dryness occurs despite discontinuation of desmopressin, authors conclude that ultimate dryness has been achieved. It is assumed that desmopressin allowed for a gradual reestablishment of the normal diurnal release of ADH, or that there has been an adjustment in the renal tubule's sensitivity to vasopressin. An interruption in a "habit" disorder should be considered to explain this phenomenon. None of these theories have been validated. Desmopressin has been used for 20 years in the treatment of central diabetes insipidus with few adverse effects. Water intoxication and hyponatremia can occur, but these effects are unlikely to occur in otherwise healthy children taking a single nighttime dose. Seizures have been reported rarely, with virtually all cases involving excessive fluid intake during the evening before the medication is taken. Overall side effects such as headaches, nausea, mild abdominal cramps, and vulvar pain have been reported at a rate of approximately 4%, but these often disappear with dosage reduction. Desmopressin does not suppress endogenous production of ADH, nor does it induce destructive antibodies. Only a few studies have compared desmopressin with other forms of therapy. However, when compared with conditioning devices, desmopressin had a more immediate benefit, but conditioning was associated with significantly more long-term results and less risk of relapse. A combination of desmopressin and conditioning has been shown to have greater long-term benefit than the latter with placebo.

Specific indications for the use of desmopressin have not been defined. This drug may be most useful in older patients whose condition has been refractory to previous therapeutic efforts. Authors have proposed the use of this agent in socially sensitive situations to ensure dryness— for example, when a youngster sleeps at a friend's house, spends time with relatives, or attends a summer camp. This approach may avoid unnecessary embarrassment for the enuretic teenager while awaiting spontaneous resolution or the benefits of other treatment. Combination therapy with other psychologic and pharmacologic interventions should be considered in difficult cases. Further studies are required to establish more definite indications.

Daytime Wetting

Adolescents with diurnal enuresis may require a more extensive medical or psychologic evaluation. If no specific cause is determined, various patterns will define the intervention. Treatment for females with urethrovaginal reflux includes advice to spread the labia when voiding and to spend adequate time to empty residual vaginally accumulated urine. Stream interception exercises, while unproven, have been helpful for "giggle" and urgency incontinence. Stress- or anxiety-related urinary frequency and urgency must involve identification and dissipation of the emotional energy and source of the stress. The use of an anticholinergic agent such as oxybutynin to relax the bladder detrusor muscle and enhance bladder capacity may be indicated and helpful in some patients.

CONCLUSION

Enuresis that continues into the adolescent years is usually difficult to treat. The best treatment regimen cannot be designed until a careful evaluation has been made and the fullest possible understanding of etiologic possibilities achieved. Since many adolescents will have had previous experience with some modalities of therapy, a reorientation to treatment must take place. Conditioning devices, which have proved effective for all age groups, should be considered as the primary approach. The benefits of conditioning can be enhanced by simultaneous administration of tricyclic antidepressants. Desmopressin has great promise and should be considered when the above combination is not adequate, when embarrassment associated with the wetting is a major concern, or when the adolescent is extremely discouraged. Some patients who respond to desmopressin may require long-term treatment. The simultaneous use of multiple forms of therapy should be considered in resistant cases.

A supportive relationship with adolescents will help the clinician to maintain their active participation and involvement especially if initial improvement is not attained. Empathy for the youngster's frustration must be demonstrated while alternative treatment approaches are designed and implemented. The cooperative approach between the clinician and the adolescent will ultimately be gratifying for both, since the patient will be extremely appreciative when dryness is finally achieved.

References

1. Fergusson DM, Horwood LJ: Nocturnal enuresis and behavioral problems in adolescence: a 15-year longitudinal study, *Pediatrics* 94:662, 1994.
2. Norgaard JP, Rittig S, Djurbuus JC: Nocturnal enuresis: an approach to treatment based on pathogenesis, *J Pediatr* 114 (suppl):705, 1989.
3. Rushton HB: Nocturnal enuresis: epidemiology, evaluation and currently available treatment options, *J Pediatr* 114 (suppl):691, 1989.
4. Olness K, Gardner GG: *Hypnosis and hypnotherapy with children,* San Diego, 1988, Grune & Stratton; p 134.
5. Moffatt MEK, Harlos S, Kirshen AJ, Burd L: Desmopressin acetate and nocturnal enuresis: how much do we know?, *Pediatrics* 92:420, 1993.

Suggested Readings

Foxman B, Valdez RB, Brook RH: Childhood enuresis: prevalence, perceived impact and prescribed treatment, *Pediatrics* 77:482, 1986.
  Reviews the results of a survey of the parents of 1750 children aged 5 to 13 regarding the presence and frequency of enuresis, its perceived impact, and physician-prescribed treatments.

Friman PC: A preventive context for enuresis, *Pediatr Clin North Am* 33:871, 1986.
  Reviews the causes of enuresis in the context of opportunities for resolution of the symptom.

Garfinkel BD: The elimination disorders. In Garfinkel BD, Carlson GA, Weller EB, editors: *Psychiatric disorders in children and adolescents,* Philadelphia, 1990, WB Saunders; p 325.
  Offers an excellent discussion of enuresis and encopresis from a psychiatric perspective.

Houts AC, Berman JS, Abramson H: Effectiveness of psychological and pharmacological treatments of nocturnal enuresis, *J Consult Clin Psychol* 62:737, 1994.
  Reviews 78 short- and long-term outcome studies of various psychologic and pharmacologic interventions.

McLorie GA, Husmann DA: Incontinence and enuresis, *Pediatr Clin North Am* 34:1159, 1987.
  Emphasizes the urologic aspects of the symptom complex.

Schmitt BD: Nocturnal enuresis: finding the treatment that fits the child, *Contemp Pediatr* 7:70, 1990.
  This comprehensive review is highlighted by practical suggestions for treatment. Handouts for parents and patients are included.

Schmitt BD: Daytime wetting (diurnal enuresis), *Pediatr Clin North Am* 29:9, 1982.
  A classic review of the causes and appropriate interventions for daytime wetters.

CHAPTER 104

Encopresis

•

Margot Davey and Leonard A. Rappaport

One of the major transitions of early childhood is the attainment of urinary and fecal continence. For most children, toileting routines are established by 4 years of age, at which time parental involvement in urination and defecation has become unnecessary. Children and adolescents with encopresis are an exception to this rule. Some adolescents have never attained total continence of stool. Others, who have achieved continence, may regress and begin to have episodes of soiling.

Societal response to these soiling episodes is usually overwhelming to both the adolescent and the family. Most families find it more difficult to tell a health professional or a family member about an adolescent's encopresis than to tell them about severe physical or emotional problems. In fact, encopresis is unique in that almost no adolescents with encopresis know of other adolescents or families with the same problem. Most families, with great shame, secretly attempt to cope alone.

Numerous studies over the past two decades have helped to define the prevalence, etiology, and treatment of encopresis in school-age children. Encopresis in adolescence, however, remains essentially unexplored. Most pediatricians, when confronted with an adolescent with encopresis, feel pessimistic about the prognosis, and this expectation clearly affects treatment and referral patterns. This attitude contrasts with that adopted toward the school-age child, for whom successful interventions have been formulated and implemented.

DEFINITION

Encopresis is generally defined as the passage of formed or semiformed stool in the underwear or other inappropriate places that occurs on a regular or semi-regular basis beyond 4 to 5 years of age. Adolescents with encopresis can be separated into subgroups. Those with *primary encopresis* have never achieved adequate control of defecation and have had soiling problems throughout their lives. Adolescents with *secondary encopresis* have achieved a long period of continence and then begin to soil. In general, the distinction made between primary and secondary encopresis has not been particularly helpful for diagnosis or treatment. A more useful separation divides adolescents with encopresis into retentive and nonreten-tive patterns. *Retentive encopresis* describes moderate to severe constipation; *nonretentive encopresis* is a condition without significant stool retention. School-age children with retentive encopresis far exceed those with nonretentive encopresis, and the former have a better prognosis.

INCIDENCE

The incidence figures for encopresis remain somewhat elusive, varying from 1% to 2% of 7-year-olds in a study in Sweden to between 1.5% and 7.5% of children of elementary school age in other studies. The incidence in adults, aged 15 to 65, is thought to be about 0.5 in 1000. The male-to-female ratio is approximately 5:1. In fact, all incidence figures regarding encopresis are severely compromised by the fact that encopresis is a "secret disorder" that is reluctantly divulged.

PROPOSED MODELS

There is a wide range of opinions concerning the cause of encopresis, from entirely physiologic to exclusively psychologic. A proposed integrated model, outlined in Figure 104-1, proposes that etiologic forces, physiologic predisposition, and exacerbating factors exist in a continuum and that their interplay determines the existence of encopresis and its severity. There may be other etiologic factors involved in nonretentive adolescent encopretics.

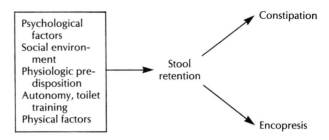

Fig. 104-1. Integrated model for encopresis.

PHYSIOLOGIC PREDISPOSITION

Physiology of Defecation

The nature of the physiologic predisposition to encopresis is unclear, and some aspects of the physiology of normal defecation are not yet understood. However, the basic anatomy and physiology can be used to help clarify the proposed mechanisms of encopresis. The rectum extends through the levator ani muscle to form the anal canal, where it develops a thick muscle layer called the internal anal sphincter. A second muscle layer, the external anal sphincter, which is striated, develops more distally. The axis of the rectum is nearly perpendicular to that of the anal canal, and this relationship is maintained by the puborectal sling.

When a fecal mass passes into and distends the rectum, sensory receptors are stimulated and afferent nerve fibers allow conscious awareness. Transient contraction of the external sphincter and the puborectal sling occur, accompanied by reflex relaxation of the internal sphincter. Relaxation of the internal sphincter is proportionate to the volume and rate of rectal distention and requires an intact myenteric plexus. For defecation to occur, the external sphincter must relax, along with the puborectal sling, thus allowing widening of the anorectal angle to facilitate the easy passage of feces. Relaxation of the external sphincter involves both reflex and voluntary pathways. Increased abdominal pressure and rectal peristalsis allow emptying of the rectum.

Pathophysiology of Defecation

Long-standing constipation results in fecal retention and stretching and dilating of the rectum, which may eventually form a megarectum. The final size of the rectum is dependent on the confining effects of adjacent organs and structures. Continued retention may extend to involve the entire colon. Chronic constipation and retention can lead to overflow incontinence, that is, leakage of liquid feces around more distally impacted stool, which results in soiling.

Anorectal manometry and surface electromyography have been used in children and adolescents to evaluate the defecation dynamics of patients with constipation and encopresis. Manometry involves a tube with balloons and side holes connected to pressure transducers being placed in the rectum. When the rectal balloon is distended, this allows assessment of the threshold volume sensed by the patient, and the amount of rectal distention required for relaxation of the internal sphincter. The placement of two other balloons more distally allows measurement of internal and external sphincter pressures. Measurement of external sphincter tone can be made during attempts at defecation. Recent studies have shown abnormal defecation dynamics in 30% to 50% of children with chronic constipation and encopresis. Reported abnormalities include decreased rectal sensation or hyposensitivity and abnormal and prolonged contraction of external sphincter during defecation (anismus).

Research into a physiologic predisposition to encopresis has been compromised by the fact that all studies are performed after the existence of encopresis or chronic constipation has been established. This makes it difficult or impossible to determine whether some of the abnormalities are secondary to chronic stool retention or are the actual cause of the problem.

EXACERBATING FACTORS

Environmental Factors

Adolescents with a physiologic predisposition to encopresis may encounter environmental stressors that make the evolution of severe constipation and encopresis more likely. For example, boys in elementary and high school rarely defecate in school bathrooms. The stall doors in school bathrooms may be missing, and boys are extremely hesitant to sit on the toilet in such an exposed position. Therefore, they may use only their home toilet, begin to ignore their body's physiologic cues, and as a result retain feces.

Psychologic Factors

Psychologic stressors also have been proposed to exacerbate and cause encopresis. Although these stressors are relatively nonspecific, most clinicians have followed up encopretic adolescents who manifest exacerbations of their problem when they enter a new or difficult school situation, or when there are stressful changes within the home. Such stressors may be distracting to adolescents and may make them pay less attention to the signals from their bodies. In addition, stress may alter eating habits and so affect bowel motility.

From a psychoanalytic perspective, encopresis is a form of oppositional behavior, and soiling is a way for the adolescent to communicate feelings of hostility. This hostility is usually directed toward the parents or primary caregivers, and it may be manifested by the adolescent who deposits feces where the parents will find them.

Physiologic Factors

In taking the history of children and adolescents with encopresis, sometimes there may be a specific physiologic event around the time of the commencement of encopresis. For example, there may have been an episode of uncontrollable diarrhea that caused soiling. The adolescent began to be nervous about defecation and started to retain feces. This stool retention led to painful bowel movements, which in turn further aggravated the problem, establishing a pain/retention cycle in which the adolescent avoided having bowel movements in order to prevent pain. This pattern can lead to chronic stool retention and subsequent overflow incontinence.

CLINICAL PRESENTATION

The clinical presentation of encopresis is relatively uniform. The adolescent usually has a history of soiling episodes occurring late in the day or early evening, typically after school. These episodes commonly occur at school and almost never at night during sleep. The adolescent claims to be unaware of the soiling episode, but parents and others find this hard to believe and feel that the adolescent "just does not care." They do not understand that the leakage of feces frequently occurs through an impacted and dilated rectum and that the normal sensation of defecation has been absent. The adolescent denies even smelling the feces. This is usually a result of the rapid habituation that occurs with exposure to a common smell in the environment. For example, when entering the home of a family with many pets, a visitor is often overwhelmed by the smell, but those who live in the house never notice it.

Infrequent bowel movements are also characteristic of adolescents with encopresis. However, parents of adolescents are, and probably should be, almost unaware of the adolescent's toileting habits, and therefore this history is difficult to elicit. Large bowel movements that block the toilet are another common presentation of children with encopresis; however, the adolescent may cope with this situation privately and not involve the parents.

When obtaining the history, the physician should spend time alone with the adolescent to elicit a clear history of the soiling pattern and toileting habits. Often a more accurate dietary history is also obtained. It is important to develop an alliance with adolescents, because ultimately they will be the ones responsible for administering and continuing their medical therapy.

DIFFERENTIAL DIAGNOSIS

The differential diagnosis for encopresis is outlined in Box 104-1. Although Hirschsprung's disease is included in this list, fecal incontinence is rarely a presenting complaint. Hirschsprung's disease is aganglionosis of the bowel that begins in the rectum and extends proximally in varying degrees. The incidence is about 1 in 5000 live births, and most cases are diagnosed in infants presenting with delayed passage of meconium, abdominal distention, and vomiting. Sometimes there are systemic symptoms secondary to the onset of enterocolitis. Older children may present with abdominal cramps and bloating. Because of increased awareness of the disease, recent studies estimate that only 6% to 15% of cases are diagnosed after 5 years of age.

Differentiating between Hirschsprung's disease and encopresis usually can be done by history and examination. Classically, adolescents with Hirschsprung's disease have a history of constipation dating back to the neonatal period and generally do not have a history of soiling. Sometimes a history of abdominal distention and poor health is elicited. On examination, these patients have an empty rectum; after withdrawal of the examiner's finger, there may be an explosive stool. In contrast, examination

of an adolescent with encopresis usually demonstrates a rectum that is dilated and loaded with stool. Ultrashort-segment Hirschsprung's disease occurs when only the distal rectum is involved. This can lead to the physiologic equivalent of encopresis, but since this condition is extremely rare, the diagnosis should be pursued only if there are unusual findings in the history and examination or if standard medical treatment fails. Possible Hirschsprung's disease should be evaluated by rectal biopsy. Anorectal manometry may also be useful diagnostically because patients fail to demonstrate relaxation of the internal sphincter after rectal distention.

PHYSICAL EXAMINATION

An adolescent with encopresis should receive a full physical examination. General growth and nutrition, along with the development of secondary sex characteristics, should be recorded. Deviation from normal growth curves warrants further investigation.

A full neurologic examination, with emphasis on the motor and sensory function of the lower extremities and careful inspection of the lumbosacral spine, is essential to rule out other causes of encopresis. A pilonidal dimple may be seen in spina bifida occulta or an associated tethered cord, and a patulous anus in other neurologic disease. Examination of the abdomen often reveals increased stool in the left lower quadrant. This finding is not universal in cases of encopresis, since stool retention may be only rectal and may not be noted on abdominal palpation. Observation of the rectal area is important to rule out exacerbating physical conditions, such as anal fissures. Extreme anterior displacement of the anus and the presence of a posterior shelf have been associated with defecation difficulties and therefore should be noted. Perianal sensation and the presence of an anal reflex or "anal wink" should be established. Digital examination allows an assessment of rectal tone and provides further information about the degree of fecal impaction.

FURTHER INVESTIGATION

An abdominal x-ray examination is often helpful in documenting the extent of fecal retention and rectal dilation. The x-ray film also can be used for educational purposes, to graphically show the adolescent exactly what is happening. It is important to exclude the possibility of pregnancy before ordering an abdominal x-ray examination in females. As part of the evaluation for encopresis in females, a urine culture should be taken, since there is a higher incidence of urinary tract infections in this population. No other evaluations are necessary at initial presentation unless an alternative cause is suggested by an atypical history and physical examination.

BOX 104-1
Differential Diagnosis
of Constipation and Encopresis

INTRAMURAL CAUSES
Congenital obstructive lesions: webs, duplications, malrotations
Acquired strictures: necrotizing enterocolitis, inflammatory bowel disease
Anorectal malformations: anterior anus, ectopic anus, anal stenosis
Painful perianal disease

MURAL CAUSES
Hirschsprung's disease

EXTRAMURAL CAUSES
Metabolic: hypercalcemia, hypokalemia, hypothyroidism, chronic dehydration (diabetes insipidus, renal tubular acidosis)
Neurologic: general central nervous system disorders (cerebral palsy, epilepsy), spinal cord lesions (myelomeningocoele, tethered cord, cauda equina lesion), autonomic neuropathy
Connective tissue disorders: scleroderma, lupus
Psychiatric disorders: depression, anorexia, sexual abuse
Drugs: analgesics (codeine containing), antacids (aluminum containing), anticholinergics, antidepressants, diuretics, hematinics (iron), metal ingestion (lead, mercury)

TREATMENT

Demystification and Education

It is essential that the adolescent learn as much as possible about the cause of encopresis and the reasoning behind the treatment plan. Often, adolescents have had encopresis intermittently throughout their life and are extremely ashamed about having this condition. Although they may have gone through periods of remission, they rarely understand the cause of the problem or how they can actually control it. They may deny that they care about these soiling episodes, but the relief of an adolescent who learns about the physiologic, as opposed to the psychologic, causes of the encopresis is usually apparent. It is important for parents to understand that the adolescent usually has not been soiling deliberately and may actually have been unaware of the accidents. Parents may feel tremendous guilt during this explanation because of previous punishments they inflicted or accusations they made about the soiling representing willful behavior by the adolescent. It is important for the physician to be sensitive and supportive to both parties during this time.

If possible, a detailed explanation about the cause and treatment of encopresis, appropriate to the adolescent's knowledge base, is indicated. Visual aids, such as drawings of the bowel at various stages of the treatment regimen, are often helpful. If an abdominal x-ray film is available, it can be used to show the adolescent something about his or her own physiology. It is essential that the adolescent understand that the bowel has been dilated over time, and that it will be necessary to remove the feces that remain in the bowel and to keep the bowel empty while the wall returns to its normal strength and size. Although the evacuation of the bowel can be done quickly, the process of normalization usually takes a minimum of 6 months. It is also essential that adolescents understand the need for this long-term intervention from the beginning so that they can take responsibility for the treatment plan and be motivated to continue following it over time. It may be prudent at this stage to warn them that exacerbations sometimes occur but that, with continued treatment and perseverance, the problem can be managed successfully.

Clean-Out Regimen

The objective of the first few weeks of intervention is to evacuate the bowel almost completely, especially in the rectal area. Multiple regimens have been proposed for the clean-out procedure for encopresis. For adolescents, it is essential that they be able to carry out this regimen themselves, although some may be comfortable obtaining help from their parents. Alternative clean-out regimens should be tailored to the needs of the adolescent and the degree of fecal retention present (Box 104-2). It is surprising how little resistance is offered by the adolescent who understands why this regimen is necessary. However, the physician needs to be flexible in designing a clean-out regimen, since it is essential that it be acceptable to the adolescent to ensure good compliance. It may be necessary to suggest alternative regimens and give the adolescent the choice after appropriate education and counseling.

Maintenance

The maintenance regimen for encopresis is difficult and is aimed at preventing reaccumulation of retained feces by means of regular soft bowel movements. Education and supportive counseling are essential for continued success, along with toileting schedules and laxative use. It is important that the adolescent use the toilet regularly, preferably twice a day (after breakfast and dinner) for 5 to 10 minutes. This timing takes advantage of the gastrocolic reflex, and the importance of this should be explained to the adolescent—to aid compliance. The goal needs to be at least one or two soft bowel movements per day. To achieve this, the adolescent is given mineral oil or another stool softener in doses sufficient to ensure normal stooling patterns. Anal leakage of mineral oil can be

---

BOX 104-2
Treatment Options
for Clean-out Regimen

MILD TO MODERATE STOOL RETENTION
Oral therapy alone
Lubricants with or without stimulants

MODERATE TO SEVERE STOOL RETENTION
Outpatient
1. Phospho-Soda enemas (Fleet enema): day 1
   Bisacodyl (Dulcolax) suppositories: day 2
   Bisacodyl (Dulcolax) tablets: day 3
   (Repeating 3-day cycles for up to 4-5 cycles)
2. Polyethylene glycol electrolyte solution (GoLYTELY) orally, starting at 40 ml/kg, over 6 hours; encopretic patients may require increased dose and duration of treatment
Inpatient*
1. Normal saline enemas, 500-700 ml bid for 3 days, in combination with oral laxatives
2. GoLYTELY administered with nasogastric tube
3. Surgical disimpaction

*Indications for inpatient management: poor compliance at home, disturbed family relationship, parents or adolescent unable to manage home treatment, failure of outpatient treatment.

controlled by decreasing the dose. For exacerbations, a stimulant medication can be added to the regimen for a few weeks. The various therapeutic agents available for use in constipation are listed in Box 104-3. A high-fiber diet is encouraged.

BOX 104-3
Therapeutic Agents in Constipation

HYDROPHILIC BULK-FORMING AGENTS

Action: Act by binding water and also act as a substrate for bacterial fermentation. Intake results in increased weight of stool and decreased transit time. Adequate fluids should be taken during administration.

Agents: Dietary (bran, cellulose), psyllium (Metamucil), semisynthetic cellulose (Citrocel).

OSMOTIC AGENTS

Action: Nonabsorbable compounds that have a direct water-binding effect. Lactulose also undergoes bacterial degradation with production of acetic and lactic acids, which may directly affect colonic motility.

Agents: Lactulose (Cephulac), magnesium sulfate (Epsom salts, milk of magnesia), sodium phosphates (Fleet enema), polyethylene glycol (GoLYTELY).

STIMULANTS

Action: Stimulate peristalsis and fluid secretion by irritant effect on mucosa of gut. Long-term usage can be associated with tolerance, and in large doses can cause significant fluid and electrolyte disturbances.

Agents: Bisacodyl (Dulcolax), senna (Senokot), phenolphthalein (Ex-Lax).

STOOL-SOFTENING AGENTS

Action: Surface active agents that increase penetration of stool by water. Also have an action on secretory activity.

Agents: Docusate sodium (Colace).

LUBRICATING AGENTS

Action: Hydrocarbon mixture that produces large frothy stools by penetrating and softening the stool. Concerns have been raised about absorption of fat-soluble vitamins. Problems include lipid pneumonia following aspiration, so contraindicated in patients with severe neurologic impairment.

Agents: Mineral oil.

Behavior Modification and Biofeedback

Over the last several years, biofeedback has been used with poor-outcome groups of patients. The objective of this intervention is to train the paradoxically contracting external anal sphincter to relax during defecation. This technique can also be used to improve the ability to sense rectal distention. Reported results from the use of biofeedback are variable but encouraging, suggesting that this may be a treatment option in adolescents with abnormal defecation dynamics who have responded poorly to traditional medical treatment.

TREATMENT OUTCOME

Multiple studies of the outcome of the treatment outlined above have shown that approximately 80% of school-age children are cured or significantly improved by 6 months to 1 year. Approximately 10% are improved but need long-term involvement of the medical provider to sustain a remission, and the remaining 10% do not appear to respond. It is unclear whether there is a difference in the physical etiology of the encopresis in this poor-outcome group or whether psychologic factors are more prominent.

Treatment response that is specific for adolescents has never been studied. Although adolescents have been included in some outcome studies, there have never been sufficient numbers to determine whether the outcome for adolescents would be the same as for the more numerous school-age children. When questioned, many pediatricians and psychiatrists believe that adolescents are a more treatment-resistant group than school-age children. However, our experience is that adolescents seem to have a similar outcome, although the intervention plan must be tailored to the specific developmental needs of an adolescent. These include privacy, establishment of autonomy and control, and a high degree of understanding of the treatment process that is to be undertaken. A supportive and trusting relationship between the adolescent and the physician is essential, especially when medical therapy may need to be continued over many months.

PREDICTORS OF POOR OUTCOME

It would be helpful for a clinician to be able to determine which adolescents might be likely to have poor outcome from medical and educational intervention. A number of studies have been performed in school-age children to identify those factors that correlate most strongly with poor success. Factors associated with good or poor outcome after medical and educational intervention are outlined in Table 104-1.

TABLE 104-1
Predictors of Outcome

Good Outcome	Poor Outcome
Late afternoon soiling	Nocturnal or early morning soiling
Stool retention on abdominal x-ray	No stool retention on abdominal x-ray
Internal locus of control	External locus of control
Good school performance	Poor school performance
Good compliance	Poor compliance
Stable family environment	Major family disruption
	Hyperactivity and poor attention
	Significant psychiatric problem
	Toilet phobia or avoidance behavior
	Abnormal defecation dynamics

ROLE OF PSYCHOLOGIC COUNSELING

Over the past two decades, care of the school-age child with encopresis has shifted from the psychiatrist and psychologist toward the pediatrician and gastro-enterologist. This trend is perhaps less applicable to the adolescent with encopresis. Although medical management has been quite effective, the role of a mental health professional as counselor remains important. First, adolescents with encopresis often feel humiliated by their condition, suffer low self-esteem, and may be punished severely by their parents. Involvement with a counselor who understands encopresis can help to attenuate the effects of the stressors. Second, some adolescents with encopresis have trouble accepting responsibility for their behavior, which appears to be essential for achieving success in the medical management of encopresis. The involvement of a counselor may be necessary for the adolescent to make this transition to accepting responsibility. Both cognitive and behavioral interventions can be helpful in this endeavor. Finally, some patients with encopresis appear to have a primarily emotional cause for their problem. They have clear psychologic difficulties, and the counselor becomes the primary caregiver in this situation. When a counselor is involved, it is essential that the medical provider and counselor work together as a team.

CONCLUSION

Our knowledge about encopresis has increased significantly since the early 1970s. Although we do not yet clearly understand the cause of this condition, models for understanding its pathophysiology have evolved, and therefore successful intervention plans can be formulated.

Unfortunately, this improvement in knowledge has not extended to adolescents. However, an evaluation and treatment protocol similar to that used with the school-age child, but adjusted and individualized to the developmental needs of the adolescent, is appropriate. Such a protocol should include extensive teaching about the cause of encopresis, tailoring the intervention to involve the adolescent maximally, and providing close follow-up and support.

Suggested Readings

Benninga MA, Buller HA, Taminiau JAJM: Biofeedback training in chronic constipation, *Arch Dis Child* 68:126-129, 1993.

Hatch T: Encopresis and constipation in children, *Pediatr Clin North Am* 35:257-280, 1988.

Ingebo K, Heyman M: Polyethylene glycol-electrolyte solution for intestinal clearance in children with refractory encopresis, *Am J Dis Child* 142:340-342, 1988.

Levine M: Encopresis: its potentiation, evaluation and alleviation, *Pediatr Clin North Am* 29:315-330, 1982.

Levine M, Bakow H: Children with encopresis: a study of treatment outcome, *Pediatrics* 58:845-852, 1976.

Loeing-Baucke V: Modulation of abnormal defecation dynamics by biofeedback treatment in chronically constipated children with encopresis, *J Pediatr* 116:214-222, 1990.

Loeing-Baucke V, Cruikshank B: Abnormal defecation dynamics in chronically constipated children with encopresis, *J Pediatr* 108:562-566, 1986.

Rappaport L, Levine M: The prevention of constipation and encopresis: a developmental model and approach, *Pediatr Clin North Am* 33:859-869, 1986.

Seth R, Heyman MB: Management of constipation and encopresis in infants and children, *Gastroenterol Clin North Am* 23:621-636, 1994.

CHAPTER 105

Sleep Disturbances

•

Mary A. Carskadon

Sleep is a complex behavioral state that, along with the other physiologic processes, changes markedly at adolescence. Basic and clinical research in the last two decades has shown that the complexities of sleep are so substantial that "intuitive clinical practice" is no longer sufficient to address sleep problems. Appropriate evaluation of sleep in adolescents requires a number of approaches, including querying the adolescent and parents, keeping sleep diaries, and in certain cases performing laboratory evaluation (nocturnal polysomnography) as a part of a full work-up at a sleep disorders center. The laboratory evaluation of sleep, which may be thought of as the physical examination of the sleeping patient, consists of continuous physiologic monitoring of several systems throughout a "normal night" of sleep. Polysomnography usually includes electroencephalography (EEG), electrooculography (EOG), electromyography (EMG), electrocardiography, and measurements of respiratory function (including airflow, effort, and oxygen saturation); a variety of other measures also may be added. In a normal adolescent, sleep, as defined through the use of polysomnography, consists of two states, each having its own physiologic and neurophysiologic substrate. These two states—REM (rapid eye movement) and NREM (pronounced non-REM) are identified and defined using EEG, EOG, and EMG. In the normal adolescent, NREM sleep occurs at the transition from wakefulness and usually persists for 80 to 120 minutes before the first REM episode occurs. (In preadolescents the delay to REM sleep is often 180 to 200 minutes.) NREM and REM sleep recur cyclically with a period length of approximately 90 minutes. Table 105-1 describes several features of these two states that are often relevant in clinical interpretation.

NREM sleep is commonly divided into four stages based chiefly on increasing EEG synchrony, which is grossly correlated with depth of sleep. Thus, stage 1 sleep, the lightest phase, is characterized by a "relatively low voltage mixed frequency pattern" of EEG.[1] Stage 2 sleep, which is somewhat deeper, is characterized by the presence of specific EEG waveforms—sleep spindles and K-complexes. In stages 3 and 4 sleep, EEG synchrony and amplitude increase and the frequency of waveforms decreases. Thus, NREM stages 3 and 4 are typified by an increasing amount of high-voltage (≥75 µV), slow-wave (≤2 cycles/sec) activity. In NREM sleep, respiratory rate is usually regular, eye movements are absent, and muscle tonus is maintained, although movement is limited. Mental activity is low during NREM, and arousals from this state provide little evidence of dreaming or other mental activity.

REM sleep, by contrast, is generally associated with a desynchronized activated EEG, bursts of rapid eye movements, suppression of postural muscle tonus, and vivid dreaming. Across the night of sleep in the adolescent, the deepest phases of NREM sleep tend to occur early in the night in the first two cycles. Although REM sleep occurs cyclically across the night in four or five discrete episodes, REM episodes tend to lengthen during the night: the first REM episode lasts perhaps several minutes, and REM episodes late in the night last as long as 30 minutes or more. Across the adolescent range, the most profound change in sleep organization and structure is an overall reduction in the amount of deep NREM sleep stages, which from age 10 to age 20 may decrease by over 40%.[2]

Another clinical test commonly used to assess sleep, particularly in patients whose sleep problem is one of excessive daytime sleepiness, is called the multiple sleep latency test (MSLT).[3] This test is ordinarily conducted at a sleep disorders center on the day after an overnight polysomnographic recording and involves a minimum of four nap opportunities at 2-hour intervals across the day. EEG, EOG, and EMG readings are recorded continuously during each nap. Patients are asked to lie quietly with eyes closed in a dark quiet bedroom and not to resist sleeping. The speed of falling asleep (sleep latency) and sleep state are determined for each approximately 20-minute nap. Faster sleep onset indicates increased sleepiness; onset into REM sleep, rather than NREM sleep, indicates

TABLE 105-1
Comparison of NREM and REM Sleep States

	NREM Sleep	REM Sleep
Timing	Occurs at sleep onset for 80-100+ min then cycles with REM sleep	Occurs after 80-100+ min of NREM sleep then cyclically at 90-min intervals
Electroencephalography	"Synchronized" sleep spindles and high-voltage slow waves	Activated, "desynchronized"
Eye movements	Slow eye movements at transitions from waking; otherwise none	Bursts of rapid, binocularly synchronous eye movement
Motor system	Intact	Pontine-generated postsynaptic hyperpolarization of spinal motor neurons leads to paralysis of postural muscles; twitches may break through this nonreciprocal inhibition (cataplexy and sleep paralysis when this component breaks into wakefulness)
Mental activity	Little coherent activity	Dreaming (hypnagogic hallucinations when this component breaks into wakefulness)

narcolepsy. The MSLT has been well validated in adolescents, and normative data are available.[2,4-6]

The functions of sleep are not fully understood, but a number of factors associated with sleep may be particularly salient in adolescence and may be associated with clinically significant conditions in these youngsters. Although the cause is unclear, the first sign of pubertal onset is an increased sleep-associated nocturnal secretion of luteinizing hormone, which persists through the pubertal maturation process. A second hormone whose secretion is tightly coupled to sleep is human growth hormone, which also shows a marked surge during sleep, specifically in association with NREM stages 3 and 4 sleep. Whether disruptions of sleep in children and adolescents may contribute to maturational delays or growth problems is not clear at present, but the relationship has not been ruled out.

Another factor most evident in regard to a function for sleep is the relationship of waking alertness to nocturnal sleep patterns. With the MSLT, it has been clearly shown that sleep deprivation and sleep restriction have an adverse effect on waking alertness in adolescents.[7-10] In adults a clear relationship between nocturnal sleep fragmentation and decreased waking alertness has also been shown, and such a relationship is also probable in adolescents with sleep fragmenting disorders.[11,12] Insofar as sleep disorders in the adolescent interfere with the normal progression of sleep states and stages, problems in these and other areas may ensue. The complexities of sleep contribute to the complexities of evaluation and treatment of sleep disorders in adolescents.

Before the sleep problems of particular relevance to adolescence are reviewed, it is important to provide a background description of normal adolescent sleep patterns. Survey data from populations in the United States and Western Europe reveal impressive changes in self-reported sleep patterns in the adolescent years. One study found that 10- and 11-year-olds in the United States normally report sleeping approximately 9.5 to 10 hours each night, with little difference between weekends and school nights. By age 14 and 15, reported sleep time is about 8 hours, with a marked increase of sleep on weekends as compared with school nights. Through the high school years (ages 16 and 17 years), sleep time is further reduced to about 7.5 hours. By freshman year in college (age 18 years), students report sleeping about 6.5 hours each school night and 8 hours or (much) longer on weekends.[13,14]

Other features that characterize the sleep patterns in adolescence are a tendency for bedtimes to shift to later hours and a distinct inclination for students to sleep late on weekends if they do not have morning jobs. Thus, for example, the bedtime of 10- and 11-year-olds on school nights was reported to be about 9:00 to 9:30 PM in one study; by senior year in high school, the mean reported bedtime was later than 11:00 PM. Rising times on school mornings, by contrast, were approximately 7:00 AM in the younger adolescents and averaged closer to 6:00 or 6:30 AM in the older groups.[14] It is interesting to note that at all ages, bedtime on weekends was reported as somewhat later than bedtime on school nights, although the youngest children tended to report waking up on weekends within 1 hour or so of their school-day rising times, thus keeping approximately the same total sleep time across the week. The older adolescents reported going to bed 1 to 3 hours later on weekends and sleeping 2, 3, or more hours later than on school days. These data reflect a clear inclination for older adolescents to be more comfortable with later bedtimes and rising times; thus, measures assessing "circadian type" generally show them to be more evening-type than morning-type. This drift appears to be a developmental evolution across adolescence; however, it is not known whether the process is mediated by physiologic or psychosocial changes, or both.

Sleep problems in adolescents span a spectrum of specific disorders, several of which are most common in younger children, some that are more prevalent in adults, and others that first emerge during the adolescent years. Few data exist to provide an estimate of the incidence or prevalence of adolescent sleep disorders, in part because the topic has received little clinical or research attention. Furthermore, geographic, racial, and gender differences are unknown. Nevertheless, sufficient clinical findings exist to allow parallels to be made from adult data. This chapter focuses on those sleep problems that are emergent or most problematic during the adolescent years. Therefore, although sleep apnea syndromes can occur during adolescence under specific circumstances, and although such developmental disorders as night terrors, sleepwalking, and sleeptalking also may persist during the adolescent years, they are not addressed here.

INSOMNIAS

Natural Short Sleeper

Perhaps the most common types of adolescent insomnia develop from problems with the scheduling of sleep. Ferber[13] describes a number of ways in which scheduling problems can lead to insomnia complaints in adolescents. The most counterintuitive type of insomnia occurs in youngsters who may be natural short sleepers or whose native sleep need is less than the amount they or their parents think that they need. Although this problem may be more common in younger children whose parents are more likely to be in control of bedtime, it also may appear in adolescents. Youngsters who truly have a short sleep need cannot be made to sleep longer simply by modifying their bedtimes; however, they can be made quite uncomfortable by inappropriate sleep scheduling.

According to Ferber,[13] this insomnia problem may be manifested in any of three ways. First, the delay in sleep onset may be very long if the youngster is going to bed too early. In general, the time the youngster falls asleep is fairly consistent, and the delay in falling to sleep is quite short on nights when a later bedtime occurs. The

teenager typically wakes up easily or spontaneously during the school week and only a little later if there is no school. Thus, total sleep is consistent from night to night, and the teenager suffers no ill consequences during the day. The second pattern Ferber describes occurs in adolescents who adjust to a too-long scheduled sleep period by falling asleep readily, but who wake very early in the morning. Again, the actual times of sleep onset and sleep offset, as well as total sleep time, are reasonably consistent across the week, and the teenager has no daytime somnolence in spite of a relatively short amount of sleep. The third manifestation of this problem occurs in adolescents who may develop a biphasic sleep pattern, in which they waken in the middle of the night and return to sleep after a prolonged period of alert wakefulness.

Given the apparently common tendency for adolescents to require more rather than less sleep than they achieve, it is unlikely that this particular type of insomnia problem is widespread in teenagers. Nevertheless, the possibility should be entertained in an adolescent who complains of insomnia but is functioning well in the daytime, with no complaints or signs of excessive somnolence or depression. In all likelihood, such a youngster also will have had signs of relatively short sleep at a younger age.

Sleep Phase Delays

In the second decade, children are given more and more control over their own schedules. This is particularly true with regard to bedtime, and changes often reflect a desire on the part of youngsters to stay up later as part of a growing sense of independence.[13-15] This pattern also may relate to an influence of biologic maturation on the neurologic system controlling the body's timing mechanisms, although data to support this hypothesis are only now emerging. Nevertheless, U.S. adolescents and their parents receive virtually no instruction or guidance regarding appropriate sleep hygiene, and decisions therefore are made in the absence of any knowledge about appropriate sleep scheduling. Another factor that contributes to certain sleep problems that arise in adolescents is that most school systems have earlier starting times for the older adolescents (senior high school students) than for younger adolescents and children. Thus, when an adolescent begins staying up later, he or she is often concurrently required to wake early in the morning to get to school.

The delayed sleep phase syndrome (DSPS) was first described in 1981.[16] This syndrome is thought to result from a flaw in the pacemaker controlling the biologic clock. The dysfunction involves an inability to shift rhythms easily to earlier hours but does not affect the ability to maintain a 24-hour rhythm. The hallmark of this problem is an often profound sleep-onset insomnia, although the actual time of sleep onset is usually quite consistent from night to night. The insomnia results from a lack of concordance between the time the body is ready to fall asleep and the time the adolescent attempts to sleep. Thus, for example, adolescents with a sleep phase delay who go to bed at midnight may be unable to fall asleep before 4:00, 5:00, or 6:00 AM. Furthermore, they find it exceedingly difficult or impossible to wake up before noon or even later. Thus, there is not only a severe insomnia but also morning hypersomnolence. Another important feature that distinguishes a sleep phase delay from the other insomnias is that adolescents who are given freedom to sleep when they wish, such as on weekends or vacations, have absolutely no difficulty, fall asleep quickly, sleep for 9 or 10 hours, and wake up spontaneously and refreshed—but at the delayed time.

When a sleep phase delay is greater than 3 or 4 hours from the desired sleeping schedule, this problem needs special treatment. The nature of the hypothesized biologic cause for DSPS is such that no matter how conscientiously the youngster and his or her parents try to enforce going to bed and waking up at more normal times, the biologic clock cannot make the change in the advancing (earlier) direction except in small increments, such as a few minutes each day. Thus, when the delay is 3 hours or more, a supervised program of "chronotherapy" may be recommended.[17] This process achieves the goal of resynchronizing to a more normal phase position because the delay mechanism of the biologic clock is apparently unimpaired. This program of chronotherapy is difficult for many families to understand and is most effective when undertaken with expert guidance.

Other treatments that offer promise include a sleep-deprivation approach in which a single night of sleep loss is used as an acute initiator of a phase change, or appropriately timed bright-light exposure is used to induce a gradual realignment of the phase position.[18,19] No such treatments should be used without supervision, and, even when successful, each suffers from one serious difficulty: none in itself can prevent the problem from recurring. In susceptible individuals, irregular sleep habits—perhaps even a day or two with a delayed sleep onset and offset—can reinitiate the phase delay. This issue is particularly problematic in adolescents for whom staying up late and oversleeping on weekends is a virtually obligatory peer group activity. To maintain entrainment to the new schedule, however, the susceptible teenager needs to avoid late nights and, perhaps even more important, needs to keep from oversleeping.

Many teenagers develop a less pathologic sleep phase delay—not sufficiently out of phase to result in a pattern that is 100% incompatible with going to school but problematic, because late sleep-onset times combined with early school start results in curtailed nocturnal sleep. Another potentially therapeutic approach that is not yet fully tested nor currently recommended for adolescents is melatonin administration. Some evidence exists to suggest that exogenously administered melatonin given on a fixed schedule may be effective to entrain the biologic clock; however, neither the dosage, timing, or efficacy have been established. Furthermore, especially in adolescents, the impact of melatonin on the reproductive system is unclear.[20]

Ferber[13] noted another sleep problem that he considers particularly difficult to treat in children and adolescents: motivated sleep phase delay. This schedule difficulty shares many of the clinical characteristics of the DSPS, with certain notable exceptions:

- Adolescents with DSPS are generally quite bothered by the condition and express a sincere desire to be able to get up in the morning and go to school; they set the alarm, and if awakened will get dressed and go to school (though they are generally unable to stay awake for their morning classes). Adolescents with a motivated sleep phase delay do not have the same affective response to missing school: they "forget" to set the alarm and, although they may wake up in the morning, they are "unable" to wake up sufficiently to get up, get dressed, and go to school.
- With DSPS, the inability to wake in the morning persists on weekends, vacations, and other nonschool days. In the motivated sleep phase delay, the youngster may have no trouble waking on days when there is no school, particularly when motivated by an interest in the planned morning activity.
- Youngsters with a motivated sleep phase delay are entirely refractory and in fact are resistant to treatment with chronotherapy or the other techniques already described.

Treatment of the motivated sleep phase delay with the chronotherapeutic strategies outlined for DSPS meets with great resistance and no success. The adolescent fails to comply with the treatment process and finds means to avoid potentially successful rescheduling efforts, such as demonstrating a further phase delay if an afternoon tutor is arranged. Failure of the chronotherapeutic approach is in itself an important diagnostic cue for the motivated phase delay; the way in which the failure presents itself also may be useful in identifying the root cause of the problem. For example, a parent may thwart the therapeutic process, thus revealing that his or her own physical or psychologic needs may have led the individual to derive secondary gain from having the teenager at home in the daytime; or the child may demonstrate behaviors suggesting a particularly impressive school resistance. Ferber[13] notes that a family issue is often involved in the motivated phase delay, and that treatment needs to be broadly based and is often laborious and challenging.

Idiopathic (Childhood-Onset) Insomnia

The International Classification of Sleep Disorders (ICSD)[21] defines idiopathic insomnia as "a lifelong inability to obtain adequate sleep that is presumably due to an abnormality of the neurological control of the sleep-wake system." Unlike the adolescents described earlier, these are youngsters who simply are unable to sleep very long or well; their difficulty is not one of the timing of the sleep schedule, but of the limited capacity to sleep well at any time. The cause of idiopathic insomnia is unknown, although an imbalance between the arousal and sleep-inducing systems is thought to underlie the disorder. This insomnia may indicate a hyperarousal or a hyposomnolence and is likely the result of a neurochemical, neuroanatomic, or neurophysiologic impairment involving the sleep-wake biologic networks. In all cases, the serious insomnia cannot be explained by other psychologic or medical problems.

According to the ICSD,[21] the chronic poor sleep experienced by persons with idiopathic insomnia is accompanied by daytime complaints of poor concentration, impaired vigilance and attention, low energy, bad mood, and increased fatigue. Furthermore, teenagers with idiopathic insomnia may have soft neurologic signs, which can appear as dyslexia or hyperactivity; they also may show EEG abnormalities that are not clinically significant, such as "ragged" alpha waves. Idiopathic insomnia is currently thought to be a rare clinical entity, with the following distinguishing diagnostic criteria: (1) there is a complaint of insomnia combined with a complaint of decreased daytime functioning that is long-standing, typically beginning in early childhood or even at birth; (2) the insomnia is unceasing and persists equally through intervals of relatively good or poor psychologic functioning; and (3) no medical or psychiatric cause can be associated with the onset of symptoms. Although not life-threatening, the prognosis for this disorder is poor, unless the patient is responsive to a hypnotic medication.

Psychophysiologic Insomnia

Psychophysiologic insomnia generally appears in young adults and is a possible, albeit unlikely, cause of insomnia in adolescents. The sleeplessness of psychophysiologic insomnia can be attributed to "learned sleep-preventing associations" and related "somatized tension."[21] The disorder generally first appears in young adulthood or later and may last for decades if untreated. Patients develop an intense and consuming preoccupation with their sleep problem that itself interferes with obtaining adequate sleep. Behavioral regimens, including such approaches as stimulus control,[22] sleep restriction,[23] and biofeedback,[24] have each shown some efficacy in

adults with psychophysiologic insomnia. Reports of therapeutic trials in adolescents are lacking.

HYPERSOMNIAS

Excessive sleepiness is quite prevalent in adolescents, many of whom sleep fewer (often considerably fewer) than 9 hours a night, the level below which a sleep deficit is thought to accrue in most teenagers. Adolescents themselves report about 9 hours when asked how much sleep they require to feel wide awake and alert,[25] and laboratory data suggest that 9 hours may be a minimal requirement for teenagers.[7] Certainly, many high school teachers are well aware of the problems of excessive sleepiness in adolescents, as they witness their students struggling to remain awake day after day in school. The more common causes of adolescent excessive sleepiness are presented below.

Delayed Sleep Phase Syndrome

This syndrome can present as a complaint of sleep-onset insomnia and with inability to wake in the morning. The latter is expressed as incapacitating sleepiness if the adolescent is awakened and transported to school. These symptoms occur in both the physiologic and motivational sleep phase delays. Daytime hypoarousal (not always manifested as sleepiness per se) often also accompanies idiopathic and psychophysiologic insomnia.

Insufficient Sleep

The most prevalent cause of hypersomnolence in adolescence appears to be insufficient sleep. The adolescent pattern of reducing and delaying sleep and sleeping late on weekends is common among students in the United States, and likely engenders a significant sleep deficit in adolescents. For example, a longitudinal laboratory study of sleep patterns across the adolescent years demonstrated that between ages 10 and 12 years and 16 and 18 years the need for sleep, as gauged by the amount of sleep obtained in a 10-hour night, remained constant at approximately 9 hours, 15 minutes. Furthermore, this study showed a decline in waking alertness that occurred at midpuberty, even in the face of this "extended" sleep in the older adolescents. One conclusion of this research, therefore, was that older adolescents do not need less sleep than younger children but in fact may need more sleep.[7]

Another piece of evidence suggesting that the "typical" amount of sleep obtained by adolescents is less than optimal comes from self-reported data in college-bound high school seniors. These students, who were questioned in the spring of their senior year of high school, reported achieving on average 74 minutes less sleep on school nights than they thought they "needed to feel refreshed." Given that they extended sleep somewhat on weekends, the nightly deficit across the week remained at approximately 45 minutes. Thus, these high school seniors were experiencing a deficit of approximately 6.5 hours across the week and making up only 1.5 hours of the deficit during the weekend nights.[25]

Adolescents in the United States today have increasingly more options and opportunities for activities that fill their days (and much of their nights). Many feel obliged to have jobs in order to fill the role of the consumer that is projected onto them by the media. My work with high school students in Rhode Island revealed that nearly 30% report working 20 or more hours per week during the school year. In association with such long work hours, these youngsters report sleeping less at night (both on school days and weekends), oversleeping and missing school more often, falling asleep in school more frequently, and experiencing difficulties staying awake while studying more often than the students who work less or not at all. Furthermore, although reported caffeine use (mostly cola drinks) was high in all adolescents in this study, those working 20 hours or more a week were more likely to drink coffee, smoke cigarettes, and drink alcohol. Thus, heavy work schedules constitute one factor that is clearly related to insufficient sleep and concomitant features in adolescents.[26]

Another factor that impinges on sleep duration in teenagers is the early start time for their days. As mentioned previously, the high school bell commonly rings earlier than for junior high and elementary school, and with busing or long commutes to school, many adolescents must routinely rise before 6:00 AM. Those with an elaborate and lengthy morning routine must rise even earlier; according to Ferber,[13] some often refuse to curtail the time they spend preparing their hair or clothing even if their daytime alertness is quite impaired. To obtain 9 hours of sleep with such a schedule, adolescents would need to retire at 9:00 PM or earlier—an unlikely scenario for the typical American teenager. Thus, it is not surprising that teachers are noticing "sleepy heads" in their classrooms.

A 1995 study followed adolescents across the transition from ninth to tenth grades with evaluations of sleep patterns, daytime alertness, and circadian phase (using dim-light salivary melatonin onset [DLSMO] as a phase marker).[27-29] In these teenagers, school start time changed from 8:25 AM in ninth to 7:20 AM in tenth grade. Figure 105-1 illustrates the sleep patterns of one girl based on wrist actigraphic monitoring for two weeks in ninth and two weeks in tenth grade. Overall, the youngsters slept approximately 40 minutes less on school nights in tenth than in ninth grade (419 minutes vs. 457 minutes),

essentially as a result of rising earlier in tenth grade (5:53 AM vs. 6:52 AM), and they were sleepier on the basis of the laboratory measure of MSLT in tenth than in ninth grade. Extreme sleepiness in the "severe" range on MSLT[27] was found in over one half of the tenth graders. Perhaps equally significant was the finding that the circadian phase position of the DLSMO (8:23 PM in ninth grade vs. 8:23 PM in tenth grade) had not advanced to accommodate to the earlier rising times.[28] In other words, no biologic adjustment had occurred in response to the earlier rising time demanded by the change in school schedule.

An after-school nap might help alleviate the sleep debt teenagers accumulate, although school club meetings, athletic team practices, and other extracurricular and social activities normally fill that time interval. The list of adolescent activities is almost endless. The Dean of Humanities of a state-of-the-art high school in Charleston, West Virginia, Jo Blackman, recently testified to the National Commission on Sleep Disorders Research: "Our school program is very active academically. It's tough competition, there are high expectations. . . . As a result we find out there's a high stress level. They have quite a bit of homework and if they do community service activities [or] if they're in extracurricular activities, . . . then our students really don't have time for [adequate sleep]." (comments to Public Hearing of the National Commission on Sleep Disorders Research, Charleston, W. Va., May 11, 1991).

Narcolepsy

Adolescence is the peak age of onset for narcolepsy, which is the second most prevalent cause of hypersomnolence in patients presenting at sleep disorders centers.[30] The full-blown narcolepsy syndrome is characterized by a number of distinctive symptoms, the most debilitating of which for most patients is excessive, intrusive daytime sleepiness. Other symptoms include cataplexy, which is characterized by brief episodes of muscle weakness often associated with an emotional precipitant; sleep paralysis, which is an atonic condition occurring at the onset or offset of sleep; hypnagogic hallucinations, which are vivid, often frightening, usually visual and auditory hallucinations occurring at the onset of sleep; and memory lapses or "blackouts," which may involve automatic behaviors.

Not all the symptoms arise concurrently in a teenager who develops narcolepsy, and adolescents rarely present with all the symptoms. In a 1994 review, Dahl and colleagues[31] reported the full symptom cluster in only one of 16 adolescent patients. As classically described, daytime sleepiness is usually the first symptom to appear, and it may interfere with the youngster's academic and social life. Unfortunately, it may be difficult to distinguish the adolescent with narcolepsy—solely on the basis of

Activity Record in an Adolescent Female

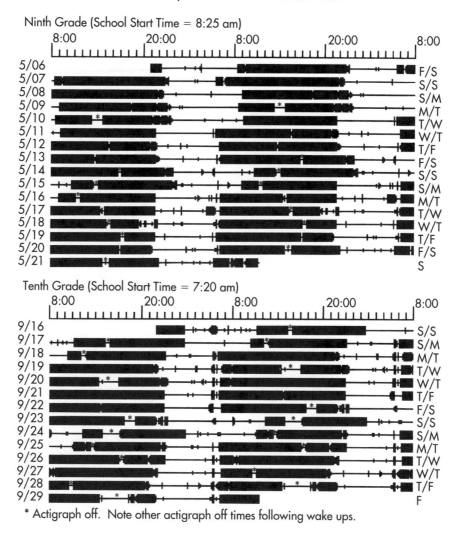

* Actigraph off. Note other actigraph off times following wake ups.

Fig. 105-1. This diagram illustrates activity and rest patterns in an adolescent girl participating in a research project over the transition from ninth to tenth grades. The data are displayed as a double plot, wherein 2 consecutive days are placed side by side and then placed over consecutive days vertically. The dark areas indicate portions of the day in which activity levels were high; light areas indicate sleep or, as designated by an asterisk, times when the activity monitor was not worn. In addition, many of the wake-up times are followed by a brief interval with the activity monitor off, particularly evident in the bottom graph. In the top graph, this girl was in ninth grade attending a junior high school that started at 8:25 AM. In the bottom graph, she was in tenth grade in a school starting each day at 7:20 AM. The average school-night sleep length in the ninth grade was 491 minutes. In tenth grade, the average school-night sleep length was 385 minutes. The difference principally resulted from an earlier rising time in tenth versus ninth grade (approximately 5:30 AM versus 7:30 AM). (From Dahl RE, Carskadon MA: Sleep and its disorders in adolescence. In Ferber R, Kryger MH, editors: *Principles and practice of sleep medicine in the child,* Philadelphia, 1995, WB Saunders; p 21.)

sleepiness—from the legions of sleepy adolescents that populate most high schools and colleges. A salient feature of the disorder, and one that may be more suggestive of the diagnosis, is what affected adolescents often refer to as their "nightmares." The young person's descriptions of these nightmares are almost unmistakenly clear-cut hypnagogic hallucinations, usually with sleep paralysis.

For example, an adolescent might report: "Most times when I'm falling asleep, I'll hear someone coming into my room and I know they're gonna kill me . . . and then I realize I can't move, and I can't scream, and I'm scared to death!" Many adolescents who have such experiences find them extremely troublesome and are fearful to talk to anyone about them since they may think they are "flipping out." Paralysis when waking up also may occur in adolescents with narcolepsy, although these episodes are less likely to be accompanied by the nightmarish hallucinations. (Non-narcoleptic individuals occasionally experience sleep paralysis, particularly when sleep-wake schedules have been seriously disrupted. Thus, the report of this symptom occurring in isolation in a teenager who has been sleep deprived or has undergone an acute sleep schedule alteration is not thought to be clinically significant.)

Cataplexy is not unknown in adolescent narcolepsy, although the symptom may be somewhat subtle. Muscle weakness with laughter, anger, and exertion are typical, and the episodes may appear as dropping a book or a glass rather than a complete collapse as in a fully established episode. Sleepiness can become a significant impediment to the educational process in adolescents with narcolepsy. In some, however, the sleepiness at a younger age appears as hyperactivity and acting out, which may represent the youngster's struggles to stay awake.

The prevalence of narcolepsy is thought to be approximately 1 in 1000, with equal numbers of males and females. One of the most troublesome aspects of the disorder is the generally lengthy delay between symptom onset and diagnosis, which has obvious ramifications for treatment. Early identification of youngsters with narcolepsy is also crucial to avoid the psychosocial stigmas and loss of educational opportunities that may affect them for years. Because most cases of narcolepsy are thought to be of genetic origin, family history may provide an additional diagnostic clue; however, the genetic transmission is thought to involve a nondominant route and perhaps varying degrees of penetrance, which may limit the extent to which family history is useful. On the other hand, if a parent, grandparent, aunt, or uncle has been diagnosed with narcolepsy (or is described to have behaviors that fit the diagnosis), the likelihood that the adolescent with the symptoms described above has narcolepsy is quite high. The presence of a specific HLA marker is also suggestive but not diagnostic.[31]

A full work-up at a sleep disorders clinic involving overnight polysomnography and daytime MSLT can provide diagnostic certainty if the syndrome is fully established.[2] In general, the overnight recording of an adolescent with narcolepsy will show somewhat disrupted sleep, though not markedly different in length or distribution of sleep stages, with the exception that the first episode of REM sleep may occur with a reduced latency from the onset of sleep. The daytime MSLT generally demonstrates a shortened latency to sleep onset, as well as the presence of two or more sleep-onset REM episodes, representing a reversal of the normal sleep-onset process. The occurrence of sleep-onset REM episodes in patients with narcolepsy is representative of what is thought to be the underlying dysfunction of the disorder: an inability of the sleep-wake mechanisms to consolidate sleep state processes (Table 105-1). Thus, the motor paralysis of the REM sleep state breaks through into the waking state as cataplexy and sleep paralysis; the dream imagery of the REM state comes to consciousness inappropriately at the onset of sleep, before the sleep state is fully established (and when NREM sleep normally occurs, with its lack of mental activation); and the somnolence characteristic of sleep also invades the waking state. The physiologic marker of narcolepsy, sleep-onset REM episodes, is therefore quite distinct.

The review of adolescent narcolepsy in 16 patients noted two other unexpected associations of the disorder: a high rate of emotional or behavioral disturbance (75%) and a high number with obesity (69%).[31] In the latter case, exclusion of obstructive sleep apnea syndrome (OSAS) should be considered. (An excellent review of pediatric OSAS and related sleep disorders is found in a 1995 publication by Carroll and Loughlin.[32-34])

No clinical trials have been performed in adolescents with narcolepsy. In adults, stimulants (methylphenidate, pemoline, amphetamine) are generally used to control daytime sleepiness, and REM sleep-suppressant medications, common antidepressants such as protriptyline, imipramine, or clomipramine, are used to control cataplexy, sleep paralysis, and hypnagogic hallucinations. Gamma-hydroxybutyrate has been reported to improve nocturnal sleep, which is thought to have a secondary positive benefit for sleepiness and cataplexy. One case report noted reduced physiologic sleepiness and fewer sleep-onset REM episodes in an older adolescent placed on a sleep-extension regimen. Prescribed brief daytime naps (15 to 20 minutes) are useful in certain patients. Close work with the school system may be as important to the adolescent with narcolepsy, particularly in terms of providing accommodations of the educational process to the youngster's symptoms. Of specific concern is the difficulty a teenager with narcolepsy has remaining vigilant during lengthy examinations, which may be of greatest consequence in taking standardized placement examinations, such as the SATs. The other notable difficulties encountered by teenagers with narcolepsy often surround their ability to cope with the life style restrictions, particularly vis-à-vis proper sleep habits and obtaining sufficient sleep. For the physician, one of the most difficult issues arises when the teenager becomes eligible to drive and safety is a concern.

SUMMARY

Teenagers are ignorant about sleep—how much they need, what the consequences of insufficient sleep are, what sleep disorders are, and how they might identify whether they or a friend have a sleep disorder. In general, they do not understand what sleep is, what is proper sleep, or what is inappropriate or abnormal sleep. Their parents, teachers, school nurses, counselors, and doctors are typically no more knowledgeable, although they have more years of lore and old wives' tales to guide their "wisdom." The sleep problems of adolescents, whether physiologically or psychologically mediated or whether a result of modern life styles, are likely to have far-reaching effects on the lives of many of them. Those who are unable to build adequate coping mechanisms to compensate for the effects of their sleep problems are vulnerable to an array of problematic outcomes. Their educational experience is likely to suffer and, as a consequence, fulfillment of their potential will be limited. Some may try to cope with the sleep problems by using alcohol, stimulants, and other chemicals. In others the sleep problem may result in frank psychopathology; depression and suicide are not inconceivable consequences. For most youngsters with excessive daytime sleepiness, there is chronic vulnerability for a "catastrophic" episode, such as falling asleep while driving an automobile. In 1990, for example, an 18-year-old Portland, Oregon, senior high school student was killed when his car missed a curve at 8:00 AM, after the boy had worked an overnight shift at a fast-food restaurant. In 1990, the United States' Safest Teenager Driver of 1989 was killed when he fell asleep behind the wheel.

The solutions for sleep disturbances involve educating children and adolescents, as well as parents, teachers, pediatricians, and others with responsibility for the health and welfare of the nation's youth, to have a proper respect for sleep-wake functioning and to understand what steps can be taken to identify and improve a problematic situation. For instance, the state medical association in Minnesota has joined the process by issuing a resolution urging school districts to consider moving the starting time later for adolescents. Increased awareness of sleep disorders and of appropriate sleep hygiene is a preliminary step to successful management of these problems.

Acknowledgements

This work was supported in part by grants to the author from NIMH (MH 45945) and NHLBI (HL44138).

References

1. Rechtschaffen A, Kales A, editors: *A manual of standardized terminology, techniques, and scoring system for sleep stages of human subjects,* Los Angeles, 1968, UCLA Brain Information Service/Brain Research Institute.
2. Carskadon MA: The second decade. In Guilleminault C, editor: *Sleeping and waking disorders: indications and techniques,* Menlo Park, CA, 1982, Addison Wesley; pp 99-125.
3. Carskadon MA, Dement WC, Mitler MM, Roth T, Westbrook P, Keenan S: Guidelines for the multiple sleep latency test (MSLT): a standard measure of sleepiness, *Sleep* 9:519-524, 1986.
4. Carskadon MA, Orav EJ, Dement WC: Evolution of sleep and daytime sleepiness in adolescents. In Guilleminault C, Lugaresi E, editors: *Sleep/wake disorders: natural history, epidemiology, and long-term evolution,* New York, 1983, Raven Press; pp 201-216.
5. Carskadon MA, Dement WC: Sleepiness in the normal adolescent. In Guilleminault C, editor: *Sleep and its disorders in children,* New York, 1987, Raven Press; pp 53-66.
6. Carskadon MA, Keenan S, Dement WC: Nighttime sleep and daytime sleep tendency in preadolescents. In Guilleminault C, editor: *Sleep and its disorders in children,* New York, 1987, Raven Press; pp 43-52.
7. Carskadon MA, Harvey K, Duke P, Anders TF, Litt IF, Dement WC: Pubertal changes in daytime sleepiness, *Sleep* 2:453-460, 1980.
8. Carskadon MA, Dement WC: Cumulative effects of sleep restriction on daytime sleepiness, *Psychophysiology* 18:107-113, 1981.
9. Carskadon MA, Harvey K, Dement WC: Acute restriction of nocturnal sleep in children, *Percept Mot Skills* 53:103-112, 1981.
10. Carskadon MA, Harvey K, Dement WC: Sleep loss in young adolescents, *Sleep* 4:299-312, 1981.
11. Carskadon MA, Brown ED, Dement WC: Sleep fragmentation in the elderly: relationship to daytime sleep tendency, *Neurobiol Aging* 3:321-327, 1982.
12. Stepanski E, Lamphere J, Badia P, Zorick F, Roth T: Sleep fragmentation and daytime sleepiness, *Sleep* 7:18-26, 1984.
13. Ferber R: Sleep schedule-dependent causes of insomnia and sleepiness in middle childhood and adolescence, *Pediatrician* 17:13-20, 1990.
14. Carskadon MA: Patterns of sleep and sleepiness in adolescents, *Pediatrician* 17:5-12, 1990.
15. Price VA, Coates TJ, Thoresen CE, Grinstead OA: Prevalence and correlates of poor sleep among adolescents, *Am J Dis Child* 132:583-586, 1978.
16. Weitzman ED, Czeisler CA, Coleman RM, Spielman AJ, Zimmerman JC, Dement WC: Delayed sleep phase syndrome. A chronobiological disorder with sleep-onset insomnia, *Arch Gen Psychiatry* 38:737-746, 1981.
17. Czeisler CA, Richardson GS, Coleman RM, Zimmerman JC, Moore-Ede MC, Dement WC, Weitzman ED: Chronotherapy: resetting the circadian clocks of patients with delayed sleep phase insomnia, *Sleep* 4:1-21, 1981.
18. Thorpy MJ, Korman E, Spielman AJ, Glovinsky PB: Delayed sleep phase syndrome in adolescents, *J Adolesc Health Care* 9:22-27, 1988.
19. Rosenthal NE, Joseph-Vanderpool JR, Levendosky AA, Johnston SH, Allen R, Kelly KA, Souetre E, Schultz PM, Starz KE: Phase-shifting effects of bright morning light as treatment for delayed sleep phase syndrome, *Sleep* 13:354-361, 1990.
20. Dahl RE, Carskadon MA: Sleep and its disorders in adolescence. In Ferber R, Kryger MH, editors: *Principles and practice of sleep medicine in the child,* Philadelphia, 1995, WB Saunders; pp 19-27.
21. Diagnostic Classification Steering Committee, Thorpy MJ, Chairman: *International Classification of Sleep Disorders: diagnostic and coding manual,* Rochester, MN, 1990, American Sleep Disorders Association.
22. Bootzin RR, Nicassio PM: Behavioral treatments for insomnia: an experimental investigation. In Hersen M, Eisler RM, Miller PM, editors: *Progress in behavior modification,* New York, 1978, Academic Press; pp 1-45.
23. Spielman AJ, Saskin P, Thorpy MJ: Treatment of chronic insomnia by restriction of time in bed, *Sleep* 10:45-56, 1987.
24. Hauri PJ: Treating psychophysiological insomnia with biofeedback, *Arch Gen Psychiatry* 38:752-758, 1981.
25. Carskadon MA, Seifer R, Davis SS, Acebo C: Sleep, sleepiness, and mood in college-bound high school seniors, *Sleep Res* 20:175, 1991.

26. Carskadon MA: Adolescent sleepiness: increased risk in a high-risk population, *Alcohol Drugs Driving* 5:317-328, 1990.

27. Carskadon MA, Wolfson A, Tzischinsky O, Acebo C: Early school schedules modify adolescent sleepiness, *Sleep Res* 24:92, 1995.

28. Tzischinsky O, Wolfson AR, Darley C, Brown C, Acebo C, Carskadon MA: Sleep habits and salivary melatonin onset in adolescents, *Sleep Res* 24:543, 1995.

29. Brown C, Tzischinsky O, Wolfson AR, Acebo C, Wicks J, Darley C, Carskadon MA: Circadian phase preference and adjustment to the high school transition, *Sleep Res* 24:90, 1995.

30. Coleman RM: Diagnosis, treatment, and followup of about 8,000 sleep-wake disorder patients. In Guilleminault C, Lugariesi E, editors: *Sleep/wake disorders: natural history, epidemiology, and long-term evolution,* New York, 1983, Raven Press; pp 87-98.

31. Dahl RE, Holttum J, Trubnick L: A clinical picture of child and adolescent narcolepsy, *J Am Acad Child Adolesc Psychiatry* 33:834-841, 1994.

32. Carroll JL, Loughlin GM: Primary snoring in children. In Ferber R, Kryger MH, editors: *Principles and practice of sleep medicine in the child,* Philadelphia, 1995, WB Saunders; pp 155-161.

33. Carroll JL, Loughlin GM: Obstructive sleep apnea syndrome in infants and children: clinical features and pathophysiology. In Ferber R, Kryger MH, editors: *Principles and practice of sleep medicine in the child,* Philadelphia, 1995, WB Saunders; pp 163-191.

34. Carroll JL, Loughlin GM: Obstructive sleep apnea syndrome in infants and children: diagnosis and management. In Ferber R, Kryger MH, editors: *Principles and practice of sleep medicine in the child,* Philadelphia, 1995, WB Saunders; pp 193-216.

Suggested Readings

Carskadon MA, Anders TF, Hole W: Sleep disturbances in childhood and adolescence. In Fitzgerald HE, Lester BM, Yogman MW, editors: *Theory and research in behavioral pediatrics,* vol 4, New York, 1988, Plenum.
> Summarizes a comprehensive perspective on pediatric sleep disorders.

Ferber R: *Solve your child's sleep problems,* New York, 1985, Simon & Schuster.
> Written for the lay public, this book gives practical recommendations regarding sleep problems, primarily of younger children, although with some insights appropriate for teenagers.

Ferber R, Kryger MH: *Principles and practice of sleep medicine in the child,* Philadelphia, 1995, WB Saunders.
> An overview of childhood sleep and sleep disorders, including several excellent review papers.

Guilleminault C, editor: *Sleep and its disorders in children,* New York, 1987, Raven Press.
> Focuses primarily on younger children, although several chapters are relevant to the adolescent age group.

Kryger MH, Roth T, Dement WC, editors: *Principles and practice of sleep medicine,* ed 2, Philadelphia, 1993, WB Saunders.
> Provides a comprehensive overview of sleep physiology and pathology.

Mindell J: Sleeping through the night, New York, 1997, Harper Collins.
> Written for parents, this book deals with sleep problems of early childhood.

CHAPTER 106

Recurrent Abdominal Pain

•

Ronald G. Barr and Siobhan M. Gormally

The assessment and management of the syndrome of recurrent abdominal pain (RAP) is a difficult challenge with children of all ages. There are no pathognomonic features to help distinguish those with organic disease from those without such disease. In addition, in those without organic disease, the cause is often obscure. In adolescents, these problems are complicated further because various characteristics of normal adolescent development may mask the signs and symptoms thought to be helpful in distinguishing organic from psychogenic (emotional) etiologies. Thus, clinicians are likely to attribute the complaint inappropriately to either organic *or* psychogenic causes. This not only compromises the accuracy of diagnosis, but also biases management decisions in ways that may seriously compromise their effectiveness.

Accounts of RAP syndrome usually describe appropriate work-ups based on the assumption that the etiologic entity is known or at least strongly suspected. In practice, however, the clinician is faced most often with an adolescent who has abdominal pain but whose condition shows no clear diagnostic direction. In this chapter, specific entities are described only insofar as they illustrate particular problems. Confirmatory diagnostic approaches for specific organic or psychiatric entities can be found in relevant chapters of this book or reviews in the literature.[1-4] A discussion of abdominal pain as a medical disorder is found in Chapter 43, "Chronic Abdominal Pain."

RECURRENT ABDOMINAL PAIN SYNDROME

RAP syndrome is typically considered to be primarily an entity of preadolescent children. The seminal work of John Apley[5] indicated that the peak prevalence occurs at 9 years of age, a pattern confirmed in a subsequent and more complete Danish study.[6] In the Danish study the declining prevalence ranged from approximately 20% to 5% between 13 and 17 years of age, respectively, making it a common adolescent concern.

Because of the prevalence profile, the classic picture of RAP syndrome is derived primarily from preadolescents. It includes attacks of pain that are paroxysmal in nature, occur frequently over an extended period (more than three episodes over 3 months or longer), and are severe enough to result in a change of activity.[5] The term *paroxysmal* refers to the unpredictable and unexpected nature of the attacks. The criterion of extended time is arbitrary—meant simply to exclude occasional, isolated, and transitory episodes of pain. The severity criterion is likewise inadequately defined, but it is meant to ensure that the pain is disruptive of the child's normal activity.

More important is the requirement that the child be well and functioning as usual between pain episodes. This feature is important in distinguishing RAP syndrome from "chronic" abdominal pain. It probably accounts for the lack of depressive symptoms in RAP that are more typically associated with chronic pain syndromes.[7] The pain of RAP syndrome is most commonly, but not necessarily, periumbilical. Usually a number of other complaints such as limb pains are involved, as well as autonomic complaints such as nausea, vomiting, pallor, perspiration, and headache.[5,6,8] In contrast, complaints usually considered as indicators of organic diseases (e.g., fever, jaundice, bloody stools, pain on urination, urgency of urination and/or stool, weight loss) are usually absent. The physical examination is typically unremarkable.

It is less clear how appropriate the classic picture is for the adolescent age group. For example, adolescents are more likely than children to be able to localize their pain despite lack of evidence of organic disease. This may indicate developmentally different mechanisms underlying the complaint, or it may simply be a function of increasing cognitive capacity to describe their complaint with accuracy. In our experience, preadolescents more frequently have spontaneous resolution of their abdominal pain than do adolescents, yet there are no specific features that differentiate adolescents with persistent complaints from those without.

It is possible that distinct clinical presentations will eventually be described that would be more common in adolescent patients than in school-age children. These include primary periumbilical pain, "nonulcer dyspepsia," and lower abdominal pain syndromes with altered bowel habits analogous to the "spastic colon" subgroup of adult irritable bowel syndrome.[1,2] The syndrome of primary periumbilical pain refers to the classic picture described for school-age children. Nonulcer dyspepsia is characterized by its upper abdominal location and by associated nausea, postprandial fullness, distention, gas symptoms (belching, hiccups), and early satiety. This clinical presentation has added interest because of the debate in recent years about the potential role of *Helicobacter pylori* gastritis and abnormal gut motility in this entity.[2,9-15] "Spastic colon" in adults is similar to RAP and is typically associated with symptoms of distention, pain relief with a bowel movement, looser and more frequent stools, mucus, a feeling of incomplete evacuation, and lower abdominal tenderness on examination. It has been suggested that most children over the age of 5 years with the symptoms of RAP fulfill the standardized criteria for irritable bowel disease.[16] Whether these or other clinical entities are more common in adolescents is yet to be demonstrated.

BIVARIATE VERSUS TRIVARIATE CLASSIFICATION

Cultural tradition and medical training predispose us to classify abdominal pain in children as having either organic or psychogenic (emotional) etiologies. However, it may be helpful to shift our thinking away from this bivariate classification to a trivariate one in which organic, dysfunctional, and psychogenic (emotional) categories are recognized. Implicit in this shift is a recognition that RAP is most often a syndrome that is managed rather than a disease that is cured.

In the traditional bivariate classification (Fig. 106-1) the problem is considered to be one of distinguishing organic from emotional pain. Ironically, this classification is inappropriately attributed to Apley,[5] who recognized a third provisional clinical category (nonorganic, nonemotional) for patients who could not be placed in either of the other two groups. The term *psychogenic* has been appropriately criticized for being nonspecific or outdated, but it is still commonly used. Usually it is meant to indicate simply that psychologic factors are etiologically important. However, the issue of proper use of the terms *psychogenic* and *organic* is not primarily a semantic one.

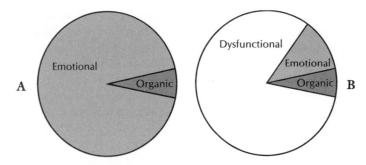

Fig. 106-1. Alternative classification systems for recurrent abdominal pain syndrome. The presence of shading indicates the assumption that "disease" is present. The size of the wedges roughly approximates prevalence according to available studies derived from series with both preadolescent and adolescent children. "Dysfunctional" RAP syndrome refers to a condition in children in whom no assumption of abnormality is made and for which evidence of organicity and psychogenicity is lacking (see text). (From Gable S, editor: *Behavioral problems in children,* New York, 1981, Grune & Stratton; p 237.)

Whatever labels are used, the bivariate classification functions in such a way that the clinician is required to make two assumptions: (1) that the pain must be *either* organic *or* psychogenic, and (2) that the symptom of disease implies the presence of disease (something wrong or abnormal) that accounts for the symptom. Neither of these assumptions has been demonstrated. In particular, evidence supporting the assumption that nonorganic cases are psychogenic is particularly weak. Series reporting higher levels of measures compatible with a psychogenic etiology seldom (1) control for referral bias, (2) agree with one another as to which factors (e.g., anxiety, depression, life stress) are significant, or (3) demonstrate a temporal relationship between the psychologic factor and the pain complaint. This does not contradict the fact that RAP can be psychogenic in an important subgroup of adolescents without an organic etiology; it means only that it does not account for all such cases. The primary argument against the second assumption is its failure to recognize that abdominal pain may be merely a symptom in an otherwise physically and mentally well adolescent. A good example is the recognition of carbohydrate intolerance as a stimulus for pain symptoms. Lactose intolerance results from an interaction between a normal developmental phenomenon (low levels of lactase activity in the small intestine) and a normal environmental phenomenon (ingestion of foods that contain lactose). The low lactase levels are not the result of a disease process (and therefore not organic), nor does the absence of organic disease imply that the complaint is psychogenic or in any other way abnormal. Since both normal physiologic and psychologic factors contribute to symptom variability, symptom reporting, and the extent to which the symptoms become a problem, it is conceptually misleading and unhelpful to classify such cases as either (1) organic or psychogenic or (2) due to disease processes.

In the recommended tripartite classification (see Figure 106-1), three major categories are recognized: organic, emotional, and dysfunctional. *Organic pain* refers to pain sensations assumed to originate intraabdominally from a specific pathologic process in an organ system or systems. Subcategories include diseases referable to the genitourinary tract, the gastrointestinal tract, and other organ systems. Compared with preadolescents, it might be expected that more causes would be genitourinary than gastrointestinal in origin in adolescents, especially females.[1]

The category of *emotional (psychogenic) pain* is reserved for those situations in which the subject experiences pain in the absence of disordered patterns originating in intraabdominal sensory nerve endings. Subcategories include pain occurring as part of a psychiatric syndrome (e.g., depression, conversion disorder, hypochondriasis) and pain complaints demonstrably linked to psychologic and behavioral events but for which full criteria for a psychiatric disorder are lacking (e.g., loss of a relative, complaint modeling, maintenance of pain for secondary gain).

In *dysfunctional pain* the pain sensations are assumed to originate intraabdominally from normal rather than disordered physiologic processes. The term *dysfunctional* is used in recognition of the fact that, even in the absence of a pathologic condition, the existence of the pain symptom itself may have secondary negative effects on peer, parent, or school relationships. There are two subcategories of dysfunctional pain. *Specific* dysfunctional pain syndromes are those in which the mechanism of pain production is recognizable. This most clearly includes entities such as carbohydrate intolerance, mittelschmerz, and pregnancy. On the basis of their ability to be recognized as distinct, nonulcer dyspepsia and irritable bowel syndrome would be included in this subcategory, although they may ultimately be defined as organic if convincing evidence of pathologic processes were demonstrable. *Nonspecific* dysfunctional pain syndromes differ in that they involve no recognizable mechanism of pain. This subcategory includes patients in whom the symptom subsides within three visits without any specific therapy (early spontaneous resolution) and those whose symptoms do not (persistent pain).

DIAGNOSIS

The tripartite classification permits one to think about the etiology more flexibly and to refrain from making assumptions that lend unnecessary bias to the investigation and treatment. First, it requires recognition of the possibility that the adolescent with RAP may be physically and mentally healthy. An example would be someone in whom no evidence of a psychopathologic condition or stress is elicited and who is classified as having nonspecific dysfunctional abdominal pain. Although not pleasant, the painful attacks are at least not abnormal.

Second, there are a number of adolescents in whom evidence of stress is clear but the etiologic relationship of the stress to the pain is not. This classification permits such patients to be understood as having a recognizable entity of nonspecific dysfunctional pain and a second problem of life stress, rather than requiring that they be treated as having psychogenic RAP. Both problems continue to be managed, but on the basis of positive data rather than the inappropriate assumption that they are causally related.

Third, this classificatory approach does not force the physician to make the untenable claim that organic disease is ruled out by an initial diagnostic phase in which a battery of tests for physical disease is performed. The ability of any such battery to accomplish this task has often been recommended but never demonstrated; nor has it been tested empirically. Furthermore, both anecdotal clinical experience and a variety of case reports attest to the danger of this practice. With the bipartite classification, an initial diagnosis of psychogenicity entails ruling out organic disease and is typically required as a precondition to management directed toward the psychologic abnormality. With the tripartite classification, the patient can be given the provisional diagnosis of nonspecific dysfunctional pain and can continue to be monitored for both underlying organic and psychologic pathologic conditions.

Although the tripartite classification may permit more diagnostic flexibility and allow fewer inappropriate assumptions to be made, neither it nor any classification makes the diagnostic process easy when conditions present behaviorally and psychologic factors are involved. Consideration of a number of these factors makes it apparent that defining their diagnostic relationship to abdominal pain in adolescents may be even more difficult.

Developmental Issues

There are two ways in which developmentally appropriate lifestyle issues may serve to complicate the diagnosis of RAP in adolescents. First, it is a rule of thumb that a number of historical features increase the likelihood that pain will be caused by organic disease: weight loss, sleep disturbance, and ability to localize pain in other than the periumbilical area. These factors make sense in preadolescents in whom such symptoms are not part of normal development. However, all three may be related to normal developmental transitions in adolescents. Patients or parents may report noting a weight loss on the basis of a perceived difference from an accumulation of truncal fat that occurred before a growth spurt. More commonly, there may be a perceived and true weight loss resulting from an individual's attempt to become more attractive that is coincidental with the presence of the pain symptom. Unfortunately, such coincidental weight changes can be problematic for both organic and psychogenic diagnoses. If the weight loss is deliberate, recognized, and admitted by the patient, the potential for inappropriately suspecting organic disease is lessened; however, the potential for inappropriately missing coexistent organic disease (e.g., inflammatory bowel disease) is increased. If the weight loss is deliberate but not recognized or admitted by the patient, the potential for inappropriately suspecting organic disease and missing psychogenic illness is increased.

Similarly, changes in sleep pattern are typical of normal adolescent development.[17] Such changes include morning fatigue, "sleeping in," and disrupted sleep schedules. These features are sometimes taken as symptoms of depression and/or organic disease, as they are in adults. As previously mentioned, nonperiumbilical pain is thought to be associated with an increased likelihood of organic etiology in school-age children. However, the ability to localize abdominal pain is a function of increasing age and therefore may be correspondingly less helpful in indicating organicity.[18] This observation seems to be confirmed by our experience, in which nonperiumbilical pain in adolescents may be, but more often is not, associated with organic disease. Lower abdominal pain is also more common in adolescents than in school-age children who meet criteria for irritable bowel syndrome.[16] Furthermore, nonperiumbilical pain is very common with the specific dysfunctional pain characteristic of lactose intolerance, an entity that is likely to be more prevalent in adolescents than in school-age children.

The second way in which developmental changes affect the diagnostic problem in adolescents is the inclusion in the differential diagnosis of abdominal pain complaints referable to the genitourinary tract, especially in females.[1] Many of these entities are related to the increasingly prevalent sexual activity typical of adolescents, and occur in all three of the main classifications of RAP. Included are specific dysfunctional entities, as occur when pain is the presentation of the normal physiologic changes associated with pregnancy, the clearly organic pathology of pelvic inflammatory disease, and the psychogenic conversion reaction providing a defense from ambivalence about sexual identity or fear of sexual abuse.[19] However, depending on age and circumstances, increased sexual activity may be both typical and healthy in adolescence. As with normal adolescent stresses, accurate diagnosis of the etiologic role of sexual activity requires detecting not only that such activity occurs but also whether and how it is related to the abdominal pain.

Sensitivity Differences

In clinical settings, complaints of abdominal pain in the absence of organic disease are often explained as being due to an increased sensitivity to otherwise normal stimuli. However attractive this rationale may seem in principle, there is little empirical substantiation for it and little evidence that such individual sensitivity can be detected in a diagnostically helpful way. Earlier concepts of specific personality profiles (particularly intense, neurotic, anxious, and high-achiever personalities) associated with RAP have not withstood the scrutiny of controlled study. In general, adolescents have a lower sensitivity to pain (as measured by anterior tibial pressure) than do preadolescents, which is consistent with the lower prevalence of reported pain complaints in adolescents.[20] Furthermore, studies attempting to demonstrate an increased sensitivity to physical stimuli in children and adolescents with RAP have shown inconsistent or negative results.[21-23] Consequently, such concepts are yet to be demonstrated to be helpful diagnostically, despite traditional assumptions.

Stress and Anxiety

Another common strategy is to search for evidence of stressful events or anxiety in adolescents to help explain the pain symptoms. Although it is reasonable to identify such factors, the diagnostic significance of such evidence is limited. An important reason is that there is a high prevalence of perceived stress in all families (three to four episodes a month, each lasting 2 to 3 days), indicating a high likelihood of coincidental association with pain episodes.[24] Furthermore, if the caricature of adolescence as a time of Sturm und Drang were true, one might expect a higher prevalence of complaints of abdominal pain in adolescence, which is contrary to the findings of available prevalence studies. Controlled studies focusing on stress factors have been contradictory in their findings; some find positive associations, but most do not. Such inconsistency makes it unlikely that perceived stress and anxiety will be diagnostically helpful, unless direct

evidence of temporal relationships with the pain attacks also can be elicited. Much of this inconsistency can be resolved if a distinction is made between anxiety that is related etiologically to the pain complaint and anxiety that is secondary to the complaint. Secondary anxiety is relatively easy to elicit and is often related to fear that the pain is due to a specific disease process, such as cancer. Even if anxiety and stress are not important diagnostically, they are always important therapeutically.

Family Factors

Typically, family factors have been thought to be relevant for two reasons: (1) because psychologic stress in the family may involve the offspring and (2) because the family may provide the model for pain behavior. However, the lack of consistent evidence of stress, anxiety, and depression in children with RAP has made the first possibility unlikely, at least as a general rule. Similarly, controlled studies have been less likely than uncontrolled ones to find evidence that patients with RAP come from "pain-prone families."[25,26] On the other hand, there is increasingly consistent evidence that the mothers and fathers of patients with RAP do report more anxiety and depression than do the parents of controls.[27,28] This might suggest that familial psychologic stress is implicated in the pain complaint, not so much as an etiologic factor, but because it increases the likelihood that family members will be taken to the physician for their complaints.[24]

Psychopathology

The relationship of various forms of psychopathology to pain complaints can be complicated and diagnostically difficult. Current classifications include hysterical conversion reaction, hypochondriasis, malingering, and psychophysiologic disorders (see Chapter 119, "Conversion Reactions and Psychosomatic Disorders"). All of these entities share the presumption that the pain symptoms are the behavioral manifestation of a disturbed psychologic state, but they differ in their postulated relationship to the pain complaint. Thus, for example, the unpleasant conflict that is being avoided in conversion reactions is unconscious and sometimes symbolic, whereas with malingering the avoidance of an unpleasant experience is conscious. With conversion reaction there may be indifference to the symptom, but with hypochondriasis there is excessive concern. In addition to the problems associated with these conceptual distinctions, diagnosis in adolescents can be difficult because many of the requisite behavioral criteria overlap with behaviors of normal adolescent development. Friedman[19] illustrates some of these difficulties with regard to conversion reaction in adolescents. For example, strict adherence to the requirement that the symptom be unconscious and have symbolic meaning may not be appropriate in adolescents, since the general area of concern (e.g., sexuality) may be identifiable or symptom selection may not necessarily involve a symbolic thought process. Relative indifference to the symptom may be characteristic of conversion reaction, represent a denial of organic disease or pregnancy, or simply be the expression of an age-typical style of increasing bravado. Behaviors characteristic of the "hysterical personality" (nonverbal communication, seductive behavior, dramatization of events) are also common in adolescents without being diagnostic of a conversion reaction. As with organic indicators, such overlap between normal adolescent development and true psychopathology increases the danger of both over- and underdiagnosis of psychogenic abdominal pain.

Organic Factors

In recent years the possibility that organic diseases are etiologically important in larger numbers of adolescents with RAP has been raised by the discovery of *H. pylori*, a gram-negative spiral organism that colonizes the gastric mucosa in humans and is the major cause of gastritis in both children and adults.[29,30] Its role in the cause of duodenal ulceration has been firmly established.[31,32] In children with duodenal ulceration, eradication of *H. pylori* results in complete healing together with resolution of any gastrointestinal symptoms due to the ulcer.[33] However, in the absence of an ulcer, both symptom and treatment studies have failed to support the role of *H. pylori* gastritis as a cause of gastrointestinal symptoms in children.[34-36] Furthermore, in pediatric studies that have specifically addressed the question of *H. pylori* gastritis in RAP syndrome with appropriate controls and/or follow-up, the evidence supporting the role of *H. pylori* in RAP has been weak or nonexistent.[37-41] Studies in adolescents and adults also suggest that *H. pylori* gastritis, in the absence of duodenal disease, is an asymptomatic condition and is not the primary cause of nonulcer dyspepsia.[12-15]

Consequently, *H. pylori* infection is relevant to RAP syndrome but only to the extent that it causes gastritis in association with duodenal ulcer. The symptoms of peptic ulcer disease are distinguishable from those of RAP and are suggested by a history of epigastric pain that is frequently associated with nocturnal awakening and vomiting.

CONCLUSION

Although traditional practice has been based on diagnosis and treatment of clearly defined medical entities, RAP represents an ill-defined syndrome in which etiologic categories are seldom clear. The traditional bivariate classification is inadequate, primarily because it demands that we act on assumptions that are unwarranted, both in general and in the management of particular cases. Furthermore, the diagnostic process may be even more problematic in adolescents because of the overlap between normal adolescent development and the symptoms and signs typically used to delineate organicity and psychogenicity.

As an alternative, the tripartite classification recognizes both classic organic and emotional (psychogenic) etiologies, but also that RAP symptoms may arise from the interaction of normal physiologic and environmental factors, some of which are identifiable (specific dysfunctional RAP) and some of which are not (nonspecific dysfunctional RAP). Furthermore, since most RAP cases are dysfunctional, it is a clinically more relevant approach to use a process strategy rather than a diagnostic strategy. In the process strategy, the complaint is seen as a symptom that must be managed rather than a disease that must be cured. The problem always has three components: (1) assessment of the symptom itself (e.g., frequency, timing, intensity), (2) assessment of the anxiety secondary to the symptom, and (3) assessment of the dysfunction secondary to being an adolescent with the symptom.

Assessment of the symptom includes a comprehensive and thorough history and examination together with traditional medical tests directed at uncovering organic disease. Investigations are handled in a staged and selective manner rather than being done with a "shotgun" approach. In contrast to traditional practice, it is neither necessary nor advisable to rule out all possibility of organic disease in order to "convince" the patient of its absence. Rather, the patient should be monitored periodically for signs of organic illness. Delineation of the meaning of the pain for the patient can be pursued after the initial visit. In our experience, attempts to elicit such information at the first visit commonly increases the patient's reluctance or denial. It is usually easier to "discover" emotionally significant feelings over time than to describe them in response to direct questioning.

Except in referral settings, no specific organic or psychogenic etiology will be defined in most adolescents with RAP. In these patients, management of anxiety secondary to the symptom is important regardless of whether the anxiety is etiologically relevant to the complaint. Such management can be facilitated directly by sensitive interviewing and counseling. It can be facilitated indirectly by having a clear commitment to follow the problem; by recruiting the patient to monitor the course of the symptom, weight changes, and temperature changes; and by having clear instructions as to the indicators of when the patient should see the physician again. Finally, prevention of dysfunction secondary to being a patient with abdominal pain ("extended RAP syndrome"[42]) through interactions with family, peers, school, and the medical care system is critical. Such effects range from inappropriate charges of malingering to prevention of unnecessary, invasive, and painful test procedures. In adolescents with dysfunctional RAP, an appropriate and achievable therapeutic goal is the reduction of three problems to one—namely, the presence of the symptom in an otherwise well and well-adjusted adolescent.

References

1. Barr RG: Abdominal pain in the female adolescent, *Pediatr Rev* 4:281-289, 1983.
2. Boyle JT: Chronic abdominal pain. In Walker WA, Durie PR, Hamilton JR, Walker-Smith JA, Walkins JB, editors: *Pediatric gastrointestinal disease,* vol 1, Philadelphia, 1991, BC Decker; pp 45-54.
3. Oberlander TF, Rappaport LA: Recurrent abdominal pain during childhood, *Pediatr Rev* 14:313-319, 1993.
4. Murphy SM: Management of recurrent abdominal pain, *Arch Dis Child* 69:409-415, 1993.
5. Apley J: *The child with abdominal pain,* London, 1975, Blackwell Scientific.
6. Oster J: Recurrent abdominal pain, headache, and limb pains in children and adolescents, *Pediatrics* 50:429-436, 1972.
7. Bennett DS: Depression among children with chronic medical problems: a metanalysis, *J Pediatr Psychol* 19:149-169, 1994.
8. Borge AIH, Nordhagen R, Moe B, Botten G, Bakketeig LS: Prevalence and persistence of stomach ache and headache among children. Follow-up of a cohort of Norwegian children from 4 to 10 years of age, *Acta Paediatr* 83:433-437, 1994.
9. Pineiro-Carrero VM, Andres JM, Davis RH, Mathias JR: Abnormal gastroduodenal motility in children and adolescents with recurrent functional abdominal pain, *J Pediatr* 113:820-825, 1988.
10. Talley NJ, Phillips SF: Non-ulcer dyspepsia: potential causes and pathophysiology, *Ann Intern Med* 108:865-879, 1988.
11. Malagelada J-R, Stanghellini V: Manometric evaluation of functional upper gut symptoms, *Gastroenterology* 88:1223-1231, 1985.
12. Gormally SM, Drumm B: *Helicobacter pylori* and gastrointestinal symptoms, *Arch Dis Child* 70:165-166, 1994.
13. Dooley CP, Cohen H, Fitzgibbons P, Bauer M, Appleman MD, Perez-Perez GI, Blaser MJ: Prevalence of *Helicobacter pylori* infection and histologic gastritis in asymptomatic persons, *N Engl J Med* 321:1562-1566, 1989.
14. Talley NJ: A critique of therapeutic trials in *Helicobacter pylori*–positive functional dyspepsia, *Gastroenterology* 106:1174-1183, 1994.
15. Bernersen B, Johnsen R, Bostad L, Straume B, Sommer A, Burhol PG: Is *Helicobacter pylori* the cause of dyspepsia?, *BMJ* 304:1276-1279, 1992.
16. Hyams JS, Treem WR, Justinich CJ, Davis P, Shoup M, Burke G: Characterization of symptoms in children with recurrent abdominal pain: resemblance to irritable bowel syndrome, *J Pediatr Gastroenterol Nutr* 20:209-214, 1995.
17. Carskadon MA: Patterns of sleep and sleepiness in adolescents, *Pediatrician* 17:5-12, 1990.
18. Heinild SV, Malner E, Roelsgaard G, Worning B: A psychosomatic approach to recurrent abdominal pain in childhood, *Acta Paediatr Scand* 48:361-270, 1959.
19. Friedman SB: Psychosocial factors in the somatic symptoms of children and adolescents. In Green M, editor: *Psychosocial aspects of the family: the new pediatrics,* Lexington, MA, 1985, Lexington Books; pp 145-156.
20. Haslam DR: Age and the perception of pain, *Psychonomet Sci* 15:86-87, 1969.
21. Apley J, Haslam DR, Tulloch G: Pupillary reaction in children with recurrent pain, *Arch Dis Child* 46:337-340, 1971.
22. Rubin LS, Barbero GJ, Sibinga MS: Pupillary reactivity in children with recurrent abdominal pain, *Psychosom Med* 29:111-120, 1967.
23. Feuerstein M, Barr RG, Francoeur TE, Houle M, Rafman S: Potential biobehavioral mechanisms of recurrent abdominal pain in children, *Pain* 13:287-298, 1982.
24. Roghmann KJ, Haggerty RJ: Daily stress, illness, and use of health services in young families, *Pediatr Res* 7:520-527, 1973.
25. McGrath PJ, Goodman JT, Firestone P, Shipman R, Peters S: Recurrent abdominal pain: a psychogenic disorder?, *Arch Dis Child* 58:888-890, 1983.
26. Faull C, Nicol AR: Abdominal pain in six-year-olds: an epidemiological study in a new town, *J Child Psychol Psychiatry* 27:251-260, 1986.
27. Hodges K, Kline JJ, Barbero G, Flanery R: Depressive symptoms in children with recurrent abdominal pain and their families, *J Pediatr* 107:622-626, 1985.
28. Hodges K, Kline JJ, Barbero G, Woodruff C: Anxiety in children with recurrent abdominal pain and their parents, *Psychosomatics* 26:859-866, 1985.
29. Warren JR, Marshall BJ: Unidentified curved bacilli on gastric epithelium in active chronic gastritis, *Lancet* 1:1273-1275, 1983.
30. Drumm B, Sherman P, Cutz E, Karmali M: Association of *Campylobacter pylori* on the gastric mucosa with antral gastritis in children, *N Engl J Med* 316:1557-1561, 1987.
31. Marshall BJ, Goodwin CS, Warren JR, Murray R, Blincow E, Blackbourn S, Phillips M, Waters T, Sanderson C: Prospective double-blind trial of duodenal ulcer relapse after eradication of *Campylobacter pylori, Lancet* 2:1437-1442, 1988.
32. Coughlan JG, Gilligan D, Humphries H, McKenna D, Dooley C, Sweeney E, Keane C, O'Morain C: *Campylobacter pylori* and recurrence of duodenal ulcers—a 12 month follow-up study, *Lancet* 2:1109-1111, 1987.
33. Israel D, Hassall E: Treatment and long-term follow-up of *Helicobacter pylori*–associated duodenal ulcer disease in children, *J Pediatr* 123:53-58, 1993.
34. Glassman MS, Schwarz SM, Medow MS, Beneck D, Halata M, Berezin S, Newman LJ: *Campylobacter pylori*–related gastrointestinal disease in children. Incidence and clinical findings, *Dig Dis Sci* 34:1501-1504, 1989.
35. Reifen R, Rasooly I, Drumm B, Millson ME, Murphy K, Sherman PM: *Helicobacter pylori* infection in children: is there specific symptomatology?, *Dig Dis Sci* 39:1488-1492, 1994.
36. Gormally SM, Prakash N, Durnin M, Daly L, Clyne M, Kierce BM, Drumm B: Association of symptoms with *Helicobacter pylori* infection in children, *J Pediatr* 126:753-756, 1995.
37. Van der Meer SB, Forget PP, Loffeld RJLF, Stobberingh E, Kuijten RH, Arends JW: The prevalence of *Helicobacter pylori* serum antibodies in children with recurrent abdominal pain, *Eur J Pediatr* 151:799-801, 1992.
38. Fiedorek SC, Casteel HB, Pumphrey CL, Evans DJ, Evans DG, Klein PD, Graham DY: The role of *Helicobacter pylori* in recurrent, functional abdominal pain in children, *Am J Gastroenterol* 87:347-349, 1992.
39. Mavromichalis I, Zaramboukas T, Richman PI, Slavin G: Recurrent abdominal pain of gastrointestinal origin, *Eur J Pediatr* 151:560-563, 1992.
40. Oderda G, Vaira D, Holton J, Dowsett JF, Ansaldi N: Serum pepsinogen I and IgG antibody in non-specific abdominal pain in childhood, *Gut* 30:912-916, 1989.
41. Macarthur C, Saunders N, Feldman W: *Helicobacter pylori,* gastroduodenal disease and recurrent abdominal pain in children, *JAMA* 273:729-734, 1995.
42. Barr RG, Feuerstein M: Recurrent abdominal pain syndrome: how appropriate are our basic clinical assumptions? In Firestone P, McGrath P, editors: *Pediatric and adolescent behavioral medicine,* New York, 1983, Springer-Verlag; pp 13-27.

CHAPTER 107

Chronic Fatigue Syndrome

•

Leonard R. Krilov and Stanford B. Friedman

Chronic fatigue syndrome (CFS) has been defined by a panel of researchers convened by the Centers for Disease Control and Prevention (CDC) to describe a group of patients with debilitating fatigue in association with a set of nonspecific symptoms.[1] The definition was revised and simplified in 1994 (see Box 107-1).[2] At present, no causative agent has been identified for this syndrome, although over the past decades a number of diseases were considered etiologic in patients with similar symptom complexes. These included chronic brucellosis, chronic candidiasis, chronic mononucleosis (chronic Epstein-Barr virus [EBV] infection), chronic human herpesvirus 6, and chronic enterovirus infection. Potential retroviral and spumavirus etiologies for CFS have been reported,[3] but the CDC was unable to reproduce either finding in a blinded study.[4] Over the years a variety of other syndromes that appear to be equivalent to CFS have been described,[5] including total allergy syndrome, hypoglycemia, myalgic encephalomyelitis, postviral asthenia, Iceland disease, Royal Free disease, and fibromyalgia.

POSSIBLE ROLE OF EPSTEIN-BARR VIRUS

Among entities that have been considered as possible causes of CFS, chronic mononucleosis and chronic EBV syndrome have been reported most often in the medical literature since the early 1980s.[6,7] A review of these reports and the subsequent doubts raised about persistent active EBV infection as the cause of CFS provides much useful insight into our present understanding of CFS.

EBV is a ubiquitous herpesvirus that persists in human B lymphocytes and salivary glands for life after acute infection, and antibody responses to the virus are also lifelong. Acute infectious mononucleosis, the primary clinical manifestation of primary EBV infection, is characterized by fatigue, lethargy, pharyngitis, and adenitis lasting 2 to 3 weeks. There are severe and/or malignant syndromes associated with EBV infection, including fatal disseminated lymphoproliferation and lymphomas in immunocompromised hosts. Given the ability of EBV to cause prolonged illnesses, the similarity of many symptoms of CFS to an acute mononucleosis that has not resolved, and the recognition that many individuals with CFS describe the onset of their symptoms in terms of a documented mononucleosis or mononucleosis-like illness, EBV has been considered a potential etiologic agent for this syndrome of prolonged fatigue. In the reports associating EBV with a syndrome of chronic fatigue, investigators have reported abnormal host antibody response to a panel of EBV antigens[6,7] (Table 107-1). However, subsequent analyses have revealed that 10% to 20% of individuals who have fully recovered from acute EBV infection have the same EBV antibody responses (i.e., elevated IgG to the viral capsid antigen [VCA] of EBV, persistence of antibody to the early antigen [EA], and lack of detectable antibody to the Epstein-Barr nuclear antigen [EBNA]).[8]

Additionally, inter-laboratory analyses of patients' sera have demonstrated great variability in results, and different laboratories have not been able to differentiate individual patients from control subjects reliably.[9] Furthermore, the prevalence and load of EBV isolated from the orpharynx and blood of patients with CFS is not different from that in the general population.[10] For a number of the other purported etiologic agents of CFS (e.g., *Brucella, Candida,* enteroviruses, and in some cases the Lyme disease organism), the same difficulties in differentiating active infection from past infection exist. Finally, a double-blind placebo-controlled trial at the National Institutes of Health demonstrated no therapeutic benefit or immunologic improvement with antiviral (acyclovir) treatment in patients defined as having chronic mononucleosis syndrome.[11] From such analyses, present understanding suggests that CFS cannot be attributed to ongoing infection but rather to postinfectious responses that can be triggered by any of a number of agents.

BOX 107-1
Case Definition of CFS*

1. New onset of persistent or relapsing fatigue (daily activity below 50% of premorbid level) for >6 months; plus
2. Exclusion of other clinical conditions causing similar symptoms based on history, physical examination, and laboratory evaluations; plus
3. At least four of the following:
   a. Self-reported impairment in short-term memory or concentration
   b. Sore throat
   c. Tender cervical or axillary lymph nodes
   d. Muscle pain
   e. Polyarthralgias without erythema or swelling
   f. Headaches (new type, pattern, or severity)
   g. Unrefreshing sleep
   h. Postexertional malaise lasting >24 hours

*Modified from Fukuda K, Straus SE, Hickie I, et al: The chronic fatigue syndrome: a comprehensive approach to its definition and study, *Ann Intern Med* 121:953-959, 1994.

TABLE 107-1
Pattern of Antibody Response to Epstein-Barr Virus Infection

	EBV Viral Capsid Antigen (VCA)		Early Antigen (EA)	Epstein-Barr Nuclear Antigen (EBNA)
	IgM	IgG		
No EBV infection	−	−	−	−
Acute mononucleosis	+	+ (≥1:320)	+/−	−
Past EBV infection	−	+ (1:80-1:160)	−	+
"Chronic EBV"*	−	+ (≥1:640)	+	−

*A similar pattern has been described in 10% to 20% of normal individuals who have recovered from infectious mononucleosis.

PSYCHOLOGIC FACTORS

Although a viral cause of CFS has been suspected for many years, it has never been demonstrated conclusively. Moreover, it has been repeatedly suggested that psychologic factors influence the natural course of EBV infection. For instance, Greenfield et al[12] reported that lack of "ego strength," as measured by the Minnesota Multiphasic Personality Inventory (MMPI), was involved in the rate of recovery among college students identified as having infectious mononucleosis. Furthermore, in a seminal study conducted at the U.S. Military Academy at West Point, Kasl et al[13] clearly indicated that psychologic factors were involved in the seroconversion rate of antibodies to EBV and also were related to the development and course of infectious mononucleosis among the 1400 cadets studied. This and other investigations have led to speculation that CFS may be the result of an interaction between EBV and psychologic factors, including the possibility that response to psychologic stress may play a major etiologic role in many instances.

However, CFS appears to have a tenuous relationship to EBV and to any single agent thus far identified as being associated with it. Therefore, it has been postulated that the search for a viral or other infectious etiologic basis will be unsuccessful. In addition, because this search is based on a simplistic assumption that many infectious illnesses are associated with fatigue, a logical extension is to consider the CFS as having an infectious etiology. However, it should be noted that fatigue is associated with many other, if not most other, disease processes. Because of the inability to identify an etiologic agent for CFS, it

has been proposed by some authors that this syndrome is actually the result of psychologic or emotional problems and therefore should be viewed as a psychosomatic (or psychiatric) disorder. It has been further suggested that many cases of CFS would have been diagnosed as neurasthenia in the past, an entity that also was never clearly defined, in terms of either etiology or clinical course.

Clinicians and investigators have noted a relationship of CFS to depressive symptoms, frank depression, and/or a family history of depression. However, there has been disagreement over whether the depressive elements are causative or the result of CFS. In fact, this may be a meaningless argument, since depression may be a psychologic factor (although not necessarily the only psychologic factor) playing a role in the etiology of the syndrome *and* be the result of having CFS. It is not necessarily an either/or situation.

In our experience, we have been impressed with the family dynamics of the adolescents with CFS we have seen. In many of these families, overprotection and overindulgence of the patient have been noted, and in some instances there has been extreme difficulty in mother-adolescent separation. We also have noted high expectations, relative to the adolescent's abilities, on the part of some of the parents, and that these expectations sometimes are superimposed on the overprotection. The complaint of chronic fatigue may result in enormous secondary gain for the adolescent, such as continuation of overprotection and provision of an excuse not to attend school. The possibility exists that in many cases the adolescent with CFS may represent a conversion reaction, perhaps based on symptoms and complaints associated with an earlier actual viral infection (e.g., EBV). The viral infection therefore serves as the model for later conversion reactions (see Chapter 119, "Conversion Reactions and Psychosomatic Disorders").

EPIDEMIOLOGY

The median age of patients with CFS described in the literature is 37 years.[14] However, some series of patients with CFS include adolescents,[15-17] and children under 11 years of age also have been described as having CFS. Up to 70% of individuals diagnosed with CFS are female, and most cases involve individuals from high socioeconomic groups. Blacks, the indigent, and Third World populations are strikingly underrepresented in reports of CFS.

CLINICAL MANIFESTATIONS

The primary symptom of CFS is fatigue-limited activity equal to less than 50% of the premorbid level of function.[1] Associated symptoms (Box 107-1) do resemble many of the findings seen in infectious mononucleosis. Most patients describe a sudden onset of the illness with an initial flulike or mononucleosis-like illness.

Up to 50% of cases may have abnormalities on physical examination, including (1) a mildly inflamed pharynx, (2) cervical adenopathy, and/or (3) low-grade temperature elevations in up to 50% of cases. However, the primary focus of the physical examination is to eliminate other known causes of the patient's symptoms. Significantly elevated temperatures, enlarged lymph nodes (>2 cm), or weight loss of more than 10% of body weight without dieting should suggest an alternative diagnosis. The differential diagnoses to be considered are outlined in Box 107-2.

LABORATORY DIAGNOSIS

There are no specific laboratory tests to aid in the diagnosis of CFS. As with the physical examination, the primary aim of laboratory evaluations is to eliminate other illnesses that may be responsible for the patient's symptoms. Laboratory evaluations to be considered in screening for CFS are outlined in Box 107-3. Investigators have described a number of immunologic abnormalities, including altered lymphocyte subsets, qualitative defects in natural killer-cell activity, abnormal lymphokine levels, decreased lymphocyte proliferation, and delayed types of hypersensitivity response. However, these findings have not been consistently observed in different groups of patients and would not adequately account for all the symptoms described in CFS.[18,19]

A 1995 report suggested that at least a subset of adolescent patients with CFS may suffer from neurally mediated hypotension as diagnosed by tilt-table testing and may respond to increased salt intake and/or drug therapy.[20] Further controlled studies are needed to determine whether these findings apply to a significant proportion of individuals with CFS.

BOX 107-2
Differential Diagnosis of CFS

Malignancy
Autoimmune disease
Localized infection (e.g., sinusitis, occult abscess)
Chronic or subacute infection (e.g., endocarditis, tuberculosis, Lyme disease)
HIV infection
Fungal disease (e.g., histoplasmosis, coccidiomycosis, blastomycosis)
Parasitic disease (e.g., toxoplasmosis, giardiasis)
Chronic psychiatric disease
Endocrine disease (e.g., hypothyroidism, Addison's disease, diabetes mellitus)
Chronic inflammatory disease (e.g., sarcoid, Wegener's granulomatosis)
Neuromuscular disease (e.g., myasthenia gravis, multiple sclerosis)
Drug dependency
Side effects of chronic medications or other toxic agent (e.g., chemical solvent, heavy metal, pesticide)
Other defined chronic pulmonary, cardiac, gastrointestinal, hepatic, renal, or hematologic disease

---

BOX 107-3
Laboratory Evaluations for CFS

Complete blood count and differential
Erythrocyte sedimentation rate (ESR)
Serum electrolyte, creantinine, BUN, glucose levels
Liver function tests, alkaline phosphatase test
Thyroid function tests
Antinuclear antibody (ANA), rheumatoid factor (RF)
HIV antibody
Tuberculin skin test with controls
Chest x-ray examination
Sinus x-ray examination

THERAPY

No specific therapy has been accepted for CFS. A trial of acyclovir in CFS patients was unsuccessful.[9] Immunomodulating therapy with liver extract–folic acid–cyanocobalamin was not effective in improving functional status or alleviating the symptoms of CFS when studied in a controlled fashion.[21] Intravenous immunoglobulin therapy for CFS is being evaluated, but studies in small numbers of patients have yielded conflicting results.[22,23] Megavitamin and/or dietary therapies have not been critically evaluated.

Our present approach to the management of adolescents with CFS is to arrange follow-up visits to explore psychosocial issues that might be contributing to the patient's symptoms, to monitor progress, and to permit identification of previous occult disease. A major role for the physician is to help the family avoid unwarranted expense, to minimize "doctor shopping," and to avoid the performance of unnecessary medical procedures. The involvement of numerous physicians, especially with a lack of communication among them, and the ordering of inappropriate laboratory tests only reinforce the illness behavior. Fortunately, long-term follow-up of adolescents with CFS suggests that the long-term prognosis is good, with most patients showing improvement and/or resolution of symptoms over 1 to 2 years.[16]

References

1. Holmes GP, Kaplan JE, Gantz NM, et al: Chronic fatigue syndrome: a working case definition, *Ann Intern Med* 108:387-389, 1988.
2. Fukuda K, Straus SE, Hickie I, et al: The chronic fatigue syndrome: a comprehensive approach to its definition and study, *Ann Intern Med* 121:953-959, 1994.
3. DeFritas E, Hilliard B, Cheney PR, et al: Retroviral sequences related to human T-lymphotropic virus type II in patients with chronic immune dysfunction syndrome, *Proc Natl Acad Sci USA* 88:2922-2926, 1991.
4. Heineine W, Woods TC, Sinha SD, et al: Lack of evidence for infection with known human and animal retroviruses in patients with chronic fatigue syndrome, *Clin Infect Dis* 18 (suppl 1):S121-S125, 1994.
5. Straus SE: History of chronic fatigue syndrome, *Rev Infect Dis* 13 (suppl 1):S2-S7, 1991.
6. Jones JF, Ray CG, Minnich LL, et al: Evidence for active Epstein-Barr virus infection in patients with persistent unexplained illnesses: elevated anti-early antigen antibodies, *Ann Intern Med* 102:1-7, 1985.
7. Straus SE, Tosato G, Armstrong G, et al: Persisting illness and fatigue in adults with evidence of Epstein-Barr virus infection, *Ann Intern Med* 102:7-16, 1985.
8. Horowitz CA, Henle W, Henle G, et al: Long-term serological follow-up of patients for Epstein-Barr virus after recovery from infectious mononucleosis, *J Infect Dis* 151:1150-1153, 1985.
9. Katz BZ, Andiman WA: Chronic fatigue syndrome, *J Pediatr* 113:944-947, 1988.
10. Sumaya CV: Serological testing for Epstein-Barr virus—developments in interpretation, *J Infect Dis* 151:984-987, 1985.
11. Straus SE, Dale JK, Tobi M, et al: Acyclovir treatment of the chronic fatigue syndrome, *N Engl J Med* 319:1692-1698, 1988.
12. Greenfield NS, Roessler R, Archer P, Crosley A: Ego strength and length of recovery from infectious mononucleosis, *J Nerv Ment Dis* 128:125, 1959.
13. Kasl S, Evans AS, Niederman JC: Psychosocial risk factors in the development of infectious mononucleosis, *Psychosom Med* 41:445, 1979.
14. Komaroff AC, Buchwald D: Symptoms and signs of chronic fatigue syndrome, *Rev Infect Dis* 13(suppl):S8-S11, 1991.
15. Smith MS, Mitchell J, Corey L, et al: Chronic fatigue in adolescents, *Pediatrics* 88:195-202, 1991.
16. Carter BD, Edwards JF, Kronenberger WG, et al: Case control study of chronic fatigue in pediatric patients, *Pediatrics* 95:179-186, 1995.
17. Bell KM, Cookafair D, Bell DS, et al: Risk factors associated with chronic fatigue syndrome in a cluster of pediatric cases, *Rev Infect Dis* 13 (suppl):S32-S38, 1991.
18. Klimas NG, Salvato FR, Morgan R, Fletcher MA: Immunologic abnormalities in chronic fatigue syndrome, *J Clin Microbiol* 28:1403-1410, 1991.
19. Straus SE, Dale JK, Peter JB, Dinarello CA: Circulating lymphokine levels in chronic fatigue syndrome, *J Infect Dis* 160:1085-1086, 1989.
20. Rowe PC, Bou-Holaigah I, Kan JS, Calkins H: Is neurally mediated hypotension an unrecognized cause of chronic fatigue?, *Lancet* 345:623-624, 1995.
21. Kaslow JE, Rucker L, Onishi R: Liver extract–folic acid–cyanocobalamin vs. placebo for chronic fatigue syndrome, *Arch Intern Med* 149:2501-2503, 1989.
22. Lloyd A, Hickie I, Wakefield O, Boughton C, Dwyer J: A double-blind, placebo-controlled trial of intravenous immunoglobulin therapy in patients with chronic fatigue syndrome, *Am J Med* 89:561-568, 1990.
23. Peterson PK, Shepard J, Macres M, et al: A controlled trial of intravenous immunoglobulin G in chronic fatigue syndrome, *Am J Med* 89:554-560, 1990.

CHAPTER 108

Substance Use and Abuse

•

Richard G. MacKenzie and Michele D. Kipke

The prevalence of alcohol and other drug use among adolescents in the United States has fluctuated over the past 20 years. During the mid-1970s and early 1980s, there was a steady increase in illicit drug use that prompted the initiation of two national surveys designed to monitor prevalence, trends in use, and changes in attitudes. The annual Monitoring the Future Study initiated in 1975 assesses use among 50,000 students in over 400 public and private secondary schools nation-wide.[1] Although this survey provides important information about trends among a general population of adolescents, it excludes those adolescents who dropped out of secondary school (as many as 30% or more of students in some urban areas) and who, ironically, may be even more heavily involved in drugs. The National Household Survey on Drug Abuse[2] attempts to overcome this deficiency by focusing on households rather than schools. Thus, it includes a broader range of young people. This survey also permits comparisons between various age groups: youths (ages 12 to 17 years), young adults (ages 18 to 25 years), and older adults (ages 26 years and older). Results from both of these surveys have revealed that illicit drug use reached its peak in the mid-1980s and then decreased. This trend was reversed in the early 1990s, showing a significant resurgence of drug use among eighth, tenth, and twelfth graders and in 12- to 17-year-olds in the National Household Survey. For example, in 1980, 65% of high school seniors reported that they had ever used an illicit substance. Eight years later, in 1988, 54% of seniors reported use of an illicit drug, a reduction of nearly 11%. In 1992, this fell to its lowest point of 41%, but it rose again to 51% in 1996. The following discussions provide a summary of the findings from these surveys, including the prevalence and patterns of alcohol and other drug use among adolescents.

For all drugs, beliefs about harmfulness predict changes in prevalence of use. The proportion of students viewing drugs as harmful continued to decline, particularly in relation to marijuana but did so much more slowly than in the previous few years. Perceived risk from use was also decreased for crack cocaine and lysergic acid diethylamide (LSD), but also less than in previous years. Other influences on drug use, such as peer disapproval, also continued to decline in the 1996 survey.

Alcohol

Alcohol is the most popular drug used by adolescents in the United States. Because of its availability and relatively low cost, it is often the first drug used by teenagers. As many as 4.6 million U.S. adolescents 14 to 17 years old are estimated to be problem drinkers. There has been a steady decline in prevalence of having "ever used" any alcohol (lifetime use) since the early 1980s, but this has leveled off in the 1990s. Approximately 80% of teenagers will have tried alcohol at least once by their eighteenth birthday, a decline of almost 10% over the last decade. In 1996, 51% of high school seniors, reported having used alcohol in the previous month, and 3.7% reported daily use. Almost 31% reported having had a recent occasion of heavy drinking (defined as five or more drinks in a row during the previous 2 weeks). Compared with 1992, all categories based on patterns of drinking showed an increase.

Males tend to initiate alcohol use when they are almost a year younger than females. They also report more frequent and heavier use. A biracial comparison of use indicates that white males have the highest rates of alcohol use. Rates of drinking in white females are comparable with those in black males.

Tobacco

Tobacco is the substance most frequently used by adolescents on a daily basis. It is also the single most important preventable cause of morbidity and premature mortality in all age groups. Experimentation with tobacco by adolescents is more likely to lead to dependence than experimentation with any other drug. Although the prevalence of daily smoking by high school students dropped from 1977 to 1981 (from 26% to 20%), there has been a distinct trend to increased prevalence of daily use by seniors (22% in 1996). Comparable increases in daily use were also noted among eighth and tenth graders. Before 1970, male adolescents smoked considerably more than females. Since 1970, rates have fallen in males and risen in females. At present, there is no appreciable sex difference in cigarette smoking, but what differences there are suggests that females are smoking more than males. For daily use of one-half pack of cigarettes per day, the rates are 12% for females and 11% for males.

Initiation of smoking usually occurs in grades 7 through 9. Very few young people initiate smoking after completion of high school. More than 90% of adult smokers therefore begin before age 20; 60% begin before age 14. In both humans and animals, tachyphylaxis may be seen after a single dose of nicotine. Therefore, the high school age cluster has become an important audience for industry advertising.

Of all the addictions, nicotine is among the most difficult to overcome, owing to a complex interaction of external and internal cues. Regular use therefore rapidly leads to compulsive use. It is estimated that over 50% of those in high school who smoke one-half pack of cigarettes or more per day will have great difficulty in stopping. Of those in high school who smoke on a daily basis, three fourths are still smoking on a daily basis 7 to 9 years later. Nicotine is considered one of the easiest chemical dependencies to establish. Nicotine addiction is such that as many as 85% of adolescents who smoke two or more cigarettes completely and overcome the initial discomfort will go on to become regular smokers. It is rare that an individual becomes an occasional user.

Cigarette smoking also bears a strong positive correlation with use of alcohol and other drugs (marijuana in particular). Of the pack-a-day smokers in high school, 95% had used an illicit substance, 81% had used an illicit drug other than marijuana, and 26% were currently daily users of an illicit drug (most commonly marijuana).[2]

Marijuana

Marijuana remains the second most frequently used drug and the most popular illicit drug used by adolescents and young adults. In the 1995 Monitoring the Future Study, it continued to show a strong resurgence of use at the eighth, tenth, and twelfth grade levels. Among eighth graders, annual prevalence of use increased from 7% in 1992 to 18% in 1996. In tenth graders, this rose from 15% in 1992 to almost 34% in 1996, a near doubling of those reporting use in the past year. Annual prevalence among twelfth graders rose from 22% in 1992 to 36% in 1996. Notable was the increase in daily use: almost 5% in seniors and 3.5% in tenth graders.

Marijuana use often progresses in a fairly predictable, stepwise fashion—from experimentation to occasional social use to regular social use. Active seeking and buying of quantities of marijuana (drug-seeking behavior) is another indicator of an increasing commitment to drug use. Of significance is the potency of the drug available to the user. The quality of the marijuana has increased over the past decade. What was previously a low-dose experimentation has become a high-potency, high-reward/reinforcement pattern of use with a predisposition to dependency. Like tobacco, marijuana may be considered a "gateway" drug because its use is often associated with a progression toward other illicit drugs. Indeed, the single most powerful predictor of cocaine use is frequent use of marijuana during adolescence.

Cocaine

Although once a favorite drug used only by the affluent, cocaine has rapidly become a preferred drug among teenagers. The price of cocaine has dropped over the last few years, and newer forms make it readily accessible to anyone. Therefore, cocaine and its congeners has become the second most frequently used illicit substance (marijuana is the first). In 1996, 7% of high school seniors reported having tried cocaine, an increase of 1% since 1995.

Cocaine's popularity with adolescents is reinforced by the sense of euphoria and self-confidence that it produces, two feelings that are greatly desired by adolescents, who by nature are less confident than they would like to be. The effects are immediate, occurring within minutes, thus providing instant positive reinforcement and gratification. The effects of cocaine peak within 20 to 60 minutes, with a gradual decline in effect over the following hours. The adolescent often feels the need to use the drug continually (runs) in an attempt to sustain the positive experience and to avoid the subsequent rebound dysphoria, depression, and fatigue.

Crack, a congener of cocaine, is inexpensive and readily available throughout the United States. It is made by "cooking" cocaine hydrochloride with ammonia or baking soda and water. When the substance hardens, it is molded and cut into approximately 100-mg chips or "rocks," which sell for $5 to $10 each. Because crack is poorly soluble in water, it is smoked. It is usually not used intranasally or injected. When crack is smoked, the vapors are inhaled deeply through a special glass pipe or a crude, homemade apparatus usually fashioned from an aluminum beverage can. Deeply inhaled crack vapors are almost immediately absorbed from the lungs into the pulmonary microcirculation. Crack reaches the dopaminergic and adrenergic neurotransmitter–mediated pleasure centers of the brain in 8 seconds and produces an immediate and intense euphoria that lasts for about 5 to

10 minutes. Euphoria is followed rapidly by an equally intense depression and cravings for more—a process that can greatly accelerate the cycle of compulsive use.

Adolescents prefer crack for several reasons. For some, smoking crack is less frightening than snorting the cocaine powder. Crack can be purchased in smaller quantities than cocaine, which is also more expensive than crack. Crack is usually contained in small vials, which makes carrying it convenient. Finally, the effects of crack are more intense than those of cocaine.

Contrary to the common belief that crack is used only by poor, urban minorities, data suggest that crack use is not uncommon among middle-class, nonminority youth. Of the high school seniors surveyed in 1996, 3.3% reported having used crack at some time in their lives, with 2% reporting use in the previous 12 months and 1% use in the 30 days before the survey. In a study of largely white, middle-class, drug-using suburban teenagers enrolled in outpatient drug treatment, 28% reported having smoked crack.[3] An analysis of use patterns revealed that 67% of the crack users were experimenters, having used crack one to nine times; 15% could be classified as intermediate users, having smoked crack 10 to 50 times; and 18% were heavy users, who reported having smoked crack more than 50 times. These youths reported a rapid onset of addiction to crack; 60% of the heavy users had progressed from initiation to use of the drug at least once a week in less than 3 months. Nearly 50% of the experimenters and almost all of the heavy users recalled preoccupation with thoughts of crack (encapsulation), rapid loss of the ability to modulate their use of the drug, and rapid development of pharmacologic tolerance. Suspiciousness, mistrust, and depressed mood were often associated with increased crack use.

Amphetamines and Other Stimulants

Amphetamine use is also popular among adolescents, particularly females. Like cocaine, amphetamines give the adolescent a sense of increased energy, self-confidence, and well-being along with a heightened awareness, loss of appetite (commonly used by females as a method of weight control or loss), and euphoria. In 1996, "having ever used" stimulants was reported by 13.5% of eighth graders, almost 18% of tenth graders, and 15% of seniors. Approximately 4% to 5% of all grade levels reported use in the 30 days before the survey.

Methamphetamine, known on the street as "speed," "crystal," "go," "crank," and most recently "ice," is potent in its psychostimulant actions. The new analog, "ice," is a pure crystaline form of D-methamphetamine that is becoming increasingly popular among adolescents. "Ice," which appears as transparent, sheetlike crystals, like crack, is smoked. One of the reasons "ice" has

become so popular is that the effects derived from smoking it are similar to those produced by an intravenous dose without the hazards of needle use. The effects of both amphetamine and "ice" last longer than those of cocaine and crack—up to several hours longer. Lifetime prevalence of use of "ice" among high school seniors was 4.4% in 1996. This reflects a continuing increase over previous years.

Use of other stimulants such as methylphenidate (Ritalin), ephedrine, and herbal mixtures have become regionally popular. Nationally, 0.8% of high school seniors in 1995 reported using methylphenidate without a doctor's prescription. Methylphenidate, commonly prescribed for attention deficit disorder, can easily find its way into the reservoir of mood-altering drugs used by adolescents. Like other stimulants, these drugs can make the user hyperexcitable, anxious, moody, and irritable.

Inhalants

This group of drugs contains a variety of chemicals, including spray and liquid paints, organic solvents and degreasers, typewriter correction fluid, spot removers, Freon, gasoline, other petrochemicals and glue. Inhalants are cheap, readily available chemicals found in almost any household and, most importantly, are not illegal. They are often the first mind-altering substance used by preadolescents who later, as adolescents, advance to other substances. Inhalants are often the only drugs used by adolescents and preadolescents in developing countries, and conspicuous street use is not uncommon. The overall proportion of high school seniors reporting lifetime prevalence of toluene and petrochemical-based inhalants (having ever used) has significantly increased since the initiation of the survey in 1975 (10.3%) to the 1996 survey (16.9%).

Amyl nitrite– and butyl nitrite–based inhalants have decreased in popularity by approximately eight- to tenfold since the mid-1980s. The anesthetic gas nitrous oxide, also known as "laughing gas," is used as a propellant for whipped cream, and also as a power booster for automobiles and motorcycles. Clusters of increased use, usually on a regional basis, are not uncommon. Physiologic dependence on these drugs appears to be uncommon, although mood and environmental reinforcers may be present, thus encouraging patterned use.

Hallucinogens

The hallucinogen class of drugs include LSD, peyote, mescaline, psilocybine (mushrooms), dimethyltryptamine (DMT), morning glory seeds, dimethoxy-4-methylamphetamine (DOM, STP), methylenedioxy-methamphetamine (MDMA, Adam and Eve, Ecstasy), jimsonweed *(Datura stramonium),* and phencyclidine

(PCP). The term *hallucinogen* is actually a misnomer, since these drugs generally produce illusions or distortion of reality rather than hallucinations. The expectation of the user and the setting in which the drug is taken greatly influence the experience. Tolerance develops rapidly, and therefore use tends to be infrequent.

Overall, the prevalence of use of these drugs decreased steadily in the 1980s from a peak level seen in the 1960s and 1970s, but recently there has been a significant increase in use. From 1990 to 1996, lifetime prevalence of use increased from 9% of seniors to almost 14%. Most of this increase was due to the use of LSD. Increase in prevalence of lifetime use was also noted in eighth and tenth graders but to a lesser degree.

Opiates

Although opiates are not commonly used by adolescents as recreational drugs, they are available throughout the United States. They tend to be favored by hard-core drug abusers. In 1996, among high school seniors, 8.2% reported having ever used an opiate; almost 2% reported having ever used heroin. Interestingly, in this survey, lifetime prevalence of heroin use by eighth graders exceeded that of tenth and twelfth graders (2.4% vs. 2.1% and 1.8%, respectively). Anecdotal reports of increased use on mainstream high school and university campuses began to appear in mid-1996 but have yet to be confirmed by systematic study.

Polydrug Use

Adolescents often use several drugs simultaneously or use drugs on the basis of market availability or what they can afford. No clear pattern of use is apparent. This is often referred to "polydrug use." The drug combination may be used to achieve a desired "high" or to modulate the experience of "coming down" from the high. For example, a depressant (e.g., alcohol, marijuana) is commonly used with a stimulant (e.g., cocaine, amphetamines) to enhance the effects of one of the drugs, to lengthen the period during which the high is experienced and to avoid the negative or "crashing" sensation common when the initial high diminishes (particularly with crack and amphetamines). Polydrug use complicates diagnosis and treatment and may put the adolescent at even greater risk for developing physical and mental health complications.

Polydrug use may also be manifested as sequential use of whatever drug is available. The specific drug used depends on availability, affordability, and the circumstance of the user. It is not uncommon for adolescents and young adults to take "drugs" that are of uncertain purity and nature, driven by peer pressure or internal dysphoric sensations.

PHYSIOLOGY AND PHARMACOLOGY

Developments in the fields of the basic neurosciences have enhanced our understanding of drug-seeking behavior and the acquisition of functional tolerance and dependence. The exact neurochemical pathways elude definition. Both excitatory and inhibitory transmitter defects have been proposed. Dopamine, a neurotransmitter, plays a significant role in addiction to stimulants, especially amphetamines and cocaine. It has also been shown to play a central role in mediating sensations of pleasure and pain. A clearer understanding of such neurotransmitters as serotonin, GABA, and norepinephrine, along with the various types of neuroreceptor, now forms the basis for comprehending addiction on a molecular basis.

Familial and genetic factors establish the setting in which biologic and social risk factors converge. The degree to which these forces interact define a "vulnerability syndrome" and thus an at-risk individual. How these various factors and influences blend together governs the decision to use drugs, and the subsequent pattern of use is governed by the unique interaction of these forces. For adolescents, the demands of psychologic and social development establish the need for problem-solving and coping responses. This challenge alone may lead to drug or alcohol use. Familial and genetic factors may now act to reinforce the drug use. The social ecology of adolescence thus reinforces the need for a problem-solving behavior. Unique neurobiologic characteristics act to sustain it.

Clinical manifestations of substance abuse appear on a spectrum of symptomatic expression that reflects, to varying degrees, the severity of the disorder. This spectrum of severity extends from the experimental user or "taster" responding to peer influence or curiosity to the individual whose genetic and neurobiologic destiny will be manifested in a drug-using life style. Those in the middle (gray) zone, who are largely social users (explorers), present the greatest challenge to the clinician in determining those at risk for developing a drug dependence or preoccupation. Fortunately, most adolescents greatly lessen or abandon drug use as they mature into adulthood.

Drugs of abuse have the common property of promoting an increased sense of well-being. This pleasure-producing sensation is often accompanied by a false sense of security and increased bravado, and confidence, and sexual prowess. These desired physical and psychologic actions may be complicated by adverse effects, toxic or idiosyncratic reactions, a temporary loss of self-control, impairment of integrative central nervous system (CNS) function, and chemical dependence.

Drugs that primarily produce a modified psychologic experience are extremely prone to external influences.

BOX 108-1
Factors Influencing Drug Effects

Dose of drug
Method of administration
Setting in which drug is taken
Expectation that user has about effects of drug
Personality and psychologic state of user
Purity of compound used
Frequency with which drug is taken

BOX 108-2
Categories of Drugs Commonly Abused

Depressants
  Alcohol
  Barbiturates
  Nonbarbiturate sedatives (especially methaqualone)
  Minor tranquilizers
Stimulants
  Amphetamines
  Cocaine
  Methylphenidate/pephedrine
  Nicotine
  Caffeine
Hallucinogens/illusionogens
  Marijuana
  Lysergic acid diethylamide (LSD)
  Mescaline
  Dimethyltryptamine (DMT)
  Phencyclidine (PCP)
  Psilocybine
  Methylenedioxymethamphetamine (MDMA)
Opiates
  Heroin
  Morphine/meperidine
  Codeine
  Methadone
Volatile agents
  Toluene-based glues and paints
  Gasoline
  Alkyl nitrites
  Triethylene chloride (in typewriter correction fluid)

Therefore, the effect that any drug has on an adolescent is dependent on a number of factors, some of which are determined by the user rather than by the drug itself (Box 108-1).

Pharmacology

A basic understanding of the pharmacologic properties of the drugs commonly used by young people helps to guide medical intervention during the acute phase but not necessarily the drug rehabilitation program. There follows a brief review of the pharmacologic issues of chemical dependence. Principles for the management of intoxication and overdose are reviewed in Chapter 75. Drugs commonly used by adolescents fall into five general categories (Box 108-2).

Alcohol

The concentration of ethanol, the active ingredient in all alcoholic beverages, determines the effect. Alcohol absorption is dependent on gastric emptying time and can be delayed in the presence of food. Alcohol is absorbed in the stomach, small intestine, and colon. Maximal serum concentration is attained over 30 to 90 minutes. This is modulated by the enzyme alcohol dehydrogenase found in both the liver and the gastric mucosa, by body size, and by metabolic tolerance. CNS adaptation also contributes to the tolerant state. The healthy liver is capable of breaking down about 10 to 12 ounces of beer per hour.

At low doses, ethanol acts as a behavioral stimulant. The well-known effects of alcohol are relaxation, euphoria, impaired coordination, and decreased inhibitions. The quality of sleep is often reduced. Toxic levels produce ataxia, decreased mentation, poor judgment, labile mood, and slurred speech. Continued ingestion may produce coma with respiratory failure.

Other than the CNS effects, the major effect of alcohol in adolescents occurs in the gastrointestinal tract. Alcohol is a direct gastric irritant that produces hyperacidity. Abdominal pain secondary to gastritis is not uncommon.

Alcohol may also produce a fatty liver, which is accompanied by a mild elevation of liver transaminase levels. Acute alcoholic hepatitis and pancreatitis are rare complications of adolescent alcohol use. Low doses may affect serum lipoproteins by increasing high-density lipoprotein (HDL); moderate and high doses may increase very-low-density lipoproteins (VLDL) and low-density lipoprotein (LDL).

The correlation between blood alcohol concentration and its effect on behavior in adolescents is not always predictable. Some may show impaired judgment and decreased ability to carry out complex tasks at a blood alcohol concentration level of less than 0.05, whereas others maintain this ability even at legally defined levels of intoxication. The disinhibition produced by alcohol leads to excitation of behavior. The triad of cerebellar signs—ataxia, slurred speech, and nystagmus—characterizes the toxic state. Blackouts, irritability during periods of abstinence, and compulsive drug-seeking behavior portend the dependent state. Pathologic intoxication is common, especially among younger adolescents who are new to the intoxicant.

FETAL ALCOHOL SYNDROME. The fetal alcohol syndrome is a complication of alcohol use during pregnancy. Heavy ingestion of alcohol during pregnancy produces an abnormal appearance of the face (microcephaly; short palpebral fissures; hypoplastic maxilla and philtrum; short, upturned nose), mental retardation, cardiac abnormalities, congenital malformations of the genitourinary system (hypospadias and labial hypoplasia), deformed kidneys, and skeletal deformities. Infants with fetal alcohol syndrome are usually small for gestational age.

Tobacco

Cigarette smoking is currently the single most important preventable cause of morbidity and premature mortality in the United States. The composition of tobacco smoke inhaled by the smoker governs the pharmacologic effect. Smoking a package of cigarettes a day for a year results in 73,000 doses of nicotine to the brain. Specific receptors have been identified in the CNS that mediate the effect of nicotine. Relaxation of skeletal muscle accompanies the mild stimulant effect. There is a decrease in anxiety and irritability. Appetite and craving for sweets are reduced, as is overall caloric consumption. Through the release of endogenous opiates, the pain threshold is increased.

Active ingredients of tobacco smoke are rapidly absorbed and reach the brain within seconds. After inhalation, significant levels of nicotine can be measured for up to 30 to 60 minutes. A clear dependence syndrome develops that is characterized by tolerance and withdrawal. Relapse rates are high after attempts at cessation.

Well-documented complications of cigarette smoking are associated with the respiratory and cardiovascular systems. Inhalation of tobacco smoke exposes the respiratory epithelium to toxins that inhibit the cilia—the fine, hairlike structures that help to maintain the tracheobronchial "toilet." Tobacco smoke also interferes with the proteolytic enzymes and immune mechanisms within the tracheobronchial tree. Intercurrent infections occur, giving rise to frequent bouts of acute and eventually chronic bronchitis and chronic obstructive lung disease. Potent carcinogens within the inhaled smoke can lead to carcinoma of the lungs, larynx, oral cavity, esophagus, bladder, and pancreas.

Smoking also produces an increased risk of premature coronary artery disease. The risk of cardiomyopathy, cerebrovascular disease, and peripheral vascular disease is also increased, since nicotine acts as a cofactor in the development of atherosclerosis. Impotence in later life has been correlated with smoking, through the development of arteriosclerosis in the pudendal artery. Nicotine also increases heart rate, blood pressure, myocardial oxygen consumption, carboxyhemoglobin levels, LDL, and free fatty acids in the plasma. Smoking also has been correlated with increased incidence of spontaneous abortion, decreased birth weight of children born to smoking mothers, increased incidence of sudden infant death syndrome (due to prematurity), and other causes of perinatal mortality. The morbidity caused by passive (downstream) smoking, particularly in infants and children, has been well described. Children who live in a household with a smoker are three times more likely to be admitted to a hospital for pneumonia and problems such as sinusitis. Eczema, hives, and skin infections are common in passive smokers, and response to therapy for respiratory infections is often delayed.

Despite the perception of many adolescents, smokeless tobacco also carries a significant risk. In addition to gum recession, periodontitis, and oral leukoplakia, carcinoma of the oral cavity, pharynx, and hypopharynx has been well documented.

Marijuana

The psychoactive ingredients of marijuana are derived from the leaf and the resin of the *Cannabis sativa* plant. Delta-9-tetrahydrocannabinol (THC) is believed to be the most active of the cannabinoids present. Increasingly potent marijuana has become available, with concentrations of up to 9% to 11% of THC. Hash oil may contain 20% to 30% THC. This high concentration of psychoactive substance is one of the reasons for marijuana's high degree of toxicity. The most common method of use is inhalation, with 50% of the active ingredients being absorbed, producing a peak plasma concentration in 10 to 30 minutes. Duration of effect is dependent on bioavailability. Oral ingestion delays in onset of action, with prolongation of effect up to 3 to 5 hours. Active ingredients are primarily metabolized by the liver. Being fat soluble, marijuana can accumulate in the body for long periods. With chronic use, urinary excretion of the drug can be detected up to almost 2 months after last use of the drug. Tolerance develops with chronic use, and a withdrawal syndrome appears when the drug is discontinued.

The primary effect of marijuana is on higher CNS function, with distortion of time sense and enhancement of the auditory and visual senses. Learning and cognitive function are impaired. Appetite is often increased. Mood fluctuations, depersonalization, and hallucinations may occur. Anxiety, panic attacks, delusions, and paranoia are common. Decreased sweating and increased body temperature may occur as a result of marijuana's effect on the thalamic and hypothalamic areas of the CNS.

A number of adverse effects from marijuana smoking have been noted. These include acute and chronic bronchitis, bronchospasm, and metaplastic changes in the tracheobronchial tree. Tachycardia, premature ventricular contractions, electrocardiographic changes, and variable increases in blood pressure have been documented. The endocrine changes usually associated with chronic use are antagonistic effects on insulin action, a decrease in fertility with an increase in abnormal sperm, variable decreases in testosterone levels, and an increase in anovulatory cycles. Impairments of vigilance, coordination, and reaction time also have been documented. In addition, marijuana produces an attention deficit, particularly when the individual is challenged with multiple stimuli. Learning and oral communication may also be impaired.

Cocaine

Stimulant use has been a common form of drug abuse among specific subgroups of adolescents. Amphetamines have been used by high school and college students to increase memory and facilitate learning; by high-risk runaway youths to overcome fatigue, despondency, and depression and to produce a false sense of bravado; by the overweight to reduce appetite; and by users of depressant drugs to counteract the sedative effects of these agents. The introduction of cocaine, in both alkaloid and hydrochloride forms, thus found a ready market. Cocaine is a stimulant made from an alkaloid contained in the leaves of the coca bush, *Erythroxylon coca.*

Cocaine may be used intranasally, orally, or intravenously or may be inhaled by smoking. It is a powerful CNS stimulant that eventually leads to blockade of the conduction of nerve impulses through the depletion of neurotransmitters at the synaptic junction. Its strong CNS effect and short half-life (30 to 50 minutes) promote bouts of intense use rather than low-dose daily use. Such a pattern is referred to as "binge use." Other pharmacologic reactions produced by cocaine include vasoconstriction of small and medium-sized arteries and a local anesthetic effect. Alkaloid cocaine is the preferred form because of its increased bioavailability after smoking. Usually sold as "crack," this smokable form is inexpensive, highly addictive, and widely available to adolescents. Owing to crack's water insolubility, intravenous or intranasal use is unlikely. Powder cocaine (cocaine hydrochloride), on the other hand, is usually absorbed through mucous membranes, by insufflation or "snorting," producing lower serum levels and shorter duration of action.

Cocaine is metabolized by the liver and plasma esterases and primarily excreted as benzoylecgonine or unaltered cocaine. The former is the sentinel compound determined in urine testing. Tolerance for cocaine develops rapidly, and withdrawal syndrome is manifest on discontinuation. The hyperalert, euphoriant effect ("high") is followed by an equally intense state of hypersomnolence and depression that often incites the user to continued use. "Cocaine babies" result from transplacental transfer of cocaine and its metabolites due to their low molecular weight and high water and lipid solubility.

Symptoms of intoxication include tachycardia, hypertension, and (possibly) arrhythmia associated with a hyperalert state, pressure of speech, restlessness, anxiety, and anorexia. Affect may be labile, and evidence of insomnia, paranoia, agitation, hallucinations, skin vermiculations, elation, and euphoria may be noted.

A number of complications relating both to the pharmacologic action of cocaine and to its mode of ingestion have been documented. Direct contact with the nasal mucosa produces intense vasoconstriction and associated inflammation. Dryness of the mucous membrane (xerostoma) may be evident, but rebound nasal congestion may occur as the effect wears off. Focal necrosis may lead to recurrent epistaxis, atrophy, and perforation of the nasal septum. Deeper inhalation has been associated with hemoptysis and black-streaked sputum. Pulmonary edema and hyperventilation have been reported. Vomiting may be associated with the use of cocaine, and in the presence of seizures it may lead to aspiration pneumonia. Cardiovascular complications, including myocardial infarction secondary to coronary artery spasm, cerebrovascular accident secondary to hypertension, and cardiac arrhythmias, have been well documented. These complications are not dose dependent but idiosyncratic. Like amphetamines, cocaine may produce anorexia and nausea leading to weight loss and malnutrition.

Aphrodisiac properties have been attributed to cocaine because of its ability to increase sensory awareness and sensuality. It also delays ejaculation and orgasm in the male. However, chronic use may lead to impotence and associated sexual dysfunction.

As a powerful CNS stimulant, cocaine may produce tonic-clonic seizures and status epilepticus. These may result in cerebral anoxia and irreversible brain damage. Psychotic behavior may be manifested as suspicious and paranoid thinking that may lead to violent acts against self and others.

Amphetamines and Related Sympathomimetics

Methamphetamine hydrochloride, known as "ice" or "croak," has become a common substitute for cocaine (crack). Crystal methamphetamine ingestion through inhalation (smoking) increases bioavailability and thus enhances the CNS effect. The stimulant effects of amphetamines and related drugs such as methylphenidate, propylhexadrine, and ephedrine are analog and dose dependent and resemble those of cocaine. The toxic effects also resemble those of cocaine but are less frequent and intense. Duration is usually longer. Most common are anxiety, paranoia, tachycardia, and mild hypertension, but arrhythmias, cerebrovascular accidents, seizures, and hyperthermia do occur. Cerebral and systemic vasculitis and renal failure have also been reported. With chronic toxicity, formications resulting in cutaneous ulcers may occur and may be a sentinel sign for detecting the user. Psychosis with auditory hallucinations is not uncommon.

Phencyclidine

Phencyclidine (PCP) is a drug with dissociative, anesthetic, analgesic, stimulant, depressant, and hallucinogenic properties. The dose that produces the desired effects is close to its toxic dose. Effects are dose dependent. Low doses are associated with euphoria and/or dysphoria and are often complicated by numbness, blank stare, nystagmus, and hyperacusis. High doses may be associated with seizures, hypertension, hyperreflexia, muscle rigidity, severe hyperthermia and rhabdomyolysis. Associated violent and aggressive behavior is not uncommon.

PCP is commonly snorted or smoked in conjunction with cigarette tobacco ("Sherms") or marijuana.[4] Despite the toxicity and risk of complications associated with PCP, the drug enjoys popularity in the Southwest and Northeast United States. Hallmark symptoms for diagnosis are vertical and horizontal nystagmus, ataxia, increased blood pressure, and increased deep tendon reflexes.

Central Nervous System Depressants

CNS depressants (barbiturates and nonbarbiturates, hypnotic sedative drugs, and minor tranquilizers) enjoy variable popularity with adolescents. These drugs are often used in conjunction with other depressants, with stimulants, or as a treatment for unpleasant reactions caused by other drugs. Short- and intermediate-acting barbiturates, having a variety of street names (reds, red devils, yellow jackets, tooies, Christmas trees), are selected according to their individual appeal. Desired effects include a laissez-faire attitude, sedation with escape from anxiety, and loosening of inhibitions. With patterned use, tolerance develops, and a clear-cut withdrawal syndrome follows discontinuation of drug use. This syndrome may be fatal, particularly if it results in grand mal seizures and circulatory collapse.

The complications of the nonbarbiturate sedative drugs are similar to those of the short-acting barbiturates. Methaqualone has the greatest potential for abuse because of its reputed aphrodisiac effects. Contrary to statements in the pharmaceutical literature, tolerance and psycho-

logic and physical dependence occur, with a withdrawal syndrome manifested on cessation of drug use.

In the class of minor tranquilizers, benzodiazepines are among the most abused group of drugs in the United States. For adolescents, their availability is modulated by limited access through either prescription or street sources. Common features of mild overdose include slurred speech, confusion, disorientation, and depressed respiration. Increasing severity of overdose may lead to cardiovascular and CNS depression as with barbiturates; withdrawal is characterized by agitation, increased excitability, tremors, increased heart rate, delirium, and seizures. Seizures may be the only clinical sign of a withdrawal syndrome. Flunitrazepam (Rohypnol), a sedative hypnotic available in Europe and Latin America, has been used much as methaqualone has been used in the past. Known as "roofies," mixed with alcohol or taken in excess, flunitrazepam produces decreased inhibitions and may cause blackouts and retrograde amnesia. It is sometimes referred to as the "date rape" drug.

Inhalants

Inhalants such as toluene-based glues and paints, alkyl nitrites (poppers), nitrous oxide, ethyl chloride, triethylene chloride (in typewriter correction fluid), and cyanomethacrylate and methymethacrylate (in contact glue) have regional popularity with adolescents, especially those less knowledgeable or experienced. All inhalants are lipid soluble and have a rapid onset of action. Low cost and ease of availability make these substances attractive alternatives to illicit drugs. Impulsive behavior is a common effect of the use of inhalant because of loss of inhibition. This often results in trauma to the adolescent or to others. During the process of inhalation, often done through a closed system such as a plastic bag, the individual may become confused and disoriented, which can lead to continued inhalation, CNS anoxia, seizures, and cardiorespiratory arrest. When an inhalant is used in conjunction with other activities, the inherent risk of the drug may be augmented by high-risk behaviors (e.g., violent acts, sexual activity, driving while intoxicated). Other reported effects include hepatic, renal, and cardiac toxicities. Inhalation of toluene-containing compounds has been associated with hypokalemia, hypophosphatemia, renal tubular acidosis, abdominal pain, weakness, and permanent neurologic damage.

Hallucinogens

The setting in which hallucinogens (e.g., LSD, mescaline, DMT, MDMA) are used greatly influences the user's experience. Although tolerance develops with the use of many of these drugs, no clear-cut withdrawal syndrome is evident. Hallucinogens, in general, are absorbed rapidly through the gastrointestinal tract, their effects being felt within minutes. Subjective experiences, which are usually dramatic, include visual and auditory illusions, synesthesias, increased sensitivity of touch, and time distortion. Injury is often experienced when the user, under the influence of the drug, misinterprets illusion for reality. In the short term these drugs may cause paranoid ideation, depression, confusion, and a loss of a sense of self (fragmentation). Long-term use has been associated with spontaneous drug-like highs (flashbacks), psychosis, depressive reactions, and personality changes. MDMA is a mild hallucinogen with its chemical roots in the amphetamine group. It has occasional regional popularity as an alternative to marijuana. The toxic effects resemble those of the amphetamines: hyperthermia, rhabdomyolysis, severe hyponatremia, and cerebral infarction.

RISK FACTORS

A number of factors have been found to increase the risk for using and abusing alcohol and other drugs.[4] The interaction of physical development with psychologic and social behaviors (the biobehavior or biopsychosocial hypothesis) plays a major role in the origin of such risk. Risk factors fall into seven general areas (Box 108-3). Investigations have attributed drug abuse to family and peer influences, behavioral deviance, problem behavior, lack of social conformity, poor academic performance, low self-esteem, depression, and stress related to life-change events. These various risk factors are not mutually exclusive. Risk in one category is often associated with risk in another. Nevertheless, the effect of these factors is thought to be cumulative. The more risk factors a youth has, the greater is the overall probability of drug use. There are also special subgroups of adolescents who are particularly vulnerable to substance abuse: those who have been physically or sexually abused; runaways; homeless youths; and gay, lesbian, or bisexual youths.

Genetic Factors and Familial Characteristics

There are two general groups of family-related risk factors that predispose to substance use among adolescents: (1) genetic factors, which may increase an adolescent's susceptibility to alcohol and drug use; and (2) familial behavioral characteristics. There is increasing evidence to suggest that alcoholism is not simply a matter of experience or learning, but that there may be significant genetic influences, particularly for the male offspring of fathers who had drinking problems in their youth. Evidence from studies of twins and adopted children has supported this. Male children of alcoholic parents are 4 to 5 times more likely to become alcoholics than are those

---

BOX 108-3
Risk Factors for Drug Use in Adolescents

GENETIC
- Alcohol or other drug use in parent

INTRINSIC
- Early initiation (<15 yr)
- Chronic illness or pain
- Runaway/homelessness
- Eating disorder
- Gay/lesbian/bisexual

PSYCHOLOGIC
- Low self-esteem
- Anxiety/depression/affective disorder
- Conduct/personality disorder
- Present/past history of abuse (physical/sexual/emotional)
- Suicidal ideation/attempt

SOCIAL/FAMILIAL
- Acceptance of drug use
- Role modeling licit/illicit drug use
- Divorce, separation, or loss of parent
- Poor relationships with parent(s)
- General family dysfunction
- Low expectation for children

PEER GROUP
- Perceived risk of harmfulness
- Peer group acceptance
- Friends' use of drugs
- Positive value to drug use
- Early delinquent behavior

SCHOOL
- Availability in school setting
- Poor academic motivation
- Failure/dropout

COMMUNITY
- Availability and norms of use
- Poor social integration/bonding
- Economic/social impoverishment

Adapted from Hawkins JD, Catalano RF, Miller JY: Risk and protective factors for alcohol and other drug problems in adolescence and early adulthood: implications for substance abuse prevention, *Psychol Bull* 112:64-105, 1992.

---

of nonalcoholic parents. Examination of neuropsychologic and physiologic precursors or markers of alcoholism in sons of alcoholics and nonalcoholics suggest possible biologic differences that may increase a person's vulnerability. It also has been suggested that children of alcoholics may be deficient in serotonin or may have an increased level of serotonin after ingestion of alcohol. The "addictive cycle"—a pattern in which a person initially drinks to feel good and then continues to drink to avoid feeling bad—may result from such a defect in serotonin metabolism. Children of alcoholics are also believed to have an increased tolerance of alcohol. The genetic link between substance abuse by parents and initiation of such abuse in their children is an intriguing one. Like other behavioral traits with genetic influence, their development depends significantly on various environmental cofactors.

Adolescents from dysfunctional families—families that are constantly disorganized, that are not cohesive, and that have a high level of conflict and/or abuse—are at increased risk for developing a substance abuse problem. Poor parenting skills, demonstrated by unclear or inconsistent rules for behavior, inconsistent reactions to the child's behavior, lax supervision or monitoring of the child's behavior, excessively severe discipline, and poor and derogatory communication patterns (e.g., constant criticism, humiliation, nagging, absence of praise), have all been found to increase the likelihood of drug use. In contrast, fulfilling relationships with parents and family members appear to discourage the initiation of alcohol use and other drug use. Bonding to families, attachment to parents, and perceived family support are protective; that is, they are negatively associated with substance use and abuse. Parents and older siblings are powerful role models for adolescents in that their drug use and their attitudes toward such use are important predictors of drug use among younger adolescents.

Thus, adolescents from families that have more encouraging or lenient attitudes toward drug use and abuse are at greater risk than those from families that do not tolerate or that discourage such use. Adolescents with parents or siblings who display antisocial behavior are also at greater risk than adolescents from families having more conventional social values.

Age of Initiation

Epidemiologic studies have shown that initial use of alcohol and other drugs at an early age, particularly before the age of 15 years, increases the risk for continued experimentation, persistent involvement in drug use, and development of a substance abuse problem. In general, adolescents who have not begun to experiment with alcohol, cigarettes, and most illicit drugs before ages 18 to 21 years are unlikely to do so. The percentage of adolescents who use illicit drugs either decreases or stays the same at age 21 years. Use of cocaine, however, is the exception to this pattern. Longitudinal studies tracking teenagers into their twenties indicate that the prevalence of cocaine use increases with each successive year after high school graduation and continues into early adulthood.

In addition, recent research indicates that frequency and duration of use positively correlate with an increased risk for school truancy, school failure, criminal behavior, and suicide. Although cause and effect cannot be presumed, this does show that drug use is quantitatively linked to other clusters of problem behaviors in youth. The more frequently adolescents use drugs, the more likely they are to experience serious problems in other areas of life.

Psychologic Characteristics

Several psychologic characteristics are associated with initiation and use of drugs. These include low self-esteem, depression (see Chapter 122) anxiety, conduct and antisocial behavior, and personality disorders (see Chapter 120). Behaviors that are part of a conduct disorder that predispose to drug use include aggression (especially when coupled with shyness in males), hyperactivity, nervousness, inattentiveness, impulsiveness, defiance, school misbehavior, weak sense of social responsibility, fighting, and sensation seeking. A reciprocal relationship exists between conduct-disordered behavior or delinquency and drug use. Just as early delinquency is associated with later drug use, early use of alcohol and other drugs increases the likelihood that an adolescent will become involved in delinquent behavior.

Students in middle school who have not adopted the dominant social values, who rebel against authority (particularly their parents and school officials), and who do not attend church tend to be at higher risk for drug abuse than those who are bonded to and respect family, school, and church. Other characteristic traits associated with drug use include lack of empathy for the feelings of others, easy and frequent lying, preferring immediate to delayed gratification, poor impulse control, and insensitivity to punishment.

PEER DRUG USE AND ATTITUDES. As adolescents separate from their family, peers become significant sources of support and influence. It is not surprising, then, that the behavior and attitudes of peers are one of the strongest predictors of drug use. Although parents greatly influence socialization before adolescence, peer norms quickly assume power afterward, modulated by family beliefs and values. Adolescents tend to select peers who have attitudes and beliefs similar to their own. Positive relationships with adults, characterized by respect and trust, experienced before 11 years of age greatly diminish the risk for deviance in general and substance abuse in particular. Drug users rely on a code of conduct established by peers rather than drawing on their own positive life experience and role models.

POOR ACADEMIC PERFORMANCE. School prevails as the most significant out-of-home environment for the socialization of children and adolescents. School failure and low level of interest in school or future employment increase the risk for drug use. Even children who underachieve in the middle to late elementary years are at risk when they reach their teens. Regardless of the reason—boredom, lack of ability, or a match with a poorly skilled teacher—school failure increases the likelihood of early experimentation with drugs and alcohol, and of their becoming regular users later in their teens.

Students who are not committed to achieving in school are more likely to use drugs. Conversely, high school students with college ambition are at significantly less risk for using the potent drugs (e.g., cocaine, stimulants, hallucinogens). Factors such as how much a student likes school, time spent on homework, and perception of the relevance of course work to present and future ambitions also have been found to be related to levels of use.

The relationship between drug use and school performance is reciprocal. This can create a vicious cycle of failure. Not only can early school failure be a precursor of later use, but drug use may result in poor school performance and dropping out. Deteriorating performance in school is frequently associated with increasing drug use. School attendance is inversely correlated with substance abuse. Teenagers who are frequent drug users are likely to skip or cut classes, arrive late, leave school early, and be truant for ambiguous reasons. Truant teenagers are also more likely to identify with the activities of adults or peers who are not attending school. Drug-using adolescents also tend to lose interest in preparing for college or vocational training.

SPECIAL HIGH-RISK POPULATIONS

Certain subgroups of adolescents may be at particularly high risk for drug abuse. Those who have experienced physical, sexual, and/or emotional abuse and neglect are vulnerable to a number of problems. Truancy and other school problems, running away from home, suicide attempts, alcohol and drug abuse, and delinquency or criminality are not uncommonly associated with a history of sexual abuse.[5] Drug use may serve as a form of "chemically induced dissociation," allowing the survivor to escape from abuse-related memories or associated mood states.[6] In one study of adolescents in psychotherapy, those with a history of sexual abuse were found to be more than twice as likely to have a history of alcoholism and 10 times more likely to report having been dependent on drugs in the past than a control group without a history of abuse.[7]

Another group at particularly high risk for abusing drugs are homeless and runaway youths. It is estimated that 750,000 to 1.3 million young people run away each year. One quarter are thought to become homeless, with no permanent residence or adult support. Recent reports suggest that these young people are a multiple-problem population with high rates of mental health, alcohol, and other drug problems. In one study, use of alcohol began in late childhood or early adolescence. These youths also experienced greater social impairment due to alcohol use, and practiced exaggerated consumption patterns in comparison with nonhomeless youths.[8] Prevalence of current alcohol use was six to eight times higher among homeless youth than among nonhomeless adolescents, and it was virtually identical to the rate for homeless adults. Homeless adolescents with a diagnosis of alcohol use had a profile of behaviors reflecting pathologic alcohol use and impaired social function similar to that of homeless alcoholic adults. Among homeless adolescents seen at an outpatient medical clinic in Los Angeles, the majority reported drug use during the 6 months before their assessment: 69%, alcohol; 53%, marijuana; 32%, stimulant use (amphetamine and cocaine derivatives); and 8%, intravenous drug use.[9] In a 1990 survey of 168 adolescents at a youth shelter in New York City, alcohol was used by 80%, marijuana by 68%, cocaine by 48%, and crack by 38%. Intravenous drug use was reported by 6%.[10]

Finally, gay and lesbian youths represent a special high-risk population. Those identified as gay are more likely to report substance abuse than are nongay youths.[11] Gay youths are also more likely to report a previous suicide attempt and current suicidal ideation, usually precipitated by interpersonal disruption.

HIV Injection and Drugs in Adolescents

Of particular concern is the fact that adolescent drug users may be vulnerable to infection with the human immunodeficiency virus (HIV).[12] AIDS is one of the leading causes of death among adolescents and young adults. As of June 1996, 2514 cases of AIDS and 3042 of HIV positivity (not AIDS) were reported in adolescents 13 to 19 years of age. Intravenous drug use, the use of nonsterile or "dirty" needles, the sharing of needles, and having sex with an IV drug user accounts for over 18% of HIV infection in this age group. Although the number of adolescents in the general population who inject drugs and engage in needle sharing is unknown, survey data indicate that a substantial number use drugs that can be injected intravenously (e.g., cocaine, heroin, amphetamines, steroids).

Use of certain drugs that do not involve intravenous injection also may increase an adolescent's risk for HIV transmission. Substance use often impairs the user's judgment, thus increasing the likelihood of risk-related behaviors, particularly unprotected sexual intercourse. The use of crack (as well as other stimulants) that increase sexual arousal may contribute to significantly impaired judgment. Crack use has been found highly predictive of HIV seropositivity among both males and females because of its strong association with HIV risk–related sexual behaviors, such as exchange of sex for crack or the money to purchase crack.

DEVELOPMENT AND PSYCHOSOCIAL CONSEQUENCES

The consequences of the first use of alcohol or another drug may be profound, although appearing trivial and inconsequential to the individual. The roles of alcohol in traffic fatalities, of cocaine in sudden death, of sedative in overdoses, and of tobacco in lung cancer and emphysema are all well known. Less dramatic, but insidious, is the role that drug abuse can play in disrupting an adolescent's healthy psychosocial development. For example, regular intermittent use of illicit drugs such as cocaine (two or three times a week over several months) is commonly accompanied by deterioration of schoolwork and loss of interest in activities such as sports. The user develops a new drug-using group of friends. Financial problems inevitably arise, and the ongoing need for money frequently leads to stealing from family and friends. The adolescent may become involved in selling drugs or may take part in other illegal activities.

Although drugs have inherent properties that are pharmacologically powerful, the expression of these properties is modulated or amplified by the user's values, motivations, life experience, personality, expectations, and social setting. Three interacting forces that influence the development of a substance abuse disorder overlap: the type of drug (agent), the psychologic make-up of the user (host), and the context or social setting (environment) in which it is used (Fig. 108-1). The interaction of

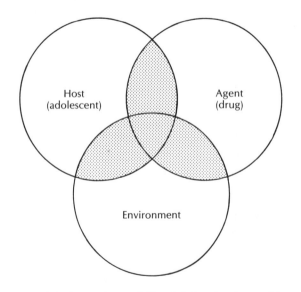

Fig. 108-1. Interacting variables defining the drug problem.

these three determinants defines the substance abuse problem. The nature of the problem is graphically represented by the shaded area. As can be imagined, each drug user's problem represented graphically will be unique, depending on the relative contribution of each force. Adolescence is a period of rapid psychosocial growth and development stimulated, in large part, by an increased interaction with societal influences. The intensity of the pressure for change and adaptation during adolescence is exceeded only by that which occurs in the fetus in utero. How a specific adolescent expresses his or her involvement with drugs is determined by individual personality and is not drug or problem specific. For this reason, the drug use may go undetected unless information and evidence are integrated from the three contributing domains.

Long-term, almost daily use of drugs is commonly associated with psychologic and psychophysiologic symptoms, and complaints such as headaches, nausea, chronic cough, palpitations, fatigue, insomnia, and chest pain are not uncommon. The associated dysfunctional psychologic state often leads to escapism, egocentrism, decision making that is easily influenced by others, poor self-image, and alienation, all of which increase the adolescent's desire to continue the drug abuse.

Dual Diagnosis

Many adolescents who are seen for treatment also manifest psychiatric symptoms.[13] Disorders of affect, conduct, attention, eating, learning, and anxiety appear to be the most common. In the National Youth Polydrug Study, 28% of this drug-using cohort reported seeking help for emotional and psychiatric problems.[14] Using a Personal Experience Inventory, a diagnostic tool based on the Diagnostic and Statistical Manual of Mental Disorders (DSM-IIIR) criteria for chemical dependency, Winters evaluated 73 teenagers attending an outpatient drug clinic.[15] Unipolar and bipolar affective disorders were most prevalent (24.7%). Other disorders included Attention Deficit Hyperactivity Disorder (20.5%), developmental disorders (15.1%), psychosis (6.8%), eating disorders (5.5%), and anxiety disorders (5.5%). In adolescents with a dual psychiatric and substance abuse diagnosis, it is not easy to determine which disorder came first.

Several relationships between coexisting substance abuse and psychologic problems have been proposed. Longitudinal research findings suggest that the antecedents of drug use appear to be similar to those linked in other studies to various forms of psychopathology. These data suggest that substance abuse and psychopathology may originate from a common vulnerability. Another explanation may be that psychiatric symptoms or disorders develop from, or are exacerbated by, the use or abuse of mood-altering substances. A third possibility is that nonprescription and illicit drugs may be used to self-medicate psychiatric symptoms or disorders; thus, substance abuse can develop as a consequence of a preexisting psychiatric disorder. Finally, the relationship between substance abuse and psychiatric disorders may be only coincidental.

Regardless of the nature of the relationship, it appears that the coexistence of a psychopathologic condition and substance abuse is common in adolescents. The following discussion is a summary of the research on coexisting affective disorders and suicidality, conduct/antisocial personality disorders, eating disorders, and drug and alcohol use in adolescents. At present, little is known about the comorbidity of anxiety disorders and substance abuse in adolescents.

Affective Disorders

It is likely that affective symptoms and disorders are the psychiatric problems most commonly coexisting with substance abuse. As many as 60% to 80% of adolescent substance abusers are diagnosed as depressed on admission to inpatient treatment programs. Many of these youths, however, experience a gradual lifting of the depression without drug therapy between 10 and 21 days after admission. In a study of adolescents seen for psychiatric evaluation in a general hospital emergency room, it was found that almost half of those having elevated blood alcohol levels (17% of the total sample) had at least one additional diagnosed psychiatric problem. The most common diagnosis was depression. Other evidence suggests that alcohol abuse is associated with major depression but not with other diagnoses. The onset of major depression had reportedly almost always preceded the alcohol or other drug abuse, thus supporting the view that depression and anxiety disorders are risk factors for subsequent substance abuse in adolescents and young adults.

Suicide

Numerous studies have found that the frequency of both suicide attempts and completed suicides is substantially higher among substance abusers than in the general population. This relationship holds true for adolescents. Suicide rates for adolescents have almost tripled in the past three decades, and suicide is the second leading cause of death in this group. Some suggest that drug use may be the single most important factor accounting for the increase in the suicide rate among adolescents in the United States. Intoxication often precedes a suicide attempt or a completed suicide in adolescents. Substance abuse also has been noted as a factor that increases the likelihood that firearms will be used as a means for committing

suicide among adolescents. Thus, when a healthcare professional is caring for a substance-abusing adolescent, it is critical that the professional initially assess and continually monitor the individual's suicidality, noting whether the youth has a plan and, if so, the lethality of the plan. Youths who are a danger to themselves should be immediately referred for crisis management.

Conduct and Antisocial Personality Disorders

Conduct and antisocial personality disorders have been strongly associated with substance abuse in both adolescents and adults for a long time (see Chapter 120, "Character Disorders"). An individual with a conduct or antisocial personality disorder is up to 21 times more likely to become an alcoholic than someone without such a disorder. Again, the nature of the relationship remains unclear. Several studies have reported that childhood behavior problems appear to be antecedents to later alcoholism. It may also be that intoxication with various substances leads to behavioral disinhibition, which decreases the threshold for antisocial behavior. However, in part, this association may be accounted for by the fact that substance abuse is one of the diagnostic criteria for antisocial personality.

Eating Disorders

Many adolescents who have an eating disorder, especially bulimia nervosa (see Chapter 32, "Bulimia Nervosa"), manifest concurrent or subsequent problems with substance abuse. Parents of youths with an eating disorder also have been found to have an increased incidence of alcohol or other drug dependence. According to one theory, bulimia is more prevalent among females than among males because it represents an expression of addiction that is specific to females. Others believe that it may be the manifestation of a compulsive disorder.

STAGES OF SUBSTANCE ABUSE

At some time, most adolescents experiment with tobacco, alcohol, or other drugs. In varying degrees, all adolescents are at risk for associated physical and mental health problems. Providing adolescents with interventions that will discourage them from initiating drug use and protect them from drug abuse is paramount in preventing these problems.

Adolescent substance abuse appears to occur in four stages: experimentation, exploration, encapsulation, and dependence (Box 108-4). Information about where an adolescent falls within these stages can be used as a guide in developing appropriate prevention or treatment inter-

---

BOX 108-4
Stages of Adolescent Drug Use

STAGE 1: EXPERIMENTATION

- Usually begins in elementary or junior high
- Often involves "gateway" drugs (e.g., alcohol, cigarettes, marijuana)
- Used in context of exploring new behaviors and experiences
- Used in setting of home or party, or while "hanging out"
- Used in response to peer norms or to feel grown-up
- Small amounts used without a definite pattern
- Helps adolescent to cope with demands of development

STAGE 2: EXPLORATION

- Progression in frequency of use, stronger drugs used
- Episodes of use may be justified as "handling stress"
- Patterned use apparent and often integrated into social situations
- Used during the week in conflict with regular activities (e.g., school)
- Problems related to drug use occur (hangover, decreased performance)
- Often dissociates from non–drug-using friends
- Deceptive behaviors to obtain drugs
- Mood swings become apparent to family and friends
- Denial often predominates

STAGE 3: ENCAPSULATION

- Tolerance develops to particular drug of choice
- More and more time spent ascertaining the drug experience
- Drugs used to maintain function and mood
- Drops out of other activities, drug use dominates life
- Other problem behaviors manifested (stealing, lying, violence, trouble with police)
- Physical withdrawal may occur
- Health problems may be manifested

STAGE 4: DEPENDENCE

- Increasing negative feelings toward self
- Deterioration of social relationships
- Social contacts limited to drug-using friends
- Denial of drug use as a problem predominates
- Involvement in illegal activity to maintain drug habit
- Life is chaotic in all domains (physical, social, psychologic, personal)
- Often self-deprecation, guilt, shame, and self-destructive behavior
- Drugs used not to feel "high" but to feel normal

---

ventions. Information collected during the risk assessment also may be used to target specific types of interventions for identified risk factors and the particular needs of adolescents.

Stage 1: Experimentation

Experimentation (testing) is the first stage of alcohol or drug use among adolescents. Younger teenagers, especially boys, are great experimenters in a number of activities, and they are especially prone to experiment with alcohol, drugs, or both. Evidence suggests that adolescents are most likely to first experiment with alcohol, cigarettes, and marijuana. For this reason, these three substances have been described as "gateway" drugs. The increasing popularity of cocaine, especially crack, among adolescents has led some to refer to this drug as a gateway drug, especially in urban impoverished communities.

Some teenagers who are experimenting with drugs decide that they do not like the effects of the first drugs they try, whereas others continue to experiment and progress to the use of other drugs such as inhalants, cocaine, and hallucinogens. The gateway drugs are usually "carried over," and use of gateway drugs is continued as new drugs (e.g., cocaine) are added to the user's repertoire. Opiates are likely to be the last drugs an adolescent will try. During this experimental stage, the common attitude of the adolescent is that it is all right to explore new behaviors and experiences.

The cognitive development of adolescents and their perceived invulnerability to harm may serve to encourage them to continue experimenting with drugs. Concrete thinking (as opposed to abstract thinking) processes make it difficult for many to understand the future consequences of their behavior. This type of thinking may profoundly limit their ability to make decisions that will prevent hazardous or dangerous drug use. If, while experimenting, adolescents perceive the substance as helping them cope with the demands of development, the use is reinforced and they are likely to continue using the substance. On the other hand, if the experience was unpleasant, they will be less likely to try it again. Adolescents at this stage can be managed in the outpatient or office setting. Several strategies may be used for primary intervention or preventive intervention (secondary prevention). Options must be chosen with the particular circumstance and individual in mind (Box 108-5). Esteem building is the most important strategy. Even though the adolescent may have only naively tried the drug, this action was carried out for a reason. The underlying motivation lies in maturational (unconscious) developmental needs, which are fueled by the tasks of adolescence. Mere curiosity may prevail, but it is more likely that either real or imagined values of the peer group or adult models played a role. Initial drug use usually

---

BOX 108-5
Methods of Changing Behavior*

Increasing self-esteem
Empowerment
Substitution
Environmental manipulation
Modeling
Peer pressure
Education
Personal crisis
Persuasion
Developmental progression (maturing out)
Rewards/coercion
Pharmacologic agents
Punishment

---

*Primary or secondary prevention.

serves to fill an emptiness, or it demonstrates a wish to be similar to or part of a perceived norm. Praise, encouragement, and empowerment integrated with a reasonable dose of education are important strategies used during this stage. If maturational development drives are identified, every effort should be made to encourage a substitute activity or behavior that will fill the same need as the drug experimentation. The issue of gateway drugs needs to be addressed and caution must be advised. Training in elementary social skills that focus on resisting peer pressure and developing individual uniqueness may be used to enhance self-confidence and arm the adolescent against possible future attacks on identity and esteem. Identification of positive role models helps to cement these new skills into a healthy sense of self.

Stage 2: Exploration

The second stage is exploration, or social use. At this stage the adolescent begins to use alcohol and/or other drugs to explore their value in social situations. On the basis of peer-group norms, the adolescent perceives it to be okay to use alcohol and other drugs within prescribed social situations. Thus, the explorer tends to develop personal and private guidelines for deciding when substance use is appropriate. The social circumstance (e.g., a party) may encourage alcohol or drug use as a means of overcoming shyness or abrogating personal responsibility for behavior. When such motivations are compounded by the adolescent need to escape from a feeling of insecurity or emotional pain (mood adjustment), the risk profile for continued and patterned use greatly increases. The problems associated with this stage may not center on the quantity and frequency of drug use but rather on the circumstances and behavioral consequences of such use. The combination of drug use and

driving, or of a risk-taking challenge, underlies the most common morbidities and mortalities in this age group.

In the case of social drug use, it is particularly important for the health professional to understand the usage in the context of the adolescent's life before developing any systematic plan for intervention. The ultimate goal is to help the young person to be separate from and yet part of the peer group. In other words, it is important to determine what role the drug is playing in this individual's life. Application of knowledge of normal development and recognition of situational expressions (i.e., drug use) of maturational crises (e.g., need for peer acceptance, fear of being different) usually provides ideas for developing a management plan. This information needs to be integrated into the drug user's total risk profile, with data gathered through an adolescent risk profile, evaluation such as that used at Children's Hospital, Los Angeles (the H.E.A.D.S.* examination),[16] and the family and genetic history. Specific information about the substances being used should be presented objectively, with clear explanations of the potential consequences of such use, and with the risks of experimenting with new substances outlined. Adolescents are not likely to stop using a drug unless they find alternative behaviors to deal with the same developmental need that the drug is fulfilling. So that a dynamic management plan can be developed, it is important for the clinician to understand that the drug use serves a purpose for the adolescent. Various possible interventions then can be identified in case the initial attempts are futile. With such an approach, the adolescent is likely to feel better understood, and this should enhance the rapport between clinician and adolescent. At this stage, some adolescents may be managed in the general ambulatory setting, but most will require a specialized intensive outpatient program.

Adolescents tend to think of themselves as invulnerable and generally underestimate their risk of developing problems associated with alcohol and drug use. Therefore, the clinician needs to present the important issues of alcohol- and drug-related deaths and other related problems (e.g., school dropout, physical health problems). They also need to understand that addiction can occur shortly after initial use. Useful strategies for avoiding harm need to be emphasized. For example, the clinician might suggest establishing a contract with the adolescent in which the youth agrees not to drive while intoxicated and to determine before going to a party who the sober designated driver will be. To prevent escalating use of alcohol, the clinician might explore controlled, manageable-use behaviors (e.g., drinking two beers at a party is okay) and what would be indications of uncontrolled or abusive behaviors (e.g., more than two beers at a party, one or more beers daily, difficulty waking

---

*See "Risk Assessment" for definition; p 841.

up in the morning because of alcohol use the previous night). This moderate approach allows the clinician to establish a contract so that the adolescent has clear guidelines for seeking help if his or her behavior starts to match what has been defined as uncontrolled or abusive. If a regular pattern of use becomes apparent, a contract for abstinence should be negotiated. Often this will empha-size to the adolescent the severity of the problem and the heightened concern of the clinician and family.

Stage 3: Encapsulation

The third stage of drug use is encapsulation, or preoccupation. The individual has now progressed from using the substance only in social situations to using it during most of his or her free time and occasionally at school. At this point, more and more time, thinking, energy, and money are directed toward being high and ensuring that a steady supply of the preferred drug(s) is available. Active drug-seeking behavior is present and the drug use becomes compulsive. Drugs become the most important thing in the adolescent's life, more important than friends, family, sports, and other activities. The focus becomes: How and when can I next get high? Few of the adolescent's daily activities will not include drug use, but this will not be perceived as a problem by the adolescent. Alcohol and/or drugs are needed to maintain function and mood. Adolescents in this stage typically begin to experience difficulties in *all* areas of their lives—with parents, school, peers, and sometimes the police. Typi-cally, dramatic behavioral changes occur to which family, teachers, and friends react. Rather than acknowledging that the drug use is the problem, the teenager commonly projects the problem upon family, teachers, and friends. This allows him or her to abrogate responsibility, deny, and cover up. Life stability seems to be more related to drugs than to human relationships.

The young person who has become preoccupied with drugs is losing control and is in need of treatment. Because of the intricate and empowering relationship that has been developed with the drug, abstinence is critical. Whether abstinence can be achieved within the setting that encouraged the drug use in the first place is a matter of the personal resources of the teenager and the skill and experience of the clinician. Further behavioral, physical, and mental health problems must be avoided, and the progression of chemical dependence must be prevented. Adolescents in this stage are likely to need counseling for depression, for combating low self-esteem, for develop-ing decision-making skills to help them avoid situations that will lead to drug use, and for training in social skills to help them learn to interact socially and appropriately in the drug-free state. For most, these needs will require a residential or day-treatment program providing medi-cally monitored intensive management.

Stage 4: Dependence

The fourth and final stage of alcohol or drug use is dependence, or addiction, in which total encapsulation has occurred. By this time, the only thing that the adolescent cares about is using drugs. Negative personal feelings toward self have been building steadily and relationships with others have deteriorated, resulting in the need for daily, sometimes hourly, relief. As a result, the adolescent is unable to distinguish drug-related behavior from non–drug-related behavior, and drug use becomes the norm. Denial becomes the catalyst for continued use, and no rational or moral argument will persuade the adolescent that there is a problem, even when there is overwhelming evidence that the drug use is out of control. The drug use is perceived as a solution to personal developmental tragedies or deprivations. El-evated levels of depression, low self-esteem, and worth-lessness are commonly experienced. Since the adolescent usually has already begun to steal from family and friends in order to purchase drugs, he or she is likely to escalate these illegal activities to continue financing the drug habit. The range of physical and psychologic problems now becomes much broader, and immediate treatment in an intensive, medically managed inpatient facility is usually required.

Prevention and treatment efforts are more likely to be effective if they (1) take into consideration the develop-mental and biopsychosocial changes that are being experienced (problem); (2) provide a healthier alternative (solution) to drug use to accomplish the particular adolescent task being addressed; (3) give the adolescent information about alcohol and other drug use and the potential dangers associated with such use; (4) empower and encourage the adolescent to make significant changes; (5) provide social and life skills training to enhance decision making, assertiveness, and communi-cation skills for resisting peer pressure; and (6) treat any associated psychiatric diagnosis uncovered. Additional interventions, including family, school, and involvement in community programs such as Alcoholics Anonymous (AA), are important adjunct measures.

IDENTIFYING SUBSTANCE ABUSERS

One of the major goals in working with adolescents is to assess their risk for substance abuse and to determine appropriate interventions. For example, adolescents who have not entered the curiosity phase and who are at relatively low risk require information and ongoing support to minimize experimentation. Those nonusers who have an at-risk profile (e.g., parents who abuse substances, chaotic childhood, absent or drug-using role models, drug-using peer group) need more intensive preventive interventions as well as ongoing peer and professional support. In contrast, adolescents who are at high risk for substance abuse and who are currently involved may need to be linked with treatment programs to help them. Performance of a risk assessment is essential to evaluating the level of risk as well as determining current use patterns. Urine screenings also may be performed to obtain an objective measure of the substances recently used and to monitor abstinence.

Risk Assessment

A risk assessment should include questions to determine (1) whether there are existing factors that put the adolescent at risk for drug use, (2) to what extent the adolescent has previously used drugs or is currently using them, and (3) whether the current use of substances is causing negative consequences or interfering with day-to-day functioning. Risk assessment or development of a risk profile does not focus only on drugs. It also must evaluate the life-risk events that are known to correlate with drug use. Therefore, it should include several general areas of an adolescent's life, including family functioning and home environment, academic performance, conduct at school, general attitudes and behaviors with adults, goals and values, daily activities and peer relationships, and psychologic or psychiatric symptoms (e.g., depression, anxiety).

A practical and efficient method of risk assessment, the adolescent risk profile interview or H.E.A.D.S. examination, has been developed in the Division of Adolescent Medicine at Children's Hospital, Los Angeles.[16] This profile is collected in conjunction with the general medical history and provides a developmental perspective. Information is gathered in a structured way that lessens the possibility of omission of important life events. The profile also provides a simple and easily updated format for documentation in the chart. This psychosocial "biopsy" gathers information initially from areas of low emotional charge and then from the often highly charged areas of sex, drugs, and physical/sexual abuse, permitting the interviewer to develop increasing rapport. Information is explored in those areas that are in dynamic change yet sensitive to adolescent development: *H*ome, *E*ducation, *E*mployment, *A*ctivities, *A*mbitions, *D*rugs, *D*iet, *S*ex (including sexual abuse), and *S*uicide (H.E.A.D.S.).

Certain warning signs can be used to "red flag" the risk. For example, in the preadolescent years, at-risk youngsters are distinguishable from others in terms of aggressive antisocial behavior, particularly the combination of shyness and aggressiveness. It is also important to recognize evidence of school adjustment and performance problems with a special emphasis on truancy. Antisocial behavior that may become a problem often

may be identified as early as kindergarten years. Care must be taken that this identification does not become the youngster's own self-fulfilling prophecy. By the late elementary grades, youngsters at highest risk are recognized by evidence of school failure in addition to aggressive behaviors. These adolescents tend to gravitate to a peer group having similar experiences, and thus they share their misery and coping responses. At this point, initial use of drugs and early acts of delinquency can be anticipated.

By adolescence, poor commitment to school and associated academic failure become evident. Other signals may be the presence of delinquent, drug-using friends; alienation from society; and rebelliousness. The adolescent drug user may drop out of school and become identified with other groups and other settings. Viewed developmentally, these adolescents are attempting to accomplish their adolescent tasks in the best way that they know how and often with limited resources available.

Diagnosis

Specific diagnostic criteria for determining whether an individual is chemically dependent have been established in the Diagnostic and Statistical Manual of Mental Disorders (DSM-IV).[17] Under the general heading Substance-Related Disorders, DSM-IV divides chemical dependence into 11 categories based on the class of substance. Substance-related disorders are further divided into Substance Use Disorders and Substance-Induced Disorders. Box 108-6 outlines the 11 classes and also includes a section Polysubstance Dependence and Other or Unknown Substance-Related Disorders (which include most disorders related to medications or toxins). Definition and diagnostic criteria for substance dependence are outlined (Boxes 108-6 and 108-7). These criteria were developed for use with adults. Unfortunately, it has not yet been determined whether the criteria can be effectively applied to adolescents who have an evolving drug use pattern so integrally intertwined into their psychologic development.

More useful criteria for diagnosing substance abuse in adolescents include objective indexes of use such as (1) quantity and frequency, (2) "symptomatic" use behaviors (e.g., intoxication, blackouts, narrowing of life style interests), and (3) areas of functional impairment presumed to be caused by substance abuse (e.g., impaired relationships with family, peers, or teachers; problems with school, police; problems associated with driving after drinking). Loss of control or an inability to limit the amount of the substance used is also a portender of a developing chemical dependence. An adolescent needs treatment (1) if the substance use is interfering with any aspect of functioning, (2) if the use is causing negative

---

BOX 108-6
Abridged Criteria
for Substance Dependence

Substance dependence: A maladaptive pattern of substance use leading to clinically significant impairment of distress. This is manifested in three (or more) of the following occurring at any time in the 12-month period:
1. Tolerance
2. Withdrawal
3. The substance is taken in increased amounts or over a longer period than was intended
4. The presence of persistent desire or unsuccessful efforts to cut down or control substance abuse
5. Large amounts of time are spent in activities to obtain substances
6. Social, recreational, or occupational activities are given up or reduced because of substance abuse
7. Use is continued despite knowledge of having a persistent or recurrent physical or psychologic problem that is likely to have been caused or exacerbated by the substance

Adapted from *Diagnostic and statistical manual of mental disorders,* ed 4, Washington, DC, 1994, American Psychiatric Association.

BOX 108-7
Diagnostic Criteria for Substance Abuse

Substance abuse: A maladaptive pattern of substance use leading to clinically significant impairment or distress, as manifested by one (or more) of the following occurring within a 12-month period:
1. Recurrent use resulting in a failure to fulfill major role obligations at school, work, or home
2. Recurrent use in circumstances in which it is physically hazardous
3. Recurrent related legal problems
4. Continued use despite having persistent or recurrent social or interpersonal problems caused or exacerbated by the effects of the substance

Symptoms have never met the criteria for substance dependence

Adapted from *Diagnostic and statistical manual of mental disorders,* ed 4, Washington, DC, 1994, American Psychiatric Association.

---

consequences, (3) if there is a loss of control of the use, or (4) if there is evidence of withdrawal symptoms. If any one of these four criteria is not present, it is difficult to motivate the adolescent, as drug use is seen not as a problem but as another life experience.

Urine and Blood Screening

Controversy continues over the nonconsenting right to random, obligatory, or involuntary screening for illicit drugs. Generally, blood and urine drug testing provides tangible evidence of drug use and, in the emergency room, supplies a valuable adjunct to patient management in adolescents involved in trauma, violence, accidents, intoxication, overdose, or bizarre behaviors. With the sophistication of technology, new, inexpensive, and reliable automated and semiautomated laboratory procedures have facilitated drug screening and identification.[18] Although urine testing is not limited to the medical environment, the physician is usually called on to interpret results, further evaluate the patient, or develop a management plan. As stated by the American Medical Association's Council on Scientific Affairs, drug testing does not provide "any information about pattern of use of drugs, abuse of or dependence on drugs, or about mental or physical impairments that may result from drug use."[19] Toxicologic testing for drugs of abuse may be carried out on specimens of blood, urine, or hair. Blood testing is particularly useful for alcohol, reflecting use during the previous 2 to 12 hours. Except in emergency situations, this narrow window of detection limits its use for most illicit drugs. Drug testing is best done by urine screening, since a specific urine aliquot represents excretory products formed over the previous 3 to 5 hours. With drugs such as marijuana that are stored in body adipose tissue, toxicologic analysis of urine may reflect drug use over the previous 1 to 2 months.

Hair and saliva have recently been used for testing and carry the advantage of being less invasive. Testing of hair also lessens the opportunity for deception by the patient and can be easily repeated if confirmation is required. Owing to its growth, a one and one-half inch piece of hair provides a chronology of drug use over the previous 90 days.

Four distinct stages are involved in urine screening: (1) preparation of the donor, (2) collection of the specimen, (3) laboratory analysis, and (4) clinical application of the laboratory results. All four stages of screening must be addressed with equal diligence. Any error may lead not only to inappropriate therapy but also to the often associated adverse legal consequences. Box 108-8 outlines the usual indications for urine drug screening in adolescents.[20] It is important to evaluate such indications on the basis of the adolescent's history. Occasionally, urine testing is requested by anxious parents or authorities whose intentions are punitive or related to a power struggle. The physician is bound by the confidentiality of the professional relationship and the limited degree of freedom that is permitted without consent. In its statement

on urine testing in children and adolescents, the American
Academy of Pediatrics states that

Voluntary screening for purposes of treatment is within the
ethical tradition of health maintenance, but the psychosocial
risks of such screening in the area of drug abuse warrant
particularly careful attention to the requirements for informed
consent and the maintenance of confidentiality. Parental consent
may be sufficient for the involuntary screening of the younger
child who lacks the capacity to make informed judgments.
Parental permission is not sufficient for involuntary screening of
the older, competent adolescent, and the Academy opposes such
involuntary screening. Consent from the older adolescent may
be waived when there is reason to doubt competency or in those
circumstances in which information gained by history or
physical examination is strongly suggestive of a young person
at high risk from substance abuse.[21]

Reasons for urine screening should be made clear to
the adolescent. Management of a positive test result
should be determined prior to the procedure itself.
Communication between adolescent and parent needs to
be encouraged and facilitated. Home testing of urine for
drugs is now available. Unless parents are prepared to
deal with the angry confrontation that usually results, this
approach may create more harm than good. Concerned
parents cannot replace a professional who is trained in
management of drug use and who has knowledge of
available community resources.

An often neglected yet critical step in a successful
screening program is the specimen collection itself.
Reliable specimen collection is of particular importance
if the result of the test will compromise the young adult's
employability, participation in sports, family relations,
hospital or recovery programs, discharge, or legal ac-
countability. Box 108-9 outlines guidelines for urine
specimen collection in drug screening.

A number of laboratory techniques are available for
effective urine screening. Individual laboratory reliability
is dependent on the inclusion of the criteria outlined by

the American Medical Association's Council on Scientific Affairs. Two categories of tests are used, screening
tests and confirmatory tests. Screening tests tend to be
simple, efficient, inexpensive, and rapid. Confirmatory
tests are used for individuals who have positive results in
the screening test; they are more complex and labor
intensive than screening tests. The director of the
toxicology laboratory usually establishes a threshold
concentration for positive values.

Four general types of methods are used in the modern
laboratory: (1) immunoassays (IAs) (enzyme IA, fluorescence polarization IA, and radio IA); (2) thin-layer
chromatography (TLC); (3) gas chromatography (GC);
and (4) gas chromatography–mass spectrometry (GC/
MS). In general, immunoassays and TLC are good
screening or first confirmation methods for certain
compounds. Gas (liquid) chromatography is used primarily for identification of volatile compounds. Gas
chromatography-mass spectrometry is used for confirmation of positive screening results, is highly sensitive
and specific, and is the only test admissible in most
courts of law. Table 108-1 summarizes the urine screening methods used for drugs commonly ingested by
adolescents.

Confronting drug abusers with objective evidence of
their drug use usually has negligible impact on behavior
or their motivation to change use patterns. Drug screening
is best integrated into contingency planning in an overall
treatment program. Such planning must incorporate a
number of negative reinforcers that will diminish the
desire for continued use. Care must be taken that such
activities do not redefine the physician's role as one of
policing rather than treating, or judging rather than
counseling.

TABLE 108-1
Urine Screening for Drugs Commonly Abused by Adolescents

Drug	Major Metabolite	Initial	First Confirmation	Second Confirmation	Approximate Retention Time
Alcohol (blood)	Acetaldehyde	GC	IA		7-10 hr
Alcohol (urine)	Acetaldehyde	GC	IA		10-13 hr
Amphetamines		TLC	IA	GC, GC/MS	48 hr
Barbiturates		IA	TLC	GC, GC/MS	Short-acting (24 hr); long-acting (2-3 wk)
Benzodiazepines		IA	TLC	GC, GC/MS	3 days
Cannabinoids	Carboxy- and hydroxymetabolites	IA	TLC	GC/MS	3-10 days (occasional user); 1-2 mo (chronic user)
Cocaine	Benzoylecgonine	IA	TLC	GC/MS	2-4 days
Methaqualone	Hydroxylated metabolites	TLC	IA	GC/MS	2 wk
Opiates					
Heroin	Morphine Glucuronide	IA	TLC	GC, GC/MS	2 days
Morphine	Morphine Glucuronide	IA	TLC	GC, GC/MS	2 days
Codeine	Morphine Glucuronide	IA	TLC	GC, GC/MS	2 days
Phencyclidine		TLC	IA	GC, GC/MS	8 days

Modified from Drugs of abuse—urine screening (physician information sheet), Los Angeles, Pacific Toxicology.
GC, gas chromatography; *IA,* immunoassay; *MS,* mass spectrometry; *TLC,* thin-layer chromatography.

TREATMENT APPROACHES

Most models for substance abuse treatment have been developed for adults. However, it is critical that treatment interventions be tailored to the unique developmental needs of adolescents inasmuch as they differ dramatically from adult substance abusers.[22] Adolescents have a shorter history of substance abuse and rarely manifest long-term physical side effects. Adolescents are also more vulnerable to peer pressure than are adults. Furthermore, the cognitive development of adolescents in their early and middle teens is not complete. They have difficulty in internalizing values, ideas, and concepts that are based partially or completely on formal operational (abstract) thinking. Consequently, they face problems in internalizing and implementing treatment concepts. Most adolescents are still in school, live at home, have achieved no (or only partial) economic independence, and need a great deal of family involvement in their treatment. Adolescents who are substance abusers are not attracted to long-term treatment goals, such as preventing liver cirrhosis from alcohol or lung cancer from cigarette smoking. Immediate and short-term goals thus need to be designed to increase their motivation.

Treatment needs are defined on the basis of stage of drug use and the matching of individuals with the appropriate level of care. This matching then facilitates the adolescent's transition through a seamless continuum of relevant services and treatment modalities. For adolescents, the American Society for Addiction Medicine has established six criteria for placement at one of four levels of care[23]: (1) acute intoxication or withdrawal potential, (2) biomedical conditions and complications, (3) emotional/behavioral conditions and complications, (4) treatment acceptance/resistance, (5) relapse potential, and (6) recovery environment. The levels of care are determined using the above criteria.

Level I: Outpatient/Office Management

There is no risk of withdrawal. Physical and mental health are stable. The adolescent is willing to cooperate after appropriate motivating and monitoring strategies. Abstinence can be maintained with minimal support and recovery goals sustainable. The adolescent has a supportive environment for recovery or has inherent skills to cope. A skilled counselor, with medical and psychologic back-up, can usually manage these types of patients. This type of setting serves the majority at stage 1, which includes almost 80% of adolescents with a drug problem.

Level II: Intensive Outpatient Management

This is suitable for those at stage 2. Risk of withdrawal is not apparent. Physically, there is no associated compromise or medical problems that would detract from ambulatory management. There may be emotional or behavioral issues that have the potential to distract from the recovery, but these are mild in severity and are manageable in an ambulatory setting. Treatment resistance mandates a structured program but is judged not to be so high as to render outpatient management ineffective. Addiction symptoms may intensify during management, and without the close monitoring and support integrated into the program may portend relapse. External environment is nonsupportive, but with program structure and support the adolescent can cope. These programs typically consist of a multidisciplinary team (medical staff, nursing, alcohol/drug counselors, activity therapists, psychologists) and are commonly located in hospitals or community-based health clinics.

Level III: Medically Monitored Intensive Inpatient Treatment

Risk of withdrawal is apparent but manageable in a medically monitored setting—usually for those in stage 3. Physical condition requires monitoring but not intensive treatment. The psychologic state requires structured 24-hour monitoring but not psychiatric intensive care. Treatment acceptance is poor with often high resistance and thus a need for constant motivating strategies that can be best accomplished in a 24-hour structured level III program. Recovery would be extremely difficult, if not impossible, in an external social environment requiring physical removal from these influences. This type of program is usually located in a free-standing residential setting that emphasizes adolescents' acceptance of responsibility for their own behavior. This may include halfway houses for those who have completed a more intensive treatment program. Day-treatment programs or overnight programs, although theoretically sound, have yet to be evaluated for effectiveness.

Level IV: Medically Managed Intensive Inpatient Treatment

Withdrawal risk is severe and the adolescent requires 24-hour medical and nursing management. Severe psychiatric problems require expert management concomitant with the addiction treatment. Resistance and relapse potential are inherent in the severity of the problem. Most adolescents in stage 4 (dependence) will need this intensity of treatment.

Inpatient treatment (level III or IV) is indicated for the following categories of adolescents:

1. Those who are severely physically dependent. Such patients need to be detoxified under medical supervision to prevent potentially life-threatening withdrawal symptoms.
2. Those who have a dual diagnosis with moderate to severe psychiatric symptoms or serious emotional problems in addition to substance abuse (e.g., suicidal behavior, anorexia nervosa, bulimia, psychosis).
3. Those who have a serious medical condition.
4. Those who have failed or do not qualify for outpatient treatment.
5. Those who need to be stabilized (i.e., homeless, runaway adolescents who do not have a supportive family or home) or removed from the family and home.

Unfortunately, affordable treatment services appropriate for adolescents are often not available. As a result, adolescents are frequently incorporated into mixed patient populations or provided with adult services that are not necessarily appropriate to their specific needs. Frequently, referral to a specific program is based on availability of space or ability to pay, as opposed to the specific needs of the adolescent.

In many treatment programs the prevailing therapeutic approach is the "shotgun" method, in which all available modalities are targeted to the adolescent. The assumption is that one or several modalities will provide the "corrective emotional experience" that will facilitate change and help the adolescent abstain. Examples of some commonly used treatment modalities include individual therapy, cognitive and behavioral therapy, family therapy, various group therapies, social skills training, and support groups for both the adolescent and family. Vocational counseling is important for school dropouts, and involvement in recreational activities is critical to fight boredom, which is closely associated with drug use and relapse among adolescents.

One of the greatest difficulties lies in helping adolescents recognize that they have a problem and need treatment. Treatment counselors are quick to point out that adolescents are typically reluctant to make a commitment to treatment that involves the goal of abstinence. Many do not voluntarily enter treatment but rather become involved because of pressure from the family, school, or legal system. Thus, the typical adolescent substance abuser who starts treatment exhibits a sense of ambivalence about drug use. Part of the adolescent's resistance to entering treatment comes from the fear that without drugs life will no longer be fun and friends will be lost. For treatment to be effective, it is critical that the adolescent recognize the need to change behavior.

One way to motivate adolescents to begin treatment is to help them understand the probable short-term negative consequences of continued use based on the current negative consequences. Then, the short-term benefits of abstinence and involvement in treatment should be emphasized. This can be done by asking adolescents what they want and then determining what privileges the parents are prepared to give and the consequences of noncompliance. It is also important to provide adolescents with specific information about treatment. They need to know what treatment program is best suited to them and for what reasons. The risks of emotional or physical discomfort need to be explained and the structure for support and alleviation emphasized. Treatment usually involves participation in twelve-step self-help recovery groups such as Alcoholics Anonymous (AA) or Cocaine Anonymous (CA).

Adolescents need to understand that they have the right to confidentiality (with some exceptions), that urine testing is likely to be required, and that treatment will include education about substance use and chemical dependency as well as education about alternatives. It is important that treatment providers indicate the minimal and maximal length of time treatment will be provided; the length and kind of sessions (group, individual, family); and the consequences of missed sessions, the inability to be abstinent, and a slip or relapse.

After-care that takes place in a drug-free, social environment that includes the usual activities of teenagers, without the use of alcohol or drugs, is critical. The clinician must act as an advocate to encourage the community to develop such programs.

The parents of substance-abusing youths may also need support and assistance. This can be done by providing them with an explanation of treatment and a referral to a parents' support group (Al-Anon, Alateen). They should enter the group at the time the adolescent enters treatment. This will give parents an opportunity to ventilate anger, frustration, and guilt. It will also provide them with support as they adopt new techniques for parenting a recovering teenager.

ETHICAL AND LEGAL CONSIDERATIONS

Within the past 20 years, the legal rights of minors have become increasingly clarified by mature-minor legislation, federal and state regulations, or legal precedents. The increased socialization of the adolescent, without mediation of parental authority, has underscored the importance of the need to be able to self-consent for health care. Most states give minors rights of self-consent if they are emancipated through age, marriage, or membership in the armed services or if they are living away from home and managing their own financial affairs. Specific circumstances, such as sexually transmitted diseases, pregnancy, contraception, and drug counseling, are also defining conditions for self-consent. More than half of the states currently have specific statutes permitting treatment for substance abuse without parental consent. Even in the absence of such statutes, it is extremely unlikely and without precedent that a state would hold a physician liable for non-negligent medical care of a minor with a drug problem without parental consent. The mere fact that the teenager has requested and given consent for such treatment would undoubtedly be judged by the court as an indication of competence for consent to such treatment.

In most jurisdictions, self-consent for medical care is accompanied by the right to confidentiality and privacy. Disclosure to parents by the professional is governed by the general rule of "what best serves the adolescent's interests." Drug and alcohol abuse in minors poses particularly complex questions. Substance abuse represents a family of disorders characterized by denial and compulsive and health-compromising behaviors. Motivation for change and treatment is usually precipitated by family members, counselors, teachers, or law enforcement authorities. However, successful treatment depends on motivation, commitment, involvement, and self-consent by the minor. The confidentiality of the physician-patient relationship allows for nondisclosure of not only socially, but also legally, unacceptable behavior. With few exceptions, in the absence of consent, information or communication about treatment issues is restricted. Despite their concern and financial responsibility, parents must negotiate early in the treatment for the greatest freedom for disclosure and involvement.

Several circumstances are usually accepted as valid reasons to supersede the constraints of physician-patient confidentiality. These particularly relate to whether the condition is life-threatening or life-endangering to self or others. Even under these circumstances, every effort should be made to involve the adolescent and secure permission for parental contact. As stated by the American Academy of Pediatrics, "In general, the principle of confidentiality is a positive good to be encouraged and supported; it is never an absolute barrier to communication." As with parents, the healthcare professional should negotiate for the greatest degrees of freedom early in the relationship. Clear disclosure of exceptional circumstances, as outlined above, should be discussed. The benefits of disclosure, while still ensuring confidentiality concerning specific information, should be presented. It is particularly important to discuss the issue of recordkeeping and the restrictions on the release of information contained therein. Adolescents must be educated about the future implications of release of sensitive substance abuse information in their medical records. When giving consent, they may exercise the option to restrict release only to that information relating to their medical condition under consideration.

The management of an adolescent who abuses drugs or alcohol is a team effort. Information may be shared among individuals who are part of this team when the sharing of this information serves the adolescent's best interest. This needs to be made clear early in the professional relationship. Failure to have this freedom would greatly compromise treatment success. Disclosure to those who are indirectly involved in the treatment program must be made only after careful evaluation. The guiding principle is that of benefit to the adolescent, who, after all, is the patient. If there is a doubt, it is prudent to seek written consent for disclosure.

Physicians are often pressured to screen for substance abuse at the request of the parents and over the objections of the patient. Failure to respect the wishes of the adolescent challenges the constructs of self-consent and confidentiality. Without consent, future successful interaction with the young person is greatly compromised because of the breach of trust. Although a substance abuse disorder is characterized by denial and nondisclosure, open communication, discussion, and expression of concern about health risk will usually lead to agreement between the adolescent and professional about treatment plans. Again, confidentiality must be ensured and explained not only to the adolescent, but also to the parents. If testing is carried out, it must be done with a clear plan of action in mind. The physician must always take a stance that promotes a helping alliance and not one that promotes a disciplinary consequence.

SUMMARY

Drug and alcohol abuse in adolescents and young adults is a disease of self-deception. In the developmental sense, it is perceived by the adolescent to serve a purpose. The intricate matrix of physical, psychologic, and social pathology created by this chemical-human interaction creates a clinical challenge that tests even the most skillful of practitioners. The necessary task of reframing the adolescent's "solution" to one of a "problem" is a critical, but often difficult first step toward intervention. Efforts at prevention, applied at vulnerable and receptive points of the brief life experience of children and adolescents, although not a panacea, will lessen this clinical burden. For those who respond to such preventive messages, much life pain will be ameliorated if these messages promote healthy developmental alternatives.

For those who succumb to the chemical life style, the options are few—to live the life of the alcoholic or drug

user or to seek change through intervention. Clinicians must be sensitized to this message for change and take appropriate action. Recognizing the syndrome through risk profile and behavior helps to create the opportunity. A methodical approach that combines knowledge, skills, and resources from a variety of disciplines will maximize the chance for success. Each step that raises self-esteem empowers the individual, detoxifies both the physical body and the social environment, and restores control to the adolescent is a step in the right direction. The crutch of clinical care must eventually be abandoned by the individual and the gift of a healthy development realized. All therapeutic interventions must have this ultimate goal.

References

1. Johnston LD, O'Malley PM, Bachman JG: Drug use, drinking and smoking: national survey results from high school, college, and young adult populations, 1975-1996: Rockville, MD, 1996, National Institute on Drug Abuse.
2. U.S. Department of Health and Human Services: National Household Survey on Drug Abuse: Population Estimates, 1994, Washington, DC, 1995, Public Health Service and Alcohol, Drug Abuse, and Mental Health Administration.
3. Schwartz RH, Luxenberg MG, Hoffmann NG: "Crack" use by American middle-class adolescent polydrug abusers, *J Pediatr* 118:1, 1991.
4. Zarek D, Hawkins JD, Rogers PD: Risk factors for adolescent substance abuse: implications for pediatric practice, *Pediatr Clin North Am* 34:2, 1987.
5. Briere J: Therapy for adults molested as children, New York, 1989, Springer-Verlag.
6. Hawkins JD, Catalano RF, Miller JY: Risk and protective factors for alcohol and other drug problems in adolescence and early adulthood: implications for substance abuse prevention, *Psychol Bull* 112:64, 1992.
7. Briere J, Runtz M: Post sexual abuse trauma: data and implications for clinical practice, *J Interpersonal Violence* 2, 1987.
8. Robertson M: *Homeless youth in Hollywood: patterns of alcohol use. A report to the National Institute on Alcohol Abuse and Alcoholism. Alcohol Research Group, School of Public Health,* Berkeley, CA, 1989, University of Southern California.
9. Kipke MD, Montgomery AS, Seils-Pascoe R, Pennbridge J, Yates G, MacKenzie RG: A comparison of health problems in homeless and non-homeless youth (unpublished manuscript).
10. Margetson N, Lipman C: *Children at risk: the impact of poverty, the family and the street on homeless and runaway youth in New York City,* Presented at the National Symposium on Youth Victimization, Atlanta, 1990.
11. Remafedi G: Adolescent homosexuality: psychosocial and medical implications, *Pediatrics* 79:331, 1987.
12. Kipke MD, Futterman D, Hein K: HIV infection and AIDS during adolescence, *Med Clin North Am* 74:5, 1990.
13. Frances RJ, Miller SI, editors: *Clinical textbook of addictive disorders,* New York, 1991, Guilford Press.
14. Friedman AS, Glickman NW: Program characteristics for successful treatment of adolescent substance abuse, *J Nerv Ment Dis* 174:669, 1986.
15. Winters K: Clinical considerations in the assessment of adolescent chemical dependency, *J Adolesc Chem Dependency* 1:31, 1990.
16. Goldenring JM, Cohen EH: Getting into the adolescent's H.E.A.D.S., *Contemp Pediatr* 5:7, 1988.

17. Diagnostic and Statistical Manual of Mental Disorders, ed 4, Washington, DC, 1994, American Psychiatric Association.

18. Saxon AJ, Calsyn DA, et al: Clinical evaluation and use of urine screening for drug abuse, *West J Med* 149:3, 1988.

19. American Medical Association, Council on Scientific Affairs: Scientific issues in drug testing, *JAMA* 257:3110, 1987.

20. MacKenzie RG, Cheng M, Haftel AJ: The clinical utility and evaluation of drug screening techniques, *Pediatr Clin North Am* 34:2, 1987.

21. American Academy of Pediatrics. Committee on Adolescence, Committee on Bioethics, and Provisional Committee on Substance Abuse: Screening for drug abuse in children and adolescents, *Pediatrics* 84:2, 1989.

22. Morehouse ER: Treating adolescent cocaine abusers. In Washton AM, Gold MS, editors: *Cocaine: a clinician's handbook,* New York, 1987, Guilford Press.

23. Hoffman NG, Halikas JA, Mee-Lee D, Weedman RD: *ASAM patient placement criteria for the treatment of psychoactive substance use disorders,* Washington, DC, 1991, American Society of Addiction Medicine; pp 109-133.

Suggested Readings

American Academy of Pediatrics: *Substance abuse: a guide for health professionals,* Elk Grove Park, IL, 1988, AAP.

George RL: *Counseling the chemically dependent: theory and practice,* Boston, 1990, Allyn & Bacon.

Legal issues for alcohol and other drug use prevention and treatment programs serving high risk youth. OSAP Technical Report 2, Department of Health and Human Services, ADMH A 1990, DHHS Pub. No.(ADM) 90-1674, Washington DC, Public Health Service.

CHAPTER 109

Risk Behaviors

•

Sheryl A. Ryan and Charles E. Irwin, Jr.

Primary care clinicians who routinely assess and treat the adolescent patient will encounter youths at risk for or actively engaging in health-compromising behaviors. All adolescents should be considered at risk for engaging in risk behaviors because of the wide prevalence of these behaviors, the developmental needs that they fulfill, and the numerous risk factors for their initiation and maintenance. Timely, comprehensive, and appropriate assessment and management of these behaviors require an understanding of the morbidity and mortality patterns of the second decade of life, knowledge of the highly prevalent risk behaviors responsible for most of this mortality and morbidity, and the developmental and environmental contexts in which these behaviors occur.

The traditional measures of morbidity and mortality used to support the view held by some that adolescents are a surprisingly healthy group are narrowly conceptualized and measured. They are both disease focused and adult focused and they underestimate aspects of health, such as functional status and specific behaviors initiated during adolescence that are responsible for short-term and long-term negative physical and psychosocial consequences.[1] Although absolute mortality rates among adolescents are low compared with those of other age groups, there is a striking increase in rates of death across the age range encompassed by adolescence. For example, 15- to 19-year-olds have an overall death rate three times that of 10- to 14-year-olds (87.2:100,000 and 28.4:100,000, respectively). This is the single largest increase in mortality rate between any two age groups, and it primarily reflects the contribution of injuries, both intentional and unintentional.[2] Adolescents of all ages experience the highest rates of mortality from injuries, including homicide, suicide, and motor vehicle accidents. Currently, these violent causes account for approximately 80% and 55% of all deaths in 15- to 19-year-olds and 10- to 14-year-olds, respectively; almost half of these deaths result from motor vehicle accidents and 15% to 35% from suicides and homicides.[3] Trend analyses have demonstrated that while motor vehicle accident death rates have remained stable since 1950, there have been major increases in the rates of homicide and suicide. Currently, suicide is the third leading cause of death among white males aged 15 to 19 years, and homicide is the leading cause of death among black males aged 15 to 19 years.[3] Subgroup analyses also consistently demonstrate striking differences in mortality rates by gender and race/ethnicity. Adolescent males of all ages experience markedly higher death rates than females for all causes, and this gap widens with increasing age; among 15- to 19-year-olds the male-to-female mortality ratio is more than 2:1.[3] Although data are limited, race/ethnic groups demonstrate important differences. For example, while death rates for most age groups in the United States have remained stable or demonstrated slight decreases, the death rate for young blacks continued to rise from 1988 to 1991.[3] This increase was particularly striking for black males aged 15 to 19 years, whose mortality rate increased 40% during this period, reflecting the contribution of homicides, as mentioned above.[3] In contrast, whites experienced suicide and motor vehicle accident death rates 2.5 times greater than those of blacks.[2]

Hospitalization and physician visit rates for adolescents are low and most adolescents experience no major medical disorders, chronic conditions, or limitations on activity. The primary causes of illness, injury, and disability in this age group, however, are behaviorally generated. More than 50% of the morbidity in adolescents stems from four behaviors: sexual activity, substance use and abuse, recreational/motor vehicle use, and interpersonal violence. These four behaviors generally have their onset in adolescence; are common among all socioeconomic, racial/ethnic, and age groups; have high probabilities for negative outcomes; and share a common theme: risk taking.[4] These activities also typically continue beyond the adolescent period and are responsible for the major types of morbidity in adults up to the age of 40 that have been targeted as important areas for prevention.[5]

DEFINITION

Risk taking can be defined as participation in potentially health-compromising activities with little understanding of, or in spite of an understanding of, the potential negative consequences.[6] This definition requires that the behavior be volitional, have an uncertain outcome (either positive or negative), and result from an interplay between the biopsychosocial processes of adolescence and the environment (see Chapter 7, "Cognitive Development"). Deliberately excluded are behaviors such as suicide and eating disorders, which are mainly psychopathologic, and homicide, a major environmental act that is beyond an adolescent's control.[7]

EPIDEMIOLOGY AND CONSEQUENCES

Specific Behaviors

In adolescents, unintentional injuries are responsible for the largest number of deaths, hospital days, and years of potential lives lost. Adolescents are also at highest risk for both nonfatal and fatal injuries related to motor vehicles, with alcohol implicated in 50% of these injuries. Falls, drownings, burns, and firearm-related events are additional relatively common causes of premature accidental death and disability. Although nonfatal injuries attract less attention, they nevertheless result in tremendous amounts of short- and long-term disability.[8] There are few data documenting the extent to which behavioral risk factors, such as life style and poor judgment, are involved in specific types of injuries, other than the association between alcohol use and motor vehicle accidents. In our studies on risk perception, we found that 29.5% of middle school students and 37.5% of high school students reported engaging in physically risky behaviors involving the use of recreational vehicles such as skateboards and bicycles. Results from the Youth Risk Behavior Surveillance System (YRBSS), which monitors priority health risk behaviors among youth and young adults through national school-based surveys, also suggest that most high school students participate in behaviors that increase their likelihood of death and disability from injury.[9] For example, 93% of students reported rarely or never wearing a bicycle helmet, 40% of students who ride motorcycles reported rarely or never wearing a motorcycle helmet, and 19% reported rarely or never using seat belts regularly.[9]

High rates of substance use among youth have been consistently documented in national surveys of secondary school students.[10] Racial/ethnic subgroups demonstrate differential rates, with non-white youths, especially Asian-American and black youths, reporting the lowest rates of use of all substances.[11] Significant declines in the use of illicit substances occurred during the 1980s, but since 1991 there have been consistent and worrying trends reflecting increased use of all illicit substances.[10] Alcohol remains the most widely used substance, with 50% of high school seniors in 1994 reporting use of alcohol within the past month, 28% reporting that more than five drinks in a row had been consumed in the previous 2 weeks, and 2.9% reporting daily use.[10] Tobacco is the second most frequently used substance, with 62% of high school seniors reporting lifetime use of cigarettes, 31% use within the past 30 days, and 19% daily use.[10] The recent rise in illicit drug use has been particularly pronounced for marijuana, the most widely used illicit substance; increases were also especially prominent for younger adolescents.[10] For example, from 1991 to 1994, annual use of marijuana (use within the previous 12 months) more than doubled for eighth grade students (from 6% to 13%); similar increases were found for tenth graders (from 16% to 25%) and twelfth graders (24% to 31%).[10] Although the long-term medical effects of substance use are much less likely than behavioral effects, adolescents are still at substantial risk for medical effects, such as injury directly resulting from alcohol intoxication (Table 109-1).

TABLE 109-1
Adolescent Health Risk Behaviors and Their Acute and Chronic Medical Consequences

	Consequence
Substance use: general	
Short-term	Acute injury due to intoxication, diminished global health status and functioning
Long-term	Addiction/habituation, multisystem organ damage
Cigarettes	
Short-term	Nicotine addiction, elevated white blood cell count, chronic bronchitis, decline in pulmonary function tests (cigarettes); periodontal disease: leukoplakia, gingival recession, caries (smokeless)
Long-term	Increase in cancer of lungs, larynx, esophagus, oral cavity; heart disease, chronic lung disease (cigarettes), oropharyngeal cancer (smokeless)
Marijuana	
Short-term	Decreased pulmonary function, chronic bronchitis, gynecomastia, decreased testosterone levels
Long-term	Increased risk of lung cancer, amotivational syndrome
Alcohol	
Short-term	Abnormal liver function tests, hepatitis, gastritis
Long-term	Chronic liver damage, malnutrition, global dementia, chronic pancreatitis
Motor/recreational vehicle use	
Short-term	Accidental death and injury
Long-term	Chronic disability/impairment
Sexual activity	
Short-term	Sexually transmitted diseases, pregnancy
Long-term	Infertility, ectopic pregnancy, AIDS, cervical intraepithelial neoplasia
Violence-related activities	
Short-term	Death and injury
Long-term	Chronic disability/impairment

Modified from Irwin CE Jr, Ryan SA: Problem behavior of adolescents, *Pediatr Rev* 10:235-246, 1989.

The National Survey of Family Growth (1988 data) indicated that 97% of black males, 85% of white males, 83% of black females, and 76% of white females have experienced sexual intercourse by age 19. Cumulative estimates from this sample also have shown that female adolescents are initiating coitus at earlier ages.[12] More recent data using the YRBSS among high school students, grades 9 to 12, have found that more than half (53%) of all students reported ever having sexual intercourse; 19% reported having had sexual intercourse during their lifetime with four or more sex partners.[9] Black male and female students reported significantly higher rates of sexual activity (89% and 70%, respectively) than white males and females (49% and 47%, respectively) or Hispanic males and females (64% and 48%, respectively).[9] Questions from this survey on condom and birth control use also document the fact that currently sexually active youths are placing themselves at risk for both sexually transmitted diseases (STDs) and unintended pregnancy; only 53% reported that they or their partner had used a condom during the most recent coitus, and only 18% reported that they or their partner had used birth control pills.[9] Epidemic rates of STDs and unintended

pregnancy have paralleled these high rates of sexual experience. From 1960 to 1988, there was a 325% increase in the prevalence of gonorrhea among 10- to 14-year-olds and a 170% increase among 15- to 19-year-olds, while young adults age 19 to 24 years experienced only a 43% increase.[2]

Adolescents are disproportionately affected by violent and abusive behaviors, including homicide and assaultive violence, child abuse, sexual assault, and firearm injury; they are more than twice as likely as other age groups to be the victims of violent crimes.[13] National statistics also document that youths are perpetrators of violent acts; adolescents account for 24% of violent offenses leading to an arrest,[14] and 67% of adolescents who were victims of a violent crime reported that their attacker was between the ages of 12 and 20 years.[13] In contrast to these official statistics, national surveys have attempted to monitor those interpersonal behaviors, such as weapon carrying and physical fighting, that increase the likelihood of an adolescent experiencing intentional injury, as either a victim or a perpetrator. Data from the YRBSS indicated that 22% and 8% of high school students reported carrying a weapon or a gun for protection, respectively, within the previous 30 days; across all age groups, males were significantly more likely than females to report weapon carrying, and black males and females (20.9% and 3.8%) were significantly more likely to report doing so than white males and females (12% and 1.2%, respectively).[9] The YRBSS also documented high rates of physical fighting and school-related violence among youths; for the 12 months preceding the survey, 42% reported being in a physical fight, 16.2% reported being in a fight on school property, and 7.3% reported being threatened or injured while at school.[9]

Covariation

Although risk behaviors traditionally have been treated as isolated phenomena by researchers, clinicians, and program planners, an accumulating body of research is showing that certain risk-taking activities are predictably associated with one another. The association between substance use, particularly alcohol, and unintentional injury involving motor vehicles, and to a lesser extent bicycles and skateboards, has been well established.[15] Millstein et al also demonstrated that early adolescents (11 to 14 years old) who were sexually active were significantly more likely to report driving or riding in a car while intoxicated than their non–sexually active peers.[16]

In general, the strongest interrelationships are concentrated in a group of health-risk behaviors that include sexual activity, cigarette smoking, alcohol use, marijuana and other illicit drug use, and delinquency. Research has consistently shown that adolescents who use one illicit substance are more likely to use others, and that there are progressive and predictable patterns of substance use and abuse.[17] Substance use is also positively correlated with early sexual debut and juvenile delinquency, and it is associated with the use of less effective means of contraception.[18,19] Longitudinal studies have found that sexual activity is both a predictor of subsequent substance use and an outcome of substance use.[20,21] In this latter case, Kegeles et al found that white adolescent females who reported both substance use and injury-related behaviors were more likely to endorse the intention to become sexually active in the subsequent year.[21]

It is not entirely clear from current longitudinal studies whether the covariation of risk behaviors reflects the causal effect of one behavior on the initiation of a second or the fact that the behaviors result from a common set of risk factors, or a general tendency toward risk taking or "deviance," as Osgood et al maintain.[19] It must be emphasized, however, that theories based on the latter explanation for covariation can account for only some of the variance in these behaviors.[19] Furthermore, the nature and strength of the covariation may differ across a variety of groups of individuals and clusters of behaviors.[19,22]

DEVELOPMENTAL CONTEXT

During adolescence there are dramatic biologic, psychologic, cognitive, and social changes that occur interdependently across multiple contexts. Inherent in each aspect of developmental change are specific milestones or needs that represent strong forces encouraging youths to take risks and engage in risk behaviors[7] (Table 109-2). When this risk taking occurs in a positive context and is limited to experimentation or taking chances, healthy development may be enhanced. More pronounced asynchronies in these developmental changes, especially in biologic and psychosocial development, may further enhance the onset of risk behaviors, such as in the early-maturing female, who may have higher needs for independence and an earlier onset of sexual activity than her normally developing peers.[23]

Risk taking may thus be viewed as a critical component of healthy adolescent development to the extent that certain risk behaviors may increase self-esteem, allow practice in taking initiative, and promote an understanding of cause-and-effect relationships. The concept of risk taking should incorporate an acknowledgment that some exploratory behaviors are adaptive and may have positive consequences, such as contributing to optimal competence or enhancing growth.[1] These behaviors, if frequent, intense, increasing over time, or associated with other high-risk activities, may become pathogenic or primarily destructive.[4,24] The personal and interpersonal resources available to youths for coping, the behavioral antecedents, and the nature of the possible consequences need to be considered in determining just how risky a specific behavior is. Unfortunately, even healthy exploration may have adverse consequences for youths, especially given possible limited cognitive capacities, lack of experience, and inability to appreciate both environmental factors and potential consequences of specific actions. Research has shown that even when teenagers are aware of the risks involved, they may be willing to participate because of a value placed on other perceived, anticipated, or experienced outcomes.[15]

A number of theories and models have been proposed to explain risk taking among adolescents and predict those at greatest risk. Some of these integrate developmental principles of adolescence with known risk factors for health-compromising behaviors. Irwin and Millstein's biopsychosocial model,[23] Jessor and Jessor's problem behavior theory,[25] and social learning theory are some of the more useful of these theoretical frameworks. None of these, however, can fully explain involvement in a wide spectrum of risky activities.[26]

TABLE 109-2
Developmental Forces and Specific Risk Behaviors Encouraged

Area of Development	Developmental Needs/ Milestones	Associated Risk Behaviors
Physiologic	Heterosocial behavior; sexuality Physical mastery	Sexual behavior, intercourse Physical risks
Psychosocial	"Tasks of adolescence" Autonomy	Physical risks/behaviors (substance use, recreational vehicle use)
	Intimacy/reciprocity in interpersonal relationships Emancipation, interdependence/ individuation from family	Social risks involving peers (substance use, sexual activity, violence-related)
	Identity formation Affiliation	Peer-associated social and physical risks (violence-related e.g., gang membership)
Cognitive	Exploration of cause and effect relationships Logical verification	Physical risks
Socioenvironmental	School transitions	Peer-associated social and physical risks

CLINICAL ASSESSMENT

Clearly, the challenge for the clinician is to distinguish between what may be normal exploratory behaviors and those that are mainly health-compromising ones. This requires (1) evaluating both the effects of these behaviors on health status and the motivation for engaging in them and (2) determining whether positive psychosocial development is being impeded. Pediatric practitioners are in a unique position to identify youths at risk for and actually engaging in risk-taking behaviors because of the wide variety of settings in which they routinely evaluate adolescents, and because they generally know the young person and the family. An open therapeutic relationship is best facilitated by establishing at the outset that the primary relationship is between the clinician and the young person. With rare exceptions (e.g., suicidal or homicidal behavior), confidentiality should not extend beyond the bounds of the clinician-adolescent relationship. Unless a relationship of trust is established with the adolescent, he or she will be uncomfortable divulging sensitive information, and the opportunity for timely assessment of and provision of appropriate information to the young person may be lost.

In any setting, a complete evaluation of the adolescent should incorporate the following: (1) an assessment of psychosocial factors placing the youth at greater or lesser risk for health-damaging behaviors; (2) an inventory of current and anticipated behaviors; (3) an assessment of the consequences of those behaviors on health status, general functioning, and psychosocial development; and (4) a physical examination and, if necessary, laboratory tests. At that point the clinician should have a clear idea of the risks facing the young person and the most appropriate intervention required: prevention, counseling, treatment, or referral.

The At-Risk Adolescent

The initial step in any comprehensive evaluation is a routine and systematic inventory of the biopsychosocial and environmental factors known to increase the vulnerability of an adolescent and encourage the initiation and maintenance of risk behaviors.[4] This information should be obtained from the teenager and the parents independently. Figure 109-1 shows the major factors predicting risk-taking behavior. It emphasizes the joint contribution of predisposing, protective, and precipitating factors; these can be further divided into endogenous biopsychosocial/behavioral factors and exogenous environmental factors. With the components of this model in mind, the clinician can inquire about a wide variety of characteristics of the young person and his or her environment in order to assess at-risk status. For example, in the biopsychosocial arena, male gender, increasing age, positive attitudes and intentions toward health-risk behaviors, and a lack of knowledge about their consequences all may increase the probability of initiating risk behaviors. Socioenvironmental factors enhancing initiation of such behaviors include family factors, such as the lack of a close relationship with parents, minimal parental supervision, and family disruption; contact with peers engaging in risk behaviors; and multiple school transitions. Likewise, the

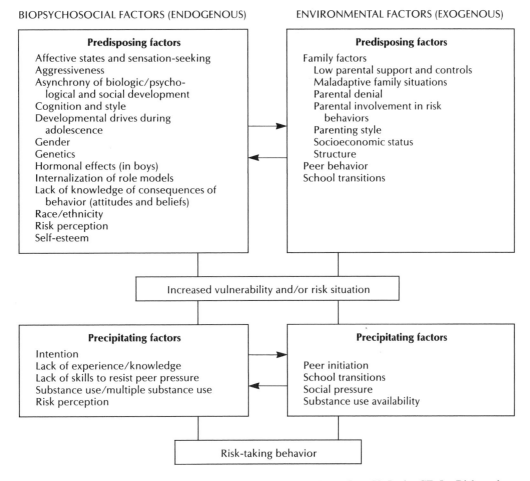

BIOPSYCHOSOCIAL FACTORS (ENDOGENOUS)

ENVIRONMENTAL FACTORS (EXOGENOUS)

Predisposing factors

Affective states and sensation-seeking
Aggressiveness
Asynchrony of biologic/psycho-
   logical and social development
Cognition and style
Developmental drives during
   adolescence
Gender
Genetics
Hormonal effects (in boys)
Internalization of role models
Lack of knowledge of consequences of
   behavior (attitudes and beliefs)
Race/ethnicity
Risk perception
Self-esteem

Predisposing factors

Family factors
   Low parental support and controls
   Maladaptive family situations
   Parental denial
   Parental involvement in risk
      behaviors
   Parenting style
   Socioeconomic status
   Structure
Peer behavior
School transitions

Increased vulnerability and/or risk situation

Precipitating factors

Intention
Lack of experience/knowledge
Lack of skills to resist peer pressure
Substance use/multiple substance use
Risk perception

Precipitating factors

Peer initiation
School transitions
Social pressure
Substance use availability

Risk-taking behavior

Fig. 109-1. Principal factors in risk-taking behaviors. (From Igra V, Irwin CE Jr: Risk and risk-taking in adolescents. In Lindstrom B, Spencer N, editors: *Social pediatrics,* New York, 1995, Oxford University Press.)

intention to refrain from initiating risk behaviors, in the context of authoritative parental control and peers who are engaging in more prosocial activities, may indicate a youth at decreased risk.

Extent of Behaviors

Once the clinician has assessed the factors placing an individual at greater or lesser risk, it is essential to inquire specifically about the nature and extent of participation in all health-risk behaviors. When the presenting complaint clearly points to a particular risk behavior, the initial questions should focus on that area. One risk behavior may serve, however, as a warning sign that the individual is engaging or intending to engage in other related risk behaviors. These behaviors may have even more serious consequences and need to be inquired about specifically.

A more difficult situation is encountered during a routine healthcare visit when the young person is unaware that certain behaviors are problematic or is reluctant to discuss or acknowledge active participation in such behaviors. In this case the clinician should still approach

the interview from the perspective that risk behaviors are common and need to be assessed routinely. We have found that inquiring about general risk taking and the adolescent's immediate circle of friends or peers before asking about the youth's own involvement in risk behaviors is a much less threatening strategy and is usually successful in promoting a frank discussion. Box 109-1 presents a summary of our approach, with recreational vehicles used as an example. Additional questions need to be asked about the frequency, intensity, and change over time of each risk behavior and whether anything is being done to minimize the risks involved, such as designating a nondrinking driver at parties where alcohol is consumed. Even in youngsters not actively engaged in risk behaviors, these questions may reveal important information about their perceptions of risk taking and intentions for the future.

Extent of Consequences

Risk behaviors, by definition, have a high potential for negatively influencing all aspects of an adolescent's

<table>
<tr><td>

BOX 109-1
Assessment of Participation
in Health-risk Behaviors

INTRODUCTORY COMMENTS
Sometimes young people do things that might be
considered risky to their health or they take
chances

GENERAL QUESTIONS
Do any of your classmates do things that you con-
sider risky or dangerous?
What kinds of activities do they do that you con-
sider dangerous?
How many of your four closest friends do things
that you consider risky?
What kinds of activities do they do that you think
are risky?
Do YOU do anything that you would consider
risky or dangerous?
Can you tell me about these activities?
If you are not doing these things now, are you
planning to start in the near future?

SPECIFIC QUESTIONS USING ACCIDENT-
RELATED BEHAVIORS AS AN EXAMPLE
How many of your friends drive? ride a skate-
board? ride bikes?
How many of them do these things recklessly?
or without helmets or protective gear?
How many of your four closest friends do these
activities?
Do any of your friends drive or ride a skateboard
after they have been drinking alcohol?
How often do your parents drive after they have
been drinking alcohol?
Have you ever driven a car or motorcycle or rid-
den a skateboard recklessly?
Have you ever driven a car or motocycle after
drinking alcohol?
Have you ever ridden a skateboard after drinking
alcohol?
When was the last time you did each of these
things?
How often do you do these things?
Have you ever hurt yourself doing any of these
things?

QUESTIONS ABOUT RELATED BEHAVIORS (FOR
EACH BEHAVIOR, ASK ABOUT FREQUENCY,
INTENSITY, AND SITUATION)
Have you ever drunk alcohol: beer, wine, wine
coolers, hard liquor?
Have you ever smoked cigarettes?
Have you ever used smokeless tobacco?
Have you ever taken any other drugs?
Have you ever had sexual intercourse?

</td></tr>
</table>

Modified from Irwin CE Jr, Ryan SA: Problem behavior of adolescents,
Pediatr Rev 10:235-246, 1989.

health status. The clinician can determine readily whether any adverse medical consequences, such as STDs, pregnancy, or injuries, have occurred by asking about the adolescent's overall sense of and satisfaction with his or her health and by obtaining a medical history and directed review of systems. Separate discussions with the adolescent and the parents about the young person's functioning in the areas of family, peers, and school or work should provide the clinician with a sense of how well that individual is meeting developmentally appropriate expectations in these contexts. Changes over time in any of these areas that indicate an escalation in the level of participation in certain behaviors also should be assessed. Box 109-2 lists some of the more common behavioral consequences that may be elicited during the psychosocial inventory.

Physical Examination

Although the psychosocial consequences are frequently of a greater magnitude than the medical consequences, a complete physical examination is indicated for any evaluation of risk behaviors. The physical examination is usually normal in an asymptomatic individual. Signs of acute trauma, such as lacerations, ecchymoses, musculoskeletal injury, and more chronic residual problems may be found in youths experiencing either intentional or unintentional injury. Assessment of physical maturation, using Tanner staging, also may help determine whether the timing of puberty, either early or late, is creating heightened asynchrony between physical and psychosocial development. A complete pelvic examinations in females or a genitourinary examination in males may indicate signs of STDs. Because the duration of effect of most substances is brief, acute effects are not usually seen unless the teenager is acutely intoxicated. The chronic effects of substance use and abuse, however, involve most systems, and the reader is referred to other texts for full descriptions of these consequences (see Chapter 108, "Substance Use and Abuse").[27]

Laboratory tests serve as an adjunct to the medical history and physical examination rather than a key tool in identifying risk behaviors. Screening tests for STDs should be obtained for all sexually active youths, whether symptomatic or not; pregnancy tests can be guided by the history and physical examination. In the setting of the emergency room, when there is acute traumatic injury, a screening for drug abuse may help determine whether substance abuse was contributory. The role of drug screening beyond use with an acutely intoxicated, comatose, or psychiatrically impaired individual is more controversial. We believe that probably little additional benefit can be obtained from routine laboratory screening of youths who may be using drugs. Highly sensitive and specific tests are rarely available; provide little informa-

BOX 109-2
**Psychosocial Inventory and Behaviors
Reflecting Possible Involvement
in Risk Behaviors**

FAMILY
Heightened conflict about rules/responsibilities
Conflicts about risk behaviors
Withdrawal/lack of communication with family
members
Decrease in family-oriented activities

PEERS
Changes to peer group where risky behaviors normative
Peer concern about adolescent's behaviors
Withdrawal from peer group/peer activities
Conflicts between parents over peer choices

SCHOOL WORK
Deterioration in school/work performance
Absenteeism
Decrease in interest/motivation
Withdrawal from extracurricular activities
Disciplinary problems

LEGAL SYSTEM
Truancy
Shoplifting
Substance abuse
Gang involvement
Court involvement/arrest/probation
Peers with criminal histories

GENERAL BEHAVIOR/RESPONSIBILITY
Dramatic swings in general mood
Overt intoxication
Depressive symptoms or equivalents (including
vegetative)
Decline in personal hygiene/habits
Decline in previous involvement with hobbies,
religion, activities

tion as to the frequency, intensity, or chronicity of use; and complicate matters with issues of confidentiality and consent. Information is best obtained directly from the adolescent.

MANAGEMENT

On completion of the comprehensive assessment, the clinician should be ready to design a management plan based on two summary clinical judgments. First, for an individual who is not engaging in risk behaviors, what are the person's intentions toward them, and what is the likelihood that he or she will initiate them in the near future? Second, for the youth who is engaging in

risk-taking activities, what are the probable trajectories of those behaviors, with the resultant negative outcomes, such as future adverse medical and psychosocial consequences?

Prevention

Primary prevention should be the key thrust of management with two general groups of adolescents not participating in high-risk behaviors. The first group includes youths who are at low risk for engaging in health-risk behaviors because of the absence of adverse risk factors or the presence of protective factors, and who have normal functioning with age-appropriate developmental attainment. A second group includes those teenagers at moderate to high risk for initiation of risk activities who are otherwise functioning and developing normally.

Basic education, the mainstay of anticipatory guidance or primary prevention in the clinical setting, includes discussions of the normative nature of some exploratory activities, the risk factors increasing participation, and the adverse consequences of specific activities. For example, parents can be informed that their own behavior, such as the use of tobacco or the wearing of seat belts, serves as a powerful message to their children. Because adolescents appreciate the present more than the future, any discussion of adverse effects of behavior should emphasize immediate, short-term results, such as compromised athletic performance with cigarette smoking, rather than the risk of lung cancer. A discussion of those aspects of normal development that encourage risk taking also may assist families in balancing the parents' needs for supervising and monitoring activities with the adolescent's needs for increased autonomy and independence through age-appropriate responsibilities and activities.

When an adolescent is at high risk for initiation of risk behaviors and the clinician is much more concerned about the possibility of future initiation, the emphasis should be on discussing the adverse consequences of particular activities. A recommendation to delay involvement in an activity, rather than to abstain for the duration of adolescence, may be the best strategy. This will be far more palatable to the youth, and any delay may enable him or her to acquire greater cognitive abilities and strategies or coping skills for resisting pressures to engage in risk behaviors. Discussion of alternative activities that serve developmental needs but do not have adverse consequences is another useful strategy. The clinician also may engage the parents in a discussion of how negative or positive risk factors may be minimized or enhanced.

Intervention

Intervention strategies are clearly indicated for adolescents already involved in risk behaviors. Depending on the situation, they may require basic counseling, treatment for any medical or psychosocial consequences, or referral to specialists or community agencies designed to deal with more extensive problems. For adolescents who are actively engaging in some risk behaviors but have neither shown any signs of escalation of these activities nor experienced any developmental impairment or adverse consequences, management should consist primarily of counseling. This may include many of the elements of prevention already discussed. However, the clinician's emphasis should be on expressing concern for the youth and engaging the adolescent in a dialogue about the roles that these risk behaviors have and whether there are other less risky activities that serve the same purpose. Realistic goals for counseling should not focus on convincing the youth to cease all risk behaviors, but rather encouraging the adolescent to modify the behaviors so that he or she is protected from the most harmful outcomes. It also should be pointed out to adolescents that their behavior may have important harmful effects on others, such as friends or family members. It is important that adolescents be actively involved in the choice of available options; otherwise, they will be less likely to adhere to any agreed-upon strategies. Hofmann[28] provides an excellent discussion of this process, which she calls guided decision making. Involving the parents of any youth involved in risk behaviors is a delicate process, given issues of confidentiality; whenever possible, such involvement should be facilitated, since the goals of intervention may be attained much more readily with parental support and understanding.

Finally, a clinician may find that the youth is heavily involved in a wide variety of risk behaviors, has experienced numerous medical or psychosocial consequences, and is at high risk for poor developmental attainment. In these situations, referral of both the youth and the family to specialized resources is probably the best approach. The clinician should be familiar with both lay resources and medical facilities available in the community and act as coordinator to these sources. The clinician, however, need not feel that his or her contribution has ended with the referral; rather, ongoing involvement, consisting of treatment of medical problems and follow-up, is a key aspect of the total management of youths engaging in health-risk behaviors.

References

1. Irwin CE Jr: Editor's notes. In *Adolescent social behavior and health,* San Francisco, 1987, Jossey-Bass.
2. Irwin CE Jr, Brindis CD, Brodt SE, Bennett TA, Rodriguez RQ: *The health of America's youth—a prelude to action,* Rockville, MD, 1991, Bureau of Maternal and Child Health Resources and Services Administration, Public Health Service, U.S. Department of Health and Human Services.
3. National Center Health Statistics: (1993) *Advance report of final mortality statistics, 1991,* Monthly Vital Statistics Report, August 31, 1991.
4. Irwin CE Jr: The theoretical concept of the at-risk adolescent. In Strasburger VC, Greydanus DE, editors: *State of the art reviews. The at-risk adolescent,* Philadelphia, 1990, Hanley & Belfus.
5. U.S. Preventive Services Task Force: *Guide to clinical preventive services: an assessment of the effectiveness of 169 interventions. Report of the U.S. Preventive Services Task Force,* Baltimore, 1989, Williams & Wilkins.
6. Irwin CE Jr, Ryan SA: Problem behavior of adolescents, *Pediatr Rev* 10:235, 1989.
7. Irwin CE Jr: Risk taking behaviors in the adolescent patient: are they impulsive?, *Pediatr Ann* 18:122, 1989.
8. Rice DP, MacKenzie EJ, et al: *Cost of injury in the United States: a report to Congress,* San Francisco, 1989, Institute for Health and Aging, University of California and Injury Prevention Center, The Johns Hopkins University.
9. Centers for Disease Control and Prevention: CDC surveillance summaries, youth risk behavior surveillance—U.S., 1993, March 24, 1995, *MMWR* 44 (no. SS-1), 1995.
10. Johnston LD: University of Michigan Institute for Social Research. Unpublished tables from the Monitoring The Future Study, 1994.
11. Bachman JG, Wallace JM, O'Malley PM, et al: Racial/ethnic differences in smoking, drinking, and illicit drug use among American high school seniors, 1976-89, *Am J Public Health* 81: 372, 1991.
12. Pratt W: *National survey of family growth, cycle III and IV for 1988,* Columbus, Ohio State University (unpublished tabulation).
13. Federal Bureau of Investigation: *Uniform crime reports for the United States,* Washington, DC, 1987, U.S. Government Printing Office.
14. U.S. Department of Justice, Bureau of Justice Statistics: *Criminal victimization in the United States, 1990 (NCJ-134126),* Washington, DC, 1992, U.S. Department of Justice.
15. Irwin CE Jr, Millstein SG: Correlates and predictors of risk taking behavior during adolescence. In Lipsitt LP, Mitnick LL, editors: *Self-regulatory behavior and risk-taking: causes and consequences,* Norwood, NJ, 1991, Ablex.
16. Millstein SG, Irwin CE Jr, Adler NE, Cohn LD, Kegeles SM, Dolcini MM: High-risk behaviors and health concerns among young adolescents, *Pediatrics* 3:422, 1992.
17. Yamaguchi K, Kandel DB: Pattern of drug use from adolescence to young adulthood: III. Predictors of progression, *Am J Public Health* 74:673, 1984.
18. Zabin LS: The association between smoking and sexual behavior among teens in the U.S. contraceptive clinics, *Am J Public Health* 74:261, 1984.
19. Osgood DW, Johnston LD, O'Malley PM, Bachman JG: The generality of deviance in late adolescence and early adulthood, *Am Sociol Rev* 53:81, 1988.
20. Mott FI, Haurin RJ: Linkages between sexual activity and alcohol and drug use among American adolescents, *Fam Plann Perspect* 20:128, 1988.
21. Kegeles SM, Millstein SG, Adler NE, Irwin CE Jr, Cohn LD, Dolcini MM: The transition to sexual activity and its relationship to other risk behaviors, *J Adolesc Health Care* 8:303, 1987.
22. Ensminger ME: Sexual activity and problem behaviors among black, urban adolescents, *Child Dev* 61:2032, 1990.
23. Irwin CE Jr, Millstein SA: Biopsychosocial correlates of risk-taking behaviors during adolescence: can the physician intervene?, *J Adolesc Health Care* 7:825, 1986.
24. Baumrind D: Familial antecedents of adolescent drug use: a developmental perspective. In Jones CL, Battjes RJ, editors:

Etiology of drug abuse: implications for prevention. NIDA Research Monograph No. 56, Rockville, MD, 1985, National Institute of Drug Abuse.

25. Jessor R, Jessor SL: *Problem behavior and psychosocial development: a longitudinal study of youth,* New York, 1977, Academic Press.

26. McCord J: Problem behavior. In Feldman SS, Elliott GR, editors: *At the threshold: the developing adolescent,* Cambridge, 1990, Harvard University Press.

27. Hofmann AE, Greydanus D: *Adolescent medicine,* Norwalk, CT, 1989, Appleton & Lange.

28. Hofmann AE: Clinical assessment and management of health risk behaviors in adolescents. In Strasburger VC, Greydanus DE, editors: *State of the art reviews. The at-risk adolescent,* Philadelphia, 1990, Hanley & Belfus.

CHAPTER 110

Runaway Youths

•

Gerald R. Adams

Adolescents have been running away since ancient days. However, a heightened concern about the incidence and implications of running away occurred in the 1970s after a series of published articles in *U.S. News & World Report.* This public concern was translated into responsive legislation, when the Runaway Youth Act (1974) authorized the Secretary of Health, Education, and Welfare to provide grants for services to runaways throughout the nation. Over the years a series of senate subcommittees on juvenile delinquency and child pornography have repeatedly provided testimony about the hardship and destitution of runaway youths.

INCIDENCE OF RUNAWAY BEHAVIOR

The actual incidence rate of runaways is difficult to determine. Investigators using probabilistic sampling and household surveys have estimated that 1:8 to 1:10 adolescents will run away from home at least once before their eighteenth birthday, with as many as three quarters of a million youths running away annually.[1,2] Furthermore, since only 3% of families in the United States experience a runaway incidence, it appears that multiple runaways are likely within the same family.[3] However, it is extremely important to realize that these families include all socioeconomic levels, both sons and daughters, married couples and divorced parents, and all regions of the United States and Canada. It should also be noted that a complete and correct incidence rate is difficult to determine because children who are 13 years of age or younger are likely to be reported as missing (possibly abducted) youths rather than as runaways in order to prompt immediate action by law enforcement agencies. Most of these agencies are likely to require the family to wait at least 48 hours before taking formal enforcement action, recognizing that many runaways return within 48 to 72 hours.

TYPES OF RUNAWAY YOUTHS

The definition of runaway behavior has been a troublesome issue. After extensive debate about alternatives, the National Statistical Survey on Runaway Youth concluded that the definition should include specifications on (1) the age of a youth, (2) the absence of parental or guardian permission, and (3) a criterion on time absent from home. The first two specifications seem to be widely endorsed, but the last one has not been rigorously or widely used. Perhaps the most common definition of runaway behavior is absence from home without permission, by youths under the age of 18 years, for more than a 24-hour period. Important distinctions can be made between various types of runaway youths.[4,5] For example, in an early observation by a clinical social worker,

Gullotta,[6] called for distinctions to be made between runaways and throwaways. Such an appeal has drawn attention to the multiple dynamics that operate in the lives of homeless children.[7]

At minimum, three classifications are needed in a typology of runaways.[8] The first type is *runaways,* who leave home because of poor family relations, alienation, and conflict.[9] The second type is *throwaways,* who are actually rejected and encouraged to leave home.[10] The third consists of societal *rejects,* who are rejected by family, peers, teachers, and even local church or social welfare service agencies.[8] Although there are variations in degree of severity and psychosocial complexity, a common theme of conflict and possible alienation in family life appears to exist among the three types of runaways.

Evidence of broad family problems in the homes of all three types of runaways has been documented.[11,12] The danger in many of these homes is reflected in the terms used to categorize the runaways: "terrified" runners, "endangered" runners, or "victim" runners. Within the three-part classification scheme, these labels are most closely associated with throwaways and societal rejects.

In a report of runaways from a sample of youths in Toronto that included 149 adolescents, the following conclusions were drawn: (1) running away is a premature separation from the home because of conflict and other poor family environmental factors; (2) runaway behavior is commonly, although not exclusively, symptomatic of an abusive home life; and (3) running away is predictive of a troubled future with heightened potential for continuing abuse and misfortune.[12] The findings in this report indicate that runaways view their homes as unresponsive, inattentive, and unsupportive to family members. In contrast, the family is viewed as manifesting higher than normal levels of anger, aggression, and conflict. When comparisons were made between runaway families that did and did not include physical abuse, this pattern became even more pronounced for the abusive runaway group. It seems likely that nonabusive homes are associated with the runaway classification and abusive homes are related to the throwaway and societal reject groups.

Brennan et al[5] used "strain" and "control" theories to build a useful and highly recommended typology and diagnosis model. According to these social scientists, the strain theory holds that deviant behavior, such as running away, is the product of socially induced pressure toward deviance. Potential sources of strain in the home, school, or peer group may function as primary agents in creating a sense of personal alienation. Feelings of estrangement from family members place a youth in a state of personal "drift," creating a setting for alienation from family norms. While in a state of alienation, the youth is likely to turn to the school or a peer setting for allegiance and commitment. If the youth is exposed to a nonconforming peer group or to a hostile or rejecting school environment, increased alienation and/or a nonconformist peer group may set the stage for flight from the home.

Control theory maintains that deviance, in the form of runaway behavior, can be accounted for by the failure of a youth to internalize social norms (or establish the necessary social linkage to conventional groups) that reinforce compliance to normative behavior. Therefore, runaways may be youths whose early socialization produced weak personal commitments to conventional norms and low levels of integration into conventional social groups and institutions. In turn, low integration of normative conduct is thought to make a person more vulnerable to deviant activities, such as running away, because weak bonds exist among the adolescent, family, school, and/or peers.

From these theories, one would expect a class of youths who run away because of conflict in the family (or other social relationship groups) that has contributed to a sense of drift and alienation. Dysfunctionality in emotional bonds, expectations, and a sense of community or union with others is likely to be the underlying dynamic force of running away. In comparison, when excessive strains (e.g., physical abuse) are present in the family and/or social groups, resulting in lowered social bonding, and the youth is affiliated with deviant subgroups or unsupportive social networks, control theory suggests that weaker bonding and lessened internalization of conventional social norms will result in a greater willingness to accept or imitate deviance (nonnormative behavior, such as running away). Therefore, delinquent peers, who provide a model for deviance, set the social environmental context for emulating and accepting deviant behavior.

Two broad categories of runaways have been confirmed as being partly explained by strain and control theories. The first category, class I: not highly delinquent, nonalienated runaways, includes three subtypes of runaways who are not highly delinquent or alienated but are relatively psychologically healthy youths who have nondelinquent or nondeviant friends. Class I runaways come from families in which the youth is socially estranged from the family, is possibly isolated from peers, or has parents who fail to provide appropriate behavioral boundaries and/or fail to supervise or monitor their adolescent's activities. These youths show no evidence of alienation and appear to be mostly psychologically healthy. Members of the second category, class II: delinquent, alienated runaways, share a common profile of parental conflict, rejecting parents, delinquent peers, school alienation, low self-esteem, and a history of personal delinquent behavior. Class II runaways are likely to include throwaways and societal rejects.

PATTERNS AND CYCLES OF BEHAVIOR

An analysis of the patterns and cycles of runaway behavior reveals that about one half of the adolescents who run away do not go far. Many stay with friends, relatives, or neighborhood families—particularly during the first or second incidence. (In fact, it is not uncommon for middle-class parents to know of the adolescent's whereabouts and provide some economic support to the youth.) Most runaways stay away for a brief time, with overnight absences most commonly noted. It is estimated that approximately 30% of runaways return home in 1 day and 50% after 3 days. Approximately 10% return in 1 month or less; another 10% are classified as missing. It has been observed that males are more likely to run away for one overnight absence or for up to 1 week and females are more likely to run away for extended periods or permanently. Nye and Edelbrock[1] indicated that about 50% of runaways report a neutral experience while away from home. Indeed, 25% report a positive adventure regarding their perceived ability to survive on their own. However, 20% report negative consequences. Janus et al[12] noted that the negative consequences are very high, particularly for youths who leave home because of physical or sexual abuse.

The most worrisome pattern of runaway behavior emerges when the incidence increases from the most common type—one or two experiences—to a repeated pattern. Youths may first enter the streets from a conflict-laden family but still be somewhat emotionally bonded to the family. However, repeat runners may be placed in foster care or group home care, which reduces perceived emotional bonding, and in a repeat incidence they enter the street from alternative home care—probably at greater risk owing to weakened bonding to the family.[13] Regardless of the point of departure, once on the street, repeat runners are likely to seek shelter in a friend's home, with extended family members, or in a crisis shelter. In sheltered contexts these runners may find a part-time job to support themselves, re-enter school, or find a social adaptation to their circumstances that results in independent living. A positive outcome is more likely with youths who are not chronic repeat runners. However, undesirable street outcomes associated with criminal acts, prostitution, and even death associated with suicide, murder, or drugs is not unlikely.[14] The risk of victimization is high. This is particularly true for youths who enter the street either from a physically or sexually abusive home or from placement in alternative foster or institutional care, through which their perceived social bonding has been reduced. For further reading about the pathways and cycles of runaway youth behavior, the work of Janus et al is recommended.[12]

There is wide agreement on the potential negative consequences of runaway behavior.[15] Confrontation with the legal system, substance abuse, coercive sexual behavior, contraction of sexually transmitted diseases, physical beatings, nutritional and general health problems, loss of educational training and employment opportunities, pregnancy, early parenthood, and even death are some of the many possible consequences.

RECOMMENDATIONS FOR PHYSICIANS

Recommendations regarding service delivery can be summarized in three general dimensions: (1) helping the parent to understand and cope with the problem, (2) intervention and treatment phases with the adolescent runaway, and (3) suggested interventions based on the type of runaway profile. These dimensions are made for convenience of presentation and should not be viewed as separate and disconnected issues.

Understanding the Problem

The problem of runaway behavior can come to the attention of the physician or the nurse through either the adolescent or the parent. It is extremely rare for a runaway on the street to come to a physician for assistance unless the latter is working with a shelter for runaways.[16] However, it is not uncommon for a physician to be asked to speak with an adolescent who has a history of running away or with parents who are seeking advice on how to deal with a current runaway incident. At such a time, it is essential that the physician determine the seriousness of the case. Evidence shows that runaways who have family histories of physical or sexual abuse are at extremely high risk. Therefore, the physician needs to attempt to determine whether such abuse is likely. Such a determination requires not only an examination of the medical records of the youth and the family but also individual interviews with the adolescent, the parents, and in some cases other family members.

What should the physician look for? First, is there any evidence suggesting previous trauma in the family that would suggest the possibility of abuse? Second, does the family show unusual guardedness, secrecy, overcontrolling behavior, or an authoritarian tendency that would suggest inaccessibility to family information? Third, does either of the parents or the adolescent show signs of a traumatic disorder? Is there any suggestion of personality disorganization, denial of feelings, or alienation that is commonly associated with experiencing traumatic life events? Finally, is there any substantial evidence to suggest that the adolescent is showing anxiety, depression, suicidal ideation, unusual anger, or antisocial behavioral tendencies? Such information[17,18] is necessary to an understanding of the "at-risk" nature of the problem.

TABLE 110-1
Seven Types of Runaways and Suggestive Intervention Directions Based on Typology Characteristics

	Subtype	Characteristic	Intervention Direction
Class I	Young temporary escapist	Overcontrolling parents: deny autonomy, not nurturant, use negative labels on child Use of social isolation, physical punishment, and rejection when disciplining child High parental conflict and family disruption; appear socially estranged Child is psychologically bonded to parents, involved and successful in school High number of friends while maintaining low commitment Positive self-concept and absence of alienation	Family therapy focusing on interpersonal conflict
	Middle-class loner	Good relationship with parents Successful, aspiring, involved in school High scores for autonomy from parents Isolated from peers and spends much time alone Parents support educational aspirations of child	Establishment of positive peer culture Social skills training
	Unrestrained, peer-oriented	Primarily youth from lower classes Family relations: low companionship levels, minimal achievement demands, high level of freedom and autonomy No expectations of succeeding in school, low educational aspirations, and dislike for school Have a few friends, but spend most of their time with them	Family therapy focusing on parent-child relations School counseling
Class II	Rejected and constrained	Parental relations include negative labeling, parental dissatisfaction, rejection, deprivation of privileges, denial of autonomy, physical punishment Parents maintain low self-esteem and high sense of alienation Unable to obtain school involvement, low grades, low extramural participation, high levels of negative labeling by teachers, and low educational or occupational aspirations High commitment to friends, who are usually delinquent Alienated and delinquent	Establishment of positive peer culture Individual counseling for parents and child focusing on personal alienation Family therapy directed at family relations School counseling
	Rebellious and constrained middle-class drop-out girls	Rejection and strain in family and at school Are angry and rebellious Parents are overprotective, deny autonomy, and are overindulgent Dislike school and have no wish to be involved as no educational ambitions Are negatively labeled by teachers Socially alienated with high commitment to personal friends who are delinquent Middle-class youth	Individual counseling directed at anger and hostile feelings Family therapy focusing on rejection and strain School counseling Establishment of positive peer culture
	Normless, rejected, unrestrained youth	Family relations include rejection, negative labeling, differential treatment of siblings, low affective reward, low levels of affiliation Uninvolved in school, no aspirations for involvement Fairly high educational aspirations but minimal occupational aspirations Have few friends and spend little time with them; friends are delinquent Spend little time with parents and much time alone Fairly delinquent Extremely normless	Family therapy focusing on relations and feelings of rejection Individual counseling directed at youth's normlessness Social skills training
	Pushouts, socially rejected youth	Extreme parental rejection with parents dissatisfied with youth, not nurturant, unconcerned, and distant Child senses emotional rejection and is seen as emotional pushout Withdrawn from school, severely negatively labeled by teachers, and no expectation of obtaining a good job High commitment to many delinquent friends Normless, powerless, and delinquent Self-esteem is very low	Family therapy Intense individual counseling for all family members School counseling

From Adams GR: Runaway youth projects: comments on care programs for runaways and throwaways; *J Adolesc* 3:321-334, 1980.

Further, it is not uncommon for middle-class parents to seek assistance and either to suggest that they do not know where their child is (to cover for abuse or neglect perceptions) or to imply that the family is a well-functioning household and that the adolescent is ungovernable. In many cases the family is aware of the child's whereabouts and is denying its contribution to the event, which is frequently related to conflict or ineffective parenting. The physician should attempt to determine whether contact is being covertly maintained, assess whether a missing person's report should be made, and arrange for social service assistance when contact is known. With this strategy the perception of blame is avoided and the rebuilding of communication between all parties is encouraged.

Intervention and Treatment Phases

The following guidelines for intervention and treatment efforts with runaways are covered in detail in another publication.[19] To summarize, the first phase consists of crisis intervention and stabilized (secure) placement. The second phase involves supportive counseling and assessment. The third phase includes long-term therapy, education/training, and supportive services. The agency (or physician) first interacting with the runaway should assume responsibility for crisis intervention and the initiation of a stabilized placement. Diagnosis and supportive counseling should be undertaken by local mental-health providers. Long-term therapy, education/training, and supportive social services should be offered through family and social welfare assistance.

Crisis intervention can diffuse existing and threatening physical, social, and emotional problems. The medical or welfare personnel accepting the initial contact should assume executive management of the problem. The most immediate need is to resolve the crisis sufficiently to ensure a secured placement. Stabilization provides the youth with some security, calms those who are frightened or anxious, and ensures the possibility of diagnosis and assessment. The assessment should provide the necessary information to enhance supportive counseling and to determine options for longer-term treatment. The umbrella goal is diminution of runaway behavior, increased skill and coping abilities, and effective reunion of the adolescent with the family and/or establishment of alternative home care.[20]

Specific Interventions

Physicians are often contacted by parents for recommendations regarding long-term treatment. In Table 110-1 the basic subtypes of class I and II runaways are identified and suggested intervention approaches are listed. Although there are many parallels between the various types of runaways, there are unique factors associated with each categorical type.

Class I includes three types of runaways. For the young adolescent, who is usually a temporary escapist, immediate attention should be directed toward family relations that promote feelings of isolation or rejection. The primary focus should be on reducing or eliminating feelings of interpersonal estrangement and conflict. For the middle-class loner, family life appears stable and supportive, but peer relations are poor. Social skills training supported by the initiation of a positive peer culture through school assistance should be considered. The unrestrained, peer-oriented runaway comes from a family with low parental involvement and accompanying school relations problems. Family therapy directed toward enhancing parental or guardian involvement, with school counseling that includes career education and individual guidance, is most likely to assist the youth in recovery. In general, class I runaways are most likely to be receptive to intervention attempts.

For class II runaways, however, the problems are more severe and require more extensive and intensive treatment interventions. These adolescents come from homes in which family relations are either rejecting or overindulgent. There is intense dislike for school, with evidence of normlessness, powerlessness, and delinquency. By experiencing the "norms" of deviance among their delinquent friends, these adolescents readily comply with peer pressures associated with antinormative behavior. Individual counseling is needed to address feelings of alienation, rejection, anger, and hostility. Family therapy is needed to restructure family communication patterns. Positive peer-culture strategies are needed to remove these youths from a deviant peer group. For many, social skills training, school counseling, and positive work experience programs are also necessary.[21]

FUTURE PERSPECTIVES

There is little evidence to suggest that the incidence of runaway behavior will decrease in the coming years. As demands on families increase the necessity of both parents to be in the full-time labor force, separation and divorce continue as a common family experience, and families necessarily often move, incidence rates actually may increase. With cutbacks in social welfare support for runaway shelters and with increasing demands for a larger homeless population, shelter and crisis intervention programs for runaways may decline in number.

It is urgent that appropriate and effective prevention programs be designed to improve parent-adolescent communication, reduce feelings of alienation by adolescents, and enhance family bonding. Likewise, effective social assistance programs are needed to facilitate positive re-entry into the home when the adolescent returns.

References

1. Nye IF, Edelbrock C: Some social characteristics of runaways, *J Fam Issues* 1:147-150, 1980.
2. Opinion Research Corporation: *National statistical survey on runaway youths,* Princeton, NJ, 1976, Opinion Research Corporation.
3. Garbarino J, Wilson J, Garbarino A: The adolescent runaway. In Garbarino J, Sebes J, editors: *Troubled youth, troubled families,* New York, 1986, Adline; pp 38-49.
4. Adams GR: Runaway youth projects: comments on care programs for runaways and throwaways, *J Adolesc* 3:321-334, 1980.
5. Brennan T, Huizinga D, Elliott DS: *The social psychology of runaways,* Lexington, MA, 1978, DC Health.
6. Gullotta TP: Runaway: reality or myth, *Adolescence* 13:543-550, 1978.
7. Windle M: Substance use and abuse among adolescent runaways: a four-year follow-up study, *J Youth Adolesc* 18:331-334, 1989.
8. Adams GR, Gullotta T, Clancy MA: Homeless adolescents: a descriptive study of similarities and differences between runaways and throwaways, *Adolescence* 20:715-724, 1985.
9. de-Man A, Dolan D, Pelletier R, Reid C: Adolescent runaways: familial and personal correlates, *Soc Behav Personality* 21:163-167, 1993.
10. Siegel M, Callesen MT: Adolescent runaway behavior from an inpatient setting, *Resid Treat Child Youth* 10:5-19, 1993.
11. Adams GR, Munro G: Portrait of the North American runaway: a critical review, *J Youth Adolesc* 8:359-373, 1979.
12. Janus M, McCormack A, Burgess AW, Hartman C: *Adolescent runaways: causes and consequences,* Lexington, MA, 1987, DC Heath.
13. Stefanidis N, Pennbridge J, MacKenzie RG, Pottharst K: Runaway and homeless youth: the effects of attachment history on stabilization, *Am J Orthopsychiatry* 62:442-446, 1992.
14. de-Man A, Dolan D, Pelletier R, Reid C: Adolescent running away behavior: active or passive avoidance?, *J Genet Psychiatry* 155:59-64, 1994.
15. Young RL, Godfrey W, Matthews B, Adams GR: Runaways: a review of negative consequences, *Fam Relations* 32:275-281, 1983.
16. Yates GL, Pennbridge J, Swofford A, MacKenzie RG: The Los Angeles system of care for runaway/homeless youth, *J Adolesc Health* 12:555-560, 1991.
17. Post P, McCoard D: Needs and self-concept of runaway adolescents, *School Counselor* 41:212-219, 1994.
18. Ward AJ: Adolescent suicide and other self-destructive behaviors: adolescent attitude survey data and interpretation, *Resid Treat Child Youth* 9:49-64, 1992.
19. Adams PR, Adams GR: Intervention with runaway youth and their families: theory and practice. In Coleman J, editor: *Working with troubled adolescents,* London, 1987, Academic Press.
20. Rotheram-Borus MJ, Bradley J: Triage model for suicidal runaways, *Am J Orthopsychiatry* 61:122-127, 1991.
21. Hohnhorst AD, Roberts MW: Evaluation of a brief work chore discipline procedure, *Behav Resid Treat* 7:55-69, 1992.

CHAPTER 111

Delinquency

•

Scott W. Henggeler

Delinquency refers to illegal activities committed by a minor. Such acts can be diverse in their seriousness and their effects on others. At the low end of the seriousness continuum are status offenses, which are behaviors that are not illegal if performed by an adult (e.g., truancy, running away). At the upper end of the continuum are serious criminal offenses such as robbery, rape, and aggravated assault. In the middle range are illegal activities such as burglary, disorderly conduct, and petty larceny. This chapter focuses on the criminal activities found in the middle to upper range of the seriousness continuum.

EPIDEMIOLOGY

The primary methods of measuring delinquency are through arrest records and adolescent self-reports. Although arrest records are used most frequently by researchers and policy makers, arrest measures are regarded as relatively unreliable for two primary reasons. First, the probability of being arrested for a particular criminal act is quite low. Second, systematic biases (e.g., gender, ethnicity) have been found in police decisions to make an arrest. Thus, it is entirely possible that an adolescent who perpetrates high rates of criminal acts will not have an arrest record. On the other hand, self-report data are favored by criminologists as more accurate indexes of offenses. Self-report methods also have limitations, however, including a tendency for minorities to underreport serious offenses and for most respondents to overreport trivial offenses.

Age

On the basis of both arrest and self-report data, prevalence rates for most crimes peak at approximately 17 years of age. At this age, for example, it was found in the National Youth Survey that during the previous year 17% of youths had sold marijuana, 18% had engaged in vandalism, and 2% had stolen an automobile. Some theorists have proposed that young adolescents engage in less crime because they are monitored more extensively by their parents and are less strongly influenced by their peers. Young adults, on the other hand, may commit fewer offenses because they are becoming involved in affiliations that are not conducive to criminal activities (e.g., marriage, career) and because they are more likely than minors to be treated harshly by the criminal justice system.

Gender

Boys have much higher rates of delinquency than do girls, especially for more serious offenses. Studies show, however, that the causes and correlates of delinquency are generally the same for both boys and girls. Explanations for gender differences have emphasized biologic factors and different socialization experiences.

Social Class

Although social class influences are highlighted in several sociologic models of delinquency (e.g., strain theory, culture deviance theory), reviewers have consistently concluded that there is only a low association between an individual's social class and delinquency when other factors are controlled. However, on a neighborhood level, social class indicators are linked with neighborhood arrest rates.

Race

African-American and Hispanic-American adolescents have much higher rates of arrest than do Caucasian adolescents. Indeed, these two minorities account for more than 50% of all youths who are incarcerated in public facilities. On the other hand, racial effects have generally failed to emerge in studies that used self-report measures of offending. Explanations for the discrepancy between findings based on arrest versus self-report data

have addressed the lower validity of self-report instruments for minorities, as well as racial discrimination in decisions to arrest and incarcerate.

Single-Parent Households

Youths from homes with one parent engage in higher rates of antisocial behavior than do youths from two-parent families. This difference in antisocial behavior is due largely to the greater autonomy, lower parental involvement, and greater susceptibility to peer pressure experienced by youths in single-parent households.

CORRELATES OF DELINQUENCY

In the social-ecological model of behavior, behavior problems, including delinquency, are viewed as products of the interplay among a child's characteristics and the child's transactions with key interpersonal systems (family, peer, school, neighborhood). This model provides the best fit for the empirical data.

Individual Characteristics

Several individual adolescent characteristics, described as cognitive factors and social competence, have been associated with delinquency. Regarding cognitive factors, consistent evidence shows that juvenile offenders score approximately one half of a standard deviation, or 7 to 8 points, lower on intelligence tests than do nonoffenders, and that this difference is independent of social class and race. Moreover, the difference between delinquents and nondelinquents is primarily a result of the relatively poor verbal performance of the former. Theorists have proposed that low verbal IQ is linked with delinquency because low intellectual abilities predispose the individual to academic difficulties, are associated with psychosocial difficulties in general, and are related to delayed development of higher-order sociocognitive processes (e.g., moral reasoning).

Several aspects of the social competence of delinquents have also been evaluated. Although delinquents are widely assumed to have deficits in social skills relative to nondelinquents, findings have been inconsistent, and most research in this area has been methodologically flawed. It also has been widely assumed that delinquents have deficits in problem-solving skills. Again, however, findings have been inconsistent, and investigators have cited numerous methodologic difficulties in this line of research. Evidence does suggest, however, that aggressive boys have an attributional bias to perceive hostile intentions from others in ambiguous situations, and that such a bias is accentuated under conditions of perceived threat. Attributional bias may be an important factor in interpersonal aggression because it increases the probability of a hostile response. Finally, delinquent adolescents generally have lower self-esteem than nondelinquents (see Chapter 120, "Character Disorders"). Although some theorists posit low self-esteem as a cause of delinquency, the empirical literature does not support such a view. Rather, the association between self-esteem and delinquency is apparently caused by the conjoint association of these variables with characteristics such as IQ, family relations, and school performance as well as the direct contribution of personal success and failure to the development of a youth's self-esteem (i.e., low self-esteem is often a realistic indicator of the offender's life difficulties).

Family Relations

Two broad dimensions of family relations have been identified by investigators: affect and control. Affect refers to parental warmth and responsivity as opposed to parental rejection and unresponsiveness. Control refers to parental discipline strategies ranging from permissive, in which parents are undemanding, to restrictive, in which parents are very controlling of their child's behavior. Evidence demonstrates that delinquency is associated with low parental warmth, low cohesion, and parental rejection. Similarly, findings show that parents of juvenile offenders tend to use lax and ineffective discipline strategies and often fail to provide sufficient monitoring of their child's behavior. Interpretations of these associations, however, must take into account the reciprocal nature of interpersonal interactions. For example, it is inappropriate to conclude that low parental warmth causes delinquency. Rather, it is just as likely that the repeated antisocial behavior of the adolescent leads to parental rejection. Finally, extensive evidence shows that delinquency is associated with parental deviance (e.g., parental criminality, drug abuse, mental illness), which most likely impedes the performance of appropriate parenting behaviors.

Peer Relations

Association with deviant peers is the most powerful and most consistent correlate and predictor of delinquency. Deviant peers model and provide social approval for antisocial behavior, and such behavior is typically part of the conforming process that occurs in adolescent friendship groups. Interestingly, however, adolescent susceptibility to negative peer pressure is attenuated by positive family relations. Thus, youths who associate with deviant peers and who also have poor family relations are at especially high risk for delinquency.

School and Academic Performance

Investigators have consistently found that delinquency is associated with poor school performance. This association may be a result of the linkages that delinquency and school performance each have with IQ and family relations. In addition, investigators have described characteristics of schools that contribute to delinquency (e.g., weak, inconsistent, and ineffective teachers and principals).

Ecologic Variables

Several ecologic variables have been examined in the literature. In contrast to the assumptions of many professionals, the empirical data suggest that employment has little or no effect on delinquency. Similarly, although low religious commitment has been associated with delinquency, this association is not independent of family relations; that is, the quality of family relations is central, not religious commitment. Finally, neighborhood characteristics, such as the existence of a criminal subculture, are also linked with delinquency.

Multidimensional Causal Models

The above discussion indicates that delinquency is associated with numerous variables. In light of the many correlates, several research groups have developed empirically based causal models to delineate the factors central to delinquency. Together, the results from these complex studies strongly demonstrate the multidimensional nature of delinquency and support the social-ecological model of behavior. Individual youth, family, peer, and school factors consistently contribute to delinquency either directly or indirectly. Thus, the most viable model of delinquency is one that includes multiple pathways from the key systems in which youths are embedded.

TREATMENT AND INTERVENTION APPROACHES

The development of effective interventions for delinquency has proved extremely difficult. In fact, the consensus among major reviewers[1,2] of the treatment outcome literature is that most treatment approaches widely used in the past were ineffective. In general, this conclusion pertains to interventions based on psychodynamic, humanistic, and behavior modification models of behavior. In light of the poor match between the primary correlates of delinquency (e.g., family relations, association with deviant peers) and the emphasis on individual psychotherapy taken in most treatment approaches, it is not surprising that such treatment models have not been successful.

Recently, several reviewers have suggested that promising new treatment strategies are in the process of emerging. Certain of these strategies continue to focus on the individual adolescent. Others address difficulties in the systems in which youths are embedded, and still others take a broad-based and comprehensive approach to intervention. The following discussion focuses on those interventions described by reviewers as promising.

Individual Treatment Interventions

Social skills training often has been used to treat juvenile offenders. This type of intervention is based on the assumed social skill deficits of delinquents (which may not be a valid assumption). Reviewers of the literature on social skills training with juvenile offenders have concluded that investigators have not demonstrated the durability of social skills acquired during training. Although offenders may show increased social facility in the therapy office or the institution, virtually no evidence shows that such changes generalize to the natural environment.

Problem-solving skills training is based on the questionable assumption that delinquents have cognitive deficits in developing and planning viable solutions for interpersonal problems. Thus, the thrust of this approach is to provide youths with highly structured cognitive strategies aimed at promoting self-control and social responsivity. Although this approach has had some limited success with elementary school children identified as aggressive, little evidence supports its effectiveness with adolescent offenders.

Combined cognitive and social skills approaches have been examined in several studies. In consideration of the difficulty in ameliorating antisocial behavior, this approach combines several types of interventions (e.g., moral education, social skills training, problem-solving skills training) with the aim of increasing the intensity and integration of treatment. Aggression replacement training, which combines training in social skills, problem-solving skills, and moral reasoning, has produced promising results in incarcerated adolescents who were later returned to the community.

Although these individually focused interventions have been generally ineffective with juvenile offenders, especially when used in isolation, such ineffectiveness should be anticipated in light of the well-documented multidetermined nature of delinquency. That is, delinquent behavior is associated with numerous individual, family, peer, and social system variables. In a given case the adolescent's behavior problems are most likely linked with a combination of pertinent variables. Thus, treatments that focus on only one variable minimize the probability of obtaining positive results.

Family Therapy

A basic assumption of family therapy is that child behavior problems are closely associated with problematic family interactions, and that, consequently, treatment must ameliorate these family difficulties. As noted earlier, the association between delinquency and family problems has been supported by numerous studies. Several reviewers have evaluated family-based treatment approaches for antisocial child behavior, and each has concluded that behavioral parent training and functional family therapy are promising interventions.

Behavioral parent training is based on findings that families of aggressive children engage in coercive exchanges that foster aversive behavior. Coercive exchanges are behavioral chains in which the negative behavior of one family member is inadvertently reinforced by the consequences provided by another family member. Thus, parent training aims at improving the parents' ability to monitor child behavior accurately and to provide consistent reinforcement for positive behavior and punishment (e.g., loss of privileges) for negative behavior. Although several studies support the efficacy of this approach for children of elementary school age, support for its effectiveness with adolescent offenders is minimal.

In functional family therapy, delinquency is assumed to reflect maladaptive interactions in the family. Intervention strategies represent a combination of behavioral and strategic approaches, including contingency contracting and training of family members to communicate more clearly. Evidence supports the effectiveness of this approach with relatively "soft" delinquents. Moreover, the positive treatment effects seem to have generalized to the siblings of these offenders.

Multisystem Interventions

Several recent reviewers have concluded that effective treatment of delinquency must recognize the multiple determinants of adolescent antisocial behavior. Consistent with this conclusion, broad-based treatment approaches intervene at multiple levels of the youth's ecology (e.g., with individual youths, family, peers, and school).

Multisystemic therapy is the ecologically based treatment that has received the most empirical attention. It represents a family-based, home-based intervention that gives considerable attention to adolescent cognitive variables and to the youth's and the family's relationships with extrafamilial systems. The components of multisystemic therapy (marital therapy, family therapy, school-based interventions, cognitive therapy, case management) are intended to meet the multiple needs of youths and families in a comprehensive, yet individualized, fashion. Randomized clinical trials of multisystemic therapy have documented its capacity to reduce long-term rates of criminal activity and incarceration in serious juvenile offenders and their multiple-need families.[3] The success of multisystemic therapy has been attributed to its emphasis on influencing the multiple determinants of antisocial behavior in real world settings (e.g., home, school, neighborhood).

INTERVENTION OF JUVENILE JUSTICE SYSTEM

The following discussion reviews the effectiveness of several intervention approaches conducted within the juvenile justice system.

Incarceration

A wide variety of interventions have been used for incarcerated adolescents. In a highly structured residential setting, problem behavior can be reduced substantially. Unfortunately, such positive changes are rarely maintained when the youth is returned to the community. This is not surprising when one considers that little therapeutic attention is devoted to altering problems within the youth's real world environment (family, peer, school, and neighborhood settings).

Boot Camps

Boot camps are currently being disseminated widely across the nation, with considerable support from the public and from policymakers. Such spread is occurring in spite of research documenting the lack of effectiveness of such programs and the open skepticism of knowledgeable professionals regarding the capacity of boot camps to reduce criminal activity.

Restitution

Restitution requires the offender to pay a sum of money or to perform a useful service for the victim. Some evidence suggests that restitution results in decreased recidivism. The mechanism for this effect may be the development of greater understanding of the effects of the crime on the victim.

Scared Straight

Although this short-term intervention, in which juveniles are confronted by adult prison inmates, has received considerable attention in the popular media, reviewers have concluded that such programs have little impact beyond their initial shock value. In one study, for example, chronic offenders who received a Scared Straight intervention showed less deviant scores on attitudes toward the police 1 week after intervention, but no differences emerged in recidivism at a 1-year follow-up (Scared Straight, 81%; control group, 67%).

CONCLUSION

Several conclusions can be drawn from the literature. First, delinquency is associated with numerous variables that pertain to the characteristics of individual adolescents and of the key social systems in which youths are involved. Second, traditional mental health and juvenile justice interventions and some currently popular programs have been largely ineffective with juvenile offenders. Third, the most promising interventions are those that are family based, pragmatic, problem focused, and multifaceted and that directly address difficulties in the youth's natural environment.

IMPLICATIONS FOR PRACTITIONERS

Findings regarding the epidemiology, correlates, and treatment of delinquency have several important implications for practitioners. The first set of implications pertains to when the practitioner should refer the adolescent and family for further evaluation. The second set pertains to the characteristics of appropriate mental-health treatment providers.

When Should Referral Be Made?

Delinquency, especially status offenses, is highly prevalent among adolescents. Thus, if minor delinquency is identified by the parents or the physician, therapeutic intervention is not necessarily warranted. In determining whether a referral for further evaluation is needed, the practitioner should assess three broad areas of adjustment: family relations, the youth's peer relations, and the youth's school performance. If significant problems are identified in any one of these areas, a referral for further evaluation is appropriate.

In light of the low probability of being arrested for committing a criminal offense, the arrest of an adolescent usually warrants further evaluation because it rarely represents isolated antisocial behavior. However, numerous adolescents are arrested who do not require therapeutic intervention—that is, the parents handle the situation appropriately, family functioning is positive, the youth has close friendships with prosocial peers, and/or the youth is performing satisfactorily in school. Involvement in serious criminal activity (e.g., sexual offenses, violent offenses, and felonies) almost always warrants referral for further evaluation.

To Whom Should Referral Be Made?

Consistent with the results of outcome research in delinquency treatment, referrals for further evaluation and possible intervention are best made to mental health professionals who have expertise in family systems or behavioral treatment approaches and who specialize in the treatment of children and families. Such professionals are more likely to implement the types of pragmatic, problem-focused interventions that have demonstrated effectiveness than are professionals who adhere to psychodynamic or humanistic treatment models. The professional degree of the mental health professional— MD, PhD, PsyD, or MSW—is less important than the individual's theoretical orientation.

Finally, referral to inpatient, residential, or other restrictive treatment facilities should be implemented only in the most extreme and dangerous cases. Despite their high expense, such facilities have no empirically demonstrated effectiveness and in the long run may do more harm than good. Again, when the causes and correlates of delinquency are appreciated (e.g., family relations, peer relations, school performance), one would expect minimal effectiveness from interventions that remove the youth from his or her family and community without addressing the factors in the natural environment that contributed to the problems.

References

1. Henggeler SW: *Delinquency in adolescence,* Newbury Park, CA, 1989, Sage.
2. Mulvey EP, Arthur M, Reppucci ND: The prevention and treatment of juvenile delinquency: a review of the literature, *Clin Psychol Rev* 13:133-157, 1993.
3. Santos AB, Henggeler SW, Burns BJ, Arana GW, Meisler N: Research on field-based services: models for reform in the delivery of mental health care to populations with complex clinical problems, *Am J Psychiatry* 152:1111-1123, 1995.

CHAPTER 112

Violence

•

Jack Gladstein, Alwyn T. Cohall, Virginia Bishop Townsend, and Renee Mayer Cohall

SCOPE OF THE PROBLEM

We, as a society, have made great strides in reducing the mortality of adolescents since the turn of the twentieth century.[1] Much of this decline can be attributed to improvements in immunization and hygiene and prompt treatment of infectious diseases. However, while the death rate from natural causes dropped 90% between 1933 and 1985, that from violence or accidental injury has remained fairly stable.[2]

In general, older adolescents are three times more likely to die a violent death than younger adolescents, and males are twice as likely as females to succumb. White males are more likely to die as a result of a motor vehicle accident; black males are more likely to die as a result of homicide, often at the hands of another black male.[2]

Homicide

Homicide is the second leading cause of death for all adolescents but the most common reason for demise among black teenagers. The rate for black teenagers and young adults (101/100,000) is more than six times the national average for young people aged 15 to 24 years.[3] In 1991, 8159 young people aged 15 to 24 years were murdered—in other words, 22 per day, almost one every hour.[4] Firearms, usually handguns, are implicated in 68% to 75% of all homicides.[5] In 15- to 19-year-olds, there was a slight 11% increase in non–firearm-related homicide rates between 1985 and 1990. However, there was an overall 141% increase in firearm-related homicide rates (5.8/100,000 to 14/100,000) and 182% among African-American males (37.4/100,000 to 105.3/100,000).[6] The

increase in homicide rates among minority males is attributable almost entirely to firearms.[7] The United States leads the pack of 21 other industrialized nations with respect to homicides among males aged 15 to 24 years, with a rate of 22.4/100,000. This rate is four times that of Scotland, which is in second place (5/100,000).[7]

Victimization

The impact of violence on adolescents is far broader than mortality statistics alone indicate. For every adolescent who is fatally injured, 41 are hospitalized with injuries and 1100 are treated in an emergency room.[8] Teenagers are twice as likely as adults and 10 times more likely than the elderly to be victims of violence.[9] For those aged 12- to 14-years, the victimization rate is 22.6/1000; for those aged 15 to 17 the rate is 27.5/1000.[10] Twenty percent of inner-city males reported being robbed or assaulted, often at gun or knifepoint. Of this sample, less than one third received supportive services. Additionally, young people often reported witnessing violent events: 36% of males had seen someone being knifed and 31% witnessed a murder taking place.[11]

School Violence

For many adolescents the violence on the street does not cease at the school door. The National Adolescent School Health Survey revealed some disturbing findings: about 20% of boys and approximately 4% of girls carried a knife to school at least once; 3% of boys carried a gun to school at least once; approximately one half of male and one third of female high school students had been in at least one fight during the school year; and 15% of both boys and girls were robbed at least once in school.[9] In another survey, ninth graders were significantly more likely than twelfth graders to have gotten into a fight during the month before the survey (50.5% vs. 33.9%).[12]

Family Violence

For many teenagers, home is no safer than the streets or the schools, and 47% of the victims of domestic maltreatment are adolescents. Teenagers are more likely than younger children to be beaten by another family member and more likely to be attacked with a gun or knife.[13]

Access to and Utilization of Weapons

One of the distinctive features of youth violence today is the frequent use of weapons to settle disputes. Thirty to 40 years ago, arguments were settled chiefly by fisticuffs; in today's environment, handguns and knives have become standard fare.

Approximately half of all homes have at least one firearm.[14] Between 1987 and 1990, 72% of weapons, including guns, confiscated from teenagers in Florida were traced back to their homes.[15] Only 22% of students surveyed in Seattle "doubted" they would ever need access to a gun.[16]

In one study of suburban/rural teenagers, 48% reported owning a gun. The average age for acquiring the weapon was 12.5 years; most often, the gun was a gift from an older male relative.[17]

Male adolescents are 13 times more likely than female adolescents to be owners of guns. White males are more likely than black males to own a long gun and less likely to own a handgun.[18] In New York City, over 2000 weapons are confiscated from students annually.[19]

In a survey of 1500 inner-city high school students, 20% had been threatened by someone carrying a gun and 12% had been shot at. Males were two to three times more likely than females to be the recipient of threatened or actual firearm-related violence.[20]

Media Violence

Television and the media play a very big part in the life of adolescents. Chapter 92, "The Media," provides a comprehensive review of this subject.

FACTORS CONTRIBUTING TO VIOLENCE

Many factors related to homicide and intentional injuries reflect societal and cultural influences. These

include racial and socioeconomic factors, developmental issues, home environment, gender issues, and neurobiology.

Poverty

Violence is linked to poverty (see Chapter 95, "Poverty"). Racial differences shown in homicide rates are greatly reduced or disappear when data are controlled by income.[21] Homicides are consistently concentrated in poorer communities and among those with high levels of income inequality and youth unemployment.[22,23]

Developmental Issues

Teenagers, facing a number of major developmental tasks, may be at risk for violent behavior.[24,25] Adolescents' preoccupation with themselves, their appearance, and their image makes them particularly susceptible to overreacting to even mild insults. Peer pressure can enhance the likelihood of violent behavior when fighting is the norm.[26]

Environment

Evidence is mounting that violence is a learned response to stress and conflict. Violence in the home has been associated with adolescent violent behavior.[27]

Gender

Predisposition to violent behavior may be based on gender-determined differences. Most males are more prone than most females to physical violence. This may be the result of hormonal influences and/or societal norms.[28,29]

Neurobiology

The role of cultural forces in either promoting or discouraging interpersonal violence is so obvious that it has been allowed to obscure the part played by biologic disorders in determining responses to endogenous and environmental challenges. Neuroscientists and clinicians have demonstrated, however, that aggression has a neuroanatomic and chemical basis, and that developmental and acquired brain disorders, as well as attention deficit hyperactivity disorder, contribute to recurrent interpersonal violence (see Chapter 128, "Attention-Deficit Hyperactivity Disorder").

Since both biologic and sociologic factors may be involved, to ignore either is to invite error and oversimplification. These observations need to be balanced by the fact that violent youths with documented neurobiologic causes of the violence represent a relatively small portion of the larger population of individuals with violence-related problems.[30]

INTERVENTIONS AND SOLUTIONS

Violence is a learned behavior that can be changed and prevented. Although intertwined with larger social issues such as racism, poverty, and employment, violence is not the innate or inevitable expression of a person in relation to his or her environment. There is no single or simple solution, however, since violent behavior is the result of the interaction of complex behavioral, economic, educational, cultural, environmental, neurobiologic, and political forces.

The Practitioner's Role

Practitioners who treat children and adolescents need to know how to screen, identify, treat, and refer violence victims. In addition, they must be familiar with community programs in place, strategies for children and adolescents, and efforts to decrease the use of weapons.

Practitioners who see adolescents need to incorporate exposure to violence into their everyday practice.[11] Stringham,[31] as director of the East Boston Neighborhood Health Center, has protocols for questions to ask families about violence from the newborn visit through and including adolescence. The program seeks to influence parents, patients, and the community. For the parents, the program advocates nonviolent approaches in childrearing, decreasing exposure to TV violence for children, and the absence of guns in the home. For the patients, the program teaches nonviolent beliefs, skills, and style and teaches respect for self, others, and the opposite sex. The physicians in this community have taken a strong public stand, and their actions have mobilized the community toward change.

The practitioner also needs to consider the impact of victimization when seeing an adolescent who is "acting out" or is at risk. In the acute setting the circumstances of suspicious injuries or wounds suffered during an altercation need to be explored so that proper action can be taken. Even in this setting, it is appropriate to suggest nonviolent conflict resolution techniques, and refer to a mental health or social work resource when appropriate.

The primary care practitioner needs to be familiar with post-traumatic stress disorder (PTSD) (see Chapter 114) to help in identification of victims and to follow a patient's progress. In this disorder, a life-threatening experience to self or others is accompanied by extreme fear and helplessness. The violence witness or victim has intrusive reexperiencing of the event, avoidance of stimuli associated with the event, generalized numbing, increased autonomic arousal (sleep disturbance, inability to concentrate), and impairment of function. Adolescents who have been victimized may present to the clinician in various ways.

They may present for triage immediately after a trauma, during the acute phase, or a while later, with PTSD symptoms, acting-out behavior, or school problems. When this diagnosis is made, referral for mental health services is mandated. The first stage of treatment, if identified immediately after a group-experienced life-threatening event, is "psychologic first aid," which can take place in the classroom or in the crisis center. This debriefing has been shown to decrease the incidence of PTSD in an exposed cohort of young people.[32] For subsequent treatment, systematic painful and exacting review of the trauma is key. In this process, the clinician clarifies the adolescent's perceptions, fantasies, misconceptions, level of exposure, and feelings of hopelessness. Cognitive-behavioral approaches, such as relaxation and breathing training, help the youngster cope with reliving the experience. If the trauma is chronic (e.g., familial sexual or physical abuse), severe psychopathology usually extends beyond PTSD symptoms. Terr therefore makes the distinction between single-incident (type I) and chronic (type II) trauma.[33] For type II trauma, longer-term counseling is indicated to treat the underlying psychopathology that often accompanies chronic exposure to violence.

In addition to a thorough understanding of the identification and treatment issues, a clinician should be aware of the community resources available to help victims of violence. With this knowledge the provider may overcome any reticence in asking about violent experiences and be able to help patients and families begin the process of healing.

Community Programs

Youth violence is a community-based problem whose resolution has gone beyond the capabilities of those agencies to which it has been traditionally delegated (juvenile and criminal justice systems).[34] Healthy People 2000[35] calls for "culturally and linguistically appropriate community health promotion for racial and ethnic minority populations." Further, the community must decide what interventions should be in place, and then monitor their effects.

Common characteristics of successful community-based programs include the formation of partnerships among different agencies and organizations within a given population. This commonality of purpose prevents duplication in this era of scarce resources. Careful planning of objectives and assessment allows for judging success and midcourse adjustments. Youth involvement in all phases of the intervention has been crucial in all successful programs.

Strategies for the General Population of Adolescents

School-based educational approaches include conflict resolution courses and programs that enhance generic interaction skills, such as self-esteem, skills training, and academic tutoring. Schools are beginning to change the physical milieu in an attempt to discourage violent occurrences on the premises. Metal detectors, uniforms, lighting, and landscaping changes are being employed to make schools a safe place for children. Good school programs use a variety of mentors, from peers to the principals, to reinforce violence prevention. Recreational interventions give adolescents an outlet for frustration, stress, and anger and allow them to spend leisure time in socially acceptable activities. Strategies also include the involvement of media campaigns, community figures, and sports/media personalities in preaching nonviolence. Community support can also be exhibited by means of job opportunities, technical assistance, and mentoring programs. A focus on decreasing the media's glamorizing of violence also should be advocated at a national level. In all these programs, a strong evaluation component is crucial in order to learn what works and what does not.

Strategies for the At-Risk Adolescent

Approaches for the high-risk adolescent may involve primary or secondary interventions. Primary interventions imply that although the youngster is at risk, he or she has not been a victim or perpetrator. Secondary interventions imply that the youth has already been exposed to violence in some way. High-risk groups deserve the highest priority. They may include[36]

1. Youths who live in geographical areas saturated with violence
2. Gang members or youths who are at risk for joining gangs
3. Youths from families who have problems with violence
4. Violent adolescents
5. Violence victims, family members of victims, and witnesses of violence

For adolescents with high-risk attributes, programs must individualize therapy for a given youth's needs, with particular emphasis on family and environment. These interventions need to be culturally relevant and realistic. They should stress conflict resolution and job training, and offer adolescents a way to gain positive feelings about themselves and their future. Of course, victims and witnesses may need a whole host of interventions to ameliorate the consequences of their experiences. These may include mentoring programs, counseling, and conflict resolution. For violent youths, realistic goals are important. Possible interventions include individual counseling, conflict resolution training, peer groups, mentoring with positive role models, and training programs that reinforce a sense of responsibility and self-worth.

Interventions for Early Childhood

Violence prevention programs need to promote nonviolent childrearing practices and to limit childhood exposure to violence at home, on television, and in the neighborhood. For the already victimized child, programs to avert aggressive behavior as an adolescent should be a priority.

Interventions in the home, school, treatment setting, and community should be coordinated to avoid duplication of services. Home visitation for families at risk have been shown to decrease child abuse and neglect.[37] Such programs for at-risk families can teach effective parenting and instill a sense of worth and dignity in parents and children. Home visits may be made by trained community workers, to increase community empowerment.

Schools can incorporate nonviolence in the preschool, lower school, and middle school curricula. Nonviolent approaches to conflict resolution as well as other social skills should be emphasized.

Treatment programs for abused and neglected children, violence victims and witnesses, and aggressive youngsters need to be intensified. The community can support families by offering crisis intervention services for families in turmoil, participating in mentoring programs, advocating public education programs, and lobbying for nonviolent schools.

Efforts to enhance civic pride and cultural identity may give a child a sense of belonging to family and community.

Interventions to Decrease the Use of Weapons

Since most youth homicides occur among people who know each other, the availability of a weapon often turns a fight into a lethal event.[38] Firearms are often purchased for perceived protection, but owners are not aware of their danger. Weapons become the tool that amplifies aggression in the aggressive. Further, firearms play a role in the drug trade: even if the drug trade moves on, the guns tend to remain.[39]

Programs cannot ignore youngsters' perceptions of protection by guns and of their right to bear arms. On a community level, a consensus needs to be reached. This is done by keeping surveillance data about firearm injuries and by organizing community forums where people can learn about the hazards of guns and debate the issues.

On all levels, efforts to curb gun-related violence should be encouraged. Many advocate to mandate firearm safety, ban the manufacture of and sale of more dangerous weapons, educate the community as to gun manufacturers' liability for the consequences of their products, increase efforts to halt illegal gun purchases, and encourage legislation to license gun owners and require them to pass proficiency tests and mandatory classes (similar to a driver's license requirement). The evaluation portion of the programs is crucial, so that the components of a program that actually decrease the magnitude and severity of weapon-related injuries can be documented.

SUMMARY

Violence in our society has reached epidemic levels, and adolescents are at very high risk for victimization. An understanding of the problem, combined with a knowledge of community resources, should help the practitioner provide for those adolescents who have been or are at risk for violence-related health problems.

References

1. Wetzel JR: *American youth: a statistical snapshot,* New York City, 1987, William T. Grant Foundation.
2. Fingerhut LA, Kleinman JC: *Trends and current status in childhood mortality, U.S. 1900-1985, Vital and health statistics series 3, no. 26,* Hyattsville, MD, 1989, National Center for Health Statistics.
3. *National Center for Health Statistics: Health U.S. 1990,* Hyattsville, MD, 1991, U.S. Public Health Service.
4. National Center for Health Statistics: *Advance report of final mortality statistics, 1991: monthly vital statistics report,* Hyattsville, MD, 42(2 suppl):21-24, 1993.
5. Division of Injury Control, Center for Environmental health and injury control, Centers for Disease Control: Childhood injuries in the United States, *Am J Dis Child* 144:627, 1990.
6. Federal Bureau of Investigation: *Crime in the United States, 1991,* Washington, DC, 1992, Department of Justice.
7. Fingerhut LA, Kleinman JC: Homicide among young males, *JAMA* 263:3292, 1990.
8. Gans JE, Blyth DA, Elster AB, et al: *American's adolescents: How healthy are they? Profiles in adolescent health,* vol 1, Chicago, 1990, American Medical Association.
9. American School Health Association, The Association for the Advancement of Health Education, and the Society for Public Health Education: *The National Adolescent Student Health Survey: A report on the health of America's youth,* Oakland, CA, 1989, Third Party Publishing.
10. National Center on Child Abuse and Neglect: *Study/Findings: Study of National Incidence and Prevalence of Child Abuse and Neglect,* 1988, Washington, DC, 1988, U.S. Department of Health and Human Services.
11. Gladstein J, Rusonis EJ, Heald FP: A comparison of inner-city and upper-middle class youths' exposure to violence, *J Adolesc Health Care* 13:275, 1992.
12. Kann L, Warren W, et al: Results from the national school-based 1991 Youth Risk Behavior Survey and progress toward achieving related health objectives for the nation, *Public Health Rep* 108 (Suppl 1):47, 1993.
13. Gelles R: Family violence and adolescents, *Adolesc Med: State of Art Rev* 1:45, 1990.
14. Christoffel KK: Towards reducing pediatric firearm injuries:

charting a legislative and regulatory course, *Pediatrics* 88(2):294-295, 1991.
15. Rollin J: *Weapons and firearms on school property. Florida Educator,* Florida School Boards Association, May/June:11, 1990.
16. Callahan CM, Rivara FP: Urban high school youth and handguns: a school-based survey, *JAMA* 267(22):3038, 1992.
17. Sadowski LS, Cairns RB, Earp JA: Firearm ownership among non-urban adolescents, *Am J Dis Child* 143:1410, 1989.
18. Price JH, Desmond SM, Smith D: A preliminary investigation of inner city adolescents' perception of guns, *J Sch Health* 61:255, 1991.
19. Northrop D, Hamrick K: Weapons and minority youth violence, *Public Health Rep* 106:274, 1991.
20. Sheley J, Wright J: Gun related violence in and around inner-city schools, *Am J Dis Child* 146:677, 1992.
21. Williams KR: Economic sources of homicide: re-estimating the effects of poverty and inequality, *Am J Soc* 49:283, 1984.
22. Block CR: Lethal violence in the Chicago Latino community. In Wilson AV, editor: *Homicide dynamics of the victim/offender interaction,* Cincinnati, OH, 1994, Anderson.
23. Sloan JH, Kellermann AL, Reay DT, Ferris JA, Koepsell T, Rivara FP, Rice C, Gray L, LoGerfo J: Handgun regulations, crime, assaults, and homicide: a tale of two cities, *N Engl J Med* 320:1256, 1988.
24. Erickson E: *Identify youth in crisis,* New York, 1968, WW Norton.
25. Jessor R, Jessor S: *Problem behavior and psychosocial development: a longitudinal study of youth,* New York, 1977, Academic Press.
26. Spivak H, Prothrow-Stith D, Hausman AJ: Dying is no accident: adolescents, violence, and intentional injury, *Pediatr Clin North Am* 35:1339, 1988.
27. Bandura A, Ross D, Ross S: Vicarious reinforcement and imitative learning, *J Abnorm Soc Psychol* 63:601, 1983.
28. Gorski RA: Sexual differentiation of the brain. In Krieger DT, Hughes JC, editors: *Neuroendocrinology.* New York, 1980, HP Publishing; pp 215-222.
29. Kagan J: Psychology of sex differences. In Beach FA, editor: *Human sexuality in four perspectives,* Baltimore, MD, 1977, Johns Hopkins University Press; pp 87-114.
30. Elliott FA: Neurology of aggression and episodic dyscontrol, *Semin Neurol* 10:303, 1990.
31. Slaby RG, Stringham P: Prevention of peer and community violence: the pediatrician's role (part 2), *Pediatrics* 4:608, 1994.
32. Yule W: Post traumatic stress disorder in child survivors of shipping disasters: the sinking of the Jupiter, *Psychother Psychosom* 57:200, 1992.
33. Terr LC: Childhood traumas: an outline and overview, *Am J Psychiatry* 148:10, 1988.
34. *Surgeon General's Workshop on Violence and Public Health. Source Book,* Leesburg, VA, 1985, National Center for Child Abuse and Neglect.
35. Office of Disease Prevention and Health Promotion: *Healthy People 2000. National health promotion and disease prevention objectives,* DHHS Publication No. 90-50212, Washington, DC, 1990, U.S. Government Printing Office.
36. Cairns RB, et al: Violence prevention strategies directed toward high-risk minority youths, *Public Health Rep* 106:250, 1991.
37. Olds D, Kitzman H: Can home visitation improve the health of women and children at environmental risk?, *Pediatrics* 86:108, 1990.
38. Cook PJ, et al: Weapons and minority violence, *Public Health Rep* 106:254, 1990.
39. National Committee for Injury Prevention and Control: *Injury prevention: meeting the challenge,* New York, 1989, Oxford University Press; pp 198-206.

CHAPTER 113

Anxiety Disorders

•

Guochuan E. Tsai and Michael Jellinek

Anxiety is an essential component of human life that provides a stimulus for individual development and a protective mechanism of species survival. However, anxiety can be excessive with fears, phobic avoidance, anticipatory anxiety, vigilance, panic attack with autonomic arousal, or (to the worst extent) overwhelming dread. Anxiety is considered pathologic when it interferes with individuals' achievement of goals, quality of life, or psychologic well-being. Pathologic anxiety is usually autonomous with minimal realistic basis. It is intense or recurrent or persists over time and can proceed to consistent behavior patterns such as phobia, avoidance, and life style constriction.

EPIDEMIOLOGY

Anxiety disorders are one of the most common adolescent clinical problems. According to community-based epidemiologic studies, about 5% to 9% of adolescents have anxiety disorders causing dysfunction and requiring treatment. Panic disorder, agoraphobia, specific phobia, social phobia, obsessive compulsive disorder, posttraumatic stress disorder, or acute stress disorder can have their onset during childhood or adulthood. These are not discussed in this chapter, which focuses on three specific anxiety syndromes identified in childhood populations: separation anxiety disorder, avoidant disorder, and overanxious disorder. The prevalence rates of separation anxiety disorder range from 2.0% to 6.8%; the avoidant disorder range is about 1.6%; the overanxious disorder onset range is 2.9% to 5.9%; the rate of social phobia is about 1%; and the simple phobia range is 2.3% to 9.1%.

Overanxious disorder in the *Diagnostic and Statistical Manual of Mental Disorders,* third edition revised (DSM-IIIR) is now diagnosed as generalized anxiety disorder with childhood onset in the fourth edition (DSM-IV). Avoidant disorder was replaced by childhood social phobia. Only separation anxiety disorder, which addresses unique childhood developmental issues, was retained as a distinct childhood anxiety disorder in DSM-IV. These major nosologic changes from DSM-III to DSM-IV reflect the concept of continuity of anxiety disorder from childhood to adulthood. It also suggests the importance of early diagnosis of anxiety disorders in childhood to reduce the morbidity and cost due to the chronicity of the disorders. The essential features of three different childhood anxiety disorders are listed in Box 113-1.

ETIOLOGY

There are multiple and complex theories concerning the origins of anxiety. Psychodynamic schools postulate that anxiety is triggered by external events that activate anxiety associated with unconscious aggressive wishes. The symbolic anxiety manifested by the adolescent serves to disguise the unconscious distortion of unacceptable wishes. For example, anger and the wish to hurt a parent would be manifested by a fear of separating from the parent and the dread that the parent will come to some harm. Behavioral and learning theorists emphasize that biologic vulnerability to anxiety is under genetic control. They explain maladaptive behavior through reinforcement such as a mother's fright every time a younger child behaves more autonomously. The correction of maladaptive reinforcement will dictate the success of treatment. For cognitive approaches, anxiety symptoms are the result of cognitive distortions. The disruption of cognitive representations of individuals' environment and experience causes anxiety. Ethologic models consider emotions as adaptive consequences of evolutionary processes resulting from natural selection. Anxiety and fear are protective of naturally occurring dangers, and also regulate social bonds that maximize survival and species reproduction. Overall, psychodynamic, learning, and

---

BOX 113-1
Diagnostic Criteria of the Major Adolescent Anxiety Disorders

SEPARATION ANXIETY DISORDER

Developmentally inappropriate and excessive anxiety concerning separation from home or from those to whom the individual is attached for more than 4 weeks, as evidenced by three or more of the following. The disturbance causes clinically significant distress or impairment in social, academic (occupational), or other important areas of functioning.

1. Recurrent excessive distress when separation from home or major attachment figures occurs or is anticipated.
2. Persistent and excessive worry about losing, or about possible harm befalling, major attachment figures.
3. Persistent and excessive worry that an untoward event will lead to separation from a major attachment figure (e.g., getting lost or being kidnapped).
4. Persistent reluctance or refusal to go to school or elsewhere because of fear of separation.
5. Persistent and excessive fear or reluctance to be alone or without major attachment figures at home or without significant adults in other settings.
6. Persistent reluctance or refusal to go to sleep without being near a major attachment figure or to sleep away from home.
7. Repeated nightmares involving the theme of separation.
8. Repeated complaints of physical symptoms (e.g., headaches, stomachs, nausea, or vomiting) when separation from major attachment figures occurs or is anticipated.

GENERALIZED ANXIETY DISORDER
(OVERANXIOUS DISORDER OF CHILDHOOD)

Excessive anxiety and worry (apprehensive expectation), occurring more days than not for at least 6 months about a number of events or activities (such as work or school performance), and the child finds it difficult to control the worry. The anxiety and worry are associated with one or more of the following six symptoms: (1) restlessness or feeling keyed up or on edge, (2) being easily fatigued, (3) difficulty concentrating or mindgoing blank, (4) irritability, (5) muscle tension, (6) sleep disturbance (difficulty falling or staying asleep, or (7) restless unsatisfying sleep). The anxiety, worry, or physical symptoms cause clinically significant distress or impairment in social, occupational, or other important areas of functioning.

SOCIAL PHOBIA (SOCIAL ANXIETY DISORDER)

The child has the capacity for age-appropriate social relationship with familiar people but has a marked and persistent fear of one or more social or performance situations in which he or she is exposed to unfamiliar or to possible scrutiny in the peer setting. The child fears that he or she will act in a way (or show anxiety symptoms) that will be humiliating or embarrassing.

Exposure to the feared social situation almost invariably provokes anxiety, which may take the form of a situationally bound or situationally predisposed panic attack or may be expressed by crying, tantrums, freezing, or shrinking from social situations with unfamiliar people. The feared social or performance situations are avoided or else are endured with intense anxiety or distress.

The avoidance, anxious anticipation, or distress in the feared social or performance situation(s) interferes significantly with the person's normal routine, occupational (academic) functioning, or social activities or relationships, or there is marked distress about having the phobia.

The duration is at least 6 months.

Adapted from *Diagnostic and statistical manual of mental disorders*, ed 4, Washington, DC, 1994, American Psychiatry Association.

---

cognitive theories differ in identifying the origin of anxiety but consider that similar mechanisms underlie both normal and pathologic conditions. In contrast, ethologic views suggest that normal fear favors species survival and that pathologic anxiety is qualitatively distinct. However, the ethologic view can account for adaptive behaviors but not the pathologic behaviors that are dysfunctional. Obviously, these theories are not mutually exclusive, and several may be operative in exacerbating anxiety.

The development of benzodiazepines and other anxiolytics have advanced neurobiologic theories of anxiety and emotional regulation. Benzodiazepines are high-affinity ligands for the receptor of the inhibitory neurotransmitter γ-aminobutyric acid (GABA). GABA receptors are enriched in the limbic system, a neuronal system that modulates environmental cues and also serves as a relay station for internal affective and visceral signals to the neocortical regions. Animal studies indicate that this limbic GABA-ergic system may play a role in modulating arousal, alertness, and behavioral inhibition. Lesion studies in nonhuman primates on the amygdala, an important limbic structure, provide compelling evidences for its involvement in emotional and social behavior. A second neurobiologic component involves the noradrenergic locus ceruleus. Fear responses can be elicited by stimulation of the locus ceruleus. The importance of the noradrenergic system is supported by the clinical efficacy of beta-adrenergic antagonists in treating anxiety disorders. In addition to the benzodiazepine and noradrenergic systems, much data have accumulated over the past decade supporting the hypothesis that cholecystokinin (CCK) plays a role in the neurobiology of anxiety and panic attacks. CCK is a normal endogenous anticipatory stress modulator in the central nervous system; enhanced sensitivity to CCK beta-receptor agonists can result in anxiety and panic attacks.

The neurobiologic theory is complemented by the temperament theory popular from the 1980s. Temperament studies indicate that inhibited children have increased risk for anxiety disorders. Inhibited temperament can be the result of genetically determined hypersensitivity of external cues due to the lowered limbic activity threshold. Theoretically, benzodiazepines are therapeutic by reducing the hypervigilance accompanied by the autonomic arousal, and the effect is mediated by correcting the threshold through inhibiting the GABA system.

CLINICAL DIAGNOSES

Adolescent anxiety disorders, as in other medical diagnoses, are diagnosed by observing the clustering of a symptom complex. There is no single symptom diagnostic of a specific anxiety disorder. For example, school refusal is a major presentation of multiple disorders: simple phobia for school, social phobia, conduct disorder, or depression. At times, dual or triple diagnoses can present simultaneously.

Adolescent anxiety is common, and most resolves spontaneously. Transient anxiety about meeting new friends, a first date, varsity tryouts, or other developmental steps toward autonomy can be expected. Clinicians should pay attention to developmental differences and severity in the presentation of anxiety disorders. For separation anxiety disorder, adolescents usually present with school refusal and somatic complaints; 9- to 12-year-olds are likely to show distress at times of separation; 5- to 8-year-olds commonly report unrealistic worry about harm to attachment figures and school refusal. For generalized anxiety disorder with childhood onset, adolescents endorse more symptoms than younger children. However, almost all children with generalized anxiety disorder have unrealistic worry about future events as their key symptom.

The spectrum of anxiety symptoms ranges from mild worry to incapacitating panic attacks. Some children have little residual symptoms, while others can relapse and exacerbate throughout childhood and into adulthood. Since children with anxiety disorders who do not receive treatment sometimes develop chronicity, it is important to have clinical assessment and intervention whenever the anxiety symptoms cause dysfunction even when the child does not meet the threshold criteria for a specific DSM-IV diagnosis of anxiety disorder. Pediatricians should act more quickly when the anxiety interferes with school or peer relationships or causes serious personal suffering.

In clinical practice, anxiety syndromes can overlap or vary considerably (Box 113-1). For example, panic attack and excessive distress are the major components of both panic disorder and separation anxiety disorder. Social phobia is characterized by a persistent fear of situations in which the patient is subjected to public scrutiny; the patient fears that situations will be humiliating and embarrassing. The social phobia may be well circumscribed (standing in front of a class) or generalized (going out with parents).

Comorbidity is a common rule of childhood anxiety disorder. About one third of children meet the criteria for two or more anxiety disorders. Major depression is also a common comorbidity, ranging from 28% to 69%, of anxiety disorder. Between 15% and 24% of children with separation anxiety disorder or generalized anxiety disorder also meet the criteria for attention deficit hyperactivity disorder.

Physical conditions including hypoglycemic episodes, hyperthyroidism, cardiac arrhythmias, caffeinism, pheochromocytoma, seizure disorders, migraine, and other central nervous system disorders (e.g., delirium, brain tumors) can mimic anxiety symptoms. Reaction to medication, including antihistamines, antiasthmatics, sympathomimetics, steroids, haloperidol and pimozide (neuroleptic-induced separation anxiety disorder), other antipsychotics (akathisia), fluoxetine, diet pills, and cold medicines all can induce anxiety symptoms. The goal of treatment for the anxiety symptoms associated with a physical condition or medication is to correct the underlying illness or remove the offending agent(s).

PREVENTION AND TREATMENT

In developing a treatment plan, overall adaptation is as important as focal symptoms that define a specific anxiety disorder. A comprehensive focus with long-term perspective in addition to short-term symptom relief is important in order to modify the maladaptive concomitants and prevent relapse. For example, the comprehensive and long-term perspective emphasizes that separation anxiety disorder can continue in adult life as agoraphobia or panic disorder; social disability and affect constriction are quite common complications of separation anxiety disorder and can persist into adulthood.

Symptom complexity, comorbidity, and chronicity

necessitate an integrated approach in treating an adolescent with anxiety disorder. Both pharmacologic and nonpharmacologic strategies are important in the treatment. Multimodal treatment is indicated as recommended by the Practice Parameters for the Assessment and Treatment of Anxiety Disorder published by the American Academy of Child and Adolescent Psychiatry. A comprehensive treatment plan should take the following components into consideration: cognitive behavioral therapy, pharmacotherapy, psychodynamic psychotherapy, family therapy when indicated, education of parents and child, and communication with school personnel and primary care physicians.

Research on pharmacologic therapies for adolescent anxiety disorders is in its infancy. Since controlled studies are limited in adolescence, clinicians treating anxious adolescents often extrapolate from adult information or make educated judgments based on information from open trials, case reports, or anecdotal experiences.

Tricyclic antidepressants may be helpful in some cases of separation anxiety disorder and school refusal, but definitive proof is lacking. Chlordiazepoxide, clonazepam, and alprazolam have been reported to be effective for separation anxiety disorder. The efficacy of benzodiazepines, serotonin uptake inhibitors, and buspirone in generalized anxiety disorder with adolescent onset has not been established, although a few open trials suggest that these agents may be effective. Many controlled studies have demonstrated that propranolol, benzodiazepines, and antidepressants are effective treatments for panic disorder, but the study is limited for adolescent panic disorder. Similarly, beta-blockers, benzodiazepines, serotonin uptake inhibitors, and monoamine oxidase inhibitors are pharmacologic treatment options in adult social phobia, but child psychiatrists have to extrapolate from the adult studies for the pediatric population.

Cognitive behavior therapy combines a behavioral approach with changes in cognition associated with anxiety. It can restructure the adolescent's thoughts into a more positive framework and adaptive behavior. In separation anxiety disorder associated with school refusal, classic condition-based systematic desensitization and exposure (operant behavioral techniques) were both reported to be effective treatments. Improvement of generalized anxiety disorder by cognitive-behavioral treatment also has been reported. In the case of simple phobia, behavioral treatment is the treatment of choice. The interventions include modeling and systemic desensitization. In psychoanalysis and psychodynamic psychotherapy anxiety is considered to be a result of maladaptive attempts to cope with internal conflicts. The approaches tie the anxiety symptoms to the adolescent's overall personality structure; symptom amelioration and modification of the personality structure are the primary goals of this treatment. The choice of different treatment modalities depends on clinical judgment and empirical results. There are no well-researched data to support specific treatment for different anxiety disorders. Thus, the pediatrician should consider the spectrum from biologic vulnerability to individual dynamics as well as family psychiatric history.

SUMMARY

Clinicians often see adolescents with anxiety disorders, as such disorders are common. Asking a shy, inhibited, or introverted adolescent questions about fear and anxiety is a good starting point for screening those at risk for anxiety disorder. A family report of separation difficulty, school refusal, poor socialization, task avoidance, or anxiety-ridden behavior should lead to further inquiry. Fortunately, most adolescents resolve their anxiety, and the treatment of more dysfunctional adolescent anxiety is often short-term. When the symptoms are severe or persistent, a referral to a child and adolescent psychiatrist for assessment and treatment is recommended.

Suggested Readings

Allen AJ, Leonard H, Swedo SE: Current knowledge of medications for the treatment of childhood anxiety disorders, *J Am Acad Child Adolesc Psychiatry* 34:976-986, 1995.

Biederman J, Rosenbaum JF, et al: Psychiatric correlates of behavioral inhibition in young children of parents with and without psychiatric disorders, *Arch Gen Psychiatry* 47:21-26, 1990.

Diagnostic and statistical manual of mental disorders, ed 4, Washington, DC, 1994, American Psychiatry Association.

Livingston R: Anxiety disorders. In Lewis M, editor: *Child and adolescent psychiatry, a comprehensive textbook,* Baltimore, MD, 1991, Williams & Wilkins; pp 673-685.

Practice parameters for the assessment and treatment of anxiety disorder, *J Am Acad Child Adolesc Psychiatry* 32:1089-1098, 1993.

CHAPTER 114

Posttraumatic Stress Disorder

•

Andrew Clark and Michael Jellinek

Under extraordinary circumstances in which an individual is faced with an inescapable threat or actual injury, normal coping mechanisms may become overwhelmed and the person experiences terror and helplessness. Such a breach of psychologic defenses, if contained, may result in moderate symptoms that wane within days or weeks. At other times, more severe symptoms develop that nonetheless remain episodic and do not interfere greatly with overall functioning. In extreme cases, however, the trauma may cause difficulties that reverberate throughout the life span, leading to a wide array of persistent and disabling symptoms, derailing development, and even distorting character formation. The formal psychiatric diagnosis of posttraumatic stress disorder (PTSD) is limited to a restricted constellation of characteristic symptoms that are directly attributable to the traumatic exposure.

Although recognized in combat veterans for over a century as "shell shock" or "battle neurosis," it is only in the last few decades that PTSD has been identified in broader populations, and even more recently that it has been recognized and studied in children and adolescents. Much of the present knowledge in the area has been gained from Terr's longitudinal study of 26 children involved in a 1976 school bus kidnapping in Chowchilla. California[1] and Pynoos et al's study of children exposed to a school yard sniper in 1987.[2] Such studies have highlighted children's vulnerability to the development of PTSD after a single traumatic event, as well as the persistence of troubling symptoms for years afterward.

The fourth edition of the *Diagnostic and Statistical Manual of Mental Disorders* (DSM-IV)[3] limits the definition of trauma to events that involve an actual threat or injury to oneself or others and that are accompanied by feelings of helplessness, fear, or horror. Such events can be either discrete episodes (such as a kidnapping or a rape) or prolonged and repetitive occurrences (such as ongoing physical or sexual abuse). Traumatic events are not limited to those that the victim experienced directly; posttraumatic symptoms can arise from witnessing an incident (e.g., a child witnessing domestic violence) and even from indirect exposure to an event (e.g., in response to a friend's suicide).

According to DSM-IV, PTSD symptoms fall into three clusters: those symptoms associated with *reexperiencing* the trauma, such as intrusive memories, nightmares, and flashbacks; those associated with *avoidance* and *numbing,* such as amnesia for aspects of the events, emotional detachment, and a foreshortened sense of the future; and those associated with *increased arousal,* such as hypervigilance, insomnia, irritability, and an exaggerated startle response.

While wars, criminal assaults, and natural disasters stand out as obvious sources of trauma, many young people experience trauma in the form of abuse and violence within their own families, or through exposure to extraordinary levels of violence within their neighborhoods. Two thirds of teenage girls in an urban adolescent medicine clinic, for example, met symptom criteria of PTSD as revealed by self-reports.[4]

The only clearly defined risk factor for the development of PTSD is exposure to the trauma itself. Studies of communities of children exposed to a common trauma such as a natural disaster have found rates of posttraumatic symptoms approaching 100%. However, factors such as social supports, a history of traumatic exposures, and comorbid psychiatric conditions probably affect the long-term outcome, including the development of PTSD. For example, children who have suffered losses such as the death of a parent or a divorce, or those with a family history or temperamental disposition to anxiety and depression, may be more vulnerable.

Frequently, even a single traumatic exposure brings in its wake additional adversities and losses. For example, abused youngsters are often taken from their parents, and natural disasters can be psychologically and financially devastating for entire families and communities. Adolescents faced with multiple adversities seem to be at elevated risk of developing not only PTSD but also depressive and anxiety disorders.

The pathophysiology of PTSD is thought to derive from the massive release of stress hormones in the face of terror and helplessness, with long-term physiologic consequences. Children and adults with PTSD, for example, in addition to their heightened responsiveness to reminders of their trauma, demonstrate an exaggerated startle response, indicating a more global disturbance of stimulus discrimination. It has been suggested that traumatic memories are different in kind from normal ones, registered in different areas of the brain and lacking the customary modulating influence of the hippocampus.[5] These traumatic memories exist primarily as visceral sensations and visual images rather than as conscious verbal recollections. Furthermore, they can be triggered by any sort of emotional arousal, and they are reexperienced even years later as vividly and powerfully as they were initially.

Adolescents respond to traumatic experiences in a variety of ways, depending in part on the nature and duration of the experience and the developmental stage of the victim at the time. Indeed, the range of other possible diagnostic outcomes following a trauma spans virtually the entirety of adolescent psychopathology, including depression, anxiety, substance abuse, conduct disorder, dissociation, and psychosis.[6] Given the diverse nature of the posttraumatic presentation, accurate diagnosis depends on a high index of suspicion coupled with an accurate history.

In the immediate aftermath of a traumatic exposure the victims generally appear still, quiet, and alert. In the following few weeks they may exhibit sleep, attention, and learning difficulties or may seem especially irritable or confused. These youngsters may appear fearful, anxious, and vigilant and may demonstrate an exaggerated startle response.

Classic symptoms of PTSD generally appear within several weeks or months of the event. By this time sleep and learning difficulties tend to resolve, but emotional constriction, specific fears related to the trauma, and intrusive memories reach their full force. For example, an adolescent assaulted in an elevator and threatened with a knife may react to a safe elevator or a butter knife at home with anxiety, flashbacks, and intrusive thoughts. Adolescents may exhibit reenactments of the trauma in which they place themselves in a position to reexperience some aspect of either the trauma or their response to it. Such reenactments may include victimizing others in some way as well, including, for example, sexualized behavior after sexual trauma.

In the aftermath of a single traumatic exposure, people tend to retain clear and extraordinarily detailed memories of discrete aspects of their experience; those memories, however, are subject to cognitive reworkings and distortions, and may not always accurately reflect the complete context of the event. Those persons exposed to ongoing or repetitive abuse are more likely to demonstrate amnesia and dissociation (a fracture of the normal integrity of identity, memory, and emotion), which can at times render their narratives fragmented and confusing.

A child's or an adolescent's long-term response to trauma frequently involves an outward appearance of relatively normal functioning. However, such persons are often beset by occult fears, ambushed by anniversary reactions, and limited by their sense of a future that holds little promise, with few expectations of surviving into a productive adult life. They may demonstrate occasional intrusive memories indiscriminately activated by emotional arousal, superimposed onto an emotional style characterized by detachment, constriction, and sadness.

There are no pathognomonic behavioral signs or conclusive test results and no useful laboratory studies to aid in the diagnosis of PTSD. Most helpful is a clear and detailed history of a person's exposure to trauma and subsequent deviation from his or her baseline level of functioning. Given the difficulty in obtaining a complete and coherent verbal account of such events, clinical data need to be carefully correlated with other sources such as medical records, police reports, and eyewitness observations.

Although many traumatic events are entirely unpredictable, some reduction in adolescents' exposure to trauma is possible through caregivers' sensitivity to evidence of ongoing abuse or domestic violence, and early involvement of the appropriate child protection agencies.

Widely experienced events, such as a natural disaster or the suicide of a peer, call for an early response from professionals to help minimize the eventual development of PTSD symptoms.[7,8] Helpful steps under these circumstances include the dissemination of clear and reliable information to quell hysteria and dispel rumors, and realistic reassurance about the children's safety. It is often helpful for professionals to meet in schools with small groups of affected youths in an effort to allow each of them to relate their experience of the event. These meetings can be helpful in calming unrealistic fears, normalizing responses that might otherwise be thought embarrassing, and providing an acknowledgment that one's experience has been shared by others. Adolescents who seem especially troubled can be identified through this process and referred for ongoing treatment.

The essential first step in the treatment of PTSD in adolescents is to ensure that they are provided with a safe environment. Second, helping to elicit and strengthen the support of family and others can go far in minimizing the long-term impact of the trauma. Family members are often in need of reassurance and support themselves, and it is essential that they be capable of actively supporting the youngster's autonomy in spite of their own anxiety and concern.

For traumatized adolescents in need of mental health intervention, psychotherapy is the mainstay of treatment.[9] Indications for referral include posttraumatic symptoms that are distressing, disabling, or persistent. Those who have suffered multiple adversities or who have suboptimal social supports should be referred early. The best time for intervention is in the acute phase of the process, when symptoms seem most amenable to change. While some persons with uncomplicated PTSD can be helped in just a few sessions, others require ongoing treatment for extended periods.

The role of medications in treating PTSD is limited to helping manage disabling symptoms, particularly those that interfere with psychotherapy. Although any number of psychotropic medications have been used in patients with some success, few controlled studies have been conducted involving children or adolescents, and no medications have demonstrated clear superiority over others. Centrally acting antihypertensive agents, such as clonidine, have proved helpful for symptoms of hyperarousal, while antidepressants and benzodiazapines have also been found useful in certain cases.

Although treatment of PTSD can clearly be helpful, the experience of trauma often leaves adolescents with permanent emotional scars. Even those persons with uncomplicated PTSD who recompensate rapidly may remain vulnerable to subsequent traumas later in life. Research on the neurobiology of trauma and on the effects of trauma on development hold promise for more effective treatments, but the most pressing need lies in helping to protect youngsters from such experiences in the first place.

References

1. Terr L: Acute responses to external events and posttraumatic stress disorder. In Lewis M, editor: *Child and adolescent psychiatry,* Baltimore, 1991, Williams & Wilkins; pp 755-763.
2. Pynoos RS, Frederick C, Nader K, et al: Life threat and posttraumatic stress in school-age children, *Arch Gen Psychiatry* 44:1057-1063, 1987.
3. American Psychiatric Association: *Diagnostic and statistical Manual of Mental Disorders,* ed 4, Washington, DC, 1994, American Psychiatric Association.
4. Horowitz K, Weine S, Jekel J: PTSD Symptoms in urban adolescent girls: compounded community trauma, *J Am Acad Child Adolesc Psychiatry* 34:1353-1361, 1995.
5. van der Kolk B: The body keeps the score: memory and the evolving psychobiology of posttraumatic stress, *Harvard Rev Psychiatry* Jan/Feb 253-263, 1994.
6. Terr L: Childhood traumas: an outline and overview, *Am J Psychiatry* 148:10-20, 1991.
7. Pynoos RS, Nader K: Prevention of psychiatric morbidity in children after disaster. In Shaffer D, Philips I, Enzer N, editors: *Prevention of mental disorders, alcohol and other drug use in children and adolescents,* OSAP Prevention Monograph-2, U.S. Department of Health & Human Services, Rockville, MD, DHHS Publication No. (ADM) 89-1646, 1989; pp 225-271.
8. U.S. Dept. of Health and Human Services, Public Health Service, Substance Abuse and Mental Health Administration, Center for Mental Health Services: *Psychosocial issues for children and families in disaster: a guide for the primary care physician,* IL, 1995, American Academy of Pediatrics, Work Group on Disaster.
9. Marmar C: An integrated approach for treating posttraumatic stress, *Rev Psychiatry* 239-272, 1993.

CHAPTER 115

Obsessive Compulsive Disorder

•

Richard M. Sarles

Obsessive compulsive disorder (OCD), once a relatively uncommon condition in the general population and extremely rare in children and adolescents, has increased dramatically since the early 1980s, partly because of greater awareness of and diagnosis of OCD by mental-health professionals but also in keeping with the earlier onset and increase of other childhood psychiatric disorders. Current epidemiology data suggest a lifetime prevalence of 2.5% and a 1-year prevalence of 1.5% to 2.1%.[1] Although comparable data are not available for children and adolescents, best estimates place the prevalence at approximately 0.5%.[2] A significant factor, however, is that 30% to 50% of adults with OCD say that their symptoms developed during childhood or adolescence.[3] Thus, pediatricians can expect that many patients will develop symptoms of OCD while under their care.

Most children and adolescents, and in fact many adults, do not self-report obsessive compulsive behaviors, and yet most children develop normal habits, superstitions, and rituals. How does the pediatrician differentiate the norm from the disorder?

NORMAL DEVELOPMENTAL RITUALS

From a developmental perspective, children begin to develop routines and a need for sameness as early as 24 to 30 months of age. Many of these routines, such as evening bathing and bedtime stories, persist well into the school-age years.

During the school-age period most children develop elaborate rules and rituals for many games such as "hopscotch," in which counting and rules are important, and "Marco Polo," a swimming game that requires ritualistic word repetition. It is also common for many school-age children to develop significant collections of various objects.

In addition to habits, rituals, and routines, children often develop many superstitions based on a magical belief or idea to ward off bad luck or misfortune or to ensure good luck. For example, to avoid bad luck children do not walk under ladders, do not step on sidewalk cracks, do not let a black cat cross their path, or do not break a mirror. To ward off bad luck, children may cross their fingers, knock on wood, carry a rabbit's foot or some other good luck charm, or hold their breath while passing a cemetery. Clearly, many of these childhood superstitions persist into adulthood and are particularly notable in competitive sports—for example, certain rituals in baseball, wearing specific items of clothing during a winning streak, blessing oneself before an athletic event, or always carrying a good luck charm.

In general, there is no evidence that normal childhood habits, rituals, or superstition form a continuum with later OCD.[4] However, patients when diagnosed with OCD were identified in retrospect by their parents as having significantly more ritualized behaviors in childhood than non-OCD patients. In addition, most childhood habits, rituals, and superstitions are culturally bound and ego-syntonic; that is, they are acceptable ideas compatible with the person and are meant to relieve tension and stress, thereby allowing the person to function better. In contrast, OCD symptoms usually create tension and stress, are usually time-consuming and wasteful, and are ego-dystonic; that is, they are unacceptable, troubling, and perplexing to the person and generally interfere with normal functioning. Lastly, OCD symptoms are charac-teristically focused on cleanliness, washing, checking, and repeating features.

Most parents welcome traits of neatness, attention to detail, tidiness, timeliness, and organization in their children, especially in adolescents. Such personality characteristics often lead to such individuations being labeled obsessive compulsive in popular parlance, which often has a pejorative connotation. However, these characteristics are adaptive and essential for mastering certain academic subjects such as science and mathematics and specific professions such as airline pilot, air traffic controller, and architect. Thus, these traits can enhance performance and productivity unless, of course, an excessive need for structure or an over-rigid, inflexible approach develops, which can stifle productivity and cripple performance.

OBSESSIVE COMPULSIVE PERSONALITY DISORDER

Obsessive compulsive personality disorder (OCPD) describes a condition in which traits normally considered to be adaptive and helpful become excessive and interfere with normal function. Patients with OCPD demand excessive attention to rules, schedules, and orderliness and have no tolerance for error. This preoccupation with minutiae is usually self-defeating in that the person is unable to finish school assignments or work projects owing to fear of error. Such people are so preoccupied with details and perfectionism that they often lose the overall major issue. The achievement of perfection is a key element in the use of time, and thus time is usually poorly allocated, deadlines are often delayed, appointments are missed, and others are usually inconvenienced and generally annoyed by the obsessive behavior.

Patients with OCPD are usually excessively conscientious to the point of being unable to justify relaxing or fun activities. Hobbies and sports are frequently serious endeavors, and relaxing play becomes a structured activity focused on mastery and perfection. These individuals are often very stubborn and rigidly believe that there is only one way to do things, which is their way. They seldom delegate or share work tasks because they believe no one else can do the job correctly. Thus, they are seldom good team players; they usually alienate peers, co-workers, friends, and often family; they seldom pay compliments; and they are often very reserved, formal, and distant.

OBSESSIVE COMPULSIVE DISORDER

Obsession refers to a persistent or inescapable pre-occupation with an idea or emotions. It is an intrusive, repetitive, unwanted mental event, generally evoking anxiety or discomfort; it usually interrupts the normal train of thought, often with an inability to turn off the intrusive idea. These intrusive thoughts often involve dirt, germs, or contamination or may represent ideas of harm befalling the patient or others, either accidentally or at the hand of the patient in horrific fashion.

Compulsions are acts or rituals that are initially unconscious to the patient; they gradually become more conscious and are intended by the patient to reduce, neutralize, or obliterate the troublesome obsessive thoughts. The patient is quite literally obliged and required to perform these compulsions in a pressured, rigid fashion. In general, however, the compulsions do little to relieve the obsessive thoughts, and the compulsions often are increased in number and complexity by the patient, consciously or unconsciously, in hopes of positively erasing the obsessions. It is common for patients to wash their hands dozens of times each day, to continuously repeat showering for up to 45 to 60 minutes at a time several times a day, or to perform touching rituals multiple times when leaving home. It is easy to see how this compulsion can significantly interfere with normal functioning, often to the point of incapacitation. Thus, the symptoms and behaviors that usually alert parents are rituals or habits far exceeding the norm. Examples include excessive numbers of showers; excessive length of time showering; multiple daily changes of underwear; repetitive hand washing; excessive trips to the bathroom at school, home, or on trips; excessive checking of doors, windows, and lights; excessive persistence in completing every detail of every project; and inability to finish reading a page of homework.

Early mental health theorists hypothesized a continuum among obsessive compulsive behaviors and character traits, OCPD, and OCD. However, current epidemiologic data show no connection with OCD and obsessive compulsive traits; in fact, when people with obsessive traits develop psychopathology, it is usually in the form of depression, paranoia, or somatic symptoms. In addition, only about 25% of patients with OCD meet the criteria for OCPD. Although the nomenclature of these disorders is similar, there are some overlapping characteristics, and both can cause considerable impairment in everyday functioning. OCPD can be easily distinguished from OCD by the absence of true obsessions and compulsions in patients with the former. Although OCPD cannot be officially diagnosed in a person below the age of 18 years, many of these characteristics, traits, and symptoms begin to develop in childhood and adolescence, and therefore the pediatrician should inquire about both OCD and OCPD symptoms.

RISK FACTORS

In addition to the clinical presentations, there are other risk factors of which the pediatrician should be aware. Comorbidity of OCD with other psychiatric (DSM-IV Axis I) disorders is common. In fact 50%, of adult patients with OCD have another Axis I disorder, most commonly anxiety or depressive disorders. In adults, 20% to 40% of patients with eating disorders, 30% of those with tic disorders, and 25% to 50% of those with Tourette's syndrome have comorbid OCD. In a National Institute of Mental Health study,[5] of 70 children and adolescents with OCD (excluding mental retardation, eating disorders, and Tourette's syndrome), only 26% had OCD as the sole disorder. Tic disorders (30%), major depression (26%), specific developmental disability (24%), simple phobia (17%), overanxious disorder (10%), adjustment disorder with depressed mood (13%), oppositional disorder (11%), and attention deficit disorder 10% were some of the most common comorbid diagnoses.

The pediatrician should be aware of the association of OCD with other conditions, and when alerted should directly inquire of the patient about intrusive thoughts and washing and checking rituals. Patients do not usually divulge their symptoms spontaneously as at one level they recognize the unrealistic nature of the obsession but are often confused and fearful of these thoughts. Patients are often embarrassed, are usually secretive, and often become anxious or depressed because of the incapacity of both the obsessions and compulsions.

Twenty percent of patients with OCD have a family member with OCD, and almost all OCD patients have a family member with either an affective, anxiety, or tic disorder. An association with rapid onset OCD and group A beta-hemolytic streptococcal infection has been reported.[6] OCD-like behaviors are frequently seen after head trauma and are associated with brain tumors, epileptic seizures, and Sydenham's chorea. Asperger's disorder, a condition with significant impairment of social interaction, is associated with restricted repetitive stereotype patterns of behavior that often resemble OCD.

TREATMENT

OCD, once believed to be a manifestation of intrapsychic or intrapersonal conflict, is now known to be a neurobiologic condition that may be exacerbated, aggravated, or complicated by psychosocial stressors. Fortunately, recent advances in neurobiology and psychopharmacology have provided important insights into the biologic basis and treatment of this condition. OCD is now known to respond well to the serotonin reuptake inhibitor clomipramine and to the selective serotonin reuptake inhibitors, including fluoxetine, sertraline, paroxetine, and fluvoxamine.[7] Medication can be very helpful to the patient with OCD. The pediatrician working with an adolescent suspected of having OCD should seek consultation with a child and adolescent psychiatrist regarding further diagnosis and treatment.

The use of medication in combination with cognitive behavioral therapy appears to provide the greatest likelihood of symptom relief and return to normalization in patients with OCD.[9] Outcome studies are few, but the National Institute of Mental Health 2- to 7-year follow-up study showed that 43% of patients still met diagnostic criteria for OCD and only 11% were totally asymptomatic.[5] In general, however, the combination of cognitive behavioral therapy and medication can provide significant improvement in patients with OCD.

References

1. American Psychiatric Association: *Diagnostic and statistical manual of mental disorders,* ed 4, Washington, DC, 1994, American Psychiatric Association.
2. Flament MF, Whitaker A, Rapoport JL, et al: Obsessive compulsive disorder in adolescence: an epidemiological study, *J Am Acad Child Adolesc Psychiatry* 27:764-771, 1988.
3. Rasmussen SA, Eisen JL: Epidemiology of obsessive compulsive disorders, *J Clin Psychiatry* 53 (suppl):10-13, 1990.
4. Leonard HL, Goldberger EL, Rapoport JL, et al: Childhood rituals: normal development or obsessive compulsive symptoms, *J Am Acad Child Adolesc Psychiatry* 29:17-23, 1990.
5. Swedo SE, Rapoport JL, Leonard H, et al: Obsessive compulsive disorder in children and adolescents: clinical phenomenology in 70 consecutive cases, *Arch Gen Psychiatry* 46:335-341, 1989.
6. Swedo S, Leonard H, Kiessling L: Speculations on anti-neuronal antibody-mediated neuropsychiatric disorders of childhood, *Pediatrics* 93:323-326, 1994.
7. March JS, Leonard HL, Swedo SE: Pharmacotherapy of obsessive compulsive disorder in children and adolescents, *Psychiatr Clin North Am* 4:217-236, 1995.
8. Rapoport JL, Leonard HL, Swedo SE, et al: Obsessive compulsive disorder in children and adolescents: issues in management, *J Clin Psychiatry* 54:27-29, 1993.
9. Berg C, Rapoport JL, Wolff R: Behavioral treatment for obsessive compulsive disorders in childhood. In Rapoport J, editor: *Obsessive-compulsive disorder in children and adolescents,* Washington, DC, 1989, American Psychiatric Press; pp 169-185.

CHAPTER 116

Developmental Disabilities

•

Theodore Kastner

Adolescents with developmental disabilities are set apart from their peers by visible and invisible functional deficits that can affect the adaptive outcome. These obstacles can complicate the normal developmental processes of adolescence. Healthcare providers must recognize adolescents with developmental disabilities so that additional supportive services can be provided and developmental goals achieved to the highest degree.

DEFINITION

Developmental disability is a term that emerged in the 1960s to describe a constellation of disorders that cause an initial impairment of function during infancy, childhood, and adolescence. This term does not describe the cause of the disorder but defines functional impairment. Although the term is often mistakenly used to describe mental retardation, it includes mental retardation and any other condition that may substantially impair function. Other conditions commonly considered to be developmental disabilities include cerebral palsy, autism, significant vision and hearing impairments, severe epilepsy, some genetic syndromes, and certain physical disabilities or chronic illnesses.

The increasingly popular use of the terminology has coincided with a growing recognition of the needs of people with developmental disabilities and an expansion of supportive services to aid them. In 1973 the Rehabilitation Act significantly expanded rehabilitation service programs. Section 504 of this act established civil rights protections for people with developmental disabilities. In

1975 the Education for All Handicapped Children Act (Pub L No. 94-142) acknowledged the rights of children with disabilities to an appropriate education, and set aside funds for states to provide educational services. In the same year the Developmental Disabilities Assistance and Bill of Rights Act (Pub L No. 94-103) expanded an earlier emphasis on the provision of community-based services for people with disabilities. The Rehabilitation, Comprehensive Services, and Developmental Disabilities Amendments of 1978 (Pub L No. 95-602) changed the definition of developmental disability to a set of functional criteria:

A severe, chronic disability of a person which (1) is attributable to a mental or physical impairment or combination of mental and physical impairments; (2) is manifested before the person attains the age of 22 years; (3) is likely to continue indefinitely; (4) results in substantial functional limitations in three or more of the following areas of major life activity: (a) self-care, (b) receptive and expressive language, (c) learning, (d) mobility, (e) self-direction, (f) capacity for independent living, and (g) economic sufficiency; and (5) reflects the person's need for a combination and sequence of special interdisciplinary, or generic care, treatment or other services that are of lifelong or extended duration and are individually planned and coordinated.

The subsequent Developmental Disabilities Act of 1984 and its reauthorization in 1994 (Pub L No. 103-230) retained this definition, with a greater emphasis on achieving independence, productivity, and integration.

In 1990 the Americans with Disabilities Act was signed into law by President Bush. This landmark legislation provides civil rights protections to an estimated 43 million Americans who were not previously protected. The law addresses five areas, including employment, public accommodation, transportation, telecommunications, and remedies/penalties. Additional information about state and national legislation and local services can be obtained from the developmental disabilities planning council or protection and advocacy agency of each state.

CAUSES

Developmental disabilities can result from genetic, pregnancy-related, and acquired causes. Genetic etiologies include chromosomal and nonchromosomal genetic disorders. Examples of chromosomal genetic disorders are Down syndrome and fragile X syndrome. Nonchromosomal inherited disorders include entities such as Tay-Sachs disease and phenylketonuria. Pregnancy-related developmental disabilities include those due to fetal exposure to teratogens such as alcohol, tobacco, or drugs. Other pregnancy-related causes of developmental disabilities are diseases transmitted to the fetus in utero, such as acquired immunodeficiency syndrome, toxoplasmosis,

syphilis, and cytomegalovirus. In approximately 50% of infants noted at birth to have developmental disabilities, the cause is unknown. Acquired developmental disabilities include those caused by trauma to the head and/or spinal column. This trauma may occur during the birth process but more commonly occurs during early childhood as a result of motor vehicle accidents or accidents in the home, as well as child abuse. Many of these are preventable causes of developmental disabilities.

PREVALENCE

The prevalence and incidence of developmental disabilities are important in planning for healthcare services. However, precise estimates of these figures are difficult to obtain because of the application of a variety of survey and estimating methods and because of a lack of accepted diagnostic characteristics and definitions. For example, if all individuals with mental retardation are included in the diagnostic category, the prevalence of developmental disabilities may be as high as 5%. If all those with learning disabilities are included in the diagnostic category, the prevalence may be as high as 10%.

Public agencies tend to have lower estimates of the prevalence of developmental disabilities because of more restrictive diagnostic criteria. In a 1988 study the New York State Office of Mental Retardation and Developmental Disabilities estimated that 1.74% of the general state population had one or more of the five categorical disabilities contained in the state definition of developmental disability, and that 0.68% of the general state population was functionally disabled.[1]

CLINICAL ASPECTS OF SELECT ASSOCIATED CONDITIONS

The examination of specific conditions associated with developmental disabilities provides some insight into the diversity of healthcare needs of adolescents with these disabilities.

Mental Retardation

Mental retardation is the most common developmental disability, affecting between 1% and 3% of the population (see Chapter 118, "Mental Retardation"). It is characterized by significantly subaverage general intellectual functioning existing concurrently with deficits in adaptive behavior manifested during the developmental period. Mental retardation is caused by a wide variety of organic factors (e.g., prenatal and postnatal infection, intoxication, trauma) and environmental factors. An effort should be made to determine the cause in order to develop a thorough understanding of the person's healthcare needs.

Cerebral Palsy

Cerebral palsy is a disorder of posture and muscle tone caused by a nonprogressive insult or injury to the brain. It is characterized chiefly by deficits in motor function and is associated with cognitive, adaptive, sensory, and other deficits. Cerebral palsy can be caused by prenatal injury, perinatal asphyxia, infectious disease, metabolic agents, and head trauma. The role of perinatal asphyxia as a cause of cerebral palsy has probably been exaggerated at the expense of prenatal factors. The prevalence of cerebral palsy varies, with estimates ranging between 1 and 4 per 1000 live births. Improved neonatal care has resulted in a reduction in athetoid cerebral palsy secondary to kernicterus.

People with cerebral palsy often have a variety of medical needs. The condition is associated with mental retardation (50% to 75%), speech and articulation problems (70%), impaired vision (35%), impaired hearing (35%), orthopedic problems (20%), behavioral and psychiatric disorders (20%), and epilepsy (20%).[2] Although nearly 50% of adolescents with cerebral palsy are intellectually impaired, the measured intelligence of one fifth of this group is average or above.[3]

Autism

Autism, a type of pervasive developmental disorder, is characterized by qualitative impairment in reciprocal social interaction, verbal and nonverbal communication skills, and imaginative or symbolic play. There is often a restricted repertoire of activities associated with sterotypic behavior. The disorder usually manifests in infancy or childhood before the age of 30 months. Autism is noted in approximately 4 to 5 children in every 10,000. The prevalence of children with autistic features, a condition generally classified as pervasive developmental disorder (not otherwise specified), is thought to be 10 to 15 children in every 10,000.[3]

Although the manifestations of autism are usually lifelong, some children experience improvements in social, language, and other skills during childhood or adolescence. Cognitive function and social skills may decline or improve independently of each other. Aggressive, oppositional, or disturbed behavior may develop. A few adolescents with autism lead independent lives, but they are often socially awkward.

Autism is associated with a variety of prenatal, perinatal, and postnatal conditions, including congenital rubella infection, untreated phenylketonuria, tuberous sclerosis, perinatal asphyxia, encephalitis, infantile spasms, and fragile X syndrome. The medical needs of the adolescent with autism usually relate to the presence of any associated conditions. For example, fragile X syndrome (X-linked recessive disorder characterized by a long narrow face, large or prominent ears, and large testicles), which occurs in approximately 1 in 1000 of the general population, is associated with mitral valve prolapse (50%), strabismus (50% to 60%), pectus excavatum (32%), height below the 5th percentile (20%), abnormal electroencephalographic picture (50%), seizures (20%), and attention-deficit hyperactivity disorder (47%) in affected males.

Adolescence often marks the onset of epilepsy in autistic individuals. Any adolescent with autism who manifests a deterioration in function should be evaluated for the presence of complex partial seizures.

Epilepsy

Epilepsy is defined as the separate occurrence of two or more apparently unprovoked seizures. Although epilepsy is a major manifestation of brain injury, it is also a serious complicating factor in people with developmental disabilities. Approximately 20% of people with developmental disabilities will at some time in their lives have seizures. Frequently, the first seizure occurs in adolescence. Generalized seizures may result from any disease that affects the entire brain, such as metabolic disorders, infection, inflammation, or degenerative disorders. Focal seizures are caused by focal lesions within the brain, including blood vessel malformations, tumors (tuberous sclerosis, neurofibromatosis), trauma, and malformations. In nearly 50% of people with epilepsy, the cause is unknown. (See Chapter 61, "Seizures.")

Classification of seizures is clinically important because it determines treatment strategies. There are two types of epileptic seizures: (1) generalized or nonfocal and (2) partial or focal. Patients who suffer partial seizures may later experience generalized seizures. Types of generalized seizures include tonic-clonic, tonic, clonic, absence, atonic/akinetic, and myoclonic. Types of partial seizures include simple partial seizures with elementary symptoms but no impairment in consciousness, and complex partial seizures with complex symptoms and impaired consciousness.

The pharmacologic management of epilepsy in people with developmental disabilities is beyond the scope of this chapter, but one point deserves attention. One study disclosed that 48% of people with developmental disabilities and a diagnosis of epilepsy remained free of seizures for an 8-year period after discontinuation of medication.[4] Clinical predictors of a seizure-free state without medication included a few documented seizures during a lifetime, no gross neurologic abnormalities, serum levels below the therapeutic range at the time of medication discontinuation, and persistently normal electroencephalographic results before and after discontinuation of medication. For an adolescent with developmental disabilities and epilepsy, tapering and withdrawal of anticonvulsant medication may be appropriate.

CHALLENGING BEHAVIOR

Mental illness generally is not considered a cause of developmental disability. However, the frequent association between developmental disabilities and psychiatric disorders has lead to the popularization of the term *dual diagnosis.* Unfortunately, this term gives the impression that the cause of the disability and the cause of the psychiatric illness are unrelated and require highly specialized separate treatments.

As many as 40% of people with developmental disabilities may experience a period of disturbed behavior and function at some time in their lives. Common maladaptive behaviors include aggression, self-injury, overactivity, and impulsiveness. Adolescence is often the time when these symptoms first appear. In many people, these symptoms are attributed to psychologic, physiologic, or hormonal changes associated with normal adolescence, and it is hoped that these symptoms will be outgrown. This belief has led to needless suffering by adolescents with developmental disabilities and their families. The three major causes of severe challenging behavior in adolescents with developmental disabilities are adaptive dysfunction, psychiatric disorders, and organic causes.

Adaptive Dysfunction

Adaptive dysfunction relates to a mismatch between the needs, abilities, and goals of the adolescent with developmental disabilities and the environment (i.e., the school and family unit). This cause of severe challenging behavior is amenable to an analysis of the person's goals and current environment to identify areas of conflict. In particular, the existence of any breakdown in communication between the family or teacher and the adolescent is sought. The communicative nature of the adolescent's behavior is also considered. For example, does head banging always occur when the adolescent is asked to do a difficult task? Environmental dysfunction can often be distinguished from mental illness or organic causes by a lack of vegetative signs (e.g., weight change or sleep disturbance) and a relationship between the behavioral disturbance and antecedent environmental events.

Psychiatric Disorders

Psychiatric illness is more common among people with developmental disabilities than in the general population. However, the standard classification text, the *Diagnostic and Statistical Manual of Mental Disorders, Fourth Edition (DSM-IV),*[3] has significant shortcomings in terms of addressing the behavior of adolescents with developmental disabilities. Therefore, alternative classification systems are often used. The most common psychiatric illnesses among adolescents with developmental disabilities are mood disorders such as depression and bipolar disorder (often in atypical forms, including rapid cycling and chronic mania). Mood disorders in adolescents with developmental disabilities can be distinguished by the presence of a sleep disturbance, change in weight or eating habits, overactivity or motor restlessness, mood lability (crying or laughing), and a behavioral history of cycling. Less common disorders include anxiety disorders, thought disorders, attention-deficit hyperactivity disorder, and obsessive-compulsive disorder. Overactivity and a short attention span seen in mania can be mistaken for the hyperactivity of attention-deficit hyperactivity disorder. When a trial regimen of stimulant medication causes a worsening of behavior, the diagnosis of bipolar disorder should be considered. Although attention-deficit disorder can be seen in all children with developmental disabilities, it is most often seen in children with mild or moderate levels of impairment.

Organic Causes

The most common organic cause of disturbed behavior in adolescents with developmental disabilities is unrecognized or partially treated epilepsy. Approximately 20% to 30% of adolescents with developmental disabilities who present to our clinic for behavior evaluation are noted to have epilepsy, usually complex partial seizures. Ictal events may be subtle and include lip smacking, eye deviation, staring, arm or leg thrusting, body jerks, or changes in mental status or affect that are not related to the environment.[5] Aggression or self-injury usually are not related specifically to the seizure.

Temporolimbic epilepsy is a common condition in which complex neurologic, behavioral, and psychiatric symptoms can be observed in the adolescent with developmental disabilities. Temporolimbic epilepsy has been associated with explosive, undirected aggression, but this behavior is rare. More commonly, it is associated with sensory alterations, motor symptoms, autonomic manifestations, hallucinations or illusions, and emotional manifestations. An electroencephalogram may be obtained if seizures are suspected. The use of nasopharyngeal and anterior temporal leads can be considered in addition to standard electrode placement. In one study of patients with complex partial seizures, standard electrode placement detected only 58% of epileptic discharges.[6] The combination of nasopharyngeal and anterior temporal leads detected 86% of spikes; when these were combined with standard electrodes, the rate of detection increased to 97%. In practice, however, problems related to patient management and the need for sedative medication substantially limit our use of electroencephalography. In some cases, clinical judgment may be the best guide to making a diagnosis and developing a treatment plan for adolescents with developmental disabilities who are suspected of having seizures.

Limbic seizures and the phenomenon of limbic kindling have been advanced as causes of mood disorders in people with developmental disabilities. This model suggests that limbic epilepsy leads to a variety of neurohormonal disturbances that can express themselves primarily in changes in affect. This theory partially explains the relatively frequent mood symptoms exhibited by people with developmental disabilities. In addition, it suggests a theoretical framework for understanding the efficacy of carbamazepine, valproic acid, and clonazepam in the treatment of adolescents with developmental disabilities and severe challenging behavior.[7]

HEALTHCARE NEEDS

Owing to changes in the guiding legislation and the financing of services for people with developmental disabilities, the residential and service sites that serve this population have shifted from the institution to the community. The number of individuals with developmental disabilities in residential facilities dropped from a peak of 194,650 in 1967 to 63,258 in 1995. This relocation has created new opportunities and hazards for people with developmental disabilities.

Gaps in healthcare services exist. Minihan and Dean[8] studied the healthcare utilization of 333 mentally retarded people over a 12-month period. Overall the group received good care from primary care physicians, with some specialty back-up. However, people with developmental disabilities experienced difficulty in obtaining home health care, preventive health services, and ancillary services such as rehabilitation therapy and adaptive equipment.

Inadequate financing was the most common and significant obstacle to the provision of adequate health care. Nearly one fourth of all subjects reported an instance in which a provider refused or was reluctant to serve them because the payment source was Medicaid. The subjects also complained of occasionally encountering negative attitudes toward individuals with mental retardation and/or the display of poor interpersonal skills by healthcare personnel with such people. These gaps in service ultimately reflect the inability of the healthcare delivery system to support adolescents with developmental disabilities adequately.

In a critique of the healthcare delivery system, Crocker and Yankauer[9] called for new priorities. They stressed that multiple options for the delivery of health care, including private practice, health maintenance organizations, community- and hospital-based clinics, and home healthcare services, should be explored as possible mechanisms. The concept of a "medical home" was emphasized. The need to establish healthcare networks with resource centers for specialty care and healthcare clearinghouses was addressed, and the development of a comprehensive record of personal health status was urged. The authors stated that fees for service must be "fair and set at the prevailing market level." In conclusion, they noted the need for improvements in healthcare training, health services research, and healthcare coordination. The usual provider of primary health care for children with special needs is the pediatrician (45% to 70%) or general practitioner (15% to 25%). In Minihan and Dean's small sample of people under the age of 22 years with mental retardation,[8] 49% received their primary health care from a pediatrician and 30% from an internist. Thus, the primary care physician, often in private practice, is on the front line of the battle to improve the health of adolescents with developmental disabilities.

In recent years, managed care has grown in popularity as a means of providing healthcare services. Currently, nearly all states offer managed health care to Medicaid recipients. At the time of this writing, most states are considering instituting Medicaid managed care programs. Many more states are planning applications to the Health Care Financing Administration for projects of this type. However, little is known about the impact of managed healthcare services on children and adolescents with developmental disabilities. While managed care may improve access to primary care services, access to specialists and preventive services may actually decrease because of efforts to contain costs. No doubt, the trend toward managed health care will accelerate as state and federal policy makers try to control healthcare costs.

As pediatricians redefine their roles and practices, it is important to remember the goals of health care for children and adolescents. Project BRIDGE of the American Academy of Pediatrics developed a statement of "Principles of Health Care for Children" that offers sound advice to physicians caring for adolescents with developmental disabilities.[10]

MULTIDISCIPLINARY APPROACH

The implementation of multidisciplinary teams to provide medical services is familiar to pediatricians and is encountered on a daily basis by most developmental pediatricians and adolescent medicine specialists. An emphasis on medical care in the context of the family and school requires an alliance among healthcare, education, social services, and other human services personnel. In the case of the adolescent with developmental disabilities, multidisciplinary teams are commonly used in the educational environment for the development of the individual education plan, and in the human services system for the development of the individual habilitation plan.

The collaborative interaction between the physician and other team members is the basis for the development and implementation of the healthcare plan. Team members are likely to include pediatricians, family practitioners, internists, psychiatrists, physiatrists, and other medical specialists working with dentists, nurses, nurse practitioners, physical therapists, occupational therapists, speech therapists, social workers, behaviorists, psychologists, special educators, and nutritionists. The formation of a team requires reaching out to individual practitioners and to agencies. Throughout this process the ongoing need is to coordinate the interaction of the team with the adolescent and the family and to monitor the treatment process. Frequently, one of the team members is identified as the primary contact coordinator; in the healthcare plan, the physician often has this role.

TRAINING

In general, a lack of familiarity with the causes, implications, and care of people with developmental disabilities is apparent. Inadequate training in medical school and residency programs in the health promotion of people with developmental disabilities is a particular problem. A 1978 survey of 7000 recent graduates of pediatric residency programs by the American Academy of Pediatrics' Task Force on Pediatric Education[11] noted that 40% had insufficient training in the area of chronic cerebral dysfunction, 51% in the area of child advocacy, and 54% in the care of patients with psychosocial and/or behavioral problems. While recent Resident Review Committee guidelines for pediatric residencies have increased the emphasis on developmental disabilities, many practicing pediatricians have had little training in regard to the needs of this population.

Numerous resources are available that enhance the skills of healthcare providers caring for adolescents with developmental disabilities. Medical journals are a regular source of current information. Foremost among these is the *Journal of Developmental and Behavioral Pediatrics,* which is the journal of the Society for Developmental and Behavioral Pediatrics. Additional journal sources include *Pediatrics, Journal of the American Academy of Child and Adolescent Psychiatry, Developmental Medicine and Child Neurology, Journal of Pediatrics, Journal of Adolescent Health Care,* and *Journal of School Health.*

Informational newsletters are a valuable adjunct to the medical journals. *Exceptional Health Care* offers a monthly review of selected developmental disability–related articles culled from a wide variety of journals in a format similar to *Pediatric Notes.* The *Habilitative Mental Health Care Newsletter* addresses psychiatric and behavioral aspects of care for people with developmental disabilities. Published on a monthly basis, it includes original articles and an informational clearinghouse. All three newsletters are an efficient means of supplementing postgraduate training.

Continuing education courses and professional society memberships can also be important sources of new information. Organizations such as the American Association on Mental Retardation and the United States Association for Retarded Citizens provide training activities. Professional societies such as the Society for Developmental and Behavioral Pediatrics and the American Academy of Developmental Medicine and Cerebral Palsy are also important vehicles for information exchange and professional camaraderie.

References

1. Health Systems Agency of New York City: Health care services plan for developmentally disabled persons in New York City, New York, 1988, New York State Developmental Disabilities Planning Council; p 8.
2. Blum RW: *Chronic illness and disabilities in childhood and adolescence,* Orlando, 1984, Grune & Stratton; p 300.
3. American Psychiatric Association: *Diagnostic and statistical manual of mental disorders,* ed 4, Washington, DC, 1994, American Psychiatric Association.
4. Alvarez N: Discontinuance of antiepileptic medications in patients with developmental disability and the diagnosis of epilepsy, *Am J Ment Retard* 93: 593-599, 1989.
5. Gedye A: Extreme self-injury attributed to frontal lobe seizures, *Am J Ment Retard* 94:20-26, 1989.
6. Goodin DS, Aminoff MJ, Laxer KD: Detection of epileptiform activity by different noninvasive EEG methods in complex partial seizures, *Ann Neurol* 27:330-334, 1990.
7. Kastner T, Friedman D, Ruiz M, Henning D, Plummer A: Valproic acid for the treatment of children with mental retardation and mood symptomatology, *Pediatrics* 86:467-472, 1990.
8. Minihan P, Dean D: Meeting the needs for health services of persons with mental retardation living in the community, *Am J Public Health* 80:1043-1048, 1990.
9. Crocker A, Yankauer A: Basic issues, *Ment Retard* 25:227-232, 1987.
10. Crocker A: Partnerships in the delivery of medical care. In Crocker A, Rubin L, editors: *Developmental disabilities: delivery of medical care for children and adults,* Philadelphia, 1989, Lea & Febiger; p 5.
11. Task Force on Pediatric Education: *The future of pediatric education,* Evanston, IL, 1978, American Academy of Pediatrics.

Suggested Readings

Bleck E, Nagel D: *Physically handicapped children: a medical atlas for teachers,* ed 2, New York, 1982, Grune & Stratton.
  A well-rounded primer for educators serving children and adolescents with developmental disabilities.

Blum R: *Chronic illness and disabilities in childhood and adolescence,* New York, 1984, Grune & Stratton.

> *An excellent overview of the effects of developmental disabilities on adolescents that includes an emphasis on the relationship between the adolescent, the family, the school, and peers.*

Crocker A, Yankauer A, Sterling D: Garrard Memorial Symposium: community health care services for adults with mental retardation, *Ment Retard* 25:189-242, 1987.

> *A concise introduction to the health care needs of people with developmental disabilities and health care delivery options; best for the feature "Basic Issues."*

Evans E, Meyer L: *An educative approach to behavior problems,* Baltimore, 1985, Paul H. Brookes.

> *A valuable overview of topics in behavioral management ranging from traditional behavior modification to an understanding of the educational and programmatic needs of people with developmental disabilities.*

Exceptional Health Care: *Developmental Disabilities Publications (60),* Morristown Memorial Hospital, Morristown, NJ 07962.

> *A monthly review of selected developmental disability–related articles culled from a wide variety of journals in a continuing medical education format.*

The Habilitative Mental Healthcare Newsletter: Psyche-Media, Inc., P.O. Box 57, Bear Creek, NC 27207.

> *A monthly newsletter including original articles and an informational clearinghouse. Previous volumes offer excellent reviews of mental health topics in developmental disabilities.*

Kinnie N: *Handling the young cerebral palsied child at home,* New York, 1974, EP Dutton.

> *An extremely practical guide for parents of a child with cerebral palsy; an excellent teaching resource.*

Pueschel S, Tingey C, Rynders J, Crocker A, Crutcher D: *New perspectives on Down syndrome,* Baltimore, 1985, Paul H. Brookes.

> *A thorough review of the most common chromosomal cause of developmental disabilities.*

Rubin L, Crocker A: *Developmental disabilities: delivery of medical care for children and adults,* Philadelphia, 1989, Lea & Febiger.

> *The standard against which to measure all other texts.*

Stark J, Menolascino F, Albarelli M, Gray V: *Mental retardation and mental health: classifications, diagnosis, treatment, services,* New York, 1988, Springer-Verlag.

> *A thoughtful review of mental health topics related to people with developmental disabilities.*

CHAPTER 117

Deafness and Psychosocial Development

•

David R. Updegraff

PSYCHOSOCIAL DEVELOPMENT OF THE DEAF CHILD

Generally the psychosocial development of the deaf child parallels that of the hearing child. In addition to general societal influences that affect all children (e.g., socioeconomic status of the family, educational attainments of the parents), several factors influence the development of the deaf child. These factors include (1) the hearing status of the parents (i.e., deaf or hearing), (2) the age of the child at the onset of hearing loss, (3) the degree of hearing loss, (4) the communication approach used, and (5) the educational program selected.

Hearing Status of Parents

The parents' hearing status has a pervasive influence. Generally, deaf children of deaf parents demonstrate the same range of psychosocial adjustment as that of hearing children of hearing parents; that is, some deaf children of deaf parents display normal adjustment, whereas others demonstrate various adjustment reactions of adolescence or may require psychiatric intervention. Overall, in comparison with deaf children of hearing parents, deaf children of deaf parents tend to develop a higher level of competence in language, learn to read and write better, have far greater success in school, and are less likely to demonstrate psychologic and social adjustment problems. On the other hand, deaf children of hearing parents tend to demonstrate a higher level of adjustment problems, especially in adolescence; tend to develop a lower level of competence in language; tend to read and write at a lower level; and generally experience less success in school and in life.

The reasons for this discrepancy are few but powerful. First, deaf children of deaf parents generally receive instant acceptance for who they are. In fact, many deaf parents ardently desire to produce deaf children, and although they love their hearing children, they may be somewhat disappointed if they do not have deaf children. Deaf parents are generally excellent parents with either deaf or hearing children. With deaf children, deaf parents can look forward to a lifetime of shared linguistic and cultural experience. With hearing children, deaf parents anticipate the time when their children's associations in the hearing world are more important than those in the deaf world. A deaf child born of hearing parents may not receive such instant acceptance and may be subject to parental grief and anger when the parents discover the child's deafness. The parents may need to work through this guilt and anger before fully accepting the child. In truth, full and unquestioned acceptance may never be achieved in some families.

Second, the child born to deaf parents is exposed to a clear, visual system of communication (generally, American Sign Language) from the moment of birth. The deaf child will likely begin to demonstrate expressive skills in sign language sooner (as early as 8 to 9 months) than a hearing child begins to speak. Early signed expressions include "mama," "milk," "dada," and other signs of significant objects in the child's environment. Such signs may be likened to "baby talk" in that the signs made by the infant will not look precisely like the formal signs the parents use. It has been suggested that deaf infants whose parents use sign language to communicate with them begin to "babble" with their hands just as hearing infants do with their voices, which is evidence of developing linguistic ability.

A deaf child born to hearing parents will more than likely not be exposed to clear visual-gestural communication from infancy. In fact, such children are often not exposed to sign language until first grade, if that early. The early educational and therapeutic efforts in many school systems are to teach such children to speak and speechread in the hope of overcoming some of the stigmatizing aspects of deafness. The effect of this effort for some children, however, is to delay the period of their beginning to become competent in any linguistic form and to increase the probability of their perceiving that they have failed to meet their parents' and teachers' expectations, thus negatively impacting their self-image. Third, deaf children of deaf parents immediately become

members of a community of deaf persons with whom they can communicate and who accept them in the same manner that their parents accept them.

Deaf children of hearing parents, on the other hand, are usually isolates in their own family and community. Generally, they are the only such child in the family and in the neighborhood. This situation may not be immediately problematic in terms of the child's adjustment, but as play with the neighbor children becomes more imbued with verbal interaction, difficulties arise. For example, the establishment of rules of games is dependent on a shared communication system. The child who cannot participate in establishing or sharing the rules of games is isolated from those who can. For those parents who do not learn to communicate with their deaf child, the school often becomes the agent of communication between parent and child, interpreting the child's wishes to the parents and vice versa. This has a devastating effect on the child's self-esteem.

Some hearing parents are also very successful in their efforts to learn how to work with their deaf child at home, supplementing the efforts of the school. Some hearing parents begin to learn to sign immediately on discovering their child is deaf, and provide the child with significant visual input from a very early age (before 1 year). Such parents often also involve neighbors and their children in learning to sign and communicate with the child. By the onset of first grade, children exposed to such influences often function at or very near expected levels. This may also be true for some children whose parents use an approach emphasizing speech development and auditory training to the exclusion of sign language (known as the oral/aural approach), but in this circumstance success is less likely.

Age at Onset of Hearing Loss

There are two primary classifications of hearing loss onset: prelingual and postlingual. Children who are born deaf or who lose their hearing because of illness or injury before the age of 2 years are generally considered prelingual; those who lose their hearing after the age of 2 are generally considered postlingually deafened. Children who did not develop a symbolic communication system before losing their hearing are at much higher risk of not becoming competent in the dominant language of their culture. Those who do not develop such competence do not then experience significant life success. Children who lose their hearing later in life may experience transitory adjustment problems, but if provided opportunities for appropriate counseling and education, such adjustment difficulties may be overcome.

In fact, persons who become deaf in childhood or early adulthood may find themselves more successful than they would have been had they not lost their hearing. A prime example of this is the personal history of a good friend and colleague of mine. This individual became deaf at the age of 8 years as a result of spinal meningitis, while his family, who came from Mexico, worked as migrant crop pickers in California. On becoming deaf, he was sent to a residential school for the deaf in California. Arriving at the school knowing only a pidgin Spanish-Mexican Indian tongue, he quickly became competent in English, American Sign Language, and Spanish. He graduated from high school at the age of 16 and matriculated at Gallaudet University. Subsequently he completed master's and doctoral degrees at universities for hearing persons and has had a distinguished career in education of the deaf. He was the first in his family to finish high school, and he subsequently facilitated the attendance of hearing members of his family at college. This individual has shared with many people his feeling that most of his life success can be attributed to the fact that he became deaf as a child and was fortunate to be sent to one of the premier schools for the deaf in this country.

Degree of Hearing Loss

There are two principal means of describing the degree of hearing loss: audiologic and behavioral. The audiologic description, based on the decibel system, is valuable as a quantifiable means of measuring the consistency of hearing loss, identifying the configuration of the hearing loss, and of prescribing hearing aids. The behavioral description allows for assessment of the deaf person's functioning in his or her environment. There are considered to be four categories of behavioral description of hearing loss:

- *Mild:* Can hear and understand most speech without the use of hearing aid(s) or other assistive devices, the use of which may or may not enhance understanding.
- *Moderate:* Can hear and understand most speech with the use of hearing aid(s) or other assistive devices, the use of which is necessary to enhance understanding.
- *Severe:* Can hear and understand some speech with the use of hearing aid(s) or other assistive devices; generally is less able to hear consonant sounds and more able to hear vowel sounds; may be able to use the telephone with an amplification switch on the headset, particularly when conversing with persons whose voices are already familiar; without the use of hearing aids, is not able to understand speech.
- *Profound:* Sense of hearing is nonfunctional for the purpose of linguistic communication; may hear loud sounds to assist with environmental monitoring (e.g., truck backfires, door slamming); the use of a hearing aid may assist with environmental monitoring but not with comprehension of speech.

Generally, the adolescents discussed in this chapter fall within the profound category, although some may fall within the severe category.

The degree of hearing loss clearly influences the manner in which an individual interacts with the hearing world and, by extension, the likelihood of success in school. Persons with profound hearing loss generally identify themselves as "deaf" and thus as members of the deaf community. Persons with mild hearing loss generally identify themselves as hearing and have no association with the deaf community.

However, persons with moderate or severe hearing loss may have difficulty establishing an identity in this regard. They must wear hearing aid(s), have telephone amplifiers, and must look at a person's face while conversing. They are obviously not "deaf" since they hear much of what transpires around them, and their speech sounds normal or almost normal, yet their hearing is obviously impaired because they require special devices to help them hear. Such individuals are identified as either "hard of hearing" or "hearing impaired."

Some hard-of-hearing persons have chosen to identify themselves as "deaf" from a sociocultural perspective and become part of the deaf community for interpersonal support. However, in recent years, hard-of-hearing persons have begun to organize in support groups just as deaf persons have been doing for years. An organization called Self-Help for Hard of Hearing Persons (SHHH), for example, gives such individuals an identity and a community.

Selection of Communication Approach

This is one of the few issues over which the family of the deaf child has any control. The main decision to be reached is whether the child is to be educated orally, with total communication (speech and speechreading plus sign language and fingerspelling), or with American Sign Language in a bilingual-bicultural approach. Although there are no hard and fast rules, generally the more severe the child's hearing loss, the more likely the child is to need a highly visual means of communication and language development, that is, a total communication approach.

Although details must be obtained from an otolaryngologist, one medical/surgical advance should be noted here. In 1990, after several years of controlled testing, the U.S. Food and Drug Administration approved the 22-Channel Cochlear Implant device for use with deaf children. This is changing the issue of communication approach for some children. The device involves surgical implantation of a 22-channel electrode in the cochlea, which stimulates the receptor cells located along the inner ear and, with other appropriate equipment, is perceived by the implant wearer as sound. The child is then taught how to interpret the sounds. Research continues on the efficacy of the implant. As with most such innovations, it appears to have a positive impact on certain children, and little impact on others. There is a great deal of controversy over the implantation in young children, which is strenuously opposed by the National Association of the Deaf and other advocacy organizations, and supported by others. The opposition is on the grounds that deafness in an individual makes that person a member of a linguistic/cultural minority, and that to attempt to take away a child's deafness is to take away his or her identity. It is most strongly suggested that deaf adolescents not receive implants unless they request it and their parents are supportive but not controlling the decision. Preadolescents and adolescents who have received the implant often reject it after a short time. The decision to recommend an implant to the parents must always be made by a team that should include at least the following professionals: a teacher who knows the child, an audiologist, a speech/language pathologist, a psychologist, and an otolaryngologist. Others may need to be included on the team in particularly difficult situations. Children who receive implants at a very early age often begin school in an oral/aural educational program.

Hearing parents of deaf children often choose to begin the child's educational exposure using an oral/aural approach to encourage the development of speech in the child. Also, professionals in audiology, speech pathology, pediatrics, and related fields often counsel parents in this direction. For this approach to be successful, a number of components must come together and be consistently present:

- Early and consistent use of appropriate amplification
- Early and continuing training of parents and other family members in the implications of hearing loss and the child's needs
- Parental participation in the school or therapy sessions the child attends so that the parents can observe the techniques used by the teachers for use at home
- Opportunity for the child's teacher to visit the home and advise the parents on structuring the home environment to facilitate the child's learning

If the child is profoundly deaf, however, the risks are high that this approach may be unsuccessful. The longer an oral approach is tried with a child who should be using sign language, the more difficulty the child will have in attempting to catch up when a sign language communication and instructional program is finally instituted.

There are several theories concerning how best to begin the deaf child's education and training. With what is now known about early language acquisition, many educators and researchers believe that it is preferable to expose children to sign language and fingerspelling as early as possible. Once initial language is established,

efforts to establish competence in speech may begin. Research indicates that early exposure to sign language does not negatively influence speech and speechreading competence.

If early efforts to teach speech and speechreading are unsuccessful and the child is unable to meet parents' and teachers' expectations in this area, severe damage to the self-concept may ensue. Profoundly deaf children do not have as much trouble learning sign language and fingerspelling as they have learning speech and speechreading. The approach most likely to lead to success should therefore be advocated.

Educational Program Selection

Educational options for deaf children, as for all disabled children, have broadened since the passage of Public Law 94-142 in 1975—The Education for All Handicapped Children Act, now known as the Individuals with Disabilities Education Act (IDEA). Among other provisions, this law requires local school districts to make available a continuum of services for handicapped children. Children are to be provided an education in the school closest to their homes that enables them to attain their educational goals.

As already noted, the major handicap that accompanies deafness is one of communication. The educational placement of deaf children must therefore take into consideration how their communication handicap will be alleviated. There are few clues to assist in predicting how a particular child will react in a particular educational setting. Such a decision is a highly important one that will influence the rest of the child's life and should be weighed carefully. Selection of an educational setting involves deciding whether the student attends a residential or day school. It also involves analyzing the extent of separation from or integration with nondisabled students, as follows:

- *Full inclusion:* A relatively new concept that involves a "merger" of special education with general education in the regular classroom the child would have attended if not disabled. Special services needed by the child (e.g., speech therapy, tutoring) are often brought into the classroom rather than having the child go to another setting to receive those services.
- *Full mainstreaming:* Placement in the local public school, either without support or with the support of an interpreter, speech therapist, and/or consulting itinerant teacher as needed. Special services are usually offered on a "pull-out" basis.
- *Full mainstreaming with resource room:* Placement in the local public school with support, with part-time placement in a classroom with a teacher of the deaf for tutoring in certain subjects.
- *Partial mainstreaming:* Placement in a self-

contained class for the deaf in a public school, with mainstreaming into the regular program for part of the day.

- *Self-contained class:* Placement in a classroom for the deaf in a public school for the full day. Lunch, recess, art, and physical education may be scheduled with children who are not disabled.
- *Day school for the deaf:* Placement in a separate school for the deaf to which the child is transported daily. Generally, only large cities are able to support a day school program. Some day school programs are located in close proximity to public schools for hearing children. In such situations, partial mainstreaming of the deaf child into the public school may occur.
- *Residential school for the deaf:* Placement in a separate school for the deaf in which the child may reside during the week because of distance from home or because of behavioral management needs. Some students also attend residential schools as commuters. The child may be partially mainstreamed from the residential school into a local public school for part of the program.

Several generalizations can be made regarding the effects of school placement decisions on the psychologic and social development of the deaf child. First, although it may sound strange, the environment of a school for the deaf can be the most normalizing and least restrictive environment for a deaf student. It is in this environment that deaf students generally feel most normal. He is surrounded by other students who are also deaf, he is able to participate in school athletics and other activities on a basis of equality, and he is able to assume leadership roles. Traditionally, the development and maintenance of the cultural norms and values of the deaf community, as well as the continuing development of American Sign Language, have taken place through the environment of the residential school for the deaf.

In the mainstreamed environment, however, a deaf child is usually the "different" student. The student may have a full-time interpreter who accompanies him everywhere—who else has their own personal adult in school?—and makes him feel very conspicuous. The student's speech is different and he has to go to speech therapy. He may not read as well as the other students and thus requires remedial reading class. Other differences may be apparent that set the deaf student apart from peers. These differences become more significant as the child ages and may be particularly difficult to deal with in adolescence.

On the other hand, if the deaf child is to have a hope of becoming successful as an adult, he will have to learn how to interact with and live with hearing people, because he will probably be seeking employment from a hearing person. Thus, for the deaf student in a separate program, extraordinary efforts must be made to ensure that he has the opportunity to learn how to interact with hearing people, particularly with hearing people who do not sign.

In terms of impact on psychologic and social development, the main concern with school placement is the damage to the self-concept and to academic development that may be done by an inappropriate placement. For this reason, mainstreaming is not advised for deaf students who are emotionally fragile for whatever reasons, or for students who are functioning below the grade level of the class in which placement is considered. Being on a par academically with the students with whom he is placed increases the deaf student's chances of being successful in that environment. Also, if the deaf child is academically behind when he enters the mainstreamed class, there is almost no chance that he will be able to catch up. For the deaf child whose achievement is commensurate with the grade level of his placement, it will be hard enough for him to keep up. Furthermore, it is helpful, although not mandatory, for the deaf child in a mainstreamed environment to have some speech and speechreading ability.

An educational model that is somewhat rare, but that is being practiced successfully in some settings, is for the deaf child's primary placement to be in a center school for the deaf, whether that be a day or residential school, and for the child to be mainstreamed into the local public school for some subjects. The child is thus able to identify with the school for the deaf as home base, with a group of deaf peers for relationship development and with the opportunity to participate fully in the life of the school, including extracurricular life. These experiences, which tend to enhance self-esteem and normal adolescent development, are balanced by the opportunity to experience the mainstreamed environment for part of the day.

The full inclusion model is thought by many educators of the deaf to be an inappropriate model of educational placement for most deaf children. There is no effective way for a deaf child to be "fully included" unless all or most individuals in that school setting can communicate directly with him. This would mean that all the other students learn sign language, and that the school administrator, counselor, teacher and teacher aides, and others learn to sign. This is not highly realistic, and such a full inclusion model would become the same as mainstreaming in which the deaf child is in, but not of, the class.

DEVELOPMENTAL ISSUES OF ADOLESCENCE

The success with which deaf youths handle developmental transitions is greatly influenced by the skills they bring to the task, including their self-esteem, the support provided by the family, and the environment in which the transition occurs.

Dating, Sexuality, and Marriage

DATING. Adolescents' experiences with dating are defined in large part by the environment in which they attend school. Historically, as many as 80% of deaf youths were educated in separate educational settings with other deaf youths. Currently, the percentage is around 20% because of the influence of the IDEA. The catch-22 for deaf youths is that there are inherent limitations on the development of their relationships with the opposite sex no matter which educational environment is experienced.

In the residential school environment, the deaf adolescent is more likely to have a choice of deaf adolescents of the opposite sex to date and with whom to develop "steady" relationships. However, the structure of many residential schools does not facilitate the independent dating that hearing high schoolers in their home communities may experience. Most dating in the residential schools is on campus and under supervision. This situation tends to protect the schools from the reactions of parents who may not want their adolescent children out in the community dating and may fulfill the "in loco parentis" role of the residential school, but it does not do much for the development of adolescent relationships or independence.

In the mainstreamed high schools in which deaf students are placed, the opposite situation may occur. A considerable amount of independence of action may be possible, but there may be few deaf youths of the opposite sex to date. Inasmuch as deafness is a low-incidence disability, occurring at the rate of about 1 per 1000 population, it is difficult to find other deaf youths with whom one might be compatible in a small city or high school. A few deaf youths successfully date hearing persons, but communication problems often preclude this.

For purposes of dating and adolescent development, the school placement of choice may be the public or private day school in a large metropolitan area. Such a placement enables the student to have a network of deaf friends at school, who may live in the metropolitan area, and to go out after school and on weekends either with a group or as a twosome. In areas in which no such program exists, the school placement of choice for most profoundly deaf adolescent students is the residential school for the deaf.

SEXUALITY. The development of sexuality in deaf youths proceeds as it does with hearing youth. One difference is that a few deaf youths in residential placement may experiment with homosexual behavior. This situation is probably similar to the experience of some hearing youths who attend boarding schools. Naïveté on sexual matters may be noted in some deaf youths and may be attributed to a paucity of exposure to sexuality education programs and to sources of information readily available to hearing youths.

MARRIAGE. Historically, some 95% of deaf persons marry other deaf persons. This is in large part due to a shared cultural and linguistic heritage and to lessened communication problems in the marital relationship. This incidence seems to hold true for deaf persons who have attended residential school as well as for those who have been mainstreamed. It now appears that mainstreaming, which became popular in the late 1970s and early 1980s, is having a negligible impact on marriage between deaf and hearing persons. There appears to be a trend for deaf students who attended mainstreamed schools to want to attend a college program designed for deaf students. In this environment, the chances of deaf young people meeting and marrying other deaf youths are enhanced.

Emancipation from Family Home

Much of the success of the process of emancipation from the family for deaf youths depends on the opportunities for independence that the deaf teenager had while growing up. For deaf youths who were educated in the residential school environment, transition from home to a college environment may be relatively easy: they are accustomed to living away from home. However, the new-found freedoms and lack of structure of college life are at times a trap into which deaf youths fall in the same manner as other teenagers. In addition, transition to full independence for these students may be limited by the fact that there tend to be fewer opportunities to experience independent living skills in the residential school environment.

For college-bound deaf youths from a day school or mainstreamed environment, who are likely to have experienced a significant level of independence of action in their communities, the transition to independent life outside the family home may be smoother than for residential school students. Parents who have not been able to work through the grief and loss often attendant on the birth of a handicapped child may have more difficulty allowing separation to occur than the young person will have. Counseling intervention may be necessary at this stage.

Higher Education Issues

Until the late 1960s, most deaf persons in the United States who continued their educations after high school did so at Gallaudet University. A few brave individuals attended college and university programs with no provision for deaf students. Postsecondary educational opportunities were available to only a few. However, in the late 1960s, additional options became available for deaf youths. The National Technical Institute for the Deaf opened at Rochester Institute of Technology in 1969. Over the next 10 years, some 150 technical-vocational programs at community colleges became available for postsecondary experiences for deaf youth. Some of the programs are quite small and serve a few deaf youths as part of a "disabled student services" office. Others are fairly large, with 50 to 100 or more students and a full complement of interpreters, note takers, tutors, and other adjunct services provided.

Deaf teenagers tend to pursue post-secondary education at a rate somewhat higher than persons with other forms of disability and somewhat lower than nondisabled persons. It is estimated that approximately 40% of the deaf high school graduates in the United States pursue post-secondary educational opportunities.

CONCLUSION

This chapter has presented an overview of some of the influences on psychosocial development in the deaf adolescent. It needs to be emphasized that just because an adolescent is deaf does not mean that psychosocial development in that young person has been arrested or is somehow awry. Clues to the psychosocial status of the young person may be gleaned from taking a thorough history from both parents and adolescent.

In taking the history, it is important to use a certified interpreter. The Americans with Disabilities Act requires physicians, as well as other professionals, to ensure such accessibility to deaf patients. A telephone call to the nearest school for the deaf or interpreter referral service will provide such a contact. Like most individuals, deaf people hesitate to show that they do not understand something. Some deaf young people may indicate that they understand what the physician is saying whether they do or not. Grave errors have been made in the medical treatment of deaf people because the physician thought that the deaf person understood what he or she was saying. Although one may be inclined to use the parents to interpret, parents are not usually qualified interpreters, particularly in the medical arena. In addition, the deaf adolescent is as protective of his or her privacy as is the hearing adolescent and may object strenuously to the presence of a parent in the examining room.

Finally, the problems imposed by deafness are not primarily medical; they are educational and communication problems. Certain deaf adolescents with additional disabilities may have medical components to their treatment plan (e.g., physical therapy). Others will experience only the routine medical involvements of nondisabled adolescents.

Suggested Readings

Benderley BL: *Dancing without music: deafness in America,* Garden City, NY, 1980, Anchor Press/Doubleday.

Cohen OP: At-risk deaf adolescents, *Volta Review* 93:57-72, 1991.

Cohen OP, Long G: An overview of adolescence, *Volta Review* 93: 1-4, 1991.

Conrad R: *The deaf school child: language and cognitive function,* London, 1979, Harper & Row.

Gjerdingen D, Manning FD: Adolescents with profound hearing impairments in mainstream education: the Clarke model, *Volta Review* 93:139-148, 1991.

Lane H: *When the mind hears: a history of the deaf,* New York, 1984, Random House.

Leigh IW, Stinson MS: Social environment, self-perceptions, and identity of hearing-impaired adolescents, *Volta Review* 93:7-22, 1991.

Meadow KP: *Deafness and child development,* Berkeley, CA, 1980, University of California Press.

Mindel ED, Vernon M: *They grow in silence: understanding deaf children and adults,* ed 2, Boston, 1987, College Hill Press.

Moores DF: *Educating the deaf: psychology, principles, and practices,* ed 3, Boston, 1987, Houghton Mifflin.

CHAPTER 118

Mental Retardation

•

Norman M. Brier

It is extremely difficult for mentally retarded individuals to resolve the developmental tasks of adolescence successfully. Despite a diminished level of cognitive and adaptive skill and difficulties with social competence, these adolescents are aware of being different at a time when the wish to be like others is extremely important. The varying expectations of the significant people in the mentally retarded adolescent's life contributes to this difficulty: at times, youngsters are viewed according to standards based on their chronologic age, whereas at other times, expectations are based on their mental age. In particular, adolescents with mental retardation have difficulties with such normative developmental tasks as the attainment of emotional independence, the establishment of an adequate self-image, and the formation and maintenance of intimate social relationships.

This chapter focuses primarily on mentally retarded adolescents with mild cognitive and adaptive impairments. These youngsters constitute the majority of adolescents who are classified as retarded, are likely to live with their families in the community, and as a result are likely to be the type of adolescent with retardation most frequently seen in a healthcare provider's office practice.

CLASSIFICATION

The most widely used definition of mental retardation is the one developed by the American Association on Mental Retardation (AAMR).[1] The term *mental retardation* refers to significantly subaverage general intellectual functioning resulting in, or associated with, impairments in adaptive behavior, with an onset before 18 years of age. Similar multidimensional definitions are found in the *Diagnostic and Statistical Manual of Mental Disorders,* fourth edition (DSM-IV)[2] and the World Health Organization's International Classification of Diseases.[3] In its latest classification and terminology manual, the AAMR made several changes in emphasis with regard to the

definition of mental retardation. Earlier definitions viewed mental retardation primarily in terms of an individual's intellectual and adaptive deficiencies. The current AAMR definition highlights the importance of the interaction between the individual and the nature of environmental demands in determining whether an individual's deficiencies become a handicap in a particular environment. Also revised was the concept of adaptive behavior from a relatively global category to ten specific adaptive skill areas (e.g., social, communication, self-care, and functional academics).

When current definitions are employed, a heterogeneous population is formed, ranging from totally dependent individuals to those almost independent. Although all retarded persons, on the basis of these definitional criteria, have some degree of deficit in intelligence and adaptive behavior, there is great variation in the degree of deficit displayed and the presence or absence of physical handicaps and stigmata. Two primary means of subclassification have traditionally been used to order the heterogeneity.

In one, retarded individuals are grouped according to their level of functioning, which is based primarily on intelligence test scores or intelligence quotient (IQ). In the other, the population is roughly grouped on the basis of the causes of their deficit and the presence or absence of signs of organic etiology.

Within the level-of-functioning classification system, retarded individuals are divided into four categories. Individuals who attain an IQ score between 50 and 70 are said to be mildly retarded; those who score below 50 are said to be moderately, severely, or profoundly retarded, depending on how much below 50 their particular score falls. Approximately 10% to 25% of retarded individuals are classified in the moderate, severe, and profound categories. The remaining 75% to 90% of retarded persons tend to be classified in the mild category. In the latest AAMR classification system, the kind and intensities of support the individual needs are used as a means of determining level of disability rather than IQ.

With the etiologic classification system, retarded individuals are divided into two categories, sometimes referred to as a "clinical" type and a "familial" type. Individuals in the clinical category have some demonstrable central nervous system (CNS) pathologic condition resulting from genetic disorders, brain trauma, or metabolic deficits and usually function in the moderate, severe, or profound range of mental retardation. Individuals in the familial category have no demonstrable CNS pathologic condition and usually function in the mild range of mental retardation.

Several reviews have questioned the validity of the clinical-familial distinction.[1] The epidemiologic studies cited have shown that more than one possible etiologic factor is involved for as much as 50% of the population of people with mental retardation, and that cumulative and/or interactive effects frequently occur (e.g., inadequate prenatal care and low birthweight).

PREVALENCE AND ETIOLOGY

Estimates of the incidence of mental retardation in the United States are usually placed at about 125,000 births per year; estimates of the prevalence of mental retardation vary somewhat. The most widely quoted prevalence figure is 3% of the general population. Studies generally support this estimate when intelligence measures are the sole criterion used to diagnose retardation. When adaptive impairment is factored in as well to make the diagnosis, consistent with most current definitions, prevalence is found to be closer to 2% to 2.5%. More males than females are retarded at every level of mental retardation.

For the mildly retarded, prevalence statistics change dramatically with age. They are highest during the school years and lower both before and after; that is, the mildly retarded individual's intellectual and adaptive deficits are most pronounced and disabling when academic demands are the major challenge to be met, and less pronounced and disabling when either sensorimotor and communication demands of early childhood or the requirements of gainful employment and social relationships after the school years have to be mastered. Prevalence statistics for mildly retarded individuals are significantly higher in lower socioeconomic classes at all ages and across all racial groups.

For about 25% of retarded individuals, a demonstrable biologic cause can be identified. These individuals, as noted, tend to be moderately to profoundly retarded. Prenatal difficulties such as infections, damage due to toxins, and genetic diseases contribute to the outcome of mental retardation at least partly in about 90% of cases. Common perinatal and postnatal causes of retardation include prematurity, hypoxia, trauma, low birthweight, infectious diseases, and nutritional disorders. Retarded individuals who have a known organic etiology also tend to have associated handicaps and stigmata, have a high mortality rate, are distributed in a roughly even manner across all socioeconomic groups, and are usually diagnosed at birth or in early childhood. About one third of this group are found to have major visual or auditory sensory impairments, motor problems (such as spasticity), or serious health problems (e.g., epilepsy or congenital heart defects).[4]

Individuals for whom there is no demonstrable biologic cause to explain the retardation do not usually have associated handicaps or stigmata and are generally first identified sometime between the beginning of formal schooling and early adolescence. Health problems for these retarded individuals are roughly similar in nature and scope to their nonretarded peers. They are found, however, to be less competent in maintaining "functional wellness behaviors,"[5] such as exercising and maintaining a proper diet, consistent with the overall mild adaptive impairments that tend to be present. Obesity in particular has been noted to be a more frequent health problem in retarded than in nonretarded populations, with rates higher for females than for males.[6] Retarded individuals may be less capable of seeing the consequences of their obesity and less capable of regulating their food intake.

Theories to account for the causes of retardation in individuals with no demonstrable biologic etiology have stressed genetics, psychosocial factors, or an interaction between the two. According to the genetic theory, mild mental retardation is not a disability but rather the lower tail of the normal distribution of genetic potential for intellectual and adaptive ability,[7] and in keeping with the perspective of the new AAMR definition, the likelihood that the genotype for intelligence will be actually expressed so that the individual functions in the mildly retarded range will depend, in large part, on the environmental demands encountered.

Psychosocial theories view mild mental retardation as an outgrowth of an adverse set of contextual factors. Consistent with this view is the fact that individuals who are mildly retarded most often come from families of low socioeconomic status, have more siblings, tend to live in poverty conditions, and have mothers who have low educational levels.[8] The interaction theory considers mild mental retardation to be a consequence of the interaction between prolonged exposure to a disadvantaged environment and a variety of subclinical biologic and/or genetic factors that as yet cannot be detected with present-day diagnostic technology.

DIAGNOSIS

According to current definitions of mental retardation, three criteria must be met for the diagnosis to be made:

(1) significantly subaverage general intellectual functioning, (2) deficits in adaptive behavior, and (3) evidence that these difficulties have been manifest during the developmental period, defined as the interval between birth and age 18 years. General intellectual functioning is determined by the youngster's performance on an individually administered test of intelligence, with "significantly subaverage" defined as an intelligence test score 2 or more standard deviations below the mean. Adaptive behavior is judged in terms of the adequacy with which an individual attains personal independence and social responsibility in relation to his or her age and cultural group. As noted, in the most recent AAMR definition, adaptive behavior is subdivided into ten skill areas: communication, self-care, home living, social skills, work, leisure, use of community resources, self-direction, functional academic skills, and health and safety.[1]

General intelligence is most often assessed by the Stanford-Binet, Kaufman Assessment Battery for Children, and Wechsler intelligence scales. Adaptive behavior is usually assessed through clinical interviews, observation, and the use of such rating scales as the Vineland Social Maturity Scale-Revised or the AAMR Adaptive Behavior Scale. Scales that measure adaptive behavior allow for quantification similar to an intelligence test score or IQ, but unlike the IQ score, they are not considered to be highly reliable or valid. Thus, some degree of clinical judgment is always included in the assessment of adaptive status, and as a result many professionals rely more heavily on the IQ score than on the adaptive rating scale score to make the diagnosis.

The nature of the test items used to measure intelligence and adaptive level varies during the developmental period. In infancy and early childhood, these items relate primarily to the achievement of sensorimotor, communication, and self-help milestones at age-appropriate times. In childhood, these items relate primarily to verbal skills and to mastery of the academic curriculum. In adolescence the adequacy of the individual's verbal skills and school performance is also assessed. Several other criteria of intelligence and adaption become important in adolescence as well: the application of basic academic competencies to everyday life situations, such as the ability to tell time and to make change; the ability to use reasoning and judgment in order to adjust to changes in the environment; the ability to participate in group activities and to develop intimate relationships; and the ability to carry out basic vocational skills.

Mildly retarded adolescents can be distinguished from more severely retarded adolescents on a variety of adaptive indices. Adolescents with mild mental retardation tend to have a history of adequate sensorimotor development or only minimal impairment in this regard, and demonstrate adequate body control and coordination. In addition, they tend to have fairly adequate social and communication skills through the preschool and early elementary school years. Academic achievement scores are usually found to be at the middle to late elementary school level, with the mildly retarded youngster typically able to read simple paragraphs and do basic mathematics. Self-care skills involved with eating, dressing, and bathing are usually adequate. In contrast, adolescents with greater degrees of intellectual impairment tend to have a higher incidence of sensorimotor impairments, display poor social and communication skills from early in life, tend not to progress beyond a second-grade level in academic achievement, and often evidence significant problems in self-care activities.

Clinically, when mildly retarded adolescents are examined, language competence tends to be the most striking indicator of their limitations. Mildly retarded adolescents tend to have a relatively limited supply of verbal labels, use descriptive words more frequently than functional or categorical words, and speak in simpler sentences than do nonretarded age-mates. Thoughts tend to be concrete and are usually focused on one dimension of an idea. When spoken to, mildly retarded youngsters tend to have difficulty following ideas that are either abstract or have multiple parts, and often at such times answer incorrectly, get "stuck," and may say, "I don't understand." Questions in which adolescents are asked to state alternatives, to describe possibilities, or delineate actions in a temporal sequence are often too difficult for them to handle adequately. Memory skills also tend to be deficient, and frequent explanation and repetition on the clinician's part are required.

The term *mental retardation* at times is confused with the terms *developmental disability* and *learning disability*. *Developmental disability* is not a diagnostic label as much as a legislative concept developed as part of entitlement statutes. In these statutes, developmental disability is usually defined as a group of conditions of a severe and lifelong nature that are attributable to a mental and/or physical impairment. The disability must be manifest before the age of 22 years and result in substantial limitations in major life activities so that a combination of long-term, multidisciplinary services are required. Most moderately, severely, or profoundly retarded adolescents meet these criteria and could be also considered developmentally disabled. Many mildly retarded adolescents, however, do not meet these criteria, and therefore the term *developmentally disabled* should not be applied to these youngsters.

The term *learning disability* is used most often to refer to a significant discrepancy between an individual's level of academic achievement in one or more academic areas and his or her overall intellectual ability. This discrepancy is considered to be primarily a result of neurologic dysfunction. A learning disability can be viewed as a "narrow-band" disorder in which the individual displays deficits in only a limited number of academic areas, whereas mental retardation can be viewed as a "broadband" disorder in which the individual displays deficits in most academic areas. Occasionally, a mildly mentally retarded individual can have a concurrent diagnosis of a learning disability. For example, a concurrent diagnosis of retardation and learning disability might apply to a 17-year-old adolescent who, on the basis of an IQ level of 65, would be expected to be reading at the third- or fourth-grade level but is unable to master reading skills beyond the first-grade level.

PSYCHOSOCIAL CORRELATES

Mentally retarded adolescents are at an increased risk for psychologic disorders. Relative to a prevalence rate of approximately 15% for the general population, about 20% to 35% of mildly retarded adolescents and 30% to 50% of moderately, severely, and profoundly retarded adolescents have significant psychologic problems. Impulse control difficulties tend to be the most frequent psychologic problem in the moderately, severely, and profoundly retarded group, with these youngsters often displaying self-injurious and stereotypic behavior, hyperactivity, and temper tantrums. For the mildly retarded adolescent, psychologic problems are evenly divided between internalizing disorders, such as anxiety and depression, and externalizing disorders, such as oppositional behavior and aggressivity. In terms of causation, the impulse problems of the more severely retarded youngsters are believed to result primarily from the same central nervous system difficulties thought to underlie the retardation of these children. For the mildly retarded youngster, adaptive and social skill deficits are thought to be critical and to result in a diminished capacity to cope with stress. Particular stressors that have been noted include social isolation and peer rejection, parental restrictions on independent behavior, and frequent failure experiences.

Mildly retarded adolescents tend to socialize significantly less often than their nonretarded peers and have few or no friends. When friendships do develop, they tend to be less stable, growing out of the adolescent's participation in an educational or training setting, and are not maintained actively once outside such a setting. Male adolescents seem to have a more difficult time relating to females than to other males. Females have a more difficult time relating to other females than to males and are found to have a more restricted set of leisure activities than nonretarded females and retarded males. Social skill deficits are common, and as a group these adolescents have difficulty initiating or maintaining a conversation and displaying empathy. Thus, they often appear to be out of synchrony with their social environment. Nonretarded adolescents often try to avoid interactions with their retarded adolescent counterparts, and when interacting with them, act in either a neutral or rejecting manner, with teasing fairly common. As a result, mildly retarded adolescents often feel lonely, see themselves as socially inept, are prone to withdraw and avoid available socialization opportunities, and tend to seek younger children as companions.

Developing a sense of independence and autonomy is also particularly problematic for mildly retarded adolescents. Their social isolation interferes with the usual developmental progression of transferring dependent feelings from parents to peers, and often results in the mildly retarded adolescent remaining overattached and dependent on his or her parents. Parents, in turn, although aware of their youngster's overdependency, are often frightened to allow greater degrees of independence, partly owing to realistic fears stemming from their youngster's adaptive deficits and partly from confusion as to what is an appropriate level of independence.

Low self-esteem is also quite common. Mildly mentally retarded adolescents have been found to have relatively low expectations for success when approaching new tasks, give up relatively easily when frustrated, and frequently display avoidant behavior. As a group, they tend to be highly dependent on the opinion of others in judging the adequacy of their performance, and as a result are highly suggestible. At times this proneness to be influenced places them at risk of sexual and criminal exploitation. When scales have been used to formally measure aspects of identity, mentally retarded adolescents display a greater degree of identity confusion than nonretarded adolescents, particularly in regard to their physical self-image, and frequently report feelings of helplessness and inadequacy. The presence of younger, nonretarded siblings sometimes contributes to their low self-esteem, as the younger siblings catch up and move past the adolescent in such areas as academic competence, household responsibilities, and the degree of autonomy allowed by the parent.

ADOLESCENT CHALLENGES AND MILD MENTAL RETARDATION

Adolescents are regularly confronted with the need to make choices in regard to such issues as sexuality, school attendance, substance abuse, and illegal opportunities. The relatively deficient cognitive and adaptive capacities of mildly retarded adolescents, along with their limited social skills, restricted opportunities for independence, and feelings of inadequacy, suggest that they may be at greater risk for making choices that result in negative consequences for themselves and others.

In one of the few investigations of sexual behavior among mildly retarded adolescents, retarded females were found to have the same desires and fantasies as their nonretarded peers and to engage in sexual intercourse at a rate comparable with that found in the general adolescent population.[9] A relatively high percentage of these youngsters were found to have been sexually assaulted, and their assailants were most often either family members or individuals well known to them. Low intellectual ability has been found to be a factor that elevates the risk for adolescent pregnancy; for example, teenagers in special education programs were found to become pregnant in disproportionate numbers compared with teenagers in regular education.[10] Thus, the relatively large percentage of sexually active mildly retarded adolescents who become pregnant suggests that contraception was either not being used or not being used appropriately.

In general, mildly retarded adolescents have been found to be less informed about human sexuality than their nonretarded peers and, in particular, display a poorer understanding of sexual anatomy, reproduction, pubertal changes, pregnancy, birth control, and venereal disease. This lack of knowledge about sexuality is consistent with their intellectual limitations and their restricted peer experiences, and, when combined with their tendency toward suggestibility, most likely contributes to the high rate of sexual exploitation and abuse noted (roughly four times higher than in nonretarded populations).[10]

With regard to school attendance, students with handicaps have been found to be more likely to drop out of school than those without handicaps.[11] This finding held true whether the student attended special education or regular education classes. When dropout rates were examined according to the type of handicapping condition, a dropout rate of about 25% was found for retarded youngsters. As the severity of the handicap increased, the dropout rate decreased, reflecting in part the more continuous presence of adult supervision and control for these youngsters. Some of the factors that have been found to distinguish handicapped youngsters who drop out from those who do not include a more negative perception of school, a lower level of participation in school-related activities, poorer school grades, and a higher frequency of grade retention. Retarded youngsters who drop out of school have been found, subsequently, to have lower rates of employment and are employed for shorter periods than retarded youngsters who complete school. A relative lack of persistence and a lower tolerance for frustration in youngsters who drop out have been seen as possible factors in that these qualities are important in completing school and in seeking and maintaining a job.

Mildly mentally retarded adolescents use less alcohol and other drugs than nonretarded peers and are less frequently found to be substance abusers.[12] Alcohol use by retarded adolescents was found in one study to result more rapidly in symptoms of alcohol dependency than alcohol use in nonretarded adolescents.[13] In addition, retarded youngsters have been found to engage less frequently in deviant or criminal behavior associated with drug use. When these adolescents do become involved with drug use, they begin at a later age than nonretarded peers.[14] The relatively low prevalence of substance abuse among mildly retarded adolescents may be a result of their greater dependence on parents, which results in less freedom from adult supervision, and may be due to the absence of a peer group, which often tends to encourage use and to provide a means of obtaining drugs.

Low intelligence has consistently been found to be a correlate of criminal behavior. In several national studies examining the number of inmates in correctional settings who are retarded, about 10% are found to meet the criteria for mental retardation relative to the 3% prevalence rate for mental retardation in the general population.[15] The overwhelming majority of these inmates tend to be classified as mildly mentally retarded. Similarly, about 10% of delinquents committed to state correctional settings are retarded.[16] The exact nature of the association between retardation and arrest, adjudication, and incarceration is unclear. In part, this association may reflect the finding that retarded individuals are more prone to confess to crimes, even ones they have not committed, and to plea-bargain.

MANAGEMENT

Parents of mildly retarded adolescents tend to seek assistance from healthcare providers when their youngster is between the ages of 8 and 14 years, usually after a period of school difficulties. They often request an explanation as to why the youngster is having difficulty, ask for ways to modify school demands, and seek advice about psychosocial expectations. The psychosocial questions during early to middle adolescence tend to center on the youngster's social isolation, confusion over what constitutes an appropriate degree of independence and responsibility for the adolescent, and ways of dealing with his or her emerging sexuality. In late adolescence, possible work or training options subsequent to formal schooling, and the likelihood of the youngster having a spouse and family, tend to be the primary concerns.

When a consultation is requested, healthcare providers need to modify their interviewing techniques when talking with retarded adolescents to try to ascertain their views and the sources of distress. Abstractions must be avoided, and questions should be divided into their component parts and presented one at a time. Repetition is often required, and several possibilities need to be offered to the adolescent if he or she appears unable to generate an answer to a question. "What" and "when" questions tend to be more effective than "how" and "why" questions. The former type of questions are less abstract and require primarily description rather than interpretation. If such subjects are not spontaneously mentioned by mildly retarded adolescents, the healthcare provider should ask about the extent and nature of their social relationships; whether family problems exist with parents and/or siblings; the degree of independence they have and the degree desired; the presence and extent of derogatory self-attitudes; knowledge of sexuality and sexual behavior; school performance, including attendance and satisfaction; and, for middle and late adolescents, plans subsequent to graduation from school.

Parents of retarded adolescents tend to view a consultation as successful if at its completion they feel clearer about their youngster's strengths and weaknesses and better prepared for developing expectations and anticipating future events. They also tend to appreciate suggestions and resources that might facilitate socialization opportunities for their adolescent, guidelines to use when allowing their child greater independence, and practical information to deal with his or her sexual feelings and behavior. As part of the consultation, additional evaluations are often needed, which usually include an up-to-date psychologic assessment of intelligence and adaptive competence and an educational evaluation to determine the adequacy of the youngster's educational progress. If special education appears warranted, the evaluator needs to indicate whether placement should be in a full-time special education program or in a part-time arrangement, with the youngster concurrently attending some special education classes and some regular education classes. During middle and late adolescence, a vocational assessment is often beneficial to determine the youngster's work readiness and to suggest possible suitable broad work categories and/or training programs. Given the mildly retarded adolescent's poor self-esteem and low expectations for success, there needs to be a continuing search for experiences that potentially can lead to feelings of mastery, so as to enhance the adolescent's determination and self-confidence.

PROGNOSIS

Long-term follow-up studies have examined the adult status of mildly retarded youngsters in regard to general psychologic adjustment, employment, and marriage. During the adult years, most youngsters diagnosed as mildly mentally retarded have been found to attain at least a moderately positive level of adjustment, with most being independent and self-supporting. For the most part, although somewhat more isolated than their nonretarded counterparts, individuals with mild mental retardation did not need assistance from mental retardation services and did not stand out from their peers. When formal diagnostic criteria have been applied, about two thirds of individuals who had earlier been diagnosed as mildly mentally retarded were no longer found to be sufficiently deficient in adaptive functioning to meet the requirements necessary for the mental retardation classification. Factors found to facilitate a better adjustment in adulthood included physical attractiveness; normal weight; adequate social skills; and the presence of a benign, nonretarded adult serving as a benefactor.

When reaching adulthood, a substantial number of mildly retarded youngsters gain and maintain regular employment, although at a rate less than that of their nonretarded peers. Most jobs are unskilled and in the service sector, such as hospital orderly, kitchen worker, and cleaning staff. As would be expected, jobs that involve predictable routines, have a clear structure, involve repetition, and de-emphasize complex judgment and academic skills tend to be carried out most adequately and be maintained longest. Approximately one half of youngsters diagnosed as mildly retarded marry as adults, with women more likely to marry than men. Those mildly mentally retarded individuals who marry tend to have relatively higher IQs. Although there are fewer marriages in the retarded than in the nonretarded population, the divorce rate of married retarded adults is nearly equal to that found in the general population. Mildly retarded females, however, are found to have more difficulties within the marriage than nonretarded females. The difference in degree of marital difficulty between retarded and nonretarded populations is less pronounced for males. Most of the offspring of these individuals make satisfactory progress in school and do not display symptoms of mental retardation.

References

1. Luckasson R, Coulter DL, Polloway EA, Reiss A, Schalock RL, Snell ME, Spitalnik DM, Stark JA: *Mental retardation: definition, classification, and systems of support,* Washington, DC, 1992, American Association on Mental Retardation.
2. American Psychiatric Association: *Diagnostic and statistical manual of mental disorders,* ed 4, Washington, DC, 1994, American Psychiatric Association.
3. World Health Organization: *Mental disorders: glossary and guide to their classification in accordance with the ninth revision of the international classification of diseases,* Geneva, 1978, WHO.
4. Baroff GS: *Mental retardation: nature, cause and management,* ed 2, Washington, DC, 1986, Hemisphere.
5. Steele S: Assessment of functional wellness behaviors in adolescents who are mentally retarded, *Compr Pediatr Nurs* 9:331-340, 1986.
6. Takeuchi E: Incidents of obesity among school children in Japan. *Am J Ment Retard* 99:283-288, 1994.
7. Zigler E: Can we "cure" mild mental retardation among individuals of the lower socioeconomic stratum?, *Am J Public Health* 85:302-304, 1995.

8. Yeargin-Allsop M, Drews CD, DeCouflé P, Murphy CC: Mild mental retardation in black and white children in metropolitan Atlanta: a case-control study, *Am J Public Health* 85:324-328, 1995.

9. Chamberlain A, Rauh J, Passer A, McGrath M, Burket R: Issues in fertility control for mentally retarded female adolescents. 1. Sexual activity, sexual abuse, and contraception, *Pediatrics* 73:445-454, 1984.

10. Levy SR, Perhute C, Nash-Johnson M, Welter JF: Reducing the risks in pregnant teens who are very young and those with mild mental retardation, *Ment Retard* 30:195-203, 1992.

11. Wolman C, Bruinks R, Thurlow ML: Dropouts and dropout programs: implications for special education, *Remed Spec Educ* 10:6-20, 1989.

12. Edgerton RB: Alcohol and drug use by mentally retarded adults, *Am J Ment Defic* 90:602-609, 1986.

13. Rychkova LS: Clinical characteristics of early alcoholism in adolescents with slight mental retardation of exogenous etiology, *Soviet Neurol Psychiatry* 20:55-63, 1986.

14. Westermeyer J, Phaobtong T, Neider J: Substance use and abuse among mentally retarded persons: a comparison of patients and a survey population, *Am J Drug Alcohol Abuse* 14:109-123, 1988.

15. Koller H, Richardson SA, Katz M, McLaren J: Behavior disturbance in childhood and the early adult years in populations who were and were not mentally retarded, *J Prev Psychiatry* 1:453-468, 1982.

16. Murphy DM: The prevalence of handicapping conditions among juvenile delinquents, *Remed Spec Educ* 7:7-17, 1986.

CHAPTER 119

Conversion Reactions and Psychosomatic Disorders

•

Gregory E. Prazar

The adolescent presenting for a brief office visit with a prolonged history of unexplained headaches, chest pain, or abdominal pain may represent a particular frustration for the primary care practitioner. From past experiences with such cases, the practitioner has learned that a brief history will contribute little to ascertaining an etiology for the symptom and that a limited physical examination addressing the specific symptom will invariably show normal results. If the adolescent's demeanor suggests little discomfort, the practitioner may conclude that the symptom indicates emotional concerns or is a sign of malingering. But what, in fact, is the accurate diagnosis? Does the patient have a psychosomatic illness such as a conversion symptom? Or is the patient a hypochondriac?

Unfortunately, the medical literature rarely aids in untangling the confusion or alleviating the frustration, since studies frequently use conflicting definitions for nonspecific symptoms. Psychosomatic problems encompass a category of situations in which a physical symptom, illness, or complaint is associated with psychosocial factors. In all cases of psychosomatic problems, biomedical findings prove insufficient to explain the problem. Specific examples of psychosomatic problems include conversion reactions, psychophysiologic symptoms, hypochondriasis, malingering and factitious illness, and somatic delusions (Table 119-1).

Conversion reactions receive the most attention in this chapter not only because this specific psychosomatic problem is often the most difficult to diagnose accurately but also because conversion reactions present complex challenges to the initiation of effective intervention. The goal of this chapter is to guide the practitioner in identifying psychosomatic problems and conversion reactions; to differentiate conversion reactions from psychophysiologic symptoms, hypochondriasis, and malingering; and to outline an approach to the treatment and referral of patients with conversion reactions. The approach to the diagnosis and treatment of conversion reactions is also applicable to other psychosomatic problems because the diagnosis of the particular problem is less important than how the evaluation proceeds and how the practitioner approaches the treatment of the patient and the family.

DESCRIPTION AND PREVALENCE OF CONVERSION REACTIONS

Engel states that conversion reactions represent "psychic mechanisms whereby an idea, fantasy, or wish is expressed in bodily rather than in verbal terms and is experienced by the patient as a physical symptom rather than a mental symptom." The idea or wish, although

TABLE 119-1
Categories of Psychosomatic Disorders

Disorder	Definition	Examples
Conversion reactions	Presence of a physical symptom that unconsciously communicates unpleasant emotions; the patient displays little or no anxiety associated with the symptom; physical findings are inconsistent with physiologic concepts	Some cases of limb paralysis and blindness, recurrent headache, recurrent abdominal pain
Psychophysiologic symptoms	Presence of a physical symptom that is precipitated by activation of biologic systems (autonomic nervous system and/or neuroendocrine system); the symptom is organic in origin and is associated with unpleasant feelings with which the patient can easily identify; physical findings are consistent with organic illness	Some cases of diarrhea and palpitations; exacerbation of inflammatory bowel disease, asthma, and peptic ulcer disease
Hypochondriasis	Presence of a physical symptom that is associated with extreme concern by the patient; the patient is preoccupied with physical disease; physical findings do not substantiate organic illness	Some cases of recurrent headaches, recurrent abdominal pain, diffuse pain
Malingering	Display of a physical symptom that the patient creates consciously to avoid unpleasant situations; physical findings often corroborate factitious illness	Some cases of skin infections, recurrent headache and recurrent abdominal pain, self-administration of excess medication
Somatic delusions	A symptom of psychosis; other signs of thought disorder are present; physical symptoms are bizarre and not substantiated by physical findings	Patients complaining of their heart shriveling up, or patients complaining of something wrong with the blood flowing through their body

completely unconscious, is unacceptable for the patient to express directly. Therefore, the conversion reaction represents the dissipation of unpleasant emotions associated with the idea through the manifestation of a somatic symptom. The patient does not relate any psychologic stigmata to this somatic complaint because the idea is unconscious. Therefore, neither the adolescent nor the family is aware of the significance of the physical symptom or complaint.

Any bodily process that can be perceived by the individual can serve as the focus for a conversion reaction. Normally, adolescents are likely to focus on body sensations, especially during an illness, which can then serve as a model for later somatic complaints. Somatic symptoms of relatives or close friends also can serve as the model for the patient's complaint. When the symptom is modeled after a symptom observed in another person, that other person is frequently an individual who evokes strong feelings in the adolescent rather than one who is distant and emotionally neutral.

Although studies have been conducted with respect to incidence rates of certain individual somatic complaints, the specific overall prevalence of conversion reactions in

adolescence is not known; available data suggest between 5% and 15%. The lack of more definitive data reflects the difficulty in ascertaining whether a somatic complaint indeed represents a conversion reaction. Conversion reactions appear to be more common in adolescent girls than in adolescent boys. Studies concur that the incidence among females increases with age.

There appears to be no correlation between the occurrence of conversion reactions and socioeconomic status. However, less sophisticated patients more often present with more blatant physiologically unexplainable symptoms.

Adolescents are more likely than children or adults to develop conversion reactions because they normally are preoccupied with their bodies. The intense and rapid physical changes that take place during adolescence, in concert with emotional changes, predispose adolescents to focus on body sensations. A normal physiologic sign that might otherwise be overlooked during another stage of life can often be misinterpreted by the adolescent as a sign of illness. Such misinterpretation is more likely to occur if there are stresses in the adolescent's life. Furthermore, there is evidence that conversion symptoms in adolescents may occur as a response to anxiety associated with the acceptability of sexual thoughts and behaviors as part of normally evolving sexual identity. Studies indicate that approximately 20% of adolescents worry about their health "all the time"; only 15% "never give their health a thought."

Conversion reactions can present as a group phenomenon. Such a situation is referred to as "epidemic hysteria" or "mass sociogenic illness." Adolescent girls swooning and fainting at rock concerts represent an easily appreciated example; in this situation the unacceptable wish relates to sexualized thoughts involving rock stars. Other examples of epidemic hysteria are less easily explained but appear to share several common characteristics: (1) audiovisual cues (e.g., watching another adolescent faint or vomit, viewing the arrival of ambulances to care for victims) appear to be important in precipitating such reactions, (2) adolescent girls are involved more frequently than adolescent boys, (3) the reaction is more likely to occur if initiated by a recognized group leader or outsider than by a member of the group, (4) participants are more likely to be less emotionally mature than peers who are not involved, and (5) episodes are likely to involve larger numbers of adolescents if the adolescents are allowed to confer among themselves without adults present. Whole school populations may be involved in cases of epidemic hysteria.

DIAGNOSIS OF CONVERSION REACTIONS

Symptoms due to conversion reactions and those attributed to organic illness can be easily confused. For this reason, when evaluating any adolescent with a somatic complaint, the practitioner should always take into consideration the diagnostic possibility of a conversion reaction. Simultaneous attention to personal history (family functioning, school performance, peer relationships) and physical functioning demonstrates to the patient and the family that the practitioner appreciates the importance of all elements that may be contributing to ill health. Such an approach communicates that there is a distinct interaction between physical and emotional functioning, an acknowledgment that will be critical when diagnostic possibilities are discussed later with the family.

The first appointment with the adolescent patient who has a suspected conversion reaction is likely to be brief, since the family assumes that the problem is a physical illness and will likely have scheduled only a brief appointment. However, despite time constraints, it is important to remember that the initial encounter is critical in determining the subsequent effectiveness of the symptom evaluation. If a conversion reaction is

suspected, the following information should be obtained: the duration of the symptom, how the symptom interferes with the adolescent's daily activity, and how the adolescent and the family react to the symptom. Nondirective interviewing proves more rewarding than direct questioning. For example, asking the patient to describe the pain ("Tell me how it feels") almost always provides insights into the emotion that the patient associates with the symptom. Suggesting how the symptom feels to the patient ("Is it a dull or sharp pain?") limits the possible responses. If the patient spontaneously offers information about recent events, the divulgence of further data related to such changes in the patient's life should be encouraged.

Care should be taken to avoid suggesting a cause-and-effect relationship between the patient's feelings and the symptoms. Because the adolescent with a conversion reaction has no conscious understanding of such an association, the suggestion of such a relationship may alienate the patient and prevent the establishment of a trusting relationship with the practitioner. Limiting the history to a symptom "shopping list" of questions may indicate to the adolescent that personal concerns are irrelevant, which is definitely not the case with conversion reactions.

After a brief history is obtained at the first appointment, a physical examination addressing the specific symptom should be performed. If the physical examination reveals no significant findings, the practitioner should briefly summarize the findings with the patient and the parents. Because the symptom is usually not of recent onset, the practitioner should indicate that a quick solution to the problem is not at hand. He or she should explain that everyone has an emotional reaction to physical symptoms and that every physical illness has an emotional component. Since adolescence is a time when emotional reactions are particularly intense, a careful evaluation will be needed to fully explore the symptom. In general, one or two extended visits in addition to a complete physical examination (even if one has previously been performed before the symptom appeared) are necessary for a complete evaluation. A summary conference is also necessary.

During the subsequent evaluation appointments with the adolescent and the family, the practitioner should be aware of several characteristics of patients who suffer from conversion reactions (Box 119-1).

Symbolic Meaning

The conversion reaction has a specific but unconscious symbolic meaning to the adolescent. The symptom often is related to an unconscious wish, and physical impairment serves to prevent the person acting out the wish. The practitioner treating adolescents is usually not aware of

---

BOX 119-1
Characteristics of Patients
With Conversion Reactions

The symptom reduces anxiety ("primary gain")
The symptom helps the patient cope with his or her environment ("secondary gain")
The symptom has symbolic meaning to the patient
The symptom has a model
History and physical findings are often inconsistent with anatomic and physiologic concepts
The patient frequently exhibits characteristic interpersonal behaviors
There is a characteristic style of reporting symptoms
Families of patients display specific interactional characteristics (e.g., overprotectiveness, problems with conflict resolution)
Symptoms occur at times of stress

Modified from Prazar GE: Conversion reactions in adolescents, *Pediatr Rev* 8:283, 1987. Reproduced by permission of *Pediatrics*. Copyright 1987.

the symbolic meaning of the symptom. Although it may be intellectually rewarding for the practitioner to be cognizant of the presence of a symbolic meaning, ignorance of specific symbolism does not prevent adequate treatment of the patient.

Modeling of Symptom

Conversion symptom presentation is based on the patient's unconscious remembrance of his or her own physical symptoms or an understanding of symptoms in others who are significant to the patient. The adolescent patient's symptom may appear dissimilar to that displayed by the other individual (often a parent or a close relative) because it is the patient's perception of disease that governs the symptoms displayed. Parents and relatives frequently withhold information about illness from an adolescent, fearing the truth would be too frightening. However, such a tactic may actually potentiate the adolescent's fantasies and result in the presentation of a symptom different from the actual one experienced by the individual serving as the model.

The choice of symptom also may be based on a previous physical illness suffered by the adolescent. Thus, patients with a history of seizures may present with a history of atypical and physiologically unexplainable seizures after many years of adequate medical control. Unfortunately, these patients typically receive only a physiologic work-up for seizures. The practitioner assumes, despite the atypical history, that the diagnosis rests on the same factors present in the past.

History and Physical Findings Inconsistent With Anatomic and Physiologic Concepts

Because the somatic complaint expressed by the patient is based on a model symptom, a physical disease often is mimicked. Most adolescents are medically unsophisticated. Close scrutiny of symptom history and description often reveals anatomic and physiologic discrepancies. The adolescent presenting with a stocking anesthesia (an anesthesia confined to a specific extremity area without a relationship to cutaneous nerve innervation) is an example of such symptom inaccuracy. The symptom is based on the patient's concept of his or her body and not on anatomic principles.

Characteristic Interpersonal Behaviors

Adolescents with conversion reactions frequently display characteristic patterns of personality, sometimes designated as those of the "hysterical personality." Such characteristics include egocentricity; labile emotional states (quick shifts from sadness to elation and from anger to passivity); dramatic, attention-seeking behavior; and sexual provocativeness (displayed in gestures and mannerisms of dress). Patients with such characteristics also tend to be demanding and to display an air of pseudomaturity. Although many aspects of the hysterical personality are seen in adolescent patients with conversion reactions, such characteristics also frequently occur in adolescents free of such symptoms. Therefore, hysterical behavior traits in isolation are not indicative of a predisposition toward conversion reactions.

Characteristic Reporting Style

The manner in which the patient with the conversion symptom describes the problem is frequently distinctive. The account is often dramatic. Patients are suggestible, so that any symptom description alluded to by the practitioner may be readily incorporated into the patient's historical repertoire and subsequently reported.

Primary Gain

As previously described, conversion reactions are unconsciously adopted in an attempt to reduce unpleasant affects, especially anxiety, depression, and guilt. Therefore, although patients may describe incapacitating pain, they often affect an air of nonchalance. Psychiatrists refer to this as *la belle indifference*. Primary gain refers to the extent to which the conversion reaction diminishes the unpleasant emotion (especially anxiety) and communicates symbolically for the patient the forbidden, but unconscious, wish. Patients with conversion reactions are often stubborn in their belief that the symptom has organic causes. This attitude reflects denial of the underlying emotional conflict or problem. On the other hand, insistence, especially by an adolescent, that the symptom is psychologic in origin may indicate denial of a physical problem. Therefore, with adolescent patients the differential diagnosis between conversion reactions and physical disease cannot rest on the patient's emotional response alone.

Secondary Gain

Conversion reactions not only effect a primary gain for patients but also serve to help them cope with the environment. In this respect, the symptom achieves a secondary gain for patients by removing them from a conflictive or uncomfortable situation. For example, the patient with a conversion reaction defending against homosexual thoughts may be excused from attending school, where anxiety may have been intensified (e.g., in the locker room). Limitations imposed by the symptom may contradict the patient's verbalized wishes to participate in activities. Nevertheless, these limitations remove the patient from potentially threatening social interactions. Interference with daily activities also provides a secondary gain to the patient in that attention and emotional support are attracted from concerned parents and friends.

Demonstration of secondary gain is not pathognomonic of a diagnosis of a conversion reaction. To an extent, all illnesses result in some secondary gain. For example, a bedridden patient must accept increased attention to cope with physical confinement. Therefore, a degree of secondary gain is necessary for adequate adaptation to a physical disability. However, in the case of a conversion reaction, secondary gain actually may encourage the continued development of somatic complaints. Because perpetuation of secondary gain is contingent on concern from others, a conversion symptom is more readily exhibited in the presence of those individuals meaningful to the patient. Unfortunately, practitioners unfamiliar with conversion reactions and issues of secondary gain may assume that the situation represents one of malingering in which the parents are being manipulated by the adolescent. Consequent practitioner insensitivity may alienate both the parents and the adolescent.

Characteristic Familial Interaction Patterns

Studies indicate that families of adolescents who experience conversion reactions often display specific characteristic patterns of interaction. First, conflict avoidance by adults in the family is common. Focusing on an adolescent's conversion symptom allows the family to avoid dealing with conflict surrounding other family issues. Second, adolescents in such families may be overprotected. Hypervigilant behavior regarding the physical well-being of each family member is prominent. Such behavior may prevent the adolescent from participating in age-appropriate activities. Third, because hypervigilance about physical well-being is a priority, somatic complaints may occupy a substantial part of daily communication among family members. Therefore, the patient's symptom may conform to the unspoken interactional rules of the family. Fourth, enmeshment may be a family characteristic in which the patient's problem is seen as a family problem and little individuality is allowed. The patient's problem is covertly reinforced by family members, who may even assume an air of unconcern with respect to the patient's symptom. In such families, adults will be reluctant to discuss emotions and conflicts with the practitioner. In some instances, family members will deny conflict even when faced with irrefutable evidence to the contrary.

Symptoms at Times of Stress

Conversion reactions may occur in association with external stresses, although the specific stress may be impossible for the practitioner to identify. A change of school, academic difficulty in school, new social experiences, competitive events, and parental conflict are examples of life events that may be temporally associated with the appearance of a conversion reaction. Unresolved grief reactions, such as those in response to the loss of a parent through death, divorce, or moving, also represent a source of stress for adolescents that may precipitate a conversion reaction. Because the association between the conflict and the symptom is unconscious, the interview with the adolescent will be helpful only if the practitioner attempts to elicit details concerning daily activities rather than trying to obtain a history aimed at uncovering stress. Direct approaches to the discussion of stressful topics may elicit denial. Often a precipitating stress event for a conversion reaction becomes apparent only after many patient visits.

It is important to remember that no one diagnostic criterion can serve as confirmatory in patients with conversion reactions. Furthermore, each patient may not display every criterion discussed. However, the diagnosis of a conversion reaction cannot be made solely on the basis of negative physical and laboratory findings. It is not a diagnosis of exclusion.

Complications of Conversion Reactions

Occasionally, there are secondary anatomic or physiologic consequences of a conversion reaction. Such consequences have been considered the *complications* of the conversion reaction. Examples include tetany as a result of blood gas changes secondary to hyperventilation (the conversion reaction), and disuse leading to muscle atrophy secondary to paralysis.

DIFFERENTIAL DIAGNOSIS OF OTHER PSYCHOSOMATIC DISORDERS

It is important to be able to differentiate conversion reactions from other psychosomatic problems in which physical symptoms and psychosocial factors are involved, as the nature of the problem carries implications on how best to intervene.

Psychophysiologic Symptoms

Patients with psychophysiologic symptoms present with an identifiable unpleasant emotion (anxiety, hopelessness, fear, anger, or sadness) of which they are usually aware. The unpleasant affect activates biologic systems (especially the autonomic nervous and neuroendocrine systems), resulting in such signs as tachycardia, sweating, vasoconstriction, or hyperperistalsis. These organic changes are experienced by the patients as palpitations, sweating, cold hands, or diarrhea. The psychophysiologic symptom is therefore of organic origin, although the original precipitating factor is emotional. Differentiation between psychophysiologic symptoms and conversion reactions is sometimes difficult because when conversion reactions fail to reduce unconscious anxiety, patients become aware of the uncomfortable emotion (i.e., the anxiety) and biologic systems are then also activated. Although all disease states may be influenced by psychophysiologic factors, some are particularly vulnerable to emotional influences. In adolescence, these diseases include inflammatory bowel disease and some cases of asthma. However, it is important to remember that these disorders are not caused by stress; rather, disease symptoms can be exacerbated by stress.

Hypochondriasis

Patients exhibiting hypochondriasis, a frequent occurrence, especially during adolescence, view their bodily functions or mild symptoms with extreme concern. There is none of the apparent indifference seen in patients with conversion reactions. Patients with conversion reactions frequently seem relieved when the possibility of an organic cause is entertained. On the other hand, patients with hypochondriasis become more concerned if an organic diagnosis is suggested because they suspect and fear serious and fatal disease. However, neither type of patient is reassured more than transiently by being informed they have no disease.

Malingering

Malingering represents a rare problem in adolescents except among those institutionalized or in restricted situations. School is the most common restricted environment for adolescents, although incarcerated youth and those in the military also may display malingering. Malingering represents a conscious effort to avoid unpleasant situations. Attempts to feign illness are often naive, especially in younger patients. Malingering adolescents with factitious illness surreptitiously create documentable physical signs associated with a symptom in an attempt to maintain the patient role.

Malingering adolescents appear aloof and hostile to the practitioner so that discovery of their deception can be forestalled. In contrast, patients with conversion reactions may act charming and garrulous when in the presence of a practitioner. Malingering should be seen as reflecting "a teenager in trouble," and the practitioner should attempt to minimize any inclination to be punitive.

Somatic Delusions

Somatic delusions are symptoms of psychosis and are not frequently confused with conversion reactions. Other signs of severe mental illness are usually present (inability to relate to peers, disorganization in communication, stereotypic behaviors). Furthermore, the symptoms are often intermittent and are frequently extremely bizarre. For example, patients with somatic delusions may verbalize the conviction that their heart is shriveling up or that there is something wrong with the blood running throughout their body.

CARE OF PATIENTS WITH CONVERSION REACTION

At the beginning of the first extended appointment with the adolescent and the family, the practitioner should review the anticipated evaluation plan, which usually requires two or three visits, a physical examination, and a summary conference. At this first appointment, the practitioner should discuss the fee with the family, who must understand that the visit fee is determined by the amount of time spent. Talking about fees rarely comes easily to the practitioner. However, whether the practitioner is a house officer, a participant in a prepaid group, or a fee-for-service provider, the fee represents an integral part of the process of comprehensive medical care. Families assess the need for care partly in terms of dollars and therefore must understand their financial commitment. If the family feels unable to assume the cost of consultation visits, alternatives must be considered, such as referral to agencies that charge on a sliding scale basis.

Although the adolescent and the parents are interviewed separately, several common considerations must be communicated during both interviews. As previously stated, the practitioner should discuss with patient and family that the cause of any disorder involves both physical and emotional factors. Simple examples should be given (e.g., most people have noticed that when they are upset, headaches are often intensified, or that when speaking before a group, they may experience an "upset stomach"). If practitioners communicate that they appreciate the role of emotions in physical disease, the family may more readily volunteer information about psychosocial functioning. Furthermore, an eventual diagnosis involving emotional aspects will be more acceptable because the family has been prepared for this possibility. Focusing only on the organic diagnosis suggests to the parents that psychologic involvement is unlikely, unimportant, and improbable. Turning to psychologic issues after all physical tests prove nondiagnostic implies to the parents that this tactic was chosen only as a last resort since the practitioner was unable to ascertain an organic cause. A concurrent physical-psychologic approach not only prepares the practitioner to assess the problem with psychotherapeutic intent but also may save time and money because multiple laboratory tests and procedures may often be avoided. Two 30-minute sessions usually suffice to obtain additional history from the teenager and the family. Sessions should be scheduled within a 2-week period to preserve continuity and rapport. It is important to see the adolescent first during counseling sessions, because adolescents distrust adults to a degree and often envision practitioners in collaboration with parents. Spending time first with the adolescent reinforces that the practitioner is the adolescent's doctor and not the parents' confidante. At the end of the parents' session, the adolescent may be briefly seen again to solidify the trust relationship with the practitioner and to determine whether the patient has questions about what the parents discussed. In general, confidentiality with the adolescent is paramount. However, exceptions should be clearly delineated at the beginning of the adolescent interview. For example, if it becomes evident that the adolescent plans to injure himself or others, parents need to be informed. Parents wishing to share confidential information with the practitioner should be apprised that the information may be discussed with the adolescent.

During the interview with the adolescent, the practitioner will need to pursue any feelings the adolescent verbalizes; feelings should be identified and acknowledged. The practitioner also should seek the adolescent's opinion concerning what may be causing the symptom, what the adolescent thinks will happen if this symptom is not relieved, and any diagnostic test or diagnoses that the patient might have considered important. The interviewer must also obtain information about the adolescent's school performance, involvement in out-of-school activi-

ties, and peer relationships. The adolescent's feelings about his or her family need to be investigated (e.g., what the parents hassle the adolescent about, whether the parents more often compliment or criticize the adolescent). While the physical examination is being performed, the practitioner must be especially sensitive to any emotional reactions displayed or verbalized by the patient.

If the adolescent lives in a two-parent family, both parents should be strongly encouraged to attend the parent interview. All the issues explored in the interview with the adolescent need also to be explored with the parents. Special attention must be given to eliciting from the parents information concerning the adolescent's merits; such information not only may help the family feel less hopeless about their adolescent's problem but also provides the practitioner with a better understanding of the adolescent's emotional, cognitive, and social resources. The practitioner should avoid offering quick advice during the first interview despite parental pressure to do otherwise. Similarly, premature reassurance from a practitioner must be avoided, especially as parents correctly may perceive such advice as based on inadequate information. Practitioners are accustomed to offering solutions and doing most of the talking during interviews, but during evaluation interviews they will find that listening and reflecting are ultimately more rewarding.

Some laboratory tests are indicated with most cases of conversion reactions, if for no other reason than to reassure the adolescent and the family that a complete evaluation is occurring. However, an exhaustive battery of laboratory tests eventually will lead to equivocal results, which then lead to the performance of more tests. One consequence will be escalating family concerns about the true diagnosis. Therefore, the practitioner must be especially prudent in selecting tests.

During the evaluation, information may be obtained that may necessitate a referral to another medical specialist. If referral is necessary, it is crucial that the consultant understand that it will be the practitioner who will review all pertinent findings and conclusions with the adolescent and the family. The consultant should never merely refer the patient to another consultant; such a maneuver encourages the family to "consultant shop" for a physical diagnosis.

At the conclusion of the evaluation sessions, the practitioner must feel satisfied with the completeness of the evaluation before holding a summary conference with the patient and the family. The practitioner's common sense should dictate the judgment that the performance of further laboratory tests is futile. Practitioner uncertainty can often be sensed by the patient and the family, especially in a situation in which the family is averse to accepting a psychologic diagnosis. Therefore, it may be prudent to solicit once again from the patient and the family any information regarding additional tests or evaluative procedures they may expect to have performed and other diagnoses they may have considered. Active involvement of the patient and the family in this diagnostic process frequently dissipates anxiety and allows progression to psychologic or other mental health counseling.

The summary conference should help the patient and the family redefine the problem so that they can begin to feel more in control of the symptom. Reviewing the adolescent's and family's strengths at the beginning of this conference starts the meeting with a positive focus. Furthermore, working with an adolescent's unique strengths will likely result in a more effective alliance between the patient and the physician in successfully addressing the conversion symptom. Next, the absence of significant organic disease must be emphasized. The practitioner should point out that all adolescents live with some conflict and that stress exists in every family. The patient and the family need to understand that the symptom is real but that it represents a signal from the patient's body that there is significant intercurrent stress. The family should be reassured that help is available but that the symptom may not quickly disappear. The goal is to help maintain normal daily functioning in school and with peers. Suggesting that the symptom will persist for a while may provide time to establish a therapeutic relationship with the patient. Moreover, this technique sometimes has a paradoxical effect. Because the probability of the symptom disappearing after two or three visits is unlikely, the practitioner's suggestion will be viewed retrospectively by the family as sound advice. Trust in the physician will be more secure and the patient may be more comfortable in communicating information about feelings. At the summary conference, the family needs to be reassured that reevaluation and reexamination of symptoms will occur if the symptom changes, and that referral to a trained mental-health professional may be necessary if progress is not made in coping with the symptom after a mutually agreed number of visits. A summary of important considerations in the initial evaluation of patients with conversion reactions appears in Box 119-2.

At the conclusion of the summary conference, the number and type of counseling sessions that the practitioner anticipates should be discussed. A contract should be flexible so that renegotiation can occur after a mutually agreed number of visits. Usually, follow-up appointments with the teenager can be limited to 15 to 20 minutes every 2 to 4 weeks. During sessions with the teenager, verbalized somatic complaints should be discouraged, although it may be productive to ask patients to keep a symptom diary or chart. The diary allows them to recall what activities were occurring concurrent with the symptom and allows the practitioner to elucidate what

---

BOX 119-2
Initial Evaluation of Patients With Suspected Conversion Reactions

From the outset, parents and patient should be told that every person has an emotional response to physical stress

Parents and patient should be encouraged to suggest diagnostic tests they may want performed and to suggest possible diagnoses for consideration by the physician

Parents and patient should understand that the symptom may persist but that the goal is to help maintain normal daily functioning in school and with peers

Parents and patient should understand that referral to a trained professional in mental health may be necessary if progress is not made in coping with the symptom

From Prazer GE: Conversion reactions in adolescents, *Pediatr Rev* 8:283, 1987. Reproduced by permission of *Pediatrics.* Copyright 1987.

---

feelings may have been associated with the activity. Such a record also helps the adolescent cope with the symptom without reporting the symptom to parents. In this way the practitioner can help the adolescent become reacquainted with how daily events and feelings are related. Encouragement should then be given to talk about intercurrent life events (e.g., school, friends, dating, family), minimizing health and illness issues. It may be necessary to reinforce that the adolescent's discomfort is real but that frequently being in an upset state can intensify or exacerbate discomfort.

Because the practitioner will serve as both therapist for the adolescent and provider of acute medical care, there may be occasions when the teenager presents with a new physical symptom or complaint. If the practitioner suspects a physical illness unrelated to the conversion reaction, he or she must perform whatever evaluation is indicated, including a full or partial physical examination.

Follow-up with parents should take place every 4 to 6 weeks. This important step in the communication process must not be ignored. During these meetings, the practitioner elicits persistent or new concerns that parents may have about their adolescent's progress and attempts to assess the parents' reaction to the continuing complaints. Positive reinforcement needs to be offered so that the parents believe they are doing what is best for their adolescent. Certain parent follow-up sessions include the adolescent. Family meetings not only demonstrate to the adolescent that confidentiality of individual sessions is not being violated but also offer the practitioner an opportunity to observe parent-adolescent interaction. Such observation may provide an important index to the effectiveness of ongoing therapy.

Hospitalization of an adolescent with a conversion reaction may occasionally be necessary, especially if the patient is significantly handicapped by the symptom (e.g., unable to attend school or participate in peer activities). Hospitalization emphasizes to the family that the symptom is significant and disabling, intensifies the concern of all involved in resolving the problem, removes the patient from the sick role in the home environment, and forces the focus on symptom resolution. Hospitalization is expensive, but when outpatient treatment has been unsuccessful, it remains less expensive than "doctor shopping" for alternative diagnoses.

Medications are rarely appropriate in treating patients with conversion reactions. Placebo medication is usually ineffective and raises questions of medical ethics. Anxiolytic medication may transiently reduce attendant anxiety in some cases, but medication as the sole therapeutic modality rarely results in lasting improvement. Because medication does not relieve the underlying conflict responsible for the symptom, another symptom may appear eventually. Furthermore, there is the risk that medication side effects may become the model for a new symptom or that new symptoms may be confused with untoward medication side effects.

Alternative therapies such as relaxation technique, biofeedback, and systematic desensitization may be of adjunctive assistance for patients with conversion reactions. However, as with anxiolytic medications, alternative therapies do not address the underlying conflict that is responsible for the symptom. Therefore, the ongoing counseling sessions remain the most important way to help patients who have conversion reactions.

Treatment goals need to be realistic. Complete disappearance of the conversion reaction seldom occurs. However, adolescents can develop effective coping skills so that daily functioning is unimpaired and dependency on secondary gain minimized. The practitioner serves a valuable role as a counselor in discouraging "doctor shopping" by the family in search of a physical diagnosis, forestalling expensive and unnecessary tests, and preventing unnecessary medical treatment or surgery.

REFERRAL

Referral to mental-health professionals is indicated when symptoms continue to interfere with the patient's daily activities or functioning or when the practitioner or school believes there has been no diminution in the adolescent's symptoms (Box 119-3). School officials can provide valuable information about the effect of the conversion reaction on school functioning and on peer interaction. Referral is, of course, mandatory if the family believes that inadequate progress has been made after an agreed duration of therapy. Parents' wishes should be

---

BOX 119-3
Indications for Referral of Patients With Conversion Reactions

The symptom continues to interfere with activities of daily functioning (school attendance, participation in extracurricular activities, involvement with peers)

Parents and/or the patient believe that no progress is being made in dealing with the symptom

Possible irreversible medical complications from conversion reaction

Practitioner feels uncomfortable with the patient's symptom or behavior (e.g., patient exhibiting seductive behavior)

Patient's family includes a social friend or relative of the practitioner

Modified from Prazar GE: Conversion reactions in adolescents, *Pediatr Rev* 8:285, 1987. Reproduced by permission of *Pediatrics*. Copyright 1987.

---

respected, even if the practitioner believes that the problem is being adequately treated. Referral also is indicated when the patient's behavior makes the practitioner uncomfortable. For example, situations involving seductive adolescent behavior in association with the symptom can interfere with the maintenance of a professional practitioner-patient relationship and can prevent effective intervention. It is as unrealistic to assume that a practitioner can adequately treat all psychologic problems as it is to assume that he or she can treat all medical problems. Cognizance of one's own limitations is an important professional attribute.

Although not a common occurrence, complications of a conversion reaction may arise. For example, aphonia, as a conversion reaction, may progress to the complication of atrophy of the laryngeal muscles. This secondary complication may eventually become irreversible, and thus demand aggressive psychiatric or behavioral intervention (e.g., aversive therapy).

Another situation requiring referral involves the patient or family member who is a close social relation or relative of the practitioner. Dealing with the emotional problems of friends' children or relatives' children is inappropriate, since obtaining intimate details of family functioning is often indicated in the evaluation and may jeopardize the social relationship. Conversely, failure or hesitancy to obtain appropriate data may jeopardize subsequent effective problem resolution.

In all instances, when referral is suggested, parental and patient compliance with the referral is improved if that possibility has been mentioned as a contingency early in the evaluation process. The practitioner should always help families understand that seeing a mental-health professional does not connote "craziness." The patient's problem needs to be restated in a way that helps the patient and parents realize why a mental-health counselor is needed. For example, the practitioner may suggest that consultation with a psychiatrist could be helpful because a professional trained in psychiatry can help teenagers understand feelings about unusual symptoms better than can a practitioner who specializes in adolescent medicine.

When the practitioner suggests a referral, one specific name of a mental-health professional should be given to the family. The practitioner will need to have previously contacted the professional to ensure that consultation time is available for the patient and to communicate the practitioner's goals in referring the patient. Choice of a mental-health professional will depend on the family's financial situation and on whether the practitioner believes that medication will be necessary. In small communities in which the number of mental-health professionals is limited and in which anonymity may be a family concern, the practitioner should determine whether the family has specific preferences regarding a referral. After the referral is made, continued practitioner contact with the family concerning the symptom helps ensure compliance with the therapy appointments, demonstrates continued practitioner interest, and helps assess progress with symptom relief.

The prognosis for patients with conversion reactions is unknown. In some studies, many patients have been judged to be improved after several years whether or not professional intervention took place. Patients with conversion reactions may indeed have an encouraging future. On the other hand, in some adolescents symptoms mark the beginning of a lifelong style of using conversion illness as a way of coping with conflict.

ANTICIPATORY GUIDANCE

Practitioners who care for children from birth through adolescence have the opportunity to offer families guidance regarding the interaction of emotions and physical symptoms. During routine physical examinations, practitioners should inquire about intercurrent stresses and changes. In this way they communicate not only that stress is an anticipated part of every family's life but also that they are interested and available to hear concerns. When a child is ill, the practitioner may wish to discuss how an individual's temperament and personality influence emotional reactions to physical illnesses. During preadolescent years, the practitioner can prepare the child and the family for the expected emotional vicissitudes of adolescence and for the intense adolescent preoccupation with body concerns. Also appropriate at this time would be a statement that adolescents often misinterpret body sensations and changes as a potential sign of illness. Although such anticipatory guidance may not prevent the development of a psychosomatic symptom or conversion reaction, it does demonstrate the practitioner's interest in both the physical and the emotional health of the patient and the family.

SUMMARY

All adolescents presenting with a long-standing somatic complaint have feelings about the symptom, even though they may initially deny any such feelings. The practitioner's initial approach to any prolonged or unusual somatic complaint in an adolescent will often influence the effectiveness of subsequent medical intervention. An evaluation should involve an inquiry into aspects of the patient's family, school performance, and peer relationships. A better understanding of the patient's baseline emotional functioning can thus be achieved. The practitioner must communicate to the parents and the patient that it is acceptable to have feelings and thoughts about somatic complaints. Both the family and the patient may be much more accepting of the importance of emotional factors if permission to discuss such feelings is given early during the practitioner-patient interaction. A diagnosis of a psychosomatic symptom, and particularly a suspected conversion reaction, should never be made solely by exclusion of an organic cause, and should follow specific diagnostic criteria.

Care of adolescent patients with a conversion reaction involves identifying and emphasizing their unique strengths, establishing a renegotiable contract for regular visits, encouraging them to discuss daily activities and related feelings, meeting with the parents regularly to provide them with emotional support and counseling, and realizing that palliation rather than cure may be the optimal goal. When the practitioner feels uncomfortable in treating a patient with a conversion reaction or when continuing follow-up appears to have made no progress in reduction of the symptom, referral to a mental-health professional should be undertaken. However, referral should not end the practitioner's contact with the patient, because sustained practitioner interest may improve patient compliance with the referral source and increases the practitioner's ability to later assume responsibility for the patient's care. The adolescent with a conversion reaction will not outgrow the symptom and will not permanently respond to placebo medication. Such patients severely tax the practitioner's sense of fulfillment in medicine, especially because much of the reward in practicing medicine lies in curing the patient's symptoms promptly. However, the practitioner who respects the interaction of emotions with somatic complaints can serve a vital role in helping patients with psychosomatic symptoms, and more particularly those with conversion reactions.

Suggested Readings

Engel GL: Conversion symptoms. In MacBryde CM, Blacklow RS, editors: *Signs and symptoms: applied physiology and clinical interpretation,* Philadelphia, 1970, JB Lippincott; pp 650-660.

Gold MA, Friedman SB: Conversion reactions in adolescents, *Pediatr Ann* 24:296, 1995.

Hodgman CH: Conversion and somatization in pediatrics, *Pediatr Rev* 16:29, 1995.

Maisami M, Freeman JM: Conversion reactions in children as body language: a combined child psychiatry/neurology team approach to the management of functional neurologic disorders in children, *Pediatrics* 80:46, 1987.

Maloney MJ: Diagnosing hysterical conversion reactions in children, *J Pediatr* 97:1016, 1980.

Moffatt MEK: Epidemic hysteria in a Montreal train station, *Pediatrics* 70:308, 1982.

Orr D: Adolescence, stress and psychosomatic issues, *J Adolesc Health Care* 9:97, 1986.

Phillips S, Sarles RM, Friedman SB: Consultation and referral: when, why and how, *Pediatr Ann* 9:269, 1980.

Prazar GE: Conversion reactions in adolescents, *Pediatr Rev* 8:279, 1987.

Stark T, Blum R: Psychosomatic illness in childhood and adolescence, *Clin Pediatr* 25:549, 1986.

CHAPTER 120

Character Disorders

•

Michael Jellinek and Steven Ablon

I take it that it is normal for an adolescent to behave for a considerable length of time in an inconsistent and unpredictable manner; to fight his impulses and to accept them; to ward them off successfully and to be overrun by them; to love his parents and to hate them; to revolt against them and to be dependent on them; to be deeply ashamed to acknowledge his mother before others and, unexpectedly, to desire heart-to-heart talks with her; to thrive on imitation of and identification with others while searching unceasingly for his own identity; to be more idealistic, artistic, generous, and unselfish than he will ever be again, but also the opposite: self-centered, egotistic, calculating. Such fluctuations between extreme opposites would be deemed highly abnormal at any other time of life. At this time they may signify no more than that an adult structure of personality takes a long time to emerge, that the ego of the individual in question does not cease to experiment and is in no hurry to close down on possibilities.

Anna Freud[1]

A character disorder is hard to define or study, yet the concept of personality encompasses much of what makes our lives meaningful and is essential clinical to an understanding of behavior. An individual's character reflects who that person is, but the complex interactions and relative contributions of genetics, constitutional factors, family life, developmental forces, and personal experience are poorly understood. Some personality traits are largely dependent on childrearing techniques, others on critical life events. Most are influenced by social class, culture, family heritage, and interpersonal relationships.

DEFINITION

A disorder of character or personality is a serious, often lifelong, distortion in an individual's understanding and approach to his or her inner feelings and to the feelings of others. An adolescent with a character disorder understands inner experiences and experiences others through an unconsciously established rigid set of beliefs and defenses. Although adolescents with these disorders are not psychotic or largely out of touch with reality, these distortions and defenses are frustrating to others, as they are not amenable to logic or to change by pointing out to adolescents their own examples of dysfunctional behavior.

Typically, there are serious consequences to character-disordered defenses and behaviors. Adolescents with character disorders develop relationships with others that conform to their own defensive systems. For example, narcissistic individuals are selfish, entitled, and arrogant and maintain relationships with others that serve their own purposes or self-aggrandizement. Such persons hurt the feelings of others well before a genuinely close relationship can develop, and this relationship failure thus confirms their view of relationships as rejecting. The inner need for closeness and the inescapable pattern of eliciting rejection result in a profound sense of loneliness.

Character-disordered adolescents often see no options and have difficulty gaining a sense of perspective. Instead, they firmly believe that their distorted, rigid, and defensive view of the world is truly valid. Despite being dysfunctional and unfulfilling, character-disordered defenses are adolescents' unconscious solution to dealing with extremely painful feelings in relation to their inner and outer worlds. Thus, adolescents with character-ologically disordered low self-esteem need to have that view confirmed; they unconsciously select others or facilitate circumstances that virtually ensure rejection and suffering.

INITIAL RECOGNITION

Some elements of personality are continuous over time, such as the relative stability of intelligence, whereas others are discontinuous, such as the role of parent.[2] These various elements of personality interact and influence one another. For example, the parental role is a distinct and unique state; however, one's approach to interpersonal relationships is a continuous element of personality that greatly influences choices in peer relationships, spouse, and quality of parenting. Other examples are the newly emergent (discontinuous) cognitive, hormonal, and emotional structures that develop during puberty and initiate a major stage of life. However, certain underlying personality features that are maintained during puberty are continuous with experiences integrated throughout infancy and childhood.

Development dramatically affects what we consider personality. The easygoing baby can become the negativistic toddler; the grade-school child will sometimes quite suddenly become more independent, interested in

facts, and concerned about right and wrong; and the preadolescent may change from being communicative and available to being secretive and introspective.

Pediatricians who observe their patients entering adolescence are aware of the many subtle discontinuities and continuities in behavior and especially of how these factors apply to the individual patient.[3] Parents routinely ask whether behaviors such as moodiness, isolation, or substance abuse are part of a "phase," a feature of adolescent "rebellion," or a forecast of lifelong distress. They want to know if the behavior is transient, essentially normal experimentation and reworking on the path toward developing a positive identity, or indicative of a deviant personality trait or a character disorder that is causing serious dysfunction and emotional suffering. Pediatricians and their personal sense of optimism, well supported by years of experience watching the overwhelming majority of adolescent patients do well medically and psychologically, usually encourage a normalizing perspective and discourage parental overreaction and guilt. However, recognition and understanding of potentially problematic or even self-destructive character patterns, although these are relatively infrequent in practice, is a necessary part of child and adolescent care.

One of the most difficult clinical tasks is to differentiate normal or expected variations in adolescent development, which sometimes are exacerbated by an acute stress, from worrisome character traits or prematurely rigid character disorders. Such diagnostic difficulties in adolescent medicine are not unique to personality issues. For example, it can be difficult to differentiate normal adolescent mood swings from clinical depression or evolving manic-depressive disorder. Given the fluidity or even lability of adolescent behavior, some have argued that the differential diagnosis of personality patterns in adolescence is impossible. Although we do not endorse this position, we do believe that a character diagnosis should be tentative, available for reconsideration, and based more on the adolescent patient's developmental dysfunction than on adherence to a particular theoretical approach. At worst, the diagnosis of a character disorder in adolescence can be an expression of the clinician's anger that often results in justifying an inadequate or punitive treatment plan.

Character disorders in adolescence cannot be diagnosed with certainty, and unless the behaviors are extreme, it is difficult to establish a diagnosis with high reliability. However, an understanding of the nature of character disorders can be helpful in organizing treatment plans, and early recognition may increase the availability of alternatives in treatment approaches, raise the likelihood that interventions will be helpful, and ease the pediatrician's sense of confusion and frustration.

CHARACTER IN CONTEXT OF DEVELOPMENT

Adolescent development is described in Chapters 7 and 8. However, it is worth reviewing some aspects of adolescent development, specifically self-confidence, investment in peer relationships, and wishes for peer acceptance and privacy, in an effort to define character pathology.[4]

One important facet of early adolescence is the process of separating emotionally from parents. Young adolescents have an expected surge of self-confidence or narcissism as part of the normal internal processes that support their separation. Parents commonly complain that all of a sudden "she knows it all" or "he thinks he can do anything." Parents are worried that given this pressure to feel confident, their young adolescent will make mistakes and may be emotionally hurt as naive hopes are dashed. Parents also fear that their child will be physically injured because feelings of invulnerability and an inflated sense of physical capabilities will lead to risk taking. As part of the narcissistic aspect of development, adolescents may also be arrogant and act distant, cold, aloof, and selfish—but still expect all the privileges and benefits possible within their family life. In addition, young adolescents may show off, be "exhibitionistic" in their clothing or accomplishments, and harbor grandiose fantasies of success in academics or athletics ("I don't have to study. I'm going to play in the NBA!"). In an adult, the aforementioned set of traits might be consistent with the diagnostic criteria for a narcissistic personality disorder. However, during adolescence, much or all of this behavior is considered normal. Adolescents need this high degree of self-confidence to support their efforts to leave the warmth and safety of their home. Feeling that they are self-sufficient and "ready for anything" helps loosen and defend against the strong feelings of attachment to their parents and to their previous adaptations during childhood.

Another feature of adolescent development is a readiness to invest heavily in peer relationships. Almost overnight, the importance of peers can rival the previously unquestioned priorities of family obligations. Scheduling of family activities, or even a special event such as a dinner for a parent's birthday, can lead to major tensions if the arrangements call for breaking plans with close or even recently acquired friends. Parents may notice certain patterns in these peer relationships. Sometimes the longings to be accepted are so strong that adolescents may not lift a finger at home but rearrange their whole day if a friend calls. Self-confidence, even inflated, is not sufficient support for adolescents to begin to separate from family. Peer relationships are a haven and a critical source of information, feedback, and encouragement. The combination of inflated self-

confidence and peer support provides support for the adolescent to loosen emotional ties to parents and develop an emerging sense of autonomy.

As a normal part of adolescence, some teenagers at times are highly dependent on peer acceptance and seem to devalue their own wishes, priorities, values, or good judgment. They appear to change their personality radically to gain a friend's praise or acceptance. If a crush is involved, parents worry that their previously reasonable child will do almost anything (e.g., lie, get drunk, have sexual intercourse) to be included or loved. Parents wonder if it is normal to be so dependent on others' judgments, a trait that could lead to being too differential toward the wishes of others or to a lifelong personality style marked by low self-esteem and a pattern of being exploited.

A common aspect of adolescent development is questioning or breaking rules. The range of misbehavior or poor conduct can include lying, cheating on a homework assignment, shoplifting, and substance abuse. Even frankly delinquent and interpersonally violent behavior, although cause for alarm and outside the normal range, is still not definitively predictive of an antisocial character disorder (criminality) in adulthood.

Privacy and the wish to be alone are a normal and expected part of adolescent development. It is not unusual for teenagers to become secretive, providing little information to adults, restricting access to their room, and even isolating themselves from peer relationships. There is a self-absorption, a turning inward, that worries parents about their child's capacity to be socially involved or close to others. Sometimes these adolescents have a secret worry about their popularity, attractiveness, or sexuality and absolutely will not share their insecurity or anxiety, instead choosing to be alone and lonely. Parents wonder why their child never goes out, stays in his or her room, refuses phone calls, and declines opportunities to go out with long-standing friends. Parents become very concerned that this pattern of behavior is predictive of a lonely life spent avoiding, rather than participating in, social relationships (schizoid personality disorder; if psychotic, schizophrenia) (see Chapter 121, "Schizophrenia").

Sometimes adolescents, like adults, present with a mixture of vague complaints, many of them somatic (see Chapter 119, "Conversion Reactions and Psychosomatic Disorders"). Again, either as a part of normal adolescence or an early indication of a personality pattern, an adolescent may complain and seem to manipulate adults by use of these somatic symptoms. In addition, some adolescents are overdramatic, frequently calling attention to themselves and acting highly emotional, oversensitive, or irritable. They are quite demanding and yet helpless. Such a combination may be reminiscent of adults who constantly use their somatic symptoms as a way of communicating or in an attempt to avoid unbearable angry or sad feelings. This behavior in adults may make others angry, but parents should be more understanding of this behavior in teenagers, who are acutely aware of their bodies and for whom everything is changing and some key functions, especially sexual, are unfamiliar, mysterious, private, and untested.

Finally, an organizing task of adolescence is that of forming an identity. During adolescence, there is an expected fluidity in self-image and identity.[5] For example, after walking out of a movie, the adolescent, more likely than most adults, entertains the notion of becoming like one of the movie characters. During adolescence, this "character identification" is normal. For adolescents, the boundaries between the character in the movie and themselves blur and become indistinct. Teenagers may dress and wish to dance like a favorite rock star, fantasize about adventures paralleling a current movie idol, or devote themselves to a philosophy espoused by a favored teacher or coach. This readiness to identify can be profound. The differences between adults' and adolescents' ability to identify with others are not always clear. Adults have the good fortune to maintain some fluidity or plasticity throughout life, and ideally, even in old age, adults can modify personality development in progressive and adaptive ways. Through identification, for example, a political leader or author can influence adults in favor of a new perspective, even to the point of taking significant action. Adults also have the capacity to identify with movie characters and derive pleasure from such fantasizing. However, for adults the boundaries are usually clearer, the impact is more subtle, and the emotional investment is less intense.

It is normal and expected for adolescents to "try on" different identities, or at least different personality features, to see how they fit. They adopt some, discard some, adapt others, and continuously work to integrate their personality with their genetically and psychologically derived identity from preadolescence. Commonly, adolescents in the midst of this process of developing an identity are certain some of the time and uncertain most of the time about who they really are and would like to be. Sometimes this insecure and unstable state of identity can be very stressful, pressuring the adolescent to behave in an extreme manner or even to appear to be paralyzed in daily functioning. The combination of this insecurity with irritability, stormy interpersonal relationships, and labile mood raises parental concerns about the very stability of their child's personality. In adolescence, confusion about one's identity can be normal, may represent a period of dysfunctional searching, or (if very prolonged) may constitute the early manifestation of more enduring ego vulnerabilities sometimes categorized as an adult borderline personality disorder.

Depression can also act to confuse the clinical picture.[6] Major affective disorder, a definable change in mood resulting in dysphoria and associated symptoms (see Chapter 122, "Depression"), or a more chronic, less profound affective disorder called dysthymia can accompany any personality trait or disorder. A 1996 study suggests that character disorders, especially those marked by interpersonal turbulence, may be a greater risk for later depression and suicide.[7]

Even more confusing is the distinction between features of affective disorders and characterologic low self-esteem. The diagnostic criteria of the fourth edition of the *Diagnostic and Statistical Manual of Mental Disorders,* (DSM-IV)[8] are descriptive (like the term "fever") and do not imply an etiology. Like the term *depression,* the term *low self-esteem* is used quite loosely; low self-esteem is not necessarily part of or synonymous with major affective disorder. A rigid, pervasive sense of low self-esteem is an underlying, central feature of all character disorders, whether or not the adolescent meets the diagnostic criteria for depression.

PSYCHIATRIC DIAGNOSIS

The DSM-IV describes the criteria for personality disorders as "an enduring pattern of inner experience and behavior that deviates markedly from the expectations of the individual's culture" in two or more of the following four areas: cognition, affectivity, interpersonal functioning, and impulse control. The DSM-IV lists three clusters of personality disorders: 1) paranoid, schizoid, and schizotypal personality disorders; 2) antisocial, borderline, histrionic, and narcissistic personality disorders; 3) avoidant; dependent and obsessive-compulsive personality disorders. These categories are complex and merit review in the DSM-IV. In Table 120-1 a number of these disorders have been selected and key characteristics have been highlighted.

DSM-IV defines subtypes of character disorder on the basis of clusters of behaviors. These criteria are not dependent on any theory of etiology or treatment but offer a basis for communication and research. Many specific symptoms are common in adolescence, and thus clinicians must use thorough interviewing techniques, clinical experience, and careful subjective judgments to support a formal DSM-IV diagnosis.

Studies of character disorder in adolescence using DSM-IV criteria have focused on diagnostic criteria, interview methodology, validity, and stability of the diagnosis over time. Mattanach et al[9] interviewed 70 hospitalized adolescents, approximately one third of whom had a character disorder. Most continued to meet these diagnostic criteria 2 years later, although some had resolved, changed subtypes, or developed additional

TABLE 120-1 Criteria for Personality Disorders				
Antisocial	**Borderline**	**Histrionic**	**Narcissistic**	**Dependent**
Grounds for arrest; deceitfulness; impulsivity. Irritability; aggressiveness; disregards safety; irresponsibility.	Fear of abandonment; unstable relationships; provocative impulsivity. Inappropriate intense anger; suicidal behavior; affective instability; chronic feelings of emptiness; identity disturbance; stress related paranoia.	Must be center of attention; seductive; power; success; suggestible; exaggerates. Intimacy; appearance to gain attention; rapid shifts in emotion; impressionistic speech; self-dramatizing.	Grandiose; self-important; fantasies of needs others to belief in being "special"; requires great admiration; marked sense of entitlement; lacks empathy. Interpersonally exploitive; marked envy; arrogant; haughty.	Requires excessive amount of advice and assurance. Takes responsibility. Fears loss of support or approval; lack of self confidence. Feels helpless when alone; urgently seeks relationships.

disorders such as depression. Bernstein et al[10] interviewed 733 young adolescents in a community-based sample. A full 17% met criteria for character disorder, although more than one half did not meet criteria 2 years later; however, although there was variability among subtypes, those who did meet the criteria over time tended to be persistent thereafter, and the diagnosis correlated with serious difficulties in school, interpersonal relationships, and family problems.[11]

Antisocial, violent, and criminal character disorders are of special societal concern. This single category may represent several subtypes, including relatively short-lived adolescent delinquent behavior (nonviolent, with peers) and persistent criminal behavior (violent, individual acting alone).[12] Clearly neuropsychologic, genetic, and environmental circumstances may cause, contribute to, or exacerbate all character disorders.

ETIOLOGY: CURRENT THEORIES

The etiology of character disorders is multidetermined. Character develops over many years and involves numerous interacting variables that influence every child's development. This multitude of variables makes character very difficult to study. There is much controversy over which particular factors should be emphasized in trying to explain the cause of character difficulties. Are genetic factors the predominant influence?[13] Does a child's temperament, either by being similar to one parent's temperament or by having a poor fit with a parent's temperament, predispose to character psychopathology? What is the extent and role of interpersonal factors such as empathy, dedication, and

ability in mastering stress, anxiety, conflict, and developmental challenges? Are there certain neurologically determined patterns of cognition and affective regulation that limit flexibility and begin a process of perceiving and interacting with the world in a narrow or increasingly rigid fashion? What is the effect of other factors such as facility with language or intelligence?

How do early childhood experiences modify genetic or temperamental factors?[10] Some children can endure a tumultuous upbringing and emerge with an intact adaptive character development or some behavioral problems but without severe character disorder, whereas others in the same circumstance suffer from serious underlying character difficulties. Other children have what superficially appears to be a normal childhood and yet display character problems that require careful analysis in order to formulate effective interventions. Further complicating the question of etiology is the role of risk and protective factors. Some children who are at risk because of a family history of psychiatric disorder, disturbed parenting, and genetic endowment seem to be partially protected from character difficulties by a positive relationship with the emotionally healthier parent or other adult; peer friendships in childhood; and special athletic, interpersonal, or academic strengths or skills. On the other hand, some children who do not appear to be at risk may develop a character disorder based solely on consistently disturbed parenting or marked social and economic stress. The overall rate of psychiatric disorder is twice as high for children raised in poverty.[14-16]

Dealing with character-disordered adolescents and their families can be stressful and irritating for the physician. The adolescent's parents, because of their own difficulties or as a response to worrying about their child, can be very anxious, demanding, and hostile.[17] An appreciation of the complexity and multifactorial nature of personality development can help the physician suppress the temptation to make rapid or pejorative judgments about the adolescent's family and about what caused the personality difficulties.

Maladaptive character behavior has particular features. For example, the pattern of the personality and behavior is usually rigid. Individuals with this disorder always rely on the same defenses, interpretations, or perspective to control their unconscious feelings. For example, those with narcissistic personality difficulties may repeatedly organize their world in a self-inflating or aggrandizing manner in an attempt to compensate for their inner, albeit often unconscious, sense of deficiency and emptiness. They may present themselves with an entitled attitude that suggests a superficial sense of self-esteem, but in truth this behavior is an unsuccessful solution to their profound sense of not being worthwhile and valued. Thus, a bad grade or athletic shortcoming is never their fault.

Since character disorders are often based on unyielding defensive structures, reality tends to have little impact. Whether a day laborer or corporate president, an individual with narcissistic difficulties never feels satisfied because money, fame, and titles do not satisfy or address the inner state of feeling deficient. In relationships, the other person may be seen as merely a series of attributes such as intelligence, success, and beauty. The individual with narcissistic difficulties believes then that "I must be a good person since this perfect person is with me and I should love this person because of these attributes." The other person's true identity is not appreciated and a sense of intimacy is not experienced.

On close examination, character disorders demonstrate a repetitive pattern of response. Logic, changing circumstances, or subtleties have little meaning for a person with a character disorder because the character structure is dedicated to avoiding the sadness, anger, emptiness, and anxiety that in childhood necessitated, or at least reinforced, the need for a particular personality pattern.

CORE FEATURES

Difficulty Relating to Others

Individuals with a character disorder have difficulty in interpersonal relationships.[18,19] Their perception of others is rigidly based on their own defensive needs. They are drawn to individuals who are congruous with their view of the world. They often cannot distinguish or differentiate the true attributes of another person from what they need that person to be. For example, an adolescent who needs to be a victim, and to see the world as a place where he or she undoubtedly will be victimized, will select a peer group and act in a manner that invites or even encourages victimization. For example, he will be caught buying liquor for his friends even though he may not have any interest in drinking himself; she may find a boyfriend who is domineering and threatens to reject her if she does not meet his needs. This behavior often extends to every aspect of life. Such an adolescent will somehow always miss the sign-up date for an apparently much desired class or activity. For vague reasons a summer job just does not work out. Efforts to give the adolescent advice not to hang out with certain peers, to resist pressure to behave in ways that will lead to getting in trouble, to be active so that a class schedule works out in the adolescent's favor, or to pick boyfriends who will be kinder and more understanding, will all be ignored. Adolescents who need to be a victim as a way of confirming their low self-esteem will be drawn to peers and situations that result in victimization.

Psychological intimacy requires the capacity to see another person as distinct, complex, and with a range of characteristics (not necessarily all positive and certainly with subtle shadings). An adolescent who chooses friends solely on the basis of their status and how they can be used to the individual's advantage does not see them as whole, complex people, but as objects or tools for gratification. Sharing, empathy, and intimacy are very limited. Sometimes a character-disordered adolescent does choose a friend who does not fit these rigid needs—a boyfriend who is kind and does not try to take advantage or a friend who refuses to victimize. The adolescent finds this refusal to victimize very stressful and the relationship is likely to end, leaving the parents and the pediatrician bewildered. To adults, losing interest in a relationship with such a caring person makes no sense. Parents may then exert pressure to force the adolescent not to see "undesirable" peers, and may invite the right kind of friend for dinner or an outing in an effort to rekindle the friendship. A character-disordered adolescent will be furious, stating, quite accurately, that "you do not understand."

Developmentally, adolescents with character disorders often have had difficulty with friends since toddlerhood. They may have been highly aggressive, withdrawn, insensitive, or unpopular (not invited to birthday parties), and may have chosen not to participate in activities that were likely to lead to friendships (e.g., neighborhood activities, sports, after-school clubs). Many did not have close friendships during elementary school and have had no one whom they could really trust, to whom they could feel close, and with whom they could share private feelings.

When counseling a repeatedly victimized adolescent, the pediatrician may suggest approaches to finding more supportive friends and recommend being more active in applying for a summer job or working out a school schedule. Despite this advice being logical and relatively simple, the adolescent will return with a further history of being victimized and unsuccessful, or of "snatching defeat from the jaws of victory." The pediatrician, corroborating what parents have shared of their own experience, will be bewildered and will probably repeat the advice to the adolescent using a slightly more frustrated and critical tone. Character-disordered adolescents are very sensitive to this change in tone and will protest that the pediatrician does not understand. This pattern may be repeated again in future visits, with building bewilderment and frustration. Even elaborate efforts to help the adolescent are unsuccessful, and the final result is that both the adolescent and the pediatrician feel that they have failed. The pediatrician will feel inadequate in his or her ability to counsel, and the adolescent will feel again a victim of an unempathetic adult.

Conduct-disordered adolescents will be loyal, at least temporarily, to their friends in a rigid manner, and will be unable to relate with any empathy or guilt to the victims of their behavior or aggression. In other types of character disorders, the quality of relating to others can be impaired in a more subtle manner. The pediatrician may feel that despite knowing the patient for many years and attempting to be supportive and understanding, there is a distinct emotional distance unlike his or her relationships with most of the other adolescent patients. Moments of sharing or closeness do not build into a relationship, but may instead result in a canceling of the next appointment or sabotage of the next productive opportunity.

Character-disordered adolescents long for closeness, but such closeness raises such inner turmoil and anxiety that intimacy is usually avoided. Adolescents in intensive psychotherapy report that closeness makes them feel too vulnerable to rejection or reminds them of what they never have had from their parents: a sense of being loved, valued, and worthy. Thus, closeness to peers or other adults can call forth a sense of loneliness or an intense rage at parents. Most frustrating are those rare times when a character-disordered adolescent has an opportunity to develop a positive and intimate relationship through a school activity. Adolescents with character disorders are sometimes pursued through letters and phone calls, invited to participate, and repeatedly asked out, but as parental hopes soar, the relationship soon sours. The character-disordered adolescent does not experience such a relationship as hopeful or fulfilling. Instead, such relationships are alien, do not meet defensive needs, and raise the anxiety about being close sexually and emotionally. Sometimes, such difficulties are related to childhood physical and/or sexual abuse, the history of which is not obvious at the initial evaluation.

Self-Esteem

Character-disordered adolescents have a low sense of self-esteem.[20] On the surface, some may appear cocky and self-confident. They may inflate their accomplishments and blame others for shortcomings or failures. Other adolescents protect their fragile sense of self-worth by lying, stealing, or being physically aggressive. These adolescents can have a profound sense of emptiness, failure, and lack of worth. The roots of low self-esteem often go back to early childhood and persist despite apparent talents and even successes.

Opportunities for success are not taken or are sabotaged because these situations are not consistent with adolescents' internal sense of low self-worth. They will not practice to make the team, will drink at a chaperoned school dance where they are almost assured of being caught, will not file a job application, and will not do a critical term paper even in an area of interest—if they do it, they will lose it or forget to hand it in. If briefly successful, the adolescent will cease participation in an activity, claiming to lose interest or to be unable to continue. In addition, these behaviors may demonstrate fears of success, aggression, competition, or failure. For someone with a character disorder, success means challenging long and rigidly held beliefs about oneself and others. The adolescent with a character disorder may think that "if now I can be successful, popular, cared for, why didn't I have that same feeling with my parents? Why didn't they consider me valuable or lovable? Why did they use me for their needs rather than let me achieve a sense of autonomy or success by my own definition?"

The pain of these feelings far outweighs the benefits of a success, so much so that any success is blocked or sabotaged. Again, both the pediatrician and the parents are bewildered. Why, for the adolescent who complains of feeling like a failure or is obviously hiding a feeling of inadequacy, is success in academic, sports, or social interaction so threatening? At the same time, when the adolescent is failing or unsuccessful, there appears to be the need to continue to do little to reverse the trend.

In contrast to most adolescents, who although insecure gradually build on their successes and avoid failures, character-disordered adolescents fail to master situations and remain in behavior patterns that guarantee failure. Efforts to reassure them that they are worthwhile or to point out their strengths or successes as part of building their self-esteem do not work. Character-disordered adolescents have a complex and multidetermined sense of failure and low self-esteem. Careful thought and planning are necessary to intervene in such a self-perpetuating, self-defeating pattern.

Loss

Character-disordered adolescents have great difficulty tolerating losses. The term "loss" can cover a wide range of experiences. For example, some such adolescents had difficulty separating from their parents on the first day of school or on a regular basis throughout early childhood.

Losses involving other people, such as a friend moving away, a family member dying, a teacher being changed, or parents divorcing, arouse a series of reactions that have some of the characteristics of normal grieving but are more intense, prolonged, and maladaptive. The adolescent does not reach the stage of acceptance or resolution. Even the process of maturing itself (a loss of one's childhood) may result in the adolescent's defenses becoming more rigid. Sometimes, adolescents have a profound reaction to what parents or the pediatrician may consider a relatively minor loss. Often, this behavior occurs because the loss reverberates with earlier losses or has important symbolic importance. Other times, serious losses elicit an almost casual response and a resistance to acknowledging any deeper feelings of sadness. Accepting a broad definition of loss, the pediatrician in taking a history can ask about expected losses the adolescent has experienced (e.g., day care, preschool, elementary school, vacations, family moves) and about serious unexpected losses (e.g., death of a family member or divorce).

All-or-Nothing Perspective

Adolescents with character disorders see the world in very clear-cut, often concrete terms. A teacher, parent, or pediatrician is either good, meaning all good, or bad, meaning all bad. These shifts, or "splitting," can occur quite rapidly: a teacher who was great one day is the worst teacher the adolescent has ever had the next. These complete turnarounds can be provoked by relatively minor events: the teacher may be critical of an essay, the parent may disagree about clothing or curfew, or the pediatrician may have gone just a little too far in pressuring for a change in behavior.

The basis for the all-or-nothing perspective is how the adolescent relates to other people. Since adolescents do not see the whole person but only those parts that agree with their own view of the world, a relatively small change in a limited area of the other person's personality can elicit a total response from character-disordered adolescents. For example, in a classroom, the teacher is seen as *either* accepting *or* rejecting. Adolescents at one level wish for acceptance and closeness but at another level cannot tolerate such closeness, as they are certain of being unworthy. When the teacher is accepting as they the adolescents crave such acceptance, the teacher is viewed as perfect. However, if at that same moment the teacher is critical, the teacher is seen as all bad. This perspective is often related to an early developmental difficulty in integrating caretakers' behavior as both gratifying and frustrating, understanding good and bad, and tolerating ambivalence and ambiguity. Adolescents with these difficulties do not view criticism as constructive or ultimately caring. These adolescents do not see the mood or multifaceted character of the teacher, and have difficulty integrating criticism in the context of a total relationship. Tragically for these adolescents, others are "only as good as their last pitch." Even if every previous "pitch" has been good, the all-or-nothing perspective of these adolescents ultimately results in rejection or a loss of interest that inhibits developing deepening personal relationships.

This all-or-nothing perspective also applies to right and wrong. Often, character-disordered adolescents are very harsh in their judgments and are unforgiving and unmerciful in their expectations concerning adult behavior. They focus on one aspect of a complex social or emotional situation and base a value judgment on that single aspect. Although there may be a good reason to change a rule (e.g., limiting driving on the night of a snowstorm), adolescents determine both that a promise has been broken and that the parent has become bad because of this "arbitrary" decision. Unfortunately, adolescents' harsh sense of right and wrong is applied equally to themselves. When they recognize something they have done as "wrong," they berate themselves and attack their already vulnerable sense of self-esteem. They may punish themselves with suicidal thoughts, poor self-care, or (if anorectic) starvation.

CLINICAL APPROACH TO DIAGNOSIS

Every pediatrician will be able to remember many adolescents with features similar to those discussed above. Certainly, in any single interview and for a relatively brief period of adolescent development, virtually every adolescent will exhibit some of the extreme behaviors discussed. There may be an overreaction to a minor loss, a period of low self-esteem, awkwardness in social relationships, and "black and white" thinking. However, on more careful reflection, pediatricians will note that of all the adolescents they have cared for, the number of those who exhibited most or all of these features consistently throughout their adolescence is quite low. For most pediatricians, these adolescents stand out as ones about whom the pediatrician had worried and had tried to counsel or refer for psychotherapy; whose parents called repeatedly because of ongoing difficulties or crises; and who had evoked in the pediatrician feelings of being helpless, inadequate, and frustrated.

The following points may be helpful in approaching the diagnosis of character disorder:

1. The diagnosis can be considered, but not confirmed, in a single interview. Character-disordered adolescents, as well as adolescents in general, usually respond better to shorter interviews (15 to 20 minutes) that review particular aspects of their development, rather than long interviews that attempt to be comprehensive. Multiple interviews

also give the pediatrician a chance to assess the quality of adolescents' relationship with them, their response to suggestions, and their ability to be reflective about their feelings and other people's reactions to them.

2. In a true character-disordered adolescent, the defensive pattern must be consistent and rigid. Such an adolescent will approach a wide variety of situations with the same underlying defensive structure. On the surface, the adolescent's responses may appear flexible, rational, and even sophisticated. However, the reasoning may not be quite right and may arouse a vague uneasiness, and the pediatrician may feel that further discussion and observation are required to understand the underlying process and motives of the adolescent's behavior.

3. The pediatrician must ascertain that the behavior patterns have been consistent over time. Character disorders form in early childhood and then become clearer at the time of school-age years and early adolescence. Some of the patterns, such as low self-esteem and difficulties with intimacy or close relationships, may be present for many years.

4. The pediatrician must approach the treatment of an adolescent with a character disorder in the knowledge that such disorders take many years to develop and many years to treat. When there is a crisis, the focus of the initial interview should be crisis intervention and support. Trying to understand the adolescent's character is a process that occurs after the crisis has calmed and the pediatrician has had the opportunity to spend several sessions interviewing the adolescent and gathering history from the family.

5. If over several interviews the adolescent, by history and clinical impression, demonstrates a pattern of difficulties in interpersonal relationships, chronic low self-esteem, unusual response to losses, and a "black and white" quality in thinking and judgments, the pediatrician has grounds to be concerned about his or her character development.

MANAGEMENT

A character disorder should be viewed as among the most serious problems in pediatric practice. Such disorders can result in intense emotional suffering and lifelong difficulties in functioning. The intensity of the pediatrician's immediate response should correspond to the degree of current dysfunction and emotional distress. Certainly a crisis may require immediate action, but usually the time course for treating a character-disordered adolescent is measured in years. Treatment requires a

thoughtful, comprehensive plan that addresses both current areas of day-to-day life as well as the establishment of a long-term relationship with a psychotherapist to address the deeper personality issues.

The first step is the pediatrician's attempt to develop a relationship and gather sufficient information so that the adolescent will accept possible interventions. Many character-disordered adolescents believe that the world is exactly as they see it, a belief that is rooted in their defensive structure and deepest emotional needs. Pediatricians face inevitable frustration because when they give advice that might contribute to adolescents' success, the latter may need to quickly give up. Sound advice leads to failure, and giving no advice leaves the pediatrician feeling helpless. Any hint of frustration distances adolescents, confirms their sense of being a failure, and supports their opinion that "you don't understand." The pediatrician can easily get caught in arguing with the adolescent about a treatment referral or intervention, and thus be regarded again as a critical and controlling adult, causing the adolescent to become uncooperative. Unless there is an acute emergency (suicide attempt, court-ordered treatment), the pediatrician should gather information by gently exploring adolescents' difficulties in functioning and inner emotional state. It is best to try to discern adolescents' goals and then assess, in a gentle and empathic manner, the quality of peer relationships, the nature of family life, and the current status of academic work. Are the adolescents satisfied with their current relationships? Do they want closer friends? Do they want girlfriends or boyfriends? Do they want to achieve a certain goal in sports or in preparation for college? Are there areas of family functioning that are disruptive, hostile, and unsatisfying? Often by being very practically focused, nonjudgmental, and working from the adolescents' perspective, the pediatrician will begin to generate a list of goals that have not been met and are unlikely to be accomplished without help. This approach will not work in a single interview.

If after several interviews the adolescent is still highly resistant, it is often useful to set up a series of contingency agreements. To avoid being seen as controlling and adversarial, the pediatrician may suggest that the adolescent, if the individual wishes, may try to accomplish selected goals on his or her own. The tone needs to be supportive and not challenging. For example, the pediatrician and adolescent could agree on limiting the use of substances such as alcohol, on ways to improve work at school, on approaches to developing closer friendships, or on ways the adolescent might try to ease some of the tensions at home. Such goals allow the pediatrician to join the adolescent, be on the "same side," and respect the adolescent's wishes but yet stay involved in terms of evaluating the outcome of these efforts. Possibly a month later there could be a second or third meeting, the goals reviewed, new goals set, and then another meeting scheduled. Over several months it will become clear whether the adolescent has the ability to make the necessary changes, and thus probably does *not* have a character disorder, or whether these efforts are unsuccessful and further professional help is required. At the end of several months and several unsuccessful plans, the adolescent may be able to see a limiting or self-destructive pattern in his or her own behavior and be willing to take the next step. At that point, the adolescent's parents probably should play an active role in trying to understand the issues, and the pediatrician should begin to look for a highly experienced, sophisticated, and dedicated psychotherapist.

The initial choice of therapist is key. Adolescents often attach to the first therapist they meet and do not tolerate meeting several in the process of "choosing." If there is a poor match, followed by a second, even more carefully selected referral is indicated. It is important to try to find an experienced therapist with whom the adolescent feels a sense of rapport. The pediatrician must be able to trust and have faith in the therapist, because the recommendations will often be complex and costly.

The therapeutic process itself is often stormy. Even under near-ideal circumstances, the psychotherapy of a character-disordered adolescent is marked by periods of slow or apparent loss of progress. The adolescent tests the therapist and parents by possibly setting up the therapist to be fired or overly revered. Sometimes the pediatrician is drawn into this behavior and enlisted in the tensions evoked by the therapy. The pediatrician should remember that the therapist is in a difficult role, constantly walking a tightrope between being too close to the adolescent and thus provoking flight, or too distant and leaving the adolescent feeling lonely and rejected. The success of therapy cannot be assessed in weeks or even months. At times the pediatrician will need to support the therapeutic plan on the basis of a discussion with the therapist and a little faith.

Treating character disorders requires a serious commitment on the part of the family in supporting the therapy and a time frame of several years. If the diagnosis is confirmed by psychiatric or psychologic evaluation, the pediatrician should support a major treatment effort. Character disorders are serious and, under the best of circumstances, very difficult to modify. At a minimum there will need to be psychotherapy (commonly more than once a week), meetings with the family by either the same or a different therapist, and a careful review of the adolescent's day-to-day life in an effort to create an environment to support the treatment. Sometimes a comprehensive outpatient program is not sufficient, and if outpatient treatment is unsuccessful, a more intensive residential treatment approach may be necessary.

CONCLUSION

Character disorders do not develop by choice but reflect adolescents' solutions to overwhelming emotions or critical, often multiple, life events experienced in early childhood. Their solution is costly because the price for adapting and surviving in the world they perceive is a poor self-image, difficulty in interpersonal relationships, a rigid approach to life choices, and a profound sense of loneliness. Treatment is difficult and lengthy. Patience, understanding, support, and referral by the pediatrician to qualified professionals can be critical to early recognition and sustained treatment of the disorder.

References

1. Freud A: Adolescence, *Psychoanal Study Child* 13:255-278, 1958.
2. Rutter M: Psychopathology and development: links between childhood and adult life. In Rutter M, Herzov L, editors: *Child and adolescent psychiatry: modern approaches,* Oxford, 1985, Blackwell Scientific; pp 720-742.
3. Parnas J, Teasdale TW, Schulsinger H: Continuity of character neurosis from childhood to adulthood, *Acta Psychiatr Scand* 66:491-498, 1982.
4. Golombek H, Marton P: Adolescents over time: a longitudinal study of personality development, *Adolesc Psychiatry* 18:213-284, 1992.
5. Korenblum M, Marton P, Golombek H, Stein B: Disturbed personality functioning: patterns of change from early to middle adolescence, *Adolesc Psychiatry* 14:407-416, 1987.
6. Marton P, Korenblum M, Kutcher S, Stein B, Kennedy B, Pakes J: Personality dysfunction in depressed adolescents, *Can J Psychiatry* 34:810-813, 1989.
7. Isometsa ET, Henriksson MM, Heikkinen ME, Aro HM, Marttunen MJ, Kuoppasalmi KI, Lonnqvist JK: Suicide among subjects with personality disorders, *Am J Psychiatry* 153:667-673, 1996.
8. American Psychiatric Association: *Diagnostic and statistical manual of mental disorders,* ed 4, Washington, DC, 1994, American Psychiatric Association.
9. Mattanach JJF, Becker DF, Levy KN, Edell WS, McGlashan TH: Diagnostic stability in adolescents followed up 2 years after hospitalization, *Am J Psychiatry* 152:889-894, 1995.
10. Bernstein DP, Cohen P, Velez CN, Schwab-Stone M, Siever LJ, Shinsato L: Prevalence and stability of the DSM-III-R personality disorders in a community based survey of adolescents, *Am J Psychiatry* 150:1237-1243, 1993.
11. Ludolph PS, Westen D, Misle B, Jackson A, Wixom J, Wiss FC: The borderline diagnosis in adolescents: symptoms and developmental history, *Am J Psychiatry* 147:470-476, 1990.
12. Moffitt TE: Adolescence and life-course-persistent antisocial behavior: a developmental taxonomy, *Psychol Rev* 100:674-701, 1993.
13. Loranger AW, Oldham JM, Tulis EH: Familial transmission of DSM-III borderline personality disorder, *Arch Gen Psychiatry* 39:795-799, 1982.
14. Schorr L: *Within our reach: breaking the cycle of disadvantage,* New York, 1988, Doubleday.
15. Anderson J, Williams S, McGee R, Silva P: Cognitive and social correlates of DSM-III disorders in pre-adolescent children, *J Am Acad Child Adolesc Psychiatry* 28:842-846, 1989.
16. Offord DR, Boyle MH, Racine Y: Ontario Child Health Study: correlates of disorder, *J Am Acad Child Adolesc Psychiatry* 28:856-860, 1989.

17. Beresin E: The difficult parent. In Jellinek MS, Herzog DB, editors: *Massachusetts General Hospital Psychiatric Aspects of General Hospital Pediatrics,* Chicago, 1990, Mosby–Year Book; pp 67-77.

18. Drake RE, Vaillant GE: A validity study of axis II of DSM-III, *Am J Psychiatry* 142:553-558, 1985.

19. Brent DA, Zelenak JP, Bukstein O, Brown RV: Reliability and validity of the structured interview for personality disorders in adolescents, *J Am Acad Child Adolesc Psychiatry* 29:349-354, 1990.

20. Mack J, Ablon S, editors: *The development and sustaining of self esteem in childhood,* New York, 1983, International Universities Press.

Suggested Readings

Freud A: Adolescence, *Psychoanal Study Child* 13:255-278, 1958.

Lewis M, Volkmar F: *Adolescence. Clinical aspects of child development,* ed 3, Philadelphia, 1990, Lea & Febiger; pp 211-252.

Rutter M, Herzov L, editors: *Child and adolescent psychiatry: modern approaches,* Oxford, 1994, Blackwell Scientific.

CHAPTER 121

Schizophrenia

•

Irving B. Weiner

Schizophrenia is a serious mental disorder that occurs in approximately 1% of the population and usually begins during the late adolescent and early adult years. About one third of people who develop schizophrenic disorder experience their first episode of breakdown before age 20. The earlier in adolescence a young person becomes overtly schizophrenic, the more likely he or she is to suffer persistent or recurrent psychologic disorder. Among individuals who first manifest schizophrenia in adulthood, the adolescent years are typically marked by prodromal adjustment difficulties. Hence, adolescence is a critical time both for diagnosing and treating schizophrenic disorder and for identifying preschizophrenic patterns of development that call for preventive intervention.

Schizophrenia consists of impaired capacities to think clearly and logically, perceive experiences realistically, relate comfortably to other people, and integrate emotions adequately. Among adolescents and adults alike, these functioning impairments result in (1) disordered thinking, which involves confused and tangential ideation and arbitrary or circumstantial reasoning; (2) inaccurate perception, which entails forming distorted or incorrect impressions of objects and events and misjudging the consequences of one's actions; (3) interpersonal ineptness, which is defined by poor social skills and concomitant difficulty in establishing and maintaining mutual relationships with other people; and (4) inappropriate affect, which constitutes ways of experiencing and expressing feelings that are not congruent with actual circumstances.

These functioning impairments give rise to the primary symptoms by which schizophrenia is diagnosed in clinical practice. Disordered thinking produces dissociation, incoherence, delusions, strange language usage, and either impoverished speech (blocking) or overly elaborate and pressured speech. Inaccurate perception gives rise to peculiar and disruptive ways of behaving, mistaken ideas that the actions of others have reference to oneself ("The President is going to speak to me on TV tonight"), odd beliefs ("People can read my mind"), and hallucinations and other unusual sensory experiences ("I sense the presence of powerful forces in the room"). Interpersonal ineptness results in marked social isolation and withdrawal from involvement with people. Inappropriate affect gives rise to exceedingly intense or extremely flat emotions and inexplicable expressions of gloom or gaiety.

ORIGIN

Schizophrenia is a disorder of uncertain origin that appears to result from an interacting combination of constitutional vulnerability and experiential stress. Substantial evidence indicates that constitutional vulnerability to schizophrenia is genetically influenced. The more closely a person is related to someone with schizophrenia, the more likely that person is to be at risk for the disorder. Compared with its 1% prevalence in the general population, schizophrenia occurs in approximately 10% of persons who have a schizophrenic sibling or schizophrenic nonidentical twin, 10% of persons with one schizophrenic parent, 35% of persons born to two schizophrenic parents, and over 45% of identical twins of schizophrenic persons.

Family studies point to a neurointegrative defect as the likely inherited characteristic that creates a constitutional vulnerability to becoming schizophrenic. Long before they become cognitively or emotionally disturbed, children who are at risk for schizophrenia by virtue of a family history of the disorder are more likely than their peers to manifest a variety of neuropsychologic and neurophysiologic abnormalities, such as delayed perceptual-motor development and low thresholds of autonomic nervous system reactivity. Defective neurointegration in schizophrenia is currently believed to derive from an imbalance in neurotransmitters.

On the other hand, because more than 50% of the identical twins of schizophrenic persons and 65% of children born to two schizophrenic parents do not become schizophrenic, it is clear that life experiences also influence who develops this disorder. In particular, research findings implicate certain patterns of deviant family communication that interfere with children forming a firm sense of reality, learning to think clearly, and becoming comfortable with close personal relationships. Parents who express themselves in confusing and impersonal ways and whose messages convey ambivalent feelings may contribute to their children learning maladaptive ways of adapting to the world.

Whereas the influence of both constitutional and experiential factors appears necessary for schizophrenia to emerge, neither are sufficient by themselves. In a widely held diathesis-stress theory of the cause of schizophrenia it is presumed that an additive interaction between a genetically transmitted neurointegrative defect and disturbed patterns of family communication are involved in producing this disorder. The stronger the genetic disposition, the more likely schizophrenia is to emerge in the context of even minimal psychologic stress. Conversely, the milder the genetic disposition, the more family disorganization and other environmental pressure a person can withstand without becoming schizophrenic.

RECOGNITION

To recognize possible schizophrenia in adolescent patients, the clinician should first listen to them to detect indications that they are thinking in a peculiar fashion or harboring far-fetched ideas. Because the thoughts of schizophrenic people are only loosely connected, their conversation is often disorganized and difficult to follow. They may lose track of what they are saying, even in the middle of a sentence, and their conversation will wander off to a different topic. They may answer questions as if they heard something different from what was asked (e.g., asked "How do your parents feel about all this?", a boy replies, "My parents are in good health," which demonstrates a subtle dissociation based on selective attention to how the parents are feeling physically rather than to the full meaning of the question). Sometimes, schizophrenic patients complain of being unable to keep their attention focused or their thoughts straight. At other times, without being aware of how their disordered thinking is affecting their language usage, they may speak in stilted or even incomprehensible phrases (e.g., "I don't converse with the female gender, because I have a disinclination for sexuality"), or may talk in a sing-song or strangely inflected manner as if they are struggling to communicate in a foreign language rather than in their native tongue.

Clinicians may at times come away from an interview with a schizophrenic patient feeling that, because they have obtained incomplete or confusing information, they have failed to ask the right questions or to ask them in the proper way. Those who have limited previous experience with such severely disturbed young people are particularly prone in such circumstances to question their interviewing skills or capacities to make adequate contact with their patients. In fact, however, a perplexing and disjointed interview with a schizophrenic adolescent is more often a consequence of the young person's disordered thinking than of the clinician's ineptness. Accordingly, marked difficulty in carrying on a coherent, logical, and informative conversation with an adolescent patient can often provide a clue to possible schizophrenic disorder.

People whose perceptions are inaccurate tend to report various kinds of unrealistic impressions of themselves and their life experiences and to show poor judgment in anticipating how one set of circumstances is likely to lead to another. They may describe themselves as brilliant and talented or as stupid and deformed when neither self-perception is justified by any objective evidence. They may feel certain that the future has extraordinarily good or bad things in store for them (e.g., "I'm going to be a famous ballerina," "I'm doomed to be an outcast for life") when the expectation does not seem at all warranted. They may report frequent occasions when, because they failed to anticipate correctly the outcome of their actions, they caused unintended physical or psychologic harm to themselves or others (e.g., "For some reason everyone ended up not liking me and saying I shouldn't come back anymore," "I didn't realize I was doing something that would make her feel so bad"). Schizophrenic patients may even misperceive the nature of the interview situation and the identity of the interviewer. For example, a schizophrenic girl, told that she was going to be asked a few questions, asked, "How many days will it take?" A schizophrenic boy, greeted at the beginning of an interview by the physician who stated, "Hello, I'm Dr. —", replied, "No, you're not; you may work here but I can tell you're not a doctor."

Aside from the content of what they are saying, the manner in which schizophrenic adolescents relate to the clinician while answering questions or volunteering information often lends an air of peculiarity or strangeness to the interview. Some of these young people, without seeming shy or anxious, keep themselves distant from the interviewer and detached from the proceedings. They sit far away with their eyes averted, appear almost oblivious to the interviewer's presence, and talk about themselves as if they were discussing a third person. Others become intensely involved in what they are saying and excessively engaged with the interviewer. They draw their chair up unusually close, keep unwavering eye contact with the interviewer, and pour out intimate concerns as if they were talking to a close personal friend. Both of these patterns are inappropriate to the actual circumstances of the interview and reflect a combination of poor judgment and limited social skills.

When a young person's conversation and interview behavior suggest strange ways of thinking, perceiving, and relating, the clinical history should be examined for three features that will increase the likelihood of a diagnosis of overt or emerging schizophrenia in an adolescent who has become behaviorally disturbed. The first risk factor is any instance of documented schizophrenia among biologic relatives. A family history never proves that the disorder is present, because the previously noted concordance data indicate that 90% of children born to a schizophrenic parent do not become schizophrenic. Nevertheless, adolescents with a schizophrenic parent are ten times more likely to develop this condition than adolescents without such a family history.

The other two risk factors are dramatic patterns of either withdrawal or misconduct. Persistent lack of peer-group relationships is one of the most reliable developmental predictors of subsequent psychologic disturbance, and growing up friendless and isolated is often a precursor to schizophrenic breakdown. Handicapped by limited social skills and usually fearful of close contact with others, young people who are progressing toward a schizophrenic disorder frequently have a premorbid history of withdrawal from interpersonal intimacy and uninvolvement in peer-group activities.

At times, pre-schizophrenic adolescents may give an illusory appearance of having an active social life or many friends. Careful investigation in such cases usually reveals that these "social" activities consist of being among groups but not really part of them, or of being around people but not really personally engaged with them. The "friends" turn out to be few rather than many in number; they are seen only occasionally rather than

regularly and in the context of only a few rather than many shared activities; and their relationship with the patient is more likely to be casual, cool, or exploitative than close, warm, and mutual.

In using withdrawal as a diagnostic clue, clinicians need to distinguish between pre-schizophrenic isolation and a diminished interest in people and activities that may be associated with a depressive disorder. Like adults, adolescents who become sad or discouraged often become disenchanted with pursuits they previously enjoyed and disengage from social activities. The distinction between pre-schizophrenic isolation and depressive loss of interest can usually be made on the basis of developmental events. The basic impairment of capacities for interpersonal relatedness that characterizes schizophrenia typically produces chronic social difficulties that can be traced to an adolescent's childhood years. In depression, by contrast, withdrawal is a consequence rather than a basic feature of the disorder. Hence, social disinterest due to depression will have begun relatively recently, in the context of depressive episodes, following a premorbid developmental history of age-appropriate social relationships.

Misconduct refers to a broad range of defiant, disruptive, and destructive behaviors exhibited by young people that hurt the feelings of others, damage property, and do harm to themselves and others. These kinds of misconduct do not bear any necessary or unique relationship to schizophrenic disorder. Often they are derived from basically antisocial attitudes (as seen in youthful conduct disorder), and often they alternatively represent neurotically determined ways of trying to exert some influence on the environment (as seen in manipulative, acting-out behavior). Occasionally, however, misconduct emerges for neither of these reasons but is instead a consequence of poor judgment and inadequate self-control. In this case, the possibility of emerging schizophrenia needs to be considered.

Behaviorally disordered adolescents who act in harmful and inconsiderate ways unintentionally, as a result of failing to appreciate the potential offensiveness of their actions or being unable to prevent themselves from exhibiting such behavior, are more likely than other troubled teenagers to be progressing toward schizophrenic disorder. The more serious the outcome of such lapses of judgment and self-control, especially when they lead to physical assaults on others or wanton destruction of property, the greater is the likelihood of emerging schizophrenia.

MANAGEMENT

For adolescents who display strange ways of thinking, perceiving, and relating on interview; whose family history is positive for schizophrenia; and who manifest markedly abnormal patterns of withdrawal and misconduct, overt or emerging schizophrenia is a definite diagnostic possibility. A definitive differential diagnosis of schizophrenia in disturbed adolescents is difficult to achieve, however. Often, extensive interviewing and psychologic test evaluation are necessary to identify the condition with certainty, especially in its early and mild stages. Hence, primary care physicians who suspect schizophrenic disorder in an adolescent patient are usually well-advised to seek diagnostic consultation with a mental-health specialist.

Parents in these instances, and sometimes the adolescents themselves, often have sensed that something more is wrong with the young person than a physical imbalance or some normal mental or emotional variation. They may well have consulted their primary care physician as an intermediate step toward seeking a mental-health evaluation, and they may be receptive to a suggested consultation with a psychologist or psychiatrist. At other times, families are totally unaware, or are doing their best to deny, that the adolescent's problems reflect a significant psychologic disturbance. In these cases the primary care physician should discuss with them as gently and supportively as possible the observation that the young person's problems seem related to having difficulty thinking clearly, seeing things accurately, and feeling comfortable around people. The physician should suggest accordingly that it would be helpful to bring in a consultant who is an expert on how teenagers think, perceive, and relate to each other.

With respect to therapy, schizophrenia is usually best treated with a judicious combination of psychotherapy, medication, and a residential milieu. The treatment is designed to minimize the basic cognitive, social, and emotional impairments that characterize this condition, with particular emphasis on helping schizophrenic adolescents to perceive their experience more realistically, which contributes to more adaptive judgment, and to handle social situations more skillfully, which contributes to more adaptive interpersonal relatedness.

For some adolescents who are pre-schizophrenic and at risk for progression of the disorder, outpatient therapy may be sufficient to arrest or reverse the progression without their having to enter the hospital. Among schizophrenic adolescents who are hospitalized, many whose disturbance is relatively mild are treated mainly on an outpatient basis after a brief period of hospitalization. Because of the specialized nature of office management of schizophrenic patients and the time investment it requires, primary care physicians ordinarily choose to refer adolescents elsewhere for therapy if their impressions and a consultant's opinion indicate schizophrenic disorder.

Suggested Readings

Costello CG, editor: *Symptoms of schizophrenia,* New York, 1993, John Wiley.

Kremen WS, Seidman LJ, Pepple JR, et al: Neuropsychological risk indicators for schizophrenia: a review of family studies, *Schizophr Bull* 20:103-120, 1994.

Lieberman JA, Koreen AR: Neurochemistry and neuroendocrinology of schizophrenia, *Schizophr Bull* 19:371-430, 1993.

McClellan J, Werry J: Practice parameters for the assessment and treatment of children and adolescents with schizophrenia, *J Am Acad Child Adolesc Psychiatry* 33:616-635, 1994.

McGue M, Gottesman II: Genetic linkage in schizophrenia: perspectives from genetic epidemiology, *Schizophr Bull* 15:453-464, 1989.

Miklowitz DJ: Family risk indicators in schizophrenia, *Schizophr Bull* 20:137-150, 1994.

Weiner IB: *Psychological disturbance in adolescence,* ed 2, New York, 1992, John Wiley.

CHAPTER 122

Depression

•

France Chaput, Donna Moreau, and Laura Mufson

Depression among adolescents is a major public health problem for two reasons: (1) it is a prevalent form of psychopathology in this population and (2) it is also an underidentified disorder. Research findings show that most adolescents do not experience major turmoil, but negative views of the self or the future and major conflictual relationships with parents are still often interpreted as part of "normal" adolescent development. Also, behavioral symptoms such as delinquency or drug abuse, often associated with depression, may deflect attention from a depressive symptomatology. Furthermore, the quiet nature of depression in many adolescents, associated with a decreased ability or desire to communicate feelings, makes the recognition of a depressive disorder difficult.

As a result of underidentification, depression remains largely undertreated. In a sample of 5596 students in ninth to twelfth grade, only slightly more than 50% of the students with a diagnosis of depressive disorder had come to clinical attention.[1] Moreover, studies of help-seeking behaviors in adolescents show that disturbed adolescents seek help from friends rather than parents and may therefore be less likely to be referred to a professional.

In addition to high prevalence and low treatment rates, several other characteristics of depression in adolescence make it a significant concern: (1) it is a major risk factor for a suicide attempt, (2) the course is typically of long duration with recurrent episodes, and (3) there are long-term effects on psychosocial functioning in adulthood.

CLASSIFICATION

It is critical to differentiate normal sadness experienced by all individuals at various points in their lives from clinical depression. The diagnostic system used in the United States (DSM-IV),[2] developed by the American Psychiatric Association, defines several categories of depressive disorders on the basis of three major types of criteria: the depressed mood has to be associated with a

set of other symptoms, the constellation of symptoms has to be present for a specified duration, and the constellation must result in significant emotional distress or functional impairment.

Despite minor variations attributable to developmental stage, the clinical presentation of adolescent depression is similar to the adult presentation and currently there are no separate diagnostic categories for depressive disorders in children and adolescents. The adult criteria are applied with a few specific modifications: depressed mood in adults may be replaced by irritable mood in children and adolescents, and a duration of 1 year, instead of 2, is required for the diagnosis of dysthymic disorder.

When the depressive syndrome appears to be induced by alcohol abuse, drug abuse, medication, or the physiological effect of a medical condition, it is no longer classified as a depressive disorder, and the following diagnoses are given, depending on the etiology: substance-related disorder, medication-induced disorder, or mood disorder due to a general medical condition.

Major Depressive Disorder

Major depressive disorder is diagnosed when there is a history of one or more major depressive episodes without a history of manic, mixed (manic-depressed), or hypomanic episodes. To meet the criteria for a major depressive episode, the adolescent must have experienced at least five of the symptoms listed in Box 122-1 nearly every day for a minimum of 2 weeks. At least one of the symptoms must be depressed/irritable mood or decreased interest/pleasure, and this condition must represent a change from previous functioning. The presence of psychotic symptoms such as delusions or hallucinations should be specified.

Dysthymic Disorder

Dysthymic disorder is a chronic form of depression with a milder presentation than major depression. The depressed or irritable mood, and two of the follow-

BOX 122-1
Criteria for Major Depressive Episode

- Depressed or irritable mood most of the day
- Significantly decreased interest or pleasure in almost all activities
- Significant change in weight or appetite
- Insomnia or hypersomnia
- Fatigue or loss of energy
- Difficulty concentrating or making decisions
- Observable psychomotor agitation or retardation
- Feelings of worthlessness or excessive guilt
- Recurrent suicidal thoughts with/without a plan or suicide attempt

Adapted from American Psychiatric Association: Diagnostic and statistical manual of mental disorders, ed 4, Washington, D.C., 1994, American Psychiatric Association.

ing symptoms, have to be present for more days than not in a period of at least 1 year: (1) appetite change, (2) sleep change, (3) low energy or fatigue, (4) low self-esteem, (5) difficulty concentrating or making decisions, or (6) feelings of hopelessness. During this 1-year period the adolescent must not have been symptom-free for more than 2 months.

Other Subtypes of Depression

ADJUSTMENT DISORDER WITH DEPRESSED MOOD. This diagnosis is given when the development of the depressive symptoms is in response to an identifiable psychosocial stressor but the episode does not meet the criteria for major depression or dysthymia. Stressors may be acute or chronic. The most common life events that may cause an adjustment disorder include divorce of parents, family illness, personal illness or injury, household relocation, change of school, pregnancy or abortion, and termination of an important relationship. To meet the criteria, the reaction must be viewed as in excess of a normal reaction to the event or must cause a significant functional impairment. The DSM-IV classification specifies that the disturbance must occur within 3 months of the onset of the stressor and must resolve within 6 months after the stressor's termination. The course is specified as acute if the duration of the episode is less than 6 months, or chronic if the duration of the episode is 6 months or longer. An initial diagnosis of adjustment disorder may be changed later to a diagnosis of major depression if the severity of the disturbance increases, or to a diagnosis of dysthymia if the disturbance follows a very prolonged course after the stressful situation has resolved.

BEREAVEMENT. This diagnosis is given when the disturbance caused by the death of a loved one does not meet the criteria for a major depressive episode. The usual

symptoms are depressed mood, insomnia, decreased appetite, and difficulty concentrating. These are considered to be part of normal grief unless they persist for more than 2 months or are accompanied by severe psychomotor retardation or agitation, excessive guilt, recurrent suicidal thoughts, marked functional impairment, or psychotic symptoms.

BIPOLAR DISORDER. If an adolescent who presents with a depressive episode has a history of one or several manic or hypomanic episodes (periods of euphoria or irritability with increased energy, increased activity, decreased need for sleep, increased talkativeness, racing thoughts, inflated self-esteem), the diagnosis is bipolar disorder, most recent episode depressed. When there is no such history, the adolescent is given a diagnosis of depressive disorder, in the knowledge that a bipolar course is possible. Some clinical features of the depression may help predict a bipolar course: acute onset, psychomotor retardation, and the presence of psychotic features.[3]

DEPRESSIVE DISORDER NOT OTHERWISE SPECIFIED. This entity is a residual diagnostic category used when a depressed individual does not meet the criteria for any of the above-mentioned disorders, either because the adolescent presents with fewer symptoms than required or because the duration is shorter than necessary. The diagnosis is also used when the depressive syndrome is superimposed on schizophrenia or delusional disorder, or when it has not been possible to determine whether it has been induced by alcohol or drug abuse or by the physiological effects of a general medical condition.

EPIDEMIOLOGY

Prevalence in Community Samples

Studies conducted in the general population to assess the prevalence of *depressed mood* or other isolated depressive symptoms have shown that rates in adolescence are quite high. In Rutter's pioneering Isle of Wight study, 42% of the boys and 48% of the girls aged 14 to 15 years reported "some appreciable misery or depression" during clinical interviews, 20% expressed feelings of self-deprecation, and 7% to 8% reported suicidal ideation. When the same adolescents were asked to complete the Malaise Inventory, 20.8% of the boys and 23% of the girls reported "often feeling miserable or depressed."

Other studies in the United States have used depression scales to measure the frequency of *depressive syndromes* in the community or in high school populations. These are self-report instruments with a cut-off score defining a significant level of depression. Rates vary greatly depending on the scale used, the informant (parent, teacher, or adolescent), and the sample.

When investigations use standardized interviews designed to provide DSM diagnoses, the prevalence rate of *depressive disorders* is much lower than that of depressive syndromes or isolated depressive symptoms. Rates of current major depression in community- or school-based samples range from 0.4% to 5.7%, and lifetime prevalence rates range from 4% to 18.4%.

Variations by Age, Gender, and Cohort

Most studies show that the prevalence rates of depressive disorders increase with age: under 12 years, when DSM criteria are applied, the rates in the general population are 1% to 2% with a sex ratio of 1:1. Throughout adolescence, the rates rise in both males and females, but more in girls than in boys, so that by late adolescence the female-to-male ratio approaches 2:1.[4]

Although the median age at onset for major depression is 25 years, data from the National Institute of Mental Health Epidemiologic Catchment Area show that the age intervals with the highest probability for onset of major depression for both males and females are 15 to 19 years and 25 to 29 years. Moreover, family studies[5] and surveys of the general population[6] suggest an increase in the rates of depressive disorders in recent cohorts over the last few decades, with a shift toward an earlier age of onset.

Finally, adolescence is also a period of major increase in suicide rates, and suicide is one of the three leading causes of death in 15- to 19-year-olds. The rates of suicide in this population tripled from 1965 to 1992 (see Chapter 123, "Suicidal Behavior and Suicide"). Recent studies of children and adolescents who have committed suicide show that two thirds of the suicides met criteria for a mood disorder.[7] For males, rates of *completed suicide* are higher than for females in all age groups, but rates of *suicide attempts* are much higher in girls than in boys.

ETIOLOGY

Genetic Factors

It has long been known that depression runs in families, and there is now strong evidence that genetic factors play an important role in this familial aggregation. However, the magnitude of their influence, the mechanisms of interaction with environmental factors, and the mode(s) of transmission remain largely unknown. Family, twin, and adoption studies in adults have shown that heritability varies across the spectrum of depressive illness. While the genetic component accounts for approximately 80% of the variance in liability to bipolar disorder and severe major depression, it accounts for only

about 20% of the variance in milder forms of major depression.[8] Children of depressed parents are at higher risk of developing depression, and of doing so at an earlier age, than are children of normal controls.[9] First-degree adult relatives of depressed children have a higher lifetime risk of having a major depressive disorder than do relatives of normal control children.[10] Finally, an early age of onset in parents has been associated with increased familial loading for both major depression and bipolar disorder, and therefore appears to be a very good index of genetic vulnerability.

Family Environment

Many family factors have been shown to be associated with a negative outcome in adolescents, a depressive condition being one such possible outcome. Parental psychopathology, such as depression, alcoholism, anxiety, and personality disorders, often results in impaired parenting skills and family dysfunction.[11] Other stressors, such as parental divorce, parental death or illness, and parental unemployment, have been related to adolescent depression. Some studies suggest that the adjustment of the parent to the stressful event has a major influence on the child's reaction.

Pubertal Development

Although the prevalence rate of depressive conditions increases during adolescence, there is limited support for the existence of a *direct* relationship between these conditions and hormonal changes.[12] However, some studies have shown that early puberty in girls is often associated with depressed affect, and an increased risk for alcohol and drug abuse due to socialization with older peers.

Other Risk Factors

Injury and physical illness place adolescents at risk for developing depression. Increased rates of depression have been found in adolescents suffering from chronic disorders such as diabetes, asthma, sickle cell anemia, Crohn's disease, cystic fibrosis, rheumatoid arthritis, and hemophilia.[13] Studies involving children and adolescents with cancer have yielded contradictory results; this may be related to denial and underreporting of depressive symptoms in this population. As with other stressors, the quality of previous individual and family functioning and the family adjustment to the illness play an important role in the adaptation of adolescents to their transitory or chronic handicap. A history of physical or sexual abuse has been found to be a significant risk factor for psychiatric disorders, including depression.[14]

Psychological Theories

Cognitive theories have postulated that depression results from a negative view of the self, the world, and the future. However, these cognitive distortions also could be a consequence of depression. In the model of learned helplessness derived from animal experimentation, the repeated occurrence of uncontrollable negative events leads individuals to believe that their behavior will have no effect on their experience, and this belief results in feelings of hopelessness and helplessness.

Behavioral theories have related depression to inadequate reinforcement in the environment, either because sources of reinforcement are rare or absent (loss or absence of a person providing positive reinforcement) or because the individual does not have the competence to elicit reinforcement (e.g., poor academic or athletic performance, poor social skills). It should be noted that depression itself often results in decreased ability to obtain reinforcement from the environment.

Psychoanalytic theories have attributed depression to repressed hostility turned inward: real or imagined object loss followed by the identification of the ego with the lost object and shifting of the hostility toward the ego. More recent formulations have emphasized the inability of the individual to live up to his or her own high aspirations, and parent-child relationships marked by an intense parental ambition in regard to the child's achievement, as factors predisposing to depression.

BIOLOGICAL CORRELATES

Studies of the biological correlates of depression in children and adolescents have attempted to replicate findings in adults. They include studies of neuroendocrine functions (hypothalamic-pituitary-adrenal axis, hypothalamic-pituitary-thyroid axis, and growth hormone secretion), studies of sleep electroencephalography, and studies of neurotransmitters. For each domain of neuroendocrine function, there is an assessment of baseline functioning or response to various challenge tests during the depressive episode and after recovery. Neurochemical studies have replicated with some success findings of disregulations of noradrenergic or serotoninergic functions in depressed adults.

These investigations represent an effort to identify "markers" of depression. Although they are of great interest as research tools to improve our understanding of the pathophysiology of depression and test the hypothesis of a continuity between the childhood and adulthood disorder, they are not useful to clinicians as diagnostic tools because their specificity is low.

Developmental changes in hormonal secretion and neurotransmitter functioning in puberty are likely to interact with other factors to increase the risk of depression in vulnerable adolescents. Some inconsistencies found across studies probably reflect the heterogeneity of depressive disorders and variations in study design.

COMORBIDITY

The co-occurrence of depression and other psychiatric disorders is very common in adolescents. The most frequent disorders associated with depression are anxiety disorders, conduct disorder, and alcohol or drug abuse. This has been found in both epidemiologic samples and clinical samples. Eating disorders and attention deficit disorder also have been found to be associated with depression in adolescents. Comorbidity has several consequences, including an increase in the severity of the symptoms, an increased suicide risk, difficult treatment, and often a worse prognosis.

ASSESSMENT

Psychiatric Interview

It is important to obtain information from various sources. Clinical experience and research have demonstrated that adolescents are better informants on their own mood and suicidal ideation or suicidal behavior than their parents. Parents provide more accurate information on behavioral problems, although they may not be aware of the extent of alcohol or substance abuse. We recommend, if possible, meeting jointly with the parents and the adolescent to obtain an overview of the presenting problems, and then meeting separately with each of them to obtain more detailed and personal information.

The clinician should assess the current depressive symptoms, including mood, sleep, appetite, concentration, fatigue, disinterest or boredom, irritability, sense of hopelessness, and possible psychotic symptoms such as auditory hallucinations or delusions. Suicidal thoughts should be carefully evaluated by direct questioning about thoughts of death, passive suicidal ideation (the adolescent may not think about "suicide" but wishes he/she were dead), thoughts of suicide, history of suicidal gesture(s) (the adolescent may have come close to hurting him or herself), history of suicide attempt(s), current suicidal plan, and seriousness of intent. The physician should also inquire about homicidal thoughts. For each symptom, duration and severity should be noted. The examination must include a search for other psychiatric problems such as· anxiety, behavioral problems like school truancy, acts of violence and trouble with the police. It is also essential to obtain information about alcohol or drug use, and risk factors for human immunodeficiency virus infection. Teenage girls should be asked about possible pregnancy.

An important part of the assessment is to gather information about current and past psychosocial functioning. Depression in adolescence has a major negative impact on the quality of interpersonal relationships and academic functioning. These problems are often what brings the adolescent to clinical attention and include school absence, school refusal, academic failure or any change in the level of achievement compared with previous functioning, difficult relationships with family or friends, decreased involvement in social life, withdrawal from usual pleasurable activities, isolation, and lack of communication. The clinician should try to obtain a sense of how much distress the adolescent experiences and how sensitive, supportive, and understanding the family appears to be. The evaluation of possible precipitants for the current episode should always include an inquiry about any history of physical or sexual abuse. When the depressive symptoms are related to a physical illness, concerns about restriction of independence, body image, peer acceptance, ability to attain professional or personal goals, and the prognosis of the illness are often present, as well as guilt or self-reproach. Some physical symptoms, such as change in appetite, sleep, or level of energy, can be part of the physical illness, and it may be difficult to distinguish which physical complaints are related to depression.

Finally, the evaluation should include inquiries about the past psychiatric history: history of psychiatric disorders and possible history of treatments (medication, counseling, psychotherapy, psychiatric hospitalizations). Of particular importance is an inquiry about hypomanic or manic symptoms; the occurrence of such symptoms in the past would preclude the use of antidepressants alone for the treatment of the current episode because these patients are at high risk for becoming manic when started on any type of antidepressant. The parents are usually better informants about the adolescent's psychiatric history, and they should be asked about the family psychiatric history as well. A family history of bipolar disorder would be a strong predictor of a bipolar course in a depressed adolescent. A history of suicide in the family should raise great concern about the depressed adolescent, especially if he or she is suicidal. The interview with the parents is also an opportunity to evaluate the presence of psychopathology in them and possible need for treatment. Parents should be asked to sign consents for release of information from teachers, school counselors, or previous therapists.

Medical Evaluation

A physical examination, including a thorough neurologic evaluation, should be performed to rule out the possibility of physical illness. Many medical conditions may present with depressive symptoms and are sometimes the primary cause of depression. These include viral or bacterial infections; epilepsy; brain tumors or injury; migraine headaches; endocrinopathies such as diabetes; adrenal, thyroid, parathyroid, or pituitary dysfunctions; electrolyte abnormalities; lupus erythematosis; rheumatoid arthritis; Wilson's disease; porphyria; and anemia. Some medications, such as anticonvulsants, contraceptives, and corticosteroids, have a depressogenic effect. This list is not exhaustive, and the clinician should inquire about all current and recent medications.

Laboratory Tests

A minimum work-up should include complete blood count with differential; electrolytes, blood urea nitrogen, creatine; liver and thyroid function tests; and an electrocardiogram (ECG). These tests are necessary before treatment with antidepressants is begun.

Psychoeducational Tests

It is helpful to request psychoeducational tests, as poor academic functioning either may be related to depression or may have preceded the occurrence of depression and be associated with a specific learning disability requiring appropriate remediation.

Other Methods of Assessment

Many assessment instruments can assist the clinician in making a diagnosis of depression. Most of these have been designed for research purposes and it is not current practice to use them in addition to a thorough clinical interview.

TREATMENT

Depression in adolescence results from the interaction between individual vulnerabilities and environmental influences. A comprehensive assessment of these factors, coupled with a careful evaluation of the depressive symptomatology and the impact on functioning, should guide the clinician in choosing the treatment modality that will best address the specific problems of the individual. This assessment should be made in collaboration with a child psychiatrist or psychologist. When the primary care physician has recognized the presence of depressive symptoms that interfere with the adolescent's functioning and have lasted for at least 2 weeks, a consultation with a specialist should be requested. Of first importance is the need to decide between inpatient and outpatient treatment. Some of the strongest indications for hospitaliza tion include psychotic features, suicidal intent, high degree of hopelessness, comorbidity with severe substance or alcohol abuse, comorbidity of severe disturbance of conduct, personal or family history of suicide attempt, lack of parental involvement or supervision, and the presence of child abuse. Whenever there is doubt about the risk of self-injury or aggression toward others, one should always be "on the safe side." After the need for inpatient treatment has been ruled out, education about the nature of depression and the available treatments is a necessary initial step in establishing a therapeutic alliance with the adolescent and the family. Each component of the treatment plan should be thoroughly discussed to ensure clear understanding, acceptance, and compliance. Finally, the clinician should emphasize that worsening of the patient's condition in the course of treatment may warrant a change in approach. The adolescent and the parents also should be advised to use emergency services if the need should arise.

Psychotherapy

Owing to a current lack of evidence concerning the superiority of antidepressants over placebo in this age group, it seems reasonable to begin with psychological treatment, particularly when the adolescent presents with a mild to moderate form of depression. Several forms of psychotherapy have been employed to treat depression and it is not yet known which form may prove superior to the others, or which form may be more appropriate in a particular case. Therefore, the choice will largely depend on the orientation of the clinician, although it is not uncommon for a therapist to combine different approaches in the course of the same treatment.

Cognitive therapies are usually structured and time limited and aim to change the negative cognitions associated with depression. Adolescents learn to identify their irrational beliefs about themselves, the world, and the future; to understand the connection between these beliefs and their own feelings and behavior; and to modify them. This goal may be achieved in individual or group therapy. Interpersonal psychotherapy focuses on interpersonal conflicts. Behavioral approaches are often combined with cognitive treatment and aim at enhancing social skills to increase adolescents' ability to generate reinforcement from the environment.

Family intervention may take the form of recommending individual treatment of a depressed parent, or marital or family therapy when dysfunctional family interactions appear to play a role in the adolescent's depression. These family interventions can be of critical importance in increasing the effectiveness of other treatments provided.

Psychodynamic therapies differ from other therapies in that they are open-ended in terms of length of treatment and in that their goal is not to identify specific cognitions or problems that may cause or perpetuate depression, but rather to explore unconscious conflicts.

Pharmacotherapy

The efficacy of tricyclic antidepressants (TCAs), selective serotonin reuptake inhibitors (SSRIs), and monoamine oxidase inhibitors (MAOIs) in depressed adults has been well established, and clinical experience suggests that some depressed adolescents respond well to these medications. However, research studies have failed to prove their superiority over placebo. In most cases, pharmacotherapy should be restricted to adolescents who have not responded to psychosocial treatment, or to adolescents who show evidence of severe impairment associated with vegetative symptoms such as insomnia or decreased appetite. There are two indications for using lithium in conjunction with an antidepressant: (1) when the adolescent has a history of a manic or hypomanic episode and (2) when the adolescent does not respond to an antidepressant alone.

Tricyclic antidepressants such as imipramine (Tofranil), nortriptyline (Pamelor), and desipramine (Norpramin) have cardiovascular effects, including slowing of cardiac conduction, arrhythmias, tachycardia, and increased blood pressure. Therefore, the ECG, pulse, and blood pressure should be monitored regularly.[15] Plasma levels should be checked whenever there are signs of cardiotoxicity, when a patient does not respond to treatment after 3 to 6 weeks, or when there is a relapse during the course of treatment and one suspects noncompliance. Owing to great interindividual variability in rates of hepatic hydroxylation, plasma levels may be very different in individuals taking the same dose. Tricyclic antidepressants also have anticholinergic side effects such as dry mouth, blurred vision, and constipation. They should be avoided in an adolescent with a seizure disorder, as they lower the seizure threshold. Finally, they are extremely toxic in overdose. Prescriptions should not exceed a 1-week supply, and parents should be advised to place the medication in a locked cabinet and to supervise administration. The dose for all tricyclics should be increased progressively from 25 or 50 mg/day to a maximum of 3 to 5 mg/kg/day in divided doses (usually twice daily). Antidepressant effects take 3 to 6 weeks to occur.

The SSRIs (fluoxetine [Prozac], sertraline [Zoloft], and paroxetine [Paxil]) have the major advantages of being much safer in case of overdose and of having fewer side effects (essentially limited to nausea and headaches). Although this class of antidepressants has not yet been approved by the Food and Drug Administration for use in younger adolescents, some clinicians give them. Again, doses should be progressively increased, normally up to 20 to 40 mg for fluoxetine or paroxetine, and 50 to 200 mg for sertraline. Fluoxetine has a half-life of 2 to 3 days and its active metabolite norfluoxetine has a half-life of 7 to 9 days; sertraline and paroxetine have a half-life of about 24 hours.

The MAOIs require compliance with a strict diet to avoid hypertensive crisis and should not be used in adolescents who are unlikely to comply.

Light therapy has been used with success in children and adolescents presenting with seasonal affective disorder.

The use of electroconvulsive therapy (ECT) in adolescents who present with a bipolar or depressive disorder has been reported as beneficial in some cases. Until more research has been done, ECT remains a last choice.

COURSE

Studies looking at the outcome of depressive disorders have suggested that episodes tend to be protracted and recurrent. Strober et al[16] found that 6.9% recovered within 12 weeks, 29.3% within 20 weeks, and 90% by 24 months. Some studies suggest that once the mood component has resolved, cognitive distortions and psychosocial impairment may persist. Childhood depression also appears to be associated with an increase of suicide risk in late adolescence or early adulthood. Finally, the adolescent onset of depression places the individual at increased risk for developing depression in adulthood.[17]

Research findings suggest that recognizing and treating depression in adolescents is not only important in the short term to provide symptom relief, improve psychosocial functioning, and help the adolescent resume his or her normal development, but also may play an essential role in preventing adult dysfunction. From animal research, it is known that repeated stressors can induce changes at the level of gene transcription that may result in enduring biochemical changes in the brain.[18] In humans, such changes could be provoked by repeated stressors and episodes, and may increase the patient's vulnerability to the occurrence of further episodes whether or not a stressor is still present.

CONCLUSION

Depression in adolescence is common and largely unrecognized. It represents a major risk factor for suicide, tends to be recurrent, and often results in significant psychosocial impairment. It is therefore critical that primary care physicians, having the most consistent contact with adolescents, be able to diagnose this disorder. The treatment is complex because these adolescents usually have multiple problems. A close cooperation between a child psychiatrist or psychologist and the primary care physician is essential for a comprehensive evaluation, formulation of an optimal treatment plan, and avoidance of inappropriate premature prescription of antidepressant medication.

References

1. Whitaker A, Johnson J, Shaffer D, et al: Uncommon troubles in young people: prevalence estimates of selected psychiatric disorders in a nonreferred adolescent population, *Arch Gen Psychiatry* 47:487-496, 1990.
2. American Psychiatric Association: *Diagnostic and statistical manual of mental disorders,* ed 4, Washington, DC, 1994, American Psychiatric Association.
3. Strober M, Carlson GA: Bipolar illness in adolescents with major depression: clinical, genetic and psychopharmacologic predictors in a three- to four-year prospective follow-up investigation, *Arch Gen Psychiatry* 39:549-555, 1982.
4. Angold A, Rutter M: Effects of age and pubertal status on depression in a large clinical sample, *Dev Psychopathol* 4:5-28, 1992.
5. Ryan ND, Williamson DE, Iyengar S, et al: A secular increase in child and adolescent onset affective disorder, *J Am Acad Child Adolesc Psychiatry* 31:600-605, 1992.
6. Lewinsohn P, Rohde P, Seeley JR, Fischer SA: Age-cohort changes in the lifetime occurrence of depression and other mental disorders, *J Abnorm Psychol* 102:110-120, 1993.
7. Shaffer D, Gould MS, Fisher P, et al: Psychiatric diagnosis in child and adolescent suicide, *Arch Gen Psychiatry* 53:339-348, 1995.
8. McGuffin P, Owen MJ, O'Donovan MC, et al: *Seminar in psychiatric genetics,* London, 1994, Royal College of Psychiatrists; pp 110-127.
9. Weissman MM, Fendrich M, Warner V, Wickramaratne P: Incidence of psychiatric disorder in offspring at high and low risk for depression, *J Am Acad Child Adolesc Psychiatry* 31:640-648, 1992.
10. Harrington RC, Fudge H, Rutter M, et al: Child and adult depression: a test of continuities with data from a family study, *Br J Psychiatry* 162:627-633, 1993.
11. Rutter M: Commentary: some focus and process considerations regarding effects of parental depression on children, *Dev Psychol* 26:60-67, 1990.
12. Buchanan CM, Eccles JS, Becker JB: Are adolescents the victims of raging hormones: evidence for activational effects of hormones on mood and behavior at adolescence, *Psychol Bull* 111:62-107, 1992.
13. Seigel WM, Golden NH, Gough JW, et al: Depression, self-esteem, and life events in adolescents with chronic disease, *J Adolesc Health Care* 11:501-504, 1990.
14. Allen DM, Tarnowski KJ: Depressive characteristics of physically abused children, *J Abnorm Child Psychol* 17:1-11, 1989.
15. Kye C, Ryan N: Pharmacologic treatment of child and adolescent depression, *Child Adolesc Psychiatr Clin North Am* 4:261-281, 1995.
16. Strober M, Lampert C, Schmidt S, Morrell W: The course of major depressive disorder in adolescents. I. Recovery and risk of manic switching in a follow-up of psychotic and nonpsychotic subtypes, *J Am Acad Child Adolesc Psychiatry* 32:34-42, 1993.
17. Harrington R, Fudge H, Rutter M, et al: Adult outcomes of childhood and adolescent depression. I. Psychiatric status, *Arch Gen Psychiatry* 47:465-473, 1990.
18. Post RM: Transduction of psychosocial stress into the neurobiology of recurrent affective disorder, *Am J Psychiatry* 149:999-1010, 1992.

CHAPTER 123

Suicidal Behavior and Suicide

•

Stephen R. Setterberg

Over the past 30 to 35 years, the suicide rate among adolescents has increased from approximately 4 per 100,000 to 12 per 100,000. Suicide is a leading cause of adolescent mortality, resulting in about 5000 deaths per year, and is second only to accidents as a cause of death among 13- to 24-year-olds. The increase in adolescent suicide has been most pronounced among white males, for whom the increase is strongly associated with substance and alcohol abuse.[1]

The increase in youth suicide does not appear to be an artifact of changing reporting practices. During these same years, the suicide rate in the general population has remained stable at around 12 per 100,000, and the overall rate of adolescent death due to other causes has declined. Nonfatal suicidal behavior also represents a major source of medical and psychiatric morbidity. The percentage of high school students who report a history of attempted suicide is as high as 9%,[2] with 2% reporting an attempt requiring medical attention in the previous year.[3] These data suggest that suicide attempts are hundreds of times more frequent than suicide completions. Suicidal impulses or acts are among the most common reasons for admitting teenagers to psychiatric hospitals.

Most studies show demographic differences between adolescent suicide "attempters" and "completers." Among adolescents the male-to-female ratio for completed suicide is approximately 4:1, whereas among suicide attempters females outnumber males by approximately the same proportion. Attempters and completers also differ diagnostically. More completers than attempters have a diagnosable psychiatric disorder, although the vast majority in both groups evidence psychopathologic disturbance.

Despite these group differences, there is evidence of continuity between attempters and completers. Psychologic autopsy studies of people who complete suicide show previous attempt rates of 30% to 50%, and follow-up studies of suicide attempters show suicide rates 50 to 60 times higher than those of the general population.

Reliable predictors of which suicide attempters will later die by suicide are not available. Even the seriousness of previous attempts does not predict subsequent suicide. Therefore, all suicidal behavior must be taken seriously and evaluated carefully.

RISK FACTORS

Psychiatric Disorders

Suicidal behavior is strongly associated with psychiatric disorders and is a sign of psychopathology that merits treatment. Psychologic autopsy studies have found diagnosable psychiatric disorders in up to 90% of those who complete suicide, and suicide attempters are far more likely to meet the criteria for a formal psychiatric disorder than are matched controls. Among those who complete suicide and seem not to have met criteria for a specific psychiatric diagnosis, some degree of symptomatic disturbance is generally uncovered during a psychologic autopsy.

The fourth edition of the *Diagnostic and Statistical Manual of Mental Disorders* (DSM-IV)[4] includes suicidal behavior in the diagnostic criteria for two psychiatric disorders: major depressive episode and borderline personality disorder. Mood disorders, especially depression, have long been linked to suicide. Several symptoms of depressive disorders—pessimism, low self-esteem, hopelessness, helplessness, excessive guilt—are conducive to suicidal ideation. The severity of suicidal ideation has been shown to correlate with increasingly severe depression.[5] About 25% of youngsters who complete suicide do so during a major depressive episode. This proportion is higher among females. Bipolar (manic-depressive) disorder is also associated with a high lifetime risk of suicide.

Psychotic disorders (e.g., schizophrenia, major depression with psychotic features) may also include suicidal impulses. Young people who are both psychotic and suicidal are at grave risk for self-harm because their judgment and impulse control may be severely compromised.

Studies that include assessments of personality disorders find high rates of borderline personality disorder in adolescents hospitalized for suicide attempts. This association remains even when suicidal behavior is not included in the criteria for assigning a borderline personality disorder diagnosis.

A high proportion of suicidal adolescents, particularly males, show evidence of conduct disturbance.[6] Conduct disorder in childhood and adolescence strongly predicts antisocial behavior in adulthood; in adults, antisocial and violent behavior are associated with suicide and suicidal behavior. Fifty percent or more of adolescents who commit suicide are found to have a mixture of depressive, aggressive, and antisocial symptoms on psychologic autopsy.

High rates of substance abuse also are found in suicidal adolescents. Autopsy data suggest that many suicides are committed during states of acute alcohol or drug intoxication. This finding is consistent with the fact that adult alcoholics have elevated suicide rates. The increasing incidence of adolescent substance abuse may be a major potentiating factor in the increased youth suicide rates of recent decades.

Many suicide attempters seen emergently are diagnosed as having an adjustment disorder, which is defined in DSM-IV as a maladaptive response to an identifiable psychosocial stress. With further evaluation, some of the patients so diagnosed are found to meet the criteria for other syndromes.

Panic disorder has also been shown to be associated with increased rates of suicidal behavior in adults. This finding underscores the heterogeneity of diagnoses associated with suicidal behavior. An estimate of suicide risk cannot be determined simply on the basis of the presence or absence of any particular psychiatric disorder.

Personality Variables

Aggressive and impulsive tendencies repeatedly have been demonstrated in adolescents who attempt suicide. This finding is consistent with the high prevalence of conduct disorder among suicide attempters, particularly males. Other personality attributes reported in suicidal adolescents include irritability, low frustration tolerance, poor self-concept, resentfulness, hostility, poor problem-solving skills, externalized locus of control, social isolation, sexual conflicts, hopelessness, and helplessness. Although many of these attributes suggest personality disorders or depressive disorders, they may be present across the full range of psychiatric disorders.

Life Events

Psychologic autopsy studies have confirmed that life events trigger suicide attempts. Often these trigger events involve shame or humiliation. Arrests, assaults, or disciplinary incidents at school are typical examples of events that can precipitate a suicide attempt in a vulnerable young person. There are also anecdotal reports that revelations of homosexuality or pregnancy have precipitated suicide attempts.

Arguments with family or boyfriends or girlfriends are frequently identified as precipitants in emergency room assessments of suicide attempters. However, such events are ubiquitous for suicidal and nonsuicidal adolescents and are therefore not sufficient to explain a suicide attempt.

Although recent loss has been considered a risk factor for suicide, this association has not been confirmed by controlled studies. However, more specific clinical phenomena, such as fantasies of a reunion through death with a deceased relative, would signal elevated suicide risk.

Familial Factors

Suicidal behavior runs in families. An estimated 40% of adolescent suicide attempters have a familial history of suicidal behavior. Families of suicidal adolescents also have an increased incidence of affective (mood) disorder and personality disorder. This familial aggregation could be due to psychosocial mechanisms such as behavioral modeling or to genetic inheritance, or to both. Twin studies suggest that suicide proneness, affective illness, and aggressive and impulsive tendencies may all be genetically transmitted. The extent to which these inherited vulnerabilities have distinct or shared underlying genetic mechanisms remains uncertain. Some twin study data support the possibility that suicide proneness is transmitted independently of associated disorders.

Exposure to suicidal behavior in the family increases the chances that an adolescent will resort to such behavior. This exposure may occur simply on the basis of identification with a suicidal parent. In some families and social networks, self-injurious behavior appears to function as a recognized communicative act for expressing extreme emotion. Stressful life events and the degree of family turmoil are elevated for suicidal adolescents, even when compared with depressed controls. Rates of physical or sexual abuse appear comparable to those for psychiatric controls.

Neurochemical Factors

Research in adults implicates the serotonin (5-HT) neurotransmitter system in suicidal behavior.[7] Low cerebrospinal fluid levels of the serotonin metabolite 5-hydroxyindole acetic acid (5-HIAA), which indicate decreased serotoninergic activity, have been associated with an increased risk of suicide in depressed patients. Low levels of brain serotonin or 5-HIAA, low cerebrospinal levels of 5-HIAA, and increased numbers of 5-HT^2 receptor sites have been demonstrated in postmortem studies of suicide victims. Decreased serotoninergic function has also been associated with violent and impulsive behavior, which can contribute to suicide risk.

ASSESSMENT OF SUICIDAL IDEATION

Whenever an adolescent is being evaluated for emotional distress, it is important to ask about suicidal thoughts or attempts. This inquiry can be made in a straightforward way during an interview. When an adolescent has revealed some degree of anxiety, depression, or rage, the subject can be prefaced and naturally introduced: "Sometimes when kids feel angry, sad, or worried, they also have thoughts about hurting themselves. Has that ever happened to you?" If a patient says no, rephrasing the question (e.g., "or sometimes they just wish they were dead or could disappear") may reveal a suicidal impulse. If suicidal impulses are detected, the risk of attempt must be evaluated. This generally involves consultation with a psychiatrist experienced in evaluating adolescents. In addition to reviewing the risk factors described above, the adolescent's responses to questions such as the following can help to gauge the present risk of attempt: "When did you last feel that way? What was happening then? Are you feeling that way now? Have you thought about how you would hurt yourself? Do you have a plan? Have you ever tried to hurt yourself in the past?"

Sometimes an adolescent will admit to suicidal ideation that on further questioning is clearly just a passing thought or of no present relevance. However, when there is uncertainty about the seriousness of the suicidal ideation, further evaluation must be arranged and the adolescent's safety ensured. Safety may require holding the patient for an emergency psychiatric consultation.

Parents or guardians must be notified if their child is potentially suicidal. Appropriate confidentiality does not extend to colluding with a suicidal adolescent. If such an adolescent is being returned to the parents for outpatient follow-up, the parents need to be told whom to call should an emergency arise.

When an abusive or dangerous family situation is uncovered along with the suicidal ideation, the appropriate child welfare agencies must be contacted. Intervention by a social agency may relieve or distress an adolescent. Ongoing monitoring of patients' mental status is important in these situations, since family upheaval can increase their suicidal feelings.

Hospitalization may be indicated for an adolescent with suicidal ideation. The mental status and situational factors that would indicate a need for hospitalization are the same as those for attempted suicide.

MANAGEMENT OF ATTEMPTED SUICIDE

Attempted suicide always constitutes a psychiatric emergency.[8] The first priority is to ensure safety. Any medical or surgical condition must be adequately stabilized and monitored. The nature of the self-inflicted harm

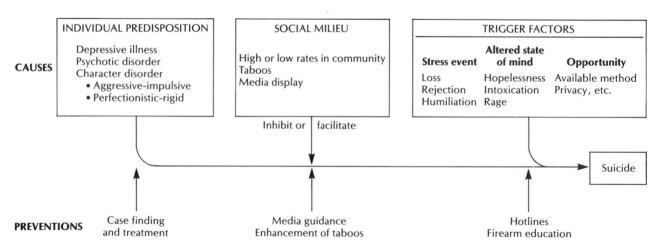

Fig. 123-1. Schematic model for suicide causation showing factors that interact to promote or inhibit adolescent suicide. The model assumes that only predisposed individuals commit suicide and that they do so in the presence of co-occurring triggering stresses and method opportunities. (Modified from Shaffer D, Garland A, Gould M, et al: Preventing teenage suicide: a critical review, *J Am Acad Child Adolesc Psychiatry* 27:675-687, 1988.)

(e.g., gunshot wound, drug overdose, carbon monoxide) will determine the appropriate medical interventions.

It is important to keep the adolescent under direct observation during the medical and psychiatric evaluations in order to prevent any further attempts at self-harm. Occasionally restraint or sedation may be required because of patient agitation or intoxication. Sedation should be avoided until the patient's toxicologic status is known.

The major psychiatric triage question during the emergency evaluation is "Does this patient need hospitalization?" In the past, any degree of self-injurious behavior constituted a sufficient indication for hospital admission. However, with the advent of crisis treatment clinics and the increasing numbers of suicide attempts, there has been a shift away from automatic hospitalization. This trend amplifies the importance of thorough, accurate, and cautious evaluations of suicide attempters. Definite indications for hospitalizing an adolescent who has made a suicide attempt are (1) persistent intent evident during interview or in the patient's behavior, (2) abnormal mental state that predisposes to suicide (e.g., depression with hopelessness) or diminishes impulse control (e.g., psychosis or intoxication), and (3) a home environment that is likely to subject the patient to extreme stress or to fail to provide monitoring and ensure follow-up care.

Lethal intent, as evidenced by a method choice other than overdose or superficial cutting (e.g., overdoses with large amounts of medication, efforts made to conceal the attempt) suggests the need for hospitalization. However, medically nonlethal methods do not reliably indicate benign intent. Young attempters especially may naively choose an objectively benign method even when their suicidal intent is extreme. Because males are more likely to complete suicide, they are generally admitted at lower thresholds of concern.

Outpatient management of suicidal adolescents requires 24-hour contingency plans. Generally, such a plan includes a promise to inform a responsible person if suicidal impulses recur and a way of reaching the therapist or bringing the adolescent to an emergency room if need be. This agreement, whether verbal or written, is often characterized as a "contract for safety." The family (or guardians) must be able to take an active role in such a plan.

Once the adolescent is medically stabilized, he or she and the family should be interviewed separately and together. Interviewing the adolescent privately yields a more accurate history of issues such as drug and alcohol use or sexual activity, and may uncover hidden family problems such as parental violence or child abuse. Interviewing the family with the adolescent provides crucial observational data on family interactions, including the degree of conflict and available support. Interviewing the family without the adolescent present may elicit information that parents otherwise might withhold. The optimal

interview sequence is generally dictated by the circumstances (e.g., clinic vs. emergency room vs. private office; who is on the scene; the patient's medical status).

Interviewing the Adolescent

After a known suicide attempt, the clinician should begin the interview by acknowledging the attempt and inviting the patient to summarize what happened. Then, before delving further into the circumstances of the attempt, the clinician should obtain a general psychosocial history and history of present problems. This approach builds rapport before the sensitive reasons for the attempt are probed in detail and provides a context in which to assess the attempt. While the psychosocial history is being obtained, special attention should be paid to assessing the risk factors. Any previous psychiatric treatment or previous attempts should be explored in detail.

It is important to understand the adolescent's mental status at the time of the attempt. This can usually be determined by asking the patient to describe very specifically what he or she was thinking and doing step by step before and during the attempt. Specific questions include "How did you try to hurt yourself?" "Where were you?" "Was anyone with you or nearby at the time?" "Did you think anyone might find you?" "How long had you been thinking of hurting yourself?" "What tipped the balance from thinking about hurting yourself to doing something?" "Had you been drinking or using any drugs?" "What were you thinking and feeling at exactly the moment you took the pills/cut yourself/etc.?" "Did you think you would die?" "Did you want to die?" "How do you feel about surviving?" If psychosis is suspected, the clinician should ask whether any voices, visions, or supernatural messages told the adolescent to harm himself or herself.

Such questions allow the interviewer to assess the severity of the suicide intent and the deliberateness or impulsiveness of the attempt, and may reveal specific interpersonal conflicts or situational factors that need to be addressed before the patient can return home. When an interview rapport has been developed with adolescents, their self-reports of suicidal thoughts or feelings are usually reliable.

Mental status findings that suggest continued high suicide risk even if current suicidal feelings are denied by the patient are (1) disturbed affective state (hostility, hopelessness, extreme pessimism, fear or anxiety), (2) impulse dyscontrol (belligerent or uncooperative attitude during interview, history of marked impulsivity), (3) impaired judgment due to psychosis (thought disorder, hallucinations, delusions, ideas of reference, paranoia), intoxication, or history of repeated intoxications.

Because a suicide attempt and the emergency interventions that follow may powerfully influence a patient's mental status or circumstances, the mental status during the evaluation may be quite different from what it was during the attempt. In some cases, the social effects of a suicide attempt will alleviate the adolescent's suicidal impulses by temporarily neutralizing even chronic family conflicts or by mobilizing support from an estranged parent, sibling, boyfriend, or girlfriend. In other instances, negative environmental responses to a suicide attempt may intensify an adolescent's suicidal impulses. For example, some families react with extreme hostility or derision rather than with support or concern. In rare instances, they even convey a wish that the attempt had succeeded.

Assessing the Family

Assessment of the family is important for a number of reasons. First, the family can provide information concerning the patient's recent behavior that may be diagnostic, or about family psychiatric history unknown to the adolescent. A family history of mood disorder or suicide is an added indication for caution. Second, the family's capacity and willingness to be involved in treatment must be assessed. The degree of this commitment is often critical in deciding whether a patient can be managed as an outpatient or whether a hospitalized patient can be discharged. Third, family conflicts need to be identified and addressed as part of stabilizing a suicidal adolescent. Fourth, parents or siblings may themselves be distressed by an adolescent's suicidal state or suicide attempt and may be in need of intervention.

Finally, the family's immediate response to the adolescent's suicide attempt needs to be addressed, and their likely future response estimated on the basis of their past behavior toward the adolescent. The family's acute, overt response to the adolescent's suicide attempt can reveal a great deal about their feelings toward him or her, their capacity to be supportive, their coping skills, and their potential reliability and judgment for participating in future treatment plans. For example, if a family reacts with frank hostility or rage toward a suicidal adolescent and shows little concern about his or her welfare, or if discussions between the family and the patient frequently degenerate into hostile arguments, it will not be safe for the patient to return home until the emotional volatility has been reduced. Other families might restrain their hostility in the emergency room or doctor's office but have a history of abusiveness or callousness toward the adolescent that warns against sending the patient home. Some communities have developed crisis beds for supervised, short-term respite while family conflicts are de-escalated. Such programs may provide an alternative intervention for suicide attempters whose psychiatric symptoms do not require inpatient stabilization.

TREATMENT

Because suicidal behavior may be superimposed on a wide range of psychopathologic conditions, there is no single treatment approach. The conventional approach is to treat the underlying psychopathologic condition and to intervene in the environmental circumstances that may have promoted the behavior. Numerous reports indicate that adolescent suicide attempters routinely end treatment after a few visits. Therefore, short-term crisis-intervention techniques emphasizing support and problem-solving strategies are preferred acutely. Family therapy is generally an integral part of this crisis management and is essential in those cases characterized by high levels of parent/child conflict. For adolescents motivated to engage in longer-term treatment, individual psychotherapy can be used to help them develop insight into the conflicts and motivations underlying the attempt. This treatment may protect against future attempts by reducing adolescents' impulsiveness in response to distress. Group therapy may be particularly useful for adolescents with socialization problems.

Psychotropic medications should be prescribed when indicated for specific disorders or syndromes but dispensed cautiously to outpatients. The risk of overdose with medications such as antidepressants needs to be weighed, and reliable parents and caregivers are needed to supervise the administration.

PREVENTION

Concern about the increase in youth suicide has given rise to suicide hotlines and school workshops designed to reach potentially suicidal adolescents before they act. Actual suicide is so rare that it is difficult to evaluate the effects of these primary prevention efforts.

Some no doubt well-meaning suicide prevention efforts leave the impression that suicidal behavior is essentially an understandable reaction to rather ordinary stresses. The intention is to encourage young people who are thinking about suicide to feel freer about revealing their problems to other people. There is some evidence that such programs may stimulate suicidal attitudes in adolescents already at risk. Programs designed to make adolescents more comfortable with revealing their suicidal feelings may inadvertently reduce their inhibitions to actual suicidal behavior.[9]

The strong association between suicide and psychopathology makes psychiatrically disturbed youths the logical target of suicide prevention efforts. Suicide prevention at this level consists mainly of improving the availability of mental-health care for adolescents, including substance abuse treatment and improved treatments for conduct disorder. Only about half of the adolescents who kill themselves have had some contact with a mental-health professional. Community screening efforts for adolescent psychopathology could be improved, and adolescents in treatment could be more thoroughly screened for suicidal impulses.

There is increasing evidence that psychologic contagion can contribute to clusters of adolescent suicides. When a student commits suicide, the school should respond in a supportive but measured way. Large group activities designed to process the event may be counterproductive. Help or counseling should be readily available, but forums for mass identification with the victim should be avoided. A responsible media can also play a preventive role by not glamorizing suicides and by emphasizing the association with mental illness. Other practical preventive efforts could include reducing adolescents' access to firearms, alcohol, and drugs. Physicians should advise such restrictions routinely to parents of adolescents at high risk for suicide.

References

1. Shaffer D, Piacentini J: Suicide and attempted suicide. In Rutter M, Taylor E, Hersov L, editors: *Child and adolescent psychiatry: modern approaches,* ed 3, Cambridge MA, 1994, Blackwell Science; pp 407-424.

2. Harkavy JM, Asnis GM, Boek M, et al: Prevalence of specific suicidal behaviors in a high school sample, *Am J Psychiatry* 144:1203-1206, 1987.

3. Centers for Disease Control: Attempted suicide among high school students—United States, 1990, *MMWR* 40:633-635, 1991.

4. American Psychiatric Association: *Diagnostic and statistical manual of mental disorders,* ed 4, Washington, DC, 1994, American Psychiatric Association.

5. Brent DA, Kalas R, Edelbrock J, et al: Psychopathology and its relationship to suicidal ideation in childhood and adolescence, *J Am Acad Child Psychiatry* 25:666-673, 1986.

6. Shaffer D: Suicide in childhood and early adolescence, *J Child Psychol Psychiatry* 15:275-291, 1974.

7. Stanley M, Mann JJ: Biological factors associated with suicide. In Frances AJ, Hales RE, editors: *Annual review of psychiatry,* New York, 1987, American Psychiatric Press; pp 334-352.

8. Pfeffer CR: Child and adolescent suicide risk. In Kestenbaum CJ, Williams DT, editors: *Handbook of clinical assessment of children and adolescents,* New York, 1988, New York University Press; pp 673-688.

9. Shaffer D, Garland A, Gould M, et al: Preventing teenage suicide: a critical review, *J Am Acad Child Adolesc Psychiatry* 27:675-687, 1988.

CHAPTER 124

Academic Achievement

•

Jeffrey L. Black

Professionals involved in adolescent health care should be concerned about their patients' academic achievement, as the adolescent's school performance is an important indicator of cognitive function, psychosocial adjustment, and developmental mastery. A decline in school performance should prompt a thorough investigation of possible contributing causes (Table 124-1). The physician's role may vary from the provision of anticipatory guidance during health supervision to the coordination of a multidisciplinary evaluation and intervention plan. Both monitoring the school progress of the academically successful adolescent and assisting him or her with underachievement in school require a basic understanding of the educational system. This includes an appreciation of evolving expectations in academic skills and changes in educational programs and support services. It is also important to recognize how school processes can detract from or contribute to a student's performance. The adolescent's physician should always be mindful of the reciprocal influences among the school, the home, and the community. Certain parenting styles, sociocultural factors, critical life events, and role models place the student at increased risk for school dysfunction. The effective physician anticipates potentially adverse influences and works to mitigate their effects.

UNDERACHIEVEMENT AND OVERACHIEVEMENT

The number of students whose academic performance falls considerably below their ability or potential is a major concern in education today. The proportion of students who could be categorized as underachieving depends on how performance and potential are defined and measured. Some authors believe the figure to be as high as 15% to 30%.[1] Students in special education with learning disabilities, a significant segment of those who underachieve, make up approximately 5% of the school population.[2] Failure to finish high school is often the result of a persistent pattern of underachievement. The national dropout rate averages about 25% and is 30% for minorities.[3] Students in urban schools have the highest dropout rates, which range from 40% to 66% in major cities.[4]

Many students succeed academically in spite of constitutional limitations, sociocultural disadvantage, or potentially stressful life events. These resilient students have a set of personality characteristics, disposition, and beliefs that foster school success.[5] They have an internal locus of control and believe they have been able to succeed because of their own choices and effort. An attitude of optimism is accompanied by realistic goals and recognition that good school performance has long-range benefits. Resilient students have adults, usually a parent and someone from the school, who have high expectations and provide support with firmness. Extracurricular activities are added sources of positive involvement with the school and opportunities for success.[6]

Some students overachieve, maintaining a level of school performance higher than their general level of intelligence would predict. While this may highlight the fallacy of using results from standardized IQ tests to predict school functioning, it also may reflect exceptional student effort, instruction, and parental support.[7] However, some pay a social or emotional cost for their overachievement. They forego socially rewarding nonacademic activities, such as hobbies, clubs, sports, or unstructured leisure time with peers, for excessive hours of study, project completion, and test preparation. If academic time is largely homework spent in isolation, the adolescent has reduced opportunities for peer interactions

TABLE 124-1
Causes of School Failure in Adolescence

Problem Area	Cause
Psychosocial problems	Adolescent developmental concerns
	Family problems
	Substance abuse
	Emotional reactions secondary to learning problems
	Intrinsic psychopathology
Sociocultural factors	Lack of academic emphasis and role models
	Nonacademic peer pressure
Pedagogic factors	Variations in school and teacher quality and standards
	Diminished individual attention and support of secondary school
Problems associated with chronic physical illness	School absence and fatigue
	Psychosocial sequelae
Sensory deficits	Hearing and visual impairments
	Refusal to use correctional aids or materials
Neurologically related disorders	Mental retardation
	Specific learning disabilities
	Attention-deficit disorders

From Black JL: Adolescents with learning problems, *Prim Care* 14:206, 1987.

that are essential for healthy psychosexual development. If overachievement is driven by upward-striving or overprotective parents, who pressure the child to get good marks and are never satisfied by what is accomplished, most adolescents eventually rebel and refuse to work to capacity.[8]

TRANSITIONS AND CHANGING EXPECTATIONS

In most schools the move to junior high school or to middle school represents a shift from a child-centered to a subject-oriented process.[9] Instead of spending most of the school day with a single caring adult, the student has multiple teachers, each of whom has a particular interest in one aspect of the curriculum. The student must adjust to a wide variety of personalities, teaching styles, and classroom routines. In addition, at this stage students have moved from an elementary school environment where they were the oldest and the most competent among schoolmates to an academic and social milieu in which they are often the youngest, smallest, and least accomplished. These changes occur with wide individual variation in physical and emotional development and ability.

Promotion to senior high school is commonly associated with a reduction in special education programs and services for the disabled that exceeds a similar loss of services that occurs between elementary school and junior high. Funding constraints, focus on early intervention, and the belief that any deficits should have been "cured" by earlier remediation often leave the student who has mild or moderate learning disabilities without

necessary resources. In addition, the educational reform movement has proposed an increase in high school graduation requirements. If such a proposal is adopted nationwide, all students would be required to take more mathematics, foreign language, science, English, and social studies and pass minimum competency tests. These changes in the nation's educational policies will make school even more difficult for adolescents with learning disabilities.

The exposure to a greater variety of academic content in junior high and senior high school offers distinct advantages as well as challenges.[10] For some, a specific subject area, such as biology or geometry, may have special interest and may generate enthusiasm for learning that spreads to other subjects. Elective courses can create a sense of control of the learning environment by allowing the adolescent to become more involved in course selection. Courses such as home economics, industrial arts, and photography can provide discouraged students who have deficits in academic skills an opportunity to experience success. Vocational education programs are offered in senior high school, but their effects are frequently limited by enrollment requirements for academic proficiency.

The educational process is structured so that certain skills are stressed at different grade levels.[11] As students proceed through middle school, junior high, and high school, there is increasing demand for encoding of thoughts and higher-order conceptualization (Table 124-2). Higher volumes of written work require strong summarization and interpretive abilities. Staging work, allocating time, and combining information from multiple sources are examples of the heightened demand for efficiency and organization. Achievement at the

TABLE 124-2
Evolution of Academic Expectation in Late Childhood

Expectation Shift	Description	Primary Academic Impact Areas
More encoding of thoughts	Growing stress on production and communication of ideas, especially on paper; higher volume output	Writing reports; taking written examinations
Increasing reliance on rapid retrieval memory (automatization)	Need to retrieve data almost instantly and with little mechanical effort or expenditure of attention	Writing; mathematics; reading comprehension; foreign language; spelling
Greater demand for attention to visual and auditory detail	Increasingly complex stimulus sets for observing and listening; less opportunity to succeed via the "big picture" exclusively	Mathematics; reading; lectures in class
Increased length of delay of gratification	Longer-range assignments; more time devoted to sustained effort with delayed rewards and feedback	All subject areas
More stress on resynthesis of ideas and skills	Process of taking in data, then restating, adapting, and applying what has been read or heard	Reading comprehension (retelling); lectures in class; studying
Growing need to integrate skills and knowledge from multiple sources	Recombining of skills and information, as from several books, from teachers, and from memory and new inputs	All subject areas
Greater stress on efficient and sophisticated language processing and production	Rapid comprehension; verbal inference; paradox, humor, irony; expressive fluency; fast, effective word finding	Understanding of verbal explanations in all areas; participation in class discussion; written language; foreign language
Heightened demand for efficiency and organization	Maintenance of notebooks; scheduling or staging work; allocating time; completing tasks; summarizing, outlining, notetaking; test taking	Study skills in general; test-taking ability; proficiency in long-range assignments
Expanded use of higher-order conceptualization	Dealing with abstraction; symbols; rules; generalizations; extrapolations; conceptual frameworks; inferential reasoning	Content courses (e.g., science, social studies); mathematics

From Levine MD, Zallen BG: The learning disorders of adolescence: organic and nonorganic failure to strive, *Pediatr Clin North Am* 31:345, 1984.

higher levels of secondary education requires the ability to abstract. As the academic curriculum increases in difficulty, strengths and weaknesses in specific skills determine the relative ease of scholastic success and preferences in subject areas.

SCHOOL: STRESS AND SUCCESS

For the adolescent, the school experience can be both a major source of stress and an arena for success. The potential for stress has escalated in recent years as schools have come under increasing pressure to raise academic requirements in response to concerns about declining scores on standardized tests of achievement and aptitude. Although some students may have profited from this trend, many others have suffered.

The role of school stress as a causative, precipitating, or exacerbating factor for psychosocial morbidity has been well substantiated.[12] Precursors of depression, and even suicidal conditions, in adolescence have been traced to the cycle of perceived failure and self-blame that many children confront in school.[13] Self-reported substance abuse in middle school students has been found to be associated with the perception of excessive academic demands and with an accumulation of stressors related to authority, peer, and academic pressures.[14] When children believe that they cannot achieve the academic success expected by their parents and teachers, they tend to lose motivation, underachieve, and (in some instances) drop out of school. The school environment has a major impact on motivation and ultimate academic performance. The quality of the educational experience for the individual student depends on how the academic setting, curriculum, and teaching styles match with the adolescent's learning style, strengths, and weaknesses.

The research of Rutter et al,[15] which involved secondary schools in London, provides some of the best evidence of which school-related factors have the greatest influence on student performance. As suggested by earlier studies, physical and administrative features of a school had limited effect on student outcome. For example, no consistent associations were found between student success and school size, class size, age of school buildings, or whether students were grouped by age or ability. Factors that did make a difference were related to the attitudes of the staff, the general school atmosphere, and the academic milieu. When teachers worked closely together, developing curriculum and discipline plans, and openly praised and displayed students' work, they facilitated better student performance. Schools that were well organized and frequently involved students in positions of responsibility (e.g., as homework monitor or assembly participant) tended to have better student outcomes. Superior scholastic attainment was found in schools that expected appropriate academic achievement, spent greater teaching time on actual lessons, and assigned more homework.

A national survey of exemplary middle schools in the United States found that academic achievement was promoted by making individual faculty members readily accessible to students.[16] In the most successful schools, in terms of the students' self-efficacy and standardized test scores, students met with a faculty advisor at least weekly for assistance that emphasized personal development and study skills.

EFFECT OF FAMILY AND HOME ENVIRONMENT

Achievement in school is the result of a complex interaction of student, school, and family factors. This interaction occurs within the context of social and environmental influences that further shape school performance. Family life events, features of the family environment, and parental psychopathology are among the major familial determinants of adolescent school achievement.

Youngsters who are depressed or worried about domestic turmoil or disruption often lack the attention and energy required for academic success. For most adolescents, a decline in school performance associated with family illness, death, and marital discord is temporary, but

for some the adverse effects are more severe and long-standing. Nearly one quarter of adolescents may have a drop in grades for 1 to 5 years after parental divorce.[17] The death of a parent or a sibling has been clearly shown to adversely affect time spent on homework, comprehension, and academic productivity.[18,19] Academic difficulties have been consistently reported among students who have a sibling with any of a variety of chronic illnesses.[20]

Schools can play an important role in helping students adjust to potentially adverse family life events. For example, children of divorced parents have better academic success if their schools provide an orderly, consistent learning environment that closely monitors their progress and offers additional direct teaching when productivity lags.[21]

Features of the home environment that have been shown to have an impact on school achievement include the parents' expectations, parental involvement in school activities, and parenting style.[22] Parents who consistently communicate to their children that they expect school success, while recognizing and praising their efforts, instill motivation and a positive attitude. By being directly involved in school activities and by having frequent contact with the child's teachers, parents help their child achieve better school performance. Involved parents are more likely to influence the school organization to take action that helps their child.[23] Although parents who are more educated tend to be more involved with schools, parental involvement improves a child's school performance regardless of parental educational status. Across a wide variety of social categories and ethnic groups, families that use authoritative parenting have children who get higher grades in school.[24] This authoritative parenting style is characterized by firm enforcement of rules and standards, open parent-child communication, and encouragement of individuality. This style can be contrasted with an authoritarian parenting style, which is more restrictive and less responsive, and permissive parenting, which allows considerable self-regulation.

The influence of siblings on school performance is commonly overlooked. An older brother or sister can make schoolwork easier by helping directly with assignments and offering valuable advice in setting study priorities and selecting courses or teachers. Competition between siblings can drive them to higher levels of achievement or cause the less competent one to give up and seek nonacademic forms of fulfillment and recognition. Discouragement can be avoided if each child is directed to an area of interest and strength where some measure of success is attainable with reasonable effort.

The personal adjustment problems of parents are sometimes the primary hindrance to a student's school achievement.[25] The school difficulties of youngsters of emotionally ill parents may include inattention, problems with peer and teacher interaction, reduced work completion, and delays in learning academic area content and skills. Academic competency declines as the severity of parental psychopathology rises. Children of parents with personality disorders and schizophrenia do less well than those whose parents suffer from disturbances of affect.[12]

COMMUNITY AND SOCIAL INFLUENCES

Adolescents are strongly influenced by their peers and by the expectations of the neighborhoods in which they live.[26] The need to conform with the norms of the desired peer clique helps determine the energy given to academic pursuits. If alliances are formed with students who are academically oriented, it is likely that schoolwork will be viewed favorably. Students who model themselves after peers or older teenagers who have not experienced school success and place no value on scholastic accomplishment have less incentive to strive for academic achievement.

Likewise, the community's emphasis on academics can act to either enhance or diminish the student's educational performance. In a neighborhood where intellectual success is exalted, the adolescent may feel frustration for not living up to this expectation. At the other extreme are communities that send a message that schoolwork and study are not relevant. Ideally, the community provides numerous role models who reach for academic excellence, it places a value on a range of activities (e.g., arts, music, sports, and mechanical and technical skills), and it recognizes that success also can be defined by progress and effort.

The positive correlation between a family's level of income and their child's school progress is well established. Still, there are instances when affluence, particularly at high levels, can be harmful. Overuse of substitute caretakers, unrealistic parental expectations, and easy access to drugs are disadvantages often associated with wealth.[27] Public schools in upper middle class neighborhoods and exclusive private schools often have overly rigid concepts of acceptable educational goals and behavior (see Chapter 94, "Affluence").

School achievement also can be strongly affected by cultural factors. A student's cultural or ethnic background is often closely related to community values that shape academic expectations. Students from minority backgrounds may face additional stress when school and community norms differ from parental standards. They may be constrained by the social stereotyping adopted by teachers and fellow students. When the student's home language or dialect differs from that of most students at the school, the school and academic challenges may be even greater.

COMMUNICATION WITH SCHOOL STAFF

It is impossible to formulate a clear and accurate description of school achievement without having some form of direct contact with the adolescent's school. The opinions of school staff and the impressions of the physician can easily be distorted by parents or students who are asked to act as intermediaries. Telephone communication, by either the physician or the medical office staff, enables a dialogue that can clarify conflicting or confusing data. If the student was referred by the school, information obtained by phone or in writing is required to determine what the school personnel see as the problem and what action they expect the physician to take.

Sometimes the school will have already completed a comprehensive assessment and will have developed an effective intervention plan so that the physician's evaluation can be focused on very specific concerns or unmet needs. Often it is helpful initially to contact the principal, who can recommend those members of the school staff who have been most involved with the student and suggest how best to reach them.

Because the adolescent has multiple teachers, the process of gathering school data can be complicated. It is common for secondary school teachers not to have discussed with one another the student's problems or shared ideas for offering assistance. Because of variations in teaching styles and differing demands of their subject areas, they often have divergent perspectives on the adolescent's school function. A questionnaire, such as the ANSER system,[28] is one method of efficiently gathering data that allows the comparison of learning and behavioral traits in different classroom settings. Adolescents usually can identify the teacher who knows them best and can serve as their school-site advocate. In many circumstances, this is the school counselor.

When sending written reports to schools, it is important to respect the adolescent's confidentiality and the educator's professional expertise. It is usually correct to assume that the student's school file is neither private nor protected. Multiple individuals have ready access to "confidential" records, and their contents are freely discussed at educational planning meetings. Potentially embarrassing or sensitive details concerning the student's background or the family's social life are best omitted from the written report. If this type of information is germane to school management, it is usually best to convey it orally to the appropriate school staff member after receiving the adolescent's and the parents' consent.

Educators regularly complain that the physician's report is not helpful or creates problems for them. Typically, the school is sent a copy of the full medical record, which is often illegible. Teachers may be especially offended when the physician makes definitive and sweeping educational recommendations without obtaining their input and without performing a comprehensive evaluation. To be most effective, the physician's report should be free of medical jargon, providing a concise summary of pertinent findings and assessment procedures, but be worded in a manner that acknowledges the school's critical role in arriving at a final diagnostic impression and management plan.

The initial report should not mark an end to the physician-school interaction. The problems that signaled the need for collaboration should be monitored and the response to the interventions assessed. Ongoing communication tends to keep all parties accountable and more likely to fulfill their roles.

INTERPRETATION OF PSYCHOMETRIC EVALUATION

When confronted with an adolescent who is having difficulty in school, the physician should request copies of teacher observations, daily work, grades, and results of group achievement tests. If the student has received an individual evaluation, copies of these test scores should be obtained as well. Although a detailed interpretation of individual diagnostic batteries is best left to those specializing in learning disorders, the adolescent's primary care physician should have general familiarity with the tests used and their limitations.

School systems administer group achievement tests at regular intervals to monitor the overall success of their programs and to screen for students at risk for academic failure. Tests available for this purpose include the Stanford Achievement Test, the Iowa Tests of Basic Skills, and the Comprehensive Test of Basic Skills. These machine-scored, multiple-choice instruments report results as grade levels and percentiles according to national norms. Occasionally, more relevant state and local district norms are available. Because these tests are group administered, students with attention-deficit disorders tend to perform below expectations. These tests give a superficial assessment of skills in academic subject areas and do not provide direct information regarding such basic abilities as writing rate, following instructions, summarizing, and organization. Students with problems in these areas often score higher than their actual classroom performance would predict.

School underachievement is the clinical problem that most frequently calls for individual psychometric testing. It is common practice to define specific learning disabilities by identifying a discrepancy of 1 to 2 standard deviations between individual achievement and intelligence test scores. The Woodcock-Johnson Psychoeducational Battery-Revised and the Wechsler Individual Achievement Test (WIAT) are the most common indi-

vidually given tests of achievement. The Wechsler Intelligence Scale for Children, third edition (WISC-III), standardized from 6-0 to 16-11 years, is regarded as the mainstay of intelligence tests for children. Wide variation among verbal and performance scores and/or subtests on the WISC-III are also frequently considered to indicate specific learning disabilities (see Chapter 125, "Psychoeducational Tests for Children").

The examiner's observations during individual assessment can overcome many of the above-noted limitations of group testing, yet too often standardized test batteries are only qualifying tools and do not yield results that are useful for planning instruction or intervention strategies. The psychometrician's report is most helpful if it contains more than a recapitulation of scores by elaborating on the student's application of academic skills, approach to problem solving, error patterns, and motivation.

There are problems with the usual individual diagnostic battery, even in the hands of an accomplished school psychologist.[29] The instruments used are often culturally biased against many ethnic minorities. Many children have significant cognitive or academic difficulties that are not detected by the standard intelligence-achievement discrepancy criteria, verbal-performance variation, or subtest score scatter. A student's learning disabilities can cause generalized depression of scores or can involve cognitive limitations not measured by the tests used. For example, commonly given tests of intelligence and achievement can easily miss critical elements of language ability.

The student's performance on the psychometric evaluation should not be the sole criterion for providing or withholding special services or for making accommodations in the regular academic program. Test scores should be handled like laboratory tests in medicine; that is, they should be interpreted in light of historical and other objective data.

IMPLICATIONS FOR ANTICIPATORY GUIDANCE

The physician's involvement in the adolescent's school achievement is often an extension of the monitoring and advice offered throughout the school years. Obtaining the student's and the family's opinions about school performance should be a routine part of the health supervision visit. Inquiries about the adolescent's school functioning should include questions about course schedules and grades, least favorite and most favorite subjects, ease or difficulty with homework, extracurricular activities, overall feelings about school, and satisfaction with school performance. Answers to these questions are usually sufficient to determine whether further evaluation is necessary (Box 124-1).

BOX 124-1
**Primary Care Assessment
for Learning Problems**

I. History (aided by questionnaires)
 A. Presenting problems
  1. Onset and course
  2. Proposed causes and solutions
  3. Past and present evaluations and interventions
  4. Behavioral and social function
 B. Areas of strength and interests as reported by student and parents
 C. Medical history
  1. Perinatal insults
  2. Later causes of central nervous system injury
  3. Early developmental milestones and temperament
  4. Conditions with academic impact
 D. Family history
  1. Academic delays and achievements
  2. Effect of presenting problems on family
  3. Dysfunctional interactions
 E. School history
  1. Current school year
   a. Counselor, teachers, subject areas
   b. Grade level and type of program
   c. Grades, performance level, attendance
   d. Teacher's descriptions of academic strengths and weaknesses
   e. Description of presenting problems and proposed solutions
  2. Previous education
   a. Past grades and schools attended
   b. Special services or programs
   c. Significant written teacher comments
   d. Achievement and psychologic/educational test scores and dates
II. Physical examination
 A. General health evaluation
 B. Vision and hearing acuity assessments
 C. Standard neurologic examination
 D. Minor neurologic signs
 E. Neurodevelopmental examination (optional)

From Black JL: Adolescents with learning problems, *Prim Care* 14:206, 1987.

The primary care physician should work with schools to anticipate factors that may increase the risk of academic difficulty and help reduce their negative impact. Students with learning disorders, chronic medical illness, and psychosocial problems are best served by a school that accommodates their special needs in the classroom and provides support services. Especially at the time of enrollment at a different school, it should not be assumed that the teachers are aware of the student's condition or are knowledgeable about their potential role in the management plan.

The physician, working with the school counselor or the school nurse, should make sure that pertinent information is disseminated to appropriate school staff. Educators often need to be alerted to the possibility of subtle or overt signs of distress that the student may manifest in response to critical life events. Students with temperamental or cognitive characteristics associated with difficulty adapting to change, such as those with attention-deficit disorders and those who are slow learners, will benefit from extended orientation and organizational skills training as they make the transition to middle school, junior high, and senior high school. Other students with developmental dysfunctions related to writing reports, assimilating information from lectures, and completing long-range assignments may have their initial experience with academic failure in secondary school, and they may require assistance to overcome or bypass their areas of difficulty. Parents, particularly those who are less educated or are members of a minority group, may need encouragement and advice to become involved in their adolescent's schooling. The physician may suggest that the school's community liaison worker reach out to those families that appear to be estranged from the educational system. Participation in extracurricular activities and peer tutoring can be used to offset any antieducation sentiment expressed by neighborhood youths by introducing the adolescent to positive role models.

Students who are already struggling academically are more likely to receive the assistance they need if their physician takes an active role in the evaluation and intervention process. The physician may be the only professional who has a longitudinal database on the competencies and vulnerabilities of the adolescent and the family. Schools tend to give high-priority status to assessments that have been initiated by outside professionals. Although the physician is usually not in a position to recommend specific educational and diagnostic tests, it is helpful to provide a general impression of factors contributing to the student's difficulty in school. Input from the physician that describes the adolescent's interests and learning style can facilitate adjustments in the curriculum that result in improved motivation and academic success.

The results of the psychometric evaluation can be used by the physician to help students better understand how their personal profile of strengths, weaknesses, life circumstances, and educational experience interact to produce their learning style and academic preferences. This type of discussion should reduce the family's and adolescent's earlier misconceptions that may have led to unnecessary guilt and blame and unrealistic expectations. Previously unrecognized or underdeveloped skills may be uncovered, particularly if the evaluation included a measure of vocational aptitude. Opportunities that enable the underachieving student to pursue athletic, mechanical, musical, or artistic strengths should be actively sought. Removal of the adolescent's only area of talent as punishment should be discouraged.

Knowing what aspects of the school milieu influence student outcome should enable the physician to advise parents on school selection and to become an advocate for reform. Policies that allow schools to set high, yet achievable performance and competency goals; require a reasonable amount of homework while offering close teacher supervision and support; and emphasize praise rather than punishment should be promoted. Underachievement in schools should not be inadvertently fostered by the schools themselves. Students should be spared inflexible practices that do not allow them to mobilize their strengths and bypass their weaknesses.

CONCLUSION

For a variety of reasons, physicians need to monitor and assess the school achievement of the adolescent patient. School performance is an important gauge of emotional health and developmental progress. School dysfunction is usually a multifaceted problem that requires physician-family-school collaboration for efficient resolution. With knowledge of the factors that commonly cause school failure in the adolescent age group, the physician can reach a diagnosis, develop a functional profile of strengths and weaknesses, and coordinate a comprehensive management plan. Schools can be influenced to provide needed services for the individual student and to institute practices that have been shown to improve the achievement levels of all students. Parents may need assistance to appreciate their child's strengths and to help him or her utilize these appropriately. If adolescents are able to see how their spectrum of talents can lead to immediate success and toward a rewarding career, the physician has played an important role in the development of a potentially happy and productive adult.

References

1. Gearhart BR, Gearhart CJ: *Learning disabilities: educational strategies,* Columbus, OH, 1989, Merrill.
2. Moats LC, Lyon GR: Learning disabilities in the United States: advocacy, science, and the future of the field, *J Learn Disabil* 26:282-294, 1993.
3. Sklarz DP: Keep at-risk students in school by keeping them up to grade level, *Am School Board J* 176:33-34, 1989.
4. Hahn A: Reaching out to America's dropouts: what to do?, *Phi Delta Kappan* 69:256-263, 1987.
5. Winfield LA: Resilience, schooling, and development in African-American youth: a conceptual framework, *Educ Urban Soc* 24:5-14, 1991.
6. McMillan JH, Reed DF: At-risk students and resiliency: factors contributing to academic success, *Clearing House,* 67:137-140, 1994.
7. Bender SL, Ponton LE, Crittenden MR, et al: For under-privileged children, standardized intelligence can do more harm than good (commentary), *J Dev Behav Pediatr,* 16:428-430, 1995.
8. Metcalf K, Gair EL: Patterns of middle-class parenting and adolescent under-achievement, *Adolescence,* 22:919-928, 1987.
9. Wright GF, Nader PR: Schools as milieux. In Levine MD, Carey WB, Crocker AC, Gross RT, editors: *Developmental-behavioral pediatrics,* Philadelphia, 1983, WB Saunders, pp 276-283.
10. Levine MD: Academic content areas. In Levine MD, editor: *Developmental variations and learning disorders,* Cambridge, MA, 1987, Educators Publishing Service; pp 371-394.
11. Levine MD, Zallen BG: The learning disorders of adolescence: organic and nonorganic failure to strive, *Pediatr Clin North Am* 1:345, 1984.
12. Elias MJ: Schools as a source of stress to children: an analysis of causal and ameliorative influences, *J School Psychol* 27:393, 1989.
13. Diener CI, Dweck CS: An analysis of learned helplessness: continuous changes in performance, strategy, and achievement cognitions following failure, *J Pers Soc Psychol* 5:541, 1978.
14. Elias MJ, Gara M, Uriaco M: Sources of stress and support in children's transition to middle school: an empirical analysis, *J Clin Child Psychol* 14:112, 1985.
15. Rutter M, Maughan B, Mortimore P, Ouston J, Smith A: *Fifteen thousand hours: secondary schools and their effects on children,* Cambridge, MA, 1979, Howard University Press.
16. George P, Oldaker L: A national survey of middle school effectiveness, *Educ Leadership* 43:79, 1985.
17. Wallestein JS: Children and divorce, *Pediatr Rev* 1:211-217, 1980.
18. Adams-Greenly M, Moynihan RT: Helping the children of fatally ill parents, *Am J Orthopsychiatry* 53:219-229, 1983.
19. Balk D: Effects of sibling death on teenagers, *J Sch Health* 53:14-18, 1963.
20. Dworkin P: Social and environmental influences on school performance. In Dworkin P, editor: *Learning and behavior problems of schoolchildren,* Philadelphia, 1985, WB Saunders; pp 212-231.
21. Guidubali J, Cleminshaw HK, Perry JD, et al: The impact of parental divorce on children: report of the nationwide NASP study, *Sch Psychol Rev* 12:300-323, 1983.
22. Hess RD, Holloway SD: Family and school as educational institutions. In Parker RD, editor: *Review of child development research,* vol 7, Chicago, IL, 1984, University of Chicago Press; pp 179-222.
23. Baker D, Stevenson D: Mothers' strategies for school achievement: managing the transition to high school, *Soc Educ* 54:156-167, 1986.
24. Dornsbusch SM, Ritter PL, Leiderman PH, et al: The relation of parenting style to adolescent school performance, *Child Dev* 58:1244-1257, 1987.
25. Forehand R, Long N, Brody GH, et al: Home predictors of young adolescents' school behavior and academic performance, *Child Dev* 57:1528-1533, 1986.
26. Levine MD: Predispositions, complications, mechanisms. In Levine MD, editor: *Developmental variations and learning disorders,* Philadelphia, 1987, WB Saunders; pp 397-444.
27. Schorr LB: Environmental deterrents: poverty, affluence, violence and television. In Levine MD, Carey WB, Crocker AC, Grass RT, editors: *Developmental-behavioral pediatrics,* Philadelphia, 1983, WB Saunders; pp 293-312.
28. Levine MD: *The ANSER system,* Cambridge, MA, 1980, Educators Publishing Service.
29. Rosenberger PB: The pediatrician and psychometric testing, *Pediatr Rev* 2:301-310, 1981.

CHAPTER 125

Psychoeducational Tests for Adolescents

•

Danielle Morris and Philip W. Davidson

In recent years, there has been a dramatic increase in the volume of psychologic tests appropriate for use with children reaching adolescent age. As more and more adolescents and their families seek professional consultations with psychologists, educators, psychometricians, and others who provide testing, it is likely that pediatricians who receive psychologic reports on their patients may encounter difficulty in recognizing the tests administered and in interpreting their results.

This chapter is designed to serve as reference to a wide range of psychosocial and psychoeducational screening and diagnostic tools commonly used by clinical and developmental psychologists, school health teams, special education specialists, and other allied health professionals. Both screening tests and diagnostic instruments should be standardized on some reference population. A screening test is designed with specificity and sensitivity to detect the presence or absence of a problem behavior or trait, but typically does not provide a scale of severity or magnitude of that condition. Therefore, few screening tests have norms. An instrument characterized as a diagnostic test should have the capacity to scale severity and therefore should be based on age-group norms.

Some screening and diagnostic tests may be designed for administration by self-report, since this method may increase the likelihood of a reliable and valid response from typically self-aware and inwardly focused adolescents. Most tests for this population are administered individually. Practice may reveal that sometimes they are inappropriately given in group settings, which may compromise their validity.

Included in Table 125-1 are tests that are usually administered by trained professionals, since these are less familiar to both parents and physicians than are the group achievement and aptitude tests usually administered in schools.

The information provided for each device is useful in identifying the general nature of each, the usual professional training of the person administering the test, and whether it is standardized or normalized. For some procedures, special features or characteristics are also noted.

Table 125-1 describes most procedures that are likely to be included in a typical consultant's report, although the list of tests is not all-inclusive. Screening procedures are presented as well as more in-depth diagnostic tests. The age ranges of the procedures presented vary, some covering all of adolescence, while others focus more on early or late adolescence, in addition to measures that cross into other age ranges.

In reviewing reports of psychologic testing, the primary care pediatrician should carefully determine the qualifications of the examiner or examiners. All tests listed in Table 125-1 are designed to be administered and interpreted by licensed psychologists or other appropriately credentialed mental-health professionals. The report should be signed by the individual who actually administered and interpreted the tests. In some evaluation settings, it may be cosigned by another professional who provided supervision during administration and interpretation.

Interpretation of screenings or complete diagnostic assessments cannot be fully accomplished without communication directly with the evaluator to clarify the results. Such contact often must be initiated by the physician, since personnel from many mental health facilities and schools may not routinely communicate with the primary healthcare provider. When initiating such communication, it is imperative to discuss the test results directly with the professional who conducted the evaluation. This strategy increases the quality of the information obtained. It also serves to establish a dialogue between professionals concerning follow-up recommendations.

TABLE 125-1
Commonly Used Tests of Educational and Psychologic Assessment

Intelligence/Achievement

Test Name	Age Range	Purpose and Description
Detroit Test of Learning Aptitude	Preschool-17 yr	Diagnostic test of learning potential, usually administered by a trained psychologist or special educator. Pre-reading, spelling, and arithmetic skills are tested. Norms are available.
Hinskey-Nebraska Test of Learning Abilities	3-18 yr	Nonverbal test of cognitive ability, generally used for deaf and hearing-impaired children. Separate norms for both deaf and hearing children are available. It is usually administed by a trained psychologist.
Leiter International Performance Scale	2 yr-adult	"Normed" diagnostic test of cognitive development, usually administered by a psychologist and particularly appropriate for evaluating speech- and hearing-impaired individuals.
Peabody Individual Achievement Test (PIAT)	5-18 yr	Measure of academic achievement, usually administered by an education specialist. The test measures word recognition, reading and math skills, and spelling. It is one of the better "normed" tests available.
Peabody Individual Vocabulary Test (PPVT)	2½ yr-adult	Screening test of receptive vocabulary, which can be administered by a speech and language specialist, teacher, or psychologist. It correlates highly with IQ tests but cannot be used in place of a more intensive test of cognitive ability.
Raven Progressive Matrices	5½ yr-adult	Diagnostic test of cognitive ability that relies heavily on visual-spatial abstract reasoning. It is claimed to be "culture free." The test is usually administered by a psychologist and is "normed."
Shipely Institute of Living Scale (SILS)	14 yr-adult	Screening test for general intellectual functioning, usually administered by a psychologist. It can aid in detecting cognitive impairment in individuals with normal intelligence.
Slosson Intelligence Test	0-27 yr	Diagnostic test of cognitive ability, usually administed by a teacher or psychologist. It is designed to be a quick assessment, is widely used in schools, and is less well "normed" than the more intensive intelligence tests.
Stanford-Binet Intelligence Test	2 yr-adult	Well-known diagnostic test of cognitive ability, administered by a psychologist. The test is not always appropriate for children with language or motor impairments. It is useful in diagnosing global intellectual level but weak for identifying specific learning disabilities.
Wechsler Adult Intelligence Scale—Revised (WAIS-R)	16 yr-adult	Most widely used test of adult intelligence. It is usually administered by a psychologist and measures verbal and performance intelligence. Subscales can be used to evaluate cognitive functioning and identify specific areas of weakness. "Normed" IQ scores result.
Wechsler Intelligence Scale for Children (WISC-III)	6-16 yr	Most commonly used school intelligence test. Usually administered by a psychologist, it measures verbal and performance intelligence. Subscales can be used to evaluate learning ability and to diagnose specific learning disabilities. "Normed" IQ scores result.

Continued

TABLE 125-1
Commonly Used Tests of Educational and Psychologic Assessment—cont'd

Intelligence/Achievement

Test Name	Age Range	Purpose and Description
Wide Range Achievement Test (WRAT)	5-64 yr	Screening test of achievement, usually administered by an educational specialist. It evaluates word recognition and math and spelling achievement.
Woodcock Reading Mastery Test	Kindergarten-12th grade	Test specific for reading skills and usually administered by an educational specialist. The test measures number and letter identification, word attack, and passage and word comprehension. "Norms" are available.
Woodcock-Johnson Psychoeducational Battery	All ages	Diagnostic test of achievement, usually administered by an educational specialist. It measures cognitive ability, achievement, and interest. The test is more reliable at the elementary than at the secondary educational level.

Psychopathology

Test Name	Age Range	Purpose and Description
Adjective Checklist	12-18 yr	Descriptive test designed to provide personality descriptions of emotionally disturbed youth. It is a self-report index of one-word adjective descriptions. It is usually administered by a trained clinician.
Beck Anxiety Inventory	Adolescence-adult	Screening test that is a self-report index for anxiety symptoms. It measures the severity of anxiety and is usually administered by a psychologist.
Beck Depression Inventory (BDI)	Adolescence-adult	Widely used diagnostic instrument designed to assess severity of depression. It has a self-report format and is usually administered by a psychologist.
Beck Hopelessness Scale	Adolescence-adult	Screening device that measures pessimistic attitudes and the extent of negative attitudes about the future as it is perceived by the individual. It is a self-report index, usually administered by a psychologist.
Beck Scale for Suicide Ideation (BSS)	Adolescence-adult	Self-report screening test designed to detect suicide ideation and measure its level of severity. It is usually administered by a psychologist.
Children's Depression Inventory (CDI)	8-17 yr	Diagnostic test that is a self-rating assessment of depression in children. It measures the presence and severity of depression and is usually administered by a psychologist.
Children's Manifest Anxiety Scale—Revised	6-17 yr, 18-19 yr	Diagnostic test that is a self-report scale that measures the level of anxiety in children and adolescents. Results are normed for two age groups. There are separate norms for males and females, and the test has a lie scale to assess the honesty of the self-report. It is usually administered by a psychologist.
Dissociative Experiences Scale (DES)	Late adolescence-adult	Screening test designed to help identify individuals with dissociative symptoms. It acts as a means of qualifying dissociative experiences. It has a self-report format and is usually administered by a psychologist.
Draw-a-House-Tree-Person	5 yr-adult	Diagnostic test of personality and cognitive status, usually administered by a trained psychologist as a projective device to evaluate self-image and other ego functions.

TABLE 125-1
Commonly Used Tests of Educational and Psychologic Assessment—cont'd

Psychopathology

Test Name	Age Range	Purpose and Description
Draw-a-Man	4-16 yr	Results of this screening test of cognitive ability give a developmental age equivalence. The test can also serve as a projective device to evaluate emotional and personality development. It can be administered by a psychologist or other trained clinician.
Gordon Personality Profile (GPP)	9th-16th grades	Diagnostic test of personality to assess different factors in the personality domain. It is an 18-item forced-choice preference questionnaire usually administered by a psychologist. "Norms" are available.
Millon Adolescent Clinical Inventory (MACI)	Adolescence	Diagnostic instrument that provides a profile of adolescent personality. It has a self-report format that measures concerns and clinical syndromes. It is usually administered by a psychologist. "Norms" are available.
Minnesota Multiphasic Personality Inventory–A (MMPI-A)	14-18 yr	Widely used diagnostic test, usually administered by a psychologist, that assesses the major patterns of personality and emotional disorders. This form is specifically for adolescents. An adult form is also available. "Norms" are provided.
Personality Inventory for Children (PIC)	3-16 yr	Screening test of personality and social development completed by parents. Areas evaluated include achievement, intellectual screening, somatic concerns, depression, family dysfunction, withdrawal, anxiety, psychosis, hyperactivity, and social skills.
Roberts' Apperception Test for Children (RAT-C)	6-15 yr	Diagnostic test administered by a trained psychologist. It assesses perceptions of common interpersonal situations. Scoring reveals adaptive profile scales, resolution styles, and clinical profiles.
Rorschach Ink Blot Test	2 yr-adult	Projective test of personality and social development specifically designed to evaluate personality structure. It is administered by a trained psychologist. Extensive scoring criteria are required to interpret the results.
Sentence Completion Tests	All ages	Projective tests of personality and social development, usually administered by a psychologist. Responses differentiating between adjustment and maladjustment can be identified. A number of different versions of the technique are in use, some of which have been validated and others in which scoring is usually achieved by clinical interpretation.
State-Trait Anxiety Inventory (STAI)	9th-16th grades	Self-report screening questionnaire that assesses anxiety as an emotional state and individual differences in anxiety proneness as a personality trait. It is usually administered by a trained psychologist.
Thematic Apperception Test (TAT)	10 yr-adult	Projective test of personality and social development measuring interpersonal relationships and usually administered by a trained psychologist. The test is useful in identifying emotional disorders. Extensive scoring criteria are applied to interpret the results.

Continued

TABLE 125-1
Commonly Used Tests of Educational and Psychologic Assessment—cont'd

Neuropsychology

Test Name	Age Range	Purpose and Description
Beery-Buktenica Developmental Test of Visual-Motor Integration	2-15 yr	Screening test of visual-motor coordination involving the copying of geometric designs. Age scores are derived from norms. It is usually administered by a psychologist.
Bender Motor Gestalt Test	4 yr-adult	Widely known and used screening test of visual-motor integration, usually administered by a psychologist. There are two "normed" scoring forms: Koppitz is appropriate for children aged 4-12 yr; Hutt is appropriate for adolescents and adults. The test also yields indicators of neurologic and emotional status.
Luria-Nebraska Neuropsychological Battery (LNNB)	8-12 yr, 15 yr-adult	There are two versions of this neuropsychologic diagnostic test: a children's version and an adolescent-to-adult version. It assesses general and specific cognitive deficits, including lateralization and localization of focal brain impairments. This test is administered by a trained psychologist. "Norms" are available.
Wisconsin Card Sorting Test (WCST)	6½-89 yr	Neuropsychologic diagnostic test that measures abstraction ability and distinguishes between a normal and clinical population. It is usually administered by a trained psychologist. "Norms" are available.

Adaptive Behavior

Test Name	Age Range	Purpose and Description
Achenbach Child Behavior Checklist	4-16 yr	Commonly used screening test for personality and social development in children and adolescents. Social competence and potential behavioral problems are inventoried through a parent questionnaire.
Adaptive Behavior Scale (ABS)	3-69 yr	Diagnostic test of adaptive behavior in children and adolescents, administered by a trained clinician. Personal independence, social maladaptation, and personal maladaptation are tested. Results of this test can be used for diagnosis, placement, and programming. The instrument has two versions: one for public school children, the other for children and adults with mental retardation.
Vineland Adaptive Behavior Scale	0-30 yr	Test of adaptive and social behavior, usually administered by an interviewer with developmental training. The test covers four major domains: communication, daily living skills, socialization, and motor development in younger children. The results yield standard scores and age equivalents.

Substance Abuse

Test Name	Age Range	Purpose and Description
Adolescent Chemical Dependency Inventory (ACDI)	12-18 yr	Screening test for adolescent substance abuse. Provides categories for risk level and contains a truthfulness scale. It has a self-report format and is usually administered by a trained clinician.
Adolescent Drinking Index (ADI)	12-17 yr	Screening test for alcohol abuse in adolescents with a self-report format, usually administered by a trained clinician.

TABLE 125-1
Commonly Used Tests of Educational and Psychologic Assessment—cont'd

Substance Abuse

Test Name	Age Range	Purpose and Description
Substance Abuse Subtle Screening Inventory (SASSI)	12-18 yr	Screening test identifying alcohol- and drug-dependent individuals. It differentiates between social users and clinical populations, and is usually administered by a trained professional.

Family Functioning

Children of Alcoholics Screening Test	School age-adult	Self-report screening measure of attitudes, feelings, and perceptions related to the individual's parent's drinking behavior. It is useful in identifying probable children of alcoholics, and is usually administered by a trained clinician.
Family Adaptibility and Cohesion Evaluation Scale (FACES III)	Family members	Self-report screening instrument designed to determine the structure of the family. It is useful in identifying patterns of interaction in the family that affect individual members. It is usually administered by a psychologist or other trained professional.
Family Environment Scale (FES)	Family members	Self-report screening test that measures the social and environmental characteristics of all types of families and of any individual family member. It assesses levels of conflict, independence, control, and other family characteristics. It is usually administered by a psychologist or other trained professional.
Family Violence Scale	Adolescence-adult	Screening instrument that measures the degree of violence present in the home during an individual's childhood. It assesses the severity of violence from least violent to most violent. It is usually administered by a trained clinician.
Kinetic Family Drawing	5 yr-adult	Diagnostic test of personality and social development that measures, in particular, family interactions. Special features of the test include identification of trends or characteristics commonly seen in various subgroups (e.g., learning disabled, developmentally disabled, or perceptual-motor-handicapped children). This test is usually administered by a psychologist or trained clinician.

Self-Esteem

Coopersmith Self-Esteem Inventories (SEI)	8-15 yr, 16 yr-adult	Screening test usually administered by a trained clinician. There is a school form and an adult form of this self-report measure of self-esteem. This instrument assesses evaluative attitudes toward the self in social, academic, family, and personal areas of expression.
Offer's Self-Image Questionnaire—Revised (OSIQ-R)	13-18 yr	Self-report screening questionnaire that measures the self-image of adolescents. It can be administered by a psychologist or other trained professional.
Piers-Harris Self-Concept Scale	8-19 yr	Screening test for personality and social development that evaluates six facets of self-concept, including physical, social, family, and school precepts. The face validity of this test appears to be quite good. It is usually administered by a psychologist or teacher.

Continued

TABLE 125-1
Commonly Used Tests of Educational and Psychologic Assessment—cont'd

Other/Miscellaneous

Test Name	Age Range	Purpose and Description
Adolescent Coping Scale (ACS)	12-18 yr	Description test that assesses different coping styles employed by adolescents in dealing with stress. It has a self-report format and is usually administered by a trained professional.
Attitudes Toward Homosexuality Scale	Adolescence-adult	Descriptive test that assesses the relationship between individual's opinions regarding sexual morality and male/female sex roles. It is self-administered and easy to score. There are two forms, one for females, the other for males. It can be useful in assessing internalized homophobia.
Bulimia Test (BUILT)	Adolescence-adult	Self-report, forced-choice measure that assesses the symptoms of bulimia. It is a screening device that identifies individuals suffering from or at risk for bulimia. It is usually administered by a psychologist.
Eating Disorder Inventory (EDI)	12 yr-adult	Self-report screening measure of psychologic features commonly associated with anorexia and bulimia. It distinguishes clinically significant profiles from "normal" dieters. It is usually administered by a psychologist.
Teenage Stress Profile (TSP)	14-20 yr	Self-report screening device that assesses sources, symptoms, and vulnerability to stress. It is usually administered by a trained professional.

CHAPTER 126

The Gifted Adolescent

•

Everett P. Dulit

WHO ARE THE GIFTED?

The term *gifted,* as used in everyday speech and in the professional literature, has various possible definitions. Two subgroups that are almost inevitably included in the overall category of the gifted are (1) children and adolescents with a very high IQ and (2) children and adolescents with outstanding special talents and abilities in such fields as art, music, or mathematics. For the first group, one can be either highly selective by setting a high cutoff figure (IQ >140) or one can be more inclusive (IQ >125). Both definitions have their merits and their areas of applicability. The more selective definition includes only the most unusual child, the outlier, who is more likely to be outside the wide range of normal in other psychologic measures beyond IQ itself. The more inclusive definition may include one half-dozen or more of the children in a classroom in communities where a majority of the parents are themselves educated and professional people. Both are legitimate but different definitions.

Even more inclusive definitions of the gifted adolescent include some or all of the following special groups: (1) the athletically gifted; (2) the theatre child, in whom the gift is less sharply defined but involves some mix of presence, talent for mimicry, and skill in areas such as song and dance; and (3) the strikingly handsome or beautiful adolescent, the "model." Then, by extension, through the common theme of *the psychology of the exception,* one can also make connection with the categories of (4) the very wealthy and (5) the disabled. All such children can come to see themselves as the exception—entitled to special treatment and exemption from the rules. Such an attitude tends to affect character development, usually adversely, although sometimes advantageously, for instance, when it sets into motion a determination to be or do something special, something especially admirable, noteworthy, or creative.

Do the gifted have more psychologic difficulties than most children? Definitely not! If anything, just the opposite is true. The results of Terman's study, supported and confirmed by other more modern studies, are that far from being in trouble psychologically, the gifted child, adolescent, and adult tends to do impressively well across a wide range of measures. This includes general physical health, social aptitude and experience, and life within the family. If there is any general trend among the gifted, it is that their lives seem favored by some mix of good fortune in both genetics and circumstances. Nonetheless, this chapter focuses on some of the special psychologic pitfalls and challenges that can arise with this special patient group. If and when the gifted do have special difficulties, they are likely to be related to one or more of the themes discussed below.

PSYCHOLOGIC DIFFICULTIES

Unevenness of Development

By definition, the gifted adolescent is far ahead of the average adolescent in some respects. For adolescents with an unusually high IQ, their mental age is well in advance of actual chronologic age. However, these same adolescents are likely to be on the regular developmental schedule in some other respects (e.g., features of psychologic development not particularly touched by the area of giftedness). At the same time, some gifted youngsters are actually behind schedule in yet other ways. Important examples would be youngsters whose giftedness draws them into a life involved mainly with adults (e.g., musical prodigy, child actor), with books and/or computers (bookworm, hacker, nerd), or with nonstop drill and practice (would-be Olympic athlete or virtuoso

instrumental soloist), and away from ordinary social interaction with other children. Such children are likely to fall behind in social skills, particularly in tolerance of the ordinary rough and tumble interactions of childhood and adolescence, and especially if their gifts have led them to be somewhat sheltered or pampered. Gifted children and adolescents can be a little like the show dog or show horse in a sense—highly refined and exceptional in some respects, but without the usual skills and desensitization acquired in everyday interactions with other dogs or horses.

That unevenness of development in the gifted adolescent—ahead in some respects, average in others, behind in still others—can make it difficult for an adult (parent, teacher, counselor, physician) to know which of those three expectations to have in mind. It is simpler to deal with the average youngster, who is usually more consistent in development. The most common error is to treat gifted adolescents as if they were as old as their IQ would suggest. This may be appropriate for matters closely tied to intellect, but it is likely to be highly inappropriate for matters not specifically related to intellect. It takes discernment and flexibility to find a good balance, and that best balance will vary greatly, depending on the area of the interaction.

Social Difficulties

Difficulties can arise for those gifted youngsters who are so sheltered from ordinary social interactions among children and adolescents that they have not developed ordinary social skills and "thickness of skin." In addition, the gifted youngster, especially the intellectually gifted one, may find the company of average same-age youngsters to have something missing, with a conversational mismatch because of the intellectual gap.

It is important to note that most often this is *not* a major problem for the gifted child because, as shown in the Terman study, that youngster is commonly able to participate in and richly enjoy all the play activities among children that do not particularly touch on intellectual level. Even though the average youngster may not be able to discuss philosophy with the gifted child, the two can enjoy being on the swings together when they are 5 years old, they can have fun roller skating together when they are 10, and they can enjoy listening to rock groups together when they are 15.

Nonetheless, that sense of something missing, associated with the intellectual gap between unusually gifted children and their more average peers, can be a problem. Parents may be able to help by searching out, engineering, or encouraging what may turn out to be a crucially welcome friendship with a particularly bright and willing older adolescent. Also, the parent may be able to find a way to set up an opportunity for the gifted child to spend some time with agemates who are also gifted, as would be an automatic outcome of placing the child in a special school or special classroom for the gifted. Usually, some time spent with gifted peers or bright older adolescents is possible, and even a little such time can be very helpful.

Match/Mismatch with Parents

Parent-child match is commonly an issue to some degree in a wide range of average families around a variety of psychologic similarities and differences. It can be particularly problematic around the issue of intellectual level and, in some families, around special talents. There is one set of potential problems associated with parent-child match and another set related to mismatch. In a parent-child match, the parents, like the child, are "way up there" in some respects (which is not uncommon, statistically, given the tendency for genetic similarities), and at least the parents and the child talk the same language and the parents "have been there" themselves. However, when difficulties arise, they tend to take the form of competitive stresses. For example, the mere existence of the successful parent and his or her career can be experienced by the adolescent as an unsettling challenge: "OK, kid—there's *my* best. Now let's see what *you* can do!" Or adolescents may feel that the path they are expected to follow (e.g., musical career, intellectual career) is chosen by others (the parents) or by fate/nature (gift similar to that of the parents), and that the only possible self-directed, independent move is to refuse to follow that path, which can lead to a strong internal resistance toward work and success.

When there is a mismatch and the parents are much more average than the child, the result may be similar to, but more pronounced than, the strains commonly seen between working-class parents and an emerging highly educated son or daughter. In such cases the young person is usually following a path that the parents have very much wanted for their child. However, in the process the child has become a very different sort of a person from the parents in some key respects. Both sides may have considerable trouble being comfortable with one another across that gap. From the parent's side, the reaction may be: "Who does he think he is, talking that way?" or "Whatsamatta—we ain't good enough for you no more?" From the adolescent's side, there is the parallel problem of negotiating the strains caused by feeling an increasing difference from the parents, which is combined with the ongoing experience of functioning at an intellectual level at which the parents cannot even join him or her, let alone help. At the same time, the child is powerfully attached to the parents and needs and wants that connection.

Grandiosity

Happily, it is the experience of most children during their first decade of life within the family to be treated by the parents as someone special, even precious, to them, the parents. That experience is very important for the individual's self-esteem forever thereafter, but then it is a part of normal and necessary development toward the end of the first decade and into the second to have to come to terms with also being just one among others from the point of view of the larger outside world. However, the gifted child may not have come to terms with that shift. Gifted children are much more likely to *continue* to be treated as very special and not just one among others, and thus come to think of themselves in the same way—as the exception. This has the potential for generating very solid self-esteem, or quite disagreeable grandiosity.

Premature Awareness of the Darker Side of Life

As people who think for themselves and have the brain power to penetrate many of the conventional bromides with which more average individuals solace themselves, gifted adolescents are exposed to inescapable confrontation with many of the painful truths about the human condition at an earlier age than is usual. These truths include universal mortality, the evil people do to each other, and life-destroying inequities—issues that can be difficult to face at 8, 10, or 12 years of age.

Drives and Passions

Some gifted people, adolescents included, find themselves virtually possessed by the drive for expression of their giftedness, which acts through them and for which they are a mere vehicle. When the gift is a passion for painting, sculpture, mathematics, or rhetoric, one can sometimes see a person in the grip of a passion or in a rage for doing, almost like one who is possessed. Vincent van Gogh, aflame with a passion to paint, provides one example. The main character in Joyce Carey's *The Horse's Mouth* offers another: a man who would stop at nothing to be able to keep on with his painting of murals, appropriating paint and walls entirely without regard for ownership because he "had to, can't you see?" Such a drive or passion can be quite unsettling for all concerned—including the parents and even the adolescents themselves.

Lopsidedness

Someone in the grip of a passion is not likely to be moved by appeals to well-roundedness: "Yes, chess is a great game, but wouldn't it also be fun to go outside and play with some of those nice children in the playground?" Indeed, some selected people, gifted adolescents included, make very good lives for themselves around one single activity (e.g., math or music, tennis or poetry) to which they are deeply devoted. Although conventional attitudes favor well-roundedness, gifted adolescents belong to a special population of people who often develop unconventional but deeply satisfying lives.

Work Inhibitions

A work inhibition is a subtle but powerful inner restraint against intellectual work, deriving from some inner conflict about doing the work. That conflict is often only partially accessible to introspection by the person affected but sometimes can be deduced from a thorough knowledge of the person's life, thoughts, and feelings. One example is the child for whom intellectual achievement means possibly outshining or at least competing with a parent. When such an outcome is feared, on the basis of fantasies of retaliation or parental hurt, the achievement is avoided. Another common example is fear by a child identified as gifted that a serious effort to turn out a really exceptional piece of work might backfire, if the work turned out to be not so exceptional after all, the child anticipating then being left feeling exposed as perhaps not really so gifted after all.

Bright children and adolescents commonly have so much spare intellectual capacity that even when they are in the grip of a substantial work inhibition, no failing may be evident, rather like a very wealthy person being able to absorb a substantial financial loss without any noticeable change in life style. Indeed, some gifted young people do not even need to learn to actually work hard until fairly late in their academic career—for example, at Ph.D. thesis time at a demanding first-class institution, when for the first time in their life the requirements of the task may force them to give everything they have. Indeed, gifted people may find such an experience to be unsettling, taking it as proof that they are not so gifted after all or making them think about the giftedness: "I've lost it! It came just like that when I was a kid. And now it's gone—just like that."

Gender Role Problems

The issue of gender role is probably less of a problem today than it was 20 years ago. However, it remains problematic when the socially expected gender role is at variance with important features of the giftedness: for example, softness of style in the young man who is a lyric poet or gentle dancer, or aggressiveness of style in the young woman who is a powerful debater or aggressive wit.

Quality of Innocence

One possible developmental outcome of a gifted childhood is the emergence by adolescence of an unusually trusting openness to experience and to people that derives from a life lived with much less of an external shield of conventional defensiveness than most people have and need. Such openness is made possible by a combination of optimal caretaking by family and inner resources for making honest, spontaneous, unique responses to others, without the armor of guarded responses most people use for most initial encounters. When this approach goes well, gifted youngsters can be seen as having, to use Phyllis Greenacre's felicitous phrase, "a love affair with the world"—with art, literature, nature, the city, music, and people. However, sometimes that same approach to life can go badly for gifted youngsters, for example when they get hurt by people who take advantage of or simply fail to recognize the tenderness and vulnerability that may go with that trusting openness.

Repudiation of Gift

By adolescence, the pleasure of being the greatly favored gifted child may give way to (1) a sense of being "stuck with" a role that has more demands in it (practice, rehearsals, training, travel, the company of adults) than pleasures; (2) an uncertainty expressed as "Who am I doing this for anyway—myself or them?" ("them" being interested and committed parents, teachers, coaches); (3) a growing sense of being "owned by" the gift rather than the other way around; and (4) an increasing wish to be like others, especially when the unusually sheltered childhood that may be associated with special giftedness has led to social awkwardness, which may become increasingly important as intimate relationships emerge. One easy way to avoid these problems and to make parents take notice is simply to repudiate the gift, at least for a while. Unfortunately, this repudiation sometimes becomes permanent.

The Odd Brilliant Kid

The odd brilliant kid is a stereotype depicted in films, novels, and comic strips. Statistically, the reality is quite the opposite, but this personality type does occur. Sometimes it represents a chance association of two very different and unconnected things: giftedness and severe mental illness. In other cases, without mental illness being involved, such behavior is a stance that adolescents find useful—to put people off; to disguise social awkwardness or displeasure with others; or even to create a needed private space behind the mask they show to the world, to get the world to move back a bit.

ADVICE FOR PARENTS

Probably the best advice that can be given to parents and physician-counselors for dealing with gifted adolescents is to (1) do as well as you can to help them put together as normal, good, fulfilling, and satisfying a life as possible outside the area of giftedness; and (2) help them fulfill themselves as much as possible in the area of giftedness through interactions with other gifted adolescents and with adults working in that area as mentors or teachers. Neither approach should be forced or imposed but comfortably attended to by caring, interested, and concerned parents. When activities in the area of giftedness interfere with "outside life" (e.g., an adolescent wants to spend a lot of time with a self-selected gifted companion who is "different" in ways that put the parents off instead of with a "regular" companion the parents would prefer), it is usually better to acquiesce and take the long view ("There's plenty of time" and "He's probably going to end up with a somewhat different sort of life anyway") than to fight over the issue.

Parents commonly have many questions about dealing with the gifted adolescent: "Is it a good idea to allow grade skipping (placing the child or adolescent one or more years ahead of agemates)?" "What about early admission to college?" "What social problems are associated with being younger than one's classmates?" "How should the substantial difficulties related to giftedness be handled?" Overall, the answers to such questions are a judgment call and hinge critically on the details and circumstances of each individual case probably best addressed in a consultation with a psychiatrist or psychologist with special experience in this area.

However, some assistance in making these judgments can come from taking into account a "typology" of gifted adolescents, introduced by Betts and Neihart in the text *Understanding the gifted adolescent.*

1. The *successful* gifted, who may "buy success" by being too conforming and perfectionistic and may need encouragement to "take chances" and become more "inner-directed."
2. The *challenging* gifted who are bored, inclined to scorn and to power struggle, who may need encouragement to become more self-aware, self-controlled, and group oriented.
3. The *underground* gifted, who tend to be shy and often are not identified as gifted by themselves or others, who may benefit from encouragement to develop self-awareness and better self-esteem.
4. Gifted *dropouts* who are angry, resentful, "burned out," explosive, and often needing therapy.
5. Those gifted who are *also handicapped* in some way, thus "doubly exceptional," who also may need therapy and, certainly, support systems.
6. The *autonomous* gifted who "have it all together."

They do well, both with adults and with agemates, and may need only some advocacy, in their struggles with conformity-encouraging systems, and in their search for opportunities to exercise their gifts.

Two important points should be made to parents. First, they can take real consolation from the fact that, in general, the lives of the gifted work out quite well. On balance, the gifted have lives as good as or better than average. Second, the average parent of the unaverage adolescent often tends to direct the adolescent toward a more conventional life than nature seems to intend. Perhaps it is best for parents simply to accept that their adolescent will have a life that is outside the wide range of normal in some significant respects, especially in relation to the area of giftedness, and to accept that this may be fine. Parents can also gracefully help create and encourage a life *outside* the area of giftedness that includes a good amount of rich, normal interactions.

If a significant problem is suspected, it is wise to seek consultation with a professional in the behavioral field, a psychiatrist or a psychologist, who is particularly experienced in working with gifted adolescents. Such a consultation can be helpful to all involved—the parents, the adolescent, the teachers, and the physician providing comprehensive health care to the adolescent.

SUMMARY

The gifted group centers on the very-high-IQ youngster and the especially talented youngster. A key theme is the psychology of the exception, including the expectation of exemption from ordinary rules. Generally, the gifted have fewer psychologic and life troubles than does the average youngster. The best overall strategy for the parents of gifted adolescents is to put together an optimal mix of (1) helping them to develop as rich a normal life as possible outside the area of giftedness and (2) assisting them to achieve as much self-fulfillment as possible within the area of giftedness. In general, parents need to accept the fact that their child's life will be different in some respects and that this can be, and usually is, a very good life.

Suggested Readings

Bireley M, Genshaft J, editors: *Understanding the gifted adolescent: educational, developmental, and multicultural issues,* New York, 1991, Teachers College Press; pp 1-32.

Getzels JW, Jackson PW: *Creativity and intelligence,* New York, 1962, John Wiley.

Hogan R: The gifted adolescent. In Adelson J, editor: *The handbook of adolescent psychology,* New York, 1980, John Wiley; pp 536-559.

Terman LM: *Genetic studies of genius, vol 1. Mental and physical traits of a thousand gifted children,* Stanford, CA, 1925, Stanford University Press.

CHAPTER 127

Learning Disorders

•

Adrian D. Sandler and Melvin D. Levine

During the past two decades there has been an explosion of interest in learning and attention-deficit disorders (see Chapter 128, "Attention-Deficit Hyperactivity Disorder") as large and increasing numbers of adolescents who fail to meet behavioral and academic expectations have been identified. Health professionals, psychologists, and educators have been compelled to identify and assist these struggling adolescents.

Extensive research points to the existence of variations in central nervous system higher cortical functioning that impede the acquisition of academic skills and lead to stress, underachievement, or outright failure at school, at home, and in the community. Moreover, learning and attention-deficit disorders are often aggravated in adolescence by the emergence of behavioral, emotional, and motivational complications. For example, the relationship of reading problems to depression, delinquency, and dropping out is of utmost importance. It is not at all uncommon to uncover a background of academic underachievement during evaluations of adolescents suffering from depression, drug abuse, and stress-related symptoms. Clearly, the identification and treatment of these disorders are of great relevance to the comprehensive health care of adolescents and young adults.

EVOLUTION OF FIELD OF LEARNING DISORDERS TREATMENT

In 1975, the Education for All Handicapped Children Act (Pub L No. 94-142) was enacted, mandating free appropriate education in the least restrictive environment for all handicapped individuals between the ages of 3 and 18 years. By 1980, this age range was extended to 21 years. This legislation was updated in 1990 as the Individuals with Disabilities Education Act (IDEA) (Box 127-1). Although more than 25 years have passed since the condition of learning disabilities (LD) was defined in federal legislation as a handicap, there remain serious questions concerning etiology, identification procedures, and eligibility criteria for special educational services. An interagency committee sponsored by the National Insti-

tute of Child Health and Human Development defined LD as "a heterogeneous group of disorders of presumed neurological origin which selectively interferes with the acquisition and use of listening, reading, speaking, writing, mathematics and social skills." The term *learning disability* does not apply to sensory impairments, mental retardation, environmental disadvantage, or primary emotional disturbance, although such problems may indeed coexist with LD. The term *learning disability* has evolved as a label and categorical entity rather than a unitary diagnosis. We subscribe to a nonlabeling, noncategorical descriptive approach and shall refer to learning disorders rather than LD. Most experts agree that there are many kinds of learning disorders, with varying characteristics and severity. There is also consensus that learning disorders may be lifelong and pervasive, selectively interfering with social interactions, self-concept, and work goals in adolescents and adults.

Attention-deficit disorders are also clouded by considerable controversy surrounding diagnostic and conceptual issues. There are divergent opinions regarding the incidence of comorbidity with other conditions, such as learning disorders, conduct disorders, and depression. Research increasingly has shown that whereas hyperactivity commonly decreases in adolescence, other symptoms of attentional dysfunction may persist or worsen. It is clear that impulsivity, inattention, and distractibility often exact a significant toll from the learning and academic achievement of affected adolescents.

INTERACTIONAL MODEL OF LEARNING DISORDERS

In the clinical evaluations of adolescents with learning disorders, it is helpful to use a paradigm that includes broad domains of neurodevelopmental function that are considered to be essential foundations of learning and academic productivity: attention, memory, visual-spatial processing, sequential processing, language, higher order cognition, neuromotor function, and social cognition.[1] Each of these functions includes constituent elemental

---

BOX 127-1
Summary of Public Law No. 94-142:
The Education For All Handicapped
Children Act

1. Full appropriate public education for all handicapped children
2. Identification and evaluation of all children with handicaps
3. Preparation and implementation of individualized education plans
4. Placement in least restrictive environment possible
5. Procedural safeguards for parents (due process)
6. Provision of "related services"
7. In-service training for teachers
8. Possibility for outside independent review

BOX 127-2
Innate and Environmental Influences

Brain disorders
Genetic predisposition
Temperament
Stress and coping ability
Motivation
Peer influence
Adult role models
School characteristics

---

functions that contribute in synergy to successful or deficient performance of academic tasks (Fig. 127-1).

Students show marked variation with respect to these elemental functions, and empiric observation reveals wide diversity in patterns of strengths and weaknesses. Some broad implications of this paradigm should be recognized:

1. An elemental function may affect the performance of multiple academic tasks. For example, poor understanding of syntax (word order) is likely to affect reading comprehension and the solution of word problems in mathematics.
2. No academic task entails only one elemental function. An individual with well-demarcated strengths or affinities of a particular type may gain access to alternative pathways to achieve task mastery.
3. The impact of weak elemental functions is modulated by interactions with biologic, temperamental, social, and emotional factors.

Some examples may serve to clarify the complex interactions between neurodevelopmental function and other innate and environmental influences (Box 127-2). The neurologic basis of learning disorders is often evident in subtle signs of minor neurologic dysfunction, such as left-right confusion or trouble with finger-thumb opposition. Adolescents with brain disorders such as epilepsy and hydrocephalus or with a history of closed head injury are more likely to have neurodevelopmental dysfunctions and learning disorders.[2] Lifelong temperamental traits may affect significantly the impact of these predispositions.[3] A tenacious and positive adolescent is more likely to achieve mastery of a challenging task than a shy and apathetic one.

Outcome may be influenced by adolescents' emotional state and coping abilities, which themselves will be shaped in part by their life's experiences in dealing with adversity. Adolescents' peer groups may have a powerful effect on overall work performance. If their friends are academically unmotivated, their grades may suffer, whereas a favorable peer work ethic may stimulate productivity. The negative influence of peers may be compounded by alcohol and marijuana use, which has been shown to impair memory and cognition.[4] Teachers and other adult role models have a powerful influence on an adolescent's disposition toward learning. Partly on the basis of these innate and environmental influences, some adolescents with learning disorders prove themselves to be malleable and resilient, whereas others suffer dire and irreversible consequences.

Another vital consideration is the influence of an adolescents' motivation, attributions, and beliefs about their own competence and learning abilities. The relationship between academic self-perceptions and subsequent motivation and school performance has been explored in Diener and Dweck's work on learned helplessness.[5] Students with learning disorders who are chronically deprived of success tend to have an external locus of control, perceiving their failure to be due to a pervasive and uncontrollable lack of ability, and they consider their rare successes to be flukes. Studies have shown that children's perceptions of their own ability become fixed by seventh grade, and for this reason loss of motivation and resignation to failure become critical issues of prevention in the early adolescent years.[6]

COMMON NEURODEVELOPMENTAL PREDISPOSITIONS

A few patterns of neurodevelopmental variation commonly encountered in adolescence are language disorders, visual-spatial processing disorders, organizational deficiencies, and passive learning styles. There are many other dysfunctions that may have impacts on learning in this age group, including memory and sequential processing disorders. It is also important to bear in mind the complex interactions between neurodevelopmental predispositions and psychosocial factors.

ELEMENTAL FUNCTIONS   PRODUCTION COMPONENTS   ACADEMIC TASKS

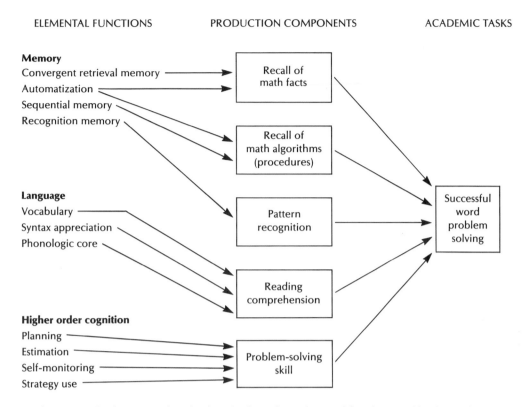

Fig. 127-1. Performance of academic tasks depends on elemental functions working in synchrony. The figure shows how language, memory, and higher order cognition elements contribute to components of solving word problems in mathematics.

Language Disorders

A broad spectrum of language disorders may be encountered in adolescents and often may lead to underachievement in a number of academic areas, including reading, writing, and content areas. Often, there is a history of delayed or atypical language development and/or speech articulation problems.[7] Language disorders may be considered primarily receptive, expressive, or mixed receptive/expressive. Receptive language problems may occur in conjunction with poor auditory attention, hearing deficits, or central auditory processing dysfunction and may impair effective interpretation of spoken or written ideas. Students may have difficulty grasping verbal concepts or appreciating figurative language, humor, and ambiguity. Expressive language problems can be equally debilitating. Some students with word-finding deficits may live in perpetual fear of being called upon in class. The slowness, imprecision, and hesitancy with which they express themselves cause frustration, both academically and socially. Deficits of verbal pragmatics (the use of language for social communication) are relatively common among adolescents with language and learning disorders, who have trouble switching codes and taking the listener's perspective in different speaker-listener interactions. Consequently, they may experience social and emotional

maladjustment. Language disorders may be associated with chronic and persistent middle ear effusions,[8] closed head injury,[2] and genetic disorders (Klinefelter's syndrome).[9]

Visual-Spatial Processing Disorders

Adolescents who have selective deficits in visual perception, spatial awareness, and/or visual-motor integration are likely to struggle in math and writing.[10] Interpreting graphs, getting oriented in geometry, and copying from the overhead projector may be daunting tasks. Commonly, there is a history of left-right confusion; difficulty in coloring, copying, and drawing; or delay in learning to tie shoes. Many adolescents develop compensatory strategies and use their language processing strengths, effectively diminishing the impact of their visual-spatial weaknesses as they grow older. Visual-spatial processing disorders are sometimes seen in adolescents of very low birth weight and are also common in Turner's syndrome,[11] neurofibromatosis,[12] and spina bifida.[13]

Organizational Deficiencies

It is not unusual to hear of an adolescent who has "organizational problems." Although sometimes considered to be trivial annoyances, such difficulties can have major impacts on academic performance and adjustment at home and in school. Several forms of organizational disarray commonly present in this age group.[14] First, there are students who exhibit material disorganization. They have problems with the "props" required for school; it is difficult for them to keep track of papers and books. They tend to forget what they need to bring home to complete assignments. Other students have impairments of temporal-sequential organization. Often they have endured a lifelong history of sequencing deficiencies. In early adolescence, they may have poor narrative skills and difficulty learning events or ideas in their proper sequence. Deadlines may be particularly hard to meet, and class schedules hard to master. Organizational problems may stem from difficulties with selective attention. Impulsivity, inattention to detail, and distractibility engender careless errors, poor planning, and fluctuating forgetfulness.

Passive Learning Styles

The volume and complexity of academic demands make the acquisition of efficiency and facilitative strategies exceedingly helpful to the adolescent student. Torgesen[15] described certain students as "inactive learners": underachievers who fail to engage in the strategies needed for effective learning. Adolescents with poor memory strategies may have difficulty knowing what they need to study for an examination, which techniques to use for the active learning of new material, and how to test themselves.

Highly proficient students not only have facilitative strategies, but also tend to have available to them multiple alternative strategies, so that if one technique fails, other options remain. Many underachieving students have one method available and apply this rigidly. When this isolated approach fails, they become discouraged, guess, and lose interest. Interestingly, it has been found that students who lack multiple alternative strategies in the cognitive domain are prone to similar problems with respect to social performance.[16] They lack flexibility in their social strategies, which can ultimately result in difficulties with peer and adult interactions.

One of the most salient developmental acquisitions in adolescence is the ability to reflect on one's own cognitive processes. This ability, metacognition, becomes a vital facilitator of learning.[17] Metacognitive development continues among college students, particularly as specific areas of expertise evolve. Most traditional views of learning disorders have included assumptions of perceptual or neurologic deficits, but it is clear that for some adolescents with learning disorders the deficit lies within their approach to solving problems.

Specific Dissonances and Affinities

Many adolescents with "learning disabilities" also exhibit significant strengths in one or more domains. For example, a boy with a language disorder may be superb at understanding and fixing machines. Such an individual is ideally suited to a variety of productive and rewarding pursuits in the adult world. His problems are largely the result of a mismatch between his prematurely specialized brain and the requirement for generalized competency in school. It is not uncommon to find struggling adolescents with clear affinities for academic and nonacademic interests and pursuits that are being underutilized in the school setting.

SPECIFIC ACADEMIC DEFICITS

Reading Disorders

In early adolescence, basic literacy skills of decoding and comprehension must be consolidated in order to be used as tools for learning in the content areas. Students are expected to acquire new information about science, social studies, and history from books. The essential task changes from learning to read to one of "reading to learn."[18] Beyond junior high school, students begin to grapple with understanding multiplicity, comparing and contrasting different points of view, appreciating irony and metaphor, and identifying recurring themes. Their reading rate must become increasingly flexible and efficient; students must know when and how to skim, scan, focus, or evoke mental images. Some adolescents do not experience reading difficulties until this age; alternatively, previously identified reading disorders take on new and complex forms.

A huge body of research on dyslexia has investigated the cognitive underpinnings and sources of individual differences in reading ability.[19] Developmental functions especially relevant to reading in adolescence include language, memory, and metacognition (Box 127-3).

BOX 127-3
Key Elements of Reading Disorders

Phonologic deficits
Weak appreciation of syntax
Deficient vocabulary
Weak sight-word recognition
Active working memory deficits
Attention deficits
Metacognitive delays

Deficits in phonologic awareness are strongly associated with decoding delays experienced in early grades, and these problems may persist beyond elementary school, interfering with reading fluency and speed. Such students may have to devote so much effort to sounding out individual words that they have few resources left for text comprehension. Weak appreciation of syntax and grammatical constructions may account for pervasive reading comprehension problems. Vocabulary is another linguistic factor contributing to reading ability among adolescents. Students are expected to understand new, specialized technical vocabulary, and studies have shown that poor readers are inferior to good readers not only in their vocabulary size, but also in their ability to derive a word's meaning from its context.

Memory plays a key role in reading. By fifth grade, for example, a student's sight recognition of frequently encountered words must be rapid and automatic. Students who recognize words slowly must resort to laborious sounding out, thereby undermining the higher level processes of reading comprehension. Some adolescents with active working memory deficits have trouble holding on to information in short-term memory. By the time they get to the end of a paragraph, they may have forgotten the beginning.

Many adolescents struggle with reading because of metacognitive deficits. Their basic reading skills are intact, but they do not have the capacity to think about their reading and modify reading strategies for different purposes. They may not be cognizant of the most salient aspects of a chapter, and summarization skills may be elusive. They may fail to pick up inconsistencies. Often, they fail to realize that they have not adequately understood a text. Such a student's plight is worsened by the fact that he or she seldom rereads, consults a dictionary, uses contextual cues, or asks for help.

Spelling Disorders

Spelling problems are a common source of annoyance in adolescence and are especially embarrassing because of their visibility. They occur in association with specific memory deficiencies and with reading or writing problems in general. One group of poor spellers have persistent problems with revisualization. Their ability to recall visual configurations is impaired, and their overreliance on phonetics leads to difficulty with irregularly spelled words, such as "pepol" for "people." Another group consists of adolescents with poor phonologic awareness, who spell words that may be visual approximations but that fail to conform phonetically, such as "pleope" for "people." Indeed, some adolescents make both error types. A common phenomenon among adolescents is the eclipse phenomenon, whereby students may spell words correctly in isolation, but with the added

demands of writing a paragraph, their brittle skills break down and misspellings abound.

Writing Disorders

Writing represents the confluence of many developmental functions and thus constitutes the most common disability of communication skills in adolescence. Because it is a visible and permanent record, it makes the struggling adolescent feel vulnerable, "on display," and therefore reluctant to write. This reluctance can aggravate the problem and result in a slow rate of writing or drastically reduced written output.

Students with writing disorders (dysgraphia) may have a history suggesting language dysfunction, with reading delays and poor oral expression. A student's oral expression and writing samples may share several common features, such as limited vocabulary and a deficient grasp of syntax and grammar. Others may have adequate basic language abilities but have trouble organizing their ideas in writing. Many adolescents have excellent oral expression but weak written expression. Some may struggle to recall the mechanics of writing, so that punctuation and capitalization are poorly automatized. Others harbor neuromotor dysfunctions that interfere with the speed and efficiency of finger movements in writing.[20] These include visual-motor integration problems, finger agnosia, motor planning deficits, and difficulty carrying out fine-motor sequences. Students with one or more of these dysfunctions are likely to adopt unusual and maladaptive pencil grasps, which lead to fatigue ("writer's cramp"). These students often avoid cursive writing because they find it consumes too much effort, and their written output is usually slow, sparse, and unsophisticated in ideation (Fig. 127-2).

Mathematics Disorders

Poor math skills in adolescence may be attributed to a variety of underlying dysfunctions (Box 127-4). Nonverbal conceptualization is essential for grasping and applying many mathematical operations. Many students with deficient nonverbal conceptualization suffer from a tenuous grasp of the subject matter. They fail to progress satisfactorily to higher levels of expertise because those essential building blocks are not set on a firm foundation. These students may have succeeded in earlier grades by relying excessively on rote memory, but heightened conceptual demands in junior high school, with emphasis on directionality, proportions, and spatial relationships, lead to declining performance. This decline may be especially acute when a student begins to study algebra. Memory dysfunctions are a serious impediment to math proficiency.[21] Many students with active working

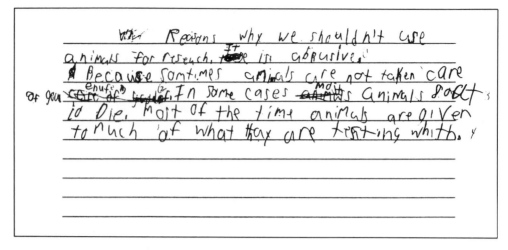

Fig. 127-2. This writing sample from a 13-year-old boy took him nearly 10 minutes to complete and shows organizational problems and graphomotor dysfluency.

BOX 127-4
Key Elements of Mathematics Disorders

Weak nonverbal problem solving
Tenuous grasp of concepts
Active working memory deficits
Poor retrieval memory
Language disorders
Attention deficits

---

memory problems tend to lose track of the components of a problem while they are solving it. Poorly automatized retrieval of basic math facts, especially multiplication tables, leads to slow and laborious computation. Many students have trouble recalling the math procedures and fail to acquire memory strategies to assist performance. Other students know these various algorithms but seem to have trouble recognizing "what to do when."

Adolescents with language disorders may have difficulty understanding the teacher's explanations of concepts or procedures. They prefer to figure things out on their own. Word problems prove especially difficult for these students. Attention deficits also have a major impact on math performance. Cognitive impulsivity, inattention to detail, and reduced self-monitoring frequently result in careless errors.

ROLE OF PEDIATRICIAN OR HEALTHCARE PROVIDER

With increased awareness of the plight of adolescents with learning and attention-deficit disorders, the pedia-

trician or adolescent healthcare provider has an opportunity to minimize the impact of endogenous dysfunction on the developing adolescent. Screening and surveillance for school problems, diagnostic procedures, appropriate referral or multidisciplinary evaluation, counseling, demystification, pharmacotherapy, and advocacy are all within the realm of clinical practice. There are many models of adolescent health care involvement in this field from private practice to school-based clinics. Optimal identification, evaluation, and management are likely to be challenging, time-consuming, and expensive for all involved. However, the price of neglect, false attributions, and excessive failure during the critical transitions of adolescence is far higher.

ASSESSMENT AND DIAGNOSIS

The first question confronting the adolescent healthcare provider concerns the early identification of the adolescent with an attention-deficit and/or learning disorder. In many adolescents, learning problems were identified earlier in childhood, but for some, changing demands and expectations trigger the emergence of problems in adolescence. Teachers may be the first to suspect underlying learning or attention-deficit disorders and may refer the student to a school psychologist for further evaluation. The results of group-administered achievement tests, such as California Achievement Tests (CATs), may be helpful in screening. Many parents become concerned about their adolescent's increasing struggles at school and discuss these concerns with healthcare providers. Problem identification is sometimes initiated by the healthcare provider, who, while managing related somatic or behavioral symptoms, begins to suspect underlying school problems. The evaluation of an adolescent with suspected learning disorders is best done through the efforts of a multidisciplinary team and should provide a comprehensive and detailed description of academic strengths and weaknesses and cognitive and neurodevelopmental abilities, as well as an overview of the student's health, emotional well-being, and social environment. Currently, in most states, eligibility for special educational services in public schools is determined by specific discrepancy formulas, which consider overall cognitive ability (measured by an intelligence test) and academic achievement (measured by standardized and individually administered achievement tests). Thorough evaluation, however, should go beyond a determination of eligibility for services. It should yield a description of the disorder that is specific enough to allow the student, parents, and teachers to understand the various problems, dispel inappropriate attributions or labels, and generate realistic recommendations (Box 127-5). Evaluating adolescents with attention deficit and learning disorders requires a thorough, sensitive, and eclectic approach that is familiar to pediatricians and adolescent healthcare providers.

History

A history should be obtained from multiple sources, including the parents, teachers, and adolescent. Major questions need to be delineated and explored. Various symptoms and attributes that cluster together should be described, including information about sleep, habits, mood, aggression, somatic complaints, responses to stress, and social behavior. Information about the family structure and function is essential. A careful family history, particularly of learning disorders and psychiatric

problems, should be obtained. It is also essential to inquire about the adolescent's medical history, paying particularly close attention to pregnancy/perinatal events, recurrent otitis media, neurologic disorders, developmental milestones, temperament, and early behavioral patterns.

Examination and Testing

There are several approaches to the direct observation and examination of adolescents. Individual educational testing allows an experienced educational diagnostician or psychologist to survey a range of academic tasks and components and to observe an adolescent's problem-solving strategies, attention, organization, efficiency, and affect. Intelligence tests may be administered to derive intelligence quotient (IQ) scores, which are related to cognitive abilities, rate of learning, and potential for future learning accomplishment. Global IQ scores are generally less valuable in the evaluation of adolescents with learning disorders than are the profiles of performance on the component subtests. Computerized Continuous Performance Tests are readily available, and preliminary evidence suggests they have some usefulness as adjuncts in the evaluation of individuals with attention-deficit disorders.[22] Some adolescents with puzzling learning disorders, especially when there is evidence of organic brain dysfunction, should be referred for more extensive or specialized neuropsychologic testing. Results of such tests may point to specific functional neurologic impairments or suggest specific areas of the brain that may be involved.[23]

A screening assessment of social and emotional functioning is an important component of the evaluation of the adolescent. Standardized self-report rating scales are a useful adjunct in this regard. If there are indications of low self-esteem, depression, or anxiety, further assessment, involving psychiatric interview and/or projective techniques, is indicated. Another form of direct ability testing used by many pediatricians and other professionals is the neurodevelopmental examination.[24,25] These tests assess broad areas of developmental functioning that are considered to be important for success at school, including attention, memory, language, visual processing, and motor function. The neurodevelopmental examinations are never used in isolation, but the findings are used in conjunction with historical data and information from educational and psychologic testing. Recurring themes that clarify an adolescent's learning problems are sought, and areas of functional strength and weakness identified.

Because it is essential not to overlook medical factors that may contribute to an adolescent's learning problems, a systematic physical examination is necessary. Throughout the examination, the clinician needs to be vigilant for dysmorphic features that might suggest fragile X syndrome, neurofibromatosis, or Klinefelter's syndrome. Minor physical anomalies, such as unusual dermatoglyphics or hair whorls, may point to possible prenatal effects but are seldom diagnostic. The existence of various conditions, such as anemia, hypothyroidism, asthma, and seizures, may need to be considered on the basis of the history, and appropriate tests ordered. Considerations of growth and pubertal maturation are important, not only to diagnose the occasional case of Turner's syndrome, but also because problems in this domain are frequently additional causes of distress for the adolescent struggling at school. Thorough neurologic examination, including assessment of minor neurologic indicators, provides helpful and supportive information.[26] The number of such signs and the degree to which they occur correlate with the presence of learning disorders and can provide further evidence that a learning problem is constitutional. Screening examinations of vision and pure tone audiometry should be done to rule out sensory deficits. Parents and teachers often voice considerable interest in having laboratory tests performed for nutritional or metabolic diagnoses. Nutritional status is not well measured by blood tests, and it is very rare that determinations of serum glucose or other substances are helpful. Likewise, there is rarely an indication for electroencephalography or brain imaging in the routine evaluation of learning disorders.

Common Diagnostic Dilemmas and Pitfalls

In the evaluation and management of adolescents with learning disorders, certain clinical dilemmas frequently arise. One such concern is the adolescent who has been labeled as a behavior problem in school. Many influential adults (e.g., teachers, parents) might be prejudiced against a student whom they perceive as a behavior problem. They are apt to mistake the adolescent's face-saving, recuperative strategies for primary behavior disorders. A negative reputation can sometimes obscure other problems such as learning disorders or emotional concerns that are amenable to interventions. In this way, the negative reputation can become a self-fulfilling prophecy, legitimizing a school's withdrawal of assistance and hastening the chain of events that leads to dropping out of school.

A related phenomenon is the trap of dichotomous thinking, whereby schools or professionals, in their efforts to apply categorical labels, think that a student who has a behavior problem cannot have a learning disorder or that a student with cultural deprivation cannot have an attention-deficit disorder. Such "either/or" thinking has little place in adolescent development, in which multiple influences converge and coexist and in which an individual cannot and should not be reduced to an abbreviation or label. Many adolescents with learning and attention-deficit disorders fail to meet traditional discrepancy formulas to receive special education services and are likely to "fall through the cracks." Many of the diagnostic instruments currently used to detect learning disabilities are limited in the range of abilities that are assessed and place few demands on precise and rapid memory, organization, concept formation, planning, or rate of production. As a result, many students lose their eligibility for assistance at school when they reach the secondary school level, and many others, who experience learning problems for the first time at the secondary school level, may go undiagnosed.

MANAGEMENT

Demystification

It would be inconceivable to manage an adolescent with diabetes without diabetes education. Similarly, it is essential to give adolescents with learning and attention-deficit disorders a thorough explanation of their strengths and weaknesses. The results of an evaluation should be communicated in nontechnical terminology, often providing concrete examples to clarify issues. Such feedback can do much more than provide information. It serves an important demystification function, dispelling misconceptions, alleviating guilt, and fostering optimism while convincing adolescents and their parents of their personal control over future outcomes. Students who understand the nature of their learning problems are more likely to feel accountable without feeling blamed. It opens the way for them to devise personal strategies to circumvent their difficulties while avoiding feelings of helplessness, futility, and denial of responsibility (Fig. 127-3).

Educational Interventions

Educational interventions are at the core of the management of learning disorders. Although a detailed discussion is beyond the scope of this chapter, there are three broad areas to consider: direct remediation, bypass strategies, and organizational skills. The therapeutics of developmental dysfunctions are controversial, especially the effectiveness of direct efforts to "fix" a dysfunction. There is evidence, however, that language therapy leads to improvement in language function and that memory strategies can be taught effectively to students with memory deficiencies.[27] It is not clear whether such improvements transfer to other learning situations or lead to broad academic gains. Further research in specific remedial interventions for specific areas of developmental weakness is urgently needed.

Any educational program for adolescents with learning disorders must include ways of bypassing areas of vulnerability. A student with graphomotor impediments to

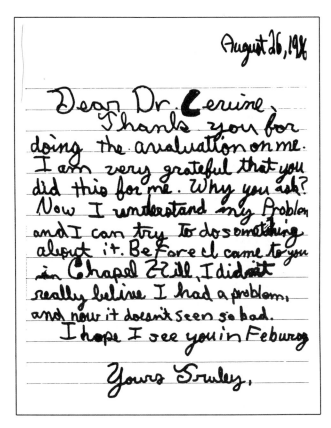

August 26, 1996

Dear Dr. Levine,
Thanks you for doing the evaluation on me. I am very grateful that you did this for me. Why you ask? Now I understand my Problem and I can try to do something about it. Before I came to you in Chapel Hill, I didn't really believe I had a problem, and now it doesn't seem so bad.
I hope I see you in Feburary.

Yours Truley,

Fig. 127-3. This letter was written by a 12-year-old boy after reluctantly undergoing an evaluation. He had been practicing a fair amount of denial, and the demystification process was especially helpful in this case.

writing, for example, should be allowed to do less copying, have some shorter assignments, and have access to word processing programs on a computer. However, teachers are apt to vary considerably in the extent to which they are prepared to make allowances and adjust expectations, curricula, and daily procedures.

Adolescents with learning problems are often in need of training in organizational skills, study skills, and test-taking strategies. Note-taking abilities and summarization skills are critical requisites for the successful mastery of increasingly complex information. Assignment books and work schedules are vitally important as students learn how to allocate time appropriately to specific tasks. Homework should be used to teach students how to study independently, and a "home office," free of distractions and conducive to thinking and productivity, should be established.

Educational Placement

The concept of "the least restrictive environment" is an important determinant in considerations of educational placement. An array of options may be available, from the regular classroom with tutorial assistance after school hours to a self-contained classroom for adolescents with

learning disorders. In between these extremes, a number of arrangements frequently are encountered in which special education services are made available to students in the form of allocated time in the resource room or consultation in the regular classrooms. Teachers are becoming increasingly aware of attention-deficit and learning disorders, and many are knowledgeable about helpful allowances and modifications in their classrooms. It is often possible to manage significant problems in regular classrooms without recourse to more restrictive placement options.

Psychologic Interventions

Social and emotional concomitants of learning problems and attention-deficit disorders often necessitate counseling, guidance, and other psychologic services. Significant emotional support can be provided by school guidance counselors working in familiar and nonthreatening school environments. Individual and group sessions can be employed to deal with issues as diverse as impulse control, parental marital breakdown, coming to terms with a learning problem, and developing social skills. Imaginative interventions by committed youth workers, such as wilderness camp experiences, can be invaluable in teaching new coping strategies and enhancing self-esteem. Sometimes there is a need for more intensive psychotherapy outside the school setting, which may include cognitive behavioral approaches and stress relaxation techniques.[28]

Vocational Considerations

There is a growing realization that for many adolescents the key to success lies in technical training and vocationally relevant education. Vocational education can be blended with a regular secondary school curriculum or take the form of innovative and cooperative work-study partnerships with industry and businesses. In other instances, vocational or technical schools offer a more intensive introduction to and preparation for the world of work. Such options frequently are not made available until too late, when motivational complications have already set in. Many young adolescents desperately need to do what they are good at for at least part of the school day, and such options should be available at an early age.

PROGNOSIS

Adolescents with learning disorders definitely have a mixed prognosis. For many, their academic failure is part of an ever-widening failure spiral. Dropping out of school, lifelong underachievement, delinquency, drug abuse, and a range of mental health complications may ensue.

The actual prognosis for a seriously underachieving adolescent is likely to depend on the balance between associated risk factors and protective factors. Among the risk factors are adolescents' own lack of insight into the nature of their learning difficulties, a home environment marked by poverty and deprivation, an educational system that has been unresponsive to the needs of the student, a history of grade retention, a lack of academically serious role models in the family or among peers, and the presence of complicating mental-health conditions, such as depression. Protective factors and influences that potentiate resiliency include enrollment in an educational program that insulates students from embarrassment and excessive criticism, the presence of recognized cognitive or athletic talents, the availability of services for students' learning difficulties, a track record of success in some domain, and adequate economic means.

Undoubtedly, complacency or a sense that the student will "outgrow it" represents a potentially dangerous attitude, one that is commonly assumed by parents, schools, some clinicians, and the students themselves. A clinician can play an important role in stressing the need for accurate diagnosis; induction of insight on the part of the student; careful educational planning; and appropriate service, guidance, and advocacy.

CONCLUSION

Management of learning and attention-deficit disorders in adolescence should be multimodal, coordinated, and individualized. Treatments may be directed at the adolescent, the classroom situation, or social and family circumstances. Early identification and vigorous intervention can interrupt a cycle of failure and disappointment, and prevent dropping out of school, drug abuse, and other calamitous outcomes of adolescence.

References

1. Levine MD, Hooper S, Montgomery, et al: Learning disabilities: an interactive developmental paradigm. In Lyon GR, Gray DB, Kavanagh JF, Krasnegor NA, editors: *Better understanding learning disabilities,* Baltimore, 1993, Paul H. Brookes.
2. Chadwick O, Rutter M, Brown G, et al: A prospective study of children with head injuries. II. Cognitive sequelae, *Psychol Med* 11:49-61, 1981.
3. Carey WB, Earls F: Temperament in early adolescence: continuities and transitions. In Levine MD, McAnarney ER, editors: *Early adolescent transitions,* Lexington, MA, 1988, DC Heath.
4. Schwartz RH, Gruenewald PJ, Klitzner M, Fedio M: Short-term memory impairment in cannabis-dependent adolescents, *Am J Dis Child* 143:1214-1218, 1989.
5. Diener CL, Dweck CS: An analysis of learned helplessness. II. The processing of success, *J Pers Soc Psychol* 39:940-952, 1980.
6. Stipek D, MacIver D: Developmental change in children's assessment of intellectual competence, *Child Dev* 50:521-538, 1989.
7. Beitchman JH, Brownlie EB, Inglis A, Wild J, et al: Seven-year follow-up of speech/language-impaired and control children: speech/language stability and outcome, *J Am Acad Child Adolesc Psychiatry* 33:1322-1330, 1994.
8. Roberts JE, Burchinal MR, Collier AM, et al: Otitis media in early childhood and cognitive, academic, and classroom performance of the school-aged child, *Pediatrics* 83:477-485, 1989.
9. Graham JM, Bashir AS, Stark RE, et al: Oral and written language abilities of XXY boys: implications for anticipatory guidance, *Pediatrics* 81:795-806, 1988.
10. Rourke BP: *Nonverbal learning disabilities: the syndrome and the model,* New York, 1989, Guilford Press.
11. Rovet J, Ireland L: The behavioral phenotype in children with Turner syndrome, *J Pediatr Psychol* 19:779-790, 1994.
12. Varnhagen CK, Lewin S, Das JP, et al: Neurofibromatosis and psychological processes, *J Dev Behav Pediatr* 9:257-265, 1988.
13. Wills KE, Holmbeck GN, Dillon K, McClone DG: Intelligence and attainments among children with myelomeningocele, *J Pediatr Psychol* 15:161-176, 1990.
14. Levine MD: *Developmental variation and learning disorders,* Cambridge, MA, 1987, Educators Publishing Service; pp 235-237.
15. Torgesen JK: The learning-disabled child as an inactive learner, *Top Learn Disabil* 2:45-52, 1982.
16. Richard BA, Dodge A: Social maladjustment and problem-solving in school-aged children, *J Consult Clin Psychol* 50:226-233, 1982.
17. Meltzer LJ, Solomon B, Fenton T, Levine MD: A developmental study of problem-solving strategies in children with and without learning difficulties, *J Appl Dev Psychol* 10:171-193, 1995.
18. Jordan NC, Reed MS: Reading disorders in early adolescence. In Levine MD, McAnarney ER, editors: *Early adolescent transitions,* Lexington, MA, 1988, DC Heath.
19. Catts HW: The relationship between speech-language impairments and reading disability, *J Speech Hear Res* 36:663-687, 1993.
20. Sandler AD, Watson TE, Footo M, et al: Neurodevelopmental study of writing disorders in middle childhood, *J Dev Behav Pediatr* 13:17-23, 1992.
21. Levine MD, Lindsay RS, Reed MS: The wrath of math, *Pediatr Clin North Am* 39:525-536, 1992.
22. Halperin JM, Matier K, Bedi G, et al: Specificity of inattention, impulsivity and hyperactivity to the diagnosis of attention deficit hyperactivity disorder, *J Am Acad Child Adolesc Psychiatry* 31:190-196, 1992.
23. Hooper SR, Willis WG: *Learning disability subtyping,* New York, 1989, Springer-Verlag; pp 109-138.
24. *Pediatric examination of educational readiness at middle childhood,* Cambridge, MA, 1985, Educators Publishing Service.
25. Sandler AD, Hooper SR, Levine MD, et al: The Pediatric Examination of Educational Readiness at Middle Childhood (PEERAMID): factor structure and criterion-related validity in a clinic-referred sample of children and adolescents, *Children's Hosp Q* 5:19-26, 1993.
26. Kandt RS: Neurologic examination of children with learning disorders, *Pediatr Clin North Am* 31:297-315, 1984.
27. Cavanaugh JL, Perlmutter M: Metamemory: a critical examination, *Child Dev* 53:11-23, 1982.
28. Kendall P, Braswell L: *Cognitive behavioral therapy for impulsive children,* New York, 1985, Guilford Press.

CHAPTER 128

Attention-Deficit Hyperactivity Disorder

•

Esther H. Wender

Attention-deficit hyperactivity disorder (ADHD) is a behavioral syndrome thought to be due to one or more variations in biologic development of the central nervous system. The defining behaviors fit into the broad categories of inattention, overactivity, and impulsivity. The severity of these behaviors occurs along a spectrum from high normal degrees of each defining behavior to degrees of severity that are definitely abnormal. The syndrome first appears in childhood, but in most patients (about 80%), symptoms persist into adolescence and adulthood. As the patient develops, however, the quality of the behaviors change in age-appropriate ways. Thus, overactivity, which in childhood is manifested by running and jumping, may be more typically demonstrated by restless, fidgety behavior in adolescence. Inattention in early childhood may be revealed in rapidly shifting from one activity to another, while in adolescence this trait may more typically show up as failing to stick with a task to completion. Impulsivity in childhood is typically manifested by interruptions and careless mistakes in school work. In adolescence, however, excessive use of alcohol and drugs and dangerous degrees of risky behavior, such as speeding in automobiles and sexual promiscuity, are more typical.

The significance of this behavioral syndrome in adolescence relates to its contribution to problems such as school failure, substance abuse, and delinquency. Substance abuse, delinquency, and school failure are not exclusively due to ADHD, but studies repeatedly show a strong association with this earlier behavioral syndrome.[1,2] Unfortunately, the connection between these adolescent problems and earlier ADHD often go unrecognized. This lack of recognition is due, in part, to the appearance of disturbing new behaviors (e.g., delinquent acts, dangerous/impulsive acts) that receive current attention while the behaviors that preceeded these in early childhood are not noticed.

The identification of ADHD in adolescence is complicated by environmental and social factors that may produce problems similar to ADHD and may significantly affect the manifestation of already existing ADHD. It becomes difficult to separate the adolescents whose current problems are due, in large part, to an earlier history of ADHD from those whose problems are due to other factors such as environmental stress or recent onset of psychiatric illness. By definition, ADHD is a disorder that begins in childhood. An absolutely essential feature of assessment is therefore a careful review of the history of behavior and school performance in childhood. However, there are several reasons why an earlier disorder may not have been identified. The adolescent with above-average intelligence may have performed age appropriately in academic tasks, thus escaping detection. Complicating social and emotional factors may have obscured the diagnosis or the family may have been resistant to identification of the problem earlier. Finally, the child with milder ADHD symptoms may have escaped notice during elementary school when there was less of an academic challenge.

PRESENTING PROBLEMS AND DEFINITIONS

ADHD is defined by the number and severity of behaviors that indicate an excessive degree of inattention, activity level, and impulsivity. The specific symptoms indicating problems in these three areas are listed in the fourth edition of the *Diagnostic and Statistical Manual of Mental Disorders* (DSM-IV).[3] These DSM-IV criteria for ADHD are listed in Box 128-1. Note that each specific behavior must occur more often than is typical of an adolescent of the same developmental age. For example, adolescents with mental retardation may also meet the criteria for ADHD if the appropriate developmental comparisons are made. These criteria allow for the occurrence of inattention without an excessive degree of hyperactivity-impulsivity (ADHD, predominantly inattentive type), and vice versa (ADHD, predominantly hyperactive-impulsive type). However, studies have repeatedly shown that most frequently all three types of symptoms are present (ADHD, combined type). These

---

BOX 128-1
Diagnostic Criteria:
Attention-Deficit Hyperactivity
Disorder

A. Inattention (6 out of 9)
Often fails to give close attention to details or makes careless mistakes
Often has difficulty sustaining attention
Often does not seem to listen when spoken to
Often does not follow through on instructions (although the instructions are understood); fails to finish tasks
Often has difficulty organizing tasks
Often shows dislike, avoidance of reluctance to engage when sustained mental effort is required
Often loses things necessary for tasks
Is often easily distracted by extraneous stimuli
Is often forgetful in daily activities

B. Hyperactivity-impulsivity (6 out of 9)
Hyperactivity
Often fidgets with hands or feet or squirms in seat
Often leaves seat in situations where remaining seated is expected
Often runs about or climbs excessively (may be limited to subjective feeling of restlessness in older individuals)
Often has difficulty in engaging quietly in leisure activities
Is often "on the go," acts as if "driven by a motor"
Often talks excessively
Impulsivity
Often blurts out answers before questions have been completed
Often has difficulty awaiting turn
Often interrupts or intrudes on others

Above behaviors present for 6 months or more
Above behaviors severe enough to be maladaptive and inconsistent with normal development
Some symptoms present before age 7 years
Some impaired function in two or more settings
Clear evidence of impairment in social, academic, or occupational functioning
Codes: Attention-deficit hyperactivity disorder, combined type (both A and B) 314.01; attention-deficit hyperactivity disorder, predominantly inattentive type (A only) 314.00; attention-deficit hyperactivity disorder, predominantly hyperactive-impulsive type (B only) 314.01

From American Psychiatric Association: *Diagnostic and statistical manual of mental disorders*, ed 4, Washington, DC, 1994, American Psychiatric Association.

---

criteria apply to adolescents and adults as well as to young children. However, some studies based on the earlier version of this nomenclature (DSM-III-R) suggested that adolescents with significant problems may have fewer positive symptoms than do younger children.[4]

Adolescents with ADHD symptoms also often have symptoms of other behavioral disorders. When the symptoms of these other disorders are sufficiently severe to meet definitional criteria for another disorder, the second disorder is said to be "comorbid" with the first. Such comorbidities constitute subgroups of ADHD that may have important implications for prognosis and treatment. The most common such comorbidities are listed in Table 128-1, along with examples of the additional behaviors that characterize these comorbid conditions. The frequency of these conditions makes it necessary to assess these conditions routinely whenever ADHD is suspected. Criteria for these comorbid disorders are contained in DSM-IV.[3] Clinicians who evaluate adolescents with ADHD must be familiar with the characteristics of these common comorbid disorders. Structured diagnostic interview tools incorporate symptoms of comorbid conditions into their format.[5]

One of the difficulties in the diagnosis of ADHD during adolescence is that the presenting clinical picture may be so complicated by emotional problems secondary to the ADHD that the true origins of the problem are obscured. In earlier childhood, ADHD is more likely to present as the classic picture of difficulty concentrating at school and rambunctious overactivity in play situations. The most common presentations during adolescence are doing poorly in school and behaving in a socially immature manner with peers and adults. The restlessness, distractibility, and inattention of earlier childhood may be less visible but are usually present when specifically assessed. Not doing well in school is often accompanied by a dislike of school and a refusal to complete school work, often leading teachers to the conclusion that the adolescent is "unmotivated." Parents often complain that the adolescent refuses to complete chores or take responsibility for homework, leading them to the conclusion that he or she is "lazy." These complaints may obscure the true origins of these behaviors in the short attention span and great difficulty sustaining effort typical of ADHD. Behavior at school often includes being silly or showing off. This social immaturity is typical of the adolescent with ADHD and appears to be due to a combination of poor social skill, which is a component of the ADHD syndrome not usually described, and attempts by the adolescent to counteract poor self-esteem through bravado or showing off.

If the adolescent has a comorbid oppositional defiant or conduct disorder, the presenting complaint is likely to be antisocial or oppositional behaviors such as defying adult authority at home and at school, or emotional

TABLE 128-1
Conditions Commonly Comorbid with ADHD and Some of Their Defining Symptoms

Conditions	Common Symptoms
Oppositional defiant disorder	Defiance of rules Negativistic behavior, e.g., talking back Temper outbursts
Conduct disorder	Violating rights of others and societal rules Excessive fighting Covert antisocial behavior, e.g., stealing, lying
Specific learning disabilities	Perceptual problems leading to significant underachievement Discrepancy between IQ and academic achievement
Depression	Persistent sadness and/or irritability Loss of interest in activities Suicidal thoughts
Anxiety	Excessive worry and fears Panic attacks Fears inhibiting normal behaviors

From American Psychiatric Association: *Diagnostic and statistical manual of mental disorders,* ed 4, Washington, DC, 1994, American Psychiatric Association.

outbursts such as temper tantrums or aggressive behaviors toward siblings or peers. The adolescent may present with truancy or even sexual misbehavior. If learning disability is present, the degree of academic underachievement may be severe, resulting in failing grades and even school refusal (see Chapter 127, "Learning Disorders").

EPIDEMIOLOGY

The prevalence of ADHD has been measured only in elementary school populations where prevalence figures of 3% to 10% of the population with the disorder are typical.[6] The condition occurs more frequently in boys, with a male-to-female ratio of 4:1. However, in the case of comorbid learning disorder with ADHD, predominantly inattentive type, a male-to-female ratio of 2:1 or even 1:1 has been found.[7]

PROGNOSIS

Long-term follow-up studies have repeatedly shown that symptoms of ADHD are likely to persist into adolescence and even adulthood. In about 40% of childhood cases the symptoms of ADHD persist into adolescence either severe enough to qualify for a diagnosis of ADHD or in milder, subclinical form. In another 40% the adolescent or young adult now carries another diagnosis of psychiatric disorder, most typically antisocial personality disorder, conduct disorder, and/or substance abuse disorder. The data suggest that these outcomes are due primarily to that subgroup of ADHD

patients with comorbid diagnoses of oppositional defiant or conduct disorder. Finally, about 20% of patients with childhood ADHD appear to be free of any diagnosis of disorder at follow-up in adolescence. However, this relatively well functioning group still reports more symptoms of distractibility and restless overactivity than in the "normal" population.[8]

ETIOLOGY

The strongest evidence for a biologic basis of ADHD comes from family studies that demonstrate a familial clustering and presumed genetic etiology for the disorder. Twin studies show a high rate of concordance for ADHD in identical twin pairs. Family studies reveal a much higher incidence of ADHD in first- and second-degree relatives of the index case than in the population as a whole. Also, cross-fostering studies show that children with ADHD in adoptive or foster care settings more closely relate to the incidence of ADHD in their biologic relatives than in the adoptive or foster care families. This evidence for a genetic, and hence biologic, etiology has not led to the identification of a specific biologic cause. The possibility that neurotransmitter dysfunction may be a cause of ADHD is based on the known effects of stimulant drugs on these neurologic chemicals, but no specific mechanism has been identified. There are also a number of specific congenital disorders that are frequently accompanied by ADHD symptoms, suggesting yet other possible biologic mechanisms producing this syndrome. Most experts expect that numerous different causes for the behavioral pattern of ADHD will be found.

DIAGNOSIS

The diagnostic process begins with a history of behavior and learning as manifested in the present and in the past, especially during preschool and elementary school years. Report cards during earlier school years can be helpful if they include descriptions of behavior: for example, descriptive statements of inattention, failure to complete work, and/or impulsive responses to classroom assignments. Results of standardized group achievement tests during childhood school years may suggest a learning disability (often accompanied by attention problems) by virtue of large discrepancies between scores in, for example, language and mathematics.

The current history of behavior and learning must also be assessed. Behavioral characteristics can be assessed more systematically through the use of standardized questionnaires that request parents and/or teachers to quantify their evaluation of specific behaviors, including those typical of ADHD.[9] Self-assessment questionnaires for adolescents have been developed.[10] Research has shown that adolescents can assess their own behavior more accurately than when they were younger.

In addition to a history of ADHD behaviors, the clinician must assess the existence of comorbid disorders, including learning disabilities, oppositional defiant and conduct disorders, anxiety disorders, and depressive disorders. The diagnosis of learning disabilities depends on both sophisticated psychologic testing and special educational testing that typically reveals a significant discrepancy between intellectual abilities and achievement in academic skills.

Finally, diagnostic assessment must include an evaluation of general medical health. Problems with vision or hearing affect academic performance. A chronic illness may lead to absences, impaired energy for learning, and a loss of self-esteem that may also affect academic performance. More acute problems such as anemia or thyroid dysfunction can also have an impact on learning and behavior.

The neurologic examination or testing has no direct relevance to making a diagnosis, either of ADHD or of related comorbid conditions. It is true, however, that a subgroup of adolescents with ADHD and with comorbid learning disability will have "soft" neurologic signs such as poor motor coordination, poor ability to distinguish right and left, and problems with what has been called "sensory integration." None of these findings are diagnostic of ADHD, and many adolescents with ADHD and/or learning disabilities have none of these problems. Neurologic tests such as electroencephalography and positron emission tomography (PET) have been employed as research tools but have no role in clinical diagnosis.

The diagnosis of ADHD is ultimately subjective and should be based primarily on a careful review of the history revealing the typical pattern of behavior over time, combined with the judgment that the behavior has significantly impaired functioning both socially and academically.

TREATMENT

Pharmacologic

Studies have revealed that at least 50% of adolescents who continue to manifest ADHD symptoms respond favorably to pharmacologic treatment with stimulant medication.[11] The favorable impact of stimulant medication in adolescents with ADHD is similar to that seen in younger children. There is an increase in the ability to sustain attention and remain focused on a task, and a reduction in impulsive responding. For adolescents with comorbid oppositional defiant or conduct disorder, there is also an increased willingness to comply and a reduction in emotional reactions to frustration.

The management of stimulant medication in the adolescent is similar to that in childhood, and typically can be prescribed and monitored by an interested primary care physician. However, there seems to be a reduction in the amount of medication per unit of body weight required in the adolescent as compared with an elementary school-age child. Table 128-2 gives typical starting doses, increases, and timing of medication during adolescence.[12]

The side effects of stimulant medication in adolescence are similar to those seen in childhood. Appetite loss, difficulty falling asleep, and a short period of irritability when the medicine is wearing off are most common. Some adolescents complain that they feel too subdued or they may report "not having any fun" when taking this medication. These feelings may be an accurate reflection of their own experience of a decrease in emotional highs that makes their behavior more acceptable to others but less agreeable to themselves. This response to medication must be distinguished from the depression that can be produced by stimulant medications. In the typical pattern, the onset of depression is insidious, often beginning after 3 to 6 months of favorable response to stimulants. The depression symptoms are seen during the peak effect of medication and often resolve quickly when the stimulant medication is discontinued. This side effect requires discontinuation of the particular medication currently being used. Often, however, a different form of stimulant will be effective without producing depression.

If stimulant medication is ineffective or produces unacceptable side effects, other medications may help. One study has demonstrated significant improvement in ADHD symptoms with tricyclic antidepressant medica-

TABLE 128-2
Stimulant Medication: Starting Doses and Titration During Adolescence

Medication	Starting Doses	Increases	Timing of Medications
Methylphenidate (Ritalin) short-acting tablets: 5, 10, 20 mg	10-mg tablets bid	5 mg per dose	AM and noon; add 4 PM dose as needed
Long-acting SR: 20 mg	20 mg SR in AM only	Add 5- or 10-mg tablets	Add tablets to AM dose and/or at 4 PM
Dextroamphetamine (Dexedrine) short-acting tablets: 5 mg	5-mg tablets bid	5-mg tablet per dose	AM and noon; add 4 PM dose as needed
Long-acting spansules: 5, 10, 15 mg	10-mg spansule in AM only	5-mg spansule in AM only or add 5-mg tablets to AM dose	Spansule AM only; add tablet to AM dose and/or 4 PM
Pemoline (Cylert) long-acting tablets: 18.75, 37.5, 75 mg	37.5 mg in AM only	18.75 mg per dose	Once in AM only; add a 4 PM dose as needed

tion in adolescents who do not respond to stimulants.[13] Recent nonblind trials have also shown some improvement in ADHD symptoms with the use of safer, nontricyclic antidepressant medications such as fluoxetine and bupropion. There are numerous anecdotal reports describing the combination of stimulant and antidepressant medications, particularly in patients whose symptoms improve with stimulants but are accompanied by unacceptable side effects. Use of such combinations cannot be recommended until studies demonstrate both safety and efficacy.

Counseling

An absolutely essential aspect of treatment of ADHD is the explanation of the condition to adolescents and their families. This helps counteract what are often firmly held attitudes that are destructive and may sabotage other treatment efforts. Such attitudes include the adolescents' belief that there is nothing wrong with them and that their problems are due to the school or the parents. Parents often see the adolescent's behavior as purposefully provocative and aimed at making them look bad. When everyone understands the biologic basis for the behavior, yet also understands that this behavior can be modified and that the adolescent can experience success, there is a change in emotional climate that can be more important than any other aspect of treatment. An important corollary of this aspect of treatment is the adolescent's understanding of medication. Without adequate explanations, adolescents may view medication as yet another example of the use of authority to control their behavior. In this situation, noncompliance often results. Successful pharmacologic treatment requires adolescents to see medication as helpful and a mode of treatment over which they

have control. In the process of titrating medication and following its effectiveness over time, the adolescent should be the primary source of information about medication effects. Adolescents should also be put in total charge of their medication as soon as possible. Fortunately, some school systems are changing their approach to allow adolescents to take their own medications, if required during school hours. This approach should be encouraged.

Traditional psychotherapy, either in the form of individual therapy for the adolescent or in the form of family therapy for the adolescent and other family members, may be indicated. This is not the treatment of choice for the primary ADHD symptoms but rather for the secondary problems that frequently develop. Examples include the adolescent who has become demoralized with a history or failures, and the dysfunctional family locked into verbal or physical interactions that are abusive.

Social skills training for the adolescent who is immature and is unable to maintain good peer relationships has become popular in recent years. Unfortunately, studies have shown that this approach is not effective outside the small group where such therapy takes place. The social problems of the patient with ADHD are usually the most difficult ones to remedy. This author finds that the most successful approaches are those that focus on the adolescent's areas of strength. For example, if the adolescent has an area of talent, any kind of social group that shares that talent should be encouraged. Also, if the adolescent prefers the company of much younger (or older) children, such associations should be encouraged. Adults often resist peer interactions between children and adolescents of disparate age on the theory that "he must learn to get along with children of his own age." Such worry is misplaced in the situation of poor social skills.

Other Treatment Approaches

Other treatments required for adolescents with ADHD are based on the comorbid conditions that may accompany the ADHD problems. The adolescent with ADHD and comorbid learning disability may need special education tutoring or special class placement, such as in a resource room. The adolescent with ADHD and comorbid anxiety disorder or depression may need treatment specific to these conditions. Adolescents with comorbid oppositional defiant or conduct disorder need to be supervised and taught by adults who are highly skilled in good behavior management techniques.

CONCLUSION

ADHD is a behavioral syndrome that begins in early childhood and most frequently persists into adolescence and adult life. Because it is a pattern of behavior that often precedes serious psychopathology in adolescence and adulthood, the condition should be recognized early and treatment should persist throughout development. With appropriate treatment, most adolescents with ADHD become productive, successful adults. However, failure to recognize and treat this condition may have serious consequences. The practitioner of adolescent medicine should become familiar with the many different manifestations of this syndrome, should be skilled at pharmacologic management, and should be able to educate adolescents and their families regarding the nature of the problem. Finally, the provider of adolescent health care should develop a network of other professionals who must provide many of the other services needed by these patients.

References

1. Brier N: Predicting antisocial behavior in youngsters displaying poor academic achievement: a review of risk factors, *J Dev Behav Pediatr* 16:271-276, 1995.
2. Lambert N, Harsough CS, Sassone D, et al: Persistence of hyperactivity symptoms from childhood to adolescence and associated outcomes, *Am J Orthopsychiatry* 57:22-32, 1987.
3. American Psychiatric Association: *Diagnostic and statistical manual of mental disorders,* ed 4, Washington, DC, 1994, American Psychiatric Association.
4. Barkley RA, Fischer M, Edelbrock CS, et al: The adolescent outcome of hyperactive children diagnosed by research criteria. I. An 8-year prospective follow-up study, *J Am Acad Child Adolesc Psychiatry* 29:546-557, 1990.
5. Herjanic B, Reich W: Development of a structured psychiatric interview for children: agreement between child and parent on individual symptoms, *J Abnorm Child Psychol* 10:307, 1982.
6. Brandenburg NA, Friedman RM, Silver SE: The epidemiology of childhood psychiatric disorders: prevalence findings from recent studies, *J Am Acad Child Adolesc Psychiatry* 29:76-83, 1990.
7. Shaywitz SE, Shaywitz BA, Fletcher JM, et al: Prevalence of reading disability in boys and girls: results of the Connecticut Longitudinal Study, *JAMA* 264:998, 1990.
8. Gittelman R, Mannuzza S, Shenker R, et al: Hyperactive boys almost grown up. I: Psychiatric status, *Arch Gen Psychiatry* 42:937-947, 1985.
9. Goyette CH, Conners CK, Ulrich RF: Normative data for Revised Conners Parent and Teacher Rating Scales, *J Abnorm Child Psychol* 6:221-236, 1978.
10. Conners CK, Wells KC: ADD-H Adolescent Self Report Scale, *Psychopharmacol Bull* 21:921-922, 1985.
11. Klorman R, Brumaghim JT, Fitzpatrick PA, et al: Clinical effects of a controlled trial of methylphenidate on adolescents with attention deficit disorder, *J Am Acad Child Adolesc Psychiatry* 29:702-709, 1990.
12. Wender EH: Attention-deficit hyperactivity disorders in adolescence, *J Dev Behav Pediatr* 16:192-195, 1995.
13. Biederman J, Baldessarini RJ, Wright V, et al: A double-blind placebo controlled study of desipramine in the treatment of ADD: I efficacy, *J Am Acad Child Adolesc Psychiatry* 28:777-784, 1989.

CHAPTER 129

School Avoidance: Excessive Absenteeism and Dropping Out

•

Carolyn Ashworth and Lorraine V. Klerman

Excessive absence from school and dropping out before receiving a high school degree are both forms of school avoidance that may negatively affect an adolescent's chances of a fulfilling adult life. Health personnel are in a unique position to influence these behaviors by stressing the importance of education when talking to their adolescent patients, and by encouraging them to attend school regularly, graduate from high school, and obtain additional education whenever possible. Health personnel should be willing to work collaboratively with the adolescent, the family, and the school in solving school avoidance problems. Also, since health personnel may be asked to evaluate adolescents who are excessively absent or in danger of dropping out for health-related reasons, they should have a knowledge of the possible causes of school avoidance, including health problems, and of the programs designed to remedy absenteeism and dropping out.

MAGNITUDE OF THE PROBLEM

Absence

School absence is usually a problem only when it is frequent, prolonged, or patterned, such as in the adolescent who regularly misses Mondays because of drinking binges. Although the term *truant* is often used to characterize students who are excessively absent, especially without an acceptable reason, the use of this term should be avoided since it places the blame exclusively on the student. Research suggests that absence and dropping out should be regarded as the result of interactions among students and their families, peers, the schools, and the community's social environment.[1]

Unfortunately, no national data source distinguishes between an occasional absence or one of short duration and frequent or prolonged absences, which are more likely to affect school achievement, but data are available on absence overall. For example, the National Center for Education Statistics (NCES) reported that in the first half of the 1990 school year, only 14.3% of tenth graders missed no school; 23.2% missed 1 to 2 days; 27.7%, 3 to 4 days; and 34.8%, 5 or more days. Among twelfth graders in the first half of the 1992 school year, the equivalent figures were 8.7%, 30.3%, 35.0%, and 25.9%, respectively. Females were more likely than males to miss 5 or more days of school; whites, Hispanics, and Native Americans more likely than blacks or Asians; those of low socioeconomic status more likely than those of middle or high status; and public school students more likely than Catholic or other private school students.[2]

For children 5 to 17 years of age, the National Health Interview Survey annually reports the number of "school-loss days" caused by an acute or chronic health condition. In 1993 there were 5.3 school-loss days per child. Again, females and whites had higher rates of absence for acute and chronic conditions than did males and blacks. Rates of absence were inversely related to income. Children in the central city of a metropolitan statistical area (MSA) had more school-loss days than those not in MSA central cities or not in MSAs.[3]

Dropping Out

Leaving school before graduation is an extreme form of school avoidance. Compulsory school attendance laws vary from state to state, but most states require school attendance only until age 16. Thus, a large number of adolescents drop out of school before high school

The preparation of this chapter was made possible, in part, by the Maternal and Child Health Bureau, U.S. Department of Health and Human Services (grant MCJ 9040).

973

graduation. The NCES reported that in 1992, 11.6% of the eighth grade class of 1988 had dropped out. However, many students who drop out before their class graduates later complete high school. Of the tenth grade class of 1980, 83.6% graduated on schedule (June 1982), 8.3% completed high school between 1982 and 1986, and 1.7% completed high school between 1986 and 1992. White and Asian students were more likely to finish on schedule than were students of other races or Hispanics; suburban students more likely than urban or rural students; and Catholic and other private school students more likely than those from public schools.

Among 16- to 24-year-olds in 1992, 11.0% were not enrolled in school and had not received a high school diploma or equivalency credential. Dropout rates were higher among those who had repeated a grade and increased with the number of grades repeated. These rates were inversely related to family income. Of students with no disability, 10.6% had dropped out, compared with 15.7% of those with a disability. Those with disabilities were also more likely to be retained in grade than those without (21.0% compared with 19.4%).[4]

CONSEQUENCES

Absence

Excessive absenteeism is associated with academic difficulty and dropping out. Many school systems will retain in grade students who have been absent 15 days or more during a 90-day term. In a 7-year follow-up of fifth grade pupils in a semirural area, frequent school absences and aggression were found to be correlated with grade retention, truancy, and dropping out of school.[5] Also, while excessive absence in the elementary years may signal a physical health problem or the school avoidance syndrome,[6] excessive absence in the middle and high school years is often a sign of disaffection with school— perhaps a more difficult problem to solve. Pupils who are frequently absent from junior and senior high school often have problems in other areas of their lives as well. Dryfoos, in her summary of studies of high-risk adolescents, noted that truancy and school misbehavior were related to substance abuse, dropping out, and delinquency.[7]

Dropping Out

A few individuals are very successful in life despite the fact that they did not graduate from high school, but recent studies show that a high school diploma and preferably some post–high school education are essential for the economic success of most individuals in American society today. In 1992, 62.8% of recent high school graduates not enrolled in college were employed, in contrast to 36.1% of recent school dropouts. This was reflected in incomes. In the same year, the median annual earning of both male and female 25- to 34-year-old whites who had not completed high school was about 75% of whites of the same age who had graduated. For blacks the earnings ratio was about 67%.[8]

HEALTH-RELATED FACTORS

Health-related factors are probably not the reasons for most cases of excessive absenteeism and dropping out in the adolescent years. Nevertheless, they are very important for a segment of middle and high school students.

Absence

A study of six Boston middle schools showed the relative importance of health, family, and school influences on absence.[9] When excessively absent pupils were asked an open-ended question about the reasons for their absences, almost half cited a health reason, almost always physical health. The remainder of the reasons were related to attitudes toward school (dislike of school, poor relationships with teachers), laziness, or missing the school bus. When offered a list of 15 possible reasons for absence, health and attitudes toward education remained important, but reasons suggesting a low priority given to school attendance by pupils or the family were checked by about two fifths of the pupils. These included bad weather, missing bus frequently, or not being awakened. In addition, about one quarter of the pupils reported missing school to care for a younger member of the household or an adult. Violence in the schools was given by 23% as a reason for absence. Parents were asked the same open-ended question and given the same list. Their spontaneous responses were similar to those of the pupils but showed somewhat more emphasis on negative attitudes toward school and less on laziness and waking up late. Using the checklist, parents were more likely than pupils to mention emotional problems, violence, and racial problems. They were less likely to mention weather conditions, no one waking up the student, or the need to care for a child or an adult in the household.

Chronic illnesses are a major cause of school absence,[10] and asthma is perhaps the most important of these. A total of 2.7 million American children under 18 years of age are estimated to have asthma, and this leads to 7.3 million days restricted to bed and 10.1 million days missed from school, or an average of 5 days per asthmatic child per year.[11] Absence due to asthma is not related exclusively to the severity of the health problem; psychosocial problems, frequent physician visits, and activity limitations may also contribute.[12]

Drug use is another significant cause of absence. A study of 300 African-American youths 9 to 15 years of age in six public housing projects found self-reported truancy to be significantly associated with selling and delivering drugs and having sexual intercourse, as well as being suspended from school.[13]

Dropping Out

The National Education Longitudinal Study of 1988 (second follow-up survey) revealed that reasons for dropping out were more often related to school than to jobs or family. Among tenth to twelfth grade dropouts, reasons given for absence were not liking school (42.9%) and failing school (38.7%). Among females, 26.8% stated that they left because they were pregnant; 7.7% of the males and 21.0% of the females said they left because they became a parent; and 6.4% of the males and 8.4% of the females said they left because they wanted to have a family.[14]

Pregnancy is still a major cause of dropping out but is less important today than it was in the 1950s. In 1958, 18.6% of those whose first birth was before 17 years of age and 51.2% of those whose first birth was at 18 and 19 had graduated high school by the time they were between 21 and 29. The equivalent figures for 1975 were 29.2% and 65.2%; and for 1986, 55.5% and 74.6%. In 1958, pregnant whites under 20 years of age were more likely than blacks to graduate; in 1986, blacks under 17 were more likely to graduate, although there was little difference for the 18- and 19-year-olds.[15]

ROLE OF THE HEALTH PRACTITIONER

Adolescent health practitioners encounter school absenteeism often, regardless of the socioeconomic, geographic, or ethnic setting within which they practice. Moreover, they are in a unique position to both prevent and manage many of the causes of excessive school absenteeism and dropping out.

Diagnosis

The practitioner may uncover a school absence or potential dropping-out problem during the course of a visit for health maintenance or when the adolescent comes to the practitioner seeking relief from one or more symptoms not thought related to absence; or a student may be referred specifically because of absences that are believed due to a health condition. A general conversation, with gentle probing and listening, can often elicit

issues with a potential for affecting school achievement and attendance—a problem with self-image or a concern about growth and sexual development, for instance. A practitioner attuned to adolescent health issues can ask further questions and uncover additional information to guide therapy.[16] A longitudinal relationship with an adolescent greatly aids this process.

Health maintenance visits represent a logical time to address school issues. If during a health maintenance visit the practitioner does not ask about adolescents' school performance and attendance, their satisfaction with school, and their peer relationships, school-related problems may go unrecognized and may eventually result in dismissal or dropping out. The purpose of the health maintenance visit is to assess all aspects of adolescent life in order to evaluate health and growth. Since adolescents spend a large part of their lives in school and since much of their intellectual and social development occurs there, the school should figure prominently in the discussion between physician and patient.[17]

Visits for symptom relief may also provide opportunities to detect school-related problems, even if they have not caused the health problem. However, when a thorough history and physical examination reveal only normal findings, a perceptive care provider should certainly ask about school functioning. A review of the medical record often reveals repeated episodes of acute illness that necessitated physician visits and school absences. When the symptoms are vague and the pattern of pain or illness occurs only on weekdays and never in the summer, the practitioner should consider the possibility of a school reluctance problem.[18] Once a school-related problem becomes a possible diagnosis, questions should be asked about the adolescent's self-image, school, and home environment. Additional information may be needed from the parents and the school in order to understand the full extent of the problem. To maintain good rapport and confidentiality, the adolescent must agree to the involvement of these individuals.

The first step in addressing school absence or potential dropping out is to identify the underlying problem. The practitioner should determine whether the absence is the result of an acute illness or whether it is part of a more chronic pattern of poor school attendance and performance. Acute episodes of absenteeism generally respond to practitioner intervention, whereas chronic absenteeism is often embedded in a complex familial and/or cultural structure that is difficult to change. Thus, chronic absenteeism is less affected by counseling and interaction with a primary practitioner. It frequently requires long-term intervention and the coordination of the efforts of many agencies.

ABSENCE DUE TO ACUTE PROBLEMS. Episodes of absenteeism caused by acute problems are best addressed as soon as recognized in order to reestablish school attendance. Attention should be focused on the events that precipitated the absences. For some adolescents, reluctance to attend school is related to anxiety about a specific situation that they perceive as a personal threat. In some cases, it may be a simple problem such as a bully on the school bus; in others, it may be more complex, involving a poor self-image or a fear of failure.

The main developmental task of adolescence is discovering one's own identity, largely by trial and error. Since adolescents are often unsure about themselves, they are frequently swayed by peers in their attitudes and feelings. For some adolescents who are "late bloomers" the move to high school, with its attendant emphasis on physical attributes and outward appearance, is excruciating. Poor physical growth characteristics can cause adolescents to feel so humiliated and rejected that they miss school to avoid this anxiety.[19] Poor school performance in the face of perceived high expectations by teachers and families can also lead to absenteeism as a means of avoiding stress.[20]

The student whose absenteeism is caused by an acute situation often develops vague somatic complaints as a way of coping with anxiety and stress. Parents and educators consider headaches, menstrual pain, abdominal pain, and fatigue as more acceptable reasons for missing school than fear of failure or being ridiculed because one is too short or underdeveloped.[21]

ABSENCE DUE TO CHRONIC PROBLEMS. Chronic forms of school absenteeism usually have a more complex etiology, often involving the adolescent's entire environment: self, school, and home. The practitioner may not become involved until there is a long-established pattern of absenteeism. This makes diagnosis and management more difficult.

Chronic diseases, such as asthma and diabetes, may cause frequent absences. If the practitioner is not aggressive about returning adolescents to school in spite of their chronic diseases, they may miss enough school to be disqualified from advancing to the next grade. Motivation to continue school may be lost if adolescents do not advance with their peer group. Pregnancy and the early postpartum period may also be a time of frequent absences. Pregnancy and parenthood can create substantial problems for adolescents in terms of their physical and emotional health. Routine obstetric appointments can become an obstacle to keeping up with class work. Parenting responsibilities after the baby is born can also interfere with school performance and attendance.

Depression is often associated with poor attendance, and in adolescents absenteeism may be the first sign. Learning disabilities and attention-deficit disorder can substantially increase an adolescent's frustration with school and, if not managed well, can lead to a number of absences.[22] (See Chapter 127, "Learning Disorders"

and Chapter 128, "Attention-Deficit Hyperactivity Disorder.")

Parents' perceptions of illnesses and of the value of education may influence the interpretation of both acute and chronic symptoms. If the adolescent is perceived as "sickly," absences may be longer than necessary.[23] For instance, it is not unusual for adolescent girls with dysmenorrhea to miss 2 or 3 days each month. As there is a recognized treatment for these symptoms, many of these absences are unnecessary. When little or no value is placed on education by the family, the adolescent may feel quite comfortable staying home for minor complaints. Other adult attitudes and behavior influence attendance. A home in which there is indifference or a lack of adult authority may allow many school days to be missed. In some families adolescents are viewed as responsible for younger siblings or aged relatives and are expected to fill the gaps in home care even if it means missing school.

The social environment also influences absenteeism. In schools where graduation rates are low and college-bound students rare, students may not realize the importance of education. A job that provides income for an extended or immediate family may seem more relevant than algebra or literature. In a poor urban high school where gangs are prominent, students' enthusiasm for staying in school may be low. Substance abuse and other high-risk behaviors play an important role in missing school, and a pattern of increasing absences may be the first clue to identifying those problems that often result from peer influence.[24] Many adolescents with histories of excessive absenteeism may make a quiet transition to high school dropout if their peers and/or their community view that as the norm.

Management

Management of the frequently absent student or the potential dropout should be tailored to the specific adolescent. Acute situations, such as the presence of a bully, that provoke anxiety should be addressed directly, with the adolescent fully involved in the decision-making process. Adolescents and their parents should be told that the vague symptoms produced by stress are real, but that addressing the root cause of the anxiety is the best way to relieve the symptoms. Often the practitioner's counseling will enable the adolescents and their families to find an acceptable solution. Support and reassurance by the practitioner may be the only resources needed. If depressive symptoms are noted, a referral to a mental-health professional for ongoing counseling is needed, regardless of whether suicidal ideation is present. When school avoidance is due to an acute anxiety-producing situation, prompt return to school is imperative.

Reassurance and education about the range of normal physical development are often helpful in cases of anxiety due to delayed development. Poor school performance can be helped by evaluation of cognitive functioning and appropriate remedial work.

When the factors affecting school attendance and success are more complex, such as chronic diseases and difficult family situations, great care must be taken to educate not only the adolescents but also their families and schools. For example, if an adolescent has an eating disorder, expectations for school attendance should be clearly stated and agreed upon by the physician, patient, and family. If the medical problem is asthma, specific guidelines for care should be determined and followed. Compliance issues, including the need for medications at school, can affect the management of a chronic condition and have a negative impact on disease control.[25] Medication schedules should be reviewed in terms of how best to reduce barriers to compliance. The timing of doses may be altered to avoid embarrassing the adolescent. The dietary limits for a diabetic must be explained and understood, affording the adolescent the opportunity to exercise control through diet exchanges. Adolescent females with dysmenorrhea should be counseled regarding treatment with prostaglandin inhibitors and placed on an appropriate treatment plan. Indications for leaving school should include uncontrollable diarrhea, severe menstrual pain, and prolonged vomiting. A physician's excuse may be required for reentry.

Education of school personnel about a particular health condition may help them understand the problems that the adolescent is facing and thus improve attendance. Fear and misunderstanding of syndromes such as Tourette's, attention-deficit disorder, and epilepsy often lead to inappropriate responses by teachers that reinforce a student's poor self-image.[26]

Sometimes the physician's role is that of a facilitator, but at other times he or she needs to be more authoritarian. The instructions for home care and the indications for missing school must be firm and reasonable. Excuse slips should always be dated and contain a definite date for return to school. Practitioners should document excuses in the medical record in case the slip is altered after the office visit.[27]

Pregnant adolescents should not be required to choose between attending school and keeping medical appointments. Prenatal visits should be scheduled after school hours. Most pregnant students can continue to attend their regular school with minor adjustments in their schedules, but some prefer to attend the special schools for pregnant students that are operated in many communities with a large number of pregnant students. Moreover, the parenting classes offered by these schools give these mothers additional tools for coping with their new responsibilities.

Child-care facilities, preferably at or near school, are essential if the new mother is to return to school after delivery. Home instruction is another alternative to absence during pregnancy but should not be used unless there is a major medical problem.

When the problem is attention-deficit disorder, learning disabilities, or similar conditions, the practitioner should be prepared for active partnership with the school. Psychometric testing by the school or a mental-health professional will be needed to determine whether specific disabilities such as dyslexia are present. Individuals with attention-deficit hyperactivity disorder may require a more structured class environment and may benefit from medication and additional instruction. In some situations, alternative educational plans may need to be developed for the adolescent.

If the problem with school attendance rests in the family's and community's attitudes toward education, the practitioner may be unable to resolve the problem in the office. Unless there is an identifiable mental or emotional health problem within the family, there may be little a practitioner can do. If a mental illness in a family member is affecting the adolescent's school attendance, referral of the entire family for counseling can be helpful. If substance abuse is a problem for either the adolescent or the family, a multidisciplinary team approach may have a positive impact. If a family is expecting an adolescent to help care for an elderly member or a younger child, state laws concerning education should be enforced, with the school and the physician assisting in finding alternative sources of care for the family member. If employment is considered more important than education, the practitioner can help the student explore community options for combining education and training.

Alternative high schools may offer more flexible hours and a vocational emphasis. In most communities, the General Education Diploma can be obtained through study in the evenings. If the community does not place a high value on education, the practitioner may spur interest by working with a parent/teacher organization and offering to serve as an adviser in efforts to improve community-wide graduation rates.

Examining the school experience from the various perspectives of adolescents, their parents, teachers, and other school personnel may provide important insights. Sometimes the avoidance of school is an appropriate student response to an inappropriate school program. The school program may be unchallenging or too challenging, there may be violence at the school, or the adolescent may encounter negative attitudes from a particular teacher or other students. Practitioners should be aware of special programs or schools in their own communities in situations such as these when an alternative educational program is necessary. A thorough evaluation of each individual's situation is essential. The health practitioner can serve as an advocate for the adolescent in the school system.

CONCLUSION

The role of the practitioner in managing school avoidance begins with efforts to prevent unnecessary school absence and to identify excessive absenteeism and potential dropouts early. Once these are identified, the practitioner must seek the cause or causes for the school avoidance. If there is a health component, the practitioner should provide the necessary therapy. For other causes, the involvement of other professionals and a knowledge of alternative programs are helpful. Working with the school is a necessary part of the management of health-related problems, as is the provision of support and counseling for adolescents and their families.

References

1. Klerman LV, Glasscock B: Features of children who do not attend school. In Berg I, Nursten J, editors: *Unwilling to school,* ed 4, London, 1996, Gaskell.
2. U.S. Department of Education, National Center for Education Statistics: *Digest of education statistics, 1994,* Washington, DC, 1994.
3. Benson V, Marano MA: Current estimates from the National Health Interview Survey, 1993. National Center for Health Statistics, *Vital Health Stat* 10(190), 1994.
4. U.S. Department of Education, National Center for Education Statistics: *The condition of education,* Washington, DC, 1994.
5. Kupersmidt JB, Coie JD: Preadolescent peer status, aggression, and school adjustment as predictors of externalizing problems in adolescence, *Child Dev* 61:1350-1362, 1990.
6. Committee on School Health: School attendance and school avoidance syndromes. In *School health: policy and practice,* Elk Grove Village, IL, 1993, American Academy of Pediatrics; pp 130-139.
7. Dryfoos JG: *Full-service schools: a revolution in health and social services for children, youth, and families,* San Francisco, 1994, Jossey-Bass.
8. U.S. Department of Education, National Center for Education Statistics: *The condition of education,* Washington, DC, 1994.
9. Klerman LV, Weitzman J, Alpert JJ, et al: Why adolescents do not attend school: the views of students and parents, *J Adolesc Health Care* 8:425-430, 1987.
10. Weitzman M: School absence rates as outcome measures in studies of children with chronic illness, *J Chronic Dis* 39:799-808, 1986.
11. Taylor WR, Newacheck PW: Impact of childhood asthma on health, *Pediatrics* 90:657-662, 1992.
12. Celano MP, Geller RJ: Learning, school performance, and children with asthma: how much at risk?, *J Learn Disabil* 26:23-32, 1993.
13. Stanton B, Romer D, Ricardo I, et al: Early initiation of sex and its lack of association with risk behaviors among adolescent African-Americans, *Pediatrics* 92:13-20, 1993.
14. McMillen MM, Kaufman P, Whitener SD: *Dropout rates in the United States: 1993,* Washington, DC, 1994, U.S. Government Printing Office.
15. Upchurch DM, McCarthy J: Adolescent childbearing and high school completion in the 1980s: have things changed?, *Fam Plann Perspect* 21:199-202, 1989.
16. Marks A, Fisher M: Health assessment and screening during adolescence, *Pediatrics* 80:135-158, 1987.
17. Berg I: Absence from school and mental health, *Br J Psychiatry* 161:154-166, 1992.
18. Schmid BD: School refusal, *Pediatr Rev* 8:99-105, 1986.
19. Committee on School Health: *School health: a guide for professionals,* Elk Grove Village, IL, 1987, American Academy of Pediatrics; pp 48-97.
20. Levine MD: Maladaptation to school. In Levine MD, Carey WB, Crocker AC, editors: *Developmental-behavioral pediatrics,* Philadelphia, 1992, WB Saunders.
21. Smith MS: Psychosomatic symptoms in adolescents. *Med Clin North Am* 74:1121-1134, 1990.
22. Buitelaar JK, van Andel H, Duyx JH, van Strien DC: Depressive and anxiety disorders in adolescence: a follow-up study of adolescents with school refusal, *Acta Paedopsychiatri* 56:248-253, 1994.
23. Green M: The "vulnerable child": intimations of mortality, *Pediatrics* 65:1042-1043, 1980.
24. MacKenzie RG: Substance abuse. In Hendee WR, editor: *The health of adolescents in San Francisco,* San Francisco, 1991, Jossey-Bass; pp 186-210.
25. Rickert VI, Jay MS, Gottleib AA: Adolescent wellness, *Med Clin North Am* 74:1085-1095, 1990.
26. Committee on School Health: Learning problems. In *School health policy and practice,* Elk Grove Village, IL, 1993, American Academy of Pediatrics; pp 161-176.
27. Committee on School Health: Children with chronic illness. In *School health policy and practice,* Elk Grove Village, IL, 1993, American Academy of Pediatrics; pp 188-195.

CHAPTER 130

School-Based Health Care

•

Julia Graham Lear

A growing trend in the delivery of adolescent health services is to "go where your patient is"—that is, health professionals are providing care to their patients in comprehensive health centers located in middle, junior high, and senior high schools. These health centers, staffed by full- and part-time medical, nursing, and mental-health personnel and linked to specialty referral care, are being developed primarily in communities in which young people are at risk for health-threatening problems and have limited access to traditional medical care.

School-based health centers are a significant innovation for a number of reasons. They are demonstrating a successful approach to connecting young people with integrated physical and mental-health services at a time when adolescents have a particular need for comprehensive care. In addition, they afford healthcare providers an opportunity to offer personal health services and to collaborate with school and community leaders in building healthier environments for adolescents.

HISTORY

The notion of providing medical services in schools is not new. The first school health programs were implemented in the late 1800s. Their purpose was to assess and, if necessary, exclude children with contagious diseases from the classroom. In 1902, New York City broadened the mission of school health services by establishing the first school nurse service to offer care and follow-up to children in schools.

Through much of the twentieth century, immunization and communicable disease control were the primary foci of school health. In the mid 1990s, 26,000 nurses were employed to provide health services in schools across the country. In most locations, their chief responsibilities are to ensure that required immunizations are complete, to screen for vision and hearing problems, and to refer children for needed health care.

As the twentieth century draws to a close, state-mandated school health services vary widely, as does the availability of nursing and other health personnel in the school environment. Recently developed services for disabled children and children enrolled in special education programs, as well as programs related to substance abuse, violence prevention, and mental-health problems, may constitute a larger portion of school health programs than traditional school nursing. Half of the states require vision and hearing testing for schoolchildren and 16 states require evidence of a physical examination, but none require evidence of treatment for problems found. In some local school systems, such as those in New York City, no school nurses are employed to provide traditional services; in others, such as the school system in Denver, all schools have nurses or nurse practitioners on staff.

Success in conquering many of the major communicable diseases of childhood and the emergence of broader concerns regarding the health of the nation's youth have sparked innovation in school health services during the past 20 years. The 1960s and 1970s saw the emergence of a new category of healthcare specialist, the school nurse practitioner, and a new multidisciplinary unit for providing health care, the school-based health center.

In 1970 the West Dallas Youth Center at Pinkston High School became the nation's first health center to offer comprehensive services on a high school campus from a multidisciplinary team of healthcare providers. Staffed by nurse practitioners, physicians, social workers, nutritionists, and health educators, this center was established by the University of Texas Health Sciences Center Pediatrics Department as part of a federally supported Children and Youth Program. A short time after the establishment of the West Dallas Youth Center, the Maternal-Infant Care Program of the St. Paul-Ramsey Medical Center opened a comprehensive clinic in Mechanic Arts High School in St. Paul, Minnesota, primarily to serve pregnant and parenting teenagers. As that program evolved, it extended its mission to provide all students with physical and

TABLE 130-1
Frequency of Diagnostic Categories Seen in Selected School-Based Health Centers (SBHCs) with Comprehensive Capacity

State	CT	NY	NY	CO	OR
Grade Level	**K-8**	**6-8**	**9-12**	**9-12***	**9-12**
Students in school	1,200	1,700	1,700	3,926*	8,858**
Enrollees in SBHC	968	668	1,000	2,595	4,336
SBHC visits/year	1,927	2,942	5,214	7,590	18,600
Diagnoses/year	2,253	2,942	5,942	7,590	23,343
Diagnostic Categories (%)					
Well child/adolescent	8	15	19	14	12
Gynecology/sexuality related	4	4	24	9	42
Mental health/social work	33	26	16	42	16
Injury/orthopedic	5	6	6	6	5
Neuroophthalmology	10	8	3	2	<1
Cardiorespiratory	8	4	4	2	3
Dermatology	6	3	3	3	4
Hematology	<1	2	3	<1	1
Gastroenterology	3	4	5	1	1
Dental	9	15	8	<1	<1
Ear/nose/throat	9	3	3	2	5
Infections	3	6	6	6	4
Drug and alcohol services	NA	NA	NA	NA	1
Other	<1	<6	<3	<1	<5

From Brellochs C, Fothergill K: *Ingredients for success: comprehensive school-based health centers. A special report on the 1993 national work group meetings,* Bronx, NY, 1995, School Health Policy Initiative, Montefiore Medical Center, Albert Einstein College of Medicine, p 27.
*Number includes two schools.
**Number includes seven schools.
NA, not available.

mental health services. Financial support for the St. Paul clinic initially came from Maternal and Child Health block grant monies. Both clinics continue to operate to this day and have served as models for the health centers established subsequently.

Physician support for the delivery of health services through the schools has grown since the mid-1980s. In a 1986 American Medical Association survey of primary care physicians, almost half of the respondents said that general medical care clinics, including those that provide contraceptive information, should be available in all high schools regardless of the school's pregnancy rate. By the end of the 1980s, the American Medical Association, the Society for Adolescent Medicine, the American School Health Association, the American Nurses Association, and other healthcare professional organizations had adopted statements in support of the continued development of school-based health centers. In 1990, through its publication *Healthy People 2000,* the U.S. Public Health Service declared that school-based or school-linked health services were appropriate vehicles for addressing the health problems of young people.

Political support for the school-based centers also increased during the same period. The waning level of controversy associated with the centers was confirmed by the health centers' inclusion in the Clinton Administra-tion's Health Security Act and bipartisan Congressional approval of the school-based health services portion of the bill. Sustained state government support for the centers, especially in the wake of the 1994 Republican election sweep, underscores the widespread acceptance of the centers.

CURRENT STATUS

In the years since the first school-based health center was established, the concept has evolved from a few scattered pilot efforts to a frequently replicated innovation occurring in almost every state in the nation. A 1996 survey found that there were 914 school-based health centers in 43 states plus the District of Columbia. The mid-Atlantic and New England states have embraced the centers most enthusiastically, with half the centers located in states between Maine and Maryland. Almost 50% of the centers are in high schools, 16% in middle schools, and 28% in elementary schools.

Typically, allowing for local variation, school-based health centers provide a standard set of services: acute medical care, physical examinations, laboratory tests, prescribing and dispensing of medications, mental health counseling, health education, nutrition education, and immunizations (Table 130-1). Some health centers also provide dental services, alcohol and drug abuse intervention and treatment, family counseling, and chronic disease management. Contraceptive services are available at some health centers, but many, under the direction of their school board or community advisory committee, do not prescribe or dispense birth control methods. An ongoing tension exists between the desire to avoid controversy and the need to reduce the continued high rates of teenage pregnancies.

Although clinic staffing patterns vary, especially in the composition of their part-time personnel, the core staff generally includes a full-time nurse practitioner or physician's assistant, a clinically trained social worker, and a receptionist/clerk. Part-time professionals typically include a pediatrician or family physician who sees students at least one session (3 to 4 hours) per week. Some centers have attempted to have an obstetrician/gynecologist on staff to see patients on site, but availability and cost issues have limited their success. Other part-time staffers have included health educators, substance abuse counselors, nutritionists, dental hygienists, pediatric or medical residents, and nursing graduate students. Frequently, part-time staff are members of community agencies who are also located in the health centers for some portion of the week.

A critical aspect of all staffing arrangements is that the clinical teams are multidisciplinary and acknowledge the important role that psychosocial issues play in adolescent health concerns. Care conferencing and consultation encourage cross-disciplinary thinking and the melding of skills to address adolescent health problems.

In addition to providing clinical care, school-based health centers contribute to other health promoting activities as well as providing training opportunities for health professionals. According to a recent survey, 86% of 228 responding school-based and school-linked health centers were engaged in classroom health education. Classroom sessions are targeted at reducing risk-taking behaviors and increasing appropriate utilization of clinical services. These efforts usually supplement the school's health education curriculum. Other health promotion work includes parent education, teacher training, school-wide health fairs, sports medicine clinics, student health clubs, and health columns for student newspapers.

Supported by the growing interest in community-based training, an increasing number of school-based health centers are also serving as training sites for physicians, nurses, social workers, and a variety of other health professionals. School-based health centers offer a unique setting in which trainees not only can learn about traditional school health practice but also gain in-depth, front-line experience in caring for adolescents within a multidisciplinary setting.

CHARACTERISTICS OF EFFECTIVE CENTERS

Although diversity characterizes the implementation of the school-based health center concept, there is a core set of attributes common to those health centers that are providing continuity care to large numbers of students successfully.

Accessibility

Like real estate, the primary characteristic of accessible adolescent services is location. Services that are next door or down the street from the school are not as accessible and will have lower student utilization rates. In addition to location, access is enhanced by generous service hours, with appointments available either before or after school. With appropriate regard for the importance of keeping students in class, the health center is available to students at most times during the day.

Acceptability

The services are attractive to students because they honor student confidentiality. The key issue of adolescent health services is addressed in several ways. Once parents have provided consent for their children to use the center, the students are assured of confidentiality in the provision of medical care. Parents not wishing their child to receive certain services are allowed to so indicate. In practice, few parents limit the services provided to their children. Neither parents, school staff, nor other health professionals may have access to medical information without the consent of the student. The health center records are maintained separately from the school health records. Clarifying the health-center policy on confidentiality for students, their parents, and school staff alike is an important early step in the establishment of a health center.

Affordability

School-based health centers have been established in low-income communities in which access to health care has been constrained by lack of both money and health insurance. Nationally, it is estimated that 4.5 million teenagers are uninsured. The school-based health centers serve primarily poor populations, with student surveys identifying between one third and one half of the population as uninsured. Only 37% of adolescents in poor families have Medicaid coverage; the financial barriers to securing care are great. Owing to the low income levels of the patients and their families, most health centers do not bill either students or their families directly for health care. Only a few centers have registration or enrollment fees.

In the past, school-based health centers have been sustained by public and private grants as well as in-kind contributions from the community. Medicaid and private insurance has covered less than 10% of the operating costs of the centers. In the future, a growing number of centers will need support from third-party payers, as well as from government agencies and private foundations, to sustain themselves. This need is leading a number of health centers to attempt to become Medicaid providers within existing fee-for-service systems and to secure a place for themselves within Medicaid-managed care networks where such have been put in place. While these new financial relationships may increase support for the centers, the negotiation of these relationships will challenge the administrative and political skills of school-based health center leadership.

RELATIONSHIP BETWEEN PRIVATE PRACTICE AND CENTERS

Many young people do not have a medical home base and indeed have not seen a healthcare provider for several years. Since school-based health centers are typically located in low-income communities that are underserved by primary care physicians, the relationships between private practice and the health centers are not well developed. A number of these health centers maintain a list of physicians who are willing to accept Medicaid or uninsured patients. The growth in managed care organizations has led to new relationships between mainstream medical care and school-based health centers. School-based centers are joining managed care networks in increasing numbers and as a result are becoming more closely linked to other participants in the healthcare system.

School-based health centers that have provided primary care to patients with chronic and critical diseases have reported developing close partnerships with specialists engaged in managing the overall care of these patients. In instances in which patients with private physicians also use the school-based health centers, relationships between the health center and the practitioner have been developed with the consent of the patient.

Finally, the school-based health centers are frequently challenged to fill far greater needs than their staffs can meet. Both through volunteering to help at the school-based health center and by offering discounted referral services at their professional offices, physicians and other health professionals can become welcome partners in these efforts to care for young people in need.

Suggested Readings

Anglin TM: Position paper on school-based health clinics, *J Adolesc Health Care* 9:526-530, 1988.
   Adopted by the Executive Council of the Society for Adolescent Medicine, this position paper not only provides the history of the school-based clinic movement but also addresses key issues: community and physician concerns, realistic expectations of the health centers, program evaluation, and long-term support. An excellent reference list identifies key documents.

Brellochs C, Fothergill K: *Ingredients for success: comprehensive school-based health centers. A special report on the 1993 national work group meetings,* Bronx, NY, 1995, School Health Policy Initiative, Montefiore Medical Center, Albert Einstein College of Medicine.
   Summarizes findings of four work group meetings that developed a consensus on guiding principles for school-based health centers, a recommended minimum core set of services, guidance for fitting school-based health centers into a managed care environment, and staffing requirements for comprehensive school-based healthcare delivery.

Council on Scientific Affairs: Providing medical services through school-based health programs, *JAMA* 261:1939-1942, 1989.
   This report, adopted by the AMA House of Delegates at its 1988 annual meeting, describes adolescent health needs, the components of school-based health centers, and evaluations of health-center effectiveness.

Juszczak L, Fisher M: Health care in schools, *AM: STARs* 7:162-325, 1996.
   A compendium of twelve articles covering diverse topics including the history of school health, the relationship of school-based primary care and managed care, college health, school nursing, and mental health services in school.

Juszczak L, Fisher M, Lear JG, Friedman SB: Back to school: training opportunities in school-based health centers, *J Dev Behav Pediatr* 16:101-104, 1995.
   Data from a 1992 survey of training activities in 18 school-based health center programs provide the foundation for a discussion of the range of training that is occurring as well as the benefits and limits of school-based training sites.

Lear JG, Gleicher HB, St. Germaine A, Porter PJ: Reorganizing health care for adolescents: the experience of the school-based adolescent health care program, *J Adolesc Health Care* 12:450-458, 1991.
   Reports on a 23-site demonstration effort by The Robert Wood Johnson Foundation to test the ability of school-based health centers to increase access to health care for low-income young people, to provide comprehensive services at school, and to secure the commitment of community institutions to participate in and sustain school-based health centers.

McKinney DH, Peak GL: *School-based and school-linked health centers: update 1994,* Washington, DC, 1995, Advocates for Youth (formerly the Center for Population Options).
   Update 1994 summarizes the characteristics of 231 school-based and school-linked centers that completed a survey of their 1992-1993 activities and operations. The 245 centers represented a 45% response rate from centers located in 35 states and the District of Columbia. Topics covered include staffing, services, student enrollment, utilization, and funding.

Schlitt JJ, Rickett KD, Montgomery LL, et al: State initiatives to support school-based health centers: a national survey, *J Adolesc Health* 17:68-76, 1995.
   A 1994 50-state survey documents numbers of school-based health centers by state and type of school, describes state funding levels and sources of support and summarizes standards adopted by ten states to guide the development of comprehensive school-based health centers.

CHAPTER 131

Literature for Adolescents

•

Roberta H. Friedman

Healthcare professionals are aware of the influence the mass media have on adolescents and therefore may attend movies, watch television shows, and listen to the music preferred by adolescents in order to understand the impact these media have on the young. They may not be as aware of the benefits to be gained by reading books written for the adolescent. Perceptive writers of adolescent fiction sensitively record the process of getting to know oneself, one of the main tasks of adolescence. Because these books mirror the adolescent world and focus on adolescent needs, emotions, and tasks, they provide insight into the adolescent character. Since all experience has to be limited, adolescent fiction can provide a valuable source of information about the lives of adolescents from a variety of backgrounds.

For example, a 50-year-old male pediatrician may recall his own distress and anxieties at 15 years of age, but what does he really understand about the feelings of a 13-year-old girl who has been sexually abused by her father? None of the books on growth and development or the clinical case studies can portray the feelings of anger, guilt, and love that this girl may feel as compellingly as the book *Abby, my love* by Hadley Irwin.[1] African-American, Hispanic-American, and Asian-American authors reflect the feelings of adolescents from different cultures who face the same developmental problems the healthcare professional did, but in a vastly different world.

Over the last two decades, hitherto taboo subjects have become common themes in adolescent literature. Serious problems such as terminal illness, death and dying, acquired immunodeficiency syndrome (AIDS), homosexuality, child abuse, incest, racism, and rape are addressed in these books, as well as the more developmental problems of divorce, teenage pregnancy, drugs, alcohol, obesity, and parental pressure. There undoubtedly has been a book written about every behavioral problem the clinician may encounter in treating adolescents. Reading such adolescent fiction will enlarge the

clinician's insights into children of the 1990s in contrast to children of the years before the 1960s.

Besides providing information about adolescents, books can serve as vehicles for discussion between the healthcare provider and the adolescent patient. The use of books in this manner is termed *bibliotherapy*. In its simplest form, bibliotherapy is the use of books to contribute to the adjustment, growth, and development of the adolescent, with an emphasis on behavioral changes. It does not require a degree in library science (or psychiatry)—all that is necessary is an ever-increasing knowledge of the books written for adolescents.

An awareness of this literature provides the clinician with a nonconfrontational tool to aid troubled teenagers and to give them examples of coping strategies in situations for which there are no easy solutions. When a reader is able to identify with a fictional character who is having problems similar to his or her own, the clinician can further help the adolescent interpret the motives of the character and understand the relationships among various characters. Bibliotherapy in this setting is not unlike play therapy with younger children. By removing the emphasis from the individual's problems, the book frees the patient to discuss the feelings of the characters in the book: for example, an alcoholic mother, a pregnant teenager, or a dying sibling.

Bibliotherapy may be particularly effective with minority groups. Often, poor patients from a minority background may be convinced that the successful clinician—of whatever race—cannot possibly understand their situation. Many of these young people are not aware that there are books written depicting minority life, and the clinician who is aware of these books may open up a new area for discussion.

Children with special needs, such as those who have learning disabilities or physical handicaps or who are gifted, may be especially receptive to such an approach. These adolescents often feel isolated and different from their peers. Books that present accurate and sympathetic portrayals of such populations can often be useful in increasing self-esteem and in helping overcome feelings of isolation.

GETTING STARTED

How does an adult acquire this knowledge of adolescent literature? Part 1 of Janice Bernstein's book, *Books to Help Children Cope with Separation and Loss,*[2] offers suggestions on how to use books with children. Ted Hipple's article "Twenty Adolescent Novels that Counselors Should Know About"[3] suggests specific books for a variety of common problems. Another approach for a busy clinician might be to start with a collection of short stories. In *Traveling On into the Light and Other Stories* by Martha Brooks,[4] teenagers face crises and gain insights. Critical incidents include being rejected by an abused mother, being wrongly accused of dealing in drugs, responding to accusations of being gay, accepting a father's being gay, adjusting to a father's suicide, and accepting an alcoholic father's death. This book gives a sample of the topics covered in teenage literature, and clinicians may see how these could be used with their patients.

The local public library can provide book lists and recommendations. The clinician can specify the subject matter of interest (e.g., anorexia nervosa, teenage pregnancy, AIDS, step families) and the librarian can make valuable suggestions. Many school-based health clinics are being established in high schools today, and the school library media specialist is a valuable source of information for the clinic staff. Another way for the clinician to acquire this knowledge is to listen to audio tapes during the commute to and from work. *Athletic Shorts* by Chris Crutcher,[5] a former family and child therapist, is a collection of short stories on tape that explore such subjects as death and dying, AIDS, friendship, abusive fathers, obesity, and gay parents. Many of these stories have multiple themes loosely connected by sports and are particularly useful for young men. The public library may have many of these tapes available. Once a book has been read, it remains part of the clinician's background, to be utilized when appropriate. One advantage is that these books do not become dated. Students are still reading *The Catcher in the Rye* by J. D. Salinger[6] and relating to this rebellious youth after 45 years. After more than 20 years, younger adolescents are still responding to Judy Blume as she discusses divorce, masturbation, religion, menstruation, obesity, and scoliosis.

Clinicians, as they read the books, may find that it is helpful to make a list of subjects, authors, and titles for future reference. If a book appears to have bibliotherapeutic possibilities, the clinician should buy one or two paperback copies and have them available on a shelf in the office or waiting room. If the books are close at hand, they are more apt to be used than if a special trip to the public library or school library is required. It also establishes clinicians' credibility, demonstrating that they believe the books to be worthy of purchasing for their own library. However, they should be prepared to lose a few books: sometimes adolescents are reluctant to admit they have an interest in these subjects (sex, alcoholism, rape, incest), and walk away with the books.

USING BOOKS WITH PARENTS

Often a patient is brought to the clinician because the parents complain that they "can do nothing" with the child. The youth has been lying, stealing, running away, doing poorly in school, or taking drugs. This young person obviously is asking for help but often has no clear idea why he or she is behaving in this fashion. There may have been a divorce, a remarriage, a new baby, problems at school, or the normal changes of puberty that can seem overwhelming. If clinicians are aware of a body of literature in which young people act in a similar manner, they may be able to draw on that knowledge and recommend books that the parents might read to gain insight into their child's actions. Parents often feel that their child is the only one who has ever had these problems, and it is helpful for them to realize that these are common conditions. For example, a mother reading *The War Between the Tates* by Allison Lurie[7] may discover that she is not the first person to have unnatural, unmotherly feelings as she reads: "It was as if she were keeping a boarding house in a bad dream and the children she had loved were turning into awful lodgers—lodgers who paid no rent, whose leases could not be terminated." A book that should be required reading for everyone dealing with adolescents is Avi's *Nothing But the Truth.*[8] With documents such as memos, phone calls, journal entries, newspaper articles, and conversations, this book documents the far-reaching consequences of one stupid action on the part of an angry young man. Discussing this book with a patient having trouble in school can raise questions about responsibility, consequences, appropriate behavior, and alternative ways of dealing with situations. It can also help parents understand the pressures adolescents are under. Adolescents also understand the value of sharing books with their parents. One eighth-grade girl remarked, "Whenever I read a good book, I give it to my mom so she can understand me better."

A nonfiction book, *Adolescence: A Survival Guide for Parents and Teenagers* by Elizabeth Fenwick and Tony Smith,[9] covers just about every important parent/teenager issue, most of it from both points of view, and would be useful to share with troubled parents and their offspring.

Parenting groups may find it useful to read and discuss some of these fiction books as a way to learn more about the adolescent mind and thus understand that others share their problems.

USING BOOKS WITH ADOLESCENTS

A feeling of trust and understanding must be established between adolescent and clinician before any suggestions of reading material can be made. Clinicians should not suggest a book they themselves have not read. It must be remembered that teenagers are in search of ideas, information, and values to incorporate into their lives, and novels are a way to reach out and explore various options without "losing face." Books can help battle peer pressure and serve as role models. Adolescents who reject the idea of actually reading a book because they "don't like to read" or have a reading problem, may be willing to listen to the audio tapes.

The clinician should be aware of the interests and reading level of the person to whom recommendations are made. If selected books are not suitable because they are too hard or too simple, the adolescent may become frustrated. Nor should the books offer simplistic and unrealistic solutions to complex problems: divorced parents seldom reunite, and dying parents do not make miraculous recoveries.

The single most important thing the clinician can do is to listen to patients as they talk about the book. Only after listening can the clinician know which concepts should be explored and expanded. Various methods of coping with the fictional problem can be explored and alternative solutions discussed. Then the clinician can perceive alterations in attitude and bring these observations to the attention of the patient. By identification and involvement, the reader will gain insight into his or her own problems and, with the help of the clinician, find solutions.

Timing is important in using books as a therapeutic tool. One approach might be to ask the patient if he or she has read any of the books available on the shelf. Contrary to popular myth, adolescents do read something besides Stephen King and *Sweet Valley High,* especially books that present situations and feelings that are relevant to their own lives. The knowledgeable clinician will be aware of the moment when the patient is ready to read and discuss books concerning his or her problems. One rape victim could not discuss her experience with her therapist but read, at the latter's suggestion, *Are You in the House Alone?* by Richard Peck[10] and was then ready to discuss the heroine's situation. Once started, she could talk about her own experience.

The clinician might suggest one or two books, but the choice should be made by the patient. Although it is anticipated that readers will identify with a character who is having problems similar to their own, sometimes they cannot face a book that mirrors their own problems. In this case, they need to read about someone overcoming difficulties of a different nature. For instance, discussing the unresponsive father in a book about the death of a mother, *There are Two Kinds of Terrible* by Peggy Mann,[11] may have more relevance for the boy with an alcohol problem than reading *The Boy Who Drank Too Much* by Shep Greene.[12]

Whichever book is chosen, it should serve to comfort teenagers who feel that only they have ever experienced these feelings or difficulties. If they can see themselves as aligned with characters, groups, or ideas presented in a book, they no longer feel isolated or abnormal.

A word of caution is in order. Getting patients to read the right books may still not make the hoped-for breakthrough in their defenses. Sometimes readers need time to reflect about what has been read, and there may be denial of the reality of their own real-life situation. Care should be taken that adolescents do not rationalize their problem by reading about it. Failure to identify with a character may serve to relieve readers of the responsibility for their own actions. Bibliotherapy is at best another tool, and it is not expected to "fix" the adolescent.

COMMON ADOLESCENT CONCERNS

Many adolescents have adjustment problems related to the divorce of their parents. Books that explore the positive and negative feelings that the characters experience, such as bewilderment, guilt, sadness, and perhaps relief, are most helpful. Over 7 million children live in blended families. Novels that consider their problems can offer support as young people in this situation attempt to cope with the feelings of anxiety, anger, or displeasure. Realistic depiction of the complexities of stepfamilies will allay the fears of many teenagers who cope with feelings of jealousy toward a stepsibling or loyalty toward their natural parent as they become attached to the stepparent.

A common disturbing experience for teenagers is that of moving to a new environment. Sometimes this move results in school phobia, acting out, withdrawal, or experiments with drugs and alcohol. The clinician who is aware of a pending move can help the family, or adolescent, by suggesting books that offer ways of coping with the situation. Although there are excellent fiction books on this subject, nonfiction books such as *Help! We're Moving* by Dianne D. Booher[13] or *The Teenager's Survival Guide to Moving* by Patricia C. Nida[14] also may be appropriate.

Weight, a problem for many teenagers, may be successfully approached through books. Following the anorexic adolescent's thought process from the start of a simple diet through the disintegration of her family, health, and daily routine in Steven Levenkron's *The Best Little Girl in the World,*[15] the reader can relate to her struggle for control and gain insight into her actions.

Quality literature with themes of death and dying allow the young reader to see the characters progress through most, if not all, of the five possible reactions to death: denial, anger, bargaining, depression, and acceptance. Automobile accidents are claiming more teenage lives every year, and the survivors must cope with guilt and remorse. A book that sends a good message to young people without preaching is *Real Life: My Best Friend Dies* by Alan Gelb.[16] Because Dave did not drink at the party, he insisted on driving his best friend home. Unfortunately he hit a patch of ice, and Walt dies in the accident. There is a realistic portrayal of family and school as Dave turns to drinking to deaden the pain. Positive adult role models (including his parents) help Dave cope.

Many young adults are struggling with issues of sexual identity, and until recently there were limited fictional resources to aid them. While in our culture one in 20 adolescents struggles with what it means to be homosexual, only recently have positive presentations of homosexual characters appeared in novels for young adults. Nancy Garden's *Annie on My Mind*[17] presents two young women exploring how to find a place for themselves in a hostile world. Garden's *Lark in the Morning*[18] combines detective work, adventure, and romance engaged in by two young female lovers. In *Toby's Lies,*[19] Daniel Vilmure presents a tragicomic story of a young Catholic high school boy who wants only to dance with his boyfriend at the prom. Books such as these demonstrate that we can provide gay students with the same resources that we give other minorities.

Although society seems unwilling to expend the resources to teach young people how to avoid and understand AIDS, the clinician may have books available that make the case for safe sexual practice. All of the facts and preaching are not as effective as stories of young people who tell what it is like to be terribly ill and scorned by family and friends, as in the nonfiction book *We Have AIDS* by Elaine Landau.[20] The lives of contemporary teenagers are touched by gay and lesbian issues, and books containing gay and lesbian characters may offset the stereotypes commonly encountered in the media.

CONCLUSION

Although clinicians may have total recall of the agony and confusion of their own adolescence, there is no way that this one experience can encompass all the various problems that beset different young people. By acquiring a broad knowledge of books written for adolescents, clinicians or other health professionals will broaden their understanding of adolescents today and acquire a tool to assist in treatment.

References

1. Irwin H: *Abby, my love,* New York, 1985, Atheneum.
2. Bernstein JE: *Books to help children cope with separation and loss,* vol 3, New York, 1989, RR Bowker.
3. Hipple T: Twenty adolescent novels that counselors should know about, *School Counselor* 32:142-149, 1984.
4. Brooks M: *Traveling on into the light and other stories,* New York, 1994, Orchard Books.
5. Crutcher C: *Athletic shorts,* New York, 1991, Greenwillow/ Charlotte Hall, Md., 1993, Recorded Books.
6. *Salinger JD: *The catcher in the rye,* New York, 1951, Bantam.
7. Lurie A: *The war between the Tates,* New York, 1974, Avon.
8. Avi (Wortis): *Nothing but the truth: a documentary novel,* New York, 1991, Orchard Books.
9. Fenwick E, Smith T: *Adolescence: a survival guide for parents and teenagers,* New York, 1995, Dorling Kindersley.
10. *Peck R: *Are you in the house alone?,* New York, 1976, Dell.
11. Mann P: *There are two kinds of terrible,* New York, 1977, Avon.
12. Green S: *The boy who drank too much,* New York, 1979, Dell.
13. Booher DD: *Help! we're moving,* Englewood Cliffs, NJ, 1983, Messner.
14. Nida PC: *The teenager's survival guide to moving,* New York, 1985, Atheneum.
15. Levenkron S: *The best little girl in the world,* New York, 1978, Warner.
16. Gelb A: *Real life: my best friend dies,* New York, 1995, Archway.
17. Garden N: *Annie on my mind,* New York, 1982, Farrah, Straus & Giroux.
18. Garden N: *Lark in the morning,* New York, 1991, Farrar, Straus, & Giroux.
19. Vilmure D: *Toby's lies,* New York, 1995, Simon & Schuster.
20. Landau E: *We have AIDS,* New York, 1990, Franklin Watts.

Selected Bibliography by Subject

Books selected here use realistic approaches dealing with problems. The characters cope as best they can with a situation as it exists and become stronger as a result. Many of the books would fit in more than one category, and many of the authors listed have written on a variety of subjects.

Abortion

Beckman G: *Mia Alone. Tr. Joan Tate,* New York, 1978, Dell.

Madison W: *Growing up in a hurry,* New York, 1970, Little, Brown.

Truss J: *Bird at the window,* New York, 1980, Harper & Row.

African-Americans

Childress A: *Rainbow Jordan,* New York, 1982, Avon.

Hamilton V: *Cousins,* New York, 1990, Putnam.

Myers WD: *Scorpions,* New York, 1988, Harper.

*Taylor M: *Roll of thunder, hear my cry,* New York, 1976, Dial.

Woodson J: *Maizon at Blue Hill,* New York, 1992, Dell.

---

*Indicates a "classic."

AIDS

Bantle L: *Diving for the moon,* New York, 1995, Macmillan.

Davis D: *My brother has AIDS,* New York, 1994, Atheneum.

Fox P: *The eagle kite,* New York, 1995, Orchard Books.

Kerr ME: *Night kites,* New York, 1986, Harper.

Anger

Crutcher C: *Ironman,* New York, 1995, Greenwillow.

*Golding W: *Lord of the flies,* New York, 1962, Coward-McCann.

Asian-Americans

Crew L: *Children of the river,* New York, 1989, Dell.

Irwin H: *Kim-Kimi,* New York, 1988, Puffin Books.

Yep L: *Child of the owl,* New York, 1977, Harper.

Death and Dying

Crutcher C: *Running loose,* New York, 1987, Dell.

Hermes P: *You shouldn't have to say good-bye,* New York, 1982, Scholastic.

Thesman J: *Nothing grows here,* New York, 1994, Harper Collins.

Divorce

Avi (Wortis): *The blue heron,* New York, 1992, Avon.

Barrett E: *Free fall,* New York, 1994, Harper Collins.

*Blume J: *It's not the end of the world,* Scarsdale, NY, 1972, Bradbury Press.

Cannon AE: *Amazing Gracie,* New York, 1991, Dell.

Danziger P: *The divorce express,* New York, 1988, Dell.

Eating Disorders

*Danziger P: *The cat ate my gym suit,* New York, 1974, Dell.

Hautzig D: *Second star from the left,* New York, 1981, Greenwillow.

Lipsyte R: *One fat summer,* New York, 1977, Bantam.

Gifted

Brooks B: *Midnight hour encore,* New York, 1986, Harcourt Brace.

*Leguin U: *Very far away from anywhere else,* New York, 1982, Bantam.

Hispanic Americans

*Anaya R: *Bless me, ultima,* Berkeley, CA, 1975, Tonatiub-Quinto Sol International.

Paulsen G: *The crossing,* New York, 1990, Dell. 1993, Recorded Books.

Soto G: *Taking sides,* New York, 1991, Harcourt Brace.

Homosexuality

Bauer MD, editor: *Am I blue? Coming out from the silence,* New York, 1995, Harper Collins.

Cohen S, Cohen D: *When someone you know is gay,* New York, 1989, M. Evans.

Herdt GH, Boxer A: *Children of horizons: how gay and lesbian teens are leading a new way out of the closet,* Boston, 1993, Beacon Press.

Heron A, editor: *Two teenagers in twenty,* Boston, 1994, Alyson Publications.

White E: *The Faber book of gay short fiction,* London/Boston, 1991, Faber & Faber.

Learning Disabilities

Banks J: *Egg-drop blues,* New York, 1995, Houghton Mifflin.

Hall L: *Just one friend,* New York, 1988, Macmillan.

Janover C: *The worst speller in jr. high,* New York, 1994, Free Spirit.

Physically Handicapped

Bowe F: *Comeback. Six remarkable people who triumphed over disability,* New York, 1984, Harper.

Calvert P: *Picking up the pieces,* New York, 1993, Scribner.

Crutcher C: *The crazy horse electric game,* New York, 1987, Dell.

Girion B: *A handful of stars,* New York, 1983, Dell.

Shreve S: *The gift of the girl who couldn't hear,* New York, 1991, Tambourine Books.

Voigt C: *Izzy, willy-nilly,* New York, 1986, Ballantine.

Sexual Abuse

Grant C: *Uncle vampire,* New York, 1993, Atheneum.

Tamar E: *Fair game,* New York, 1993, Harcourt Brace.

Voigt C: *When she hollers,* New York, 1994, Scholastic.

Substance Abuse

*Childress A: *A hero ain't nothin' but a sandwich,* New York, 1986, Dell.

Koertge R: *The boy in the moon,* New York, 1990, Avon.

Rodowsky C: *Hannah in between,* New York, 1994, Farrar, Straus, & Giroux.

*Scoppettone S: *The late great me,* New York, 1986, Dell.

---

*Indicates a "classic."

PART FOUR

Gynecologic, Urologic, and Sexual Issues

CHAPTER 132

Physiology of Menstruation and Menstrual Disorders

•

Joseph S. Sanfilippo and S. Paige Hertweck

PHYSIOLOGY OF MENSTRUATION

The earliest physiologic beginnings of the menstrual cycle occur during fetal development 10 to 12 weeks after conception. In humans, sexual dimorphism begins at this point, resulting in male and female sexual differentiation. The hypothalamic-releasing hormone is a decapeptide that has been noted in the fetal circulation at 10 weeks' gestation.[1] The development of the hypothalamic-pituitary-ovarian axis from neonate to initiation of puberty is further discussed in Chapters 5 and 6.

The exact "trigger" for the onset of puberty remains a point of controversy. Whether this represents a change in sensitivity to negative feedback at the hypothalamic level; the presence of a critical lean body mass; or enhanced (i.e., increased) pulsatile secretion of GnRH, with subsequent increases in both follicle-stimulating hormone (FSH) and luteinizing hormone (LH), remains to be determined.[2-4] Interestingly, the onset of adrenarche, which is clinically manifested at around 9 to 10 years of age, actually begins at approximately 6 years of age.[5] The usual sequence of pubertal milestones includes thelarche, adrenarche, peak growth velocity, and ultimately menarche.

Hormonal Patterns of First Menstrual Cycles

Hypothalamic development, as it pertains to reproductive neuroendocrinology, primarily involves the development of the median eminence and the medial preoptic area. Neurons containing gonadotropin-releasing hormone (GnRH) are present in both of these segments of the hypothalamus. The gonadostat, the physiologic structure made up of the hypothalamic median eminence and medial preoptic area, serves as the primary site of GnRH release. This region of the brain is associated with the pulsatile efflux of GnRH (every 60 to 90 minutes). Hypothalamic output is delicately balanced, in such a way that neural input into this region is received from serotoninergic, noradrenergic, and dopaminergic pathways. GnRH (a decapeptide) is released into the portal system; the releasing hormone is then delivered to the anterior pituitary gland, with a resultant release of the glycoprotein hormones FSH and LH. Both gonadotropins exit the pituitary and enter the bloodstream, through which they ultimately are delivered to the ovarian follicle apparatus, with resultant stimulation of preantral follicles. A composite view of the relationship between FSH, LH, and estradiol is presented in Figure 132-1. Oocytes are recruited, after which a dominant follicle is selected to provide primary governance during that particular menstrual cycle. Once ovulation occurs, a corpus luteum is formed on the ovary at the site where the ovum was extruded. Formation of the corpus luteum is characterized by production of progesterone.

The circulating gonadotropin levels throughout a woman's life from conception to adolescence are highlighted in Figure 132-2. A nadir of circulating gonadotropin (FSH and LH) levels occurs at 4 to 8 years of age, followed immediately by a prepubertal pattern of gonadotropin production[6] (Fig. 132-3). This prepubertal period is characterized by unique nocturnal LH surges,[7] in large part associated with rapid eye movement (REM) sleep.

Knowledge of this preliminary information enables the clinician to understand how persistent endocrine patterns

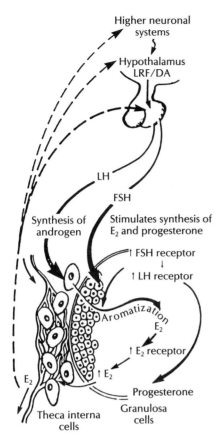

Fig. 132-1. Composite view of the relationship between FSH, LH, and estradiol (E_2) during the menstrual cycle. *LRF,* leuteinizing hormone–releasing factor; *DA,* dopamine. (From Yen SSC, Jaffee RB: The human menstrual cycle. In Yen SSC, Jaffee RB, editors: *Reproductive endocrinology: physiology, pathophysiology and clinical management,* Philadelphia, 1978, WB Saunders.)

observed in the course of early puberty (i.e., anovulation) may explain pathologic conditions during adult life such as polycystic ovarian disease.[8,9]

Figure 132-4 depicts a comparison of the hypothalamic-pituitary-ovarian axis of the fetus with those of the prepubertal as well as the late pubertal patient. Apter and Vihko[10] noted that under normal circumstances the first endocrinologic change recorded in the immediate premenarchal period at 7 years of age is an increase in serum dehydroepiandrosterone concentrations, complemented by an elevation of testosterone levels (Fig. 132-5). In the immediate postmenarcheal period there is a predominance of FSH in the circulation.[11] Once regular ovulatory cycles are established, an adult FSH-to-LH ratio evolves. FSH appears to be the primary hormone involved in ovum recruitment, with the selection of a dominant follicle usually around cycle day 6 or 7 and a subsequent rapid increase in the circulating concentration of estradiol. Serum testosterone and androstenedione levels closely parallel that of estradiol throughout the menstrual cycle.[12]

The frequency of ovulation after menarche is an interesting and somewhat perplexing phenomenon. Table 132-1 presents the frequency of ovulation as correlated with chronologic age beginning in adolescence. Ultimate synchronization of the hypothalamic-pituitary-ovarian axis results in further coordination of circulating serum gonadotropin levels as well as those of estradiol and progesterone (Fig. 132-6).

Regulation of the Menstrual Cycle

The menstrual cycle, in essence, is composed of three components: the follicular, ovulatory, and luteal phases.

FOLLICULAR PHASE. During this phase, primordial follicles progress through the stages of preantral, antral, and preovulatory follicle development. The primordial follicle, surrounded by a single layer of granulosa cells, is characterized by an oocyte, which appears to be arrested in the dictyotene phase of the diplotene stage of meiotic prophase. It progresses to the preantral stage, during which oocyte enlargement occurs and the zona pellucida develops. The granulosa cells proliferate, complemented by the development of the thecal layer during this developmental phase. Growth of the preantral follicle appears to be directly dependent on FSH and LH and correlates with increased production of estrogen.[13] The key events in preantral follicle development are (1) initial recruitment and growth independent of gonadotropin influence, (2) response to FSH stimulation as the follicle begins to grow, and (3) FSH-induced aromatization of androgens in the granulosa cells, which appear to be transported from the thecal cells in response to FSH stimulation. The end product is estradiol production; growth-stimulating hormone (GH) and estradiol induce FSH receptors on the preantral follicle.[13]

The next stage of development is the formation of the antral follicle. This segment of the ovarian mechanism has a characteristic follicular fluid with a predominant estrogen component and is surrounded by well-developed granulosa and thecal cell layers. The dominant follicle is "selected" from the 1000 original primordial follicle cohort, which is initiated each cycle before antral follicle development. Exactly how the dominant follicle is selected remains a question of continued research and fascinating inquiry. Once the dominant follicle is selected, usually on cycle day 6 or 7 in the typical 28-day cycle, this follicle becomes responsible for production of large quantities of estradiol, further induction of FSH receptors on the thecal and granulosa cells, and continued stimulation of the enzyme aromatase in granulosa cells, which is primarily affected by FSH and associated with the development of LH receptors. All this activity enhances the dominant follicle's response to both FSH and LH. Simultaneously, at the pituitary level, steroid modulation appears to occur, which enables the pituitary

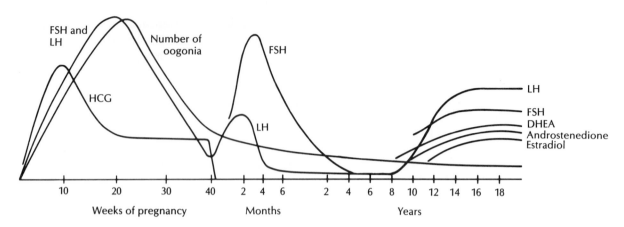

Fig. 132-2. Serum levels of FSH, LH, human chorionic gonadotropin (hCG), dehydroepiandrosterone (DHEA), androstenedione, and estradiol in females from prenatal state to 18 years of age. (From Speroff L, Glass RH, Kase NG: *Clinical gynecologic endocrinology and infertility,* ed 4, Baltimore, 1989, Williams & Wilkins; p 83. Copyright © by Williams & Wilkins, 1989.)

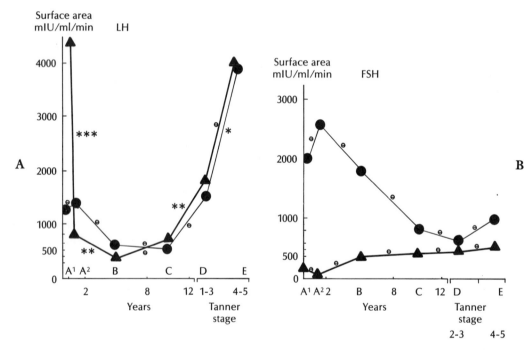

Fig. 132-3. Changes with age in hormonal response to bolus intravenous injection of 150 μg GnRH. Pituitary mobilized reserves of LH (**A**) and FSH (**B**) were estimated by calculating the surface area of the response curve for 90 minutes after stimulation and expressed in mIU/ml/min. *Filled circles,* females; *filled triangles,* males. Subjects were divided according to age: **A¹,** 0 to 6 months; **A²,** 7 to 24 months; **B,** 2 to 8 years; **C,** prepubertal children 8 to 12 years old. Groups **C** and **D** correspond to Tanner pubertal stages 2 and 3 and 4 and 5, respectively. Statistical analysis between subsequent age groups showed * = p <.005, ** = p <.025, *** = p <.005, and 0 = no significant difference. In infants (group **A¹**) a marked sex difference was also observed: the pituitary reserve of LH was significantly higher in males than in females, whereas the reverse was true for FSH. (Modified from Plauchu H, Claustrat B, Bétend B, et al: Le test à l'hormone hypothalamique synthétique LHRH chez l'enfant normal de la naissance à l'âge adulte, *Pediatrie* 35:119-131, 1980.)

to further respond to GnRH. In response to exposure to large quantities of estradiol (≥200 pg/ml for at least 36 hours), the hypothalamus releases a surge of GnRH. The GnRH surge then causes a large LH surge and a smaller FSH release, which results in ovulation within approximately 36 hours of the GnRH surge. The remaining cohort

of original follicles undergo atresia, primarily as a result of the predominant androgenic steroidal milieu.

The dominant follicle appears to be dependent on FSH as it completes the transition from preovulatory follicular phase to ovulatory phase. It may well be that the greater number of FSH receptors on the dominant follicle allows

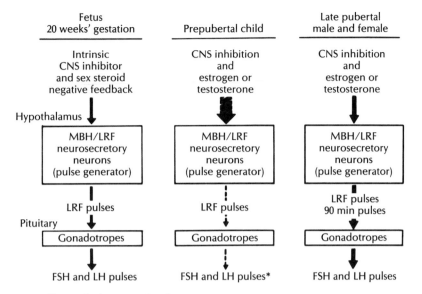

Fig. 132-4. Changes in activity of the medial basal hypothalamic pulse generator during development, and the effect on pituitary gonadotropes. It is hypothesized that functional GnRH insufficiency of a prepubertal child is a consequence of central nervous system (CNS) restraint by sex steroid–dependent and sex steroid–independent mechanisms. *MBH,* medial basal hypothalamus; *LRF,* luteinizing hormone–releasing factor. (From Warren MP: Metabolic factors and the onset of puberty. In Grumbach MM, Sizonenko PC, Aubert ML, editors: *Control of the onset of puberty,* Baltimore, 1990, Williams & Wilkins. Copyright © by Williams & Wilkins, 1990.)

it to "survive" while the cohort of follicles tends to undergo demise. As the mass of granulosa cells continues to proliferate, thecal vasculature matures, and by day 9 the thecal vasculature in the dominant follicle is twice as advanced as that of the antral follicles.[14] The polypeptide prolactin appears to be present in follicular fluid and is associated with a circulating increase of prolactin at midcycle. However, its role in ovulation remains a point of conjecture.

In addition, a number of growth factors are involved with follicle development. These include epidermal growth factor (EGF) and transforming growth factor alpha (TGF-α), which have the same receptor. Their primary influence occurs at the level of the granulosa cells; thus, these cells are involved in the autocrine aspects of follicle development.[9] In addition, transforming growth factor beta (TGF-β) has a receptor distinct from that of EGF/TGF-α and belongs to the same gene family as inhibin, a substance that primarily inhibits FSH release. Somatomedin-C (insulin-like growth factor I) has receptors on granulosa cells and plays a role in the ovarian follicle apparatus response to FSH, GH, and estradiol.[13] Somatomedin-C enhances FSH stimulation of steroidogenesis, LH receptors, and granulosa cell proliferation. Fibroblast growth factor, a potent mitogen, and platelet-derived growth factor also play a role, the latter apparently modifying cyclic adenosine monophosphate activity as FSH stimulates production of adenosine triphosphate, which is a mani-

festation of FSH linkage to its receptor on the cell membrane. When adenyl cyclase is stimulated and ATP production occurs, protein kinase is activated; it is this enzymatic catalyst that allows cholesterol to undergo a number of chemical changes within the thecal cell apparatus, with resultant androgen production (i.e., androstenedione or testosterone). FSH stimulation at the receptor level also plays an integral role in adenyl cyclase activation and conversion of androgens to estrogens within the granulosa cell in the presence of aromatase. Angiogenic growth factor appears to be involved in the enhanced vascularization of the follicle, especially at the thecal level.[15]

Thus, the events in the antral follicle include (1) follicular phase—estrogen production by the thecal-granulosa cell apparatus, which responds to FSH and LH; (2) selection of the dominant follicle between cycle days 6 and 7, with significant increase in estradiol production; (3) increase in estradiol levels, which provides positive feedback with GnRH and resultant LH and FSH surges; (4) increase in LH levels during the late follicular phase, which is responsible for thecal androgen production and serves as a prerequisite for conversion to estradiol in the granulosa cell apparatus, development of FSH receptors induced by estradiol, and development of LH receptors in response to both estradiol and FSH; and (5) the involvement of a number of growth factors in the follicular response to gonadotropins and further cellular multiplication of the thecal-granulosa cell apparatus.[13]

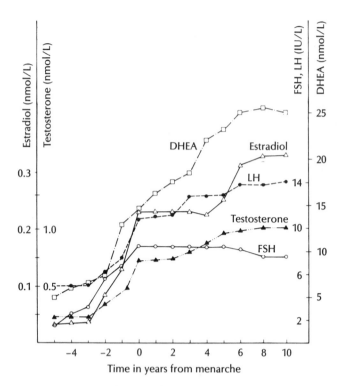

Fig. 132-5. Serum concentrations of FSH, LH, dehydroepiandrosterone (DHEA), estradiol, and testosterone in relation to time since menarche (no. of observations = 410). First points at −5 years include all subjects 7.3 to 5 years before menarche. Last points at 10 years include all subjects from more than 8 to 12.7 years since menarche. Postmenarchal specimens were drawn on days 6 to 9 of the cycle. (From Apter D, Vihko R: Hormonal patterns of the first menstrual cycles. In Flamigni C, Venturoli S, Givens JR, editors: *Adolescence in females,* Chicago, 1985, Mosby–Year Book; p 218.)

Ovulation is as a direct response to the LH surge, which occurs between midnight and 3 AM in two thirds of women.[16] Furthermore, ovulation occurs in the morning during spring and primarily in the evening during autumn and winter.[17] From July to February, 90% of women ovulate between 4 PM and 7 PM; during spring, 50% ovulate between midnight and 11 AM.[16] As LH levels in the circulation rise and the quantity of the glycoprotein hormone in the ovarian apparatus increases, LH overcomes the local inhibitory action of oocyte maturation inhibitor and luteinization inhibitor, both of which facilitate extrusion of the ovum. Progesterone contributes to enhanced distensibility of the follicle wall.[13] This distensibility is complemented by smooth muscle contraction at the level of the ovary. Digestion of collagen takes place in the follicular wall in response to the proteolytic enzymes collagenase and plasmin. In addition, histamine has been associated with ovulation in animal models, although its role in humans remains to be defined.[17] The level of prostaglandins in the follicular fluid peaks just before the release of the ovum.[17] Furthermore, prostaglandin synthetase inhibitors have an adverse effect on ovum release.[18]

TABLE 132-1
Frequency of Ovulation in Adolescent Menstrual Cycles in Relation to Chronologic Age

	Ovulatory Cycles (%)*	
Chronologic Age (yr)	Of All Cycles	Of Cycles With Specimen Drawn <10 Days Before Next Bleeding
12.2-13.9	38	54
14.0-14.9	41	47
15.0-15.9	50	53
16.0-16.9	58	74
17.0-17.9	56	63
18.0-18.9	67	77
19.0-19.9	71	83
20.0-25.8	95	95

From Apter D, Vihko R: Hormonal patterns of first menstrual cycles. In Flamigni C, Venturoli S, Givens JR, editors: *Adolescence in females,* Chicago, 1985, Mosby–Year Book.
*A serum progesterone concentration of >6.4 nmol/L (2 ng/ml) was considered to signify an ovulatory cycle, and a concentration of <1.6 nmol/L (0.5 ng/ml) in specimens drawn on days 20 to 23 of the cycles and later was considered to indicate an ovulatory cycle.

LUTEAL PHASE. The luteal phase is characterized by the release of progesterone in response to LH stimulation. Luteinizing hormone is released from the pituitary in a pulsatile manner, and progesterone levels appear to reflect this pattern in response: pulsatile release of progesterone has been reported.[19] In addition, low-density lipoprotein (LDL)-cholesterol provides the precursor for progesterone production. The enzymatic machinery of the corpus luteum allows cholesterol to be converted to pregnenolone and ultimately to progesterone. Peak levels of progesterone occur on cycle days 20 to 22 of the 28-day cycle. In general, the luteal phase lasts 14 days; however, a range of 12 to 17 days is considered normal.[20]

The corpus luteum appears to decline approximately 10 days after ovulation. The exact mechanism that initiates this decline is not understood. If fertilization does occur, human chorionic gonadotropin (hCG) appears to continue to stimulate the LH receptors, since there seems to be one receptor that responds to either LH or hCG.[21]

Body Composition and Effect on Onset of Puberty

Demographic data attest to the finding that menarche may indeed be affected by nutritional, environmental, and genetic factors. Age at menarche has decreased over the past 150 years in industrialized nations along with improvements in nutrition and life style[22] (Figs. 132-7 to 132-9).

The popular theory has held that a critical percentage of body composition, especially of body fat, is associated

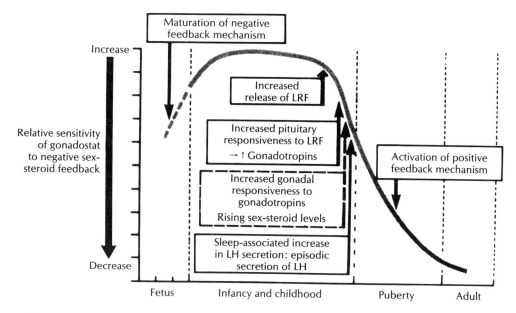

Fig. 132-6. Change in the set point of hypothalamic (GnRH) luteinizing hormone–releasing factor (LRF) and in pulse-generator pituitary gonadotrope unit (gonadostat) (denoted by dashed and solid line) and maturation of negative and positive feedback mechanism from fetal life to adulthood in relation to normal changes of puberty. (From Grumbach MM, Roth JC, Kaplan SL, Kelch RP. Hypothalamic-pituitary regulation of puberty in man: evidence and concepts derived from clinical research. In Grumbach MM, Grave GD, Mayer FE, editors: *Control of the onset of puberty,* New York, 1974, John Wiley; pp 115-166.)

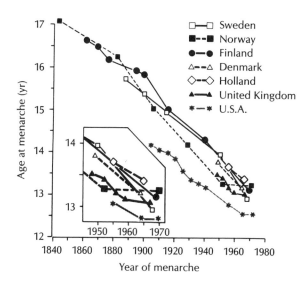

Fig. 132-7. Changes in age at menarche between 1840 and 1978 in seven countries. (Modified from Tanner M, Eveleth PB: Variability between populations in growth and development at puberty. In Berenberg SR, editor: *Puberty, biologic and psychosocial components,* Leiden, Netherlands, 1975, HE Stenvert Kroese, BV; p 256. Reprinted by permission of Kluwer Academic Publishers.)

with the age of onset of menarche. Lean body mass is more critical than total body fat, although the two appear to be related.[23] Figure 132-9 demonstrates the correlation between percentage body fat and age, with attention focused on the onset of puberty in both men and women.

Controversy continues with regard to athletic endeavors and pubertal aberration. Evidence suggests that a child who engages in physical activity may well experience delayed onset of menarche compared with the inactive or bedridden child, because an active child has a lower level of body fat than one who is less active[24] (Figs. 132-10 and 132-11) (Table 132-2).

AMENORRHEA

Menarche is an important milestone for the female adolescent. Amenorrhea, the absence of menses, may cause serious concern to the patient, family, and physician in that the condition may be indicative of a host of pathologic entities requiring medical attention.

Amenorrhea is divided into two clinical subgroups. Primary amenorrhea, with an incidence of 0.1%, is defined as absence of menses in a female with secondary sexual characteristics who has never menstruated by the age of 16.5 years, or as the lack of secondary sexual characteristics and the absence of menarche by age 13 years.[25] Secondary amenorrhea, with an incidence of 0.7%, is defined as the loss of menses for an arbitrary period, usually 6 months or longer.[25] By definition, primary amenorrhea affects adolescents, and on many occasions secondary amenorrhea occurs in this same population.

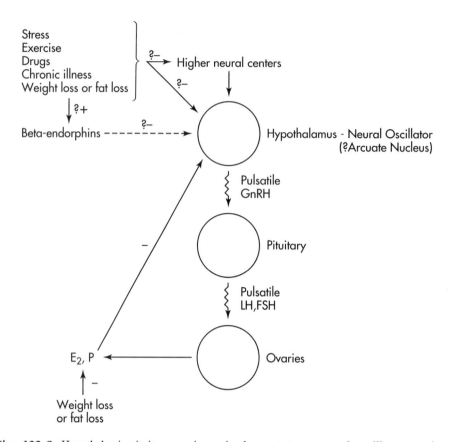

Fig. 132-8. Hypothalamic-pituitary-ovarian axis demonstrates a neural oscillator, causing a pulsatile secretion of GnRH with resultant pulsatile secretion of FSH and LH. The figure also demonstrates the possible roles of stress, exercise, drugs, chronic illness, and weight loss in menstrual dysfunction. (From Neinstein LS: Menstrual dysfunction in pathophysiological states, *West J Med* 143:476-484, 1985.)

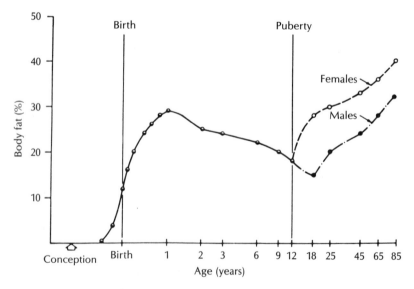

Fig. 132-9. Changing body composition from gestation through adult life. (From Bray GA, editor: The obese patient. In *Major problems in internal medicine,* vol 9, Philadelphia, 1976, WB Saunders; p 23.)

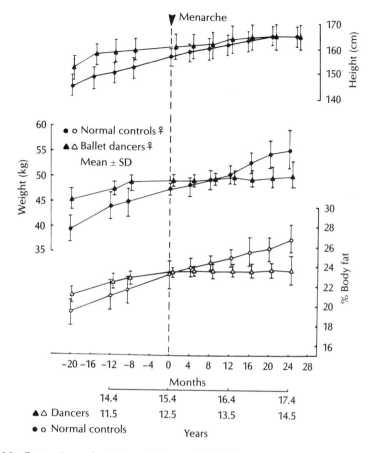

Fig. 132-10. Comparison of heights, weights, and body fat values and age in ballet dancers and normal controls, with menarche as the point of reference. Weights and body fat values are significantly higher for dancers before menarche ($p <.01$). Weight is slightly higher for dancers at menarche ($p <.05$), but body fat does not differ. (From Warren MP: The effects of exercise on pubertal progression and reproductive function in girls, *J Clin Endocrinol Metab* 51:1150, 1980. Copyright © by The Endocrine Society.)

PRIMARY AMENORRHEA

Menarche is a late event of puberty (median age 12.8 years),[13] occurring approximately 1 to 2 years after pubarche and less than 1 year after the onset of peak growth velocity.[26] Thelarche is usually the initial visible sign of pubertal onset. The mean interval between breast budding and menarche is 2.3 ± 1 year. Although this interval from the onset of puberty to menarche may be up to 5 years, the absence of breast budding or menses by the fourteenth birthday should prompt an evaluation, since these patients are not likely to menstruate by 16.5 years of age.[25]

There are many causes of primary amenorrhea, some of which overlap with those of secondary amenorrhea. Menstruation is dependent on several factors: (1) an intact central nervous system (CNS) with appropriate hypothalamic pituitary function, (2) proper end-organ or gonadal responsiveness, and (3) an intact outflow tract. The easiest clinical manner in which to evaluate the first two factors

is to assess patients regarding the presence or absence of secondary sexual characteristics (breasts)[27] and female internal genitalia (uterus). This classification process emphasizes the importance of a general physical and pelvic examination in these patients and allows accurate diagnosis and treatment with only essential laboratory testing (Box 132-1).

Primary amenorrhea must be distinguished from delayed puberty. Obviously the latter is associated with absence of secondary sex characteristics by 13 years of age, and frequently is associated with growth-retarding and/or growth-attenuating disorders, in part manifested by delayed bone age. The most common cause of delayed puberty has a constitutional nature, but other metabolic disorders associated with chronic disease must be considered. Evaluation should include obtaining a complete blood count, erythrocyte sedimentation rate, SMAC, serum for thyroxin, thyroid-stimulating hormone (TSH), and somatomedin-C. A GnRH stimulation is often helpful in the evaluation. Skeletal assessment for bone age, as

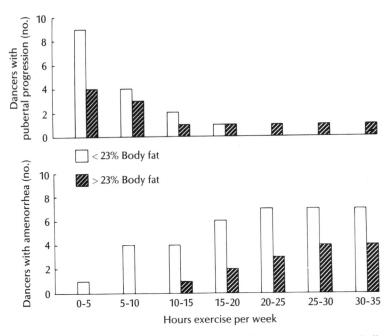

Fig. 132-11. Relationship of exercise to pubertal progression and amenorrhea in ballet dancers. Cumulative data on 15 ballet dancers over a 13-year period were accumulated on a quarterly basis. The exercise level for the preceding 4 months was averaged on a weekly basis. Differences in weight and body fat were calculated for each quarter preceding and during the event (pubertal progression). Values did not differ significantly. Pubertal progression was defined as a change in Tanner stage for breast development or achievement of menarche. (From Warren MP: The effects of exercise on pubertal progression and reproductive function in girls, *J Clin Endocrinol Metab* 51:1150, 1980. Copyright © by The Endocrine Society.)

TABLE 132-2
Typical Daytime Normal Ranges for Gonadotropins and Sex Steroids During Puberty

	E2 (pg/ml)	Estrone (pg/ml)	17-OH-PROG (ng/dl)	A (ng/dl)	T (ng/dl)	DHAS (µg/dl)
Umbilical cord	5,000-15,000	15,000-39,000	1200-4200	15-170	5-50	50-260
0.1-1.0 yr	<75	<20	<200	<80	<20	<40
1.0-4.0 yr	<10	<40	<60	<70	<15	<40
4.0-8.0 yr	<10	<40	<80	<50	<15	<40
Prepubertal >8 yr	<10	<40	<90	<100	<20	10-95
Pubertal	5-125	10-95	15-110	15-150	5-80	40-400
Postmenarchial†	25-250	15-100	25-120	55-200	15-80	60-500

From Rosenfield RL: The ovary and female sexual maturation. In Kaplan SA, editor: *Clinical pediatric endocrinology*, ed 2, Philadelphia, 1990, WB Saunders, p 285.
*Actual values in any laboratory vary with assay method. *17-OH-PROG*, 17-hydroxyprogesterone; *A*, androstenedione; *T*, testosterone.
†Follicular phase adult, exclusive of preovulatory period.

well as a skull film to rule out entities such as craniopharyngioma (calcifications on skull film), remain useful. The response to the GnRH stimulation test, whether it be LH dominant (indicative of late pubertal development) or FSH dominant (indicative of a prepubertal state), becomes particularly important with respect to prognosis in that constitutional delay of puberty is a "presumptive diagnosis" and thus a diagnosis of exclusion.

Primary Amenorrhea with Absent Breast Development

Lack of breast development is a clinical finding indicative of insufficient estrogen production as a result of lack of CNS stimulation of end-organ steroid production or gonadal failure. The two main classes of this clinical presentation are hypergonadotropic hypogonadism (gonadal failure) and hypogonadotropic hypogonadism.

HYPERGONADOTROPIC HYPOGONADISM. Failure of gonadal development is the most common cause of primary amenorrhea, occurring in almost half of these patients.[25] It is usually the result of a genetic enzymatic defect or a chromosomal disorder.

Turner syndrome and Turner mosaicism. Typically, patients with Turner syndrome present with delayed pubertal development, first- or second-degree amenorrhea, short stature, webbed neck, and a shieldlike chest with widely spaced nipples. The incidence is 1 per 2700 live newborns but is as frequent as 0.8% of all zygotes and is the most common human chromosomal abnormality. Interestingly, overall only 3% of all 45,X conceptuses survive to term.[28]

Another variant of Turner syndrome is Turner mosaicism, which also results in gonadal dysgenesis. The most common form is 45,X/46,XX, but it can occur as 45,X/47,XXX or 45,X/46,XX/47,XXX karyotypes. These patients are not always of short stature; on occasion some may ovulate, experience menses, and even conceive.

46,X, Abnormal X. Although these patients are sex-chromatin positive, their defect lies in a structurally abnormal X chromosome. The most frequent abnormality is a deletion of a portion of the X. Deletion may be of either the short arm (p) or long arm (q) of the chromosome. Those patients with short-arm deletion resemble patients with a 45,X karyotype, being of short stature with webbed neck. Patients with long-arm deletion have normal stature and few characteristics similar to those of Turner's syndrome patients. Either deletion defect can cause primary amenorrhea, although those with Turner's syndrome characteristics are often diagnosed before puberty. Other variants include ring X chromosome and isochromosome of the (q)Y.[28]

Pure 46,XX and 46,XY gonadal dysgenesis. These patients have streak gonads and lack secondary sexual characteristics but have normal stature. Primary amenorrhea may be the presenting complaint. Swyer's syndrome patients have a Y chromosome and normal female internal genitalia. They may develop gonadal malignancies and therefore require gonadectomy at puberty owing to a propensity of their intraabdominal gonadal tissue to develop into gonadoblastomas or dysgerminomas.[13]

17α-Hydroxylase deficiency 46,XX. Although a rare disorder, this cause of hypoestrogenism and amenorrhea has important clinical consequences (Fig. 132-12). As a result of a 17α-hydroxylase deficiency (46,XX), there is a deficiency of C21 and C19 steroids. Therefore, these patients have decreased cortisol levels and increased adrenocorticotropic hormone (ACTH) release. The elevation of mineralocorticoid levels resulting from increased progesterone release associated with this enzymatic deficiency gives rise to sodium retention and potassium excretion, with resultant hypertension and hypokalemia.[13,28]

HYPOGONADOTROPIC HYPOGONADISM. Those patients who have amenorrhea resulting from this disorder have no secondary sex characteristics owing to a central defect and therefore have low levels of gonadotropins and serum estrogen. These findings may be a result of CNS lesions, inadequate levels of gonadotropins, decreased GnRH levels, or inability of the pituitary to respond to GnRH. These entities can be distinguished by GnRH stimulation testing.

Central nervous system lesions. This category includes pituitary neoplasms (prolactin- and non–prolactin-secreting) and intrasellar masses (e.g., tuberculoma, gumma, craniopharyngioma). These intrasellar masses cause local destruction of the pituitary gland, resulting in varying degrees of hypopituitarism and therefore hypogonadism. By far the most common cause is the prolactin-secreting pituitary adenoma. Despite the associated increase in prolactin, a minority of such patients have galactorrhea. Certainly all amenorrheic patients with low to normal FSH levels should have their prolactin level measured. Less common pituitary adenomas include those that secrete ACTH or GH, which are associated with symptoms of Cushing's disease or acromegaly, respectively.

Inadequate GnRH release. This cause of hypogonadotropic hypogonadism has only recently been identified. Administration of GnRH to patients with this disorder gives rise to an increase in FSH and LH. This entity is indicative of a hypothalamic defect, caused by either insufficient GnRH secretion or a neurotransmitter defect. When this condition is associated with anosmia, it is referred to as female Kallmann's syndrome. The patient with Kallmann's syndrome presents with primary amenorrhea, infantile secondary sexual characteristics, female karyotype, and anosmia. The clinical manifestation is a result of a congenital anatomic defect, including hypoplastic or absent olfactory sulci in the rhinencephalon.[13,29]

Isolated gonadotropin deficiency. This group of patients manifests no increase in gonadotropin levels after GnRH stimulation testing. This condition has been related to thalassemia major. A proposed mechanism in thalassemic patients is mild to moderate siderosis with a decrease in the number of pituitary gland cells.[30,31]

Primary Amenorrhea with Breast Development and Absence of Uterus

Patients with breasts and primary amenorrhea but no uterus have either a congenital absence of internal genitalia or complete androgen insensitivity (testicular feminization).

CONGENITAL ABSENCE OF UTERUS. This is the second most common cause of amenorrhea and is a result of partial or complete müllerian agenesis.[32] The defect can range from uterine agenesis with a blind-ending vagina to complete absence of the uterus and vagina. Amenorrhea associated with complete müllerian agenesis is called Mayer-Rokitansky-Küster-Hauser syndrome[13] and occurs in 1 in 4000 to 1 in 5000 female births.[28] Diagnosis is rarely established in infancy but is usually first suspected at puberty. The patient is noted to have normal breast development as well as pubic and axillary hair growth. However, these patients have amenorrhea secondary to either end-organ absence with uterovaginal agenesis or outflow tract obstruction in association with vaginal agenesis. The latter may present with cyclic abdominal pain at puberty. At the time of diagnosis, an intravenous pyelogram should be obtained, since approximately 30% of these patients may have associated renal anomalies. Further radiologic studies can help detect associated skeletal anomalies, which occur in 12%.[33] Further management is discussed below.

COMPLETE ANDROGEN INSENSITIVITY (TESTICULAR FEMINIZATION). This disorder is a failure of proper sexual differentiation, the result of target-organ insensitivity to androgen—a genetically transmitted condition for which two thirds of those affected are X-linked recessive and the remainder X-linked dominant.[28]

The incidence ranges from 1 in 20,000 to 1 in 624,000.[34] As with congenital absence of the uterus, the diagnosis is not established until puberty, when amenorrhea results. In contrast to patients with uterine agenesis, however, these patients have scant or no pubic or axillary hair and are genotypically males with a normal 46,XY karyotype.

The gonads of patients with androgen insensitivity are primarily testes that produce normal male levels of testosterone; however, as a result of androgen insensitiv-

ity there is a lack of male differentiation of external and internal genitalia. The testes also produce müllerian-inhibiting substance (MIS), which acts to repress the normal müllerian structures (uterus, fallopian tubes, upper vagina). Therefore, these patients have normal female external genitalia with an absent or blind vagina and no internal genitalia except for gonadal tissue. Normal to enlarged breast development occurs secondary to estrogen production by the gonads and adrenal glands without androgen inhibition. The incidence of malignancy in the gonads of these patients is as high as 20%.[35,36] Neoplasia is rare before puberty, and the presence of a gonad ensures smooth pubertal changes with complete androgen insensitivity. The gonads usually are left in place until completion of sexual maturation. At that time, the patient should undergo gonadectomy to prevent formation of gonadoblastomas or dysgerminomas. Postoperative hormonal replacement is required.

Primary Amenorrhea with Absence of Breasts and Uterus

Possible etiologies for this rare cause of amenorrhea include a sex-steroid enzyme deficiency or agonadism. A 17,20-desmolase deficiency affects androgen and estrogen production. Therefore, a 46,XY individual without androgen production would develop female external genitalia with a vaginal pouch and have no müllerian structures, owing to MIS production with atypical or complete absence of male internal genital structures. The lack of estrogen production due to the enzyme deficiency is the apparent cause of breast absence.[37]

Another enzyme deficiency resulting in the lack of uterus and breast development is 17α-hydroxylase deficiency in a 46,XY "male." The mechanism is similar to that of 17,20-desmolase deficiency. In the former patient population there is also a decrease in cortisol production with an increase in mineralocorticoid levels that results in hypertension and hypokalemia. Cortisol replacement in addition to hormonal therapy is necessary just as in the 46,XX patient with the same enzyme deficiency.

True agonadism is the absence of any gonadal tissue. In this circumstance, MIS functions to inhibit müllerian structures at 8 to 10 weeks' gestation (testosterone formation occurs at 12 weeks' gestation). These patients have normal female external genitalia, indicating a lack of androgen production; in addition, they have no internal female genitalia, indicating functional MIS.

Primary Amenorrhea with Breast Development and Uterus

Amenorrhea with overt physical evidence of estrogen production and female genitalia (external and internal) indicates either an outflow tract obstruction or a CNS mechanism responsible for the menstrual dysfunction.

Defects of the hypothalamic-pituitary-ovarian axis also can cause secondary amenorrhea and are addressed in the discussion of secondary amenorrhea. Outflow tract defects include imperforate hymen, transverse vaginal septum, cervical atresia, and the previously described müllerian agenesis (Mayer-Rokitansky-Küster-Hauser syndrome).

IMPERFORATE HYMEN. An imperforate hymen results from a failure of perforation of the hymenal plate, providing no connection between the vestibule and the vaginal vault. Although this canalization usually occurs in utero, often its absence is not discovered until puberty when cyclic abdominal pain and pressure are noted at the time of expected menarche. Examination reveals a bulging hymen and frequently an associated palpable pelvic and suprapubic mass, occasionally resulting in acute urinary retention. This problem is easily corrected by surgical incision of the hymenal ring, thereby creating an unobstructed outflow tract.

TRANSVERSE VAGINAL SEPTUM. A transverse vaginal septum presents in the same manner as an imperforate hymen and is also the result of incomplete canalization of müllerian structures. The septum is usually in the middle third of the vagina, forming a short lower vagina that ends

in a blind pouch. Since the cervix has no outflow tract, a hematocolpos occurs as menstrual flow collects behind the septum. This condition is surgically corrected by means of incision or excision of the vaginal septum.

CERVICAL DYSGENESIS. An uncommon condition, cervical atresia is defined as congenital absence or hypoplasia of the cervix. A vagina and uterus are present on examination, but no cervix is identified. Surgical canalization results in menstrual flow and cessation of symptoms of outflow obstruction, but cervical incompetency may be a future issue with respect to fertility.

Initial Evaluation and Management

Evaluation should include plotting of the patient's height and weight on a growth curve, with continued monitoring and documentation during the course of treatment and follow-up. A routine history and physical examination should be completed, with special attention paid to ophthalmologic, neurologic, and pelvic examination. With this information it should be possible to coordinate patient management (Fig. 132-12).

Those amenorrheic patients presenting with a uterus and no breast development can be classified according to

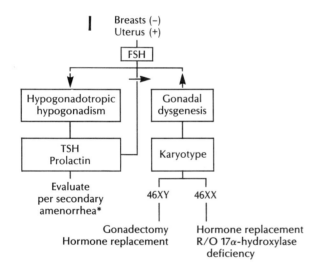
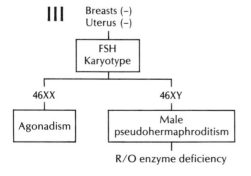
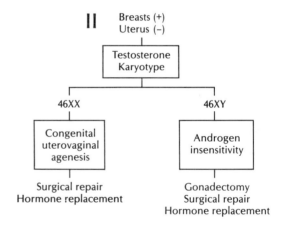
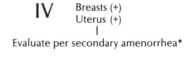

Fig. 132-12. Evaluation and management strategies for primary amenorrhea. *FSH,* follicle-stimulating hormone; *TSH,* thyroid-stimulating hormone; *R/O,* rule out. (*See Fig. 132-14).

whether serum FSH levels are elevated. An elevated FSH level (>40 mIU/ml) indicates first-degree hypogonadism (gonadal failure). The differential diagnosis includes both congenital and acquired disorders. Disorders causing congenital primary hypogonadism can have an anatomic basis, such as gonadal dysgenesis, or a functional basis. Patients with increased FSH levels should have a karyotype performed. Because of a 20% incidence of gonadoblastoma and dysgerminoma, individuals with 46,XY must undergo gonadectomy, usually at the completion of puberty.[35,36] These patients then must receive estrogen replacement therapy on a permanent basis. The patient with a normal female karyotype (46,XX), in addition to cyclic hormonal therapy screening, must be evaluated for a functional cause of hypogonadism such as a high steroidogenic block such as 17α-hydroxylase deficiency. Measurement of serum electrolyte, cortisol, and progesterone levels should reveal hypernatremia and hypokalemia, hypocortisolism, and increased serum progesterone levels (>0.2 ng/ml) as well as elevated serum deoxycorticosterone (>17 ng/dl).[38] These patients require cortisol replacement. Patients with Turner syndrome or other forms of gonadal dysgenesis should receive physiologic hormonal therapy (see Chapter 28, "Disorders of Puberty"). Acquired disorders causing amenorrhea include oophorectomy- or radiotherapy- or chemotherapy-induced ovarian failure, and these also require hormone replacement therapy. Premature ovarian failure is discussed in more detail under secondary amenorrhea below.

A diagnosis of hypogonadotropic hypogonadism is established on the basis of a normal to low FSH level in a patient without breast development in the presence of a uterus. It is difficult to distinguish between idiopathic gonadotropin deficiency and constitutional pubertal delay. Pubertal delay is discussed in detail in Chapter 5. These patients may have a pituitary lesion and as a result should undergo screening for prolactin and TSH levels. An increased TSH level indicative of hypothyroidism requires supplementation of thyroid hormone. The remainder of these hypogonadal individuals require either hormonal replacement or GnRH stimulation testing if fertility is desired. Hormonal replacement should mimic the normal cycle (e.g., conjugated estrogens, 0.625 mg, or comparable exogenous estrogen replacement therapy on days 1 to 25 with medroxyprogesterone acetate, 10 mg, on days 16 to 25 of the cycle). Adequate estrogen replacement therapy helps to avert osteoporosis.

A serum testosterone level and karyotype readily distinguish androgen insensitivity syndrome from müllerian agenesis. Patients with androgen insensitivity require gonadectomy with surgical reconstruction of the vagina and estrogen replacement therapy. Congenital uterovaginal agenesis likewise may necessitate surgical formation of a functional vagina. In some cases in which a vaginal dimple is noted, successive dilators may be used to create a vagina in lieu of surgery, in which case a referral to a specialist in adolescent gynecologic surgery is indicated. These patients do not require hormonal replacement, as their ovarian function is normal. In patients presenting without breast or uterine development, a karyotype will provide appropriate information regarding management. Individuals with 46,XY require gonadectomy. Both 46,XX and 46,XY patients need estrogen replacement therapy. Evaluation of endocrine and genetic parameters is usually coordinated by specialists to assist in a proper diagnosis.

Primary amenorrhea in the presence of breasts and uterus entails differential diagnosis and management similar to that for secondary amenorrhea.

Secondary Amenorrhea

Physiologic menstrual cycles are dependent on uninterrupted signals between the CNS and end organs of the ovary and uterus. Therefore, any disruption at the hypothalamic, pituitary, ovarian, or uterine levels will result in amenorrhea. With the exception of intrauterine adhesions, all the causes of secondary amenorrhea also may produce primary amenorrhea in a phenotypic female with a normal uterus and breast development (Box 132-2).

BOX 132-2
Differential Diagnosis of Secondary Amenorrhea

CENTRAL NERVOUS SYSTEM CAUSES
Hypothalamic local lesions
　　Craniopharyngiomas
　　　　Granulomatous disease
　　　　Encephalitis sequelae
　　　　Empty sella syndrome
Pituitary neoplasm
　　Prolactinoma
Nonneoplasm
　　Pituitary damage (Sheehan's syndrome or
　　　　Simmonds' syndrome)
Drug-induced neurotransmitter alterations
Hypothyroidism
Hypothalamic-pituitary dysfunction
　　Stress and exercise
　　Weight loss and anorexia
　　Hyperprolactinemia

UTERINE CAUSES
Intrauterine adhesions (Asherman's syndrome)

OVARIAN CAUSES
Ovarian failure
Polycystic ovary syndrome

CENTRAL NERVOUS SYSTEM CAUSES. Central nervous system etiologies for amenorrhea include lesions such as craniopharyngiomas, granulomatous disease, and prolactinomas; drug-induced neurotransmitter alterations; and various causes of hypothalamic-pituitary dysfunction such as stress, excessive exercise, anorexia, and hypothyroidism.

HYPOTHALAMIC LOCAL LESIONS. Local lesions of the hypothalamus-pituitary such as craniopharyngiomas and granulomatous disease (tuberculosis, sarcoidosis) interfere with GnRH release and cause local pituitary destruction, resulting in low FSH and LH production and subsequent amenorrhea.[39] In a similar fashion, empty sella syndrome secondary to absence or distortion of the pituitary gland results in decreased pituitary function and amenorrhea, which may be manifested as delayed puberty and short stature, depending on the time of onset and extent of pituitary deficiency.[40] There is also a 5% association between empty sella syndrome and hyperprolactinemia.[41]

NONNEOPLASM. In rare cases, secondary amenorrhea may be a result of pituitary necrosis secondary to a hypotensive event (Simmonds' syndrome). When associated with a peripartum hemorrhage, this condition is termed Sheehan's syndrome. The pituitary damage results in varying degrees of hypopituitarism and thereby interferes with normal menses.

DRUG-INDUCED NEUROTRANSMITTER ALTERATIONS. Certain tranquilizers and antihypertensives may interfere with dopamine synthesis or action. As dopamine is the regulating neurotransmitter of prolactin, a decrease in dopamine secretion increases prolactin release, thereby resulting in galactorrhea as a direct effect, and amenorrhea in association with the inhibitory effect of prolactin on GnRH. The largest category of medications that interfere with this mechanism are phenothiazines, including fluphenazine, thioridazine, and trifluoperazine. Table 132-3 lists other common medications associated with amenorrhea or galactorrhea.[42]

HYPOTHYROIDISM. In hypothyroidism, a low-circulating thyroid hormone level results in an increase in thyroid-releasing hormone (TRH). Because TRH acts as a prolactin-releasing factor, it increases prolactin secretion, with a resultant inhibition of GnRH production through a mechanism similar to that of drug-induced amenorrhea or galactorrhea.[43]

STRESS AND EXERCISE. Stress resulting from major life style changes, such as a recent divorce or the death of a loved one, can be associated with amenorrhea. In a survey of adolescent women in a private school, Wilson et al[44] noted that almost 30% of students with previous regular menses developed oligomenorrhea during the same year they entered boarding school.

Excessive exercise also can cause amenorrhea. Mansfield and Emans,[45] using the presence or absence of

menstrual cycles as a definition of amenorrhea, estimated the prevalence of amenorrhea in runners to be between 6% and 51%. If significant athletic endeavor occurs during the premenarcheal period, menarche can be delayed 0.4 years for each year of athletic training.[46] In an attempt to control stress factors involved with exercise, Warren[47] compared the menstrual history of preprofessional ballet dancers with that of music students, both groups being under presumably equal competitive stress. In this study, ballet dancers experienced delayed menarche, whereas the musicians did not, thus indicating the involvement of factors other than stress. Warren theorized that the "energy drain" of exercise was a factor because dancers unable to dance as a result of injury often noted menses without a body weight change.[47] This

TABLE 132-3
Centrally Acting Drugs That Cause Galactorrhea or Prolactin Increase

Medication	Proprietary Name(s)
Rauwolfia derivatives	
Rauwolfia	Raudixin, Rauval, Hyperloid, Rauja, Rautina, Wolfina
Alseroxylon	Rauwiloid
Reserpine	Serpasil, Serfin, Sandril, Lemiserp, Reserpoid, Resercen, Rau-Sed (plus many combinations)
Phenothiazine derivatives	
Butaperazine	Repoise
Carphenazine	Proketazine
Chlorpromazine	Thorazine
Fluphenazine	Prolixin, Permitil
Mesoridazine	Serentil
Methotrimeprazine	Levoprome
Pericyazine	
Perphenazine	Trilafon, Triavil,* Etrafon*
Piperacetazine	Quide
Prochlorperazine	Compazine
Promazine	Sparine
Thiopropazate	Dartal
Thioridazine	Mellaril
Trifluoperazine	Stelazine
Trimeprazine	Temaril
Substituted thioxanthenes	
Chlorprothixene	Taractan
Thiothixene	Navane
Substituted butyrophenone	
Haloperidol	Haldol
Tricyclic antidepressants	
Amitriptyline	Elavil, Etrafon†
Imipramine	Tofranil
Protriptyline	Vivactil
Methyldopa	
Methyldopa	Aldomen
Opiates	
Codeine	Numerous proprietary names
Morphine	Morphine
Thyroid-releasing hormone	

Modified from Dickey RP, Stone SC: Drugs that affect the breast and lactation, *Clin Obstet Gynecol* 18:96, 1975.
*Combined with amitriptyline.
†Combined with perphenazine.

theory is supported by the fact that exercise amenorrhea is more common in sports such as running, ballet, and gymnastics, all energy-intensive sports. Those patients with stress- or exercise-induced amenorrhea were all associated with a diagnosis of hypothalamic amenorrhea, since the pathophysiology primarily affects the hypothalamus. Hypothalamic amenorrhea is characterized by a loss of GnRH pulse amplitude and frequency.[48]

Various neurotransmitters are involved in GnRH regulation. For example, norepinephrine stimulates GnRH release, whereas dopamine inhibits GnRH and prolactin release. There is growing evidence that endogenous opiates (endorphins) inhibit GnRH and LH secretion.[45,48,49] In fact, the administration of naloxone, an opiated antagonist, to women with hypothalamic amenorrhea results in increased LH pulse frequency and amplitude, further defining this mechanism of action.[49] Small pulsatile doses of GnRH have been used to activate cyclic pituitary ovarian function in hypogonadotropic "acyclic women." The result has been induction of ovulation, resulting in pregnancy and live birth.[50]

WEIGHT LOSS AND ANOREXIA. Weight loss of 10% to 15% below ideal body weight or loss of 50% of total body fat stores causes amenorrhea in most women.[51] With mild weight loss, there is direct and indirect hypothalamic dysfunction, whereas severe weight loss of more than 25% of ideal body weight results in additional pituitary dysfunction.[25]

Frisch and McArthur[52] devised a nomogram indicating the minimal weight per given height necessary for a female to experience normal menarche (Fig. 132-13). The lowest diagonal line indicates the minimal weight per height for menarche; the second lowest diagonal line corresponds to the weight needed for restoration of menses in an adolescent with weight loss and secondary amenorrhea.

Anorexia nervosa is a psychiatric disorder characterized by severe weight loss and subsequent amenorrhea. It is a fairly common entity, affecting 1 in 100 to 1 in 1000 females in the population most at risk—adolescent girls and women under 25 years of age in the middle to upper socioeconomic segment of society.[25,45] Patients with anorexia nervosa have a hypothalamic disorder that interferes with GnRH secretion. The LH secretion pattern in this group of patients is similar to that of premenarcheal patients in that LH pulses are absent. Studies on the use of naloxone in anorexic females revealed an increase in LH after opiate blockade, indicating a possible role of endogenous opiates in the mechanism of LH inhibition in anorexia nervosa.[53]

HYPERPROLACTINEMIA. Prolactin regulation primarily revolves around a hypothalamic inhibition through secretion of a prolactin-inhibiting factor. Prolactin-inhibiting factor is thought to be dopamine or a dopamine-like substance. Medications such as phenothi-

azines and diazepam either deplete hypothalamic dopamine or block dopamine receptors. Reserpine and alpha-methyldopa deplete dopamine by blocking synthesis. As a result, these medications increase prolactin release via its GnRH inhibition, thus producing amenorrhea.

There are many causes of hyperprolactinemia, including prolactin-secreting pituitary tumors that produce acromegaly and Cushing's disease. In addition, hypothalamic disease (craniopharyngioma, granulomatous disease), chronic renal disease (with decreased glomerular filtration rate), chronic breast stimulation, chest trauma, hypothyroidism, pharmacologic agents, pregnancy, exercise, stress, and bronchogenic or renal carcinoma can be associated with hyperprolactinemia.

The presenting complaint may be galactorrhea, delayed puberty, or primary or secondary amenorrhea. The absence of galactorrhea is not unusual and should not influence the decision to evaluate prolactin. Any amenorrheic patient with low to normal serum FSH and LH levels, even with a positive progesterone challenge test for withdrawal bleeding, should have the serum prolactin level measured.

Approximately 50% of females with hyperprolactinemia have prolactinoma.[54] This is the most common pituitary tumor associated with an elevated prolactin level. Prolactinomas are classified as microadenomas if the diameter is less than 1 cm, and as macroadenoma if larger. Microadenomas are the most common presentation. Hyperprolactinemia occurs in about 25% of patients with acromegaly and 10% of those with Cushing's disease, indicating that these pituitary tumors can secrete prolactin in addition to GH and ACTH. The incidence of prolactinoma is higher in patients with evidence of profound hypothalamic-pituitary-ovarian dysfunction indicated by hyperprolactinemia, galactorrhea, and secondary amenorrhea with low estrogen levels. In one study, 70% of such patients showed radiologic evidence of a pituitary adenoma, whereas only 20% to 30% of hyperprolactinemic patients with normal menses, oligomenorrhea, or secondary amenorrhea with a positive progesterone challenge test showed evidence of tumor radiologically.[54]

UTERINE CAUSES. Intrauterine adhesions (IUAs), also termed Asherman's syndrome, present as partial or complete obliteration of the uterine cavity. Of patients with IUA, 37% present with amenorrhea that may be associated with infertility and habitual abortion.[55]

The most common cause of IUA is induced abortion or curettage after spontaneous abortion.[55] Intrauterine manipulation is the primary mechanism. The second most common cause is postpartum curettage, occurring in 20%. Other less common etiologies are fibrosis occurring after cesarean section, molar pregnancy evacuation, myomectomy, and diagnostic curettage. Genital tuberculosis is a rare cause of IUA. Miliary spread of extragenital

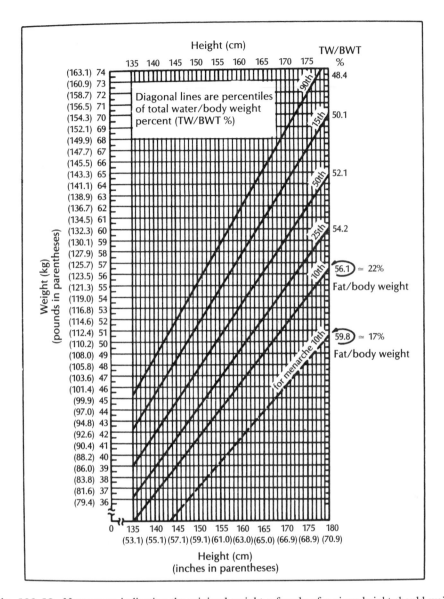

Fig. 132-13. Nomogram indicating the minimal weight a female of a given height should weigh to be likely to have normal menses. The lowest diagonal line is the tenth percentile of total water/body fat for menarche. The second lowest diagonal line is the tenth percentile for 18-year-old adolescents; this diagonal often corresponds to the weight needed for restoration of menses in an adolescent with weight loss and secondary amenorrhea. (From Frisch RE, McArthur JW: Menstrual cycles: fatness as determinant of minimum weight for height necessary for their maintenance or onset, *Science* 185:949, 1974. Copyright © 1974 by the American Association for the Advancement of Science.)

tuberculosis or drainage of tuberculosis salpingitis causes a chronic inflammation of the endometrium that in many cases results in total atresia of the uterine cavity.[56]

The diagnosis of IUA should be suspected in patients who have a history of manipulation of a pregnant uterus. The diagnosis can be confirmed radiographically with hysterosalpingography, or by hysteroscopy.

OVARIAN CAUSES. Ovarian failure by any mechanism results in decreased ovarian estrogen output and hence decreased endometrial stimulation. Menstrual irregularity and amenorrhea can follow. This failure can

be caused by ovarian damage or premature ovarian failure (POF).

Ovarian damage may be seen in patients who gradually become amenorrheic after medical treatment of a tuboovarian abscess, a surgical procedure of the pelvis that may compromise ovarian blood supply, or surgical excision of bilateral ovarian cysts.

POF is defined as ovarian failure occurring in women under 40 years of age with elevated circulating serum FSH and LH levels.[57] It usually is accompanied by amenorrhea but occasionally manifests with oligomenorrhea. The entity of POF can be classified further as gonadotropin-resistant ovary syndrome, autoimmune ovarian failure, follicular ovarian failure (premature menopause), or idiopathic ovarian failure. Initially these distinctions were based on ovarian biopsy results: gonadotropin-resistant ovaries had primordial follicles with no progression beyond antral stage and no evidence of autoimmune disease. However, it is now recognized that ovarian biopsy is not required for the diagnosis of POF, because the biopsy result will not change management and there is a low probability of subclassifying the diagnosis of ovarian failure with biopsy.

POF has been associated with various autoimmune disorders in 20% to 50% of cases.[58] These include hypoparathyroidism, Hashimoto's thyroiditis, Addison's disease, myasthenia gravis, Crohn's disease, systemic lupus erythematosus, and the presence of antimicrosomal antibodies.[25,51,58] An infectious etiology of POF, causing oophoritis in 5% of infected patients, is mumps.[58]

POF also can be the result of ovarian exposure to radiation or systemic chemotherapy used in cancer treatment. Stillman et al[59] reported that, in long-term survivors of childhood malignancy, the ovarian failure rate was 68% in patients who had both ovaries within abdominal radiotherapy fields, 14% in patients with ovaries at the edge of the treatment field, and 0% in those with one or both ovaries out of field. The likelihood of ovarian failure is dosage related: higher doses and advanced age are associated with an increased risk of ovarian damage.[41] Chemotherapy-induced ovarian failure is more likely to occur in postpubertal than in prepubertal females and is also dose related.[60]

In some cases of POF, more often in patients with gonadotropin-resistant ovaries, the effects may be transient; occasionally, patients are able to ovulate and conceive. However, the probability of this is very low, and the pregnancy rate has been estimated by Aiman and Smentek[57] to be 1 in 9200.

POLYCYSTIC OVARY SYNDROME. Polycystic ovary syndrome is a common cause of amenorrhea in adolescents. Although this syndrome was originally described as Stein-Leventhal syndrome in 1935, characterized by polycystic ovaries, amenorrhea, hirsutism, and obesity, it now is recognized to be actually a spectrum of disorders resulting in chronic anovulation.[54a] Polycystic ovary syndrome is discussed in more depth in Chapter 133, "Hirsutism."

Evaluation and Management

Any patient with complaints of secondary amenorrhea should be evaluated, particularly those who experience abrupt cessation of menses for several months after the onset of regular cycles or those with persistent oligomenorrhea. It is important to remember that normal adoles-

cents may have irregular menses for up to 18 months after menarche.

The initial evaluation requires a thorough history and physical examination. As pregnancy is the most common cause of amenorrhea, a proper menstrual history, sexual history, and assessment of pregnancy symptoms should be incorporated appropriately in the history. One must not assume that the patient is not pregnant merely on the basis of a stated negative sexual history.

The history also should focus on issues of stress; recent changes in environment; weight changes; amount and level of athletic activity; history of medication use, including oral contraceptives; and history of previous pregnancy or instrumentation of the uterus.

The physical examination should include a height and weight check plotted on a growth curve; visual field evaluation; thyroid gland assessment; breast examination with check for galactorrhea; and evaluation for signs of hirsutism, virilization, clitoromegaly, and acne. During the pelvic examination, estrogen status, uterine size, and adnexal masses, i.e., ovarian enlargement, should be assessed.

The full evaluation sequence for secondary amenorrhea is schematically diagrammed in Figure 132-14. In addition to the initial history and physical examination, a sensitive pregnancy test should be obtained before any evaluation of the outflow tract with a progesterone challenge. If the pregnancy test is negative, either progesterone in oil, 50 to 100 mg administered intramuscularly, or oral medroxyprogesterone acetate (Provera), 10 mg for 5 days, may be prescribed. If the circulating estradiol level is 40 pg/ml or more, withdrawal bleeding will occur within 2 weeks after the medication regimen is completed. Any spotting or vaginal bleeding is considered a positive response to the progesterone challenge test.

In patients with IUA, hypothalamic-pituitary failure, ovarian failure, or severe weight loss, the progesterone challenge test is usually negative as the result of either an obstructed outflow tract or a lack of an estrogen-primed endometrium. Since Asherman's syndrome is a rare finding in adolescent patients, those individuals with a negative progesterone challenge test need further evaluation for a possible hypoestrogenic state. If the patient history suggests IUA and if cyclic administration of conjugated estrogens and medroxyprogesterone acetate is without response, a full uterine evaluation with uterine sounding, as well as a hysterosalpingogram, should be performed. However, in an adolescent with a history not suggestive of IUA, the administration of higher doses of estrogen for several months may be required. Certainty of patient compliance is necessary before the uterine cavity is further evaluated.

If a patient has a negative progesterone challenge test and a normal to low serum FSH level, prolactin and TSH

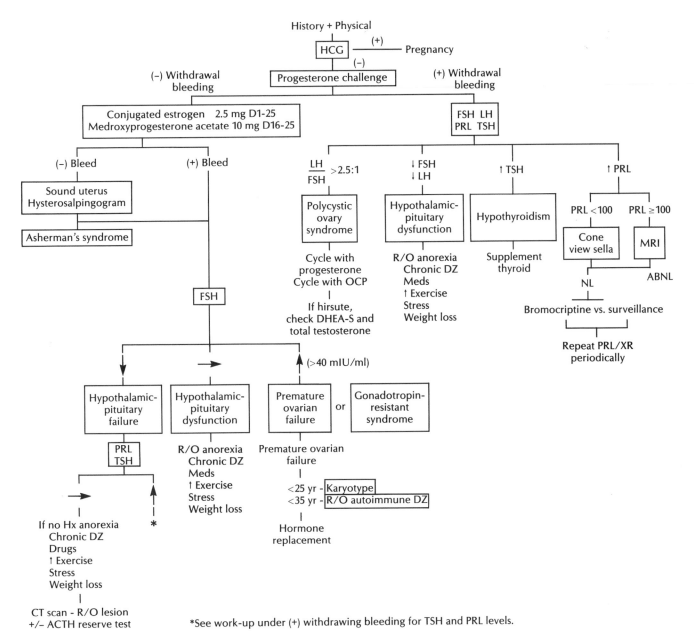

Fig. 132-14. Evaluation and management strategies for secondary amenorrhea. *HCG,* human chorionic gonadotropin; *PRL,* prolactin; *TSH,* thyroid-stimulating hormone; *R/O,* rule out; *DZ,* disease; *OCP,* oral contraceptives; *DHEAS,* dehydroepiandrosterone sulfate; *NL,* normal; *ABNL,* abnormal; *XR,* radiographic evaluation; *Hx,* history; *ACTH,* adrenocorticotropic hormone; ↓, decreased level; →, normal level; ↑, increased level.

levels should be measured to rule out a pituitary etiology. If these levels are normal and there is no history of stress, strenuous exercise, or severe weight loss, radiologic evaluation, such as computed tomography (CT) of the hypothalamic-pituitary area, should be obtained to rule out a central abnormality. If the patient has a lesion or a history consistent with pituitary anoxia (Sheehan's or Simmonds' syndrome), an ACTH reserve test should be completed.[25] If all these tests are negative, the diagnosis is hypothalamic-pituitary failure of uncertain etiology.

These patients need to receive cyclic hormonal therapy with either 0.625 mg conjugated estrogen from days 1 to 25 and 10 mg medroxyprogesterone acetate from days 15 to 25, or oral contraceptives. Such patients occasionally resume normal menstrual cycles without treatment.

An elevated FSH level is indicative of ovarian failure. In patients without a history of ovarian destruction, the possibility of an autoimmune disease should be considered. If the patient is under 35 years of age, antinuclear and antithyroid antibodies should be evaluated. If the patient is under 25, a karyotype also should be completed to rule out mosaicism.[21] These patients should receive cyclic estrogen-progestin therapy.

Patients with a positive progesterone challenge test are usually normal but require evaluation of FSH, LH, prolactin, and TSH, hypothalamic-pituitary dysfunction, including prolactinoma and hypothyroidism. An elevated LH level (>30 mIU/ml) with a normal FSH level or an LH-to-FSH ratio greater than 2:1 is suggestive of polycystic ovary syndrome. Owing to the association with hyperandrogenism, dehydroepiandrosterone sulfate and testosterone levels should also be evaluated. These patients can be treated with cyclic hormonal therapy, either with 10 mg medroxyprogesterone acetate per day for 13 to 14 days every 1 to 3 months, or oral contraceptives, to prevent endometrial hyperplasia associated with unopposed estrogen stimulation. If pregnancy is desired, clomiphene citrate can be used to stimulate ovulation, with a starting dose of 50 mg.

The nonspecific diagnosis of hypothalamic-pituitary dysfunction is made in the presence of low FSH and LH levels; the influence of excessive exercise, anorexia, stress, chronic disease, and use of hypothalamic interactive medications needs further evaluation. Usually a decrease in exercise level, an increase in weight, or cessation of interactive medications will allow resumption of normal cyclic menses. Patients with a 2-year history of amenorrhea who refuse to comply with these restrictions require calcium carbonate, 1.5 g/day, and hormonal supplementation to reverse the hypoestrogenic effect on bone density.

Patients with prolactin-secreting microadenomas eventually become estrogen deficient but initially have enough circulating estrogen to have a positive progesterone challenge test.

In patients with hyperprolactinemia, pregnancy, hypothyroidism, renal and hepatic disease (decreased prolactin clearance), medication interaction, and cocaine use should be ruled out. Under these circumstances the prolactin level usually ranges between 30 and 100 ng/ml.[45] In patients with a prolactin level less than 100 ng/ml and no other predisposing factors as noted above, an evaluation of the sella turcica with a coned-down view is appropriate. If results are normal, treatment with bromocriptine (a dopamine agonist) or surveillance is offered, with periodic measurement of prolactin levels.

If an abnormality of the sella is detected on the coned-down view or if the prolactin level is 100 ng/ml or more, magnetic resonance imaging (MRI) can rule out empty sella syndrome, suprasellar abnormality, or a microadenoma or macroadenoma. The presence of a microadenoma is an indication for treatment with bromocriptine in adolescent patients, because most girls of this age with this lesion eventually become estrogen deficient and need normal estrogen levels to establish peak bone mass.[51] Patients receiving this treatment usually resume normal menses and, as applicable, restoration of fertility.

Treatment of macroadenomas is controversial. Surgical treatment carries a cure rate less than 40%, and therefore many authors advocate medical management with bromocriptine. If such management is instituted, prolactin level monitoring and CT evaluation must be performed on a regular basis.

Bromocriptine therapy is initiated at a dose of 1.25 mg at bedtime, increasing to 2.5 mg at bedtime the ensuing week, and finally to 2.5 mg twice daily. This gradual increase in dosage seems to alleviate a number of side effects, including nausea, orthostatic hypotension, and dizziness. The dosage of 5 mg/day usually is adequate to control mild to moderate hyperprolactinemia.[51]

DYSMENORRHEA

Dysmenorrhea is defined as recurrent abdominal pain, crampy in nature, and is often associated with nausea and vomiting occurring around the time of menses. Additional symptoms include increased pain with defecation, headaches, and muscular cramps during menses.[61]

Incidence

Approximately 30% to 50% of the more than 40 million women of childbearing age in the United States suffer from painful menstruation. Of women 19 years old, over 70% have reported experiencing dysmenorrhea, and over 50% reported loss of time from school or work.[62,63] Approximately one third of all women experience dysmenorrhea during the first 6 months after menarche.[63]

Dysmenorrhea is a leading cause of recurrent short-term school absenteeism in adolescent girls.[61,64] Of 2699 menarcheal adolescents 12 to 17 years old assessed in the National Health Examination Survey, 59.7% indicated they experienced dysmenorrhea; 14% said they frequently missed school because of it. Socioeconomic status correlated with the incidence of dysmenorrhea: economically disadvantaged students missed school because of dysmenorrhea more often than did those from affluent families—23.6% versus 12.3%, respectively.[61]

Prevalence and Evaluation

The prevalence of dysmenorrhea in adolescents has been addressed by Wilson,[64] who noted that 86% (76 of 88) of adolescents experienced dysmenorrhea that caused school absenteeism. It appears that the adolescents in this series had little insight into the problem and little knowledge of where to obtain such information.

A number of factors appear to be associated with menstrual pain, including an increased frequency of upper respiratory tract infections. In addition, sedentary

TABLE 132-4
Chronic Pelvic Pain and Diagnosis

Author	No. of Patients	Endometriosis	Pelvic Adhesions	Uterine Anomaly	Normal Pelvis
Goldstein et al (1980)	140	52	7	11	18
Strickland et al (1988)	100	10	29	0	46
Vercellini et al (1990)	47	38	13	9	40

adolescents and those who imbibe alcoholic beverages or who smoke have more menstrual pain.

Distinction must be made between primary dysmenorrhea in which there is no underlying anatomic abnormality and secondary dysmenorrhea in which there is evidence of a specific cause for the dysmenorrhea. Evaluation of the adolescent with dysmenorrhea includes obtaining a history, inquiring about the character of the pain as well as the interval between episodes. Certainly, a history of previous pelvic surgery, pelvic inflammatory disease, or a gastrointestinal or genitourinary condition should alert the clinician to the underlying cause of the pelvic pain. In all probability, this pain will not be of a cyclic manner and does not qualify for the definition of dysmenorrhea (Table 132-4).

The physical examination must include a pelvic examination to identify any anatomic abnormality, tenderness, or pelvic mass. A rectovaginal examination is an integral part of the overall assessment.

Physiology and Pathophysiology

In the 1930s, researchers hypothesized that increased uterine activity caused dysmenorrhea.[65] In 1957, Pickles[66] described the prostaglandin cascade and its effect on the menstrual cycle. Prostaglandins, especially E_2 and $F_{2\alpha}$, are associated with inhibition of uterine blood flow, with resultant ischemia and pelvic pain.[67] Endometrial prostaglandin $F_{2\alpha}$ content appears to be greater in the secretory than in the proliferative phase of the menstrual cycle.[68] An estrogen-induced decrease in progesterone during the luteal phase is mirrored by a rise in prostaglandin $F_{2\alpha}$.[68] It is believed that dysmenorrhea is a direct result of prostaglandin effects on uterine musculature.

Psychosocial Factors

Data from several researchers attest to a much greater incidence of chronic pelvic pain in patients who were physically or sexually abused during their childhood.[69-71] Indeed, a number of psychologic and personality factors can predispose the patient to dysmenorrhea.[72] Increased anxiety, overconformity, insecurity, immaturity, neurosis, dependency, oversensitivity, introversion, underachieve-

ment, and perfectionism all have been suggested as risk factors for dysmenorrhea.[73,74]

Treatment

NONSTEROIDAL ANTIINFLAMMATORY DRUGS. Nonsteroidal antiinflammatory drugs (NSAIDs) have proved to be a most efficacious method of treatment for primary dysmenorrhea. Pickles[66] found that the lowering of serum prostaglandin levels during anovulatory cycles was associated with a decrease in dysmenorrheic pain. NSAIDs inhibit production and/or action of prostaglandins; they are best administered several days before the onset of menses and continued for an average of 3 days after onset.

ORAL CONTRACEPTIVES. Oral contraceptives appear to have a significant effect on uterine activity with primary dysmenorrhea. Hauksson et al.[74] noted that oral contraceptives containing 30 µg ethinylestradiol with 150 mg levonorgestrel affect uterine activity and reactivity to lysine, vasopressin, and prostaglandin $F_{2\alpha}$ metabolism. Intrauterine pressure recordings showed an intense increase in pressure with lysine and vasopressin infusion, and prostaglandin $F_{2\alpha}$ stimulation is associated with increased contractile activity and discomfort. The effect of this oral contraceptive was to decrease intrauterine pressure and reactivity and lessen uterine response to vasopressin and prostaglandin $F_{2\alpha}$.[74] Thus, the implication is that gestagen-dominated oral contraceptives have a therapeutic effect in primary dysmenorrhea. This was interpreted to mean that hysterometric (i.e., assessment of uterine pressure) activity showed that oral contraceptive therapy resulted in less uterine hyperactivity, as well as less vessel compression and uterine ischemia, all of which produced less pelvic pain (i.e., dysmenorrhea).[74]

It has been noted that oral contraceptives decrease prostaglandin content in menstrual fluid.[75,76] Approximately 90% of adolescents with primary dysmenorrhea experience some degree of relief with oral contraceptive therapy.[71]

Progestins have been shown to decrease prostaglandin $F_{2\alpha}$ secretion. It is possible that this is one additional mechanism by which oral contraceptives alleviate primary dysmenorrhea.

OTHER MEDICAL THERAPIES. Calcium channel blocking agents, also termed calcium antagonists, have been used to treat primary dysmenorrhea. Nifedipine is one such calcium antagonist. A dose of 30 mg administered on the first day of menstruation provides prompt relief of menstrual cramps. It has a prominent tocolytic effect, which decreases uterine activity, thus relieving dysmenorrhea.[77]

SURGICAL THERAPY. Lichten and Bombard[78] described a series of patients with primary dysmenorrhea who apparently responded to laser uterosacral nerve ablation. They noted that approximately 24% of dysmenorrheic patients showed no improvement with NSAIDs. These authors reported a double-blind study of 21 patients with primary dysmenorrhea, 81% of whom had significant relief from dysmenorrhea postoperatively. Laser uterosacral nerve ablation was performed laparoscopically. Although there was significant improvement, not all patients were pain free. A number of those who still experienced dysmenorrhea were able to respond to NSAIDs postoperatively. The authors concluded that uterosacral nerve interruption may prove to be an effective alternative treatment for primary dysmenorrhea. This procedure does not appear to be efficacious as a primary form of therapy for adolescent females.

Presacral neurectomy for chronic pain also has been advocated.[79,80] Fifty presacral neurectomies were performed at Madigan Army Medical Center. Each patient included in the study had been refractory to NSAIDs. Of the total number, 73% experienced relief from dysmenorrhea, 77% from dyspareunia, and 63% from other pelvic pains. The authors concluded that bilateral uterosacral ligament resection did not appear to increase the success rate compared with the presacral neurectomy surgical procedure. For adolescents a surgical approach for treatment of dysmenorrhea should be considered only in very extenuating circumstances.

Secondary Dysmenorrhea

It should be apparent that for adolescents with chronic pelvic pain refractory to medical therapy, careful consideration should be given to proceeding with the appropriate evaluation, which often includes diagnostic laparoscopy.[81-83] Table 132-4 conveys information regarding the predominant findings of endometriosis and pelvic adhesions in this population of adolescents. Uterine anomalies also should be considered in the evaluation of pelvic pain in adolescent females, and therefore müllerian tract anomalies must be included in the differential diagnosis of secondary dysmenorrhea in adolescents.[84] Psychiatric considerations with respect to chronic pelvic pain also must be studied.[85] In a series of 25 patients, each had a normal gynecologic evaluation. A psychiatric assessment identified the most frequent diagnosis to be "significant pathology with borderline syndrome and hysterical character disorder." A significant incidence of early childhood family dysfunction and incest was noted in the series.[85] Clear differentiation between organic and psychogenic functional pelvic pain is, of course, hard to establish. In general, however, organic pain frequently presents with sharp, crampy discomfort, waking the patient at night with intermittent periods of radiating pain. Psychogenic pain usually is absent during sleep.

ENDOMETRIOSIS. The patient who presents with dysmenorrhea refractory to ovulatory suppression and NSAIDs and with chronic pelvic pain of 6 months' duration or more merits an evaluation for endometriosis. Endometriosis is discussed in Chapter 138 "The Uterus and Adnexa."

MITTELSCHMERZ. Pain at the time of ovulation is termed mittelschmerz. It is believed to be the result of peritoneal irritation associated with the release of follicular fluid, and it often can be alleviated by use of NSAIDs or oral contraceptives.

PREMENSTRUAL SYNDROME

Premenstrual syndrome (PMS) was described first by Frank[86] in 1931. A host of physical and emotional changes were noted consistently each menstrual cycle preceding the onset of menses. In 1953, Greene and Dalton[87] further elaborated on such PMS manifestations as fluid retention, bloating, breast tenderness, headaches, irritability, fatigue, anxiety, hostility, and/or depression. These symptoms are often complemented by a craving for sweets (especially chocolate), salty foods, and alcoholic beverages. "I feel like I'm a different person before my period" or "My life seems entirely out of control during this time of the month" are comments often heard from patients with PMS.

Diagnosis

A careful history often attests to the changes in physical condition, generalized discomfort, water retention, fatigue, and autonomic physical changes. Mood-behavioral changes, such as impaired social functioning, accompanying depression, and frequently impulsive behavior, are characteristic. Adolescents often seem to have more severe symptoms when they also have untreated dysmenorrhea.[88]

Treatment

Initially, adolescents should be managed with reassurance along with dietary and exercise modifications rather than with medications.[89] A host of medical therapies have been prescribed, especially for adults, including the use of progesterone.[90] Greene and Dalton's work[87] attested to the efficacy of progestin and progesterone in the treatment of PMS. The problem is that a number of double-blind crossover studies question the effectiveness of progesterone.[91,92]

Other medical therapies have included use of diuretics such as spironolactone, 25 mg four times daily, during the luteal phase.[93] Vitamin B$_6$ also appears to be efficacious, although the dose is critical, since toxic levels have been reported.[94] Pyridoxine, 50 mg daily, appears to be somewhat more effective than placebo in reducing PMS symptoms. Bromocriptine also has been used, although the only real effectiveness of this particular choice of therapy appears to be improvement of mastodynia.[95] In addition, use of alprazolam (Xanax) in adult women with PMS has been reported by Smith et al,[96] who concluded that this agent appeared to be more effective than placebo. Treatment with essential fatty acids, especially τ-linoleic acid, as noted in work reported at the 1983 International Symposium on Dysmenorrhea and Premenstrual Tension, has been described.[97]

Newer treatment modalities now include serotonin reuptake inhibitors. One such agent is fluoxetine hydrochloride (Prozac). This therapy appears to be especially effective if the predominant PMS symptoms are depression and anxiety. In one placebo-controlled study involving 405 women randomized either to fluoxetine, 20 or 60 mg per day, or placebo, the researchers concluded that fluoxetine was useful at a dose of 20 mg (or greater) in alleviating premenstrual symptoms.[98] Clinicians must be aware when counseling patients on fluoxetine that sexual dysfunction may occur as a side effect of such therapy.[99]

DYSFUNCTIONAL UTERINE BLEEDING

Dysfunctional uterine bleeding (DUB) is defined as excessive, prolonged, or irregular bleeding from the uterine endometrium that is unrelated to anatomic lesions of the uterus.[100] As anovulation or disruption of normal ovarian function accounts for more than 75% of cases,[97] some authors have advocated referring to DUB as anovulatory uterine bleeding.

Normal menstrual cycles have been defined as having a mean interval of 28 days (± 7 days) with a mean duration of 4 days (± 2 to 3 days). Normal menstrual flow is approximately 30 ml/cycle,[101] with an upper limit of normal at 60 to 80 ml.[102] Therefore, bleeding of more than 80 ml occurring at intervals of 21 days or less for more than 7 days is considered abnormal. Definitions for various uterine bleeding abnormalities are listed in Box 132-3.

DUB affects 10% to 15% of all gynecologic patients and occurs most commonly in adolescents.[97] The etiologic factors center around the slow maturation of the hypothalamic-pituitary-ovarian axis in female adolescents, leading to anovulatory cycles. Although menarche

---

> **BOX 132-3**
> **Primary Coagulation Disorders Associated with Abnormal Uterine Bleeding**
>
> Idiopathic thrombocytopenic purpura
> von Willebrand's disease
> Glanzmann's disease
> Fanconi's anemia
> Thalassemia major

---

occurs on average at 12.87 years of age in the United States, the establishment of orderly ovulatory bleeding may take up to 5 years. However, it usually occurs within 18 months after menarche.[103] McDonough and Ganett[104] observed anovulation in 55% to 82% of the cycles from menarche to 2 years post menarche, in 30% to 55% of the cycles from 2 to 4 years post menarche, and in 0% to 20% of cycles from 4 to 5 years post menarche. Jones[105] reported abnormal bleeding in more than 500 adolescent females followed for 5 years, 75% of whom were anovulatory, thus indicating a relatively high association of anovulation with DUB in the adolescent patient.

Normal ovulation involves a regular cyclic production, first of estradiol, initiating ovarian follicular growth and endometrial proliferation, then of ovulation, which produces a significant increase in the progesterone level, which acts as a stabilizer of the endometrial matrix. Without ovulation and subsequent progesterone production, a state of unopposed estrogen occurs, which dilates the spiral arteries supplying the endometrium and causes endometrial growth, resulting in an endometrium with abnormal height and without structural support that can suffer spontaneous superficial breakage with random synchronous bleeding.[101] Eventually, this increased estrogen level will have a negative feedback to the hypothalamus and result in a decrease in GnRH, FSH, LH, and estrogen levels, causing vasoconstriction and collapse of a thickened hyperplastic endometrial lining and heavy and prolonged bleeding.[106]

Although anovulation is the most common finding associated with DUB, a number of ovulatory patients have intermenstrual bleeding. The mechanism surrounding this event is uncertain. Also, a condition of prolonged progesterone excretion due to a prolonged corpus luteal cyst after ovulation can give rise to 6 to 8 weeks of amenorrhea followed by irregular menstrual flow with an associated persistent corpus luteal cyst (Halban's syndrome) on examination.[107]

Diagnosis

DUB is a diagnosis of exclusion. Initial attempts at diagnosis of anovulation as the cause of irregular bleeding should be directed toward eliminating the possibility of organic lesions in the reproductive tract as well as coagulation disorders. Organic disorders that resemble simple anovulatory bleeding include intrauterine benign neoplasms, reproductive tract malignancies, bleeding with early pregnancy as in threatened abortion, ectopic pregnancy, and hydatidiform mole. Associated blood dyscrasias include thrombocytopenic purpura, von Willebrand's disease, platelet defects, and platelet storage pool diseases (Box 132-3).

Despite extensive possibilities,[103] the usual diagnosis in an adolescent patient remains anovulation. As previously stated, the most common cause of anovulation in the adolescent is hypothalamic-pituitary-ovarian axis immaturity. However, it is important to recognize that any hypothalamic dysfunction associated with stress, exercise, weight loss, or systemic diseases also can affect ovulation. In particular, congenital adrenal hyperplasia, Cushing's syndrome, and hepatic dysfunction all can interfere with the process.[100] In some of these situations the interaction is not well understood, but the hormonal derangement associated with adrenal dysfunction interferes with central regulating mechanisms of ovulation, and it is thought that thyroid abnormalities and liver dysfunction result in a derangement of the metabolic clearance rate of estrogen.[97]

The second most common cause of abnormal bleeding in adolescents is a coagulopathy. Claessens and Cowell,[108] in their 9-year review, examined all admissions for acute menorrhagia at a children's hospital and determined that 19% were the result of primary coagulation disorders. These disorders are outlined in Box 132-3. Of the nine patients in this study who presented with acute menorrhagia at menarche, 55% were found to have a coagulation disorder. These girls constituted 45% of all patients in the study determined to have blood clotting abnormalities. This association illustrates the importance of excluding a hematologic problem whenever menorrhagia occurs at menarche. An underlying coagulation disorder can be noted in one of four girls with severe menorrhagia and with a hemoglobin level of less than 10 g/dl and in one out of two adolescents presenting at the time of menarche.[109] Of those patients with bleeding dyscrasias, 10% present with cyclic hypermenorrhea. Probably the most common hematologic disorder in adolescents is idiopathic thrombocytopenic purpura.[103] Platelets and fibrin play a direct part in the hemostasis achieved in a bleeding menstrual endometrium; therefore, deficiencies in these constituents, as evident in thrombocytopenia and von Willebrand's disease, cause the associated increased blood loss with menses.[101] In a similar fashion, there have been case reports of menorrhagia in individuals with platelet storage pool diseases—a defect in which there is an inability of platelets to aggregate.[109]

Evaluation

Evaluation for abnormal bleeding is initiated with a detailed gynecologic history (menarche, frequency, duration, last menstrual period) as well as a sexual history. A list of medications being taken by the patient also should be obtained, as certain medications can interfere with normal menses and/or interfere with proper metabolism of oral contraceptives. Any medication that increases the cytochrome P-450 mechanism in the liver (i.e., seizure medications) also will increase the metabolism of oral contraceptives. In addition, patients taking oral contraceptives must be questioned extensively concerning proper compliance, without which irregular bleeding can occur. A careful review of systems should be made—in particular, evaluation of bleeding disorders (easy bruising, epistaxis, gingival bleeding) and endocrine disorders (hirsutism, galactorrhea, thyroid symptoms). The physical examination provides an opportunity to assess Tanner staging and signs of endocrine abnormalities, and a pelvic examination can detect the possibility of pregnancy, the presence of a foreign body, or an anatomic source of the bleeding.

Essential laboratory tests include a complete blood count with platelet evaluation, blood smear, serum pregnancy test, and coagulation profile including prothrombin and partial thromboplastin time, as well as bleeding time (Box 132-4). In sexually active patients, testing for sexually transmitted diseases such as chlamydial infection and gonorrhea should be obtained, as cervicitis may be the cause of DUB. These coagulation tests should be completed before any transfusion or hormonal treatment is begun. Endocrinologic evaluation should be completed by obtaining thyroid function tests; usually the measurement of thyroxine and TSH levels is sufficient. In cases of menorrhagia at menarche or severe anemia associated with DUB, a work-up for von Willebrand's disease is warranted, including an assay for von Willebrand factor and ristocetin cofactor. As these levels may fluctuate, repeat testing may need to be computed if tests return normal and suspicions are increased for a bleeding dyscrasia.

BOX 132-4
Evaluation of Abnormal
Uterine Bleeding

Pregnancy test
Complete blood count with platelet evaluation
Coagulation profile
Thyroid functions (as warranted)

Treatment

Management of DUB is based on the presenting signs and symptoms; examination findings; and the presence, absence, or severity of associated anemia (Box 132-5). Treatment for mild cases (defined as irregular intervals of bleeding at 20 to 60 days with a hematocrit >30) should be supportive reassurance. Education should focus on proper diet, exercise, stress management, and maintenance of a proper menstrual calendar. Usually these situations resolve after 1 to 2 years with the onset of spontaneous ovulation. If contraception is needed, an oral contraceptive pill could be initiated. These patients need reevaluation on a 6-monthly basis. In patients with severe, recurrent DUB or in whom it is associated with anemia, hormonal therapy is indicated. Most commonly, this is accomplished by the initiation of cyclic medroxyprogesterone acetate or a combination oral contraceptive pill. Progesterone or progestins are antiestrogenic when given in a pharmacologic dosage.[110] Progesterone induces an enzyme, 17-hydroxysteroid dehydrogenase, in endometrial cells that converts estradiol to estrone. Progestins also diminish the estrogenic effect on target cells by inhibiting augmentation of estrogen cytosol receptors that ordinarily modulate estrogen action. These influences account for the antimitotic, antigrowth impact of progestins in the endometrium. In the treatment of oligomenorrhea, withdrawal flow can be initiated by administration of a progestational agent such as medroxyprogesterone acetate, 10 mg daily for 10 days a month.[111] To treat metrorrhagia or polymenorrhea, medroxyprogesterone acetate, 10 mg daily, is prescribed for 10 days per month to induce stomal stability, which is followed by withdrawal flow. This can be used cyclically every month for 3 to 6 months, after which it can be discontinued and the condition observed. If the adolescent needs contraception, an oral contraceptive can be used alternatively. These have the added benefit of cyclic regulation in that oral contraceptives have been noted to decrease the amount of menstrual blood by at least 60% in patients with a normal uterus. Because the mechanism of action of oral contraceptives is that of ovulation suppression, the underlying anovulatory problem is not alleviated in these patients. Therefore, they should be informed that most individuals will have spontaneous ovulation with maturation of the HPO axis. In a significant number, however, anovulation persists.

An acute anovulatory bleeding episode can be controlled with a 35-µg estrogen-progestin oral contraceptive. Therapy consists of one pill every 6 hours until the bleeding stops (usually within 1 to 5 days). If this does not stop the flow, causes other than anovulation must be ruled out, including the presence of myomas, polyps, or bleeding diathesis. If flow diminishes significantly or abates predictably, the oral contraceptives should be tapered to one pill every day. The once-a-day regimen should then be continued for the 21-day cycle, after which withdrawal flow will occur. The patient should be warned to anticipate a flow after therapy, and may continue on oral contraceptives for an additional 3 months for treatment purposes or longer if necessary for birth control. In addition to the normal therapy, these adolescents should be placed on iron therapy to compensate for decreased iron stores. Persistent oligomenorrhea 1 to 2 years after the initial evaluation will necessitate further evaluation with an assessment of LH and FSH levels for possible polycystic ovary syndrome, and prolactin and TSH to rule out a central cause for anovulation. This bleeding pattern with an LH-to-FSH ratio of 2:1 to 3:1 provides evidence for a clinical diagnosis of polycystic ovary syndrome.

Intermittent vaginal bleeding frequently is associated with lower circulating estrogen levels that result in breakthrough bleeding. In this circumstance, progestins do not control this bleeding. This is commonly seen in adolescent patients in whom there has been prolonged

---

BOX 132-5
Management of Dysfunctional Uterine Bleeding

Hemoglobin >12 g/dl
  Reassurance
  Menstrual calendar
  Iron supplements
  Periodic reevaluation
Hemoglobin 10-12 g/dl
  Reassurance and explanation
  Menstrual calendar
  Iron supplements
  Cyclic progestin therapy or oral contraceptives
  Reevaluation in 6 mo
Hemoglobin <10 g/dl
  No active bleeding
    Explanation
    Transfusion/iron supplements
    Oral contraceptives
    Reevaluation in 6-12 mo
  Acute hemorrhage
    Transfusion
    Fluid replacement therapy
    Hormonal hemostasis (intravenous conjugated estrogen)
    Intensive progestin therapy
    D & C when hormonal hemostasis fails
    Oral contraceptives for 6-12 mo

From Muram D, Sanfilippo SJ, Hertweck SP: Vaginal bleeding in childhood and menstrual disorders in adolescence. In Sanfilippo JS, editor: *Pediatric and adolescent gynecology*, Philadelphia, 1994, WB Saunders; pp 222-232.

anovulation leading to persistent desquamation, leaving little residual endometrial tissue. Therefore, estrogen therapy must be administered before progestin therapy. In cases of acute or heavy bleeding, hospitalization with possible transfusion may be indicated. Intravenous conjugated estrogen, 25 mg, may be administered every 4 to 6 hours until bleeding ceases.[112] Conjugated estrogen appears to have multiple direct effects on clotting, including platelet aggregation, increased fibrinogen levels, increased factors V and IX, and decreased effectiveness of bradykinin, thereby causing hemostasis.[113] After the bleeding ceases, the patient may be prescribed cyclic progestational dominant oral contraceptives such as Ovral, Lo/Ovral, or cyclic progestin. The oral contraceptives should be used as one tablet four times a day for 4 days, then three times a day for 3 days, then twice a day for 2 weeks. The patient should be given the oral contraceptives cyclically for an additional 2 months.

In acute cases a response to hormonal therapy usually is seen in 24 to 48 hours. If this does not occur, the patient needs reevaluation for a coagulopathy or an anatomic disorder. Curettage is the last line of attack in the adolescent and is rarely necessary. In those circumstances, without response to hormonal therapy, a dilation and curettage (D&C) and hysteroscopy is advisable for diagnostic and therapeutic purposes followed by appropriate medical and hormonal therapy. If bleeding persists, one must suspect an anatomic abnormality not identified by the D&C. Although this unresponsiveness is rare in adolescents, its occurrence should be a sign for necessary reevaluation. Neoplasia is also rare in adolescents but does occur, as reported by Davis and Reindollar in their description of two adolescents aged 17 and 13 with adenomatous hyperplasia, the former with severe atypia diagnosed by D&C, the latter diagnosed through an endometrial biopsy.[114]

One other method of treating severe acute bleeding is the use of desmopressin (dDAVP). This has been classically used in the treatment of central diabetes insipidus but is not advocated for abnormal uterine bleeding in patients with different types of hemophilia and von Willebrand's disease, as well as in patients without a coagulation abnormality.[115-118] There are two modes of administration, through the intranasal route and through the more efficient parenteral route. The intravenous dose is 0.3 µg/kg diluted in 50ml of normal saline administered over 15 to 30 minutes. The dosage results in a rapid rise of coagulation factor VIII, with peak levels at 90 to 120 minutes and a duration of approximately 6 hours. Repetitive doses administered in 12 and 24 hours reproduce the incremental effect but with a diminishing response over time. The intranasal dose is 300 µg repeated every 8 to 12 hours as needed. However, as with the intravenous dosing of dDAVP, prolonged use of the intranasal dose for more than 3 or 4 days increases the risk of tachyphylaxis.

Irregular bleeding is frequently encountered in patients on long-standing oral contraceptives or on depomedroxyprogesterone acetate. Irregular bleeding occurring in the first part of the cycle may be secondary to inadequate estrogen production and may result in an unstable atrophic endometrial lining. Cyclic estrogen in the form of conjugated estrogen, 2.5 mg daily for 7 days during the cycle of therapy, should control this problem.

Antiprostaglandins act on the endometrial vasculature. The concentrations in PGE_2 and $PGF_{2\alpha}$ increase progressively in the endometrium during the menstrual cycle. The prostaglandin synthetase inhibitors appear to decrease menstrual blood loss.[119,120] This may result from altering the balance between platelet proaggregating vasoconstrictor thromboxane and antiaggregating vasodilator prostacyclins, and by inhibiting prostaglandin endoperoxidase synthetase decreasing the total amount of prostaglandin levels. Whatever the exact mechanism, prostaglandin inhibitors diminish menstrual bleeding in normal women as well as the bleeding associated with chronic endometritis as seen with intrauterine devices. Numerous preparations are available, none with superiority over the others. These compounds may be prescribed in conjunction with cyclic hormonal therapy. Commonly, they are initiated at the first sign of menses or with the first cramping episode at the time of menses, and continue throughout the menstrual cycle.

In rare situations in which hormonal therapy is contraindicated or bleeding is excessive and uncontrollable, the use of GnRH analogs has been recommended. Their administration suppresses gonadotropin secretion and subsequent estradiol secretion, which results in arrest of menstruation; therefore, they not only decrease menorrhagia but also produce amenorrhea.[108,121] McLaughlan et al reported that after 12 weeks of administration of intranasal GnRH treatment in four women with menorrhagia, the total menstrual blood loss decreased from 95 to 198 ml per month to 4 to 30 ml per month in the second and third treatment cycles. Limitations to long-term GnRH agonist use are osteoporosis and undesirable lipoprotein changes. Whereas these alternatives are thought on the basis of limited data to be reversible, the risks of this form of therapy far outweigh the benefits for long-term treatment.

Failure to respond to medical therapy usually is seen when progestins are used to control bleeding in patients with a hypoestrogenic or desquamated endometrium. Curettage is the last remaining option to treat anovulatory irregular bleeding in adolescent patients and is rarely necessary except in patients with a known bleeding diathesis. Under these circumstances, bleeding should be controlled by every effort being made to normalize coagulation studies, followed by D&C, after which appropriate medical therapy should be initiated. If bleeding persists, one must suspect an anatomic abnormality not identified during the surgical procedure.

Further diagnostic evaluation such as hysteroscopy should be considered.

Treatments that eliminate reproductive potential, such as hysterectomy or endometrial ablation, are indicated rarely in adolescent patients. The long-term prognosis for adolescents with irregular bleeding can be described as guarded at best. About 5% continue to have severe episodes of anovulatory bleeding and merit endocrinologic evaluation. The importance of continued follow-up is illustrated by the results of a 25-year prospective evaluation of adolescents with DUB.[122] In 291 patients, 60% had continued bleeding for 2 years after initial onset. Persistent problems were evident in 50% of patients after 4 years and in 30% after 10 years. Except in cases of blood dyscrasias, patients with normal menses before the start of irregular bleeding had a more favorable prognosis.

References

1. Kaplan S, Grumbaugh M: Physiology of puberty. In Flamigni C, Givens J, editors: *The gonadotropins: basic science and clinical aspects in females,* New York, 1982, Academic Press; p 167.

2. Grumbach MM, Roth JC, Kaplan SL, et al: Hypothalamic-pituitary regulation of puberty in man. Evidence and concepts derived from clinical research. In Grumbach MM, Grave GD, Mayer FE, editors: *Control of the onset of puberty,* New York, 1974, John Wiley; p 115.

3. Freisch RE, McArthur J: Menstrual cycles: fatness as a determinant of minimum weight for height necessary for their maintenance or onset, *Science* 185:949, 1974.

4. Neinstein LS: Menstrual problems in adolescence, *Med Clin North Am* 74:1181, 1990.

5. Rosenfield RL, Lucky AW: Acne, hirsutism and alopecia in adolescent girls: clinical expressions of androgen excess, *Endocrinol Metab Clin North Am* 22:507, 1993.

6. Roth J, Kelch R, Kaplan S, Grumbach M: FSH and LH response to luteinizing hormone–releasing factor in prepubertal and pubertal children, adult males, patients with hypogonadotropic and hypergonadotropic hypogonadism, *J Clin Endocrinol Metab* 37:68, 1973.

7. Foster DL, Root A: *Problems in pediatric endocrinology,* New York, 1980, Academic Press.

8. Yen SSC: The polycystic ovary syndrome, *Clin Endocrinol* 12:177, 1980.

9. Rosenfield R: The ovary and female sexual maturation. In Kaplan SA, editor: *Clinical pediatric and adolescent endocrinology,* Philadelphia, 1982, WB Saunders.

10. Apter D, Vihko R: Hormonal patterns of the first menstrual cycles. In Flamigni C, Venturoli S, Givens J, editors: *Adolescence in females,* Chicago, 1985, Mosby–Year Book.

11. Apter D, Pakarien A, Vihko R: Serum prolactin, follicle stimulating hormone and luteinizing hormone during puberty in girls and boys, *Acta Paediatr Scand* 67:417, 1978.

12. Apter D: Serum steroids and pituitary hormones in female puberty: a partly longitudinal study, *Clin Endocrinol* (Oxf) 12:107, 1980.

13. Speroff L, Glass RH, Kase NG, editors: *Clinical gynecologic endocrinology and infertility,* ed 4, Baltimore, 1989, Williams & Wilkins; p 409.

14. Zeleznik A, Schuler H, Reichert L: Gonadotropin binding sites in the rhesus monkey ovary: role of the vasculature in the selective distribution of human chorionic gonadotropin to the pre-ovulatory follicle, *Endocrinology* 109:356, 1981.

15. Frederick J, Shimanuki T, deZerega G: Initiation of angiogenesis by human follicular fluid, *Science* 224:389, 1984.

16. Speroff L, Glass RH, Kase NG: Regulation of the menstrual cycle. In Speroff L, Glass RH, Kase NG, editors: *Clinical gynecologic endocrinology and infertility,* ed 4, Baltimore, 1989, Williams & Wilkins; pp 91-119.

17. Lumsden M, Kelly R, Templeton A, van Look P, Swanston I, Baird D: Changes in the concentrations of prostaglandins in pre-ovulatory human follicles after administration of hCG, *J Reprod Fertil* 177:119, 1986.

18. O'Grady J, Caldwell B, Auletta F, Speroff L: The effects of an inhibitor of prostaglandin synthesis (indomethacin) on ovulation, pregnancy and pseudopregnancy, *Prostaglandins* 1:97, 1972.

19. Saracoglu OF, Aksel S, Yeoman RR, Wiebe RH: Endometrial estradiol and progesterone receptors in patients with luteal phase defects and endometriosis, *Fertil Steril* 43:851, 1985.

20. Lenton E, Langren B, Sexton L: Normal variation in the length of the luteal phase of the menstrual cycle: identification of the short luteal phase, *Br J Obstet Gynaecol* 91:685, 1984.

21. Rao CV, Griffin LP, Carman FR Jr: Gonadotropin receptors in human corpora lutea of menstrual cycle and pregnancy, *Am J Obstet Gynecol* 128:146, 1977.

22. Bullough V: Age at menarche: a misunderstanding, *Science* 213:36, 1981.

23. Frisch R, Wyshak G, Vincent L: Delayed menarche and amenorrhea in ballet dancers, *N Engl J Med* 303:17, 1980.

24. Osler D, Crawford J: Examination of the hypothesis of a critical weight at menarche and ambulatory and bedridden mentally retarded girls, *Pediatrics* 51:674, 1973.

25. Mishell DR Jr: Amenorrhea. In Droegemueller W, Herbst AL, Mishell DR Jr, Stenchever MA, editors: *Comprehensive gynecology,* St. Louis, 1987, Mosby–Year Book; p 966.

26. Reindollar RH, McDonough PG: Etiology and evaluation of delayed sexual development. Symposium on Pediatric and Adolescent Gynecology, *Pediatr Clin North Am* 28:2, 1981.

27. Marshall WA, Tanner JM: Variations in the pattern of pubertal changes in girls, *Arch Dis Child* 44:291, 1969.

28. Jaffe RB: Disorders of sexual development. In Yen SSC, Jaffe RD, editors: *Reproductive endocrinology: physiology and clinical management,* Philadelphia, 1986, WB Saunders; p 283.

29. Klingmullen D, Dewes W, Krake T, Brecht G, Schweikert H: Magnetic resonance imaging of the brain in patients with anosmia and hypothalamic hypogonadism, *J Clin Endocrinol Metab* 65:581, 1987.

30. Kletzky OA, Costrin G, Morris RP, et al: Endocrine abnormalities in thalassemia major, *Am J Dis Child* 133:497, 1979.

31. Costrin G, Kogert M, Hyman CB, et al: Endocrine abnormalities in thalassemia major, *Am J Dis Child* 133:497, 1979.

32. Mashchak CA, Kletzky OA, Davajan V, Mishell DR Jr: Clinical and laboratory evaluation of patients with primary amenorrhea, *Obstet Gynecol* 57:715, 1981.

33. Harkins JL, Gysler M, Cowell CA: Anatomical amenorrhea: the problems of congenital vaginal agenesis and its surgical correction. Symposium on Pediatric and Adolescent Gynecology, *Pediatr Clin North Am* 28:345, 1981.

34. Griffin JE, Wilson JD: The androgen resistance syndromes: 5α-reductase deficiency, testicular feminization and related disorders. In Scriver CR, Bendet AL, Valer D, editors: *The metabolic basis of inherited disease,* ed 6, vol 2, New York, 1989, McGraw-Hill; pp 1919-1944.

35. Scully RE: Tumors of the ovary and maldeveloped gonads. In *Atlas of tumor pathology,* 2nd series, fascicle 16, Washington DC, 1974, Armed Forces of Pathology.

36. Scully RE: Gonadoblastoma. A review of 74 cases, *Cancer* 25:1340, 1970.

37. Foster D, Olster D, Yellon S: Neuroendocrine regulation of puberty by nutrition and photoperiod. In Flamigni C, Venturoli S,

Givens J, editors: *Adolescence in females,* Chicago, 1985, Mosby–Year Book; p 19.

38. Purcell A, Bumpos F, Husain A: Rat ovarian angiotensin II receptors: characterization and coupling to estrogen secretion, *J Biol Chem* 262:7076, 1987.

39. Jenkins JS, Gilbert CJ, Ang V: Hypothalamic pituitary function in patients with craniopharyngiomas, *J Clin Endocrinol Metab* 43:394, 1976.

40. Radwanska E: Primary amenorrhea, *Obstet Gynecol Ann* 10:313, 1981.

41. Gharib H, Frey HM, Laws ER Jr, et al: Coexistent primary empty sella syndrome and hyperprolactinemia: report of 11 cases, *Arch Intern Med* 143:1383, 1983.

42. Dickey RP, Stone SC: Drugs that affect the breast and lactation, *Clin Obstet Gynecol* 18:95, 1975.

43. Speroff L, Glass RH, Kase NG: The breast. In Speroff L, Glass RH, Kase NG, editors: *Clinical gynecologic endocrinology and infertility,* ed 4, Baltimore, 1989, Williams & Wilkins; p 292.

44. Wilson C, Emans SJ, Mansfield J, et al: The relationship of calculated percent body fat, sports participation, age and place of residence on menstrual pattern in healthy adolescent girls at an independent New England high school, *J Adolesc Health Care* 5:248, 1984.

45. Mansfield MJ, Emans SJ: Adolescent gynecology: anorexia nervosa, athletics and amenorrhea, *Pediatr Clin North Am* 36:533, 1989.

46. Frisch RE, Gotz-Welbergen AV, McArthur JW, et al: Delayed menarche and amenorrhea of college athletics in relation to onset of training, *JAMA* 246:1559, 1981.

47. Warren MP: The effects of exercise on pubertal progression and reproductive function in girls, *J Clin Endocrinol Metab* 51:1150, 1980.

48. Kase NG: The neuroendocrinology of amenorrhea, *J Reprod Med* 28:251, 1983.

49. Lui JH: Hypothalamic amenorrhea: clinical perspectives, pathophysiology and management, *Am J Obstet Gynecol* 163:1743, 1990.

50. Miller DS, Reed RR, Cetal NS, Rebar RW, Yen SC: Pulsatile administration of low-dose gonadotropin-releasing hormone: ovulation and pregnancy in women with hypothalamic amenorrhea, *JAMA* 250:2937, 1983.

51. Emans SJ, Goldstein DP: Delayed puberty and menstrual irregularities. In Emans SJ, Goldstein DP, editors: *Pediatric and adolescent gynecology,* ed 3, Boston, 1990, Little, Brown; pp 145-242.

52. Frisch RE, McArthur JS: Menstrual cycles. Fatness as determinant of minimum weight for height necessary for their maintenance or onset, *Science* 185:949, 1974.

53. Baranowska B, Rozbicka G, Jeske W, Abdel-Fattah MH: The role of endogenous opiates in the mechanism of inhibited luteinizing hormone secretion in women with anorexia nervosa: the effect of naloxone on LH, FSH, prolactin and β-endorphin secretion, *J Clin Endocrinol Metab* 59:412, 1984.

54. Mishell DR Jr: Hyperprolactinemia, galactorrhea, and pituitary adenoma. In Droegemueller W, Herbst AL, Mishell DR Jr, Stenchever MA, editors: *Comprehensive gynecology,* St. Louis, 1987, Mosby–Year Book; p 994.

55. Schenker JG, Margalioth EJ: Intrauterine adhesions: an updated appraisal, *Fertil Steril* 37:593, 1982.

56. Gwynne J, Strauss J: The role of lipoproteins in the steroidogenesis and cholesterol metabolism in steroidogenic glands, *Endocrinol Rev* 3:299, 1982.

57. Aiman J, Smentek C: Premature ovarian failure, *Obstet Gynecol* 66:9, 1985.

58. Morrison JC, Givens JR, Wiser WL, Fish SA: Mumps oophoritis: a cause of premature menopause, *Fertil Steril* 26:655, 1975.

59. Stillman JR, Schinfeld JS, Schiff T, et al: Ovarian failure in long term survivors of childhood malignancy, *Am J Obstet Gynecol* 139:62, 1981.

60. Rivkees SA, Crawford TD: The relationship of gonadal activity and chemotherapy-induced gonadal damage, *JAMA* 259:2123, 1988.

61. Klein H, Litt I: Epidemiology of adolescent dysmenorrhea, *Pediatrics* 68:661, 1981.

62. Smith R: Primary dysmenorrhea in the adolescent patient, *Adolesc Pediatr Gynecol* 1:23, 1988.

63. Andersch B, Milsom I: An epidemiologic study of young women with dysmenorrhea, *Am J Obstet Gynecol* 144:655, 1982.

64. Wilson EA: *Endometriosis,* New York, 1987, Alan R. Liss; p 1.

65. Krohn L, Lackner J, Soskin S: The effect of the ovarian hormones on the human (non-puerperal) uterus, *Am J Obstet Gynecol* 34:379, 1937.

66. Pickles V: A plain muscle stimulant in the menstruum, *Nature* 180:1198, 1957.

67. Akerlund M: Pathophysiology of dysmenorrhea, *Acta Obstet Gynecol Scand Suppl* 87:27, 1979.

68. Auletta F, Agins H, Scommegna A: Prostaglandin F mediation of the inhibitory effect of estrogen on the corpus luteum of the rhesus monkey, *Endocrinology* 103:1183, 1978.

69. Rapkin AJ, Kames LH, Darke LL, et al: History of physical and sexual abuse in women with chronic pelvic pain, *Obstet Gynecol* 76:92, 1990.

70. Harrop-Griffith J, Katon W, Walker E, Holm L, Russo J, Hickok L: The association between chronic pain, psychiatric diagnoses and childhood sexual abuse, *Obstet Gynecol* 71:589, 1988.

71. Walker E, Katon W, Harrop-Griffith J, Holm L, Russo J, Hickok L: Relationship of chronic pelvic pain to psychiatric diagnoses in childhood sexual abuse, *Am J Psychiatry* 145:75, 1988.

72. Lawlor C, Davis A: Primary dysmenorrhea: relationship to personality and attitudes in adolescent females, *J Adolesc Health Care* 1:208, 1981.

73. Lawlor C, Jay MS, Durand R: The patient with dysmenorrhea, *Postgrad Med* 73:103, 1983.

74. Hauksson A, Ekstrom P, Juchnicka E, Laudanski T, Akerlund M: The influence of a combined oral contraceptive on uterine activity and reactivity to agonists in primary dysmenorrhea, *Acta Obstet Gynecol Scand* 68:31, 1989.

75. Chan W, Dawood M: Prostaglandin levels in menstrual fluid of nondysmenorrheic and dysmenorrheic subjects with and without oral contraceptive or ibuprofen therapy, *Adv Prostaglandin Thromboxane Res* 8:1443, 1980.

76. Dawood M: Dysmenorrhea, *Clin Obstet Gynecol* 26:719, 1983.

77. Ulmsten U: Calcium blockade as a rapid pharmacological test to evaluate primary dysmenorrhea, *Gynecol Obstet Invest* 20:78, 1985.

78. Lichten E, Bombard J: Surgical treatment of primary dysmenorrhea with laparoscopic uterine nerve ablation, *J Reprod Med* 32:37, 1987.

79. Lee R, Stone K, Magelssen D, Belts R, Benson W: Presacral neurectomy for chronic pelvic pain, *Obstet Gynecol* 68:517, 1986.

80. Black WT: Use of presacral neurectomy sympathectomy in treatment of dysmenorrhea, *Obstet Gynecol* 9:16, 1964.

81. Goldstein D, DeCholnoky C, Emans J: Adolescent endometriosis, *J Adolesc Health Care* 1:37, 1980.

82. Strickland DM, Hauth JC, Strickland KM: Laparoscopy for chronic pelvic pain in adolescent women, *Adolesc Pediatr Gynecol* 1:31, 1988.

83. Vercellini P, Fedele L, Molteni P, Arcaini L, Bianchi S, Candiani GB: Laparoscopy in the diagnosis of gynaecologic chronic pelvic pain, *Int J Gynaecol Obstet* 32:261, 1990.

84. Sanfilippo J: Strassman procedure for correction of a class II müllerian anomaly in an adolescent, *J Adolesc Health* 12:63, 1991.

85. Gross R, Doerr H, Caldirola D, et al: Borderline syndrome and incest in chronic pelvic pain patients, *Int J Psychiatry Med* 10:79, 1980.

86. Frank R: The hormonal causes of premenstrual tension, *Arch Neurol Psychiatry* 26:1052, 1931.

87. Greene R, Alton K: The premenstrual syndrome, *Br Med J* 1:1007, 1953.

88. Fisher M, Trieller K, Napolitano B: Premenstrual syndrome in adolescence, *J Adolesc Health Care* 10:369, 1989.

89. Coupey S, Ahlstrom P: Menstrual disorders, *Pediatr Clin North Am* 36:551, 1989.

90. Gray L: The use of progesterone in nervous tension states, *South Med J* 34:1004, 1941.

91. Sampson G: Premenstrual syndrome: a double-blind controlled trial of progesterone and placebo, *Br J Psychiatry* 135:209, 1979.

92. Chakmakjian Z: A critical assessment of therapy for the premenstrual tension syndrome, *J Reprod Med* 28:532, 1983.

93. O'Brien P: The premenstrual syndrome: a review of the present status of therapy, *Drugs* 24:140, 1982.

94. Abraham G, Hargrove J: Effect of vitamin B$_6$ on premenstrual symptomatology in women with premenstrual tension syndrome—a double-blind crossover study, *Infertility* 2:315, 1980.

95. Andersen A, Larson J, Steenstrup O, et al: Effect of bromocriptine on the premenstrual syndrome. A double-blind clinical trial, *Br J Obstet Gynaecol* 84:270, 1977.

96. Smith S, Rinehart JS, Ruddock VE, Schiff I: Treatment of premenstrual syndrome with alprazolam: results of a double-blind, placebo-controlled, randomized crossover clinical trial, *Obstet Gynecol* 70:37, 1987.

97. Horrobin D, Brush M: Premenstrual syndrome (PMS) and essential fatty acid (EFA) metabolism. Presented at the International Symposium on Dysmenorrhea and Premenstrual Syndrome, Kiawah Island, SC, September, 1983.

98. Steiner M, Steinberg S, Stewart D, et al: Fluoxetine in the treatment of premenstrual dysphoria. Canadian Fluoxetine/Premenstrual Dysphoria Collaborative Study Group, *N Engl J Med* 332:1529, 1995.

99. Pearlstein TB, Stone AB: Long-term fluoxetine treatment of late luteal phase dysphoric disorder, *J Clin Psychiatry* 55:332, 1994.

100. ACOG Technical Bulletin no. 134: *Dysfunctional uterine bleeding,* 1989.

101. Speroff L, Glass RH, Kase NG: Dysfunctional uterine bleeding. In Speroff L, Glass RH, Kase NG, editors: *Clinical gynecologic endocrinology and infertility,* ed 4, Baltimore, 1989, Williams & Wilkins; p 265.

102. Hallberg L, Hogdahl AM, Nilsson L, Rybo G: Menstrual blood loss—a population study: variations at different ages and attempts to define normality, *Acta Obstet Gynecol Scand* 45:320, 1966.

103. Gidwani G: Vaginal bleeding in adolescents, *J Reprod Med* 29:419, 1984.

104. McDonough PG, Ganett P: Dysfunctional uterine bleeding in the adolescent. In Barrom BN, Belisle BS, editors: *Adolescent gynecology and sexuality,* New York, 1982, Masson.

105. Jones GS: Endocrine problems in the adolescent, *Maryland State Med J* 16:45, 1967.

106. Spellacy WN: Abnormal bleeding, *Clin Obstet Gynecol* 26:702, 1983.

107. Dunnihoo D: Abnormal uterine bleeding. In Dunnihoo D, editor: *Fundamentals of gynecology and obstetrics,* New York, 1989, JB Lippincott.

108. Claessens EA, Cowell CA: Acute adolescent menorrhagia, *Am J Obstet Gynecol* 139:277, 1981.

109. Walker RW, Gustavson LP: Platelet storage pool disease in women, *J Adolesc Health Care* 3:264, 1983.

110. Nilsson L, Rybo G: Treatment of menorrhagia, *Am J Obstet Gynecol* 110:713, 1971.

111. Hertweck SP: Dysfunctional uterine bleeding, *Obstet Gynecol Clin North Am* 19:129, 1992.

112. DeVore GR, Owens O, Kase N: Use of intravenous Premarin in the treatment of dysfunctional uterine bleeding—double-blind randomized controlled study, *Obstet Gynecol* 59:285, 1982.

113. Livio M, Mannucci PM, Vigano G, et al: Conjugated estrogens for the management of bleeding associated with renal failure, *N Engl J Med* 315:731, 1986.

114. Davis A, Reindollar R: Adolescent endometrial hyperplasia associated with hyperinsulinemia in non-androgenized patients (abstr), Ft. Lauderdale, 1991, North American Society for Pediatric and Adolescent Gynecology.

115. Kubrinsky NL, Tulloch H: Treatment of refractory thrombocytopenic bleeding with desamino-8-D-arginine vasopressin (desmopressin), *J Pediatr* 112:993, 1988.

116. Neissner H, Korninger C: 1-Desamino-8-D-arginine vasopressin: an alternative in the management of mild haemophilia A and von Willebrand's disease, *Wien Klin Wochenschr* 95:753, 1983.

117. Richardson DW, Robinson AG: Desmopressin, *Ann Intern Med* 103:228, 1985.

118. Lethagen S, Harris AS, Nilsson IM: Intranasal desmopressin (dDAVP) by spray in mild hemophilia A and von Willebrand's disease type I, *Blut* 60:187, 1990.

119. Anderson ABM, Haynes PJ, Gnillebaud J, et al: Reduction of menstrual blood loss by prostaglandin synthetase inhibitor, *Lancet* 1:774, 1976.

120. Fraser IS, Svearman RP, McIlvern J: Efficacy of mefenamic acid in patient with a complaint of menorrhagia, *Obstet Gynecol* 58:843, 1981.

121. McLauchlan RI, Nealey DL, Burger HG: Clinical aspects of LHRH analogs in gynecology: a review, *Br J Obstet Gynaecol* 93:431, 1986.

122. Southam AL, Richart RM: The prognosis for adolescents with menstrual abnormalities, *Am J Obstet Gynecol* 94:637, 1966.

CHAPTER 133

Hirsutism

•

Joseph S. Sanfilippo

Hirsutism can be of significant concern to the female adolescent. Its impact on body image, peer interaction, and self-esteem often has a profound effect on the patient. Consultation is frequently sought for an adolescent who has become socially withdrawn and the subject of ridicule, as well as a great concern to herself and her parents. It should be the clinician's first responsibility, however, to rule out an androgen-producing neoplasm, the hallmark for serum androgen assessment being of paramount importance.[1]

PHYSIOLOGY

Androgen Production

The pathway from cholesterol to androgen production is outlined in Figure 133-1. The clinician should be aware that the primary areas of androgen synthesis include the ovary, the adrenal glands, and extraglandular conversion. Each site supplies different quantities of each androgen. The ovary contributes 25% of total testosterone production; another 25% is produced by the adrenal gland, and 50% is derived from peripheral conversion of androstenedione and estradiol.[1] Traditionally, serum testosterone is utilized as a marker of ovarian androgen production, since it is known that excessive testosterone production may be adrenal in origin.

The primary adrenal androgens are dehydroepiandrosterone (DHEA) and its sulfate (DHEA-S); 70% of DHEA is produced by the adrenals and 30% by the ovaries.[1] In the case of DHEA-S, 95% has an adrenal source and the other 5% an ovarian source.[1] Consequently, DHEA-S is a convenient marker of adrenal androgen production.

Fifty percent of total androstenedione production is of ovarian origin. It is peripherally converted to estrone, a weak estrogen found at increased levels in hormonal states such as polycystic ovarian syndrome (PCO) and menopause. Sex hormone–binding globulin (SHBG) is an important factor in the bioavailability of circulating androgens. In normal women, 80% of total testosterone is bound to SHBG, 19% is bound to albumin, and 1% exists as free steroid.[1] Only the albumin-bound and free portions are biologically active. SHBG levels are affected by many factors; androgens and obesity independently lower SHBG concentration, whereas estrogen and dexamethasone elevate SHBG.

Pubertal Ovarian Physiology

The fetal ovary is functional in utero. It is stimulated by pituitary gonadotropin-releasing hormones (GnRH), follicle-stimulating hormone (FSH), and luteinizing hormone (LH). The number of oocytes present in the ovary varies with age. At 20 weeks' gestation, there are 6 to 7 million oocytes. Owing to subsequent atresia, there are 1 million at birth and 300,000 at puberty.[1] These primordial follicles can produce androgens and estrogens in response to pituitary gonadotropin stimulation.

The onset of puberty appears to be due to a combination of increasing hypothalamic sensitivity to circulating estrogens and a progressive decline in SHBG levels throughout preadolescence.[2] Increased gonadotropin output takes place with a gradual recruitment of ovarian follicles and resultant production of ovarian steroid hormones. Follicles are hormonally active even before true ovulatory cycles occur. Increasing steroid concentrations along with greater bioavailability due to decreasing SHBG levels leads to the development of breasts, and pubic and axillary hair; uterine growth; and eventually menses. The chronologic order of these early events depends on the relative sensitivity of the target tissues.

Adrenal Physiology

During normal development, the adrenal gland undergoes its own pubertal hormonal increase. This process is

---

This chapter is based in part on Sanfilippo JS, Bailey-Pridham DD: Hirsutism in the adolescent female, *Pediatr Clin North Am* 36:581-599, 1989. Adapted with permission.

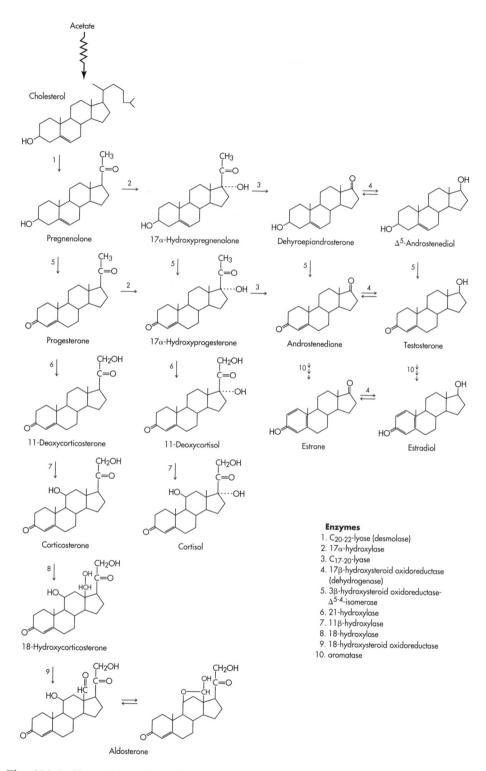

Fig. 133-1. The pathway from cholesterol to androgen production, showing biosynthesis of androgens, estrogens, and corticosteroids. (From Stanczyk FZ: Biosynthesis of androgens, estrogens, and corticosteroids. In Mishell OR, Davajan B, Logo RA, editors: *Infertility, contraception, and reproductive endocrinology,* ed 3, London, 1979, Blackwell Scientific; p 58.)

commonly termed *adrenarche* and is manifested by the appearance of pubic and axillary hair *(pubarche)*. The exact impetus causing increased adrenal androgen production, usually around 7 years of age, is not well understood.

Theoretical factors, such as adrenal androgen–stimulating hormone (AASH) or corticoadrenal-stimulating hormone (CASH), have been proposed as initiators of adrenal androgen production.[2] The identity of AASH or CASH is unknown. Hypotheses have included melatonin and adrenocorticotropic hormone (ACTH) as the initiators. Whatever the trophic event, adrenarche is characterized by significant increases in DHEA and DHEA-S.

HAIR GROWTH

Physiologic understanding of hair growth requires knowledge of the various stages and types of human hair. These are outlined in Box 133-1. Androgens appear to act at the level of the pilosebaceous unit, as androgen receptors are located in this region. Testosterone is converted to dihydrotestosterone (DHT) by the enzyme 5α-reductase at the peripheral level. Growth hormone also appears to act synergistically in producing hair growth, thus having an effect on the pilosebaceous unit. There is also evidence that insulin-like growth factors play an integral role in hair follicle development.

Therefore, hirsutism is a manifestation of increased density of terminal hair growth. It is important to differentiate between hirsutism and hypertrichosis in the hirsute patient. The latter is represented as a generalized increase in vellus hair, particularly along the extremities. This type of hair growth is especially manifested with endocrinologic problems such as Cushing syndrome.

BOX 133-1
Hair Growth

TYPES OF HAIR
Vellus: fine, soft, unmedullated, rarely pigmented, less than 2 cm long, unnoticeable
Terminal: coarse, medullated, pigmented, visible
Nonsexual: vellus or terminal, does not change original type, unresponsive to androgens
Sexual: vellus or terminal, usually midline, responds to androgen stimulation

STAGES OF HAIR GROWTH
Anagen: growth phase
Catagen: rapid involution phase
Telogen: resting phase

From Bailey-Pridham DD, Sanfilippo JS: Hirsutism in the adolescent female, *Pediatr Clin North Am* 36:581-599, 1989.

PATHOPHYSIOLOGY

When the physician is presented with an adolescent concerned with excess hair growth, the differential diagnosis must be considered, followed by an exclusionary work-up before initiation of therapy. This requires an understanding of the cause of hirsutism and the clinically available tests that may distinguish the various etiologies. Several diseases that may present with hirsutism can be life threatening to the patient, quite apart from their effect on personal appearance. Therefore, it is important to determine the pathogenesis of the hirsutism accurately. Box 133-2 conveys possible causes of hirsutism.

Peripheral Factors

IDIOPATHIC HIRSUTISM. Idiopathic hirsutism is the most common diagnosis established after evaluation of the hirsute patient. It is defined as normal total circulating androgen levels in the presence of hirsutism. This condition represents an interesting contrast to "cryptic hyperandrogenemia," in which androgens are elevated but no hirsutism is present. Clearly, a difference in sensitivity to circulating androgens must be involved. Many patients with idiopathic hirsutism may in reality have one of the conditions discussed below; the true pathogenesis may not be apparent without extensive testing, which usually will not affect management.

The relationship of mild hirsutism or acne in women to androgen concentrations has been studied by Reingold and Rosenfield.[3] In an investigation of 62 white females aged 18 to 21 years, an attempt was made to relate hirsutism and acne to plasma free testosterone, the main circulating determinant of increased androgenicity. Women with mild hirsutism as well as those with mild acne had a significantly elevated *mean* free testosterone compared with the mean of normal controls. Of interest is the variability in the relationship between pilosebaceous overactivity and free testosterone levels. In the mildly hirsute group, plasma free testosterone was normal in one half of the subjects. Variation in skin sensitivity to the level of circulating androgens (increased conversion to DHT) seemed to contribute equally to the pathogenesis of mild hirsutism and acne. The clinician should assume that hyperandrogenemia will be found in about one half of women with mild cases of hirsutism and in approximately one third with minor acne. Actual measurement of free testosterone is not clinically essential in the work-up or follow-up of hirsutism.

Even if basal circulating androgen levels are normal, there may be an abnormal response to stimulation. Many cases of cryptic and adult-onset congenital adrenal hyperplasia (CAH) show evidence of normal resting serum androgen levels but at the same time abnormal responses to an ACTH stimulus. Patients with subtle PCO may also have normal baseline androgens but reveal an abnormal pituitary LH and FSH response to stimulation with GnRH. Thus, dynamic testing may identify some patients who have an adrenal or ovarian pathogenesis for their condition, which was otherwise labeled "idiopathic hirsutism."

SHBG levels may be decreased in hirsute patients, allowing a higher fraction of bioactive androgens despite normal *total* serum androgen levels. SHBG levels are affected by several factors. Androgens, specifically testosterone, cause a fall in SHBG, whereas estradiol and

dexamethasone elevate SHBG levels.[1] A decline in SHBG levels is noted with increasing age, especially from prepuberty to adolescence. Body weight has an inverse correlation with SHBG levels independent of circulating androgen levels.

The activity of 5α-reductase in the skin of hirsute patients may be different from that in similar nonhirsute females. Direct measurements of the enzyme from skin cultures[8] and measurements of 3α-diol-glucuronide[4] (a metabolite of DHT) have a direct correlation with the degree of hirsutism. Hirsute women may convert testosterone to DHT at rates similar to those of normal males; normal women have one fourth this rate (Box 133-3).

ANDROGEN INSENSITIVITY AND ANDROGEN RECEPTOR DEFECTS. A rare condition that is usually suspected on physical examination is androgen insensitivity. This involves an androgen receptor defect that during fetal development causes a lack of development of male external genitalia despite the presence of normal testes and a 46,XY karyotype. Normal female genitalia are present, but the cervix and uterus are absent. Sexual hair is diminished or absent. There is a variant of this condition in which the enzyme is partially active, often increasing in activity at puberty. Activity levels can reach peak values in the range of those for normal males, and cause the patient of female phenotype and rearing to develop inappropriate hirsutism at adolescence. Treatment of this type of male pseudohermaphroditism includes gonadectomy because of the high risk of dysgerminoma and gonadoblastoma.

The role of nuclear androgen receptor levels in hirsutism is controversial. Eil et al[5] found no difference in receptor levels in normal women, hirsute women, and normal men regardless of plasma androgen levels or incubation with DHT. These researchers believe that androgen receptors are probably not induced directly by androgens. Schmidt, in a similar series of experiments, found a trend toward a greater percentage of hirsute women having androgen receptors present than patients with alopecia or acne, but did not measure actual receptor levels or include a control group of normal women. 5α-Reductase activity is probably more important than nuclear receptor levels.

BOX 133-2
Causes of Hirsutism

PERIPHERAL
Idiopathic
Partial androgen insensitivity (5α-reductase deficiency)
HAIR-AN syndrome (hirsutism, androgenization, insulin resistance, and acanthosis nigricans)
Hyperprolactinemia

GONADAL
Polycystic ovarian syndrome (PCO, chronic anovulation)
Ovarian neoplasm (Sertoli-Leydig cell, granulosa cell, thecoma, gynandroblastoma, lipoid cell, luteoma, hypernephroma, Brenner's tumor)
Gonadal dysgenesis (Turner mosaic with XY, or H-Y antigen positive)

ADRENAL
Cushing's syndrome
Adrenal hyperresponsiveness
Congenital adrenal hyperplasia (classic, cryptic, adult onset)
   21-hydroxylase deficiency
   11-hydroxylase deficiency
   3β-ol-dehydrogenase deficiency
   17-ol-dehydrogenase deficiency
Adrenal neoplasm (adenoma, cortical carcinoma)

EXOGENOUS
Minoxidil   Danazol
Dilantin   Acetazolamide sodium
Cyclosporine   Androgenic steroids
Anabolic steroids   Psoralens
Acetazolamide sodium   Diazide
Penicillamine   Phenothiazines
Oral contraceptives (progestin dominant)

CONGENITAL ANOMALIES
Trisomy 18 (Edwards' syndrome)
Cornelia de Lange's syndrome
Hurler's syndrome
Juvenile hypothyroidism

From Bailey-Pridham DD, Sanfilippo JS: Hirsutism in the adolescent female, *Pediatr Clin North Am* 36:581-599, 1989.

BOX 133-3
Clinical Evaluation of Hirsutism

Age of onset   Quantitative hair growth
Rapidity of onset   Other signs of virilization
Medications   Physical findings
Family traits

From Bailey-Pridham DD, Sanfilippo JS: Hirsutism in the adolescent female, *Pediatr Clin North Am* 36:581-599, 1989.

5-ALPHA REDUCTASE DEFICIENCY. Imperato-McGinley et al reported a series of patients in the Santa Domingo area of the Dominican Republic who developed a "penis at 12."[6] The disorder is autosomal recessive and especially common when there is consanguinity. This cohort of patients at the time of birth have normal-appearing female external genitalia but male internal reproductive organs. As puberty is reached, and hence the inability to convert testosterone to DHT, the result is virilization in association with testosterone-responsive tissues—thus, the presence of a male habitus, voice deepening, and clitoromegaly. These individuals are fertile males in that spermatogenesis occurs.

HAIR-AN syndrome is an association of hirsutism, androgen excess, insulin resistance, and acanthosis nigricans. The complete pathogenesis of the syndrome is unknown, but there appears to be a defect in membrane insulin receptors (as determined by binding studies on circulating monocytes). This process leads to a reactive hyperinsulinemia that may be the direct cause of the androgen excess. Studies using insulin infusions with glucose lock have shown that elevated insulin levels lead to a 25% to 35% increase in plasma androstenedione concentrations in normal patients. Elevated androgens may in turn contribute to the development of acanthosis; in one patient with bilateral androgen-producing ovarian tumors and acanthosis nigricans, the skin condition resolved after excision of the androgen source.

HAIR-AN syndrome affects 2% to 5% of hirsute women and is associated with insulin resistance and elevated insulin levels, as well as acanthosis nigricans and hyperandrogenemia. A number of medical therapies have been advocated, including GnRH agonist suppression. This mode of treatment results in suppression of free testosterone, an increase in SHBG, and subjective improvement with regard to hair growth.

Hyperprolactinemia

Hyperprolactinemia, although a central disorder, has been included here as it is an occasional cause of hyperandrogenemia not primarily of ovarian or adrenal origin. Approximately 40% of patients with hyperprolactinemia may exhibit androgen abnormalities. Laboratory findings in hyperprolactinemia are not uniform among patients and may include elevated free testosterone levels due to decreased SHBG, possibly altered function of 5α-reductase, and increased adrenal production of 17-OH-progesterone (17-OHP) and androstenedione after ACTH stimulation, with normal efficiency of adrenal enzymes. Many of these changes are normalized by dexamethasone suppression.

GONADAL FACTORS. Polycystic ovarian syndrome (PCO, Stein-Leventhal syndrome, chronic anovulation) is the most commonly diagnosed ovarian cause of hirsut-ism. Like patients with idiopathic hirsutism, many patients diagnosed with PCO may actually have other underlying defects not detected by routine baseline studies.[7] Dynamic testing may reveal other conditions such as adult-onset (late) CAH. The underlying biochemical cause of PCO is not known, and controversy exists over whether the basic defect is central (abnormal hypothalamic or pituitary regulation of gonadotropins) or ovarian (defect in a peptide hormone, perhaps inhibin, with resultant abnormal feedback to the pituitary). The usual hormonal pattern of PCO begins with altered LH release elevated total serum levels, an LH-to-FSH ratio of $\geq 2:1$, shortened pulse frequency, and slightly increased pulse amplitude. The result is abnormal development of ovarian follicles (increased rate of atresia, no dominant follicle, anovulation) and increased stromal androgen production. Increased androgens are converted peripherally by aromatase to estrone, causing a feedback effect on the pituitary-enhancing LH release, and completing the cycle.

It has been theorized that PCO occurs at the time of puberty.[7] Strong consideration of this entity should be provided in the hirsute adolescent who continues to have irregular menses beyond the first 18 months after menarche (it may take 18 months to establish normal ovulatory cycles). In adolescents, hyperandrogenic states for which an androgen-producing neoplasm has been ruled out are often best treated with oral contraceptives as well as medications such as spironolactone or cimetidine.

The clinical utility of low-dose oral contraceptives has been repeatedly demonstrated.[8] Hyperandrogenemia in association with acne, obesity, and hirsutism, especially when associated with PCO, shows improvement as the amount of free testosterone is decreased: that is, increasing SHBG with oral contraceptive therapy.

Other more recent medical treatments have included GnRH agonist as well as cyproterone acetate. In one study, 45 adolescents with PCO were randomly selected for either of two study groups, one of which was treated with ethinyl estradiol/cyproterone acetate and the other with a GnRH analog.[22] No significant changes were detected with regard to body mass index and waist/hip circumference. A significant improvement in the hirsutism was noted in both patient groups. Authors have concluded that either form of therapy appeared to be safe and effective in the management of PCO in adolescents.

Simultaneous ovarian and adrenal vein catheterization suggests that the androgen overproduction seen in PCO is indeed of ovarian origin, even though it may be suppressible with dexamethasone. Increased androgen levels are detectable in ovarian tissue from PCO patients. Although granulosa cells still produce mainly estradiol, testosterone levels in follicular fluid may be 30 to 200 times higher than in normal ovaries. In patients with PCO, thecal cells may produce two to six times the levels of androgens as normal thecal tissue, whereas the ovarian stroma may demonstrate a marked increase in testosterone production of 50 to 250 times normal.

Although the changes described above are typical of PCO patients, the final clinical presentation is variable. Mild obesity is common and oligomenorrhea is usually reported. Although serum testosterone and DHEA-S levels are often mildly elevated, they may be in the normal range and hirsutism may or may not be present. Peripheral factors contribute to this equation: SHBG tends to be suppressed in PCO patients with hirsutism, whereas SHBG levels are normal in patients with anovulation but "cryptic androgenemia." Additionally, 5α-reductase may be more active in PCO patients with hirsutism than in those without.

Ovarian hyperthecosis that can be familial may well be a variant of PCO. Hyperthecosis is defined as isolated islands of luteinized cells within the ovary contributing to increased androgen production. The ovarian androgen production and peripheral effect are similar to that in PCO.[9]

Ovarian neoplasms, although uncommon, do occur in the adolescent age group. These are most often germ cell tumors, but occasionally ovarian stromal tumors, usually steroid producing, are reported. These include granulosa-theca cell, Sertoli-Leydig cell (arrhenoblastoma, hilar cell), thecoma, luteoma, gynandroblastoma, lipoid cell, hypernephroma, and Brenner's cell tumors.[10] Patients may present with either primary or secondary amenorrhea, and usually (but not always) are more severely virilized (i.e., loss of breast tissue, frontal balding, clitoral enlargement, deepening voice) than are patients with benign causes of hirsutism.

Lastly, an ovarian source of hyperandrogenism may occur in patients with gonadal dysgenesis (Turner syndrome) who have some component of a Y chromosome present. This can include mosaics of 45,X/46,XY, 45,X/45,X, i(Yq), and 45,X with positive H-Y antigen.[11] In all these cases it is common to find some remnant of testicular tissue, which should be surgically excised.

Adrenal Factors

Hirsutism is a symptom in about 85% of cases of Cushing syndrome and may be the only presenting complaint. Signs and symptoms may resemble PCO, including obesity, amenorrhea, hirsutism, and mildly elevated androgens. The clinician should look for additional findings, including striae, moon facies, or abnormal adipose distribution ("buffalo hump") to suggest the diagnosis. Further laboratory testing can establish the diagnosis of Cushing's syndrome. Table 133-1 provides an orderly method of evaluating patients with Cushing syndrome. In Chapter 26, "Adrenocortical Disorders," Cushing syndrome is discussed further.

Studies of hirsute women undergoing ACTH stimulation testing have revealed an abnormal adrenal response in up to one half of the subjects. The condition in a number of patients was consistent with Cushing syndrome or variants of CAH; however, between one third and one half of the abnormal responders seemed to have a generalized hyperplasia of the zona reticularis (androgen-producing zone) with an "exaggerated adrenarche." At least one study has identified a familial occurrence of this exaggerated adrenarche and adrenocortical hyperresponsiveness. This condition does not seem to be the result of an enzyme deficiency, but rather may be either X-linked dominant or autosomal in its inheritance pattern.

Late-onset CAH also may masquerade as PCO. Several possible enzyme defects can occur; the one most commonly recognized is 21-hydroxylase deficiency. The block in this deficiency occurs on the cortisol arm of the steroid pathway, causing excessive precursor just before the block, in this case 17-OHP (Fig. 133-1). This can occur in the classic juvenile form, cryptic form, and adult-onset form. The full clinical features of each condition are seen with homozygosity for its specific allele. Patients also may be heterozygous for any allele, with variable expression. Estimates of the incidence of this defect in hirsute women vary from 6% to 33%.[12,13]

TABLE 133-1
Evaluation for Cushing's Syndrome or Disease

	Cushing's Disease	Adrenal Hyperplasia	Adrenal Neoplasm	ACTH-Producing Neoplasm
Serum ACTH	Sl Elevated	Normal	Low	High
Dexamethasone suppression test				
Low dose	NS	NS	NS	NS
High dose	S	S	NS	NS

From Bailey-Pridham DD, Sanfilippo JS: Hirsutism in the adolescent female, *Pediatr Clin North Am* 36:581-599, 1989.
ACTH, adrenocorticotropic hormone; *NS,* no suppression; *S,* suppression.
Low dose = 0.5 mg PO every 6 hr for 4 days.
High dose = 2.0 mg PO every 6 hr for 4 days.

Some reports of this condition may overestimate its prevalence if testing for 11-hydroxylase deficiency (which also produces elevated 17-OHP with ACTH stimulation testing) is not performed. Patients with adult-onset (late) CAH may have normal baseline androgen, cortisol, and 17-OHP levels, and only with provocative testing reveal the true picture. The overall incidence in the population is small (0.3% in the general population, 3% in Jews of European ancestry), but the suggested incidence in hirsute females may make screening in specific populations worthwhile. Association with HLA antigens B14 and Aw33 has been noted. Of patients with known adult-onset 21-hydroxylase deficiency, about 40% present with a PCO pattern, 40% with hirsutism alone, and 20% with anovulation and cryptic (nonhirsute) hyperandrogenemia.

Determination of levels of 11-deoxycortisol, cortisol, and 17-OHP during an ACTH stimulation test can identify an 11-hydroxylase deficiency. In one series of eight hirsute women, a partial block of this enzyme was found in all eight. This may suggest either that 11-hydroxylase deficiency is a common defect in hirsute women, or perhaps that the efficiency of this enzyme is altered by elevated androgen levels.

Several authors have reported 3β-ol-dehydrogenase deficiency as a cause of late-onset (adolescent) adrenal hyperplasia. In several incidence studies among hirsute women, the defect was identified in 14% to 60% of patients, all of whom demonstrated elevated 17-OHP and DHEA after following ACTH stimulation. This may be an important causal factor in patients previously classified as having PCO or idiopathic hirsutism.

Another very rare enzyme deficiency is lack of 17β-ol-dehydrogenase, noted in a familial cohort. This is the enzyme that converts androstenedione to testosterone, and it seems to be regulated by LH rather than by ACTH. The deficiency results in high levels of androstenedione.

The occurrence of adrenal adenomas or adrenocortical carcinomas in adolescents is rare. Several case reports with associated hirsutism have appeared in the literature.[14,15] Virtually all patients complained of hirsutism and/or virilization.

Exogenous Factors

Several medications are associated with hirsutism, including minoxidil, phenytoin, cyclosporine, androgenic and anabolic steroids, danazol, progestin dominant oral contraceptives, acetazolamide sodium, diazide, phenothiazines, penicillamine, and psoralens. Radiation and chronic irritation such as placement of a cast can initiate localized, nonendocrinologic hair growth. A careful history taking should eliminate any possible exogenous cause of hirsutism.

CONGENITAL FACTORS. Several congenital anomalies, such as trisomy 18 (Edwards' syndrome), Cornelia de Lange's syndrome, Hurler's syndrome, and juvenile hypothyroidism are associated with hirsutism.

EVALUATION OF THE HIRSUTE PATIENT

The objectives are to determine the primary source(s) of androgens for excessive hormone output and further discern whether it is due to a state of hyperplasia or neoplasm. The history and physical examination are of tremendous importance and are highlighted in Box 133-3.

Distinction between hirsutism and virilization must be established. The latter involves frontal balding, increased muscle mass, loss of normal female fat deposits (hips and breasts), deepening of the voice, clitoromegaly, and increased libido. It is important to determine the extent of hair growth whether the patient primarily has a problem with hirsutism or with virilization. The classification system of Ferriman and Gallwey has been designed to facilitate evaluation and documentation of hirsutism.[14]

In pursuing the evaluation of the hirsute or virilized patient, the objective remains to determine the underlying cause of the increased androgen production. In addition to androgen-producing tumors, entities such as Cushing syndrome or disease, as well as CAH that may be of adult onset, should be considered. Laboratory diagnosis in the hirsute patient is outlined in Table 133-2. It has been advocated that in the hirsute patient a morning fasting serum 17-OHP level should be determined. This in essence serves as a screening for adult-onset CAH. Elevation of 17-OHP, either as a baseline level or with ACTH stimulation, is indicative of a heterozygous state of 21-hydroxylase deficiency. Specifically, 17-hydroxyprogesterone is the precursor of 11-deoxycortisol in that 21-hydroxylase is responsible for this conversion. Thus, if a patient presents with any form of 21-hydroxylase deficiency (e.g., adrenal hyperplasia), the appropriate diagnosis should be established.

Ideally, in hirsute or virilized patients the serum level of total testosterone should be tested, which will reflect ovarian as well as adrenal androgen production and DHEA-S sulfate, primarily representing an adrenal origin, as well as 17-OHP levels, the latter in a morning sample or one obtained after ACTH stimulation.

Determination of free testosterone levels has little clinical role and tends to be more expensive than total testosterone testing; therefore, this test is not advocated, especially for screening purposes. Entities such as Cushing syndrome can initially be ruled out with the overnight dexamethasone suppression test, which involves administration of 1 mg dexamethasone, ideally at

TABLE 133-2
Laboratory Diagnosis in Hirsutism

Initial Evaluation	Normal Levels	Tumor Range
Total testosterone	<1.1 ng/ml	>1.5 ng/ml
DHEA-S	<430 µg/dl	>700 µg/dl
Prolactin	<25 ng/ml	>100 ng/ml
Consider:		
FSH and LH		
Elevated in PCO (LH > FSH)		
ACTH stimulation test		
Pre- and post-17-OH-progesterone, cortisol, and DHEA-S		
Overnight dexamethasone suppression test		
1 mg at bedtime*		
Further evaluations		
If overnight dexamethasone suppression test is >5 µg/dl, proceed to high-dose suppression test (4 days, 2 mg q6h, measure urinary free cortisol and creatinine levels in 24-hr collections)		
If ovarian or adrenal tumor suspected, obtain abdominal CT or MRI		

Modified from Bailey-Pridham DD, Sanfilippo JS: Hirsutism in the adolescent female, *Pediatr Clin North Am* 36:581-599, 1989.
*False-positive with obesity or depression.
DHEA-S, dehydroepiandrosterone sulfate; *FSH,* follicle-stimulating hormone; *LH,* luteinizing hormone; *PCO,* polycystic ovarian syndrome; *CT,* computed tomography; *MRI,* magnetic resonance imaging.

11 P.M., followed the next morning by determination of the serum cortisol level. In a patient who is negative for Cushing, the levels are less than 5 to 7 µg/dl. A false-positive result can occur with obesity for which higher doses of dexamethasone (2 mg) appear to be adequate, or with depression. If there is an abnormal response to the overnight dexamethasone suppression test, a more elaborate dexamethasone suppression assessment is indicated. Low-dose dexamethasone suppression requires administration of 0.5 mg orally every 4 to 6 hours for 4 days; high-dose suppression requires 2 mg orally every 6 hours, also administered for 4 days. Determination of urinary levels of 17-hydroxyprogesterone as well as the creatinine level provide the end point for assessment. If there is suppression with high-dose dexamethasone, Cushing disease, with resultant adrenal hyperplasia, must be strongly considered.

Serum ACTH levels that prove to be slightly elevated are also indicative of Cushing disease, whereas if the level is markedly elevated it is primarily indicative of an ACTH-producing neoplasm such as an oat cell carcinoma.

Abdominal computed tomography (CT) or magnetic resonance imaging (MRI) now have resolutions of under 5 mm, allowing accurate detection of adrenal tumors. Selective retrograde venous catheterization has been used to determine differential effluent peripheral vein androgen gradients.[15] Steroid-producing ovarian neoplasms may be quite small, and a normal pelvic ultrasound examination does not exclude a neoplasm. Exploratory surgery is indicated if androgen levels or rapid onset of virilization suggest an ovarian neoplasm.

It is possible to perform measurements of many other androgens along with their precursors and metabolites in both basal and dynamic testing. SHBG can be estimated or measured directly. Apart from its academic interest, however, the practical use of such testing is limited. Regardless of pathogenesis, the treatment of hirsutism follows one of several approaches (Table 133-3) once the possibility of serious disease is excluded.

TREATMENT

As mentioned previously, management of the patient with hirsutism must address the underlying cause. In addition, the psychologic sequelae associated with hirsutism must be considered. Careful documentation and treatment of the degree of hirsutism are important in the evaluation phase of patient management. The patient must be counseled regarding the goal of treatment, which is *prevention* of new hair growth; little relief is to be offered for manifestations of hirsutism already present, short of electrolysis.

Treatment alternatives for idiopathic hirsutism and PCO are outlined in Table 133-3. If an oral contraceptive is prescribed, an estrogen-dominant pill such as one containing ethynodiol, desogestrel, or norethindrone as the progestin is preferable.

Hirsutism secondary to hyperprolactinemia is best treated with bromocriptine. The initial dosage is 2.5 mg daily for 1 week followed by 2.5 mg twice daily. The more common side effects include nausea, orthostatic hypotension, and fatigue. Bromocriptine should not be

TABLE 133-3
Treatment of Hirsutism: Idiopathic and Polycystic Ovarian Syndrome

Medication	Dosage*	Comments
Oral contraceptives (estrogen dominant)	35 µg	Decrease in plasma testosterone, androstenedione, and DHEA-S
Spironolactone	100 mg bid	Decreased androgen production and androgen receptor competition
Medroxyprogesterone acetate (Depo-Provera)	150-250 mg q 2-4 wk	Decreased testosterone production and 17-ketosteroid levels
Cyproterone acetate	Diane, 2 mg Androcur, 100 mg	Decreased plasma testosterone, androstenedione, SHBG, induces "insulinemia"
Dexamethasone	0.25-0.5 mg	Dose adequate if plasma free testosterone <15 pg/ml
Cimetidine	200-300 mg tid-qid	Decreased serum testosterone, increased serum estradiol
GnRH agonist	1000 µg	Decreased testosterone and androstenedione
Finasteride	5 mg	5α-reductase inhibitor

Modified from Bailey-Pridham DD, Sanfilippo JS: Hirsutism in the adolescent female, *Pediatr Clin North Am* 36:581-599, 1989.
*Dosage for 70-kg female; daily dosage unless otherwise specified.
DHEA-S, dehydroepiandrosterone acetate; *SHBG,* sex hormone–binding globulin.

used in patients under 15 years of age. A follow-up serum prolactin level should be obtained 6 weeks after initiation of therapy.

Cushing disease, by definition, is due to a pituitary tumor secreting excess ACTH. Treatment is primarily surgical, involving excision or radiation therapy. Cushing's syndrome requires determination of the pathogenesis. Treatment of a neoplasm is surgical, whereas adrenal hyperplasia is best treated with exogenous glucocorticoid suppression such as with prednisone. In treating the exogenous causes of hirsutism, it is necessary to eliminate the implicated medication. This approach usually results in elimination of further hirsutism.

References

1. Speroff L, Glass RH, Kase NG: *Clinical gynecologic endocrinology and infertility,* ed 4, Baltimore, 1994, Williams & Wilkins.
2. Grumbach MM, Richards HE, Conte FA, et al: Clinical disorders of adrenal function and puberty: an assessment of the role of the adrenal cortex in normal and abnormal puberty in man and evidence for an ACTH-like pituitary adrenal androgen stimulating hormone. In Serio M, editor: *The endocrine function of the human adrenal cortex (Serono Symposium),* New York, 1977, Academic Press.
3. Reingold S, Rosenfield R: The relationship of mild hirsutism or acne to androgens, *Arch Dermatol* 123:209-212, 1987.
4. Kirschner MA, Samojlik E, Szmal E: Clinical usefulness of plasma androstanediol glucuronide measurements in women with idiopathic hirsutism, *J Clin Endocrinol Metab* 65:597-601, 1987.
5. Eil C, Cutler GB Jr, Loriaux DL: Androgen receptor characteristics in skin fibroblasts from hirsute women, *J Invest Dermatol* 84:62-65, 1985.
6. Imperato-McGinley J, Peterson RE, Sturla E, et al: Primary amenorrhea associated with hirsutism, acanthosis nigricans, dermoid cysts of the ovaries and a new type of insulin resistance, *Am J Med* 65:389-395, 1978.
7. Rosenfield RL, Luckay AW: Acne, hirsutism and alopecia in adolescent girls: clinical expressions of androgen excess, *Endocrinol Metab Clin North Am* 22:507-532, 1993.
8. Mamamoto T, Okata H: Clinical usefulness of low-dose oral contraceptives for the treatment of adolescent hyperandrogenemia, *Asia Oceania J Obstet Gynaecol* 20:225-230, 1994.
9. Aiman J, Edman CD, Worley RJ, et al: Androgen and estrogen formation in women with ovarian hyperthecosis, *Obstet Gynecol* 51:1-9, 1978.
10. Greenblatt RB, Mahesh VB, Gambrell RD: Arrhenoblastoma: three case reports, *Obstet Gynecol* 39:567-576, 1972.
11. Rosen GF, Kaplan B, Lobo RA: Menstrual function and hirsutism in patients with gonadal dysgenesis, *Obstet Gynecol* 71:677-680, 1988.
12. Emans SJ, Grace E, Fleischnick E, et al: Detection of late-onset 21-hydroxylase deficiency congenital adrenal hyperplasia in adolescents, *Pediatrics* 72:690-695, 1983.
13. Lobo RA, Goebelsmann U: Adult manifestation of congenital adrenal hyperplasia due to incomplete 21-hydroxylase deficiency mimicking polycystic ovarian disease, *Am J Obstet Gynecol* 138:720-726, 1980.
14. Ferriman D, Gallwey JD: Clinical assessment of body hair growth in women, *J Clin Endocrinol Metab* 21:1440, 1961.
15. Surrey ES, deZiegler D, Gambone JC, et al: Preoperative localization of androgen-secreting tumors: clinical, endocrinologic, and radiologic evaluation of ten patients, *Am J Obstet Gynecol* 158:1313-1322, 1988.

CHAPTER 134

Breast Disorders

•

Reuben D. Rohn

During adolescence, breast examination should be a routine part of the physical examination for both boys and girls. In girls, it is often not done because of concern about causing the patient undue anxiety or in deference to the patient's sense of modesty.[1] It even has been argued that breast examination is not cost effective and therefore should not be performed routinely.

Since adolescents are usually highly concerned about their body image, even slight deviations from what they consider normal may cause them significant anxiety. Therefore, the physician caring for adolescent patients should use the breast examination as an opportunity to desensitize and educate these patients and thus to allay their fears.

BREAST EXAMINATION

Breast examination should be undertaken at thelarche, or the beginning of breast development, which usually occurs between ages 8 and 12 years. Since in today's society considerable emphasis is given to women's breasts, girls may have undue anxiety about the size and shape of their breasts as pubertal changes occur. Breast examination offers a good opportunity to inform the adolescent about the wide variation in timing of breast development and to reassure her that differences in breast size and shape are quite normal.

By the time the girl has reached Tanner stage 5 in physical development and shows appropriate emotional maturity (approximately age 16), it is recommended that she learn breast self-examination. At least one study has indicated that this is a useful technique.[2] A contrary opinion is that breast self-examination is either inadequate in identifying lesions or raises too much anxiety in a young girl in view of the fact that cancer in adolescence is extremely rare.[1] However, the major purpose of teaching breast self-examination is to establish the habit and to demystify this part of the female anatomy. Any anxiety on the part of the patient can be reduced by reassuring her that if any lumps are detected, it is highly unlikely that they will be cancerous.[2] The physician should emphasize to the patient that the importance of self-examination lies in the habituation and increased familiarity with her own body.

Girls who manifest breast development before age 8 years have either premature thelarche, which is isolated breast development without increased secretion of luteinizing hormone, follicle-stimulating hormone, and estrogen, or true precocious puberty, which is the onset of hypothalamic-pituitary-ovarian axis function with increased secretion of these hormones. Girls whose breast development is delayed beyond the age of 12 years should be evaluated for the possibility of endocrinopathies, genetic disorders such as Turner's syndrome or gonadal dysgenesis, systemic illness, or eating disorder.

As described by Reynolds and Wine[3] and by Tanner,[4] breast development proceeds through five distinct stages: stage 1, no development; stage 2, breast bud with tissue under the areola only; stage 3, breast mound with tissue growth well beyond the areolar border; stage 4, double mound with an areolar hump above the breast mound; and stage 5, adult with only the fully developed nipple protruding above the breast mound.

A tape measure should be used for each breast. Such measurements are made to assess breast asymmetry or to determine possible breast overgrowth.[5] Since a high degree of ambiguity exists in the last two stages of breast development, nipple measurement becomes useful in distinguishing between these two stages (Table 134-1). Breast size and areola size are strongly dependent on genetic factors. Nipple size is distinctly a function of the physiologic and hormonal changes that accompany puberty.[6]

Unusual but normal variations in the breasts may be identified during the examination. Occasionally an extension of breast tissue, known as the tail of Spence, may occur at the lateral border of the pectoralis major muscle through the axillary fascia and into the axilla. This extension may enlarge in conjunction with the hormonal changes of puberty or pregnancy, but it usually regresses spontaneously. There are glands located on the areola,

TABLE 134-1
Nipple Diameter in Relation to Tanner Breast Stage

Stage	Diameter (mm)
1	2.9 (0.8)*
2	3.3 (0.9)
3	4.1 (1.4)
4	7.7 (1.5)
5	9.9 (1.4)

From Rohn RO: Nipple (papilla) development in puberty: longitudinal observations in girls, *J Pediatr* 79:745-777, 1987.
*Numbers in parentheses show ± standard deviation.

called the glands of Montgomery, that may secrete a discharge.[7] This discharge, which is normal and does not emanate from the nipple, is opalescent or brown in color. However, such a discharge needs to be distinguished from that of galactorrhea, which is usually white, originates from the nipple, and can be pathologic. Some females, usually those of Mediterranean or Latin descent, may have a variable amount of areolar hair. These patients should be advised not to pluck the hairs, since infection or abscess may result. Excessive friction caused by wearing a bra that does not fit properly, or not wearing any bra during physical exercise, can lead to a condition known as "jogger's nipples."[8] Although this condition consists of scaling that might be confused with Paget's disease, it is truly benign. Chafing to the point of bleeding also may occur. Adequate bra support and the use of a lubricant such as lanolin can help to resolve this problem.

When breast development occurs very rapidly, stretch marks may result. They can also occur in association with rapid weight gain or pregnancy. The possibility of virginal breast hypertrophy may need to be determined. Initially, stretch marks may be disconcerting to the adolescent because of their reddish coloration and prominence. Although these marks will never disappear completely, the adolescent should be reassured that they will fade and become much less apparent, a process that may take 2 to 3 years.

Breast asymmetry is an annoying but usually benign condition. Careful measurement of breasts in girls and women almost always indicates that one breast is somewhat larger than the other. In general, this size difference is minor and does not cause concern,[3] but a considerable difference in size of breasts sometimes occurs. Occasionally, the asymmetry is merely an indication of the dissociation in pubertal growth of the two breasts. Breast measurement is often necessary in adolescents who have scoliosis, since a diagnosis of breast asymmetry may be made mistakenly. No treatment is indicated unless the discrepancy between the size of the breasts is substantial. If treatment is necessary, it should not be started until breast development has been com-

pleted. The most accurate indicator of adult development is nipple size. Although the breasts may be asymmetric in size, both nipples usually measure more than 9 mm when adult development has been reached (Table 134-1). One breast may show less volume growth than the other for as long as 6 months to 1 year.

CONGENITAL ANOMALIES

Polythelia, or the presence of supernumerary nipples, is quite common in both sexes. The extra nipples may occur anywhere along the embryonic milk line, from the axilla to the groin. This anomaly has been noted in up to 5% of the population. The only significance of supernumerary nipples is their reported association with abnormalities of the cardiovascular or urologic system.[9] Polymastia, or the presence of supernumerary breasts, occurs much less frequently and is rarely associated with any problems (except for cosmetic ones). Aplasia of the breasts, or amastia, is very rare and may be hereditary. The absence of a nipple, athelia, usually is associated with amastia, but this condition also may occur alone. Most commonly, amastia is seen in Poland's anomalad, which is characterized by absence of the pectoralis muscle, upper limb defects, and rib deformities[10] (Fig. 134-1).

Another cause of amastia is inadvertent surgical removal of a breast bud—in asymmetric thelarche—that was thought to have been a breast tumor. Hypoplasia of the breast usually results from delayed puberty or slow breast development in an otherwise normal female. Breast hypoplasia associated with primary amenorrhea may indicate endocrinopathy, gonadal dysgenesis, systemic illness, or an eating disorder. With this condition, nipple development will be minimal. Breast hypoplasia in females who have normal adult nipple development and normal menses is presumed to result from end-organ breast tissue that is not responsive to hormones. In our breast-oriented culture, psychologic problems associated with small breast size are often encountered. In some instances, the wearing of a padded bra may suffice to solve the problem; in others, breast augmentation may be necessary.

Inverted nipples are a fairly common finding in females and are usually only a cosmetic concern. Adolescents can be taught to use traction exercises to draw out the nipple. The only clinical significance of this condition is the fact that an inverted nipple may cause problems with suckling. In addition, it is important that an inverted nipple be distinguished from a depressed nipple, in which nipple tissue is absent. With a depressed nipple, the lactiferous ducts open directly into an area that forms a depression in the center of the areola, which can make suckling impossible.[9]

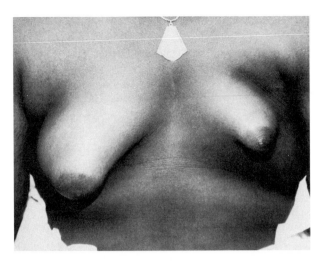

Fig. 134-1. Amastia associated with Poland's anomalad in a 14-year-old obese girl. Note the nipple development.

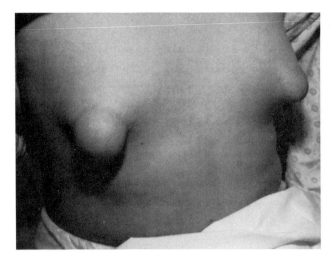

Fig. 134-2. Tuberous breast anomaly in a 13-year-old girl.

The massive overgrowth of the breast (hyperplasia) that occurs during puberty or adolescence is termed *virginal breast hypertrophy.* The word *virginal* frequently is used to distinguish this type of overgrowth from that which sometimes occurs during pregnancy. *Macromastia* and *gigantomastia* are alternative terms for this condition. Breast overgrowth can be unilateral and usually commences shortly after thelarche. Although the cause is unknown, it is possible that this condition may result from oversensitivity of the breast to estrogen.[11] Some cases have been linked to the use of oral contraceptives; others seem to have a familial association. The major clinical problem is psychologic because of the disproportionately large breast size. However, associated physical complaints, including breast, neck, or back pain and poor posture, may occur with extreme breast growth. When unilateral breast enlargement occurs, the possibility of a giant fibroadenoma must be considered. The histologic appearance of virginal breast hypertrophy is that of an exaggeration of normal breast structure. Although medications have been used in an attempt to suppress the breast growth (e.g., danazol, medroxyprogesterone, dydrogesterone), reduction mammoplasty is often necessary either for treatment of the physical condition or for alleviation of the associated psychologic difficulties. It is advisable to postpone this surgery until maximal growth has been attained. A surgical procedure that is performed prematurely may be unsatisfactory, since regrowth of breast tissue may occur later.

Another unusual anomaly is breast tuberosity. Tuberous breasts are typified by limited horizontal and vertical dimensions; forward projection of tissue growth; and often a highly overdeveloped, large nipple-areola complex (Fig. 134-2). The appearance of the breast may mimic an exaggeration of the double-mound stage of breast development (Tanner stage 5), but with the areola complex almost overwhelming the base mound. Surgical correction is usually necessary for treatment of this condition.

Atrophy of the breasts may occur during adolescence in females who undergo severe weight loss resulting from chronic illness, anorexia nervosa, or severe dieting. The breasts take on a senile appearance, becoming flattened, wrinkled, and ptotic. Improvement in diet, especially increased protein consumption, may restore the breasts to a more normal appearance.

MASSES

In the adolescent age group, fibroadenoma is by far the most common breast mass, accounting for 50% to 95% of breast tumors.[12,13] Fibroadenomas are more common in the black population. Peak incidence occurs in late adolescence (17 to 20 years of age). Commonly asymptomatic, fibroadenomas are usually rubbery, hard, nontender, freely mobile, and clearly demarcated from the rest of the breast tissue. Oval or irregular in shape, they may enlarge slowly over weeks or months. Although fibroadenomas are typically unilateral, in 25% of patients they are bilateral or multiple (fibroadenomatosis). Some evidence indicates that these tumors may be sensitive to estrogen.[14] They often increase in size during pregnancy.[9] Most fibroadenomas (approximately 60%) are found in the upper outer quadrant. Their histologic appearance is similar to that of virginal breast hypertrophy or male gynecomastia. Large lesions may be associated with erythema or dilated veins overlying the lesions or even peau d'orange (skin dimpling that resembles that of an orange). Differential diagnosis includes other causes of breast masses (Box 134-1).

Because carcinoma of the breast is exceedingly rare, and since up to one fourth of fibroadenomas may regress

---

BOX 134-1
Causes of Breast Masses

COMMON
Virginal breast hypertrophy
Fibroadenoma (and juvenile fibroadenoma)
Cystosarcoma phylloides
Intraductal papilloma
Cysts (various etiologies)
Trauma (contusion, hematoma, fat necrosis)
Abscess
Lipoma

LESS COMMON
Breast cancer
Ductal adenocarcinoma
Angiosarcoma
Dermatofibromatosis
Granular cell myoblastoma
Hemangioma
Hemangioendothelioma
Interstitial fibrosis
Intraductal granuloma
Keratoma of the nipple
Liposarcoma
Lymphangioma
Mammary duct ectasia
Metastatic disease
Nipple adenoma
Neurofibromatosis
Papilloma sarcoidosis
Papillomatosis
Sclerosing adenosis
Tuberous mastitis

---

with time, observation for 2 to 4 months is suggested. Some physicians may even choose to observe these tumors for as long as 6 months. However, anxiety on the part of the patient or family may lead to a request for excisional biopsy. Fine-needle aspiration (FNA) may provide an excellent means to diagnose the nature of such a lesion. While most FNA studies have been performed in adults, the sensitivity, specificity, and predictive proficiency of this procedure has been validated in a meta-analysis of several thousand women.[15] Two 1994 studies investigated the long-term risk of breast cancer in women who had fibroadenoma. It was concluded that there is a small but statistically significant risk of approximately twice that of the control group[16] or a cumulative risk of 2.2% 12 years after the diagnosis of fibroadenoma.[17] Both studies were performed in adults and thus it is difficult to extrapolate a risk in adolescents. Ultimately, the decision whether to excise such a lesion that persists for longer than 6 months rests upon the adolescent and her family's wishes once they are provided with appropriate information. FNA has its limitations. Some studies imply that in some cases it is

very difficult to distinguish between benign and cancerous lesions.[18]

New techniques may further help in the decision-making process regarding excision of fibroadenomas. One study detected chromosomal abnormalities in three of 25 fibroadenoma specimens analyzed. These anomalies may herald an increased risk of cancer.[19] Future research may define the clinical effectiveness of such techniques.[20] If a fibroadenoma is excessively large, it may need to be removed before growth leads to a more difficult cosmetic surgical procedure. In 5% to 10% of patients, rapid growth of a fibroadenoma may lead to remarkable tumor size. Such lesions, referred to as giant juvenile fibroadenomas, have been known to double in size in a span of 3 to 6 months. A typical giant fibroadenoma has a less well defined edge than a smaller fibroadenoma and is often softer in consistency.[14] Breast distortion and superficial venous distention are common. The presence of fibroadenomas may be confused with unilateral virginal breast hypertrophy or with cystosarcoma phylloides. Because of their size and rapid growth, excision of giant fibroadenomas is usually necessary.

Cystosarcoma phylloides is a tumor that is closely related to fibroadenoma. It is distinguishable from the latter only by its histologic appearance, which shows a greater degree of stromal cellularity that is most pronounced adjacent to the ducts.

Fibroadenoma and cystosarcoma are distinguishable by means of polymerase chain reaction and DNA sampling techniques. Fibroadenomas are polyclonal for both the epithelial and stromal cellular components. Cystosarcomas are polyclonal for the epithelial components but monoclonal for the stromal components. Fibroadenoma is hyperplastic in nature and not a neoplasm, while cystosarcoma is a neoplastic lesion.[21] Cystosarcoma is a much rarer tumor in adolescents; it accounts for only about 2% of lesions reported in the pediatric literature and is the type most frequently disposed to malignancy. Cystosarcoma is usually a slow-growing tumor that is often large at the time of discovery, has a firm consistency on palpation, and has a discrete mass to its borders.[14] When the lesion is large, the overlying skin may be stretched and shiny, with distended veins. Skin ulcers, overlying erythema, parenchymal necrosis, nipple retraction, and even bloody nipple discharge may be present. Enlargement of axillary lymph nodes is reported in up to 20% of patients. When axillary enlargement does occur, it is usually secondary to necrosis and infection rather than to metastases. Nipple discharge does not imply malignancy. The diagnosis is dependent on excisional biopsy.[9]

Intraductal breast papilloma is a very rare and usually benign tumor in adolescence. It is most often detected as a small subareolar lesion that produces a brownish or bloody discharge from the nipple. Diagnosis is aided by cytologic examination of nipple discharge, ultrasound examination, or FNA.[12] Local excision is curative. Additional rare tumors are listed in Box 134-1.

In adolescents, cysts of the breast are relatively uncommon.[13,22] Solitary cysts may be filled with different fluidlike materials of varying color. The cause of these cysts is unknown. They are often confused with, and may be difficult to distinguish from, fibroadenomas. Cysts may follow fat necrosis due to trauma, or they may be associated with ductal ectasia; however, they are not part of the controversial "fibrocystic breast disease." Ultrasound examination may be used to distinguish a cyst from a solid mass. Observation over several menstrual cycles may help to distinguish a cyst from other lesions, since a cyst frequently may change in size according to the time of the cycle. For treatment of large persistent cysts, some physicians advocate FNA. Others prefer excisional biopsy, especially if the fluid is bloody or if the cyst recurs.[23]

Two populations of gross breast cysts occur: apocrine and attenuated. Apocrine cysts tend to be bilateral, multiple, and prone to recurrence. They are lined by full columnar epithelial cells. Biochemical analysis indicates that they have Na:K ratios of less than 3:1, and they have high levels of apocrine protein, epidermal growth factors, dehydroisoandrosterone, and 11S secretory IgA. Attenuated cysts are lined by flattened epithelial cells and contain a Na:K ratio of greater than 3:1, plus albumin, low levels of apocrine protein, and secretory 7S immunoglobulin.[24] In another study, those cysts containing a low Na:K ratio tended to accumulate large amounts of other steroids, including DHEA-sulfate, estrone-sulfate, androstane-3α, 17β-diol glucuronide, androsterone glucuronide, testosterone, and dihydrotestosterone. Women with apocrine cysts have a greater cancer risk than women with attenuated cysts or women without cysts.[25]

The consistency of adolescent breast tissue is often quite nodular. Cyclic swelling and tenderness and even overt breast pain (mastalgia or mastodynia) are common. During different phases of the menstrual cycle and throughout the aging process, physiologic changes occur that affect the texture of the breasts. Breast pain may be associated with the menstrual cycle, but it sometimes may occur noncyclically. The term "fibrocystic breast disease," often used to describe textural changes and associated breast pain, is now being abandoned.[9,26] It is important that breast pain be differentiated from cervical root disease, other referred pain, and osteochondritis (Tietze's syndrome).

Mild analgesics and good bra support can be used to alleviate breast pain. The use of vitamin E and the restriction of methylxanthines, dairy products, and chocolate are unproved strategies in the treatment of breast tenderness or pain. Sometimes a direct association

between breast pain and certain drugs (e.g., reserpine, phenothiazines, exogenous hormones) is noted. If this can be determined, the offending medication should be removed. Diuretics may be useful if excessive pain and swelling are part of a general premenstrual syndrome.

Breast cancer is exceedingly rare among adolescents. Fewer than 100 cases have been reported in the past 100 years.[12,14,27] Breast cancer may be detected as a hard, nontender, indurated, solitary mass with indistinct margins. This mass may be fixed to the chest wall or breast tissue. Associated conditions may include skin or nipple retraction, skin edema (peau d'orange), nipple discharge, Paget's disease, and lymphadenopathy. Since malignant breast disease is so rare in adolescents, the general approach to breast masses is conservative. If there is any doubt about the nature of the mass after physical examination has been performed, frequent reexamination, especially during different phases of the menstrual cycle, may help to clarify the diagnosis. Masses that remain significantly unchanged or significantly enlarged over three or four cycles may be excised for further histologic examination.

Trauma to the breast may lead to the development of breast masses. Contusion may result in a firm, tender, and poorly defined mass. Hematomas, which are more sharply defined and tender, usually are found in association with ecchymosis of the skin. Resolution of the hematoma may be hastened by the use of ice or cold compresses on the first day, with warm pads and compression applied for several days subsequently. Complete resolution of the trauma may take several months, and a small mass of scar tissue often remains. Fat necrosis sometimes follows trauma and may present as a distinct, painless mass that is quite firm but well circumscribed and mobile. Since the mass is usually not noticed until several months after the injury, it may be somewhat difficult to differentiate it from other breast masses. Excisional biopsy is often necessary because a history of trauma is either vague or absent.[27]

INFECTIONS

Mastitis may occur in the adolescent. Lactational mastitis occurs in about 2% of women, usually post partum but occasionally pre partum. Obstruction of milk ducts due to plugging plus mild stasis leads to secondary infection. Mastitis is characterized by sudden swelling, erythema, warmth, and tenderness. Occasionally, the mass may be fluctuant. Trauma to the areola-nipple complex or duct ectasia may predispose to infection. Although *Staphylococcus aureus* and streptococci are the most frequent organisms found, other bacteria may be the etiologic agents.[9] Initial treatment consists of soaks and antibiotics, but incision and drainage are indicated if the mass is fluctuant. Manually stripping pus from the infected breast of women with lactational mastitis is effective in preventing breast abscess formation.[28] Since significant damage to the breast may occur, early and aggressive treatment is encouraged.

Nonlactational mastitis may follow trauma, duct ectasia, epidermal cysts, or superficial skin infections. Treatment is the same as for lactational mastitis. Differential diagnosis includes Mondor's disease (superficial phlebitis); mammary duct ectasia, a rare entity that is seen more often in menopausal women and is associated with nipple discharge; trauma; and carcinoma.[9]

GYNECOMASTIA

Gynecomastia is defined as any visible or palpable development of breast tissue in males.[29] The tissue may be as small as 1 cm and disk-like in form, or as large as that of a normal woman's breast (Fig. 134-3). For gynecomastia to become noticeable, the breast must reach a size of greater than 2 cm. Many clinicians divide gynecomastia into two broad types characterized by tissue less than 3 to 4 cm (type I) and tissue greater than 3 to 4 cm (type II).[30] The former is referred to as pubertal gynecomastia and the latter as pubertal macromastia.

Type I gynecomastia is common, with an incidence of 60% to 70%.[31] It is characterized as transient and correlates best with Tanner stages 3 and 4 of genital development. This type of gynecomastia is characterized by a small, disk-like subareola mass, which is often quite tender. Characteristically, the mass resolves spontaneously within several months to 2 years. In one study, more than two thirds of the type I masses resolved within 2 years, and more than 90% resolved within 3 years.[32] Many male adolescents complain of discomfort during various activities or because of rubbing of the nipple against clothing. Extreme discomfort can be treated with mild analgesics or with cold compresses applied to the breast. Rarely, nipple discharge may occur as a result of attempts to reduce the gynecomastia by massage. This discharge needs to be distinguished from galactorrhea.[33]

Macromastia, or type II gynecomastia, which occurs much less frequently (4.5% estimated incidence), may be much more distressing. The degree of breast development sometimes becomes extreme, with a configuration not unlike that of Tanner stage 3 (or greater) female breast development. Although most cases of macromastia are idiopathic, a careful history should be obtained to rule out other causes, including medications and drugs, endocrinopathies and tumors, systemic infections, or (occasionally) familial tendency (Box 134-2). Careful physical examination is important and should include measurement not only of breast size, but also of the patient's height, weight, blood pressure, and sexual maturity

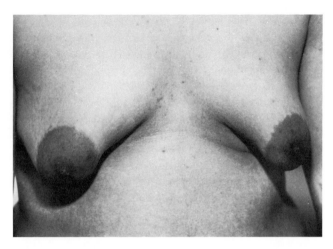

Fig. 134-3. Macromastia in a 16-year-old obese boy.

rating. Genital size and testicular size should be evaluated carefully to rule out endocrinopathies and genetic disorders such as Klinefelter's syndrome and pseudohermaphroditism.

In general, the cause of gynecomastia is unknown. Several reports implicate changes in estrogen metabolism or in estrogen-to-testosterone ratios. Studies detecting such changes have either been long-term longitudinal investigations that compared testosterone with estradiol levels, or 24-hour profiles indicating a relative estrogen dominance and submaximal testosterone production.[19,34-36] Other studies failed to find convincing changes in these hormone levels.[37] Since gynecomastia, both types I and II, often occurs as a unilateral phenomenon, the relationship of any of these hormonal changes to breast tissue enlargement is still in question. Local tissue factors have been considered as a way of understanding the cause of types I and II gynecomastia and the phenomenon of unilateral gynecomastia. However, to date, studies of estrogen and progesterone receptors in pubertal macromastia have not been enlightening.[38]

The laboratory work-up of gynecomastia depends on the history and physical examination findings. Since no clear-cut endocrinologic cause is evident in most cases, endocrine studies are not necessary. If Klinefelter's syndrome or certain forms of pseudohermaphroditism are suspected, karyotyping and testosterone biosynthetic pathway studies are appropriate. Other studies pertinent to a specific hypothesized cause may be undertaken if necessary: for example, thyroid or liver function studies.

Although type I gynecomastia usually requires no specific treatment, pubertal macromastia may be a significant emotional burden for an adolescent male. Chemical treatments have been attempted, including clomiphene (an estrogen antagonist), danazol (an antigonadotropic), tamoxifen (an antiestrogen), and dihydrotes-

---

BOX 134-2
Causes of Type II Gynecomastia

Idiopathic
Familial
    Endocrine/hormonal (e.g., Reifenstein's syndrome)
    Nonendocrine syndromes
Primary testicular failure: radiation, chemotherapy, cryptorchidism, orchitis, hydrocele, varicocele, spermatocele, trauma, tuberculosis, leprosy, leukemia, hemophilia
Malnutrition/starvation
Endocrine: hyperthyroidism, hypothyroidism, congenital adrenal hyperplasia/cryptogenic adrenal hyperplasia
Chronic illness: cirrhosis; ulcerative colitis; rheumatic fever; pulmonary, renal, neurologic diseases
Tumors: seminoma, choriocarcinoma, Leydig's cell and embryonal cell tumors, teratoma, androblastoma, hepatoma, adrenal adenoma and carcinoma

Drugs
    Estrogen-like: clomiphene citrate, diethylstilbestrol
    Antihypertensives: guanabenz, reserpine, propranolol, hydralazine
    Cardiac: amiloride, digoxin, calcium channel blockers
    Chemotherapeutic: busulfan, procarbazine, vincristine
    Neuroleptics: phenothiazines, benzodiazepines, tricyclic antidepressants
    Diuretics: spironolactone, thiazide
Anabolic steroids
Opiates: heroin, methadone
Others: amphetamines, penicillamine, ergotamine, cimetidine, isoniazid, teratoma, ketoconazole, leuprolide, marijuana, methyldopa, metronidazole, sulindac, tamoxifen, theophylline, alcohol, clofibrate, ibuprofen, vitamin E

---

tosterone (nonaromatizable androgen).[39] However, their efficacy remains to be proved. The issue of the side effects of these drugs also needs to be clarified. At present, the most successful form of treatment is cosmetic surgery. Appropriate psychologic evaluation is necessary to assess the patient's intrinsic self-esteem and to make sure that surgery will be beneficial. Self-esteem and body image often are distorted, especially in adolescent males with large, pendulous breasts. Comments by peers can be devastating at this vulnerable stage. Adolescents who show significant anxiety and depression should receive both counseling and surgical intervention for the best possible outcome.[30]

GALACTORRHEA

Any amount of persistent discharge or material expressible from the breast that looks like milk, and that either does not occur in relation to parturition or continues post partum in the absence of nursing for more than 6 months, is defined as galactorrhea.[40] Discharge may be seen in one or both breasts. Since breast discharge often comes in various colors and consistencies, the surest way to corroborate the diagnosis of galactorrhea objectively is to stain a smear of the discharge for fat globules. Fat-laden macrophages seen under the microscope represent strong evidence of milk production, and hence galactorrhea. The incidence of nonpuerperal lactation ranges widely, from 0.6% to 50%.[33] The incidence in adolescents has not been determined definitely, but it is

not considered insignificant. The most effective means of eliciting galactorrhea is the technique known as breast stripping. The causes of galactorrhea can be classified into six major categories: neurogenic, hypothalamic, pituitary, endocrine/hormonal, drug-induced, and idiopathic (Box 134-3). Neurogenic causes of galactorrhea are relatively uncommon except for those that occur in association with manipulation of the breasts and nipples. Hypothalamic disorders are also relatively unusual causes of galactorrhea. Pituitary lesions, especially pituitary tumors, are far more numerous. Prolactinomas, the most common type of pituitary tumor associated with galactorrhea, are thought to be the most common secretory pituitary tumors. The incidence of prolactinoma associated with galactorrhea has been reported to range from 13% to more than 85% of women.[33] Of the endocrine/hormonal causes, contraceptive pills and pregnancy are by far the most common. Drug-induced galactorrhea is not uncommon. Idiopathic galactorrhea appears to be the single most common cause.[41] A significant number of adolescent cases have been described in the literature, most of which have been either pituitary or endocrine and hormonal in nature.[33]

Any female adolescent presenting with galactorrhea should have a history taken carefully, with specific concentration on any symptoms suggestive of pituitary disease or medication or drug usage. Symptoms such as headaches, visual disturbance, arrested sexual maturation, oligomenorrhea and/or amenorrhea, polyuria, or polydipsia may be suggestive of a hypothalamic or pituitary lesion. Attention should also be paid to any possible drug ingestion, including estrogen or oral

---

BOX 134-3
Causes of Galactorrhea

NEUROGENIC
Chest wall: burns, crutch-bearing, thoracotomy
Breast: chronic inflammatory disease, nipple manipulation, reduction mammoplasty
Psychoses: pseudocyesis, pseudonursing, psychosomatic disorders
Others: laparotomy, laminectomy, hysterectomy, spinal cord injury

HYPOTHALAMIC
Tumors: craniopharyngioma, meningioma, metastatic, pineal
Phakomatoses: neurofibromatosis, tuberous sclerosis
Diffuse: coma, encephalitis, pseudotumor cerebri
Others: histiocytosis X, aneurysms, stalk section, uremia, sphenoethmoid sinus mucocele

PITUITARY
Tumors: prolactinoma, other adenomas
Others: cysts, empty sella syndrome, Sheehan's syndrome

ENDOCRINE/HORMONAL
Tumors: adrenal, hypernephroma, teratoma, chorionepithelioma
Estrogens: contraceptive pills, pregnancy, starvation/refeeding
Others: hypothyroidism, hypogonadism, growth hormone isoform excess

DRUG-INDUCED
Neuroleptics: phenothiazines, haloperidol, metoclopramide, sertraline
Tricyclic antidepressants: amitriptyline, imipramine
Opiates: codeine, heroin, morphine
Others: methyldopa, amphetamines, cimetidine, tamoxifen, atenolol

IDIOPATHIC
Benign: normoprolactinemic, hyperprolactinemic
Others: acute intermittent porphyria, myeloma, Hodgkin's disease

---

prolactin level to rule out hyperprolactinemia. The most thorough way to determine hyperprolactinemia is to obtain three blood samples over the course of 1 hour. Each sample can be determined separately or combined into one pooled specimen. The purpose of collecting prolactin in this manner is to minimize the chance of a spuriously low level due to the episodic nature of prolactin secretion. If hyperprolactinemia is documented, the work-up is then focused on ruling out a pituitary tumor, especially if oligomenorrhea or amenorrhea exists and there is no history of drug ingestion.

If hyperprolactinemia is detected and galactorrhea is associated with oligomenorrhea or amenorrhea, magnetic resonance imaging or computed tomography may be necessary to rule out a microadenoma. Lack of hyperprolactinemia should lead to a search for other causes of galactorrhea. If galactorrhea occurs in association with amenorrhea but without hyperprolactinemia, appropriate work-up of the amenorrhea is necessary. Long-term management and treatment of galactorrhea depends on the cause. Increasingly, patients with microprolactinoma are being treated with dopamine agonists such as bromocriptine. Many centers continue to employ transsphenoidal adenomectomy. Larger tumors are difficult to treat, since response to the conventional regimen of surgery and radiotherapy is poor. A few studies have reported that dopamine agonist therapy alone has been more efficacious.[42]

Management of other causes that are part of a clearly identified etiology should be directed toward that etiology. For example, in drug-induced galactorrhea, the offending drug should be discontinued (if possible) and a substitute drug administered. If no clearly defined cause is evident, the work-up is negative, and galactorrhea is occurring without hyperprolactinemia or amenorrhea, there is little likelihood of significant pathology. Yearly follow-up is probably sufficient. The adolescent female with galactorrhea/amenorrhea who has normoprolactinemia requires more careful follow-up, with prolactin levels measured yearly. In the adolescent female who has hyperprolactinemic galactorrhea and oligomenorrhea or amenorrhea without prolactinoma, dopamine agonist therapy may help reduce galactorrhea or restore normal menstrual cycles.

contraceptives. Questioning should help to exclude the possibility of a previous pregnancy or the presence of any symptoms of thyroid or adrenal dysfunction. The breast discharge should be examined for color, consistency, and fat globules (via microscopic examination of a stained smear). A thorough neurologic examination should be performed in association with examination of visual fields, extraocular eye movements, ocular fundi, thyroid size, and sexual maturity rating, as well as examination of the skin for texture, pigmentation, or hirsutism. The cornerstone of the work-up is determination of the

References

1. Goldbloom RB: Self-examination by adolescents, *Pediatrics* 76: 126, 1985.
2. Hein K, Dell R, Cohen MI: Self-detection of a breast mass in adolescent females, *J Adolesc Health Care* 3:15, 1982.
3. Reynolds EL, Wine JV: Individualized differences in physical changes associated with adolescence in girls, *Am J Dis Child* 75:329, 1948.
4. Tanner JM: *Growth at adolescence*, ed 2, Oxford, 1962, Blackwell Scientific.
5. Capraro VJ, Dewhurst CJ: Breast disorders in childhood and adolescence, *Clin Obstet Gynecol* 18:25, 1975.

6. Rohn RD: Nipple (papilla) development in puberty: longitudinal observations in girls, *Pediatrics* 79:745, 1987.

7. Heyman RB, Rauh JL: Areola gland discharge in adolescent females, *J Adolesc Health Care* 4:285, 1983.

8. Levit F: Jogger's nipples, *N Engl J Med* 297:1127, 1977.

9. Greydanus DE, Parks DS, Farrell EG: Breast disorders in children and adolescents, *Pediatr Clin North Am* 36:601, 1989.

10. Jones KL: *Smith's recognizable patterns,* Philadelphia, 1988, WB Saunders, p 260.

11. Griffith JE: Virginal breast hypertrophy, *J Adolesc Health Care* 10:423, 1989.

12. Schydlower M: Breast masses in adolescents, *Am Fam Physician* 25:141, 1982.

13. Daniel WA, Matthews MD: Tumors of the breast in adolescent females, *Pediatrics* 41:743, 1968.

14. Oberman HA: Breast lesions in the adolescent female, *Pathol Annu* 14:175, 1979.

15. Vetroni A, Fulcinitti F, DiBenedetto G, et al: Fine-needle aspiration biopsies of breast masses, *Cancer* 69:736, 1992.

16. Dupont WD, Page DL, Parl FF, Vnencak-Jones CL, Plommer WD, Rados MS, Schuyler PA: Long-term risk of breast cancer in women with fibroadenoma, *N Engl J Med* 331:10, 1994.

17. Levi F, Randimibison L, Te V-C, LaVecchio C: Incidence of breast cancer in women with fibroadenoma, *Int J Cancer* 57:681, 1994.

18. Rogers LA, Lee KR: Breast carcinoma simulating fibroadenoma or fibrocystic change by fine-needle aspiration, *Am J Clin Pathol* 98:155, 1992.

19. Ozisik YY, Meloni AM, Stephenson CF, Peier A, Moore GE, Sandberg AA: Chromosome abnormalities in breast fibroadenomas, *Cancer Genet Cytogenet* 77:125, 1994.

20. Odagiri E, Kanda N, Jibiki K, Demura R, Aikawa E, Demura H: Reduction of telomeric length and C-cvb B-2 gene amplification in human breast cancer, fibroadenoma and gynecomastia, *Cancer* 73:2978, 1994.

21. Noguchi S, Motomura K, Inajc H, Imaoka S, Koyama H: Clonal analysis of fibroadenoma and phyllodes tumor of the breast, *Cancer Res* 53:4071, 1993.

22. Stone AM, Shenker IR, McCarthy K: Adolescent breast masses, *Am J Surg* 134:275, 1977.

23. Pietsch J: Breast disorders. In Lavery JP, Sanfilippo JS, editors: *Pediatric and adolescent obstetrics and gynecology,* New York, 1985, Springer-Verlag; p 96.

24. Fiorica JV: Fibrocystic changes, *Obstet Gynecol Clin North Am* 21:445, 1994.

25. Angeli A, Dogliotti L, Naldoni C, et al: Steroid biochemistry and categorization of breast cyst fluid: relation to breast cancer risk, *J Steroid Biochem Mol Biol* 49:333, 1994.

26. Hutter RVP: Goodbye to "fibrocystic disease," *N Engl J Med* 312:179, 1985.

27. Seashore JH: Breast lesions in children. In Gallager HS, Leis HP, Snyderman RK, Urban JA, editors: *The breast,* St. Louis, 1978, Mosby–Year Book; p 497.

28. Bertrand H, Rosenblood LK: Stripping out pus in lactational mastitis: a means of preventing breast abscess, *Can Med Assoc J* 145:299, 1991.

29. Knorr D, Bidlingmaier F: Gynecomastia in male adolescents, *J Clin Endocrinol Metab* 4:157, 1975.

30. Schonfeld WA: Gynecomastia in adolescence: effect on body image and personality adaptation, *Psychosom Med* 24:379, 1962.

31. Carlson HE: Gynecomastia, *N Engl J Med* 303:795, 1980.

32. Nydick M, Bustos J, Dale JH, Rawson RW: Gynecomastia in adolescent boys, *JAMA* 178:449, 1961.

33. Rohn RD: Galactorrhea in the adolescent, *J Adolesc Health Care* 5:36, 1984.

34. Lee PA: The relationship of concentrations of serum hormones to pubertal gynecomastia, *J Pediatr* 86:212, 1975.

35. Moore DC, Schlaepfer LV, Paunier L, Sizonenko PC: Hormonal changes during puberty. V. Transient pubertal gynecomastia: abnormal androgen-estrogen ratios, *J Clin Endocrinol Metab* 58:492, 1984.

36. Large DM, Anderson DC: Twenty-four-hour profiles of circulating androgens and estrogens in male puberty with and without gynecomastia, *Clin Endocrinol* 11:505, 1979.

37. Marynick SP, Nisula BC, Pita JC, Loriaux DL: Persistent pubertal macromastia, *J Clin Endocrinol Metab* 50:128, 1980.

38. Lee KO, Chua DYF, Cheah JS: Estrogen and progesterone receptors in men with bilateral or unilateral pubertal macromastia, *Clin Endocrinol* 32:101, 1990.

39. Eberle AJ, Sparrow JT, Keenan BS: Treatment of persistent pubertal gynecomastia with dihydrotestosterone heptanoate, *J Pediatr* 109:144, 1986.

40. Frantz AG: The breasts. In Wilson JE, Foster DW, editors: *William's textbook of endocrinology,* ed 7, Philadelphia, 1985, WB Saunders; p 406.

41. Klienberg DL, Noel GL, Frantz AG: Galactorrhea: a study of 235 cases including 48 with pituitary tumors, *N Engl J Med* 296:589, 1977.

42. Carter JN, Tyson JE, Tolis G, et al: Prolactin-secreting tumors in hypogonadism in 22 men, *N Engl J Med* 299:847, 1978.

CHAPTER 135

The Pelvic Examination

•

Roberta K. Beach

The ability to perform a sensitive and thorough pelvic examination is an essential skill for healthcare providers who treat adolescents.[1] Up to one half of medical visits by young women aged 15 to 19 years are for gynecologic or obstetric conditions. In general, adolescent girls have considerable anxiety about the pelvic examination, and their experiences in this area will sensitize them, positively or negatively, toward future healthcare encounters.

INDICATIONS

The indications for an adolescent pelvic examination are extensive (Box 135-1). An initial pelvic examination for routine health screening is recommended for all young women at approximately the age of 16 to 18 years. The examination should be performed earlier (1) if the patient is, or plans to become, sexually active; or (2) anytime upon request. The initial visit for birth control purposes is perhaps the most common time for the first pelvic examination. Other indications include evaluation of most gynecologic signs or symptoms, such as delayed puberty or delayed menarche, severe dysmenorrhea, irregular or heavy menstrual bleeding, amenorrhea, vaginal discharge, exposure to sexually transmitted diseases (STDs), suspected pregnancy, suspected pelvic mass, pelvic pain, or unexplained abdominal pain.

Certain situations require special examination techniques that are not addressed in this chapter. Maternal exposure to diethylstilbestrol (DES) necessitates pelvic examination of the daughter at age 14 by an experienced expert. However, the use of DES was essentially halted in 1971, and so children born subsequently are unlikely to have been exposed. The forensic examination of victims of alleged sexual assault or sexual abuse must be performed in exact compliance with state and local legal requirements by examiners who are familiar with specific procedures.

BASIC ISSUES

Relationship and Setting

The relationship between the adolescent and her caregiver changes with the introduction of the pelvic examination. The realities of the individual's progressing from childhood to young womanhood, her emerging sexuality, and her growing independence create a need for a patient-centered approach that is nonjudgmental, sensitive, and based on honest communication. Although adolescent girls usually express a strong preference for female examiners, a successful pelvic examination can be accomplished by a gentle, respectful healthcare provider of either sex. The setting should reflect a concern for the patient's comfort, dignity, and privacy. The office staff should be carefully trained, since the sensitivity and sense of caring expressed by the staff are major determinants in how the teenager perceives the experience.

Consent and Confidentiality

Parental involvement in and consent to a minor child's gynecologic care is the ideal and should be sought whenever possible. For many teenagers, however, trust in the provider's ability to ensure confidentiality is an essential prerequisite to confiding their needs for birth control, pregnancy testing, or treatment for STDs. Legal requirements and standard practices for confidential care vary by state, and they should be reviewed and thoroughly understood by the physician and staff (see Chapter 18, "Legal and Ethical Concerns"). If confidential care is being provided, the minor's own consent should be obtained.

Chaperones

The presence of a female chaperone is recommended for adolescent pelvic examinations for several reasons: to

---

BOX 135-1
Indications for Pelvic Examination

1. For routine health assessment beginning at age 16 to 18 years, depending on community norms; repeated annually if the teenager is sexually active
2. When the teenager is sexually active (or about to be) for:
   Birth control
   Sexually transmitted disease check (every 12 months if asymptomatic)
3. For any gynecologic complaints
   Delayed menarche
   Vaginal discharge
   Menstrual disorders
   Dysmenorrhea unresponsive to NSAIDs
   Abdominal or pelvic pain
   Suspected pregnancy
4. On request
5. Referral to a specialist for:
   DES exposure
   Forensic rape examination

DES, diethylstilbestrol; *NSAIDs,* nonsteroidal anti-inflammatory drugs.

maximize the patient's comfort, to assist the examiner, and to address medicolegal considerations. A young teenager may wish her mother to be present; older teenagers often prefer an office assistant to be in the examining room.[2] The patient's preferences should be honored to the greatest extent possible.

The First Pelvic Examination

Most women remember their first pelvic examination for the rest of their lives. This examination may determine, for better or worse, a young woman's attitudes toward future medical examinations, physicians, and gynecologic concerns. It is essential to take the time necessary to prepare the patient, explain all procedures, and demonstrate the instruments.[3] The use of plastic models, videotapes, or booklets may be helpful. Typical concerns or fears should be addressed (Will it hurt? Will I still be a virgin?). The examination should proceed slowly, with the examiner showing patience and allowing the patient as much control as possible. The initial pelvic examination may require 30 to 45 minutes of office time. Subsequent examinations may take only 10 to 15 minutes.

Patients Who Refuse Examination

Most adolescents cooperate fully with the pelvic examination if they have received careful preparation. Cultural attitudes toward female modesty or privacy may need sensitive attention. Resistance or refusal is most

often a sign of fear. Occasionally, refusal may result from a power struggle between an insistent parent and a reluctant teenager. Excessive anxiety is sometimes seen in victims of sexual abuse. Questions, fears, or previous negative experiences with examinations should be discussed patiently. Reflective listening can be very useful, as can turning control over to the patient by allowing her to decide what to do next. A rectal or bimanual examination without the speculum may suffice in some cases. If the patient is unwilling to proceed, the examiner should do as much as the patient will allow and reschedule the remainder of the examination. Restraints, sedation, or anesthesia should not be used in nonemergency situations.

GYNECOLOGIC INTERVIEW

Hidden Agendas

Confidence and rapport are often best established while taking a thorough and sensitive history. The interview should take place before the examination, with the adolescent still dressed and comfortable. The stated reason for the visit will determine the initial focus of the interview, but the caregiver should then gently try to discover any hidden agendas. For example, it is common for an adolescent to deny initially a history of sexual intercourse, especially if a parent is present, when in fact an underlying fear of pregnancy may be the adolescent's chief concern. The history should be taken (or retaken) in private and with assurance of confidentiality.

History Taking

The information needed for the adolescent gynecologic history is shown in Box 135-2. The order in which the information is gathered may vary according to the situation. A history form filled out in advance by the patient (and parent, if appropriate) can be helpful, but pertinent details should be reviewed during the interview.

Helpful Techniques

Adolescent sexuality is controversial in our society, and teenagers are very cautious about revealing information that may result in disapproval. Several interview techniques are especially helpful in obtaining an accurate sexual history:
- Privacy, with the caregiver's full attention
- Reassurances of confidentiality (nothing shared without permission)
- A nonjudgmental and respectful attitude, avoiding assumptions, with sensitivity to cultural needs and expectations

---

BOX 135-2
Gynecologic History

1. *Reason for visit* (patient's view, which may differ from parents')
2. *Menstrual history*
   - Last menstrual period
   - Age at menarche
   - Typical duration, pattern
   - Associated symptoms (dysmenorrhea, premenstrual syndrome)
   - Previous treatment
   - Recent changes, problems
3. *Gynecologic history*
   - Last pelvic examination
   - Last Pap test
   - Vaginal discharge
   - Abdominal or pelvic pain
   - Urinary tract symptoms
   - Virilization, endocrine symptoms
   - Previous gynecologic diagnoses
   - Previous surgical procedures
4. *Sexual and contraceptive history*
   - Dating history (sexual preference)
   - Sexual activity/intercourse
   - Use of contraception/condoms
   - HIV risk factors
   - History of sexually transmitted diseases
   - History of sexual abuse
   - Specific concerns or worries
5. *Obstetric history*
   - Pregnancies and outcomes (type of delivery, abortions, miscarriages)
   - Desire for pregnancy, childbearing
   - Current concern about being pregnant
   - Concern about infertility
6. *Medical and family history*
   - Allergies
   - Growth, puberty
   - Previous medical history
   - Previous psychosocial history
   - Maternal diethylstilbestrol exposure
   - Maternal obstetric/gynecologic history
   - Breast or gynecologic cancer history
   - Other family medical history
7. *Related health issues*
   - Smoking
   - Alcohol use
   - Drug use
   - Nutrition, weight
   - Eating disorders
   - Emotional symptoms, depression

BOX 135-3
Equipment and Supplies for Pelvic Examination

Room with warm running water
Examination table with stirrups
Light source (gooseneck lamp, halogen lamp, headlight)
Gloves, water-soluble lubricant
Gowns, drapes
Tissue, tampons, or pads
Hand mirror
Cotton swabs, small and large
Vaginal specula (metal or disposable)
  Narrow Pederson (virginal)
  Medium Pederson
  Medium Graves (obese or pregnant patients)
Pap smear materials
  Cytology brush
  Ayers wooden spatula
  Frosted-tip glass slide
  Fixative
pH (nitrazine) paper
Infection test materials
  Gonorrhea test
  Chlamydia test
  Wet-mount prep supplies (plastic tube, normal saline, 10% KOH)
  Optional: viral test for herpes simplex, HPV
Microscope
Pregnancy test kit

HPV, human papillomavirus; *KOH*, potassium hydroxide.

- Clear, straightforward language, avoiding both medical jargon and street vernacular (clarify terms if in doubt)
- Open-ended questions at the beginning of the interview (Tell me what your periods are like? What do you think caused your problem?)
- Direct questions asked later in the interview (Do you think you could be pregnant? Would you like information about birth control?)
- Careful listening (observe body language, interrupt rarely, do not lecture)

PREPARATION FOR EXAMINATION

Equipment and Supplies

The list of equipment for the adolescent pelvic examination is shown in Box 135-3. Vaginal specula come in several sizes. The two most useful sizes are the narrow Pederson (½″ × 4½″) for virginal examinations and the medium Pederson (1″ × 4½″) for most sexually active teenagers. The short, narrow Huffman speculum (½″ × 3″) can be used for prepubertal girls. The medium Graves speculum (1¾″ × 4″) has wider blades, which may be helpful for obese or pregnant patients. Metal specula must be sterilized after each use. Disposable plastic specula in various sizes are also available.

Screening Tests

Careful attention to obtaining accurate screening tests is an essential part of the examination. Supplies needed depend on the specific tests selected. Technology is rapidly expanding in this area and many options are available. Typically the tests for gonorrhea and *Chlamydia,* viral cultures for herpesvirus, and the Papanicolaou (Pap) test are sent to a referral laboratory. The laboratory's specific instructions for collection and transport should be followed exactly (see Chapter 140, "Sexually Transmitted Diseases"). Some screening tests, such as the pregnancy test, may be done on site, in which case the manufacturer's directions should be followed.

GONORRHEA TESTS. Culture for *Neisseria gonorrhoeae* on modified Thayer-Martin medium under anaerobic conditions is standard. Newer, nonculture enzyme immunoassay and DNA probe tests with sensitivities of 97% to 99% are now available but require technical expertise.[4]

CHLAMYDIA TESTS. Although cell culture remains the "gold standard" for *Chlamydia trachomatis,* rapid nonculture screening tests are widely used, including direct fluorescent antibody, enzyme immunoassay, and isotopic DNA probes. Nonculture tests have variable reliability and sensitivities of 68% to 88%, no specific method being clearly superior.[5] Collection techniques vary, and the directions of the manufacturer and referral laboratory should be followed precisely.

OTHER CULTURES. A viral culture for herpes simplex virus may be indicated if suspicious lesions are present. A sterile swab is saturated in the transport medium in the viral culture tube, rubbed firmly on the lesion, placed back in the tube, and broken off inside. The culture tube must be transported immediately to the laboratory. If a fungal infection is suspected, Nickerson's or Biggy agar medium can be inoculated for culture. Testing for human papillomavirus (HPV) currently relies on nucleic acid hybridization techniques (ViraPap, ViraType), is expensive, and is usually reserved for research studies, although testing of selected high-risk populations may become useful in the future.[6]

WET-MOUNT SMEARS. The wet "prep" may be examined immediately under a microscope as a simple office procedure. A drop of vaginal secretions is mixed with a drop of normal saline on a clean, dry slide and scanned under ×10 and ×40 magnification for motile trichomonads and the characteristic clue cells of bacterial vaginitis (vaginal epithelial cells coated with bacteria). A drop of 10% potassium hydroxide (KOH) is then added to search for the hyphae and spores of *Candida* organisms. The release of a fishy amine odor upon addition of KOH (the positive "whiff" test) suggests bacterial vaginosis (see Chapter 140, "Sexually Transmitted Diseases"). White blood cells indicating cervicitis may also be visible in a wet prep.

pH (NITRAZINE) TEST. A sample of vaginal discharge can be tested with pH paper, or the pH paper may be pressed against the vaginal wall. The normal vaginal pH is acidic at pH 4.5 or less. Increased pH may suggest bacterial vaginosis or trichomoniasis.

FERN TEST. "Ferning" of the cervical mucus is a simple test of ovarian function that confirms adequate estrogen status during the first half of the menstrual cycle, and may denote unopposed estrogen in dysfunctional uterine bleeding. Progesterone produced after ovulation abolishes the ferning for the remainder of that cycle. A small amount of cervical mucus is taken from the external os, deposited on a glass slide, and allowed to air dry. The slide is examined under low to medium microscopic magnification to detect the fern pattern.

PAPANICOLAOU (PAP) SMEARS. Frosted-tip glass slides should be prelabeled with the patient's name. Collection of an accurate sample from the squamocolumnar junction of the cervix is essential. Two specimens are usually obtained, one from the ectocervix and one from the endocervix. An Ayers wooden spatula is used to scrape the ectocervix. The use of a cytology brush, instead of a swab, for endocervical sampling produces the most reliable specimen of endocolumnar cells and is the standard practice.[7] Combining the two samples on a single slide is now preferred to the use of two slides to aid in technician productivity when the slides are read. The slides must be fixed immediately with spray of liquid fixative to prevent drying artifact. The specific instructions of the referral laboratory for correct slide preparation should be followed carefully. See Chapter 137, "Cervical Findings and The Pap Smear," for more detailed discussion.

PREGNANCY TESTS. A pregnancy test is often an important part of the gynecologic evaluation. Simple, accurate, rapid office test kits are available that can detect as little as 50 mIU/ml of β-human chorionic gonadotropin (β-hCG) in the urine, resulting in a positive test about 14 days after conception. Several kits include self-contained controls for quality assurance.

PROCEDURES FOR EXAMINATION

After the history has been taken and the procedures have been fully explained, the adolescent changes into a gown for the examination. Vital signs for height, weight, blood pressure, or temperature may be taken, depending on the reason for the visit. The patient should have an empty bladder, be positioned comfortably on the table with her head elevated, and draped as she desires. If this is an annual examination, the thyroid should be palpated and the heart auscultated. The examiner continues with a careful breast examination. The abdomen is then palpated and the groin checked for inguinal nodes. Any hirsutism or other signs that might be indicated for evaluation of

STEPS IN PELVIC EXAMINATION*

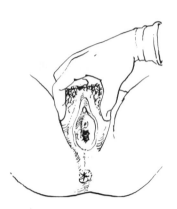

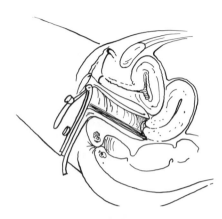

1. *Inspect external genitalia.* With a gloved hand, inspect the vulvar structures for lesions, warts, lacerations, or fissures and any signs of inflammation. Palpate the periurethral and Bartholin's glands for masses or discharge. Note the Tanner sexual maturity rating (see Chapter 13, "Physical Examination"). Check for clitoromegaly. Note the configuration of the hymen.

2. *Inspect internal genitalia.* Select the appropriate-size speculum, warm it with water (use no lubricant), and touch it to the patient's thigh to check temperature for comfort. Explain what the patient will feel, then spread the labia widely and insert the speculum slowly while pressing downward toward the perineum. Be careful to avoid pressure on the sensitive anterior wall and urethra. Advance the closed speculum horizontally, aiming downward, until fully inserted. Gently open the blades, slowly sweeping upward until the cervix comes into view. Inspect the cervix for ectropion, inflammation, lesions, discharge. Note any vaginal discharge. Press a strip of pH paper against the side of the vaginal wall and read the pH level.

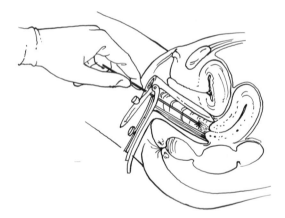

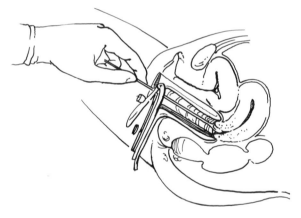

3. *Obtain cytologic smear.* The Pap smear should be done first, before the cervical cells are disturbed by other tests. Use the specific method recommended by the laboratory. To obtain endocolumnar cells, one standard method is to rotate a cytology brush (or cotton-tipped swab) in the endocervical os in one direction, withdraw it, and plate the cells by rotating the brush in the opposite direction on one half of a glass slide. Apply fixative to that half of the slide.

4. *Scrape cells from squamocolumnar junction.* Using an Ayers wooden spatula, lightly scrape the cervix in a 360-degree rotation, maintaining enough pressure to scrape the epithelial cells from the mucosal surface. Smear the sample on the other half of the slide. Fix immediately (drying artifact will invalidate the Pap smear). A well-prepared smear should contain endocolumnar cells, squamous cells, and little or no blood. A Pap smear should not be taken if the patient is menstruating. Likewise, obvious infection or cervicitis should be treated first and cervical cytology postponed for at least 6 weeks.

---

*All illustrations in this section have been modified from Routine gynecologic examination and cytologic smear, *CA* 25:281-286, 1975. Copyright © 1975 *CA—A Cancer Journal for Clinicians* and the American Cancer Society, Inc.

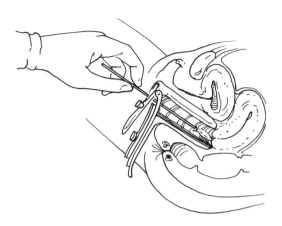

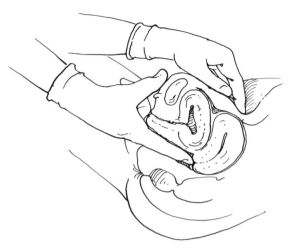

5. *Obtain infection tests.* Specific techniques depend on the test methods used. In general, for the gonorrhea test, insert a swab in the endocervical canal for 10 to 15 seconds to absorb secretions, then plate on the culture medium. For the *Chlamydia* test, rotate the swab from the test kit vigorously in the endocervical canal to pick up endocolumnar cells, then place in the tube or on the slide as directed. For the wet prep, collect a sample of the vaginal pool on a swab and place in a plastic tube with a few drops of normal saline, or prepare the slide itself. When tests are completed, gently rotate the speculum blades to inspect the vaginal wall. Close the blades and withdraw the speculum.

6. *Perform bimanual palpation.* Have the patient breathe deeply to relax her abdominal muscles. Lightly lubricate the gloved fingers and insert one or two fingers slowly, then palpate the pelvic structures. Press on the cervix to check for pain (significant pain on cervical motion is a sign of pelvic infection). Place the opposite hand on the abdomen and press down while gently pushing the uterus upward with the internally placed fingers. Note the uterine size and shape. Press firmly on the uterus to check for pain. Patients may normally note a crampy, uncomfortable feeling. Significant pelvic pain is usually marked by involuntary guarding.

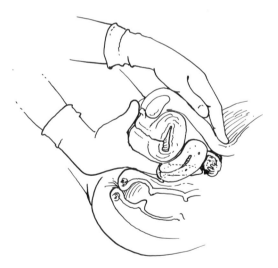

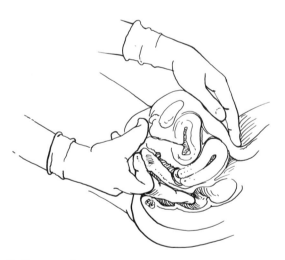

7. *Palpate the adnexa.* Move your fingers laterally to one side of the fornix, press down deeply with the hand that is on the abdomen, and palpate the adnexal structures. Pressure on the ovary is somewhat painful; the patient usually can tell you when you have located it. Check for enlargement, cysts, masses, or severe pain, then repeat on the opposite side. The normal adnexa is smooth and walnut-sized, composed of the ovary, fallopian tubes, and ligaments. These structures usually cannot be distinguished separately.

8. *Perform rectal examination.* A rectovaginal examination of the septum for nodules is rarely indicated in teenagers. A simple one-finger rectal examination is indicated to check for hemorrhoids, to check tenderness of the posterior uterus, or to confirm a retroverted uterus. Check for occult blood if the visit is for abdominal pain. When the examination is completed, reassure the patient if the examination is normal and allow her to dress before the final discussion.

specific symptoms, as recorded in the history, should be noted. The patient then should be assisted into the lithotomy position, with the stirrups adjusted for comfort. She should be asked to stretch her thighs into a frog-leg position, which helps relax the pelvic muscles.

A very helpful technique is to talk to the patient throughout the examination, briefly explaining what you are doing and why it is necessary, and offering reassurances about normal findings. The examination can be used as an opportunity for education. As much as possible, the teenager should be actively involved in helping with the examination.

Although many variations are possible, the basic steps illustrated on pages 1040 and 1041 are usually included in a full gynecologic examination. Specific instructions from the referral laboratory should be followed in collecting specimens for the Pap test and STD tests.

ADDITIONAL DIAGNOSTIC STUDIES

Laboratory Studies

If the visit is with a new patient or for a periodic health appraisal, additional screening tests may be indicated. For a complete adolescent gynecologic evaluation, these may include hemoglobin and hematocrit, urinalysis, urine culture if indicated, syphilis serology, rubella titer, and hepatitis B antigen and human immunodeficiency virus (HIV) screening for patients with risk factors (see Chapter 14, "Laboratory Testing"). For specific disorders, a wide spectrum of hematologic studies, endocrine studies, serum chemistries, and other tests may be necessary.

New Technology

Routine office assessment of gynecologic complaints, once confined to the pelvic examination and a few basic laboratory tests, has entered a new realm of high-technology options. Pelvic ultrasonography, enhanced by the use of vaginal probes, has become a standard office procedure to evaluate pelvic pain, suspected masses, or complications of pregnancy. Colposcopy (discussed in Chapter 137, "Cervical Findings and the Pap Smear") represents the next step in evaluating abnormal cervical cytology. Computed tomography and magnetic resonance imaging may be useful for further evaluation of anatomic abnormalities of the genital tract. Laparoscopy remains the most accurate means of confirming endometriosis or pelvic adhesions.[8] These technologies require technical expertise and in-depth experience for accurate use and interpretation. Adolescent healthcare specialists in some settings, such as training centers, may become expert in the use of these modalities. In other settings, referral to an experienced colleague is appropriate.

COUNSELING PATIENTS AFTER EXAMINATION

The adolescent should be allowed to dress in private before the final consultation. The findings and the assessment should be clearly explained, treatment plans discussed, and questions answered. If parents or a support person are waiting, they may be included at the end of the discussion, with the patient's permission and to the extent she prefers.

Anticipatory Guidance

If the findings are normal, the adolescent will appreciate strong verbal reassurance that she is healthy. Depending on the initial concern, specific direct comments may be helpful ("You are not pregnant," "You do not appear to have any infection," "You do not have a tumor."). Since the adolescent's anxiety level is reduced once the examination is over, the postexamination discussion is a useful setting for addressing the issues of sexual decision making, contraception, prevention of STDs, or any other concerns the young woman may have. Anticipatory guidance can be reinforced with brochures or patient handouts.

Compliance with Treatment

If a specific diagnosis has been made, sufficient time must be allowed to explain the treatment plan in detail. After this explanation, the patient should be encouraged to repeat the plan in her own words and to ask questions. Many common gynecologic treatments may be new and unfamiliar to the teenager, such as the use of vaginal creams, the specific instructions for contraceptive methods, or the need to treat sexual partners for STDs. Nothing should be assumed and everything should be explained in order to ensure patient compliance.

"Door-Knob" Syndrome

Just as the patient is leaving, she may finally express the hidden agenda by asking a special question. Such a divulgence is a sign of trust in the professional and it should be treated seriously. The question should be welcomed and the issue explored if possible. If time is not available, an appointment can be scheduled to continue the conversation later. The last-minute question may be the adolescent's way of testing the caregiver's true interest in her, and she will be acutely aware of the response.

Follow-up Care

Since some test results may be pending, follow-up plans need to be confirmed. The return appointment, if needed, should be scheduled before the patient leaves. A reliable contact telephone number or address is especially important for patients who request confidentiality. For certain ongoing problems, such as menstrual irregularity or recurrent pain, a calendar or symptom diary for the return visit may be useful. If subspecialty care is needed, appropriate referrals should be made. The adolescent, and her family with her permission, should be encouraged to call promptly if any questions or concerns arise.

The pelvic examination represents an important milestone in a young woman's health care. It offers an opportunity for education and anticipatory guidance on many significant aspects of decision making, self-responsibility, and healthy sexuality. When approached with sensitivity and attention to the special needs of the adolescent, the initial pelvic examination will be a positive experience for the adolescent, her family, and the caregiver.

References

1. Tolmas HC: Adolescent pelvic examination: an effective practical approach, *Am J Dis Child* 145:1269-1271, 1991.
2. Phillips S, Friedman SB, Seidenberg M, et al: Teenagers' preferences regarding the presence of family members, peers, and chaperones during examination of the genitalia, *Pediatrics* 68:665-669, 1981.
3. Leppert PC: The adolescent's first pelvic exam, *Contemp Adolesc Gynecol* 1:12-19, 1994.
4. Kellogg JA, Orwig LK: Comparison of GonoGen, GonoGen II, and MicroTrak direct fluorescent-antibody test with carbohydrate fermentation for confirmation of culture isolates of *Neisseria gonorrhoeae, J Clin Microbiol* 33:474-476, 1995.
5. Schubiner HH, Lebar W, Jemal C, et al: Comparison of three new non-culture tests in the diagnosis of *Chlamydia* genital infections, *J Adolesc Health Care* 11:505-509, 1990.
6. Cox JT, Lorincz AT, Schiffman MH, et al: Human papilloma virus testing by hybrid capture appears to be useful in triaging women with a cytologic diagnosis of atypical squamous cells of undetermined significance, *Am J Obstet Gynecol* 172:946-954, 1995.
7. Neinstein LS, Church J, Akiyoshi T: Comparison of Cytobrush with Cervex-Brush for endocervical cytologic sampling, *J Adolesc Health Care* 13:520-523, 1992.
8. Howard FM: The role of laparoscopy in chronic pelvic pain: promise and pitfalls, *Obstet Gynecol Surv* 48:357-387, 1993.

Suggested Readings

Emans SJ: Pelvic examination of the adolescent patient, *Pediatr Rev* 4:307-312, 1983.

Emans SJH, Goldstein DP: *Pediatric and adolescent gynecology,* ed 3, Boston, 1990, Little Brown.

Goldstein DP: Pediatric and adolescent gynecology. In Ryan KJ, Berkowitz R, Barbieri RL, editors: *Kistner's gynecology: principles and practice,* ed 5, Chicago, 1990, Mosby–Year Book; pp 610-670.

Graydanus DE, Shearin RB: *Adolescent sexuality and gynecology,* Philadelphia, 1990, Lea & Febiger.

Lichtman R, Papera S: *Gynecology: well-woman care,* Norwalk, CT, 1990, Appleton & Lange.

Strasburger VC, editor: *Basic adolescent gynecology: an office guide,* Baltimore, 1990, Urban & Schwarzenberg.

Wilson MD, Joffe A: Step-by-step through the pelvic exam, *Contemp Pediatr* 5:92-104, 1988.

CHAPTER 136

Perineal and Vaginal Findings

•

Roberta K. Beach

Although examination of the external genitalia is recommended as part of routine physical assessment starting in infancy, many young women will not have had careful genital inspection until they present for pelvic examination as adolescents. Developmental anomalies may be initially diagnosed at this time. In addition, puberty or sexual activity may result in signs or symptoms that require evaluation. In this chapter, disorders of the female external genitalia are divided into perineal findings and vaginal findings.

PERINEAL FINDINGS

The external female genitalia include the tissues of ectodermal origin from the mons pubis to the coccyx between the lateral groin creases. The entire area is called the perineum. The structural anatomy of the external genitalia is shown in Figure 136-1. The wide variety of perineal lesions that may be encountered during the pelvic examination will be discussed in three categories:

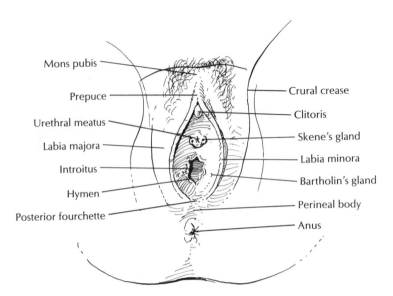

Fig. 136-1. Structural anatomy of the female external genitalia. The perineum extends from the mons to the coccyx between crural creases. The vulva includes the mons pubis, labia majora, and vestibule. The vestibule is made up of mucosal surfaces with the clitoris, urethral meatus, labia minora, introitus, and posterior fourchette.

developmental anomalies, benign vulvar lesions, and malignant vulvar lesions. It is not the intention of the author of this chapter to discuss medical treatment for these disorders but rather to provide a differential diagnosis for consideration when lesions are found.

DEVELOPMENTAL ANOMALIES

Major defects of the external genitalia are encountered rarely; in large studies the prevalence ranges from 1:2000 to 1:8000 examinations.[1] However, such defects may not be detected until menarche, unless a careful genital inspection was made earlier.

Ambiguous Genitalia

This condition rarely goes unnoticed beyond childhood. Chromosomal abnormalities that may produce vulvar defects include true or pseudohermaphroditism, androgen insensitivity, and gonadal dysgenesis.[2] Anomalous development of female external genitalia can also result from prenatal exposure to androgens by way of maternal ingestion, congenital adrenal hyperplasia, or androgen-producing maternal tumors during pregnancy.[3] Early detection and correction of anatomic defects are important in order to conform to the sex of rearing, which will usually be female to meet functional criteria.

Labial Anomalies

LABIAL AGGLUTINATION. A fibrinous exudate secondary to chronic vulvitis may cause the labia minora to

adhere to each other. The process typically begins at the fourchette and progresses ventrally. Although the condition is usually found in children under the age of 6 years, it may begin later and persist until puberty. Long-standing adhesions in older children may require surgical separation performed with the patient under local or general anesthesia.

LABIAL FUSION. True fusion of the labia may result from intrauterine or chronic perinatal inflammation of the vulva. It should be differentiated from a urogenital sinus of virilized external genitalia. The fusion is usually of the lower labia, which allows urinary outflow but may cause obstruction of menstrual outflow, thus precipitating diagnosis at puberty. Surgical correction is indicated.

HYPERTROPHY OF LABIA MINORA. Prominent labia minora protruding beyond the labia majora are a normal variant. This condition may be unilateral or bilateral, and the tissue may be hyperpigmented. No causal relationship to masturbation or chronic friction has been demonstrated. Surgical revision is advised if the hypertrophy is excessive or irritated by walking or exercise.

Supernumerary Nipples (Groin)

The mammalian nipple line extends to the upper thigh, and occasionally an accessory nipple is found in the groin area. It should be differentiated from a nevus or a new lesion such as a melanoma.

Clitoral Anomalies

CLITOROMEGALY. The clitoris is normally 2 to 5 mm in breadth. Clitoromegaly is usually defined as clitoral breadth of more than 6 mm, although some authors define it as more than 10 mm.[4] Clitoromegaly in adolescents suggests a hyperandrogenic effect, which may have many causes, including congenital adrenal hyperplasia, female hermaphroditism, male pseudohermaphroditism, and asymmetric gonadal dysgenesis. If none of these conditions is found, other possible causes include neurofibromatosis, transient clitoromegaly from chronic severe vulvovaginitis, and idiopathic clitoromegaly. Treatment consists of surgical recession with preservation of the glans for future orgasmic response. Clitoral edema from nephrotic syndrome may mimic clitoromegaly. Clitorism is a painful, persistent erection of the clitoris, sometimes seen with hematologic disorders such as leukemia. Clitoral tourniquet syndrome, which results from a hair wrapped around the base of the clitoris, has been reported.

CLITORAL HYPOPLASIA. Agenesis of the clitoris is extremely rare. A bifid clitoris may be noted as part of a fusion deformity.

CLITORAL HOOD. An extension of the prepuce that forms a hood over the clitoris is a nonspecific congenital variant. It may become inflamed or abscessed and thus be brought to medical attention. Rarely, labial adhesions may begin at the prepuce, resulting in a preputial fusion that mimics a clitoral hood.

Clitoridectomy (Female Circumcision)

Recent worldwide attention has been directed toward the cultural practice of excising the clitoris and/or vulva of young girls in some African cultures. The surgical procedures range from clitoridectomy (excision of all or part of the clitoris) to infibulation (excision of the clitoris and labia and stitching the raw surfaces together to leave only a small posterior opening for passage of urine and menstrual blood). Female circumcision is thought by many to constitute a public health issue with short- and long-term physical complications and psychologic effects.[5] Short-term complications reported include hemorrhage, severe pain, fatal shock, severe anemia, wound infection, abscesses, septicemia, tetanus, and gangrene. Long-term complications from infibulation result from obstructed urine and menstrual flow and include chronic pelvic and urinary tract infections, dysmenorrhea, infertility, and kidney damage.

Excisional scars are associated with dermoid cysts, keloids, and entrapment neuromas. Infibulated women are at higher risk for complications of childbirth. There is little available scientific research on the psychologic and sexual effects of female circumcision.

It is estimated that at least 100 million women worldwide are circumcised. Increased refugee immigration from Africa in the past decade requires that health professionals be familiar with the practice and its medical ramifications.

BENIGN VULVAR LESIONS

The external genitalia, being composed of ectodermal skin, are subject to an extensive array of dermatologic conditions. The lesions commonly encountered during adolescence are presented here, categorized by their visual appearance on examination.

Vulvar Abrasions and Traumatic Injuries

Abrasions and lacerations of the vulva may be caused by sexual intercourse, instrumentation, masturbation, and trauma. Accidental trauma, typically straddle injuries, may be accompanied by bruising and hematoma formation. Injuries that are suspected to be the result of alleged sexual assault require forensic examination and reporting (see Chapter 102, "Sexual Assault").[6] In an adolescent couple, voluntary sexual intercourse may commonly result in abrasions if the episode is hurriedly or awkwardly performed. Vulvar abrasions usually become painful within 1 to 2 days. On examination, linear abrasions around the posterior fourchette may be noted when the tissue is stretched. Lacerations typically occur in the 6 o'clock position. A yellow exudate from superficial bacterial overgrowth may be seen. Abrasions should be differentiated from the painful ulcerations of herpes simplex infection. Treatment is supportive, with careful hygiene, sitz baths, and application of a topical antiseptic ointment. The abrasions heal in 10 to 14 days. Similar traumatic abrasions may be found on the rectal, anal, or urethral mucosa, depending on the type of sexual intercourse.

Dermatoses

SEXUALLY TRANSMITTED GROWTHS AND LESIONS. The conditions discussed in this section are described in further detail in Chapter 140, "Sexually Transmitted Diseases."

Genital warts. Condylomata acuminata are among the most common external lesions found in adolescents. Variable in size from small solitary lesions to large confluent clusters, the warts are identifiable by their whitish-gray, cornified, "cauliflower" surface. They are of significant interest because of the relationship of the causative human papillomavirus (HPV) to cervical disease.

Bowenoid papulosis. Bowen papules are small (2 to 5 mm), shiny, mahogany-brown elevations on the external genitalia found most often in sexually active adolescents and young adults. Usually referred to as "atypical genital warts," they are associated with HPV type 16 and present an increased risk for cervical neoplasia.[7]

Molluscum contagiosum. Caused by a poxvirus, molluscum is sexually transmittable. The round, pink, umbilicated lesions are small (3 to 7 mm), are filled with a cheesy central core, and tend to cluster on the upper thighs and pubis.

Ulcerative lesions. Most ulcerating sores found on the genitalia are from sexually transmitted diseases (STDs), such as herpes genitalis, syphilis, chancroid, granuloma inguinale, and lymphogranuloma venereum. Other causes of ulcerative lesions include Behçet's disease, Crohn's disease, cutaneous amebiasis, and some staphylococcal lesions.

Contagious skin infestations. These include pediculosis pubis and scabies.

PUSTULAR LESIONS

Folliculitis. This bacterial infection of the sebaceous ducts of the hair follicles is most often caused by *Staphylococcus* organisms. Friction from tight clothing and irritation from shaving the "bikini" area are frequent predisposing factors. Conservative management includes the use of antibacterial soap, avoidance of irritants, and observation. Occasionally a course of oral antibiotics is needed.

Impetigo. Secondary bacterial spread from an infected follicle or a lesion such as a mosquito bite may result in impetigo. The course follows the usual progression from vesicle to pustule to honey-colored, crusting scales. The treatment with oral antibiotics is the same as for impetigo in other parts of the body.

Hidradenitis suppurativa. Skin bacteria (staphylococci, streptococci) can cause infection of the apocrine sweat glands. Sometimes described as "heat rash out of control," the nodular lesions can be widespread and extensive and have foul-smelling, purulent drainage. As with axillary hidradenitis, the condition may be resistant to treatment, but it ultimately undergoes spontaneous resolution, often with residual scarring.

Vaginal varicella. The presentation of chickenpox may include typical pustular lesions on the vulva.

ERYTHEMATOUS SCALING LESIONS

Psoriasis. A psoriatic lesion may appear on the vulva as an erythematous plaque with a violaceous hue. In moist areas, it may or may not have a silvery scale. Diagnostic clues include recurrence in the same spot, lesions elsewhere on the body, and family history. As with psoriasis elsewhere, treatment is difficult. Small lesions may respond to topical steroids. A patient with extensive lesions should be referred to a specialist.

Seborrhea. Seborrheic dermatitis can be found in any area with numerous sebaceous glands. "Dandruff of the vulva" manifests as a mildly pruritic scaling or flaking rash and intertrigo, with redness and cracking of the labial or inguinal skinfolds. It tends to be a chronic, recurrent inflammation. Low-dose topical steroids may be useful on a short-term basis.

Candida *infections.* Usually associated with vaginitis, yeast infections also may cause vulvitis, especially in diabetic patients. *Candida albicans* and

other *Candida* strains are the usual pathogens involved. The eruption is often intensely pruritic, with confluent patches; somewhat discrete, nonelevated margins; and satellite lesions. A wet-mount prep with KOH (potassium hydroxide) may show budding yeast and pseudohyphae. Treatment involves topical application of the same antifungal creams used for vaginal yeast (e.g., miconazole, butoconazole, clotrimazole, terconazole, nystatin).

Tinea cruris. "Jock itch" presents as a confluent red rash with elevated, well-demarcated borders. The crural creases and upper thighs are often involved. The fungal infection may be caused by several dermatophytes, including *Trichophyton*, *Microsporum*, and *Epidermophyton*. The diagnosis is generally made by clinical appearance. Scales obtained by scraping the border of the rash may be prepared as a wet mount with KOH and examined under a microscope for branching hyphae. Several antifungal creams can be used for treatment, including clotrimazole, miconazole, and tolnaftate.

WHITE LESIONS

Lichen sclerosis. The vulva may be affected by several conditions characterized by white patches. Formerly termed "leukoplakia," these disorders are now referred to as dystrophic lesions (hyperkeratosis and lichen sclerosis).[8] Although usually seen in perimenopausal women, lichen sclerosis occasionally may be found in childhood and persist into adolescence. The vulva typically shows a patchy, white bilateral lesion surrounding the vestibule. The epidermis appears atrophic and thin (parchment-like).[9] There may be subepidermal vesicles or lesions that bleed with friction, scratching, or wiping. Histology reveals a chronic underlying inflammatory infiltrate. The cause is unknown; there may be a genetic predisposition, and chronic irritation or scratching may precipitate the onset. Although the lesion may be asymptomatic, adolescents usually complain of pruritus, dysuria, and occasionally vulvar bleeding. Biopsy confirms the clinical diagnosis. There are little data on effective treatment in adolescents. Avoidance of irritants, tight clothing, and scratching; short-term use of topical steroids for pruritus; and trials of topical progesterone cream, as used in postmenopausal women, have been suggested.[8,9]

Vitiligo. Vitiligo, which often begins in adolescence, may cause vulvar depigmentation. The lesions are well-circumscribed white macules similar to those found elsewhere on the body.[8] The cause of the loss of melanin is not known, but it may be associated with an autoimmune process. The vulvar lesions are asymptomatic, may be transient, and do not require treatment.

Vulvitis and Vulvodynia

VULVITIS. Vulvitis is an inflammation of the vulva. Its presenting symptoms include erythema, pruritus, and occasionally a rash, which may be papular, vesicular, or scaling. Often the external vulvitis is associated with vaginitis, but isolated vulvar inflammation may occur. Vulvovaginitis that is caused by infectious organisms is discussed in Chapter 140, "Sexually Transmitted Diseases." Many noninfectious causes of vulvitis exist, as shown in Box 136-1. A thorough history is essential for diagnosis. Because the possible causes are so extensive, it may be expedient to have the patient use a checklist or self-assessment form to gather the history. Physical examination may help identify dermatoses and systemic disease. The main purpose of a careful laboratory evaluation is to rule out specific infections. After sexually transmitted infections, yeast infections, and dermatoses have been excluded, the most likely causes of vulvar inflammation in adolescents are either local irritants or contact irritants.

Local irritants. Vulvar inflammation may result from a combination of excessive moisture, friction of the skin, and bacterial overgrowth by local organisms.[10] Poor hygiene, obesity, and hot weather may precipitate the condition. Excessive cleansing may do the same. Treatment includes careful instructions about perineal hygiene, use of cotton underwear, wearing of loose clothing, application of cornstarch powder to absorb moisture, and short-term use of topical low-dose steroid cream for acute itching or discomfort.[11]

Contact irritants. Contact dermatitis is probably the most common benign disorder of the female genitalia. Numerous substances can produce contact dermatitis of the vulva.[10] The diagnosis is made by identifying the offending chemical. A temporal connection between the use of a new product and the appearance of the rash may simplify the diagnosis. More often the process is one of

---

BOX 136-1
Noninfectious Causes of Vulvitis

LOCAL IRRITANTS
Poor hygiene
Overcleansing
Heat, sweating
Obesity
Intertrigo
Synthetic underwear
Excessive friction
Daily use of minipads

CONTACT IRRITANTS
Bath soaps
Bubble bath, bath oil
Colored toilet paper
Contraceptive foams, gels, inserts
Deodorant sprays
Deodorant tampons, pads
Douches
Dyes (dark clothing)
Hair removers
Latex condoms
Lubricants
Laundry detergents
Laundry bleaches
Perfumes
Shaving cream
Spermicides

PHYSIOLOGIC LEUKORRHEA
Bacterial vulvitis (non-STD)
Coliform bacteria
Streptococci
Staphylococci
Lactobacilli overgrowth

DERMATOSES
Candidiasis
Tinea cruris
Psoriasis
Seborrheic dermatitis
Atopic dermatitis
Lichen sclerosis
Folliculitis
Hidradenitis
Cellulitis
Pinworms
Insect bites
Dermatitis medicamentosa
Allergic reactions (antibiotics)
Stevens-Johnson syndrome

SYSTEMIC DISEASES
Varicella
Measles
Kawasaki disease
Scarlet fever
Crohn's disease
Behçet's disease
Diabetes mellitus
Hypovitaminosis (vitamin A)
Leukemia
Severe anemia

NEURODERMATITIS
Anxiety states
Psychogenic pruritus vulvae
Compulsive masturbation
Vulvodynia

OTHER MISCELLANEOUS CAUSES

elimination, with the patient excluding possible irritants one by one. Patch testing may be tried. Consultation with a dermatologist may be useful in persistent cases. Once the substance is known, treatment consists of avoidance. Manufacturers are increasingly offering household products that are free of irritants, dyes, and perfumes. Young women should be given anticipatory guidance about avoiding bubble baths, feminine deodorant sprays, and other possible irritants to the delicate vulvar area. For acute contact vulvitis, topical steroid creams are very effective. Adolescents must be warned against chronic long-term use, which can cause tissue thinning or systemic reactions.

VULVODYNIA. Many terms have been used for the complaint of persistent vulvar pain that occurs in the absence of any underlying physical findings of infection, contact irritants, or dermatoses. The chronic discomfort is typically described as "burning," "stinging," or "irritating." It has been called psychogenic pruritus vulvae, burning vulva syndrome, psychosomatic vulvitis, and neurodermatitis. McKay[12] recommends the term *vulvodynia* and has identified at least five subgroups: (1) vulvar dermatoses, (2) cyclic vulvitis, (3) vulvar papillomatosis, (4) vulvar vestibulitis, and (5) essential vulvodynia. Since the mid-1980s, there has been a dramatic increase in the number of young women seen with vulvodynia, including adolescents.[13] A meticulous search for causative agents is recommended, including *Candida* cultures, "acetowhitening," and colposcopy to look for evidence of HPV, and biopsy of any questionable areas.

Vulvar papillomatosis (see Plate 1). Vulvar (or vestibular) papillomatosis describes the condition of multiple papillae that may cover all or part of the labia minora. Visible with or without magnification, the appearance is enhanced by application of dilute acetic acid (acetowhitening). The significance of vulvar papillomatosis is unclear, but in some studies it has been associated with HPV infection.[14] Most investigators suggest that no treatment is needed,[15] but patients should be followed for increased risk of cervical neoplasia.

Essential vulvodynia. Essential (or psychogenic) vulvodynia, a diagnosis of exclusion, is uncommon in adolescents, but it may be associated with sexual abuse, sexual guilt feelings, reproductive anxieties, or school phobia.[10] The diagnosis is suggested by chronic symptoms that are unresponsive to therapy and frequent visits in the absence of pathogens. A sympathetic approach includes listening well, searching the patient's history for past trauma, office counseling, and referral for more intensive therapy (if indicated). Biofeedback, stress management techniques, or low-dose antidepressants may be useful.[12] Anatomic causes of pain should be carefully excluded. Membranous hypertrophy of the posterior fourchette, with consequent stricture of the vaginal introitus, has been identified as a cause of dyspareunia and vulvodynia in young women, with complete resolution of symptoms after excision of the posterior vestibular tissue.[16]

Vulvar Masses

Vulvar neoplasms are categorized as either cystic or solid. Most lesions in adolescents are benign, but several malignant variants are known (Box 136-2). Comments on the most common masses found in adolescents are included here.

CYSTIC LESIONS

Bartholin's gland lesions. The glands are located in the 4:30 and 7:30 o'clock positions at the introitus. Inflammation may be acute or chronic. An acute abscess is hot and tender, with pus or erythema at the duct opening. *Neisseria gonorrhoeae* is the classic causative organism, but *Escherichia coli, Proteus mirabilis,* and mixed flora may be cultured. Systemic symptoms such as chills and fever may be present. Treatment includes antibiotics for patient and partner, hot packs, and sometimes incision and drainage.[17] The gland may become a chronic nontender cyst in the wall of the posterior labia minora. Bartholin's cysts, the most common type of vulvar cyst in adolescents, are usually asymptomatic. Recurrent cysts can be treated surgically with a marsupialization procedure. Skene's gland cysts have a similar clinical etiology and clinical presentation (Plate 2).

Papillary hidradenoma. Hidradenomas are benign epidermal cysts arising from the epithelium of the sweat glands. They are most commonly found on the inner

---

BOX 136-2
Vulvar Masses

CYSTIC	
Bartholin's gland cyst	Leiomyoma
Papillary hidradenoma (cystic)	Granular cell tumor
	Lipoma
Epidermal inclusion cysts	Fibroma
Sebaceous cysts	Neurofibroma
Mucinous cysts	Granuloma
Cyst of canal of Nuck	Fibroepithelial polyp
Hydroceles	
Syringomas	MALIGNANT
Lymph node hyperplasia	Melanoma
	Sarcoma
SOLID	Adenocarcinoma
Papillary hidradenoma (solid)	Malignant lymphoma
Hemangioma	

aspect of the labia majora. The typical lesion is small (<1 cm), mobile, well demarcated, painless, and asymptomatic. Occasionally the cyst ulcerates and bleeds if irritated. Simple excision is curative.

Other epithelial cysts. A variety of benign cystic lesions may be found on the vulva.[8] Epidermal inclusion cysts (sebaceous cysts) appear as single or multiple small (2- to 10-mm) firm nodules. They are often found along surgical repair sites (episiotomy, vaginal lacerations), where they may form as a result of entrapment or occlusion of small gland ducts. These cysts are also common along the outer edges of hypertrophied labia minora, perhaps resulting from excessive friction or irritation. No treatment is necessary. Mucinous cysts are typically found on the mucosal surface of the inner labia minora or around the introitus. Like oral mucinous cysts on the inner lip, mucinous cysts form from blocked mucoid glands. They are usually small and transient. These cysts may become large (1 to 3 cm) and painful, in which case surgical excision is curative.

Cysts of canal of Nuck (hydroceles). The canal of Nuck is a rudimentary peritoneal structure that lies in the upper aspect of the labia majora in the middle vulvar area. A hydrocele may form, presenting as a painless, small (1- to 2-cm) swelling in the inguinal region. It is homologous to the hydrocele in males. The cyst should be differentiated from a hernia. Asymptomatic small hydroceles do not require surgery, but cosmetic excision may be considered.

SOLID LESIONS. Solid vulvar neoplasms are rare in adolescents, although virtually all forms of benign neoplastic lesions have been reported.[18] Usually the patient complains of a lump. A careful history, noting onset, growth, changes in appearance, and associated symptoms, should be documented. Solid lesions require biopsy for accurate diagnosis. The differential list of solid tumors is shown in Box 136-2.

Hemangioma. The most common benign, solid vulvar tumor in adolescents is the hemangioma ("strawberry mark"). The lesion may be of either the capillary or cavernous type. Capillary hemangiomas sometimes improve with time. The growth of pubic hair may mask the appearance of either type after puberty; hence, observation over time may be recommended. Surgical and sclerosing treatments should be avoided, since the resultant scars may be disfiguring. Occasionally a hemangioma may be mistaken for a traumatic hematoma if a past history has not been elicited.

Fibroepithelial polyps. These common skin tags are soft, skin colored, and pedunculated and range in size from 2 to 12 mm. They are usually found in skinfolds or inguinal creases that are subject to friction from movement or tight elastic underwear bands. Typically asymptomatic, these polyps may become swollen, painful, or ulcerated, in which case they should be removed.

Leiomyomas and neurofibromas. These benign subepithelial tumors are firm, discrete, slow-growing masses, most frequently occurring in the labia majora. One half of patients with vulvar neurofibromas have von Recklinghausen's disease.[19] Lipomas can be distinguished by their softer fatty tissue feel. Excision is diagnostic and should be considered for larger growths that may be unsightly or may cause discomfort.

Granular cell tumors. Although granular cell myoblastomas are rare, 5% develop on the vulva.[20] The lesion presents as an asymptomatic, solitary, well-defined mass. Although such lesions are benign, wide excision is recommended to prevent recurrence.

URETHRAL LESIONS

Urethral caruncle. This is the most common benign tumor of the female urethra. It presents as a bright-red polypoid growth protruding from the meatus. It is usually asymptomatic, but on occasion it may cause symptoms of urethritis such as hematuria, dysuria, or urinary frequency. The differential diagnosis includes urethral hemangioma, papilloma, or polyp.

Urethral prolapse. Most often seen in prepubertal girls, this condition presents as a circumferential eversion of urethral mucosa protruding through the meatus. Typically, it resolves spontaneously and rarely requires surgical resection.

MALIGNANT VULVAR LESIONS

True vulvar malignancies are uncommon in children and adolescents, but the physician must be watchful for them during examination. Biopsy of suspicious lesions will help to prevent misdiagnosis. Two types of malignant lesions deserve mention: malignant melanoma and sarcoma.

Malignant Melanoma

The incidence of melanoma has been increasing over the past 30 years, and 3% to 7% of cases involve a vulvar lesion. Melanoma is the second most common vulvar malignancy in women.[21] Adolescent and young adult patients are reported in most clinical case studies.[21,22]

Melanoma tends to have an unpredictable but often aggressive course in young patients. In most cases vulvar lesions are found on the labia, introitus, or clitoral area. The lesion is usually black, blue-black, or brown, but it may be mottled or have an atypical appearance. The surface is smooth and slightly elevated, with notched margins. Four histologic types are reported: superficial spreading melanoma (50%), nodular melanoma (22%), lentigo maligna melanoma (14%), and acral lentiginous type (14%), which is most commonly found in Asian and black patients.[21-23] Prognosis depends on the thickness of the lesion and the depth of invasion at diagnosis. Patients with lesions less than 1 mm thick have an excellent prognosis when wide excision is performed; those with more than 1 mm have only a 33% survival rate at 2 years.[8]

Sarcoma

Sarcomas, although rare, are the most common vulvar malignancy in teenagers.[20] The lesion often presents as a tender labial swelling similar in appearance to a Bartholin's gland infection, but it is unresponsive to antibiotic treatment. Exploratory incision reveals the solid neoplasm. Rhabdomyosarcomas disseminate quickly and are usually fatal despite aggressive radical vulvectomy, regional node dissection, and chemotherapy. Slower-growing fibrosarcomas and liposarcomas have a better prognosis.

Other Vulvar Malignancies

Vulvar intraepithelial neoplasia, also called vulvar carcinoma in situ or Bowen's disease, is typically found in women in the third and fourth decades of life. This condition is associated with HPV types 6 and 11, and its incidence is increasing in younger age groups. Variable in appearance, the lesions range from asymptomatic dark-colored papules to pruritic lumps or scaly white, red, or pigmented patches. Invasive carcinoma of the vulva rarely occurs before age 40. Paget's disease, or carcinoma of the apocrine glands, occurs mainly in 50- to 70-year-old women.

A number of other lesions can occur on the vulva, including almost all dermatologic conditions that affect skin elsewhere on the body.

VAGINAL FINDINGS

The vagina (a term derived from the Latin word for "sheath") is composed of four walls of smooth muscle (anterior, posterior, and two lateral walls) that lead from the introitus to the cervix. It is lined with stratified squamous epithelium. In the pubertal adolescent the walls are deep pink with smooth rugae. The spaces between the vaginal walls and the cervix are called fornices.

The vagina is subject to fewer disorders than the skin of the external genitalia. This section reviews vaginal findings that may be encountered during the adolescent pelvic examination in three categories: congenital anomalies, benign vaginal lesions, and malignant lesions. The most common vaginal complaint in teenagers is vaginal discharge, the causes of which may range from physiologic leukorrhea to serious sexually trans-

mitted infection. (The diagnosis and treatment of specific vaginitis is discussed in detail in Chapter 140, "Sexually Transmitted Diseases.") Comments on noninfectious causes of vaginal discharge complete the following discussion.

CONGENITAL ANOMALIES

Hymenal Variations

The hymen is a thin membrane located within the introitus. Although embryonically it is formed from the urogenital sinus and thus is technically part of the external genitalia, the hymen is usually discussed as a vaginal component.

IMPERFORATE HYMEN (PLATES 3, 4, 5). The hymen is a remnant of the urogenital diaphragm, which normally undergoes central degeneration to become patent. If it remains imperforate, it will block the outflow of mucus in childhood and menstrual blood at menarche. Mucocolpos, the presence of mucus in the obstructed vagina, is usually asymptomatic and often remains undetected unless a careful vaginal inspection made in childhood reveals the bulging hymen. At menarche the obstructed menstrual outflow produces hematocolpos, the presence of blood in the blocked vagina, and the symptom of primary amenorrhea. Because of its elasticity, the vagina may fill with 500 to 1000 ml of blood or mucus before symptoms develop, often causing a delay in diagnosis. After six to eight menstrual cycles, the girl may start complaining of pelvic pain. On examination, the bulging membrane will appear blue-black from the retained blood. Treatment is simple hymenectomy. A microperforate hymen has a very small opening, usually found high on the anterior aspect. Menstrual flow also remains obstructed. Slight irregular spotting may be the only symptom.

HYMENAL CONFIGURATIONS. Excellent studies describing hymenal variations in prepubertal children have been published to provide guidelines for evaluation of childhood sexual abuse.[24-26] Descriptive studies on hymenal findings in adolescent women have also become available.[27] At present, there are no longitudinal studies of the hymen throughout puberty. Estrogenization at puberty alters the configuration of the hymen: the membrane thins, the opening enlarges, the anterior portion may regress or disappear so that only a posterior rim remains, and other changes occur.[28] Despite the changes, it is useful to borrow the standardized terminology for prepubertal hymenal configurations and apply it to findings in the adolescent. Thus, the old terms of "virginal" or "marital" introitus can be replaced with objective descriptions (Fig. 136-2).

The circumferential or annular ring hymen is typical of

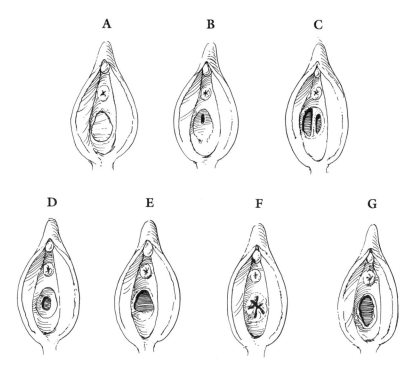

Fig. 136-2. Variations of the hymen. **A,** Imperforate. **B,** Microperforate. **C,** Septate. **D,** Circumferential (annular ring). **E,** Posterior rim. **F,** Fimbriated. **G,** Hymenal remnants.

the younger child. The posterior rim configuration is often found in pubertal girls. Scalloping is a normal variant, producing a fimbriated (or denticular) hymen. Occasionally, septate bands are found across the introitus. These may break spontaneously, through the use of tampons, or from other trauma. If an intact hymen is subject to sufficient stretching, from sexual intercourse or other causes, breaks or lacerations occur that eventually heal as hymenal remnants. With extreme stretching of the vaginal orifice, typically from childbirth, nubbins of hymenal tissue called myrtiform caruncles may form.[28] A rigid hymen, composed of firm, inelastic tissue, may result in a painful speculum examination or dyspareunia. Treatment consists of progressive dilation performed at home by the patient or hymenectomy for extreme cases.

Cautious adolescent specialists advise parents or patients that there is no objective way to determine "virginal status" by a pelvic examination. After puberty the well-estrogenized female has increasing elasticity of the introitus, which can stretch to accommodate a medium Pederson speculum (or small penis) without disrupting the hymen. Conversely, there are many explanations other than sexual intercourse for an apparently "broken" hymen, including congenital variations, childhood injuries, self-exploration, masturbation, and pelvic examinations. Hymenal findings in virginal adolescents who use tampons are not significantly different from findings in those who use pads.[27]

Vaginal Anomalies

Rock and Azziz[1] present an excellent review of vaginal anomalies. Although malformations are not common, they may compromise fertility. Early diagnosis provides an opportunity for both treatment and reproductive counseling. Embryologically, anomalies stem from (1) müllerian duct agenesis, (2) disorders of vertical fusion, or (3) disorders of lateral fusion (Fig. 136-3). Lesions are often part of a multifactorial picture. Approximately 20% to 30% of patients have associated renal anomalies (e.g., renal agenesis, malrotation, double collecting system), so that careful evaluation is essential, including cystogenitography and pelvic magnetic resonance imaging (MRI). Since approximately 80% of girls with major genitourinary malformations also have anomalies of other systems (gastrointestinal, musculoskeletal, respiratory, central nervous, cardiac), a meticulous total physical examination is important.[3]

ABSENT VAGINA (MÜLLERIAN AGENESIS). The müllerian system evolves into the uterus and the upper third of the vagina. Müllerian agenesis (Mayer-Rokitansky-Küster-Hauser syndrome) therefore results in absence of the uterus and part of the vagina. It occurs in 1 in 2500 to 1 in 5000 females and is the second leading cause of primary infertility (after gonadal dysgenesis).

The young woman usually presents for care because of

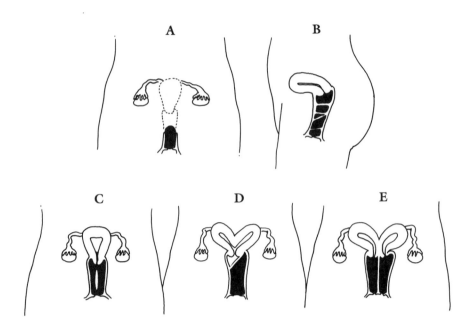

Fig. 136-3. Vaginal anomalies. **A,** Müllerian agenesis (absent upper third of vagina and absent uterus). **B,** Transverse vaginal septa (multiple). **C,** Partial longitudinal vaginal septum (nonobstructive). **D,** Obstructive longitudinal septum (with hemivagina and bicornuate uterus). **E,** True double vagina with double cervix (uterus didelphys).

primary amenorrhea. Occasionally, a sexually active older adolescent may present for a pregnancy test, and only after careful questioning does the history of primary amenorrhea emerge. Approximately one of five cases of primary amenorrhea is caused by müllerian agenesis.[29] Secondary sexual characteristics are present, including normal breasts and pubic hair. The pelvic examination reveals a blind vaginal pouch and no palpable uterus. Ultrasonography confirms the absence of the uterus. Ovaries are normal in müllerian agenesis. Karyotyping and laparoscopy are recommended to differentiate absent vagina from testicular feminization (androgen insensitivity syndrome), a 45,XY end-organ defect with intraabdominal testicles that should be removed to prevent risk of malignant changes. Pelvic MRI, ultrasonography, and intravenous pyelography (IVP) may be recommended, since 15% of patients with müllerian agenesis have some associated renal anomalies. Another 12% of patients have skeletal anomalies, usually of the thoracic and lumbar spine. Vaginoplasty to lengthen the vagina may be needed to reduce dyspareunia. The adolescent and her family should be counseled about infertility issues and options. Since the ovaries function normally, gamete retrieval for transfer into a surrogate uterus is possible.

Very rarely, an isolated fusion defect of the urogenital sinus results in an absent vagina accompanied by a functional uterus.[30] The adolescent patient will have primary amenorrhea and cyclic pelvic pain from retrograde reflux of menstrual blood into the fallopian tubes.

Vaginoplasty and surgical creation of an outflow exit should be attempted as soon as the condition is diagnosed in order to prevent endometriosis.

TRANSVERSE VAGINAL SEPTA (DISORDERS OF VERTICAL FUSION). Normally, the caudal ends of the fused müllerian ducts, called the müllerian tubercles, progress downward to join the upward progression of the urogenital sinus, and canalization of the resultant solid tube forms the vagina. Disorders of this vertical fusion or canalization may produce transverse vaginal septa. These septa are rare, occurring in 1 in 80,000 females. The septum is a plate of fibromuscular tissue that partially or completely obstructs the vagina. It may occur at any level: high transverse septa are the most common (46%), followed by middle (35%) and low (19%) septa.[1] Occasionally, there are multiple septa.

Often unnoticed in childhood, unless vaginal patency is tested for some reason, an obstructive transverse septum produces hematocolpos and primary amenorrhea after menarche, similar to imperforate hymen. Pelvic pain may result from distention or from backflow into the fallopian tubes. On speculum examination, the septum is usually bulging and blue-black from retained blood. Ultrasonography reveals a normal uterus, distinguishing the condition from müllerian agenesis. IVP should be performed to rule out ureteral anomalies. Treatment consists of surgical resection performed as soon as the condition is diagnosed. Prolonged obstruction of menstrual flow may cause subsequent endometriosis and compromised fertility.[31]

LONGITUDINAL VAGINAL SEPTA (DISORDERS OF LATERAL FUSION). Failure of the two müllerian ducts to fuse can produce longitudinal septa continuing down a portion of the length of the vagina. In nonobstructive lesions the patency of the cervix is maintained and menstruation is normal. A complete longitudinal septum, or a partial septum in the upper vagina in opposition to the cervix, usually is associated with uterine fusion defects (uterus didelphys, septate uterus, or bicornate uterus).[29] A longitudinal septum is termed "obstructive" if it results in a blind vaginal pouch ("hemivagina") with no visible cervix. This variant usually is associated with a double uterus and renal agenesis.[32] Pain from obstructed menstrual outflow may cause the adolescent to seek medical care. Surgical incision and resection will establish patency.

DOUBLE VAGINA. A true double vagina is accompanied by a double cervix and a double uterus. Each vagina is anatomically complete and each ends in a separate cervix. On pelvic examination a separate set of cultures and Pap smears should be taken from each side. No corrective surgery is necessary, since the obstetric risk is usually low.

BENIGN VAGINAL LESIONS

Condylomata Acuminata

Genital warts are the most common lesions found on examination of the vagina of an adolescent patient (see Plate 6). Vaginal condylomas are less common than external vulvar lesions, but they grow more rapidly and are harder to manage (see Chapter 140). They may be associated with condylomas of the cervix or vulva, or may appear only as vaginal lesions.

Vaginal Cysts

MESONEPHRIC CYSTS (GARTNER'S DUCT CYSTS). Remnants of the embryonic wolffian ducts within the vaginal walls form small sacs that may fill with serous fluid to produce a Gartner's duct cyst. The swelling is palpable on the lower anterolateral vaginal side wall. Small cysts are usually asymptomatic, may be single or multiple, and require only observation. Larger cysts may bulge into the introitus, causing discomfort. On initial visualization the cyst may look like an imperforate hymen or a low transverse septum, yet the examiner's finger can probe past the bulge.[33] Large cysts may be treated with a marsupialization procedure. A section of cyst wall should be excised and sent for biopsy to rule out other neoplasms.

PARAMESONEPHRIC DUCT CYSTS. Remnants of the müllerian ducts may produce cysts in the upper third of the vaginal walls or in the fornices. These sacs are lined with endometrium-like cells that bleed cyclically with menstruation, thus becoming symptomatic after menarche.[33] Incision and drainage produce old blood. Treatment consists of excision of the cyst, with care taken to protect the nearby ureter. As with all müllerian duct lesions, an IVP is recommended to exclude renal anomalies.

EPITHELIAL INCLUSION CYSTS. Small, firm epithelial cysts can present in the hymenal area of the introitus as well as on the labia (see discussion of vulvar lesions on p 1049).

CYSTOCELES AND RECTOCELES. If the elastic and muscular support of the vaginal walls weakens, a cystocele or rectocele may develop. Although these conditions are more common in middle-aged women, when elastic tissue normally deteriorates, they may occur in adolescents as a result of trauma or childbearing. The cystocele bulges downward from the anterior wall, especially when the patient coughs or strains. A rectocele bulges upward from the posterior wall (for visualization, the patient is asked to bear down). In teenagers, treatment involves Kegel exercises to strengthen the vaginal walls. Surgical correction is rarely necessary.

Polypoid Lesions of Pregnancy

Vaginal polyposis is characterized by numerous small fibroepithelial polyps throughout the vagina and the portio of the cervix; the lesions are usually associated with pregnancy. A pregnant 15-year-old was reported to have polyposis vaginalis that disappeared spontaneously by 6 weeks post partum.[34] The benign polyps of vaginal polyposis must be differentiated from sarcoma botryoides. In general, a biopsy should be performed for any vaginal polyp to rule out neoplastic lesions.

MALIGNANT VAGINAL TUMORS

Vaginal cancers account for less than 2% of gynecologic cancers at any age, and such cancers were very rare in adolescents until the rise in incidence of diethylstilbestrol (DES)-related clear cell adenocarcinoma in the 1970s.

Adenosis

Disorders related to the use of DES are becoming of only historical interest in adolescents. DES was widely used between 1942 and 1971 for threatened abortion or high-risk pregnancies. Several million pregnant women were exposed. Since the use of DES during pregnancy ceased in the early 1970s, most offspring of these women are now aged 20 to 50. Up to 90% of the offspring exposed before 10 weeks of gestation may have vaginal adenosis, cervical or vaginal malformations, or slightly increased fetal wastage due to lower tract anomalies.[35] A pelvic examination by experienced experts was recommended for DES-exposed daughters at age 14.[36] Typical conditions found included the following: *adenosis,* tall mucus-secreting endocolumnar glands on the ectocervix or the upper vagina; *cervical hood or cervical collar,* a prepuce-like ring of vaginal mucosa projecting around the cervix; *cervical cockscomb,* a firm, scalloped ridge arising from the upper vagina and extending over the cervix; and *beefy-red granular epithelial tissue,* appearing as patchy spots on the upper vagina or ectocervix.[36] The Pap smear might contain suspicious-looking cells if a vaginal specimen were obtained. Colposcopy defines the borders of the lesions, and biopsy confirms the diagnosis of adenosis.[37] Fortunately, the feared epidemic of adenocarcinoma from DES exposure did not develop. About 1 in 1000 exposed offspring have been found to develop clear cell adenocarcinoma. The DES registry contains over 500 cases, detected at an average age of 19 years.[35] The neoplasm is malignant and can be fatal.[38] It is not yet known what will happen when the cohort reaches older age, but a potential association with squamous cell carcinoma and breast cancer has been theorized.[39,40] It also has been suggested that an increase in adenosis may be seen again because of the current widespread use of clomiphene citrate, a drug very similar to DES, in the treatment of infertility.[39] Once diagnosed, adenosis is observed without institution of therapy. Most cases of adenosis resolve spontaneously.[33] Because of the malignant potential, vigilant long-term follow-up of DES-exposed women and offspring is recommended.[41]

Sarcoma Botryoides

Until DES-related adenocarcinoma became common, sarcomas were the most common vaginal malignancy in adolescents. Sarcoma botryoides is a mixed mesodermal tumor, the polypoid variety of rhabdomyosarcoma. Vaginal locations are most common in children under age 5 years. The cervical location is more common in adolescents. Vaginal sarcoma botryoides presents as a mass at the introitus that has a grapelike appearance. Treatment is with chemotherapy and conservative surgery.[39,42]

Malignant Melanoma

The initial presentation of melanoma may occur in the vagina or in the vulvar area (see discussion on p 1049). Although the incidence of vaginal melanoma is less than vulvar (0.03 per 10,000 compared with 0.1 per 10,000), the prognosis is even worse (19% 5-year survival compared with 50% for vulvar). Black race is an adverse prognostic factor.[43]

Primary Vaginal Squamous Cell Carcinoma

Vaginal intraepithelial neoplasia almost always occurs in older women (median age 50 years). Only 10% of squamous cell carcinoma occurs in women under 40 years old. An extensive literature review reported only five well-documented cases found in adolescents aged 11 to 20.[44]

NONINFECTIOUS CAUSES OF VAGINAL DISCHARGE

Physiologic Leukorrhea

Physiologic leukorrhea refers to normal vaginal discharge found in estrogenized females. At any given time, 10% of postmenarcheal girls complain of vaginal discharge; hence, it is important to distinguish physiologic secretions from specific causes of vaginitis.[45]

At puberty, females produce vaginal secretions in response to fluctuating levels of hormones. Normal discharge follows a typical cyclic pattern of scant clear secretions early in the menstrual cycle, sticky ("egg-white") mucus around the time of ovulation, and cloudy mucoid secretions in the second half of the cycle. The discharge is nonirritating, has no objectionable odor, and has no noticeable color, although it may dry yellow on the underwear. The amount of discharge normally increases at ovulation, before menstruation, with sexual arousal or increased stress, and in response to hormone stimulation from oral contraceptives or pregnancy. Physiologic leukorrhea is composed primarily of mucus produced by the cervical glands that is mixed with secretions from sebaceous, sweat, and Bartholin's glands and with desquamated squamous epithelial cells.

The normal flora of the vagina has been called "a dynamically changing eco-system" and includes a wide range of indigenous microorganisms that vary among individuals and by age, hormonal status, hygiene, and other factors.[46] Lactobacilli (Döderlein's bacilli) are the predominant species. These "healthy bacteria" metabolize sloughed-off squamous cells to produce lactic acid, which maintains the normal acidic vaginal pH of 3.5 to 4.5.[45] The acidic environment is protective, since most vaginal infections require a pH greater than 4.8 for growth. Other common facultative organisms, including *Corynebacterium* (diphtheroids), *Staphylococcus epidermidis,* and streptococci, can be found, along with numerous anaerobes.

The diagnosis of physiologic leukorrhea is confirmed

by (1) a wet-mount prep showing only an abundance of mucus, epithelial cells, and large nonmotile rod bacteria (lactobacilli); (2) an acid pH; and (3) negative tests for STDs. Treatment involves reassurance and education. Anticipatory guidance about normal physiologic discharge as part of routine well-child care would be helpful for many peripubertal girls.

Nonspecific Vaginitis

Nonspecific vaginitis is a term now used to refer to a symptomatic overgrowth of normal flora.[47] It is distinguished from bacterial vaginosis, a specific infection of mixed pathogens including *Gardnerella vaginalis, Mobiluncus, Mycoplasma* spp., *Ureaplasma* spp., and others (see Chapter 140, "Sexually Transmitted Diseases"). In nonspecific vaginitis, coliform bacteria from the rectal area are the most common organisms found (68%), producing a brown or greenish discharge with fecal odor. Coliform vaginitis may result from bacterial migration or from anal sexual practices if scrupulous hygiene is not maintained.[48] The second most common organisms are streptococci and staphylococci, which may be transferred from the respiratory tract or may be found indigenously. A symptomatic overgrowth of lactobacilli has been reported to cause a pasty yellow discharge with a slight stinging or burning sensation, presumably from excessive lactic acid produced by the large numbers of bacteria.[49] Vaginitis symptoms also may result from many of the contact irritants noted in the discussion of vulvitis (Box 136-1). Treatment of nonspecific vaginitis focuses on good perineal hygiene and avoidance of sources of contaminating bacteria. To prevent vulvovaginitis, adolescents would benefit from being taught the following ten healthy habits for perineal hygiene:

1. Avoid vulvar and vaginal irritants.
2. Wipe from front to back (to decrease the chance of fecal contamination).
3. Wash the genital area daily with warm water and bland soap. Rinse and dry thoroughly.
4. Wear absorbent (100% cotton) underwear with loose-fitting elastic bands.
5. Do not share intimate clothing, washcloths, or towels.
6. Change sanitary pads or tampons frequently (every 6 hours). Do not use tampons overnight (to prevent toxic shock syndrome).
7. If sexually active, use condoms each and every time sexual intercourse takes place.
8. Be sure sexual partners practice good hygiene.
9. Avoid anal intercourse.
10. See a medical caregiver promptly for any genital symptoms (discharge, odor, sores, pain, discomfort).

Infectious Vaginitis

Vaginitis that is caused by specific organisms, including *Candida* spp., *Trichomonas* spp.; the mixed pathogens of bacterial vaginoses; and sexually transmitted infections are discussed in detail in Chapter 140.

In differentiating normal from abnormal vaginal discharge, it is helpful to note that normal discharge is largely asymptomatic with an acid pH (3.5 to 4.5), whereas abnormal discharge is symptomatic (itching, burning, odor, color) and often has a pH greater than 4.5 if bacteria or *Trichomonas* spp. are involved.

Vaginal Foreign Bodies

Numerous foreign bodies may be retained in the vaginal cavity and eventually produce symptoms that bring the patient to medical attention. Toilet tissue in children and tampons in teenagers are the most commonly found foreign bodies. Forgotten contraceptive diaphragms or vaginal sponges are not unusual. Self-inserted objects may be found more commonly in mentally limited adolescents. (Deliberately inserted foreign objects in young children should raise a suspicion of sexual abuse.)

Presenting symptoms include atypical menses (light menses or persistent spotting due to obstruction or heavier bleeding due to mucosal erosion), a serosanguineous discharge, and a strong odor. The pronounced foul odor is a symptom highly suggestive of a foreign body. On examination the object may be difficult to see if it is lodged in the posterior fornix. It can sometimes be felt on bimanual or rectal examination. Removal is usually accomplished by inserting long forceps through an open speculum placed in the vagina. After removal of the object, a fulminant odor may fill the room, requiring a strong deodorizer and several hours of waiting before the room can be used again. The adolescent should be warned of the possibility of such an odor in advance in order to decrease any embarrassment. Removal of the object is curative, but an acidifying vaginal cream may be used daily for 1 week to soothe the mucosa.

References

1. Rock JA, Aziz R: Genital anomalies in childhood, *Clin Obstet Gynecol* 30:682-696, 1987.
2. Reindollar RH, Tho SPT, McDonough PG: Abnormalities of sexual differentiation: evaluation and management, *Clin Obstet Gynecol* 30:697-713, 1987.
3. Quigley MM, Gwatkin RBL: Embryology and developmental defects of the female reproductive system. In Scott JR, DiSaia PJ, Hammond CB, Spellacy WN, editors: *Danforth's obstetrics and gynecology,* ed 6, Philadelphia, 1990, JB Lippincott.
4. Rimsa ME: An illustrated guide to adolescent gynecology, *Pediatr Clin North Am* 36:639-663, 1989.
5. Toubia N: Female circumcision as a public health issue, *N Engl J Med* 331:712-716, 1994.

6. Bays J, Jenny C: Genital and anal conditions confused with child sexual abuse trauma, *Am J Dis Child* 144:1319-1322, 1990.

7. Stafford EM, Greenberg H, Miles PA: Cervical intraepithelial neoplasia III in an adolescent with bowenoid papulosis, *J Adolesc Health Care* 11:523-526, 1990.

8. DiSaia PJ, Woodruff JD: Disorders of the vulva and vagina. In Scott JR, DiSaia PJ, Hammond CB, Spellacy WN, editors: *Danforth's obstetrics and gynecology,* ed 6, Philadelphia, 1990, JB Lippincott.

9. Carli P, Bracco G, Taddei G, et al: Vulvar lichen sclerosis: immunohistologic evaluation before and after therapy, *J Reprod Med* 39:110-114, 1994.

10. Rosenfeld WD, Clark J: Vulvovaginitis and cervicitis, *Pediatr Clin North Am* 36:489-511, 1989.

11. Sanfilippo JS: Adolescent girls with vaginal discharge, *Pediatr Ann* 15:509-519, 1986.

12. McKay M: Vulvodynia: a multifactorial clinical problem, *Arch Dermatol* 125:256-262, 1989.

13. Reid R, Omoto KH, Precop SL, et al: Flashlamp-excited dye laser therapy of idiopathic vulvodynia is safe and efficacious, *Am J Obstet Gynecol* 172:1684-1696, 1995.

14. Welch JM, Nayagam M, Parry G, et al: What is vestibular papillomatosis? A study of its prevalence, aetiology, and natural history, *Br J Obstet Gynaecol* 100:939-942, 1993.

15. Dennerstein GJ, Scurry JP, Garland SM, et al: Human papillomavirus vulvitis: a new disease or an unfortunate mistake? *Br J Obstet Gynaecol* 101:992-998, 1994.

16. Barbero M, Micheletti L, Valentino MC, et al: Membranous hypertrophy of the posterior fourchette as a cause of dyspareunia and vulvodynia, *J Reprod Med* 39:949-952, 1994.

17. Aghajanian A, Bernstein L, Grimes DA: Bartholin's duct abscess and cyst: a case control study, *South Med J* 87:26-29, 1994.

18. Gallup DG, Talledo OE: Benign and malignant tumors, *Clin Obstet Gynecol* 30:662-670, 1987.

19. Horbelt DV, Delmore JE: Benign neoplasms of the vulva. In Sciarra JJ, editor: *Gynecology and obstetrics,* vol I, revised ed, Philadelphia, 1995, JB Lippincott.

20. Underwood PB, Kreutner A: Neoplasms and tumorous conditions of the lower genital tract and uterus. In Kreutner AK, Hollingsworth DR, editors: *Adolescent obstetrics and gynecology,* Chicago, 1978, Mosby–Year Book; pp 479-490.

21. Brand E: Vulvovaginal melanoma, *Gynecol Oncol* 33:54-60, 1989.

22. Ronan SG, Eng AM, Briele HA, et al: Malignant melanoma of the female genitalia, *J Am Acad Dermatol* 22:428-435, 1990.

23. Wright TC, Richart RM: A pigmented vulvar lesion: malignant melanoma, *Contemp Obstet Gynecol* 36:129-142, 1991.

24. Emans SJ, Woods ER, Flagg NT, et al: Genital findings in sexually abused, symptomatic and asymptomatic girls, *Pediatrics* 79:778, 1987.

25. Pokorny SF, Kozinerz C: Original studies: configuration and other anatomic details of the prepubertal hymen, *Adolesc Pediatr Gynecol* 1:97-103, 1988.

26. McCann J, Wells R, Simon M, Voris J: Genital findings in prepubertal girls selected for nonabuse: a descriptive study, *Pediatrics* 86:428-439, 1990.

27. Emans SJ, Woods ER, Allred EN, Grace E: Hymenal findings in adolescent women: impact of tampon use and consensual sexual activity, *J Pediatr* 125:153-160, 1994.

28. Pokorny S: The physical examination of the reproductive systems in female children and adolescents, *Curr Probl Obstet Gynecol Fertil* 13:202-213, 1990.

29. Buttram VC: Müllerian anomalies and their management, *Fertil Steril* 40:159-163, 1983.

30. Lichtman R, Duran P: The vulva and vagina. In Lichtman R, Papera S, editors: *Gynecology: well-woman care,* Norwalk, CT, 1990, Appleton & Lange; p 183.

31. Rock JA, Zacue HA, Dlugi AM, et al: Pregnancy success following surgical correction of imperforate hymen and complete transverse vaginal septum, *Obstet Gynecol* 59:448, 1982.

32. Shibata T, Nonomura K, Hidehiro K, et al: A case of unique communication between blind-ending ectopic ureter and ipsilateral hemi-hematocolpometra in uterus didelphys, *J Urol* 153:1208-1210, 1995.

33. Delmore JE, Horbelt DV: Benign neoplasms of the vagina. In Sciarra JJ, editor: *Gynecology and obstetrics,* vol 1, revised ed, Philadelphia, 1995, JB Lippincott.

34. Tobon H, McIntyre-Seltman K, Rubino M: Polyposis vaginalis of pregnancy, *Arch Pathol Lab Med* 113:1391-1393, 1989.

35. Emans SJ, Goldstein DP: *Pediatric and adolescent gynecology,* ed 3, Boston, 1990, Little, Brown; pp 411-413.

36. Robboy SJ, Moller KL, Kaufman RH, et al: Prenatal DES exposure: recommendations of the DES-adenosis project for identification and management of exposed individuals, NIH Publ. No. 81-2049, reprinted March 1981.

37. Helmerhorst TJ, Wijnen HJ, Kenemans P, et al: Colposcopic findings and intraepithelial neoplasia in DES-exposed offspring, *Am J Obstet Gynecol* 161:1191-1194, 1989.

38. Melnick S, Cole P, Anderson D, Herbst AL: Rates and risks of diethylstilbestrol related to clear cell adenocarcinoma of the vagina and cervix, *N Engl J Med* 316:514-518, 1987.

39. Gallup DG, Talledo OE: Benign and malignant tumors, *Clin Obstet Gynecol* 30:662-670, 1987.

40. Bibbo M, Haenszel WM, Wied GL: A twenty-five year follow-up study on women exposed to diethylstilbestrol during pregnancy, *N Engl J Med* 298:763-767, 1978.

41. Mittendorf R, Herbst AL: Managing the DES-exposed woman: an update, *Contemp Obstet Gynecol* 39:62-80, 1994.

42. Raney RB, Hays DH, Tefft M, Triche TJ: Rhabdomyosarcoma and the undifferentiated sarcomas. In Pizzo PA, Poplack DG, editors: *Principles and practice of pediatric oncology,* ed 2, Philadelphia, 1993, JB Lippincott.

43. Weinstock MA: Malignant melanoma of the vulva and vagina in the United States, *Am J Obstet Gynecol* 171:1225-1230, 1994.

44. DiDomenico A: Primary vaginal squamous cell carcinoma in the young patient, *Gynecol Oncol* 35:181-187, 1989.

45. Chantigan PD: Vaginitis: a common malady, *Prim Care* 15:517-547, 1988.

46. Cook RL, Vincente RL, Sobel JD: The vaginal microflora of normal women. In Sobel JD, editor: *Vulvovaginal infections. Current concepts in diagnosis and therapy,* New York, 1990, Academy Professional Information Services.

47. Vandeven AM, Emans SJ: Vulvovaginitis in the child and adolescent, *Pediatr Rev* 14:141-147, 1993.

48. Cohall AT, Warren A: Persistent vaginal discharge in a sexually active adolescent female, *Adolesc Health Care* 12:58-59, 1991.

49. Burnhill MS: Sorting out the major vaginal infections, *Contemp Obstet Gynecol* 29:47-62, 1987.

CHAPTER 137

Cervical Findings and the Pap Smear

•

Roberta K. Beach

The uterine cervix is the site of a significant number of pathologic conditions and its evaluation is an important focus for reproductive health care.[1] Two of the primary reasons for performing an adolescent pelvic examination are to screen for cervical cancer and to obtain cervical specimens to test for sexually transmitted infections. In this chapter the cervical findings that may be encountered during the examination are described in three categories: anatomic variations, benign cervical lesions, and malignant cervical lesions. Some findings are apparent on visual inspection (Fig. 137-1). Others are determined by cytology, colposcopy, or biopsy. The Papanicolaou (Pap) smear and management of abnormal cytologic findings are discussed in detail.

CERVICAL FINDINGS

ANATOMIC VARIATIONS OF THE CERVIX

The cervix, often described as the neck of the uterus, enlarges with estrogen stimulation at puberty to become a 2- to 2.5-cm protrusion from the posterior vaginal wall. The visible portion, or ectocervix, has an anterior and a posterior lip. The endocervix contains the endocervical canal, which has an external os that is visible on speculum examination and an internal os that opens into the uterus. The external os on a nulliparous cervix appears as a small, round opening ("dimple"). After childbirth, it widens into a transverse slit ("smile"). The internal os is normally closed and resists pressure from a swab or probe. A freely patent or open os may signal a spontaneous abortion in a pregnant patient. On bimanual examination, the cervix feels firm, similar to the cartilage at the tip of the nose. Numerous endocervical glands secrete a clear or cloudy mucus in response to hormone stimulation. With estrogen stimulation alone, the mucus has a clear, egg-white consistency that can be drawn into

long strings (spinnbarkeit) and dries on a glass slide in a fernlike pattern under the microscope (the "fern" test). With the production of progesterone, the mucus turns cloudy and does not show the fernlike pattern.

Variations in Appearance

ECTROPION (PLATE 7). Formed from the müllerian system, the cervix is initially covered with endocolumnar cells. During childhood and adolescence, the endocolumnar cells are gradually replaced with squamous cells in an orderly progression from the vaginal walls toward the cervical os. The border between the smooth, dull-pink squamous cells and the dark-red, granular endocolumnar cells is called the squamocolumnar junction. During early and middle adolescence, the squamocolumnar junction still may be visible with a ring of deep-red endocolumnar cells surrounding the external os, a condition known as ectropion. The ring is typically 5 to 10 mm wide, has a smooth regular border, and does not bleed to touch. By adulthood, the endocolumnar cells usually have regressed into the endocervical canal and are no longer visible. Hormone stimulation from oral contraceptives or during pregnancy may slow cellular replacement and prolong the visible ectropion.[2] The squamocolumnar junction, as an area of metaplasia, and the exposed endocolumnar cells are vulnerable to a variety of infectious organisms, including *Neisseria gonorrhoeae, Chlamydia trachomatis,* and human papillomavirus (HPV). The presence of this vulnerable ectropion may partially explain why sexually active teenagers are at highest risk for contracting sexually transmitted infections and for increased rates of later cervical neoplasia.[3]

EROSION. Cervical erosion is a manifestation of chronic inflammation or trauma. It appears around the os as a patch of beefy-red tissue with irregular borders and usually bleeds easily when rubbed with a swab (friability). It may be accompanied by mucopurulent cervical discharge and generalized cervical hyperemia. The term *erosion* is nonspecific but is useful in differentiating

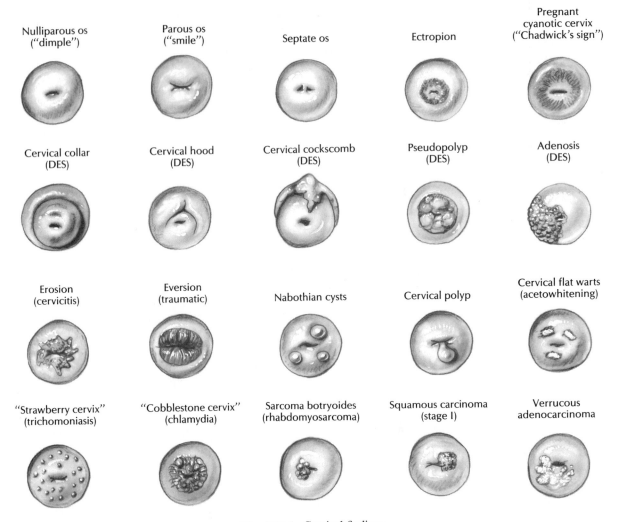

Fig. 137-1. Cervical findings.

inflammation from normal ectropion. Cervical erosion is a sign of chronic cervicitis[2] (Plate 8) (see Chapter 140, "Sexually Transmitted Diseases").

Cervical motion tenderness, which is significant pain felt by the patient when the cervix is pressed or moved during the bimanual examination ("chandelier sign"), is also a sign of cervical and intrauterine infection.

EVERSION. Another somewhat vague term, cervical *eversion* in adolescents is best used to describe the protrusion of granular red vascular membrane from the endocervical canal as a result of cervical laceration or trauma. In young children, some authors use the term *eversion* interchangeably with *ectropion* to describe endocolumnar tissue covering the cervix.[4]

CHANGES IN EARLY PREGNANCY. At approximately the fourth week of pregnancy, the consistency of the cervix softens to become similar to that of the lips (Hegar's sign), rather than being firm like that of the nose, and this change is often the earliest physical sign of pregnancy noted on pelvic examination. The cervix of the gravid uterus acquires a bluish or purple color termed *cervical cyanosis* (Chadwick's sign) starting around the sixth to eighth week of pregnancy.

Diethylstilbestrol-Related Structural Anomalies

Significant anomalies of the vagina and the cervix may be found in 30% of diethylstilbestrol (DES)-exposed offspring, and cellular changes may be noted in up to 90%.[5] Although DES has been the most widely used compound to cause defects, over 75 DES-type hormone preparations have been prescribed, and some, such as clomiphene citrate, remain in current use for women who are presumed to be nonpregnant. Caregivers who perform pelvic examinations should remain aware of possible findings.[6] Vaginal findings related to DES exposure include partial longitudinal and transverse vaginal septa; absence, fusion, or other abnormalities of the vaginal fornix; and vaginal adenosis (see Chapter 136, "Perineal and Vaginal Findings").

Cervical structural abnormalities have been variously

described by different authors. The diethylstilbestrol-adenosis (DESAD) project, sponsored by the National Cancer Institute since 1974, uses the following descriptive terminology[6]:

Cervical hood. Markedly enlarged folds of cervical stroma and epithelium protrude over the anterior cervical lip to create a prepuce-like hood.

Cervical collar. Lower and broader folds of cervical stroma rim the cervix, either partially or completely.

Cervical cockscomb. A firm, raised, scalloped transverse ridge of cervical stroma, usually anterior in position, hangs over the cervix in a manner similar to its namesake. When viewed under colposcopy, it has a grapelike glandular appearance.

Cervical pseudopolyp. A circumferential constricting groove (sulcus) around the ectocervix causes a protrusion of thickened or hyperplastic stroma from the endocervical canal, which may be polypoid in appearance. The presence of the os at the center of a cervical pseudopolyp differentiates it from a true polyp.

Adenosis of ectocervix. A particularly large cervical ectropion (>1 cm) in an older adolescent, especially if it extends to the vaginal fornix, should raise the suspicion of DES-type hormone exposure. Adenosis is confirmed by biopsy, which reveals tall, secretory (mucus-secreting) columnar glands. On visual inspection, the cervix may have a "strawberry" appearance with red granular spots of variable size. On bimanual examination, the cervix may feel grainy. Adenosis does not stain with acetic acid or iodine solution.

No treatment is indicated for DES-related structural changes of the cervix. Adenosis may regress over time. Rates of infertility or obstetric complications appear to be slightly higher in DES-exposed offspring, although the data are inconclusive as to the cause. Counseling is appropriate in individual cases. All women exposed to DES-type hormones in utero should be kept under surveillance for potential, but rare, clear cell adenocarcinoma. Annual Pap screening is sufficient. The value of routine colposcopy is still undetermined.[7] DES-grandchildren (the daughters of DES-daughters) are now reaching adolescence. Although no genital or reproductive anomalies have been reported to date, screening and follow-up of this third generation are recommended.[8,9]

Other Congenital Anomalies

Congenital anomalies of the cervix, if not DES related, are primarily the result of disorders of lateral fusion of the müllerian ducts.

SEPTATE CERVIX. A septum may be located only in the cervix, or it may extend downward into a longitudinal vaginal septum or upward into a septate uterus. A solitary cervical septum is usually asymptomatic, but it may obstruct entry of the cotton swab or cytology brush during the pelvic examination, thus leading to its diagnosis. The septum may rupture during childbirth, causing hemorrhage. The condition is amenable to surgical correction by hysteroscopic incision of the septum.[10] Cervical anomalies suggest uterine anomalies, and further evaluation is indicated.

DOUBLE CERVIX. Lack of fusion of the müllerian ducts may result in a double reproductive system. The double cervix is typically associated with a double vagina and double uterus (uterus didelphys). The condition is compatible with normal fertility, although there is a risk of preterm delivery.[10] As with uterine anomalies, cervical anomalies may be difficult to define visually. Definitive diagnosis may require hysterosalpingography, ultrasonography, magnetic resonance imaging, or laparoscopy.

BENIGN CERVICAL LESIONS

Nabothian Cysts (Plate 9)

A secretory cervical gland (nabothian gland) may become obstructed with mucus, forming a retention cyst (nabothian cyst). The cyst typically appears as a pearl-like nodule on the ectocervix. Retention cysts may be variable in size; single or multiple; and clear, yellow, or blue in color. They can be associated with chronic cervicitis. Small cysts require no treatment. Rarely, a cyst may be large enough to simulate an adnexal mass on ultrasonographic imaging.[11]

Endometriomas

An endometrioma is a submucosal cyst caused by endometriosis. Although rare, on the cervix it appears as a 2- to 3-mm dark-red or reddish-blue round spot ("powder-burn"). Usually asymptomatic, cervical endometriomas may produce intermenstrual or postcoital spotting or bleeding.[12]

Cervical Polyps

Cervical polyps are common benign lesions usually found in menstruating women. Formed from an overgrowth of epithelial tissue, a polyp usually arises in the endocervical canal and protrudes through the external os. Polyps are typically painless, bright-red, and soft and may be pedunculated. If traumatized, the polyp may bleed. Women with cystic fibrosis are at risk for endocervical polyps, and may have a dry viscous cervical mucus that may inhibit sperm migration.[13] Polyps can be removed through a simple office procedure. The polyp is grasped with forceps and twisted off; the base of the lesion is then cauterized with a silver nitrate stick.[14] The specimen should be sent for pathologic examination to rule out sarcoma botryoides.

Cervical Stenosis

The cervical os or endocervical canal may become stenotic from scar tissue after chronic infection, extensive cauterization, cryosurgery, radiation, or deep surgical cone biopsy (conization). Backflow from obstructed menses may cause dysmenorrhea, or the patient may present because of infertility. On examination, probing of the cervical os is difficult or painful. Treatment consists of repeated dilation, usually done with the patient under general anesthesia to minimize pain.

Inflammatory Lesions

Cervicitis. Because it is frequently exposed to trauma resulting from sexual intercourse, childbirth, masturbation, or douching, the cervix is often inflamed. Mild noninfectious inflammation is a very common microscopic finding of no clinical consequence. If a specific organism is suspected as the cause, the term *cervicitis* is generally used.[15] Cervicitis from infectious causes has significant clinical consequences for the adolescent and requires vigorous attention. All the organisms that can cause vaginitis, and most of those associated with sexually transmitted infections, can cause cervicitis. The cervix is red with patchy erosion and has a mucopurulent discharge that makes a white swab appear yellow. The primary symptom of acute cervicitis is leukorrhea. The inflamed ectocervix and the endocervical canal are friable and bleed easily when rubbed. A wet mount and standard tests for infection should be obtained.[16] Treatment varies according to the suspected organism. In particular, *C. trachomatis* has been associated with mucopurulent cervicitis.[2] Presumptive treatment is warranted pending test results.[17] (See Chapter 140, "Sexually Transmitted Diseases.")

"Strawberry" cervix. Classically, the *Trichomonas vaginalis* organism causes petechiae in the vagina or on the cervix. The tiny, bright-red raised dots with underlying cervical hyperemia produce a stippled appearance termed "strawberry" cervix.

"Cobblestone" cervix. The *C. trachomatis* organism may produce a pattern of raised, edematous, follicular-appearing, hypertrophic ectopy on the cervix. A similar follicular appearance on the conjunctivae is known to ophthalmologists as "the cobblestones of Boston."

Condylomata acuminata (plate 10). Genital warts caused by HPV may be found on the vulva, vagina, or cervix. Cervical warts are usually subclinical ("flat condyloma") and difficult to detect with the naked eye. After acetowhitening, they may be visible with colposcopy. Otherwise, the diagnosis may be suggested by cervical cytologic examination. A prominent, warty-looking "cauliflower" growth on the cervix should be viewed with suspicion and carefully evaluated to rule out verrucous adenocarcinoma.[14]

Herpetic lesions (plate 11). Type 2 herpesvirus hominis (herpes progenitalis) can cause lesions on the cervix similar to those on the vulva. These lesions may appear as multiple, small, superficial ulcers with or without vesicles, often surrounded by diffuse inflammation and edema. Cervical lesions may be associated with leukorrhea, abnormal spotting, and pain.[18] Treatment is the same as for vulvar herpes. (See Chapter 140, "Sexually Transmitted Diseases.")

MALIGNANT CERVICAL LESIONS

Cervical cancer is rare in adolescence. Among all women, 90% of cervical cancers are squamous cell carcinomas, 5% are endocervical adenocarcinomas, 2% are clear cell adenocarcinomas, and the remainder are sarcomas and lymphomas.[19] In the last three decades the predominant cervical cancer among adolescents has been clear cell adenocarcinoma related to in utero exposure to DES,[20] followed by infrequent occurrences of cervical sarcoma botryoides and adenocarcinoma.

There is growing concern that the rates of true cervical squamous cell carcinoma will rise for women under age 25, because the rates of abnormal cervical cytologic findings and the incidence of precursor lesions (cervical intraepithelial neoplasia) in adolescents have increased significantly in recent years.[21-23] Traditional risk factors associated with cervical cancer—early age of first intercourse, multiple sexual partners, high parity, and low socioeconomic class—are now interpreted in the context of sexually transmitted etiologic agents such as HPV.[23] Prevention of cervical carcinoma will depend on changing the sexual practices of adolescents and young adults.

Clear-Cell Adenocarcinoma

Clear-cell adenocarcinoma related to DES exposure has been the most common malignancy of the lower genital tract in adolescents for the last 30 years, with over 500 cases listed in the Registry for Research on Hormonal Transplacental Carcinogenesis. The age range is 7 to 34 years, with peak incidence of diagnosis at age 19.[24] Approximately 40% of lesions involve the cervix. About one third of patients with clear-cell adenocarcinoma have no history of in utero exposure to hormones. As Emans and Goldstein[20] observe, these patients are more likely to have cervical than vaginal lesions. Since clear-cell adenocarcinoma of the cervix was well known even before the widespread use of DES, some additional etiologic factor is presumed to be involved. The epidemiology differs from squamous cell carcinoma in that patients are more likely to be nulliparous, single, and of higher social class.[23,25]

The lesion usually starts within the endocervix and grows silently in a papillary manner. In an advanced stage, the tumor will be clinically evident as a polypoid, ulcerated, or granular lesion on the cervix alone or extending to the vaginal fornix.[18] Abnormal cells on cytologic examination may be reported. Cervical clear-cell adenocarcinoma is classified as stages I to IV, with an 85% 5-year survival rate for stage I lesions and no survival with stage IV disease.[20]

The differential diagnosis of clear-cell adenocarcinoma includes atypical forms of benign microglandular hyperplasia of the cervix. Glandular epithelium of the cervix may proliferate with the hormone stimulation associated with pregnancy, oral contraceptives, or progestin. The usual histologic features of microglandular hyperplasia are now well known, but atypical patterns still may be confused with clear-cell adenocarcinoma.[26] With the increasing use of long-acting progestins (Depo-Provera, Norplant) as contraceptive agents in adolescents, pathologists need to be aware of such features to avoid misinterpretation of this condition as a malignancy.

Sarcoma Botryoides

The cervix is the most common location of sarcoma botryoides (polypoid rhabdomyosarcoma) when it occurs in adolescents. Initially the tumor may appear as a small polypoid lesion that may be mistaken for a benign cervical polyp. Gradually it progresses into the classic grapelike cluster at the cervical os. Traditional treatment has been radical hysterectomy and postoperative chemotherapy, but current recommendations are for conservative surgery plus combined chemotherapy with vincristine, actinomycin-D, and cyclophosphamide.[27]

Mesonephric Adenocarcinoma

Adenocarcinomas (other than clear-cell types) are rare in teenagers. When present, they are usually of mesonephric origin. These adenocarcinomas are asymptomatic until bleeding occurs in the advanced stage; hence, diagnosis is often delayed in young adolescents or those who are not sexually active, who would not undergo routine pelvic examination. Treatment is with radical hysterectomy, partial vaginectomy, and pelvic node dissection, sparing the ovaries. Prognosis is usually poor because of the late diagnosis.[28]

Squamous Cell Carcinoma

In common usage, *cancer of the cervix* refers to squamous cell carcinoma. Squamous cell carcinoma of the cervix is a progressive disease that begins as cervical dysplasia, develops into carcinoma in situ, and finally becomes invasive cancer. The scope of histologic changes from dysplasia through carcinoma in situ were previously referred to as *cervical intraepithelial neoplasia* (CIN). Although the 1991 revised Bethesda system for Pap smear classification uses the term *squamous intraepithelial lesion* (SIL), for this discussion CIN will be used, to be consistent with the studies reported. Early cytologic detection and treatment of the precursory cervical dysplasia can essentially eliminate the risk of progression to invasive cancer. Since cervical dysplasia may first appear in adolescence, screening for cervical changes is an important component of the pelvic examination of an adolescent patient.

The role of HPV in cervical neoplasia is covered in Chapter 140, "Sexually Transmitted Diseases." The clinical aspects of CIN that are relevant to adolescents are discussed here.

INCIDENCE. For the United States in 1996, the National Cancer Data Base estimates an incidence of 50,000 new cases of cervical carcinoma in situ, 15,700 new cases of invasive cancer, and 4900 deaths from advanced disease.[29] The average age at diagnosis is now 35 years for carcinoma in situ and 45 years for invasive cancer. The age range for cervical cancer has declined steadily over the past 20 years, and the incidence of precancerous cervical dysplasia in adolescents has been rising.[21-23,30,31] Rates vary widely, depending on the population studied. The frequency of cervical dysplasia in sexually active teenagers in the United States who were screened from 1984 to 1991 ranges from 2% (large national databases) to 18% (inner city teenage mothers).[21,22] The rate of biopsy-proven carcinoma in situ in this age group is about 2.6 in 1000.[21] Invasive cervical cancer is still rare in adolescence.[31]

ETIOLOGY. CIN can be considered a sexually transmitted disease (Plate 12). It is virtually nonexistent in females who have never had intercourse. It is highly associated with early age of first coitus, multiple sexual partners, and the partner's number of additional sexual partners. Although the causative agent is not known, HPV, particularly types 16 and 18, is strongly associated with increased risk of CIN.[32] Women with HPV infection are 10 to 15 times more likely to develop CIN than women without HPV infection,[33] and young women who develop an HPV infection before age 25 are 40 times more likely to progress to carcinoma in situ.[34] Dysplasia begins in the transformation zone of the squamocolumnar junction. Adolescents are presumed to be at greater risk because this zone is often still exposed on the ectocervix (as ectropion) and hence vulnerable to the etiologic agent.

Other risk factors include a history of other sexually transmitted diseases (STDs), nonuse of barrier contraceptive methods, use of oral contraceptives, high number of pregnancies, smoking, race, and low socioeconomic class.[22,35] Isolation of independent risk factors is difficult because the behavioral patterns are interwoven and result in a complexity of confounding variables. Cervical neoplasia is most likely a multifactorial process in which sexually transmitted viruses play a key role.

DISEASE PROGRESSION. Cervical cancer develops relatively slowly. The average time for mild dysplasia to progress to carcinoma in situ is 7 years. It is important to realize that dysplasia may not progress at all. In large studies, up to 60% of cases of mild dysplasia return to normal over 3 years of observation, especially in younger women.[36] On the other hand, if dysplasia does progress, there is concern that it may do so more aggressively in younger women. Small studies indicate a worse prognosis in young women, but this finding has not yet been confirmed by large population-based studies.[23,37] The progression from carcinoma in situ to invasive cancer takes an average of 10 years, but in 5% of women it may take less than 3 years.[38] Invasive carcinoma, that which has broken through the basement membrane, then proceeds through four stages, classified by depth of invasion. Five-year survival rates range from 85% for stage I lesions (invasion confined to cervix) to less than 20% for stage IV lesions (extension to adjacent organs and distant metastases).[29]

DIAGNOSIS. Screening, classification of lesions, management of abnormal Pap smears, and the use of colposcopy and cervicography are discussed in the Pap Smear section of this chapter.

TREATMENT. CIN is a curable lesion that should have no serious sequelae if treated early. If cervical cytologic examination and colposcopic evaluation reveal a high-grade squamous intraepithelial lesion (encompassing moderate and severe dysplasia and carcinoma in situ), treatment is indicated. Cone biopsy (conization) of the cervix is no longer recommended in adolescents because of the unnecessary risk of complications such as hemorrhage and cervical stenosis.[39] Ablative therapies are currently standard practice, including cryosurgery in many settings or laser therapy with the CO_2 laser or the neodymium:yttrium-aluminum-garnet (Nd:YAG) laser in referral centers.[40] Cryotherapy for CIN in adolescents also carries a small risk of cervical stenosis with unknown implications for future fertility.[41] Loop electrosurgical excision procedure (LEEP) also shows promise as an alternative low-cost, effective treatment.[42] It is judicious to refer adolescents with cervical neoplasia to medical centers that have advanced equipment, patient volume, and expertise for definitive treatment. Management of low-grade squamous intraepithelial lesions is somewhat controversial, depending on the perceived risk of progression versus the likelihood of regression. (See discussion of abnormal Pap smears, p 1066.)

PREVENTION. Like other STDs, cervical cancer is a preventable condition, and adolescence is the ideal time to encourage protective sexual behaviors. It is appropriate to advise the adolescent patient about abstinence, delayed onset of first coitus, monogamy, limited sexual partners, consistent use of condoms, and the "safer sex" practices that have been well defined.

THE PAP SMEAR

The Pap smear is the basic screening test for cervical cancer. It is also called the cervical smear or the cervical/vaginal cytologic examination. Its widespread use has been associated with a significant reduction in death rates from invasive cervical carcinoma over the past 40 years. Criticism of ambiguous terminology, and the need to strengthen quality assurance measures in cytopathology, led to the 1988 Bethesda System for reporting cervical and vaginal cytologic findings. Revised and simplified in 1991, the Bethesda System has now replaced older classification systems and is used by over 80% of cytology laboratories in the United States.[43,44] It is essential to understand that the cervical smear is only a screening device to detect the presence of abnormal cells. Further evaluation, usually with colposcopy and biopsy, is necessary for diagnosis of precancerous or cancerous lesions. Sexually active teenagers are an important population for cervical screening. In this section aspects of screening, collection technique, interpretation of findings, and follow-up of abnormal tests that are relevant to adolescents are discussed. Controversy exists in all these areas, and careful attention is necessary to stay abreast of rapid advances in knowledge and changing recommendations.

VALUE OF CERVICAL CYTOLOGY

George Papanicolaou and Herbert Traut published their classic work *The Diagnosis of Uterine Cancer by Vaginal Smear* in 1943, based on observations of cervical cytology that began in 1924. The Pap smear gradually achieved widespread use, and in 1957 the American Cancer Society (ACS) began recommending annual screening. Since its endorsement by the ACS and the National Cancer Act of 1974, the Pap test has become a well-established standard of care in preventive health protocols. During this time the death rate from invasive cervical cancer has decreased by 70% and the 5-year survival has increased to 80% owing to earlier diagno-

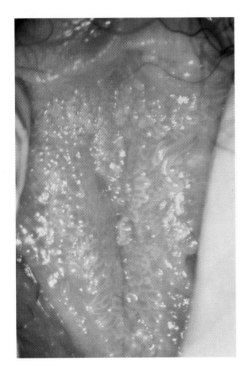

PLATE 1

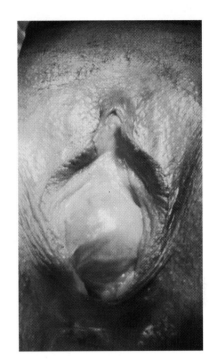

PLATE 2

PLATE 1   Vestibular physiologic papillomatosis

PLATE 2   Right Skene's gland cyst

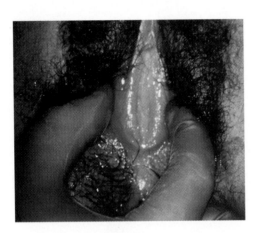

PLATE 3

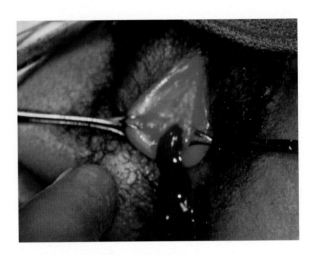

PLATE 4

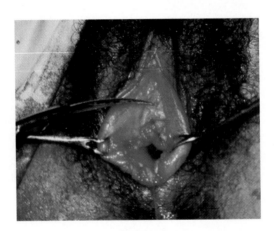

PLATE 5

PLATE 3   Imperforate hymen (preoperative)

PLATE 4   Imperforate hymen (intraoperative)

PLATE 5   Imperforate hymen (postoperative)

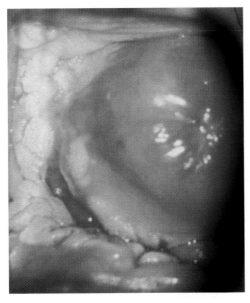

PLATE 6

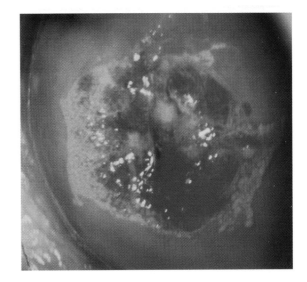

PLATE 7

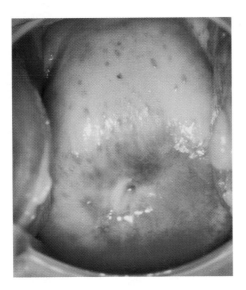

PLATE 8

PLATE 6   Condylomata acuminata with traumatic laceration of the vagina (1½ years after 2 cryosurgeries on the cervix shown in Plate 12)

PLATE 7   Exocervix, squamocolumnar junction and transformation zone after application of acetic acid

PLATE 8   Chronic cervicitis, chlamydia

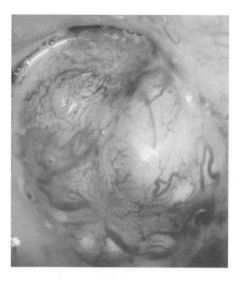

PLATE 9

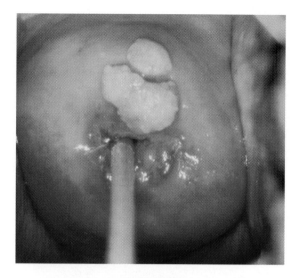

PLATE 10

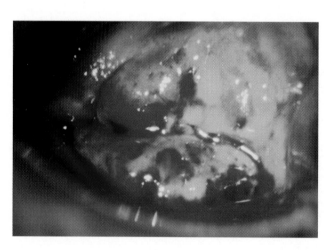

PLATE 11

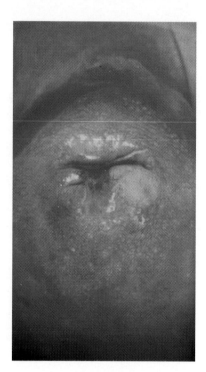

PLATE 12

PLATE 9   Nabothian cysts

PLATE 10   Condylomata acuminata of the cervix

PLATE 11   Acute cervicitis, herpes simplex virus type II

PLATE 12   Cervical intraepithelial neoplasia grade II-III, mosaic (patient, age 15, para 0010)

sis.[33,45] Because it affords early detection of precancerous lesions, which can be cured with virtually 100% success, the Pap test is perhaps "the only truly effective cancer screening test known today."[46]

Although precise data on the sensitivity and specificity of the Pap smear are lacking because of methodologic problems, its specificity is probably greater than 90%.[47] Sensitivity remains one of the controversial areas, with false-negative results currently reported to be 10% to 40%.[48] Even in the best of certified laboratories in 1991, false-negative diagnoses were made in 5.1% of smears with CIN.[49] Test-retest reliability is likewise undependable. For reasons that are unclear, if the original smear is abnormal, a repeat test several days or weeks later may be read as normal in up to 60% of patients with significant neoplastic lesions.[46] Human error appears to be the primary cause of erroneous readings.[49] The Bethesda System, better collection techniques, and reductions in workloads of cytotechnologists should improve these statistics. Targeted rescreening with the use of new computerized technology (such as PAPNET/Auto Pap 300QC)—combining image analysis with sophisticated neural nets—may detect up to 92% of false-negative smears.[49,50]

Despite the methodologic issues, the Pap test is highly regarded as a safe, effective screening test that should be made accessible to all women at risk.[48] Cervical cancer continues to be a significant cause of cancer death in women because of the failure to reach enough of the target population: half of the women diagnosed with invasive cervical cancer have never had a Pap test.[45,46] Adolescence is an ideal time for young women to become familiar with the value of preventive well-woman health care.

SCREENING RECOMMENDATIONS

There has been significant variation in opinion and practice regarding who should be screened, how often, and at what ages. Lack of consensus stems from debate over the natural history of cervical cancer, reliability of repeat screening, and priorities placed on costs, mathematical models, medicolegal considerations, ethics, and other factors. Pap smear controversy peaked in the mid-1980s, but some degree of consensus has now been achieved.

In 1996, the revised Guide to Clinical Preventive Services, second edition, published by the U.S. Preventive Services Task Force, recommended "routine Papanicolaou (Pap) testing for all women who are or have been sexually active, beginning with the onset of sexual activity (or at age 18 if the sexual history is unreliable) and repeated at least every 3 years."[51]

The new guidelines are consistent with the American Cancer Society's 1990 recommendations: "All women who are, or have been, sexually active, or have reached age 18, should have an annual Pap test and pelvic examination. After a woman has had three or more consecutive satisfactory normal annual examinations, the Pap test may be performed less frequently at the discretion of her physician."[52]

This guideline represents a consensus recommendation adopted in 1988 by the ACS, the National Cancer Institute, the American College of Obstetricians and Gynecologists, the American Medical Association, the American Nurses Association, the American Academy of Family Physicians, and the American Medical Women's Association.[53]

The interval of 1 to 3 years "at the physician's discretion," instead of the older recommendation of annual Pap tests for all women, is related to the slow progression of cervical cancer and the desire for cost effectiveness. The high-risk factors justifying more frequent annual screening are listed in Box 137-1. It is well accepted that sexually active teenagers are a high-risk group in need of screening for both cervical cytology and STDs. The risk factors of early age of first coitus (18 years or younger) and multiple partners apply to most U.S. teenagers, since the average age of first intercourse is 16 years, with most teenagers reporting two or more partners at the time of survey (see Chapter 9, "Development of Sexual Behavior"). These current patterns of sexual behavior indicate that pelvic examinations should be a routine aspect of care for many early and middle adolescents and that it would be prudent to repeat examinations annually. For some urban clinic settings, on the basis of patient risk factors, it is appropriate to recommend annual pelvic examinations starting at age 16.

Specific screening recommendations for adolescents have been published by the American Medical Association as part of its Guidelines for Adolescent Preventive

---

BOX 137-1
Risk Factors for Cervical Cancer
(Indications for Annual Pap Screening)

First coitus before age 18
Multiple partners (two or more)
Partners with multiple sexual contacts
History of sexually transmitted disease (including
    human papillomavirus infection)
Previous abnormal Pap smear
Diethylstilbestrol exposure in utero
Smoking
Oral contraception (or lack of barrier contraceptive) possibly

---

Based on recommendations of the American Cancer Society (1988) and the U.S. Preventive Services Task Force (1989).

Services (GAPS) and by the American Academy of Pediatrics.[54,55] Both recommend annual Pap screening for sexually active adolescents and routine screening starting at age 18, whichever comes first. The cost effectiveness of screening teenagers has been questioned, because of older studies indicating that most abnormal Pap findings in adolescents are minor, that 65% of cases of adolescent cervical dysplasia eventually revert to normal without intervention, and that the 15% of cases that progress to carcinoma in situ do not do so before age 21.[56] It is suggested that routine Pap screening of sexually active teenagers is not justified and could be delayed until age 20. However, most reviewers note that for adolescents the annual gynecologic examination also provides the opportunity for STD screening, discussion of contraceptive needs, health risk assessment, anticipatory guidance, and other preventive measures.[54] Since an annual examination for sexually active teenagers should be carried out for these reasons, neither major expenditure nor reorganization is required to incorporate Pap screening into existing clinical practice.[57] Because no definitive recommendations apply to all women, decisions on age of screening and frequency should be individualized on the basis of patient profiles.

CERVICAL (PAP) SMEAR TECHNIQUE

To increase the accuracy of screening, significant changes have occurred over the past few years in recommendations for how the Pap smear should be performed.[49,50] The quality of the cervical smear depends on the sampling method used. Correct technique is essential to produce a slide that can be accurately interpreted. An optimal specimen from an adolescent contains cells from three areas: (1) the endocervix, evidenced by the presence of endocervical columnar (glandular) cells; (2) the squamocolumnar junction (also called the transformation zone), which is the site where cervical neoplasia first develops; and (3) the ectocervix, evidenced by the presence of squamous epithelial cells. In peri- or postmenopausal women, a vaginal wall sample from the fornix is also obtained to help detect cancer cells shed from the endometrium or ovaries.[45,46] The presence of endocervical columnar cells is important for accurate screening, since cervical intraepithelial neoplasia is detected two to three times more frequently in smears with endocervical cells than in those without them.[59] The 1991 Bethesda System now requires evidence of an endocervical component for the slide to be rated "satisfactory" without limitations.

Collection Devices

Since the mid-1980s, several new cellular collection tools have been introduced that enhance the quality of the Pap slide. In the past the most common technique recommended involved the use of a cotton swab for endocervical sampling and an Ayers wooden spatula for ectocervical sampling. Many controlled studies have demonstrated the superiority of an endocervical brush over the cotton swab for the preparation of endocervical samples and the detection of CIN, and hence the combination of brush plus spatula is now the recommended technique.[60] In these studies the presence of adequate endocervical material increased from 60% to over 80% when the endocervical brush was used. Newer wide brushes with elongated tips (e.g., Cell-Sweep, Papette) that allow excellent combined ectocervical and endocervical cell samples from a single device have been introduced,[61,62] but their cost effectiveness remains to be shown.

Slide Preparation

Another recent change in technique is the recommendation that both ectocervical and endocervical samples be plated on a single slide rather than on two separate slides (Fig. 137-2). The primary stimulus for this change is to lessen the cytotechnologist's fatigue by reducing the number of slides to be read. The use of a single slide requires agility in applying fixative to the specimens. Ideally, one sample should be plated on half the slide and fixed immediately with a carefully aimed aerosol fixative. A piece of cardboard can be used to protect the unplated half. Then, the second sample is plated on the remaining half of the slide and fixed. If there is any fixative on the

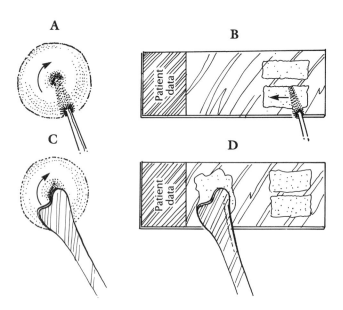

Fig. 137-2. Single-slide method for plating a cervical smear. **A,** Endocervical specimen. **B,** Plating is done with reverse rolling motion. Fixation is done immediately with the unplated half covered. **C,** Ectocervical specimen (includes the transformation zone). **D,** Plating is done on the remaining half of the slide. Fixation is done immediately.

slide before application of the specimen, it will prevent adherence of cells; hence, careful technique is needed. Alternatively, both specimens may be obtained first, then immediately applied to the slide and fixed with a single application of fixative. The slide should be drenched until the fixative drips freely. Commercially prepared aerosol or spray cytofixatives are widely used, replacing the older method of immersion of slides in a jar of 70% to 95% alcohol. Ideally, aerosols should be sprayed from a distance of 25 cm. Immediate fixing is essential. Air drying will cause cellular distortion and artifacts, resulting in an unsatisfactory specimen (Box 137-2).

Patient Data

Frosted-tip glass slides are used for Pap smears. Patient identification is written on the frosted end in pencil, since ink "bleeds" when the slides are processed. The Bethesda System requires specific data on the accompanying forms for proper interpretation of the smears: last menstrual period, type of specimen (cervical, endocervical, vaginal), and patient history (pregnant, postpartum, use of intrauterine device [IUD], hysterectomy, irradiation). Box 137-3 lists the steps required to obtain an optimal cervical smear.

Value of Wet Mounts

Preparation of wet mounts and cervical cultures at the time of the Pap smear in asymptomatic young women helps in the interpretation of minimally abnormal smears and probably decreases the need for repeat smears and colposcopy.[63] This is especially true for smears showing atypical cells of undetermined significance, which in adolescents have been associated with bacterial vaginosis and chlamydial infection. In 83% of patients with an initial abnormal Pap smear and evidence of infection, a normal Pap smear is noted after the infection is cleared.[63]

BOX 137-2
Reasons for Unsatisfactory Specimen

Scant cellularity
Poor fixation or preservation
Presence of foreign material (e.g., lubricant)
Obscuring inflammation
Obscuring blood
Excessive cytolysis or autolysis
No endocervical component (if intact uterus)
Not representative of anatomic site listed
Other causes

Based on 1991 Bethesda System for reporting results of cervical cytologic examination. Limitations should be described in the report.

INTERPRETATION OF CERVICAL SPECIMEN

Over the past 50 years, several different classification systems have been used to report screening results. Papanicolaou originally used a set of five Roman numerals to define class I (negative for cancer cells) through class V (positive for cancer cells.) This numerical system was replaced by a descriptive classi-

---

BOX 137-3
Steps for a Satisfactory Cervical (Pap) Smear

1. The patient should not be bleeding from the cervix or have a significant vaginal infection. If frank infection is noted, delay the Pap smear procedure until after treatment. (Blood or inflammation obscures cells.)
2. Ideally, the patient should not have douched, had sexual intercourse, or used vaginal medications or spermicides within the preceding 24 hours. (All may disturb integrity of the cervical cells.)
3. Prepare clean frosted-tip glass slide(s) with patient identification written in pencil. (Ink "bleeds" when slides are processed.)
4. Prepare accompanying forms with full patient data required by the laboratory. (Without data, the specimens cannot be correctly interpreted.)
5. Properly position the patient, use good illumination, and visualize the cervix with a warm speculum, using only water for lubrication if needed. (Lubricants may cause cell lysis or obscure reading.)
6. Excessive cervical mucus should be gently removed with a swab. The Pap smear should be obtained before other tests are done. (Vigorous swabbing of the cervix or endocervical canal will destroy cell integrity.)
7. Obtain the endocervical sample. Insert the cytology brush to 2 cm into the endocervical canal and rotate 180 degrees (90 degrees if pregnant) only once. Remove and plate carefully onto slide. Fix immediately.
8. Obtain ectocervical/transition zone specimen. Place long tip of Ayers spatula in os, press firmly, and rotate 360 degrees around the cervix. Plate onto glass slide. Fix immediately.
9. When plating specimens, roll out a thin, even layer of cells. Do not rub on slide or overlap layers. (Rubbing will cause cell distortion.)
10. Fix immediately by drenching with aerosol or spray fixative, or immerse slides in 70% to 95% alcohol. (Even momentary air drying will cause artifacts and cell lysis.)

fication in the 1970s, in which results were reported as negative, atypia, dysplasia (mild, moderate, severe), carcinoma in situ, and invasive carcinoma. In the 1980s, Richart's proposed classification, based on findings of CIN (CIN 1, 2, 3), gained widespread acceptance. Because the different terminologies were ambiguous and confusing, the National Cancer Institute (NCI) convened a major consensus workshop in Bethesda, Maryland, in 1988 to make recommendations for effective reporting. The resultant 1988 Bethesda System was then revised and simplified in 1991 by the National Cancer Institute Workshop,[43] and it is now accepted by certified laboratories as the standard reporting classification.

Accurate interpretation of cervical smears is one of the most challenging areas of microscopy. Initial screening of cervical slides is done by trained cytotechnologists. All abnormal smears are then reviewed by a pathologist for final interpretation. For quality control, the Centers for Disease Control and Prevention (CDC) recommends rescreening of 10% of all negative smears. The final interpretation of the cytologic specimen must then be reported to the clinician for patient follow-up.

Bethesda System

The basic premise of the Bethesda System is that the cytology report is a medical consultation that should provide effective communication between the cytopathologist and the referring physician through uniform terminology that is useful for patient management. The rationale for the new classification is to provide a uniform format and standardized nomenclature based on a current understanding of cervical disease. The format of the report in the 1991 Bethesda System includes three elements: (1) a statement of adequacy of the specimen, (2) a general categorization of the diagnosis as within normal limits or not, and (3) a descriptive diagnosis. Compared with previous classification systems, the Bethesda System helps distinguish between benign cellular changes associated with inflammation and infection and those that indicate squamous cell atypia and dysplasia. The specific nomenclature used is summarized in Box 137-4. A complete description of the 1991 Bethesda System is included in the reference list.[44]

Specimen Adequacy

For adolescents with an intact uterus, the presence of endocervical cells or squamous metaplastic cells from the transformation zone are necessary for the specimens to be satisfactory for examination. An unsatisfactory smear should be repeated, with careful attention to technique.

Benign Cellular Changes

INFECTIONS AND CERVICAL CYTOLOGY. The cytology report may note benign cellular changes "consistent with" various vaginal infectious organisms, such as *Trichomonas, Candida,* or bacteria. Definitive diagnosis depends on confirmatory clinical and laboratory findings. As previously discussed, obtaining a wet mount and cervical cultures at the same time as the Pap smear is taken will help the clinician interpret the significance of the cytology report. Infections should be treated and followed with a repeat Pap smear in 3 to 6 months.

INFLAMMATION AND CERVICAL CYTOLOGY. The cytology report may note "reactive changes associated with inflammation." Inflammatory changes may actually be due to infectious agents such as *C. trachomatis* that lack diagnostic features reported as infection in the Bethesda System.[64] Noninfectious causes of inflammation of the cervix include trauma to the cervix due to recent childbearing, masturbation (use of vibrators), or possibly excessive friction from frequent intercourse (see discussion of cervicitis, p 1060). If no infection is found clinically, benign inflammation may be followed with an annual Pap smear.

Epithelial Cell Abnormalities

ATYPICAL SQUAMOUS CELLS OF UNDETERMINED SIGNIFICANCE. Once considered benign, atypical Pap smear results in adolescents are becoming more common, and current research confirms a frequent association with precancerous lesions; therefore, more aggressive evaluation of atypia is now recommended.[22,65] The cytology report of atypical squamous cells of undetermined significance (ASCUS) was one of the confusing components of the 1988 Bethesda System. The category encompasses any nuclear abnormality that is not clearly benign inflammation but is insufficient to warrant the label of dysplasia. The 1991 Bethesda System further clarified the responsibility of the cytopathologist to communicate whether the cells favored a reactive or a premalignant process. Standardization of the use of ASCUS by applying strict criteria is still under way, and acceptable rates for ASCUS diagnoses are currently being defined.[66] Inconsistent reporting can result in enormous variations in the prevalence rates of abnormal Pap smears as well as dilemmas for patient follow-up.

If an infection was identified when the Pap smear was taken, such as chlamydial or gonorrheal cervicitis, the patient should be treated and reevaluated with a repeat smear in 3 months. Abnormal Pap smears due to infection typically revert to normal after treatment. If no cause of ASCUS is identified, observation and a follow-up Pap smear in 6 months is reasonable for adolescents, to allow time for regression or progression to become apparent.

BOX 137-4
The 1991 Bethesda System

ADEQUACY OF THE SPECIMEN
- Satisfactory for evaluation
- Satisfactory for evaluation but limited by . . . (specify reason)
- Unsatisfactory for evaluation

GENERAL CATEGORIZATION (OPTIONAL)
- Within normal limits
- Benign cellular changes: *See* Descriptive diagnoses
- Epithelial cell abnormality: *See* Descriptive diagnoses

DESCRIPTIVE DIAGNOSES
BENIGN CELLULAR CHANGES
INFECTION
- *Trichomonas vaginalis*
- Fungal organisms morphologically consistent with *Candida* spp.
- Predominance of coccobacilli consistent with shift in vaginal flora
- Bacteria morphologically consistent with *Actinomyces* spp.
- Cellular changes associated with herpes simplex virus
- Other

REACTIVE CHANGES
Reactive cellular changes associated with:
- Inflammation (includes typical repair)
- Atrophy with inflammation ("atrophic vaginitis")
- Radiation
- Intrauterine contraceptive device (IUD)
- Other

EPITHELIAL CELL ABNORMALITIES
SQUAMOUS CELL
- ASCUS (atypical squamous cells of undetermined significance): Qualify*
- LSIL (low-grade squamous intraepithelial lesion) encompassing HPV,† mild dysplasia, CIN 1.
- HSIL (high-grade squamous intraepithelial lesion) encompassing moderate and severe dysplasia, CIS/CIN 2, and CIN 3.
- Squamous cell carcinoma

GLANDULAR CELL
- Endometrial cells, cytologically benign, in a postmenopausal woman
- AGUS (atypical glandular cells of undetermined significance): Qualify*
- Endocervical adenocarcinoma
- Endometrial adenocarcinoma
- Extrauterine adenocarcinoma
- Adenocarcinoma, not otherwise specified

OTHER MALIGNANT NEOPLASMS: SPECIFY HORMONAL EVALUATION (APPLIES TO VAGINAL SMEARS ONLY)
- Hormonal pattern compatible with age and history
- Hormonal pattern incompatible with age and history: Specify
- Hormonal evaluation not possible due to: Specify

---

*Atypical squamous or glandular cells of undetermined significance should be further qualified as to whether a reactive or a premalignant/malignant process is favored.
†Cellular changes of human papillomavirus (HPV)—previously termed koilocytosis, koilocytotic atypia, or condylomatous atypia—are included in the category of LSIL.
CIN, cervical intraepithelial neoplasia; *CIS,* carcinoma in situ.

A second ASCUS report indicates a need for colposcopy. Patients with an initial report of "atypia favoring dysplasia" should be referred for colposcopy. The ASCUS category of the Bethesda System will undoubtedly undergo continuing refinement and clarification over time.

LOW-GRADE SQUAMOUS INTRAEPITHELIAL LESION. The cytology report of "low-grade squamous intraepithelial lesion" (LSIL) includes cellular changes associated with HPV infection, and the changes previously called mild dysplasia or CIN 1. The epithelial cell effects induced by HPV may be indistinguishable from early neoplastic changes on the continuum progressing to invasive cervical cancer. Approximately 60% of these lesions regress spontaneously, but some progress to true invasive cancer over a period of 20 months to 9 years.[23,67] Progression may be more rapid in younger women, although not all studies have confirmed this finding.[23] Women with LSIL are typically referred for colposcopic evaluation.

HIGH-GRADE SQUAMOUS INTRAEPITHELIAL LESION. The cytology report of "high-grade squamous intraepithelial lesion" (HSIL) encompasses the previous classifications of moderate or severe dysplasia, CIN 2 or 3, and carcinoma in situ. These lesions (Plate 12) are more likely to progress than are LSIL lesions, and subcategorization is not considered clinically relevant. Patients are referred for colposcopy, directed biopsy, and endocervical curettage. If HSIL is confirmed histologically, treatment in adolescents is typically with ablative techniques.

ATYPICAL GLANDULAR CELLS OF UNDETERMINED SIGNIFICANCE. The category of "atypical glandular cells of undetermined significance" (AGUS) refers to uterine endometrial cells that may be associated with uterine polyps, chronic endometritis, an IUD, endometrial hyperplasia, or uterine cancer. Typically problems of older women, these conditions and the AGUS classification rarely apply to adolescents.

HUMAN PAPILLOMAVIRUS AND CERVICAL CYTOLOGY

HPV may be the most common STD in adolescents, with a prevalence rate of 15% to 38%.[22,68] HPV is closely associated with precancerous lesions of the cervix[69,70] (see Chapter 140, "Sexually Transmitted Diseases"). The cytologic finding of hollow squamous cells, termed *koilocytotic atypia,* is indicative of HPV. Strict criteria to define koilocytotic atypia, including nuclear enlargement, perinuclear halos, and staining intensity, are recommended to reduce overdiagnosis.[71] In the Bethesda System the finding is reported as "LSIL, cellular changes associated with HPV." On biopsy, approximately 50% of Pap smears containing koilocytosis are associated with a confirmed LSIL, 30% are not confirmed, and significantly 20% are associated with an HSIL that would have gone undetected. Older protocols suggested observation of the patient and repeating the Pap smear in 3 to 6 months, on the assumption that lesions might regress. Current recommendations suggest that such a finding in adolescence requires further clinical evaluation with colposcopy to detect high-grade lesions.[69]

The availability of office methods for HPV DNA testing (e.g., Vira-Pap test) raises the question of whether routine HPV testing when the Pap smear is taken could be helpful for clinical management. Patients with atypical cytology (ASCUS or LSIL) and a positive HPV test could be considered high risk and referred for colposcopic evaluation, and those with negative HPV tests could be considered low risk and followed with repeat Pap smears.[72] Although this is theoretically sound, the concern is cost effectiveness. Approximately 80% of adolescents have normal Pap smears, and no treatment is currently recommended for a positive HPV test in the presence of a normal Pap smear.[73] Hence, most routine HPV tests would not be clinically useful. At present, HPV DNA testing is still considered an investigational technology and is not recommended for routine annual screening in adolescents. Large-scale studies sponsored by the CDC and the NCI are under way to determine whether HPV testing can reliably triage ASCUS and LSIL

lesions and may help elucidate specific clinical roles for HPV testing.[73]

MANAGEMENT OF ABNORMAL CERVICAL (PAP) SMEARS

Interim Guidelines

The Bethesda System does not include guidelines for patient management, but such guidelines are desirable. The NCI convened a workshop in 1992 to develop interim guidelines until additional research and clinical trials resolve certain unanswered questions, especially in terms of management of ASCUS and LSIL.[65] Consensus guidelines specific for adolescents are not yet available. Management of adolescents with abnormal Pap smears should focus on preventing invasive cancer by the most conservative and cost-effective means possible. Controversy exists because at present the natural progression of precursor lesions is unclear, it is not possible to determine which dysplastic findings have carcinogenic potential, and the time frame for malignant transformation is variable. Clinical protocols that emphasize prevention as an essential component of cervical cancer screening are advocated.[74] The algorithm for managing abnormal Pap smears shown in Figure 137-3 reflects the NCI interim guidelines and the 1991 Bethesda System terminology. The clinician can justify observation, rather than further diagnostic tests, if patient follow-up is reliable. The management plan should be individualized to the patient according to clinical judgment of risk factors, compliance, and past history.

The Role of Colposcopy

The purpose of cervical screening is to detect any abnormal cells that may be precursors to invasive carcinoma. When the cytopathologist reports abnormal findings, further clinical evaluation is needed to make a definitive diagnosis. Colposcopy is the primary tool for investigating potential lesions.

The colposcope is a low-power magnifying instrument used to view the cervix under tenfold to fifteenfold magnification. The procedure is similar to a standard pelvic examination, with a Graves speculum used to visualize the full cervix. The cervix is swabbed with 3% or 5% acetic acid to remove mucus and dehydrate surface cells, producing acetowhitening of dysplastic cells or flat condyloma warts.

The colposcopist examines the squamocolumnar junction for white lesions, hyperkeratosis, punctuation, mosaic lesions, and atypical blood vessels. Suspicious lesions are biopsied. A magnified colpophotograph may be taken for later evaluation. Endocervical curettage is

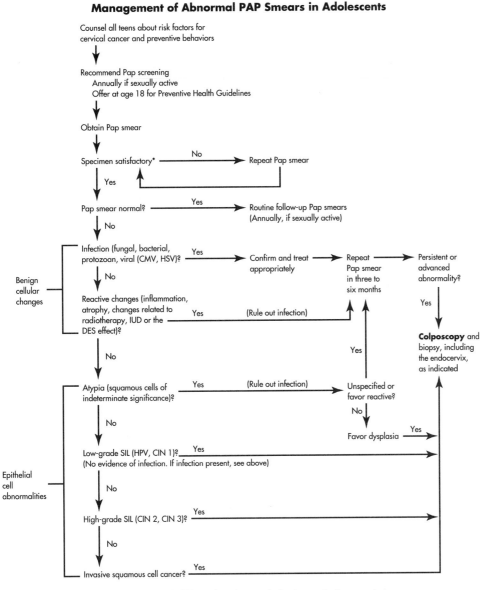

Management of Abnormal PAP Smears in Adolescents

Fig. 137-3. Algorithm using the 1991 Bethesda System and 1992 Interim Guidelines for Management of Abnormal Cytology.[65] Adapted from Shepherd JC, Fried RA: Preventing cervical cancer: the role of the Bethesda system, *Am Fam Physician* 51:434-440, 1995. *CIN,* cervical intraepithelial neoplasia, with CIN I signifying dysplasia, CIN 2 signifying moderate dysplasia, and CIN 3 signifying severe dysplasia; *CMV,* cytomegalovirus; *DES,* diethylstilbestrol; *HPV,* human papillomavirus; *HSV,* herpes simplex virus; *IUD,* intrauterine device; *Pap,* Papanicolaou; *SIL,* squamous intraepithelial lesion.

* In adolescents with an intact uterus, specimens should be read as adequate only if endocervical cells or metaplastic components are seen.

performed to obtain material from the portion of the canal that is beyond the colposcopist's view. The combination of colposcopy, directed biopsy, and endocervical curettage allows definitive diagnosis of areas of suspected malignancy.[75] Accurate interpretation of the visual examination requires a well-trained, experienced colposcopist. The procedure is time-consuming and moderately expensive.

Colposcopy is required for any finding of HSIL.[65] For patients with LSIL, numerous studies confirm the superiority of colposcopy to repeat Pap smears for detecting undiagnosed high-grade lesions (CIN 2 and 3), using biopsy histology as the "gold standard."[75,76] If followed cytologically, many patients with LSIL will need colposcopy eventually, and because of the risk that adolescents will be lost to follow-up, immediate referral for colpos-

copy may be prudent. Cost effectiveness is a concern, but it may be better addressed by increasing technical training and making colposcopy more widely available in primary care settings.

A diagnosis of ASCUS "favoring dysplasia" is managed in the same way as LSIL. For a diagnosis of ASCUS, when not qualified further or when it favors a reactive process, follow-up by repeat Pap smears without colposcopy is acceptable. A second ASCUS report within the 2-year follow-up period should be considered for colposcopy[65] (Box 137-5).

Other Modalities for Evaluation

CERVICOGRAPHY. Introduced by Stafl in 1981, the cervigram has been recommended as an intermediate step

---

BOX 137-5
**Indications for Colposcopy
in Adolescents**

1. Abnormal Pap smear report
   - Any HSIL (high-grade intraepithelial lesion)
   - LSIL (low-grade intraepithelial lesion)
     (unless untreated cervical infection was
     present: treat and repeat in 3 months)
   - ASCUS (atypical cells of undetermined sig-
     nificance)
     If report favors dysplasia
     If this is second ASCUS within 2 years
   - Benign cellular changes
     If persistent or advancing abnormality on
     repeat Pap smear in 3 to 6 months
2. Abnormal cervigram (if done)
3. Abnormal cervical findings on visual inspection
4. DES exposure (possibly)

---

before colposcopy for atypia or low-grade lesions.[77,78] As with colposcopy, the cervix is visualized and 3% or 5% acetic acid applied. Next, a cerviscope, an adapted 35-mm camera with bright light (1/2000 second electronic blitz) and fast speed (1/30 second), is used to take two photographs of the cervix. Because no magnification is used, the cervigram is extremely sharp, with excellent detail and clarity. The cervigram is then sent to a certified cervicographic evaluator for interpretation. Findings are reported on a standardized form as negative (repeat cytology in 1 year), atypical (no significant lesion, no colposcopy necessary, repeat cytology and cervigram in 6 months), positive (colposcopy required, suggestive of HPV or CIN 1 to 3 or SIL in the Bethesda System), or technically defective (unsatisfactory, needs repeat). There are several advantages of cervicography over colposcopy for evaluation of atypical cervical smears: (1) the cervigram may be taken by a nonphysician after brief training, (2) the procedure can be done in any office where the equipment is present, (3) the procedure can be performed quickly (90 seconds to take the photographs), (4) it is more cost efficient, (5) the cervigram provides a permanent record, and (6) the interpretations are highly reliable and consistent because of the certification and quality assurance procedures required for evaluators. However, cervicography does not visualize the endocervix, does not provide biopsy material, and is not a substitute for colposcopy done for advanced lesions. Used primarily in referral centers where certified interpreters are available, cervicography has not been widely accepted.

NAKED EYE INSPECTION OF THE CERVIX. Application of acetic acid to the cervix is a standard part of the colposcopic examination and it helps direct biopsy samples. During the pelvic examination, the clinician can also apply 5% acetic acid to the cervix and observe with the naked eye for any acetowhite lesions that may indicate HPV infection or low-grade lesions. It has been suggested that naked eye inspection of the cervix (NIC) may enhance the interpretation of Pap smear reports and help detect false-negative results.[79] A negative NIC and a negative Pap smear provide reassurance of a healthy cervix. However, up to 75% of young women may have abnormal NIC findings.[79] If the Pap report is normal, the clinician faces a dilemma of whether to refer for colposcopy. At present, NIC is not recommended as a standard component of the pelvic examination or routine Pap screening visit.

Special Populations

THE PREGNANT ADOLESCENT. The American College of Obstetricians and Gynecologists recommends a Pap smear at the time of the initial prenatal examination and a repeat smear after delivery, preferably 12 weeks post partum, after the cervix has healed. Interpretation of the cytologic smear is more difficult in pregnancy. Endocolumnar cells are difficult to obtain because they retreat high into the endocervical canal during pregnancy. Use of the Cytobrush is recommended, but it should be limited to one 90 degree rotation to minimize irritation of the canal. In addition, atypical cells or dysplastic changes are more common because of hormonal stimulation. The management of abnormal findings follows the same protocol as for nonpregnant patients. Colposcopically directed biopsy has proved to be a safe and reliable method of evaluating pregnant patients with abnormal cervical cytology.[80] Endocervical curettage is avoided during pregnancy.

THE HIV-POSITIVE ADOLESCENT. Studies of adults have shown an increased rate of cervical dysplasia in HIV-infected women.[81] It is not clear whether this is related to life-style risk factors, a result of immunosuppression, or a combination of factors. Comparable studies are not yet available in HIV-positive adolescents. The increasing HIV-seroprevalence in adolescent females is well documented; these young women likely represent a very-high-risk group for cervical neoplasia. Frequent cervical screening of HIV-positive adolescents is recommended.[22]

Counseling the Adolescent with Abnormal Cytology

Abnormal findings on cervical cytologic examination are becoming more common among sexually active adolescents. Learning about abnormal results can trigger significant emotions in the young woman and her family and strain her relationship with her partner. Loss of confidentiality can be a serious issue if parental consent is necessary for biopsy or treatment. Even though the patient can be reassured that a precursor state is not the same as invasive cancer, and that the condition is curable with preservation of fertility, the psychologic stress should not be underestimated. Sensitive counseling should be offered to the teenager, her partner, and her family (if appropriate).

Limitations of Pap Smear Screening

As with all screening tests, the limitations of the method need to be recognized.

LOW POSITIVE PREDICTIVE VALUE. The primary purpose of the Pap smear is to screen for cervical cancer or its precursor lesions. Since the incidence of cervical cancer in the United States is low (about 5 cases per 100,000 women per year), any screening test tends to have a low positive predictive value.[74]

DETECTION OF BENIGN LESIONS. In using the screening tool the physician assumes that precursor lesions will progress to invasive disease, but studies on the natural history of dysplasia suggest that 20% to 60% of low-grade lesions resolve spontaneously.[23] The unpredictable nature of dysplasia forces cytologists to categorize its stages arbitrarily.[74] Lesions that in fact would be benign are therefore subject to overdetection and overtreatment.

FALSE-NEGATIVE PAP SCREENS. Published false-negative rates range from 1% to 80% and may realistically be 5% even in the best circumstances. Errors may arise from inadequate sampling, processing, or interpretation or incorrect use of results.

FALSE-POSITIVE PAP SCREENS. Published false-positive rates range from 0% to 8%. Erroneous readings stem primarily from variability in laboratory interpretation. Cervical cytology is subjective and depends on human judgment. Both the medical and emotional consequences of false-positive results are significant.

IMPACT ON RECOMMENDATIONS FOR MANAGEMENT. The disparity of Pap smear accuracy and efficacy makes it difficult to reach consensus on guidelines for management, as recognized by the NCI 1992 workshop that developed "Interim Guidelines." The effect of Pap smear screening on healthcare utilization and costs needs additional research, to develop a rational approach that neither under- nor overtreats.

Despite its limitations, the benefits of Pap smear screening for early detection of and reduced mortality from cervical cancer are unquestioned. As experience grows, enhanced options for screening and treatment will become available. Prevention of cervical cancer in the United States depends on preventive counseling and appropriate screening of adolescent females.

References

1. Chacko MR, Rosenfeld WD: The uterine cervix: diagnostic opportunities, *Pediatr Ann* 24:317-323, 1995.
2. Critchlow CW, Wolner-Hanssen P, Eschenbach DA, et al: Determinants of cervical ectopy and of cervicitis: age, oral contraception, specific cervical infection, smoking, and douching, *Am J Obstet Gynecol* 173:534-543, 1995.
3. Moscicki AB: Reproductive growth and development in the female adolescent. In Rudolph A, editor: *Rudolph's pediatrics,* ed 19, Norwalk, CT, 1991, Appleton & Lange; p 52.
4. Greydanus DE, Shearin RB: *Adolescent sexuality and gynecology,* Philadelphia, 1990, Lea & Febiger; p 34.
5. Helmerhorst TJ, Wijnen JH, Kenemans P, et al: Colposcopic findings and intraepithelial neoplasia in diethylstilbestrol-exposed offspring, *Am J Obstet Gynecol* 161:1191-1194, 1989.
6. Jeffries JA, Robboy SJ, O'Brien PC, et al: Structural anomalies of the cervix and vagina in women enrolled in the diethylstilbestrol adenosis (DESAD) project, *Am J Obstet Gynecol* 148:60, 1984.
7. Noller KL: Role of colposcopy in the examination of diethylstilbestrol-exposed women, *Obstet Gynecol Clin North Am* 20:165-176, 1993.
8. Mittendorf R, Herbst AL: DES exposure: an update, *Contemp Pediatr* 11:59-79, 1994.
9. Wilcox AJ, Umbach DM, Hornsby PP, Herbst AL: Age at menarche among diethylstilbestrol granddaughters, *Am J Obstet Gynecol* 173:835-836, 1995.
10. Quigley MM, Gwatkin RBL: Embryology and developmental defects of the female reproductive system. In Scott JR, DiSaia PJ, Hammond CB, Spellacy WN, editors: *Danforth's obstetrics and gynecology,* ed 6, Philadelphia, 1990, JB Lippincott; p 50.
11. Janus C, Wagner L: Nabothian cysts simulating an adnexal mass, *Clin Imaging* 13:157-158, 1989.
12. Muse K: Clinical manifestations and classification of endometriosis, *Clin Obstet Gynecol* 31:813-822, 1988.
13. Greydanus DE, Hofmann A: The lower respiratory tract. In Hofmann A, Greydanus DF, editors: *Adolescent medicine,* ed 2, Norwalk, CT, 1989, Appleton & Lange; p 95.
14. Smith ML, Scott JC: Benign neoplasms of the cervix. In Sciarra JJ, editor: *Gynecology and obstetrics,* vol 1, revised ed, Philadelphia, 1995, JB Lippincott; p 1.
15. Rosenfeld WD, Clark J: Vulvovaginitis and cervicitis, *Pediatr Clin North Am* 36:489-511, 1989.
16. Regard MM, Chacko MR, Kozinetz CA, et al: Reliability of cervical findings and endocervical polymorphonuclear cells in detecting chlamydial and gonococcal cervicitis in young women receiving contraceptive services, *Adolesc Pediatr Gynecol* 6:129-134, 1993.
17. Treatment of Sexually Transmitted Diseases, *Med Lett* 37(964): 117-122, 1995.
18. DiSaia PJ: Disorders of the uterine cervix. In Scott JR, DiSaia PJ, Hammond CB, Spellacy WN, editors: *Danforth's obstetrics and gynecology,* ed 6, Philadelphia, 1990, JB Lippincott; p 992.
19. Perez CA, DiSaia PJ, Knapp RC, Young RC: Gynecologic tumors. In DeVita VT, Hellman S, Rosenberg SA, editors: *Cancer: principles and practice of oncology,* Philadelphia, 1985, JB Lippincott.
20. Emans SJ, Goldstein DP: *Pediatric and adolescent gynecology,* ed 3, Boston, 1990, Little, Brown; pp 413-417.
21. Sadeghi SB, Hsieh EW, Gun SW: Prevalence of cervical intraepithelial neoplasia in sexually active teenagers and young adults, *Am J Obstet Gynecol* 155:741, 1986.
22. Roye CF: Abnormal cervical cytology in adolescents: a literature review, *J Adolesc Health Care* 13:643-650, 1992.
23. Crowther ME: Is the nature of cervical carcinoma changing in young women?, *Obstet Gynecol Surv* 50:71-82, 1994.
24. Melnick S, Cole P, Anderson D, et al: Rates and risks of diethylstilbestrol-related clear cell adenocarcinoma of the vagina and cervix, *N Engl J Med* 316:514, 1978.
25. Peters RK, Chao A, Mack TM, et al: Increased frequency of adenocarcinoma of the uterine cervix in young women in Los Angeles County, *J Natl Cancer Inst* 76:423-428, 1986.

26. Young RN, Scully RE: Atypical forms of microglandular hyperplasia of the cervix simulating carcinoma, *Am J Surg Pathol* 13:50-56, 1989.

27. Bell J, Averette H, David J, et al: Genital rhabdomyosarcoma: current management and review of the literature, *Obstet Gynecol Surg* 41:257, 1986.

28. Gallup DG, Talledo OE: Benign and malignant tumors, *Clin Obstet Gynecol* 30:662-670, 1987.

29. Parker SL, Tong T, Bolden S, et al: Cancer statistics: 1996, *CA Cancer J Clin* 46:5-28, 1996.

30. Russo JF, Jones DED: Abnormal cervical cytology in sexually active adolescents, *J Adolesc Health Care* 5:269, 1984.

31. Piver MS, Baker TR: Cervical cancer in the adolescent patient, *Pediatr Ann* 15:536-541, 1986.

32. Rosenfeld WD, Vermund SH, Wentz SJ, Burk RD: High prevalence rate of human papillomavirus infection and association with abnormal Papanicolaou smears in sexually active adolescents, *Am J Dis Child* 143:1443-1447, 1989.

33. Mandelblatt J: Cervical cancer screening in primary care: issues and recommendations, *Prim Care* 16:133-155, 1989.

34. Spitzer M, Krumholz BA: Pap screening for teenagers: a lifesaving precaution, *Contemp Obstet Gynecol* 30:33-42, 1988.

35. Winkelstein W: Smoking and cervical cancer—current status: a review, *Am J Epidemiol* 131:945-957, 1990.

36. Nasiell K, Roger V, Nasiell M: Behavior of mild cervical dysplasia during long term follow-up, *Obstet Gynecol* 67:665-669, 1986.

37. Buckley CH, Beards CS, Fox H: Pathological prognostic indicators in cervical cancer with particular reference to patients under the age of 40 years, *Br J Obstet Gynaecol* 95:47-56, 1988.

38. Richart RM, Barron BA: Screening strategies for cervical cancer and cervical intraepithelial neoplasia, *Cancer* 47:1176, 1981.

39. Richart RM: Causes and management of cervical intraepithelial neoplasia, *Cancer* 60 (suppl 8):1951-1959, 1987.

40. Ferenczy A: Laser treatment of patients with condylomata and squamous carcinoma precursors of the lower female genital tract, *CA* 37:334-347, 1987.

41. Hillard P: Complications of cervical cryotherapy in adolescents, *J Reprod Med* 36:711-716, 1991.

42. Wright TC, Gagnon MD, Richart RM, et al: Treatment of cervical intraepithelial neoplasia using the loop electrosurgical excision procedure, *Obstet Gynecol* 79:173-178, 1992.

43. Broder S: Rapid communication—the Bethesda System for reporting cervical/vaginal cytological diagnoses: report of the 1991 Bethesda workshop, *JAMA* 267:1892, 1992.

44. Kurman RJ, Solomon D: *The Bethesda System for reporting cervical/vaginal diagnoses: definitions, criteria and explanatory notes for terminology and specimen adequacy*, New York, 1994, Springer-Verlag.

45. Dewar MA, Hall K, Perchalski J: Cervical cancer screening: past success and future challenge, *Prim Care* 19:589-605, 1992.

46. Koss LG: The Papanicolaou test for cervical cancer detection: a triumph and tragedy, *JAMA* 261:740-743, 1989.

47. Tawa K, Forsythe A, Cove JK, et al: A comparison of the Papanicolaou smear and the cervigram: sensitivity, specificity, and cost analysis, *Obstet Gynecol* 71:229-235, 1988.

48. Shingleton HM, Patrick RL, Johnson WW, et al: The current status of the Papanicolaou smear, *CA Cancer J Clin* 45:305-320, 1995.

49. Koss LG: Cervical (Pap) smear: new directions, *Cancer* 71:1406-1412, 1993.

50. Mango LJ: Computer-assisted cervical cancer screening using neural networks, *Cancer Lett* 77:155-162, 1994.

51. U.S. Preventive Services Task Force: *Guide to clinical preventive services*: ed 2, Washington DC, 1996, U.S. Government.

52. American Cancer Society: Recommendations for the early detection of cancer, *CA* 40:77-101, 1990.

53. Fink DJ: Change in American Cancer Society checkup guidelines for detection of cervical cancer, *CA* 38:127-128, 1988.

54. American Medical Association: *AMA guidelines for adolescent preventive services (GAPS): recommendations and rationales*, Baltimore, 1993, Williams & Wilkins.

55. American Academy of Pediatrics: *Recommendations for preventive pediatric health care*, Elk Grove Village, IL, 1995, American Academy of Pediatrics.

56. Olamijulo J, Duncan ID: Is cervical cytology screening of teenagers worthwhile?, *Br J Obstet Gynaecol* 102:515-516, 1995.

57. White LN: An overview of screening and early detection of gynecologic malignancies, *Cancer* 71:1400-1405, 1993.

58. Miller K: The Bethesda System and Pap smear screening, *Am Fam Physician* 51:331-332, 1995.

59. Mauney M, Eide D, Sotham J: Rates of condyloma and dysplasia in Papanicolaou smears with and without endocervical cells, *Diagn Cytopathol* 6:18-21, 1990.

60. Neinstein LS, Rabinovitz S, Racalde A: Comparison of Cytobrush with cotton swab for endocervical cytologic sampling, *J Adolesc Health Care* 10:305-307, 1989.

61. Tyau L, Hernandez E, Anderson L, et al: The Cell-Sweep. A new cervical cytology sampling device, *J Reprod Med* 39:899-902, 1994.

62. Ferenczy A, Robitaille J, Gurainick M, et al: Cervical cytology with the Papette Sampler, *J Reprod Med* 39:304-310, 1994.

63. Eltabbakh GH, Eltabbakh GD, Broekhuizen FF, et al: Value of wet mount and cervical cultures at the time of cervical cytology in asymptomatic women, *Obstet Gynecol* 85:499-503, 1995.

64. Eckert LD, Koursky LA, Kiviat NB, et al: The inflammatory Papanicolaou smear: what does it mean?, *Obstet Gynecol* 86:360-366, 1995.

65. Kurman RJ, Henson DE, Herbst AL, et al: Interim guidelines for management of abnormal cervical cytology, *JAMA* 271:1866-1869, 1994.

66. Howell LP: Cervical pathology: the Bethesda System and the "atypical squamous cells of undetermined significance" controversy, *West J Med* 162:446-447, 1995.

67. Ostor AG: Natural history of cervical intraepithelial neoplasia: a critical review, *Int J Gynecol Pathol* 12:186-192, 1993.

68. Jamison JJ, Kaplan DW, Hamman R, et al: Spectrum of genital human papillomavirus infection in a female adolescent population, *Sex Transm Dis* 22:236-243, 1995.

69. Levine AJ, Harper J, Hilborne L, et al: HPV DNA and the risk of squamous intraepithelial lesions of the uterine cervix in young women, *Am J Clin Pathol* 100:6-11, 1993.

70. Schiffman MH, Bauer HM, Hoover RN, et al: Epidemiologic evidence showing that human papillomavirus infection causes most cervical intraepithelial neoplasia, *J Natl Cancer Inst* 85:958-964, 1993.

71. Crum C: Koilocytosis in Pap smears: how useful a finding?, *Contemp Obstet Gynecol* 35:66-77, 1993.

72. Rosenfeld WD, Rose E, Vermund SH, et al: Follow-up evaluation of cervicovaginal human papillomavirus infection in adolescents, *J Pediatr* 121:307-311, 1992.

73. Cole HM: Human papillomavirus DNA testing in the management of cervical neoplasia, *JAMA* 270:2975-2981, 1993.

74. Shepherd JC, Fried RA: Preventing cervical cancer: the role of the Bethesda System, *Am Fam Physician* 51:434-440, 1995.

75. Wright VC, editor: Contemporary colposcopy, *Obstet Gynecol Clin North Am* 20:1-260, 1993.

76. Higgins RV, Hall JB, McGee JA, et al: Appraisal of the modalities used to evaluate an initial abnormal Papanicolaou smear, *Obstet Gynecol* 84:174-178, 1994.

77. August N: Cervicography for evaluating the atypical Papanicolaou smear, *J Reprod Med* 36:89-94, 1991.

78. Ferris DG, Payne P, Frish LE, et al: Cervicography: adjunctive cervical cancer screening by primary care clinicians, *J Fam Pract* 37:158-164, 1993.

79. Frish LE, Milner FH, Ferris DG: Naked-eye inspection of the cervix

after acetic acid application may improve the predictive value of negative cytologic screening, *J Fam Pract* 39:457-460, 1994.

80. Economos K, Veridiano NP, Delke I, et al: Abnormal cervical cytology in pregnancy: a 17-year experience, *Obstet Gynecol* 81:915-918, 1993.

81. Schrager LK, Friedland G, Maude D, et al: Cervical and vaginal squamous cell abnormalities in women infected with human immunodeficiency virus, *J Acquir Immune Defic Syndr* 2:570-575, 1989.

CHAPTER 138

The Uterus and Adnexa

•

Elizabeth M. Alderman

The uterus is a pear-shaped, fibromuscular, midline organ that is normally $8 \times 6.5 \times 3.5$ cm. It is divided anatomically into two parts: the fundus, which is the body of the uterus, and the cervix, which is 3.5 cm in length and partially intravaginal. The adnexa consists of the ovaries, fallopian tubes, round ligaments, and ovarian ligament.

The position of the uterus in the pelvis is usually anteverted and anteflexed, although it may be axial or retroverted or retroflexed. The adnexa is palpable on bimanual examination but may be difficult to evaluate in an obese adolescent.

THE UTERUS

Congenital Anomalies

Congenital anomalies of the uterus are a result of incomplete or abnormal fusion of the paired müllerian ducts.[1] The most common defect results in a bicornuate uterus. Other types of uterine anomalies include a rudimentary uterine horn and unicornuate, didelphic, or septate uterus.[2] If there are two uterine cavities, one of the two sides is usually more developed than the other. Abnormal uteri may or may not be associated with single or double cervices.

Many patients with congenital anomalies of the müllerian duct are asymptomatic; therefore, the true incidence of these conditions is not known. Infertile females have a six times greater incidence of uterine abnormalities than the general obstetric population.[3]

Adolescents with uterine anomalies usually present with pelvic pain.[4] Other symptoms may include infertility, recurrent miscarriages, abnormal vaginal bleeding or discharge, endometriosis, and menstrual disorders. Women who were exposed to diethylstilbestrol in utero are also at risk for uterine anomalies such as hypoplasia, T-shaped abnormalities, uterine constriction, and uni- and bicornuate uteri.

The diagnosis of uterine anomalies is best made by ultrasonography. Computed tomography (CT), hysterosalpingography, hysteroscopy, and laparoscopy may be useful adjuncts to delineate a more complicated uterine anatomy. Surgical intervention may be necessary to treat severe dysmenorrhea or endometriosis and to improve the reproductive outcome. If one of the uterine cavities has no external opening, or if the opening is obstructed, a resultant unilateral hematometrocolpos may need to be surgically drained.

Müllerian anomalies may be associated with congenital renal anomalies, most notably renal agenesis. Skeletal or cardiac malformations may also be present. It is therefore important to evaluate the patient for these concomitant congenital anomalies.[5]

Uterine Masses

In adolescent females a uterine mass is usually a pregnancy. Other types of uterine masses are uncommon, although a study of nonovarian female genital tract tumors in children showed that 21% were uterine cancers,[6] and such cancers were associated with a high mortality rate. The most common cancers were botryoid, mixed mesenchymal, and rhabdomyosarcoma. Surgery; radiation; and chemotherapy with vincristine, actinomycin, and cyclophosphamide are the most effective treatments for uterine malignancies.[7]

A uterine myoma is a benign, discrete, firm mass in the uterus that may be either in the myometrium, within the endometrium, or on the surface of the uterus. Myomas may be single or multiple. Infarction or infection may cause lower abdominal pain. Uterine myomas may be a cause of secondary dysmenorrhea. Bleeding from small myomas is rare in adolescent females. Myomectomy is not usually warranted.

Endometriosis

Although in the past endometriosis was viewed as a problem only of women in their twenties and thirties, it is now known to occur in teenagers and is among the most common causes of chronic pelvic pain in adolescent females.

ETIOLOGY. Endometriosis is the presence of endometrial tissue anywhere in the pelvis from the ovaries, the most common site, to the bladder and rectum.[8] The pathophysiologic origin of endometriosis is thought to be retrograde menstruation with endometrial cells regurgitated through the fallopian tubes and seeded throughout the pelvis. There also may be lymphatic and hematogenous spread of this tissue to the lungs, extremities, bowel, and skin.[9] Endometriosis also may be secondary to structural anomalies of the müllerian duct causing uterine outflow obstruction.[10]

Studies of adolescent girls with chronic pelvic pain revealed that 20% to 50% had had endometriosis.[11,12] As such, endometriosis is not an uncommon problem in adolescent girls, although its presentation differs from that in older women, in whom it is usually discovered during an evaluation for infertility. Girls at increased risk for endometriosis include those with structural abnormalities of the genital tract, former intrauterine device users, and those with a family history of endometriosis. Girls with a first-degree relative who has endometriosis appear to have a sevenfold increased risk for this disorder.[13]

DIAGNOSIS. In adolescents, endometriosis usually presents as chronic pelvic pain that may or may not coincide with the menstrual cycle. Most girls have cyclic pain just before or during menses that may be confused with primary dysmenorrhea. The pain is usually severe enough to prevent normal activities such as school attendance. Less commonly, the pain may have no relation to the menstrual cycle or may occur in midcycle. Other gynecologic symptoms of endometriosis in adolescents include irregular menses, dyspareunia (usually with deep penetration), brownish vaginal discharge, and infertility. Infertility is less common as a symptom in adolescents than in adults. Gastrointestinal complaints such as constipation, nausea, vomiting, diarrhea, or pain on defecation before or during menstruation are also common. The pelvic pain is rarely relieved by antiprostaglandins used for the treatment of dysmenorrhea.

The pain of endometriosis is caused by swelling and bleeding of the endometrial implants consequent to hormonal stimulation during the menstrual cycle. When endometrial implants occur on the ovary (so-called "chocolate" cysts), the cysts may burst, causing severe acute abdominal pain.

On physical examination, three fourths of girls with endometriosis have generalized abdominal tenderness, and most also show evidence of localized pain.[11] The pain most commonly occurs the week before menses begins or with the onset of menses. Other findings common to the pelvic examination of these teenagers include a tender adnexal mass, nodularity of the cul-de-sac, nonspecific thickening of the adnexa, and fixed uterine retroflexion. However, in a minority of girls the pelvic examination is normal.

MANAGEMENT. Any adolescent female with persistent pelvic symptoms should be considered for laparoscopy to search for signs of endometriosis. Laparoscopy not only facilitates making a diagnosis of endometriosis but also allows for staging of the disease, the performance of confirmatory biopsies, and treatment. The importance of early diagnosis is to permit treatment of chronic pain and preservation of fertility.

The most commonly used system for classifying endometriosis at the time of laparoscopy was proposed by the American Fertility Society.[14] This system defines four states of disease: minimal, mild, moderate, and severe. Staging is based on a weighted point system that describes the size and position of the endometrial implants in the peritoneum and ovaries. It also describes the size and position of adhesions on the ovaries and fallopian tubes. Endometriosis of the bowel, urinary tract, vagina, cervix, skin, and other organs is designated additional endometriosis.

In a 1980 study of 66 adolescents diagnosed as having endometriosis at the time of laparoscopy involving the use of an earlier system of classification, 58% were found to have minimal disease—that is, one or more implants less than 0.5 mm in diameter and localized to the pelvic peritoneum.[11] An additional 23% had ovarian or pelvic adhesions; 15% had more extensive ovarian disease with larger implants; and less than 5% had extensive disease with endometriosis found on the ovaries, fallopian tubes, bladder, and rectum. This study suggests that minimal disease is responsible for the pelvic symptoms in most teenagers. Adults who may have had endometriosis from the time of menarche typically present with infertility caused by peritubal endometriosis and adhesions resulting in tubal obstruction or impaired tubal mobility. Adults with mild or minimal disease usually have no decrease in fertility.[9]

TREATMENT. There are both pharmacologic and surgical treatments for endometriosis. Surgical therapy includes lysis of adhesions and fulguration of lesions at the time of laparoscopy, or a more extensive intervention at laparotomy. Either initially or subsequent to surgery, pharmacologic treatment may be implemented. The goals of pharmacologic therapy are to shrink the endometriomas by lowering the estrogen level, and to reduce the opportunity for retrograde seeding by decreasing the menstrual flow. These goals can be accomplished by using monophasic oral contraceptives to create a pseudopregnancy. Gonadotropin-releasing hormone agonists, such as intranasal nafarelin (400 to 800 µg daily), and intramuscular leuprolide also may be used to create a low estrogen state by decreasing follicle-stimulating hormone and luteinizing hormone.[15] Side effects of nafarelin and leuprolide therapy are the same as the symptoms of menopause (hot flashes, osteoporosis, decreased libido, vaginal dryness).[16] To counteract these side effects, additional estrogen may be necessary. Alternative treatment regimens, although unpopular with adolescents because of the side effects, are androgens, such as danazol, and synthetic progestins. These agents cause atrophy of endometrial implants and interrupt ovarian follicle development by creating an antiestrogen state. Side effects of androgens include irregular menses, virilization with hirsutism, acne, deep voice, and weight gain. The side effects of progestins include irregular menstrual bleeding and weight gain.

In severe or persistent disease, laparotomy may be necessary to lyse adhesions and remove implants. Additional possible interventions include presacral neurectomy to relieve pain and uterine suspension to correct retroversion. In a study by Goldstein et al on adolescents with endometriosis,[11] more advanced disease was treated by laparotomy to lyse adhesions and fulgurate masses, whereas minimal disease was treated by ovulation suppression after laparoscopy.

Girls with endometriosis require periodic reevaluation at approximately 6-month intervals to monitor progress and assess the side effects of medication. A serologic marker, CA-125, may correlate with disease activity in endometriosis and may be useful in monitoring response to treatment.[17]

PROGNOSIS. The prognosis for control of disease and future fertility of adolescent girls with endometriosis is quite good. Most adolescents have minimal disease that is responsive to available therapies. In the study by Goldstein and his colleagues,[11] 65% of teenagers treated had a good response to medical or surgical treatment without recurrent disease. Of the 35% in whom treatment failed, 12% were noncompliant to treatment because of side effects, 8% did not have an initial response to treatment, and 15% had recurrence of symptoms after completion of therapy. Those who underwent conservative laparotomy with ovulation suppression had the best chance of cure, and those undergoing operative laparoscopy had the next best prognosis.

Endometriosis in adolescent girls is a potentially curable disease. The challenge for the clinician is to make the diagnosis early so as to prevent chronic pelvic pain and preserve future fertility. In working with the adolescent, the clinician must be mindful of the side effects of the medications used to treat endometriosis, since compliance may be the key to attaining a cure.

THE ADNEXA

Ovarian Cysts

The normal ovarian follicle is less than 3 cm in diameter.[18] Ovarian cysts develop as a result of accumulation of fluid and distention of the preformed ovarian cavities. Functional ovarian cysts are common in postmenarcheal adolescents. Girls in early or middle puberty may have enlarged ovaries with multiple small cysts. This is a variant of normal.

Most ovarian cysts are follicular and are a result of the failure of the maturing follicle to ovulate and involute.[19] Such cysts contain clear fluid and may resolve spontaneously. Follicular cysts may be small and asymptomatic, or may enlarge to 6 to 8 cm and thus twist the adnexa or rupture, causing acute abdominal pain.[9] Other types of functional ovarian cysts include postovulatory corpus luteum cysts that rarely exceed 5 cm in diameter but tend to be more symptomatic than follicular cysts, and theca luteum cysts that are usually multiple.[20]

Symptoms of ovarian cysts include acute or chronic abdominal pain due to torsion, rupture or hemorrhage, menstrual abnormalities, constipation, and/or urinary symptoms. An adnexal mass may be palpated on bimanual examination. A pelvic ultrasound examination to determine the size and appearance of the cyst is important for subsequent management. On ultrasound, nonhemorrhagic cysts appear to be smooth and unilocular.[18] Hemorrhagic cysts contain internal debris. The size and appearance of the cyst should be correlated to the menstrual cycle.

Most follicular cysts resolve spontaneously within a few months.[9] Large cysts are those greater than 5 cm in diameter. If a patient has an asymptomatic cyst determined to be simple on ultrasound examination, the patient should be given oral contraceptive pills (OCPs) for 2 to 3 months.[20] The low-dose estrogen/progestin formulation of OCPs suppresses the hypothalamic-ovarian axis, and thus growth of the cyst. A monophasic OCP should be prescribed, as there have been unconfirmed reports that triphasic pills increase the incidence of cysts. Progestin-only pills also increase functional cyst formation.[21] The patient should be examined monthly, and a repeat ultrasound examination 8 to 10 weeks into treatment is recommended.

If the cyst is greater than 5 cm, laparoscopic drainage of the cyst or cystectomy is necessary to reduce the risk of torsion. These patients are then placed on monophasic OCPs to prevent future cyst development.

Adnexal Tumors

DERMOID CYST (BENIGN MATURE TERATOMA). Dermoid cysts or teratomas are the most common ovarian germ cell neoplasm in adolescent girls.[22] These benign tumors contain virtually any descendant of endoderm, ectoderm, or mesoderm enclosed in a thick capsule of squamous epithelium. Common components of dermoid cysts include hair, thyroid tissue, teeth (which can be visualized on a plain radiograph), sebaceous glands, sebum, and choroid plexus. As their average size is 10 cm in diameter, dermoid cysts may present as an abdominal mass, abdominal pain due to torsion of the ovarian pedicle, or (rarely) rupture of the thick capsule. Alternatively, they may be asymptomatic. Teratomas do not have one distinct appearance on ultrasonography, which is the best radiographic study to determine the diagnosis.[23] Pelvic CT or magnetic resonance imaging may further characterize the cyst. Dermoid cysts should be resected from the ovary, if possible, to preserve future reproductive function. As 15% of all ovarian teratomas appear bilaterally, the opposite ovary should be visually inspected, but biopsy or removal of the unaffected ovary is not necessary.[24]

OVARIAN MALIGNANCY. Sixty percent of all gynecologic malignancies in children and adolescents are ovarian neoplasms. Ovarian tumors are more likely to occur in the right ovary.[25] The first step in treating ovarian carcinoma is a staging laparotomy. If the tumor is localized to one ovary, unilateral salpingooophorectomy is performed with removal of the paraaortic and ipsilateral lymph nodes. Diagnostic cytologic washings of the diaphragm and peritoneum, as well as omentectomy, are also performed at this time. Box 138-1 describes the staging system for ovarian cancer.[26]

Ovarian dysgerminomas are the most common malignant tumors. Dysgerminomas are analogous to seminoma of the testes in males. Most are unilateral (85%).[6] Dysgerminomas have no specific tumor markers, but patients may have elevated human chorionic gonadotropin (hCG) and lactic dehydrogenase levels. Treatment includes staging laparotomy. Postoperative chemotherapy with bleomycin, etoposide, and cisplatin (BEP) has produced the best results with preservation of future fertility. Radiation therapy has been virtually abandoned because of subsequent infertility and tissue scarring.

The second most common ovarian tumor is the endodermal sinus tumor that originates from extraembryonic germ cells. This tumor produces alpha-fetoprotein (AFP), which can serve as a useful tumor marker in the course of therapy. Endodermal sinus tumors are radioresistant, so after resection of the tumor and lymph nodes

---

> **BOX 138-1**
> **Staging of Ovarian Carcinoma**
>
> Stage I   Limited to one ovary
> Stage II   Beyond ovary but not involving trans-abdominal structures
> Stage III   All the above but with tumor nodules in omentum, retroperitoneal lymph nodes, or mesentery
> Stage IV   Distant metastases (lung, liver, bone)

Adapted from Kottmeiier HL: Classification and staging of malignant tumors in the female pelvis, *Int J Gynaecol Obstet* 9:172-180, 1971.

> **BOX 138-2**
> **Gynecologic Causes of Acute Abdominal Pain in Adolescent Females**
>
> Rupture of ovarian cyst
> Pelvic inflammatory disease
> Torsion of ovary
> Ectopic pregnancy
> Threatened abortion
> Intrauterine pregnancy
> Ovarian tumor
> Endometriosis

---

and peritoneal sampling, chemotherapy with BEP is usually the treatment of choice.

Other ovarian carcinomas that may be found in adolescent girls include the immature teratoma, embryonal carcinoma, mixed germ cell carcinoma, and juvenile granulosa cell tumors. Embryonal carcinoma usually occurs in prepubertal girls or young adolescents. Beta-hCG and AFP are useful tumor markers for embryonal carcinoma and mixed germ cell tumors. Again, after surgical resection, chemotherapy with BEP has been shown to produce the best outcome.

Pelvic Pain

Pathologic processes of the uterus or adnexal organs are major causes of acute and chronic pelvic pain in adolescents. The differential diagnosis of acute pelvic pain includes the gynecologic as well as the gastrointestinal and urologic organ systems. Box 138-2 lists the gynecologic causes of acute pelvic pain. Many of these entities have been discussed in detail throughout this chapter. Pelvic inflammatory disease is described in Chapter 140. Pregnancy and its complications are discussed in Chapter 142.

It is important when eliciting a history of the acute pain to determine the sequence of events and include a thorough menstrual, sexual, and contraceptive history.

BOX 138-3
Gynecologic Causes of Chronic
Abdominal Pain in Adolescent Females

Ovarian cyst
Mittelschmerz
Dysmenorrhea
Endometriosis
Genital tract malformation
Chronic pelvic inflammatory disease
Pelvic serositis
Pelvic congestion

Every sexually active female with abdominal pain requires a physical examination with special attention to the abdomen, pelvic organs, and rectum. The diagnostic work-up for acute pelvic pain usually includes a complete blood count with differential, sedimentation rate, urinalysis, urine culture, pregnancy test, and gonorrhea and *Chlamydia* tests if the girl is sexually active. Often, a pelvic ultrasound examination is helpful. If not, laparoscopy may be the only method to determine the appropriate diagnosis.

In a study at Boston Children's Hospital, 121 adolescent girls were evaluated by laparoscopy for acute abdominal pain.[27] The most common diagnoses were ovarian cyst, acute salpingitis, no pathology, appendicitis, and ovarian torsion. Thus, rupture, infection, and torsion involving the ovary and adnexa are leading causes of acute abdominal pain in adolescent girls.

Diagnosing chronic pelvic pain in adolescent girls is often a source of frustration for both the adolescent and the physician. The work-up is similar to that for acute abdominal pain, although laparoscopy may be invaluable to enable the definitive diagnosis when all other diagnostic tests are unfruitful.[28] Box 138-3 lists the gynecologic causes of chronic abdominal pain. A study of adolescent girls undergoing laparoscopy for chronic pelvic pain revealed endometriosis, no organic disease, postoperative adhesions, serositis, and ovarian cysts to be the most prevalent causes of pain.[27]

References

1. Moore KL: *The developing human,* ed 3, Philadelphia, 1982, WB Saunders; pp 272-281.
2. Freeman MF: Uterine anomalies, *Semin Reprod Endocrinol* 4:39, 1986.
3. Sanfilippo JS, Yussman MA, Smith O: HSG in the evaluation of infertility. A six year review, *Fertil Steril* 30:636, 1978.
4. Pinsonneault O, Goldstein DP: Obstructing malformations of the uterus and vagina, *Fertil Steril* 44:241, 1985.
5. Edmonds DK: Sexual developmental anomalies and their reconstruction: upper and lower tracts. In Sanfilippo JS, Muram D, Lee PA, Dewhurst J, editors: *Pediatric and adolescent gynecology,* Philadelphia, 1994, WB Saunders; pp 535-566.
6. La Vecchia C, Draper GJ: Childhood nonovarian female genital tract cancers in Britain, 1962-1978. Descriptive epidemiology and long-term survival, *Cancer* 54:188-192, 1984.
7. Hicks ML, Piver MS: Oncologic problems. In Sanfilippo JS, Muram D, Lee PA, Dewhurst J, editors: *Pediatric and adolescent gynecology,* Philadelphia, 1994, WB Saunders; pp 601-616.
8. Jenkins S, Olive DL, Haney AF: Endometriosis: pathogenetic implications of anatomic distribution, *Obstet Gynecol* 67:335-338, 1986.
9. Emans SJH, Goldstein DP: *Pediatric and adolescent gynecology,* ed 3, Boston, 1990, Little, Brown; pp 284-291.
10. Metzger DA, Haney AF: Etiology of endometriosis, *Obstet Gynecol Clin North Am* 16:1-14, 1989.
11. Goldstein DP, de Cholnoky C, Emans SJ: Adolescent endometriosis, *J Adolesc Health Care* 1:37-41, 1980.
12. Gidwani GP: Endometriosis: more common than you think, *Contemp Pediatr* 6:99-110, 1989.
13. Simpson JL, Elias S, Malinak LR, et al: Heritable aspects of endometriosis. I. Genetic studies, *Am J Obstet Gynecol* 137:327, 1980.
14. American Fertility Society: American Fertility Society classification of endometriosis, *Fertil Steril* 43:351, 1985.
15. Henzl MR, Corson SC, Moghissi K, et al: Administration of nasal nafarelin as compared with oral danazol for endometriosis, *N Engl J Med* 318:485-489, 1988.
16. Lu PT, Ory SJ: Endometriosis: current management, *Mayo Clin Proc* 70:453-463, 1995.
17. Barbieri RL: CA-125 in patients with endometriosis, *Fertil Steril* 45:767-769, 1986.
18. Surratt JT, Siegel MJ: Imaging of pediatric ovarian masses, *Radiographics,* 11:533-548, 1991.
19. Murray S, London S: Management of ovarian cysts in neonates, children, and adolescents, *Adolesc Pediatr Gynecol* 8:64-70, 1995.
20. Stegner HE: Hormonally related non-neoplastic conditions of the ovary, *Curr Top Pathol* 78:11-39, 1989.
21. Tayob Y, Adams J, Jacobs H, et al: Ultrasound demonstration of increased frequency of functional ovarian cysts in women using progestogen only oral contraception, *Br J Obstet Gynaecol* 92:1003, 1985.
22. Jones HW: Germ cell tumors of the ovary. In Jones HW, Wentz AC, Burnett LS, editors: *Novak's textbook of gynecology,* ed 11, Baltimore, 1988, Williams & Wilkins.
23. Laing FC, Van Dalsem VF, Marks WM, et al: Dermoid cysts of the ovary: their ultrasonographic appearances, *Obstet Gynecol* 57:99-104, 1981.
24. Woodruff JD, Protos P, Peterson WF: Ovarian teratomas, *Am J Obstet Gynecol* 102:702, 1968.
25. Raney RB, Sinclair L, Uri A, et al: Malignant ovarian tumors in children and adolescents, *Cancer* 59:1214-1220, 1987.
26. Kottmeiier HL: Classification and staging of malignant tumors in the female pelvis, *Int J Gynaecol Obstet* 9:172-180, 1971.
27. Goldstein DP: Acute and chronic pelvic pain, *Pediatr Clin North Am* 36:573-580, 1989.
28. Howard F: The role of laparoscopy in chronic pelvic pain: promise and pitfalls, *Obstet Gynecol Surv* 48:357-387, 1993.

CHAPTER 139

Male Genitalia: Examination and Findings

•

Reuben D. Rohn

COMPONENTS OF EXAMINATION

During adolescence the male genitalia undergo maturational changes that should be observed and documented. Sexual maturation scales such as Tanner staging are used to rate both pubic hair and genital development.[1] The Tanner genital scale is a composite rating of penile, scrotal, and testicular development. It is therefore more accurate to assess each component (penis, scrotum, and testes) separately. The orchidometer measures testicular size. Penile measurements also can be assessed.[1,2] In general, scrotal and testicular enlargement changes take place before penile enlargement, and penile lengthening occurs before an increase in girth.

Adolescents are highly concerned about their body image, and even slight deviations from their perception of normal development may cause anxiety. The physician may use the examination of the genitalia as an opportunity to educate as well as allay any fears and reassure the adolescent.

The male with delayed pubertal development often suffers psychologically because of the delay and the relatively small genital size. Our society places much emphasis on the size of a man's penis, the size of the phallus being equated with the degree of sexual satisfaction.

The physician should be aware of the normal range for penile size and should reassure the adolescent about the lack of relationship between size and sexual potency. The genital examination allows the physician to introduce the concept of testicular self-examination. When the adolescent has reached Tanner stage 5, he is at the appropriate emotional maturational level to be taught this procedure. Some argue that testicular self-examination causes anxiety in adolescent males and that it is neither medically nor financially cost effective.[3] However, educating males and giving them the ability to have some control over their bodies by performing self-examination probably reassures them.

The physical examination consists of inspection of the penis and the scrotum, palpation of the scrotum and its contents (including the testes), and rectal examination for palpation of the prostate gland. Prepubertally the prostate is extremely small and cannot be palpated. With the onset of puberty, the prostate gradually enlarges. Although disorders of the prostate are uncommon in most adolescents, prostatitis can occur, especially as a result of sexually transmitted disease (STD). Prostatic examination may be important for diagnostic purposes in certain cases.

PHYSICAL FINDINGS

Penis

Most congenital anomalies of the penis are discovered before adolescence. Penile agenesis, hypospadias (ventral displacement of the urethral meatus) and epispadias (dorsal deviation of the urethral meatus), diphallia, and accessory penis are usually discovered early.[4] Micropenis, or small penile size, however, may be brought to the attention of the physician during adolescence. Concern about adequate size may be an issue. Schonfeld and Beebe published data on normal penile size according to age (Table 139-1). Length must be evaluated when the penis is in the stretched state, with measurement made from the symphysis pubis to the tip. Often the perineal fat pad may be quite large in obese males, causing concern about inadequate penile length. Appropriate measurement and reassurance is needed in such cases. If penile length is below age standards, evaluation for primary or secondary hypogonadism or isolated deficiency of growth hormone should be undertaken with the appropriate stimulation studies.

Torsion of the penis as an isolated finding is uncommon. It typically occurs in association with hypospadias or chordee. Torsion is a twisting of the penis around its

TABLE 139-1
Normal Penile Length Measurements

	Penile Length (cm)		
Age (yr)	10th Percentile	Median	90th Percentile
9	4.9	6.3	7.6
10	4.9	6.2	7.6
11	4.7	6.6	8.7
12	4.9	7.1	11.3
13	6.1	8.7	12.2
14	6.6	9.8	13.5
15	9.1	11.8	14.8
16	10.8	12.5	15.3
17	10.8	13.3	15.3
18-19	10.8	13.1	15.5
20-25	11.3	13.0	15.5

From Schonfeld WA, Beebe GW: Normal growth and variation in male genitalia from birth to maturity, *J Urol* 48:759, 1942. Williams & Wilkins, 1942, Copyright ©.

length, usually in a counterclockwise fashion, with the median raphe usually spiraling obliquely around the shaft. The penis is otherwise normal in development and configuration. In most instances intervention is not required, but if the condition is severe, surgical correction may be made.[5]

Chordee involves ventral or dorsal bending of the penis, the former being much more common. Although usually associated with hypospadias, chordee can be an isolated phenomenon and may therefore not be recognized until adolescence.[6] Downward flexion occurs because of insufficient skin on the ventral surface of the organ. The extent of the flexion is usually worse during erection. Surgical correction may be needed if the condition is severe.

Lateral curvature of the penis due to a congenital asymmetric development of the corpora cavernosa is another relatively rare condition.[7] Usually the penis is normal in its flaccid state but bends laterally on erection. If the condition is severe, surgical correction may be needed.

Penile skin lesions of fairly minor significance include mucosal subcutaneous cysts and dermoid cysts, which are usually found along the median penile raphe.[5] In contrast, pink pearly papules, approximately 1 to 3 mm in diameter, are found along the penile corona.[8] These lesions need to be differentiated from condylomata acuminata. Surgical excision may be necessary to remove large lesions.

Balanitis (inflammation of the glans penis) and balanoposthitis (infection of the glans or prepuce) are seen occasionally in uncircumcised adolescents. Prevention consists of appropriate personal hygiene.[9] These infections sometimes occur because of phimosis. They usually respond to antimicrobial therapy but need to be distinguished from an STD. Occasionally, when the condition is severe, surgical drainage and incision of the prepuce is needed. Penile skin lesions resulting from STD, including syphilitic chancres, herpetic vesicles, venereal warts (condylomata acuminata), and soft chancres, may be detected. Monilial balanitis may occur, producing a characteristic red pruritic inflammation, with white, curdlike discharge from the prepuce. STDs are discussed in Chapter 140.

Priapism (persistent painful penile erection) commonly occurs in association with local irritation, but it may occur in other conditions such as urethritis, urethral or bladder stones, blunt perineal trauma, spinal cord injury, sickle cell anemia, leukemia, thrombosis of the corpora cavernosa, mumps, and Fabry's disease.[10] Conservative management includes ice packs and analgesics; if this approach is unsuccessful, surgical intervention, including needle aspiration and irrigation procedures, may be required.

Undescended Testicle

There is no universally accepted definition of undescended testis. One definition of an undescended or maldescended testis is of one that lies less than 4 cm below the pubic tubercle[11]; however, most believe that a description of the testicular location is the best way to define the problem.[12] A retractile testis is one that is intermittently retracted out of the scrotum, as a function of the cremasteric muscle reflex. Such a testis can be manipulated into the scrotal sac. An ectopic testis is one that has descended through the inguinal canal but has not reached the scrotum; is situated in the superficial inguinal pouch; does not have an associated hernia; and may be in a pubic, penile, femoral, or peroneal position. A cryptorchid testis is one that lies along the normal route of descent but has not passed through the external inguinal ring. Finally, anorchia refers to complete absence of the testicle.

INCIDENCE. Cryptorchidism occurs in 2% to 6% of full-term infants and decreases by 1 year of age to 0.7% to 2%.[13] Regardless of this variability, the consistent finding is that the incidence remains constant beyond 1 year of age. Thus, cryptorchidism is one of the most frequent developmental abnormalities of the human male. Furthermore, spontaneous descent after 1 year of age is rare. An increased incidence of cryptorchidism is seen in various conditions or syndromes. There appears to be a genetic predisposition, since cryptorchidism is present in 1% to 4% of siblings and 6% of fathers of children with undescended testes.[14]

EMBRYOLOGY OF DESCENT. Until 6 to 8 weeks of gestation, the fetal gonad is indeterminate. In the seventh week of embryologic development, the gonad begins to differentiate into a testis under the influence of the SRY gene (present on the short arm of the Y chromosome). Sertoli cells of the testis begin to release müllerian inhibitory factor, which causes regression of the müllerian structures. Under the influence of testosterone production, which begins by the eighth week of gestation, the mesonephric (wolffian) duct develops into the male ductular system (epididymis, vas deferens, seminal vesicles). Dihydrotestosterone formed through peripheral conversion of testosterone by the enzyme 5α-reductase promotes the external genitalia to develop between 10 and 16 weeks of fetal development. At about 11 weeks, the processus vaginalis is recognizable, located at the level of the internal inguinal ring. The processus vaginalis is in contiguity with a gelatinous material—gubernaculum—that inserts on the mesonephric duct. The first of the two separate stages of this particular descent then takes place transabdominally. By the seventeenth week, the testis is at the internal inguinal ring and begins to elongate in its vertical axis. This phase of descent is androgen independent.[15] The testis remains at the level of the internal inguinal ring until approximately the twenty-eighth week of gestation, when the inguinal scrotal stage of descent (second phase) begins. This stage is dependent on gubernacular regression.[16] The precise mechanism for the inguinal scrotal descent is unclear. Various hormonal factors (descendin, müllerian inhibitory factor, and estrogen) have possible roles to play.[15-18] The roles of nerves (genitofemoral) and intraabdominal pressure have also been investigated and may be involved in testicular descent.[17-19] At this point, the mechanism of testicular descent is yet to be fully elucidated.

The etiology of maldescent includes many anatomic, hormonal, and genetic abnormalities, including pituitary absence, intersex, dysgenetic testis, and anatomic obstruction. Evaluation of the patient includes a careful history taking to ascertain whether testes have ever been present, or noted on physical examination in the past.

Physical examination should be done in a warm room with the patient lying supine. If cryptorchidism is suspected, the patient should also be examined in a cross-legged position, allowing a retractile testis to descend spontaneously into the scrotum without manipulation.

One third of boys with true cryptorchidism have bilateral cryptorchid testes, while two thirds are unilateral (right-sided 70%, left-sided 30%). In the same study, abdominal cryptorchidism occurred in 8%, inguinal cryptorchidism in 72%, maldescent in 20%, and testicular aplasia or anorchia in 2.6%.[20]

Hormonal treatment for cryptorchidism has been in use since the 1930s, but its use remains controversial. Human chorionic gonadotropin (hCG) has been the primary hormonal treatment in the United States. Treatment regimens vary from 4 days to 6 weeks, with dosage varying from 500 IU daily for 1 week up to 1500 IU every other day. Response rate is highest in the older child. Therefore, adolescents presenting with cryptorchidism would be expected to have the highest success rate with this form of therapy. Unfortunately, germ cell damage is well established by 2 years of age, with 40% of testes demonstrating azoospermia.[21,22] Luteinizing hormone–releasing hormone (LHRH) administered through nasal spray has been studied in Europe but is not readily available in the United States. A very well-performed control study showed no statistical difference in the success rate of LHRH compared with placebo.[23] In general, hormonal treatment appears to work best in boys with low-lying testes (maldescended). It has even been argued that much of the success rate in many studies is predicated upon a high rate of retractile testes in the subjects studied. In one clinical situation, hormonal treatment is invaluable. A teenage male with totally nonpalpable testes should undergo hormonal testing. A lack of significant testosterone rise in response to hCG even after a short course of 4 or 5 days of treatment suggests a lack of any testicular tissue. In these circumstances, surgical exploration would be unwarranted.

Surgical treatment is thus the choice for boys under 2 years of age for preservation of germinal cell function. It is also recommended for postpubertal men under 32 years of age, determined by a statistical evaluation of cancer risk.[24] The goal of surgery in adolescence is to avoid the complications of psychologic maladjustment, testicular malignancy, possible longer-term endocrine deficiency, vulnerability to trauma, and inguinal hernia.

Testicular cancer is the major sequela of cryptorchidism in adolescent males. Of all cases of testicular cancer, 7.3% have a history of cryptorchidism.[24] The risk of cancer is greater in intraabdominal testes than in lower-lying gonads: an overall 22.2-fold increase in risk compared with adolescent males with scrotal testes.[21] Interestingly, in unilateral cryptorchidism, testicular cancers occur in the contralateral normally descended testis in 20% of all cases of testicular cancer.[25]

Despite histologic damage, the rate of fertility, as determined through either semen analysis or paternity, is not as devastating as one might expect. In 21 reports since 1935, azoospermia or oligospermia was noted in 44% to 100% of patients studied. Many studies imply that one fourth to as many as one half of men with previous bilateral cryptorchidism may be fertile. This appears to be further confirmed by reports that 43% to 62% of married men with bilateral cryptorchidism have fathered children. In all cases, variability appeared to be less critical with regard to the age of surgical repair as long as it was done at the time of adolescence or earlier.[13]

Scrotum

Appropriate examination of the scrotum and its contents involves inspection, palpation, and transillumination. Inspection and palpation should be done with the adolescent in both the standing and supine positions.

Palpation of the scrotum is best managed systematically. The testis, epididymis, and spermatic cord should be palpated separately. The testis lies vertically in the hemiscrotum, is ovoid, and is firm to palpation. The epididymis is closely attached to the posterolateral border of the testis. The head of the epididymis (globus major) is at the superior portion of the testis, and the tail of the epididymis (globus minor) is at the inferior pole of the testis. The vas deferens emerges from the tail of the epididymis as a relatively hard cord lying in the posteriomedial portion of the spermatic cord. The spermatic cord itself emerges from the testis and runs the length of the scrotum upward into the inguinal canal.

Several congenital anomalies may affect the scrotum and its contents. Most should have been detected before puberty. These include bifid scrotum, in which each hemiscrotum is separate from the other; penoscrotal transposition, in which the penis lies partially or entirely behind the scrotum; and ectopic scrotum.[10] These uncommon conditions are often associated with other genitourinary anomalies. Surgical treatment may be necessary, depending on the degree of deformity in each of the conditions. Hypoplasia of the whole scrotum or the hemiscrotum is a sign of cryptorchidism or monorchidism, respectively.

SCROTAL WALL SWELLINGS

Swellings of the scrotum may occur as a result of conditions involving the scrotal wall or the internal structures of the scrotum. Scrotal wall swellings tend to be less frequent than intrascrotal content swelling. However, at times there may be confusion and difficulty

in differentiating the margin, and hence location, of a painful swelling.

Acute Idiopathic Scrotal Wall Edema

This condition may affect one or both sides of the scrotum and is characterized by a violaceous coloration that may spread to the perineum or to the abdominal wall.[26] Usually, the testis and epididymis are palpable separately from the swelling and are themselves nontender. This helps to differentiate this condition from more serious intrascrotal disorders. The cause of acute idiopathic scrotal wall edema is unknown, although occasionally it can be associated with insect bites and contact allergies. Spontaneous resolution of this condition is the rule.[27]

Acute Vasculitis

Henoch-Schönlein purpura, which may cause acute pain and swelling, can mimic testicular torsion. Usually, swelling is confined to the wall itself, but in 15% of cases testicular swelling also occurs.[28] The scrotal findings may precede the characteristic rash of Henoch-Schönlein purpura. The scrotal wall is purpuric, erythematous, and tender to palpation. To further complicate the issue of differential diagnosis, spermatic cord torsion has been reported in Henoch-Schönlein purpura.[29] Thus, a high index of suspicion of this condition must exist to confirm the diagnosis of acute vasculitis. In most instances, spontaneous resolution without significant sequelae is the rule in this uncommon condition.

Idiopathic Fat Necrosis

Idiopathic fat necrosis is unusual. Although most often it results from trauma, the preceding history is often difficult to elicit.[30] The condition may present with unilateral or occasionally bilateral tenderness. Sometimes a mass may be palpated, but this is usually separate from the testis. Scrotal sonography may be indicated to clearly distinguish this mass from the testis proper. Testicular torsion must be excluded, and when there is doubt, surgical exploration is indicated.

Spontaneous Gangrene

Spontaneous gangrene is a rare condition most often seen in neonates. Acute swelling, edema, and necrosis may appear. This condition is associated with fever and frank toxemia. A portal of entry is often identifiable (e.g., circumcision).[31] Treatment consists of intravenous antibiotics, soaks, and (if necessary) incision and debridement.

Cutaneous Cysts and Tumors

Midline inclusion dermoid cysts may occur anywhere along the scrotal raphe.[10] They result from implantation of cell rests during fusion of the genital swellings. Occasionally, calculi or infection may develop and lead to a discharging sinus. Sometimes, they may be so deep as to be difficult to differentiate from intrascrotal structures. Scrotal sonography may be required to confirm the diagnosis. Sebaceous and epidermal inclusion cysts may occur but are uncommon. These latter two conditions tend to be subcutaneous and are usually easy to distinguish from other scrotal conditions. Surgical excision may be necessary for any of these cysts.[27]

INTRASCROTAL NONPAINFUL MASSES

Hernias and Hydroceles

Hernias and hydroceles occur as a result of failure of fusion and obliteration of the processus vaginalis (Fig. 139-1). They are usually nonpainful and may be only intermittently palpable. Most are detected in early infancy, but some may persist to be detected only in later childhood and adolescence. Pain occurs as the hernia is incarcerated or strangulated. Strangulation requires immediate admission and surgical intervention. Incarcerated hernia should also be tended to immediately. An attempt may be made to reduce the hernia manually after sedation. Should this fail, surgery is required. Asymptomatic masses that are reducible may be handled on an elective basis.[27] Complete opening of the processus vaginalis is almost always seen in infancy. Those that are delayed are found in children or adolescents who have a patent

processus vaginalis proximally with the processus obliterated distally (Fig. 139-1). Controversy exists regarding the need for surgical exploration of the contralateral side. In boys with a history of inguinal hernia, 59% up to the age of 16 years were found to have a contralateral patent processus vaginalis.[32] In another study, McGregor et al found that if a boy had had a previous left-sided hernia repair, he had a 41% chance of a right-sided hernia. However, if a right-sided lesion had been repaired, there was only a 15% chance of a left-sided hernia.[33] At the present time, there is a significant divergence of opinion regarding the approach to exploration of the contralateral side. It appears that 80% of pediatric surgeons surveyed routinely perform contralateral side explorations.[34]

A hydrocele occurs when there is persistence of the processus vaginalis with partial or complete fusion in the proximal portion (Fig. 139-1). Almost all of these lesions are communicating in nature, and therefore intermittently enlarge. Because such hydroceles do not spontaneously close beyond age 2 years, such a lesion found in an adolescent requires surgical repair. If an associated hernia is present, surgical intervention should be more immediate. A spermatic cord (loculated) hydrocele may occur anywhere along the cord. It arises from distal closure of the processus vaginalis, with the more proximal ends still patent. These may occur anywhere along the cord and tend to be more firm in nature. They are often difficult to distinguish from an independent or a paratesticular rhabdomyosarcoma on physical examination. Transillumination and, if necessary, sonography can help confirm the diagnosis. Such a lesion usually requires surgical exploration. The rarest of all hydroceles is an isolated scrotal hydrocele, which occurs with absence of proximal patency of the processus vaginalis. Such a lesion may be the presenting sign of a serious condition such as a

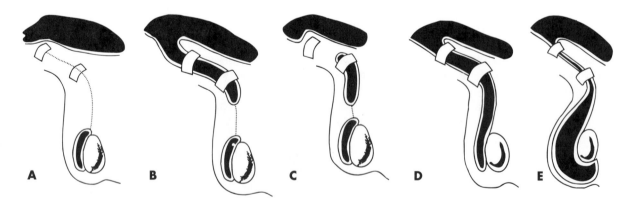

Fig. 139-1. Diagrammatic representation of persisting patent processus vaginalis. **A,** Normal obliteration of the patent processus. **B,** Patent processus proximally with inguinal bulge; the processus is obliterated distally. **C,** Closure proximal and distal with loculated hydrocele of the cord. **D,** Complete patency with the hernia sac extending into the scrotum. **E,** Partial proximal closure, resulting in scrotal hydrocele and proximal patent processus. (From Lewis JE Jr: *Atlas of infant surgery,* St. Louis, 1967, Mosby–Year Book; p 89.)

testicular tumor or chronic epididymitis. Surgical exploration is usually mandatory.[27]

Varicocele

Varicocele is one of the more misdiagnosed and misunderstood causes of scrotal swelling of childhood, adolescence, and adulthood.[35] Gross distention of multiple veins and the spermatic cord, which are visible and palpable, is easily recognized. It is assumed that these dilated veins result from venous incompetence, but the latter may occur in the absence of dilated veins, and dilated veins may occur in the absence of venous incompetence. Furthermore, it is difficult to identify lesser forms of varicoceles. In 1988, Hudson[36] developed a classification criteria for varicoceles as follows:

Subclinical: Not palpable or visible, even with Valsalva maneuver, but demonstrable on Doppler examination or other special test
Grade I: Palpable only during Valsalva maneuver
Grade II: Palpable at rest but not visible
Grade III: Palpable and visible at rest

Despite the above classification criteria, confusion and disagreement may occur between physicians. One study found disagreement in 36 of 138 cases between two doctors who previously had agreed on criteria for the varicocele.[37] There is a great degree of subjectivity in the diagnosis, especially between grade I and II varicocele. Evaluation of outcome studies based on clinical examination must be interpreted with caution. The incidence of varicocele ranges from 9% to 26% of adolescent males. Collation of four published series revealed that 2123 of 10,669 patients (20%) had a varicocele.[38-41] A similar frequency of varicocele was noted in the adult male population.[27] The cause or mechanism for formation of varicoceles has been debated for some time. Ninety percent are left-sided, which supports one theory that varicoceles develop because of incompetence of the spermatic vein, which drains directly into the renal vein on the left side at right angles to it. On the right side the spermatic vein drains obliquely and directly into the inferior vena cava; hence, right-sided incompetence varicocele is much less frequent. Additional possible causes, including alterations in temperature and local hormonal concentrations, relative testicular hypoxia, and reflux of vasoactive substances and steroids in retrograde fashion from the renal vein to the testes, have all been postulated but not proved.[42] In a study of 659 patients, Braedel et al[43] demonstrated that retrograde flow of blood through persistent intracardinal anastomoses secondary to disordered involution of the venous system during embryogenesis is the probable cause of varicocele.

The physical examination for varicocele is subjective in nature. There are objective ways of making the diagnosis. These include (1) venography, which is the gold standard but very expensive, invasive, and requiring skilled radiologic technique; (2) Doppler probe, which is noninvasive, is relatively inexpensive, and correlates reasonably well with other tests and clinical examination; and (3) contact thermography strips, thermometry, and ultrasonography, which have also been used with varying degrees of accuracy.[35] Should there be a need for objective assessment of questioned clinical varicocele, tests done with the combination of ultrasound and Doppler give results close to those of venography, with lesser expense and without invasiveness.

Varicoceles have been associated with a decrease in volume of the ipsilateral testis. The larger the size of the varicocele, the greater is the degree of testicular volume loss and of testicular atrophy. In adults, there is a higher rate of infertility in individuals with varicocele. For most adolescent boys, palpation of the testes in a standing position, together with measurement of volume of both testes, should be sufficient to confirm the diagnosis of varicocele and to determine the degree of its clinical effect on the individual. One study has indicated that horizontal lie of the testis is a useful clinical sign that should alert the examiner to the possibility of varicocele.[44] If there is concern regarding fertility, hormonal testing may be of further assistance. Elevated follicle-stimulating hormone (FSH) in comparison with the norm usually indicates damage to spermatogenesis. Increased LH levels occur only in severe bilateral testicular atrophy, signaling a very poor prognosis.[27] Lower levels of testosterone have been noted in men with varicocele as opposed to normal men, but this is usually seen in older men.[35]

Varicoceles should be treated if they are exceedingly large, if there is a significant change in testicular consistency, or if there is symptomatic pain or discomfort.[45] Treatment of varicocele for prevention of infertility is not generally acceptable.[27,38,45] The treatment of varicocele is surgical ligation or percutaneous testicular vein embolization. Complications of treatment include a 5% rate of persistence of testicular atrophy, a 6% rate of hydrocele formation, and a 1% rate of varicocele recurrence.

Macroorchidism

Macroorchidism may occur as a result of compensatory hypertrophy in males who have had an undescended testis or a rudimentary testis on the contralateral side. A rudimentary testis may result from inappropriate fetal development, vascular impairment, or degeneration after orchitis. Unilateral compensatory hypertrophy is often associated with elevated FSH secretion and sometimes with oligospermia, suggesting that hypertrophy may result in abnormality of function as well.[46] The unilaterally enlarged testis that is very hard upon palpation and heavier than the other testis may indicate malignant tumor. Bilateral macroorchidism is usually a benign condition that is not associated with any pathologic problem (idiopathic).[13,47] In this situation, the testes feel normal in texture and consistency. Bilaterally enlarged testes in an adolescent with significant mental retardation necessitates evaluation for fragile X syndrome.[48] Although much less common, leukemia may be associated with bilateral enlargement of the testes along with hardness upon palpation. Congenital adrenal hyperplasia may present with bilateral testicular enlargement, usually with considerable testicular nodularity, resulting from adrenal rest tissue hyperplasia.[49] Unilateral enlargement of the testis or left-sided scrotal swelling has been noted with accessory spleen attachment to the upper pole of the testis, but this is rare.[50]

Microorchidism

The finding of unusually small testes for the degree of pubertal development needs further investigation. By age 14, testicular volume should be greater than 4 ml as a result of increased gonadotropin secretion. Complete lack of sexual maturation (i.e., no pubic hair, no scrotal vascularization, and small penis and testes) requires appropriate investigation of the whole hypothalamic-pituitary-testicular axis. If small testicular size is associated with normal scrotal, penile, and pubic hair development, the possibility of Klinefelter's syndrome, mumps orchitis, or other testicular failure must be considered.[51] Bilateral testicular hypoplasia also has been described in males after diethylstilbestrol (DES) exposure in utero.[10]

Spermatocele

A spermatocele is a painless cystic mass that contains spermatozoa and feels like a small, round, nontender bulb. The specific cause is unknown. It appears that the cysts arise as dilations of the afferent ductules that connect the rete testis to the head of the epididymis. They tend to be located at the head of the epididymis, and thus above and posterior to the testis. They are usually small, 1 cm in size or less, but can be as much as ten times that size. Transillumination may help to differentiate the condition from a testicular tumor. Ultrasonography may be used to confirm the location and hence the diagnosis. Spermatoceles are usually of no significance; they occasionally grow large enough to cause discomfort or pain. Surgical excision may be indicated to relieve the pain, discomfort, or excessive swelling. Sclerotherapy has also been used as an alternative form of treatment.[52]

Malignant Neoplasms

Testicular malignancy is the most common solid tumor occurring in males between the age of puberty and 40

years. Even though the incidence is still rare—overall about 2 to 3 per 100,000—the risk of malignancy in undescended testis is anywhere from five to 48 times the risk in a normally descended testis.[53-55] In one of the more extensive studies, it appears that the overall risk of testicular cancer in cryptorchid testis—regardless of its surgical repair—is 9.7 times the risk of a never cryptorchid testis.[23] Etiologically, germinal cell tumors are the rule (96%). Approximately 25% of tumors are composed of multiple cell types, the most common mixture being embryonal carcinoma with teratoma. Non–germ cell tumors account for 3% to 4% of all primary testicular tumors (Box 139-1).

Almost 20% of all testicular malignancies in men with unilateral undescended testes occur in the normal scrotal testis (this is about twice the incidence as compared with bilaterally descended testes). Also, the possibility of a second testicular tumor in a patient who has had one such tumor is extremely high. The chances are even higher if the patient had bilateral nondescent of the testis.[12] A testicular tumor may be a firm to hard mass or nodule palpated within the testis. Such an abnormality must be considered to be a tumor until proved otherwise. The examiner must be careful to differentiate between the epididymis and the testis itself to ensure that the mass is

---

BOX 139-1
**Histologic Classification
of Primary Neoplasms**

A. Germinal neoplasms (demonstrating one or more of the following components)
  1. Seminoma
    a. Classic (typical) seminoma
    b. Anaplastic seminoma
    c. Spermatocytic seminoma
  2. Embryonal carcinoma
  3. Teratoma (with or without malignant transformation)
    a. Mature
    b. Immature
  4. Choriocarcinoma
  5. Yolk sac tumor (endodermal sinus tumor; embryonal adenocarcinoma of the pubertal testis)
B. Nongerminal neoplasms
  1. Specialized gonadal stromal neoplasms
    a. Leydig cell tumor
    b. Other gonadal stromal tumor
  2. Gonadoblastoma
  3. Miscellaneous neoplasms
    a. Adenocarcinoma of rete testis
    b. Mesenchymal neoplasms
    c. Carcinoid
    d. Adrenal rest "tumor"

truly within the tunica albuginea. The mass is usually painless, but a dull ache may be felt in 40% of individuals. A dragging sensation or a feeling of heaviness may be noted. Occasionally, acute pain and swelling occur if there is a hemorrhage within the tumor. Painful presentation may delay diagnosis, if it is presumed that torsion of the testis or orchitis is the cause of the pain. If the diagnosis is delayed, metastatic symptoms may predominate. Metastatic disease may present as back pain, abdominal mass, or inguinal or supraclavicular adenopathy. Occasionally, reactive hydroceles may form in the scrotum. With estrogen production by the tumor, feminization may take place, producing gynecomastia, breast tenderness, loss of libido, or loss of the male escutcheon of pubic hair. Other presenting symptoms may result from metastatic disease (neck mass, respiratory symptoms, gastrointestinal disturbance, or lumbar back pain). Infertility is a rare presenting complaint. Unfortunately, there is usually a delay in diagnosis in most patients. Therefore, the importance of teaching adolescent males the technique of testicular self-examination cannot be stressed enough.

Serologic markers have proved very useful in detection and characterization of testicular tumors. More than 70% of such tumors elaborate one or another marker. The most commonly used are serum hCG and serum alpha-fetoprotein (AFP). hCG is derived from the syncytiotrophoblast, while the AFP is produced by yolk sac cells. Of further diagnostic assistance is ultrasonography, which helps localize the mass as intratesticular rather than extratesticular in nature. This technique differentiates varicoceles and spermatoceles, and also distinguishes between solid and cystic lesions. Failure to identify the nature of a mass satisfactorily by physical examination, transillumination, and ultrasonography requires surgical exploration for diagnosis. If not obtained previously, hCG and AFP levels should be obtained before any surgical procedures are undertaken. These markers serve as monitoring techniques as well as indicators of response to therapy.[56]

Histologically, tumors are divided into seminomatous and nonseminomatous germ cell tumors (NSGCTs). Each broad type has its own nuance of clinical and surgical/pathologic staging. There remains controversy over staging, since different systems are in use in different parts of the world and even in different institutions within the United States. Surgical staging, however, is critical to determine the degree of metastatic spread to lymph nodes. It is still more accurate and sensitive than clinical staging even with the use of magnetic resonance imaging (MRI) or computed tomography (CT). Treatment depends on the surgical/pathologic stage as well as the type of germ cell involved. Pure seminomas are very radiosensitive, and low-stage seminoma responds well to this mode of therapy. Higher-stage seminoma and other NSGCTs are given chemotherapy as the primary mode of therapy, with

surgical intervention for any residual disease. In low-stage seminoma, a higher than 95% cure rate is achievable with radiation therapy.[57] Cure rates and salvage rates have improved with the higher-stage seminomas and other NSGCTs.

The outcome for NSGCTs has improved because of improvements in clinical staging procedures and chemotherapy. Stage I NSGCT averages an approximately 98% 2- to 5-year survival with simple orchiectomy and a radical lymph node dissection procedure. The outcomes for higher stages have improved over the years with more aggressive chemotherapy and surgery. Exact statistics vary, with certain centers having more experience and better outcomes than others.[57]

With the success of newer treatments and a higher rate of survival, there is an increasing rate of long-term complications, including a high rate of infertility (secondary to cancers) and ejaculatory dysfunction (secondary to lymph node dissection procedures). Hypogonadism of the remaining testicle may also occur because of radiation therapy. Vascular complications, myocardial infarction, pulmonary fibrosis, and secondary malignancies are other late sequelae of treatment.[57] Pretreatment sperm banking is available to preserve future reproductive prospects for adolescents.

PAINFUL MASSES

Testicular Torsion

Testicular torsion represents one of the most serious urologic emergencies. Urgent and accurate diagnosis is needed. The time that has elapsed before the diagnosis is made is critical. Studies in rats indicate that the testis can survive 4 to 6 hours after experimental torsion. In humans, it appears that about 12 hours is the maximal length of survival before damage occurs, according to studies indicating 70% survival if surgery occurs within 12 hours. In general, the success rate for testicular survival subsequent to surgery has increased, probably as a result of recognition of the urgent nature of the condition. Testicular torsion occurs in about one in 4000 males below 25 years of age. Two thirds of all cases appear to occur in the pubertal age range of 12 to 18 years. Boys with absent testes (unilateral or bilateral) probably had previous undetected testicular torsion.[58]

Testicular torsion results from a "bell-clapper" deformity caused by the peritoneal investiture of the testis lying on the cord rather than on the lower pole of the testis (Fig. 139-2). The two most critical issues regarding the outcome of this disorder are the confusion involved in making the diagnosis in the first place, and a delay in seeking surgical intervention after establishing the diagnosis. The degree of testicular torsion appears to influence the degree of ischemia: Usually, 720 degrees is required

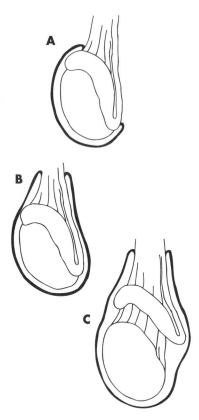

Fig. 139-2. Diagrammatic representation of the anatomy of spermatic cord tosion. **A,** Normal anatomy. The tunica vaginalis does not envelop the epididymis. **B,** "Bell-clapper" deformity. The tunica vaginalis extends high on the spermatic cord, enveloping the epididymis and allowing the testis to twist within. **C,** Testis suspended from the epididymis, allowing a twist to occur between the testis and the epididymis.

to produce ischemia. The classic presentation of acute scrotal pain, and associated nausea and vomiting and lack of urinary symptoms or findings, may not occur, and 10% of torsion may actually be painless. Pain may begin in the abdominal area and then be referred to the iliac fossa or groin before being localized to the scrotum. In up to one third of cases the history may indicate that one or more previous episodes of acute pain occurred and subsided spontaneously, with long intervening asymptomatic periods, sometimes lasting for weeks. It must be remembered that testicular torsion is the most common cause of acute scrotal pain. In one large series of males with acute scrotal pain, testicular torsion was the cause in 40%.

On physical examination, with the patient in the standing position, the affected testis may ride higher in the scrotum than the unaffected testis. The epididymis may be palpated in an abnormal location. Fever is not commonly present. The urinalysis usually shows normal results. Doppler flow studies or radionuclide scanning with intravenous technetium may be helpful in differentiating testes with normal or increased blood flow from those with torsion and decreased perfusion. However, one

must not place blind faith in these studies. When in doubt, surgical exploration is mandatory in order not to cause further delay and possible loss of testicular viability. Delay in diagnosis is not unusual, since the adolescent or his family may not have sought immediate treatment to begin with.

Manual derotation may be attempted by those who have experience. Sedation is required. The technique is to derotate toward the thigh, remembering, however, that derotation provides only temporary relief and does not obviate the need for surgical intervention and repair. Moreover, the surgical procedure requires treatment of a contralateral unaffected testis, since there is a higher rate of deformity in that one also.

Overall outcome has improved, with a 90% survival of the testes currently. Atrophy was reported in one third to two thirds of cases previously, probably secondary to the saving of poorly viable testes. Animal studies, primarily in rats and mice, have detected histologic changes in the contralateral testis of animals undergoing repair of torsion.[60] Elevated antibodies and diminished fertility have been found in these animals. Clinical studies in humans have also identified histologic changes in the contralateral testis. In some cases, this has been associated with abnormal semen analysis.[61] However, there is controversy over whether these changes are preexistent to the torsion, as claimed by Hadziselimovic et al,[62] or a consequence of the torsion, as claimed by Anderson et al.[63]

Torsion of the Testicular Appendages

Torsion of the vestiges of the müllerian and mesonephric ducts may occur and may mimic many of the findings of torsion of the spermatic cord and testis. The vestige known as the appendix testis or the hydatid of Morgagni is the most common appendage to be affected.[10] In one series, this disorder accounted for one fourth of all cases of acute testicular pain and swelling.[59]

Pain may be sudden or gradual in onset. It may vary from moderate to severe in nature, may occur without any precipitating event, and may be localized in the upper pole of the testis. Sometimes, if examination is made early, a firm, exquisitely tender, and relatively mobile pea-sized nodule may be noted in the upper scrotum attached to the testis or epididymis. Occasionally, the nodule may be perceived as a blue dot underneath the scrotal skin. Sometimes a nodule may be detected by transillumination. If the diagnosis can be made with confidence, observation without intervention may be pursued. On the other hand, the situation may be confusing and difficult to differentiate from true torsion of the testis, thus requiring surgery.

Torsion of portions of the epididymis or paradidymis is less frequently encountered. However, since males exposed to DES in utero have a higher incidence of epididymal cysts, the possibility of such torsion must be kept in mind.[10]

Epididymitis

Epididymitis is more common than usually believed. In one study, it accounted for 31% of all cases of scrotal pain and swelling.[59] It is seen commonly in boys who have urinary tract infections or structural lesions of the urinary tract, or who have previously undergone reconstructive surgery with indwelling urethral catheters present. Pathophysiologically, it appears that retrograde spread from the urinary tract infection, STD, postsurgical construction, or structural abnormality may be responsible for the epididymitis. Acute epididymitis is characterized by more gradual onset of pain, which is usually localized to the scrotum. Nausea and vomiting are uncommon; there is a greater likelihood of associated urinary tract symptoms. The patient is often febrile, with a fever greater than 101° F. Examination of the scrotal contents may detect that the pain is localized to the epididymis itself. The epididymis may enlarge and become tender and firm. The testicle is often normal. Elevation of the scrotal contents in epididymitis often leads to diminution of the pain (Prehn's sign). Doppler flow studies or radionuclide scanning may show increased or normal flow to the involved testis, thus helping to differentiate this entity from torsion of the spermatic cord.

Epididymitis is more commonly seen in the sexually active adolescent. The most common etiologic pathogens of the epididymitis are *Chlamydia trachomatis* or gonorrhea.[64] Pyuria and bacteriuria occur frequently. Unfortunately, two studies have indicated a 27% to 40% rate of pyuria in patients with spermatic cord torsion.[65,66] If epididymitis has been documented without the presence of an STD, the patient should probably undergo sonography of the kidneys and pelvis to rule out any abnormalities of the upper urinary tract system.

Orchitis

Orchitis is usually a secondary event after viral infection or epididymitis. Mumps, varicella, infectious mononucleosis, and coxsackieviruses have been implicated in this condition. A 30% incidence is reported with mumps, but anywhere from a 3% to 100% occurrence has been reported in the literature. Mumps orchitis sequelae include a risk of testicular atrophy in 33% of cases and an increased risk of infertility. Some authors have postulated the possibility of an increased risk of cancer after an episode of mumps orchitis. As in acute epididymitis, the pain is usually gradual in onset. A history of any of the previously mentioned illnesses may

help differentiate this entity from torsion of the testis. Other signs and symptoms are fairly similar to those of epididymitis.[67]

DIFFERENTIAL DIAGNOSIS

Painful Scrotal Swelling

The key to making the diagnosis (Table 139-2) is usually the history and physical examination. On the latter the consistency, nodularity, transillumination characteristics, localization, and reducibility, as well as the ability to palpate a normal testis separately, all help to pinpoint the cause of the pain. Chronic persistent scrotal swellings should be surgically explored. Acute scrotal swelling whose cause cannot be conclusively determined on physical examination also should be surgically explored within the 12-hour window of testicular viability associated with testicular torsion.

Ancillary tests such as technetium scanning may be helpful. Inflammatory processes lead to increased vascularity and therefore increased flow, while ischemia produces decreased flow or cold spots. Similarly, Doppler ultrasonography may be helpful. Both techniques, unfortunately, produce significant false-positive and false-negative results, and thus both necessitate requisite skill by the user. False-positive results occur because of overlying hernias, hydroceles, or epididymitis. False-negative results have been found in abscess formation, late torsion with hyperemia, and detorsion/retorsion anomalies. Technetium scanning and ultrasound examination are helpful when the diagnosis is indeterminate. It cannot be emphasized too strongly that when there is any doubt whatsoever, surgery is mandatory.

Prostatitis

Prostatitis consists of four clinical disease entities: (1) acute bacterial prostatitis, (2) chronic bacterial prostatitis, (3) nonbacterial prostatitis, and (4) prostatodynia. Although prostatitis refers to inflammation of the prostate gland, in actual clinical practice prostatitis is used to describe any unexplained symptom or condition that might originate with the prostate. At one point, this entity was described as "the wastebasket of clinical ignorance."[68] All this confusion is thought to be the result of imprecise diagnostic methods.[69] The entities of acute and chronic bacterial prostatitis need to be differentiated from nonbacterial prostatitis and prostatodynia. The latter two are poorly defined because etiologies are vague. Of the four entities, nonbacterial prostatitis is the most common. Chronic bacterial prostatitis is relatively uncommon, and acute prostatitis is rare. In general, prostatitis is more an adult than an adolescent disease. It has been stated that

TABLE 139-2
Differential Diagnosis of Acute Scrotal Swelling in Childhood

	Spermatic Cord Torsion	Epididymoorchitis	Appendiceal Torsion
Age	**1st Year and Adolescence**	**Adolescence and After**	**Adolescence**
Symptoms and signs			
Pain	Acute, severe onset	Gradual localization to upper or posterior testis	Usually gradual
	Frequent antecedent similar pains	Uncommon	Occasional
	Localized to testis, radiates to groin and lower abdomen	Usually localized to epididymis and testis, sometimes to groin	Localized to appendix or general scrotal region
Fever	Rare	Common	Rare
Vomiting	Frequent	Rare	Rare
Dysuria	Rare	Common	Rare
Physical examination	Testis may be high-riding, swollen, exquisitely tender	Testis and epididymis are firm, tender, swollen	Testis usually normal; firm mass may be seen and felt at upper pole; distinct from epididymis
Laboratory examination			
Pyuria, urinary infection	Rare	Common	Rare
Blood flow (Doppler, isotope scrotal scan)	Diminished	Increased	Normal or increased

50% of adult men experience prostatitis at some point in their lives.[70]

ACUTE BACTERIAL PROSTATITIS. This is the easiest of the four entities to diagnose but is the rarest. Acute fever, urinary tract–type symptoms, dysuria, obstruction, low back pain or perineal pain along with malaise, myalgia, and occasionally arthralgia are the typical signs and symptoms. Diagnosis is made by urinalysis showing increased white blood cells (WBCs). Prostatic massage should be avoided in this entity. Trimethoprim-sulfa or fluoroquinoline are the antibiotics of choice on an outpatient basis. If the symptoms are severe, hospitalization is necessary, and aminoglycosides plus intravenous ampicillin or ciprofloxacin are then the drugs of choice. Thirty days of treatment is required. Should there be acute urinary retention, suprapubic urinary drainage may be necessary. Bed rest, hydration, analgesia, antipyretics, and stool softeners complete the regimen. Gram-negative rods, commonly *Escherichia coli,* are the agents causing this disorder.[71]

CHRONIC BACTERIAL PROSTATITIS. Etiologically, gram-negative bacteria predominate. The role of gram-positive cocci such as *Staphylococcus* and *Streptococcus* organisms is controversial, at best. Gonorrhea and *Chlamydia* urethritis may progress to prostatitis. It

appears that an ascending infection is the likely mechanism for disease.

The male urinary tract is remarkably resistant to colonization. Furthermore, there are particular antibacterial properties of the prostatic fluid that protect the male from prostatitis. Prostatic antibacterial factor (PAF) is a zinc-containing polypeptide that appears to be an important antimicrobial agent. It may inhibit gonorrhea, yeast, viruses, *Trichomonas,* and *Chlamydia trachomatis.* Spermine, the major constituent of prostatic fluid, has been demonstrated to have activity against gram-positive bacteria. Finally, IgG and IgA are secreted as part of the immune response of the prostate against bacterial invasion. It has been demonstrated that men with chronic bacterial prostatitis have decreased levels of PAF, magnesium, zinc, calcium, spermine, cholesterol, and lysozymes in the prostatic fluid. Therefore, bacterial prostatitis is not a random event.[70]

For the most part, chronic bacterial prostatitis is seen in older males and is much less common in adolescents. In general, the symptoms are less dramatic and more subtle or even absent compared with those of acute prostatitis. The diagnosis of chronic prostatitis cannot be made on clinical grounds alone or by examination of expressed prostatic secretion (EPS) alone.

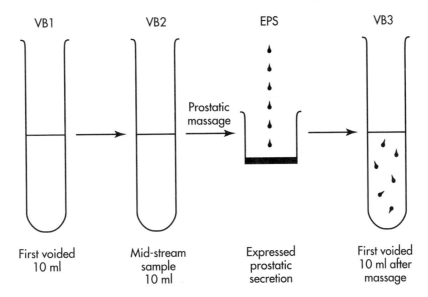

VB1 VB2 EPS VB3

Prostatic massage

First voided
10 ml

Mid-stream
sample
10 ml

Expressed
prostatic
secretion

First voided
10 ml after
massage

Fig. 139-3. Stamey localization procedure.

To make the diagnosis, the Stamey localization procedure should be used.[68] This consists of three voided bladder (VB) specimens (VB1, VB2, VB3) before and after prostatic massage to obtain EPS. At the present time, the consensus diagnostic significance value for EPS is 10 or more WBCs per high-power field (hpf). This would also include findings of greater than two lipid-laden macrophages per hpf. However, there are confounders to the use of EPS. Some authors say that more than 20 WBC/hpf are necessary to make the diagnosis. Normal EPS may be seen in chronic bacterial prostatitis patients who have been on antibiotics. Up to 10% of normal males may have more than 10 WBC/hpf. Recent ejaculation may interfere with the interpretation, since spermatogonia may be misinterpreted as WBCs.[70]

The finding of bacteriuria does not necessarily prove chronic bacterial prostatitis, nor is a positive EPS culture alone sufficient for a diagnosis of chronic bacterial prostatitis. False-negative cultures may occur in chronic bacterial prostatitis. Thus, the Stamey localization procedure provides the best technique to rule out the confounding issues (Fig. 139-3). To consider that an organism is the etiologic agent of the prostatitis, the colony count in EPS and VB3 is required to be greater than that in VB1 and VB2 by a factor of at least 10 (Fig. 139-3).[69] Also, the urine should be sterile, but if not, 5 days of treatment with an antimicrobial agent that is fully concentrated in the prostate is advised. The Stamey procedure should then be repeated.

Chronic bacterial prostatitis is the most common cause of recurrent urinary tract infections in men. A history of a good response to previous antimicrobial treatment is a good clue to chronic bacterial prostatitis.[71]

NONBACTERIAL PROSTATITIS. The cause of nonbacterial prostatitis is unknown. Various bacteria, other

microbes, fungi, and viruses have been almost totally eliminated as causes. Either an agent is as yet unidentified or multiple agents must be involved in the etiology.[72] Previous studies indicating that *C. trachomatis* or *Ureaplasma urealyticum* are responsible for nonbacterial prostatitis have not been confirmed. The diagnosis is made by history, transient response or no response to antimicrobials, or response to nonspecific treatment.

PROSTATODYNIA. Etiologically, this condition is related to pelvic floor tension myalgia or neuromuscular dysfunction of the bladder outlet or external sphincter. Meares[73] studied 64 males with prostatodynia and found that 70% had bladder neck spasm, 17% had bladder neck spasm plus tension myalgia, and 9% had tension myalgia alone. Prostatodynia is associated with a high frequency of stress or emotional instability. Nonspecific prostatitis and prostatodynia both occur more often in young men or adolescents.[73]

INFERTILITY

Failure of a couple to conceive in the first year of unprotected sex is the most widely accepted definition of infertility, since 80% of couples usually achieve pregnancy in that span of time. Sterility implies an intrinsic inability to achieve pregnancy. Primary infertility indicates that a couple has never achieved pregnancy. Secondary infertility is infertility in a couple who previously have conceived. Fecundability refers to the 25% to 30% per month chance of any couple achieving pregnancy.[74]

There has been an exponential increase in the numbers of infertile couples since the mid-1980s. The reason for this is not fully understood. A male factor is involved in 30% to 33% of infertile couples. The work-up of the male factor infertility follows the usual model of medical investigation. A good health history and complete physical examination are the cornerstones of the initial evaluation. Laboratory analysis can then further identify specific abnormalities. These laboratory studies include sperm analyses, hormonal studies, specialized studies, testicular biopsy, and posttesticular work-up. The causes of infertility can be classified as pretesticular, testicular, and posttesticular. From 70% to 75% of all causes remain unidentified; 1% are hypothalamic-pituitary in origin, 10% to 15% testicular in origin, 4% to 6% due to sperm autoimmunity, 8% to 10% posttesticular genital diseases, and 1% copulatory/ejaculatory dysfunctions. The history taking should focus on the wide variety of possible factors that could lead to infertility (Box 139-2). A complete physical examination is necessary to determine the general health of the adolescent as well as the presence of signs of specific single or multiorgan diseases and/or endocrine dysfunction. The extent of masculinization and the general body appearance and body habitus should be assessed. The physical examination primarily focuses on a thorough genital examination.

Laboratory Tests

SPERM ANALYSIS. Sperm analysis serves only as a rough indication of a patient's fertility. Sperm analyses vary with time because there is seasonality to spermiogenesis. Sperm sample handling is also a factor. Samples should be obtained after a minimum of 2 to 3 days' abstinence to a maximum of 7 days. Samples should arrive at the laboratory within 2 hours of having been obtained. For these reasons, as well as other technical ones, a minimum of two samples should be obtained before any conclusions can be made.

The sperm sample is routinely analyzed for volume, sperm count, motility, viability, and morphology. A sperm volume of less than 1 ml could well indicate obstruction of ejaculatory ducts. A volume greater than 6 ml indicates hyperspermia, which is often associated with decreased fertility or may indicate prolonged abstinence. The physical properties of the sample hold little diagnostic significance. Liquefaction takes place within 5 to 30 minutes after ejaculation. Impairment of liquefaction may indicate prostatitis. On the other hand, increased viscosity may make accurate counting of the sperm difficult. Increased pH of the semen may be associated with acute prostatitis; decreased pH may be associated with chronic prostatitis. However, changes in liquefaction and pH are uncertain causes of infertility.

A sperm count of less than 20 million is considered oligospermia.[75] A low sperm count alone is not necessarily indicative of infertility. Sperm viability, motility, and morphology must also be evaluated. Motility refers to the percentage of sperm actively moving: less than 50%

motility is considered abnormal. Directionality of movement is also assessed; one classification system uses a scale of 0 to 4, with 0 being no movement and 4 indicating excellent movement with forward direction. This scale is based on an assessment of the majority of the spermatozoa. Computer-assisted micrography and other more sophisticated attempts at enhancing the objectivity of sperm motility are highly controversial.[75] Sperm morphology is also evaluated, but detailed evaluations serve very little predictive value.

The etiology of oligospermia or azoospermia can be divided into three major causes: (1) disturbed spermato-

---

BOX 139-2
Infertility History

History of infertility
  Duration
  Previous pregnancies
    Present partner
    Another partner
  Previous evaluations, treatments
Sexual history
  Potency, libido
  Lubricants
  Timing, frequency
  Habits, preferences
Childhood and onset of puberty
  Surgery (undescended testicles, orchiopexy, herniorrhaphy, Y-V plasty of bladder)
  Testicular torsion, trauma
  Malignancy (chemotherapy, radiation)
Medical history
  Systemic illness (diabetes, obesity, ulcer, liver or lung diseases)
  Malignancy
  Cystic fibrosis
Surgical history
  Retroperitoneal surgery
  Pelvic surgery
Infections
  Viral
  Mumps orchitis
  Sexually transmitted diseases
  Systemic (tuberculosis)
Toxins
  Chemicals, pesticides
  Drugs (chemotherapeutic, cimetidine, psychotropic, antibiotics, alcohol, marijuana, hormones)
  Heat
  Radiation
  Review of systems
    Anosmia
    Galactorrhea
    Impaired visual fields

genesis, (2) ejaculatory duct obstruction, and (3) retrograde ejaculation. Specific etiologies of each of these are noted (Box 139-3). Chemical analysis for semen have also been determined, and these include fructose concentration, alpha-glucosidase, and creatine kinase (CK). Decreased fructose is associated with seminal vesicle disease or obstruction of the ejaculatory tracts. This test is now much less useful because of the advent of transrectal ultrasonography.[76] Alpha-glucosidase and CK tests have been so specialized as to need independent verification of their general applicability.[75]

HORMONAL STUDIES. Gonadotropin levels along with testosterone and prolactin levels are helpful in assessing the cause of infertility (Table 139-3).

Specialized studies of the sperm have been applied to varying degrees, but most of these studies are equivocal

---

BOX 139-3
Etiology of Oligospermia
and Azoospermia

1. Disturbed spermatogenesis
   a. Genetic and chromosomal disorders (e.g., Klinefelter's syndrome, Noonan's syndrome)
   b. Hypothalamic and pituitary disorders (e.g., hypogonadotropic hypogonadism)
   c. Testicular disease
      Developmental (e.g., cryptorchidism)
      Infectious (e.g., mumps)
      Iatrogenic (e.g., cancer chemotherapy)
      Idiopathic (e.g., germinal cell aplasia)
2. Obstruction or aplasia of ductal system
   Congenital (e.g., aplasia of vas deferens)
   Inflammatory (e.g., sexually transmitted diseases)
   Traumatic/iatrogenic (e.g., vasectomy, torsion)
3. Retrograde ejaculation (e.g., autonomic disturbances, ganglionic blockers)

---

or controversial, at best. They include immune agglutination, zona-free hampster, oocyte penetration, acrosome test, mucus migration test, and hypoosmotic swelling test.[75]

Open surgical testicular biopsy may be undertaken if the sperm findings are not explained by any endocrine abnormalities or by the clinical features of specific syndromes. The morphology of the gland is evaluated, with emphasis on seminiferous tubules and Leydig's cells. Several scoring systems have been used for this evaluation.[75] Testicular biopsy is also important in azoospermia to rule out obstruction from ablative testicular changes. The testicular biopsy represents only qualitative data.[77]

Posttesticular studies are indicated when an obstruction of the excretory ducts or retrograde ejaculation is suspected. These studies follow all of those previously mentioned. That is, when an individual who has severe oligospermia or azoospermia has a normal testicular biopsy, suspicion turns to the posttesticular arena. Retrograde ejaculation may be documented by finding a high proportion of spermatozoa in the postejaculate urine, with no or very little sperm in the semen analysis. When azoospermia or oligospermia occur in the face of a normal testicular biopsy and in the face of lack of retrograde ejaculation, studies to rule out obstruction are necessary. Vasography has been the primary modality for this determination. Transurethral ultrasonography has been used successfully in recent years and may ultimately replace the more invasive technology.[78]

Some authors advocate that testicular biopsy is no longer useful since FSH levels together with testicular volumetric measurements can just as accurately predict damage to spermatogenesis.

All analyses of fertility and/or testicular function must be taken with a grain of salt, except in the face of complete azoospermia with very elevated FSH levels (indicating true damage of spermatogenesis). In all other circumstances, the only true way to measure fertility is through the outcome of pregnancy. That is, men with low

---

TABLE 139-3
Hormonal Profiles of Infertile Men with Azoospermia
or Oligozoospermia

Testosterone	LH	FSH	PRL	Possible Diagnosis
Low	Low	Low	Low	Hypothalamic or pituitary hypogonadism; pituitary tumor
Low	Low	Low	High	Prolactinoma
Normal	Normal	High	Normal	Germ cell aplasia
Normal	Normal	Normal	Normal	Idiopathic infertility

FSH, follicle-stimulating hormone; *LH,* luteinizing hormone; *PRL,* prolactin.

sperm counts, abnormalities of motility, and failure of other sperm function studies have successfully fathered children. Thus, there is no exact correlation between sperm measurements and fertility rates.[35]

IMPOTENCE

Impotence may be divided into six broad categories of disorders: (1) neurologic, (2) vascular, (3) endocrine, (4) surgical/traumatic, (5) drug-associated or drug-induced, and (6) psychogenic.

Neurologic Disorders

PERIPHERAL NEUROPATHY. Diabetic neuropathy is one of the more common organic causes of impotence. There is controversy over whether diabetic neuropathy is truly a primary neurologic manifestation or is a secondary effect of vascular-enhanced microangiopathic changes associated with the disease. There is an increased incidence of impotence in diabetic males as they age; 7.5% of males under 45 years of age reportedly suffer from impotence, characterized by a gradually decreasing rigidity or firmness that progressively worsens. There is disagreement regarding whether this impotence is related to the degree of control of the diabetic condition or not. Men with diabetes usually have normal libido despite the impotence, at least initially, although after a while depression may depress libido as well. Those individuals who develop impotence with diabetes tend to have other associated somatic and autonomic manifestations as opposed to those males who have no problems with penile tumescence.[79] Abnormal sacral reflexes[80] and true microscopic neuromorphologic changes have been described in this disorder.[81] Unfortunately, the prognosis is poor. Hormonal abnormalities do not seem to play a prominent role.

Uremic neuropathy as a result of chronic renal failure may lead to impotence, which may not be primarily neurologic but may be hormonal in nature. Increases in gonadotrophins (FSH, LH) with a decrease in testosterone levels are not unusual in uremic men with impotence. Hyperprolactinemia has also been described in chronic renal failure. Uremia has also been associated with spermatogenic changes and damage upon microscopic evaluation of the testis.

Spinal Cord Lesions/Diseases

Spinal cord injuries have been shown to produce sexual dysfunction. Erectile function is frequently preserved in the presence of higher lesions, although this may be short-lived. Coitus is thus possible; however, seminal emissions and orgasm are rare, since there is true ejaculatory dysfunction. In lower spinal cord lesions, erections as a result of reflex stimulation are usually absent, but psychogenically induced erection is common (up to 90% of patients). Ejaculation with orgasm is more common in lower cord lesions. After traumatic spinal cord damage, it is often difficult to predict the future effects until many weeks or months have passed. Thus, prediction of final outcome is uncertain.[82]

Multiple sclerosis may cause impotence. Although impotence may happen early in the disease, the longer the duration, the more likely it is to occur. Sexual potency often remits and relapses. Other spinal cord diseases may also affect potency as well.[82]

Vascular Disorders

Most vascular disorders affecting erectile function occur later in life. Thrombotic obliteration, atherosclerosis, fibrosis, and calcification all occur with increasing age and may result in impotence.

Endocrine Disorders

In a prospective study of 256 men, 17.5% were found to have hypothalamic-pituitary-gonadal axis abnormalities leading to impotence.[83] Findings consistent with dysfunction of the hypothalamic-pituitary axis include change in body habitus, development of gynecomastia, and decrease in volume of the testes. Some of these changes may be associated with other etiologies that impinge upon the axis. Therefore, measurement of gonadotropin and testosterone levels is important. One should pay attention to distinct dysmorphisms that might alert the examiner to various syndromes (e.g., Kallmann's, Prader-Willi, Laurence-Moon-Biedl, cerebellar ataxia, Klinefelter's). Hyperprolactinemia may lead to impotence; it tends to suppress the hypothalamic-pituitary-gonadal axis. The hyperprolactinemia may be primary from a pituitary tumor or may be secondary in nature, the result of various medications, illicit drug use, or other conditions including uremia. There is some controversy regarding the role of hyperprolactinemia in impotence, since some authors have concluded that impotence is not related to hyperprolactinemia.[84] Hyperthyroidism has been associated with impotence. As previously discussed, uremia has been associated with impotence, but the underlying mechanism remains unclear.

Traumatic and Surgical Disorders

Trauma, specifically fractured pelvis associated with bladder or urethral injury, may be associated with impotence. Major surgery in the prostate for testicular cancer (radical lymph node dissection), rectal or bladder sphincter surgery, and even surgery for lower bowel disease have all been implicated as causes of impotence.

Drug-Induced Impotence

Drug-induced impotence is thought to be the single most common cause of sexual dysfunction.[85] The mechanisms appear to be many, although not all are proven, and include (1) central nervous system depression, (2) drug-induced hyperprolactinemia, (3) antiandrogen effects, (4) anticholinergic effects, and (5) antiadrenergic effects.[86] The two most common classes of medications leading to impotence are psychiatric/antidepressant or antihypertensive agents.

Psychogenic Disorders

Approximately one third of patients, if not more, are found to have psychogenic impotence.[83] Impotence is not the only psychogenic sexual dysfunction. Premature ejaculation and ejaculatory incompetence may also have psychologic origins. Psychogenic impotence is divided into primary and secondary forms. Men with the primary form may have some form of sexual repression in their background because of specific family or religious issues in which they were raised. Such men may associate sexuality with sinfulness or immorality.[87] Secondary psychogenic impotence is thought to arise from diverse antecedents that lead to performance anxiety, which then precipitates the impotence. A combination of temperamental, emotional, familial, affective, cognitive, cultural, maturational, and biologic factors of various sorts in manifold combinations have been hypothesized as some of these antecedents.

In today's society, men are expected to be virile and never have any sexual performance problems, which leads to unrealistic self-expectation. Especially in view of the titillation provided by literature, television, and the movies, it is not surprising that many adolescent males find themselves questioning their virility to the extent that it may interfere with sexual performance. This form of psychogenic impotence is also known as excitement inhibition. It is more successfully treated than the other form, known as desire inhibition, or deficiency of desire. Specific techniques (according to Masters and Johnson), including that of sensate focus, are often used to treat this condition.[88] Desire inhibition is considered by some to be more common than the other form of impotence. Specific systemic diseases, the use of some medications or drugs, and overt depression must be ruled out before the diagnosis of desire inhibition is made.

Evaluation of the patient with impotence or sexual dysfunction requires much education. Penile erectile dysfunction is a complex situation. Patients usually desire a quick remedy; this is not usually possible, since the etiology may be fairly complex. The patient needs to understand that organic difficulties may lead to secondary psychologic issues, just as psychogenic problems result in erectile dysfunction.[82]

A careful history and physical examination, as in most other medical conditions, is critical. It is necessary to determine the duration and nature of onset of the impotence. Organic causes of impotence usually result in a slow, but progressive erectile dysfunction. Psychogenic impotence is usually more abrupt in nature. It is important to determine whether morning erections and erections in other circumstances (outside of that with a sexual partner) are occurring. These latter issues are clues to a psychogenic cause. On the other hand, loss of libido is more common with a hormonal enhanced organic etiology. One should elucidate symptoms compatible with organic illnesses or etiologies previously described. All oral medications that the patient is using, both licit and illicit, should be documented.

Physical examination is then directed toward identifying any specific neurologic, hormonal, vascular, or genital abnormalities. A complete genital and rectal examination, including evaluation of rectal tone and bulbocavernous reflex, should be undertaken. Evaluation of body habitus, sex hair distribution, and gynecomastia completes the examination.

Laboratory Testing

Laboratory testing includes evaluation of gonadotropin, testosterone, and prolactin levels as well as thyroid function studies, as indicated by the history and physical examination. More complex neurologic testing and urodynamics may be necessary in certain circumstances. Specialized studies of penile blood flow using special pneumatic cuffs, ultrasonography of pelvic and iliac vessels, and arteriography may be indicated if a vascular cause is suspected. A number of devices to measure nocturnal penile tumescence—specialized transducers and recorders—are often advised, since the presence of nocturnal penile erections is strong evidence of a psychogenic cause of the impotence. However, other reports indicate that such studies have an uncertain validity and therefore more limited usefulness.[90-92] More involved dynamic studies, including intracorporal injection, cavernosography, and cavernosonometry, are newer techniques used by some to determine blood flow into and out of the penis.

Specialized neurologic testing has also been performed by many. Its efficacy is limited by two caveats: (1)

if a specific neurologic lesion is demonstrated, it does not necessarily mean that it is responsible for the impotence; and (2) the integrity of the autonomic nervous system control of penile erection cannot be directly measured by neurologic studies.

Therapy

Various therapies, including medications, intracorporal injection, vacuum devices, penile prostheses, penile revascularization, and venous ligation, may be needed to treat the impotence. Details of these are beyond the scope of this chapter.

OTHER SEXUAL DYSFUNCTIONS

Although impotence has been emphasized in this discussion of sexual dysfunction, there are other forms of dysfunction. Probably the most common sexual dysfunction in sexually active teenagers is premature ejaculation. It has been estimated that three quarters of all men ejaculate less than 2 minutes after the start of intercourse.[92] Specific exercises described by Masters and Johnson have proved helpful in overcoming premature ejaculation. These include the so-called "squeeze" technique.[92]

Sexual dysfunction is only one aspect of the larger issue, namely, sexual counseling. Sexual counseling in general is of prime importance to physicians dealing with adolescents. The rate of sexual activity among adolescents increases with increasing age. Each adolescent is an individual, and each may or may not be participating in some form of sexual activity whether auto-, hetero-, bi-, or homosexual. Sexual counseling should also include the issues of responsibility in sexual relations between partners. The approach to the male should include emphasis on participation in protecting himself and his partner from STDs, from possible pregnancy, or from both. Despite the societal double standard, significant numbers of older adolescent boys are not sexually active and need to be supported in their decision to be abstinent. Although abstinence for many is an impossible ideal, it is nevertheless the only guaranteed choice of action that ensures absolute protection from STDs and pregnancy. Other chapters in this book discuss these and other aspects of adolescent sexuality in greater detail.

References

1. Rohn RD: Penile diameter during puberty in boys, *J Adolesc Health Care* 10:250, 1989.
2. Schonfield WA, Beebe GW: Normal growth and variation in male genitalia from birth to maturity, *J Urol* 48:759, 1942.
3. Goldbloom RB: Self-examination by adolescents, *Pediatrics* 76:126, 1985.
4. Johnston JH: Abnormalities of the penis. In Williams DI, Johnston JH, editors: *Paediatric urology,* London, 1982, Butterworth; p 435.
5. Pomerantz P, Hanna M, Levitt S, et al: Isolated torsion of the penis: report of 6 cases, *Urology* 11:37, 1978.
6. MacKinney CC, Uhle CA: Congenital chordee without hypospadias, *J Urol* 84:343, 1960.
7. Fitzpatrick TJ: Hemihypertrophy of the human corpus cavernosum, *J Urol* 115:560, 1976.
8. Neinstein LS, Goldenring J: Pink pearly papules. An epidemiologic study, *J Pediatr* 105:594, 1984.
9. Govan DE, Kessler R: Urologic problems in the adolescent male, *Pediatr Clin North Am* 27:109, 1980.
10. Klauber GI, Sant GR: Disorders of the male external genitalia. In Kelalis PP, King LR, Belman AB, editors: *Clinical pediatric urology,* Philadelphia, 1985, WB Saunders; p 825.
11. Scorer CG, Farrington GH: *Congenital deformities of the testis and epididymis,* New York, 1971, Appleton-Century-Crofts.
12. Cilento BG, Najjar SS, Atala A: Cryptorchidism and testicular torsion, *Pediatr Clin North Am* 40:1133, 1993.
13. Lee PA: Fertility in cryptorchidism: does treatment make a difference?, *Endocrinol Metab Clin North Am* 22:479, 1993.
14. Hadziselimovic F: *Cryptorchidism: management and implications,* New York, 1993, Springer-Verlag; pp 20, 47, 66, 89, 94, 113.
15. Hutson JM, Donahue PK, MacLaughlin DT: Steroid modulation of müllerian duct regression in the chick embryo, *Gen Comp Endocrinol* 57:88, 1985.
16. Wensig CJG: The embryology of testicular descent, *Horm Res* 30:1444, 1988.
17. Hutson JM, Beasley SW: Embryologic controversies in testicular descent, *Semin Urol* 6:68, 1988.
18. MacLaughlin DT, Hutson JM, Donahoe PK: Specific estradiol binding embryonic müllerian ducts: a potential modulation of regression in the male and female chick, *Endocrinology* 113:141, 1983.
19. Mininberg DT: The epididymis and testicular descent, *Eur J Pediatr* 146 (suppl 2):28, 1987.
20. Kleinteich B, Hadziselimovic F, Hesse V, et al: *Kongenitale Hodendystopien.* Leipzig, Germany, 1979, VEB George Thieme.
21. Hadzielimovic F: Cryptorchidism. In Gillenwater JY, Grayhack JT, Howards SS, Pucket JW, editors: *Adult and pediatric urology,* ed 2, Chicago, 1991, Mosby–Year Book; p 2217.
22. Mengel W, Heinz HA, Sippe WG, et al: Studies on cryptorchidism: a comparison of histological findings in the germinative epithelium before and after the second year of life, *J Pediatr Surg* 9:445, 1974.
23. DeMuinck Keizer-Schrama SMPF, Hazebroek WJ: Hormonal treatment of cryptorchidism: role of pituitary gonadal axis, *Semin Urol* 6:84, 1988.
24. Farrer JH, Walker AH, Raifer J: Management of the postpubertal cryptorchid testis: a statistical review, *J Urol* 134:1071, 1985.
25. Saenger P, Reiter EO: Management of cryptorchidism, *Trends Endocrinol Metab* 3:249, 1992.
26. Kaplan GW: Acute idiopathic scrotal edema, *J Pediatr Surg* 12:647, 1977.
27. Kogan SJ: Acute and chronic scrotal swellings. In Gillenwater JY, Grayhach JT, Howards SS, Ducket JW, editors: *Adult and pediatric urology,* ed 2, Chicago, 1991, Mosby–Year Book; p 2189.
28. O'Regan S, Robitaille P: Orchitis mimicking testicular torsion in Henoch-Schönlein's purpura, *J Urol* 126:834, 1981.
29. Loh HS, Jalan OM: Testicular torsion in Henoch-Schönlein syndrome, *Br Med J* 2:96, 1974.
30. Donohue R, Utley WLF: Idiopathic fat necrosis in the scrotum, *Br J Urol* 47:331, 1975.
31. Redman JF, Yamauchi T, Higginbothom WE: Fournier's gangrene of the scrotum in a child, *J Urol* 121:827, 1979.
32. Minton JP, Clatworthy HW: Incidence of patency of the processus vaginalis, *Ohio State Med J* 57:530, 1961.

33. McGregor DB, Halverson K, McVay CB: The unilateral pediatric inguinal hernia: should the contralateral side be explored?, *J Pediatr Surg* 15:33, 1980.

34. Rowe MI, Marchildon MB: Inguinal hernia and hydrocele in infants and children, *Surg Clin North Am* 61:1137, 1981.

35. Hargreave TB: Varicocele—a clinical enigma, *Br J Urol* 72:401, 1993.

36. Hudson RW: The endocrinology of varicoceles, *Fertil Steril* 49:199, 1988.

37. Hargreave TB, Liakatar J: Physical examination for varicocele, *Br J Urol* 67:328, 1991.

38. Oster J: Varicocele in children and adolescents, *Scand J Urol Nephrol* 5:27, 1991.

39. Steeno O, Knops J, Declerck L: Prevention of fertility disorders by detection and treatment of varicocele at school and college age, *Andrologia* 8:47, 1976.

40. Berger OG: Varicocele in adolescence, *Clin Pediatr* 19:810, 1980.

41. Pozza D, D'Ottavio G, Masci P, et al: Left varicocele at puberty, *Urology* 22:271, 1983.

42. Turner TT: Varicocele: still an enigma, *J Urol* 129:695, 1983.

43. Braedel HU, Steffens J, Ziegler M, Polsky MS, Platt ML: Possible ontogenic etiology for idiopathic left varicocele, *J Urol* 151:62, 1994.

44. Coveney EC, Fitzgerald RJ: Varicocele and the horizontal testis: a change in position?, *J Pediatr Surg* 29:452, 1994.

45. Goldstein M: Adolescent varicocele (editorial), *J Urol* 153:484, 1995.

46. Laron Z, Dickerman Z, Ritterman I, et al: Follow-up of boys with unilateral compensatory hypertrophy, *Fertil Steril* 33:297, 1980.

47. Breen DH, Braunstein GD, Neufeld N, et al: Benign macroorchidism in pubescent boys, *J Urol* 125:589, 1981.

48. Turner G, Daniel A, Frost M: X-linked mental retardation macro-orchidism and the Xq 27 fragile site, *J Pediatr* 96:837, 1980.

49. Kirkland RT, Kirkland JL, Keenan BS: Bilateral testicular tumors in congenital adrenal hyperplasia, *J Clin Endocrinol Metab* 44:369, 1977.

50. Johnston JH: Abnormalities of the scrotum and testes. In Williams DI, Johnston JH, editors: *Paediatric urology,* London, 1982, Butterworth; p 451.

51. Zornow DH, Landers RR: Scrotal palpation, *Am Fam Physician* 23:150, 1981.

52. Tammela TLJ, Hellstrom PA, Mattila SI, Ottelin PJ, Malinen LJ, Makarainen HP: Ethanolamine oleate sclerotherapy for hydroceles and spermatoceles: a survey of 158 patients with ultrasound follow-up, *J Urol* 147:1551, 1992.

53. Gilbert JB: Studies in malignant testis tumors. V. Tumors developing after orchidopexy: report of 2 cases and review of 63, *J Urol* 46:740, 1941.

54. Campbell HE: The incidence of malignant growth of the undescended testicle: a reply and re-evaluation, *J Urol* 81, 663, 1959.

55. Collins DH, Pugh RCB: *The pathology of testicular tumours,* Edinburgh, 1964, Livingstone.

56. Rowland RG, Donahue JP: Scrotum and testis. In Gillenwater JY, Grayhock JT, Howards SS, Ducket JQ, editors: *Adult and pediatric urology,* ed 2, Chicago, 1991, Mosby–Year Book; p 1565.

57. Einhorn LH, Richie JP, Shipley WU: Cancer of the testis. In DeVita VT, Hellman S, Rosenberg SA, editors: *Cancer: principles and practice of oncology,* ed 4, Philadelphia, 1993, JB Lippincott; p 1126.

58. Kogan SJ, Gill B, Bennett B, et al: Human mono-orchidism: a clinicopathological study of unilateral absent testes in 65 boys, *J Urol* 135:758, 1986.

59. Knight PJ, Vassy LE: The diagnosis and treatment of the acute scrotum in children and adolescents, *Ann Surg* 200:664, 1984.

60. Nagler HM, DeVere White R: The effect of testicular torsion on the contralateral testis, *J Urol* 128:1343, 1982.

61. Thomas WEB, Cooper MJ, Smith JHF, et al: Sympathetic orchidopathia following acute testicular torsion, *Br J Surg* 71:380, 1984.

62. Hadziselimovic F, Snyder H, Duckett J, Howards S: Testicular histology in children with unilateral testicular torsion, *J Urol* 136:208, 1986.

63. Anderson MJ, Dunn JK, Lipshultz LI, Coburn M: Quality and endocrine parameters after acute testicular torsion, *J Urol* 147:1545, 1992.

64. Berger RE, Alexander R, Monda GD: *Chlamydia trachomatis* as a cause of acute "idiopathic" epididymitis, *N Engl J Med* 298:301, 1978.

65. Stage KH, Schoenvogal R, Lewis S: Testicular scanning: clinical experience with 72 patients, *J Urol* 125:334, 1981.

66. Abu-Sleiman R, Ho JE, Gregory JG: Scrotal scanning; present value and limits of interpretation, *Urology* 13:326, 1979.

67. Scorer CG, Farrington GH: Congenital anomalies of the testes. In Harrison JH, Gittes AD, Perlmutter AD, et al, editors: *Campbell's urology,* ed 4, Philadelphia, 1978, WB Saunders; p 1549.

68. Stamey TA: *Pathogenesis and treatment of urinary tract infections,* Baltimore, 1980, Williams & Wilkins.

69. Doble A: Chronic prostatitis, *Br J Urol* 74:537, 1994.

70. Fowler JE. Prostatitis. In Gillenwater JY, Grayhack JT, Howards SS, Duckett JW: *Adult and pediatric urology,* ed 2, Chicago, 1991, Mosby–Year Book; p 1395.

71. Moul JW: Prostatitis, *Postgrad Med* 94:191, 1993.

72. Dairiki-Shortliff LM, Sellers RG, Schacter J: The characterization of non-bacterial prostatitis: search for an etiology, *J Urol* 148:1461, 1992.

73. Meares EM Jr: Prostatodynia: clinical findings and rationale for treatment. In Weidner W, Brunner H, Krause W, et al, editors: *Therapy of prostatitis.* Munich, 1986, W Zucksschwerdt Verlag Gmbh; p 207.

74. Mann MC: Infertility. In DeCherney AA, Pernoll ML, editors: *Current obstetric and gynecologic diagnosis and treatment,* ed 8, Norwalk, CT, 1994, Appleton Lange; p 996.

75. Damjanov I: *Pathology of infertility,* Chicago, 1993, Mosby–Year Book; p 7.

76. Abbitt PL, Watson L, Howards S: Abnormalities of the seminal tract causing infertility: diagnosis with endorectal sonography, *Am J Radiol* 157:337, 1991.

77. Lipshultz LI, Howards SS, Buch JP: Male infertility. In Gillenwater JY, Grayback JT, Howards SS, Duckett SW, editors: *Adult and pediatric urology,* ed 2, Chicago, 1991, Mosby–Year Book; p 1425.

78. Kuligowska E, Baker CE, Oates RD: Male infertility: role of transrectal US in diagnosis and management, *Radiology* 185:353, 1992.

79. Campbell IW: Diabetic autonomic neuropathy, *Br J Clin Pract* 3:153, 1976.

80. Ellenberg M: Impotency in diabetics: a neurologic rather than an endocrinologic problem, *Med Aspects Human Sex* 7:12, 1973.

81. Ruzbarsky V, Michael V: Morphologic changes in the arterial bed of the penis with aging, *Invest Urol* 15:194, 1977.

82. Benson GS, McConnell JA, Lipshultz LI, et al: Neuromorphology and neuropharmacology of the human penis, *J Clin Invest* 65:506, 1980.

83. Nickel JC, Morales A, Condra M, et al: Endocrine dysfunction in impotence: incidence, significance, and cost-effective screening, *J Urol* 132:40, 1984.

84. Miller JB, Howards SS, McLeod RM: Serum prolactin in organic and psychogenic impotence, *J Urol* 123:862, 1980.

85. Slag MF, Morley JE, Elson MK, et al: Impotence in medical outpatients, *JAMA* 29:1736, 1983.

86. Horowitz JD, Gobel AJ: Drugs and impaired male sexual function, *Drugs* 18:206, 1979.

87. Marmor J: Impotence and ejaculatory disorders. In Kaplan H, Sadock D, Freedman A, editors: *Sexual experience,* Baltimore, 1976, Williams & Wilkins.

88. Masters WH, Johnson VE: *Human sexual inadequacy,* Boston, 1970, Little, Brown.

89. Kinsey AC, Pomeroy BW, Mortin CE: *Sexual behavior in the human male,* Philadelphia, 1948, WB Saunders; p 580.

90. Karacan I, Goodenough DR, Shapiro A, et al: Erection cycle during sleep in relation to dream anxiety, *Arch Gen Psychiatry* 15:183, 1966.

91. Fisher C, Gross J, Zuch J: Cycle of penile erection synchronous with dreaming (REM) sleep, *Arch Gen Psychiatry* 12:29, 1965.

92. Seagraves RT, Madsen R, Carter CS, et al: Erectile dysfunction associated with pharmacological agents. In Seagraves RT, Schoenberg HW, editors: *Diagnosis and treatment of erectile disturbances,* New York, 1985, Plenum Press.

CHAPTER 140

Sexually Transmitted Diseases

•

Walter D. Rosenfeld and Nathan Litman

The significance of sexually transmitted diseases (STDs) in adolescence is related to the fact that this age group has some of the highest prevalence rates for each entity considered. Moreover, many of the infections can produce major lifelong adverse sequelae. Most young people who have begun sexual activity engage in serial monogamous relationships and thus are exposed to a wide variety of pathogens. Therefore, when signs or symptoms suggest the possibility of an STD, even when the patient believes this possibility to be inconceivable, the clinician should perform the appropriate physical examination and laboratory tests.

Certain principles that apply to all STDs are useful to review. First, human immunodeficiency virus (HIV) infection (see Chapter 67, "HIV Infection and AIDS") should be considered, with counseling and testing offered to all patients and especially those with multiple sexual partners. At a minimum, any patient who has had an STD should be informed about HIV and its consequences. Second, patients need to be informed that infection with sexually transmitted pathogens does not confer immunity from reinfection. Third, unlike most other situations in medicine in which one is encouraged to be parsimonious with diagnoses, even when the patient has a variety of complaints, it is typical for patients to present with multiple concurrent STDs. Thus, the clinician should not be satisfied with finding *the* answer but should search for other infections. Among groups at high risk for STDs, such as those who trade sex for drugs, a serologic test for syphilis should be performed when any new STD is discovered. Fourth, in most circumstances sexual partners should not only be examined and tested for infection but also treated on an epidemiologic basis. Patients and partners should be encouraged to complete their full course of oral an-

tibiotics, since symptomatic relief may occur rapidly without true eradication of the infection. Fifth, counseling regarding STDs and pregnancy prevention go hand in hand. The two issues are so obviously linked that it behooves clinicians to seek information and attempt to achieve behavioral change in both areas even when only one of the issues seems to be of current concern to the adolescent. Of course, sensitivity and balance need to be exercised, as many adolescents may be overwhelmed, unprepared, or simply unable to deal with even one major life problem. Helping young people work through these very difficult problems almost never takes place all in one encounter. Finally, prevention of STDs through education, encouraging the use of condoms, and helping young people make decisions about their sexual behavior in a way that minimizes the risk for these infections is essential in order to reduce the rates of STDs among adolescents.

INFLAMMATORY CONDITIONS

NEISSERIA GONORRHOEAE AND *CHLAMYDIA TRACHOMATIS* INFECTIONS

Currently, *Neisseria gonorrhoeae* and *Chlamydia trachomatis* are the two most common sexually transmitted bacterial infections in the United States. Both agents primarily infect squamocolumnar epithelial cells and cause the same type of local infections (urethritis, cervicitis, proctitis, conjunctivitis) and complications of local infection (epididymitis, salpingitis, perihepatitis) and similar systemic syndromes (disseminated gonococ-

1097

cal infection and Reiter's syndrome). Indeed, both organisms often coexist in the same patient.

Gonococci are aerobic, gram-negative diplococci that grow best in an atmosphere supplemented with 5% carbon dioxide. They have complex growth requirements, including a chocolate agar or similar medium. Unfortunately, other less fastidious organisms found at sites of gonococcal infection grow readily on these media and may obscure the presence of gonococci. The commonly used selective medium for gonococci (e.g., Thayer-Martin medium) incorporates antibiotics that suppress the normal flora but not *N. gonorrhoeae* organisms. Gonococci must be differentiated from other pathogenic and nonpathogenic species of *Neisseria* by biochemical and/or immunologic tests. DNA probe technology is now available for the detection of gonococci. Before 1976, all gonococci were viewed as susceptible to penicillin. Since 1976, there has been widespread development of plasmid- or chromosome-mediated resistance to penicillin and/or tetracycline. By 1990, almost 9% of isolates in the United States were antibiotic-resistant strains.

Chlamydia organisms are obligate intracellular parasites that cannot be cultured on artificial media. There are three species of *Chlamydia* that cause human disease: *C. psittaci* (the agent of psittacosis), *C. pneumoniae* (TWAR agent causing community-acquired, atypical pneumonia), and *C. trachomatis*. *C. trachomatis* includes several serovars, classified according to disease association: serovars A, B, Ba, and C, causing trachoma; serovars D, E, F, G, H, I, J, and K, causing inclusion conjunctivitis and common sexually transmitted syndromes such as urethritis, cervicitis, and salpingitis; and serovars L^1, L^2, and L^3, causing lymphogranuloma venereum. Only serovars D to K are the subject of this section. (Serovars L^1, L^2, and L^3 are discussed with lymphogranuloma venereum. Serovars A to C, *C. psittaci,* and *C. pneumoniae* are not discussed further.) The *C. trachomatis* organism can be grown in specially treated tissue culture, but this technique is not available for routine use except at major medical centers. In most clinical situations the methods used for detection of this organism are direct immunofluorescent staining of smears using monoclonal antibodies to the outer membrane protein of the organism, enzyme-linked immunosorbent assay (ELISA), DNA probes, or ligase chain reactions. Since *Chlamydia* organisms are intracellular, specimens for culture and/or antigen detection should include epithelial cells from the affected site, not exudate or mucus. All techniques have high sensitivity and specificity when compared with tissue culture; however, they are subject to false-positive results and therefore should not be used alone in cases with potential medicolegal implications such as sexual abuse. Although in vitro *C. trachomatis* is susceptible to a variety of antimicrobial drugs, only macrolides, tetracyclines, ofloxacin, and sulfonamides have proved clinical efficacy.

Gonorrhea is the second most common of the notifiable diseases in the United States. Reported cases peaked at approximately 1 million per year from 1975 to 1980, but the rate declined to 393,000 cases in 1995. However, it has been estimated that only about one third of the cases are reported. There is a marked discrepancy in the rates of gonorrhea among different populations within the United States. Among blacks there are approximately 1200 cases per 100,000 population; among whites, 30 per 100,000; and among Hispanics, 100 per 100,000. The age-specific attack rate is only slightly lower for 15- to 19-year-olds than for 20- to 24-year-olds, the age group with the highest attack rate. Although gonorrhea is noted throughout the United States, the highest incidence is found in the Southeast, where the rates are two to three times the national average.

Chlamydial infection is the most common bacterial STD, with an estimated 3 to 5 million new cases occurring annually. Among sexually active teenagers, surveys of the inner-city populations and on college campuses have revealed a 5% to 25% prevalence rate of *C. trachomatis* infection.

URETHRITIS

Dysuria and/or urethral discharge are the usual complaints of teenage boys with symptomatic urethritis. Although there is a clinical overlap in findings, there are some distinguishing features between gonococcal and nongonococcal urethritis. The incubation period for the development of gonococcal urethritis is usually 2 to 7 days, the discharge is typically profuse and purulent, and most patients complain of dysuria. With nongonococcal urethritis (NGU) the incubation period is approximately 1 to 3 weeks; the onset of symptoms is insidious, with only scant mucoid discharge; and dysuria is present in only half of those affected. *C. trachomatis* is the cause of NGU in approximately 50% of patients. *Ureaplasma urealyticum* (T-strain mycoplasma) is a less common cause. *Trichomonas vaginalis* and herpes simplex virus are rare causes of urethritis. *Mycoplasma genitalum* is a recently recognized agent of NGU. Postgonococcal urethritis is NGU that develops after treatment of gonorrhea with a beta-lactam antibiotic or spectinomycin; this condition represents coinfection with two urethral pathogens. Up to 50% of patients with gonorrhea have simultaneous infection with *C. trachomatis.* Although usually viewed as causing symptomatic infection, both *N. gonorrhoeae* and *C. trachomatis* may cause asymptomatic urethritis.

Adolescent males presenting with complaints of urethral discharge and/or dysuria almost always have sexually transmitted urethritis and should be examined before a urine sample is requested for analysis and culture. (The urine stream may temporarily flush out the urethral discharge and other signs of inflammation.) Adolescent males rarely have bacterial urinary tract infection unless they have an underlying anatomic or neurologic abnormality or recently have undergone urethral instrumentation. In patients without obvious discharge, the meatus should be examined for crusts and the underwear inspected for staining. Sometimes discharge can be expressed by gentle milking of the urethra from the base of the penis to the meatus. Occasionally, boys may mistake semen from masturbation or nocturnal emission for urethral discharge.

If urethral discharge is present, it should be cultured for *N. gonorrhoeae,* and Gram's stain should be applied. White blood cells with gram-negative intracellular diplococci are diagnostic of gonococcal urethritis; the absence of organisms is highly specific for exclusion of gonococcal infection. A smear demonstrating atypical or extracellular organisms is inconclusive. If there is no discharge, the presence of urethritis can be determined by examination of a urethral smear or the first 10 ml of voided urine. A calcium alginate swab passed 1 to 2 cm into the urethra and rotated can be used to obtain cells for examination with Gram's stain; four or more white blood cells (WBCs) per oil immersion field indicates urethritis. The presence of more than 15 leukocytes per high-power field (×400) in centrifuged urine is also diagnostic of urethritis in adolescent males.

Adolescent girls with complaints of frequency and dysuria often have bacterial urinary tract infections. If urine cultures are negative, such patients should be diagnosed as having acute urethral syndrome. The patient may be able to differentiate external from internal dysuria. Internal dysuria often indicates urethral infection by *C. trachomatis* or *N. gonorrhoeae* organisms; signs of urethritis (e.g., urethral discharge) are infrequent, but cervicitis is often present. External dysuria may be secondary to yeast or herpetic vulvitis or trichomonal vaginitis.

Culture of discharge or urethra for *N. gonorrhoeae* should be taken in all cases of urethritis, since interpretation of Gram's stain may not be reliable, and also to determine antibiotic susceptibility. Ideally, tests for the *C. trachomatis* organism also should be obtained; however, since drug resistance has not yet been reported and the standard regimens for treatment of presumed gonococcal and nongonococcal urethritis are effective for chlamydial infection, these tests are not mandatory. Even asymptomatic sexually active adolescents should be screened for infection. In males, a urinary leukocyte esterase test performed on the initial 10 ml of voided urine is a good screening test for urethritis. If this test is positive, the same urine specimen can be submitted for *N. gonorrhoeae* culture and *C. trachomatis* antigen detection. In females, endocervical specimens can be submitted for culture or antigen detection testing.

The recommended regimen for the treatment of uncomplicated gonococcal infection is ceftriaxone, 125 mg administered intramuscularly once, and doxycycline, 100 mg orally twice daily for 7 days. Doxycycline is not considered adequate for treatment of gonorrhea, but it is added as therapy for the frequently coexisting chlamydial infection. The alternatives to ceftriaxone are ciprofloxacin, 500 mg orally once; ofloxacin, 400 mg orally once; cefixime, 400 mg orally once; azithromycin 2 g orally once; and ceftizoxime, 0.5 g intramuscularly once; spectinomycin, 2 g intramuscularly once, may be administered to those who cannot tolerate cephalosporins or quinolones. Ciprofloxacin and ofloxacin are quinolone antibiotics that are contraindicated during pregnancy or nursing and not licensed for use in adolescents under 16 years of age. Alternatives to doxycycline are azithromycin, 1 g in a single oral dose (not in pregnant or lactating women); ofloxacin, 300 mg orally twice daily for 7 days; erythromycin base, 500 mg or erythromycin ethylsuccinate, 800 mg, each administered orally four times a day for 7 days; or sulfisoxazole, 500 mg four times a day for 10 days. Patients with gonorrhea should receive a serologic test for syphilis. The treatment regimens that include ceftriaxone, erythromycin, or tetracyclines will cure incubating syphilis; patients with clinical or serologic evidence of syphilis must be specifically treated for syphilis.

Treatment failures rarely occur after the ceftriaxone/doxycycline regimen. Infection that is present after treatment is likely a result of reinfection and indicates the need for patient education and treatment of the patient's sex partner(s).

The drug regimen for NGU is doxycycline or its alternatives (as described for treatment of gonococcal urethritis). Specifically for chlamydial infection, sulfisoxazole, 500 mg orally four times a day for 10 days, is another choice.

EPIDIDYMITIS

Epididymitis may result from three different pathogenetic processes. In adolescent males the most common mechanism is retrograde migration of sexually transmitted pathogens from the urethra by way of the vas deferens to the epididymis. *C. trachomatis* and *N. gonorrhoeae* are the etiologic agents. Reflux of infected urine into the epididymis occurs in young males with anatomic or functional abnormalities or in older men with prostatism; hematogenous infection of the epididymis may occur with bacterial or viral agents. Epididymitis secondary to a sexually transmitted pathogen has an insidious onset characterized by a dull, aching pain in the scrotum;

dysuria; and urethral discharge. Most affected adolescents are afebrile and have no toxic effects. The scrotum on the affected side is erythematous and swollen. The epididymis is in its normal posterolateral position in relationship to the testis and is enlarged and tender. The ipsilateral vas deferens is often tender to palpation.

The diagnosis of sexually transmitted epididymitis usually can be made on the basis of the characteristic history and clinical findings. Urinalysis reveals pyuria; Gram's stain of urethral discharge or urethral smear should demonstrate leukocytes and suggest whether the process is gonococcal or nongonococcal. Epididymal aspirate cultures can be useful in guiding therapy when the pathogen cannot be identified by other techniques, and in treatment failures. The differential diagnosis includes testicular torsion and trauma, although the latter is usually excluded on the basis of history. Torsion should be suspected with acute onset of pain, abnormal position of the involved gonad, and absence of evidence of urethritis. Despite the differences cited, the presenting symptoms and signs often do not permit distinction between torsion and epididymitis. Urological consultation or Doppler ultrasonographic or radionuclide scans can be used to detect diminished blood flow as evidence of testicular torsion and the need for surgical exploration.

Empiric therapy for sexually transmitted epididymitis is ceftriaxone, 250 mg administered intramuscularly once, and doxycycline, 100 mg twice daily for 10 days. Ofloxacin, 300 mg orally twice daily for 10 days, is an alternative.

SYSTEMIC MANIFESTATIONS OF GONORRHEA AND *CHLAMYDIA*

Disseminated gonococcal infection (DGI), or gonococcal arthritis-dermatitis syndrome, usually follows asymptomatic local infection and is therefore much more common in teenage girls than in boys. The illness can be divided into an initial bacteremic phase and a subsequent suppurative stage. During the initial phase the patient may be febrile, show signs of toxicity, and have leukocytosis; or may be afebrile, show no signs of toxicity, and have a normal WBC count. A migratory polyarthritis and tenosynovitis involving primarily the large joints of the extremities are present. The synovial fluid has a low WBC count, normal glucose level, negative Gram's stain, and negative culture. Skin lesions appear over the extensor surface of the distal extremities and range in number from three to 20. The lesions start as erythematous macules and progress to papules and then vesicopustules or purpura with necrosis. Blood cultures are positive for *N. gonorrhoeae* in less than 50% of cases, but cultures of the cervix or urethra, rectum, and throat yield the agent in almost all patients. The bacteremic phase continues for 7 to 10 days,

at which time the symptoms may totally resolve or develop into the suppurative stage, in which the organism localizes to a single site, usually a joint. At that time the patient is febrile, has a toxic appearance, and has leukocytosis; arthrocentesis reveals purulent fluid with a low glucose level and positive Gram's stain and culture. Gonococcal bacteremia may result in meningitis or endocarditis.

The recommended regimen for DGI is ceftriaxone, 1 g administered intravenously or intramuscularly every 24 hours (or equivalent third-generation cephalosporin); patients allergic to beta-lactams may be started on spectinomycin, 2 g intramuscularly every 12 hours. Twenty-four to 48 hours after symptoms resolve, patients with uncomplicated disease may be switched to cefixime, 400 mg orally twice daily; or ciprofloxacin, 500 mg twice a day—to complete a week of therapy. Longer courses of intravenous therapy are indicated for patients with meningitis or endocarditis, who should be managed in consultation with an expert in infectious disease. Patients with recurrent DGI should be evaluated for complement deficiencies.

In the United States, Reiter's syndrome of urethritis, arthritis, and conjunctivitis appears to be an abnormal host response to a preceding chlamydial urethritis. In other countries, Reiter's syndrome has been described as following bacterial gastroenteritis. It is a disease predominantly of young men. NGU is usually the first manifestation of the syndrome. Within a few weeks, arthritis develops. Initially the knees, ankles, and small joints of the feet are involved, but later sacroiliitis and spondylitis develop. Conjunctivitis, iritis, or uveitis develops in up to 50% of patients. Keratoderma blennorrhagicum, hyperkeratotic papules that resemble psoriasis, occurs predominantly on the soles of the feet and less frequently on the palms of the hands. Serpiginous dermatitis of the glans penis, which is painless, is called circinate balanitis. Treatment with tetracycline as for NGU usually resolves the urethritis but generally has no effect on the arthritis. Nonsteroidal antiinflammatory drugs are the most effective therapy for the arthritis. The initial episode of Reiter's syndrome usually lasts up to 6 months, but the disease recurs in up to 70% of patients, with resultant disability in nearly half of these individuals.

VAGINITIS

Any disturbance of the normal vaginal physiologic milieu is loosely defined as vaginitis, including some conditions that do not involve a true inflammatory process. Such processes occur when the balance of bacterial flora is disturbed, when the hormonal environment is altered, or when pathogens are introduced through sexual contact. Alternatively, it is not uncommon to find adolescents concerned about the possibility of having an abnormal discharge, which varies in quantity with the menstrual cycle, who actually have physiologic leukorrhea. This is so partly because with a younger gynecologic age (i.e., chronologic age minus age at menarche) and the presence of an eversion, a more copious but nonmalodorous discharge often occurs. The almost constant wetness that may be present can give rise to vulvar pruritus. The patient can be reassured about the normalcy of this complaint if she is virginal and the discharge has the characteristics already described.

Yeast Vaginitis

Candida albicans and other yeastlike organisms, which are part of the normal flora of many women, can overgrow, thus causing vaginitis. Diabetes mellitus, hormonal factors such as pregnancy and the use of oral contraceptives, systemic antibiotics that disturb the balance of bacteria present in the vagina, and disruption of the immune system are some of the important predisposing influences for yeast vaginitis. Although it is by no means the most common mode of acquisition, sexual transmission of yeast vaginitis is an often overlooked and significant mechanism for infection. This possibility should be considered in the sexually active patient with yeast vaginitis if the infection seems resistant to treatment or when there are frequent recurrences. In such circumstances, examination of the patient's sexual partner usually reveals a dry, mildly erythematous, scaly, pruritic rash on the penis, scrotum, or perineal area.

Patients with vulvovaginal yeast infection may complain of pruritus, burning, "external" dysuria, and discharge. The discharge is nonmalodorous and often has a creamy appearance. The classic thick, nonhomogeneous discharge that has the appearance of cottage cheese is not always present.[1] On microscopic examination of a wet-mount specimen, yeast buds or hyphae may be seen. Addition of 10% potassium hydroxide to the slide aids in visualization, but even then findings may be missed. Since *Candida albicans* is often found as part of the normal vaginal flora, cultures on Nickerson's or Sabouraud's medium should be reserved for symptomatic patients if the wet-mount specimen is nondiagnostic and the patient appears to have resistant or recurrent problems.

A variety of medications are available in cream or suppository form for 1-day, 3-day, and 7-day treatment regimens (Table 140-1). Nystatin has largely been replaced by miconazole, clotrimazole, butoconazole, and terconazole, all of which can be used once a day.[2] These agents tend to be effective, but it is not uncommon for persistent or recurrent infection to require a second course of treatment. Also available is single-dose, oral treatment with fluconazole. The fact that many patients prefer the convenience of this regimen to the use of intravaginal products must be weighed against the relatively common occurrence of gastrointestinal side effects (about 15%) and the infrequent reports of serious systemic reactions associated with this medication. Recurrences are common after any of the topical or oral regimens. Many clinicians use oral fluconazole once weekly or once monthly in patients with recurrent or persistent vulvovaginal yeast infection.

Trichomoniasis

Trichomonas vaginalis is a flagellated protozoan that is a common cause of vaginitis in sexually active adolescents. It may produce a yellow-green, frothy

---

TABLE 140-1
Once-Daily Treatment Options for Yeast Vaginitis

Medication	Formulation	Treatment Course
Intravaginal		
Butoconazole	Cream, 2%, 5 g	3 days
Clotrimazole*	Suppository, 100 mg	7 days (or 2 suppositories × 3 days)
Clotrimazole*	Cream, 50 mg	7 days
Clotrimazole	Suppository, 500 mg	Single dose
Miconazole	Suppository, 200 mg	3 days
Miconazole*	Suppository, 100 mg	7 days
Miconazole*	Cream, 2%, 5 g	7 days
Terconazole	Suppository, 80 mg	3 days
Terconazole	Cream, 20 mg	7 days
Oral		
Fluconazole	Oral tablet, 150 mg	Single dose

*Nonprescription drug.

discharge that is malodorous and associated with intense pruritus and dyspareunia.[3] Infection may involve Skene's glands and the urethra, resulting in dysuria and urinary frequency. Cervical involvement produces the classic "strawberry cervix" caused by punctate hemorrhage and erythema. Alternatively, trichomoniasis is most often asymptomatic in males and is seen commonly in females who have no associated complaints but are having a routine pelvic examination.

The diagnosis is usually made by microscopic examination of a wet-mount smear of the vaginal discharge in which motile trichomonads can be seen. Less commonly the organisms are described in a urinalysis or Papanicolaou (Pap) smear report. Treatment involves administration of metronidazole, 2 g taken orally all at once. An alternative regimen is metronidazole, 500 mg twice daily for 7 days. Metronidazole is contraindicated in the first trimester of pregnancy, but after this time it is recommended that patients should be given the single-dose regimen, as trichomoniasis has been associated with adverse pregnancy outcomes. Since the diagnosis is extremely difficult to make in males, sexual partners also should be treated to preclude the possibility of reinfection.

Bacterial Vaginosis

Bacterial vaginosis, the most poorly understood form of vaginal infection, is caused by *Gardnerella vaginalis, Mycoplasma hominis, Mobiluncus,* and a variety of anaerobes. This condition is no longer called "nonspecific vaginitis" because the responsible infectious agents are known (at least in part). It is considered a "vaginosis" rather than a "vaginitis" because inflammation is usually not a prominent feature of this infection. Sexual activity plays some role in the development of bacterial vaginosis, but whether this is the exclusive, or even the principal, mode of acquisition is unclear. Of great concern are data suggesting that this condition may be linked with development of pelvic inflammatory disease, puerperal infections, and premature labor.[4]

The cardinal symptom of bacterial vaginosis is a fishy, malodorous discharge that tends to be gray to white in color and thin in consistency. Dysuria, pruritus, and dyspareunia are infrequent complaints, and although the quantity of the discharge may vary, it tends to be scant. The pH of the vaginal fluid is usually greater than 4.5, and on microscopic examination relatively few leukocytes are present but "clue cells" are seen. Clue cells are vaginal epithelial cells in which the cytoplasm is so loaded with coccobacillary organisms that the nucleus and the cell border are obscured. A positive "whiff test" confirms the diagnosis: potassium hydroxide is mixed with a droplet of vaginal fluid and a strong amine (fishy) odor is liberated. Metronidazole, 500 mg orally twice daily for 7 days, is

the treatment of choice. Metronidazole, 2 g as a single dose, although less effective, may be used to improve compliance. Other effective choices include clindamycin cream, 2%, one applicator (5 g) intravaginally at bedtime for 7 days; metronidazole gel, 0.75%, one applicator, (5 g) intravaginally, twice a day for 5 days; or clindamycin, 300 mg orally twice a day for 7 days. Clindamycin cream is recommended for use throughout pregnancy, although oral metronidazole or the gel preparation may be used after the first trimester. Routine treatment of male sexual partners is not indicated, as no equivalent clinical disease is recognized in men. Furthermore, treatment of the partner does not influence the woman's response to initial therapy, nor does it have any bearing on the relapse or recurrence rate.

Miscellaneous Conditions

In the differential diagnosis of vulvovaginal abnormalities in adolescents, a number of causes unrelated to sexual activity also need to be considered. A common cause is a foreign body, such as a forgotten tampon or a misplaced piece of toilet paper, that may produce a bloody or purulent discharge. A variety of dermatologic conditions, including eczema, seborrhea, contact dermatitis, psoriasis, and Behçet's syndrome, may involve the external genitalia. Signs and symptoms suggesting the presence of these conditions elsewhere on the body often can be elicited in affected patients and may be an important clue to the diagnosis.

CERVICITIS

Definition and Etiology

Two varieties of cervical infection may occur: ectocervicitis and endocervicitis. Ectocervicitis, an infection limited to the outer portion of the cervix, may be caused by *T. vaginalis* or yeast and does not progress to involve the upper genital tract. Endocervicitis, an inflammation of the cervix, results from *N. gonorrhoeae, C. trachomatis,* or herpes simplex virus infection and has potential for causing more extensive disease. Although many other bacteria and viruses have been investigated, these are the only ones proved to be etiologic agents of this condition. Nonetheless, it is common to find a true endocervicitis that requires treatment when none of these specific pathogens can be found. The term *mucopurulent cervicitis* is used when yellow mucopus is seen coming from the cervical os, often in conjunction with erythema and friability. Microscopic evidence of infection includes the presence of 10 or more polymorphonuclear leukocytes per oil immersion field of a specimen from the endocervix that has had Gram's stain applied to it. Use of the diagnostic term *mucopurulent cervicitis* is helpful because it emphasizes the need to identify and treat all cases of infection, regardless of whether a specific etiologic agent can be identified.

Although cervicitis may be associated with unpleasant symptoms, the condition is often asymptomatic and by itself does not result in major morbidity. Nonetheless, there are several reasons why this disorder merits serious attention. First, cervicitis is most often, and perhaps exclusively, an STD. Hence, the public health considerations inherent to any STD apply—that is, it involves the potential of spreading to others in the community. Second, the proximal progression of endocervicitis to the endometrium and fallopian tubes, which often occurs in untreated cases, is associated with significant short- and long-term morbidity. Third, infection during pregnancy may result in postabortion endometritis, chorioamnionitis, premature labor, or puerperal and neonatal infections. Therefore, early recognition and treatment of cervicitis are important.

Epidemiology

Rates of infection have ranged from 1% to 18% for gonorrhea[5,6] and 14% to 26% for *Chlamydia*[7,8] among various populations of adolescents. The frequency of mucopurulent cervicitis is unknown, partly because it is often asymptomatic or is associated with nondescript manifestations that go unrecognized. As a result of both behavioral and physiologic factors, the highest rates of cervicitis are believed to be found among adolescents. Experimentation with sexual activity, which is typical of many adolescents, and inadequate use of barrier methods of contraception undoubtedly contribute to the high rates of infection observed. Furthermore, infection with *C. trachomatis* is facilitated by the presence of a cervical eversion, an anatomic variant that occurs most frequently during the peripubertal years and among users of oral contraceptives and in pregnant women.

Diagnosis

The diagnosis of cervicitis should be considered under a variety of circumstances: (1) when a vaginal discharge is present with or without foul odor, urinary frequency, urinary urgency or dysuria, or vaginal bleeding; (2) when a male sexual partner shows signs of urethritis; (3) on screening examination, when the patient is found to have a positive test for gonorrhea or *Chlamydia* infection; or (4) on routine examination, when signs of cervical inflammation are present.

Since cervicitis is a localized infection, systemic symptoms do not occur. Thus, any patient with complaints of a new or abnormal vaginal discharge who is a nonvirgin should have a speculum examination performed. Also, it should not be assumed that lower urinary tract symptoms in a sexually active female are caused by cystitis, since sexually transmitted cervicitis or urethritis may present in this manner. The examination findings may be somewhat confusing, because an eversion can be mistaken for an erosion. A cervical eversion (i.e., the presence of columnar cells on the portion of the cervix exposed to the vagina, or the portio vaginalis) is positively correlated with early gynecologic age, use of oral contraceptives, and pregnancy. Thus, an eversion is commonly present in female adolescents. Although there is evidence that an eversion also occurs more frequently with concurrent or recent cervicitis, an eversion needs to be distinguished from an erosion, since the latter represents one diagnostic component of cervical infection. The determination of whether a purulent discharge is present at the cervical os is made by inserting a white swab into the endocervical canal, rotating it to remove some of the secretions, and then holding the swab against a white background such as a sheet. Friability is defined as bleeding that occurs after the first or second swab is inserted, not the bleeding that regularly results from use of a cytology brush or after the cervix has been traumatized by insertion of multiple swabs.

If mucopus and friability are not both present or are equivocal, a Gram's stain should be taken. After the mucus and vaginal secretions have been wiped away from the os, an additional specimen is obtained for microscopic examination. Various studies have defined a minimum significant number of polymorphonuclear leukocytes (PMNs) as ranging from 5 to 30 per ×1000 magnification.[9] Furthermore, if gram-negative diplococci are present within the cytoplasm of the PMNs, this situation is highly suggestive of gonococcal cervicitis. Specific tests for *N. gonorrhoeae* and *C. trachomatis* organisms should be performed even though there is no need to withhold treatment pending the results of these tests.

Treatment

Establishing a clinical diagnosis for mucopurulent cervicitis and not relying on microbiologic tests is of great advantage because it allows the clinician to begin treatment at the time of the patient's initial visit. It also helps avoid the pitfall of denying treatment for patients with infection when cultures or other test results are negative. Such false-negative results occur for a variety of reasons, including (1) improper handling of media before or after specimens are collected (e.g., Thayer-Martin culture medium is not brought to room temperature after removal from the refrigerator); (2) test sensitivity that is less than 100%, particularly for the nonculture methods used to detect gonorrhea or *Chlamydia;* and (3) as is the case in males with urethritis (the equivalent of female cervicitis), the distinct possibility that other infectious etiologic agents are involved that cannot be identified by current diagnostic methods.

The treatment of choice for patients with mucopurulent cervicitis is identical to that recommended for patients with chlamydial infections. Treatment for gonorrhea also should be initiated when working with patient populations in which the prevalence rate of gonorrhea is high, when the Gram's stain is suggestive of this condition (i.e., gram-negative intracellular diplococci are present), when the gonorrhea culture result is positive, or when it is known that the patient's sexual partner had gonorrhea.

PELVIC INFLAMMATORY DISEASE

Definition and Etiology

The terms *pelvic inflammatory disease* (PID) and *acute salpingitis* are often used interchangeably, even though the former actually includes infection of any part of the proximal genital tract resulting from ascension of microorganisms from the cervix. Since subacute and chronic infections of the upper genital tract occur infrequently in adolescents, this discussion will focus on sexually transmitted acute PID. *C. trachomatis* and *N. gonorrhoeae* are often etiologically linked to acute PID, but in many cases, particularly in repeat episodes of PID, genital tract flora—including anaerobes, gram-negative rods, streptococci, and *Mycoplasma hominis*—attain a pathogenic role resulting in a polymicrobial infection[10] (Box 140-1). The cervicitis that precedes an episode of PID is typically asymptomatic or only mildly bothersome and can be present for months before the onset of symptoms associated with upper tract disease.

Pelvic peritonitis, Fitz-Hugh-Curtis syndrome (perihepatitis), and tuboovarian abscess represent the most severe end of the spectrum of PID. Although these conditions result from progression of infection beyond the fallopian tubes, they often occur simultaneously with the first signs of acute salpingitis, or present de novo when signs or symptoms of earlier disease have been absent. Adolescents are at the very beginning of their years of fertility. Thus, PID, with its potentially severe long-term consequences, has tremendous importance.

Epidemiology

Adolescents appear to be at greater risk for PID than any other group. Weström[11] calculated that sexually active 15-year-olds have a 1:8 risk of developing acute salpingitis compared with a 1:10 risk for 16-year-old nonvirgins; he estimated that there is a 1:80 risk of this disease occurring in 24-year-old women. Although it is undoubtedly true that some young people have a greater

---

BOX 140-1
Microbiologic Etiology of Acute PID

SEXUALLY TRANSMITTED PATHOGENS
Chlamydia trachomatis
Mycoplasma hominis
*Mycoplasma genitalium**
Neisseria gonorrhoeae
*Ureaplasma urealyticum**

FACULATIVE GENITAL TRACT FLORA†
AEROBES
Enterobacter cloacae
Escherichia coli
Gardnerella vaginalis
Haemophilius influenzae
Klebsiella pneumoniae
Proteus mirabilis
Streptococcus spp.
ANAEROBES
Bacteroides spp.
Peptococcus spp.
Peptostreptococcus spp.

*The role of these organisms is unclear.
†Sexual activity also may play a role in the transmission of these organisms.
PID, pelvic inflammatory disease.

---

number of sexual partners than their adult counterparts, a variety of other behavioral and physiologic factors have been postulated to explain the high rates of infection observed among adolescents. Potentially relevant elements include differences in the host immune response; an increased degree of cervical ectopy; and the likelihood that the youngest adolescents may have a tendency to engage in more dysfunctional sexual behavior, such as having a high-risk (for STDs) partner and being less likely to use an effective contraceptive method.

Although in the 1980s the incidence of PID in the United States and elsewhere seemed to be increasing over that in earlier decades,[5] the overall hospitalization rate for acute PID declined by 36%. Unfortunately, the rate for 15- to 19-year-old women dropped by only 10% during this period, and this group had the highest hospitalization rate in 1987 to 1988.

Any factor that increases the probability of exposure to STDs, such as involvement in a nonmonogamous relationship, inadequate use of a barrier contraceptive, or substance abuse, indirectly promotes the development of PID (Table 140-2). Other factors, such as use of an intrauterine device, not seeking care when symptoms of cervicitis appear, and poor compliance, more directly facilitate PID. Vaginal douching has been demonstrated to be associated with a higher risk for PID. It is unknown whether this behavior plays a cause-and-effect role or represents the greater likelihood that women with vaginal

TABLE 140-2
Risk Factors for STDs and PID and Its Sequelae*

Risk Factor	Acquisition of STD	Development of PID	Development of PID Sequelae
Demographic and social			
Age	+	+	−
Socioeconomic status	+	+	•
Marital status	+	+	•
Residence (rural or urban)	+	•	•
Sexual behavior			
Number of partners	+	•	•
Age at first sexual intercourse	+	•	•
Frequency of sexual intercourse	+	•	•
Rate of acquiring new partners	+	•	•
Contraceptive practice			
Barrier method	−	−	−
Hormonal drug	+	−	•
Intrauterine device	•	+	+
Healthcare behavior			
Evaluation of symptoms	+	+	+
Compliance with treatment	+	+	+
Partner notification	+	+	+
Other			
Douching	•	+	•
Smoking	+	+	•
Substance abuse	+	•	•
Menstrual cycle	+	+	•

Modified from Centers for Disease Control: Pelvic inflammatory disease: guidelines for prevention and management; purified protein derivative (PPD)–tuberculin anergy and HIV infection: guidelines for anergy testing and management of anergic persons at risk of tuberculosis, *MMWR* 40(RR-5):1-25, 1991.
Bullets indicate no known association.

symptoms (e.g., discharge due to cervicitis) are more likely to douche.

The role of oral contraceptives in PID has been the subject of much controversy. Their use has been linked with a higher risk for chlamydial cervicitis[12] and possibly also for gonococcal infection. Although the cervical ectopy that occurs with oral contraceptive use probably serves to facilitate the development of cervicitis, other factors related to sexual activity, which may be observed more often in those who take oral contraceptives, may be confounding this observation. Most important, it appears that oral contraceptives actually reduce the probability of PID,[13] particularly nonchlamydial PID, and are protective against symptomatic PID in women with chlamydial infection of the distal genital tract. In contrast, the use of an intrauterine device increases the risk for PID, although this does not appear to have as great an effect as originally believed.

Diagnosis

The diagnosis of PID should be considered in any nonvirginal female adolescent with abdominal pain of any intensity. Even when a sensitive and skillfully obtained history has been recorded, the risk factors for and the symptoms of this sexually transmitted infection are often not volunteered by the patient, or may be atypical. Most important, PID is a clinical diagnosis. Waiting for a positive culture or other test for gonorrhea or *Chlamydia* infection, which is actually confirmatory only of cervicitis, causes unnecessary delay in treatment and thus has great potential for doing harm.

Most patients complain of discomfort in the lower abdomen, and although the pain may seem to be localized to one side, the tenderness is most often bilateral. With gonococcal salpingitis, the onset of pain is likely to occur within 1 week of menses, although when *C. trachomatis* is the etiologic agent, and certainly when neither gonorrhea nor *Chlamydia* is found, symptoms may begin at any time.[14] Patients may have dysuria, probably indicative of concomitant urethral infection with gonorrhea, *Chlamydia,* or another organism. New or increased vaginal discharge, a history of recent urethritis in a sexual partner, and right upper quadrant pain (indicative of perihepatitis) are variably found, but are suggestive of PID. Increased menstrual flow and cramps as well as metrorrhagia are often present. Superficial dyspareunia is pain experienced with initial penetration during intercourse and usually indicates vulvovaginitis or lack of lubrication. On the other hand, adolescents with deep dyspareunia complain of a pain felt deeper in the abdomen during thrusting. This pain is usually the result of PID or other significant pelvic pathology. Clinicians should avoid reliance on temperature elevation in making the diagnosis of acute PID. Although fever may occur more often in patients with gonococcal salpingitis than in those with other etiologies, many studies have demonstrated that patients with PID are more likely to be afebrile.[15]

The pelvic examination is of paramount importance in cases of PID. Cervical motion tenderness and direct adnexal tenderness are present in almost all patients with acute PID. When other diagnoses, such as acute appendicitis or ectopic pregnancy, can be excluded, these two findings, along with lower abdominal tenderness, should be used as minimal criteria for treatment (Box 140-2). A positive culture or other test for *N. gonorrhoeae* or *C. trachomatis* in the patient or her partner, or signs of mucopurulent cervicitis, are highly suggestive supplementary findings. On bimanual examination, a fullness or a mass in the adnexa may be noted in patients with acute salpingitis. When an adnexal mass is present, it should be made certain that this does not represent a tuboovarian abscess. Although patients with the latter tend to have a longer duration of pain, greater temperature elevation, and a higher erythrocyte sedimentation rate (ESR) than those with uncomplicated PID, there is considerable overlap in symptoms.[16]

The WBC count is usually not helpful, because it is inconsistently elevated in PID and may be high with many of the other conditions being considered in the differential diagnosis. Similarly, the ESR is often elevated, but this finding is so variable that it is not of great use clinically. In patients with acute salpingitis, the sonogram may be entirely normal or may show nonspecific findings such as fluid in the cul-de-sac or a slightly enlarged adnexa.[17] Ultrasonography is most useful when other diagnoses are considered possible, such as an ectopic or intrauterine pregnancy or an ovarian cyst or neoplasm. In addition, it should be used when the clinical presentation is more complicated than usual, particularly (1) in patients with a prolonged history of pain or a markedly elevated ESR, (2) when marked improvement does not occur within 24 to 48 hours after initiation of antibiotics, or (3) when the disease course is prolonged. Endometrial biopsy can provide histopathologic evidence

---

BOX 140-2
Criteria for Clinical Diagnosis of PID

Minimum Criteria
 Lower abdominal tenderness
 Bilateral adnexal tenderness
 Cervical motion tenderness
Additional useful criteira*
 Readily available
  Oral temperature >38.3° C
  Abnormal cervical or vaginal discharge
  Elevated erythryocyte sedimentation rate
   and/or C-reactive protein
  Cervical infection with *n. gonorrhoeae* or
   C. trachomatis†
 More expensive, invasive, and not routinely available
  Histopathologic evidence on endometrial biopsy
  Tuboovarian abscess on sonography
  Laparoscopy

From Centers for Disease Control and Prevention: 1993 Sexually transmitted diseases treatment guidelines, *MMWR* 42:77, 1993.
*Use of these criteria will increase the specificity of the diagnosis, which is suggested in patients with more severe presentations when an incorrect diagnosis is more likely to result in severe morbidity.
†All patients should have culture or other tests performed for *N. gonorrhoeae* and *C. trachomatis,* although there is no need to delay initiation of treatment pending available results. Negative results do not imply an incorrect diagnosis.

BOX 140-3
Rationale for Inpatient Management of PID

GENERAL ADVANTAGES
Close, direct observation of patient is possible, allowing confirmation of diagnosis and exclusion of other serious possibilities (e.g., ectopic pregnancy, tubo-ovarian abscess)
Treatment with high-dose parenteral antibiotics is possible
If nausea or vomiting occurs (from either disease or medications), treatment may proceed uninterrupted with parenteral antibiotics
Medication side effects can be identified quickly and appropriate changes made

SPECIFIC ADVANTAGES FOR ADOLESCENTS
Compliance with oral medications may be more difficult
Long-term consequences (e.g., infertility), which are more likely to occur in noncompliant patients, can be disastrous given that adolescents have the greatest number of fertile years to risk
Fears regarding maintenance of confidentiality, resistance to accepting seriousness of infection or potential for severe sequelae, or other factors may make it less likely for adolescents to return for required progress update within 72 hours of initiation of treatment
Although not applicable to all teenagers with PID, opportunity may be missed to identify those at-risk adolescents as in whom episode of PID represents only one of many dysfunctional behaviors

of endometritis, but this test is invasive and not always available. In addition, waiting for test results causes a delay in treatment. Laparoscopy allows one to directly visualize the fallopian tubes and obtain cultures from the site of infection; it is considered the "gold standard" for diagnosis. Unfortunately, this procedure is invasive and costly and requires general anesthesia and an experienced surgeon, all of which preclude its routine use.

Treatment

There are no controlled studies of outcome comparing patients with PID who are treated as outpatients and those who are hospitalized for treatment. The traditional indications for hospitalization include an uncertain diag-

---

> **BOX 140-4**
> **Treatment Regimens for Acute PID**
>
> INPATIENT TREATMENT
> Regimen A
>   Cefoxitin, 2 g IV every 6 hr, or cefotetan, 2 g IV
>   every 12 hr
>   *plus*
>   Doxycycline, *100 mg PO or IV every 12 hr
> Regimen B
>   Clindamycin, †900 mg IV every 8 hr
>   *plus*
>   Gentamicin, IV or IM 2 mg/kg (loading dose),
>   folowed by 1.5 mg/kg (maintenance dose)
>   every 8 hr
>
> OUTPATIENT TREATMENT
> Regimen A
>   Cefoxitin, 2 g IM plus probenecid, 1 g PO in a
>   single dose concurrently, or ceftriaxone,
>   250 mg IM, or other parenteral third-
>   generation cephalosporin (e.g., ceftizoxime
>   or cefotaxime)
>   *plus*
>   Doxycycline, *100 mg PO two times a day for
>   14 days
> Regimen B
>   Ofloxacin, 400 mg PO 2 times a day for 14 days
>   *plus*
>   Either clindamycin, 450 mg PO 4 times a day, or
>   metronidazole, 500 mg PO 2 times a day for
>   14 days

*Doxycycline and other tetracyclines are contraindicated during pregnancy. Tetracycline, 500 mg four times a day, also may be used, but this has disadvantages of more frequent dosing and possible interference with intake of dairy products. Erythromycin, 500 mg four times a day, may be substituted in pregnant patients and in those for whom a tetracycline is otherwise contraindicated.
†A tetracycline is the drug of choice for chlamydial infections, although some data suggest that clindamycin also may be effective.

---

nosis or the possibility of a surgical abdomen, the presence of a pelvic abscess, a concurrent pregnancy, or the failure of outpatient management. Patients with PID who are HIV positive may have a more complicated disease course, including development of a tuboovarian abscess, and should be treated with antibiotics administered parenterally. Furthermore, there are compelling reasons why most, if not all, adolescents should be treated as inpatients (Box 140-3).

No one combination of antibiotics has been demonstrated to be ideal, but several regimens are recommended by the Centers for Disease Control and Prevention (CDC) as logical empirical choices, given the organisms known to be etiologic in PID (Box 140-4). Treatment for infection with *C. trachomatis* should be included in any regimen, since this bacteria is commonly found with PID, its presence may be more difficult to document, and patients who do not receive such treatment may appear to be cured despite ongoing infection and tubal damage. Any regimen should be modified or a different diagnosis should be given renewed consideration if the patient does not show significant improvement within 24 to 48 hours. Practical constraints, including the high cost of inpatient treatment and the sometimes inflexible rules of managed care companies, must be balanced against the very likely long-term adverse costs and consequences of inadequate treatment of a teenager with PID. Intravenous medication should be continued for at least 48 hours after the patient shows substantial improvement, and then oral doxycycline should be continued for a total of 14 days. Clindamycin, 450 mg orally four times a day, may be an acceptable alternative to doxycycline. The sex partners of patients with PID should be examined and empirically treated with a regimen effective against both *N. gonorrhoeae* and *C. trachomatis*.

Infertility and ectopic pregnancy are the two most serious complications of PID, although chronic pelvic pain, dyspareunia, and possible increased risk for repeat episodes of PID are also significant problems. One estimate for infertility due to tubal occlusion in women 15 to 24 years old at the time of their first episode of PID shows the risk to be about 9% after a single episode, 21% after two episodes, and 52% after three or more. Most teenagers understand that the only way to test fertility is to try to become pregnant. Thus, another not uncommon event is an "unintended" pregnancy in an adolescent after an episode of PID.

ENTERIC INFECTIONS

Sexual activity can result in an enteric infection caused by either classic sexually transmitted pathogens or typical gastrointestinal infectious agents. Although such infections most commonly occur among homosexual males, it is the pattern of sexual activity (i.e., multiple anonymous sexual partners) and the opportunity for fecal contamination or rectal penetration, and not the sexual orientation per se, that puts the individual at risk for acquisition of these infections. The typical gastrointestinal organisms may be transmitted through anilingus or from a fecally contaminated penis in fellatio. Both gastrointestinal and sexually transmitted agents can be acquired through genital-rectal intercourse. In women, the anorectal sexually transmitted infections also may arise from contiguous spread of infection from the genitalia.

There are three relatively distinct sexually transmitted enteric infection syndromes, each with its own characteristics and etiologies. Proctitis refers to inflammation limited to the rectal mucosa. This condition may be asymptomatic or may cause severe anorectal pain, itching, burning, tenesmus, hematochezia, and constipation; mucopurulent discharge may be misinterpreted as diarrhea. Endoscopic examination reveals ulcerations, friability, or "cobblestoning" of the rectal mucosa. Gram's stain of rectal swabs will reveal inflammatory cells. The organisms most commonly causing proctitis are the conventional STD pathogens: herpes simplex virus, *N. gonorrhoeae*, *Treponema pallidum,* and *C. trachomatis* (both lymphogranuloma venereum [LGV] and non-LGV serovars).

If the mucosa is inflamed more than 12 cm above the anal verge, the condition is classified as proctocolitis. In addition to the symptoms described for proctitis, diarrhea is present. *Campylobacter* spp., *C. trachomatis* (LGV serovars), *Shigella* spp., and *Entamoeba histolytica* are the agents most frequently causing this syndrome.

Inflammation that is limited to the small intestine without signs of proctitis or proctocolitis is called enteritis. Diarrhea is the major symptom, with associated abdominal cramps and bloating or flatulence; rarely, fluid loss may result in dehydration and electrolyte imbalance. *Giardia lamblia* is most often associated with sexually transmitted enteritis; *Salmonella* spp. and *E. histolytica* are less frequently identified. In HIV-infected patients, *Mycobacterium avium-intracellulare,* cytomegalovirus, *Cryptosporidium,* and *Isospora belli* must be considered as possible causes of diarrhea.

Comprehensive evaluation for sexually transmitted enteric infection should include endoscopy; rectal culture for *N. gonorrhoeae, C. trachomatis,* and herpes simplex virus; stool culture for routine bacterial enteric pathogens; stool examination for ova and parasites; and serologic tests for syphilis. While the laboratory test results are awaited, empiric therapy for proctitis may be initiated with ceftriaxone, 250 mg intramuscularly once, and doxycycline, 100 mg twice daily for 7 days.

Specific therapy can be offered when an infectious agent is identified.

GENITAL LESIONS

HUMAN PAPILLOMAVIRUS INFECTION

Definition and Etiology

Human papillomavirus (HPV) is a double-stranded DNA virus that cannot be grown in cell culture and has no known serologic markers. Molecular hybridization techniques have allowed classification of this virus into various DNA types. The list of known HPVs continues to grow, since new types are being discovered on a regular basis. When the DNA base-pair sequence is less than 50% homologous with a known HPV type, this is considered to be a new HPV type. Specific types tend to have a predilection for infection of certain tissues (Table 140-3). Furthermore, within categories (e.g., anogenital types, skin types), there are differences in the virulence or disease-producing capability. HPV is of importance to clinicians for a number of reasons. First, as a sexually transmissible agent, HPV is associated with the public health implications common to all STDs. Second, HPV plays an important role in the production of neoplastic disease of the genital tract. Third, vertical transmission of the virus from mother to offspring may have adverse health effects (e.g., condyloma acuminatum, laryngeal papillomatosis) for the infant. Fourth, other circumstances in which there is spread of infection from an adult to a child, including sexual abuse, have injurious health and psychosocial consequences for the child and the family. A discussion of HPV infection in infants and children is beyond the scope of this chapter, but reviews of this subject are available elsewhere.[18]

The anogenital HPVs are believed to be acquired most often through intimate sexual contact, although there is strong evidence that this is not the exclusive mode of transmission.[19] A wide range of presentations are produced by the genital HPVs. Condyloma acuminatum (venereal warts) is an obvious and usually easily recognizable manifestation of infection. Specific abnormalities found in cervical epithelial cells obtained through Pap smear screening are pathognomonic of HPV infection. HPV also has been found with great regularity within invasive cervical cancer tissue and in squamous intraepithelial neoplastic lesions of the cervix. Thus, it is believed that HPV is one of the crucial elements serving a causal role in the development of cancer of the cervix.[20] At the other end of the spectrum, HPV infection may be asymptomatic, without any visible manifestations, and

TABLE 140-3
HPV Types and Their Clinical Manifestations

Type	Clinical Manifestations
1, 4	Plantar warts
2	Common warts (verrucae vulgaris)
3, 10, 28	Juvenile flat warts (verrucae plana)
5, 8, 9, 12, 19-25, 36, 40	Epidermodysplasia verruciformis with progression to skin cancer
7	Butcher's warts
13, 32	Focal epithelial hyperplasia of oral cavity (Heck's disease)
26-29, 34	Bowen's disease (nongenital)
6, 11, 42	Anogenital condyloma acuminatum
	Low-grade squamous intraepithelial lesions of cervix
	Laryngeal papillomatosis
16, 18, 31, 33, 35, 39	Anogenital condyloma acuminatum
	High-grade squamous intraepithelial lesions of cervix
	Squamous cell carcinoma

discovered only through the use of sophisticated molecular diagnostic techniques.

Epidemiology

The diagnostic methods used to detect HPV infection vary widely in sensitivity. Documentation of visible lesions (e.g., condylomata acuminata) or detection of abnormalities by Pap smear will fail to reveal subclinical infections that may or may not have potential for producing disease in the future. In contrast, molecular techniques (e.g., Southern blot test, polymerase chain reaction [PCR]) are highly sensitive but can uncover HPV infections that may have no clinical significance. Given these limitations, reports of condyloma acuminatum seen by physicians in fee-for-service office-based practices in the United States demonstrate a more than fourfold increase from 1966 to 1981, with over 65% of the consultations among 15- to 29-year-old patients.[21] When molecular genetic techniques are used, prevalence rates of genital HPV infection as high as 38% to 46% have been observed among populations of sexually active urban youths and college women, arguably making this the most common STD.[22]

Diagnosis

To a large extent the location and type of lesion produced determine the manner in which a patient with HPV infection presents. Condylomata acuminata, which are exophytic warts, have a cauliflower-like appearance and may be observed on the vaginal mucosa, vulva, urethra, perineal skin, and (occasionally) cervix of female patients. In males, these warts can occur anywhere on the penis or urethra and also may be seen on the scrotum. Direct anal-genital contact may give rise to lesions in the perianal area, although such lesions are not uncommon in

female patients who have engaged in only vaginal intercourse. Papular warts, which have a more attenuated appearance, are more likely to occur on the labia majora, perineal skin, or shaft of the penis. All the above lesions may be painless unless they become large or are subject to friction, in which case they may bleed and become uncomfortable. Flat condylomas are visible only after application of 3% or 5% acetic acid to an infected area for several minutes and observation of the site with a colposcope or other magnifying device. The lesions appear white and roughened compared with the normal pink or tan surrounding tissue of the mucosa or skin.

Normal anatomic variants may be confused with HPV lesions. These include parallel rows of 1- to 3-mm papillae grouped along the corona of the penis, termed "pink pearly papules," found in one study among 16% of pubertal male adolescents.[23] White or yellowish sebaceous glands that may occur on the penis or the vulva also should not be mistaken for warts. Other STDs, such as condyloma latum (a manifestation of secondary syphilis) and molluscum contagiosum, need to be distinguished from HPV infection.

The Bethesda System of classification for cervical cytology or some modification of this system is widely in use throughout the United States and around the world and has largely replaced the "class I, class II" terminology previously used to categorize Pap smears.[24] The presence of koilocytosis or other forms of atypia within cervical cells is diagnostic of HPV infection and is probably indistinguishable from low-grade squamous intraepithelial lesion (SIL). HPV infection of the cervix, particularly HPV types 16, 18, 31, 33, 45, and others, has been regularly associated with high-grade SIL and invasive carcinoma.[25] Fortunately, although low-grade SIL is observed frequently among sexually active adolescents, high-grade lesions and malignancy occur much less frequently.

Molecular diagnostic techniques include PCR, Southern blot test, hybrid capture, dot blot test, and in situ hybridization. PCR, a method whereby minimal amounts of genetic material can be amplified, is the most sensitive and most specific of these methodologies, but it has been fraught with technical difficulties. Therefore, the Southern blot remains the "gold standard" for diagnosis in most research laboratories. Hybrid capture utilizes RNA probes and permits the amount of HPV DNA present to be quantified. This technique is also not currently in use in clinical settings. HPV detection kits using the dot blot are commercially available. However, simply knowing that infection is present is of questionable value, since within any adolescent population far more patients have HPV infection than have cervical disease. Furthermore, data from longitudinal studies suggest that most patients with subclinical HPV infection and normal Pap smears do not develop significant neoplastic disease.

Treatment

The choice of treatment is in part dependent on the location and number of lesions present. Patients with few condylomata acuminata of nonmucosal surfaces of the genitalia or perianal area can be treated with either trichloroacetic acid or a 20% to 25% solution of podophyllin resin, both of which usually require multiple applications. When podophyllin is used, the surrounding normal skin first should be protected through an application of petroleum jelly. Podofilox, a 0.5% solution of purified podophyllotoxin, has the advantage of being the only treatment available by prescription for patients to self-apply at home. The initial application should always take place in the clinician's office to make certain that the correct diagnosis has been made and so that the patient can be instructed in its proper use. With more extensive lesions or when mucosal surfaces are involved, alternative options must be used (Box 140-5). Unfortunately, none of these options provides consistently superior initial results or lower recurrence rates. All three agents may cause severe local reactions, and podophyllin can result in neurologic or bone marrow toxicity if large amounts are absorbed. Podophyllin and podofilox are also teratogenic in laboratory animals and should not be used during pregnancy. Imiquimod (Alsara) cream is also now available. Disadvantages of the surgical treatment options are that they are inconsistently successful and often require general anesthesia. The use of systemic or intralesional interferon, although greeted with great enthusiasm when it was first introduced, is effective in some patients but is also limited by its side effects and the associated incidence of recurrent lesions. Loop electrosurgical excision procedure (LEEP) involves using a wire loop that, like cautery, will remove a circular band of tissue from the cervix. The advantage of this procedure is that it provides

---

BOX 140-5
Treatment Modalities for HPV Infections

MEDICAL REGIMENS
  Trichloroacetic acid
  Podophyllin
  Podofilox
  5-Fluorouracil
  Interferon (systemic or intralesional)
  Imiquimod

SURGICAL REGIMENS
  Loop electrosurgical excision procedure (LEEP)
  Excision
  Cryotherapy
  Electrocautery
  Laser

HPV, human papillomavirus.

---

tissue for histologic analysis while simultaneously removing abnormal areas. It also has the limitation that it is quite easy for excessive tissue to be excised. It is not uncommon for patients with conditions that produce various degrees of compromised cell-mediated immunity (e.g., pregnancy, diabetes mellitus, systemic lupus erythematosus, HIV infection) to have extensive lesions that are resistant to all available treatments.

Cervical lesions that have been discovered through Pap smear screening or colposcopy must be evaluated by histopathologic examination to determine the degree of disease present. Low-grade neoplastic lesions are often treated with localized excisional biopsy, cryosurgery, or laser therapy. High-grade lesions usually require conization of the cervix or treatment with LEEP. There is no clear answer as to how a patient should be managed when HPV infection is discovered through one of the molecular genetic tests. Certainly, if there are concurrent abnormalities of the Pap smear, colposcopy with biopsy of the suspicious areas should be performed. However, when the Pap smear is normal, the value of ablative treatment is uncertain. All the treatment options are not without risk, expense, and substantial failure and recurrence rates. Moreover, there is ample evidence that most HPV infections are not likely to result in cervical disease, especially in adolescents. Although colposcopy is a reasonably benign test, it is not always available and is more expensive than Pap smear screening. Considering that cervical cytologic sampling has a false-negative rate as high as 50% even in high-quality laboratories, a prudent approach is to obtain Pap smears more often (every 4 to 6 months) in patients with HPV infection in whom the initial cytologic specimen was normal.

Counseling efforts regarding HPV infection should be informative but not dogmatic. Sexual partners of patients found to have any variety of HPV infection should be examined to determine whether treatable HPV lesions are present and to screen for other STDs. However, the clinician must be cautious in counseling patients regarding when or from whom they acquired infection. The incubation period for HPV may vary from less than 1 month to over 2 years, and condylomata acuminata often recur spontaneously despite treatment that results in apparent resolution of the infection. Moreover, infection may be asymptomatic, with overt manifestations occurring months to years later, a situation that occurs frequently in patients with abnormal cervical cytologic specimens.

GENITAL HERPES

Definition and Etiology

Genital herpes is an acute and recurrent infection of the skin and mucous membrane of the genitalia. Herpes simplex virus type 2 (HSV-2) is responsible for approximately 90% of genital infections; type 1 (HSV-1) accounts for the remainder. It is the most common cause of genital lesions in sexually active adolescents in the United States.

Epidemiology

Although genital herpes is not a reportable disease, the incidence appears to be markedly increasing. In 1989, there were approximately 150,000 initial visits to physicians' offices for genital herpes, compared with 20,000 in 1966. HSV-2 seroprevalence rates in the general U.S. population range from 20% to 60%, being higher in lower socioeconomic groups and nonwhites. Genital infection with HSV is almost always sexually acquired, although autoinoculation from infectious oral secretions via the hands may occur infrequently.

Diagnosis

Three presentations of genital disease are recognized: primary, nonprimary initial, and recurrent infection. Primary genital herpes infection develops in individuals with no preexisting herpes antibody. A person who is experiencing his or her first clinical evidence of genital herpes but has preexisting herpes antibody is having a nonprimary initial episode. Recurrent genital herpes is diagnosed when an individual has a history of similar previous genital infection.

Primary genital herpes develops 2 to 12 days after sexual exposure to the virus. Local pruritus and tingling may precede the genital lesions. Erythematous maculopapules rapidly progress to grouped vesicles or pustules on an erythematous base; individual vesicles are 2 to 3 mm in diameter. The vesicles and pustules rupture, producing multiple superficial ulcers that may coalesce to form erosions that are 2 cm in diameter and exquisitely painful. The eruption may spread in a wavelike fashion to involve the entire perineum, with new crops of lesions developing for up to a week. The most common site of involvement in males is the penis, and one quarter of affected men have urethral discharge; in women, the vulva, perineum, vagina, and cervix are the sites affected with vaginal discharge in 85%. At this stage severe dysuria may result in urinary retention, sexual contact produces dyspareunia, and even the minor friction of walking exacerbates the discomfort. With dry crusting and underlying reepithelialization, cutaneous lesions heal in 2 to 3 weeks; ulcers in moist areas become macerated, tend to heal slowly, and may develop secondary bacterial infection. Bilateral, firm, tender, nonfluctuant inguinal adenopathy is present. Systemic complaints accompanying primary genital herpes include fever, anorexia, headache, malaise, and myalgia. Symptomatic pharyngitis due to HSV is seen in about 20% of patients. Clinical aseptic meningitis requiring hospitalization is seen in 6% of women and 2% of men; subclinical cerebrospinal fluid (CSF) pleocytosis occurs more frequently than clinically evident meningitis. Extragenital herpetic lesions occur in 26% of affected women and 8% of affected men.

Patients with nonprimary initial episodes have statistically fewer lesions, less pain, less constitutional symptoms, shorter duration of viral shedding, and an overall shorter course of illness. However, without knowledge of the patient's antibody status, it may not be possible clinically to differentiate primary from nonprimary first episodes.

Recurrent genital herpes is caused by reactivation of latent endogenous herpesvirus in the sacral sensory ganglia. Triggering factors for the recurrent episode identified by many patients include fever, trauma, emotional stress, menses, and sexual intercourse. Recurrences may be noted as often as monthly or as infrequently as once a year. The frequency and severity of recurrence diminishes as the time interval from the first episode increases. A prodrome of localized paresthesia, itching, or burning at the site of the subsequent lesion is experienced by half of the patients. Grouped vesicles on an erythematous base tend to reappear at the same location with each episode. The overall course of each recurrence is much milder than that of the first episode of infection, with less pain and shorter duration, lesions remaining localized to one site, only one quarter of patients having tender adenopathy, absence of systemic manifestations, and overall duration of 7 to 10 days. Recurrent genital herpes occurs in 90% of individuals after a first episode and is more frequent with HSV-2 than with HSV-1.

Patients with active genital lesions are highly contagious; however, even during asymptomatic intervals they may shed virus in genital secretions and infect sexual partners. Newborn infants may acquire devastating herpetic infection from contaminated maternal genital secretions in the birth canal.

Genital ulceration due to HSV enhances the risk of acquisition of HIV infection. HIV-infected patients, as well as those immunocompromised from treatment of malignancy or transplantation, have more severe and chronic genital and perianal mucocutaneous ulcerations due to HSV.

Herpes simplex is the most common cause of genital ulcer disease. If the patient describes (or the physician sees) grouped vesicles on an erythematous base, the diagnosis is almost certainly genital herpes. After the vesicles have ruptured and ulcers are coalesced or scabbed, the major differential diagnoses are syphilis, chancroid, scabies, pediculosis, and trauma. Isolation of the virus is the most sensitive and most specific technique used to confirm the diagnosis. The lesions can be cultured directly for virus; intact vesicles should be unroofed before obtaining the specimen. A Tzanck preparation of the base of the lesion can be made and stained with Giemsa or Wright's stain to find multinucleate giant cells, or the preparation can be stained with fluorescein-conjugated antibodies to locate herpesvirus antigens. Cervical Pap smears also can be used to demonstrate the presence of herpesvirus. Serology is of limited value in the diagnosis of genital herpes.

Treatment

Treatment of genital herpes with antiviral agents reduces the pain, speeds healing, and shortens the duration of viral shedding, especially in first clinical episodes. Acyclovir 200 mg taken five times a day for 5 to 10 days is the usual regimen for outpatients; valacyclovir, a prodrug of acyclovir, is also effective for recurrent genital herpes at a dose of 500 mg twice daily for 5 days. Therapy has no effect on the frequency or the severity of recurrences after the drug has been discontinued.

Individuals with frequent recurrences may benefit from daily suppressive therapy; acyclovir, 400 mg taken twice a day, has been demonstrated to be safe and effective in reducing recurrences by more than 75% for 1 year or longer. Prophylactic acyclovir should be periodically discontinued so that the patient's recurrence rate can be reassessed.

Adolescents must be informed of the recurrent nature of the infection and the potential for contagion even when they are asymptomatic. An adolescent girl may be seen with genital herpes at a time when she is not pregnant; however, if she becomes pregnant months or years later, her obstetrician should be informed of her history of genital herpes.

SYPHILIS

Definition and Etiology

Because of its protean presentations and the wide spectrum of diseases that syphilis may mimic, Sir William Osler stated: "Know syphilis in all its manifestations . . . , and all other things clinical will be added unto you." A century later, that statement remains true. Although the initial sign of syphilis is a self-limited genital lesion, the diverse manifestations of the later stages reveal the systemic involvement of the disease.

The etiologic agent of syphilis is a spirochete, *Treponema pallidum.* The organism cannot be grown in an artificial medium; the only reliable way to cultivate the organism outside of man is by intratesticular inoculation of the rabbit. The organism cannot be seen with either hematoxylin and eosin stain or Gram's stain, but it can be demonstrated through dark-field microscopy, silver staining, or fluorescent-antibody techniques. Thus, scientific study of this spirochete and its resultant disease has been difficult.

Epidemiology

After the post–World War II decline in the incidence of primary and secondary syphilis in the United States, there was a resurgence of the disease in the 1960s and 1970s to approximately 20,000 cases per year. There has been a much sharper increase since 1985, peaking at 50,000 new cases reported in 1990, and a subsequent decline to 17,000 in 1995. Throughout the 1970s, syphilis was predominantly a disease of homosexual men, with an approximately 3:1 male-to-female ratio of infection in 1982. The epidemiology changed in the 1980s, with altered patterns of sexual behavior among homosexual men in response to the AIDS epidemic and the development of the crack-cocaine subculture of sex for drugs. By 1995, the male-to-female ratio had dropped to 1.2:1. Accompanying this change has been the return of epidemic levels of congenital syphilis. Within the 15- to 19-year-old age group, the incidence of syphilis is actually higher in girls than in boys. Although syphilis is seen throughout the United States, the highest incidence is in the Middle Atlantic and Southeastern states. In 1993, the rate for blacks (approximately 75 per 100,000 population) was far greater than among Hispanics (8 per 100,000 population) or whites (<2 per 100,000 population).

Syphilis is transmitted by sexual contact, exposure to infected blood, or the transplacental route. All blood products are prescreened to exclude units with positive serology, and the usual processing of blood inactivates spirochetes. Nonetheless, intravenous drug abusers who share needles can transmit syphilis by way of contaminated needles and syringes. Transmission by sexual contact requires exposure of mucous membranes or abraded skin to moist mucosal or cutaneous lesions. The spirochetes cannot penetrate unbroken keratinized skin. The rate of acquisition of syphilis after intercourse with an infected partner is approximately 33% to 50%.

Diagnosis

Syphilis is traditionally divided into five stages: incubation, primary, secondary, latent, and tertiary (or late). Within hours to days after infection with *T. pallidum,* the organism enters the lymphatic system and the bloodstream and is disseminated throughout the body. The incubation period after exposure averages 3 weeks, but it may range from 10 to 90 days. The primary stage is characterized by the development of a chancre at the site of inoculation; however, the lesion may be inconspicuous and go unnoticed or it may be absent. The classic primary chancre begins as a single papule that quickly erodes to an indurated ulcer. Multiple chancres are infrequently seen, except in HIV-infected persons. The chancre base is smooth and clean, and the borders are raised. The size of the chancre ranges from a few millimeters to 2 cm in diameter. Although chancres occur most commonly on the external genitalia, they also may be found on the cervix, in the mouth, or in the perianal area. The ulcer is painless; when abraded for dark-field examination, it is only minimally tender and exudes serum rather than blood. Regional lymphadenopathy, manifest through moderately enlarged, rubbery, painless, nonfluctuant lymph nodes, accompanies the chancre. No fever or constitutional manifestations are present during the primary stage, and thus adolescents may ignore the findings. Secondary bacterial infection of the chancre, especially in the oral or anal area, can result in a painful lesion. If untreated, chancres heal spontaneously in 1 to 6 weeks. Any genital lesions should raise the suspicion of syphilis. Primary syphilis must be differentiated principally from genital herpes, chancroid, traumatic abrasions, other STDs, and other genital dermatoses.

Secondary syphilis begins approximately 6 weeks (range, 2 weeks to 6 months) after the primary lesion has appeared. This generalized condition, having constitutional, mucocutaneous, and visceral manifestations, occurs at a time when the greatest number of treponemes are present in the body, and persists until the host has developed an immune response that exerts some control over the infection. Systemic symptoms, found in up to 70% of patients, include fever, malaise, anorexia, sore throat, headache, and musculoskeletal complaints. Generalized lymphadenopathy, especially involving the epitrochlear nodes, occurs in two thirds of patients. Skin and/or mucous membrane findings are present in 90% of patients. Macular, maculopapular, papular, papulosqua-

mous, and pustular lesions all may be present; vesicular lesions are never seen in acquired syphilis. The rash usually begins on the trunk with erythematous macules, 0.5 to 1 cm in diameter, and progresses to a papular or pustular eruption involving the whole body but characteristically including the palms and the soles, where the rash is usually squamous. In moist intertriginous areas, such as the perineal or perianal region, the papules enlarge and erode to form white to erythematous plaques called condylomata lata. Involvement of the hair follicles can result in areas of patchy scalp alopecia, or hair thinning and loss of eyebrows and beard. Mucous patches are silvery erosions seen on the oral mucous membranes. All the skin and mucosal lesions are teeming with organisms and therefore highly infectious. Secondary syphilis may infrequently present as aseptic meningitis, hepatitis, glomerulonephritis, uveitis, arthritis, or osteitis. Without therapy, the secondary phase resolves in 1 to 8 weeks. Secondary syphilis is most often misdiagnosed as pityriasis rosea, psoriasis, tinea versicolor, drug eruptions, scabies, pediculosis, acute viral exanthemata, infectious mononucleosis, condyloma acuminatum, and lichen planus.

The latency period occurs after secondary syphilis, when there are no clinical manifestations of disease but the presence of infection can be documented by serologic testing. Latency may last a lifetime or may be followed years later by lesions of late (tertiary) syphilis. About one third of untreated patients develop the late destructive lesions of syphilis in the heart (10%), central nervous system (8%), or elsewhere (gummas, 17%). Since these disorders occur almost exclusively out of the adolescent spectrum, they are not discussed here.

The diagnosis of syphilis can be confirmed by demonstration of the presence of the *T. pallidum* organism or by serologic testing. Serous fluid for examination may be obtained by abrading a chancre or a skin lesion with saline-soaked gauze and squeezing it, or through aspiration of a lymph node. Dark-field microscopy reveals the coiled and undulating spirochete; alternatively, the specimen may be examined through the use of fluorescein-conjugated antitreponemal antibody. Previous systemic or topical antibiotic therapy can lead to false-negative test results.

Serologic investigation consists of a screening (nontreponemal) test and a confirmatory (treponemal) test. The screening tests—Venereal Disease Research Laboratory (VDRL), rapid plasma reagin (RPR), and automated reagin test (ART)—detect antibody to reagin, a cardiolipin-cholesterol-lecithin antigen. These tests are rapid, inexpensive, and relatively easy to perform and correlate with disease activity, but biologic false-positives (BFPs) occur frequently. The tests are only 70% sensitive during the primary stage (therefore, dark-field examination of the lesion must be performed), but they are over

99% sensitive during secondary syphilis if a dilution is done to exclude the possibility of a negative test due to prozone phenomena because of high antibody levels. The nontreponemal tests are quantitative; BFPs rarely exceed a titer of 1:8. BFPs are noted most commonly with intravenous drug use, collagen vascular disease, pregnancy, other spirochetal infections (e.g., leptospirosis, nonvenereal treponematoses), tuberculosis, endocarditis, Epstein-Barr virus, HIV, and other infections. The treponemal confirmatory tests consist of the fluorescent treponemal antibody-absorbed (FTA-abs) test, *T. pallidum* hemagglutination assay (TPHA), and microhemagglutination assay for *T. pallidum* (MHA-TP). These tests are more difficult to perform but are less subject to BFPs than the nontreponemal tests, and they are about 85% sensitive during primary syphilis and 100% sensitive during later stages; they are not, however, quantitative. After treatment of primary syphilis, the VDRL result reverts to negative within 1 year; after treatment of secondary syphilis, the VDRL reverts to negative within 2 years; duration of syphilis for longer than 1 year will result in a decline in the VDRL titer, but there may be a persistent low titer positivity (serofast state). Thus, the VDRL is a good test to follow to monitor efficacy of therapy. Once the specific treponemal tests are positive, they remain positive despite therapy and cannot be used to assess disease activity (Table 140-4).

Treatment

The drug of choice for the treatment of all stages of syphilis has been and still is penicillin. The current CDC and American Academy of Pediatrics recommendation for the treatment of primary or secondary syphilis is 2.4 million units of benzathine penicillin G administered intramuscularly in one dose; alternative regimens for the nonpregnant, penicillin-allergic patient are doxycycline (100 mg twice daily), tetracycline (500 mg four times a day), or erythromycin (500 mg four times a day), each given for 2 weeks; another regimen is ceftriaxone (250 mg intramuscularly once daily for 10 days). Pregnant teenagers should be treated with penicillin; tetracyclines are contraindicated during pregnancy, and erythromycin carries a high risk of failure to cure infection in the fetus. If the pregnant patient is allergic to penicillin, skin testing and desensitization should be accomplished in a referral center. Within hours after treatment with penicillin, the patient may develop the Jarisch-Herxheimer reaction, consisting of abrupt onset of fever, chills, myalgia, tachycardia, and vasodilation resulting from the antibiotic therapy, which causes a sudden release of pyrogen from the spirochetes. A VDRL test should be done during follow-up visits at 3, 6, 12, and 24 months. If the nontreponemal antibody titer has not declined fourfold by 3 to 6 months, or has not reverted to negative by 1 to 2 years, the patient should be reevaluated and undergo further treatment.

Patients with a positive VDRL test of more than 1 year's duration or unknown duration, or with HIV infection, should undergo a CSF examination consisting of cell count, protein, and VDRL determinations. If these study results are normal, the patient should be treated with benzathine penicillin G, 2.4 million units administered intramuscularly once weekly for three doses; alternative regimens for penicillin-allergic patients are doxycycline, 100 mg twice daily, or tetracycline, 500 mg four times a day, each for 4 weeks. If the patient has clinical or CSF findings indicative of neurosyphilis, the recommended regimen is aqueous crystalline penicillin G (2 to 4 million units every 4 hours intravenously for 10 to 14 days) or procaine penicillin (2.4 million units intramuscularly daily) and probenecid (500 mg four times a day), both for 10 to 14 days. Such patients should be managed and have follow-up in consultation with an expert.

All patients with syphilis should be offered, and encouraged to undergo, tests for HIV antibody, because syphilis enhances the transmission of HIV, and HIV infection is associated with the rapid development of syphilitic central nervous system infection and reduced efficacy of penicillin therapy.[26]

The recognition of a 30% isolation rate of *T. pallidum* from the CSF in patients with primary and secondary

	Untreated Patients with Positive Test (%)		**Test Response in Treated Patients During Early Syphilis**	
Test	**Primary**	**Secondary**	**Primary**	**Secondary**
Screening (e.g., VDRL)	70	99	Reverts to negative within 1 yr	Reverts to negative within 2 yr
Confirmatory (e.g., FTA-abs)	85	100	Remains positive	Remains positive

TABLE 140-4
Serologic Testing for Syphilis

FTA-abs, fluorescent treponemal antibody-absorbed test; *VDRL*, Venereal Disease Research Laboratory.

syphilis, and the previous knowledge of the low levels of penicillin achievable in the CSF with benzathine penicillin G, has called into question the current treatment regimens.[27] New regimens are likely to be developed soon.

MOLLUSCUM CONTAGIOSUM

Molluscum contagiosum is a common and benign skin infection that can be transmitted either sexually or nonsexually. The etiologic agent is a DNA virus that is a member of the poxvirus family.

There is a paucity of statistical information on the epidemiology of molluscum contagiosum, since infected people usually do not seek medical attention; this condition is generally discovered incidentally during a routine physical examination or during evaluation for another problem. It is not a reportable disease, but longitudinal surveys indicate that there has been a severalfold increase in this diagnosis over the last 20 years. The infection is spread by direct contact with infected lesions or with fomites; the degree of infectivity is low. Nonvenereal transmission occurs primarily in children, whereas venereal spread is common among adolescents and adults. Autoinoculation also occurs. The incubation period averages 1 to 2 months but may extend to 6 months.

The lesions begin as pinhead-sized discrete papules that enlarge, over a period of days to weeks, to a diameter of 3 to 10 mm. As the papules grow, the characteristic central umbilication becomes apparent. The lesions are firm and flesh-colored and typically range in number from two to 20. When sexually transmitted, the infection tends to involve the normal skin of the lower abdominal wall, pubis, and inner thighs and (less commonly) the skin and mucous membranes of the genitalia. The lesions are generally asymptomatic. Caseous material can be expressed from the molluscum.

Bacterial superinfection may complicate molluscum contagiosum in up to 40% of patients. Eczematous dermatitis 3 to 10 cm in diameter may encircle one or more lesions in 10% of patients. Individuals with impaired cell-mediated immunity, especially those with AIDS or those undergoing immunosuppressive therapy, may develop hundreds of lesions.

Molluscum contagiosum is usually diagnosed clinically on the basis of the characteristic flesh-colored, umbilicated lesions from which caseous material can be expressed. In questionable cases the diagnosis can be confirmed through microscopy. Staining of material expressed from the lesion with Wright's or Giemsa stain will demonstrate epithelial cells with intracytoplasmic molluscum bodies that compress the nuclei to the periphery. Characteristic viral particles can be visualized by electron microscopy. At present, there is no role for viral isolation or serology.

The lesions resolve spontaneously, generally within several months. However, it may be advisable to eliminate lesions, both to prevent transmission and for cosmetic purposes. Curettage or expression of the core followed by cauterization of the base with silver nitrate, electrodesiccation, or cryotherapy is the therapy most frequently employed. Bacterial superinfection should be treated with systemic antibiotics; topical steroids are administered for eczematoid dermatitis.

LYMPHOGRANULOMA VENEREUM

Lymphogranuloma venereum (LGV) is an acute and chronic infection with primary, secondary, and tertiary stages. Painful inguinal lymphadenitis is the most commonly recognized form of the disease. *C. trachomatis* serovars L^1, L^2, and L^3 cause the syndrome.

Although LGV is a sporadic disease in North America, it is prevalent in tropical and subtropical areas. Approximately 300 infections are reported annually in the United States; most cases involve a history of travel to an endemic region. Infection is diagnosed much more frequently in males, because females develop inguinal adenitis less often.

After sexual exposure to an infected person, a primary lesion may develop in 3 days to 2 weeks. Usually unnoticed or ignored, the lesion is a painless vesicle, papule, or ulcer. The lesion is recognized on the penis in fewer than one third of men and even less commonly in women, in whom it may appear on the labia, fourchette, cervix, or vaginal wall. If the lesion occurs intraurethrally, nonspecific urethritis results. Males may develop lymphangitis on the dorsum of the penis. If untreated, the primary lesion heals rapidly and does not leave a scar.

The secondary stage begins 2 to 6 weeks after exposure, when inflammation and swelling of regional lymph nodes develop. Inguinal and femoral nodes are usually affected, with initial infection of the penis or the vulva; the spread is to perirectal and pelvic nodes from vaginal or anorectal infection. Inguinal adenopathy is bilateral in one third of patients. Concomitant femoral node involvement separated by Poupart's ligament results in the "groove sign" characteristic of LGV. As the nodes enlarge, they become matted, the pain increases, and the overlying skin becomes red and adherent. Approximately one third of inguinal buboes rupture, draining thick pus and relieving pain. Most nodes form firm inguinal masses without draining. The secondary phase in women and homosexual men is more commonly an acute hemorrhagic proctocolitis. Initial manifestations of anal pruritus and tenesmus rapidly progress to bloody or mucopurulent discharge, left lower quadrant tenderness, and rectal pain.

The rectal mucosa is friable with ulcerations, resulting in a picture similar to that of inflammatory bowel disease. Systemic symptoms accompanying the second stage include fever, malaise, myalgia, nausea, and headache. The third stage occurs months to years later, when persisting inflammation and scarring produce rectal stricture, fistula, or chronic edema and ulceration of the external genitalia.

The primary lesion and the inguinal adenitis of LGV must be differentiated from syphilis, genital herpes, and chancroid; the inguinal component alone, from routine bacterial adenitis, lymphoma, and incarcerated hernia; and the anorectal syndrome, from viral, bacterial, or protozoal proctocolitis and inflammatory bowel disease.

The diagnosis of LGV can be confirmed serologically with either the complement fixation or the microimmunofluorescent test. The latter is both more sensitive and more specific but is not widely available. Both tests suffer from cross-reactions caused by other chlamydial infections. *Chlamydia* organisms can be isolated from bubo pus in fewer than one third of patients.

Doxycycline, 100 mg twice daily for 21 days, is the treatment of choice for all stages of LGV. Alternatives are erythromycin and sulfisoxazole, each in a dose of 500 mg given four times a day for 21 days. Fluctuant nodes should be aspirated through adjacent areas of healthy, noninvolved skin.

CHANCROID

Chancroid is an acute, painful, ulcerative genital infection caused by the *Haemophilus ducreyi* organism. The disease is recognized 10 times as often in males as in females. Recent epidemics in the United States have resulted in 5000 cases reported annually. This disease is a major public health problem in many underdeveloped nations. In Africa, for example, chancroid appears to increase the risk of both acquiring and transmitting HIV infection.

After an incubation period of 3 to 10 days, the genital lesion begins as a tender papule that rapidly erodes to a painful ulcer. The base of the ulcer is covered with necrotic exudate and bleeds easily when abraded; the border is erythematous with undermined edges and is not indurated. Fifty percent of men have a single ulcer, whereas women usually have multiple lesions. The ulcers range in size from a few millimeters to 2 cm. Lesions are most often found on or around the foreskin in males and at the introitus in females. Tender unilateral inguinal adenopathy is present in half of the patients; if untreated, this condition progresses to bubo formation and rupture.

The genital lesions of syphilis, herpes, and LGV must be differentiated from chancroid by serologic testing,

dark-field microscopy, Tzanck preparation, and/or culture. Gram's stain of a specimen from the undermined edge of a chancroidal ulcer will demonstrate gram-negative coccobacilli, but this test is not specific. *H. ducreyi* organisms can be grown from the base of the ulcer in most patients when cultured on chocolate agar; however, bubo pus is sterile. The microbiology laboratory should be informed of the presumed diagnosis to ensure optimal processing of the specimen.

The recommended treatment regimens for chancroid are azithromycin, 1 g orally in a single dose; ceftriaxone, 250 mg intramuscularly once; or erythromycin, 500 mg four times a day for 1 week. Alternative regimens are Augmentin (amoxicillin, 500 mg, and clavulanic acid, 125 mg) administered three times a day for 1 week; and ciprofloxacin, 500 mg twice daily for 3 days. Ulcers due to chancroid improve within 3 to 7 days of successful treatment. The lymphadenopathy resolves more slowly and may require needle aspiration through adjacent noninvolved skin.

GRANULOMA INGUINALE

Granuloma inguinale (donovanosis) is a chronic ulcerative disease of the genitalia. It is rare in the United States, with less than 100 cases reported annually, but common in New Guinea and parts of Africa, India, and the Caribbean. *Calymmatobacterium granulomatis,* a gram-negative bacillus, is the etiologic agent.

The initial lesion, an indurated subcutaneous nodule, appears 8 to 80 days after sexual exposure. It erodes to produce an ulcer with exuberant granulation tissue. The lesion is painless, bleeds easily on contact, and slowly enlarges. Ninety percent of patients have genital lesions, which appear on the foreskin or glans in males and on the labia in females. Lesions may extend to the inguinal area in 10% of patients, producing a pseudoadenopathy.

The clinical features of the syndrome are usually characteristic enough to allow the diagnosis to be made. However, other STDs, especially chancroid and syphilis, and carcinoma and cutaneous amebiasis should be considered in the differential diagnosis. The organism is not cultivable on routine laboratory media. Intracytoplasmic Donovan bodies can be demonstrated through Wright's, Giemsa, or hematoxylin and eosin staining of a crush preparation or biopsy. Tetracycline, 500 mg four times a day, is the initial drug of choice. Ampicillin, 500 mg four times a day; erythromycin, 500 mg four times a day; and trimethoprim-sulfamethoxazole, 160 mg/800 mg twice daily, are alternative regimens. The duration of treatment is a minimum of 3 weeks. Clinical response should be seen within 1 week; complete healing, within 3 to 5 weeks. Chloramphenicol, 500 mg three times a day, or gentamicin, 1 mg/kg twice daily, is reserved for use in disease unresponsive to initial oral therapy.

PEDICULOSIS PUBIS

Pediculosis is infestation with one or three species of lice: *Pediculus humanus capitis,* the head louse; *Pediculus humanus corporis,* the body louse; and *Phthirus pubis,* the pubic or crab louse. Crab lice are so called because of their resemblance to crabs. They are visible to the naked eye as brown creatures about 1 mm in diameter, usually clasping a hair shaft. Although body lice serve as vectors for serious infections such as typhus, head and pubic lice are not major health hazards. Only pubic lice are sexually transmitted.

Although head lice are limited to scalp hair, pubic lice can infest eyelashes, eyebrows, and axillary, chest, and perianal hair in addition to pubic hair. The main symptom associated with pubic lice is intense pruritus of the involved area. The itching leads to scratching, which results in excoriations and secondary bacterial infection. Maculae ceruleae, blue macules approximately 1 cm in diameter, are seen on the skin as the result of crab louse bites. The average infestation consists of fewer than ten lice; however, the lice are identifiable in almost all patients who have not received previous treatment. The nits or eggs are silvery oval structures, approximately 0.5 mm long, that are tightly adherent to the hair shaft near the skin.

The diagnosis of pubic lice is readily made by visual inspection. If there is any question, the presumed louse or nit can be examined through low-power microscopy for confirmation.

Permethrin 1% cream rinse (Nix) is pediculicidal and ovicidal; residual activity persists on the hair for 2 weeks. It is the most effective and least toxic treatment for head lice, the only indication for which it is currently licensed. Permethrin is applied as a 10-minute shampoo. This agent should prove to have equal or better efficacy for pubic lice than the currently licensed products: pyrethrin with piperonyl butoxide (RID, A-200), lindane (gamma benzene hexachloride, Kwell), and malathion 0.5% (Ovide). A single treatment with permethrin or malathion is adequate; with the other agents, a second application 1 week after the initial therapy is recommended. All infested areas must be treated, not just the pubic area. Careful examination of the patient and an explanation of the sites to be treated are required if failures are to be avoided. Clothing and bedding should be washed and dried on a hot cycle to kill lice or nits. Oral antibiotic therapy should be administered for secondary bacterial infection. Pruritus resolves quickly with effective treatment; if it persists, reevaluation is required to exclude treatment failure or reinfection. Itching may also continue because of a local hypersensitivity reaction; oral antihistamine and/or topical steroids can be used. For crab lice infestation of eyelashes, petrolatum ointment can be applied twice daily for 1 week, and any nits can be removed mechanically.

SCABIES

Scabies is a common superficial skin infestation caused by the mite *Sarcoptes scabiei.* The gravid female mite burrows into the skin and lays eggs, which subsequently develop through larval and nymphal stages to adulthood to complete the life cycle. The mite is transmitted through close physical contact with an infected person, either sexually or nonsexually. In persons without previous scabies infection, the incubation period is about 4 to 6 weeks, since many of the manifestations of infestation are caused by sensitization to the mite. Symptoms develop within a few days of exposure in individuals with previous episodes of scabies.

Intense pruritus, which worsens at night, is the chief complaint of most affected individuals. The characteristic linear burrow is infrequently identified. Individual or grouped erythematous papules, often excoriated and secondarily infected, are the most commonly recognized lesions. After sexual transmission, the genitalia, buttocks, and thighs are the sites most commonly involved; however, there is often spread to the typical nongenital sites, including the interdigital webs, flexor surface of the wrists, extensor surface of the elbows, anterior axillary fold, umbilicus, and legs. Nodular lesions occasionally occur on the genitalia. Lesions may be difficult to find in individuals who bathe frequently.

Scabies should be suspected on the basis of a history of nocturnal itching and the presence of lesions in the typical locations. The mite is approximately 0.35 mm in size, thus at or below the level of detection with the unaided eye. Scabies can be confirmed microscopically by demonstration of the mite, its eggs, or fecal pellets in a skin scraping or shaving taken, under mineral oil, from a fresh, unexcoriated papule or burrow. In the burrow ink test, a suspected papule is covered with ink and then the excess ink is wiped from the surface with an alcohol pad; in scabies, the ink will track down into the mite burrow, forming a dark line leading away from the papule. Because both these techniques can give false-negative results, a therapeutic trial may be indicated. Scabies is most commonly confused with insect bites, pyoderma, contact dermatitis, atopic dermatitis, and papular urticaria.

Permethrin 5% cream (Elimite) is the drug of choice for the treatment of scabies on the basis of its efficacy and lower potential for toxicity than that of more traditional therapy.[28] The cream is massaged into the skin from the neck to the soles of the feet. It should be washed off after 8 to 14 hours. Lindane 1% (Kwell), an alternative to permethrin, is administered with the same instructions. Crotamiton 10% (Eurax) is less effective and requires multiple applications. Ivermectin, in a single oral dose of 200 μg/kg, has been reported to be effective in the treatment of scabies in both healthy and HIV-infected persons.[29] Local hypersensitivity reaction will cause the pruritus and especially the papular lesions to persist after adequate scabicidal therapy; topical steroids and oral antihistamines can be used to provide symptomatic relief. Oral antibiotic therapy directed at staphylococci and streptococci should be employed if secondary bacterial infection is present. Clothing and bed linen should be washed and dried on the hot cycle.

References

1. Paavonen J, Stamm WE: Lower genital tract infections in women, *Infect Dis Clin North Am* 1:179-198, 1987.
2. Reef SE, Levine WC, McNeil MM, et al: Treatment options for vulvovaginal candidiasis, 1993, *Clin Infect Dis* 20:S80-S90, 1995.
3. Wolner-Hanssen P, Krieger NJ, Stevens CE, Kiviat NB, Koutsky L, Critchlow C, DeRouen T, Hillier S, Holmes KK: Clinical manifestations of vaginal trichomoniasis, *JAMA* 261:571-576, 1989.
4. Hillier S, Holmes KK: Bacterial vaginosis. In Holmes KK, Mardh PA, Sparling PF, Wiesner PJ, editors: *Sexually transmitted diseases,* ed 2, New York, 1990, McGraw-Hill; pp 547-559.
5. Centers for Disease Control: Gonorrhea and salpingitis among American teenagers, 1960-1981, *MMWR* 32:25ss-30ss, 1983.
6. Alexander-Rodriguez T, Vermund SH: Gonorrhea and syphilis in incarcerated urban adolescents: prevalence and physical signs, *Pediatrics* 80:561-564, 1987.
7. Fisher M, Swenson PD, Risucci D, et al: *Chlamydia trachomatis* in suburban adolescents, *J Pediatr* 111:617-620, 1987.
8. Chacko MR, Lovchik J: *Chlamydia trachomatis* infection in sexually active adolescents: prevalence and risk factors, *Pediatrics* 73:836-840, 1984.
9. Moscicki B, Shafer MA, Millstein SG, Irwin CE, Schachter J: The use and limitations of endocervical Gram stains and mucopurulent cervicitis as predictors for *Chlamydia trachomatis* in female adolescents, *Am J Obstet Gynecol* 157:65-71, 1987.
10. Thompson SE, Hager WD, Wong KH, Lopez B, Ramsey C, Allen SD, Stargel MD, Thornsberry C, Benigno BB, Thompson JD, Shulman JA: The microbiology and therapy of acute pelvic inflammatory disease in hospitalized patients, *Am J Obstet Gynecol* 136:179-186, 1980.
11. Weström L: Incidence, prevalence, and trends of acute pelvic inflammatory disease and its consequences in industrialized countries, *Am J Obstet Gynecol* 138:880-892, 1980.
12. Louv WC, Austin H, Perlman J, Alexander WJ: Oral contraceptive use and the risk of chlamydial and gonococcal infections, *Am J Obstet Gynecol* 160:396-402, 1989.
13. Rubin GL, Ory HW, Layde PM: Oral contraceptives and pelvic inflammatory disease, *Am J Obstet Gynecol* 144:630-635, 1982.
14. Fried Oginski W, Rosenfeld WD, Bijur PE: Acute pelvic inflammatory disease in adolescents, *Adolesc Pediatr Gynecol* 5:243-247, 1992.
15. Cromer BA, Heald FP: Pelvic inflammatory disease associated with *Neisseria gonorrhoeae* and *Chlamydia trachomatis:* clinical correlates, *Sex Transm Dis* 14:125-129, 1987.
16. Cromer BA, Brandstaetter LA, Fischer RA, Brown RT: Tubo-ovarian abscess in adolescents, *Adolesc Pediatr Gynecol* 3:21-24, 1990.
17. Golden N, Cohen H, Gennari G, Neuhoff S: The use of pelvic ultrasonography in the evaluation of adolescents with pelvic inflammatory disease, *Am J Dis Child* 141:1235-1238, 1987.
18. Davis AJ, Emans SJ: Human papilloma virus infection in the pediatric and adolescent patient, *J Pediatr* 115:1-9, 1989.
19. Pacheco BP, DiPaola G, Ribas JMM, Vighi S, Rueda NG: Vulvar infection caused by human papilloma virus in children and adolescents without sexual contact, *Adolesc Pediatr Gynecol* 4:136-142, 1991.
20. Koutsky LA, Galloway DA, Holmes KK: Epidemiology of genital human papillomavirus infection, *Epidemiol Rev* 10:122-163, 1988.
21. Centers for Disease Control: Condyloma acuminatum—United States, 1966-1981, *MMWR* 32:306-308, 1983.
22. Rosenfeld WD, Vermund SH, Wentz SJ, Burk RD: High prevalence rate of human papillomavirus infection and association with abnormal Papanicolaou smears in sexually active adolescents, *Am J Dis Child* 143:1443-1447, 1989.
23. Neinstein LS, Goldenring J: Pink pearly papules: an epidemiologic study, *J Pediatr* 105:594-595, 1984.
24. Broder S: Rapid communication: the Bethesda System for reporting cervical/vaginal cytological diagnoses: report of the 1991 Bethesda Workshop, *JAMA* 270:2975, 1993.
25. Wright TC Jr, Richart RM: Review: role of human papillomavirus in the pathogenesis of genital tract warts and cancer, *Gynecol Oncol* 37:151-164, 1990.
26. Tramont EC: Syphilis in the AIDS era, *N Engl J Med* 316:1600, 1987.
27. Musher DM: How much penicillin cures syphilis?, *Ann Intern Med* 109:849, 1988.
28. Schultz MW, Gomez M, Hansen RC, et al: Comparative study of 5% permethrin cream and 1% lindane lotion for the treatment of scabies, *Arch Dermatol* 126:167, 1990.
29. Meinking TL, Taplin D, Hermida JL, et al: The treatment of scabies with ivermectin, *N Engl J Med* 333:26-30, 1995.

Suggested Readings

Centers for Disease Control and Prevention: 1993 sexually transmitted diseases treatment guidelines, *MMWR* 42 (RR-14):1-102, 1993.

This supplement to Morbidity and Mortality Weekly Reports *is updated every 3 to 4 years. It provides current recommendations for treatment by authorities in the field.*

Holmes KK, Mardh PA, Sparling PF, Wiesner PJ, editors: *Sexually transmitted diseases,* ed 2, New York, 1990, McGraw-Hill.

This multiauthored text covers the epidemiology, behavioral aspects, microbiology, clinical syndromes, and treatment of sexually transmitted diseases. As the "bible" on the subject, it should be readily available to professionals treating patients with such infections.

CHAPTER 141

Contraceptive Technology and Practice

•

Richard R. Brookman

Few adolescents expect or want pregnancy to result from sexual intercourse. Most are aware of the hazards of sexually transmitted infections and the possibility of AIDS. Nevertheless, few use any method of contraception for the first 6 to 12 months of coital activity.[1] Initial contraceptive efforts such as douching or withdrawal may be relatively ineffective. Adolescents may use effective methods incorrectly or sporadically. They may attempt periodic abstinence, the "rhythm method," without accurate knowledge of reproductive physiology and the timing of ovulation. Consulting a reliable medical source for contraceptive information and methods tends to be a late event. At the time of the first visit for family planning services, many teenagers are already pregnant.

Adolescents fail to use contraception for many reasons, often a combination of these.[2] Young adolescents may believe that they are invulnerable to harmful consequences and deny the possibility of pregnancy or infection even in the presence of obvious symptoms. They are susceptible to myths and misinformation from their peers about the risks of sexual activity and the safety or reliability of contraceptive methods. They hesitate to reveal or even acknowledge their sexual involvement by consulting a health professional or other adult. Although today few teenagers are unaware of contraceptive methods or how to obtain them, obstacles to family planning services include facility hours, location, and cost of services. Some may fear the necessary physical examination and tests.

Healthcare providers may add barriers by neglecting to inquire about sexual activity or failing to offer assistance with family planning needs, especially to minors. Some providers hold personal beliefs that no teenager should be engaging in sexually intimate behavior. Those providers who have cared for adolescents since early childhood may feel disloyal to the parents if they offer services that may be opposed by the parents. Some fear that provision of contraceptives to teenagers will encourage sexual activity, despite the lack of empirical evidence to support this fear. State laws allow minors to seek family planning services on their own consent, except for sterilization.

Parental notification requirements affect minors' access to pregnancy termination in some states but do not extend to contraception.

Motivation for contraception may be affected by numerous aspects of psychosexual development, and varies among subgroups of adolescents. For many teenagers, sexual intimacy is a means of establishing self-identity, acquiring peer approval, or enhancing self-esteem, especially when life options appear extremely limited. Teenagers who seek emotional gratification through sexuality and are unable to form stable, lasting relationships often experience a series of sexual partners over short intervals. This increases their risk of exposure to sexually transmitted diseases and/or pregnancy and decreases the likelihood of contraceptive use. Discussion of responsibility for prevention of consequences tends to be a late event in these short-term relationships and usually follows several episodes of unplanned intercourse. The high value placed by some teenagers on romantic spontaneity contributes to this lack of planning.

Adolescents most likely to use contraception have high levels of scholastic achievement, are highly motivated to complete their education, and have strong religious beliefs supporting virginity. At highest risk for nonuse of contraception are the truly promiscuous teenagers—runaways who support themselves by sexual activity, male and female prostitutes, and those with a constellation of problem behaviors, including substance abuse and delinquency. These teenagers are often victims of physical and/or sexual child abuse, have a very poor self-image, and have little or no motivation to prevent the consequences of their behaviors. Judgment altered by drugs or depression compounds the risk.

COUNSELING FOR CONTRACEPTION

Adolescents in need of contraception may request this service directly or at the suggestion or insistence of a parent or partner, or they may have the need identified by the provider during the course of a healthcare visit.

1119

Counseling teenagers about contraception tends to be more complicated than counseling adults. Attention must be paid to a variety of developmental and psychosocial issues. Use of contraceptives by adolescents is less influenced by education and knowledge than by cognitive developmental stage, personal beliefs, life style, sociocultural background, and external support systems. A high value placed on fertility by the adolescent, partner, peers, or even family, together with ambivalence about pregnancy, may create unconscious interference with conscious decisions to use contraception. Recognition of potential psychologic barriers may be more critical than attention to informational or economic barriers.[3]

General Principles

The following general principles should be considered when counseling adolescents and their families about reproductive health care:

1. The most effective way to prevent both pregnancy and sexually transmitted infections is to avoid sexual intercourse. The biologic pressures of puberty and psychosexual development, and the sexually stimulating messages pervasive in society, make it difficult for teenagers to abstain from all forms of sexual intimacy. To avoid coitus, it may be necessary to permit and even encourage forms of sexual expression that are developmentally appropriate, such as "petting"—even to orgasm—and masturbation. It is important for providers and parents to convey the message that the teenager is not expected to have sexual intercourse until a more appropriate age and should be able to control his or her behavior in a sexually arousing situation. Each adolescent and each family will be comfortable with various degrees of sexual expression as a result of differing religious beliefs and cultural traditions, and the influence of former generations. The "right time" for first sexual intercourse may be defined by chronologic age, developmental age, or marital status. This decision is best left to young adults and families.

2. When sexual intercourse occurs, any preventive method is better than none; however, not all methods that prevent pregnancy will prevent infections. The most effective means of preventing pregnancy are implanted and injected hormonal contraceptives. The most effective way to prevent the spread of the greatest variety of sexually transmitted infections is the consistent combined use of a condom and a vaginal spermicide containing nonoxynol 9.

3. There is no ideal contraceptive method. None is 100% effective in preventing both pregnancy and infections, completely acceptable to all users, free of any side effects or risks, inexpensive, and unrelated to the act of coitus.

4. The best contraceptive method for the individual adolescent is the one that the adolescent and his or her partner will use correctly and consistently.

5. Prevention of consequences at different times and under different circumstances, with the same or different partners, may require the use of different methods. Teenagers should receive education about, and be prepared to use, all methods of contraception suitable for them.

Specific Guidelines

The following guidelines are suggested for approaching the individual adolescent about contraception:

1. Determine the need for prevention. Some teenagers are brought by anxious parents to the physician for birth control before they have ever had sexual intercourse. Instituting contraception too soon may communicate the unintended message that early coital activity is acceptable as long as pregnancy is avoided. There may be increased pressure for sexual involvement from peers or prospective partners who know that a girl is "on the pill." A dilemma is raised by the practitioner's enthusiasm for the planning of prevention before risk-taking behavior occurs, and the possibility that this support for planning will promote risk-taking behavior at too early an age.

   Some teenagers have had intercourse only once and affirm a decision to avoid it for a long time. Others may have frequent sexual intercourse but at unpredictable intervals. Some who have not yet had coitus may be judged at high risk for a "sexual debut" in the near future: for example, a 14-year-old with poor school performance, few extracurricular interests, concerns about her sexual attractiveness, and one or more sisters who were pregnant as teenagers. The practitioner must explore carefully all risk factors and make a decision about when to advocate contraception and which method is appropriate for the expected frequency of intercourse.

2. Support a decision for abstinence at the outset. Teenagers who are virgins can be assisted in remaining virginal, supported in their choice, and helped in learning how to resist pressures and recognize the advantages of postponing first intercourse. The concept of delay until a more appropriate time of life may be more acceptable than a strict prohibition against sex until marriage, an event that may be 10 to 15 years in the future for many. Teenagers who have had intercourse once or

twice and decide to avoid it for a time can be supported in this decision.

3. Determine any obstacles to effective use of prevention. The practitioner may identify factors that will inhibit motivation for consistent prevention of the consequences of sexual intimacy. Careful attention should be paid to improving self-esteem, enlisting the support of the sexual partner and/or supportive adults, and dispelling myths and misinformation about specific methods and their side effects. The practitioner should discuss the costs and logistics of obtaining contraceptives, and offer practical advice such as inexpensive sources and the obligation of the partner to share expenses. A history should be obtained about the patient's previous experiences and the experiences of partners, parents, peers, and siblings with specific methods. Negative reactions to any method from a significant other may discourage the patient from continuing or even trying that method.

4. Determine any contraindications to specific methods. Careful history taking, including family history, physical examination, and selected laboratory studies based on history, should reveal any medical reasons to avoid a specific method. Barrier methods may be recommended for almost all teenagers except those with a history of allergic reactions to such products. Hormonal contraception rarely is contraindicated for the normal healthy teenager, but it should be avoided, at least temporarily, when any condition is present that predisposes to venous or bile stasis. Use of hormonal contraception in teenagers with specific chronic diseases requires individual evaluation and consideration of the risk of pregnancy versus the risk of hormonal administration, as well as the potential for correct use of nonhormonal methods.[4]

5. Educate the adolescent about conception and infection and their consequences. Emphasize the risks of sexual intercourse without prevention. The teenager should be helped to understand the many options that are available, including avoidance of coitus and use of alternative means of responding to psychosexual needs.

6. Educate in detail about contraceptive methods, especially the one selected by the teenager. This may, and perhaps should, require a second visit. The first visit often overloads the patient with information about reproductive anatomy and physiology, pregnancy, infections, and methods of contraception, along with what may be the first pelvic or detailed genital examination. At a second visit education can focus on the method(s) selected and questions can be answered. Between the first and second visits the teenager may read printed materials provided by the practitioner. The teenager should be encouraged to discuss prevention options with her or his partner and with a parent or other trusted adult.

Special attention must be given to young adolescents with immature cognitive development. Education should involve simple, clear, concrete messages and should include anatomic diagrams and demonstrations of actual contraceptive methods. The practitioner should ask the adolescent to repeat information to determine what has been comprehended. An invitation may be extended for partners and/or parents to participate in the educational discussions at initial or subsequent visits.

7. Obtain consent when needed and document the information provided. If there is concern about legal liability, especially for the use of a new technologic device, it is advisable to document that the adolescent has given informed consent and to obtain the minor's signature. A parent or guardian should provide written consent when hormonal contraceptive implants or injections are given to a minor deemed incapable of informed consent.

8. Arrange for close follow-up. First-time contraception users, especially teenagers, tend to lose motivation quickly, especially when their social situation changes and they experience long intervals between intercourse. They may discontinue a method, then meet a new partner, resume coital activity, and finally decide that contraception is again desirable. Frequent brief visits, supplemented as needed by telephone calls, permit the practitioner to reinforce motivation, assess compliance, and anticipate and quickly address minor side effects before the patient discontinues the method. New users of hormonal methods and those with a history of poor compliance should have a follow-up visit every 3 months for at least the first year. Older teenagers, those who demonstrate excellent motivation for prevention, and those who select barrier methods should be seen every 6 months. For those at high risk of infection, this may be a desirable interval for pelvic examination, screening for gonorrhea and *Chlamydia* infection, and obtaining a Papanicolaou (Pap) smear.

HORMONAL CONTRACEPTION

Oral Contraceptives

Most female adolescents who consult a health professional about birth control request "the pill." The oral contraceptive is believed to be the most effective way to prevent pregnancy. However, few adolescents understand that the pill's effectiveness depends on daily correct use or realize that the pill offers little if any protection from sexually transmitted infections. The safety of oral contraceptives for adolescents has been stated emphatically.[5,6]

Many oral contraceptives are on the market, some combining an estrogen and a progestin, others containing only a progestin as the active ingredient. Combined oral contraceptives prevent ovulation by suppressing the release of gonadotropin-releasing hormone from the hypothalamus and possibly by blocking the release of follicle-stimulating hormone and luteinizing hormone from the pituitary gland. This prevents the midcycle surge in gonadotropin secretion that triggers ovulation. Combined pills also thicken cervical mucus, slow tubal motility, and alter the endometrium, thus interfering with fertilization and implantation if ovulation should occur. Progestin-only pills mainly interfere with implantation by affecting cervical mucus, tubal function, and the endometrium, but they may inhibit ovulation, especially after months of use.

Combined oral contraceptives contain one of two estrogens, ethinyl estradiol or mestranol. Mestranol is demethylated in the liver to the bioactive ethinyl estradiol with approximately two thirds its potency. Since 1992, all formulations with 35 μg or less of estrogen have used only ethinyl estradiol. The combined forms contain one of several progestins: norethindrone, norethindrone acetate, norgestrel, levonorgestrel, norethynodrel, ethynodiol diacetate, desogestrel, or norgestimate. The net result of each combination is a balance of estrogenic and progestogenic effects. Pill selection may include a consideration of the relative estrogenicity, progestogenicity, or neutrality of a pill in avoidance of side effects and improvement of user acceptability. Combined oral contraceptives may have the same formulation for each pill in the 21-day hormonal cycle, with or without seven inert pills. These placebo pills allow for an artificial menstrual cycle of 28 days and a regularly spaced withdrawal flow simulating a menstrual period. Triphasic pills vary the dose of estrogen and progestin at different intervals during the 21-day hormonal cycle and also include the seven inert pills. Advertised as "more natural," triphasic pills are not necessarily better than other combined pills, especially for the adolescent. Triphasic pill packages contain four different colored pills in either equal or unequal numbers. The advantages of a lower total progestin dose and fewer metabolic effects on lipids, blood pressure, and carbohydrate metabolism must be weighed against the disadvantages of a more confusing pill package, limited flexibility in making up a missed pill, and a reported increase in break-through bleeding.

While the array of available oral contraceptives can be confusing to the healthcare provider and certainly to the consumer, most adolescents do well with any of the combined pills. In fact, side effects are related more often to incorrect usage than to the hormonal balance in the pill. The provider should become familiar with several oral contraceptives that offer a selection of low-, moderate-, and high-potency estrogenic, balanced, and progestogenic effects, and at least one triphasic option (Table 141-1).

Combined oral contraceptives are contraindicated when there is a history of thromboembolic disorders, cerebrovascular disease, breast cancer, or any estrogen-dependent neoplasia. They should be avoided or discontinued when prolonged immobilization is necessary (e.g., with body cast, long leg cast, or extended bed rest), with acute impairment of liver function, or when pregnancy is diagnosed or suspected. Combined and progestin-only pills should not be prescribed in the presence of undiagnosed abnormal vaginal bleeding because they will mask symptoms and may further confuse the diagnostic evaluation.

Relative contraindications to combined oral contraceptives include vascular or migraine headaches, collagen vascular diseases, severe hypertension, chronic heart disease, sickle cell disease, severe renal disease, and diabetes mellitus. Whenever possible, adolescents with these chronic diseases should be counseled and assisted in effective use of nonhormonal contraception. However, both provider and patient must weigh the risk of hormonal contraceptive use against the medical risks of pregnancy as well as the psychosocial implications of childrearing with a serious chronic or even terminal illness. Depression, asthma, and epilepsy may worsen or improve with oral contraceptive use, and patients should be observed closely for individual responses. Tobacco smoking has been associated with increased risk of cardiovascular complications in women over 30 years of age who use oral contraceptives. While this association has not been observed in younger women, all users of oral contraceptives should be strongly encouraged to never start smoking, or advised to stop smoking and offered assistance in doing so.

Gynecologic immaturity no longer is considered a contraindication to oral contraceptive use. In most adolescents, growth is nearly completed at the time of menarche (or soon after it), and sexual debut, or first sexual intercourse, usually follows menarche by 1 or more years. Mature ovulatory cycles and the ability to implant and sustain a fertilized ovum may be expected by 2 or more years after menarche, but these may take up to 5 years to become established. Most providers prefer to withhold oral contraceptives until 6 to 12 months after menarche in sexually active teenagers to observe for some regularity of the menstrual cycle and to avoid masking a dysfunction of reproductive maturation.

Prediction of poor compliance is a relative contraindication to oral contraceptives of any kind, since daily motivation is required. However, poorly compliant patients may fare no better with other methods. In fact, a method that is independent of the act of coitus may

TABLE 141-1
Oral Contraceptives—Selected Examples

	Estrogen (µg)	Progestin (mg)
Single-Phase Pills		
Loestrin 1.5/30	Ethinyl estradiol 30	Norethindrone acetate 1.5
Lo/Ovral	Ethinyl estradiol 30	Norgestrel 0.3
Norinyl 1/35	Ethinyl estradiol 35	Norethindrone 1
Ortho-Novum 1/35		
Ortho-Cept	Ethinyl estradiol 30	Desogestrel 0.15
Ortho-Cyclen	Ethinyl estradiol 35	Norgestimate 0.25
Ovral	Ethinyl estradiol 50	Norgestrel 0.5
Triphasic Pills		
Triphasil	Ethinyl estradiol	Levonorgestrel
Day 1-6	30	0.05
Day 7-11	40	0.075
Day 12-21	30	0.125
Ortho-Novum 7/7/7	Ethinyl estradiol	Norethindrone
Day 1-7	35	0.5
Day 8-14	35	0.75
Day 15-21	35	1.0
Ortho-Tricyclen	Ethinyl estradiol	Norgestimate
Day 1-7	35	0.18
Day 8-14	35	0.215
Day 15-21	35	0.25

involve less forgetfulness or ambivalence on their part, especially if some form of daily reminder can be used, such as a calendar, a chart, or even a parent. When poor compliance is anticipated or when a patient expresses concern about side effects, it may be prudent to avoid progestin-only pills and even triphasic pills to minimize the chance of pill discontinuation due to irregular menstrual bleeding.

Adolescents using oral contraceptives for the first time usually do best with a "balanced" pill containing 35 µg of ethinyl estradiol and a moderate progestin such as desogestrel, with the same formulation for 21 days. Those who request renewal of a prescription obtained elsewhere, or those who wish to resume use after a period of nonuse, should continue the pill that was most acceptable to them. An estrogen-dominant pill may be selected for adolescents with an androgenic profile (i.e., moderate to severe acne, hairiness, small breasts, short and scanty menstrual periods), even if these are symptoms of a hyperandrogenic state due to an ovarian or adrenal disorder. Progestin-dominant pills may best suit the estrogenic profile (i.e., large breasts, heavy leukorrhea, premenstrual edema and/or weight gain, long and heavy menstrual flow).

Adolescents will be least confused by a 28-day package containing four rows of seven pills arranged in a calendar format. They can be advised to begin the package on the first Sunday after the start of a normal menstrual period and to match their pills with the weekdays. Because there are so many variations in packaging and because manufacturers may change the packaging of the same pill, providers should have current samples on hand for demonstration. The provider should discuss with the adolescent where to store the pills, methods for remembering to take them, and how to schedule pill consumption into a daily routine (e.g., as a part of preparation for bedtime). The need for consistency should be emphasized.

Side effects such as nausea, headaches, and breast tenderness occur most often with the first cycle of use and generally improve within three cycles. Premature switching to other pills should be discouraged, because different side effects may be experienced with each change. If physical symptoms develop, the adolescent may not associate them with obvious causes such as low back pain after heavy exercise or indigestion from excessive snacking on spicy foods. New users of oral contraceptives may blame such symptoms on the pill, abruptly discontinue use, and even have unprotected intercourse before contacting a healthcare provider to discuss their concerns. Above all, they must be strongly advised not to discontinue using the pill if they experience any symptoms that they believe indicate a side effect; they should be told to call the provider as soon as possible to determine whether there is cause to stop using the pill or to change brands.

The provider should investigate all side effects and not alarm the patient.[7] Side effects caused by estrogen may require a pill that is lower in estrogen. Nausea and vomiting may be relieved by taking the pill with food.

Headache and fatigue may have psychosocial causes, including anxiety and guilt related to pill use without parental knowledge or in the face of partner disapproval or pressure for pregnancy. Weight gain may respond to decreased caloric intake and increased exercise. Changes in vaginal discharge may be induced by estrogen but more often represent a vaginal or endocervical infection that requires appropriate screening.

Changes in menstrual function are common with pill use but seldom are pronounced. Amenorrhea or oligomenorrhea and/or galactorrhea warrant evaluation for pregnancy or endocrine abnormality. Potent pills such as Ovral may decrease or stop menses. Heavier than usual menstrual flow or cramping would not be expected and may be symptomatic of infection. Irregular bleeding between withdrawal flows usually is due to cervicitis or incorrect pill use, despite the patient's report. Regular break-through bleeding may be treated with a pill higher in estrogen if it occurs early in the hormone cycle (before day 15) or with a pill higher in progestin if it is late in the cycle (days 15 to 21). Irregular bleeding is common with progestin-only pills, but it cannot be managed without adding estrogen and may not be tolerated by many adolescents.

Oral contraceptives should be discontinued if the patient experiences blurred vision, loss of vision, paresthesias, paralysis, severe headaches, worsening migraines, thrombophlebitis, suspected embolic phenomena, severe hypertension, hyperlipidemia, hepatitis from any cause, or depression that appears to be related to pill use. Patients should be educated about and advised to use a back-up method during the first month of pill use, or if they decide to discontinue use or are advised to do so during a cycle.

Adolescents frequently forget to take one or more pills and may even misplace a package while in the middle of a cycle. Missing placebo pills will have no effect, but missing two or more hormone pills early in the schedule could result in break-through bleeding and even ovulation. If one pill is missed, it should be taken as soon as remembered within the same 24 hours. If two or more pills are missed, they can be taken twice a day, morning and evening, until the patient is back on schedule; a second contraceptive method should be added for the rest of that cycle.

Adolescent users of oral contraceptives should be seen frequently to review correct use, to reinforce compliance, and to anticipate and try to prevent side effects. First-time pill users, especially the very young or those who are immature, may be prescribed only two packs and seen during the second cycle. Others should be seen in 3 months. All adolescent patients should see the provider every 3 months for at least a year until patterns of use are established. Blood pressure and weight should be checked at each visit, but a complete physical examination is not required unless the patient has specific complaints. A pelvic examination with Pap smear is recommended yearly but may be required more often for those at high risk for sexually transmitted infections. A page of simple instructions with phone numbers for 24-hour response to concerns may be provided to all new users, and given again on subsequent visits. Commercially available pamphlets and posters may help reinforce basic information about oral contraceptives.

Postcoital Contraceptives

Implantation of a fertilized ovum may be prevented by hormones administered within 72 hours of sexual intercourse. If the patient has had intercourse during midcycle and if there is no question of pregnancy from previous intercourse, four Ovral tablets may be administered in doses of one tablet every 3 hours or two tablets repeated in 12 hours. Ethinyl estradiol, 5 mg a day for 5 days, is an alternative method. Nausea and vomiting are common side effects and may require concomitant antiemetics. These methods have a very low failure rate (<0.5%) with correct use; however, the patient should be advised to seek medical attention if no menstrual flow occurs at the expected time. Thrombosis or hypertension is a contraindication to postcoital estrogen use; alternatives include danazol, three 200-mg tablets repeated in 12 hours, or insertion of a copper intrauterine device (IUD).

Hormonal Injections

Injections of medroxyprogesterone acetate (Depo-Provera) and norethindrone enanthate (Noristerat) have been used throughout the world for contraception and have proved to be more effective, and probably safer, than oral contraceptives.[8] In the United States, the Food and Drug Administration did not approve these hormonal injections for use as contraceptives until 1992, after extensive study. Medroxyprogesterone acetate injection is administered as 100 to 150 mg every 3 months; norethindrone enanthate, as 200 mg every 7 to 10 weeks. These hormones appear to inhibit ovulation, alter cervical mucus, and cause atrophy of the endometrium. The last effect usually produces oligohypomenorrhea or amenorrhea, which may not be tolerated by some women but may be desirable for others.

Adolescent girls with severe mental or physical disabilities may be restricted from school attendance and other social and recreational opportunities during their menstrual periods if they are unable to handle menstrual hygiene. Adolescents with sickle cell disease or other severe anemia may have recurrent blood loss with menstrual periods that compromise their underlying disease. Long-acting injectable progestins may improve the quality of life and health status of such adolescents while affording contraception.

Long-acting progestins appear to provide protection against pelvic inflammatory disease as well as ovarian and endometrial cancer. They rarely have been associated with thromboembolic or cardiovascular complications and do not alter blood pressure or clotting function. They may decrease high-density lipoprotein cholesterol levels. Anovulation and amenorrhea may persist for several months after discontinuation of injections, but 60% of users are likely to conceive within 12 months and 90% by 24 months after the last injection. Break-through bleeding can be managed by increasing the dose or reducing the interval between injections. Patients should have blood pressure and weight checked at the time of each injection, and pelvic examinations and Pap smears done yearly.

Subdermal Implants

Norplant subdermal implants are nonbiodegradable polymeric silicone (Silastic) capsules or rods that slowly release levonorgestrel into the bloodstream. The amount of release is 50 to 80 μg daily in the first year, tapering to 30 to 35 μg daily by the fifth year. Experience to date indicates a high degree of contraceptive effectiveness for several years, with little or no effect on liver function, carbohydrate metabolism, blood pressure, or body weight.[9] The side effect of irregular menstrual bleeding is common and may be unacceptable to many teenagers. The site of implantation of the requisite five rods is noticeable, but it can be concealed by clothing. Subdermal implants offer a reliable long-term means of pregnancy prevention that is independent of coitus and immune to noncompliance. Removal requires a visit to a clinician and minor surgery. Adolescents at risk for infection would still require barrier methods for complete safety. Studies to date have reported no significant difference between teenagers and adults in acceptance or continuation of Norplant, but teenagers with low tolerance for side effects or ambivalence about pregnancy are likely to request removal of Norplant after a few months of use. Teenagers considering Norplant may benefit from a trial of progestin-only pills or medroxyprogesterone acetate injection to determine their experience with, and response to, side effects of progestins.

NONHORMONAL METHODS

Barrier Methods

Barrier methods currently include condoms; spermicidal foams, jellies, and suppositories; diaphragms; and cervical caps. All prevent fertilization by keeping sperm from reaching the ovum through physical obstruction or chemical destruction. To be reliable, barrier methods must be readily available for use with every act of coitus. They are the only contraceptives that offer a reasonable degree of protection against the transmission of infection and the factors that increase the risk of cervical cancer. This type of contraception has few side effects, although a topical allergic reaction (vulvovaginitis or balanitis) to the spermicidal chemical or the latex rubber may develop in some individuals. Barrier methods involve low cost unless intercourse is a very frequent event. They are recommended for couples who are motivated to prevent pregnancy, concerned about transmission of infection, and willing to postpone intercourse if the method is not readily accessible. They are recommended as a form of back-up during the first month's use of a hormonal method, and whenever a hormonal method is interrupted or stopped prematurely.

CONDOMS. The use of condoms alone or with any other barrier method can greatly reduce the risk of exposure to all sexually transmitted infections; however, instructions for use must be followed correctly, and the condom must be used with each act of sexual intercourse. Condom use reinforces the participation of the male in responsible sexual behavior. Surveys of adolescents indicate that both males and females misperceive their partners' feelings about condom use and that many couples fail to discuss condoms, each assuming that the other would object to this method.

Latex condoms are available in various textures, colors, and shapes; some include a lubricant and some contain the spermicide nonoxynol 9. Condoms made of animal skin are more expensive than other types, but these may be used if allergy to latex is a consideration. Condoms are available in pharmacies, large grocery stores, and discount department stores, usually located near other nonprescription barrier method and menstrual hygiene products.

Adolescents must be given explicit, concrete instructions about condoms. Pictures or anatomic models may help to demonstrate correct usage. Sample supplies may be given to adolescents of either sex with information about purchase sites, suggested brands, and costs.

The following points should be emphasized:

1. The condom should be applied before the penis makes any contact with the perineal area, to avoid transmission of infectious organisms or any sperm that may be present in preejaculate penile secretions.
2. Space must be left at the end of the condom to hold the ejaculate and to avoid rupture during use.
3. A vaginal spermicide or personal lubricant may aid in lubrication and enhance sensation. Petroleum products such as petroleum jelly or mineral oil should not be used because they will damage latex condoms.
4. Adolescent males may fear decreased sensation with condom use. However, this can be presented as a benefit in delaying orgasm and increasing pleasure for both partners.

5. The condom should be held in place during withdrawal of the penis from the vagina, with care taken not to spill the contents anywhere on the perineum.
6. Condoms should never be reused. They should not be stored in warm areas, such as automobile glove compartments in the summer or back trouser pockets, for prolonged periods. Attractive condom holders are available for both male and female use.

Teenagers today should be advised to use condoms every time they have intercourse, even if other methods are used for pregnancy prevention.

VAGINAL SPERMICIDES. When used correctly and consistently, spermicidal foams, jellies, and suppositories protect against pregnancy and cervical infections. However, they do not prevent inoculation of the perineum or the vagina with infectious agents such as herpesvirus, papillomavirus, and *Trichomonas vaginalis*. Vaginal spermicides are most effective if they are placed deep in the vagina near the cervix. The spermicidal chemical, usually nonoxynol 9 or octoxynol 9, is contained in an inert base that is dispersed over the cervix within a few minutes of insertion. The reported high pregnancy rate, 20% to 30% per year, among users of vaginal spermicides is due mainly to inconsistent use. Many females do not fully accept this method because of reluctance to touch their genitals and insert their fingers into their vagina; some consider vaginal spermicides too messy.

Adolescents who plan to use these products alone or with condoms should be advised as follows:
1. Spermicidal foams are preferred because they disperse best and have the longest efficacy in killing sperm.
2. Suppositories, although easy to insert, are least effective because they may not dissolve properly or may be placed too far away from the cervix. Spermicidal suppositories must not be confused with preparations intended to be used only as vaginal deodorants.
3. Spermicides must be inserted no more than 10 to 20 minutes before sexual intercourse, and douching should be done 6 to 8 hours after intercourse.
4. A new application of spermicide must be made before each act of coitus.

DIAPHRAGM AND CERVICAL CAP. These devices provide some physical barrier to the entry of sperm into the cervix. However, they mainly provide placement of a spermicide close to the cervix. Since they can be inserted well ahead of coitus and removed many hours later, they do not interfere with foreplay or coitus. These barrier devices require touching of the genitals and proper placement to be effective. They protect the cervix from infection and agents that increase the risk for cervical cancer, but they do not protect the perineum or the vagina. Disadvantages of these devices include the possibility of topical allergic reaction. In addition, the diaphragm's pressure on the urethra has been implicated in recurrent urinary tract infections. The diaphragm has been associated with toxic shock syndrome when left in place too long, and it is unclear whether correct use presents an increased risk for this syndrome. It should be noted that the risk of death from pregnancy greatly exceeds the risk of death from toxic shock syndrome.

The diaphragm and the cervical cap must be fitted and prescribed by a healthcare provider. Clinicians who seldom see sexually active adolescents and rarely receive a request for either of these methods should refer such patients to an appropriately experienced professional. In offices where many adolescents are seen for reproductive health care, at least one clinician should be trained in fitting patients for these methods.

Users of these methods should be advised as follows:
1. The cervical cap is not yet approved for marketing as a contraceptive method in the United States.
2. The diaphragm should always be used with a spermicidal jelly or cream applied around the edge and on the center side that fits against the cervix.
3. If coitus is repeated, the diaphragm must not be removed, but additional spermicide should be applied vaginally.
4. The diaphragm should not be removed for at least 6 hours after sexual intercourse.
5. Water-soluble lubricants will not affect the diaphragm, but petroleum products may damage the latex.
6. A new diaphragm is recommended after 2 years of use, and a new size may be needed after pregnancy or a weight change of 15 or more pounds.

It should be noted that the contraceptive sponge was withdrawn from the market by the manufacturer in 1995.

INTRAUTERINE DEVICES

When first developed, the IUD seemed to be the solution to problems of compliance in sexually active adolescents, and was both widely recommended and used.[10] Differently shaped devices made from steel, plastic, or plastic and copper, when inserted into the uterine fundus, prevent implantation of a fertilized ovum by altering the endometrium through low-grade inflammation and the production of prostaglandins. Tubal motility also may be affected. Recent devices that contain progestin for slow release also suppress endometrial proliferation and thicken the cervical mucus.

During the years of their widespread use, IUDs were associated with a pregnancy rate of 1% to 3%, although many users requested removal after a short time because of increased menstrual cramps and/or heavier menstrual flow. Pregnancy occurring with an IUD in place carried an increased risk of being ectopic or resulting in spontaneous abortion. In addition, concern arose because of the association of septic abortion with one brand of IUD, and the occurrence of pelvic inflammatory disease in IUD users who were exposed to sexually transmitted infections. Because of lawsuits, most manufacturers have ceased production and distribution of these devices.

Owing to the risk of serious reproductive tract infections and resultant infertility, most clinicians now advise against the use of IUDs in patients who have not yet completed their families, especially nulliparous women and all adolescents. The IUD certainly is contraindicated for adolescents at high risk for infection because of multiple partners, sex with high-risk partners, unwillingness to use concurrent barrier methods, and/or a history of sexually transmitted infections. If an IUD is the only acceptable method for a specific teenager and if the risk of infection is believed to be low, the individual should be referred to a physician with experience in the use of the IUD. Previous screening for infection and treatment of any detected gonorrhea or *Chlamydia* infection is essential.

VOLUNTARY STERILIZATION

Permanent contraception through vasectomy or tubal ligation is strongly discouraged for the adolescent age group because of the low chance of reversibility and the unlikelihood that an adolescent is ready to make an irrevocable decision regarding his or her reproductive future. Most state laws restrict access to sterilization for persons younger than 21 years unless they follow judicial process.

When childbearing and parenthood are highly undesirable, as in individuals with severe mental impairment or with certain severe physical disabilities, parents of adolescents may pursue the statutory process for sterilization. This entails a complete diagnostic evaluation and multidisciplinary review of the situation. After the procedure, counseling of the parents and the adolescent is necessary to deal with attendant feelings. Comprehensive sexuality education may be indicated to handle any continuing risk of sexual exploitation and infection, even if pregnancy is impossible. An effective method such as Depo-Provera may be instituted while awaiting and immediately following the sterilization of females.

References

1. The Alan Guttmacher Institute: *Sex and America's teenagers,* New York, 1994, Alan Guttmacher Institute.
2. Morrison DM: Adolescent contraceptive behavior: a review, *Psychol Bull* 98:538, 1985.
3. Davis AJ: The role of hormonal contraception in adolescents, *Am J Obstet Gynecol* 170:1581, 1994.
4. Neinstein LS, Katz B: Contraceptive use in the chronically ill adolescent female: Parts I and II, *J Adolesc Health Care* 7:123, 350, 1986.
5. American College of Obstetricians and Gynecologists: Safety of oral contraceptives for teenagers, *J Adolesc Health* 13:333, 1992.
6. Tyrer LB: Oral contraception for the adolescent, *J Reprod Health* 29:551, 1984.
7. Block M, Rulin MC: Managing patients on oral contraceptives, *Am Fam Physician* 32:154, 1985.
8. Cromer BA: Depo-Provera: wherefore art thou?, *Adolesc Pediatr Gynecol* 5:155, 1992.
9. Liskin LS, Blackburn R: Hormonal contraception: new long-acting methods, *Popul Rep* K-3:1, 1987.
10. Treiman K, Liskin LS: IUDs—a new look, *Popul Rep* B-5:1, 1988.

Suggested Readings

Harlap S, Kost K, Forrest JD: *Preventing pregnancy, protecting health: a new look at birth control choices in the United States,* New York, 1991, Alan Guttmacher Institute.

Hatcher RA, Guest F, Stewart GK, et al: *Contraceptive technology 1992-1994,* ed 16 (revised), New York, 1994, Irvington.

Joffe A: Adolescents and condom use, *Am J Dis Child* 147:746, 1993.

Rosenfeld WD, Swedler JB: Role of hormonal contraceptives in prevention of pregnancy and disease in adolescents, *Adolesc Med: State of Art Rev* 3:207, 1992.

Sikand A, Fisher M: The role of barrier contraceptives in prevention of pregnancy and disease in adolescents, *Adolesc Med: State of Art Rev* 3:223, 1992.

Educational Materials for Patients

American Academy of Pediatrics
Department of Publications
141 Northwest Point Blvd.
P.O. Box 927
Elk Grove Village, IL 60007-0927
  Offers pamphlets on abstinence and birth control.

American College of Obstetricians and Gynecologists Resource Center
409 12th St., SW
Washington, DC 20024-2188
  Offers pamphlets on all methods of contraception.

Channing L. Bete Co., Inc.
200 State Rd.
South Deerfield, MA 01373-0200
  Supplies illustrated booklets on contraception in general and on specific methods.

Network Publications
P.O. Box 1830
Santa Cruz, CA 95061-1830
  Offers many pamphlets, books, and videos about sexual responsibility, abstinence, and all contractive methods.

Planned Parenthood Federation of America, Inc.
810 Seventh Ave.
New York, NY 10019
  Offers pamphlets on specific methods of contraception.[1]

Healthcare providers interested in these pamphlets should request catalogs and samples from the publishers. After previewing materials and selecting those most appropriate for the clinical setting, the provider should order bulk quantities for waiting-room display or direct distribution in patient-counseling sessions.

CHAPTER 142

Adolescent Pregnancy

•

Nelson W. Davidson

EPIDEMIOLOGY

The rates of pregnancy, abortion, and births have been relatively stable among adolescents in the United States in the past decade, but teenage pregnancy remains a serious problem. Since the consequences of adolescent pregnancy are complex, including physical, psychologic, social, economic, and educational sequelae, all clinicians who care for adolescents need to be aware of these issues.

The pregnancy rate is defined as the number of live births plus induced abortions per 1000 women within a particular age group. Spontaneous abortions or stillbirths may or may not be included in this statistic. The birth rate refers only to the number of live births per 1000 women in an age group.

Data on trends in pregnancy, abortion, and birth rates have generally been available only since the early 1970s. Although pregnancy rates increased in the 1970s for both younger (<15 years of age) and older (15- to 19-year-old) adolescents, they leveled off during the 1980s. During the 1970s, birth rates declined and abortion rates increased, but both rates generally stabilized during the 1980s. The pregnancy rates remained relatively stable in the 1980s, but from 1986 to 1990 the U.S. birth rates increased by 20%.[1] In 1991, there were 1.1 million pregnancies among teenagers aged 15 to 19 years. There were approximately 57,000 pregnancies in adolescent girls aged 14 years or under. It is estimated that about 80% of these pregnancies were unintended.[2] Approximately 14% of these pregnancies ended in miscarriage and 35% in induced abortions.[3]

Figure 142-1 shows the trends in the rates of pregnancy, birth, and abortion among older teenagers from 1970 to 1990. It is apparent that the trends during the first decade of increased pregnancy rate and abortion rates and decreased birth rates have stabilized during the 1980s. As Figures 142-2 to 142-4 indicate, in the adolescent age group the United States has the highest pregnancy, birth, and abortion rates among all industrialized nations.[4-8] Although pregnancy occurs in teenagers from all racial and socioeconomic groups, racial differ-

ences are evident in the pregnancy, birth, and abortion rates among adolescents. Figure 142-5 shows that all these rates are higher for black than for white teenagers. Among Hispanic teenagers, the birth rate rates are almost twice that of whites, but birth rates are increasing more sharply among young whites (<15 years of age) than in any other racial group.[5]

Another factor in the pregnancy rates is the delay of younger teenagers in starting effective contraceptive practices. About 40% of 15-year-old adolescents wait more than 1 year after first intercourse before starting any type of contraception. The percentages decrease to 35% in 15- to 17-year-olds and 15% in 18- to 19-year-olds. Sixty percent of adolescents under 15 years of age fail to use contraception with first intercourse.[9]

The economic impact of adolescent pregnancy is also of great concern. About 50% of these costs are for Aid to Families with Dependent Children (AFDC), 35% for food stamps, and about 15% for Medicaid.[9] About three out of four women under 30 receiving AFDC funds had their first child as an adolescent. In 1990, $25 billion in aid (AFDC, food stamps, and Medicaid) was given to women whose first child was born while they were still an adolescent.[2]

DIAGNOSIS

The diagnosis of pregnancy begins with certain signs and symptoms that may prompt the adolescent or the healthcare provider to request a pregnancy test. However, the results of a single laboratory test must not be relied on solely in an evaluation for pregnancy. The diagnosis is based on the patient's history, physical examination, and laboratory test results and (when applicable) on sonographic information.

The adolescent usually presents with some signs or symptoms of pregnancy, but not always. In fact, some pregnant teenagers may not even realize that they are pregnant and may report only vague complaints. The

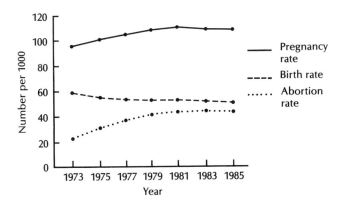

Fig. 142-1. Abortions, births, and pregnancies per 1000 women aged 15 to 19, United States, 1970-1989. (From Hatcher RA, et al: *Contraceptive technology,* ed 16 [revised], New York, 1994, Irvington.)

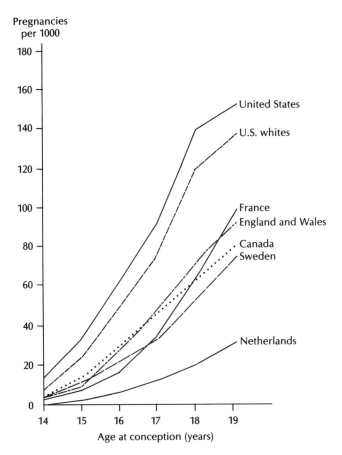

Fig. 142-2. Pregnancies per 1000 women by single year of age, 1980. (From Jones EF, Forrest J, Goldman N, Henshaw SK, Lincoln R, Rosoff J, Westoff C, Wulf D: *Teenage pregnancy in industrialized countries,* New Haven, CT, 1986, Yale University Press. Copyright © 1986 by Yale University Press.)

most common presenting complaint is a missed or abnormal menstrual period. A complete menstrual history should be obtained, including age of menarche, frequency and length of menses, history of previously missed periods, dates of previous and last menstrual periods, and

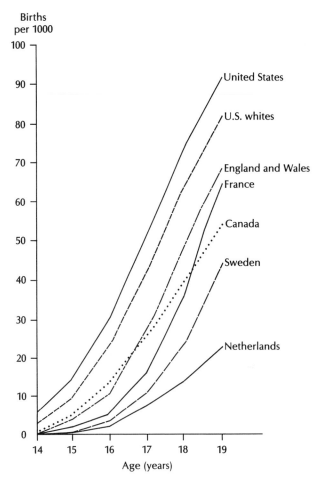

Fig. 142-3. Births per 1000 women by single year of age, 1980. (From Jones EF, Forrest J, Goldman N, Henshaw SK, Lincoln R, Rosoff J, Westoff C, Wulf D: *Teenage pregnancy in industrialized countries,* New Haven, CT, 1986, Yale University Press. Copyright © 1986 by Yale University Press.)

any abnormalities of the last period (shorter, lighter, or heavier than normal). Recent or current use of contraceptives and recent sexual practices should be explored. The frequency of intercourse, the number of sexual partners, and the date of the most recent intercourse should be obtained. This information will help the clinician estimate the probability and the gestational age of the pregnancy, which should be corroborated by the physical examination.

Common symptoms of pregnancy include breast tenderness or fullness and nipple sensitivity, which usually appears 1 to 2 weeks after conception. Fatigue, nausea, vomiting, abdominal pain, and frequent urination are symptoms that may occur beyond 2 weeks in the pregnant patient. Fetal movement (quickening), which begins at 16 to 20 weeks, may be noted by the adolescent. Vaginal bleeding, which may be light or heavy, or spotting may occur after conception. A history of heavy bleeding may indicate an ectopic pregnancy or a missed or

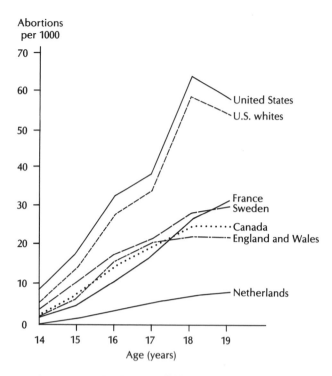

Fig. 142-4. Abortions per 1000 women by single year of age, 1980. (From Jones EF, Forrest J, Goldman N, Henshaw SK, Lincoln R, Rosoff J, Westoff C, Wulf D: *Teenage pregnancy in industrialized countries,* New Haven, CT, 1986, Yale University Press. Copyright © 1986 by Yale University Press.)

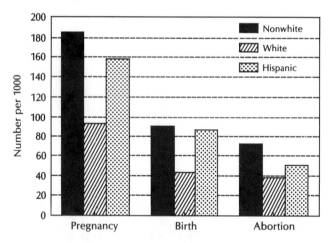

Fig. 142-5. Racial and ethnic differences in pregnancy, abortion, and birth rates among older adolescent women: 15- to 19-year-olds. (From Henshaw SK, Kenney AM, Somberg D, Van Vort J: *Teenage pregnancy in the United States: the scope of the problem and state responses,* New York, 1989, Alan Guttmacher Institute.)

threatened abortion. Pregnancy must be considered as a diagnosis when the previously listed complaints are noted, even if the adolescent reports a normal menstrual history. Since adolescents often fear being pregnant and deny that possibility, they may relate a completely normal menstrual history.

In the physical examination, the clinician should look for breast fullness, tenderness, nipple discharge, protrusion or fullness on abdominal examination, and any cervical changes. Uterine enlargement may be noted on abdominal examination. At about 12 weeks' gestation the uterus can be felt above the pelvic rim. By 16 weeks the upper boundary of the uterus is at a midpoint between the symphysis pubis and the umbilicus. By 20 weeks the uterus is located at the umbilicus, and at 28 weeks it will be between the umbilicus and the xiphoid process. Hegar's sign (upper cervical segment softening), Goodell's sign (cervical softening), and Chadwick's sign (bluish discoloration of cervix) may be noted on pelvic examination as early as 6 weeks' gestation.

The diagnosis of pregnancy by laboratory methods is based on the presence of human chorionic gonadotropin (hCG) in either serum or urine samples. hCG is made up of two subunits, an alpha chain and a beta chain. The alpha subunits of hCG, luteinizing hormone, follicle-stimulating hormone, and thyroid-stimulating hormone are almost identical to one another. The beta subunits are different, although there is enough similarity with the subunits of hCG and luteinizing hormone to cause cross-reactivity with less sensitive and less specific pregnancy tests.

With the implantation of the morula, trophoblastic cells begin secreting hCG. At less than 24 hours after implantation, hCG levels are 5 mIU/ml or less. Figure 142-6 shows the changes in hCG levels during a normal pregnancy, a molar pregnancy, and an abnormal or ectopic pregnancy. By 1 week after conception, hCG levels range from 70 to 100 mIU/ml. After 2 weeks, these levels will be more than 250 mIU/ml in a normal pregnancy. hCG levels peak (100,000 mIU/ml) at approximately 10 to 12 weeks' gestation and then decrease to levels of 3000 to 10,000 mIU/ml for the remainder of the pregnancy. hCG will still be present after termination of the pregnancy. Seven to 10 days after an abortion that occurs in the first or second trimester, most routine urine tests are negative. However, ultra-sensitive urine tests or serum radioimmunoassay still may be positive within 10 days. These tests should be negative by 14 to 21 days after abortion.

All pregnancy tests are based on the use of either immunoassay (IA), radioimmunoassay (RIA), or enzyme-linked immunosorbent assay (ELISA). The most sensitive, most specific, and most frequently used test for quantitative measurements of hCG is RIA of serum. The IA tests used most commonly in offices are also very sensitive, with low levels of hCG. Levels of hCG may be detected between 5 and 50 mIU and therefore are positive as early as 3 to 4 days after implantation or 7 to 10 days after conception. These tests have up to a 98% positivity rate after 7 days of implantation or at 7 to 10 days after

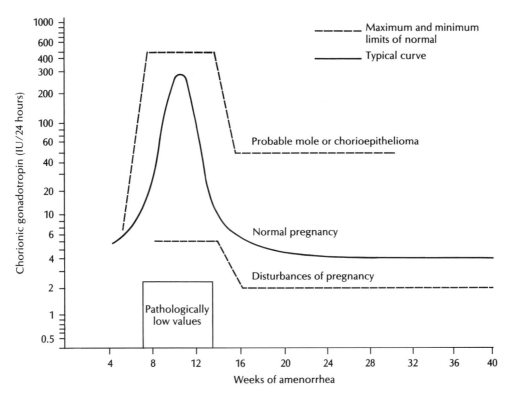

Fig. 142-6. Urinary human chorionic gonadotropin levels during normal pregnancy. (From Hatcher RA, et al: *Contraceptive technology 1988-1989,* New York, 1988, Irvington.)

conception. Urine slide or tube tests are generally not as sensitive as the RIA tests on serum. However, some of the newer ELISA tests for urine detection may be sensitive to as low as 20 to 50 mIU of hCG. However, many of the home kits measure total hCG and are not specific for the beta subunit. Table 142-1 lists most of the tests currently available, their sensitivity, and the time required to perform the test. Some of the causes of false-negative or false-positive results in pregnancy testing are listed in Box 142-1.

The issue of home pregnancy testing is important. When this testing is done correctly, its accuracy is similar to that of urine tests performed in the clinician's office. However, home pregnancy test kits are not recommended for use by adolescents, for several reasons. First, the instructions may be confusing, and so the adolescent may not perform the test properly. Second, the adolescent may not understand how to interpret the results or accept the possibility of false-positive or false-negative results. Third, she may delay seeking a pregnancy evaluation because of an incorrectly performed test. The adolescent may not realize that an apparently true negative test needs to be repeated in 7 to 14 days. She may panic at a false-positive result and, out of fear or denial, delay seeking evaluation. An area of concern, with both home and office tests, is the possibility of false-negative results in ectopic pregnancies or threatened abortions.

Finally, when the patient's clinical picture is confusing and the hCG results are negative, two procedures are indicated. If the hCG result was only a *qualitative* test, a *quantitative* serum beta-hCG test may be performed. If the clinical presentation indicates that the patient seems to be pregnant, may have an ectopic pregnancy, or is threatening spontaneous abortion, a pelvic ultrasonographic examination should be performed.

PREGNANCY COUNSELING

All pregnant adolescents need counseling. Informing an unmarried adolescent that she is pregnant usually precipitates both a personal and a family crisis. At this difficult time, a host of practical matters must be addressed, including medical, emotional, psychologic, economic, familial, legal, and confidentiality issues. The clinician needs to understand the cognitive and psychosocial stages of development in adolescence and recognize where the patient falls in that continuum. For example, younger adolescents often lack the cognitive and emotional maturity to cope adequately with the many ramifications of being pregnant. The practitioner also must be familiar with state laws involving parental notification and confidentiality, especially if abortion is being considered. The clinician must provide nonjudgmental counseling on all relevant issues so that the

TABLE 142-1
Commonly Used Clinic and Office Pregnancy Tests

Name (Manufacturer)	Sensitivity (mIU/ml)*	Time Required (min)	No. of Steps/Comments
Immunometric Tests			
Specific for beta hCG; no LH, FSH, or TSH cross-reaction. Reliably detect pregnancy 7-10 days after conception.			
Cost: $2.30-$7.00†			
CARDS (Pacific Biotech)	25	3	1 step/urine
Clearview hCG (Wampole)	50	5	1 step/urine
Icon II hCG (Hybritech)	20	5	5 steps/serum
	25	4	5 steps/urine
Nimbus (Biomerica)	10-25	5-15	Serum or urine sensitivity depends on time
One Step (Wampole)	25	7	1 step/serum
	25	5	1 step/urine
PregnaGen (Biogenex)	40	4	1 step/urine
Precise (Becton Dickinson)	25	4	1 step/urine
Pro-Step hCG (Disease Detection Intl)	25	4	1 step, dip/serum
	25	3	Urine
Quick Vue (Quidel)	25	3	1 step/urine
Surcell hCG (Kodak)	30	2	2-3 steps/serum
	30	1	2-3 steps/urine
	50	1	2-3 steps/urine
Tandem Icon QSR (Hybritech)	<5	7	Serum
Target (V-Tech)	50	4	Urine
		5	Serum
Testpack plus hCG (Abbott)	50	5	1 step/urine
Testpack plus hCG combo (Abbott)	25	7	1 step/urine
	50	4	Urine
Agglutination Inhibition Slide Tests			
Test antibody reacts to whole hCG, not specific for beta-hCG; cross-reaction with LH, FSH, and TSH is possible. Reliably detect pregnancy 18-21 days after conception (32-36 days after last menstrual period).			
All require urine specimen.			
Cost $1.30-$2.30†			
Pregnosticon (Organon)	1000-2000	2	
Pregnosis (Roche)	1500-2500	2	
Wampole UCG (Wampole)	1500-2500	2	

*Sensitivity specified as the lower limit of reliable hCG detection in product literature. Test results may be positive at lower hCG in some cases.

†Bulk or nonprofit agency discount purchase may reduce costs significantly.

Source: Manufacturer's product literature (1993).

Note: Intermediate sensitivity slide tests that detect hCG levels of approximately 500 mIU/ml are also available but cost as much as immunometric tests. Immunometric kits are more sensitive and easier to use.

hCG, human chorionic gonadotropin; *LH,* luteinizing hormone; *FSH,* follicle-stimulating hormone; *TSH,* thyroid-stimulating hormone.

---

adolescent can explore all her options. Ideally, pregnancy counseling takes place before a pregnancy occurs. The issues of effective contraception and the risks of ineffective contraception should be addressed as soon as an adolescent becomes sexually active. Unfortunately, most pregnancy counseling sessions take place after pregnancy has been diagnosed.

Once the diagnosis of pregnancy has been made, the adolescent must be told her options: delivery and parenting, delivery with adoption, or induced abortion. The adolescent's choices may be narrowed by moral, cultural, or religious beliefs, and she may be pressured to make a specific decision by friends, family, or the father

of the baby. However, it is important that she make a decision that takes into account her own fears and needs. If time allows, the health care provider often can facilitate this decision through individual and family counseling. Difficulties arise when the adolescent presents in the 18- to 22-week range of gestational age. In such a situation, if an abortion is being considered, time is limited for the adolescent and family to fully explore all options. Once a decision has been made, follow-up should continue to determine how well the adolescent and her family are coping with the decision. If the pregnancy is to continue, follow-up contact during the prenatal period is important for continuity. Whatever decision is made by the adolescent, counseling in regard to sexuality, contraception, and the physical and psychologic effects of pregnancy and/or abortion should be continued.

Care must be taken to assure the adolescent of confidentiality based on the standards in each state. In most states adolescents may obtain information, diagnosis, and treatment for family planning, pregnancy, and sexually transmitted diseases (STDs) without parental consent. Since the *Roe v. Wade* Supreme Court decision in 1973, which legalized abortion, there have been numerous challenges and attempts to legislate access to abortion services. A number of states have passed laws requiring either parental notification or consent in cases of abortion involving a minor. There has been much debate over the constitutionality of such laws and their impact on teenagers, their parents, and society in general. Parental notification laws challenged in the U.S. Supreme Court generally have been upheld as long as a judicial bypass mechanism has been in place. Proponents of parental notification laws contend that parents have the right to be involved in a major decision such as pregnancy, regardless of the adolescent's wishes. Often there is concern about whether a minor is mature enough to give informed consent for a surgical procedure. Opponents of such laws believe that these laws will not enhance communication between adolescents and their parents. Since a majority of adolescents do discuss decisions regarding their pregnancy with their parents, it is believed that laws requiring notification are unnecessary. Finally, there is the fear that by requiring notification or consent of parents, certain teenagers may seek illegal abortions or self-induce abortions to avoid confrontation with a parent.[10-12] Clinicians involved in the counseling of adolescents regarding pregnancy must be aware of pertinent laws in their states and understand the extent to which these are enforced.

All adolescents, regardless of age, should be strongly encouraged to discuss their decisions about pregnancy with their parents. If the clinician notices reluctance or fear in the adolescent, the reasons for this attitude should be explored. Because very young adolescents often lack the maturity to make a decision of this magnitude alone, the clinician may need to involve a parent or adult relative even when the adolescent is reluctant to do so. When the adolescent knows what the clinician needs to do and why, a trusting relationship with her can be maintained. The adolescent will feel better when she has some options about whom to involve and how to inform the adult of the pregnancy. Frequently, she will feel more secure about revealing the pregnancy to a parent in the presence of the physician. In clinics or practices with adolescent family planning programs, the counseling may be done by the practitioner, but more often it is done by a nurse or social worker. Whoever does the counseling must be familiar with the resources available in the community. If prenatal care and/or abortion services are not available within the clinic or practice, a referral base must be generated. When abortion is requested, there is wide variability as to whether a patient can be seen at a particular place. Financial status, gestational age, waiting lists, and location are common barriers to finding an appropriate referral site (see Chapter 144, "Abortion").

PRENATAL CARE

Despite the obvious need for early and comprehensive prenatal care, many adolescents receive little or late prenatal care. This is probably related to delay in seeking a diagnosis. Although some consider all pregnant adolescents as high-risk patients, recent studies have shown that pregnant adolescents who undergo diagnosis early and receive early and consistent prenatal care tailored to their needs are not at any higher risk for complications than are adults from the same race or socioeconomic levels. Factors other than age account for some of the higher morbidity seen among pregnant adolescents. The exception may be the youngest adolescents (14 years of age or younger), whose age may be associated with increased morbidity.

More recent research has shown that there probably is not an increased incidence of anemia, toxemia, pregnancy-induced hypertension (PIH), prematurity, and perinatal and maternal mortality when properly matched controlled studies are used. As long as there is good and consistent prenatal care, outcomes are very similar to those of older women. Adolescents account for up to 25% of premature births in the United States. In addition, there is a higher percentage of low birthweight (LBW) (<2500 g) infants born to adolescents than to adult women. This LBW factor contributes to a rate of neonatal mortality among some adolescent populations that is higher than the national average. Again, age is not considered to be the sole factor for these differences. Other factors are socioeconomic status, education, physical size (younger adolescents may not have reached full adult size), weight gain during pregnancy, prenatal care, and substance use.

Comprehensive care for the pregnant adolescent is essential for a good outcome. It has been clearly shown that adolescents who receive prenatal care in interdisciplinary settings have better medical and psychosocial outcomes during and after pregnancy. The interdisciplinary team usually includes an obstetrician, a pediatrician, a nutritionist, a social worker/counselor, and a nurse. Comprehensive prenatal care may be provided in different types of settings: a special adolescent obstetrics clinic within a community family planning clinic, a health department obstetrics clinic, a university obstetrics clinic, or sometimes, a school-based clinic. Some models have been developed that are joint obstetrics-pediatric/adolescent medicine programs, and these have shown excellent outcomes.

Because of the complex nature of pregnancy in adolescence, all staff must be sensitive to the special needs of the patient. It is particularly important to have counseling support services available to help the adolescent and her family cope with the emotional, psychosocial, physical, and economic stressors associated with the pregnancy. In some cases an adolescent may not receive much support from family and friends during the pregnancy. The father of the child may not be emotionally or financially supportive. Whenever possible, counseling and support should also be available to the father of the baby.

Nutritional assessment and supportive services are critical in adolescent pregnancy, since adolescents often have poor nutritional habits that contribute to increased nutritional difficulties during pregnancy. The consumption of adequate calories, protein, vitamins, and minerals is important for both the adolescent's health and the development of the fetus. Poor weight gain (less than 24 to 28 pounds) during pregnancy contributes to having an LBW infant. Caloric intake should be between 2400 and 2700 cal/day. Protein intake must be increased to about 75 g/day. Multivitamins with iron supplementation of 30 to 60 mg/day of iron salts are also necessary. Table 142-2 shows the recommended requirements for nonpregnant and pregnant teenagers, with significant increases noted for the latter in caloric, protein, calcium, phosphorus, iron, and folic acid requirements.

As part of comprehensive care, peer groups may be helpful. Exposure to other adolescents having similar experiences is often reassuring to adolescents. Prenatal classes also should be offered to focus on nutrition, pregnancy, labor and delivery, contraception, and STDs.

The initial medical evaluation of the pregnant adolescent should encompass a complete history, including medical, family, and drug use histories. A thorough physical and pelvic examination should be performed. The pelvic examination helps in estimating gestational age and in assessing evidence of cephalopelvic disproportion. In addition, the clinician should screen for STDs. Routine laboratory tests that should be obtained on an initial visit include (1) hematocrit or complete blood count, (2) urinalysis, (3) blood type and group, (4) rapid plasma reagin (RPR) or venereal disease research laboratory (VDRL) test, (5) hepatitis B screen, (6) sickle cell screen (in black patients), (7) rubella titer, (8) Papanicolaou (Pap) smear, (9) gonorrhea culture, (10) *Chlamydia* culture, and (11) KOH/wet prep of vaginal fluid.

The frequency of visits for prenatal care varies, depending on the problems and needs of the adolescent as well as the facilities and staffing of the clinic, but adolescents generally need more visits than do adults. A typical schedule includes visits every 2 to 4 weeks up until 28 weeks, every 1 to 2 weeks from 28 to 32 weeks, and then each week beyond 32 weeks. These visits are for both medical follow-up and education. Issues to be discussed include the process of pregnancy, nutrition, activity levels and/or restrictions, warning signs (e.g., abdominal pain and vaginal bleeding, which might indicate problems), medication and drug use, care of the newborn, preparation for childbirth and contraception, and familial and psychologic coping with the pregnancy.

Family planning counseling also must be a part of prenatal care. Appropriate contraception; proper use of contraceptive methods; and counseling and education through schools, health centers, hospitals, and the com-

TABLE 142-2
Nutritional Needs of Nonpregnant and Pregnant Adolescents

Nutrients	Nonpregnant		Pregnant
	Ages 11-14	Ages 15-18	Ages 11-18
Energy (kcal/day)	2200	2200	2500
Protein (g/day)	46	44	60
Minerals			
Calcium (mg/day)	1200	1200	1200
Phosphorus (mg/day)	1200	1200	1200
Magnesium (mg/day)	280	300	300
Zinc (mg/day)	12	12	15
Iron (mg/day)	15	15	30
Iodine (mg/day)	150	150	175
Fat-Soluble Vitamins			
Vitamin A (IU/day)	800	800	800
Vitamin D (IU/day)	10	10	10
Vitamin E (IU/day)	8	8	10
Vitamin K (mg/day)	45	55	65
Water-Soluble Vitamins			
Vitamin C (mg/day)	50	60	70
Vitamin B_6 (mg/day)	1.4	1.5	2.2
Vitamin B_{12} (mg/day)	2	2	2.2
Folate (mg/day)	150	180	400
Niacin (mg/day)	15	15	17
Riboflavin (mg/day)	1.3	1.3	1.6
Thiamine (mg/day)	1.1	1.1	1.5

From *Recommended dietary allowances*, ed 10. Copyright 1989 by the National Academy of Sciences, National Academy Press.

munity will be the foundation for preventing repeat pregnancies.

COMPLICATIONS OF PREGNANCY

The clinician should be aware of some common complications of adolescent pregnancy, such as ectopic pregnancy, threatened or incomplete abortion, pregnancy-induced hypertension (PIH), and premature delivery.

Ectopic Pregnancy

The adolescent presenting with abdominal or pelvic pain, amenorrhea, and/or irregular vaginal bleeding must be evaluated carefully. One of the most serious considerations is ectopic pregnancy, the incidence of which has been increasing since 1970. The Centers for Disease Control and Prevention (CDC) reported that rates increased from 17,800 (4.5 per 1000 live births) in 1970 to 88,000 (16.8 per 1000 live births) in 1987 for women aged 15 to 44. In general, there are higher rates in older women (20.5 per 1000 live births in women aged 35 to 44) than in younger women (6.3 per 1000 live births in women aged 15 to 24).[13] Ectopic pregnancy is a leading

cause of maternal mortality, accounting for 10% to 15% of maternal deaths. The risk of death is higher in blacks than in whites, partly because of a common delay in seeking prenatal care in the first trimester. In general, adolescents are at particularly high risk for mortality because they frequently delay in seeking prenatal care and may have limited access to health services. Risk factors for ectopic pregnancy include previous or current use of an intrauterine device (IUD), previous pelvic inflammatory disease (PID), previous ectopic pregnancy, previous pelvic surgery, and use of progestin-only oral contraceptive pills.

The classic presentation of ectopic pregnancy is pelvic pain, amenorrhea, and vaginal bleeding. However, this triad is found in only about half of the patients. Table 142-3 lists the common signs and symptoms of ectopic pregnancy. The most common site is the fallopian tubes (95% to 97%), with two thirds based in the ampulla. Other sites include the ovaries, cervix, and abdominal cavity. It may be difficult to obtain an accurate history of menstrual pain and bleeding from the adolescent. However, because the consequences of missing the diagnosis are severe, any adolescent with a positive pregnancy test, abdominal pain, and bleeding should be considered as having a possible ectopic pregnancy or threatened abortion until it

TABLE 142-3
Signs and Symptoms of Ectopic Pregnancy

	Patients (%)
Signs	
Adnexal tenderness	95
Unilateral	60
Bilateral	40
Adnexal mass	35-50
Normal uterine size	71
6- to 8-wk uterine size	26
Shock	20
Fever	<5
Symptoms	
Pain	99
Diffuse	40-50
Unilateral	33
Acute (<24 hr before presentation)	45-50
1 wk before presentation	30
>1 wk before presentation	25-30
Amenorrhea	65-80
Abnormal uterine or vaginal bleeding	70

is proved otherwise. Patients with a tubal pregnancy that ended in rupture usually present with a history of recurrent, sharp, fleeting pain that led to an episode of sudden, sharp, unilateral pain at rupture. Patients who have had a tubal abortion present with crampy, intermittent pain lasting over a longer time. Episodes of pain usually are accompanied by vaginal spotting or bleeding. Profuse bleeding is not common.

Diagnostic evaluation is based on the use of hemoglobin or hematocrit testing, quantitative beta-hCG level, ultrasonography, culdocentesis, and finally laparoscopy or laparotomy. A hematocrit level of less than 30 is seen in about 25% of patients with ectopic pregnancy. The use of serial quantitative beta-hCG tests can be helpful. Serum beta-hCG tests can be sensitive to 5 mIU/ml and may be positive 8 to 10 days after conception. A negative quantitative beta-hCG is essentially 100% accurate in ruling out a gestational cause for the pain or bleeding. In normal pregnancy the production of beta-hCG doubles every 2 days for the first 6 to 8 weeks of gestation; afterward, it takes about 4 days to double. After 48 hours, an increase of less than 66% from the initial beta-hCG level suggests an abnormal gestation: either an ectopic pregnancy or an abortion. The value of the beta-hCG test is also noted when it is used in conjunction with pelvic ultrasonography. At about 6 weeks' gestation the beta-hCG will be approximately 6500 mIU/ml. This level also correlates with the presence of a gestational sac on ultrasonography. A beta-hCG of 6500 mIU/ml and the absence of an intrauterine gestational sac are considered

diagnostic for an ectopic pregnancy. However, if transvaginal ultrasound is available and used, the cutoff for seeing a gestational sac is at a beta-hCG level of 2000 mIU/ml. After one ectopic pregnancy, the patient is at risk for more. All adolescents who have a history and physical examination suggestive of an ectopic pregnancy must have an immediate obstetrics/gynecology consultation.

Threatened or Spontaneous Abortion

The incidence of threatened or spontaneous abortion among adolescents is not known. There are probably many adolescents who do not seek medical care for missed periods with subsequent vaginal spotting, bleeding, and eventual resumption of menstruation. The causes of spontaneous abortion are multiple and may be related to the fetus, the mother, or the father. It has been estimated that about 150 of every 1000 pregnancies will result in spontaneous abortion, with 60% related to chromosomal aberrations in the fetus.[14] Besides chromosomal aberrations, factors such as maternal infections, malnutrition, ABO incompatibility, and maternal cigarette or alcohol use may play a role in spontaneous abortion.

Abortions occur in four clinical stages: threatened, inevitable, incomplete, and complete. A patient with threatened abortion presents with slight vaginal spotting and abdominal cramping that may subside in 1 to 2 days or may worsen over the course of 1 to 2 weeks. No changes occur in the cervix with a threatened abortion. A patient with inevitable abortion presents with more severe bleeding and cramping. Fetal tissue may be passed in the form of clots. The cervix effaces and dilates, with subsequent bulging of fetal membranes. A patient with incomplete abortion usually presents at 8 to 14 weeks' gestation with severe cramping and bleeding. The bleeding may lead to anemia and may result in shock or even death. A complete abortion usually occurs in the first 6 weeks of gestation or after week 16. The uterus is completely evacuated of fetal and placental tissue.

Missed abortion, which is classified separately, involves retention of the products of conception for longer than 8 weeks after fetal death. A patient with missed abortion usually presents in the early part of the second trimester. The presentation is most similar to that of a threatened abortion without the signs and symptoms of pregnancy. Patients who have a history and physical examination consistent with a spontaneous abortion should receive a consultation with an obstetrician.

Pregnancy-Induced Hypertension, Preeclampsia, and Eclampsia

Disturbances of blood pressure (BP) are common in pregnancy, abnormalities ranging from mild to severe. Various reports estimate the incidence of PIH in adolescents to be 10% to 30% (compared with 6% to 10% in adults). Eighty-five percent of the cases occur in primigravidas. Although the cause of PIH is unknown, the pathophysiology involves a generalized arteriolar vasoconstriction that especially affects the uterus, kidneys, and central nervous system.

PIH is defined as BP of more than 140/90, or a rise in systolic BP of more than 30 or a rise in diastolic BP of more than 15 after week 24 of gestation. Mild preeclampsia is PIH in association with persistent proteinuria and edema. Severe preeclampsia includes PIH, proteinuria, edema, and one or more of the following: systolic BP more than 160 mm Hq, diastolic BP more than 110 mm Hq, elevated liver function test results, thrombocytopenia, oliguria, pulmonary edema, abdominal pain, and coma. Clonus also may be present. Management of PIH varies from bed rest at home with frequent BP checks and urine dipsticks for mild cases to hospitalization for more severe cases. The use of an antihypertensive (e.g., hydralazine) and an anticonvulsant (e.g., magnesium sulfate) may be necessary. In severe cases, the precipitation of a premature delivery may be necessary. Once the infant is delivered, resolution of the presenting signs and symptoms will occur over a period of days to a few weeks.

Premature Delivery

Adolescents under 15 years of age have a higher risk of premature delivery (before 37 weeks) and delivery of infants with LBW (<2500 g). Black adolescents in this age group have the highest neonatal mortality rate, almost double the national average of 7.6 in 1000 live births. Young adolescents are also more likely to have infants who are born weighing less than 2500 g (14% of births to teenagers vs. 6% of births to women aged 25 to 29).[15,16]

The association between young age at pregnancy and perinatal outcome is not necessarily related to biologic factors. Demographic and social variables also play a significant role in determining the pregnancy risk for the adolescent. The factors associated with premature delivery and/or LBW infants are shown in Box 142-2. Of note is the fact that there does not appear to be an increased risk for premature delivery in adolescents who have had previous abortions in the first trimester unless the cervix is damaged. With early and comprehensive prenatal care, the risk for premature delivery or LBW infants among adolescents is greatly reduced. Some studies have shown that with repeat teenage pregnancy there is an increased risk of neonatal mortality and LBW infants. Other studies have noted similar rates of LBW infants despite the interval between pregnancies.

The increased risk of premature delivery and neonatal morbidity and mortality has consequences for both the adolescent and society. Premature newborns have an

---

BOX 142-2
Risk Factors for Premature Delivery

Delayed prenatal care
Inadequate prenatal care
African-American race
Lower socioeconomic class
Low prepregnancy weight
Anemia
Smoking
Narcotic use/abuse
Primigravida
Poor nutrition
Obstetric history including any of the following:
   Multiple gestations
   Premature cervical dilation
   Previous preterm delivery
   Previous second trimester abortion or pregnancy
     loss

---

increased number of health problems, and they require longer hospitalization, often in intensive care units. This is psychologically costly to the adolescent and economically costly to the adolescent and society. The increased time and care required by premature infants may make the adjustment to motherhood even more difficult for the adolescent. Adequate social and medical supports are necessary to help the adolescent adjust to the role of mother.

Effects of Illicit Drugs, Medications, and Cigarettes

The need to obtain a complete drug history of a pregnant adolescent cannot be overemphasized. Such a history has important implications for the mother's health—increased risk of complications, effects on fetal development, and effects on the health of the newborn. Even when there is no such history, the healthcare provider must counsel the adolescent about the risks of drug use in pregnancy. All too often physicians fail to explore this area adequately and appropriately. When a positive history of abuse is found, difficulties often arise. For example, many drug detoxification centers will not accept pregnant women or adolescents. The pregnant adolescent who is a substance abuser presents a special challenge to the clinician, who is responsible for coordinating care directed toward both the drug abuse and the pregnancy.

Studies have estimated that 8% to 20% of women of childbearing age report use of an illicit drug within the previous month.[17,18] One survey of 36 hospitals, both public and private, reported that 11% of women undergoing delivery had used illicit substances at some point during their pregnancy.[19] A study by Almaro et al[20] reported on substance use by 253 pregnant adolescents. Within the preceding year, 65% had used alcohol, 41% marijuana, and 17% cocaine. The percentages decreased during pregnancy but are still alarming, with 52% using alcohol, 32% marijuana, and 14% cocaine.[19] With self-reports and drug screening used, studies focusing on drug use among pregnant adolescents have shown prevalence rates of 11% to 32%.[20,21]

All substances or medications that cross the placenta pose a potential risk to the fetus. The newborn is at risk from any drugs transmitted through the breast milk. Despite the fact that most substance-abusing mothers do not breast-feed their babies, they should be counseled regarding the hazards of drug use. Some young mothers are willing to obtain drug counseling during pregnancy for the sake of the infant.

The use of tobacco by an adolescent during pregnancy is an important consideration. Although the prevalence of smoking among the general population has declined over the past 20 years, smoking among older female adolescents has increased. One study reported that 35% of adolescents between 12 and 19 years of age who gave birth during a 5-year period reported that they smoked during the pregnancy.[22] It has been shown that smoking during pregnancy can cause intrauterine growth retardation, increased risk of spontaneous abortion, and premature delivery. The prenatal care of the adolescent who smokes should include education about the harmful effects that smoking may have on the developing fetus.

Many medications commonly used should be avoided by the pregnant adolescent. Because of potential harm to the developing fetus, medications such as aspirin, sodium bicarbonate, amino glycoside antibiotics, metronidazole, tetracycline, doxycycline, diazepam, phenytoin, and retinoic acid should be avoided. Table 142-4 lists illicit substances and other drugs that have been shown to have a negative effect on the fetus or the newborn.

TABLE 142-4
Teratogenic Drugs and Chemicals That Affect the Fetus

Drug	Effect
Alcohol	Fetal alcohol syndrome: IUGR, mental retardation, craniofacial abnormalities (microcephaly, cleft palate, micrognathia), cardiac defects
Tobacco	IUGR, high risk of spontaneous abortion or premature delivery
Marijuana	Chromosomal breaks, IUGR, irritability, restlessness, poor feeding
Heroin/methadone	IUGR, high risk of hepatitis, HIV exposure; neonatal abstinence syndrome: irritability, tremors, vomiting, high-pitched cry, hypertonicity, hyperactivity, seizures and sweating
Cocaine	High risk of spontaneous abortion, premature delivery, abruptio placentae, IUGR; neurobehavioral changes: irritability, tremulousness, lethargy, inappropriate response to stimulation; poor feeding
LSD (lysergic acid diethylamide)	Hydrocephalus, myelomeningocele, spina bifida
PCP (phencyclidine)	Teratogenicity; neonatal withdrawal syndrome
Amphetamines	Limb deformities, biliary atresia; neonatal withdrawal syndrome
Antacids	Malformations
Antibiotics	
Acyclovir	Safety unclear
Aminoglycosides	Ototoxicity
Cephalosporins	No definite risks
Erythromycin	Safe
Erythromycin estolate	High risk of cholestatic hepatitis in mother
Isoniazid	Safety unclear
Metronidazole	Chromosomal damage
Penicillin	Safe
Sulfonamides	Displaces bilirubin from albumin; may cause kernicterus if used late in pregnancy
Tetracycline	Limb deformities and tooth staining
Anticonvulsants	
Carbamazepine	Risks unknown
Diazepam	Cleft lip
Phenobarbital	Learning difficulties
Phenytoin	IUGR < cardiac defects, craniofacial abnormalities, limb deformities
Aspirin	Hydrocephalus, cardiac defects
Phenothiazines	Cleft palate, cardiac, hypospadias, clubfoot
Retinoic acid	Craniofacial and cardiac malformations

IUGR, intrauterine growth retardation.

ELECTIVE ABORTIONS

The choice of having an elective abortion is a difficult one for adolescents, their families, the medical community, and society. Accurate data on adolescent abortions are difficult to obtain owing to the variable statistics from each state. Abortion ratios (number of legal abortions per 1000 live births) and abortion rates (number of legal abortions per 1000 women aged 15 to 44) increased from 1970 to 1980, but they remained relatively stable in the 1980s and early 1990s. In 1992, 1,359,145 legal abortions in women aged 15-44 were reported to the CDC.[23] The true number of abortions is higher, since it does not include abortions obtained by adolescents under 15 years of age. Up to 50% of unintended pregnancies end in abortion. Studies comparing those adolescents who choose abortion over childbearing show that they are younger, Caucasian, still in school, and in appropriate grade levels.[24]

Appropriate counseling must be offered to the adolescent who is considering an abortion. All pregnancy options must be discussed, including the possibility of adoption. Parental consent and notification laws as they pertain to a particular state must be reviewed. With younger adolescents, encouragement and assistance with involving the parent(s) or another adult family member in the decision-making process is crucial. The estimated gestational age is an important factor in guiding the adolescent and her family in the timing of decisions. Obviously the earlier the adolescent is in her pregnancy, the less is the urgency in making a quick decision. See Chapter 144, "Abortion," for a detailed discussion.

PSYCHOSOCIAL ISSUES IN PREGNANCY

The impact of the pregnancy often depends on both the chronologic age and the developmental stage of the adolescent. The girl's family, the infant's father, and the father's family may be devastated. The availability of support systems at home, in school, and in the community is an important factor in determining how the adolescent and her family cope with the pregnancy and make decisions about it.

The adolescent may be afraid to reveal the pregnancy to a parent. She may feel alone, scared, depressed, or angry. In some instances she may be in a state of denial. Other adolescents may be happy with the diagnosis. Their reasons for wanting to become pregnant are varied. The adolescent who feels alone or abandoned by family or friends may see a baby as a way to gain love and attention. She may have a sister or a friend with a new baby, and may want to mimic that person's behavior. There may be pressure from a boyfriend to become pregnant. Since adolescents vary widely in their response to the diagnosis of pregnancy, it is common clinical practice to impart this information in person rather than by phone.

Whether the pregnancy was desired or not does not diminish the need for adequate support systems. If the adolescent elects to continue the pregnancy to term, she needs emotional and physical support from her family. The biologic father may or may not be involved, either emotionally or financially. Lack of support from the father places an additional burden on the pregnant adolescent and her family. The type and level of support from the family, the father, and friends is often related to the extent to which they agree with the adolescent's decision to continue the pregnancy. Ideally, this decision has been made with the support and advice of the family and with the aid of nonjudgmental counseling from her clinician.

Family and friends may respond to the news of the pregnancy in various ways; some feel hurt or angry; others are joyous. Friends may be either supportive or distant at this crucial time. Regardless of these reactions, the adolescent and her family both need support to face the emotional turmoil and the difficulty in making decisions about the pregnancy. After these decisions have been made, the adolescent will need follow-up to ensure compliance with prenatal and postnatal care or postabortion counseling and subsequent family planning.

Pregnancy may have a dramatic effect on an adolescent's education. In some school systems, pregnant adolescents are asked to leave school for the duration of the pregnancy. Other schools have developed separate sites designed for them to continue their education. These schools often provide specialized education and support in the areas of prenatal care, child care, and child development; some even have nurseries. Such schools have been very successful in helping pregnant adolescents to continue their education. This type of support is important for many adolescents, since they tend to view the pregnancy as an end to education. Adolescent parents, both young women and young men, may not continue school for economic reasons. Hence, vocational counseling and job training are important so that the new parents can support themselves and their infant. It has been found that some teenage girls who drop out of school often resume their education when their children are toddlers and their lives have become more stable.

The role of the infant's father should not be overlooked. Unfortunately, the father often takes no responsibility for the pregnancy and abandons the girl; this may be devastating to her. However, many young fathers do choose to be involved in the pregnancy. If the pregnant adolescent approves, the father should be welcomed as a participant in prenatal care settings. In some areas of the United States, nearly half of the fathers of infants born to minor mothers are over 21 years old. The relationship between the mother and the father of the infant needs to be explored carefully to rule out unlawful intercourse, rape, or incest. Some young couples may decide to marry as a result of the pregnancy; for them, counseling may be helpful. A marriage that is based on the pregnancy alone is not usually long-lasting.

POSTNATAL FOLLOW-UP

The completion of pregnancy results in many physiologic and psychologic changes. Many factors play a role in how the adolescent recovers from childbirth. It is important to have early and comprehensive follow-up so that both immediate and long-term needs are met. Complications during pregnancy, the difficulty and length of labor, the type of delivery, blood loss or complications during delivery, the health of the newborn, the method of feeding the newborn, the temperament of the newborn, and sleep and feeding schedules are all issues to be considered and addressed in follow-up care.

The length of hospital stay for delivery varies according to the hospital, the obstetrician, and sometimes the insurance coverage. However, vaginal deliveries typically require 1 to 3 days in the hospital, and cesarean sections require 3 to 5 days. Any complications involving the mother or the newborn may add extra days to the hospital stay. The time of hospitalization offers an opportunity to ensure that the adolescent understands basic infant care and proper feeding methods, and knows when to call the pediatrician for illness in the infant and when to contact the obstetrician about illness or complications related to her own health. Follow-up appointments for the mother and the infant should be made before discharge. Many centers that have comprehensive adolescent obstetrics clinics have special appointment times for combined follow-up of mother and newborn. The centralization of services appears to help with compliance in follow-up appointments. Medical and counseling services also should be available in these settings.

The first follow-up appointment should take place 2 weeks after discharge from the hospital. The purpose of this visit is to make sure that the mother or the infant have no medical or psychologic problems. The infant usually receives a brief examination at this time. In general, the mother is not examined during this visit unless there are specific problems or unless suture/staple removal is required because of cesarean section. Again, issues related to care of the infant, recovery of the mother, and adjustment of the adolescent to her role as a mother are discussed. At 6 to 8 weeks a complete physical examination of the mother, including a pelvic examination, is performed. By this time the anatomic changes in the vagina, cervix, and uterus associated with the pregnancy should be resolved. The vagina usually returns to normal size by the third postpartum week. Lactating mothers may have a thin, pale vaginal epithelium with diminished rugation during the nursing period. The cervix will continue to show some increased vascularity, glandular hypertrophy, and hyperplasia for about 7 to 10 days and then slowly return to normal by 6 weeks. The uterus returns to its normal size over the course of about 6 weeks, changing from a weight of approximately 1000 g to 50 to 100 g.

The return of menses depends on whether the mother is nursing. In lactating mothers, elevated prolactin levels suppress ovulation for up to 4 to 6 months. Prolactin levels remain elevated for about 6 weeks and then decrease to normal levels; however, transient elevations are associated with feedings. In lactating women, the appearance of the first postpartum menses varies, depending on the duration of nursing. In nonlactating women, prolactin levels fall to prepregnancy levels in 3 to 4 weeks, and the first menses usually occurs 6 to 9 weeks post partum. Clinicians should be aware that in both nursing and nonnursing mothers the first menses may be delayed because of another intrauterine pregnancy. It is important to note that breast-feeding does not necessarily protect against a repeat pregnancy.

Postpartum complications or complaints may arise before the first follow-up visit. In adolescent patients, the most common complaint is vaginal bleeding and/or discharge. Lochia, which is normal, is mild vaginal bleeding that is initially bright red, then becomes light brown, and slowly diminishes 2 to 3 weeks after a vaginal delivery (3 to 4 weeks after a cesarean section). The adolescent should be reassured that lochia is to be expected but advised against using tampons at this time owing to the risk of toxic shock syndrome (see Chapter 70, "Toxic Shock Syndrome"). Appropriate warnings must be given about excessive bleeding, prolonged heavy bleeding, continued bright-red bleeding, fever, pain, abdominal tenderness, malaise, or foul-smelling lochia.

Endometritis may occur after either vaginal or cesarean delivery. Risk factors include prolonged rupture of membranes (i.e., more than 12 to 24 hours), anemia, multiple vaginal examinations during labor and delivery, and a history of infection just before or during delivery. The cause of endometritis is usually cervical or vaginal flora. Leukocytosis may be present, but a white blood cell count above 20,000 may be seen normally in the postpartum female. Prognosis is good if treatment is begun early. Complications include the development of a pelvic abscess. Wound infections may occur after an episiotomy or a cesarean section. Risk factors include diabetes, obesity, poor nutrition, poor hygiene, immunosuppressant therapy, prolonged operating time, or emergency delivery. Instructions on wound care must be given, and the signs and symptoms of infection explained to the patient. Mastitis is a possible complication in lactating mothers. It may develop during the hospital stay or later at home; in either situation it is usually caused by incomplete evacuation of the breast. The adolescent may present with fever, localized breast tenderness, erythema, induration, or frank abscess.

Prolonged or excessive hemorrhaging also may occur. Typical blood loss from a vaginal delivery is 500 ml; with a cesarean section, the loss is 1000 ml. Excessive loss of blood is usually related to delayed or incomplete contraction of the myometrium after delivery or in association with uterine atony. Risk factors include uterine overdistention, prolonged or dysfunctional labor, infection (chorioamnionitis), cervical/vaginal laceration, incomplete placental separation, retained placental fragments, uterine rupture, and coagulopathy. Again, the adolescent must be cautioned about continued heavy bleeding or ongoing bright-red bleeding. Questions about postpartum bleeding should be addressed at the 2-week check-up.

Other possible postpartum complications include backache, hemorrhoids, pubic separation, vaginitis, cervicitis, and urinary tract infection.

Since family planning counseling needs to be part of postpartum care, contraceptive options should be discussed with the adolescent. Appropriate contraception; proper use of contraceptive methods; and counseling and education through schools, health centers, physicians, and the community will provide the foundation for preventing repeat pregnancies. Just as comprehensive care by an interdisciplinary team helps to create the right setting for prenatal care, comprehensive and convenient family planning services are necessary to reduce the number of undesired repeat pregnancies.

References

1. Centers for Disease Control: *Teenage pregnancy and birth rates—United States, 1990, MMWR* 42:3, 1993.
2. Hatcher RA, et al: *Contraceptive technology*, ed 16 (revised), New York, 1994, Irvington.
3. Goldenberg R, Klerman L: Adolescent pregnancy—another look, *N Engl J Med* 332:1161, 1995.
4. Alan Guttmacher Institute: *Teenage pregnancy: the problem that hasn't gone away*, New York, 1981, Alan Guttmacher Institute.
5. Henshaw SK, Kenney AM, Somberg D, Van Vort J: *Teenage pregnancy in the United States: the scope of the problem and state responses*, New York, 1989, Alan Guttmacher Institute.
6. Henshaw SK, Van Vort J: Teenage abortion, birth and pregnancy statistics: an update, *Fam Plann Perspect* 21:85, 1989.
7. Jones EF, Forrest J, Goldman N, Henshaw SK, Lincoln R, Rosoff J, Westoff C, Wulf D: *Teenage pregnancy in industrialized countries*, New Haven, CT, 1986, Yale University Press.
8. Hayes C, editor: *Risking the future: adolescent sexuality, pregnancy and childbearing*, vol 1, Washington, DC, 1987, National Academy Press.
9. Elster A, Kuznets N: *AMA guidelines for adolescent preventive services (GAPS)*, Baltimore, 1994, Williams & Wilkins.
10. Blum RW, Resnick MD, Stark T: Factors associated with the use of court bypass by minors to obtain abortions, *Fam Plann Perspect* 22:158, 1990.
11. Worthington EL, Larson DB, Lyons JS, Brubaker MW, Colecchi CA, Berry JT, Morrow D: Mandatory parental involvement prior to adolescent abortion, *J Adolesc Health Care* 12:138, 1991.
12. Crosby MC, English A: Mandatory parental involvement/judicial bypass laws: do they promote adolescents' health?, *J Adolesc Health Care* 12:143, 1991.
13. Centers for Disease Control: Ectopic pregnancy in the United States 1970-1987, CDC surveillance summaries, *MMWR* 39:9, 1990.
14. Boué J, Boué A, Lozar P: Retrospective and prospective epidemiological studies of 1500 karyotyped spontaneous human abortions, *Teratology* 12:11, 1975.
15. Santelli JS, Jacobson MS: Birth weight outcomes for repeat teenage pregnancy, *J Adolesc Health Care* 11:240, 1990.
16. Slap GB, Schwartz JS: Risk factors for low birth weight to adolescent mothers, *J Adolesc Health Care* 10:267, 1989.
17. *NIDA household survey of drug abuse 1988, population estimates, ADM 89-1636*, Rockville, MD, 1989, National Institute of Drug Abuse, Department of Health and Human Services.
18. Chasnoff IJ, Landress H, Barrett M: The prevalence of illicit drug or alcohol use during pregnancy and discrepancies in mandatory reporting in Pinellas County, Florida, *N Engl J Med* 332:1202, 1990.
19. Chasnoff IJ: Drug use and women: establishing a standard of care, *Ann N Y Acad Sci* 562:208, 1989.
20. Amaro H, Zuckerman B, Cabral H: Drug use among adolescent mothers: a profile of risk, *Pediatrics* 84:144, 1989.
21. Kokotailo PK, Adger H, Joffe A, et al: Substance use by pregnant adolescents: prevalence, detection, and associated risk factors, Presented at the 17th Annual Research Meeting of the Society for Adolescent Medicine, Atlanta, March 1990.
22. Davis RL, Tollestrup K, Milham S: Trends in teenage smoking during pregnancy: Washington State: 1984-1988, *Am J Dis Child* 144:1297, 1990.
23. Centers for Disease Control: Abortion surveillance: preliminary data—United States, 1992, *MMWR* 43, 1994.
24. Cartoof V: Adolescent abortion: correlates and consequences, *Adolesc Med STARS* 3:2, 1992.

CHAPTER 143

Adolescent Parenthood

•

Linda Juszczak

Adolescent parenthood and its impact on the young parents and their child is a phenomenon that has been described in public health statistics, national surveys, and research studies dealing with early childbearing and its consequences. The data suggest multiple negative outcomes for these young parents and their offspring. In 1993 the birth rate in the 15- to 17-year-old age group was 37.8 per 1000.[1] This was a decline after the rate had steadily increased from 1986 to 1991. The financial costs of this problem can be substantial, as exemplified by the total of $21.5 billion spent by the federal government in 1989 for welfare programs designed to support families started by teenagers.[2] The impact of adolescent childbearing on young parents, their children, their families, and the public has made efforts to ameliorate the effects of this event a high priority for healthcare professionals, educators, employers, and public policy makers alike.

Although this chapter focuses on the consequences of teenage parenthood and efforts to reduce its negative effects on the young parents, primary prevention remains the most effective intervention. Clinicians need to concentrate their efforts on prevention of teenage pregnancies through encouragement of abstinence, delayed sexual activity, and use of contraceptives. The goal is postponement of the pregnancy and parenting experience until the individual has reached his or her own physical, emotional, and vocational maturity, thereby reducing the risks of a negative outcome.

IMPACT ON ADOLESCENT MOTHER

Early motherhood has effects on the educational, vocational, psychosocial, marital, and subsequent childbearing future of the adolescent. The adolescent mother is more likely than her nonparenting peers to come from a disadvantaged background. Although differences such as race, socioeconomic status, and family background influence the attainment of educational and economic goals, there is a negative effect independent of these factors that results from too early childbearing.

Educational, Vocational, and Financial Impact

The most immediate and obvious sequela of pregnancy is the interruption of schooling. Pregnancy is one of the most common reasons girls cite for failing to complete high school. Previous academic difficulties may play a role in the pregnant teenager's decision to drop out of school, but the importance of this factor is unclear. It has been noted that these adolescents are more likely to have had educational difficulty and low vocational aspirations and to have engaged in more problem behaviors than those who have not become parents.[3]

After the birth of their infant, many young mothers express the desire to return to school, but limited options for child care and other factors prevent them from doing so. Although there has been an increase in the number of young mothers completing high school in the past decade (as high as 75% in some groups), being black, disadvantaged, and younger in age at first birth continue to be risk factors for dropping out.[4] Although young mothers may return to school and make progress in their education, they often do not catch up completely with their peers. As a whole, the number of years that these young women would otherwise spend in school—high school, college, and graduate school—are abbreviated compared with those of their peers who delay childbearing until adulthood.[4-6]

Closely related to a disruption in education are the often decreased employment opportunities open to adolescent mothers. With decreased education come poor job skills, less job satisfaction, and overall dismal prospects in the employment market. Adolescent mothers, who are likely to come from a background of poverty, are also likely to remain in poverty. They perpetuate the cycle and turn to public assistance, which does not seem to serve as an economic incentive to childbearing but as a means of subsistence. Forty-two percent of all families receiving Aid to Families with Dependent Children at any given time were begun by a mother who was under 20 when she gave birth.[7] Many of these young women are unmarried and dependent on their families for support. In some cases their families also may be financially stressed. The baby's father, although he may be in social contact with the mother, is rarely a source of significant financial support.

Family Relationships and Psychologic Impact

Parenthood during adolescence is associated with a disruption of social and emotional growth in all but the most exceptional cases. Young mothers are vulnerable not only to education and financial problems but also to difficulties with their families, social relationships, and parenting skills. At a time in their life when independence, identity formation, development of future plans, and establishment of social relationships are tasks that they are trying to achieve, the competing demands of parenthood create an additional set of stressors.

Those parenting adolescents who remain in the family home are more likely to offset the negative effects of too early childbearing. They are more likely to stay in school and advance economically than those who choose to move out of their home or are forced to do so.[8] The family can provide important support to the young mother by offering parenting role models, childcare help, and emotional and financial assistance, thus making her transition to adult parenthood somewhat easier. Remaining in the family, however, may present an additional set of stressors. For example, the adolescent's parenting style and new role in relation to her elders and her siblings may result in problems. For adolescents who are struggling to achieve independence from the family, parenthood often does not provide the release they might have imagined. Their dependency on the family may be increased by their financial and childcare needs. In addition, their attempts to take control of decision making for their child may be thwarted by parents who do not trust them or feel that they "know better." On the other hand, the adolescent's attempts to relinquish childcare duties can be met by reminders that the child is her responsibility. The young mother's attempts to sever or maintain relationships with the child's father may be dictated by the family's anger toward him. The father's contact with the mother and the child may be prohibited. Alternatively, because of family pressure, demands on his involvement may increase, despite the wishes of the mother.

Clinicians who work with young mothers need to be aware that to provide care for these young mothers and their infants they must address the often conflicting advice being given in the family. It is usually advisable to meet with the adolescent mother and other significant decision makers and caregivers together so that workable solutions can be devised to reduce stress. The goal is to foster the adolescent's own development as well as her mothering role.

Although there is scant empirical evidence to support a high incidence of mental health problems among adolescent mothers, the mental health needs of this population are of great concern. Young mothers are identified as at high risk not only for diminished future potential—in education, employment, and income earning—but also for a host of mental health problems, including depression, anxiety, psychosomatic complaints, substance use, and family difficulties. Adolescent mothers may be more likely to exhibit problems with postpartum affective disorders, impaired maternal sensitivity and responsiveness, and poor social support.[9] Postpartum teenagers with high stress and conflict and low levels of support should be considered at high risk for depressive symptoms.[10] Since they often deny the effects of early parenthood on their life plans, it may be difficult for the clinician to engage them in counseling. The denial may be a result of obstacles that seem insurmountable and a lack of orientation toward the future. However, over time, as a sense of trust is established between the clinician and the adolescent, counseling may become possible. Counseling services need to be presented in a nonthreatening, concrete manner and directed toward the achievement of realistic goals.

Marital Stability and Subsequent Childbearing

It is increasingly uncommon for adolescents to elect to marry in order to legitimize a pregnancy. This trend is associated with significant deterioration in the well-being of young mothers and their children; for example, families in which the fathers are officially absent are far more likely to be poor than are married couples. Even so, adolescent marriages are generally identified as highly unstable, and they frequently end in separation and divorce. Many of those who remain married report having severe marital problems. Teenagers who do marry are less likely to continue their education and are more likely to have a rapid repeat pregnancy than those who do not marry. Increased rates of marital instability, higher levels of completed fertility, and lower levels of educational attainment make these young women at especially high risk for continued poverty.[11,12]

Subsequent pregnancies in adolescent mothers are a major concern: 20% of 15- to 17-year-olds have a repeat pregnancy within 2 years of the first birth, and 41% within 3 years. The rates are slightly higher for those under age 15.[13] Any assumption that the pregnancy and parenting experience and its effects will act as a deterrent to unprotected intercourse and repeat pregnancy is erroneous. Young mothers, like their nonparenting peers, need information about contraceptive methods, easy access to contraceptive services, and a wide array of support services to help them delay subsequent pregnancies until adulthood.

Interventions

There is evidence to suggest that over time many young mothers recover from the effects of too early parenthood, but there remains a significant proportion who do not do well.[3,14] Interventions designed to reduce the impact of early parenthood on young mothers should be comprehensive and interdisciplinary, offering a wide array of services—medical, social, psychologic, and health educational. They also should provide or have close ties with support services such as child care, public assistance, education, and vocational training.

Little is known about what is most beneficial to adolescent mothers. What constitutes a well-designed program and what effects are produced by separate service components are also unclear.[15] There are, however, promising interventions directed toward alleviating the effects of early parenthood. Quality child care that includes programming to address the young mother's deficits in knowledge of child development and parenting skills has the potential to benefit both mother and child.[16,17] Programs to increase the teenage mother's financial independence are also receiving attention. A demonstration welfare-to-work project showed that clear participation expectations and strong case management services can promote employment and earnings gains for young parents at a reasonable cost.[18]

The clinician needs to maintain an ongoing assessment of the impact of parenthood on the young mother, including her educational progress, financial status, family relationships, relationship with the child's father, childcare arrangements, mental health status, risk of repeat pregnancies, and needs for parenting education. The provider needs to develop strong working relationships with community resources available to these young mothers and to facilitate appropriate referrals for further assessment or service. Recognition of the magnitude of the challenge of teenage parenting and the need to address the many associated problem areas can be overwhelming to the individual provider. In fact, the needs of teenage mothers may be better served by a comprehensive program that is well supported by an interdisciplinary staff.

IMPACT ON ADOLESCENT FATHER

The impact of adolescent parenthood on the father is less dramatic than on the mother. Much less is known about teenage fathers and the consequences of fatherhood. In part, the differences stem from the young father's greater ease in walking away from the responsibility of parenthood, less opportunity to assume responsibility because of traditional beliefs that the woman is responsible for child care, and negative social sanctions against an unmarried father's participation in childcare responsibilities. Although the results are less severe, the teenage father does suffer negative effects on the realization of his educational, vocational, marital, and psychosocial potential. Adolescent fathers represent a much smaller group than do adolescent mothers. In 1988, 50% of 15- to 17-year-old mothers reported that the father of their child was age 20 or older, and 19.7% reported that the father was under age 18.[19] Their relatively small numbers, and their lack of willingness or opportunity to assume the father role, has made teenage fathers less of a priority than teenage mothers and their infants.

Educational, Vocational, and Financial Impact

Like the teenage mother, the teenage father is more likely than his peers who have postponed fatherhood to come from an economically disadvantaged environment and to have poor academic skills. Teenage fathers are more likely to drop out of school and to have lower income-earning potential than nonfathers. The cause-and-effect relationship between fatherhood and academic achievement is not clear; however, whether teenage fathers fail to complete schooling as a result of fatherhood or because they are unsuccessful in school and therefore look to other roles for achievement, these young men have academic, vocational, and income-earning difficulties before and after fatherhood. Teenage fatherhood, like teenage motherhood, reinforces the cycle of poverty and disadvantage. Even if teenage fathers are willing to contribute financially to the support of their partner and child, they are poorly prepared to do so.[20,21]

Involvement with Adolescent Mother

Falling marriage rates and increases in out-of-wedlock births combine to decrease the potential impact of early fatherhood on the young male. The extent to which the teenage father declines to accept responsibility for parenthood may minimize the effect of early paternity. He must decide whether marriage, living together outside of marriage, an even less formal arrangement, or no commitment at all is the degree of responsibility he is willing to accept. It has been noted that young men whose first child was conceived after marriage have the poorest high school completion rates.[20]

Although adolescent fathers are often absent from the household of their partner and child, many remain involved. Although the extent of an adolescent father's involvement is highly variable, the picture of a father who is unconcerned or uncaring is not typical. A father's active involvement in prenatal care and labor and delivery has been reported as a predictor of later involvement with the children of teenage mothers.[22] The young father is often in prolonged social contact with the mother and the child. Even though he is rarely a significant source of child care or financial assistance, he often reports strong emotional ties to the mother and the child and concern for their welfare. Owing to ignorance, denial, or refusal to accept the responsibilities of parenthood, a minority of fathers do not admit paternity.[21]

Early fatherhood is often a catalyst for change in the adolescent's relationships. If the father chooses to marry or to live with the mother and the child, he may be faced with premature emancipation from his family. On the other hand, he may have increased dependence on his own family if they continue to be involved and want to share in the responsibility. Like the adolescent mother, the father can be caught in a conflict between the competing role requirements of adolescence and fatherhood. He also is often faced with conflicts in his relationships with the family of the mother as well as with his own family. Many young fathers report difficulty in dealing with the anger and demands of their partners' families. Some common concerns are the health of the mother and the child, the need to find a job that will allow the fathers to contribute financially, completing school, maintaining their personal freedom, and learning to behave as a father. A young father often may question the paternity of the child he has been told is his. This uncertainty may be justified, or it may be an expression of his ambivalence about accepting a responsibility he is ill equipped to meet.

Child Support

The issue of formal establishment of paternity and child support for the children of teenage mothers is receiving renewed interest. The long-term financial outlook for the adolescent mother and her infant remains poor, and it is reasonable to assume that the burden of premature childbearing should not be hers alone. The solution is not the prosecution of young men who are unable to meet their responsibility, however, and creative solutions to this dilemma are beginning to appear. Linking enforcement of child support with educational and training opportunities as well as training in parenting skills is one promising trend.[21]

The benefits of the formal establishment of paternity may outweigh the young father's and the clinician's fear of establishing child support. The benefits to the child include access to the father's future resources, including employment and social security benefits, and to family history, with the potential for establishment of familial ties. For the teenage father the benefits include establishment of his legal rights and a possible psychosocial benefit for both him and the child.[23] Young fathers and clinicians alike are often woefully uninformed on issues related to the official child support system. The knowledgeable clinician can offer support and information to

the young father regarding his rights and responsibilities under the law.

Interventions

Programs designed to lessen the impact of teenage parenthood need to include services for teenage fathers. All aspects of service delivery should encourage the involvement of the fathers and foster the feeling that they have an important contribution to make to the social, emotional, and financial well-being of their offspring. Like teenage mothers, teenage fathers need access to job training services, education in child care, and contraceptive services. Aggressive efforts are needed to recruit teenage fathers into service programs. Providers need to be sensitive to meeting the needs of a population whose involvement in fathering is highly variable. In addition, young fathers need assistance with their own problems as well as help in caring for and supporting their children.

IMPACT ON CHILD

The impact of early parenthood on the children of adolescents echoes the themes of the effects of too early childbearing on young parents. In an extensive review of the literature, Hofferth[24] concluded that the children of young parents are at greater risk than their peers for a variety of health, social, and economic problems. The strongest evidence for these differences is indirect—a result of coming from a disadvantaged environment, where lower socioeconomic status, less stable family structure, larger family size, and less educational attainment are more likely.[24,25] There is less evidence to support the idea that the long-term problems for these children are a result of having young mothers, who are not well equipped emotionally to become parents and not experienced in parenting.

Health and Medical Consequences

There is an increased risk of poor pregnancy outcomes among adolescent mothers. The risk of having low-birthweight babies is higher for adolescent mothers than for older mothers, and this risk increases with younger age of the mother.[26] The infants of adolescent mothers have been reported to have higher rates of mortality and morbidity, including accidents, burns, poisoning, and superficial injury.[27,28] These reductions in the optimal health appear to relate less to the age of the young mother and more to health and environmental factors. In special hospital populations that receive quality prenatal and postnatal care, there seems to be little difference in perinatal outcomes, and the provision of adequate medical care continues to reduce the environmental influence on children's health over the first year of life.[24]

Psychosocial Development

Assessment of the risk of developmental, cognitive, and social problems among the children of young parents includes evaluating the impact of social and environmental factors, and the influence of the potential conflict between the developmental tasks of adolescents and the responsibilities of parenthood. In general, children of adolescent mothers are at a developmental disadvantage compared with children of older mothers. Results of studies show a negative effect on intelligence scores, cognitive tests, retention in grade, and parental and teacher evaluations of performance. In addition, adverse effects on the socioemotional development of these children have been noted, but these appear to be weak (e.g., mild behavior disorders). Small but consistent differences in cognitive functioning appear in early childhood and continue throughout the school years. Success in schooling increases with corresponding increased educational attainment by the mother. Which factors account for the cognitive and socioemotional developmental outcomes for the children of teenage mothers is unclear. However, the results appear to be indirect effects of adverse social and economic environments rather than being associated with the age of the mother per se.[24]

There is little evidence to support the idea that inadequate parenting on the part of teenage parents is the basis for the problems these children may develop. There are no significant differences in mothering behaviors at birth among mothers of different ages. Although teenage mothers may be less knowledgeable about child development than older mothers, the differences are relatively small.[24] There is also no consistent relationship between the mother's age and child abuse and neglect.[29] The main reason for a link, if any exists, is the socioeconomic status of families; both adolescent parenthood and child abuse and neglect are more common among the disadvantaged.[24] Adolescent mothers who live apart from related adults may be at higher risk for maltreatment of their children.[30]

In summary, differences in the development of children of young parents exist, but the outcomes are not markedly different from those in children of older parents. The outcomes for children of the youngest parents may be slightly improved, which suggests that assistance from the extended family may ameliorate some of the adverse effects.

Long-Term Effects

Of great concern to clinicians who work with adolescent parents and their children are the long-term effects of too early childbearing. These children have been viewed as being at especially high risk for pregnancy and parenting once they reach adolescence. In fact, it is not uncommon to hear clinicians describe family units with grandparents in their early thirties, although there are relatively little data to support the assumption that too early childbearing will be repeated in subsequent generations. In a 22-year follow-up of children of teenage parents, it was found that although these children were not doing well in comparison with the children of older mothers (23% of the children of teenage parents dropped out of school, 17% were in correctional institutions, and 32% experienced symptoms of depression), the differences were not as great as might have been predicted, and two thirds of the daughters delayed their first birth until age 19 or later.[31] The authors did express concern that young women who became teenage parents might be less likely than their parents to overcome the handicaps associated with adolescent parenthood, thus perpetuating a cycle of poverty.

Interventions

Services directed toward improving the outcomes for the children of adolescent parents, like those for their parents, need to be based on the recognition that adolescent parenthood is a complex problem with numerous potential difficulties in the areas of health, development, education, and financial stability. Health and social service providers need to consider interventions that target teenage mothers and their infants for follow-up care. This care must directly address the provision of services for child care, child development, family support, and family health. The goals of these programs need to be long-term ones, aimed not only at improving the outcome for the adolescent mother but also at prevention of the cycle of premature childbearing into another generation.

References

1. National Center for Health Statistics: Advance report of final natality statistics, 1993, *Monogr Vital Stat Rep* (suppl) 44:3, 1995.
2. Armstrong E, Waszak C: *Teenage pregnancy and too early childbearing: public costs, personal consequences,* ed 5, Washington, DC, 1990, Center for Population Options.
3. Abrahamse AF, Morrison PA, Waite LJ: Teenagers willing to consider single parenthood: who is at greatest risk?, *Fam Plann Perspect* 20:1, 1988.
4. Upchurch DM, McCarthy J: Adolescent childbearing and high school completion in the 1980s: have things changed?, *Fam Plann Perspect* 21:5, 1989.
5. Hofferth S: Social and economic consequences of teenage childbearing. In Hofferth S, Hayes C, editors: *Risking the future: adolescent sexuality, pregnancy, and childbearing,* vol 2, *Working papers and statistical appendixes,* Washington, DC, 1987, National Academy Press.
6. Mott FL, Marsiglio W: Early childbearing and completion of high school, *Fam Plann Perspect* 17:5, 1985.

7. U.S. General Accounting Office: *Families on welfare: teenage mothers least likely to become self sufficient,* GAO/HEHS-94-115, Washington, DC, 1994, U.S. General Accounting Office.

8. Furstenburg F: Burdens and benefits: the impact of early childbearing on the family, *J Soc Issues* 36:1, 1980.

9. Trad PV: Mental health of adolescent mothers, *J Am Acad Child Adolesc Psychiatry* 34:2, 1995.

10. Barnet B, Joffe A, Duggan AK, Wilson MD, Repke JT: Depressive symptoms, stress, and social support in pregnant and postpartum adolescents, *Arch Pediatr Adolesc Med* 150:1, 1996.

11. Furstenburg F: The social consequences of teenage parenthood, *Fam Plann Perspect* 8:4, 1976.

12. Card JJ, Wise RR: Teenage mothers and teenage fathers: the impact of early childbearing on the parents' personal and professional lives, *Fam Plann Perspect* 10:4, 1978.

13. Pittman K, Adams G: *Teenage pregnancy: an advocate's guide to the numbers,* Washington, DC, 1988, Adolescent Pregnancy Prevention Clearinghouse.

14. Furstenberg FF: As the pendulum swings: teenage childbearing and social concern, *Fam Relat* 40:4, 1991.

15. Hayes C, editor: *Risking the future: adolescent sexuality, pregnancy, and childbearing,* Washington, DC, 1987, National Academy Press.

16. McAnarney ER, Lawrence RA: Day care and teenage mothers: nurturing the mother-child dyad, *Pediatrics* 91:1, 1993.

17. Furstenberg FF, Brooks-Gunn J, Chase-Lansdale L: Teenaged pregnancy and childbearing, *Am Psychol* 44:2, 1989.

18. Aber JL, Brooks-Gunn J, Maynard R: Effects of welfare reform on teenage parents and their children, *Future Child* 5:2, 1995.

19. Landry DJ, Forrest JD: How old are U.S. fathers?, *Fam Plann Perspect* 27:4, 1995.

20. Marsiglio W: Adolescent fathers in the United States: their initial living arrangements, marital experience and educational outcomes, *Fam Plann Perspect* 19:6, 1987.

21. Sullivan M: *The male role in teenage pregnancy and parenting: new directions for public policy,* New York, 1990, Vera Institute of Justice.

22. Cox JE, Bithoney WG: Fathers of children born to adolescent mothers: predictors of contact with their children at 2 years, *Arch Pediatr Adolesc Med* 149:8, 1995.

23. Savage B: *Child support and teen parents,* Washington, DC, 1987, Adolescent Pregnancy Prevention Clearinghouse.

24. Hofferth S: The children of teen childbearers. In Hofferth S, Hayes C, editors: *Risking the future: adolescent sexuality, pregnancy, and childbearing,* vol 2, *Working papers and statistical appendixes,* Washington, DC, 1987, National Academy Press.

25. Baldwin W, Cain V: The children of teenage parents, *Fam Plann Perspect* 12:1, 1980.

26. National Center for Health Statistics: Advance report of final natality statistics, 1982, *Monogr Vital Stat Rep* (suppl) 33:6, 1984.

27. Lawrence RA, Merritt TA: Infants of adolescent mothers: perinatal, neonatal and infancy outcome, *Semin Perinatol* 5:1, 1981.

28. Taylor B, Wadsworth J, Butler NR: Teenage mothering, admission to hospital, and accidents during the first five years, *Arch Dis Child* 58:1, 1983.

29. Massat CR: Is older better? Adolescent parenthood and maltreatment, *Child Welfare* 74:2, 1995.

30. Flanagan P, Coll CG, Andreozzi L, Riggs S: Predicting maltreatment of children of teenage mothers, *Arch Pediatr Adolesc Med* 149:4, 1995.

31. Furstenberg F, Levine JA, Brooks-Gunn J: The children of teenage mothers: patterns of early childbearing in two generations, *Fam Plann Perspect* 22:2, 1990.

CHAPTER 144

Abortion

•

Lynn Borgatta

INCIDENCE OF INDUCED ABORTION AMONG ADOLESCENTS

Adolescent women who become pregnant are more likely than older women to choose abortion. In the United States, most adolescent pregnancies are unintended and about half, more than 400,000 yearly, are terminated by abortion.

Birth rates to adolescent women have been declining for most of the twentieth century, with leveling of the rate in the 1980s. Abortion rates rose steadily in the 1970s after legalization in several large states and the *Roe v. Wade* Supreme Court decision. Rates stabilized in the 1980s and may be declining slightly. Therefore, the abortion ratio, the proportion of births terminated by abortion, has been stable or declining. Younger adolescents have lower pregnancy rates but higher abortion ratios. Pregnancy rates are higher in Hispanic and African-American women than in white women, higher in lower socioeconomic groups, and higher in older adolescents. Once pregnancy occurs, African-American women and white women are equally likely to choose abortion. Pregnant adolescents of high socioeconomic groups are more likely to choose abortion than to give birth. Consequently, the highest birth rates remain in minority women of low socioeconomic class.

Industrialized, high-income countries such as those in Western Europe, Canada, and Japan have pregnancy rates much lower than those in the United States. Abortion ratios are similar or lower in general; both birth and abortion rates are much lower than those in the United States. The major factor in the different rates appears to be the use of effective contraception, as rates of sexual activity are similar.

Half of all abortions occur among women who are not using any form of contraception. Adolescents are less likely than older women to use effective contraception, particularly in the first 6 months after initiation of sexual activity. Many young women feel or fear that they are infertile. Medical advice, including a previous negative pregnancy test or infection reduction counseling, may unwittingly reinforce this belief. Some women may seek pregnancy but realize after conception that conditions are not what they had anticipated; a relationship may end or family support may not materialize. The pregnancy may also have a desired effect of precipitating a family crisis or reorganization.

Adolescents also have higher rates of pregnancy than adults while using contraceptives. A higher failure rate of barrier methods of contraception is related to increased frequency of coitus, younger age, and unmarried marital status. Oral contraceptives also have a higher failure rate in adolescents than in older women. Postcoital contraceptives may be unfamiliar or inaccessible.

TERMINOLOGY

Induced abortion refers to termination of a pregnancy by medical or surgical intervention, as distinguished from *spontaneous abortion*. With the use of ultrasonography, abnormal pregnancies may be identified before the onset of spontaneous abortion. These pregnancies, which would result in spontaneous abortion without any intervention, may be included in induced abortion statistics.

Elective abortion may be chosen by a woman who does not want to continue a pregnancy for personal reasons, while some abortions are indicated because of fetal abnormality or risk to the woman's health. *Nontherapeutic abortion* refers to one induced by nonmedical people and includes self-induced abortions.

Techniques of induced abortion are used to terminate both normal and abnormal pregnancies, and are also used to treat spontaneous or incomplete abortion.

COUNSELING AND EDUCATION

Adolescents generally seek diagnosis later in pregnancy than do older women; reasons include denial, lack of access to care, and financial and confidentiality concerns. Some insurance plans may release records of medical visits to parents; thus, the adolescent must seek care on her own, without insurance, if she wishes to maintain confidentiality.

Once ectopic pregnancy and spontaneous abortion have been excluded as outcomes, three options remain. The pregnancy can continue with the baby accepted, it can continue with the baby released for adoption, or it can be terminated by induced abortion. The medical, socioeconomic, and psychologic outcomes of each path need consideration. Some women enter a counseling session with previous knowledge of the pregnancy and have already considered the options. Others may be uncertain of (or deny) the pregnancy or its impact, and require much more education and open-ended support. The younger adolescent may need more concrete and specific education and counseling than the older teenager, as well as more guidance and direction. Whether the counselor is a medical professional or a trained lay person, counseling should include discussion of the immediate situation as well as planning for future social and personal behavior.

PARENTAL INVOLVEMENT

Most adolescents voluntarily inform one or both parents about plans for abortion. The younger the adolescent, the more likely she is to notify a parent before making any contact with the healthcare system. Some young women will notify a parent if assistance in talking to the parent is offered. Some would rather make all arrangements without parental involvement, either because of fear of parental reaction or as an expression of personal responsibility.

In the United States, approximately half of the states have parental notification laws for women under 18 years of age. Where parental notification is in force, judicial bypass must be available for women who choose not to notify their parents. The effect of parental notification laws has generally been to increase the gestational age at which abortion occurs and to change the location of abortions to neighboring states. It is unclear how much effect such laws have on either the total number of abortions or family communication.

MEDICAL PREPARATION

Pregnancy must be confirmed by pregnancy testing or ultrasound examination. The size and location of the pregnancy and the position of the uterus need to be established. During the first trimester, menstrual history and physical examination are often sufficient. However, ultrasound should be used for confirmation if examination is difficult because of apprehension, obesity, or uterine position. Ultrasonography should always be used before second trimester termination.

Rh typing and anemia screening are indicated if previous results are not available. Rh-immune globulin should be given whenever an Rh-negative woman has a spontaneous or induced abortion.

SURGICAL ABORTION

Suction Abortion

The most common technique of abortion in the first trimester is suction abortion under local anesthesia by paracervical block. The cervix is grasped with a tenaculum or clamp to straighten the cervical canal. The cervix is dilated with graded metal dilators until sufficient dilation is attained or until resistance is encountered. A suction cannula appropriate for the size of the pregnancy is passed through the internal os of the cervix and attached to suction. The suction cannula is rotated to detach the placenta and decidual lining. At the end of the procedure, a sharp curette may be used to confirm completion, but excessive sharp curettage will increase the chance of trauma. A skilled operator can perform most early abortions in less than 10 minutes and with minimal blood loss (10 to 20 ml), but variations certainly occur.

Variations of Surgical Abortion

Menstrual extraction refers to early aspiration of the uterine contents, before 6 weeks, and does not require cervical dilation; early surgical abortion is a more accurate term. When early surgical abortion is performed, pregnancy tissue must be definitely identified, or the rate of continuing pregnancy will be higher than that with later procedures.

Cervical osmotic dilators absorb water after placement in the cervical canal, increasing their diameter and dilating the cervix over a number of hours. This technique results in greater dilation than could be safely achieved with graded mechanical dilators used for several minutes, and decreases the length of the operative procedure. Use of osmotic dilators during the first trimester is a matter of preference but is indicated for second trimester surgical abortion, which is usually termed dilation and evacuation (D&E). Depending on the size of the pregnancy, several or many osmotic dilators may be used. Multiple insertions of dilators allow more dilation than a single session; for

late second trimester pregnancies, dilation may take several days.

After adequate dilation has been achieved, the dilators are removed and counted and the amniotic sac is ruptured. The fetus and placenta are removed with tissue forceps and large-bore suction. Transabdominal ultrasound guidance is frequently used to direct the instruments.

D&E is the preferred method of abortion in the second trimester up to 16 weeks. After 16 weeks, the selection of technique may be determined by the facilities available and the expertise of the physician, as well as patient preference.

MEDICAL ABORTION

Currently, all medical abortions in the United States represent "off-label" use or clinical trials of the medications involved. Some of the procedures most commonly performed, which represent community standards of care, use medications that are not labeled as indicated for abortion by the Food and Drug Administration.

Almost all first trimester medical abortions in the United States have been done with mifepristone or methotrexate. Mifepristone (RU 486) is used widely in several European countries and has had clinical trials in the United States. This agent blocks progesterone-binding sites, resulting in placental separation in pregnancies of 9 weeks or less. Although a small percentage of women abort with mifepristone alone after 48 hours, administration of a prostaglandin such as misoprostol will result in abortion within 4 hours in about 75% of women. Of the women remaining, most will abort within the next 2 weeks, for an overall failure rate of 2% to 4%. In addition, a few women have incomplete abortions. In spring 1997, the FDA was considering approval of mifepristone.

The second method involves a single injection of the folic acid antagonist methotrexate, followed 5 to 7 days later by misoprostol. In contrast to mifepristone, the percentage of women who abort shortly after prostaglandin administration is much lower, with the majority of abortions occurring at home, and an overall abortion rate of 90% to 95% within 2 weeks.

During the second trimester, uterine contractions may be induced with several medications. In the United States, prostaglandin E_2 vaginal suppositories; intraamniotic infusion of prostaglandin, urea, or saline; intravenous oxytocin; and vaginal misoprostol have all been used. The interval from administration of drug to abortion may be as long as 48 hours, generally requiring hospitalization. A significant minority of women expel the fetus but not the placenta, necessitating surgical curettage.

In addition to the methods outlined above, there are many individual variations and combinations of techniques. For example, osmotic dilators may be employed before the use of prostaglandin in second trimester abortion.

FERTILITY AND CONTRACEPTION AFTER ABORTION

Ovulation may occur as early as 1 week after first trimester medical abortion, and usually occurs without delay after early abortion. After second trimester abortion, ovulation occurs 2 to 4 weeks later in most women. Women should be advised against vaginal sexual activity until the uterus has involuted and bleeding has stopped, which may take several days or several weeks. Resumption of sexual activity at that point without contraception may result in another pregnancy.

Barrier methods of contraception that do not require fitting, such as condoms, can be resumed immediately. Diaphragms and cervical caps can be fitted after several weeks when uterine involution is complete, although most women do not change size after an abortion. Hormonal contraception, including oral contraceptives, implants, and injections, may be started immediately after first trimester abortion. After late second trimester abortion, many clinicians delay estrogen use for 2 to 3 weeks, but progestin-only methods such as implants, injections, and progestin-only oral contraceptives may be started immediately.

First trimester suction abortion has not been shown to have an adverse effect on subsequent fertility, even when multiple procedures have been performed. First trimester medical abortion is also unlikely to have adverse consequences, but long-term studies have not been performed. Women seeking second trimester abortion are more likely to have other characteristics associated with risk for infertility, such as a history of sexually transmitted disease (STD), although second trimester abortion performed with current methods has not been shown to have a significant effect on fertility. Repeated abortion by sharp curettage, as is the practice in some countries, is associated with cervical weakening.

Despite the relative safety of the procedure, many lay and professional people assume abortion to have deleterious effects on fertility, and the perception of impaired fertility may discourage contraceptive use and place the woman at risk for repeat unintended pregnancy. However, unintended pregnancy is more likely than abortion to result in complications with adverse effects on fertility. Childbirth is more likely to result in serious infection or hysterectomy. Ectopic pregnancy, which occurs in about 1% of pregnancies, may also result in relative or absolute infertility. Overall, the most important contributors to impaired fertility are the sequelae of sexually transmitted infections and age. To preserve fertility, women need to avoid STDs and unintended pregnancy.

RISKS AND COMPLICATIONS

Overall, abortion is a safe procedure when performed properly. The mortality rate for all abortions in the United States is approximately 5 per million, contrasted to rates hundreds of times higher in places where legal abortion is inaccessible. Overall, mortality from childbirth is 10 to 20 times higher than that from abortion.

The lowest incidence of complications occurs in the (early) first trimester, prior to 10 menstrual weeks. The risks of abortion can be decreased by an early decision and access to medical care, treatment of coexisting infections, and the technical skill of the practitioner. When complications do occur, most can be treated with full resolution if they are promptly recognized.

Incomplete abortion occurs in 1% or less of women undergoing surgical abortion but is more frequent with any type of medical abortion. Incomplete abortion may be indistinguishable from retained blood clot, which is equally common. Either situation may result in continued spotting or bleeding, which may be minimal or heavy. Treatment may consist of medication to contract the uterus and expel the contents, such as methylergonovine, or suction curettage.

Cervical trauma may result from the tenaculum, dilation, or removal of tissue. Uterine trauma, including perforation, may result from dilators or intrauterine instruments. Uterine injury is less likely with the use of local anesthesia and with adequate cervical dilation. The rate of serious uterine injury is approximately 1 per 1000, but small perforations may be asymptomatic. Suspected uterine injury requires evaluation of the risk of injury to other organs, such as bowel or ureter. Evaluation and treatment may range from observation to laparoscopy or laparotomy, depending on the site and extent of the injury. Serious injuries are more likely at advanced gestational ages.

Infection rates may be less than 1% to 2%. Infection is less likely when prophylactic antibiotics are used in groups at increased risk for sexually transmitted infections, including adolescents. Bacterial vaginosis, *Trichomonas* infections, and cervicitis should be treated at the time of abortion. Even among women colonized with gonorrhea or *Chlamydia,* postabortal infection is uncommon if they have been given antibiotics at the time of the abortion.

When mild postabortal endometritis does occur, outpatient antibiotic treatment is usually sufficient if instituted promptly, with good compliance and follow-up. If concurrent incomplete abortion is present, suction curettage is indicated after antibiotics have been started. If infection occurs despite antibiotics covering most common sexually transmitted infections, drugs with good coverage of anaerobic bacteria should be added: e.g., clindamycin and metronidazole.

Anesthetic complications can also occur, particularly with general anesthesia. Local anesthesia is adequate for most early abortion procedures. Medical abortions, particularly in the first trimester, require less pain medication.

NONTHERAPEUTIC ABORTION

Self-induced abortion and abortions induced by non-medical persons are now uncommon in the United States, but are common where abortion is illegal, inaccessible, or restricted. See Chapter 4, "International Health." Placement of a foreign body such as a catheter in the cervix or uterus may cause dilation of the cervix, bleeding, or uterine contractions, which may be followed by a complete or incomplete abortion. Instrumentation of the uterus may accomplish the same end. Vaginal instillation of caustic solutions is rarely effective but potentially harmful. Misoprostol alone has some effectiveness in high doses. Any method of nontherapeutic abortion has a higher rate of both failure and complications than legal medical abortion. In some countries, up to one third of gynecologic admissions are of women with complications of nontherapeutic abortion, the most common being infection and uterine and cervical injury. Where abortion is illegal, nontherapeutic abortion remains a leading cause of maternal death.

CONTRAINDICATIONS

In general, factors that increase the risk of abortion in an individual woman, such as systemic illness, also increase the risk of continuing a pregnancy. Therefore, there are no absolute medical contraindications to abortion, although there may be technical reasons to select a particular method, which might in turn necessitate a delay. Uterine anomalies may require individual planning. Active pelvic infection may necessitate a delay until treatment has started. However, despite the medical safety of abortion, it should not be undertaken when the woman is obviously ambivalent, when it appears that she will be unable to cope emotionally with her decision, or when she appears to be heavily pressured. The adolescent who is pressured into having an abortion may immediately seek another pregnancy if none of the underlying conflicts or desires have been resolved. In these situations, additional counseling and

support are needed and may appropriately take precedence over an early decision.

EMOTIONAL REACTIONS

Women of all ages have a variety of psychologic reactions to abortion. The most common reaction reported is relief of psychologic distress, and the absence of distress or guilt should not in itself be regarded as abnormal. Attention should be focused on possible changes in behavior that will improve social and medical well-being. However, many women experience sadness or grieving and may benefit from a supportive counseling session.

The incidence of severe psychologic distress is higher after childbirth than after abortion, and there does not appear to be any specific syndrome of postabortion psychologic dysfunction. However, several groups of women may require additional attention. Women with serious underlying psychiatric disease need continued follow-up. The younger pregnant adolescent is more likely to have been coerced directly or indirectly into sexual activity, and needs more extended support. Similarly, strong pressure to conceive or to continue or abort a pregnancy, contrary to the wishes of the young woman, indicates family dysfunction. Pregnancy may elicit family attention, which is withdrawn when the pregnancy ends.

SUMMARY

Abortion represents an outcome of an unwanted, complicated, or abnormal pregnancy. Optimal safety may be obtained with early access to education, counseling, and experienced and well-trained providers. The incidence of abortion could be safely decreased by changes in sexual practices, including increased use of effective contraceptives.

Suggested Readings

American College of Obstetrics and Gynecologists: Methods of midtrimester abortion, *ACOG Technical Bulletin* 109:1-4, 1987.

Griffen-Carlson MS, Mackin KJ: Parental consent: factors influencing adolescent disclosure regarding abortion, *Adolescence* 28:1-9, 1993.

Grimes DA: Surgical management of abortion. In Thompson JD, Rock JA, editors: *Te Linde's operative gynecology,* ed 7, Philadelphia, 1992, JB Lippincott; pp 317-342.

Hatcher RA, Trussell J, Stewart F, et al: *Contraceptive technology,* ed 16, New York, 1994, Irvington.

Henshaw S, Kost K: Parental involvement in minors' abortion decisions, *Fam Plann Perspect* 24:196-213, 1992.

Jones EF, Forrest JD, Goldman N, et al: *Teenage pregnancy in industrialized countries,* New Haven, CT, 1986, Yale University Press.

Melton GB, editor: *Adolescent abortion,* Lincoln, NB, 1986, University of Nebraska Press.

Stone R, Waszak C: Adolescent knowledge and attitudes about abortion, *Fam Plann Perspect* 24:52-57, 1992.

Stotland NL: Induced abortion. In Stewart DE, Stotland NL, editors: *Psychologic aspects of women's health: the interface between psychiatry and obstetrics and gynecology,* Washington, DC, 1993, American Psychiatric Press; pp 207-225.

Zabin LS, Hirsach MB, Emerson MR: When urban adolescents choose abortion: effect on education, psychologic status and subsequent pregnancy, *Fam Plann Perspect* 21:248-254, 1989.

Zabin L, Hirsch M, Emerson M, Raymond E: To whom do inner-city minors talk about their pregnancies? Adolescents' communication with parents and parent surrogates, *Fam Plann Perspect* 24:148-173, 1992.

Zabin L, Sedivy V: Abortion among adolescents: research findings and the current debate, *J School Health* 62:319-324, 1992.

PART FIVE

Surgery

CHAPTER 145

Ophthalmology

•

Brian N. Campolattaro, Jeffrey L. Berman, and Frederick M. Wang

OPHTHALMOLOGIC ASSESSMENT

Adolescence is a time of great ophthalmic importance. Although the eye undergoes most of its growth during the first 3 years of life,[1] dynamic changes occur during adolescence as ocular maturation is completed. Many of the common pathologic processes of adolescence have significant ocular manifestations. Furthermore, many of the behaviors and activities of adolescents put their eyes at risk for a host of difficulties.

Medical History

Ophthalmologic assessment should begin with a thorough history. The history of present illness should include all ocular and systemic symptoms related to the chief complaint. Many ocular disorders are manifestations of other systemic illnesses, and related symptoms should be sought. For example, a previous rash and joint pain may be important clues to a more widespread disease such as systemic lupus erythematosus. It is important to note whether the symptoms occurred acutely or progressed insidiously and whether one or both eyes are affected. A history of trauma should be elicited, and the possibility of child abuse may need to be addressed.

The ocular history should be explored by the clinician. A history of occlusion patching may indicate amblyopia. A history of ocular surgery should be obtained. Previous episodes of redness and itching associated with seasonal variation may indicate ocular allergy. A history of spectacle and contact lens use should also be elicited.

A list of medications taken recently and drug allergies should be obtained. Many teenage patients may not regard eyedrops as medication, so their use should be inquired about specifically. The duration of usage is important, as is the response of the symptoms. Many ocular problems are the result of the use or overuse of eyedrops. For example, patients may experience allergic reactions to the preservatives such as benzalkonium or they may develop contact dermatitis secondary to neomycin allergy.

Systemic medications also can cause ocular symptoms. For example, symptoms of keratoconjunctivitis sicca (dry eyes) may be associated with antihistamine use. Allergies to systemic medications, especially antibiotics, also may result in serious ocular illness. Oral contraceptives may trigger migraine headaches.

A family history should be taken, with particular attention to family members who have a history of blindness, strabismus, glaucoma, refractive error, retinal disease, or migraine headache.

A social history regarding sexual activity and illicit drug usage may be indicated. It may be necessary to question the patient alone, without the parents present, to obtain this sensitive information. The teenage patient is susceptible to many sexually transmitted diseases (STDs) that can affect the eye (e.g., *Chlamydia* infection, herpes simplex, gonorrhea).

A travel history may be important at times (e.g., a visit to endemic areas of Lyme disease). Finally, if the patient is suspected of malingering, possible underlying psychosocial problems should be explored. For example, teenagers may complain to their parents of visual loss or of difficulty seeing to prevent embarrassment from poor performance at school or even from an inability to read.

Physical Examination

ACUITY. The common incidence of refractive errors in the adolescent population necessitates routine visual screening. The ocular examination should begin with an assessment of visual function. The eyes should be tested monocularly, with and without corrective lenses. The patient should be tested with a Snellen acuity wall chart to assess visual acuity, standing 20 feet, or 6 meters, from the chart. The vision is recorded as a numerator, which represents the viewing distance, over a denominator, which represents the distance at which one should be able to distinguish that particular sized figure. For example, individuals with 20/40 vision can see a particular sized Snellen figure at 20 feet that they should be able to distinguish at 40 feet. A 1.2-mm pinhole may be used to eliminate refractive errors. Poorer vision can be recorded as an ability to see "finger counting" or "hand motion," or "light perception" or "no light perception."

OCULAR ALIGNMENT. Before the techniques that the clinician may use to investigate ocular alignment are discussed, a brief comment on nomenclature and theory is warranted. A spontaneously present or constantly manifested deviation of the eyes is a heterotropia or "-tropia." A latent deviation of the eyes is a heterophoria, or "-phoria," and is elicited by interrupting normally present fusional mechanisms, for example, by covering one eye. Terminology referring to inturned eyes is prefaced "eso-" and outturned eyes are indicated by the prefix "exo-." Vertical misalignments are usually referred to according to the higher eye and are called "hypertropias."

Children with ocular deviations (strabismus or "squint") learn to suppress the image of the deviating eye to avoid diplopia. This adaptive mechanism occurs if the deviation occurred before age 9 years and may result in amblyopia, which is visual loss due to the dropout of cells in the visual pathways secondary to disuse.[2] Ocular misalignments beginning in adolescence, such as cranial nerve palsies, result in diplopia.

An ocular misalignment can be detected by observing the position of corneal light reflexes. The patient is asked to look at a fixation target while the examiner shines a penlight onto both eyes. The light reflex should be from corresponding parts of both corneas. If a deviation is present, the light reflex in the nonviewing eye will be displaced in the opposite direction of the deviation. This is known as the Hirschberg test (Fig. 145-1). The degree of deviation can be estimated by the degree of light reflex displacement.

A cover test can more accurately disclose misalignment. While the patient is viewing a target, one eye is covered by the clinician while the uncovered eye is observed for movement. If there is no movement of the uncovered eye, the uncovered eye is not deviated if the visual system is intact. The test is then performed on the opposite eye. If no movement is observed in the opposite uncovered eye, the patient's eyes are considered straight or orthotropic (Fig. 145-2, A). If, upon covering

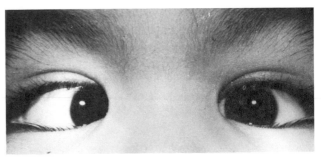

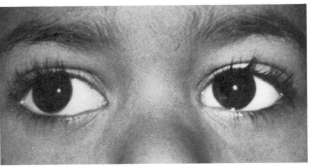

Fig. 145-1. **A,** Hirschberg test demonstrating esotropia. Note the temporal displacement of the corneal light reflex in the right eye. **B,** Exotropia. Note the nasal displacement of the corneal light reflex in the right eye. (From Wang FM: Eye problems. In Shelov SP, Mezey AP, Edelemann CM Jr, Barnett HL, editors: *Primary care pediatrics: a symptomatic approach,* Norwalk, Conn., 1984, Appleton-Century-Crofts.)

an eye, the uncovered eye moves to pick up fixation, it was deviated and a "-tropia" exists (Fig. 145-2, B). If the eyes are orthotropic but the eye under cover moves to refixate when the occluder is removed, a "-phoria" exists. The degree of deviation can be measured by neutralizing the movement with prisms while alternately covering the eyes.

Childhood tropias that persist into adolescence do not cause diplopia. The presence of amblyopia is indicative of a preadolescent strabismus. Furthermore, childhood strabismus usually does not change with the position of gaze (i.e., comitant) and is painless with extraocular movement. Conversely, ocular misalignments occurring in adolescence or adulthood usually cause diplopia. They may change with the position of gaze (i.e., incomitant) and be accompanied by a limitation of ocular motility and occasionally by pain. Extraocular motility always should be tested and limitations noted.

GLOBE AND PERIOCULAR STRUCTURES. One should be familiar with the basic anatomy of the eye and its nearby structures (Fig. 145-3). The globe and periocular structures can be examined with a penlight. The eyelids, lashes, and lacrimal apparatus should be assessed. Lymphatic drainage of the eyelids occurs through the submandibular and superficial preauricular lymph nodes. These nodes may become enlarged in cases of viral

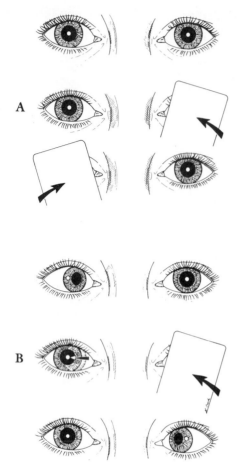

Fig. 145-2. A, Cover test demonstrating orthotropia. Note that there is no movement of the uncovered eye when either eye is covered. **B,** Cover test demonstrating alternating esotropia. Note that the deviated eye moves to pick up fixation when the fixing eye is covered. (From Wang FM: Eye problems. In Shelov SP, Mezey AP, Edelemann CM Jr, Barnett HL, editors: *Primary care pediatrics: a symptomatic approach,* Norwalk, Conn., 1984, Appleton-Century-Crofts.)

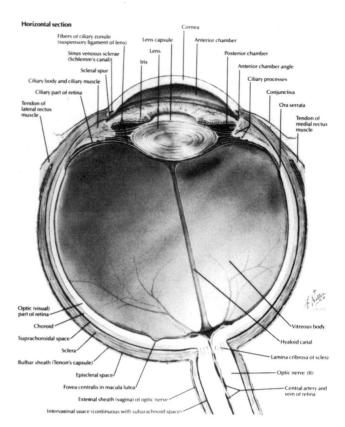

Fig. 145-3. Horizontal section of the globe. (From Colacino S, editors: *Atlas of human anatomy,* West Caldwell, NJ, 1989, Ciba-Geigy Corp. Copyright © 1989 Ciba-Geigy Corporation. Reprinted with permission from *Atlas of human anatomy,* illustrated by Frank H. Netter, M.D. All rights reserved.)

conjunctivitis and preseptal cellulitis, for example, and should be palpated.

The conjunctiva and underlying sclera should be examined and patterns of injection noted.

The cornea should be inspected carefully and should be clear. Opacities may indicate serious ocular infection, especially if accompanied by injection of the conjunctiva. Corneal sensitivity should be noted, since it may be decreased by certain infections such as herpes zoster. One or two drops of topical anesthetic (e.g., proparacaine hydrochloride 0.5%) can be instilled into the lower fornix, and fluorescein staining can be used to look for epithelial defects (e.g., corneal abrasions). The epithelial defect will fluoresce green under an ultraviolet light such as a Wood's lamp or under cobalt-blue light. The patient should remove contact lenses for examination, since fluorescein will stain the lenses. Foreign bodies in the

cornea should also be noted; if these are present, the patient should be referred to an ophthalmologist.

The anterior chamber of the eye can be seen behind the cornea and should be clear. Blood in the anterior chamber (hyphema) may commonly result from blunt trauma to the globe. Pus in the anterior chamber (hypopyon) is a marker of serious ocular inflammation.

The pupils should be carefully evaluated, especially in cases of suspected visual loss. A relative afferent pupillary defect usually indicates optic nerve disease. This sign is elicited with the swinging flashlight test. When the penlight is shone into the normal eye, both pupils react briskly (direct and efferent consensual responses intact). However, when the penlight is swung back to the abnormal eye, there is a paradoxic dilation of the pupils.

The lens can also be easily observed with a penlight. In the adolescent, a newly acquired white pupil (leukocoria) is most commonly caused by a cataract, *Toxocara* infection of the retina, or isolated retinal telangiectasia (Coats' disease).

The posterior pole of the retina can be evaluated with a direct ophthalmoscope through the undilated pupil. The direct ophthalmoscope provides a real image of the retina with ×15 magnification.[3] The optic nerve can be visualized by having the patient fixate on an object in the distance, with the clinician directing the ophthalmoscope at an angle of 15 degrees temporal to the visual axis. The macula can be visualized by asking the patient to fixate on the light of the ophthalmoscope. The pupils can be dilated with one or two drops of tropicamide 1% with phenylephrine 2.5% if the fundus is not well visualized through the undilated pupil. The cycloplegic effect of tropicamide usually lasts 4 to 8 hours.

EYE TRAUMA

Trauma to the globe and periocular tissues can result in serious injury that must be recognized, and the patient should be treated or referred to an ophthalmologist promptly. Whereas marked eyelid swelling and ecchymosis may hide an otherwise intact globe, seemingly minimal eyelid damage may be associated with serious ocular injury.

The cause of ocular injury should be quickly assessed. Chemical burns require immediate irrigation with copious amounts of saline solution or water before full evaluation. In suspected cases of perforating injuries to the globe, vomiting and severe coughing should be controlled to avoid expulsion of the intraocular contents.

Sports-related injuries, knife wounds, injuries inflicted by shards of glass or pointed objects such as darts and pencils, fireworks accidents, and gunshot or BB-gun wounds are common mechanisms of ocular trauma in the adolescent population. Child abuse should always be suspected, especially in younger teenagers and with recurrent injuries.

A detailed history should be taken to determine the nature and extent of the injury for medical and legal purposes. In cases of perforating injuries, the tetanus immunization should be updated if necessary. A history of drug allergies should be elicited. The patient should be questioned about food consumption in the previous 8 hours, and should not be given any food or liquids by mouth if general anesthesia administration is considered during surgical repair.

Patients with decreased visual acuity, suspected perforating injuries to the globe, and eyelid lacerations involving the lid margin or lacrimal drainage system should be quickly referred to an ophthalmologist for evaluation and treatment. Other subspecialty services such as neurology and otolaryngology may need to be consulted to help assess possible associated neurologic, bony facial, and dental trauma.

Eyelids

Trauma to the eyelid can be secondary to perforating or blunt injuries. Blunt trauma to the orbit usually causes

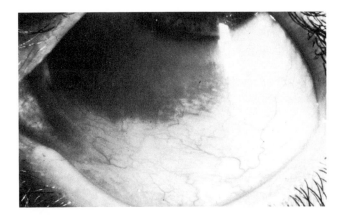

Fig. 145-4. Inferior subconjunctival hemorrhage after blunt trauma. (Courtesy of Martin Mayers, M.D., New York.)

eyelid ecchymosis and edema. Initial management consists of cold compresses or ice for the first 24 to 48 hours to reduce swelling, with warm compresses applied thereafter. Superficial skin abrasions are cleansed and treated with bacitracin ointment to prevent secondary infection.

Penetrating injuries of the eyelid are particularly worrisome when the lid margin or lacrimal drainage system is involved. Superficial lid lacerations not involving the lid margin may be sutured primarily, using basic plastic surgical principles. Deeper penetrating injuries of the central upper eyelid need careful evaluation of the levator muscle to prevent future ptosis. Lid lacerations involving the eyelid margin must be carefully apposed to prevent notching that could later compromise normal movement of tear film over the cornea. The lacrimal drainage system may be damaged in lacerations involving the medial canthal area. Patients with such lacerations should be referred for probing and possible intubation with silicone tubing to prevent future epiphora (excessive tearing).

A gauze soaked in sterile saline solution may be placed over the lid laceration to keep the tissue moist until surgical repair is possible.

Adolescents suffer burns to the eyelids from fires, curling irons, or chemicals (e.g., battery acid). Antibiotic ointments such as bacitracin may be applied to burns to prevent secondary infections. Severe burns may require initial treatment in a hospital burn unit, with lubrication of the exposed cornea to prevent epithelial breakdown. Temporary surgical closure of the eyelids (i.e., tarsorrhaphy) may be necessary if the cornea cannot be protected by lubrication alone. Some patients require secondary repair with skin grafting.

Subconjunctival Hemorrhages

Trauma to the globe can cause subconjunctival hemorrhages (Fig. 145-4). These hemorrhages usually appear bright red initially but change color as the blood subsequently breaks down and resorbs over weeks. No treatment is required (if there is no other ocular injury) because they resolve spontaneously without sequelae.

Nontraumatic subconjunctival hemorrhages may result from the pressure caused by diving or excessive coughing or straining. Although rarely associated with bleeding disorders, isolated episodes of subconjunctival hemorrhage need not be investigated.

Corneal Abrasions

The cornea is a richly innervated, multilayered structure covered by nonkeratinized epithelium.[4] Trauma to the corneal epithelium usually causes pain, foreign body sensation, tearing, injection of the conjunctiva, and photosensitivity.

Abrasions of the cornea result in epithelial defects that may be seen easily under ultraviolet light after the instillation of fluorescein. One or two drops of topical anesthetic will temporarily relieve the patient's discomfort and facilitate examination. The anesthetic effect of proparacaine hydrochloride 0.5% usually lasts 15 to 20 minutes. Topical anesthetics should never be prescribed for symptomatic relief, since long-term use is toxic to the cornea and may produce persistent epithelial defects and severe keratitis.[5-7]

The corneal epithelium usually heals in 24 to 36 hours. Since the epithelium represents the cornea's normal barrier to infection, prophylactic topical antibiotics such as gentamicin, tobramycin, or 10% sulfacetamide should be administered. Two or three drops of antibiotic solution or ½ inch of antibiotic ointment should be instilled, and the eyelids should be closed and patched tightly with two eye pads over the eye, secured with paper tape (Fig. 145-5). Pressure patching eliminates blinking, which reduces the denuding of the newly formed epithelial cells. The patient should be reexamined every 24 to 36 hours until the epithelium heals completely.

An alternative to pressure patching in uncooperative patients or those with very small abrasions is to prophylactically instill antibiotic ointment or solution four times a day until the epithelial defect resolves. Because of the high risk of corneal ulceration, any corneal abrasion associated with contact lens wear should not be patched until a thorough slit-lamp examination by an ophthalmologist has been performed.[8]

Burns

The corneal epithelium may be damaged by thermal, ultraviolet, and chemical burns. Ultraviolet and chemical burns are more common in the adolescent population. Patients may present with ultraviolet burns after pro-

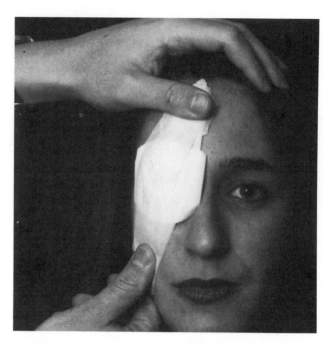

Fig. 145-5. Pressure patching technique for corneal abrasions.

longed exposure to reflected sunlight (e.g., "snow blindness" in skiers) or to ultraviolet sunlamps. Symptoms may not be manifested until several hours after the exposure when corneal edema and epithelial breakdown ensue. These burns should be treated as corneal abrasions.

Chemical burns are ocular emergencies and should be irrigated immediately. Irrigation can be performed more easily after the instillation of a topical anesthetic. Saline solution, 1 or 2 liters, may be administered by way of intravenous tubing with the patient lying on his or her back. Alkali burns are more dangerous than acid burns, as acids precipitate proteins in the cornea, which then act as a barrier against further penetration.[9] Alkalis cause saponification and cell membrane damage and allow continued penetration and destruction of the corneal stroma. Markers of more serious ocular injury are blanching of the perilimbic vasculature (the circumcorneal vessels are necessary for corneal healing), corneal haziness,[10] and elevated intraocular pressure (usually from scleral shrinkage). Extensive eyelid and corneal scarring is a major late complication of severe alkali burns. Common substances that cause alkali burns are lye, plaster, and calcium hydroxide (lime used to mark baseball and football fields).

Foreign Bodies

Superficial corneal foreign bodies may sometimes be removed with irrigation or a cotton-tipped swab after the instillation of a topical anesthetic. On examination, metallic foreign bodies may be surrounded by a brownish

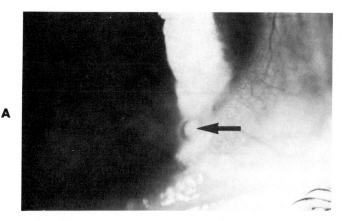

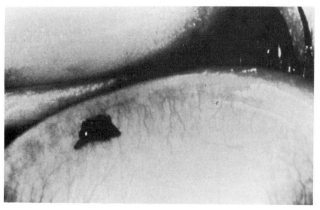

Fig. 145-6. A, Peripheral superficial corneal metallic foreign body *(arrow)* with surrounding rust ring. **B,** Everted upper eyelid revealing an occult conjunctival foreign body. (Courtesy of Peter Hersh, M.D., New York.)

"rust ring" (Fig. 145-6, *A*). Patients with corneal foreign bodies not easily removed with a cotton-tipped swab should be referred for slit-lamp examination to assess the depth of penetration. These foreign bodies may be removed under slit-lamp magnification with a 25-gauge needle or a battery-powered burr. After removal of the foreign body, the patient usually has an epithelial defect that should be treated as a corneal abrasion. Residual rust rings may be burred after 24 hours of pressure patching with topical antibiotic coverage. Administration of one or two drops of homatropine 5% or cyclopentolate 1% for cycloplegia may be necessary to relieve symptoms of associated iritis.

Conjunctival foreign bodies can present with redness, irritation, tearing, and a foreign body sensation. They can usually be seen with a penlight and removed with irrigation or a cotton-tipped swab after the installation of a topical anesthetic. Foreign bodies under the upper lid may cause vertically oriented linear abrasions of the cornea. The upper lid should be everted to locate and remove these foreign bodies (Fig. 145-6, *B*).

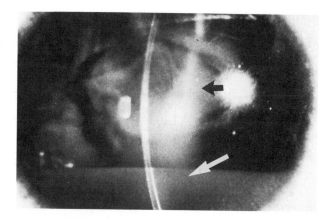

Fig. 145-7. Hyphema: slit-lamp photograph demonstrating inferiorly layered blood in the anterior chamber *(white arrow)* and clot obscuring the pupil *(black arrow)*. (Courtesy of Martin Mayers, M.D., New York.)

Traumatic Iritis

Any trauma to the globe can result in traumatic iritis. Symptoms and signs include pain, tearing, photosensitivity, visual loss, perilimbic redness, and miosis (small pupil). Mydriasis (large pupil) may be seen, especially if tears of the iris sphincter are present. Slit-lamp examination usually reveals evidence of protein exudation ("flare") and white blood cells in the anterior chamber. Iritis may occur hours to days after the initial injury. Treatment usually involves the administration of cycloplegic agents to relieve the pain of ciliary spasm. Homatropine 5% or cyclopentolate 1% may be given four times a day. In some cases, topical corticosteroids are also administered.

Hyphema

Vessels of the iris and ciliary body may bleed into the anterior chamber after trauma, causing hyphema (Fig. 145-7). The blood may be grossly visible as it layers inferiorly, or may be subtle and detected as circulating red blood cells seen only on slit-lamp examination. Hyphemas are usually associated with traumatic iritis and other ocular injury and may be quite painful. Nausea, vomiting, and somnolence are common secondary to the oculovagal reflex.

The patient is at major risk for rebleeding 2 to 5 days after the initial hyphema.[11] Corneal blood staining and elevation of intraocular pressure are serious concerns during the first week. Glaucoma can also develop weeks to months after the incident secondary to damage to the filtering mechanism of the eye located in the anterior chamber angle (see discussion of glaucoma). The risk of rebleeding and the overall prognosis are related to the size of the hyphema.

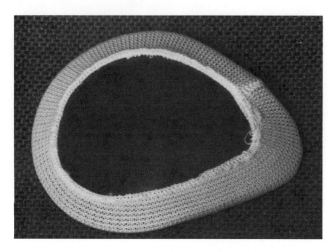

Fig. 145-8. Plastic eye shield used to protect the globe.

Patients with sickle cell disease or trait are at greater risk for glaucoma after hyphema, since the stiffened sickled red blood cells are poorly filtered.[12,13] Sickle cell preparation or hemoglobin electrophoresis should be performed in all black patients with hyphema.

A plastic or metal eye shield (Fig. 145-8) should be placed over the eye to avoid further trauma, which could cause rebleeding. Bed rest for the first 5 days after injury is recommended, with or without hospitalization, depending on the age of the patient, the size of the hyphema, and the dependability of the patient and parents. Bilateral patching[14] has been used in the past but is usually not necessary. Reading should be discouraged, but patients may watch television. The head of the bed should be elevated 30 to 45 degrees so that the blood layers inferiorly, away from the pupil, lowering the pressure in the ocular vasculature and clearing the visual axis.

Acetaminophen should be given as an analgesic, since salicylates may inhibit platelet function and increase the risk of rebleeding.[15] Antiemetics may be used to control nausea and vomiting. ε-Aminocaproic acid (50 to 100 mg/kg/dose every 4 hours) is given orally as an antifibrinolytic agent to prevent rebleeding,[16] although intraocular pressure spikes have been reported after discontinuation of the drug.[17] The maximal daily dosage should not exceed 30 g. Common side effects are nausea, vomiting, and diarrhea. More serious side effects include generalized thrombosis and hepatic necrosis.

Atropine 1% is a topical cycloplegic agent used to reduce pain from ciliary spasm, prevent the development of adhesions between the iris and the lens (posterior synechiae), and keep the iris at rest. Intraocular pressure should be monitored and pressure elevations should be controlled initially with topical beta blockers. Oral carbonic anhydrase inhibitors may be given to control severe intraocular pressure spikes, except in patients with sickle cell trait or disease, since metabolic acidosis may

worsen the sickling.[18] Surgical management may be necessary if the intraocular pressure cannot be controlled medically.

When possible, the eye should be thoroughly examined for damage to the lens and retina.

Lens

Trauma to the globe can cause dislocation of the lens or cataract formation. Traumatic cataracts require removal if the vision is significantly decreased. Monocular aphakia ("without lens") cannot be corrected by spectacles, because the image magnification of aphakic spectacle correction (25%) will create diplopia because of the unequal image sizes (aniseikonia). The aphakic refractive error can be corrected by contact lenses, intraocular lenses, or refractive corneal procedures (e.g., epikeratophakia).

Retina

The retina is prone to damage from blunt and penetrating damage to the globe. Contrecoup injury to the globe caused by blunt trauma is often associated with a disruption of the photoreceptor layer without extracellular edema (commotio retinae).[19] When commotio retinae involves the macular region (Berlin's edema), it may cause decreased visual acuity. Subretinal hemorrhages, choroidal ruptures, and vitreous hemorrhages are other sequelae of blunt trauma to the retina.

Visual complaints of flashing lights, floaters, or shadows should raise the suspicion of retinal traction with possible holes, tears, or detachments. Patients with these symptoms should be referred to an ophthalmologist for a complete examination of the retinal periphery. Holes are treated with laser or cryotherapy. Tractional detachments may require vitrectomies by skilled vitreoretinal surgeons. Other detachments may be repaired by buckling the sclera inward to reattach the choroid and overlying retinal pigment epithelium to the retina.

Ruptured Globes

Penetrating injuries of the cornea may be obvious or subtle. Important clues to the presence of corneal lacerations include a shallow anterior chamber and distortion of the pupil ("peaking") secondary to the iris being trapped in the wound (Fig. 145-9, *A*).

Possible penetrating injuries of the cornea or sclera must be considered and explored, especially in cases of blunt trauma and subconjunctival hemorrhages or conjunctival lacerations located over the recti muscle insertions or near the limbus, where the sclera is thinnest (Fig. 145-9, *B*). All patients with suspected ruptured globes must be referred to an ophthalmologist quickly for

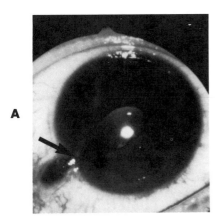
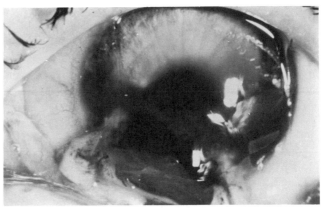

Fig. 145-9. A, Corneal-scleral laceration with "peaking" of the pupil *(arrow)* secondary to entrapped iris within the wound. **B,** More obvious ruptured globe occurring at the limbus where the sclera is thinner and more susceptible to rupture from blunt trauma. (From Shingleton BJ, Hersh PS, Kenyon KR, editors: *Eye trauma,* St Louis, 1991, Mosby–Year Book.)

evaluation and repair. An eye shield (not a patch) should be taped over the bony face to avoid further trauma or manipulation of the globe. Broad-spectrum antibiotics such as cefazolin and gentamicin should be administered intravenously as soon as possible in cases of obviously ruptured globes.

Occasionally, a plain film or computed tomographic (CT) scan of the globe and orbit may be indicated to detect occult radiopaque foreign bodies, such as metal and leaded glass. Magnetic resonance imaging (MRI) should not be performed, since intraocular metallic foreign bodies may move under the magnetic forces and cause further damage to the eye. Some metallic foreign bodies, such as copper and iron, are toxic to the eye and must be removed as soon as possible.[20] Other foreign bodies, such as glass, are inert.

If no scleral rupture is present, larger conjunctival lacerations should be closed with absorbable suture; the patient should be anesthetized topically and prophylactic topical antibiotics given.

Orbital Fractures

The orbital and surrounding facial bones are susceptible to fracture from blunt trauma. The orbital rim should be palpated and appropriate radiologic studies obtained to rule out fractures. Most commonly, the orbital floor is fractured as part of a "blow-out" fracture.[21] Infraorbital hypesthesia is common secondary to trauma to the infraorbital nerve. Orbital contents may prolapse through the fracture into the maxillary sinus and become entrapped. Plain films with Waters views can be used to visualize large floor fractures with tissue prolapse and opacification of the maxillary sinus, but they are generally not indicated since CT scans show far more detail.[22]

Indications for surgical investigation and repair include sinking of the globe into the orbit due to the loss of

orbital fat (enophthalmos) and restriction of extraocular muscles with diplopia.[23] Fractures longer than 15 mm on CT may need to be repaired to prevent the occurrence of late enophthalmos. Associated facial fractures also may need to be repaired.

Retrobulbar hemorrhage with elevated intraocular pressure is an ophthalmic emergency. A lateral canthotomy should be performed as soon as possible by cutting the lateral canthus down to the lateral orbital wall, allowing the eye to move forward and relieve the pressure.

Blunt trauma can indirectly contuse the optic nerve, usually in the bony optic canal. This injury is evidenced by marked visual loss and a relative afferent pupillary defect. Some authorities advocate high-dose steroids to reduce edema.[24,25] Optic nerve decompression may be necessary if there is bony impingement on the optic nerve as evidenced by CT.[26-28]

HEAD TRAUMA

Trauma to cranial nerves III (oculomotor), IV (trochlear), and VI (abducens) may result in paralytic strabismus and diplopia. Traumatic third cranial nerve palsies are associated with significant head trauma.[29] The fourth cranial nerve is especially vulnerable to trauma where it passes beneath the free tentorial edge after crossing dorsally in the roof of the fourth ventricle. Head trauma, with rapid acceleration and deceleration, usually with loss of consciousness, such as that which occurs in motorcycle accidents, may cause bilateral fourth cranial nerve palsies. Sixth cranial nerve palsies may be due to indirect trauma to the nerve fascicle or may be seen with increased intracranial pressure. The sixth cranial nerve is particularly susceptible to damage where it ascends from the pons toward the cavernous sinus. Other vertical ocular deviations may also occur with brain stem injury secondary to head trauma (skew deviation). Child abuse should be considered in cases of cranial nerve palsies associated with other signs of trauma without obvious cause. Papilledema secondary to increased intracranial pressure may be seen with any severe head trauma.

Cavernous sinus-carotid fistulas may develop after trauma, with orbital signs of proptosis, injection and chemosis (edema) of the conjunctiva, and restriction of extraocular motility. Patients with this condition must be observed closely for optic nerve dysfunction, in which case balloon embolization or neurosurgical intervention may be indicated to close the fistula.[30]

Closed head trauma can result in damage to the occipital lobes and subsequent visual loss with retention of normal pupillary reflexes. Homonymous visual field deficits and even total cortical blindness may ensue.

SPORTS INJURIES AND PREVENTION

Adolescents involved in sporting activities are particularly prone to ocular trauma. Basketball, racquetball, handball, squash, hockey, and baseball are examples of such high-risk athletic activities.[31] Fingers, fists, racquets, sticks, and balls are common offending agents that cause direct injury to the globe. Protective eyewear should be mandatory for all monocular patients and for all adolescents participating in sports in which the ball or puck moves at relatively high velocity in an enclosed space.

Protective frames or goggles should be fitted with lenses made of relatively impact-resistant plastic, such as polycarbonate. Helmets with impact-resistant visors can be worn in hockey and football.

PTOSIS

Blepharoptosis, or ptosis, describes a droop of the upper eyelid. Ptosis may be congenital or acquired. The position of the ptotic lid in downgaze will differentiate the congenital from the acquired etiologies. The congenital ptotic lid is higher in downgaze than the contralateral, normal lid; the acquired ptotic lid remains ptotic in all positions of gaze.

Ptosis may be classified on the basis of its underlying abnormality; myogenic, neurogenic, mechanical, or traumatic. Variability in the degree of ptosis should alert one to consider myasthenia gravis and synkinetic causes.

Treatment options include nonsurgical modalities, such as eyelid crutches attached to the eyeglass frames or lid taping during times when visual demands warrant. Surgical treatment is often undertaken; the choice of procedure is often determined by the amount of levator muscular function present.

PROPTOSIS

Proptosis is a forward displacement of the globe usually resulting from a mass, a vascular abnormality, or an inflammatory process. It is usually measured with an exophthalmometer, although it is often obvious by inspection alone when an examiner looks over the patient's forehead and brows from above. There is a noticeable difference in exophthalmometry readings measured in occidental and black patients: blacks have greater average exophthalmometry values.

Proptosis, when unilateral, is often caused by orbital cellulitis, although mass lesions such as rhabdomyosarcoma must always be considered. Bilateral proptosis may be caused by leukemia, pseudoproptosis, or thyroid-related orbitopathy.

Pseudoproptosis may be caused by any of the following: enlarged globe, extraocular muscle paralysis, contralateral enophthalmos, asymmetric orbital size, or asymmetric palpebral fissures. The diagnosis of pseudoproptosis should not be made until the possibility of a mass lesion has been ruled out.

"RED" EYE

Apparent injection (redness) of the normally "white" portion of the eye most commonly represents limited conjunctival inflammation, such as that seen in conjunctivitis. However, other more serious etiologies should be sought and excluded before empirical treatment is begun. Primary inflammation of the eyelids, cornea, and uvea is usually accompanied by conjunctival inflammation and must be differentiated from primary conjunctivitis. Patterns of injection and corneal involvement are useful differentiating signs. Any patient with a corneal opacity associated with ocular inflammation (keratitis) must be quickly referred to an ophthalmologist for evaluation.

Inflammation of the Eyelids

Lid margin colonization by staphylococcal bacteria may lead to inflammation (blepharitis) and "styes." Staphylococcal blepharitis may be associated with conjunctivitis and marginal infiltrates of the cornea, which are thought to represent an inflammatory response to the staphylococcal exotoxins released.[32,33]

Treatment is directed toward decreasing the colonization of the lid margin by performing lid hygiene and applying appropriate topical antibiotics. The patient should be instructed to debride the lid margins with a cotton-tipped swab and a dilute solution of baby shampoo and warm water. Bacitracin or erythromycin ointment should be applied to the lid margins twice a day. Treatment may need to be continued for several months.

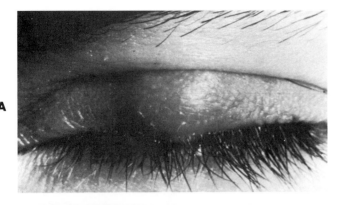

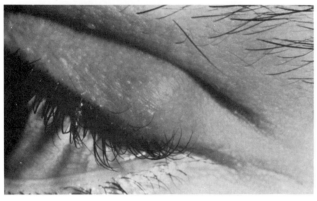

Fig. 145-10. A, Acute stye, or hordeolum, of the central upper eyelid. **B,** Less inflamed, more chronic stye, or chalazion, of the lateral upper eyelid. (Courtesy of Peter Hersh, M.D., New York.)

In more severe cases, mild steroids may be added to the regimen to reduce the inflammatory response incited by the exotoxins.

Styes of the eyelid are often associated with staphylococcal infections. When acute, this condition is known as *hordeolum* and may be directed internally or externally, depending on the eyelid glands involved (Fig. 145-10, *A*). Pain, redness, and purulent discharge are common. Hot compresses and appropriate topical antibiotics should be prescribed. Incision and drainage by an ophthalmologist may be necessary.

Chronic styes, or chalazia, are usually granulomatous inflammatory reactions to obstruction of the meibomian glands of the eyelids (Fig. 145-10, *B*). Hot compresses, lid hygiene, and massage may resolve the lesions. Incision and curettage from the conjunctival side, with removal of the fibrotic capsule, may be necessary.

Preseptal and Orbital Cellulitis

It is extremely important to differentiate inflammation anterior to the orbital septum—preseptal cellulitis—from true orbital cellulitis.[34,35] Orbital cellulitis is a potentially vision- and life-threatening condition requiring immediate attention.

Preseptal cellulitis is characterized by moderate eyelid edema and erythema without proptosis or restriction of ocular motility. It most commonly occurs after trauma to the eyelid or in association with upper respiratory infections. *Staphylococcus aureus* is the most common offending organism associated with preseptal cellulitis in the adolescent population. *Streptococcus pneumoniae* is another common organism that causes this condition.

Any ocular discharge should be cultured before antibiotic therapy is begun. Incision and drainage of the preseptal space are sometimes necessary to reduce the pus and resultant edema. Dicloxacillin or cephalexin can be given orally for 7 to 10 days to provide good coverage for gram-positive organisms.

Orbital cellulitis is an infection of the space behind the orbital septum. The vital contents of this orbital space include extraocular muscles, the optic nerve, and other cranial nerves that innervate the eye. Symptoms and signs of orbital cellulitis include pain, headache, fever, diplopia secondary to limitation of extraocular movements, erythema and edema of the eyelids and conjunctiva, and proptosis (Fig. 145-11). Decreased visual acuity and color vision and a relative afferent pupillary defect signal optic nerve dysfunction.

Orbital cellulitis occurs most commonly secondary to paranasal sinusitis, usually of the ethmoid sinuses, or after penetrating orbital trauma. *S. aureus, Streptococcus pyogenes,* and *S. pneumoniae* are the most common offending organisms in adolescence. Mucormycosis and other fungi should be suspected in diabetic and immunocompromised patients.

Suspected orbital cellulitis should be investigated with CT scans of the orbits and paranasal sinuses. A complete blood count, blood cultures, and a Gram's stain and culture of any discharge from the eye or nasopharynx should be obtained. Penicillinase-resistant antibiotics such as methicillin should be given parenterally, and close follow-up should be provided to observe for signs of visual loss. Warm compresses and nasal decongestion obtained with inhaled phenylephrine hydrochloride are often helpful. Surgical decompression of the orbit and paranasal sinuses may be necessary. Subperiosteal abscesses seen on CT necessitate prompt surgical exploration and drainage. Otolaryngologic consultation is usually necessary.

Dangerous ocular complications include exposure keratitis secondary to proptosis, secondary glaucoma, and blindness from optic nerve compression or central retinal artery occlusion. Meningitis, brain abscess, and cavernous sinus thrombosis are life-threatening complications.

ACUTE FOLLICULAR CONJUNCTIVITIS

Some common conditions associated with acute follicular conjunctivitis are shown in Box 145-1.[36]

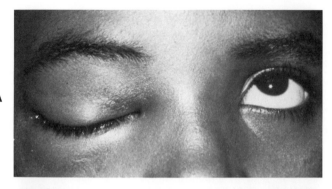

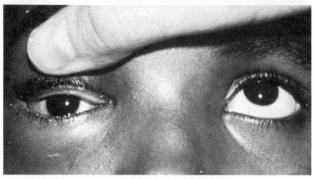

Fig. 145-11. A, Right orbital cellulitis with the eyelid closed secondary to marked periorbital edema. **B,** Conjunctival chemosis and injection and limitation of upward gaze. (From Wang FM: Eye problems. In Shelov SP, Mezey AP, Edelemann CM Jr, Barnett HL, editors: *Primary care pediatrics: a symptomatic approach,* Norwalk, Conn., 1984, Appleton-Century-Crofts.)

Common causes of this condition in adolescence are outlined below.

Viral Conjunctivitis

Viral conjunctivitis is the most common form of conjunctivitis in the adolescent population. An upper respiratory illness often precedes its appearance. If there are other family members with "pink eye" a viral etiology is suggested, also.

The symptoms and signs usually begin in one eye and then spread to the contralateral eye, presumably by hand-to-eye contact. Redness, itching, and watery discharge associated with a follicular reaction of the tarsal conjunctiva are common. Follicles are small elevations of tissue consisting of aggregates of avascular lymphoid tissue. A nonspecific papillary reaction of the tarsal conjunctiva may accompany the follicular reaction. Papillae are small elevations of hyperemic tissue with a central fibrovascular core. Lid edema and preauricular lymphadenopathy also often occur. Iritis may accompany severe cases of conjunctivitis.

The adenovirus is the most common cause of viral conjunctivitis. Certain strains of adenovirus can cause keratoconjunctivitis, a more severe form of conjunctivitis

---

BOX 145-1
Conditions Associated With Acute Follicular Conjunctivitis

Pharyngoconjunctival fever
Epidemic keratoconjunctivitis
Herpesvirus hominis (herpes simplex type 1) keratoconjunctivitis
Inclusion conjunctivitis
Other chlamydial infections
Acute hemorrhagic conjunctivitis

Modified from Dawson CR, Sheppard JD: Follicular conjunctivitis. In Tasman W, Jaeger EA, editors: *Duane's clinical ophthalmology,* vol 4, Philadelphia, 1990, JB Lippincott.

---

with transient corneal involvement. Epidemic keratoconjunctivitis (EKC) is caused by adenovirus types 8 and 19. It is associated with subepithelial infiltrates thought secondary to an immune reaction to the viral antigen.[37] Although EKC is usually self-limited, these corneal opacifications may persist for months or years.

Pharyngoconjunctival fever is a self-limited infection most commonly caused by adenovirus type 3. The typically nonpurulent, follicular conjunctivitis is accompanied by pharyngitis and fever.

Although these diseases are self-limited, lasting from 2 to 4 weeks, patients should be told that the symptoms may worsen before they improve. The highly contagious nature of the infection should be stressed, especially in suspected cases of EKC. The mode of transmission should be explained and hand washing emphasized. Towels and washcloths should not be shared. Depending on the severity of disease, the patient may need to be kept out of school for 1 to 2 weeks to prevent an epidemic.

Treatment of these entities is symptomatic. Cold compresses can be used for comfort along with a corneal lubricant such as artificial tears. Topical antihistamines such as naphazoline hydrochloride may be used to relieve some of the redness and itching. A cycloplegic agent should be prescribed in cases of concurrent iritis.

When the subepithelial opacities of EKC interfere with vision, the administration of topical corticosteroids may be considered. It should be emphasized that the lesions may recur after cessation of the steroid therapy.

Herpes Simplex

An acute follicular conjunctivitis usually accompanies primary and recurrent ocular herpes simplex infections. Severe keratitis may occur with recurrent attacks.

Allergic Conjunctivitis

Allergic or atopic conjunctivitis is common in the adolescent population. It is mediated by the release of vasoactive substance from mast cells activated by IgE antibodies, in response to airborne antigens such as pollen.[38] A history of allergic rhinitis or asthma may be elicited, as well as a family history of atopy. Symptoms occur rapidly and include marked itching; lid swelling; redness; and watery, mucoid discharge.

Vernal keratoconjunctivitis is a type of atopic keratoconjunctivitis. The inflammation is seasonal, recurrent, and bilateral. Itching, blinking, photosensitivity, and mucoid discharge are common. Large "cobblestone" papillae on the upper tarsal conjunctiva are characteristic. The inflammation is mediated by basophil and mast cell–IgE antibody complexes.[39] Scrapings of the upper tarsal conjunctiva reveal many eosinophils and eosinophilic granules. Horner-Trantas dots are white concretions, composed of eosinophils, occasionally seen at the superior border of the conjunctiva and cornea.

The treatment of allergic conjunctivitis includes cold compresses and application of topical antihistamines. Topical 4% cromolyn sodium solution may be used for more severe cases to inhibit mast cell release prophylactically. Topical steroids, topical nonsteroidal antiinflammatory agents, and oral antihistamines may be used; referral to an allergist may be necessary.

Related syndromes seen in contact lens wearers (especially those who wear soft contact lenses) are contact lens–induced papillary conjunctivitis and the more severe giant papillary conjunctivitis.[40] The clinical picture of giant papillary conjunctivitis is similar to that of vernal conjunctivitis, but fewer eosinophils are seen in scrapings.[41] Thimerosal preservatives in contact lens solutions have been implicated, as well as other irritative agents (e.g., increased coatings on worn contact lenses).[42]

CHRONIC FOLLICULAR CONJUNCTIVITIS

Some causes of chronic follicular conjunctivitis are outlined in Box 145-2.[36] The more common causes in adolescents are detailed below.

Chlamydia

Chlamydiae are obligate intracellular organisms containing both RNA and DNA and a bacterial cell wall. Serotypes D to K of *Chlamydia trachomatis* can cause chronic follicular conjunctivitis with preauricular lymphadenopathy in young adults.[43] The disease is sexually transmitted and can be associated with a "nonspecific" urethritis or cervicitis. Peripheral corneal infiltrates are common, and iritis may occur in the later stages. Conjunctival scrapings reveal typical chlamydial inclusions and give positive results on the rapid, direct chlamydial immunofluorescent antibody test (Micro-Trak).[44] Chlamydiazyme[44] is an enzyme-linked immunoassay that can also detect chlamydial antigens. Serum

---

> **BOX 145-2**
> **Conditions Associated With Chronic Follicular Conjunctivitis**
>
> Trachoma
> Inclusion conjunctivitis and other chlamydial infections
> Toxic follicular conjunctivitis
>   Molluscum contagiosum
>   Topical eye medication
>   Eye make-up
> Bacterial (*Moraxella lacunata*)
> Morax-Axenfeld chronic follicular conjunctivitis
> Chronic follicular keratoconjunctivitis of Thygeson
> Parinaud's oculoglandular syndrome
> Lyme disease

Modified from Dawson CR, Sheppard JD: Follicular conjunctivitis. In Tasman W, Jaeger EA, editors: *Duane's clinical ophthalmology,* vol 4, Philadelphia, 1990, JP Lippincott.

---

chlamydial antigen–complement fixation titers may be elevated. Treatment consists of oral erythromycin, tetracycline, or doxycycline for 3 to 4 weeks. Sexual partners should be notified and treated.

C. trachomatis serotypes A, B, and C cause trachoma, a potentially blinding chronic keratoconjunctivitis.[45] This inflammatory condition may be accompanied by scarring of the conjunctiva, late lid scarring, and misdirection of the lashes inward (trichiasis), causing corneal damage. Trachoma is uncommon in the United States except in areas with poor sanitation and low standards of living. If detected before extensive scarring occurs, this condition responds to oral tetracycline, doxycycline, and erythromycin. In cases of severe scarring, surgical repair of the eyelids may be necessary.

Molluscum Contagiosum

Chronic follicular conjunctivitis may occur with molluscum contagiosum infections. This DNA-carrying poxvirus causes smooth, raised molluscum nodules on the eyelid. Lesions on the lid margins spill viral proteins into the conjunctival fornix, inciting an inflammatory reaction mimicking trachoma. Treatment involves removal of the lid lesions by excision, electrocautery, or freezing with liquid nitrogen.[46]

Eye Make-up

Chronic follicular conjunctivitis is sometimes produced in adolescent girls by eye make-up. This condition can be caused by a direct toxic effect of the make-up on the conjunctiva, or less commonly it may develop secondary to infection with *Moraxella lacunata* spread by way of shared eye make-up.

Topical Eye Medications

Chronic use of various topical eye medications, such as gentamicin solution, may also result in chronic follicular conjunctivitis. Treatment consists of discontinuation of the offending medication.

Parinaud's Oculoglandular Syndrome

Parinaud's oculoglandular syndrome is a unilateral, follicular mucopurulent conjunctivitis associated with a focal granulomatous lesion of the conjunctiva and preauricular and submandibular lymphadenopathy. Fever and malaise are common. Parinaud's oculoglandular syndrome is one ocular manifestation of cat-scratch disease, a disorder believed to be caused by *Bartonella* spp.[47] Other manifestations of cat-scratch disease include papillitis, serous retinal detachment, and neuroretinitis.[48,49] Typically, a cat scratch or close contact with cats, especially kittens, precedes the illness by a few days to several weeks. Serologic diagnosis of patients with cat-scratch diseases can be performed by means of an indirect fluorescent antibody assay for *Bartonella* spp.[50] Treatment requires systemic antibiotics, including tetracycline.

BACTERIAL CONJUNCTIVITIS

Staphylococcus Aureus

S. aureus is the most common offending organism in bacterial conjunctivitis. It is usually accompanied by a mucopurulent discharge and lid margin involvement (blepharitis). Corneal involvement (marginal infiltrates) is also common. Treatment usually involves the application of topical erythromycin or 10% sodium sulfacetamide solution or ointment for 5 to 7 days.

Neisseria Gonorrhoeae

Gonococcus is the most feared cause of bacterial conjunctivitis. Infection usually occurs secondary to inoculation of the conjunctiva from infected genital secretions.[51,52] It is characterized by a hyperpurulent inflammatory response with lid edema, marked conjunctival injection and swelling (chemosis), and occasionally the development of an inflammatory membrane or pseudomembrane on the tarsal conjunctiva. Preauricular lymphadenopathy is usually present.

Gonococcus is highly invasive, and corneal ulceration may ensue. Disseminated disease, including meningitis, can result from spread to the bloodstream.

Conjunctival Gram's stains typically show many polymorphonuclear leukocytes and gram-negative diplo-cocci. Cultures should be performed on chocolate agar and Thayer-Martin media in all suspected cases of gonococcal conjunctivitis. Serologies for syphilis should be obtained and the possibility of other STDs excluded.

Treatment should include the administration of systemic ceftriaxone, penicillin, or ampicillin and the application of topical ophthalmic bacitracin ointment. Oral tetracycline or erythromycin should also be administered because of the high incidence of concurrent chlamydial infections. The eye should be irrigated frequently to remove the harmful purulent inflammatory material. Topical cycloplegic agents may be useful in cases of associated iritis. Sexual partners should be contacted and treated.

CORNEAL INFLAMMATION

Inflammation of the cornea, or keratitis, may occur as a primary process or it may be secondary to conjunctival and eyelid inflammatory processes, as described earlier. The risk of visual loss due to corneal scarring mandates prompt referral of all patients with active corneal inflammation to an ophthalmologist.

Symptoms of keratitis can include minimal to moderate pain, redness, foreign body sensation, tearing, and decreased vision. Signs include infiltration and neovascularization of the normally clear, avascular cornea. Accompanying conjunctival injection and iritis are common. Peripheral or marginal corneal infiltrates more commonly occur with sterile immune reactions to microbial antigens released from organisms such as *S. aureus* or *C. trachomatis*,[33] whereas central corneal infiltrates are more commonly seen with direct microbial infection.

Herpes Simplex

Keratitis secondary to infection with the DNA-carrying *Herpesvirus hominis* may be seen in adolescence. It is a common cause of corneal scarring and visual loss in the United States. Except in cases of neonatal herpetic infections, ocular disease is most commonly due to infection with herpes simplex virus (HSV) type 1. Although HSV type 2 can cause ocular disease, this serotype is more commonly associated with genital herpes infections.[53,54]

Disease may occur with primary infection or with recurrences after asymptomatic latent periods. Primary infection is usually secondary to direct contact with particles shed from an individual with active lesions; however, the virus occasionally can be transmitted by asymptomatic individuals. Latent virus is thought to be localized in the trigeminal ganglia, with clinical recurrences usually precipitated by mild trauma, exposure to sunlight, respiratory or gastrointestinal infections, and other stressful events.[55,56]

Ocular infection is usually associated with acute follicular conjunctivitis with preauricular lymphadenopathy. Primary infections are often accompanied by systemic symptoms of malaise, myalgia, and fever. Herpetic vesicles may be seen on the eyelids and may be accompanied by edema.

The classic corneal lesion is the branching dendrite (Fig. 145-12), which represents a coalescence of epithelial vesicles. Early corneal involvement may be detected with rose bengal, which stains the devitalized, swollen epithelial cells. Associated iritis is common. Corneal sensitivity is typically decreased with recurrent episodes, and this lack of pain may mask serious infection.

The diagnosis can be confirmed by isolating the virus from untreated vesicles in culture. Giemsa stain of scrapings of the base of cutaneous vesicles may reveal typical viral multinucleated giant cells (Tzanck test). Rising serum antibody titers may be helpful.

Treatment involves the administration of antiviral agents.[57,58] Trifluridine solution is applied to the eye every 2 hours, up to nine times a day. The dendritic lesions may need to be debrided mechanically to reduce the viral load. Oral acyclovir may be prescribed, although its true benefit in ocular disease is still unknown.[59] Topical steroids are contraindicated. Close slit-lamp observation by an ophthalmologist is necessary. Cycloplegic agents can be given to relieve the pain of ciliary spasm associated with iritis. The patient should be followed closely, and antiviral agents should be continued until the corneal lesions resolve. Dendritic keratitis typically lasts for 2 to 3 weeks.

Complications include secondary bacterial superinfection of the conjunctiva and periocular skin. Topical antiviral medications may cause secondary follicular conjunctivitis and keratitis. Extensive corneal scarring can occur, especially in the form of disciform lesions of the deeper corneal tissue, presumably secondary to cell-mediated immune responses to viral antigens.

Bacterial Keratitis

The normally intact epithelium of the cornea provides a good barrier against microbial infection. When the corneal epithelium is disrupted, bacteria can enter the cornea and cause inflammation and destruction. Although bacterial keratitis is often preceded by trauma, even minute epithelial defects, such as with contact lens wearing or dry eyes, can lead to bacterial infiltration. The most common organisms cultured from previously healthy corneas include *Pseudomonas aeruginosa, S. pneumoniae, Moraxella* spp., beta-hemolytic streptococci, and *Klebsiella pneumoniae.*[60] Previously diseased corneas also can be opportunistically infected by *S. aureus* and *Staphylococcus epidermidis,* alpha-hemolytic streptococci, and *Proteus* organisms. Immunocompromised patients can be infected by an even wider variety of more exotic organisms.

Although certain clinical features of bacterial keratitis are more common with gram-positive or gram-negative organisms, it is extremely difficult to distinguish the offending agent on clinical grounds alone. Any patient who has a whitish, corneal infiltrate with an overlying epithelial defect and associated ocular inflammation must be referred to an ophthalmologist immediately for evaluation and treatment (Fig. 145-13). Associated iritis is very common, and layered pus in the anterior chamber (hypopyon) may be seen with more severe infections.

In general, gram-positive organisms, such as *S. aureus,* produce yellow-white, well-demarcated focal infiltrates with overlying epithelial defects. The associated anterior chamber reaction is usually not severe with staphylococ-

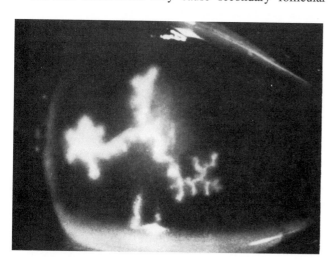

Fig. 145-12. Typical corneal dendrite occurring with herpes simplex keratitis, as demonstrated by fluorescein stain. (Courtesy of Martin Mayers, M.D., New York.)

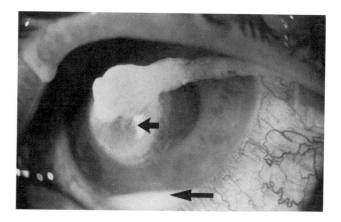

Fig. 145-13. Central corneal infiltrate *(short arrow)* in *Pseudomonas aeruginosa* keratitis. Note the overlying mucus and inferiorly layered pus *(long arrow)* in the anterior chamber (hypopyon). (Courtesy of Martin Mayers, M.D., New York.)

cal infections. As previously discussed, more peripheral staphylococcal marginal infiltrates are usually sterile immune reactions to bacterial exotoxins. *S. pneumoniae* infections are generally more extensive, with more severe inflammatory reactions, including hypopyon.

Gram-negative organisms typically cause a rapidly evolving, diffuse, gray-white, deep stromal infiltrate with an overlying epithelial defect. Inflammation is usually marked, and sterile hypopyon is common. The classic gram-negative corneal ulcer is caused by *P. aeruginosa* and is seen in soft contact lens wearers.[61,62]

Fungal keratitis occurs most commonly in the southeastern region of the United States and often results from a corneal abrasion involving a tree branch or piece of wood. *Fusarium, Aspergillus,* and *Penicillium* spp. are the common offending filamentous organisms. Yeasts, such as *Candida* spp., commonly are found in immunocompromised individuals. The ulcers typically are gray, irregular lesions with smaller, surrounding satellite lesions.[63] Hypopyon is often present.

The management of all corneal ulcers begins with diagnostic studies involving scraping the infiltrate for identification of the offending organism. Scrapings should be plated directly onto culture media, and slides should be prepared for Giemsa and Gram's stains. Swab cultures of both conjunctivae should be obtained to help establish the baseline ocular flora. Administration of topical cefazolin and fortified gentamicin drops should be started empirically for broad-spectrum coverage if no organism is identified on the initial stains.[64,65] Each drop should be given hourly, alternating the two medications so that the patient receives one drop every half-hour. Alternatively, the newer topical fluoroquinolone antibiotics (e.g., ciprofloxacin) may be used (initial dosage of 2 drops every 15 minutes for the first 6 hours of treatment and then every 30 minutes for the first day).[66] A cycloplegic agent should be given to reduce pain from associated iritis and to prevent posterior synechiae. The antibiotic regimen can be modified as culture results become known. Fungal infections may be treated with topical polyene antibiotics. Some authorities use topical collagenase inhibitors such as 10% acetylcysteine to limit corneal tissue destruction. Therapeutic soft contact lenses, collagen shields, or conjunctival flaps may be needed for more severe tissue destruction and impending perforations. The use of topical corticosteroids to reduce inflammatory scarring remains controversial.[67]

Corneal ulcers resistant to treatment may represent infections with *Acanthamoeba* spp.[68] These protozoans cause chronic, classically painful keratitis. Infection has been linked to contamination of soft contact lenses by storage or irrigating solutions.[69] Treatment is with topical propamidine isethionate and neomycin.

Complications of corneal ulceration include permanent scarring, perforation, and endophthalmitis. Corneal transplantation is required in instances of severe visual loss secondary to scarring.

Interstitial Keratitis

Interstitial keratitis is an inflammatory condition of the cornea involving the deeper corneal tissues (stroma). Ghost vessels and corneal scarring are common sequelae of interstitial keratitis. The major infectious etiologies include congenital syphilis and tuberculosis. Syphilitic interstitial keratitis is usually seen in adolescence in association with anterior uveitis as a late manifestation of congenital infection. It is thought to be secondary to an immune reaction to the treponemal antigen. Acute episodes of inflammation should be treated with topical corticosteroids, although systemic penicillin may be required. Herpes simplex, varicella zoster, *Borrelia burgdorferi*,[70,71] and mumps are other potential infectious agents. Treatment should be directed at the underlying cause, with topical corticosteroids given to reduce the inflammation and cycloplegic agents administered to help treat associated uveitis.

Uveitis

Inflammatory conditions involving the iris, ciliary body, and choroid (Fig. 145-3) cause pain, redness, photosensitivity, and tearing. Whereas iritis strictly defines inflammation of the iris, anterior uveitis encompasses inflammation of the iris and ciliary body. By definition, acute anterior uveitis lasts less than 6 weeks, whereas chronic uveitis can last months to years.

The classic pattern of injection is circumcorneal, giving the perilimbic sclera a violaceous color or "flush." The hallmark of anterior uveitis is increased vascular permeability, giving rise to protein exudation ("flare") and the presence of inflammatory cells in the anterior chamber, which can be seen by slit-lamp biomicroscopy. Severe inflammation may lead to a fibrin reaction in the anterior chamber. Cells may accumulate on the corneal endothelial surface, giving rise to keratic precipitates, and iris nodules may be seen. Adhesions (posterior synechiae) may form between the iris and anterior surface of the lens, and spontaneous hyphema may develop secondary to bleeding from the inflamed iris vessels.

Most cases of acute, unilateral anterior uveitis remain idiopathic despite extensive laboratory investigations. The work-up should be tailored to the systemic and ocular findings in the individual patient.

Cycloplegic agents should be administered to prevent pain from ciliary spasm and limit posterior synechiae formation. Topical corticosteroids should be given to reduce inflammation. Periocular or oral steroids may be added to the treatment regimen for more severe or refractory cases. Underlying causes should be addressed and treated when possible.

Trauma is probably the most common cause of acute anterior uveitis in the adolescent population. It is usually self-limited, although cycloplegic agents are helpful. There is no direct evidence that corticosteroids are beneficial.

Ankylosing spondylitis, Reiter's syndrome, and inflammatory bowel diseases also have a high incidence of associated acute iritis. These spondyloarthropathies share the histocompatibility locus antigen HLA-B27.[73,74]

Behçet's disease occurs most commonly in young Japanese men and is characterized by acute iritis with hypopyon, oral and genital aphthous ulcers, synovitis, cutaneous and retinal vasculitis, and superficial thrombophlebitis.[75] It is associated with a high incidence of the HLA-B5 antigen.[76,77]

Chronic uveitis may have an insidious onset and the patient may not present to the clinician until the development of late sequelae. Visual loss is common secondary to the deposition of calcium in the cornea (band keratopathy), glaucoma, cataract formation, and fluid in the macular region of the retina (cystoid macular edema).

Juvenile rheumatoid arthritis is the classic cause of chronic uveitis in adolescents. Ocular involvement is more common in young women with pauciarticular or monoarticular disease. These patients tend to be antinuclear antibody positive and rheumatoid factor negative.[78,79]

Other causes of chronic uveitis include sarcoidosis, tuberculosis, Lyme disease,[67,80] and syphilis, although these conditions may also present acutely.

Toxoplasma gondii is an obligate intracellular protozoan parasite that commonly causes focal, necrotizing retinitis associated with posterior, and sometimes anterior, uveitis. Serum IgG and IgM antibodies to *Toxoplasma* organisms may be detected by the enzyme-linked immunosorbent assay (ELISA) or indirect fluorescent antibody and agglutination tests. Treatment of active toxoplasmosis should include the administration of pyrimethamine and triple sulfonamides. Peripheral leukocyte and platelet counts should be monitored and folinic acid given to prevent bone marrow suppression. Alternative therapeutic agents are clindamycin and tetracycline.

AIDS

AIDS secondary to HIV in children may have many ophthalmic manifestations. The retina appears to be the most common site of ocular HIV infection, and cotton-wool spots, which are infarcts at the level of the nerve fiber layer, seem to be the most commonly noted finding in patients infected with HIV.

One of the more common retinal disorders that may lead to blindness in patients with AIDS is cytomegalovirus (CMV) retinitis. Therapies to treat CMV retinitis and prolong useful vision in affected individuals include intravenous regimens of ganciclovir or foscarnet; use of both agents simultaneously is currently under investigation.

GLAUCOMA

Glaucoma is a condition in which elevated intraocular pressure causes optic nerve damage and resultant, progressive visual field loss. Intraocular pressure is dependent on the equilibrium between fluid production and fluid egress from the eye. Fluid (aqueous humor) is produced by the ciliary body in the posterior chamber of the eye. The aqueous humor flows around the iris into the anterior chamber of the eye to escape through the trabecular meshwork, to Schlemm's canal, and into the episcleral venous system (Fig. 145-14). The trabecular meshwork is situated in the junction between the cornea and the iris, which is referred to as the anterior chamber angle. Because of the phenomenon of total internal

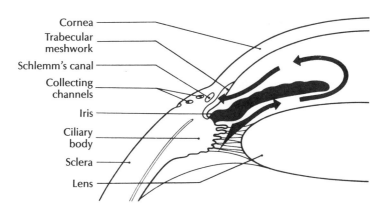

Cornea
Trabecular meshwork
Schlemm's canal
Collecting channels
Iris
Ciliary body
Sclera
Lens

Fig. 145-14. Schematic drawing of the anterior segment of the eye demonstrating the flow of aqueous humor from the posterior chamber, where it is produced in the ciliary body, into the anterior chamber, where it escapes through the trabecular meshwork. (From Spalton DJ, Hitchings RA, Hunter PA, editors: *Atlas of clinical ophthalmology,* London, 1984, Gower Medical Publishing.)

reflection of light emanating from the eye, the trabecular meshwork and other structures contained in the anterior chamber angle can be examined only through gonioscopy, which involves indirect visualization through a slit lamp with a special contact lens.

Although "normal" intraocular pressure is considered to be between 10 and 20 mm Hg,[81] there is no absolute pressure at which glaucomatous damage begins. Elevated intraocular pressure may occur without optic nerve damage. Furthermore, there can be wide individual fluctuations in intraocular pressure.

Glaucoma can be classified as primary open-angle, primary closed-angle, or secondary. Open-angle glaucoma is associated with elevated intraocular pressure in the presence of a normal-appearing anterior chamber angle. It is usually idiopathic and asymptomatic. Although primary open-angle glaucoma can occur in adolescence, it is unusual to see this disease in patients under the age of 40. It is the most common type of glaucoma in the adult population.

Angle closure occurs when the peripheral iris blocks the egress of aqueous humor through the trabecular meshwork. Symptoms of acute closed-angle glaucoma include eye pain, tearing, decreased vision, headache, nausea, and vomiting. The patient may complain of seeing halos around lights secondary to associated corneal edema. Signs include marked firmness of the globe on palpation, redness, haziness of the cornea, and a sluggishly reactive or nonreactive, partially dilated pupil. Primary closed-angle glaucoma is also very rare in the adolescent population.

Secondary glaucoma occurs as a result of acquired blockage of the fluid exit from the eye. This may be produced by structural changes in the anterior chamber angle, although it more commonly involves blockage of the trabecular meshwork by cells or organic debris.

Primary congenital glaucoma is usually related to developmental abnormalities of the anterior chamber angle.[82] Juvenile glaucoma refers to primary congenital glaucoma that appears in late childhood or adolescence. Dysgenesis of the iris and anterior chamber angle may be associated with glaucoma, as well as with other ocular and systemic abnormalities. Patients with excessive tearing, abnormal-appearing irides, or cloudy corneas should be referred to an ophthalmologist for evaluation.

Blunt trauma to the globe may cause secondary glaucoma by a variety of mechanisms. Pressure elevations may occur with hyphema due to blood clots obstructing the outflow of aqueous humor through the trabecular meshwork. Patients with sickle cell disease or trait are particularly susceptible to glaucoma in association with hyphema.[12,13] In addition, old, rigid red blood cells ("ghost cells") can enter the anterior chamber after vitreous hemorrhage and can clog the trabecular meshwork.

Blunt trauma may also produce angle recession, a widening and disruption of the anterior chamber angle. The angle recession is only a marker of the previous trauma to the anterior chamber angle that may lead to intraocular pressure elevations. Glaucomatous damage may occur years after the initial injury.

Pigmentary glaucoma is a form of secondary open-angle glaucoma seen in young, Caucasian, myopic men.[83] In this clinical entity, pigment from the iris is dispersed throughout the anterior chamber, reducing aqueous outflow facility.

Sturge-Weber syndrome and von Recklinghausen's disease, two types of phakomatosis, are also often associated with secondary glaucoma, especially with involvement of the upper eyelids. The elevated intraocular pressure in Sturge-Weber syndrome is thought to be secondary to elevated episcleral venous pressure and anomalous development of the anterior chamber angle.[84]

Secondary glaucoma also may be seen in some individuals who have used topical corticosteroids for a long time. Glucocorticoid creams or lotions applied to the face and systemic corticosteroids may also produce intraocular pressure elevations.[85] Patients using any corticosteroids chronically should be monitored for elevations in intraocular pressure and potential glaucomatous damage.

Treatment of childhood glaucoma should be directed toward the underlying abnormality when possible. Disease progression can be monitored by subsequent visual field examinations and evaluation of the optic nerve head for progressive cupping. Intraocular pressure should be lowered medically by reducing aqueous humor production with topical beta blockers or carbonic anhydrase inhibitors. Aqueous humor outflow may be facilitated by topical application of cholinergic agents such as pilocarpine and perhaps by epinephrine derivatives. In cases of pigmentary and other open-angle glaucomas, laser burns can be applied to the trabecular meshwork (argon laser trabeculoplasty) to improve aqueous humor outflow.[86] Juvenile glaucomas are often poorly controlled with only medical therapy, and surgery (e.g., trabeculectomy) is usually required to create new pathways for the aqueous humor to leave the eye.

PAPILLEDEMA

Optic disc edema can be called papilledema only when it is both bilateral and a result of increased intracranial pressure. Optic nerve function is typically normal in papilledema. Other than an increase in intracranial pressure, causes of bilateral optic disc edema include diabetic papillopathy as well as a variety of entities that more typically cause unilateral edema. These include optic neuritis; ischemic optic neuropathy; and leukemic, metastatic, or infectious infiltrative disorders.[87] Neuroimaging studies are vital to exclude mass lesions as the cause of bilateral disc edema in adolescents.

In assessing a swollen disc, one must determine whether the appearance is that of papilledema or pseudopapilledema. In pseudopapilledema, there is no edema, and thus no obscuration of vessels at the disc margin.[88] Pseudopapilledema is most commonly produced by optic disc drusen.[89] High hyperopia with a small scleral opening is another possible cause.

REFRACTIVE ERRORS

The eye is an optical system that functions to focus light on the retina, which sends visual impulses to the occipital cortex of the brain. The cornea is responsible for 70% of the refractive power of the eye in its relaxed, unfocused state (unaccommodated). The remainder of the refractive power is supplied by the lens.[90] The lens can add additional focusing power through the process of accommodation, which involves contraction of the smooth muscle surrounding the lens. The unaccommodative refractive state of the eye is determined by the fixed corneal refractive power, determined by the curvature of the corneal surface, the power of the relaxed lens, and the axial length of the eye.

In patients with no refractive error, parallel rays of light are focused on the retina without accommodative effort. For myopic patients, images at a distance are blurred; parallel rays of light focus in front of the retina. The optical power of the eye can be considered "too strong" in myopia. This condition can be secondary to steep axes of curvature of the cornea or a long axial length of the eye. In hyperopic patients, parallel rays of light focus "behind" the retina. This circumstance can be due to flat axes of curvature of the cornea or a short axial length. Astigmatism is produced when the refractive power of the cornea or lens varies in different meridians. In astigmatic eyes, the central cornea resembles an ellipsoid more than a sphere.

Mild hyperopia usually can be overcome by accommodation in young patients. Headaches and visual complaints while reading (asthenopia) may be caused by uncorrected, larger hyperopic errors. Hyperopia can also cause esodeviation secondary to excessive convergence with accommodative effort.

There is a normal progression from hyperopia toward myopia during adolescence.[91] This progression is probably genetically determined, although environmental influences have been debated.[92] High degrees of myopia may be associated with retinal abnormalities that may limit visual acuity.

Anisometropia is a difference in refractive errors of the two eyes and may be associated with amblyopia.

Spectacle correction of large differences may not be tolerated owing to the difference in retinal image sizes (aniseikonia), and contact lenses may be required (e.g., for unilateral aphakia). Occlusion therapy may be attempted to reverse amblyopia even in adolescence.[93]

Keratoconus is a corneal disorder that causes markedly irregular astigmatism. If the corneal distortion cannot be corrected with spectacles or contact lenses, a corneal transplant may be necessary.

Correction

The cosmetic concerns of adolescents should be considered in their eye care. Personal appearance and self-image should be balanced with vision and safety. Refractive errors may be corrected by spectacles, contact lenses, or surgical procedures. The choice of correction should be tailored to the individual's needs.

SPECTACLES. Spectacles can be prescribed in a variety of materials. Plastic lenses are lighter and safer than glass lenses but are scratched more easily. Various colored tints and densities are available for both plastic and glass. Thin coatings can be added to reduce surface reflections. Photochromatic material, which darkens when exposed to ultraviolet light, can be incorporated into glass spectacles. Ultraviolet-absorbing sunglasses can be prescribed according to the standards set by the Ophthalmic Standards Committee of the American National Standards Institute.[94] Impact-resistant lenses prescribed for occupational purposes should be mounted in appropriate safety frames.

CONTACT LENSES. The use of contact lenses carries a significant commitment to proper care by the patient and physician because of the risk of corneal injury and infection, especially with soft contact lenses.[95] Patients must be suitable candidates in terms of motivation and reliability. They must be properly instructed on lens insertion, removal, and hygiene. Most contact lenses need to be removed and cleaned daily owing to the increased risk of infection with extended wear.

Contact lenses are available in various materials to fit the patient's needs. Hard contact lenses can be made of hard polymethylmethacrylate or various gas-permeable, rigid materials. The gas-permeable lenses allow oxygen to pass through to the cornea and are generally better tolerated than the more conventional polymethylmethacrylate lenses. Gas-permeable lenses also cause fewer allergic reactions and last longer than soft contact lenses. Hard contact lenses have the advantage of correcting corneal distortions and astigmatism by modifying the corneal surface.

Soft contact lenses are generally more comfortable and better tolerated than hard contact lenses because of their increased hydration and pliability.[96] They are the most common contact lenses prescribed for the correction of myopia. Because they mold to the eye, ordinary soft contact lenses do not correct astigmatism. Toric soft contact lenses, which correct mild astigmatism, are available. Soft contact lenses stay on the eye more easily than hard contact lenses and are therefore generally better for athletes.

A large variety of soft contact lenses are available and vary in water content, oxygen transmission, shape, size, and type of polymer used. Soft contact lenses that can remain on the eye for extended periods are available.[97] Extended-wear lenses are generally thinner and have a higher water content than daily-wear lenses. The extended-wear lenses also need to be replaced more often than daily-wear lenses and are more prone to accumulate lens deposits on their surface. These lenses need to be removed at regular intervals for cleaning and disinfection. Many authorities recommend the daily removal and cleaning of all soft contact lenses, given the higher degree of morbidity and risk of serious ocular infection, especially *Pseudomonas* keratitis, with extended-wear lenses.[98-101] The advent of disposable soft contact lenses has helped to circumvent some of the problems associated with extended soft contact lens wear; however, the use of these lenses is still not without risk.

Tinted hard and soft contact lenses are available for cosmetic alteration of iris color. Translucent or opaque images can be safely imprinted into soft contact lenses. Only opaque images have the ability to change dark irides to light colors, since translucent images are modified only by whatever color is behind them. Cosmetic contact lenses should not be worn without careful consideration, given the risks of complications associated with any contact lens wear.

Hard contact lenses are generally cleaned with various soaking solutions. Soft contact lenses may be cleaned by chemical or heat disinfection. Cleaning solutions for soft contact lenses include surface-acting cleaners (surfactants), hydrogen peroxide cleaners, and enzyme cleaners. Heat cleaning methods are less expensive than chemical methods, but they leave more lens deposits and require a higher rate of lens replacement.[102,103] A variety of rinsing and storage solutions are available.

Fluorescein and topical medications should not be used while patients are wearing soft contact lenses because of the risk of lens staining.

SURGICAL CORRECTION. Radial keratotomy is the most common surgical technique to correct myopic refractive errors.[104] Small, partial-thickness radial incisions are made in the peripheral cornea to induce flattening of the central cornea. Refractive errors may not be totally eliminated, and patients often still need other modes of correction. Radial keratotomy is most successful with mild myopia. This elective procedure should be undertaken only with great consideration in view of vision-threatening complications.

Other surgical procedures can be undertaken to correct various refractive errors. Epikeratophakia can be used to correct aphakia and high hyperopia. In this procedure, a lamellar graft is mounted on the central cornea like a "living contact lens."[105,106] Excimer lasers have been developed that can cut corneal tissue and reduce refractive errors without causing thermal damage.[107] The efficacy of this procedure is still under investigation.

AESTHETIC CONSIDERATIONS

Congenital or acquired drooping of one or both eyelids (ptosis) should be referred to an ophthalmologist for evaluation and possible surgical repair. Ocular misalignments also may be surgically repaired in adolescence.

Patients with opaque corneas can be fitted with an opaque contact lens. Blind and disfigured eyes may also be covered with a cosmetic, opaque contact lens or scleral shell, or they may be surgically removed (enucleation) if painful. After enucleation, good postoperative motility can be obtained by suturing the extraocular muscles to hydroxyapatite orbital implants covered by donor sclera. Prostheses are individually made and fitted to match the fellow eye to provide excellent cosmetic results.

EYE MAKE-UP

Many girls learn to use eye make-up during adolescence. Most products are tested by ophthalmologists and dermatologists for quality and allergenic potential before marketing. Individuals may still be sensitive to so-called hypoallergenic products.[108]

The use of eye make-up has been associated with many ocular complications. Styes can occur from obstruction of the openings of the glands in the eyelid. Pigment from mascara can be permanently incorporated into periocular tissues, and corneal abrasions can occur from contact with mascara brushes. Chronic follicular conjunctivitis secondary to the use of eye make-up can also result.

VISUAL DISABILITY

There are many causes of visual dysfunction in the United States[109] and even more worldwide.[110] Major causes of visual deficits in childhood include congenital abnormalities, cataracts, and retinopathy of prematurity.[111] It is important to establish a diagnosis in all cases of visual dysfunction in order to determine the prognosis for further visual loss and to allow for special education and training at an early age.

U.S. regulations define legal blindness as best corrected visual acuity of 20/200 or less or a visual field of

20 degrees or less in the better eye.[112] Total blindness usually connotes the absence of light perception. Although some state variations exist, low vision is usually considered 20/70 to 20/200. The evaluation of visual disability should include measures of impairment of the whole person rather than merely central acuity or field. Many classification schemes have been designed to include other visual deficits.[113] Approximately one in every 500 schoolchildren is partially sighted.[114]

Color deficiencies are transmitted on the X chromosome and are not a major visual handicap. In 5% to 6% of boys there is some form of color deficiency.

After psychologic adjustment to the loss of one eye, monocular individuals function quite well. Although stereopsis is lost, young individuals adapt very well to the use of other visual clues, such as relative size, for depth perception. Constriction of the binocular visual field on the blind side of a monocular patient is another limitation.

Registries of the blind are available to provide services for, as well as compile statistics on, the legally blind. Registries tend to underreport the number of patients with visual deficits.[115] All legally blind patients should be registered in their state. A directory can be found in a current edition of the *Physician's Desk Reference for Ophthalmology*.[116]

Other state and federal agencies are designed for the education and support of the visually handicapped. Furthermore, many optical aids are available through the American Foundation for the Blind or the New York Association for the Blind. An application to join the Talking Books Program can be sent to the National Library Science for the Blind and Physically Handicapped. The addresses of these agencies also can be found in the *Physician's Desk Reference for Ophthalmology*.[116]

Vision standards exist for driving a motor vehicle, becoming a pilot, and joining the armed forces. State variations exist in standards for motor vehicle operation. Most states require a best corrected vision of 20/40 in the better eye. Visually handicapped individuals should be counseled on such regulations.

PSYCHOLOGIC ADJUSTMENT TO VISUAL LOSS

The adjustment to the loss of vision in one or both eyes can be physically and emotionally devastating to teenagers and their families. The disfigurement or physical loss of an eye adds an additional psychologic burden. Whereas partially sighted children tend to develop—emotionally, socially, and physically—similarly to sighted children,[117] the adjustment to the loss of vision in adolescence can be extremely difficult, because the goals of adolescence become even more difficult. Gaining independence and autonomy and dealing with issues of identity and sex become nearly insurmountable tasks.[118]

Denial is often an early response to new blindness, followed by a stage of mourning.[110,119] Depression often follows next, with the patient becoming passive and closed. New coping strategies must be developed for the patient to regain self-esteem and ultimately recover.

Family interactions are severely affected by the loss of vision in adolescence. Blind adolescents are extremely dependent on their families for physical and emotional support.[120] This sudden dependence can be even more difficult for the newly blind adolescent, who has been trying to emerge from this dependence in order to gain self-identity and autonomy. Parents should learn about their child's disability so they can better understand his or her potential as well as limitations. A positive parenting style is extremely important to the growth and development of the adolescent.[121]

Primary care physicians should be aware of the potential physical, psychologic, and emotional problems of visual loss. These difficult issues must be approached thoughtfully. Feelings of guilt in family members of the newly blind may need to be addressed. Counseling and participation in appropriate support groups may be necessary.

References

1. Flynn JT: Neonatal ophthalmology: evaluation of visual function in the neonate and infant. In Harley RD, editor: *Pediatric ophthalmology,* ed 2, Philadelphia, 1983, WB Saunders; p 6.
2. Burian HM: Pathophysiologic basis of amblyopia and its treatment, *Am J Ophthalmol* 67:1, 1969.
3. Duke-Elder S, Abrams D: Clinical instruments. Ophthalmic optics and refraction. In Duke-Elder S, editor: *System of ophthalmology,* London, 1970, Henry Kimpton; p 846.
4. Waltman SR, Hart WM: The cornea. In Moses RA, Hart WM, editors: *Adler's physiology of the eye. Clinical application,* St. Louis, 1987, Mosby–Year Book; p 36.
5. Burns RP, Forster RK, Laibson PR, Gipson IK: Chronic toxicity of local anesthetics on the cornea. In Leopold IH, Burns RP, editors: *Symposium on ocular therapy,* vol 10, New York, 1977, John Wiley; p 31.
6. Willis WE, Laibson PR: Corneal complications of topical anesthetic abuse, *Can J Ophthalmol* 5:239, 1970.
7. Rosenwasser GOD, Holland S, Pflugfelder SC, et al: Topical anesthetic abuse, *Ophthalmology* 97:967, 1990.
8. Clemons CS, Cohen EJ, Arentsen JJ, et al: *Pseudomonas* ulcers following patching of corneal abrasions associated with contact lens wear, *CLAO J* 13:161, 1987.
9. Slansky HH: Mechanical and nonmechanical injuries. Acid burns. In Fraunfelder FT, Roy FH, editors: *Current ocular therapy 3,* Philadelphia, 1990, WB Saunders; p 312.
10. Lemp MA: Cornea and sclera, *Arch Ophthalmol* 92:158, 1974.
11. Wilson FM: Traumatic hyphema: pathogenesis and management, *Ophthalmology* 87:910, 1980.
12. Goldberg MF: Sickled erythrocytes, hyphema, and secondary glaucoma. 1. The diagnosis and treatment of sickled erythrocytes in human hyphemas, *Ophthalmic Surg* 10:17, 1979.

13. Goldberg MF: The diagnosis and treatment of secondary glaucoma after hyphema in sickle cell patients, *Am J Ophthalmol* 87:43, 1979.

14. Edwards WC, Layden WE: Monocular versus binocular patching in traumatic hyphema, *Am J Ophthalmol* 76:359, 1973.

15. Crawford JS, Lewandowski RL, Chan W: The effect of aspirin on rebleeding in traumatic hyphema, *Am J Ophthalmol* 80:543, 1975.

16. Crouch ER Jr, Frenkel M: Aminocaproic acid in the treatment of traumatic hyphema, *Am J Ophthalmol* 81:355, 1976.

17. Dieste MC, Hersh PS, Kylstra JA, et al: Intraocular pressure increase associated with epsilon-aminocaproic acid therapy for traumatic hyphema, *Am J Ophthalmol* 106:383, 1988.

18. Finch CA: Pathophysiologic aspects of sickle cell anemia, *Am J Med* 53:1, 1972.

19. Sipperly MJO, Quigley HA, Gass JDM: Traumatic retinopathy in primates: the explanation of commotio retinae, *Arch Ophthalmol* 96:2267, 1978.

20. Deutsch TA, Feller DB, editors: *Paton and Goldberg's management of ocular injuries,* ed 2, Philadelphia, 1985, WB Saunders; p 72.

21. Smith B, Regan WF Jr: Blow-out fracture of the orbit. Mechanism and correction of internal orbital fracture, *Am J Ophthalmol* 44:733, 1957.

22. Gilbard SM, Mafee MF, Lagouros PA, Langer BG: Orbital blowout fractures. The prognostic significance of computed tomography, *Ophthalmology* 92:1523, 1985.

23. Deutsch TA, Feller DB, editors: *Paton and Goldberg's management of ocular injuries,* ed 2, Philadelphia, 1985, WB Saunders; p 37.

24. Anderson RL, Panje WR, Gross CE: Blindness following blunt forehead trauma, *Ophthalmology* 89:445, 1982.

25. Lam BL, Weingeist TA: Corticosteroid-responsive traumatic optic neuropathy, *Am J Ophthalmol* 109:99, 1990.

26. Guy J: Surgical treatment of progressive visual loss in traumatic optic neuropathy, *J Neurosurg* 70:799, 1989.

27. Joseph MP, Lessel S, Rizzo J, Momose KJ: Extracranial optic nerve decompression for traumatic optic neuropathy, *Arch Ophthalmol* 108:1091, 1990.

28. Kennerdell JS, Amsbaugh GA, Myers EN: Transantral-ethmoidal decompression of an optic canal fracture, *Arch Ophthalmol* 94:1040, 1976.

29. Burde RM, Savino PJ, Trobe JD: *Clinical decisions in neuro-ophthalmology,* St. Louis, 1985, Mosby–Year Book; p 185.

30. Keltner JL, Satterfield D, Dubin AB, et al: Dural and cavernous sinus fistulas. Diagnosis, management and complications, *Ophthalmology* 94:1585, 1987.

31. Larrison WI, Hersh PS, Kunzweiler T, Shingleton BJ: Sports-related ocular trauma, *Ophthalmology* 97:1265, 1990.

32. Smolin G, Okumoto M: Staphylococcal blepharitis, *Arch Ophthalmol* 95:812, 1977.

33. Thygeson P: Marginal corneal infiltrates and ulcers, *Trans Am Acad Ophthalmol Otolaryngol* 51:198, 1946.

34. Gillady AM, Shulmon ST: Periorbital and orbital cellulitis in children, *Pediatrics* 61:272, 1978.

35. Goldberg F: Differentiation of orbital cellulitis from preseptal cellulitis by computed tomography, *Pediatrics* 62:1000, 1978.

36. Dawson CR: Follicular conjunctivitis. In Tasman W, Jaeger EA, editors: *Duane's clinical ophthalmology,* vol 4, Philadelphia, 1989, JB Lippincott.

37. Dawson CR, Hanna L, Togni B: Adenovirus type 8 infections in the United States. IV. Observations on the pathogenesis of lesions in severe eye disease, *Arch Ophthalmol* 87:258, 1972.

38. Allansmith MR, Ross RN: Allergic conjunctivitis (atopic conjunctivitis, hay fever conjunctivitis). In Fraunfelder FT, Roy FH, editors: *Current ocular therapy 3,* Philadelphia, 1990, WB Saunders; p 400.

39. Allansmith MR: Vernal conjunctivitis. In Tasman W, Jaeger EA, editors: *Duane's clinical ophthalmology,* vol 4. Philadelphia, 1989, JB Lippincott.

40. Allansmith MR, Korb DR, Greiner JV: Giant papillary conjunctivitis in contact lens wearers, *Am J Ophthalmol* 83:697, 1977.

41. Allansmith MR, Baird RS, Greiner JV: Vernal conjunctivitis and contact lens–associated giant papillary conjunctivitis compared and contrasted, *Am J Ophthalmol* 87:544, 1979.

42. Allansmith MR, Ross RN: Giant papillary conjunctivitis. In Fraunfelder FT, Roy FH, editors: *Current ocular therapy 3,* Philadelphia, 1990, WB Saunders; p 411.

43. Dawson CR: Inclusion conjunctivitis (paratrachoma, chlamydia). In Fraunfelder FT, Roy FH, editors: *Current ocular therapy 3,* Philadelphia, 1990, WB Saunders; p 50.

44. Hammerschlag MR: Chlamydial infections, *J Pediatr* 114:727, 1989.

45. Darougar S, Viswalingam N: Trachoma. In Fraunfelder FT, Roy FH, editors: *Current ocular therapy 3,* Philadelphia, 1990, WB Saunders; p 51.

46. Curtin BJ, Theodore FH: Ocular molluscum contagiosum, *Am J Ophthalmol* 39:302, 1955.

47. Wear DJ, Malaty RH, Zimmerman LE, et al: Cat scratch disease bacilli in the conjunctiva of patients with Parinaud's oculoglandular syndrome, *Ophthalmology* 92:1282, 1985.

48. Dalton MJ, Robison LE, Cooper T, et al: Serologic diagnosis of cat scratch disease at CDC, *Arch Intern Med* 155:1670, 1995.

49. Zacchei AC, Newman NJ, Sternberg P: Serous retinal detachment of the macula associated with cat scratch disease, *Am J Ophthalmol* 120:796, 1995.

50. Szelc-Kelly CM, Goral S, Perez-Perez CI, et al: Serologic responses to *Bartonella* and *Afipia* antigens in patients with cat scratch disease, *Pediatrics* 96:1137, 1995.

51. Ullman S, Roussel RJ, Forster RK: Gonococcal keratoconjunctivitis, *Surv Ophthalmol* 32:199, 1987.

52. Wan WL, Farkas GC, May WN, Robin JB: The clinical characteristics and course of adult gonococcal conjunctivitis, *Am J Ophthalmol* 102:575, 1986.

53. Neumann-Haefelin D, Sundmacher R, Wochnik G, Bablok B: Herpes simplex virus types 1 and 2 in ocular disease, *Arch Ophthalmol* 96:64, 1978.

54. Binder PS: Herpes simplex keratitis, *Surv Ophthalmol* 21:313, 1977.

55. Baringer JR: The biology of herpes simplex virus infections in humans, *Surv Ophthalmol* 21:171, 1976.

56. Baringer JR: Recovery of herpes-simplex virus from human trigeminal ganglions, *N Engl J Med* 288:648, 1973.

57. McGill J, Fraunfelder FT, Jones BR: Current and proposed management of ocular herpes simplex, *Surv Ophthalmol* 20:358, 1976.

58. Pavan-Langston D: Diagnosis and management of herpes simplex ocular infection, *Int Ophthalmol Clin* 15:19, 1975.

59. Schwab IR: Oral acyclovir in the management of herpes simplex ocular infections, *Ophthalmology* 95:423, 1988.

60. Abbott RL, Abrams MA: Bacterial corneal ulcers. In Tasman W, Jaeger EA, editors: *Duane's clinical ophthalmology,* vol 4, Philadelphia, 1989, JB Lippincott.

61. Wilson LA, Schlitzer RL, Ahearn DG: *Pseudomonas* corneal ulcers associated with soft contact-lens wear, *Am J Ophthalmol* 92:546, 1981.

62. Galentine PG, Cohen EJ, Laibson PR, et al: Corneal ulcers associated with contact lens wear, *Arch Ophthalmol* 102:891, 1984.

63. Jones DB: Fungal keratitis. In Tasman W, Jaeger EA, editors: *Duane's clinical ophthalmology,* vol 4, Philadelphia, 1989, JB Lippincott.

64. Jones DB: Initial therapy of suspected microbial corneal ulcers. II. Specific antibiotic therapy based on corneal smears, *Surv Ophthalmol* 24:105, 1979.

65. Baum J: Therapy for ocular bacterial infection, *Trans Ophthalmol Soc UK* 105:69, 1986.

66. Leibowitz HM: Clinical evaluation of ciprofloxacin 0.3% ophthalmic solution for treatment of bacterial keratitis, *Am J Ophthalmol* 112:345, 1991.

67. Leibowitz HM, Kupferman A: Topically administered corticosteroids. Effect on antibiotic-treated bacterial keratitis, *Arch Ophthalmol* 98:1287, 1980.

68. Cohen EJ, Buchanan HW, Laughrea PA: Diagnosis and management of *Acanthamoeba* keratitis, *Am J Ophthalmol* 100:389, 1985.

69. Moore MB, McCulley JP, Luckenbach M, et al: *Acanthamoeba* keratitis associated with soft contact lenses, *Am J Ophthalmol* 100:396, 1985.

70. Baum J, Barza M, Weinstein P, et al: Bilateral keratitis as a manifestation of Lyme disease, *Am J Ophthalmol* 105:75, 1988.

71. Winterkorn JMS: Lyme disease: neurologic and ophthalmic manifestations, *Surv Ophthalmol* 35:191, 1990.

72. Rosenbaum JT, Wernick R: The utility of routine screening of patients with uveitis for systemic lupus erythematosus or tuberculosis, *Arch Ophthalmol* 108:1291, 1990.

73. Ohno S, Kimura GR, O'Connor GR: HLA antigens and uveitis, *Br J Ophthalmol* 61:62, 1977.

74. Keat A: Reiter's syndrome and reactive arthritis in perspective, *N Engl J Med* 309:1606, 1983.

75. Chajek T, Fainaru M: Behçet's disease. Report of 41 cases and a review of the literature, *Medicine* 54:179, 1975.

76. Michelson JB, Chisari FV: Behçet's disease, *Surv Ophthalmol* 26:190, 1982.

77. James DG, Spiteri MA: Behçet's disease, *Ophthalmology* 89:1279, 1982.

78. Kanski JJ, Shun-Shin GA: Systemic uveitis syndromes in childhood. An analysis of 340 cases, *Ophthalmology* 91:1247, 1984.

79. Kanski JJ: Anterior uveitis in juvenile rheumatoid arthritis, *Arch Ophthalmol* 95:1794, 1977.

80. Steere AC, Malawista SE, Bartenhagen NH, et al: The clinical spectrum and treatment of Lyme disease, *Yale J Biol Med* 57:453, 1984.

81. Shields MB: *Textbook of glaucoma*, ed 2, Baltimore, 1987, Williams & Wilkins; p 45.

82. Shaffer RN, Weiss DI: *Congenital and pediatric glaucomas*, St Louis, 1970, Mosby–Year Book; p 37.

83. Speakman JS: Pigmentary dispersion, *Br J Ophthalmol* 65:249, 1981.

84. Weiss DI: Dual origin of glaucoma in encephalotrigeminal hemangiomatosis, *Trans Ophthalmol Soc UK* 93:477, 1971.

85. Alfano JE: Changes in the intraocular pressure associated with systemic steroid therapy, *Am J Ophthalmol* 56:346, 1963.

86. Thomas JV, Simmons RJ, Belcher CD: Argon laser trabeculoplasty in the presurgical glaucoma patient, *Ophthalmology* 89:187, 1982.

87. Beck RW, Smith CH: *Neuro-ophthalmology: a problem-oriented approach*, Boston, 1988, Little, Brown; p 18.

88. Erkkila H: Optic disc drusen in children, *Acta Ophthalmol* 55:7, 1977.

89. Rosenberg MA, Savino PJ, Glaser JS: A clinical analysis of pseudopapilledema. I. Population, laterality acuity, refractive error, ophthalmoscopic characteristics and coincident disease, *Arch Ophthalmol* 97:65, 1979.

90. Katz M: The human eye as an optical system. In Safir A, editor: *Refraction and clinical optics*, New York, 1980, Harper & Row; p 81.

91. Milder B, Rubin M: *The fine art of prescribing glasses without making a spectacle of yourself*, Gainsville, FL, 1978, Triad Publishing, p 59.

92. Rubin M, Milder B: Myopia—a treatable disease?, *Surv Ophthalmol* 21:65, 1976.

93. Kushner BJ: Functional amblyopia: a purely practical pediatric patching protocol. In Reinecke RD, editor: *Ophthalmology annual*, New York, 1988, Raven Press, p 173.

94. *Requirements for nonprescription sunglasses and fashion eyewear*, New York, 1977, American National Standards Institute; p 7.

95. Rao GN, Saini JS: Complications of contact lenses. In Aquavella JV, Gullapalli GN, editors: *Contact lenses*, Philadelphia, 1987, JB Lippincott; p 195.

96. Thomas J: Hydrogel lenses: cosmetic. In Aquavella JV, Gullapalli GN, editors: *Contact lenses*, Philadelphia, 1987, JB Lippincott; p 70.

97. Coon LJ, Miller JP, Meier RF: Overview of extended wear contact lenses, *J Am Optom Assoc* 50:745, 1979.

98. Binder PS: Complications associated with extended wear of soft contact lenses, *Ophthalmology* 91:630, 1981.

99. Hassman G, Sugar J: *Pseudomonas* corneal ulcer with extended wear soft lens for myopia, *Arch Ophthalmol* 101:1549, 1983.

100. Baum J, Boruchoff SA: Extended-wear contact lenses and pseudomonal corneal ulcers, *Am J Ophthalmol* 101:372, 1985.

101. Koch JM, Refojo MF, Hanninen LA, et al: Experimental *Pseudomonas aeruginosa* keratitis from extended wear of soft contact lenses, *Arch Ophthalmol* 108:1453, 1990.

102. Stein JM, Stark RL, Randeri K: Comparison of chemical and thermal disinfection regimens: a retrospective data analysis, *Int Eyecare* 2:570, 1986.

103. Greco A: A review and update of contact lens care systems, *Int Contact Lens Clin* 11:266, 1984.

104. Bores LD: Historical review and clinical results of radial keratotomy, *Int Ophthalmol Clin* 23:93, 1983.

105. Kaufman HE: The correction of aphakia, *Am J Ophthalmol* 89:1, 1980.

106. Morgan KS: Visual rehabilitation of aphakia. IV. Epikeratophakia, *Surv Ophthalmol* 34:379, 1990.

107. Cotlier S, Schubert H, Mandel E, et al: Excimer laser radial keratotomy, *Ophthalmology* 92:206, 1985.

108. Wang FM, Marmor M: Ophthalmic problems during adolescence. In Boley SJ, Cohen MI, editors: *Surgery of the adolescent*, Orlando, FL, 1986, Grune & Stratton; p 122.

109. Kahn HA, Moorehead MB: *Statistics on blindness in the model reporting area, 1969-1970*, U.S. Department of Health, Education, and Welfare Pub. No. 73-427, Washington, DC, 1973, U.S. Government Printing Office.

110. World Health Organization: Blindness information collected from various sources, *Epidemiol Vital Stat Rep* 19:437, 1966.

111. Foster A: Patterns of blindness. In Tasman W, Jaeger EA, editors: *Duane's clinical ophthalmology*, vol 5, Philadelphia, 1989, JB Lippincott.

112. *Vision standards and low vision. Physician's desk reference for ophthalmology*, ed 18, Oradell, NJ, 1990, Medical Economics Books; p 46.

113. Genesky SM: A functional classification system of the visually impaired to replace the legal definition of blindness, *Am J Optom Arch Am Acad Optom* 48:631, 1971.

114. Wang FM, Marmor M: Ophthalmic problems during adolescence. In Boley SJ, Cohen MI, editors: *Surgery of the adolescent*, Orlando, FL, 1986, Grune & Stratton; p 120.

115. Goldstein H: Magnitude and causes of blindness: sources and limitations of data. In Tasman W, Jaeger EA, editors: *Duane's clinical ophthalmology*, vol 5, Philadelphia, 1989, JB Lippincott.

116. *Vision standards and low vision. Physician's Desk Reference for Ophthalmology,* ed 18, Oradell, NJ, 1990, Medical Economics Books; p 47.
117. Tuttle DW: *Self-esteem and adjusting with blindness,* Springfield, IL, 1984, Charles C Thomas.
118. Katz EH: On becoming blind: the loss and the change in the family—a case study, *Fam Systems Med* 5:89, 1987.
119. Cholden LS: *A psychiatrist works with blindness,* New York, 1958, American Foundation for the Blind.
120. Schulz PJ: *How does it feel to be blind: the psychodynamics of visual impairment,* Los Angeles, 1980, Muse-Ed.
121. Sommers V: *The influence of parental attitudes and social environment on the personality development of adolescent blind,* New York, 1944, American Foundation for the Blind.

Suggested Readings

Fraunfelder FT, Roy FH, editors: *Current ocular therapy 3,* Philadelphia, 1990, WB Saunders.

Harley RD: *Pediatric ophthalmology,* ed 2, Philadelphia, 1983, WB Saunders.

Tasman W, Jaeger EA, editors: *Duane's clinical ophthalmology,* Philadelphia, 1989, JB Lippincott.

Taylor D: *Pediatric ophthalmology,* Oxford, 1990, Blackwell Scientific Publications.

CHAPTER 146

Otolaryngology

•

Mark N. Goldstein

The onset of adolescence causes a shift in the focus of head and neck healthcare problems. The childhood diseases of otitis media and upper respiratory infections are replaced in adolescence by illnesses resulting from nasal obstruction, sinusitis, and sinus-related headache. These maladies are attributed to the growth and development of the anatomic structures, as well as to reactions of the nasal and paranasal mucosa to inflammation due to allergies and/or infection.

In the adolescent the eustachian tube has matured anatomically and functionally, and the middle ear function has improved. There is a regression of the adenotonsillar tissue, and tonsillitis becomes less of a problem except in a small percentage of adolescents. Voice strain or improper voice projection techniques result in laryngeal problems presenting as hoarseness, which is secondary to inflammation, and occasionally in the form of nodules.

EXAMINATION OF THE HEAD AND NECK

Beginning with the external aspect of the nose, the clinician should note whether a horizontal crease appears in the lower portion, indicating constant wiping of the nose. A persistent discharge from the nose frequently causes erythema and crusting around the nares. The internal nose is examined for congestion, edema, and erythema of the mucosa. The mucosal lining in patients with allergies that affect the nose appears gray or bluish in color. The position and appearance of the nasal septum and turbinates should be noted to determine whether a deviated septum or enlarged turbinates are causing obstruction. Enlarged boggy turbinates are consistent with allergic rhinitis. Enlarged turbinates with a clear discharge are consistent with pregnancy. Discharge near the turbinates, either clear or purulent, unilateral or bilateral, also should be examined to determine whether there is an infection in the paranasal sinuses. A vasoconstricting agent should be placed on the mucosa and allowed to absorb for several minutes so that the mucosal lining will contract. Subsequent examination will reveal the degree of mucosal congestion and underlying bony hypertrophy. In addition, the repeat examination may enable visualization of the posterior aspect of the nasal cavity to detect anatomic deformities or purulent discharge. Posterior rhinoscopy may be performed either with a flexible endoscope through the anterior nares or by a mirror examination looking at the nasopharynx from the oropharynx. In addition, nasal polyps, a posterior spur of the septum, or adenoidal hypertrophy may be diagnosed by rhinoscopy.

During otologic examination, the color and thickness of the external canal skin should be noted. Tenderness upon pulling the pinna implies otitis externa; tenderness upon palpation of the tragus and the anterior canal wall implies temporomandibular joint syndrome. Wax should normally be present in the lateral, hair-bearing aspect of the external auditory canal, and the tympanic membrane should be examined to detect any discoloration, scarring, retractions, or loss of mobility. Pneumatic otoscopy is performed to assess the movement of the tympanic membrane while tuning forks (256 and 512 Hz) are used to assess the patient's hearing status. The extraocular motions of both eyes are noted to rule out nystagmus, which is rhythmically repetitive movement of the eyes.

The oral cavity and oropharynx are examined for signs of infection involving the mucosa, teeth, or opening of the salivary ducts. Tonsillar size and symmetry and the presence of erythema, exudate, and inspissated food are recorded as abnormalities. Tenderness of the ptyergoid muscles is frequently associated with temporomandibular joint pain.

The hypopharynx and larynx are examined by indirect laryngoscopy or by further advancing the flexible endoscope from the nose through the oropharynx and hypopharynx. The larynx is examined for mobility, color, and thickness of the vocal cords, as well as for abnormalities such as nodules or polyps. The neck is palpated for enlarged lymph nodes, the size and location of which are noted, and the major salivary glands and the temporomandibular joint are palpated. Thyroid position and size are noted. Palpation of the carotid vessels, including the bifurcation, and the larynx completes the initial examination.

NASAL OBSTRUCTION

The primary functions of the nose include humidification, filtration, heat exchange, olfaction, and speech. Except for olfaction and speech, the autonomic nervous system controls most of the functions of the nose. The nasal cavities process approximately 10,000 L of air per day, and they normally contribute 30% of the airflow resistance to the lungs. The specific resistance of each side of the nose varies owing to the alternating swelling and constriction of the mucosa over the nasal turbinates. This variation in resistance is cyclic, occurring every 45 to 90 minutes, and is known as the nasal cycle. Rhinologic obstruction can be the result of the nasal cavity anatomy itself. Whereas the external nose is formed of an upper portion consisting of bone and a lower portion of cartilage, the internal nose is divided in the midline by the cartilaginous septum anteriorly and bony septum posteriorly. Inferior and middle turbinates form the lateral wall of the internal nose, and the superior turbinate forms the posterior aspect. Deviation of the septum becomes more pronounced as the child grows, and the turbinates may hypertrophy, causing unilateral or bilateral obstruction.

Patients presenting with nasal obstruction frequently complain of airway "stuffiness," which may be seasonal, acute, or chronic. This sensation may be unilateral or bilateral, and it is important to determine changes with the nasal cycle. These patients also complain of a dry mouth and frequently have recurrent sore throats as a result of mouth breathing. Headaches develop from referred pain to other areas in the paranasal region, and sleep disturbance may be secondary to the nasal obstruction. A careful history must be obtained to rule out antecedent trauma. Allergy symptoms, including rhinorrhea, postnasal discharge, sneezing, headaches, and itching, should be thoroughly investigated. Exposure to specific irritants, such as fumes or smoke, and the use of medications or illegal drugs should be determined. During history taking, the patient should be specifically questioned about excessive use of nasal sprays, which is a common cause of nasal obstruction.

Physiologic causes of nasal obstruction include the nasal cycle, the nasopulmonary reflex, paradoxical obstruction, and hormonal alterations. The nasopulmonary reflex occurs when increased nasal resistance produces increased pulmonary resistance and decreased pulmonary compliance, causing abnormal blood gases. This phenomenon may explain why an active upper respiratory infection causes breathlessness. Paradoxic nasal obstruction results from a long-standing anatomic deformity such as septal deviation. The normally patent side of the nose intermittently obstructs, leading to complaints of difficulty in breathing from the patent side. Puberty causes changes in the mucosal lining of the nasal cavity, which are mediated by increases in the estrogen hormone levels in both sexes. Intermittent nasal obstruction may be secondary to hormonal changes during menses. Normal vasomotor reaction to external stimuli, such as temperature, humidity, dust, and smog, frequently causes nasal obstruction. However, the most common cause of acute nasal obstruction is the common cold. Persistent acute rhinitis (for longer than 7 to 10 days) associated with significant nasal or nasopharyngeal discharge suggests sinusitis. Table 146-1 summarizes the more common causes of rhinitis.

After a thorough physical examination, appropriate laboratory tests should be performed and should include cultures of any thickened secretions or purulent material. Nasal cytology showing greater than one neutrophil per high-power field correlates with an 80% radiographic diagnosis of sinusitis. The presence of eosinophils on a nasal smear suggests allergy. With nasal cytology there is a false-negative incidence of 11%, which should be considered when basing therapeutic decisions on the results.

Rhinomanometry is used to calculate airway resistance by measuring airflow and pressure differences across the nasal cavity. This technique is useful in documenting the

TABLE 146-1
Rhinitis

Etiologies	Comments	Management
Infectious		
Viral	Upper respiratory infection	Decongestants
	HIV	Saline irrigations
Bacterial		Antibiotics
Fungal	Asthmatics	Antifungals
	Immunocompromised	Drainage
		Debridement
Allergic		
Polyps		Steroids/oral, nasal antibiotics
		Excision
Fungal		Antifungals
Rhinitis Medicamentosum		
Irritants		Oral steroids
		Saline irrigations
Medication		
Oral contraceptive pills		Adjust medicine
Antihypertensives		
Pregnancy		Saline irrigations
Drugs		
Smoking		Saline irrigations
Cocaine	Perforation/necrosis	
Constitutional		
Cystic fibrosis		Antibiotics, irrigations
Immotile cilia		
Immune deficiency		

amount of obstruction and recording the changes of resistance with the use of vasoconstrictors. The testing of olfaction has now been standardized by a scratch-and-sniff technique that forces the patient to choose one of four answers. It documents the degree of olfactory loss and is effective in unmasking malingerers.

Inflammation of the nose is the most common cause of nasal obstruction and is produced by bacterial, viral, allergic, or toxic agents. Adenoidal hypertrophy, an anatomic problem, is exacerbated by any inflammatory reaction. Metabolic abnormalities that cause obstruction include cystic fibrosis, diabetes mellitus, thyroid disease, and immune deficiency disease. In adolescent men the most common neoplasm causing obstruction is juvenile angiofibroma.

SINUSITIS

Sinusitis may complicate the treatment of nasal obstruction by causing inflammation of the adjacent nasal mucosa. This diagnosis should be considered when a patient fails to respond to medical management of nasal obstruction. The clinical manifestations of sinusitis in adolescents are different from those in children. By adolescence, most of the sinuses are developed. Malodorous breath and a persistent cough, as well as headache in the periorbital area, facial pain, and dental pain, may indicate sinusitis. In evaluation of patients with headache of possible sinus origin, it should be noted that 4% of patients have aplasia of the frontal sinuses and 16% have hypoplasia of the frontal sinuses. The complication of periorbital swelling is a common manifestation of sinusitis and may be the initial presenting symptom of the sinus infection. A tenderness to palpation of the face is a more reliable symptom of sinusitis in adolescents than in children.

Transillumination does not add significantly to the diagnosis, but radiographic films are generally used. Standard radiographs include the Waters view for the maxillary sinus, the Caldwell view for the frontal and ethmoid sinus, and the submental vertex and lateral views for the sphenoid sinuses. The lateral view also assists in

BOX 146-1
Orbital Complications from Sinusitis

Periorbital inflammatory edema
Orbital cellulitis
Subperiosteal abscess
Orbital abscess
Cavernous sinus thrombosis

BOX 146-2
**Intracranial Complications
from Sinusitis**

Meningitis
Epidural abscess
Subdural abscess
Venous sinus thrombosis
Brain abscess

visualizing the ethmoid and frontal sinuses. When the sinus radiographs are reviewed, an air-fluid level, complete opacification, or mucosal thickening of 4 mm or more, is correlated with pus in the sinus. Computed tomography (CT) and magnetic resonance imaging (MRI) have been used more frequently than routine radiographs to diagnose and monitor sinusitis. When plain films are compared with CT scans, there is up to an 84% discrepancy in findings. The plain films are useful in monitoring acute disease using the criteria of opacification, air-fluid levels, or mucosal thickening. CT scans are superior for monitoring chronic disease (infection of 4 weeks or longer) in which the ethmoid sinuses are most frequently involved. CT provides a significant amount of detail, particularly when performed in the coronal plane, because on CT the osteomeatal complex of the sinuses is better defined. This superior definition on CT is especially important for determining the cause of recurrent sinusitis. Orbital complications are clearly demonstrated when the two planes of the CT view are compared. The scans are also used in preparation for endoscopic sinus surgery involving the osteomeatal complex and the ethmoid sinuses, in which diseased mucosa is removed using telescopic lenses and instruments. MRI is useful for noting the inflammatory process and areas of opacification, but bony detail is better visualized by CT.

It is important to recognize the relationship between nasal obstruction, sinusitis, and asthma and to obtain the appropriate diagnostic studies. Medical and/or surgical treatment of sinus infection frequently helps to manage asthma. Effective treatment of sinusitis in asthmatic adolescents improves pulmonary function and frequently permits reduction of the asthma medication.

Cystic fibrosis is another special case in which extensive sinusitis is involved. Nasal polyposis occurs in 6% to 9% of children with cystic fibrosis and is more common in adolescents with this disease than in younger children. A sweat chloride test should be obtained for all children who have nasal polyps before surgery for removal of the polyps is contemplated. Excision of the polyps and appropriate drainage of the involved sinuses lead to a significant disease-free interval, with less nasal obstruction and/or sinusitis.

Treatment of nasal or sinus infection consists of the administration of antibiotics; topical and systemic decongestants; and, when allergy is a possible underlying etiology, antihistamines, intranasal and/or oral steroids. The most common bacterial organisms are *Streptococcus pneumoniae, Haemophilus influenzae,* and *Branhamella catarrhalis.* Anaerobic organisms account for approximately 40% of the bacteria isolated. The initial oral antibiotic therapy should involve either amoxicillin, amoxicillin-clavulanate, trimethoprim-sulfamethoxazole, or erythromycin-sulfazoxisol. Intranasal and/or oral decongestants reduce mucosal swelling and aid sinus drainage. Antihistamines reduce mucosal reactivity to environmental factors. Steroids can be used in severe inflammatory states, but antibiotic administration is necessary if there is any possibility of an infection. The possibility of fungal infections, although rare, should be considered in patients with long-standing sinus infections (i.e., asthmatics) or those who have compromised immune function. The treatment regimen of antibiotics and decongestants usually takes 10 days, with several weeks of treatment necessary in some cases.

The patient usually responds within the first 2 to 3 days of medical treatment. Intranasal lavage of the sinus is recommended for patients with persistent symptoms, documented radiographic findings, or therapeutic failure. Lavage clears disease from the sinus, and an accurate culture of the infected sinus can be obtained. Hospitalization with administration of intravenous antibiotics is recommended for patients who fail to respond to medical management, suffer recurrent episodes of sinusitis, or develop a complication. Orbital complications are the most common, intracranial complications being the second most common (Boxes 146-1 and 146-2).

Once the patient has been treated for the acute nasal or paranasal sinus condition, a full evaluation, with special attention to the possibility of allergic rhinitis or anatomic deformities, should be performed. If the patient has medical problems, including allergic rhinitis, desensitization or the use of oral or intranasal medications to control the disease is appropriate. Surgical intervention is used acutely to drain an infected sinus and adjacent area if a complication has developed. Surgical management is also used to correct nasal obstruction due to a deviated septum or enlarged turbinates. These procedures are usually performed on an outpatient basis. Postoperative visits to the clinician are necessary to clear the nasal cavity of crusts until the mucosa has healed. The patient also may undergo sinus drainage as an outpatient procedure. The removal of any anatomic abnormalities and the opening of the sinus ostia permit appropriate drainage from the sinuses to the nasal cavity. Patients require follow-up care for the next few weeks to remove crusts from the surgical sites. Occasionally, the endonasal procedures fail owing to blockage of the ostia or recurrent infection, and external procedures are necessary. These external procedures generally require hospitalization for several days and a subsequent recuperative period at home for an equal amount of time.

EPISTAXIS

Evaluation of epistaxis should always include the history of whether the bleeding is unilateral or bilateral, the amount of bleeding (e.g., the patient stained a tissue, filled a cup), the time and duration, and whether it was a posterior bleed (went down the back of the throat while the patient was sitting up) or an anterior bleed (all blood comes anteriorly). Systemic problems relating to blood loss should be recorded (diaphoresis, tachycardia, orthostatic hypotension, perfusion of the skin, petechiae).

Most epistaxis is from the anterior septum, and only 10% is thought to be from the posterior septum or nasal cavity. The patient should sit up and lean forward to clear the airway, and blood should be collected in a basin to estimate the amount of blood lost. If blood goes down the back of the throat, this is believed to indicate a posterior bleed requiring hospital evaluation and management. Vital signs indicate the amount of blood lost. Tachycardia can result from blood loss or the patient's mental status. Normal blood pressure indicates less than 10% blood loss; postural hypotension indicates greater than 10% blood loss. If the blood pressure is low and the pulse rapid, the loss of blood is causing impending shock. Elevated blood pressure may be a contributing factor or may be related to the patient's mental status.

Treatment consists of packing the nose with Neo-Synephrine 0.5% or Afrin Nasal spray, or the equivalent, on a piece of cotton. Hold the nostrils closed for several minutes. If bleeding continues or is profuse, pack the nose with expandable packing or gauze and call for consultation. Transferring the patient to the hospital is appropriate so that an intravenous line can be started and blood samples obtained for complete blood count, type, and cross-match, as well as coagulation screening.

If the bleeding subsides, replace the cotton with the constricting agent with a cotton soaked in 4% lidocaine.

Remove this cotton after several minutes and cauterize the bleeding area with silver nitrate applicators. Place a third cotton, this time mixed with antibiotic ointment, in the nose after the cauterization and keep it in place for several hours. The patient should refrain from hot foods for 2 or 3 days. No excessive activity should be allowed for 5 days, although the patient may go to school. Antibiotic ointment should be applied to the nose twice daily to cover the cauterized area for 5 to 7 days.

Bleeding that is severe, necessitating admission to the hospital, requires team management to monitor the need for blood or blood products. A posterior pack may be necessary, and sinus radiographs or a CT scan should be obtained when this type of pack is placed to examine the anatomy. Antibiotics are given because of the possibility of sinusitis. Supplemental oxygen is given via a mask. If the bleeding is controlled, the packing is advanced after 48 hours and removed shortly thereafter. If the bleeding continues, the patient is evaluated for either angiographic embolization or surgical ligation of the appropriate arteries.

TONSILLITIS

The incidence of all upper respiratory infections diminishes in adolescence. However, recurrent tonsillitis remains a significant problem in a small portion of this population and is frequently associated with adenoiditis. At puberty the tonsils and adenoids regress further, having previously reduced in size between the ages of 6 and 8 years. Persistence of large tonsils and adenoids causes problems with the upper airway, such as mouth breathing, snoring, occasional snorting, and some difficulty eating, since the mouth cannot be closed to chew properly. Poor sleeping may lead to morning tiredness with excessive daytime sleepiness and poor attention span in school. Occasionally, an adolescent presents for evaluation because of halitosis that does not respond to antibiotics. The patient may have cryptic tonsils that trap food and lead to malodorous breath. Other causes of bad breath include chronic adenoiditis and sinusitis.

In the adolescent who has recurrent problems with tonsils and adenoids, a careful examination of both nasal cavities must be performed to rule out purulent discharge, intranasal pathologic conditions, or sinusitis. The adenoids are visualized by flexible endoscopy to observe the size, degree of erythema, and presence of any purulent exudate on their surface. The oropharynx and hypopharynx are examined endoscopically to see whether the hypertrophied tonsils are impinging on the airway. The larynx is examined to ensure that the lingual tonsils are not part of the obstructing complex. Oropharyngeal examination is performed to determine the exact relationship between the tonsils and the palate. The palate is palpated for the presence of a submucous cleft. The neck is palpated for persistent cervical adenopathy.

Serous otitis media is a frequent presentation of adenoidal hypertrophy. Cervical adenopathy associated with adenotonsillar hypertrophy points to an infectious etiology. Laboratory evaluation for Epstein-Barr virus and, if suspected, human immunodeficiency virus should be included. Surgery for drainage of serous fluid or for adenotonsillar hyperplasia is deferred if the patient has an acute viral infection (Box 146-3).[15] Infection of the tonsils occurs frequently during upper respiratory infections. In addition to pain, patients have erythema, possibly exudate, and cervical adenopathy. Fever may be present. It is important to take a throat culture to rule out group A beta-hemolytic streptococci. Assymetry of the tonsils may indicate a peritonsillar abscess; this is associated with trismus, voice changes ("hot potato voice") with fullness, and erythema of one tonsillar pillar more than the other.

Infectious mononucleosis mimics tonsillitis but is frequently more severe with both tonsils enlarged with exudate and the characteristic posterior cervical adenopathy. Therapy is directed at reducing the upper airway obstruction with the use of steroids and antibiotics (ampicillin is not used since this is associated with a rash in a high percentage of patients). Owing to airway obstruction, it may be necessary either to provide a nasopharyngeal airway or to intubate the patient.

If intervention is indicated, treatment is generally surgical. If an abscess is suspected, local anesthesia is administered to the anterior pillar of the tonsil. The tonsillar pillar is aspirated; if this is unsuccessful the pillar is incised with a No. 15 blade through the mucosa, and the area of the tonsillar capsule is exposed, the incision being enlarged with a tonsil clamp.

Tonsillectomy is performed as ambulatory surgery in an outpatient setting of a hospital or ambulatory surgical facility. In older patients, recuperation takes 7 to 14 days. The lengthy recuperative time is due to the large surface area at the site of excision. Postoperative pain, frequently referred to the ears, is controlled with analgesics. A healing white eschar fills the tonsillar fossae and is often considered to represent infections. The eschar separates after 1 week, occasionally causing some bleeding. By the seventh postoperative day the patient generally returns to school, with athletics permitted on the seventeenth to twenty-first postoperative days. The complication of bleeding generally occurs in less than 1% of patients, so blood typing is usually not performed preoperatively.

ORAL CAVITY LESIONS

The most common types of nontraumatic ulcerative lesion in the oral cavity are the aphthous ulcers. Immunologic factors have been implicated in the etiology. The lesions may be minor, major, or herpetiform. There is usually a tingling or burning sensation before the eruption of the ulcer. Over-the-counter medications can provide good control of the disease, and prescription medications are not usually necessary. Topical or systemic steroids are occasionally used for severe cases.

Gonorrhea also presents with multiple ulcerations, but more commonly there is a general erythema with the ulcers, along with cervical adenopathy. After appropriate cultures, antibiotics are prescribed.

Smokeless tobacco presents as white lesions in the oral mucosa where the tobacco is usually kept. The mucosa has a granular, irregular appearance. The lesions are painless and asymptomatic initially. Cessation of the tobacco use leads to regression. If the lesion persists or becomes larger or more ulcerative, malignancy should be suspected and appropriate referral and biopsy recommended.

OTOLOGIC PROBLEMS

Otologic problems that occur during adolescence are usually either a progression of ear disease that presented during infancy or a manifestation related to noise exposure. The child who has recurrent ear infections with frequent perforations, or has had the tympanic membrane surgically manipulated, may develop softening of the tympanic membrane with a retraction of the membrane toward the medial aspect of the middle ear space or onto the ossicular chain. Frequently this condition progresses, causing potential ossicular disruption with hearing loss. If hearing loss exists, amplification to improve the hearing

---

BOX 146-3
Tonsil and Adenoid Surgery: Indications

OBSTRUCTION
Hypertrophy of tonsils or adenoids
Obligate mouth breathing not attributed to other
  causes
Sleep apnea
Speech abnormalities
Chronic otitis media with effusion
Recurrent or chronic otitis media with perforation
Chronic or recurrent nasopharyngitis

INFECTION
Recurrent tonsillitis despite adequate medical
  therapy
Peritonsillar abscess
Recurrent tonsillitis with cardiac disease
Recurrent tonsillitis with persistent streptococcal
  carrier state
Halitosis

level or surgical treatment is recommended. The surgery is planned to repair the tympanic membrane and/or to repair the ossicular chain. Overnight hospitalization is usually necessary, with return to school or work within a week.

For the ear that continues to be infected, the infectious process should first be controlled medically or surgically before any reconstructive procedures are performed. Cholesteatoma is a possibility that should be considered with all ongoing infections that do not clear within a 4- to 6-week period. A discharge from the ear associated with otitis externa may represent a chronic infection of the middle ear. The outer ear must be treated first to permit good visualization of the tympanic membrane. Preoperative radiographic evaluation consists of a CT scan to visualize any bony abnormalities of the mastoid and to determine the extent of the disease.

Otitis externa tends to be extremely painful and is common during the summer months. The use of expandable wicks has reduced the difficulty in treating this disease. Spongelike wicks are inserted into the swollen ear canal with little difficulty, and the topical drops then cause the wick to expand, reducing the edema, minimizing the pain of the ear canal, and ensuring that the medication stays in contact with the skin surface. The wick is usually removed in 24 to 48 hours and the ear canal cleansed thoroughly, enabling visualization of the tympanic membrane. To avoid otitis externa, the patient can use most commercial preparations of acetic acid and alcohol to dry the ear and prevent infections. This solution is used regularly at the end of the day, with cotton placed on the outside for 15 to 20 minutes.

A sensorineural hearing loss noted in adolescence may be related to noise exposure or a sequela of persistent otitis media of childhood. Loud music, even when listened to through headphones, has been known to cause unsafe levels of sound. It is especially advisable for adolescents who use headphones to keep the volume level low to avoid causing hearing problems. Frequently, the first sign of a hearing problem is a temporary threshold shift after exposure to loud noises. If exposure occurs regularly, a permanent threshold shift will be experienced.

All patients who have ear complaints should undergo a complete audiogram, including the testing of acoustic reflexes, to determine whether a hearing loss exists and to measure its significance. The audiogram should include pure tone testing from 250 to 8000 Hz. Air and bone conduction should be examined to determine whether conductive loss, as opposed to sensorineural loss, has occurred. The normal hearing range is 0 to 25 dB; above 25 dB, one notices a hearing problem. The audiogram also examines speech discrimination—the ability to understand phonetically balanced words at a given decibel level. Tympanometry is used to measure tympanic membrane mobility. Acoustic reflexes test the integrity of the cochlear nerve to elicit a stapedial reflex (governed by cranial nerve VII) when a loud noise is present. The reflex is both ipsilateral and contralateral. At high frequency (above 8000 Hz), audiometry can identify unsuspected sensorineural hearing loss not apparent during routine screenings. Using the tones available from the audiometer, one can try to match the tinnitus tone that the patient senses. If a unilateral hearing loss exists, further evaluation should include vestibular function tests and specialized audiometric tests to rule out retrocochlear pathologic conditions such as a tumor. MRI is extremely useful in identifying the cochleovestibular complex in order to visualize any pathologic conditions in this area.

Sensorineural hearing loss due to noise exposure is frequently in the upper frequencies, corresponding to the basal turn of the cochlea near the oval window where sound enters. Acute sensorineural hearing loss usually affects many frequencies. Because of the emergent nature of this loss, treatment is directed at possible causes, including inflammation (bacterial, viral) and poor circulation to the inner ear (sludging of blood or vasoconstriction). Treatment with antibiotics, oral steroids, vasodilating agents, and anticoagulants (aspirin, dipyridamole [Persantine]) is common. The results of treatment depend on the degree of the patient's preexisting hearing loss before the acute loss occurred. If a hearing loss existed previously, the prognosis is less favorable.

Tinnitus is frequently associated with hearing loss. Causes of tinnitus in adolescents also include eustachian tube dysfunction, temporomandibular joint disease, allergy, and metabolic problems. There is no specific treatment, but a thorough understanding of the problem helps the patient. Specific psychosocial stress factors associated with adolescence should be identified. Helpful suggestions include the use of competing noise as the child attempts to go to sleep, and the avoidance of any loud noises that may aggravate the tinnitus or hearing problems. Treatment of underlying medical problems should help. Biofeedback has been used with some success.

Vertigo is relatively uncommon in adolescents and is usually related to an inner ear infection or trauma to the head, causing an inner ear problem. It is important to distinguish vertigo from dizziness. The patient should be questioned specifically concerning aural symptoms; if there are no associated hearing problems, it is unlikely that there is end-organ (vestibular) disease. A thorough head and neck examination should be performed, including pneumatic otoscopy, which may unmask a fistula of the inner ear. A full neurologic test is also important, including cerebellar testing. Having the patient hyperventilate for 30 seconds frequently produces the symptom complex and identifies hyperventilation as the etiology. A full audiologic evaluation is necessary. Should any of the initial clinical tests prove abnormal, an electronystagmogram, and possibly CT or MRI, should be performed. If no specific cause is found and the examination is clinically normal, Cawthorne exercises, designed specifically to strengthen balance function, can be used by the patient to help compensate for the sensation of imbalance. These exercises are done twice daily for approximately 15 minutes. The patient is reevaluated at 2-week intervals to check on progress. Laboratory tests, including hematologic evaluation with tests for infectious and metabolic abnormalities, should be performed.

LARYNGEAL PROBLEMS

Laryngeal problems in the adolescent are usually related to either acute infections affecting the vocal cords or vocal abuse, which leads to persisting hoarseness. The acute infections are frequently viral in origin, causing edema of the cords and hoarseness. The patient is usually treated with decongestants, humidification, and voice rest with good resolution. Persistence of the hoarseness or an attempt to use the voice during the acute episode frequently leads to irritation of the vocal cords at the junction of the anterior and middle thirds of the vocal cord. Persistent irritation or vocal abuse can lead to the development of small nodules at this location. The nodularity can also develop from chronic vocal abuse, shouting, or use of poor technique in an attempt to project the voice to large audiences. Any hoarseness that persists for more than 4 to 6 weeks should be evaluated by a specialist, and if vocal cord nodules are present, voice rest and instruction on the proper use of the voice should be the primary therapy. Evaluation by a speech pathologist is generally indicated to diagnose the specific problems patients are having with their voice, and therapy is usually performed once or twice a week. Occasionally adolescents who are using their voice in a professional manner, as in singing or acting, may need instruction from a voice coach on a regular basis. Once they have improved speech habits, the persistent nodules may be excised in an outpatient procedure under microscopic control to avoid damage to the delicate surrounding structures. Postoperatively, 4 to 6 weeks of voice rest are required, with continued speech therapy to solidify the gains the patient made during the initial treatment. Surgical intervention is not indicated as the primary treatment because poor vocal habits cause recurrence of the nodules. With good speech therapy, surgical intervention can frequently be avoided.

Suggested Readings

Graney DO: Paranasal sinuses, anatomy. In Cummings CW, Fredrickson JM, Harker LA, et al, editors: *Otolaryngology—Head and neck surgery,* St. Louis, 1986, Mosby–Year Book; p 845.

Hibbert J: Tonsils and adenoids. In Mackay IS, Bull TR, editors: *Scott-Brown's otolaryngology,* vol 6, London, 1987, Butterworth; p 368.

King HC, Mabry RL: *A practical guide to the management of nasal and sinus disorders,* New York, 1993, Thieme.

Leonard G, Owen Black F, Schramm VL: Tinnitus in children. In Bluestone CD, Stool SE, editors: *Pediatric otolaryngology,* vol 1, Philadelphia, 1983, WB Saunders; p 271.

Mackay I, Cole P: Rhinitis, sinusitis and associated chest disease. In Mackay IS, Bull TR, editors: *Scott-Brown's otolaryngology,* vol 4, London, 1987, Butterworth; p 61.

CHAPTER 147

Dentistry

•

Bryan J. Williams, Lezley P. McIlveen, and Donald J. Forrester

The masticatory apparatus is of great importance to the adolescent not only for basic health but also for the key role of the appearance of the dentition in the adolescent psyche. There are a number of important dental health issues in the adolescent, including: dental and facial development and the role of orthodontic treatment, dental caries and its sequelae, dental impact of bulimia nervosa, periodontal disease, soft tissue lesions, dentoalveolar trauma, and mandibular fractures.

DEVELOPMENT OF DENTITION

During adolescence the transition from mixed (primary and permanent teeth) to permanent dentition is completed. Generally, most of the permanent teeth erupt by the age of 12 to 13 years, with the exception of the third molars (wisdom teeth), which do not erupt until 17 to 25 years of age (Table 147-1). During a period of 3 to 4 years beginning at age 9 years, 12 primary teeth are exfoliated and 16 permanent teeth erupt. Delayed eruption is associated with certain conditions such as Down syndrome, ectodermal dysplasia, osteogenesis imperfecta, achondroplasia, and cleidocranial dysplasia. Premature loss of a posterior primary tooth due to dental caries or trauma can disrupt eruption and lead to alignment and space problems in the permanent dentition.

There is controversy over routine extraction of third molars. Generally if these teeth can be accommodated in the arch and are used in function, extraction is contraindicated. However, if the teeth are impacted (Fig. 147-1) or if there are pathologic conditions such as recurrent pericoronitis, dental caries, cystic degeneration, or periodontal problems, the third molars should be extracted. The myth that eruption of third molars contributes to anterior tooth crowding has been dispelled and is not an indication for extraction. As the roots of third molars often show unusual structure, surgical removal during adolescence before completion of root formation is generally less complicated than in adulthood.

FACIAL GROWTH AND DEVELOPMENT

Facial growth contributes to significant changes in appearance during adolescence. The convex facial profile of the child develops into the more straight facial profile of the adult, and the height of the face increases. Craniofacial growth is focused on the lower two thirds of the face, producing a downward and forward displacement of the maxilla and mandible. The amount and direction of mandibular or maxillary growth can be unpredictable and can be so significantly different that changes in occlusion and facial appearance occur over time. The rate of skeletal jaw development parallels that of the body as a whole; therefore, changes are maximal during the adolescent growth spurt.

ORTHODONTIC ISSUES IN THE ADOLESCENT

The specialty of orthodontics is concerned with optimal function of dentition and the masticatory apparatus, the aesthetics of the dentition, and harmony and balance of facial proportions. A problem in the alignment and fit of the teeth is called malocclusion and can be acquired (e.g., from trauma or early loss of a primary tooth) or congenital. Underlying patterns of jaw length disharmony are usually inherited. Both tooth alignment and structural relations of the jaw are addressed in orthodontic assessment and treatment (Fig. 147-2).

Particularly in patients with jaw length discrepancy it is critical that orthodontic referral be made before the cessation of jaw development. In many of these patients the orthodontist can, to a degree, differentially manipulate jaw development as well as tooth alignment in order to achieve an optimal aesthetic and functional result (Fig. 147-3). Once growth has ceased, orthognathic surgery in conjunction with orthodontics may be necessary to achieve the best results (Fig. 147-4). Also, certain skeletal disharmonies are optimally correctable only with a

TABLE 147-1
Chronology of the Human Dentition

Tooth	Hard Tissue Formation Begins	Amount of Enamel Formed at Birth	Enamel Completed	Eruption	Root Completed
Primary Dentition					
Maxillary					
Central incisor	4 mo in utero	Five sixths	1½ mo	7½ mo	1½ yr
Lateral incisor	4½ mo in utero	Two thirds	2½ mo	9 mo	2 yr
Cuspid	5 mo in utero	One third	9 mo	18 mo	3¼ yr
First molar	5 mo in utero	Cusps united	6 mo	14 mo	2½ yr
Second molar	6 mo in utero	Cusp tips still isolated	11 mo	24 mo	3 yr
Mandibular					
Central incisor	4½ mo in utero	Three fifths	2½ mo	6 mo	1½ yr
Lateral incisor	4½ mo in utero	Three fifths	3 mo	7 mo	1½ yr
Cuspid	5 mo in utero	One third	9 mo	16 mo	3¼ yr
First molar	5 mo in utero	Cusps united	5½ mo	12 mo	2¼ yr
Second molar	6 mo in utero	Cusps tips still isolated	10 mo	20 mo	3 yr
Permanent Dentition					
Maxillary					
Central incisor	3-4 mo		4-5 yr	7-8 yr	10 yr
Lateral incisor	10-12 mo		4-5 yr	8-9 yr	11 yr
Cuspid	4-5 mo		6-7 yr	11-12 yr	13-15 yr
First bicuspid	1½-1¾ yr		5-6 yr	10-11 yr	12-13 yr
Second bicuspid	2-2¼ yr		6-7 yr	10-12 yr	12-14 yr
First molar	At birth	Sometimes a trace	2½-3 yr	6-7 yr	9-10 yr
Second molar	2½-3 yr		7-8 yr	12-13 yr	14-16 yr
Mandibular					
Central incisor	3-4 mo		4-5 yr	6-7 yr	9 yr
Lateral incisor	3-4 mo		4-5 yr	7-8 yr	10 yr
Cuspid	4-5 mo		6-7 yr	9-10 yr	12-14 yr
First bicuspid	1¾-2 yr		5-6 yr	10-12 yr	12-13 yr
Second bicuspid	2¼-2½ yr		6-7 yr	11-12 yr	13-14 yr
First molar	At birth	Sometimes a trace	2½-3 yr	6-7 yr	9-10 yr
Second molar	2½-3 yr		7-8 yr	11-13 yr	14-15 yr

After Logan and Kronfeld: *J Am Dent Assoc* 20, 1933 (slightly modified by McCall and Schour). Copyright by the American Dental Association. Reprinted by permission.

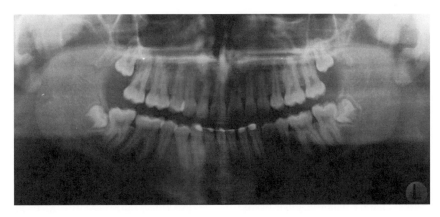

Fig. 147-1. Panoramic radiograph of a 16-year-old postorthodontic patient (note the fixed retainer lower anterior). Third molars (wisdom teeth) are present with inadequate space for eruption.

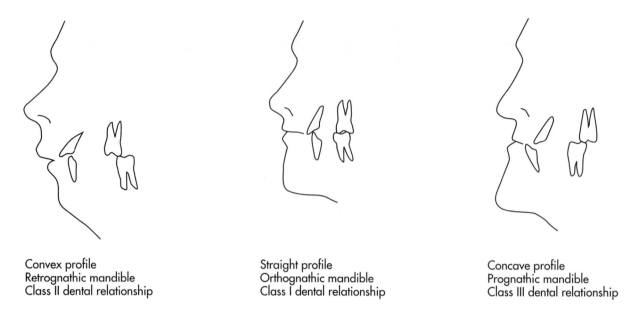

Convex profile
Retrognathic mandible
Class II dental relationship

Straight profile
Orthognathic mandible
Class I dental relationship

Concave profile
Prognathic mandible
Class III dental relationship

Fig. 147-2. Common facial patterns and usual underlying occlusal relations.

combination of orthodontics and orthognathic surgery (e.g., mandibular overgrowth or prognathism, skeletal open bite) (Fig. 147-5).

DENTAL CARIES

Currently, dental caries is increasingly thought of as an infective disease with multifactorial etiology. Although its incidence has demonstrated a well-documented decline, this microbial infection of the dental hard tissues still affects many children. A 1986 National Institute of Dental Research study indicated that 50% of children between the ages of 5 and 17 years were caries free compared with 37% in 1980 and 28% in the early 1970s.

However, although the results of this study are encouraging, it must also be remembered that 50% of children and adolescents do have dental caries. Adolescence represents a period of significant cariogenic activity. Irregular eating habits, frequent snacking, and consumption of retentive foods with a high cariogenic potential, especially if combined with poor oral hygiene, place newly erupted permanent teeth at high risk for dental caries. In severe cases, extensive destruction of the dentition can occur. This condition, termed *rampant caries,* presents a considerable challenge to the dental practitioner.

Sequelae of Dental Caries

Untreated dental caries can have major health impacts. Once the caries reaches the dental pulp, the pulpal tissues begin to degenerate. The patient usually has significant pain by this point. As the pulp continues to necrose, the infectious organisms and necrotic by-products can extend to adjacent tissues, both bone and soft tissues (Fig. 147-6). If the process continues to extend, serious complications can result (Fig. 147-7).

Prevention

Because of the increased carious activity during adolescence, periodic dental evaluation is essential. The emphasis of these professional visits should be on maintenance of optimal oral hygiene, use of topical fluorides, and dietary management.

ORAL HYGIENE. Oral hygiene recommendations should be realistic. As with many other issues in adolescent life, nagging by a parent usually leads to a negative response. The goal should be one thorough cleaning daily, including dental flossing. Bedtime is the preferred time for thorough brushing and flossing because of reduced salivary flow during sleep.

Waxed or unwaxed dental floss should be used either manually or with the assistance of a floss holder. Although a wide variety of toothbrush designs are available, the preferred toothbrush design possesses a small, straight brush head and contains soft-textured, multitufted nylon bristles. Clinical studies indicate that electrically powered toothbrushes are equally effective, and for disabled individuals who have difficulty cleaning their teeth, these are more effective than manual toothbrushes. Currently, some electric brushes emit ultrasonic waves that seem to be particularly effective in dislodging plaque.

WATER FLUORIDATION AND FLUORIDE. Since its introduction in 1945, public water fluoridation has repeatedly proved to be the most economic, safe, convenient, and effective measure available to prevent

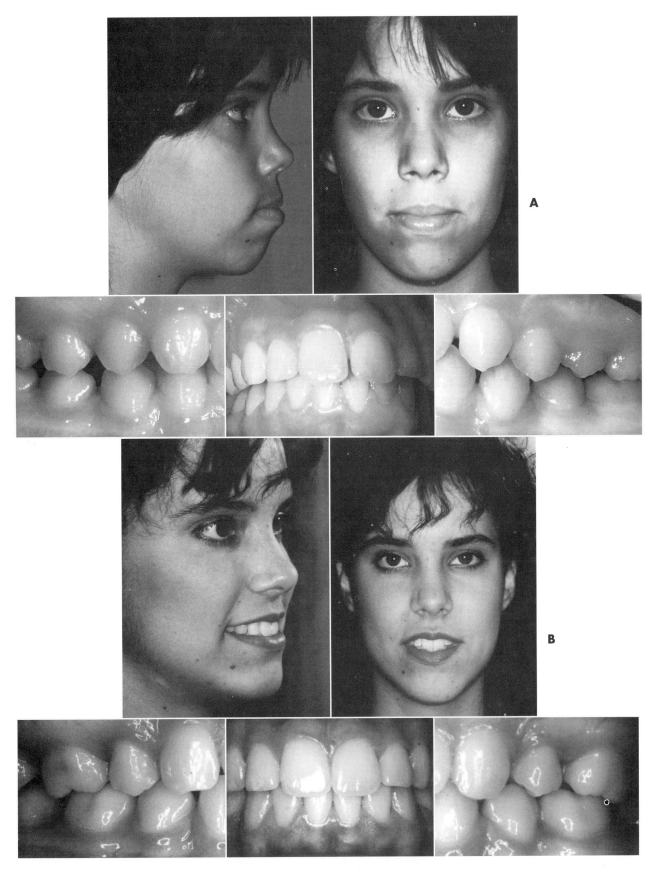

Fig. 147-3. **A,** Preorthodontic treatment demonstrating convex facial profile and dental protrusion. **B,** After treatment involving extraction of the first bicuspid teeth and orthodontics to align and retract the teeth. Improvements are evident in the facial profile, the alignment of the teeth, and the posterior occlusion.

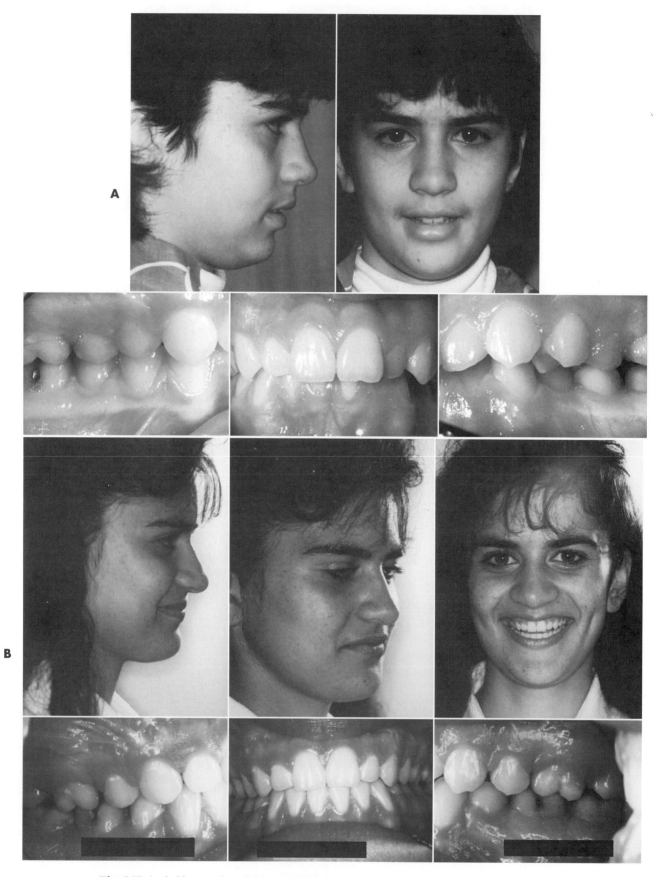

Fig. 147-4. A, Nongrowing adolescent with a convex facial pattern, mandibular retrognathia, and class II malocclusion. **B,** Results after treatment involving orthodontic alignment and surgical mandibular advancement.

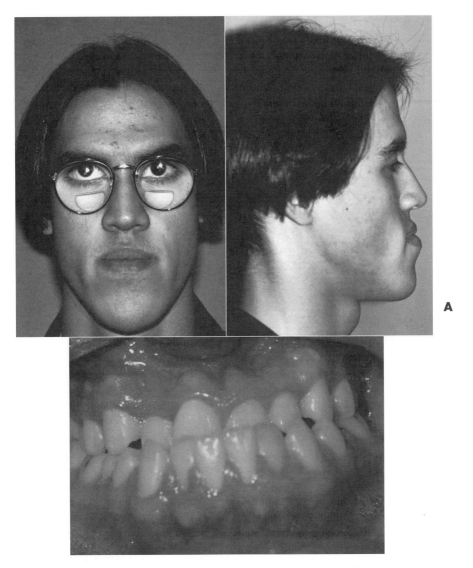

Fig. 147-5. A, Adolescent with severely concave facial profile, maxillary deficiency, and mandibular prognathism.

dental caries. Unfortunately, only 50% of the American population now ingests drinking water containing fluoride at optimal levels. It is therefore appropriate for the physician providing health care to children and adolescents in nonfluoridated areas to develop a fluoride supplement regimen. In 1995 the guidelines were modified to reflect the additional amounts of fluoride that children and adolescents receive from sources such as ingested toothpaste (Table 147-2).

The need for fluoride supplements beyond regular brushing with a fluoride dentifrice should be carefully evaluated in all children and adolescents. Successful results from fluoride supplements depend primarily on parents reinforcing in their children the habit of taking fluoride supplements. In this regard, compliance can be greatly improved by the physician's emphasis on the need for daily fluoride supplementation and by the inclusion of clear instructions. If the fluoride content of the drinking

water is unknown, fluoride supplement recommendations should be determined by the results obtained from fluoride analysis of the water source in question. This is critical, since levels of fluoride beyond the optimum can have detrimental aesthetic effects on the dentition.

Dentifrices. Parents and their children should be encouraged to use a fluoride dentifrice that has American Dental Association (ADA) approval. At present, the ADA is the only national agency that objectively evaluates the therapeutic claims of dental products. Used regularly, a fluoride dentifrice inhibits dental caries by 20% to 30%.

Mouth rinses. The use of over-the-counter 0.05% fluoride mouth rinses has been well documented as an accepted, safe, and inexpensive dental caries–inhibiting procedure. Whether used in a community with optimally fluoridated water or in an unfluoridated community, it has been shown to provide 35% to 40% protection against caries. Fluoride mouth rinses are recommended for use by

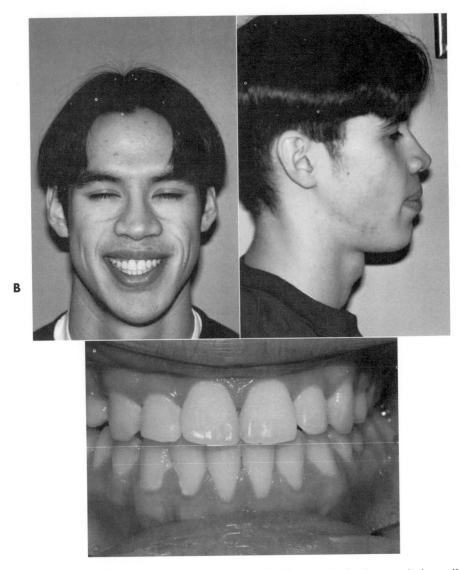

Fig. 147-5, cont'd. B, Results after treatment involving orthodontics, surgical maxillary advancement, and mandibular setback.

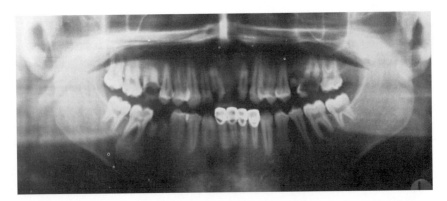

Fig. 147-6. Panoramic radiograph demonstrating carious destruction of adolescent dentition. Note the area of condensing osteitis associated with the roots of a pulpally involved mandibular right second molar.

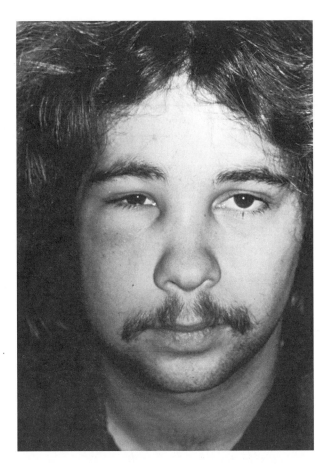

Fig. 147-7. Adolescent with severe facial cellulitis involving the orbital area. Dental caries with pulpal necrosis in a maxillary bicuspid was the underlying cause.

individuals using orthodontic appliances and by those with medical or physical disabilities–in short, by all who have an increased susceptibility to dental decay.

Gels. Self-applied, prescription-dispensed fluoride gels are recommended for individuals with severe or rampant caries. As much as 70% to 80% reduction in the incidence of caries has been reported with the daily application of fluoride gel in dentist-fabricated, custom-fitted oral trays. Daily application of fluoride gel by toothbrushing will result in an approximately 20% reduction in the incidence of caries.

Professionally applied topical solutions. The annual or semi-annual dental office application of topical fluoride solutions or gels is a well-established caries preventive procedure that inhibits the incidence of caries by 30% to 40%. The target populations for this form of fluoride application are children and young adults with oral conditions that increase dental caries susceptibility.

Toxicity. Ingestion of lethal doses of fluoride is rare. The ADA recommends that no more than 264 mg sodium fluoride (120 mg fluoride ion) be prescribed at any one time. This dosage is safe even for young children. In the event of accidental overdose, the risk of toxicity is greatly reduced by the ingestion of large quantities of milk, milk of magnesia, or other aluminum hydroxide preparations in order to complex the fluoride and to delay and reduce its absorption.

Enamel fluorosis. Because its cause is frequently misunderstood, it must be remembered that enamel fluorosis (mottling of tooth enamel) is caused by the disruption of enamel formation and only occurs preeruptively when the enamel matrix of the tooth is calcifying. Fluorosis can be caused only by the ingestion of fluoride at levels exceeding the recommended systemic dosage. Topical fluoride, whether professionally or self-applied, does not cause enamel fluorosis. The severity of enamel fluorosis ranges from barely noticeable white specks covering a small percentage of the enamel surface to confluent pitting of the enamel surface, usually accompanied by dark brown staining (Fig. 147-8).

Pit and fissure sealants. As the prevalence of dental caries continues to decline, the distribution of caries on different tooth surfaces has markedly changed. Whereas interproximal caries is approaching eradication, almost two thirds of all dental carious lesions involve the developmental pits and fissures on the occlusal (chewing) surface of the posterior teeth. Because fluoride exerts its maximal benefit on the smooth enamel surfaces, it is very desirable to protect the developmental pits and fissures from dental decay. Sealants are plastic resins that protect these pits and fissures. When sealants are fully retained, dental caries does not occur (Fig. 147-9).

Most teeth treated with a single application of pit and fissure sealants remain completely sealed for periods up to 7 years. When one realizes that the average life span of a silver amalgam restoration is 4 to 8 years, sealant longevity compares very favorably. In addition, sealant treatments have a tremendous advantage over restorative procedures because they are noninvasive and allow the healthy tooth to remain intact. They provide effective caries protection to adolescents in fluoridated and non-fluoridated communities during their caries-susceptible ages. With the smooth-surface protection provided by fluoride supplements and the pit and fissure protection from sealants, the technology now exists to largely prevent the pain, expense, and destruction associated with dental caries.

DENTAL IMPACT OF BULIMIA NERVOSA

Bulimia nervosa is a complex problem that involves binge eating followed by attempts to lose weight by severely restricted diets, self-induced vomiting, use of laxatives or diuretics, or excessive exercise. Diagnosis can be difficult owing to the secretive nature of the activity. In patients who binge and purge by self-induced

TABLE 147-2 Supplemental Fluoride Dosage Schedule (mg/day)			
Age	<0.3 ppm*	0.3-0.6 ppm*	>0.6 ppm*
Birth-6 mo	0	0	0
6 mo-3 yr	0.25 mg	0	0
3 yr-6 yr	0.50 mg	0.25 mg	0
6 yr-16 yr	1.0 mg	0.50 mg	0

*Fluoride in water supply (ppm).
Recommended by the Council on Dental Therapeutics of the American Dental Association and by the Committee on Nutrition of the American Academy of Pediatrics (1995).

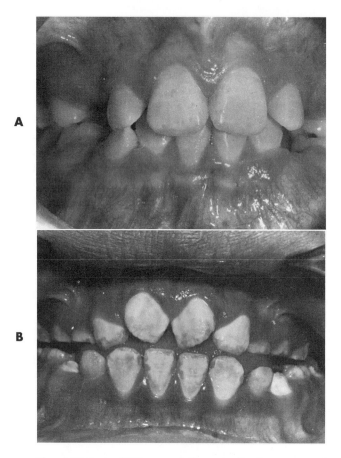

Fig. 147-8. A, Mild enamel fluorosis. **B,** Severe enamel fluorosis in an adolescent from West Texas, where the fluoride content of well water can approach 8 ppm.

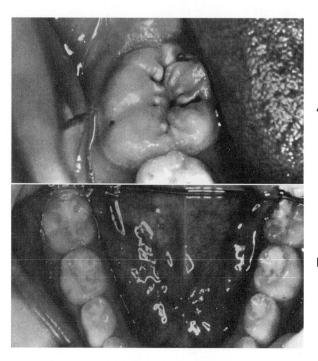

Fig. 147-9. A, Pit and fissure caries in a mandibular permanent first molar. **B,** Sealants in place on the occlusal surfaces of permanent and primary molars in the mixed dentition.

vomiting, the repeated exposure to gastric acid can have deleterious effects on the dentition. The most common effect is an erosion of the enamel from the palatal surfaces of the maxillary incisor teeth. Since this is an area rarely affected by enamel destruction from other causes, the presence of erosion should trigger further investigation.

Patients in whom bulimia nervosa has been diagnosed should have a dental consultation, since measures such as home-applied fluoride in trays will reduce the amount of enamel erosion while therapy is under way. Restoration of this type of enamel erosion is both difficult and expensive. Accordingly, every effort should be directed toward prevention of erosion in patients with this diagnosis.

PERIODONTAL DISEASE

The periodontium consists of the periodontal ligament, tooth root, and alveolar socket. The tooth is suspended in the alveolar socket by collagen fibers (periodontal ligament) embedded in the alveolar bone and the cementum. Overlying these structures are the gingiva and alveolar mucosa (Fig. 147-10). Gingivitis is characterized clinically by swelling, redness, change in position of the gingival margin, and bleeding associated with tooth brushing or flossing. Periodontitis describes the condition in which the inflammatory process extends into the periodontal ligament and bone, leading to destruction of both ligament and bone and eventual loss of the tooth. As the destruction of bone progresses, the gingiva migrates along the root surface to form periodontal pockets.

The clinical manifestations of gingival and periodontal disease in adolescents are similar to those in adults. In

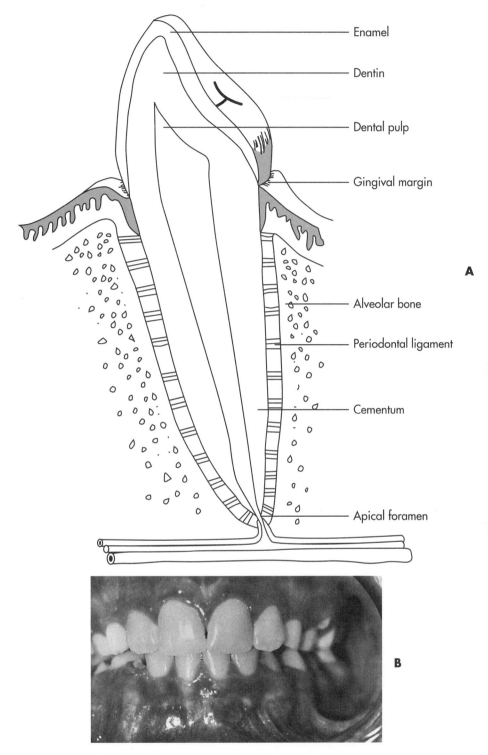

Fig. 147-10. **A,** Basic dental anatomy. **B,** Healthy gingiva in an adolescent.

children, progression from gingival to periodontal disease is uncommon. However, studies have shown that adult periodontal disease is commonly initiated before the age of 20 years. Thus, adolescence is a period of critical importance for establishing habits that may prevent the development of periodontal disease in later years.

Puberty Gingivitis

Gingivitis is a common occurrence during puberty. When combined with local irritants such as plaque or calculus, hormonal exacerbation of tissue response produces a more severe gingivitis than that expected from local factors alone. Therapy is local in nature and consists of professional removal of calculus and plaque followed by daily brushing and flossing. After 7 to 10 days, most cases show considerable improvement. In cases refractory to this regimen, fibrosis of the enlarged gingival tissue may ensue and necessitate surgical intervention.

Effect of Oral Contraceptives

Individuals taking oral contraceptives may demonstrate gingivitis similar to puberty gingivitis. This condition is thought to be a result of the interaction of hormones and local irritants (plaque and calculus). Treatment consists of professional cleaning and improvement of oral hygiene. If the condition is untreated, periodontitis may ensue.

Eruption Gingivitis

During tooth eruption, the gingiva around the tooth may become inflamed. Eruption of the tooth through the gingiva evokes an inflammatory response. The discomfort associated with tooth eruption often leads to inadequate oral hygiene in that area, with accumulation of dental plaque and exacerbation of the inflammation. When the tooth attains normal occlusal position, the gingivitis resolves. Good oral hygiene is the treatment of choice for eruption gingivitis.

Acute Necrotizing Ulcerative Gingivitis

This acute form of gingivitis is characterized by fetid odor, pain, and necrosis of the interdental papillae and gingival margin (Fig. 147-11). It is also referred to as trench mouth or Vincent's infection. Acute necrotizing ulcerative gingivitis (ANUG) most commonly affects adolescents and young adults. In underdeveloped countries, children under the age of 10 years are most com-

monly affected. The cause is complex. The bacteria presently implicated in the etiology of ANUG are spirochetes, fusiform bacteria, and *Bacteroides intermedius,* which appear to function as opportunistic pathogens. Other etiologic factors are poor oral hygiene, smoking, emotional stress, decreased host resistance, and certain systemic diseases involving depression of leukocyte numbers or function. These conditions are thought to be associated with underlying tissue changes that allow these organisms to produce the clinical manifestations of ANUG.

Such manifestations include pseudomembrane, fever, lymphadenopathy, malaise, increased salivary flow, and a metallic taste. Treatment of ANUG involves (1) professional debridement of all local irritants, (2) good oral hygiene and the use of an oxygenating mouth rinse such as 1.5% hydrogen peroxide solution (Peroxyl), (3) administration of systemic antibiotics such as penicillin or metronidazole, (4) administration of analgesics such as acetaminophen or ibuprofen, and (5) later surgical correction of any tissue destruction.

Pericoronitis

Pericoronitis refers to inflammation of the tissues surrounding an erupting tooth. The mandibular third molars are most commonly affected. Food or plaque accumulation under the operculum (soft tissue flap overlying the crown of the tooth) leads to gingival inflammation and swelling (Fig. 147-12). As the operculum enlarges, the opposing tooth may cause additional trauma and ulceration of the operculum. Treatment of minor cases is usually palliative in nature and consists of irrigation under the operculum, saline solution mouth rinses, and reduction of the opposing tooth. In more severe cases with facial swelling, lymphadenopathy, or limitation of opening, antibiotic therapy is indicated. If the tooth is impacted, extraction is indicated after resolution of the acute phase of this condition.

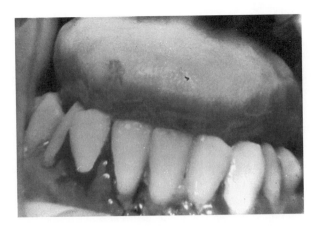

Fig. 147-11. Lower anterior gingiva demonstrating destruction caused by acute necrotizing ulcerative gingivitis.

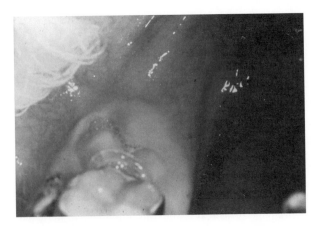

Fig. 147-12. Operculum (tissue flap) over an erupting second permanent molar demonstrating low-grade pericoronitis.

Drug-Related Gingival Overgrowth

Gingival enlargement has been reported in association with administration of phenytoin, cyclosporine, valproate sodium, and nifedipine. Gingival overgrowth occurs in approximately 50% of individuals for whom phenytoin is the sole antiepileptic medication. When phenytoin is taken in combination with other antiepileptic agents, the prevalence of gingival overgrowth is higher. Teenagers and young adults are more commonly affected. Sometimes early clinical signs, such as gingival tenderness and soreness, are reported 2 to 3 weeks after phenytoin therapy is initiated.

During the first 6 to 9 months, gingival overgrowth is clinically detectable. The increase in gingival mass is due to an increased connective tissue component. The interdental papillae form large, firm triangular masses (Fig. 147-13), which may fuse over the next 1 to 2 years to form a continuous ridge of gingival overgrowth. The gingival lesions associated with cyclosporin and nifedipine are clinically similar to those resulting from phenytoin administration, although nifedipine tends to affect the anterior sections of the dentition more severely. Maintenance of oral hygiene becomes increasingly difficult, and inflammatory gingivitis often exacerbates the gingival overgrowth.

Treatment becomes necessary to improve aesthetics, facilitate maintenance of oral hygiene, and eliminate occlusal trauma due to severe gingival overgrowth. If an alternative drug is substituted for phenytoin, spontaneous regression may occur in 12 months. In less severe cases, frequent professional cleaning coupled with excellent oral hygiene will allow resolution of the inflammatory component of the gingival enlargement. Rigorous home care helps prevent or delay the initiation of gingival overgrowth and prevent its recurrence after periodontal surgery.

Early-Onset Periodontitis

Early-onset periodontitis is periodontal disease that affects young, otherwise healthy individuals. Two forms are recognized: localized and generalized.

The localized form (also called localized juvenile periodontitis) occurs in teenagers and young adults and appears to be self-limiting. The first molars and incisors are most commonly affected. The gingiva may appear healthy on visual inspection and there is often little plaque or calculus present. However, clinical and radiographic examination reveals extensive bone loss around the first permanent molars and incisors (Fig. 147-14). Bacteria of likely etiologic significance include virulent strains of *Actinobacillus actinomycetemcomitans*. In addition, neutrophils from affected individuals show impaired chemotaxis and bactericidal activity. Treatment of localized juvenile periodontitis consists of local treatment and appropriate antibiotic therapy. Tetracycline has traditionally been the drug of choice. However, more recently, amoxicillin, penicillin, and a combination of amoxicillin and metronidazole has been shown to be effective.

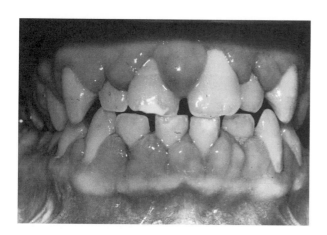

Fig. 147-13. Moderate gingival hyperplasia associated with dilantin use.

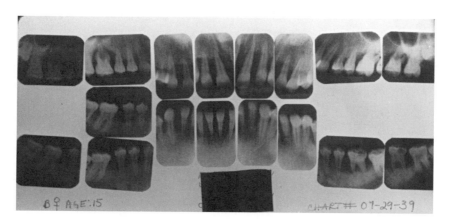

Fig. 147-14. Intraoral radiographs demonstrating bone loss associated with juvenile periodontitis in a 15-year-old girl.

The generalized form is manifested at or around puberty. Marked clinical inflammation and large amounts of plaque and calculus are present. Neutrophil function is abnormal as in localized juvenile periodontitis. Successful treatment depends on diagnosing the condition early and directing therapy toward the infecting microorganisms.

Periodontitis Associated With Systemic Disease

Periodontal disease is associated with certain systemic diseases in children and adolescents, including Papillon-Lefèvre syndrome, cyclic neutropenia, Down syndrome, type I diabetes mellitus, and leukocyte adhesion deficiency (Fig. 147-15). It is most likely that neutrophil defects associated with these conditions contribute to an increased susceptibility to periodontal disease.

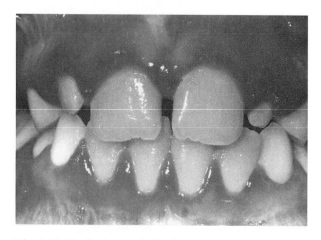

Fig. 147-15. Severe gingival inflammation in the absence of local factors in a patient with cyclic neutropenia.

Acquired Immunodeficiency Syndrome: Gingival and Periodontal Disease

The pathogenesis of HIV-associated periodontal disease (HIV-P) and HIV-associated gingivitis (HIV-G) remains unclear. In healthy individuals the development of periodontal disease depends on the interaction between the host response and the resident microflora. Compromises in the host's immune system may play a significant role in the development of HIV-P and HIV-G; however, the influence of changes in oral microflora and host response may also be of significance.

Characteristic clinical features of HIV-G include a distinct red linear band on the gingival margin and spontaneous bleeding, especially in the interproximal area. Unlike conventional gingivitis, the gingival inflammation is not specifically associated with dental plaque and is refractive to conventional therapy. A unique feature of HIV-G is the involvement of the attached gingiva. Red petechiae may be seen as isolated lesions uniformly spread over the attached gingiva, or occasionally they may coalesce to form a diffuse red band. An additional distinctive feature of HIV-G is the bright red appearance of the vestibular mucosa. The whole mouth is generally affected, although in some cases only certain isolated areas may be affected (Fig. 147-16).

Diagnosis of HIV-G is important, since it is often the first indication of an individual's HIV status. Also, available clinical data indicate that it may be the first step in the progression to HIV-P. Lesions of HIV-P occur in areas of preexisting HIV-G. Severe cases can affect the entire dentition, although it is more common for HIV-P to affect several localized areas.

In contrast to individuals with HIV-G, individuals with HIV-P often have other oral manifestations of HIV infection such as candidiasis, hairy leukoplakia, or Kaposi's sarcoma. Initially, HIV-P resembles ANUG in

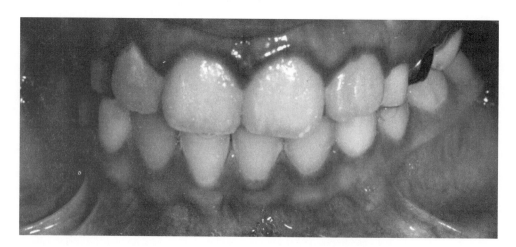

Fig. 147-16. Gingival changes of HIV gingivitis.

that affected individuals demonstrate interproximal necrosis and cratering, spontaneous bleeding, pain, and fetid odor. However, in contrast to ANUG, soft tissue involvement may extend beyond the gingival margin and the pain tends to be deep-seated in nature, often localized to the bone itself rather than to the gingiva. HIV-P soft tissue lesions closely resemble those of HIV-G. However, in HIV-P, tissue destruction rapidly extends into the adjacent bone, often leading to loss of the teeth or denudation and sequestration of bone if the rate of soft tissue destruction exceeds that of hard tissue destruction.

Both these conditions are refractive to conventional periodontal therapy. At present, acute management consists of in-office irrigation of affected tissue with povidone-iodine followed by professional debridement. Home use of povidone-iodine four or five times daily is continued for several weeks. For long-term maintenance, 0.12% chlorhexidine gluconate mouth rinse is used. In general, antibiotic therapy is not indicated for management of HIV-P because of the potential for candidal overgrowth.

SOFT TISSUE LESIONS

Herpes Simplex Virus (HSV) Type 1

Eighty percent of Americans have antibodies to type 1 herpesvirus that indicate previous infection. The primary infection normally occurs in childhood and can result in significant fever and malaise.

Recurrent herpetic infection occurs in one third of those who have had a primary infection with HSV-1. Although the lesions can occur intraorally on keratinized tissues, the lips are the most common site for recurrent lesions. The virus can be reactivated by fever, exposure to sunlight, hormonal influences, or stress, which are all common conditions in adolescence. Patients usually have a prodromal phase of infection with itching or tingling at the site. Vesicles then develop, usually in small groups

(Fig. 147-17). The vesicles generally rupture quickly and heal without scarring in 7 to 10 days. Treatment is symptomatic only, although some patients find that acyclovir 5% topical ointment is beneficial. Recurrent HSV-1 infections are occasionally confused with aphthous ulceration, but the latter does not start as a vesicular lesion. Other differential diagnosis are erythema multiforme, pemphigus, and pemphigoid.

Aphthous Ulceration

Aphthous lesions frequently occur in teenage patients and are found in the unattached tissues (Fig. 147-18). These ulcerations are of undetermined origin but are possibly the result of a small mechanical break in the mucosa followed by a localized autoimmune response. Predisposing factors are stress, trauma, endocrine alterations, and certain foods. Minor aphthae (canker sores) are shallow ulcerations covered by a gray membrane and surrounded by a narrow erythematous halo. The discomfort is out of proportion to the size of the lesion, and the presence of more than one area of ulceration can be debilitating to the patient. Patient comfort can be increased by the topical use of triamcinolone in Orabase.

Angular Cheilitis

Angular cheilitis is characterized by painful moist fissured lesions in the corners of the mouth (Fig. 147-19). It is caused by a mixed infection of candidae, staphylococci, and streptococci. Predisposing factors include local habits, drooling, decreased lower facial height and lip support, and anemia. Treatment involves identification and correction of the predisposing factors. Nystatin-triamcinolone ointment is usually of benefit when applied to the areas.

Effects of Smokeless Tobacco

It is estimated that approximately 10% of boys aged 12 to 17 years use smokeless tobacco on a regular basis. Gingival and periodontal tissues show gingivitis, gingival recession, exposure of the root surface, or hyperkeratosis

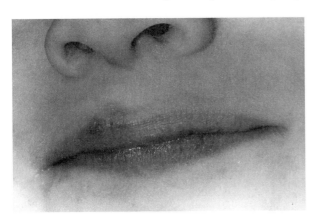
Fig. 147-17. Herpes labialis.

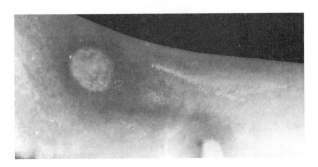
Fig. 147-18. Aphthous ulceration on mucosa of the cheek.

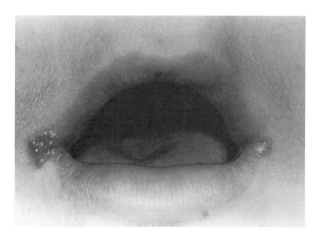

Fig. 147-19. Angular cheilitis in an adolescent patient with severe vertical overclosure.

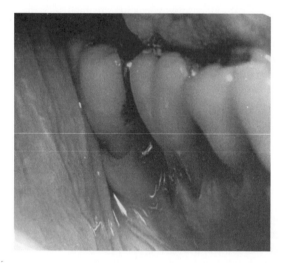

Fig. 147-20. Intraoral changes with smokeless tobacco use in an adolescent patient. There is hyperkeratosis on cheek mucosa and severe recession of buccal gingiva.

of the mucosa adjacent to the site where tobacco is most commonly placed (Fig. 147-20). Hyperkeratosis is often reversible on cessation of the habit. These individuals are also thought to be at increased risk for oral carcinoma.

DENTOALVEOLAR TRAUMA

Injury to the permanent dentition occurs twice as often in males as in females and is usually the result of a fall, fight, automobile accident, or sports injury. Other less common causes of dental trauma include seizures, child abuse, and severe clenching of teeth associated with drug abuse. There are seasonal variations in the frequency of traumatic dental injuries; an increased number of cases occur during the warmer months. Individuals with protruding upper incisors and insufficient lip closure are at increased risk. Ideally, these individuals should be targeted for early orthodontic correction of the malocclusion. In both conditions the teeth most commonly affected are the maxillary incisors, followed by the mandibular central incisors and maxillary lateral incisors.

The incidence and severity of sports-related dental trauma can be significantly reduced by the use of mouth protectors. These devices can be custom-made by the dentist or purchased from a sporting goods store. The custom-made variety offer greater protection but are more costly. Alternatively, a "mouth-formed" type of mouth protector can be used, made of thermoplastic material that can be heated and molded to the shape of the dental arch. Special mouth protectors are available for individuals with fixed orthodontic appliances that allow continued tooth movement.

Dentoalveolar injuries can be classified as hard tissue and pulp injuries, injuries to the periodontium, or alveolar fractures. Table 147-3 provides a simplified summary of management of the most common dental injuries.

TABLE 147-3
Simplified Management of Common Dental Injuries

Injury		Primary	Permanent
Coronal fracture	Minor	Polish or restore	Polish or restore
	Pulp exposure	Root canal or extract	Root canal
Root fracture		Extract	Splint, root canal (Ext.?)
Luxation	Minor	Observe	Reposition and splint
	Major	Extract	Reposition and splint
Intrusion	Minor	Observe	Reposition and splint
	Major	Extract	Reposition and splint
Evulsion		Verify and call tooth fairy	*Preserve, reimplant, splint

*Permanent Tooth Evulsion: time to reimplantation critical to prognosis; do not handle root; store in "save a tooth" or milk.

Hard-Tissue and Pulp Injuries

These injuries are classified as complicated or uncomplicated depending on whether the dental pulp is exposed (complicated) or not exposed (uncomplicated) (Fig. 147-21). Management of uncomplicated fractures is aimed at protecting the pulp even though it has not been exposed. The patient often complains of sensitivity to cold liquids or air. A protective base of calcium hydroxide is placed over the exposed sensitive dentin followed by a temporary restoration as soon as possible. An aesthetic restoration is performed at a later date (Fig. 147-22). The prognosis for uncomplicated fractures is usually favorable. Complicated fractures by definition demonstrate hemorrhaging from the central area of the tooth (dental pulp). The prognosis depends on the size of the exposure and the length of time the pulp has been exposed. Bacterial contamination of the dental pulp can lead to infection and necrosis. Therefore, to preserve pulp vitality, therapy should be instituted immediately. Small exposures (less than 1 mm in diameter) carry the best prognosis. In light of the potential for pulpal necrosis after these injuries, periodic evaluation by a dentist familiar with their management is recommended.

Root fractures may involve the dentin, enamel, or cementum and are more common in the maxillary central incisor area of 11- to 20-year-olds. In the younger age group, incomplete root formation of permanent teeth coupled with the various stages of eruption predisposes to luxation injuries. The location of the root fracture determines the degree of mobility of the coronal fragment, with fractures in the coronal half of the root showing greater mobility and displacement than fractures in the apical segment. The affected tooth tends to be lingually displaced and extruded. However, wide individual variation in tooth position and eruption can complicate the diagnosis of displacement injuries. As a result, root fractures are easily overlooked during clinical evaluation. Intraoral dental radiographs are required to determine the exact location of the fracture (Fig. 147-23). Most root fractures are in the middle third of the root. If this type of injury is suspected, dental consultation should be obtained immediately. Permanent teeth require rigid fixation with an acid-etch resin splint, coupled with radiographic observation and pulp vitality tests to detect pulpal necrosis.

Injuries to the Periodontium

The tooth is supported in the socket by the periodontal ligament, which consists of elastic collagen fibers. These fibers can be broken by trauma to the tooth and result in increased mobility, displacement, or heightened sensitivity. Luxation injuries represent 15% to 40% of cases of trauma to the permanent dentition. The most commonly

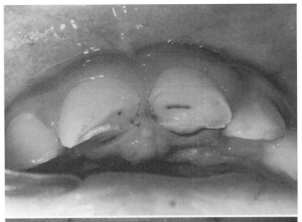

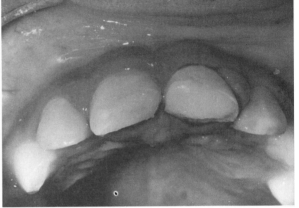

Fig. 147-21. A, Traumatic fracture of maxillary central incisors demonstrating pulpal exposures. **B,** Initial protective dressings covering pulpal treatments.

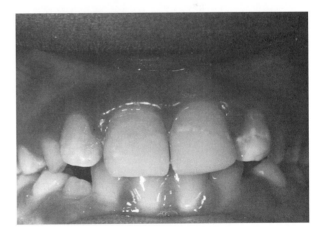

Fig. 147-22. Aesthetic restoration of the fractured teeth seen in Figure 147-21.

involved teeth are the maxillary incisors. The force and direction of impact and the age of the patient significantly influence the type of luxation injury.

CONCUSSION. In this type of injury, the periodontal ligament has sustained only minor injury and no loosening or displacement occurs. The tooth may be sensitive

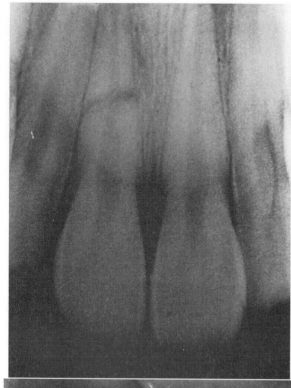

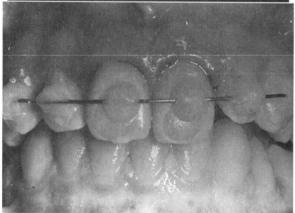

Fig. 147-23. A, Intraoral radiograph demonstrating root fracture. **B,** Rigid splint to stabilize the root fracture.

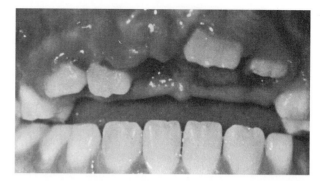

Fig. 147-24. Clinical appearance of permanent tooth intrusion. (Courtesy of the American Academy of Pediatric Dentistry.)

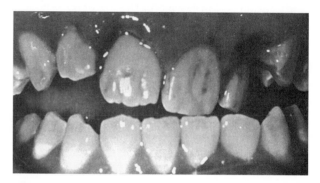

Fig. 147-25. Clinical appearance of permanent tooth extrusion. (Courtesy of the American Academy of Pediatric Dentistry.)

and a marked reaction to percussion is elicited. These teeth generally do not require any intervention; however, because of the potential for pulpal necrosis, they should be monitored radiographically for 1 year.

SUBLUXATION. This type of injury generally results in abnormal mobility and sensitivity to percussion and occlusal forces, but the normal position in the dental arch is retained. Hemorrhage may be observed at the gingival margin and is a result of damage to the periodontal tissues. If mobility is noticeable, patients with these injuries should be referred for immediate therapy. An acid-etch resin splint may be placed to immobilize the tooth and facilitate healing of the periodontal tissues. These teeth should be monitored radiographically for 1 year.

INTRUSIVE LUXATION. In this type of injury, teeth are displaced into the alveolar bone, leading to comminution or fracture of the socket (Fig. 147-24). If the tooth is completely intruded, it may give the appearance of being avulsed. To rule out the possibility of avulsion and to confirm intrusion, an intraoral dental radiograph is required. Intrusion injuries have a very poor prognosis, especially if root formation is complete. Revascularization is more easily established in immature teeth with an open apex, thereby increasing the probability of pulp survival. Waiting for spontaneous reeruption of intruded mature permanent teeth is contraindicated. Immediate dental consultation and initiation of surgical or orthodontic repositioning are necessary.

EXTRUSIVE LUXATION. These teeth are partially displaced out of the socket, appearing elongated and displaced on clinical examination. Hemorrhage around the gingival margin is also noted (Fig. 147-25). Primary teeth with this kind of injury are usually extracted. Permanent teeth can be repositioned by digital pressure and immobilized only if the patient seeks immediate medical or dental attention. Otherwise, the teeth become consolidated in their new position and should be repositioned orthodontically. Early dental intervention and close follow-up are essential, because many of these teeth

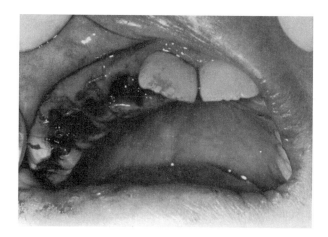

Fig. 147-26. Clinical appearance of evulsion of a maxillary permanent lateral incisor, primary cuspid, and permanent first bicuspid. The patient was hit by a golf club.

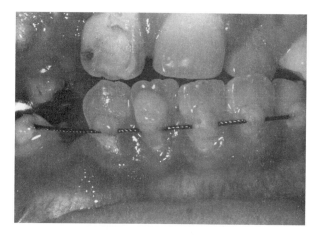

Fig. 147-27. Acid-etch resin splint to stabilize luxated lower anterior teeth. The patient has a right-sided cleft lip, alveolus, and palate.

undergo pulpal necrosis. The prognosis is more favorable if root formation is incomplete.

LATERAL LUXATION. In this type of injury the tooth is displaced in a nonaxial direction. The crown is usually displaced lingually and an associated fracture of the socket wall is present. In individuals with rotations and unusual inclination of the maxillary incisors, evaluation of lingual displacement is often difficult. Management of these injuries is similar to that for intrusive luxation. The prognosis is more favorable than for extrusive luxation injuries.

AVULSION. This term describes injuries in which a tooth is completely displaced from the alveolus (Fig. 147-26). The teeth most commonly involved are the maxillary incisors, and 7- to 10-year-old children are most often affected. However, this type of injury can occur at any age. Reimplantation of teeth has been considered a temporary measure because many of these teeth develop root resorption and are eventually lost, although they can remain functional for many years. As with intrusive injuries, teeth with incomplete root formation have a better prognosis.

The prognosis of this type of injury is significantly affected by the length of the extra-alveolar period and the conditions under which the tooth has been stored. If the extra-alveolar period is greater than 2 hours, the prognosis is considerably reduced, with 95% of the teeth demonstrating resorption. However, if the tooth has been out of the socket for 30 minutes or less, only 10% have been reported to undergo root resorption. The manner in which the tooth is stored is also highly significant in terms of the tooth's survival. Drying of the periodontal ligament fibers attached to the root surface is associated with a less favorable prognosis. The tooth should be kept moist. Appropriate storage media include saliva, milk, or saline solution; milk is best.

If the tooth cannot be located, the possibility of aspiration should be ruled out. Tetanus prophylaxis

should also be considered, because many of these teeth and wounds are soil contaminated. After reimplantation, an acid-etch resin splint should be placed immediately. Dental follow-up is essential, because pulpal therapy is generally required.

Alveolar Fractures

This injury tends to be more common in older age groups and is often associated with other dental injuries such as extrusive or lateral luxations or root fractures. The fracture may be located apical to the apices of the teeth but often involves the alveolar socket. Clinical diagnosis of this injury is relatively simple owing to the displacement of the fragment. In addition, when mobility of a single tooth is tested, adjacent teeth attached to the fractured segment are seen to move simultaneously. Radiographic examination may not reveal the fracture despite strong clinical evidence.

Treatment of these fractures usually involves the placement of a splint for 4 weeks; in children, this time can be reduced to 3 weeks. Several different methods of stabilization are available: arch bars, wire, or acrylic splints. One that closely approximates the ideal method of fixation is the acid-etch resin splint technique (Fig. 147-27). Other splinting modalities have significant disadvantages but may be necessary if inadequate adjacent teeth are present, in order to impart stability to the displaced tooth or alveolar segment.

MANDIBULAR FRACTURES

Most mandibular fractures occur in males. The adolescent age group (10 to 20 years) is the second most commonly affected after 20- to 30-year-olds. Despite the many variables associated with the etiology of mandibular fractures, vehicular accidents and assaults are the

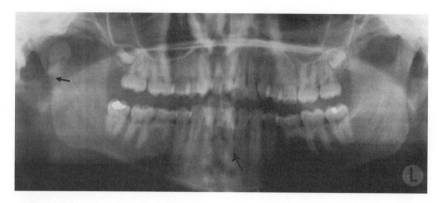

Fig. 147-28. Panoramic film of a 15-year-old girl. An angled blow to the left parasymphyseal area resulted in left parasymphyseal fracture and right subcondylar fracture.

primary cause. The body of the mandible, condyle, and angle are the most common locations for fractures, followed by the symphysis, ramus, and coronoid process. Approximately 50% of individuals present with more than one mandibular fracture.

Diagnosis

The type and direction of the force causing the fracture can be helpful in diagnosis. The magnitude of the force in motor vehicle accidents is severe, and as a result these individuals tend to have multiple compound, often comminuted fractures. Knowledge of the direction of the force allows prediction of concomitant fractures. For example, an anterior blow directly to the chin can cause bilateral condylar fractures that are often undetected, or an angled blow to the parasymphyseal area may result in a contralateral condylar or angle fracture (Fig. 147-28).

Clinical Examination

Signs and symptoms of mandibular fractures are as follows:

1. *Change in occlusion.* The patient often volunteers the information that the "bite feels different." Any change in occlusion has to be considered the primary diagnostic sign of a fracture. For example, an occlusal step deformity occurs with displaced fractures of the body of the mandible; an anterior open bite deformity occurs with bilateral condylar or angle fractures; and a unilateral crossbite occurs with a unilateral condylar fracture.
2. *Pain and swelling.* A change in facial contour may be masked by swelling; however, the face and mandible should be examined for abnormal contours that may be the result of an underlying fracture. The presence of a step deformity at the inferior border of the mandible indicates a fracture. If palpation elicts point tenderness, an underlying fracture is suspected.

3. *Crepitus.* Palpation of the mandible is accomplished using both hands, with the thumb on the teeth and the fingers on the lower border of the mandible. When pressure is slowly and carefully placed between the two hands and crepitation is noted, a fracture exists.
4. *Paresthesia or anesthesia.* Numbness in the distribution of the inferior alveolar nerve is pathognomonic of a fracture distal to the mental foramen. However, most nondisplaced fractures do not cause paresthesia.
5. *Hematoma or ecchymoses.* The presence of a hematoma in the floor of the mouth indicates a symphyseal or body fracture.

If a mandibular fracture is suspected, immediate referral for management is indicated. In the developing adolescent, this involves both immediate management of the fracture and long-term follow-up relating to the impact of the fracture on future jaw growth.

TEMPOROMANDIBULAR DISORDERS

The term *temporomandibular (TM) disorders* has been adopted by the ADA to describe all disorders related to function of the masticatory system. Factors such as stress, occlusal disharmony, bruxism, trauma, certain systemic conditions, and malocclusions have all been implicated, although the exact etiology remains elusive. These disorders are most likely multifactorial in nature. Considerable emphasis has been placed on the prevalence and management of TM disorders in the adult population. However, there is a paucity of data pertaining to pediatric and adolescent populations. Signs and symptoms of TM disorders most commonly described in the literature include TM joint sounds, TM joint pain, tenderness or pain of the masticatory muscles, impaired mobility of the mandible, irregular path of movement of the mandible, and headaches (particularly bitemporal). Pain is the most common reason for seeking treatment. It is estimated that although approximately 10% of the adult population experiences some masticatory difficulties, only 5% seek treatment.

A number of epidemiologic studies have been conducted to evaluate the prevalence of signs and symptoms of TM disorders in children and adolescents. These studies suggest that the prevalence of TM disorders ranges from 20% to 74%, whereas the prevalence of signs is between 22% and 68%. The wide range in findings can be accounted for by the lack of unanimity in definition of symptoms and examination methods, and by the poor correlation between the information reported by the subject and the results of clinical examination. Despite these limitations, it has been clearly demonstrated that the signs and symptoms of TM disorders are not uncommon in childhood, and that the incidence increases during adolescence and early adulthood.

Although a wide range of treatments have been advocated for TM disorders, few data are available to support their effectiveness. It appears that conservative reversible therapy is effective for approximately 80% of adults. Studies conducted in children appear to support this finding. Initial management consists of analgesic administration, elimination of heavy chewing (such as chewing gum), physical therapy (heat, massage), and occlusal appliances. The use of occlusal appliances involves dental impressions and custom fabrication with adjustment to the patient's occlusion. Because of the potential limitation of growth and development of the dental arches, appliance therapy should be carefully monitored.

Suggested Readings

American Academy of Oral Medicine: *Clinicians' guide to treatment of common oral conditions,* ed 3, New York, 1993, American Academy of Oral Medicine.

Anderson M, Bales D, Omnell K: *Modern management of dental caries, J Am Dent Assoc* 124:37-44, 1993.

Andreason Jo, Andreason FM: *Textbook and color atlas of traumatic injuries to the teeth,* ed 3, Copenhagen, 1994, Munksgaard.

Burt BA, editor: Proceedings for the workshop: cost-effectiveness of caries prevention in dental public health, *J Public Health Dent* 49:250-352, 1989.

Council on Dental Therapeutics: *Accepted dental therapeutics,* ed 40, Chicago, 1984, American Dental Association.

Council on Dental Therapeutics: American Dental Association: Intervention: fluoride supplementation, *J Am Dent Assoc* 126:195, 1995.

Genco R, Goldman HM, Cohen DW: *Contemporary periodontics,* St. Louis, 1990, Mosby–Year Book.

Jack S, Bloom B: *National Center for Health Statistics. Use of dental services and dental health, United States, 1986. Vital health statistics,* Series 10, No. 165, DHHS Publication No. 88-1593 (PHS), Washington, DC, 1988, U.S. Government Printing Office.

Kaban LB: *Pediatric oral and maxillofacial surgery,* Philadelphia, 1990, WB Saunders.

McDonald RE, Avery DR: *Dentistry for the child and adolescent,* ed 6, St. Louis, 1994, Mosby–Year Book.

Okeson JP: Temporomandibular disorders in children, *Pediatr Dent* 11:325-329, 1989.

Scully C, Flint S: *Color atlas of oral diseases,* Philadelphia, 1989, JB Lippincott.

Symposium on appropriate uses of fluoride in the 1990s, *J Public Health Dent* 51:20-63, 1991.

Wood NK, Goaz PW: *Differential diagnosis of oral lesions,* ed 4, St. Louis, 1991, Mosby–Year Book.

Zarb GA, Carlsson GE: *Temporomandibular joint—function and dysfunction,* Copenhagen, 1979, Munksgaard.

Zeng Y, Sheller B, Milgrom P: Epidemiology of dental emergency visits to an urban children's hospital, *Pediatr Dent* 16:419-423, 1994.

CHAPTER 148

Central Nervous System Trauma

•

James Tait Goodrich

Head injuries remain one of the leading causes of significant morbidity and mortality in the adolescent population. Most result from motor vehicle accidents, but in urban areas, missile injuries (gunshot wounds, stabbings, injuries with blunt instruments such as with baseball bats) predominate. Since 50% to 60% of deaths in these cases occur within the first 24 hours after injury, this time frame is the window within which aggressive management must occur if long-term morbidity and mortality are to be reduced.[1-5]

INITIAL NEUROLOGIC EVALUATION

On arrival in the emergency room, a patient who has sustained a serious head injury requires a thorough evaluation. The evaluation is similar to the standard emergency room examination and is performed in stepwise fashion.

Provision for Adequate Airway and Ventilation

Patients with severe head injury tend to be obtunded, with altered mental status; a seizure may have resulted from the initial injury. Vomiting with aspiration is a not uncommon sequela to head injury (particularly closed blunt injury). Injury to the brain stem can significantly alter breathing regulation. For these reasons, an open and secured airway must be established and maintained. Any patient with altered mental status should be intubated and hyperventilated to reduce the potential for increased intracranial pressure (ICP).

Observation of Vital Signs

The vital signs must be documented, monitored closely, and recorded at least every 15 minutes. By doing so, the physician can detect trends and try to predict and avoid an impending catastrophe. The well-known Cushing's phenomenon—systemic hypertension with bradycardia—occurs when ICP is significantly increased. Cushing's phenomenon is an ominous sign and an indication for immediate efforts to reduce increased ICP.

Determination of State of Consciousness

The patient's level or state of consciousness must be documented to provide a baseline for measuring changes. If the patient is brought in by family members or ambulance, it is critical to question the family or paramedics about the mental status of the patient before arrival, along with any changes, and to document this information. Most emergency room personnel now use the Glasgow Coma Scale (GCS) for this purpose.

Neurologic Examination

The neurologic examination need not be a thorough and complete assessment of all twelve cranial nerves and all motor groups. Rather, it should document the level of consciousness and the function of the third, fifth, sixth, seventh, and tenth cranial nerves. The physician must determine and document the pupillary responses and extraocular function (are the pupils reactive? is pupillary response symmetric?). The corneal reflex can be quite sensitive; its loss is a grave prognostic sign. The eyes should be ophthalmologically examined for retinal hemorrhages; if present, this is an ominous finding. Is there facial symmetry? Does the patient have an intact gag response? Motor and sensory function is evaluated simply: is there withdrawal from pain and is this withdrawal symmetric? Decorticate or decerebrate posturing is a clinical sign of injury to the brain stem and severe compression of the neural axis. The presence of either of these signs may be associated with Cushing's phenomenon and is an ominous prognostic indicator.

History of Trauma

It is distressing to know how often the history of the trauma is not obtained in the emergency room. In most cases the history can be obtained from the family members, police, or ambulance crew. This information is extremely important, since it determines how the neurosurgical team will treat the patient. A history of blunt injury can require a surgical protocol entirely different from that for a penetrating injury.

Glasgow Coma Scale

In recent years it has become standard practice in most emergency rooms to determine the GCS score. Over the years, trauma services have correlated this score with the eventual neurologic outcome. As a result, it has become a useful grading system, not only for acute evaluation, but also for the neurosurgical team's determination of long-term prognosis. The score is standardized and should be available to all physicians (Table 148-1).

Typically, a patient who arrives with a GCS of 15 will do well unless there is an acute change. However, a patient with a GCS of only 8 has a severe neurologic injury, and the injury may become permanent if not managed promptly. A patient who arrives in the emergency room with a GCS of 3 to 5 is severely injured and carries an extremely poor prognosis.

MANAGEMENT OF ELEVATED INTRACRANIAL PRESSURE

Since elevated ICP is observed in over half of all head injuries, any patient who arrives in the emergency room with a significant head injury must be evaluated for this condition. In a number of series it has been found that for patients with an ICP greater than 20 mm Hg that is not controlled, the mortality rate exceeds 80%. Early recognition and treatment are therefore critical.[2,3]

Management of the head-injured patient depends on a key principle: maintenance of cerebral perfusion pressure (CPP) within an acceptable range. The CPP is the

TABLE 148-1
Glasgow Coma Scale

	Score
Eyes	
Open spontaneously	4
Open to verbal command	3
Open to pain	2
No response	1
Best Motor Response	
To verbal command	
Obeys	6
To painful stimulus	
Localizes pain	5
Flexion—withdrawal	4
Flexion—abnormal	3
Extension	2
No response	1
Best Verbal Response	
Oriented and converses	5
Disoriented and converses	4
Inappropriate words	3
Incomprehensible sounds	2
No response	1

difference between the mean arterial blood pressure (MABP) and the ICP:

$$CPP = MABP - ICP$$

If CPP falls below the acceptable range, oxygenation of brain tissue is compromised and permanent brain injury will result if CPP is not promptly restored. Box 148-1 classifies ICP levels according to their clinical significance.

Position of Head

The simple technique of raising the patient's head above the heart level (approximately 30% Gatch, or head elevation) increases venous return from the head and in turn lowers ICP.

Hyperventilation

Hyperventilation through an endotracheal tube can lead to a rapid, and even dramatic, decrease in ICP. The reduction of a patient's Pco_2 level from the normal level of 40 mm Hg to 20 mm Hg results in an immediate 50% reduction in ICP. Hyperventilation reduces the Pco_2 level and in turn causes cerebral vasoconstriction. This vasoconstriction reduces the blood volume in the intracranial cavity and in turn lessens ICP.

BOX 148-1
Intracranial Pressure Levels*

Normal	1-10 mm Hg
Slightly increased	11-20 mm Hg
Moderately increased	21-40 mm Hg
Severely increased	41 mm Hg

*Patients with ICP greater than 20 mm Hg need immediate and aggressive management to lower ICP.

Hyperosmolar Agents

A number of useful agents can be used to produce effective diuresis. Mannitol, the one most commonly used by neurosurgeons, decreases extracellular water in the brain by osmosis, which leads to diuresis and results in a reduction in ICP. The typical dose is 0.25 to 0.5 g/kg given every 6 hours. Mannitol does have a number of adverse side effects that must always be considered. It can cause substantial changes in fluid balance, altered serum osmolarity, secondary rebound in ICP, and seizures. Whenever mannitol or a diuretic agent is being used, the fluid balance must be closely monitored. The patient should be closely followed up, particularly if diuresis occurs, to ensure that the electrolytes, especially sodium and potassium, remain in the normal range. The serum osmolarity can be a helpful indicator; a range of about 290 to 295 is satisfactory. Mannitol can safely be used for no more than 48 to 72 hours. After this interval, it may enter brain cells, and an effect opposite to that desired occurs: brain cells swell as a result of internal osmolar effects. Every patient with a head injury should also receive some type of anticonvulsant medication. Seizures occur frequently after head injury; the incidence is higher in those receiving mannitol.

Diuretics

An excellent adjunct to osmolar agents is a diuretic such as furosemide (Lasix). Such agents can induce rapid, profuse diuresis and are useful in the early management of head-injured patients. The unwanted side effects are the same as those of osmolar agents.

In the past, the use of barbiturates and steroids was recommended in the treatment of head-injured patients, but later studies showed that the morbidity associated with their use exceeds the benefit. For this reason, trauma centers no longer routinely use either of these drugs in the management of head injuries.[6-13]

Removal of Cerebrospinal Fluid

A rapid method for ICP control is the removal of cerebrospinal fluid (CSF) by means of an intraventricularly placed catheter system. These systems are easily placed when the patient is in the emergency room and are also useful for pressure monitoring.

MONITORING INTRACRANIAL PRESSURE

Neurosurgical services use ICP monitoring devices in the care of people with head injuries. Numerous devices are available, but the principle for each is the same: to provide accurate, simple, and low-risk constant monitoring of ICP. Devices now in use are the intraventricular catheter, epidural monitor, subarachnoid bolt, and subdural catheter.

Intraventricular Catheter

The most common means of monitoring ICP is the intraventricular catheter. It is placed within the ventricular system by means of a frontal burr hole and coupled to a transducer that gives a constant readout of ICP. The advantages of this system are the ability to monitor constantly, the ability to remove CSF for pressure reduction, and highly accurate pressure readings. The catheter may be readily placed in the intensive care unit, and the procedure usually requires less than 10 minutes with either a burr hole or a twist drill technique. The primary disadvantage is the risk of infection. The catheter cannot be left in place for longer than 72 hours (if the catheter tract is subcutaneously tunneled some distance away from the burr hole, it can remain in situ for up to 1 week). The catheters are sometimes difficult to secure and can be dislodged by routine nursing care. There is also a risk of bleeding during the passage of the catheter, although this risk is usually less than 5%.

Epidural Monitor

In recent years the epidural monitor technique has become a frequently used method of monitoring ICP. The monitor is a small, thin disk that can be easily placed between the dura and the skull through a burr hole. Since the dura is left intact, the risk of infection is much lower. A number of sophisticated digital monitors are available for reading ICP at the bedside. The main disadvantage of the epidural monitor is the inability to remove CSF for pressure reduction.

Subarachnoid Bolt

The subarachnoid bolt system is not currently in widespread use. It is a monitoring system with a transducing element placed within the subarachnoid space. It does not work well when the ICP is high and it has a tendency to clog.

Subdural Catheter

Once commonly used, the subdural catheter has been replaced by either the intraventricular catheter or the epidural monitor. The subdural system can be unreliable when ICP is high, giving false low readings.

INTRACRANIAL HEMORRHAGE IN HEAD TRAUMA

There is a high incidence of intracranial hemorrhage in serious head injury. Knowledge and recognition of the type of hemorrhage are critical for optimal management. Essentially, three types of intracranial hemorrhages are seen in adolescents: (1) acute subdural (50% mortality); (2) acute intraparenchymal (30% to 60% mortality); and (3) acute epidural (10% to 20% mortality).

Acute Subdural Hematoma

Subdural hematoma (Fig. 148-1), a common injury in the adolescent population, carries a poor prognosis. It occurs when direct injury to the brain results in a torn bridging vein or artery or injury to a pial vessel. Greater force is required to cause injuries of this type in adolescents, since most of them do not have brain atrophy, such as that seen in adults. It is essential to recognize this injury early, because it is a surgical emergency requiring immediate evacuation of the clot.

Acute Intraparenchymal Hematoma

The most common sites of intraparenchymal injury are the frontal and temporal lobe tips (Fig. 148-2). This most commonly occurs as a result of motor vehicle injuries in which the victim is thrown forward. The other common cause of intraparenchymal trauma is a penetrating injury, such as a gunshot wound (Fig. 148-3). These grave injuries almost always carry a long-term morbidity. In most cases, craniotomy is required for removal of the intraparenchymal clot and surrounding devitalized tissue.

Acute Epidural Hematoma

This injury results from hemorrhage in the potential space between the dura mater and skull (Fig. 148-4). Often, injury of the middle meningeal artery causes an acute epidural hematoma. In my experience this lesion is the most common type overlooked in the emergency room. Typically, the patient receives some sort of head blow, in many cases a mild one. In the emergency room the patient walks, talks, and seems fine, so is sent home, only to be brought back obtunded, with a fixed and dilated pupil. What is observed in the emergency room is the

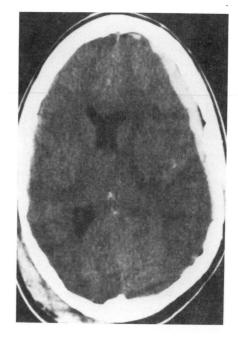

Fig. 148-1. Computed tomography (CT) scan showing a subdural hematoma over the left hemisphere. Fresh blood is seen between the cerebral cortex and skull. Brain shift is present, with the ventricles moved to the right of the midline. Evidence of this type of mass effect is ominous and requires surgical evacuation of blood clot on an emergent basis.

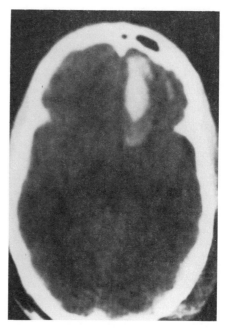

Fig. 148-2. CT scan of an intraparenchymal hemorrhage resulting from a blow to the head. The left frontal lobe has an extensive recent hemorrhage.

so-called lucid interval. Because the hematoma expands slowly, a period of minutes to hours can elapse during which the patient appears well. Only when the hematoma expands does the patient become obtunded and exhibit an

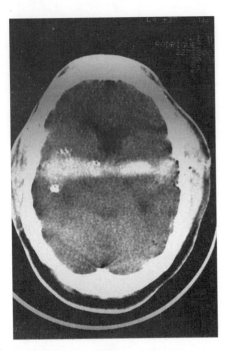

Fig. 148-3. CT scan of a 16-year-old who committed suicide by placing a gun to the temporal region. This is a devastating "through-and-through" type of injury which results in a very poor prognosis.

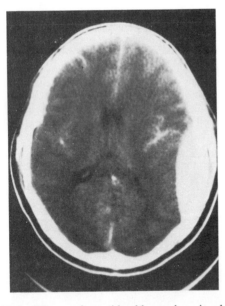

Fig. 148-4. CT scan of an epidural hemorrhage involving the left temporal parietal region. The location of this epidural hemorrhage is typical in that it is near the middle meningeal artery, the most common site for an epidural hemorrhage.

altered mental status. If these injuries are recognized early and surgically treated, the long-term morbidity is low. Since the brain is only compressed, prompt removal of the blood clot is sufficient to ensure a good prognosis.

SKULL FRACTURES AND MANAGEMENT

One of the most common head injuries seen in adolescents is a fracture of the skull. Some skull fractures require surgery, whereas others can be managed conservatively. The types of skull fractures and guidelines for managing them are listed in Boxes 148-2 and 148-3.

A number of criteria guide the decision of the trauma and neurosurgical teams to operate on a skull fracture. In any skull fracture with bone fragments driven into the brain, the fractures and the bone fragments need to be elevated (Fig. 148-5). Typically, any depressed skull fracture greater than 1 cm in diameter, or in which the outer bone table is below the inner bone table as detected on computed tomography, needs to be elevated (Fig. 148-6). If an underlying hematoma is compressing the brain or if a neurologic deficit is suspected, exploration and elevation are indicated. If CSF is seen issuing through the wound, the dura mater has been torn. Under such circumstances, there is a significant increase in the risk of meningitis. Therefore, such wounds are explored, the fracture is elevated, and the dura is repaired. Similarly, if air is present in the subarachnoid space, the dura has been torn, and in most cases exploration is necessary.

Fractures over the paranasal and mastoid sinuses are often repaired to prevent otorrhea or rhinorrhea, the incidence of which is otherwise high. In adolescents, there is a high incidence of basilar skull fractures, usually manifested by Battle's sign, an area of ecchymosis behind

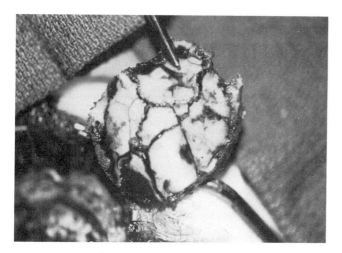

Fig. 148-5. An adolescent girl struck on the head with a ball-peen hammer during a rape attempt suffered a stellate fracture, with bone fragments driven into the brain. The fracture has been elevated and the inner table of the bone can be seen.

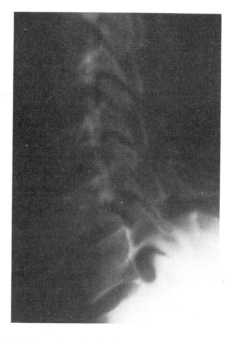

Fig. 148-7. Lateral cervical spine radiograph showing a C7-T1 subluxation in a high school football player. This subluxation was initially missed because of the patient's large shoulders. The repeat radiograph taken with the shoulders pulled down showed the subluxation.

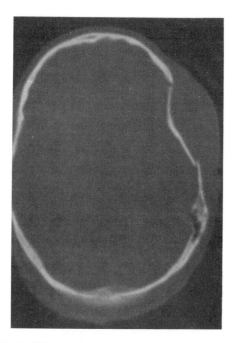

Fig. 148-6. CT scan of the patient in Figure 148-5 showing the degree of bone depression and soft tissue swelling over the injury site.

the ear around the mastoid prominence. There is a CSF leak in many cases, but fortunately most leaks resolve spontaneously and require no surgery. In the 5% or so that do not resolve, placement of a lumbar spinal drain with negative pressure over a 7-day period usually suffices. The need for intracranial exploration to repair the fracture is rare, occurring in less than 2% of patients treated by our service.

As a final caution, when managing the patient with a head injury, the emergency room team must not forget to assess the cervical region. The incidence of cervical spine

injuries is high in this population. Therefore every patient with a head injury should be stabilized with a neck collar and treated as though a spine injury is present until it is proved otherwise. It is critical that all cervical vertebrae be evaluated, including those down to C7. The most commonly missed cervical injury in the emergency room is the C7-T1 injury, which is overlooked because of a failure to pull the shoulders down during the radiograph examination (Fig. 148-7).

SEQUELAE OF HEAD TRAUMA

Posttraumatic Epilepsy

Posttraumatic epilepsy in the adolescent with a head injury is a not uncommon sequela with a 2.5% to 7% incidence in reported series.[14-16] The risk of seizure is directly related to the type and mechanism of injury. Injuries resulting in subdural or parenchymal injury (i.e., penetrating injury) have the highest risk of seizures: 30% to 36%. Epidural and skull fractures have an incidence of 9% to 13%, and even in minor head injury without neurologic sequelae there is a reported incidence of 1% to 2%. A question always arises about the use of anti-epileptic medications in early posttraumatic epilepsy (i.e., within the first week of injury). If the patient has only one early seizure, there is no evidence that prophylaxis will have any effect on long-term outcome; therefore, for a single seizure treatment is not recommended. Late post-traumatic seizures (occurring a week or later after trauma) carry a more ominous prognosis. If these seizures occur in a patient with only closed head trauma, they can be followed to see what pattern (i.e., frequency) develops. In patients with penetrating injury, particularly those who develop focal neurologic symptoms, there is a high risk of development of permanent epilepsy that will require medication.

Long-Term Management

Late posttraumatic seizures greatly affect an adolescent in learning and development and need to be aggressively managed. In adults, it has been shown that late seizures greatly lessen the chance of gainful employment after treatment. The single most ignored factors in the adolescent who has sustained a head injury are the psychologic sequelae. After a head injury has occurred, particularly in an assault case, adolescents can become fearful, with retrograde amnesia, and a loss of learning skills is not uncommon. If these conditions are recognized early and treated, the outcome will be much improved.

Posttraumatic Syndrome

General sequelae following a head injury include the following:

1. Headache (mild to excruciating), typically in the occipital region, which can often persist for up to 6 to 12 months after the injury.
2. Irritability, which often affects social interactions and school performance.
3. Forgetfulness: retrograde amnesia is common, and school performance can be affected in that these patients have difficulty acquiring new knowledge.
4. Postural vertigo (dizziness).
5. Enuresis.
6. Disturbance in sleep patterns.
7. Episodic aggressive behavior, particularly in adolescent males.
8. Decline in school performance: teachers typically note impaired concentration skills.

It should also be borne in mind that whenever there is a medicolegal coincident situation, patients may not do well until the legal matters are resolved.

The posttraumatic syndrome is one of the most ignored sequelae in the adolescent population. This is particularly the case in adolescent males, in whom a bravado attitude tends to lead the family and school to ignore the problem. In adolescent females, particularly those who are victims of assault, the psychologic sequelae can be devastating and need to be closely monitored. Typically, the earliest subtle signs in both girls and boys changes in school performance. Fortunately, a persistent posttraumatic syndrome is uncommon in adolescents and almost always resolves with time. This does not negate the fact that these patients need close monitoring in the first 6 months after the injury.

References

1. Alberico AM, Ward JD, Choi SC, et al: Outcome after severe head injury. Relationship to mass lesions, diffuse injury, and ICP course in pediatric and adult patients, *J Neurosurg* 67:648-656, 1987.
2. Becker DP, Miller JD, Ward JD, et al: The outcome from severe head injury with early diagnosis and intensive management, *J Neurosurg* 47:491-502, 1977.
3. Saul TG, Ducker TB: Effect of intracranial pressure monitoring and aggressive treatment on mortality in severe head injury, *J Neurosurg* 56:498-503, 1982.
4. Seelig JM, Becker DP, Miller JD, et al: Traumatic acute subdural hematoma: major mortality reduction in comatose patients treated within four hours, *N Engl J Med* 304:1511-1518, 1981.
5. Fackler ML: Wound ballistics. A review of common misconceptions, *JAMA* 259:2730-2736, 1988.
6. Piatt JH Jr, Schiff SJ: High dose barbiturate therapy in neurosurgery and intensive care, *Neurosurgery* 15:427-444, 1984.
7. Ward JD, Becker DP, Miller JD, et al: Failure of prophylactic barbiturate coma in the treatment of severe head injury, *J Neurosurg* 62:383-388, 1985.
8. Eisenberg HM, Frankowski RF, Contant CF, et al: High-dose barbiturate control of elevated intracranial pressure in patients with severe injury, *J Neurosurg* 69:15-23, 1988.
9. Giannotta SL, Weiss MH, Apuzzo MLJ, Martin E: High dose glucocorticoids in the management of severe head injury, *Neurosurgery* 15:497-501, 1984.
10. Braakman R, Schouten HJA, Dishoeck MB, Minderhoud JM: Megadose steroids in severe head injury, *J Neurosurg* 58:326-330, 1983.
11. Deardon NM, Gibson JS, McDowall DG, et al: Effect of high-dose dexamethasone on outcome from severe head injury, *J Neurosurg* 64:81-88, 1986.
12. Molofsky WJ: Steroids and head trauma, *Neurosurgery* 15:424-426, 1984.
13. Braughler JM, Hall ED: Current application of "high-dose" steroid therapy for CNS injury, *J Neurosurg* 62:806-810, 1985.
14. Gennarelli TA, Ghibault LE: Biomechanics of head injury. In Wilkins RH, Rengachary SS, editors: *Neurosurgery,* Baltimore, 1985, Williams & Wilkins; pp 1531-1536.
15. Rivera FP, Alexander B, Johnston B, Soderberg R: Population based study of fall injuries in children and adolescents resulting in hospitalization or death, *Pediatrics* 92:61-63, 1993.
16. Young B: Sequalae of head injury. In McLaurin R, et al, editors: *Pediatric neurosurgery,* ed 2, Philadelphia, 1989, WB Saunders; pp 1688-1693.

CHAPTER 149

Brain Tumors

•

James Tait Goodrich

Despite the complexity of brain tumors in the adolescent population, their clinical characteristics are straightforward. The physician must keep in mind that different tumor varieties favor certain sites in the brain, that tumors differ in their predilections as to age at onset, and that their symptoms are referable to the anatomic location of the tumor. As for treatment, adolescent patients with brain tumors are always managed in a multimodal fashion; the treatment possibilities include surgery (Box 149-1), radiotherapy, chemotherapy, and immunotherapy.

INCIDENCE

The general incidence of brain tumors in all age groups is about 2%, with some 17,000 new primary brain tumors diagnosed per year in the United States. There is a biphasic peak occurrence in brain tumors, with the highest incidences among children and adults over 55 years of age. The frequency in adolescents averages about 2 per 100,000 per year.

DIAGNOSIS

The diagnosis of a brain tumor rests on two major factors: signs and symptoms due to tumor location and intracranial pressure (ICP). A tumor mass competes for space already filled by the brain. Since the brain is tightly enclosed within the skull vault, some of the earliest signs of a brain tumor are symptoms of ICP: headache, vomiting, papilledema, and diplopia. Headache is usually the earliest symptom, with the type of headache classic. The patient usually gives a history of an intermittent, nocturnal, dull, throbbing headache persisting over a period of days to weeks. The headaches seldom lateralize and are usually frontal or occipital; they worsen with coughing or straining. Vomiting is not usually associated with nausea or meals. Adolescent patients often resume eating after

vomiting, in contrast to their behavior during an episode of gastroenteritis or viral illness. The vomiting can eventually become intractable and unrelenting. Papilledema is a chronic finding, indicating that the patient has been subjected to increased ICP for some time. Examination of the retinal fields shows swelling of the optic disc with loss of the physiologic cup, blurring and elevation of the disc margins, venous distention, and often peripapillary hemorrhage. Visual acuity is usually normal. Diplopia results from stretching of the sixth cranial nerve, causing a typical inturning of the eye (i.e., an unopposed third cranial nerve). The patient often holds the head at a tilt to correct for the double vision.

Other signs and symptoms can be subtle but helpful in diagnosis. In teenagers an often early diagnostic sign is a change in personality. Frequently the parents or a schoolteacher will be the first to note such changes. Typically, the affected adolescent manifests a lack of energy, a lack of attention to school work, and oversleeping; these behaviors can all be early, subtle signs of increased ICP. Focal neurologic findings caused by the displacement of brain tissue can also be manifested. Ataxia in an otherwise healthy athlete is often seen. The adolescent develops a broad-based, staggering, drunken gait. Long-track motor findings such as a mild limp or weakness can occur. A subtle but useful examination finding to seek is a motor "drift": the patient is asked to hold both arms and hands outstretched with the palms rotated upward and then to close the eyes. The examiner notes whether one arm "drifts" downward. If this occurs, it indicates a lesion on the contralateral side. Seizures, a common presentation in brain tumors, are due to the local irritation of brain tissue by tumor, and can be focal or generalized. The new onset of seizures in an otherwise healthy adolescent is an ominous sign. Such a patient should be considered to have a brain tumor until it is proved otherwise.

Meningismus is often a useful early diagnostic sign. Tumors—particularly those in the posterior fossa that cause increased pressure around the upper cervical and occipital nerves—can lead to signs of meningitis such as a stiff neck. Endocrine abnormalities are also common, particularly in patients with midline tumors (e.g., in the pituitary and pineal regions). Growth delay, loss of secondary sexual characteristics, diabetes insipidus, and hypersomnia are all commonly observed in patients with midline brain tumors.

EVALUATION

Several general but helpful studies can be ordered early in the evaluation of a brain tumor. Skull radiographs remain a useful diagnostic tool. Suture separation can occur with the growth of a brain tumor, even in a mature skull. The sign of "beaten metal" (i.e., convolutional markings on the inner table) is evidence of increased ICP. An eroded sella, particularly a loss of posterior clinoid process, is diagnostic. A number of adolescent tumors form calcifications within the tumor that are visible on skull radiographs.

Evaluation of visual acuity and visual fields is helpful in diagnosing tumors along the midaxis of the brain. Since loss of visual acuity is often ignored by the adolescent, this symptom can be easily overlooked. Changes in the visual fields, in particular, suggest a tumor in and around the sella turcica.

Lumbar puncture is never recommended for the initial evaluation of a patient with a brain tumor. Because of the associated increased ICP, the risk of downward cerebral herniation is significant. Lumbar puncture should be deferred until computed tomography (CT) or magnetic resonance imaging (MRI) has been performed and increased ICP has been ruled out. CT and MRI are now the main diagnostic tools for localizing a brain tumor. MRI is particularly sensitive for the detection of low-grade tumors. Occasionally, it is possible to speculate as to tumor type on the basis of location and signal characteristics as evidenced on MRI or CT. However, since these diagnostic procedures are not infallible, tissue diagnosis is almost always indicated.

TUMOR TYPES AND THEIR MANAGEMENT

Adolescents, being midway between children and adults, share the tumor types of both age groups (Table 149-1).[1-6] Unfortunately, the tumors that are common in adolescence often have a poor prognosis.

Astrocytoma

Astrocytomas arise from the glial support cells of the brain. Most are benign and have low-grade characteristics. In the general population the incidence ranges from 0.81 to 2.6 per 100,000, depending on the study cited.[6,7] Despite their benign characteristics, these tumors are associated with a poor long-term prognosis; only 50% of patients survive 5 years from the time of diagnosis (Fig. 149-1). In Cushing's initial series in 1931,[8] the 5-year survival was only 37%. With adjuvant chemotherapy, survival is improved, but total cure has yet to be achieved. The primary reasons for surgery are to enable a tissue diagnosis and to "debulk" the tumor to the extent that its anatomic location permits. Because of the infiltrative nature of astrocytomas, complete and total removal can rarely be accomplished without grave morbidity. Furthermore, because of the similarity of normal brain tissue to a low-grade astrocytoma, it is often not possible for the neurosurgeon to differentiate normal tissue from tumor. In such situations, most surgeons are conservative in terms of excision.

The one subgroup in which survival is excellent is the cerebellar astrocytomas. These tumors arise in either the hemisphere or the vermis of the cerebellum. In most cases they are pilocystic, and they often consist of a nodule with a surrounding cyst component (Fig. 149-2). The surgical goal is removal of the nodule and drainage of the cyst. Accomplishment of this goal provides an excellent 5-year survival rate of more than 85%. Although more common in children, these tumors do occur in adolescents.

Medulloblastoma

Medulloblastomas account for about 20% of all adolescent brain tumors. Males are affected 1.3 times as often as females. Medulloblastoma is one of the most biologically aggressive and malignant tumors in the

TABLE 149-1
Distribution of Brain Tumors in Adolescents

Type	%
Astrocytoma	30
Medulloblastoma	20
Ependymoma	10
Craniopharyngioma	10
Glioblastoma	
Germ cell	
Chordoma	
Papilloma	
Teratoma	30
Hamartoma	
Neurofibroma	
Pituitary tumor	

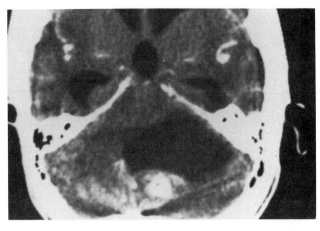

Fig. 149-2. CT scan with contrast material showing a cerebellar astrocytoma with a contrast-enhancing nodule in the posterior fossa and surrounding cyst. A common finding, due to tumor compression of the aqueduct of Sylvius, is hydrocephalus. Note the dilated third and lateral ventricles.

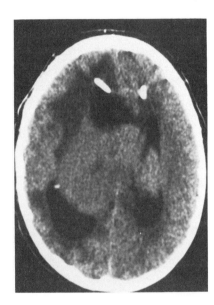

Fig. 149-1. CT scan of a 16-year-old boy who presented with progressively severe headaches and mental status changes. This scan was taken after placement of emergency ventricular drains. A large intraventricular astrocytoma causing both mass effect and surrounding edema can be seen. The tumor occupies both lateral ventricular systems, with the right system more involved than the left.

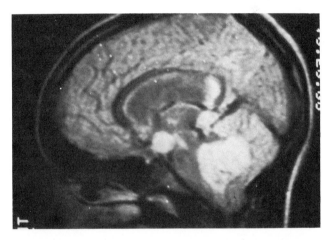

Fig. 149-3. A 14-year-old girl presented with headaches, vomiting, and a staggering gait. MRI shows a large mass in the posterior fossa compressing the brain stem and occupying the cerebellar vermian region. Subsequent surgical diagnosis showed this mass to be a medulloblastoma.

brain. It arises from embryonic tissue and has the ability to disseminate throughout the neural axis via cerebrospinal fluid (CSF) pathways. These tumors tend to present in the midline along the cerebellar vermian axis. A posterior fossa craniotomy is performed with total removal of tumor. Occasionally, the tumor invades the brain stem or is intimately involved with local critical structures, thereby not allowing complete removal (Fig. 149-3). Even after gross total removal of the tumor, patients need follow-up radiation therapy and chemotherapy. With combined treatment modalities, the 5-year survival is 40% to 50% and up to 70% in some series. In patients

with dissemination of tumor into the subarachnoid space, the 5-year survival drops to 25%.[9-18]

Collin's law is often used as a prognostic indicator in these cases. This law involves adding 9 months to the patient's age at diagnosis; if there is no tumor recurrence within this period (i.e., the age of the patient plus 9 months, the sum expressed as a number of months), the patient is "cured." Although this predictor holds in most cases, there are still a few late recurrences. Collin's law is based on the premise that medulloblastomas are embryonic tumors with a constant growth rate. Once the tumor has been surgically removed, the bulk of the remaining tumor, if any, grows at a constant rate, and recurrences must therefore take place within the predicted time. Because of the location in which these tumors occur (in and around the fourth ventricle, where they can block

CSF outflow), patients not uncommonly present with an acute case of hydrocephalus. This is a life-threatening emergency requiring immediate and direct action. The simplest treatment is to admit the patient to the intensive care unit (ICU), where the neurosurgical team places a ventricular catheter to reduce the CSF pressure to normal levels. Typically, the patient is kept in the ICU postoperatively, and an externalized ventricular drain remains in place. The drain pressure and CSF flow are monitored to determine whether the drain can be removed. In about one third of patients a permanent ventriculoperitoneal shunt is necessary.

Ependymoma

An ependymoma is another type of highly malignant tumor that occurs primarily in the posterior fossa. The growth characteristics of this tumor are such that symptoms are usually more subtle than those of other tumors discussed thus far. Patients have a high incidence of vomiting, thought to be due to the tumor's location next to the floor of the fourth ventricle, by the obex and the hypoglossal and vagal trigones (Fig. 149-4). Dysarthria and difficulties with eating and swallowing are not uncommon. Since the tumor is close to or in the floor of the fourth ventricle, hydrocephalus is also common and often acute. Ependymomas can also occur at any location within the ventricular system because they arise from the cells in the ventricle wall lining. Another typical location is the lateral ventricles, particularly in the area of the trigone.

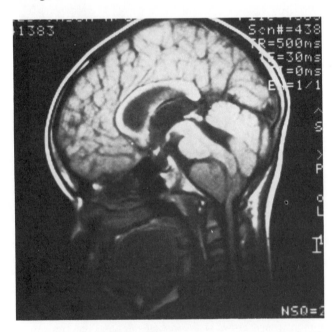

Fig. 149-4. MRI showing a large lesion occupying the fourth ventricle and extending down through the foramen magnum. At surgery an ependymoma that originated from the floor of the fourth ventricle and extended out through the lateral recess was found.

Age is an important consideration—the younger the patient, the worse is the prognosis. Aggressive tumor removal is performed, the goal being to reduce the tumor burden to the essential minimum. Every patient receives subsequent adjuvant chemotherapy. Despite aggressive management with both surgery and adjuvant therapy, the 3-year survival rate is only 17% and the 5-year survival rate only 14%—truly dismal results.[16-18]

Postoperatively, patients must be closely monitored. The tumor's location in the posterior fossa can lead to significant problems with airway management, aspiration pneumonia, and swallowing difficulties. As these tumors often invade the brainstem nuclear complexes (cranial nerves IX, X, and XII) that control the ability to speak and swallow, patients often have complicated postoperative courses that challenge the skills of ICU personnel.

Craniopharyngioma

Craniopharyngiomas represent about 10% of the brain tumors that occur in adolescents. These slow-growing tumors are usually in the sella and parasellar region. Their presentation in the adolescent population is variable. The clinical findings are usually due to increased ICP (81%), visual field anomalies (54%), or endocrine disturbances (35%).[19-21] The visual findings in adolescents with craniopharyngiomas are usually visual field cuts; the type depends on the site at which the tumor compresses the optic chiasm. The proximity of the tumor to the pituitary gland and hypothalamus gives rise to various endocrine abnormalities. Typical endocrinopathies result in diabetes insipidus, short stature, loss of secondary sexual characteristics, hypersomnia, and obesity (Fig. 149-5).

The surgical goal is total removal of tumor, if possible. The transnasal/transsphenoidal approach is used if the

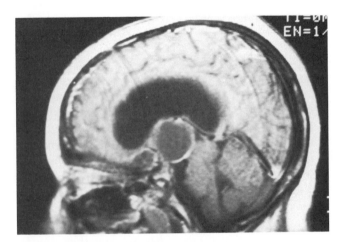

Fig. 149-5. A 14-year-old boy presented with obesity and diabetes insipidus. MRI showed a large cystic lesion in the parasellar region extending up into the third ventricle. As a result of the third ventricle extension of the tumor, the foramen of Munro had become occluded, and hydrocephalus resulted. At surgery, a craniopharyngioma was found.

tumor lies within the sella. The subfrontal craniotomy approach is used for tumors in the parasellar region that do not extend up into the third ventricle. For tumors in the third ventricle, either an interhemispheric/transcallosal or a transcortical/intraventricular approach is used. The choice of approach depends on the location of the tumor, its relationship to the third ventricle, and the presence or absence of hydrocephalus. The absence of hydrocephalus makes the transcortical approach more difficult. A number of studies have shown that long-term survival is directly related to the amount of tumor resected. In patients with total resection the 5-year survival is 77% and the 10-year survival 47%. In contrast, the 5-year survival after subtotal resection is only 14% and 10-year survival only 7%. Most patients in these series received adjuvant radiation therapy, which enhanced the duration of survival.[22,23]

The postoperative course can be complex. Diabetes insipidus is common and requires control with vasopressin or desmopressin acetate; it usually resolves spontaneously over 2 to 3 weeks. It is rare for a patient to need long-term pharmacologic supplementation to control diabetes insipidus. Endocrinologic abnormalities should be anticipated, and the endocrine service should always be involved in monitoring such patients in the postoperative period. If the transcortical approach is used, postoperative seizures are a risk; every patient should receive anticonvulsant agents before and after surgery.

Germ-Cell Tumors

Essentially five types of germ-cell tumors occur in adolescents: germinoma (65%), teratoma (18%), embryonal carcinoma (5%), endodermal sinus tract (7%), and choriocarcinoma (5%).[24] They almost always occur along the midline brain structures, ranging from the suprasellar cisterna to the pineal gland. An abrupt surge in incidence among adolescents in the early pubertal years suggests a strong hormonal influence. The peak age of occurrence is 10 to 12 years; 68% of all germ-cell tumors occur between the ages of 10 and 21 years.[24]

Because of their location, germ-cell tumors often cause diabetes insipidus, visual field deficits, hypothalamic and pituitary dysfunction, and finally hydrocephalus, if the CSF pathways are occluded by tumor. In the posterior third ventricle region, along the pineal area, midbrain compression can result if the tumor is large enough, causing Parinaud's syndrome (Fig. 149-6). Symptoms of this syndrome are paralysis of the conjugate upward gaze, lack of pupillary constriction, retraction nystagmus, and blepharospasm.

Many germ cell tumors have markers that are assayed in the diagnostic evaluation. These include carcinoembryonic antigen, alpha-fetoprotein, and human chorionic gonadotropin. CSF cytology from the lumbar subarachnoid space is positive for markers in at least 33% of cases.

Serial CSF studies (up to six) increase the sensitivity of detection by up to almost 100%.[25-27]

Because of the complexity of treating germ-cell lines, positive tissue diagnosis is essential in every case. The typical midline location of germ-cell tumors allows for easy surgical access. The morbidity associated with these operations is low (under 5%), and for this reason surgery is advocated for both tumor debulking and tissue diagnosis. The most common germ-cell tumors, germinomas, are quite radiosensitive and are associated with a good 5-year survival rate. The prognosis for patients with other types of germ-cell tumor (the incidence of which is fortunately rarer) is much poorer.

Optic Glioma

Optic gliomas have become more diagnostically evident with the advent of MRI. The optic glioma is common in patients with neurofibromatosis; its occurrence in these patients accounts for about 30% of its incidence.[28,29] Typically, the tumor is a benign pilocystic astrocytoma with a very slow course (Fig. 149-7). The decision regarding when to operate is complex. If the patient's vision is normal and no exophytic tumor component is evident radiographically, surgery is not indicated. Tumor that invades the optic chiasm or follows the optic radiations is considered inoperable. However, if the lesion occurs anterior to the chiasm and if visual acuity is markedly impaired, an operation is performed to remove the involved segment. The worst case is that of the patient with the diencephalic variant, who has glioma involvement extending into the hypothalamus and diencephalon.

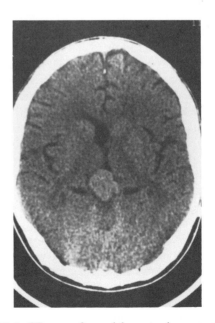

Fig. 149-6. CT scan of an adolescent who presented with Parinaud's syndrome. A lesion of increased density can be seen in the pineal region. Surgical diagnosis showed this tumor to be a germinoma of the pineal region.

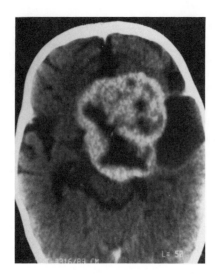

Fig. 149-7. CT scan showing a large cystic lesion occupying the parasellar region and extending laterally. To the left side of the lesion is a large cyst. Surgical exploration showed this tumor to be a benign optic glioma with a large exophytic component.

The prognosis is extremely poor. Often such patients exhibit severe visual, endocrine, and metabolic disturbances—all manifestations of the diencephalic syndrome. Symptoms of the diencephalic syndrome are emaciation despite nutrition, hypokinesis, vomiting (which can be severe and unrelenting), pallor (typically a pasty white skin), hypoglycemia, and hydrocephalus (frequent symptoms due to third ventricle obstruction).

Chordoma

Chordoma is very rare in adolescents, representing only about 1% of intracranial tumors. It typically arises in the clivus or in the sacral region (Fig. 149-8). Derived from remnants of the notochord, it is a very slow-growing extradural tumor. In adolescents, it not uncommonly presents as a nasopharyngeal mass. Because of its location, it has been a surgical challenge until recently. With the new craniofacial-, midfacial-, and skull-based approaches, these tumors can be resected much more safely than in the past. Chordomas are notoriously unresponsive to radiation therapy and there is no known effective chemotherapy regimen. The only treatment is attempted total surgical resection.

Fibrous Dysplasia

Fibrous dysplasia is not a true brain tumor but rather a lesion of the skull. However, because of its growth patterns, it can mimic the findings of a brain tumor. Fibrous dysplasia occurs as a result of an accumulation of fibrous connective tissue within one (monostotic) or more (polystotic) bones. It is thought to arise from a developmental mesenchymal defect; no known hereditary asso-

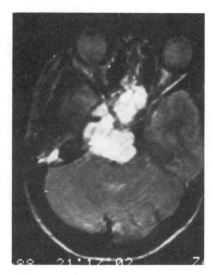

Fig. 149-8. MRI of a patient who presented with swallowing difficulties. Evaluation revealed a large destructive lesion arising from the clivus and extending up to the sella and to both cavernous sinuses. This chordoma resulted in complete destruction of the clivus and, in turn, compression of the mesencephalon.

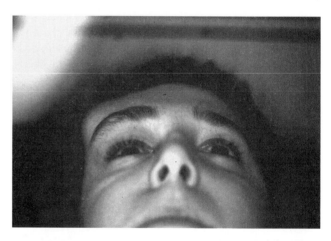

Fig. 149-9. Clinical photograph of a 13-year-old boy who presented at age 4 with a "swelling" over the right eye. This remained unchanged in size until he was 12, when it became acutely painful and doubled in size. This lesion turned out to be fibrous dysplasia with an acute hemorrhage that involved the right orbital rim and roof and extended back to the optic chiasm.

ciations have been reported. There is a well-known tendency for fibrous dysplasia to accelerate during intervals of rapid skeletal growth; hence, its increased frequency in adolescents (Fig. 149-9). The radiographic findings of fibrous dysplasia consist of a diffuse sclerosis and thickening of the involved bones (Fig. 149-10). The areas most involved in adolescents are the frontal fossa floor, the sphenoid wing, the orbit, and the periorbital regions. Those lesions that occur in the facial region can cause significant cosmetic deformities. More important, lesions in the skull base and sphenoids can threaten the orbital

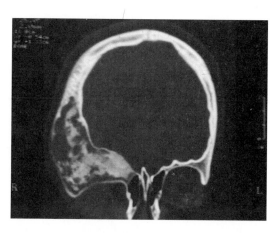

Fig. 149-10. Coronal MRI of the patient in Figure 149-9 showing the typical characteristics seen on radiologic examination of fibrous dysplasia. The involvement of the orbital roof and skull expansion can be appreciated from this view.

complex, causing serious risk to vision and extraocular movement.

As there are no known successful hormonal or chemotherapeutic treatments, surgery remains the therapy of choice. Radiation therapy was advocated in the past, but the occurrence of malignant degeneration was very disheartening, so that radiation therapy is now rarely, if ever, used. There have also been a number of cases of spontaneous malignant sarcomatous degeneration occurring in fibrous dysplasia, making this a potentially devastating lesion. When there is evidence of a rapidly growing fibrous dysplastic lesion, sarcomatous degeneration has to be ruled out by biopsy and followed by a wide surgical excision. While many cases of fibrous dysplasia appear to remain self-limited in growth, those that progress and show neurologic impairment (e.g., visual loss, optic atrophy) or orbital proptosis require surgical correction. The involved bone is removed back to normal margins. If the optic foramina are involved, these must be decompressed by craniotomy and by unroofing the optic nerve. MRI has proved helpful in determining the extent of abnormal bone involvement. The development of three-dimensional reconstructions has remarkably enhanced the surgical team's ability to determine what is normal and what is not.

POSTOPERATIVE COMPLICATIONS: MEDICAL AND SURGICAL MANAGEMENT

The frequency of postoperative complications from brain tumor surgery is low. The accepted complication rate in routine tumor surgery is about 5%. When they do occur, complications must be recognized immediately and treated aggressively to prevent permanent morbidity and mortality.

> **BOX 149-2**
> **Management of Postoperative Hemorrhage**
>
> CT scan (if time permits)
> Hyperventilation (Pco_2 reduced to 25 mm Hg)
> Hyperosmolar or diuretic agents (mannitol, furosemide [Lasix], or both)
> Steroids (dexamethasone)
> Anticonvulsant agents

Many brain tumors are quite vascular. Despite careful surgical closure with no intraoperative evidence of surgical site bleeding, the patient can rapidly deteriorate postoperatively, with loss of consciousness and respiratory arrest due to acutely raised ICP. Hemorrhage and acute ICP elevation are medical emergencies (Box 149-2). Removal of the tumor can cause severe, reactive edema around the tumor bed. This edema and swelling can mimic an acute hemorrhage. For this reason, CT is performed urgently, if time allows, to differentiate between hemorrhage and edema. In either case, whether hemorrhage or edema, the patient must be hyperventilated to reduce the Pco_2 to around 25 mm Hg. Diuretic agents are given (mannitol, 0.5 g/kg; furosemide [Lasix], dose calculated for age and weight) to remove the extracellular free water. The administration of steroids (dexamethasone) helps reduce the extent of reactive edema. In patients who become acutely obtunded, the possibility of a seizure having occurred must be considered. It is essential to ensure that anticonvulsant serum concentrations are at therapeutic levels. All the above measures, administered promptly and efficiently, can prevent or mitigate serious postoperative morbidity.

Cerebral Edema

In the era before steroids and CT scans, 10% to 15% of patients operated on for brain tumors were returned to the operating room within 8 to 10 hours for evaluation of neurologic deterioration. Rarely was a hemorrhage found; most patients had severe swelling due to the surgery and tumor resection. Since the institution of steroid administration 25 years ago, the incidence of this complication has been markedly reduced. Now all patients receive steroids preoperatively, and administration is continued for at least 1 week, after which the dose is slowly tapered.

Infection

In routine craniotomies in the absence of underlying systemic disorders (e.g., AIDS), the incidence of infection and meningitis is approximately 2% to 5%. The adolescent population is by and large a healthy group, and so the infection risk is low. The typical infectious organisms are the skin contaminants such as *Streptococcus* and *Staphylococcus* organisms. If infections due to these agents are recognized early and treated aggressively, complications are rarely long term. The major complication is infection of the bone flap. If the bone flap becomes involved with osteomyelitis, it must be discarded; cranioplasty is performed some 6 months later.

Posterior Fossa Syndrome (Aseptic Meningitis)

This well-known syndrome can develop in the adolescent patient who has undergone a posterior fossa craniotomy for tumor resection.[30] The patient initially does well, and then between the fifth and seventh postoperative days fever, malaise, bulging of the craniotomy site, and meningismus develop—classic findings of infectious meningitis. Lumbar puncture evaluation shows an increased inflammatory cell count, a low glucose level, and an increased protein level. However, microorganisms cannot be detected, and none grow in culture. The diagnosis is posterior fossa syndrome or aseptic meningitis. Patients are given a long-term course of steroids and eventually do well. The syndrome is thought to occur because of the location of the operative site, the normal surgical debris that is left behind, and the exposure of the nuchal muscles to CSF. Fortunately, in most instances the syndrome resolves without permanent sequelae. The physician must be aware of the possibility of this syndrome developing so that the patient is not subjected to an unnecessary antibiotic regimen.

Medical and Psychologic Effects of Treatment of Brain Tumors

Often overlooked by the adolescent medical team are the psychologic and medical sequelae of brain tumor treatment protocols. Most of these patients undergo chemotherapy and radiation therapy, the sequelae of which can be devastating both mentally and physiologically. Early in the treatment phase the most common change is a lower academic performance in school. This is most commonly due to the psychologic distraction of the treatment. Walking about with an indwelling catheter reduces the activities in which the adolescent can participate and also provides a psychologic reminder that something serious is going on. As the treatment progresses, there is hair loss (alopecia), which can have dire emotional consequences in both males and females. Not uncommonly, steroids are used, so weight gain is common. The side effects of chemotherapy for nausea and vomiting can affect social relationships and increase the stress level at home and within the family.

Adolescents vary markedly in maturity and hence in the ability to handle the diagnosis of a brain tumor. "Am I going to die?" is a comment often thought of but rarely expressed by the patient. It is extremely important that all forms of treatment be discussed, along with the expected complications and side effects, so that the patient is forewarned as to what to expect. Support groups of similarly affected patients who have been through similar treatments are extremely helpful. The parents and siblings should not be ignored, as they also need to be educated about the possible medical and psychologic sequelae. Both radiation therapy (particularly the high doses of 55 Gy) and the chemotherapy protocols are known to have long-term effects on the brain. Changes in school performance (e.g., worsening grades), deterioration in interpersonal relations, lack of attention and motivation, all can and do develop in adolescents undergoing therapy. Recognition of these problems and addressing them with the patient and family will go a long way to alleviate the long-term outcome.

References

1. Hammill JF, Carter S: Brain tumors in childhood. In Brenneman-Kelley, editor: *Practice of pediatrics,* vol 4, Hagerstown, MD, 1964, WF Prior; pp 1-19.
2. Laurent JP, Cheek WR: Brain tumors in children, *J Pediatr Neurosci* 1:15-32, 1985.
3. Dohrmann GJ, Farwell JR, Flannery JT: Astrocytomas in childhood: a population based study, *Surg Neurol* 23:64-68, 1985.
4. Kornblith PL, Walker MD, Cassady JR, editors: *Neurologic oncology,* Philadelphia, 1987, JB Lippincott.
5. Shapiro WR: Treatment of neuroectodermal brain tumors, *Ann Neurol* 12:231-237, 1982.
6. Hirschfeld A, Kornblith PL: Uncommon tumors of the nervous system. In Williams CJ, Krikorian JG, Green MR, Ragavan D, editors: *Textbook of uncommon cancer,* New York, 1988, John Wiley; pp 529-630.
7. Wallner KE, Gonzales MF, Edwards MSB, et al: Treatment results of juvenile pilocystic astrocytoma, *J Neurosurg* 69:171-176, 1988.
8. Cushing H: The surgical mortality pertaining to a series of two thousand verified intracranial tumors. Standards of computation, *Trans Am Neurol Assoc* 456-463, 1931.
9. Farwell JR, Dohrmann GJ, Flannery JT: Medulloblastoma in childhood: an epidemiological study, *J Neurosurg* 61:657-664, 1984.
10. Tomita T, Mclone DG: Medulloblastoma in childhood: results of radical resection and low-dose neuraxis radiation therapy, *J Neurosurg* 64:238-242, 1986.
11. Allen JC, Epstein JC: Medulloblastoma and other primary malignant neuroectodermal tumors of the CNS. The effect of patients' age and extent of disease on prognosis, *J Neurosurg* 57:446-451, 1982.
12. Harisiadis L, Chang CH: Medulloblastoma in children: a correlation between staging and results of treatment, *J Radiat Oncol Biol Phys* 2:833-841, 1977.
13. Epstein F: Pediatric posterior fossa tumors—Part I, *Contemp Neurosurg* 8:1-6, 1986.
14. Park TS, Hoffman HJ, Hendrick B, et al: Medulloblastoma: clinical presentation and management, *J Neurosurg* 58:543-552, 1983.
15. Carmel PW: Role of neurosurgery in tumors of the posterior fossa and posterior third ventricle tumors in children. In *Tumors of the central nervous system,* New York, 1980, Masson.

16. Kornblith PL, Walker MD, Cassady JR: Treatment of tumors of the posterior fossa—astrocytomas, medulloblastomas, ependymomas, and hemangioblastomas. In Kornblith PL, Walker MD, Cassady JR, editors: *Neurologic oncology,* Philadelphia, 1987, JB Lippincott.

17. Goodrich JT, Kornblith PL: Chemotherapy for pediatric brain tumors. In Long DL, editor: *Current therapy in neurological surgery,* Toronto, 1989, Mosby–Year Book; pp 95-97.

18. Humphreys RP: Posterior cranial fossa brain tumors in children. In Rengachary S, Wilkins R, editors: *Neurosurgery,* Baltimore, 1987, Williams & Wilkins; pp 2733-2757.

19. Fischer EG, Welch K, Beilli JA, et al: Treatment of craniopharyngioma in children: 1972-1981, *J Neurosurg* 62:496-501, 1985.

20. Carmel PW, Antunes JL, Chang CH: Craniopharyngiomas in children, *Neurosurgery* 11:382-389, 1982.

21. Matson DD, Crigler JF Jr: Management of craniopharyngioma in childhood, *J Neurosurg* 30:377-390, 1969.

22. Sung DI, Chang CH, Harisiadis L, Carmel PW: Treatment results of craniopharyngiomas, *Cancer* 47:847-852, 1981.

23. Sweet WH: Radical surgical treatment of craniopharyngiomas in children, *Clin Neurosurg* 27:206-229, 1980.

24. Jennings MT, Gelman R, Hochberg F: Intracranial germ-cell tumors: natural history and pathogenesis, *J Neurosurg* 63:155-167, 1985.

25. Allen JC, Nisselbaum J, Epstein F, et al: Alpha-fetoprotein and human chorionic gonadotropin determination in cerebrospinal fluid. An aid to the diagnosis and management of intracranial germ-cell tumors, *J Neurosurg* 51:368-374, 1979.

26. Arita N, Ushio Y, Hayakawa T, et al: Serum levels of alpha-fetoprotein, human chorionic gonadotropin and carcinoembryonic antigen in patients with primary intracranial germ cell tumors, *Oncodev Biol Med* 1:235-240, 1980.

27. Brodeur GM, Howarth CB, Pratt CB, et al: Malignant germ cell tumors in 57 children and adolescents, *Cancer* 48:1890-1898, 1981.

28. Spitzer D, Goodrich JT: Neurosurgical management of optic gliomas, *Neurofibromatosis* 1:223-232, 1988.

29. Cheek WR, Riccardi VM, Laurent JP: Neurofibromatosis of childhood: neurosurgical implications, *Concepts Pediatr Neurosurg* 4:319-334, 1983.

30. Carmel PW, Fraser RAR, Stein BM: Aseptic meningitis following posterior fossa surgery in children, *J Neurosurg* 41:44-48, 1974.

CHAPTER 150

Intracranial Vascular Malformations

•

James Tait Goodrich

Few lesions of the brain have a more devastating impact than hemorrhage from an intracranial vascular malformation. Some vascular malformations present with warning signs, allowing an alert physician to make an early diagnosis. The most common vascular malformations in adolescents that lead to intracerebral and subarachnoid hemorrhage in the brain are aneurysms, arteriovenous malformations (AVMs), and cavernous angiomas.

ANEURYSMS

Intracerebral aneurysms were originally thought to be uncommon in adolescents, but with the introduction of magnetic resonance imaging (MRI) and more sophisticated angiography, aneurysms have been shown to occur somewhat frequently in this age group. In several series the incidence ranged from 0.5% to 4.6%.[1-7] Such lesions are associated with a high mortality rate in this population, 43% within the first week of diagnosis. The locations of aneurysms in adolescents are different from those seen in adults. The most common sites in adolescents are the internal carotid artery bifurcation (26% to 54%) (Fig. 150-1), anterior communicating artery (20%), and middle cerebral artery (5%).[1,2] Aneurysms of the posterior fossa circulation are rare in adults but relatively common in adolescents. Interestingly, adolescents tend to have a higher incidence of giant aneurysms (>2.5 cm in diameter). As many as 25% of adult aneurysm patients have multiple aneurysms (e.g., more than one aneurysm of the circle of Willis), whereas only 5% of adolescent aneurysm patients have more than one aneurysm. The male-to-female ratio in adolescent aneurysm patients is 3:2.[6,7]

Etiology

Unlike adult aneurysms, which are arteriosclerotic in etiology, adolescent aneurysms are congenital in origin. In addition, adolescents with aneurysms are at risk for a number of associated syndromes: coarctation of the aorta, polycystic kidney disease, connective tissue disorders, mycotic infection, and traumatic injury.

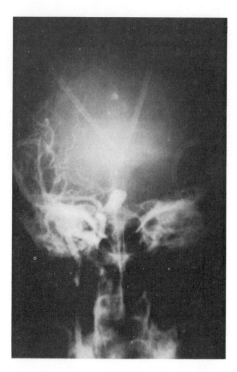

Fig. 150-1. Angiogram of a 16-year-old boy with coarctation of the aorta, showing a large internal carotid bifurcation artery aneurysm filled with contrast material pointing up and medially.

Coarctation of the aorta has long been recognized as being associated with a heightened risk of intracranial aneurysms based on accompanying arterial hypertension. The frequency of ruptured aneurysms, however, remains low—under 5%. Both children and adolescents with polycystic kidney disease are at an increased risk of cerebral aneurysms. Like those with coarctation of the aorta, patients with polycystic kidney disease are at low risk for hemorrhage.

The nature of the underlying pathologic alterations in aneurysms has long given rise to speculation that their incidence must be elevated in patients with connective tissue disorders (e.g., Ehlers-Danlos, Marfan's, Rendu-Osler-Weber syndromes). Although this association has been much discussed, no large statistical series are currently available to document the incidence and prevalence of aneurysms among adolescents with connective tissue disorders.

Of patients with bacterial endocarditis, 3% to 15% have cerebral aneurysms.[1] As opposed to congenital aneurysms, which form at bifurcations, mycotic aneurysms form on the distal vessels or branches of the cerebral circulation. They most commonly occur in patients with rheumatic heart disease. Other populations at risk include patients with right-to-left intracardiac shunts, those with prosthetic heart valves, and—the most recent addition—people involved with intravenous drug use. Within this last group is a subgroup of adolescents who regularly use cocaine, among whom an epidemic of ruptured intracranial aneurysms has recently developed.

As adolescents have become sophisticated in the use of high-power and high-velocity weapons, the incidence of intracerebral traumatic aneurysms has increased. In any individual who has sustained a penetrating injury of the head in which there may be an associated injury to the underlying vessels, an angiogram should be performed to rule out a traumatic aneurysm. Such aneurysms are as lethal as congenital and acquired aneurysms and require appropriate surgical treatment.

Pathology

The primary etiologic mechanism in aneurysm formation, and accordingly a key pathologic finding, is the fragmentation or absence of the internal elastic membrane and muscularis layer of the arterial wall. A congenital defect combined with ongoing hemodynamic injury to the internal elastic membrane can cause an aneurysm to develop at a bifurcation. Aneurysms typically form in the direction of normal blood flow.

Diagnosis

The recognition of aneurysm rupture is straightforward when the treating physician appreciates the presenting signs of subarachnoid hemorrhage. Typically, patients (if awake) complain of a sudden, severe, explosive headache, more severe than any headache pain they have previously experienced. Often associated with this headache are vomiting, meningismus (stiff neck), photophobia, and alteration in mental status that can range from mild confusion to a comatose state with fixed and dilated pupils. Seizures are not uncommon; they tend to be focal motor seizures or can evolve into a grand mal episode. Other neurologic deficits often occur, such as dilated pupils and hemiparesis. Over 90% of patients with aneurysms have no earlier history of symptoms.[4,5] The patient in whom diagnosis is the most difficult is the one who presents with severe headache but without any other pertinent signs and symptoms. Other subtle findings, such as extraocular dysfunction (diplopia being the most common), can help point to the diagnosis of aneurysms. Large aneurysms can manifest with mass effect, giving rise to focal neurologic findings.

Diagnostic evaluation should begin with a lumbar puncture to obtain spinal fluid, the examination of which will disclose the presence of subarachnoid blood. A "bloody tap" (spinal fluid that does not clear) is a reliable indicator of subarachnoid hemorrhage. Computed tomography (CT) also shows subarachnoid blood in most cases (Figs. 150-2, 150-3). A severe hemorrhage may create a casting of the ventricular system and basal cisterna visible on CT. Intracerebral clots can also occur but are less common.

MRI is also a useful diagnostic tool because blood from a freshly ruptured aneurysm produces a high signal

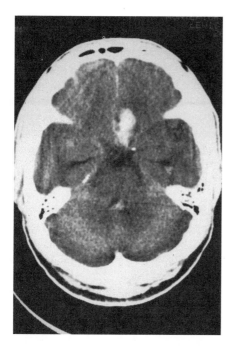

Fig. 150-2. Axial CT scan of an 18-year-old girl with polycystic kidney disease, showing an acute rupture of an anterior communicating artery aneurysm with diffuse subarachnoid blood.

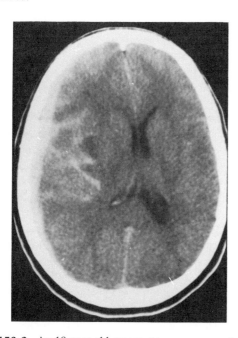

Fig. 150-3. An 18-year-old pregnant teenager presented with the "worst headache of my life." A CT scan was ordered and showed a diffuse subarachnoid hemorrhage, with most of the hemorrhage in the right temporal region. A resultant right-to-left shift of the brain occurred secondary to edema and subdural blood hematoma.

> **BOX 150-1**
> **Grading System for Aneurysms**
>
> Grade 0: Unruptured aneurysm (usually inciden-
> tally found)
> Grade 1: Alert with no deficit
> Grade 2: Alert with minimal deficit or meningis-
> mus signs
> Grade 3: Drowsy or confused with or without
> deficit
> Grade 4: Stuporous or semicomatose
> Grade 5: Deep coma, moribund

From Hunt WE, Hess RM: Surgical risk as related to time of intervention in the repair of intracranial aneurysms, *J Neurosurg* 28:14-20, 1968.

vascular system without the need for invasive intravascular techniques.

Neurosurgeons now routinely classify the clinical status of patients with a subarachnoid hemorrhage to help distinguish patients who are likely candidates for early operation (within the first 48 hours of hemorrhage) from those in whom late surgery is indicated (usually 10 to 14 days from aneurysm rupture) (Box 150-1). Typically, patients with a grade 0 to 2 classification will be offered early surgery. Most surgical teams delay surgery for patients in grade 3 or higher. Surgery is rare in patients who remain in grade 5.

Differential Diagnosis

In the patient who has had a subarachnoid hemorrhage, the diagnosis is easy to make. Unfortunately, the patient with an unruptured aneurysm may not be so easy to detect. Since these patients have a significant risk of hemorrhage (3% per year), early diagnosis is critical. Migraines usually can be identified by the history and type of headache. Subtle signs of a progressive neurologic defect, such as extraocular dysfunction (e.g., double vision) or hemiparesis, can be an early indication of an expanding giant aneurysm causing cranial nerve compression.

Management

The treatment of choice for an intracranial aneurysm remains the placement of a metal spring clip on the aneurysm neck to achieve occlusion. Occasionally, the aneurysmal structure is such that there is no definable neck. In such circumstances, a number of other techniques are available, including "wrapping" the aneurysm in material such as muslin or acrylic (a method rarely used today) and "sharing" or ligating the aneurysm at its neck. Occasionally, the aneurysm can be trapped, that is, occluded on both sides and then bypassed with a vein graft. In addition, interventional neuroradiologists can

visible on MRI; in some cases the signal void of an aneurysm dome can be detected. More medical centers will be able to provide MRI angiography within the next several years. Using computer subtraction techniques, the MRI angiographer can now image the intracranial now use intravascular techniques to place balloons and thrombotic material, like copper coils, within the aneurysm to occlude it.

Mycotic aneurysms remain one of the most difficult management problems for neurosurgeons. Fortunately, most mycotic aneurysms regress with appropriate antibiotic therapy. The indication for surgery is continued aneurysm growth despite antibiotic administration. Mycotic aneurysms are friable and rarely have a suitable neck for clipping.

Prognosis

The prognosis for the patient who has survived an aneurysm rupture is good, provided that the hemorrhage has not been devastating. Adolescents who suffer such a rupture have a good potential for recovery because of their youth. The mortality rate in aneurysm rupture remains high: 15% of patients die at the time of the initial hemorrhage, 28% die during hospital admission, and 14% experience rebleeding before surgery, for a combined mortality rate of 57%.[1-5]

The question often arises of what to do with the asymptomatic patient found to have an incidental aneurysm. Various cooperative studies have shown that the risk of bleeding is 3% per year. On the basis of these data and the typical adolescent life expectancy, most neurosurgeons advocate aneurysm surgery at the time of detection.

ARTERIOVENOUS MALFORMATIONS

If an adventurous young surgeon cuts into the body of a tumour of tortuous veins and arteries, he has vessels throwing out their blood over both his shoulders. But if he keeps wide of the diseased mass, he perhaps cuts across one artery which throws out its blood with no uncommon velocity.
Sir Charles Bell (London 1812)

With the advent of MRI and improved CT scanning, AVMs, once thought to be very rare, are being diagnosed much more frequently. The prevalence ranges from 1.5% to 4% in the pediatric and adolescent population; in the general autopsy population it is about 0.14%. It is now recognized that AVMs are the most common vascular malformation in adolescents; they are ten times more common than aneurysms in this age group. The peak age for bleeding is between 15 and 20 years. The risk of death from rupture is about 30%. The morbidity risk is also high: 23% after rupture. As with aneurysms, the risk of rupture is about 2% to 3% per year in incidentally found AVMs.[8-16]

AVMs are congenital lesions of the vascular system, a persistence of embryonic blood vessels. During the development of the vascular system, the intermediate capillary bed does not form and so an arteriovenous shunt develops. In the arterial vessels the pathologic alteration consists of a poorly developed media and elastica. The distal vessels are very thin walled and are transitional between arterial and venous channels. These areas are at the greatest risk for hemorrhage. Interestingly, the tissue within the AVM varies from normal brain, showing only gliosis, to edema, calcifications, small cysts, and (usually) evidence of both old and recent hemorrhages.

Diagnosis

Hemorrhage with an intraparenchymal clot is the most common presenting feature of an AVM (55% to 76%).[8-15] The most devastating hemorrhage is the one in which the AVM bleeds directly into the ventricles. AVMs are typically triangular in shape, with an apex that angles toward the ventricle; this apex is also the weakest area and the area at greatest risk for hemorrhage.

The second most common clinical finding in a patient with an AVM is a seizure, which occurs in approximately 20% of the population with AVMs. The seizure type is typically related to the location of the AVM. Partial complex motor seizures are common. Other symptoms are progressive but slow mental deterioration and neurologic deficit, thought to be caused by a steal syndrome, in which the high-flow AVM diverts blood supply away from normal brain tissue.

Despite the amount of discussion about them, intracranial bruits are actually quite rare in AVMs except in traumatic dural AVMs; the overall incidence is well under 5%. Occasionally, the patient complains of a roaring noise in the head. The other common symptom, which is probably the most difficult to classify, is a migrainous headache, which is reported in about 20% of AVM patients. These individuals are typically treated as migraine patients.

On CT the physician typically sees an irregular, slightly hyperdense area with an area of bright density, indicating a recent hemorrhage (Fig. 150-4).[17] Like CT, MRI shows an increased signal from blood and a signal void where there is high blood flow within the AVM. With MRI it is now easy to locate AVMs without the need for invasive angiography. In the adolescent patient with an atypical headache presentation, MRI is indicated, but the diagnostic test of choice remains the angiogram (Fig. 150-5). A thorough four-vessel study is needed to localize both the arterial feeder vessels and the venous drainage system (Fig. 150-6).

Management

Since the risk of hemorrhage from an unruptured AVM is 2% to 3% per year, most surgeons recommend AVM excision, except in cases in which the AVM is situated too

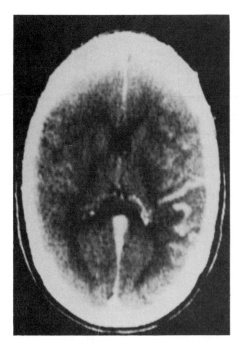

Fig. 150-4. CT scan of an arteriovenous malformation occupying the left temporal occipital region. With the introduction of contrast material, the rich vascularization of the hemispheres can be appreciated.

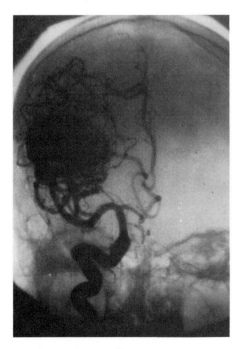

Fig. 150-5. Angiogram of a large left arteriovenous malformation with feeder vessels coming from the middle cerebral artery complex. There is also feeding from the anterior cerebral artery.

deeply or located in a critical structure such as the brain stem (although these AVMs are operated on occasionally). As neuroradiologists have become more adept in placing catheters within brain vessels, they have gained the ability to embolize the various feeding vessels.

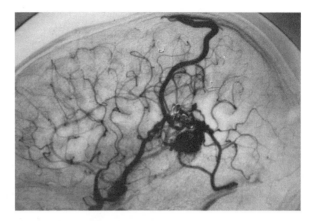

Fig. 150-6. Lateral carotid angiogram of a 13-year-old girl who presented with an acute, sudden severe headache; speech arrest; and loss of consciousness. The angiogram shows a large left middle cerebral artery complex AVM with a large draining vein emptying into the sagittal sinus.

However, an AVM has the ability to "steal" or recruit vessels from around its nidus. For these reasons and because of the technical limitations involved in cannulating smaller vessels, it is not yet possible to obliterate AVMs completely through intravascular approaches.

Several medical centers have advocated the use of high-energy external radiation to treat AVMs, particularly smaller, deeper AVMs less than 2.5 cm in diameter.[18] Early studies showed successful reduction, if not obliteration, of small AVMs by means of this technique. The only remaining question concerns the effect of radiation and the potential for subsequent tumor development, a well-known phenomenon that occurs after ionizing radiation therapy.

Prognosis

Prognosis varies with the severity of the initial injury caused by an intracerebral AVM hemorrhage. Since AVMs develop without normal brain tissue within them, they can be removed safely with low morbidity and almost no operative mortality. Considering the risk of hemorrhage in AVMs and the adolescent patient's age, it is recommended that excision at least be considered for any AVM.

CAVERNOUS ANGIOMAS

Before the advent of MRI, cavernous angiomas were thought to be extremely rare. They are difficult to see on CT and are rarely detected on angiograms. In the past, the typical patient with a cavernous angioma presented with a severe intracranial hemorrhage. The neurosurgeon removed the clot and often no pathologic changes could be detected in the surgical specimen. It appeared as if the

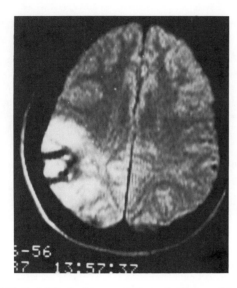

Fig. 150-7. MRI of a 14-year-old boy who had a sudden onset of headaches and seizures. This scan shows the typical "bullet-ring" appearance of a cavernous angioma in the right occipital region. Surrounding edema from a recent hemorrhage is also present.

lesion self-destructed. The diagnosis—reached by exclusion of other possibilities—was usually AVM. Now, with the increased sensitivity of MRI, cavernous angiomas are being detected more frequently.

Incidence and Frequency

The male-to-female ratio in terms of incidence of cavernous angioma is about equal in most series. These lesions tend to be located in the periphery of the brain at the hemispheres following the subcortical plane. They are rare in adolescents, representing about 5% to 8% of all vascular malformations detected clinically.[19] Most cavernous angiomas appear to remain asymptomatic; the incidence of clinically silent lesions in autopsy series is 4% to 5%. Multiple cavernous angiomas (i.e., two or more lesions) are found in about 6% of patients.[20-25]

Pathology

Cavernous angiomas are congenital malformations composed of thin-walled sinusoidal space lined with endothelium. There is no elastic or muscular layer, nor is there any intervening neuronal tissue.[20] It is not unusual to find thrombosis and hyalinization of the angioma wall. These angiomas are difficult to identify on angiography because of the lack of large feeding vessels and the diminished venous draining pattern; these features do not allow for a good angiographic image.

Clinical Presentation

There are three main clinical presentations of angiomas: seizures (54%), hemorrhage (31%), and focal neurologic findings (15%).[21] The typical patient with a cavernous angioma presents with a recent onset of seizures; evaluation reveals a normal CT image and a nonfocal electroencephalogram. MRI then discloses the lesion. Usually the evidence of a previous hemorrhage gives rise to the "bullet-ring" appearance of these lesions on MRI (Fig. 150-7). A follow-up angiogram (which is no longer indicated in the evaluation of these lesions if angioma is suspected) is usually normal.

About one third of patients with cavernous angiomas present with an intracerebral hemorrhage associated with loss of consciousness and severe neurologic defect. In these patients, CT indicates a recent hemorrhage. Because of the fresh clot, the diagnosis of angioma is difficult to make. In an emergency situation in which the clot is causing a mass effect, the patient is taken to the operating room for removal of the clot. In my experience, no pathologic changes are found in most cases, as the lesions tend to self-destruct. Evaluation with MRI can help localize multiple lesions.

In fewer than one third of patients, there is a small hemorrhage or an increase in hemorrhage size, causing a mass effect on the surrounding brain tissue; in these cases, the patient presents with a focal neurologic deficit. As these lesions are typically in the cerebral hemisphere, focal motor or sensory findings are most common.

The risk of hemorrhage in the incidentally found angioma is still unknown. In the few reports of series in which this problem has been investigated, the risk of hemorrhage has been found to be about 30% over the lifetime of the patient.[21] Because of this high risk, most neurosurgeons recommend that cavernous angiomas be removed as long as their location allows for acceptable operative morbidity.

Surgical Management and Prognosis

The cavernous angioma is a slow-flow vascular lesion that is well demarcated from surrounding brain. As noted above, the lesions tend to occur in the cerebral hemispheres and are peripheral. These locations make for relatively simple surgical excision without injury to the surrounding brain. Once removed, they do not recur, making for an excellent long-term prognosis. Interestingly, a number of studies have suggested that cavernous angiomas can be safely removed even from within the brain stem (Fig. 150-8). Removal from these delicate structures is possible because of the lesion's pathologic nature: a discrete, well-circumscribed mass with minimal potential for active hemorrhage.

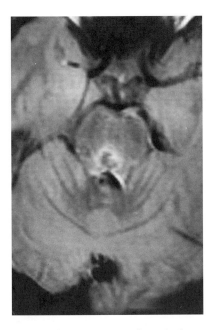

Fig. 150-8. MRI of a cavernous angioma in the mesencephalon of a 15-year-old girl. She presented with acute headache and double vision (diplopia). A spinal tap was positive for acute blood, but CT showed only some speckling of blood in this region. This follow-up MRI view shows much more clearly the lesion and its relationship to the brain stem.

References

1. Meyer FB, Reeves AL: Pediatric and adolescent aneurysms, *Contemp Neurosurg* 12:1-6, 1990.

2. Amacher AL: Subarachnoid hemorrhage in children and adolescents, *Contemp Neurosurg* 6:1-6, 1984.

3. Amacher AL, Drake CG: The results of operating upon cerebral aneurysms and angiomas in children and adolescents. 1. Cerebral aneurysms, *Childs Brain* 5:151, 1979.

4. Heiskanen O: Ruptured intracranial arterial aneurysms of children and adolescents: surgical and total management results, *Childs Nerv Syst* 5:66, 1989.

5. Humphreys RP: Intracranial arterial aneurysms. In Edwards MSB, Hoffman H, editors: *Cerebral vascular disease in children and adolescents,* Baltimore, 1989, Williams & Wilkins; pp 247-254.

6. Meyer FB, Sundt TM Jr, Fode NC, et al: Cerebral aneurysms in childhood and adolescence, *J Neurosurg* 70:420, 1989.

7. Storrs BB, Humphreys RP, Hendrick EB, Hoffman HJ: Intracranial aneurysm in the pediatric age-group, *Childs Brain* 9:358, 1982.

8. Martin NA, Edwards MSB, Wilson CB: Management of intracranial vascular malformations in children and adolescents, *Concepts Pediatr Neurosurg* 4:264-290, 1983.

9. Gutierrez FA, McLone DG, Naidich TP: Cerebrovascular malformations in children, *Concepts Pediatr Neurosurg* 5:136-153, 1985.

10. Garza-Mercado R, Cavazds E, Tamez-Montes D: Cerebral arteriovenous malformations in children and adolescents, *Surg Neurol* 27:131-140, 1987.

11. Graf CJ, Perret GE, Torner JC: Bleeding from cerebral arteriovenous malformations as part of their natural history, *J Neurosurg* 58:331-337, 1983.

12. Fults D, Kelly DL Jr: Natural history of arteriovenous malformations of the brain: a clinical study, *Neurosurgery* 15:658-662, 1984.

13. Humphreys RP: Aneurysms and arteriovenous malformations of the brain. In Hoffman HJ, Epstein F, editors: *Disorders of the developing nervous system: diagnosis and treatment,* Boston, 1986, Blackwell Scientific; pp 769-793.

14. Wilkins RH: Natural history of intracranial vascular malformations: a review, *Neurosurgery* 16:421-430, 1985.

15. Brown RD Jr, Wiebers DO, Forbes G, et al: The natural history of unruptured intracranial arteriovenous malformations, *J Neurosurg* 68:352-357, 1988.

16. Lemme-Plaghos L, Kucharczyk W, Brant-Zawakzki M, et al: MRI of angiographically occult vascular malformations, *AJNR* 146:1223-1228, 1986.

17. Kucharczyk W, Lemme-Plagnos L, Uske A, et al: Intracranial vascular malformations: MR and CT imaging, *Radiology* 156:383-389, 1985.

18. Kjellberg RN, Hanamura T, Davis DR, et al: Bragg-Peak proton therapy for arteriovenous malformations of the brain, *N Engl J Med* 309:269-273, 1983.

19. McCormick WF: The pathology of angiomas. In Fein J, Flamm EG, editors: *Cerebrovascular surgery,* vol 4, New York, 1985, Springer-Verlag; pp 1073-1095.

20. New PFJ, Ojemann RG, Davis KR, et al: MR and CT of occult vascular malformations of the brain, *Am J Radiol* 147:985-993, 1986.

21. Tagle P, Huete I, Mendez MD, del Villar S: Intracranial cavernous angioma: presentation and management, *J Neurosurg* 64:720-723, 1986.

22. Becker DH, Townsend JJ, Kramer RA, et al: Occult cerebrovascular malformations. A series of 18 histologically verified cases with negative angiography, *Brain* 102:249-287, 1979.

23. Giombini S, Morello G: Cavernous angiomas of the brain. Account of fourteen personal cases and review of the literature, *Acta Neurochir* 40:61-82, 1978.

24. Savoiardo M, Strada L, Passerini A: Intracranial cavernous hemangiomas: neuroradiological review of 36 operated cases, *AJNR* 4:945-950, 1983.

25. Voigt K, Yasargil MG: Cerebral cavernous haemangiomas or cavernomas. Incidence, pathology, localization, diagnosis, clinical features and treatment. Review of the literature and report of an unusual case, *Neurochirurgia (Stuttg)* 19:59-68, 1976.

CHAPTER 151

Orthopedics

•

Neil J. Macy

A number of orthopedic disorders predominantly affect the adolescent population or commonly occur during adolescence. Because skeletal growth continues through adolescence, skeletal injuries or disorders in this age group necessitate accurate assessment and immediate treatment. Idiopathic scoliosis directly affects this age group and must be recognized early to effect appropriate therapy. When an adolescent experiences hip pain, the possibility of a slipped capital femoral epiphysis must be considered, since complete skeletal maturity has not been attained. Knee pain as a result of intraarticular disorders of the knee (meniscal injury, cruciate ligament tears) is common in this population, especially among teenage athletes. Bone tumors do not occur with greater frequency in this age group, but the consequences of a misdiagnosis or a delay in arriving at the correct diagnosis can be dire. Although infection (osteomyelitis, septic arthritis) and trauma can occur at any age, these disorders may require special treatment modalities in adolescents.

ADOLESCENT IDIOPATHIC SCOLIOSIS

The word *scoliosis* originates from the Greek word meaning crooked and indicates a lateral curvature and rotation of the vertebral column. Depending on the type and severity of the curve, this condition can lead to deformity of the ribcage and may adversely affect pulmonary and cardiac function. Cosmesis is also an important consideration. Through early diagnosis and proper treatment, most of the serious consequences of scoliosis can be prevented. Public education and screening programs facilitate early diagnosis.

The etiology of adolescent idiopathic scoliosis seems to be multifactorial. A study by Wynne-Davies demonstrated a twentyfold increased incidence of scoliosis among the families of girls with this condition. Neither nutritional deficiencies nor endocrine abnormalities have been demonstrated. Aberrations in the central nervous system (abnormal balance in the labyrinth system) have also been implicated, but a specific cause remains unknown. The incidence of scoliosis, defined as a vertebral curvature of 10 degrees or greater, is 1% to 2%. Those with more severe curvature and who require active treatment are typically female. Patients with scoliosis usually seek medical attention because someone noticed "a high shoulder," poor posture, breast or waist asymmetry, or the curvature itself. Scoliosis is being detected more and more often during routine physical examination and school screening programs.

Information obtained during history taking should include onset of the deformity, mode of presentation, awareness of progression, family history, menarche, symptoms of neurologic abnormalities, and evidence of cardiopulmonary compromise. The history of the development of secondary sexual characteristics is important in assessing potential future growth, which can affect the prognosis. Idiopathic scoliosis is almost always asymptomatic, and a history of pain or rapid progression of the curvature should alert the physician to a possible underlying pathologic condition. A complete physical examination should be performed. General observations should include the patient's height, Tanner stage of development, and abnormal skin pigmentation. A patient with scoliosis who has a heart murmur, a high-arched palate, a dislocated ocular lens, and long thin fingers has

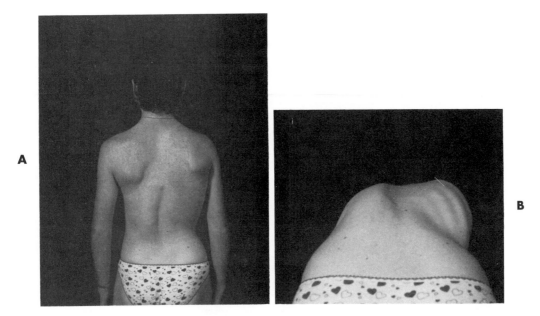

Fig. 151-1. Scoliosis. **A,** Posterior view demonstrating scapulae and flank asymmetry. **B,** Forward-bending view demonstrating the thoracic and lumbar elevations caused by the rotational component of scoliosis.

Marfan's syndrome with associated scoliosis. A thorough neurologic assessment is essential to exclude serious underlying pathologic conditions. The possibility of spinal tumors and neuromuscular diseases must be considered. The combination of foot deformity and spinal deformity should lead the physician to suspect a neurologic disorder (e.g., diastematomyelia, intraspinal lipoma). Examination of the spine begins by having the patient undress sufficiently for the entire back to be visualized. The skin over the spine should be examined for lipomas, dermal sinuses, hairy patches, hemangiomas, or nevi, which suggest congenital anomalies.

With the patient in an erect posture, the spinal alignment is inspected from the front, side, and back (Fig. 151-1, *A*). The height measurements of the right and left iliac crests are compared to detect possible discrepancies in leg length. Scapulae or flank asymmetry is also noted. The anatomic areas and the magnitude of the deviation of the spine from the midline are assessed. The most sensitive clinical parameter for the detection of scoliosis is the abnormal spinal rotation that accompanies the abnormal lateral curvature. The rotation is best visualized by examining the spine with the patient bending forward (Fig. 151-1, *B*) and comparing the height of the paravertebral regions on the patient's right and left sides. Anteriorly, one should evaluate for rib flare and asymmetric breast appearance. The quantity of breast tissue is equal; however, as the spine rotates, the attached ribs also rotate, causing one hemithorax to be more prominent and hence causing the overlying breast to appear larger.

Roentgenographic Evaluation

Because screening programs have been successful in screening large numbers of schoolchildren for spinal deformity, the number of patients undergoing roentgenographic evaluations has increased. Those patients requiring long-term treatment need further periodic radiographic studies. As a result, these individuals are at greater risk for radiation exposure. To minimize this risk, initial screening studies should be limited to a single anteroposterior (AP) radiograph of the entire spine on a scoliosis cassette. A lateral radiograph is ordered only if a deformity in the AP plane (kyphosis, lordosis) is clinically apparent.

Breast tissue has been shown to be at the highest carcinogenic risk from radiation. Using posteroanterior rather than AP exposure for subsequent evaluations reduces the radiation burden to the breasts. Gonadal shielding is important. In addition, the use of higher-speed film, greater collimation, shielding screens, and anthropomorphic filtering further minimizes radiation exposure.

Differential Diagnosis

The diagnosis of idiopathic scoliosis requires the exclusion of known causes. The main considerations include congenital scoliosis, which can be detected by radiographic evaluation; functional scoliosis caused by a leg length discrepancy; neuromuscular scoliosis, which can be detected by a thorough neurologic examination;

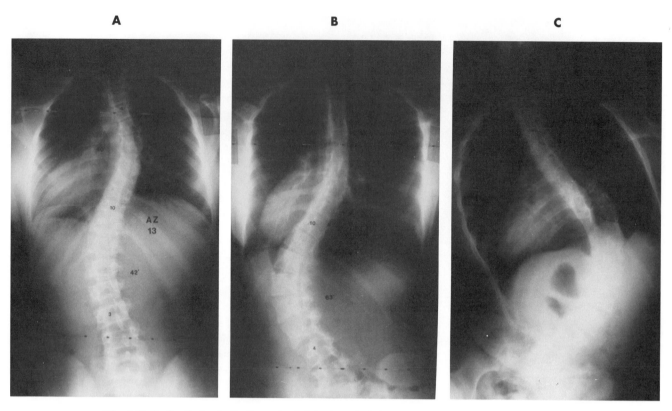

Fig. 151-2. Scoliosis. **A,** Radiograph of right thoracic left lumbar pattern. **B,** Radiograph of left lumbar pattern. **C,** Radiograph of right thoracolumbar pattern.

and painful scoliosis (e.g., discogenic, osteoid osteoma), which can be detected through the patient history and further studies as required.

Treatment

To develop a rational method of treatment, one must be aware of the natural history of the condition. Not all curves progress. The probability of curve progression can be assessed by the following criteria: potential for further growth (age, height, menarche, secondary sexual characteristics, and radiographic markers), curve pattern (Fig. 151-2) and magnitude of the curve on initial presentation. The younger the patient and the greater the curve magnitude, the greater is the chance of progression. Thoracic and double primary curves progress to a greater degree than single lumbar or thoracolumbar curves. There are currently only three treatment alternatives for idiopathic scoliosis: observation, bracing, and surgery. A fourth alternative, electric stimulation, is no longer considered an effective form of treatment.

The primary goal of observation is to determine whether the curve is progressive and will require active treatment. Observation is indicated for skeletally immature patients who have curves of less than 20 degrees. In growing patients, curves with documented progression,

whether less or greater than 20 degrees, require active treatment.

Exercise treatment alone has no proven value. Bracing remains the nonoperative treatment of choice. The object of bracing is to prevent progression of the curve, not to correct it. The major difficulty with brace treatment is poor patient compliance in this rebellious, self-conscious, and appearance-oriented group of patients. Studies are being conducted on the use of nighttime bracing in comparison with full-time bracing, which is currently employed. Bracing is used until there is evidence of spinal skeletal maturation.

Surgical management is reserved for patients whose curves progress despite brace treatment and for those with curves of 50 degrees or greater; in the latter group, surgery is necessary because the curve is likely to progress even after skeletal maturity. Concerns with self-imaging and appearance may be another indication for operative treatment.

The main objective of surgical management in scoliosis is to perform a solid fusion of all the involved vertebrae in order to halt curvature progression. Concomitant with this goal is correction of the abnormal curvature(s) and maintenance of the physiologic curvatures (lumbar lordosis, thoracic kyphosis) in order to improve the cosmetic appearance and enhance the success rate of the fusion. The posterior approach to the spine is the one most commonly used for exposing the involved vertebrae. Correction can be obtained with a variety of instrumentations that apply both distractive and compressive forces as dictated by the curve pattern. The success or failure of this operation depends on the creation of a solid fusion. Autogenous bone from the posterior iliac crest is most commonly used to augment the fusion. Failure to accomplish solid fusion leads to a loss of correction and to pain associated with the most common long-term complication—the development of a pseudarthrosis (false joint)—and eventually culminates in breakage of the instrumentation.

SCHEUERMANN'S KYPHOSIS

The term *kyphosis* or *roundback* refers to a curvature of the spine in the sagittal plane with the convexity of the curve directed posteriorly. Kyphosis is normally found in the thoracic and sacral regions. Only when the magnitude of the curvature exceeds normal limits is this considered abnormal. Unlike scoliosis, kyphosis does not usually compromise pulmonary function, but it can lead to neurologic compromise. Cosmesis and pain relief are also major considerations. Through early diagnosis and proper treatment, permanent deformity can be prevented and pain relief achieved.

The cause of Scheuermann's disease is unknown. Some authors believe this condition to be a form of osteochondrosis. A mechanical theory involving increased pressure of the anterior aspect of the vertebral body has been suggested to explain the finding of disk material herniated through the cartilaginous end plate into some of the affected vertebral bodies. This could alter the orderly endochondral ossification and affect their growth. A hormonal theory has also been suggested. One study reported an autosomal dominant transmission with variable expressivity.

The incidence of Scheuermann's kyphosis probably varies between 1% and 2% of the population. There is no definite sex predilection. Patients commonly present between 12 and 17 years of age because of parental concerns of "bad posture" or complaints of back pain. The pain is localized to the back without radiation to the extremities, and is relieved by lying down.

A complete physical examination is essential, and evaluating for kyphosis should be a natural extension of a comprehensive spinal screening process. During the forward-bending examination, the spine is viewed from the side. Normally there is a gentle, smooth, dorsally directed curve. In Scheuermann's kyphosis there will be an increased curvature and, depending on the severity, there may be marked dorsal angulation. In addition, these patients frequently have increased lumbar lordosis.

The diagnosis is confirmed by radiographic evaluation that demonstrates anterior wedging of 5 degrees or more of the affected vertebral bodies in association with irregularity of the vertebral end plates and disk protrusions into the vertebral bodies (Schmorl's nodes).

The main differential diagnosis of Scheuermann's kyphosis is postural roundback deformity or "sloppy or lazy posture." The latter spine demonstrates a smooth contour and full correction when patients are asked to hyperextend their spine voluntarily. Congenital kyphosis and Scheuermann's kyphosis are rigid and can be distinguished by the radiographic evaluation. Other causes of kyphosis include traumatic compression fractures, infection, and postlaminectomy or postirradiation status.

Treatment alternatives include observation, bracing, casting and bracing, and surgery. An exercise regimen alone will not be sufficient to correct the vertebral wedging but is beneficial in conjunction with bracing. Bracing requires sufficient growth remaining to be effective. Surgery is reserved for curves that progress despite bracing or for curves that are too rigid to permit bracing. Surgery may be performed posteriorly, anteriorly, or both, depending on the individual circumstances of the patient.

HIP PAIN

Limping is a common presenting complaint in the adolescent. When this problem is associated with pain in the anterior thigh or groin, a hip disorder is likely. However, hip disorders may present with referred pain about the anteromedial aspect of the distal thigh or knee and thereby obscure the correct diagnosis. In all adolescents presenting with knee complaints, the hips must be examined also.

The most common hip disorder among adolescents is slipped capital femoral epiphysis. Stress fractures, septic arthritis, nonarticular rheumatoid disease, neoplasms, ischemic necrosis, and congenital hip dysplasia are also encountered. The following discussion is limited to slipped capital femoral epiphysis.

Slipped Capital Femoral Epiphysis

This condition was first described by Ambroise Paré in 1572 when he noted the possibility of confusing this condition with dislocation of the hip. E. Müller in 1888 called this condition "bending of the femoral neck in adolescence." The disorder consists of an anterior and lateral movement of the femoral neck in relation to the femoral head. The femoral head maintains its normal anatomic relationships with the acetabulum.

The incidence of slipped capital femoral epiphysis is reported to be between 1 and 3 per 100,000. Males are more frequently affected than females. Black adolescents are at greater risk than Caucasian or Hispanic teenagers. The age of onset coincides with periods of rapid growth. In males, the age range is 10 to 16 years, with incidence peaking at 12 to 14 years; in females, onset occurs from 8 to 14 years, with incidence peaking at 11 to 12 years. The younger the age at presentation, the greater is the association with endocrine abnormalities. This disorder is noted bilaterally in 25% to 50% of patients at initial presentation or subsequent evaluation.

ETIOLOGY. The etiology of slipped capital femoral epiphysis appears to be multifactorial. Proposed mechanisms include mechanical, endocrine, metabolic, traumatic, and inflammatory processes. The femoral head is attached to the femoral neck by means of the growth plate. The anatomic stability of this region is dependent on many factors: perichondrium, perichondrial ring, transphyseal collagen, height of the hypertrophic zone, mamillary processes, and angle of inclination of the growth plate. Any process that results in weakening of this structural complex will allow the shear stress present with normal weight bearing to disrupt the anatomic integrity, resulting in a slipped capital femoral epiphysis.

The perichondrial ring is a peripheral fibrous band composed of collagen fibers that span the growth plate and provide resistance to shear stress. During adolescence this structure normally decreases in thickness, providing less mechanical stability. Transphyseal collagen fibers also provide a counter to shear stress. In lathyrism, the collagen cross-linking is decreased, resulting in reduced collagen tensile strength and less resistance to shear stress.

The growth plate has distinctive zones. The hypertrophic zone is characterized by a relatively decreased proportion of intercellular matrix around the cell compared with other zones. Since the intercellular matrix contains the collagen, which is the main structural support, the hypertrophic zone represents the weak link in the growth plate and is the predominant area through which the disruption occurs in slipped capital femoral epiphysis. Processes that increase the height of the hypertrophic zone adversely affect resistance to shear stress. Growth hormone—directly or through somatomedin—stimulates cartilage metabolism, with a resultant increase in height of the hypertrophic zone. Estrogens and androgens suppress the proliferation of cartilage and thereby decrease the height of the hypertrophic zone. Therefore, a relative imbalance in the growth hormone–sex hormone quantitative relationship may account for this condition, although no specific abnormality has been documented.

Metabolic disorders such as rickets and particularly renal osteodystrophy are associated with an increased hypertrophic zone and may predispose the patient to a slipped capital femoral epiphysis. Patients with renal osteodystrophy also frequently develop secondary hyperparathyroidism and may sustain pathologic fractures rather than a true slipped capital femoral epiphysis. Thyroid hormone deficiency delays closure of the growth plate and allows it to be subject to shear stress beyond the normal physiologic time limit. Treatment with thyroid hormone induces a rapid increase in the cartilagenous portion of the growth plate, also increasing the risk.

Patients who have received radiotherapy that included the femoral head within its portal may be at increased risk for a slipped epiphysis. The irradiation causes an arrest of chondrogenesis and, when combined with actinomycin D, enhances the toxic effects.

The growth plate develops in a horizontal direction during childhood, and the angle of inclination increases to an oblique orientation during adolescence, creating a mechanical disadvantage. If this change in orientation is coupled with obesity, as is often the case in this patient population, the shear stress may overcome the normal anatomic integrity.

EVALUATION. The clinical manifestations on presentation are dictated by the duration of the pathologic processes and can be classified as chronic, acute on chronic, and acute traumatic. In the chronic slip the presenting complaint is a limp associated with pain in the groin, or pain referred to the anteromedial aspect of the distal thigh or knee. The pain is characterized as an ache, which is exacerbated by activity and has been present for weeks or months. The patient walks with an antalgic gait and the affected limb is externally rotated. The most notable clinical findings are decreased hip abduction and internal rotation. The more severe the slip, the greater are the physical limitations. Limb shortening may also be noted. Patients with an acute on chronic slip present with a history similar to that of those with a chronic slip, but they then develop the sudden onset of severe pain and an inability to bear weight as the process is exacerbated by relatively minor trauma. The least common presentation is in the patient with an acute traumatic slip who experiences only the sudden onset of severe pain and the inability to bear weight.

Radiographic assessment of these patients must include AP and lateral views of both hips (AP and frog pelvis views). The earliest finding is a widened and irregular growth plate. The femoral head-neck relationship is unchanged. The next step in assessment depends on the magnitude of the displacement. On AP view, minimal slips can be detected by extending a line along the superior aspect of the femoral neck (Fig. 151-3, *A*). This line should pass through a portion of the femoral head at a point identical to that for the opposite leg (beware of bilateral involvement). The lateral radiograph is the most sensitive view for detection of small degrees of displacement (Fig. 151-3, *B*). Massive slips are easily recognized on both views (Fig. 151-3, *C*).

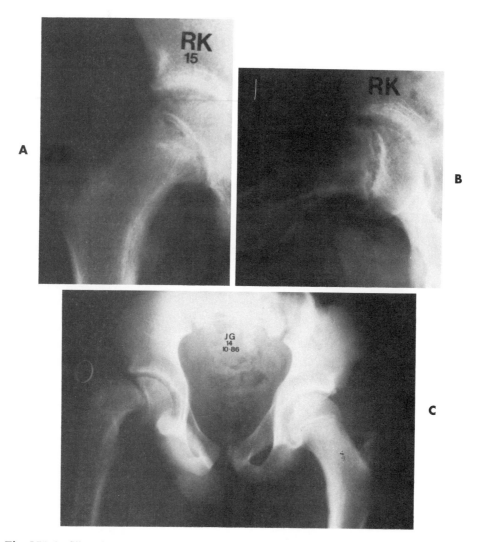

Fig. 151-3. Slipped capital femoral epiphysis. **A,** Anteroposterior view of the hip demonstrating a mild slip. **B,** Lateral view demonstrating posterior displacement. **C,** A massive slip is easily detected in this AP view.

TREATMENT. The most important aspect of treatment is early diagnosis and immediate cessation of weight-bearing activity to prevent further displacement. The patient should be admitted to the hospital for traction to relieve the muscle spasm and associated synovitis. The next step is surgical stabilization, the main objective of which is closure (fusion) of the growth plate and therefore elimination of the weak link.

The two most common treatment methods currently used are screw fixation and epiphysiodesis. Proponents of screw fixation choose this method because of its ability to rapidly stabilize the epiphysis and avoid hip spica cast immobilization. Surgically, the lateral or anterolateral aspect of the proximal femur is approached and, under fluoroscopic control, the fixation device is placed through the femoral neck and across the growth plate into the epiphysis (Fig. 151-4). This method is technically difficult to perform without penetration of the articular surface. Furthermore, the patient has to restrict his or her activity level until growth plate closure occurs; this takes 6 months to 1 year on average but is difficult to predict. The need for removal of the fixation device is controversial; if the patient chooses this procedure, another operation is required. Proponents of epiphysiodesis select this method because it is done under more direct conditions, and the time to growth plate closure is shorter and more predictable. The hip is usually approached anteriorly, a portion of the growth plate is curetted out, and a bone graft is placed across the area to stabilize the epiphysis and shorten the time to fusion. However, these patients must be placed in a hip spica cast for 6 to 8 weeks and then must begin rehabilitation.

COMPLICATIONS. The two major complications that may occur are chondrolysis and avascular necrosis. Chondrolysis is an acute necrosis of the articular cartilage of unknown etiology. This condition, which is reportedly

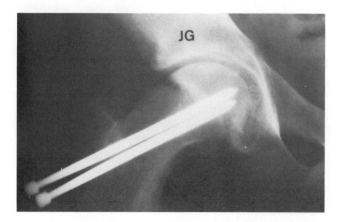

Fig. 151-4. Anteroposterior view demonstrating internal fixation to stabilize the slip.

more common among blacks and among females, adversely affects the prognosis. Avascular necrosis of the femoral head may be partial or total and should be suspected when there is persistent pain and limitation of motion in the postoperative period. The extent of the necrosis determines the severity of the resultant degenerative arthritis that develops.

KNEE PAIN

Knee pain is a common presenting complaint in adolescents and the list of possible etiologies is enormous. A complete history is key to establishing a presumptive diagnosis. In any patient presenting with knee pain, the hip must also be examined to rule out referred pain.

Acute traumatic disorders include ligamentous and meniscal injury, patellar dislocations, and fractures. The mechanism of injury and the site of maximal pain are noted. The presence of swelling or ecchymosis suggests a significant injury. The knee needs to be examined in a systematic fashion, and the evaluation can be divided between the tibiofemoral and patellofemoral areas.

The tibiofemoral articulation is assessed by testing for medial, lateral, and anteroposterior stability. To test the collateral ligaments, the knee is held in the extended position, and varus and valgus stresses are applied to test the integrity of the lateral and medial collateral ligaments, respectively. A 1 cm or greater separation of the joint line compared with that of the contralateral leg is significant and represents damage to the collateral ligament and cruciate ligaments. If there is no stability in extension, the knee is flexed to 30 degrees and the test repeated. Instability at 30 degrees represents injury isolated to the collateral ligament.

The next step is to evaluate the integrity of the cruciate ligaments. The knee is flexed to 15 degrees and the tibia is pulled forward on the femur (Lachman's test).

Normally a sharp end point is encountered. Increased anterior excursion of the tibia or lack of a sharp end point compared with the opposite knee suggests a deficient anterior cruciate ligament. The knee is then flexed to 90 degrees, and anterior forces followed by posterior forces are applied to the tibia while the presence of increased tibial excursion in relation to the femur is observed. Increased anterior excursion confirms damage to the anterior cruciate ligament; increased posterior excursion or "drop back" suggests damage to the posterior cruciate ligament.

Radiographs of the knee should be obtained, because growth plate injuries may simulate medial or lateral collateral ligament injuries, and fractures of the intercondylar eminence may resemble cruciate ligament injuries. The knee should be immobilized and weight-bearing activity prohibited. If necessary, a large effusion may be aspirated for comfort. A hemarthrosis substantially increases the likelihood of a significant ligamentous injury, particularly of the anterior cruciate ligament. The method of management depends on the degree of loss of structural integrity and can range from cast immobilization to surgical reconstruction.

Meniscal injuries are frequently associated with twisting injuries. Repetitive deep squatting is another mechanism known to cause meniscal damage. The patient complains of pain, swelling, and episodes in which the knee becomes "locked" in a flexed position, requiring manipulation to fully straighten out the knee. Physical examination is characterized by an effusion and joint line tenderness overlying the damaged area. McMurray's test can be performed to support the diagnosis. The patient's knee is fully flexed, the lower leg internally rotated, and the knee then extended. The test is repeated with the lower leg externally rotated. An audible or palpable click represents a positive test.

A suspected meniscal injury should be treated with immobilization and cessation of weight-bearing activity. Magnetic resonance imaging (MRI) has become the most frequently used noninvasive form of investigation to confirm the clinical diagnosis. The location and nature of the tear within the meniscus determine the subsequent management. Nondisplaced peripheral tears are capable of healing and are treated with immobilization. Displaced tears may require arthroscopic repair or partial excision. A meniscus should never be removed in its entirety.

Patellar dislocations are the result of direct trauma or of a vigorous quadriceps contracture with a flexed knee. The dislocation may reduce spontaneously. The patient presents with marked pain and swelling. Physical examination reveals marked tenderness of the soft tissues along the medial aspect of the patella. Attempts to gently move the patella laterally will cause a great deal of pain. Radiographs are necessary to detect osteochondral fractures that might have occurred during the dislocation or more commonly during the relocation of the patella. Conservative treatment of pure patellar dislocations consists of immobilization in a cylinder cast to allow the soft tissues to heal. Osteochondral fractures require operative intervention to either remove or replace the fragment. Surgical repair of the acute patellar dislocation is controversial.

A fracture of the intercondylar eminence is the bony counterpart to anterior cruciate ligament disruptions. This fracture may occur as a small flake of bone or may be large enough to disrupt the articular surface of the tibia. The patient presents with a painful and swollen knee. Treatment consists of immobilization for nondisplaced fractures and surgical correction for displaced fractures.

The most common nontraumatic causes of a painful knee are Osgood-Schlatter disease and osteochondritis dissecans. Osgood-Schlatter disease is characterized by pain and swelling in the region of the tibial tubercle. It is commonly seen in boys between 11 and 16 years of age and in girls between 9 and 14 years. Boys are much more commonly affected than girls. The onset frequently coincides with a rapid growth spurt and is associated with active participation in athletics. It is caused by the tensile forces acting on the tubercle, which are generated by repetitive quadriceps contractures, resulting in the detachment of cartilaginous particles from the tibial tubercle. This detachment stimulates an inflammatory and reparative process, causing tenderness and swelling in the region. The pain is exacerbated by activity and alleviated with rest. The "disease" is self-limited and spontaneously arrests when the tibial tubercle apophysis fuses with the tibia. Treatment consists of performing quadriceps-stretching exercises as well as tailoring the patient's level of activity to the level of discomfort. Rarely, a loose ossicle develops within the patellar ligament and may be sufficiently symptomatic to require a simple excision of the loose portion.

Osteochondritis dissecans of the knee is a condition in which segments of articular cartilage and subchondral bone progressively separate from the surrounding articular cartilage (Fig. 151-5). The lesion may remain in situ, may partially separate, or may detach fully and act as a loose body in the joint. The most common location for this lesion is the lateral aspect of the medial femoral condyle. No definite cause has been elucidated, although a history of injury is frequently noted. Histologic assessment of these lesions reveals avascular necrosis of the subchondral bone. Males are more frequently affected than females. Clinically, the patient complains of intermittent pain, swelling, clicking, buckling, and "locking" of the knee. Physical examination may detect an area of localized tenderness on the femoral condyle. Another means of locating this tenderness is to flex the knee to 90 degrees, internally rotate the tibia fully, and then extend the knee. The patient will complain of pain at approxi-

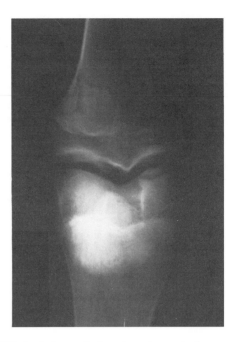

Fig. 151-5. Anteroposterior view demonstrating an osteochondritis dissecans lesion of the lateral aspect of the medial femoral condyle.

mately 30 degrees of flexion, and the pain is relieved with external rotation (Wilson's sign). AP and lateral radiographs reveal a fragment of subchondral bone demarcated by sclerosis from the femoral condyle. The tunnel view is particularly helpful in visualizing this lesion. Treatment depends on the stage of detachment. In situ lesions are usually treated with immobilization in a cylindric cast to protect against weight-bearing forces. Partially or fully detached lesions require operative management.

BONE TUMORS

Bone tumors and lesions simulating bone tumors are not common occurrences in adolescents. Many lesions are discovered fortuitously in conjunction with radiography for a recent injury or are detected when a fracture occurs with relatively minor trauma. At other times patients note the insidious onset of pain, which is progressive in severity to the point of awakening them from sleep. This presentation should prompt the physician to search vigorously for a lesion. Less often the patient reports a mass. Physical examination is usually nondiagnostic.

When a bone lesion is suspected, plain radiographs of the affected area should be obtained; these are effective in detecting most lesions. However, if no lesion is found, a bone scan is recommended to increase the yield in localizing small and occult lesions (e.g., osteoid osteoma) (Fig. 151-6), particularly in difficult areas such as the spine and pelvis. Computed tomography (CT) and MRI

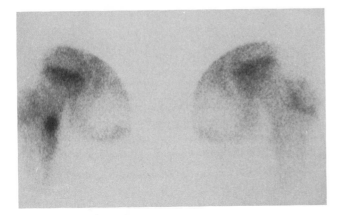

Fig. 151-6. Bone scan demonstrating increased uptake in the medial aspect of the femoral neck at the site of an osteoid osteoma.

may be necessary later for diagnostic and staging purposes. The most definite evaluation is a biopsy of the lesion.

Tumorlike Lesions

NONOSSIFYING FIBROMA. A nonossifying fibroma is a fibrous tissue-filled area that, if of sufficient size, may cause structural weakness and result in a pathologic fracture, leading to pain and swelling. The lesion is a well-demarcated, eccentric, radiolucent, multilocular defect with a sclerotic rim in the metaphyseal area of a long bone (Fig. 151-7). The most common sites are the distal tibia and femur. Pathologic fractures heal normally. Rarely is curettage and grafting necessary to prevent recurrent fractures in large lesions.

UNICAMERAL (SIMPLE) BONE CYST. This lesion is a true liquid-filled cyst that may lead to pain and swelling as a result of a pathologic fracture. The cyst is a well-demarcated, expansile, centralized, radiolucent lesion in the metaphyseal-diaphyseal region of a long bone (Fig. 151-8). The cyst initially develops below the growth plate and moves away from it with further growth. Pathologic fractures heal normally with standard fracture treatment. Large lesions, which make the patient prone to recurrent pathologic fractures, are treated with aspiration and the instillation of corticosteroids, which may be repeated two to three times at 6-month intervals. Rarely does this lesion require curettage and bone graft for eradication.

ANEURYSMAL BONE CYST. An aneurysmal bone cyst is a richly vascular lesion with a honeycomb architecture of blood-filled spaces that presents with pain and swelling and frequently a pathologic fracture. The lesion is a well-demarcated, eccentric, markedly expansible, radiolucent defect with a "soap-bubble" or "blown-out" appearance. The containing cortex is eggshell thin. Periosteal elevation and new bone formation are common. The lesion most frequently occurs in the metaphysis

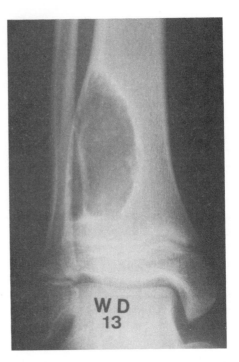

Fig. 151-7. Nonossifying fibroma. Anteroposterior view of the distal tibia demonstrates a well-demarcated, eccentric, radiolucent lesion in the metaphyseal region.

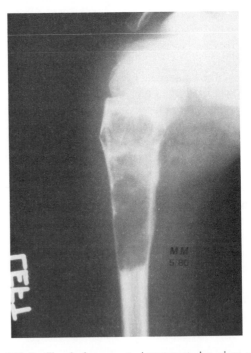

Fig. 151-8. Simple bone cyst. Anteroposterior view of the proximal humerus demonstrates a well-demarcated, centralized, expansible, radiolucent lesion in the metaphyseal-diaphyseal region.

of long bones or the posterior elements (neural arch) of the spine.

An aneurysmal bone cyst may be a primary lesion that arises de novo or a secondary occurrence that develops in association with other primary bone lesions such as osteosarcoma, osteoblastoma, and fibrous dysplasia. Therefore, the diagnostic studies must be carefully evaluated for evidence of a primary lesion that has developed an aneurysmal bone cyst component.

The aneurysmal bone cyst is a benign but locally aggressive lesion that is best treated surgically with either excision or curettage and bone graft, depending on the site. There is a definite incidence of recurrence.

EOSINOPHILIC GRANULOMA. Eosinophilic granuloma is a form of histiocytosis X restricted to bone lesions comprised of a round cell infiltrate (histiocytes, eosinophils, and plasma cells). The presenting complaint is usually pain experienced over weeks or months. The radiographic appearance depends on the site of involvement. In the spine the vertebral body is affected, predominantly in the thoracic region, and the lesion presents initially as a purely lytic defect that, on compression and collapse, results in a markedly flattened vertebral body—vertebra plana. In the long bones there is a well-demarcated, radiolucent, expansile lesion in the diaphysis. Periosteal new bone formation in response to the slowly growing expansile lesion may create an onionlike appearance similar to Ewing's sarcoma and osteomyelitis, and may require a biopsy for a definitive diagnosis.

Patients with spinal lesions frequently respond to rest and immobilization, with a partial restoration of the vertebral height. Long bone lesions may be self-limited as well. Persistent symptoms may require intralesional injection of steroids to facilitate lesion resolution. Rarely is surgical curettage and bone grafting necessary.

FIBROUS DYSPLASIA. Fibrous dysplasia is a lesion that occurs in a monostotic and polyostotic form. The monostotic form is more common and is more likely to be confused with other solitary lesions. This lesion consists of fibroosseous tissue characterized by a radiolucent defect described as having a "ground-glass" appearance and endosteal erosion involving the diaphyseal and metaphyseal regions of bone. Large lesions may be associated with pathologic fractures, which are treated by standard fracture care. Persistent symptoms may require curettage and bone graft.

Benign Tumors

OSTEOID OSTEOMA. An osteoid osteoma is a benign lesion consisting of a nidus of osteoid that evokes reactive sclerosis in the surrounding host bone. This lesion is characterized by pain that worsens at night and may be dramatically relieved with aspirin. If the lesion is located near a joint, pain and a sympathetic effusion may mimic septic arthritis. An osteoid osteoma that affects the spine may cause painful scoliosis. The classic radiographic appearance is that of a small radiolucent area (the nidus) surrounded by dense sclerotic bone. Linear or computed tomography may be required to demonstrate the nidus.

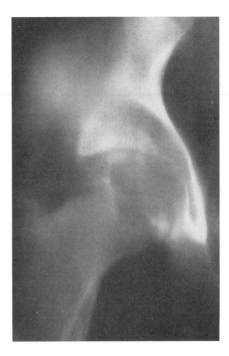

Fig. 151-9. Chondroblastoma. Anteroposterior tomographic view of a proximal femur with a well-demarcated, radiolucent lesion in the epiphysis.

Bone imaging with technetium-99m (^{99m}Tc) shows a markedly increased uptake in the lesion. The lesion is most often treated with surgical excision, although cases of spontaneous arrest after 3 to 5 years have been reported.

OSTEOBLASTOMA. An osteoblastoma is a benign growth with histologic features similar to those of an osteoid osteoma, but it is larger in size and is occasionally locally aggressive. The neural arch of the spine is a common site, and the lesion may be associated with localized pain, neurologic symptoms, and painful scoliosis. The metaphyseal or diaphyseal regions of long bones reveal a radiolucent, expansile defect. This lesion is best treated by surgical excision. It is important not to misdiagnose this lesion as an osteosarcoma.

CHONDROBLASTOMA. A chondroblastoma is a benign neoplasm that is characterized by its location in the epiphyseal ends of long bones. It may be locally aggressive and can break out of the bone into the joint. Symptoms consist of pain, swelling, and joint effusions. It is primarily found in the proximal humerus, distal femur, and proximal tibia. The radiograph reveals an eccentric radiolucent defect with a sclerotic border (Fig. 151-9). Punctate calcifications may be seen within the lesion. The diagnosis must be confirmed by biopsy before definitive treatment is instituted, to rule out a clear cell chondrosarcoma. For a chondroblastoma confined to bone, treatment consists of curettage and bone graft.

CHONDROMYXOID FIBROMA. The chondromyxoid fibroma is a benign neoplasm composed of chondroid, fibrous, and myxomatous tissues in variable proportions.

It is usually located in the lower limb, the tibia being the most frequently affected site. The femur, fibula, calcaneus, and metatarsals can also be affected. On radiography, chondromyxoid fibroma is a large, eccentric, expansible, radiolucent lesion with a lytic or "soap-bubble" appearance confined to the metaphyseal end of the bone. This lesion must not be confused with malignant chondrosarcoma. The chondromyxoid fibroma is best treated by en bloc excision if possible because of the high recurrence rate after curettage.

SOLITARY ENCHONDROMA. Enchondromas are benign growths composed of lobules of cartilage surrounded by lamellar bone that develops in the medullary cavity of both short and long tubular bones. In the phalanges, metacarpals, and metatarsals, patients report progressive swelling of the area that then suddenly becomes painful because of a pathologic fracture. In adolescents, lesions in long tubular bones are usually incidental findings. Radiographs of lesions in the hands or feet reveal a centrally located, well-demarcated, expansible, lytic lesion with stippled calcific densities within the lesion. Lesions in long bones show well-defined, punctate, ringlike densities to short linear densities, which represent calcified cartilage.

Enchondromas of the hands and feet are treated with curettage and bone graft. Lesions in the long tubular bones must be carefully observed because of the possibility of malignant transformation (chondrosarcoma) in adult life. Malignant change is manifested by the onset of pain in a previously asymptomatic lesion, radiographic evidence of erosion (scalloping) of the adjacent cortex, and evidence of bone destruction beyond the confines of the stippled densities.

Malignant Tumors

OSTEOSARCOMA. Osteosarcoma is the most common primary malignant tumor of bone. Although there are various types of osteosarcomas, this discussion is limited to the classic intramedullary osteosarcoma. This lesion is characterized by the presence of anaplastic stromal cells that directly produce osteoid or primitive bone. They may also produce malignant cartilage. The peak incidence of tumor formation occurs between 10 and 20 years of age. Local pain and swelling are the most common complaints. There are generally no systemic complaints on presentation. Laboratory testing is remarkable for an elevated alkaline phosphatase level. The lesion occurs in the metaphyseal region, the distal femur and proximal tibia being the most common sites. The proximal humerus (Fig. 151-10) and femur are also common sites.

The radiographic appearance is of a combination of host bone destruction and tumor bone formation eccentrically located within the metaphysis and with ill-defined borders. The tumor frequently breaks through the cortex to form a soft tissue mass associated with fluffy tumor bone deposition. The periosteum forms reactive new bone in the form of Codman's triangles or sunburst patterns.

The differential diagnosis includes myositis ossificans, exuberant callus formation from a stress fracture, osteomyelitis, osteoblastoma, and Ewing's sarcoma. The definitive diagnosis rests on the inspection of an adequate biopsy specimen. Bone and CT scans are important to detect "skip" lesions within the affected bone as well as to assess the degree of soft tissue extension. Pulmonary CT is essential to search for small lung metastases. MRI is also helpful in staging the lesion.

Once the diagnosis is histologically confirmed, treatment consists of adjuvant chemotherapy and ablative surgery. Preoperative chemotherapy reduces the size of the tumor, making limb salvage surgery a more likely possibility. After the definitive surgical procedure, additional adjuvant chemotherapy is administered. The choice of agents depends on the tumor's histologic response to the initial agents as determined by study of the resected specimen.

The choice of a definitive surgical procedure is between amputation and limb salvage. Limb salvage offers such alternatives as prosthesis, allografts or autografts, and procedures such as the van Ness rotationplasty.

EWING'S SARCOMA. Ewing's sarcoma is the second most common primary malignant tumor of bone occurring in childhood. The lesion is characterized by sheets of

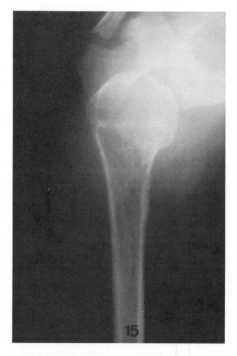

Fig. 151-10. Osteosarcoma. Anterposterior view of the proximal humerus demonstrates an ill-defined radiolucent lesion at the junction of the metaphysis and diaphysis. The periosteal reaction is evident medially.

small round cells widely infiltrating the medullary canal. Ewing's sarcoma usually manifests when the patient is between 10 and 15 years of age. This lesion may be associated with systemic involvement, as evidenced by the patient appearing ill and febrile in addition to complaints of localized bone pain, swelling, and a soft tissue mass. A single bone is initially involved, with multiple sites noted after pulmonary and visceral metastases become evident.

The radiographic appearance of Ewing's sarcoma is characterized by an ill-defined lacy pattern of permeative bone destruction ("moth-eaten" appearance) in the diaphysis associated with a laminated "onion-skin" periosteal reaction (Fig. 151-11). A soft tissue mass overlying the area of bone destruction is common.

The differential diagnosis includes osteomyelitis, lymphoma, osteosarcoma, eosinophilic granuloma, and metastatic neuroblastoma. The definitive diagnosis rests on study of the biopsy specimen. A bone scan is the best method of detecting skeletal metastases. CT or MRI may be used to delineate the local extent and spread of the sarcoma.

Treatment consists of a combination of irradiation, chemotherapy, and surgical ablation. The particular combination depends on the anatomic location of the primary lesion and the extent of bony and visceral metastases. Implementation of this combined approach has markedly improved the 5-year survival rate.

CHONDROSARCOMA. The type of chondrosarcoma that affects adolescents is almost exclusively restricted to the malignant transformation of benign cartilaginous

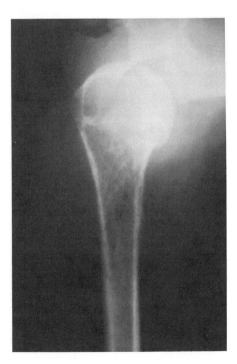

Fig. 151-11. Ewing's sarcoma.

lesions of childhood—osteochondromas or enchondromas—into chondrosarcomas. Malignant transformation is more common in hereditary multiple exostoses and multiple enchondromatosis than in their solitary disease counterparts. Exostoses about the shoulder and pelvic girdle and enchondromas of the long tubular bones more frequently undergo malignant transformation. The onset of pain in a previously asymptomatic lesion or the growth of a previously quiescent osteochondroma should alert the physician to this problem. Diagnosis is confirmed by biopsy. After appropriate staging of the lesion, surgical ablation, with limb preservation if possible, is the treatment of choice.

INFECTION

Pyogenic infections of bones and joints are more common in young children than in adolescents. These disorders result in lifelong complications if not recognized early and treated vigorously. In addition, the arthritis that accompanies this condition and the emergence of Lyme disease make diagnosis more difficult.

Osteomyelitis

Osteomyelitis is a pyogenic inflammation of bone. It is usually hematogenous, but it may also occur as a result of direct extension from surrounding tissues or by the direct entrance of organisms from the environment, as in open fractures. In patients with open growth plates, the bacteria initially lodge in the metaphysis, initiating an inflammatory response characterized by edema, vascular engorgement, abscess formation, and bone necrosis. The infection then spreads through the haversian system and Volkmann's canals to the exterior surface of the bone, elevating the periosteum. If the periosteum ruptures, the infection spreads to the surrounding soft tissues. If the metaphysis is intracapsular, as in the proximal femur, the infection will spread into the joint, resulting in septic arthritis as well as osteomyelitis.

Clinically, there may be an antecedent history of trauma, and the physician must question the patient regarding any recent history of infection. The patient presents with acute septicemia, high fever, chills, and bone pain. There is marked localized tenderness to palpation of the affected metaphysis. Swelling and increased warmth may also be noted.

The initial laboratory studies should include a complete blood count, erythrocyte sedimentation rate (ESR), and blood cultures. The white blood cell (WBC) count will be elevated with a left shift, the erythrocyte sedimentation rate will be substantially elevated, and the blood cultures may discern the infecting organism. The early radiographic findings will be limited to swelling of the deep soft tissues adjacent to the bone. The physician must request a soft tissue study rather than standard bone radiographs to detect this finding. The bone will not show changes for 7 to 10 days. At that time, a radiolucent area will develop in the metaphysis, followed by periosteal new bone formation. These are late changes, and treatment must be initiated long before their manifestation.

A bone scan with ^{99m}Tc will usually be positive (increased uptake) 24 hours after symptoms present. Bone scans are nonspecific and should be used as an adjunct to the clinical diagnosis. Bone scans are most effective in assessing areas such as the pelvis and spine, which are difficult to examine, or in cases in which multiple sites of involvement are suspected. If a bone scan cannot readily be performed, treatment must not be delayed. Other imaging modalities such as CT, MRI, and gallium or indium scans can be employed if there is still uncertainty after the initial studies are completed.

When there is a high clinical suspicion of osteomyelitis, the next step is aspiration of the affected site to obtain a bacteriologic specimen for Gram's stain and culture to determine whether an abscess is present. Canale and Tolo have shown that it is not necessary to delay the aspiration while awaiting a bone scan, because needle aspirations do not adversely affect the scan. *Staphylococcus aureus* is the most frequently encountered organism in adolescents. *Pseudomonas* organisms must be considered if a puncture wound through a shoe or sneaker has occurred. *Salmonella* spp. must be suspected in patients with sickle cell disease; however, even in adolescents with this condition, *Staphylococcus* spp. occur most often.

The most important aspect of treatment is early diagnosis and the institution of parenteral antibiotic therapy. Antibiotics are initially prescribed on the basis of clinical suspicion and the Gram's stain. Their administration should be modified once culture and sensitivity results are available.

The need for operative intervention is determined by whether or not an abscess is present. An abscess is best treated by decompression and drainage. Occasionally, patients may not present with an abscess and yet fail to improve within 24 to 48 hours with antibiotic therapy alone. These patients benefit from early operative intervention.

Septic Arthritis

Acute septic arthritis is a pyogenic inflammation of a joint. The infection most commonly occurs through a hematogenous route, but may also arise by direct extension from an adjacent site (e.g., osteomyelitis) or from an external entry point (e.g., a puncture wound).

The onset of symptoms is acute. Pain about the involved joint is associated with systemic complaints of fever and general malaise. Examination of the involved joint reveals swelling, increased warmth, and a marked pain response to gentle joint motion. The patient will hold the joint in a position that maximizes the capsular volume to minimize overall joint pressure. Laboratory studies demonstrate an elevated WBC count and increased ESR.

Radiographs reveal an effusion and soft tissue swelling. Careful scrutiny is necessary to be certain there is no osteomyelitis of the adjacent bone. Ultrasonography, if readily available, is another good method of detecting increased joint fluid. When acute arthritis is suspected, joint aspiration should be performed under fluoroscopic control. A large-bore needle is introduced under sterile conditions and the joint is aspirated. If no fluid is retrieved, sterile nonbacteriostatic saline solution is injected and the joint is then aspirated. The aspirate must be cultured and Gram's stain taken; if there is sufficient fluid, a cell count and chemistries (glucose and protein), as well as counter immunoelectrophoresis, must be performed. The injection of a radiographic dye (e.g., Hypaque) is recommended before the needle is removed to verify that the joint has been properly studied. Results of aspirations may provide false-negative results because the needle never entered the joint.

In acute septic arthritis the WBC count of the aspirate is usually greater than 60,000 and may be as high as 200,000; the WBCs are mainly polymorphonuclear cells. Joint glucose level will be substantially lower than peripheral blood glucose level drawn at the same time, and joint protein level will be increased. The culture must include aerobic and anaerobic studies, preferably in blood culture bottles, and direct inoculation onto Thayer-Martin media if clinically indicated.

Gram's stain may or may not reveal the organism. The combination of joint aspirate cultures, blood cultures, and counterimmunoelectrophoresis increases the likelihood of identifying the organism.

Once the appropriate cultures have been obtained, parenteral antibiotic therapy should be quickly initiated. The choice of antibiotics is facilitated if the organism is identified on Gram's stain. If it cannot be identified, a "best guess" coverage should involve the administration of a penicillinase-resistant penicillin or a second-generation cephalosporin until culture and sensitivity results are available. If the patient is sexually active, gonococcal infection is possible and penicillin should be added to the initial antibiotic regimen.

The need for surgical intervention is determined by the specific joint involved, quality of the aspirate, and clinical response to antibiotic therapy. A deep joint such as the hip is difficult to monitor and reaspirate; therefore, once the diagnosis is established, surgical drainage should be part of the initial treatment. When the aspirate reveals frank pus, the likelihood of adhesions and loculations is high, and surgical drainage will facilitate clinical improvement. Surgical drainage may consist of anthroscopic debridement or arthrotomy, depending on the joint involved.

Furthermore, if there is no significant improvement after 24 to 48 hours of parenteral antibiotic therapy as witnessed by clinical parameters and reaspiration of the joint, surgical drainage should be performed.

TRAUMA

Major advances in the basic science of fracture and soft tissue healing and the diagnostic assessment and surgical stabilization of these injuries have occurred since the mid-1980s. This knowledge has led to a dramatic change in the approach to the care of these injuries in the adolescent population. For example, the operative stabilization of femoral shaft fractures in the older adolescent (Fig. 151-12) using the new closed rodding techniques allows the patient to return home and to school in 7 to 10 days, rather than remain in traction for 6 weeks and then undergo cast immobilization for an additional 6 to 10 weeks before beginning a rehabilitation program. The functional difference, as well as the psychologic and economic benefits derived from a shortened hospitalization period, can be readily appreciated.

Classification

In general, the growth plate is the weak link in bone, and ligaments are stronger than the growth plate.

Therefore, injuries that could result in a torn ligament in an adult may produce a fracture of the growth plate in the adolescent, and this diagnosis should be considered in adolescent patients who present with "sprains." The classification of growth plate injuries was first described by Salter and Harris in 1963. Since that time, Ogden has vastly expanded upon their work, but for the sake of simplicity, this discussion will use the Salter-Harris classification as its framework and add Ogden's type VI classification.

A type I fracture is a fracture through the growth plate that causes a separation of the epiphysis from the metaphysis. This fracture occurs predominantly through the zone of provisional calcification, with the growth region remaining with the epiphysis. Often a type I fracture is misdiagnosed as a sprain unless there is displacement or a slight widening of the growth plate. A stress radiograph can be used for clarification (Fig. 151-13). Growth is usually not disturbed. This fracture is treated with closed reduction and cast immobilization.

A type II fracture begins as a separation as in a type I fracture, but rather than continue across the growth plate, it deviates toward and exits through the metaphysis (Fig. 151-14). Type II is the most common pattern of growth plate fractures. The metaphyseal fragment created by this fracture is usually triangular in shape, varying in size, and referred to as the Thurston-Holland sign. The growth region of the plate is usually spared, and growth dis-

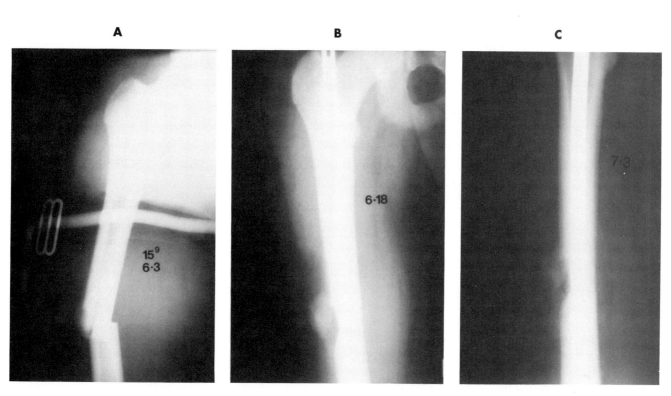

Fig. 151-12. A to **C,** Operative stabilization of a femoral shaft fracture. Note the rapidity of the healing process after surgery (**A** taken June 3, **B** June 18, and **C** July 3).

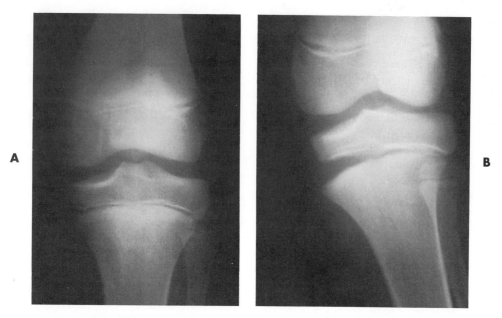

Fig. 151-13. Type I fracture. **A,** Plain x-ray film. **B,** Stress radiograph. Note the normal appearance in **A** versus the evident fracture in **B.**

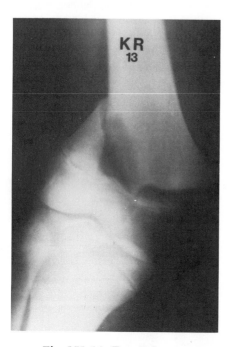

Fig. 151-14. Type II fracture.

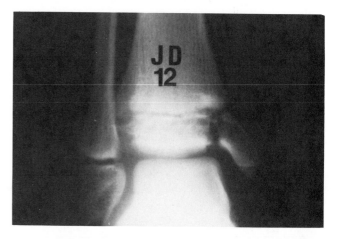

Fig. 151-15. Type III fracture.

turbance is infrequent. Type II fractures of the distal femur are the exception, and a growth disturbance in this situation is not uncommon. The magnitude of the force necessary to create this injury and the anatomic configuration of this region may explain this propensity. Most type II fractures are amenable to closed reduction and cast immobilization. Displaced type II fractures of the distal femur can usually be reduced closed, but optimal immobilization requires a spica cast. The latter treatment option can be avoided by limited internal fixation and a long leg cast, which allows the adolescent to return to

school sooner and makes personal hygiene less anxiety provoking.

A type III fracture is an intraarticular fracture that begins at the joint surface, extends to the growth plate, and then passes through it as it exits at the periphery (Fig. 151-15). The major considerations in the care of this fracture are anatomic restoration of the congruity of the joint surface and realignment of the zones of the growth plate. Surgical intervention is frequently required. Failure to reestablish joint congruity predisposes to degenerative changes, and growth plate malalignment predisposes to partial premature growth plate closure and deformity with further growth.

A type IV fracture is an intra-articular fracture that begins at the joint surface, fully traverses the growth plate, and continues into and exits through the metaphysis (Fig. 151-16). This fracture results in a disruption in all

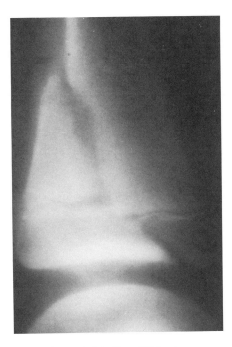

Fig. 151-16. Type IV fracture.

the zones of the growth plate. The considerations for fracture care are the same as those for type III fractures. Displaced fractures are best treated with surgical restoration of the anatomy.

Type V fractures are characterized by the causal agent: a crushing force that causes an excessive compression of the growth plate. Detection of this injury in the acute phase is extremely difficult. Growth arrest frequently occurs, but fortunately this pattern of injury is uncommon.

A type VI fracture involves an injury to the perichondrial ring at the periphery of the growth plate, specifically the zone of Ranvier. This injury may not be associated with a fracture per se but can result from a deep burn or deep laceration such as in a lawn mower injury. Type VI injuries can lead to localized growth plate closure, and a resultant angular deformity develops with further growth of the uninjured portion of the plate.

Prognosis

Once the correct diagnosis has been made, the following factors are used to formulate a prognosis: age, mechanism of injury, specific anatomic site, Salter-Harris classification, type of injury (open or closed), and method of treatment.

Age. The younger the patient, the greater is the amount of expected future growth, and therefore the greater the risk of significant deformity.

Mechanism of injury. A fracture that results from a fall and a fracture that results from being struck by a car may have very different prognoses despite similarity in

radiographic appearance if one takes into account the amount of energy absorbed, and therefore the amount of damage to the growth mechanism.

Specific anatomic site. The distal growth plate accounts for approximately 70% of the longitudinal growth of the femur, and therefore injury to this site has greater consequences relative to a leg-length discrepancy than injury to the proximal femoral growth plate. Similarly, the proximal humeral and distal radial growth plates contribute significantly more growth than the distal humeral or proximal radial growth plates, and thus injury to the former involves potentially more serious consequences.

Salter-Harris classification. This classification is intended to contribute to the formulation of a prognosis in concert with consideration of other factors mentioned, and is not meant to be used in isolation. The higher the classification, the greater is the likelihood of subsequent growth disturbance.

Open versus closed injury. Open fractures (fractures that communicate with the external environment) can be assumed to have absorbed a greater degree of energy than closed fractures, as evidenced by the degree of associated soft tissue disruption. Therefore, open fractures involve a greater risk of growth disturbance in addition to the risk of infection.

Method of treatment. Reduction of these injuries must be performed as gently as possible to prevent further damage during manipulation. A general anesthetic should be used if possible. Displaced types III and IV fractures require anatomic restoration of the joint surfaces to prevent degenerative changes, and anatomic restoration of the growth plate to prevent growth disturbance. These fractures frequently require surgical treatment, and the remodeling potential of youth should not be relied upon.

Should complete growth arrest occur, a limb length discrepancy will develop if there is sufficient future growth remaining in the contralateral limb. There has been a marked advancement in the understanding and technology involved in limb lengthening of both the upper and lower extremities, and these procedures represent a viable choice for the care of affected patients.

Partial growth arrest can also result in a limb length discrepancy if it occurs in the central portion of the growth plate. Partial growth arrest occurring in the peripheral portion of the plate will result in an angular deformity. Areas of premature growth arrest affecting less than 40% of the area of the growth can be treated with resection of the affected area and insertion of fat or Silastic, allowing resumption of normal growth.

MYOSITIS OSSIFICANS. This is a condition in which there is damage from blunt trauma to a large muscle such as the quadriceps, resulting in heterotopic calcification and ossification in the muscle tissue. This diagnosis should be suspected in patients who have a history of trauma with symptoms that initially improved but have recurred, and who have persistent pain, swelling, and limitation in joint motion. The differential diagnosis is osteosarcoma.

Suggested Readings

Canale ST, Tolo VT: Fractures of the femur in children, *AAOS Instructional Course Lectures* 40:255-273, 1995.

Crawford AH: Current concepts review. Slipped capital femoral epiphysis, *J Bone Joint Surg* 70A(9):1422-1427, 1988.

Fulkerson JP, Shea KP: Current concepts review. Disorders of patellofemoral alignment, *J Bone Joint Surg* 72A(9):1424-1429, 1990.

Hensinger RN: Acute back pain in children, *AAOS Instructional Course Lectures* 40:111-126, 1995.

Keller RB: Nonoperative treatment of idiopathic scoliosis, *AAOS Instructional Course Lectures* 38:129-135, 1989.

Kennedy JCS: *The injured adolescent knee,* Baltimore, 1979, Williams & Wilkins.

Kostuik JK: Current concepts review. Operative treatment of idiopathic scoliosis, *J Bone Joint Surg* 72A(7):1108-1113, 1990.

Morrisy RT: Acute hematogenous osteomyelitis: a model with trauma as an etiology, *J Pediatr Orthop* 9:447-456, 1990.

Ogden JA: *Skeletal injury in the child,* Philadelphia, 1982, Lea & Febiger.

Weinstein SL: Adolescent idiopathic scoliosis: prevalence and natural history, *AAOS Instructional Course Lectures* 38:115-128, 1989.

CHAPTER 152

Sports Medicine

•

Michael A. Nelson and William L. Risser

Sports medicine is a huge field, covering much more than the diagnosis and management of musculoskeletal problems. This chapter can only introduce some topics, giving references for further reading. A well-informed clinician can help young athletes to participate in sports safely and successfully and can have fun in the process.

PREPARTICIPATION EXAMINATION

Goals, Frequency, and Timing

Preparticipation examinations are screening evaluations to identify factors that may lead to injury, illness, or death during athletic participation. They are imperfect, because not enough is known about the risks of many medical conditions; the examination is not sufficiently sensitive to identify all conditions that might put an athlete at risk; and there is uncertainty and controversy about the significance of some findings.

Many school systems require complete examinations yearly, but the available evidence indicates that this is excessive.[1] A reasonable approach is to examine athletes fully at entry into junior and senior high school and college programs. Between these evaluations, before each new sports season, the athlete should complete an interim history form (Fig. 152-1) describing any medical problems and injuries that have occurred since the last complete examination. A healthcare provider can review this form and refer the athlete for full evaluation if the interim history indicates the need.

The examination or history review should take place long enough before the season to allow time for evaluation or treatment of any significant medical problems. An interval of at least 6 weeks is desirable.

Format

Despite the logistical problems of finding adequate staff and facilities, the station examination[2] offers the advantages of low cost, which enables indigent athletes to participate in sports; and of speed and convenience, allowing evaluation of a large number of athletes in one place in a short time. If the examining clinicians are knowledgeable about sports medicine and reasonable about their goals, referrals and disqualifications can be minimized. The station examinations typically include registration, blood pressure, height and weight, vision, and medical assessment, which can be performed by the same individual, or divided into parts: for example, the general and the musculoskeletal examinations. Coaches, school nurses, and other volunteers can staff some

SPORTS PARTICIPATION HEALTH RECORD

This evaluation is only to determine readiness for sports participation. It should not be used as a substitute for regular health maintenance examinations.

NAME _____ AGE _____(YRS) GRADE _____ DATE _____

ADDRESS _____ PHONE _____

SPORTS _____

The Health History (Part A) and Physical Examination (Part C) sections must both be completed, at least every 24 months, before sports participation. The Interim Health History section (Part B) needs to be completed at least annually.

PART A — HEALTH HISTORY:
To be completed by athlete and parent

		YES	NO
1. Have you ever had an illness that:			
a. required you to stay in the hospital?		____	____
b. lasted longer than a week?		____	____
c. caused you to miss 3 days of practice or a competition?		____	____
d. is related to allergies? (ie, hay fever, hives, asthma, insect stings)		____	____
e. required an operation?		____	____
f. is chronic? (ie, asthma, diabetes, etc)		____	____

2. Have you ever had an injury that:
   a. required you to go to an emergency room or see a doctor? ____ ____
   b. required you to stay in the hospital? ____ ____
   c. required x-rays? ____ ____
   d. caused you to miss 3 days of practice or a competition? ____ ____
   e. required an operation? ____ ____

3. Do you take any medication or pills? ____ ____

4. Have any members of your family under age 50 had a heart attack, heart problem, or died unexpectedly? ____ ____

5. Have you ever:
   a. been dizzy or passed out during or after exercise? ____ ____
   b. been unconscious or had a concussion? ____ ____

6. Are you unable to run 1/2 mile (2 times around the track) without stopping? ____ ____

7. Do you:
   a. wear glasses or contacts? ____ ____
   b. wear dental bridges, plates, or braces? ____ ____

8. Have you ever had a heart murmur, high blood pressure, or a heart abnormality? ____ ____

9. Do you have any allergies to any medicine? ____ ____

10. Are you missing a kidney? ____ ____

11. When was your last tetanus booster? _____

12. **For Women**
   a. At what age did you experience your first menstrual period? _____
   b. In the last year, what is the longest time you have gone between periods? _____

EXPLAIN ANY "YES" ANSWERS _____
_____
_____
_____

I hereby state that, to the best of my knowledge, my answers to the above questions are correct.

Date _____

Signature of athlete _____

Signature of parent _____

PART B — INTERIM HEALTH HISTORY:
This form should be used during the interval between preparticipation evaluations. Positive responses should prompt a medical evaluation.

1. Over the next 12 months, I wish to participate in the following sports:
   a. _____
   b. _____
   c. _____
   d. _____

2. Have you missed more than 3 consecutive days of participation in usual activities because of an injury this past year?
   Yes _____ No _____
   If yes, please indicate:
   a. Site of injury _____
   b. Type of injury _____

3. Have you missed more than 5 consecutive days of participation in usual activities because of an illness, or have you had a medical illness diagnosed that has not been resolved in this past year?
   Yes _____ No _____
   If yes, please indicate:
   a. Type of illness _____

4. Have you had a seizure, concussion or been unconscious for any reason in the last year?
   Yes _____ No _____

5. Have you had surgery or been hospitalized in this past year?
   Yes _____ No _____
   If yes, please indicate:
   a. Reason for hospitalization _____
   b. Type of surgery _____

6. List all medications you are presently taking and what condition the medication is for.
   a. _____
   b. _____
   c. _____

7. Are you worried about any problem or condition at this time?
   Yes _____ No _____

   If yes, please explain: _____
   _____
   _____
   _____

I hereby state that, to the best of my knowledge, my answers to the above questions are correct.

Date _____

Signature of athlete _____

Signature of parent _____

Fig. 152-1. Sports participation history and interim history. (Reprinted with permission. "Sports Participation Health Record." Copyright © 1990 American Academy of Pediatrics.)

stations. This format is well suited to easy communication between the coaching staff and the medical team.

One potential problem is the lack of continuity of care. If follow-up is needed, written instructions can be given to parents who are present, or else mailed to the athlete's home, and the coaching staff (and athletic trainer if available) can be given a list of the athletes who have significant problems and their follow-up needs.

Because studies have determined that 80% to 90% of adolescent athletes seek routine health care only to obtain clearance for sports participation,[1,3] some clinicians have argued that preparticipation evaluations should be done by the athletes' private physicians during regular office visits. This format offers the opportunity for the physician to address the psychosocial issues that are often the major health concerns relevant to adolescents and to deal with common medical problems, such as acne, that are not relevant to sports participation. The private physician is likely to have good medical and family histories to clarify the significance of existing medical problems and can perform or coordinate any needed follow-up. However, focusing on psychosocial issues may distract the evaluator from issues relevant to sports participation, for example, obtaining a sports-related history; such examinations are expensive and time-consuming; adequate appointment time may not be available during the periods of peak need in late summer; indigent athletes may not have a private physician or the money to pay for such an evaluation; and insurance companies may not provide reimbursement.[3]

All experts condemn the "line-up" examination in which a single clinician performs a fast, superficial evaluation of a group of athletes. It can be justified only if there is no alternative.

Expected Outcome

In published studies, the disqualification rate is usually less than 1%.[1,3] Referral rates for further evaluation before participation are higher, but after this evaluation almost all athletes are cleared to play.

Medical History

Studies have shown that approximately 75% of significant problems that may affect sports participation are mentioned in the history.[1,3] The preparticipation history is different from the conventional medical history (Fig. 152-1). Younger athletes may have medical problems such as asthma whose impact on sports participation has not yet been evaluated, whereas older high school and college athletes are most likely to have problems resulting from recent or previous musculoskeletal injuries. Although they almost always are false-positives, symptoms of possible cardiac disease are of concern in all age groups. The clinician should probably repeat the important questions even if the self-reported history is negative, because some questions may be misunderstood or purposely answered incorrectly.

Ideally, a parent should collaborate with the athlete in completing the history. One study showed that only 39% of histories provided by athletes agreed with those supplied independently by parents.[1] However, requiring participation by parents may at times interfere with the completion of the evaluation, for example, when clinicians in a station setting are evaluating a group of athletes whose parents have failed to return the questionnaires that were sent home, or when a clinician is evaluating athletes in a school-based health center. In some areas, there is a high illiteracy rate in both students and parents.

Physical Examination

The cardiovascular examination is of obvious importance because of concern about sudden death in young athletes. Many adolescents have innocent pulmonary flow murmurs, whereas others have innocent Still's murmurs, venous hums, or carotid bruits. These murmurs all have characteristics that often make them recognizable; they are usually not diagnoses of exclusion. Athletes who have mild forms of most congenital heart lesions can play all sports; the 26th Bethesda Conference has defined what constitutes mild disease.[4]

The most common cardiac problem is mitral valve prolapse (MVP). If the diagnostic midsystolic click at the apex is followed by a late systolic murmur, mitral regurgitation is present. Asymptomatic athletes who have mitral valve prolapse may play any sport unless they have evidence of mitral regurgitation or have a family history of sudden death associated with MVP. The latter two groups need further evaluation, as do symptomatic athletes (chest pain, palpitations, dysrhythmia, near syncope, syncope).[5]

All clinicians worry about missing occult heart disease that may lead to sudden death, although probably only about 1 in 200,000 athletes has such a lesion.[6] The most common of these is hypertrophic cardiomyopathy, an autosomal dominant disease that may have insignificant or absent auscultatory findings.[3]

Although the incidence of Marfan's syndrome is only 1 in approximately 10,000, this disease is often a concern in tall athletes. A variety of ocular, skeletal, and musculoskeletal findings (e.g., myopia, ectopia lentis, MVP, aortic regurgitation, arachnodactyly, decreased upper/lower segment ratio, pectus deformity, hyperextensible joints) are consistent with, but not pathognomonic of, this diagnosis. The most definitive tests are echocardiography, to look for aortic root dilation, and an ophthalmologic examination, to look for laxity of the suspensory ligaments of the lenses. A good family history of cardiac and visual problems is also important, but since 25% of patients have new mutations, and the variability of expression of the abnormalities is great, this history may be benign.[7]* (See Chapter 36, "Cardiac Infection and Inflammation: Rheumatic Fever, Endocarditis, and Myocarditis.")

Experts agree that only secondary or severe essential hypertension must be evaluated or treated, or both, before sports participation. The Second Task Force on Blood Pressure Control in Children defined severe hypertension as values exceeding the 98th percentiles for age. These are: ages 6 to 9 years, 130/86 mm Hg; ages 10 to 12, 134/90; ages 13 to 15, 144/92; and ages 16 to 18, 150/98.[8] A recent Task Force update (*Pediatrics* 98:649-658, 1996) leaves these recommendations in place. (See Chapter 57, "Hypertension.")

Some patients have diastolic pressures below these values but systolic pressures above them. If these individuals show no evidence of end-organ damage, as they almost certainly will not, they can be considered to have less than severe hypertension.[8] The Task Force recommended dynamic (aerobic) exercise programs for persistently hypertensive youths, and these exclude weight training.[8] Not all experts agree with this restriction.[4]

Many athletes have occasional premature ventricular contractions. These are not of concern if they are simple (unifocal, and never two or more occurring consecutively), disappear when exercise increases the heart rate to 150 to 160 beats per minute (bpm), and are not associated with underlying heart disease or previous cardiac surgery. The American Academy of Pediatrics (AAP)[9] and the 26th Bethesda Conference[4] have published guidelines for participation of athletes who have dysrhythmias.

The sports-related reason to evaluate male genitalia is to identify athletes who have a single testis, because this needs extra protection during some sports.[10] Tanner staging of athletes is advocated by some clinicians, because they believe that athletes should be matched by level of development rather than chronologic age, or that immature athletes should be counseled to avoid contact sports in which they will play against more mature youth. There are no convincing data that smaller athletes are at significantly increased risk of injury when matched with larger athletes, or that they will heed advice to change sports, and few programs match athletes by stage of development. Therefore, Tanner staging is not a necessary part of the usual preparticipation examination.

Visual acuity testing is very important. The American Academy of Ophthalmology and the AAP have recently approved a joint policy statement recommending that athletes whose best corrected vision in the worse eye is less than 20/40, and those who have had previous eye surgery or trauma that leaves them at increased risk for severe eye injury, must use appropriate eye protection in high-eye-risk sports (Box 152-1).[11] This recommendation follows from the fact that, if the better eye is seriously injured, the athlete will be unable to obtain a driver's license in many states and will be handicapped in many jobs and leisure activities. Unfortunately, when indigent athletes are examined, those with decreased visual acuity may be unable to afford eye examinations, and so they will never receive clearance to participate even though their visual acuity is correctable to 20/40 or better. An inexpensive device called a "pinhole occluder," available from companies

---

BOX 152-1
Sports Having High Risk of Eye Injury

LOW-RISK SPORTS

Diving	Water skiing
Track and field, cross-country	Swimming
Gymnastics	Weight and power lifting
Skating	Curling
Aerobic dancing	Archery
Crew	Riflery

HIGH-RISK SPORTS: ADEQUATE PROTECTION NOT POSSIBLE
Boxing
Wrestling
Full contact martial arts

HIGH-RISK SPORTS: PROTECTION POSSIBLE

Field hockey (both sexes)	Squash
Football	Handball
Ice hockey	Raqcquetball
Lacrosse (both sexes)	Fencing
Soccer	Tennis
Baseball	Badminton
Basketball	Swimming/Pool sports
Volleyball	Street hockey
Softball	

SOME-RISK SPORTS: PROTECTION DESIRABLE
Table tennis
Golf
Bicycling
Horseback riding
Skiing (cross-country and downhill)
Rodeo

Adapted from Risser WL: Sports medicine, *Pediatr Rev* 14:428, 1993.
Prepared with the help of Dr. John B. Jeffers.

---

*Diagnosis of this disorder has recently been reviewed by the American Academy of Pediatrics, *Pediatrics* 98:978-982, 1996.

selling optometry supplies, for example, the Brunell Corporation in South Bend, Indiana, can be used by primary care physicians to determine if visual acuity defects are correctable. If athletes need eye protection, they and their parents must be counseled that this equipment is not 100% effective, although it may reduce the risk by at least 90%.[11]

General recommendations for eye protection are in Box 152-2. Not all eye protectors fit all athletes well, and so the participant should have the opportunity to try different styles, all of which should meet the appropriate standards of the American Society for Testing and Materials or the American National Standards Institute. Lens material should be polycarbonate with a center thickness of at least 2 mm; "CR-39" plastic with a center thickness of at least 3 mm is used for strong prescriptions (above − 8.00 sphere and − 4.00 cylinder).[11]

There is controversy over what constitutes an appropriate orthopedic examination for a young athlete. It is clearly important for clinicians to be expert in performing standard orthopedic evaluations of areas of recent and old

---

BOX 152-2
Eye Protection for Athletes

AVAILABLE PROTECTORS
1. Sturdy streetwear frame and polycarbonate lenses with center thickness of 2 mm and a posterior lip in the frame to prevent dislodgement back into the eye*
2. Molded polycarbonate frame and lenses with 3-mm center thickness†
3. Face mask (usually attached to a helmet)

RECOMMENDATIONS FOR ATHLETES WHO HAVE UNCORRECTABLE VISION <20/40 IN ONE EYE
1. Avoid boxing, wrestling, and full contact martial arts (eye protection not possible).
2. For day-to-day use and eye-safe sports, use protector No. 1, even if glasses are not required for improved vision.
3. For all other sports, use protector No. 2. In addition, use the face mask in those sports that require one. In baseball, wear a helmet with polycarbonate eye protector and protector No. 2 for batting and base running. While fielding, use protector No. 2.
4. In football, a polycarbonate eyeguard can be added to the face mask for extra protection, and protector No. 2 should also be worn.

Adapted from Risser WL: Sports medicine, *Pediatr Rev* 14:427, 1993.
*Must meet American National Standards Institute (ANSI) standard Z 87.1 for safety glasses for daily wear.
†Must meet American Society for Testing and Materials (ASTM) or Canadian Standards Association (CSA) standards for racquet sports.
Prepared with the help of Dr. John B. Jeffers.

---

injury. The examiner should be alert to evidence that the injury has not been properly rehabilitated, because this is a proven risk factor for further injury, and may also interfere with the athlete's ability to enjoy the sport and perform as well as possible. Persistent pain, limitation of function, reduced range of motion, and reduced strength or muscle mass are symptoms and signs suggesting incomplete rehabilitation.

One commonly recommended screening evaluation for the entire musculoskeletal system is the "90-second" or "2-minute" orthopedic examination developed by Garrick: this is a rapid screen that replaces the joint-by-joint orthopedic testing, which is time-consuming and unproductive except in areas of previous injury.[2] Garrick's examination was found to have problems of sensitivity and specificity when it was evaluated in a college program in which the prevalence of orthopedic problems was high; the investigators recommended modifications.[12] This examination has never been evaluated in the junior or senior high school setting, and its usefulness is unclear.

Some clinicians advocate expanded evaluations that include measurement of such factors as body composition, flexibility, strength, and cardiovascular fitness. No convincing evidence indicates that abnormal measurements are accurate predictors of injury risk, and many secondary school athletic programs lack the resources to provide follow-up interventions to remediate these problems in specific athletes.

Laboratory Tests

Experts agree that no laboratory test need be a standard part of the examination. In a variety of studies, urinalyses do not provide useful information in asymptomatic youth, and the prevalence of iron deficiency anemia severe enough to definitely affect sports performance is low.[13] There is controversy over whether either iron deficiency without anemia or mild iron deficiency anemia can affect performance in endurance athletes; in females competing at the elite level, enough evidence supports an effect, and the prevalence of both is high enough, that evaluation of serum ferritin and hemoglobin concentrations is probably reasonable if economically feasible.[13]

MEDICAL CONDITIONS AFFECTING SPORTS PARTICIPATION

Clinicians who care for athletes should be familiar with the AAP's policy statement concerning medical conditions that affect sports participation (Table 152-1).[10] Current evidence supports the participation in most athletic activities of children and adolescents who have chronic health conditions.

TABLE 152-1
Medical Conditions Affecting Sports Participation

Condition	May Participate?
Atlantoaxial instability (instability of the joint between cervical vertebrae 1 and 2)	Qualified Yes
Explanation: Athlete needs evaluation to assess risk of spinal cord injury during sports participation.	
Bleeding disorder	Qualified Yes
Explanation: Athlete needs evaluation.	
Cardiovascular diseases	
Carditis (inflammation of the heart)	No
Explanation: Carditis may result in sudden death with exertion.	
Hypertension (high blood pressure)	Qualified Yes
Explanation: Those with significant essential (unexplained) hypertension should avoid weight and power lifting, body building, and strength training. Those with secondary hypertension (hypertension caused by a previously identified disease), or severe essential hypertension, need evaluation.	
Congenital heart disease (structural heart defects present at birth)	Qualified Yes
Explanation: Those with mild forms may participate fully; those with moderate or severe forms, or who have undergone surgery, need evaluation.	
Dysrhythmia (irregular heart rhythm)	Qualified Yes
Explanation: Athlete needs evaluation because some types require therapy or make certain sports dangerous, or both.	
Mitral valve prolapse (abnormal heart valve)	Qualified Yes
Explanation: Those with symptoms (chest pain, symptoms of possible dysrhythmia) or evidence of mitral regurgitation (leaking) on physical examination need evaluation. All others may participate fully.	
Heart murmur	Qualified Yes
Explanation: If the murmur is innocent (does not indicate heart disease), full participation is permitted. Otherwise the athlete needs evaluation (see "Congenital heart disease" and "Mitral valve prolapse" above).	
Cerebral palsy	Qualified Yes
Explanation: Athlete needs evaluation.	
Diabetes mellitus	Yes
Explanation: All sports can be played with proper attention to diet, hydration, and insulin therapy. Particular attention is needed for activities that last 30 minutes or more.	
Diarrhea	Qualified No
Explanation: Unless disease is mild, no participation is permitted, because diarrhea may increase the risk of dehydration and heat illness. See "Fever" below.	
Eating disorders	Qualified Yes
Anorexia nervosa	
Bulimia nervosa	
Explanation: These patients need both medical and psychiatric assessment before participation.	
Eyes	Qualified Yes
Functionally one-eyed athlete	
Loss of an eye	
Detached retina	
Previous eye surgery or serious eye injury	
Explanation: A functionally one-eyed athlete has a best corrected visual acuity of <20/40 in the worse eye. These athletes would suffer significant disability if the better eye was seriously injured, as would those with loss of an eye. Some athletes who have previously undergone eye surgery or had a serious eye injury may have an increased risk of injury because of weakened eye tissue. Availability of eye guards approved by the American Society for Testing Materials (ASTM) and other protective equipment may allow participation in most sports, but this must be judged on an individual basis.	

This table is designed to be understood by medical and nonmedical personnel. In the "Explanation" section, "needs evaluation" means that a physician with appropriate knowledge and experience should assess the safety of a given sport for an athlete with the listed medical condition. Unless otherwise noted, this is because of the variability of the severity of the disease or of the risk of injury among the specific sports, or both.

Continued.

TABLE 152-1
Medical Conditions Affecting Sports Participation—cont'd

Condition	May Participate?
Fever	No
Explanation: Fever can increase cardiopulmonary effort, reduce maximal exercise capacity, make heat illness more likely, and increase orthostatic hypotension during exercise. Fever may rarely accompany myocarditis or other infections that may make exercise dangerous.	
Heat illness, history of	Qualified Yes
Explanation: Because of the increased likelihood of recurrence, the athlete needs individual assessment to determine the presence of predisposing conditions and to arrange a prevention strategy.	
HIV infection	Yes
Explanation: Because of the apparent minimal risk to others, all sports may be played that the state of health allows. In all athletes, skin lesions should be properly covered, and athletic personnel should use universal precautions when handling blood or body fluids with visible blood.	
Kidney: absence of one	Qualified Yes
Explanation: Athlete needs individual assessment for contact/collision and limited contact sports.	
Liver: enlarged	Qualified Yes
Explanation: If the liver is acutely enlarged, participation should be avoided because of risk of rupture. If the liver is chronically enlarged, individual assessment is needed before collision/contact or limited contact sports are played.	
Malignancy	Qualified Yes
Explanation: Athlete needs individual assessment.	
Muscoloskeletal disorders	Qualified Yes
Explanation: Athlete needs individual assessment.	
Neurologic	
History of serious head or spine trauma, severe or repeated concussions, or craniotomy.	Qualified Yes
Explanation: Athlete needs individual assessment for collision/contact or limited contact sports, and also for noncontact sports if there are deficits in judgment or cognition. Research supports a conservative approach to management of concussion.	
Convulsive disorder, well controlled	Yes
Explanation: Risk of convulsion during participation is minimal.	
Convulsive disorder, poorly controlled	Qualified Yes
Explanation: Athlete needs individual assessment for collision/contact or limited contact sports. Avoid the following noncontact sports: archery, riflery, swimming, weight or power lifting, strength training, or sports involving heights. In these sports, occurrence of a convulsion may be a risk to self or others.	

Condition		Participation
Obesity		Qualified Yes
	Explanation: Because of the risk of heat illness, obese persons need careful acclimatization and hydration.	
Organ transplant recipient		Qualified Yes
	Explanation: Athlete needs individual assessment.	
Ovary: absence of one		Yes
	Explanation: Risk of severe injury to the remaining ovary is minimal.	
Respiratory		
Pulmonary compromise including cystic fibrosis		Qualified Yes
	Explanation: Athlete needs individual assessment, but generally all sports may be played if oxygenation remains satisfactory during a graded exercise test. Patients with cystic fibrosis need acclimatization and good hydration to reduce the risk of heat illness.	
Asthma		Yes
	Explanation: With proper medication and education, only athletes with the most severe asthma will have to modify their participation.	
Acute upper respiratory infection		Qualified Yes
	Explanation: Upper respiratory obstruction may affect pulmonary function. Athlete needs individual assessment for all but mild disease. See "Fever" above.	
Sickle cell disease		Qualified Yes
	Explanation: Athlete needs individual assessment. In general, if the status of the illness permits, all but high exertion, collision/contact sports may be played. Overheating, dehydration, and chilling must be avoided.	
Sickle cell trait		Yes
	Explanation: It is unlikely that individuals with sickle cell trait (AS) have an increased risk of sudden death or other medical problems during athletic participation except under the most extreme conditions of heat, humidity, and possibly increased altitude. These individuals, like all athletes, should be carefully conditioned, acclimatized, and hydrated to reduce any possible risk.	
Skin: boils, herpes simplex, impetigo, scabies, molluscum contagiosum		Qualified Yes
	Explanation: While the patient is contagious, participation in gymnastics with mats, martial arts, wrestling, or other collision/contact or limited contact sports is not allowed. Herpes simplex virus is probably not transmitted via mats.	
Spleen, enlarged		Qualified Yes
	Explanation: Patients with acutely enlarged spleens should avoid all sports because of risk of rupture. Those with chronically enlarged spleens need individual assessment before playing collision/contact or limited contact sports.	
Testicle: absent or undescended		Yes
	Explanation: Certain sports may require a protective cup.	

This table is designed to be understood by medical and nonmedical personnel. In the "Explanation" section, "needs evaluation" means that a physician with appropriate knowledge and experience should assess the safety of a given sport for an athlete with the listed medical condition. Unless otherwise noted, this is because of the variability of the severity of the disease or of the risk of injury among the specific sports, or both.
From American Academy of Pediatrics, Committee on Sports Medicine and Fitness: Medical conditions affecting sports participation, *Pediatrics* 94:757-760, 1994.

The impact of some medical problems depends on whether sports involve contact; Table 152-2 classifies sports by this parameter.[10] Because of incomplete epidemiologic data, and the fact that serious injuries can occur even in noncontact sports, this table reflects imperfectly the relative likelihood that participation in different sports will result in acute traumatic injury. Data are often inadequate to determine the actual risk to an athlete with a specific problem who wishes to play a particular sport, and one must make an educated guess. Recent court decisions have affirmed the right of young athletes with medical problems to play risky sports, as long as they and their families understand the dangers. In this situation, the clinician should obtain written consent documents from the athletes and the family indicating that the risks have been explained and that all family members chose to accept them.

Acute Illness

Acute illnesses most commonly are respiratory or gastrointestinal illnesses or viral illness with fever but no localizing signs. Fever can increase cardiopulmonary effort, reduce maximal exercise capacity, and increase orthostatic hypotension during exercise. It may increase the risk of dehydration and heat illness, especially if diarrhea is present. Rarely, fever may accompany myocarditis or other illnesses that may make exercise dangerous. Viral infection occasionally inflames skeletal muscle, compromising performance. Respiratory infections, even those in the upper tract, may affect pulmonary function. These facts support the common sense approach of restricting strenuous exercise during all but the mildest acute illnesses.[14]

Spontaneous or traumatic splenic rupture is a rare complication of infectious mononucleosis. Spontaneous rupture has been estimated to occur in no more and probably less than 0.1% of patients with this disease. The incidence of traumatic rupture is unknown. Almost all the rare cases of spontaneous rupture have occurred within 3 weeks of the onset of symptoms. Most experts recommend that light conditioning activities can resume after 3 weeks, if the athlete feels well enough. Return to full activity can begin after about 1 month if the athlete feels able and if the spleen size is normal on palpation and percussion. Even though clinical examination is known to be somewhat inaccurate, no convincing evidence indicates that safety is enhanced by using a radiologic method to confirm that the spleen is at least nearly normal in size.[14]

Nasal Allergies and Asthma

Allergic rhinitis is probably the most common chronic illness that may interfere with sports participation.[14] Athletes need good therapy, which often includes environmental controls, antihistamine/decongestant combinations, nasal steroids or cromolyn sodium, and sometimes desensitization. Sympathomimetic decongestants are banned in National Collegiate Athletic Association, Olympic, and most other elite competition.

In the 1984 Olympic Games, 11.25% of U.S. athletes had exercise-induced bronchospasm. Most asthmatics have this problem, as do many individuals with nasal allergies and some athletes with no known allergic disease. As many as 40% of affected people do not know that they have exercise-induced bronchospasm. The symptoms include shortness of breath, choking, coughing, chest tightness, chest pain, fatigue with exercise, or wheezing. A late recurrence of symptoms sometimes occurs 2 to 8 hours after initial recovery.[14]

Bronchospasm is induced by continuous effort for at least 5 to 6 minutes. Running is the most common trigger. Cold, dry, polluted air or inhaled allergens may worsen the response. The bronchospasm usually becomes evident 5 to 10 minutes after stopping exercise, with recovery requiring 45 to 60 minutes. This is followed by a

---

TABLE 152-2
Classification of Sports by Contact

Contact/Collision	Limited Contact	Noncontact
Basketball	Baseball	Archery
Boxing*	Bicycling	Badminton
Diving	Cheerleading	Body building
Field hockey	Canoeing/kayaking	Bowling
Football	(white water)	Canoeing/kayaking
Flag	Fencing	(flat water)
Tackle	Field	Crew/rowing
Ice hockey	High jump	Curling
Lacrosse	Pole vault	Dancing
Martial arts	Floor hockey	Field
Rodeo	Gymnastics	Discus
Rugby	Handball	Javelin
Ski jumping	Horseback riding	Shot put
Soccer	Racquetball	Golf
Team handball	Skating	Orienteering
Water polo	Ice	Power lifting
Wrestling	Inline	Race walking
	Roller	Riflery
	Skiing	Rope jumping
	Cross-country	Running
	Downhill	Sailing
	Water	Scuba diving
	Softball	Strength training
	Squash	Swimming
	Ultimate Frisbee	Table tennis
	Volleyball	Tennis
	Windsurfing/	Track
	surfing	Weight lifting

*Participation not recommended.
From American Academy of Pediatrics, Committee on Sports Medicine and Fitness: Medical conditions affecting sports participation, *Pediatrics* 94:757-760, 1994.

refractory period of approximately 1 hour during which bronchospasm will be absent or reduced if exercise is resumed.

Diagnosis can be confirmed with exercise testing, but a trial of a bronchodilator such as albuterol is often diagnostic as well as therapeutic. Athletes must be trained in inhaler use, and the medication should be used at least 20, and preferably 30, minutes before exercise. Cromolyn sodium can be substituted or added. More severe asthmatics may also need daily maintenance medications such as inhaled corticosteroids or oral theophylline.

An active warm-up period can induce exercise-induced asthma, after which the athlete can use an inhaler and then rest for 5 to 10 minutes. Trouble-free exercise is often possible for the next 3 to 4 hours. An occasional athlete may have to choose a sport that requires less continuous exercise.

Adults often inappropriately restrict the participation of children who have exercise-induced asthma, and sometimes no one recognizes that the problem is present. The physician often must educate the child and the parents, coaches, teachers, and school nurse concerning the possibility of unrestricted exercise and the proper use of medications.

Seizure Disorders

Epilepsy that is well controlled should not preclude participation in most sports.[10] Until an adequate seizure-free period is demonstrated, participation in sports in which a significant injury could occur during a convulsion should be avoided. These include underwater swimming; diving; mountain climbing; and some gymnastic activities involving equipment such as rings, parallel bars, or high bars. With the exception of those who have frequent seizures, participation in contact/collision sports such as football and wrestling is permissible for adolescents with epilepsy. The participation decision should be based on not only the seizure-free interval but also the likelihood of recurrent seizures. The likelihood of recurrence is determined on the basis of etiology, age, medical compliance, and the duration of a seizure-free interval. For instance, a patient who has experienced a seizure because of electrolyte imbalance associated with acute gastroenteritis would be unlikely to have any adverse outcome from participation in sports. Determining a minimal seizure-free interval for sports participation is often a subjective and difficult judgment, but most states allow a driver's license after a 1- or 2-year seizure-free period. It is reasonable that the patient should not be excluded from any sport for any period longer than that designated for obtaining a driver's license. Current recommendations allow participation in some sports even if the seizures are poorly controlled. Those sports not allowed if a patient's seizures are poorly controlled

include contact/collision sports, swimming, weight lifting, archery, and riflery.

Concussion

Concussion is a common injury in sport, affecting as many as 25% of football players per year. Accumulating evidence indicates that even mild concussions can affect central nervous system functioning for many weeks, and that second concussions soon after the first may be associated with more severe symptoms and even longer periods of disability. Rarely, a second head injury following soon after a concussion may result in life-threatening cerebral injury. These considerations have led some experts to recommend conservative return-to-play rules after concussions and to consider advising against continued participation in contact sports when the number of concussions has mounted.[15] Box 152-3 lists the

---

BOX 152-3
Concussion and Sports Participation

- Grade 1 (mild): Confusion without amnesia; no loss of consciousness
  Return to play if asymptomatic at rest or exertion after observation for 20 minutes
  Participation
      After three grade 1 concussions:
          Terminate season
          Consider further participation in contact sports after 3 months if asymptomatic at rest and exertion
- Grade 2 (moderate): Confusion with amnesia; no loss of consciousness
  Return to play after 1 week if asymptomatic at rest and exertion and neurologic examination is normal
  Participation
      After two grade 2 concussions:
          After 1 month if asymptomatic at rest and exertion
          Consider termination of season
      After three grade 2 concussions:
          Terminate season
          Discourage return to contact sports
- Grade 3 (severe): Loss of consciousness
  Return to play after 1 month if asymptomatic for at least 2 weeks at rest and exertion and neurologic examination is normal
  Participation
      After two grade 3 concussions:
          Terminate season
          Seriously discourage return to contact sports

Modified from *Guidelines for the management of concussion in sports*, Colorado Medical Society, May 1990.

recommendations of the Colorado Medical Society, which have been endorsed by the AAP. Slightly modified recommendations have been published as a practice parameter of the American Academy of Neurology. The only significant difference is less restriction after a grade 3 concussion.[35] These are controversial because of the lack of conclusive supporting research, but until better information becomes available they may be appropriate for athletes at the amateur level of competition.

HIV and Hepatitis B and C Infections

All organizations associated with sports, including the AAP, the National Collegiate Athletic Association (NCAA), and the U.S. and International Olympic Committees, agree that HIV-positive athletes should be allowed to participate in all sports that their state of health allows.[16] No documented case of HIV transmission has occurred in the athletic setting, and the theoretical risk is judged by experts to be very small, much less than the risk from percutaneous exposure among health workers of approximately one infection per 300 exposures. The Supreme Court has never ruled on this subject, but it has ruled that exclusion must be based on "reasonable medical judgments given the state of medical knowledge."[17] It is clear that clinicians are not legally liable if they fail to warn an uninfected opponent of an HIV-positive athlete, even if the athletic contact leads to infection. A few high schools have canceled basketball games against a rival team that has a player known to be HIV positive. Lower federal courts on a few occasions have banned an HIV-positive athlete from playing contact sports, without citing medical authorities or other supporting evidence of risk. These judgments appear to be inconsistent with the Supreme Court's stand.[17] It is clear that school athletic programs must follow prudent guidelines to limit exposure of athletes and staff to blood-borne pathogens; recommendations are available in recent publications.[16] Schools may be required to adhere to Occupational Safety and Health Administration (OSHA) guidelines for limiting employees' exposure to blood-borne pathogens,[18] or to state or local regulations; regulations differ among states.

Hepatitis B is more readily transmitted (one third of percutaneous exposures among healthcare workers),[16] and there is a documented episode of transmission from an e-antigen–positive carrier to five teammates on a Japanese high school sumo wrestling team.[19] Although no other expert bodies have gone this far, the NCAA has suggested that "it is prudent to consider removal" of athletes with acute hepatitis B infection from "combative, sustained, close contact sports (e.g., wrestling)" until they are no longer contagious, and that chronic carriers of hepatitis B should "probably be removed from competition indefinitely."[20] Clinicians should immunize athletes

(and others) with hepatitis B vaccine. Although the epidemiology of hepatitis C transmission is less well understood, it also probably carries a low risk of transmission in the athletic setting that is similar to that of HIV.[16]

Sickle Cell Trait

One study has shown an apparent increased risk of sudden death during basic training among young black recruits who had sickle cell trait,[21] and there are anecdotal reports of deaths of affected athletes during sports participation. Better data are needed (e.g., through a national registry of athletes who experience sudden death), but experts currently suggest that these black athletes are unlikely to have an increased risk of sudden death except under "the most extreme conditions of heat, humidity, and possibly increased altitude. These athletes, like all others, should be carefully conditioned, acclimatized, and hydrated to reduce any possible risk."[10]

Diabetes Mellitus

Diabetic adolescents notoriously have difficulty with control of their disease. For the adolescent who is motivated to participate in sports, provisional clearance based on good control of the disease may provide an incentive for improved management. For safe, successful sports participation, most diabetic adolescents need to maintain good control of their disease, to have supportive families, to express a willingness to increase the frequency of home glucose monitoring, and to give themselves additional insulin and alter the amount and timing of food consumption. The enhanced self-esteem achieved through sports participation should make the extra effort required by the adolescent and physician worthwhile. These two should have frequent contact as the adolescent is adapting to sports participation.

If a patient has reasonably good diabetic control, prolonged exercise will lower the blood glucose level; the larger the amount of circulating insulin, the faster is the decline. Athletes who are hyperglycemic or ketotic, or who have a low insulin level often experience an elevation of glucose level and may even develop ketoacidosis.

Initially, the adolescent should increase the frequency of glucose monitoring during practices and games to measure the impact of participation on diabetic control. During the first few days of the season, frequent monitoring of glucose every 30 to 60 minutes before, during, and after practices and games is required. Nocturnal glucose levels should be checked, since significant numbers of patients may experience delayed-onset hypoglycemia during sleep.

Attempts should be made through manipulation of diet and insulin administration to maintain pre-practice and competition glucose levels between 100 and 250 mg/dl. Food intake should be timed consistently in relation to practice and competition, which may necessitate eating at other than usual mealtimes. It is usually best to inject insulin doses in the anterior abdominal wall, thereby avoiding rapid absorption secondary to injection in exercising arms and legs.

THE ATHLETE WITH A DISABILITY

With the help of modern technology, adolescents with disabilities can ski, swim, bicycle, ride horses, play wheelchair sports, and participate in almost any activity. They may need the clinician's help in getting involved and in choosing a suitable activity.

School physical education programs are one possible place for activity for adolescents with disabilities. Their participation has been mandated in Public Law 94-142. Adults at the school may need advice about what the athlete can and cannot do.

Many organizations sponsor sports programs for these adolescents (Box 152-4). The best known and most available is probably the Special Olympics for people with mental retardation, including the subset who have disabilities. Riding and water sports are particularly good activities for youths with disabilities. Local park and recreation departments and Mental Health/Mental Retardation Associations should have information about such programs.

The physician faced with the task of evaluating a child with a disability may find the following facts helpful. Almost all children with mental retardation can participate in the Special Olympics. Behavioral problems are usually more of a limiting factor than are physical ones. With brief training, physical therapists can check orthoses for fit and durability and assess the need for physical or occupational therapy before participation. Many of these

---

BOX 152-4
National Organizations

1. Special Olympics International, 1325 G. Street N.W., Suite 500, Washington, DC 20005; (202) 628-3630
2. Disabled Sports U.S.A., 6060 Sunrise Vista Dr., Suite 3030, Citrus Heights, CA 95610; 1-800-989-0478
3. Wheelchair Sports, U.S.A., 3595 E. Fountain Blvd., Suite L-1, Colorado Springs, CO 80910; (719) 574-1150
4. American Alliance for Health, Physical Education, Recreation and Dance, 1900 Association Dr., Reston, VA 2091; (703) 476-3400

---

athletes need protective eyewear because of visual problems, and others who have seizure disorders may need special precautions, including supervision of medication use during trips. Participants who have an increased risk of heat illness should be identified. These include athletes with mental retardation, who will be less likely than others to drink enough fluid during exercise.

NUTRITION

Problems

Problem areas in athletes' diets are many.[2,22,23] They and their coaches are often ill educated and misinformed about good nutrition practices. Many athletes have counterproductive dietary notions (e.g., that red meat or milk is bad for them) or are vegetarians but do not know how to make their diet adequate. Many athletes, particularly females, do not eat enough on a regular basis, even if they are not dieting. This may lead to deficits in muscle glycogen that interfere with performance, or to deficiencies in vitamin or mineral intake, particularly iron. To obtain 75% of the Recommended Daily Allowance of iron of 14 mg, girls need to eat 1750 kcal of a balanced diet, since the average iron content of this diet is 6 mg/1000 kcal. Many do not, and few take an iron supplement.

Many athletes, especially females, consider themselves to be overweight when they are not. This perception is often related to concern about appearance rather than a desire to improve performance. Sometimes the concern results from a conviction of the athlete or coach about the optimal percentage body fat for performance, although this value in most sports is unknown. Male athletes are more likely to consider themselves to be underweight, often inappropriately.

Many athletes, usually females, diet during the season in ways that may interfere with performance. This is particularly likely in sports in which thinness is thought to be important to success or in which there are weight classes: body building, cheerleading, dancing, distance running, diving, figure skating, gymnastics, horse racing, rowing, swimming, weight-class football, and wrestling. Some athletes in these sports (and others) may use abnormal weight-control practices that include fasting; purging; use of laxatives or diuretics; and use of rubber suits, steam baths, or both. The term "disordered eating" has been coined to describe these behaviors, which usually do not meet the criteria for anorexia nervosa or bulimia nervosa. These two psychiatric disorders are also relatively common among athletes.[23]

The negative effects of disordered eating include impaired athletic performance when rapid dehydration is used, particularly in sports that require strength and endurance. Amenorrhea in girls may lead to loss of bone mineral mass (disordered eating, amenorrhea, and osteoporosis have been named the "female triad").[23] Chronic dieting and weight loss during the season may compromise performance.

Athletes are sometimes encouraged to gain weight for sports such as football. They need proper education and supervision so that they gain appropriate amounts of both fat and lean-body mass.

Despite their irrelevance, nutritional supplements for athletes have become a multimillion dollar industry in the United States. Protein supplements and other special nutritional products are not necessary unless the athlete is on an inappropriately restrictive diet. Such athletes may need the help of a nutritionist to define and correct dietary inadequacies, which should be corrected through intake of normal foods.

Interventions

Interventions include nutrition education for athletes and the coaching and medical staffs. The NCAA has prepared a videotape with accompanying written materials for use in education. For athletes who are training hard or are in endurance sports, inadequate muscle glycogen stores may limit performance. The older adolescent or adult athlete in rigorous training needs at least 400 g/day of carbohydrates. These can be simple or complex. The latter have the advantages of supplying other nutrients and of being digested slowly; however, complex carbohydrates are bulky, and many athletes have difficulty eating enough, so that simple sugars have a place in the athlete's diet.

Athletes are educable about nutrition. The diet should emphasize appropriate numbers of servings from the basic food groups to provide necessary protein, vitamins, and minerals. This diet will not have enough calories; these should come mainly from carbohydrate-rich low-fat

---

BOX 152-5
Skinfold Calipers Technique

Grasp the skinfold and underlying fat with thumb and forefinger. Do not pick up underlying muscle.

Place caliper jaws ¼ to ½ inch from fingers at a depth equal to thickness of fold.

Release caliper jaws.

Read dial to closest 0.5 mm. Read within 2 seconds.

Anatomic sites for measurement (Jackson-Pollock formula):

Chest: a diagonal fold one third of distance from anterior axillary line and nipple

Abdomen: a vertical fold 1 inch to side of umbilicus

Triceps: a vertical fold on posterior midline of upper arm halfway between acromion and olecranon

Suprailium: a diagonal fold above crest of ilium at or lateral to anterior axillary line

Thigh: with weight supported on nondominant leg and knee of dominant leg slightly bent: a vertical fold on front of dominant thigh halfway between hip and knee

Data from Jackson AS, Pollock ML: Practical assessment of body composition, *Phys Sportsmed* 13:85, 1985.

TABLE 152-3
Percentage Body Fat Estimate

Sum of Skinfolds (mm)	Fat (%)	Sum of Skinfolds (mm)	Fat (%)
Men*		**Women†**	
8-10	1.3	23-25	9.7
11-13	2.2	26-28	11.0
14-16	3.2	29-31	12.3
17-19	4.2	32-34	13.6
20-22	5.1	35-37	14.8
23-25	6.1	38-40	16.0
26-28	7.0	41-43	17.2
29-31	8.0	44-46	18.3
32-34	8.9	47-49	19.5
35-37	9.8	50-52	20.6
38-40	10.7	53-55	21.7
41-43	11.6	56-58	22.7
44-46	12.5	59-61	23.7
47-49	13.4	62-64	24.7
50-52	14.3	65-67	25.7
53-55	15.1	68-70	26.6
56-58	16.0	71-73	27.5
59-61	16.9	74-76	28.4
62-64	17.6	77-79	29.3
65-67	18.5	80-82	30.1
68-70	19.3	83-85	30.9
71-73	20.1	86-88	31.7
74-76	20.9	89-91	32.5
77-79	21.7	92-94	33.2
80-82	22.4	95-97	33.9
83-85	23.2	98-100	34.6
86-88	24.0	101-103	35.3
89-91	24.7	104-106	35.8
92-94	25.4	107-109	36.4
95-97	26.1	110-112	37.0
98-100	26.9	113-115	37.5
101-103	27.5	116-118	38.0
104-106	28.2	119-121	38.5
107-109	28.9	122-124	39.0
110-112	29.6	125-127	39.4
113-115	30.2	128-130	39.8
116-118	30.9		
119-121	31.5		
122-124	32.1		
125-127	32.7		

Excerpted from Jackson AS, Pollock ML: Practical assessment of body composition, *Phys Sportsmed* 13:76-90, 1985.
*Sum of chest, abdomen, and thigh measurements.
†Sum of triceps, suprailium, and thigh measurements.

foods eaten with meals and as snacks. These foods can be chosen from the bread-cereal and fruit-vegetable food groups. The overall diet should contain about 15% protein, 25% to 35% fat, and 50% to 60% carbohydrate (70% in athletes training to exhaustion on a daily basis).

Athletes who have warning signs of eating disorders should have psychiatric evaluations. Such athletes can be screened with questionnaires such as the Eating Attitudes Test or the Eating Disorders Inventory, but underreporting occurs. Athletes can be followed with serial weight and body fat determinations, using skinfold calipers; diet histories in athletes who have declining or disappointing performances; and similar evaluations of amenorrheic athletes.

To assess levels of body fat and monitor changes, the practitioner should become familiar with the proper use of skinfold calipers (Box 152-5). To determine percentage body fat using calipers, skinfold measurements are performed at three sites: in males at the anterior axillary line, paraumbilical area, and anterior thigh; and in females at the triceps, suprailium, and anterior thigh. There are many formulas for determining percentage body fat, but they are population specific for ethnicity, age, and sex. The Jackson-Pollock formula (Table 152-3) for young adults has been validated in adolescent populations. Although the ideal weight or percentage body fat for women in sports has not been determined, the data are included for the interested practitioner. The overall error in skinfold assessment of body fat is approximately 10%, including about 5% for precision of measurement and 5% for accuracy in comparison with underwater weighing. This error may be greater if the athlete is fat (skinfolds > 15 mm) or lean (< 5 mm), and varies with the population and the prediction equation.[24]

PERFORMANCE-ENHANCING DRUGS

Stimulants

Stimulants clearly enhance the performance of athletes in most sports. Therefore, the use of stimulant medications such as methylphenidate and dextroamphetamine has been banned by the United States Olympic Committee and the NCAA. Once they leave high school athletics, adolescents with attention-deficit (hyperactivity) disorder (AD [H] D) who need these medications to function in the school environment and frequently in the athletic world are not able to use them in collegiate or Olympic sports. This situation is indeed a tragedy, as there are some very good student athletes who might be able to compete at the collegiate level if allowed to continue legitimate medical treatment for AD(H)D. However, it is doubtful that this situation will change in the foreseeable future because of the difficulty in precisely defining diagnostic criteria for AD(H)D and the performance enhancement action of stimulants.

Anabolic Steroids

Current surveys in high school adolescents have shown a 5% to 11% prevalence of anabolic steroid (AS) use,[2,25] including up to 2.4% of girls. Trends in these surveys indicate that increasing numbers of adolescents, including younger ones, are using AS for cosmetic reasons. AS users may share needles and use other illicit drugs.

Virtually no athlete is immune from the temptation to use AS to improve performance. Previously it was thought that these drugs were not effective in increasing strength. Data now clearly indicate that AS used in conjunction with a proper diet and intense strength training will result in increases in lean body mass and strength beyond those obtained with diet and training alone. In addition, AS appears to counteract the catabolic effect of intense training, resulting in more effective training cycles for endurance sports.

Table 152-4 lists the possible side effects of AS. Much of this information is anecdotal or comes from data about problems associated with therapeutic use of AS, so that its applicability to use by athletes is unknown. Of particular concern in young athletes is premature closure of the epiphyses, but this probably happens very rarely.

Many alleged changes in mental status or behavior have been ascribed to AS use, including irritability, aggressiveness, euphoria, depression, mood swings, altered libido, psychosis, and withdrawal and dependency disorders. There are disturbing reports of depression and suicidal ideation severe enough to require hospitalization in chemical dependency treatment centers after discontinuance of AS use.

Given their high cost and fallibility, tests for AS do not appear to be a viable way of recognizing users, who are not likely to share this information with clinicians. The clinician is most likely to recognize use AS through side effects such as rapid gains in muscle mass, bulk, and definition; increased aggressiveness or emotional lability; severe acne; gynecomastia; early male-pattern baldness; other evidence of virilization in girls; testicular atrophy; and elevations in blood pressure. If AS use is suspected, the clinician should be nonjudgmental and conduct a balanced discussion of risks and benefits, not use scare tactics, and remember that AS may have beneficial effects on performance. An attempt can be made to convince athletes that it is possible and desirable to meet their goals without AS use.

No published data indicate that educational programs deter AS use. Athletic programs that give a clear message to their athletes that steroid use will not be tolerated have been effective in reducing AS use at the collegiate level.

TABLE 152-4
Possible Anabolic Steroid Toxicities

Cardiovascular

    Hypertension
    Thrombosis
    Increased low-density lipoprotein cholesterol
    Decreased high-density lipoprotein cholesterol
    Increased total cholesterol

Endocrinologic

    Acne
    Amenorrhea
    Male-pattern baldness
    Testicular atrophy
    Priapism
    Impotence
    Gynecomastia
    Oligospermia, azoospermia
    Decreased sperm motility
    Masculinization in women
    Prostatic hypertrophy, carcinoma

Musculoskeletal

    Muscle strains/ruptures
    Epiphyseal closure

Hepatic

    Hepatocellular damage
    Cholestatic jaundice
    Peliosis
    Hepatocarcinoma, hepatoma

Behavioral

    Aggressiveness
    Increased libido
    Increased energy
    Irritability
    Mood swings
    Depression
    Withdrawal, dependency disorders
    Psychosis

Infectious

    HIV infection
    Hepatitis B and C infection (from shared
      needles)

Adapted from Risser WL: Sports medicine, *Pediatr Rev* 14:430, 1993.

Until better strategies are devised, the most practical intervention is for everyone associated with sports to send a clear and concise message to adolescent athletes that AS use is a form of cheating and may have negative long-term consequences.

Growth Hormone

Human growth hormone (hGH) is potentially attractive because it may increase muscle strength without being detectable in the urine. Anecdotal information indicates that hGH is available on the black market, although some preparations of alleged hGH have been found not to contain this hormone. Athletes and their parents may find hGH particularly appealing because of its ability to accelerate height velocity and increase stature in short athletes, although final adult height is apparently not increased.

Erythropoietin

Erythropoietin is becoming increasingly available and may eventually replace "blood doping" as a performance enhancer in endurance sports. Blood doping (autologous transfusion of previously harvested red cells) appears effective for enhancing performance in endurance athletes and its practice is virtually undetectable. Theoretically, erythropoietin use would be as effective for increasing red cell mass and would be equally undetect-

able. The adverse effects of erythropoietin use have not been completely identified because of the short history of the drug's availability. Although use in adolescent athletes at this time is exceedingly rare, it is likely to be one of the most popular performance enhancers of the future.

ATHLETIC AMENORRHEA

Amenorrhea may occur in adolescent athletes for a variety of reasons unrelated to sports: for example, pregnancy, endocrine disorders, and anorexia nervosa. Before intense exercise and limited diet are assumed to be causative, pregnancy and other medical conditions should first be ruled out through a thorough history, physical examination, and appropriate laboratory tests. In the absence of evidence of other problems in the history and physical examination, the important tests are for pregnancy, hypothyroidism (thyroid-stimulating hormone), and a prolactin-secreting adenoma (prolactin level).[26] Anorexia nervosa and bulimia nervosa should be ruled out, especially in sports in which thinness is considered important. If these evaluation results are normal and bleeding occurs after a course of progesterone (progesterone in oil, 200 mg intramuscularly, or medroxyprogesterone acetate, 10 mg orally daily for 5 days), it is reasonable to assume that the athlete has anovulation. She can be treated with medroxyprogesterone acetate, 10 mg orally for the first 10 days of each month, or with contraceptive hormones if she is sexually active.[26]

An athlete who is amenorrheic as a result of intense exercise and poor nutritional intake may have hypothalamic amenorrhea because of the loss of pulsatile secretion of gonadotropin-releasing hormone from the hypthothalamus. This is confirmed if there is no bleeding after a progesterone challenge; serum follicle-stimulating hormone and luteinizing hormone are normal or low; and an imaging study of the sella turcica (e.g., a coned-down view on plain radiography) is normal.[26] Low levels of body fat, psychologic stress, and high energy expenditure seem to play independent roles in causing this problem. Some affected athletes have disordered eating, and a few have anorexia nervosa or bulimia nervosa. Girls with hypothalamic amenorrhea are at risk for loss of bone mineral mass. Maximization of bone mineral mass during the second decade of life is probably important for avoiding osteoporosis later in life, and so factors that interfere with this process in adolescence are potentially detrimental.[27]

Changes in lifestyle, in particular increased caloric intake, a reduction of stress, less rigorous training, or a combination of these, can result in the resumption of menses. If not, or if the athlete is unwilling to make such changes, experts recommend hormonal therapy. This can be a combination of estrogen and progesterone, either individually (e.g., 0.625 mg conjugated estrogen on days 1 to 25 of the month, with 10 mg medroxyprogesterone acetate on days 16 to 25); or oral contraceptive pills if the athlete is sexually active. If an athlete wishes not to menstruate, she can be given this dose of estrogen and 2.5 mg medroxyprogesterone acetate or an active low-dose oral contraceptive pill daily without a break.[26] Although none of these regimens has been proved to prevent or reverse loss of bone mineral mass,[27] experts recommend hormonal therapy, because studies to date have not been definitive.[26,27]

Not all athletes accept hormonal therapy because of fears of weight gain or other concerns. These girls should be urged to consume the Recommended Daily Allowance for adolescents of 1500 mg calcium per day, even though it is not clear that this protects bone density.[27] For those with inadequate dietary intakes of calcium, supplementation is easily accomplished through the use of over-the-counter antacids containing calcium carbonate (40% calcium).

SPORTS PSYCHOLOGY

The important area of sports psychology is generally given scant attention, even though a large body of research provides useful information. One of the most important areas is the interaction of coaches and parents

with athletes. Bad experiences with coaches and inappropriate behavior by parents are common reasons why many young people drop out of sports programs. Some of the elements of successful coaching and parenting are detailed here. Athletes should be helped to master the skills of the sport to the extent possible given their developmental levels and innate abilities. Each should be given specific performance goals. Young athletes do not enjoy playing even for likeable coaches who are unable to teach them effectively. When athletes make mistakes, they should receive both emotional support and corrective instruction. Coaches and parents should make it clear that the athletes' worth does not depend on winning; they are to participate, have fun, and improve their skills. At least among preadolescents, playoffs, all-star contests, and award ceremonies for individuals should be discouraged.[28]

Courses for coaches are available, as well as materials for self-study. The most well developed are those offered by Human Kinetics in Champaign, Illinois.

PHYSICAL ACTIVITY AND FITNESS

Epidemiologic studies have shown that a sedentary life style among adults is a risk factor for many significant common chronic diseases such as coronary artery disease and diabetes mellitus.[29] Experts have begun to emphasize moderately vigorous physical activity that does not necessarily improve maximal aerobic capacity, because both have health benefits for adults. A goal of activity programs for youth is therefore the promotion of physically active life styles that will be carried into adulthood. Research on the effects of physical activity in childhood and adolescence is limited but suggests that fit and active adolescents are more likely to remain active as adults; that exercise can help to treat obesity, hypertension, depression, and other chronic diseases, at least in short-term programs; and, in cross-sectional studies, that higher levels of activity are associated with lower levels of body fat, increased bone mineral mass, and lower levels of tobacco and alcohol use and other problem behaviors. Some intervention programs have been implemented in the school setting.[29,30]

Much remains to be learned about the most effective ways to help children and adolescents become more physically active. Currently recommended interventions[29] include daily, high-quality physical education in schools that emphasizes at least moderately vigorous physical activity and activities that can be continued into adulthood; school-based health education that teaches the value of physical activity and that helps students gain the behavioral skills necessary to sustain a physically active life style; family exercise programs that involve children in fun, age-appropriate activities; role modeling of an active life style by parents, teachers, and other adults; limitations on the time that youths are allowed to watch television; after-school programs for children of working parents that emphasize physical activity; and anticipatory guidance from clinicians about how families can become more active.

TRAINING

Aerobic, endurance, and strength training and acclimatization before the first practice of the season are thought to help prevent injury and illness, improve performance, and decrease the athlete's degree of physical discomfort early in the season. The adolescent who impulsively decides to participate in a sport without the benefit of preseason conditioning is particularly susceptible to overuse injuries.

Aerobic and Endurance Training

Workouts should be pain-free and progressive in nature, beginning at least 6 weeks before the start of the season. For instance, in cross-country running the competitive distance is approximately 2½ miles. However, as part of the preseason conditioning, a coach may require athletes to run distances of 3 to 5 miles. In the preseason, the athlete should start a running program on a daily basis, beginning with a distance as short as ½ mile and gradually increasing the distance to 3 to 5 miles; pain on running may indicate that the increase has been too fast, and the distance should be temporarily decreased.

Athletes who play another sport before the current season may injure themselves if they do not start a training program appropriate for the new sport. The coach may assume that the athletes are already well conditioned, but the new sport may require strength, endurance, and flexibility in muscle-tendon units that were not much used in the previous activity. This concept is called specificity of training.

Strength Training

Strength training is valuable for virtually all athletes, including those participating in endurance sports such as long-distance running, to improve performance and probably prevent injury. Strength-training programs should be run by a coach who has participated in certification programs such as those offered by the National Strength and Conditioning Association in Lincoln, Nebraska, or through university continuing education courses.[31]

To begin a strength-training program, common sense should guide the determination of the amount of weight to lift. The athlete should be able to complete three sets of 10 to 12 repetitions with a given weight. For instance, it would be unreasonable for a 110-pound prepubertal boy to begin individual arm curls with a 40-pound weight. If the athlete begins with 20 pounds and is able to lift the weight ten times in the first set, eight times in the second set, and three times in the third set, the amount of weight should be reduced at the next session. Conversely, if ten repetitions were accomplished during all three sets, the weight should be increased at the next session. Incremental progression in the amount of weight lifted during subsequent workouts should not exceed 10%. A knowledgeable coach can help the athlete select specific exercises appropriate to the sport being played; useful books are available for self-education.[32]

Strength training should be differentiated from the sports of weight or power lifting. The first involves the use of lighter weights lifted repetitively, and the latter two involve making a single lift using the maximal amount of weight possible. Body building is another competitive sport in which participants may train with large amounts of weight. The AAP recommends that single maximal lifts be avoided until the athlete is skeletally mature (Tanner stage 5). This recommendation seems reasonable, because athletes will have passed their period of maximal velocity of height growth, during which their epiphyses may be especially vulnerable to injury.[31] Unfortunately, many coaches unnecessarily use maximal lifts to determine the progress of growing athletes involved in strength-training programs.

Several types of lifts using free weights have been shown to be associated with significant injuries. These include the power clean, the snatch, the incline and overhead presses, the clean and jerk, the dead lift, and the squat lift. These should be undertaken only by mature athletes who have mastered the proper techniques and, for some of these lifts, in the presence of spotters who can grab the bar if the lifter loses control. Adult supervision in the weight room can ensure that athletes use proper technique and other safety practices.

Acclimatization

Heat illness[33] is a preventable consequence of physical activity. Children are more susceptible to this problem than adults; adolescents have an intermediate risk. Some medical conditions put the athlete at increased risk: mental retardation, obesity, gastroenteritis with dehydration, fever, cystic fibrosis, anorexia nervosa, chronic heart failure, diabetes mellitus and insipidus, malnutrition, and sweating insufficiency and neurocardiogenic syndromes. The following interventions should be used to prevent heat illness in all young athletes.

They need to increase their activity level gradually over a 10- to 14-day period when beginning strenuous exercise or after moving to a warm climate. Because dehydration is an important contributor to heat illness, and because they often do not voluntarily drink enough fluids to replenish losses, young athletes should have scheduled water breaks at least every 30 minutes during which they are required to drink specified amounts (e.g., 150 ml for a child weighing 40 kg, 250 ml for one weighing 60 kg). They should begin practice fully hydrated. Clothing should be replaced when it becomes saturated with sweat, and it should be light in weight and only one layer thick. When air temperature, relative humidity, and solar radiation are above critical levels, the intensity of activity should be reduced.[33] The success of the program in keeping athletes well hydrated can be assessed by nude weights before and after practice.

Cold water is an excellent fluid for hydrating athletes. However, research has shown that flavored drinks (especially grape) with a small amount of added sodium chloride (15 to 20 mmol/L) are preferred by some children, who will therefore drink more.[34]

References

1. Risser WL, Hoffman HM, Bellah GG: Frequency of preparticipation sports examinations: are the University Interscholastic League's guidelines appropriate?, *Tex Med* 81:35-39, 1985.
2. American Academy of Pediatrics, Committee on Sports Medicine and Fitness: *Sports medicine: health care for young athletes,* ed 2, Elk Grove Village, IL, 1991, American Academy of Pediatrics, pp 49-74, 84-146.
3. Harris SS: The preparticipation examination. In Reider B, editor: *Sports medicine: the school-aged athlete,* ed 2, Philadelphia, 1996, WB Saunders; pp 95-114.
4. 26th Bethesda Conference: Recommendations for determining eligibility for competition in athletes with cardiovascular abnormalities, *J Am Coll Cardiol* 24:845-899, 1994.
5. American Academy of Pediatrics, Committee on Sports Medicine and Fitness: Mitral valve prolapse and athletic participation in children and adolescents, *Pediatrics* 95:789-790, 1995.
6. Epstein SE, Maron BJ: Sudden death and the competitive athlete: perspectives in preparticipation screening studies, *J Am Coll Cardiol* 17:220-230, 1986.
7. Pyeritz RE, McKusick VA: The Marfan syndrome, diagnosis and management, *N Engl J Med* 200:772-779, 1979.
8. National Heart, Lung, and Blood Institute: Report of the Second Task Force on Blood Pressure Control in Children—1987, *Pediatrics* 79:1-25, 1987.
9. American Academy of Pediatrics, Committee on Sports Medicine and Fitness: Cardiac dysrhythmias and sports, *Pediatrics* 95:786-788, 1995.
10. American Academy of Pediatrics, Committee on Sports Medicine and Fitness: Medical conditions affecting sports participation, *Pediatrics* 94:757-760, 1994.
11. American Academy of Pediatrics, Committee on Sports Medicine and Fitness: Protective eyewear for young athletes, *Pediatrics* 98:311-313, 1996.
12. Gomez JE, Landry GL, Bernhardt DT: Critical evaluation of the 2-minute orthopedic screening examination, *Am J Dis Child* 147:1109-1113, 1993.
13. Risser WL, Risser JMH: Iron deficiency in adolescents and young adults, *Phys Sportsmed* 18:87-101, 1990.
14. Risser WL: Exercise for children, *Pediatr Rev* 10:131-139, 1988.
15. Colorado Medical Society, Sports Medicine Committee: *Guidelines for the management of concussion in sports,* Denver, CO, 1991, Colorado Medical Society.
16. American Medical Society for Sports Medicine, American Academy of Sports Medicine: Joint position statement: human immunodeficiency virus and other blood-borne pathogens in sports, *Clin J Sports Med* 5:199-204, 1995.
17. Mitten MJ: Editorial: athletic participation with a contagious blood-borne disease, *Clin J Sports Med* 5:153-154, 1995.
18. American Academy of Pediatrics: *OSHA,* ed 2, Elk Grove Village, IL, 1994, American Academy of Pediatrics.
19. Kashiwagi S, Hayashi J, Ikematsu H, Nishigori S, Ishihara K, Kaji M: An outbreak of hepatitis B in members of a high school sumo wrestling club, *JAMA* 248:213-214, 1982.
20. NCAA Committee on Competitive Safeguards and Medical Aspects of Sports: Blood-borne pathogens and intercollegiate athletics. In *NCAA sports medicine handbook,* Overland Park, KS, 1994, National Collegiate Athletic Association, pp 24-28.
21. Kark JA, Posey DM, Schumacher HR, Ruehle CJ: Sickle-cell trait as a risk factor for sudden death in physical training, *N Engl J Med* 317:781-787, 1987.
22. Berning JR, Steen SN: *Sports nutrition for the 90s: the health professional's handbook,* Gaithersburg, MD, 1991, Aspen Publishers.
23. American Academy of Pediatrics, Committee on Sports Medicine and Fitness: Promotion of healthy weight-control practices in young athletes, *Pediatrics* 97:752-753, 1996.
24. Lukaski HC: Methods for the assessment of human body composition: traditional and new, *Am J Clin Nutr* 46:537-556, 1987.
25. American Academy of Pediatrics, Committee on Sports Medicine and Fitness: Adolescents and anabolic steroids: a subject review (in press).
26. Speroff L, Glass RH, Kase NG: *Clinical gynecologic endocrinology and infertility,* ed 5, Baltimore, MD, 1994, Williams & Wilkins; pp 401-456.
27. Hergenroeder AC: Bone mineralization, hypothalamic amenorrhea, and sex steroid therapy in female adolescents and young adults, *J Pediatr* 126:683-689, 1995.
28. American Academy of Pediatrics, Committee on Sports Medicine and Fitness: Organized athletics for preadolescent children, *Pediatrics* 84:583-584, 1989.
29. Centers for Disease Control and Prevention: Guidelines for school and community programs to promote lifelong physical activity among young people, *MMWR* 46(RR-6):1-36, 1997.
30. Bar-Or O: Childhood and adolescent physical activity and fitness and adult risk profile. In Bouchard C, Shephard RJ, Stephens, editors: *Physical activity, fitness, and health: international proceedings and consensus statement,* Champaign, IL, 1994, Human Kinetics Publishers; pp 931-942.
31. American Academy of Pediatrics, Committee on Sports Medicine and Fitness: Strength training, weight and power lifting, and body building by children and adolescents, *Pediatrics* 86:801-803, 1990.
32. Fleck SJ, Kraemer WJ: *Strength training for young athletes,* Champaign, IL, 1993, Human Kinetics Publishers.

33. Committee on Sports Medicine and Fitness, American Academy of Pediatrics: Climatic heat stress and the exercising child, *Pediatrics* 69:808-809, 1982.
34. Wilk B, Meyer F, Bar-Or O: Effect of electrolytes and carbohydrate drink content on voluntary drinking and fluid balance in children, *Med Sci Sports Exerc* 26:S205, 1994.
35. American Academy of Neurology, Quality Standard Subcommittee: Practice parameter: the management of concussion in sports, *Neurology* 48:581-585, 1997.

Suggested Reading

The manuals and books cited above have much useful information. The American Academy of Pediatrics' manual *Sports Medicine* is free to Fellows of the Academy. Any of its policy statements can be ordered from the AAP's Publication Department (1-800-433-9016). The Colorado Medical Society guidelines on concussion are also available from the Academy. Human Kinetics in Champaign, Illinois has published many useful books on fitness, coaching, and sports psychology.

CHAPTER 153

Cervical Masses

•

John S. Rubin and Angela Damiano

Neck masses in adolescents are extremely common. Almost all individuals experience cervical adenopathy at some time during their childhood or adolescence. Most cervical masses resolve without the need for surgical intervention. Masses that require biopsy are most usually benign, with the malignancy rate variably reported to be between 2% and 16%. This chapter outlines an approach to the diagnosis and management of cervical masses.

HISTORY

Information gained upon questioning the patient or parent is of great importance in determining the cause of a neck mass. The diagnosis is reached on history alone up to 50% of the time. The history taking should be directed toward elucidating the chief complaint, severity, duration, time, progression, and onset of symptoms. It is important to obtain the history of any associated symptoms, such as fever or pain.

Cervical masses occur in several different pathologic conditions, each with its own characteristics. Congenital masses usually present at birth or can present as slow-growing masses. For example, a thyroglossal duct cyst may increase in size only when it becomes secondarily infected or fills with cystic fluid. It is at this time that the young person seeks medical attention.

Inflammatory neck masses can be chronic or acute in nature. Granulomatous diseases are characterized as chronic infection accompanied by low-grade intermittent fever. Acute inflammatory masses are more common. These are typically associated with pain, discomfort, fever, and inflammatory signs such as erythema and tenderness to palpation. Neoplastic masses, however, can grow rapidly without causing significant symptoms. If pain is associated with a neoplastic process, it is usually

due to either acute bleeding causing distention, or neural invasion. Neck masses need to grow significantly before they cause obstruction to the air and food passages.

Most neck masses are inflammatory in origin, and the clinician should determine any history of recent infection. Viral infections of the upper respiratory tract are the most likely causes of cervical adenopathy. Many viral agents, including adenovirus, rhinovirus, and others, cause cervical adenopathy as well as flu-like symptoms. Adenopathy secondary to these infections should resolve within a few weeks.

Bacterial infections can also cause cervical adenopathy, and the medical history may disclose the location of the primary infection. *Staphylococcus* organisms and β-streptococci are the most common etiologic agents. In one study, neck aspirate cultures of 65% of the patients showed *Staphylococcus aureus,* and 41% of patients with neck masses exhibited immune response to one or more extracellular antigens of group A streptococcus.

Other medical history that may help elucidate the origin of a mass includes previous exposure to radiation, which has an association with thyroid cancer. Symptoms of fatigue, weight loss, or night sweats may also be clues to an underlying malignant process. It is important to determine whether medications are being taken; phenytoin (Dilantin), for example, has an association with cervical lymphadenopathy that may resemble a neoplastic process. It is essential to obtain a history of other possible vectors of infection. The presence of a cat in the house may indicate cat-scratch fever. Recent exposure to friends with infectious mononucleosis may aid in diagnosis. Multiple areas of adenopathy in the neck or in other areas of the body may suggest the possibility of AIDS or underlying malignancy.

Depending on the geographic location of the patient, the physician may consider tropical diseases that may also be associated with cervical lymphadenopathy. Tuberculous cervical adenitis is more likely to be found in residents of metropolitan areas. Tularemia is ubiquitous in the northern hemisphere between 30 degrees and 70 degrees north latitude. In the United States, it occurs in the southern and western states, especially in Arkansas, Missouri, Oklahoma, and Texas. *Yersinia pestis* is still rarely encountered on Indian reservations in the western United States.

PHYSICAL EXAMINATION

Physical examination should begin with inspection of the neck in good light. The inspection phase should identify all normal landmarks such as the jaw, sternocleidomastoid muscle, and laryngeal framework. The inspection should then attempt to identify abnormal findings such as abnormal pulsations, a neck mass, any vascular markings, or skin discoloration. Next, it is important to characterize the location of the mass. The neck can be subdivided conveniently into regions, and each region can be considered with regard to the specific masses encountered in that location (Fig. 153-1). For example, thyroglossal anomalies tend to occur in the midline, whereas branchial cleft anomalies tend to be in the lateral neck. The presence of scars and fistulous tracts, and the relationship of the mass upon swallowing, tongue protrusion, or lowering of the head, should be noted. For example, masses involving the thyroid gland have a tendency to move upon swallowing; thyroglossal anomalies move upon protrusion of the tongue. Upon lowering of the head, there is an increase in venous congestion, ultimately causing an increase in the size of cavernous hemangiomas.

Next in the examination process is palpation of the mass. It is best to palpate with the palmar surface of the fingertips, while the other hand stabilizes the head. Upon palpating the mass, it is important to note such aspects as mobility, consistency, and tenderness. For example, sebaceous cysts are intimately attached to the epidermis, and it is not possible to roll these masses underneath the skin. Benign lesions are typically freely mobile upon palpation, whereas malignant lesions are frequently fixed to the skin and surrounding tissue.

It is also important to note the regularity and shape of the mass. Irregular lesions are more often associated with malignancy. Lesions can also be localized or diffuse. The consistency of the mass (rubbery, firm, indurated, or cystic) provides useful information to the diagnostician regarding the etiology. Congenital lesions are often cystic, and transillumination may be performed to detect fluid. Lipomas tend to be soft and localized independent of the surrounding tissues. Benign reactive lymph nodes tend to be firm, mobile, and rubbery with well-defined borders. Malignancies tend to be woody and hard, secondary to rapid growth. Also, the compressibility of the mass can give clues to the cause. Cavernous hemangiomas and laryngoceles are compressible masses. Tenderness is an important symptom to assess, since

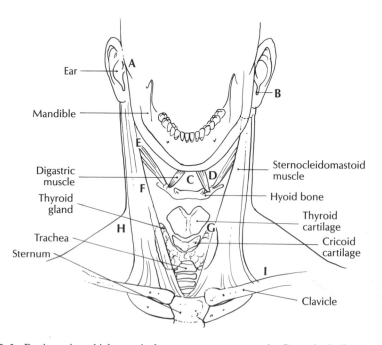

Fig. 153-1. Regions in which cervical masses can occur. **A,** Preauricular/intraparotid; **B,** postauricular/occipital; **C,** submental; **D,** submandibular; **E,** upper jugular; **F** and **G,** middle and lower jugular; **H,** posterior triangle; and **I,** supraclavicular.

inflammatory processes represent the most common neck masses seen.

As most neck masses are inflammatory, a primary source of infection should be sought. It is crucial to perform a complete head and neck examination in all instances. The teeth and floor of the mouth should be carefully examined for caries, gum disease, or other inflammatory processes. The tonsils and oropharynx must be examined for infection or exudates. Wharton's and Stensen's ducts should be inspected for evidence of inflammation or purulent secretions. The range of motion of the jaws should be ascertained. Trismus might indicate an inflammatory process involving the peritonsillar or parapharyngeal spaces or the muscles of mastication. The ears should be examined for evidence of related otitis media, serous otitis media, or other aural pathologic conditions. For example, a first branchial cleft anomaly may be connected through its tract to the external ear canal; discharge from the cyst may well present as recurrent otitis externa. The nose should be examined for purulence or polypoid changes. Infection or chronic irritation within the nares could lead to enlarged nodes in the neck.

LABORATORY EVALUATION

Beyond routine evaluations such as a complete blood count and a differential white blood cell (WBC) count, further testing is directed by the history and physical examination. Such tests might include a culture from an identified primary site of infection, an erythrocyte sedimentation rate (ESR), a test for mononucleosis, or a tuberculin test. A chest radiograph may be necessary when hilar adenopathy or other chest pathologic conditions are suspected.

A needle aspiration biopsy may be indicated at the initial visit; alternatively, a course of antibiotic therapy may serve as both a diagnostic and a therapeutic tool. If the mass does not shrink after treatment with antibiotics, further testing, including biopsy, may be required. If the diagnosis of a neck abscess is being entertained, a lateral radiograph of the neck will rapidly and inexpensively confirm the presence of free air or increased prevertebral soft tissues. Currently, however, the study of choice for deep infections of the neck is computed tomography (CT) for differentiation between cellulitis, abscess, and other pathologic conditions. Cellulitis appears as soft tissue swelling with obliteration of the fat planes; an abscess can be detected as a low attenuation area within a phlegmon. Contrast dye may be injected intravenously on CT studies of the neck to further identify vascular structures. CT scanning is also useful for the evaluation of noninflammatory masses such as thyroglossal duct cysts or branchial cleft cysts. The role of magnetic resonance

imaging (MRI) in the evaluation of neck masses is increasing. The major disadvantage of MRI is that it cannot image bone and thus is not helpful in determining tumor invasion. It is, however, particularly useful in differentiating inflammatory processes from neoplastic disease.

If the mass is believed to represent a thyroglossal duct cyst, thyroid scanning, ultrasonography, or CT should be performed to confirm the presence of viable thyroid tissue in the thyroid gland. These tests are also useful in differentiating intrathyroid pathologic conditions. If the mass is considered to be malignant, fine-needle aspiration biopsy is the initial diagnostic modality of choice. A study of 135 fine-needle aspiration biopsies in 123 children reported a sensitivity of 90.6% and a specificity of 100%, with no false-positive diagnoses and only four false-negative results.

Imaging modalities, including CT and MRI, help to identify a primary lesion. Should these studies not elucidate the pathologic nature and/or source of the tumor, endoscopy and possibly open biopsy are indicated. Endoscopy should be performed first. If the primary tumor is identified endoscopically, appropriate tissue can be obtained for a pathologic diagnosis. An open biopsy should be performed only if less invasive methods have failed to obtain adequate tissue for a pathologic diagnosis. If malignancy is strongly suspected preoperatively, fresh tissue is given to the pathologist at the time of surgery for immunologic studies and to detect markers and receptors.

SPECIFIC PATHOLOGY

The evaluation of a neck mass in an adolescent should be performed systematically on the basis of location. Inflammatory processes are the leading cause of lymph node enlargement within this age group; malignancy, either primary or metastatic, is much less common but certainly more sinister in prognosis. The evaluation of a neck mass begins with an understanding of the patterns of lymphatic drainage in the head and neck.

There are approximately 300 lymph nodes in the head and neck. All the lymphatic drainage ultimately ends in the thoracic duct. The lymph nodes vary in size from 1 to 25 mm in diameter. Any description of the patterns of drainage to these regional lymph nodes (Table 153-1) is by necessity an oversimplification, because exceptions to usual pathways do occur and on occasion a metastatic lesion will bypass nodes and first be manifested in a more distant site. Thus, no one drainage area is pathognomonic for a primary site of tumor. When the pattern of lymph node drainage is understood, neck masses can be evaluated on the basis of anatomic location.

TABLE 153-1
Patterns of Lymph Drainage from Head and Neck

Regional Lymph Node Group	Areas Drained
Preauricular/intraparotid	External ear, upper face, parotid gland, temporal scalp, posterior teeth
Postauricular/occipital	Temporoparietal scalp, posterior scalp, mastoid, external ear
Submental	Floor of mouth, anterior lip, buccal mucosa, anterior teeth
Submandibular	Floor of mouth, anterior tongue, lips, nose, buccal mucosa, teeth, submandibular gland
Upper jugular (anterior border of SCM)	Nasopharynx, anterior tongue, base of tongue, palatine tonsil, parotid gland, ear, floor of mouth
Middle and lower jugular, including thyroid (anterior border of SCM)	Larynx, hypopharynx, thyroid gland, cervical esophagus
Posterior triangle (posterior border of SCM)	Nasopharynx, posterior neck and scalp, thyroid gland, cervical esophagus
Supraclavicular	Thyroid gland, lungs, breasts, gastrointestinal tract
Retropharyngeal (Rouviere's)	Nasopharynx, posterior nose, paranasal sinuses

SCM, sternocleidomastoid muscle.

NON–SITE-SPECIFIC MASSES

Inflammatory Lesions

LYMPHADENITIS. Lymphadenopathy caused by bacterial or viral inflammatory processes is undoubtedly the most common cause of a neck mass in adolescents and can present in any region of the neck. Nodes increase in size acutely at the time of infection and most often gradually subside. Since most of these infections are self-limited, they rarely require biopsy or incision and drainage. They usually resolve within 5 to 10 days and require only supportive therapy such as antipyretics, decongestants, and analgesics. Varicella, mumps, herpes simplex, and rubeola cause cervical adenopathy, however, with a clinical course prolonged for up to 14 days. Rubella is associated with postauricular as well as cervical adenopathy. Bacterial cervical adenitis caused by *S. aureus* and group A streptococcus still remain the most common bacterial pathogens. Bacterial adenitis is usually preceded by an upper respiratory infection, which in itself can lead to fever, swollen glands, feeding difficulties, and lethargy. The relatively low incidence of reactive adenopathy in reported large series of neck masses is attributable to the likelihood that most patients with reactive adenopathy never seek medical attention.

CAT-SCRATCH DISEASE. Cat-scratch disease is a common cause of chronic cervical adenopathy. It is a self-limiting lymphadenitis following a primary skin lesion that occurs in children or young adults as a result of a scratch or bite by a cat. Initially considered to be rickettsial in etiology, it is presently regarded as being of unknown cause. However, on Warthin-Starry silver impregnation stain a gram-negative bacillus is generally seen, which is considered by some to be the cat-scratch bacillus. Cat-scratch disease has been known to occur in all parts of the world. It is most commonly seen in temperate climates and between the months of September and February. Eighty percent of cases have been diagnosed in patients under the age of 20; 95% of these patients have had contact with or been scratched by a cat. The disease has also been reported in people having been bitten by a dog or monkey. There are no reported cases of person-to-person transmission.

The pathologic appearance of the lymph nodes includes a progression from a reticulum cell hyperplasia to a tubercle-like granuloma with Langerhans giant cells and formation of microabscesses. All of these stages may occur in one lymph node. The patient with cat-scratch disease presents with primary skin lesions (seen in 50% of affected patients) approximately 10 days after innoculation. Tender, cervical lymphadenopathy occurs 3 to 30 days after exposure in association with fever, headache, and malaise. This is followed by a 2- to 3-month indolent course. To diagnose cat-scratch disease, three of the following four criteria should be fulfilled: (1) history of cat contact, scratch/bite, and/or primary cutaneous lesion; (2) sterile, purulent material from the involved node; (3) pathologic characteristics of the involved lymph node; and (4) a positive skin test (Hangar-Rose).

No specific treatment is necessary unless the patient is acutely ill, in which case a course of antibiotics against

Staphylococcus and *Streptococcus* organisms is indicated. Incision and drainage is not wise, as this may lead to the development of a drainage sinus tract that persists for months. Recurrent needle aspirations are a more sensible approach from both diagnostic and management standpoints.

INFECTIOUS MONONUCLEOSIS. This condition is caused by the Epstein-Barr virus. Generalized cervical adenopathy is encountered, although it is predominantly found in the nodes surrounding the jugular chain. Waldeyer's ring may be markedly enlarged to the point of upper airway embarrassment; exudative tonsillitis can be present with an irregular white membrane. Hepatosplenomegaly is frequently encountered. The patient often presents with weakness, malaise, and fever. Atypical lymphocytes are identified in the peripheral blood smear; agglutination test results, such as Paul-Bunnell, are positive. Management is supportive, including hydration, bed rest, and analgesics. Recovery should occur within 2 to 4 weeks, but cases with hepatomegaly may take up to 6 weeks. A brief course of steroids frequently causes rapid improvement in symptoms and may be indicated to ameliorate difficulty with swallowing or breathing. (See Chapter 66, "Infectious Mononucleosis and Epstein-Barr Virus Infections.")

KAWASAKI DISEASE (MUCOCUTANEOUS LYMPH NODE SYNDROME). Kawasaki disease is a vasculitis of unknown cause affecting multiple organ systems. The disease has multiple head and neck manifestations, including stomatitis, pharyngitis, and cervical adenopathy. It is accompanied by high spiking fevers, bilateral conjunctivitis, dry erythematous lips, strawberry tongue, and skin lesions. Many patients may also have serious cardiac problems; in fact, Kawasaki disease has surpassed acute rheumatic fever as the leading cause of acquired heart disease among young children in the United States.

Laboratory abnormalities associated with Kawasaki disease include anemia, leukocytosis, and thrombocytosis. There is no specific laboratory test, and so the diagnosis is usually made from a compilation of clinical features. It must be distinguished from various other diseases such as poststreptococcal disease and Stevens-Johnson syndrome.

Involvement of deep cervical lymph nodes produces large hypodense lesions on CT scan, which may lead to the misdiagnosis of a deep neck abscess and subsequent unnecessary surgery.

Treatment consists of early administration of salicylates and immune globulin to prevent cardiac sequelae. This treatment has proved effective in several studies. Recovery usually occurs in patients who do not develop cardiac complications, although rare second attacks do occur.

Granulomatous Processes

TUBERCULOSIS AND ATYPICAL MYCOBACTERIAL INFECTIONS. Both of these diseases are encountered in adolescents, especially in human immunodeficiency virus (HIV)-positive patients, and may present as a fluctuant or draining cervical mass. Enlargement of the superficial lymph nodes is an integral element of primary tuberculosis. Tonsillar and submandibular nodes most commonly are affected, probably as an extension from peritracheal nodes and not from the tonsil (as was previously thought). Enlargement of the supraclavicular nodes can accompany primary pulmonary lesions in the upper lung fields.

The lymph nodes are initially rubbery, painless, and discrete. Thereafter, gradual enlargement of the glands occurs, with matting, caseation, and sinus tract formation. In addition to tuberculosis, atypical mycobacterial infection in adolescents is commonly manifested by cervical lymphadenitis. The diagnosis and treatment of tuberculosis are addressed in Chapter 68, "Tuberculosis."

SARCOIDOSIS. Sarcoidosis is a multisystem granulomatous disorder of unknown etiology; however, it has been speculated that it could be infectious, immunologic, or an abnormal reaction to tubercular disease. It is characterized by widespread epithelioid granulomas, usually of the lymphoreticular tissue; histologically, noncaseating epithelioid tubercles are the hallmark along with mononuclear cells, giant cells of Langerhans with inclusion bodies, Schaumann's and asteroid bodies. Also noted is depression of the delayed-type hypersensitivity reaction, impaired T-cell function, and lymphoproliferation. It usually presents in the older adolescent. It affects people in various parts of the southern United States and Australia; it is more commonly seen in African-Americans and Puerto Ricans, and the female-to-male ratio is 2:1. Cervical lymph nodes are affected most often, but other sites such as nose, nasopharynx, paranasal sinuses, larynx, pharynx, salivary glands, auditory system, and cranial nerves are further manifestations of sarcoid in the head and neck region. The cervical nodes are discrete, rubbery, and movable. Systemic involvement is widespread and can include the eye, parotid gland, lung, spleen, liver, and other organs. Hilar lymphadenopathy as identified on the chest film is an early sign. Low-grade fever, parotid gland swelling, uveitis, and facial palsy may be seen. The patient often complains of malaise and weight loss.

On laboratory examination, the serum protein concentration is often abnormally high. Eosinophilia is noted in over 50% of patients. Other nonspecific abnormalities may include elevation of the ESR and alkaline phosphatase levels and a depressed WBC count. The Kveim test is frequently positive, but a false-positive rate of 1% to 2% is seen in patients with leprosy, Crohn's disease, ulcerative colitis, celiac disorders, and various lymphad-enopathies. Fifty percent of patients fail to react to Kveim antigen within 5 years of onset of disease. Angiotensin-converting enzyme (ACE) titers are elevated in 80% to 90% of patients with active disease, but in treated or inactive disease it is normal or only slightly elevated. There is no specific treatment, but steroids have been used to treat respiratory involvement.

Neoplastic Lesions

Approximately 10% of neck masses that undergo biopsy are malignant. Lymphoma is by far the most common malignancy encountered, followed by thyroid carcinoma and rhabdomyosarcoma.

LIPOMA. Lipoma is a benign process that can occur anywhere in the neck. Needle aspiration is frequently nondiagnostic. The lesion is very slow-growing and can be followed clinically. Indications for surgery are an increase in size or a suspicious needle aspirate.

LYMPHOMA. Lymphoma is the third most common malignancy in children under the age of 14 years. It is the most common nonepithelial tumor and the most common malignant tumor of the head and neck. In children aged 8 years and older, such neoplasms are equally divided between Hodgkin's and non-Hodgkin's lymphomas.

Hodgkin's lymphoma. There is a high incidence of Hodgkin's lymphoma during the adolescent years, reaching a peak in adults in their late twenties. In 80% to 90% of patients the presentation is of an asymptomatic cervical mass consisting of nodes that are typically nontender, mobile, and rubbery in consistency. Extranodal presentation in the head and neck is uncommon. About one half of patients present with localized disease. Roughly one third present with systemic symptoms, including weight loss, night sweats, and fever. When lower cervical nodes are involved, mediastinal adenopathy is frequently present. At biopsy, marked infiltration of the lymph node is noted with progression to granuloma formation. Pleomorphism and large multinucleated giant cells with abundant cytoplasm (Reed-Sternberg cells) can usually be identified. Hodgkin's lymphoma must be differentiated from granulomatous disease.

Non-Hodgkin's lymphoma. Cervical lymphade-nopathy as the primary symptom is less common in non-Hodgkin's lymphoma than in Hodgkin's lymphoma. However, most patients with non-Hodgkin's lymphoma present with systemic signs. The non-Hodgkin's form is more likely than Hodgkin's to be found extranodally and to be disseminated at the time of presentation. Most extranodal lesions of the head and neck are in Waldeyer's ring; the tonsil is the most common site of involvement. In general, non-Hodgkin's lymphoma in adolescents is a more malignant process than that in adults. Staging is essential before initiation of a specific therapy, which

consists of chemotherapy, radiotherapy, or a combination of the two. (See Chapter 51, "Malignant Solid Tumors.")

RHABDOMYOSARCOMA AND NEUROBLASTOMA. Rhabdomyosarcoma and neuroblastoma, although common in children, are far less common during adolescence and even more rarely present as a neck mass.

SITE-SPECIFIC MASSES (FIG. 153-1)

Preauricular/Intraparotid Region

FIRST BRANCHIAL CLEFT ANOMALIES. These cysts and sinuses are remnants of the branchial apparatus that is related embryologically to the gill slits. They are very uncommon, representing only about 1% of all branchial cleft anomalies. They have been recognized since the first case report by Sir James Paget in 1878. Formation of first branchial cleft sinuses is thought to be due to failure of obliteration of the corresponding branchial cleft and pouch.

Mounsey et al (1993) described the 7-year experience at the Hospital for Sick Children at Toronto, identifying nine cases. Recurrent periauricular or angle of mandible erythema, swelling, and/or drainage was seen in all patients. Two had recurrent aural drainage. Of interest, most patients had undergone multiple limited procedures before diagnosis.

As the sinus tract can have an unpredictable relationship to the facial nerve, the definitive surgical procedure is superficial parotidectomy with definite identification of the facial nerve and the tract of the fistula, followed by excision of the sinus and fistula.

Inflammatory Lesions

PAROTITIS. There are three types of parotitis: mumps, bacterial parotitis, and benign lymphoepithelial disease of the parotid. With mumps, swelling of the salivary glands occurs, usually bilaterally. Sensorineural hearing loss and meningoencephalitis may also be present. Of importance to the adolescent male is the possibility of mumps orchitis, which potentially can cause sterility. Management is supportive and nonsurgical.

Bacterial parotitis is uncommon in healthy adolescents, and generally this process is seen only in immunocompromised patients. The usual infecting organism is *S. aureus*. Management includes hydration, an appropriate antibiotic regimen, and sialagogues.

Benign lymphoepithelial disease of the parotid is common in HIV-positive patients. It presents as unilateral or bilateral multicystic swelling of the parotid glands. Treatment is debatable. In a series from Columbia Presbyterian Medical Center in New York, Huang et al (1991) reviewed their own patients as well as 19 other series of 118 HIV-positive patients with parotid masses. Of the cystic lesions, only 1% were malignant; of the solid lesions, 40% were malignant. The authors' recommendation is to perform recurrent needle aspirations on all cystic lesions and follow them with watchful waiting. Tissue must be obtained in all cases, as lymphoma, tuberculosis, and Kaposi's sarcoma are common in the HIV population. All patients with solid parotid masses should undergo surgical removal if medically stable.

NEOPLASTIC LESIONS. Salivary tumors are uncommon in children, representing only 1.7% to 3% of all such tumors. Parotid tumors are most frequently encountered. A review of salivary gland tumors at Children's Hospital in Boston (Lack, 1988) identified 80 patients aged 18 or younger with a diagnosed epithelial or nonepithelial lesion of salivary origin. In accordance with older studies, the most common tumor overall was a capillary hemangioma (34%). Of the epithelial tumors (which represented only 31% of the series), pleomorphic adenoma (benign mixed tumor) was the most common tumor identified. The most common malignant tumor was mucoepidermoid carcinoma.

Postauricular/Occipital Region

Congenital first branchial cysts may be encountered. Neoplasms are uncommon in the adolescents, but sebaceous cysts are found not infrequently in this location. It must be recalled that mastoiditis, even in the era of antibiotics, may present as a subperiosteal abscess with induration, erythema, and fullness in the postauricular region, with the pinna pushed forward. Management consists of appropriate antibiotic coverage and adequate surgical drainage. Histiocytosis X may also present in this fashion. Although uncommon, it must be considered, especially if associated with a draining ear, a skin rash, or an enlarged spleen.

Submental Region

THYROGLOSSAL DUCT CYSTS. Thyroglossal duct cysts (TDCs) are the most common nonodontogenic cysts occurring in the neck. They account for 70% of all congenital neck cysts. TDCs represent remnants of thyroid tissue that have remained after embryonic descent of the thyroid from a point between the tuberculum impar and cupula, which in later life becomes the foramen cecum linguae, to the lower neck. The cysts can occur anywhere along this pathway but most commonly are identified in the midline of the neck adjacent to the hyoid bone. They usually present as painless, midline lesions that are mobile and (unlike dermoids) move with tongue protrusion. Some present with a sudden increase in size after an upper respiratory tract infection; under these circumstances, they may be acutely inflamed.

In a recent series of 230 children with preoperative diagnosis of TDCs, 70% had histologically proved thyroglossal duct cysts. The most common error in diagnosis was of a dermoid, which was noted on histologic evaluation 17% of the time, followed by a hyperplastic lymph node (8%).

Surgical excision includes resection of the cyst in contiguity with the central portion of the hyoid and a tract of tissue toward the tongue base. Inclusion of the central hyoid bone (the Sistrunk procedure) has reduced recurrences from approximately 30% to less than 4%. Careful pathologic review of the specimen is required, as thyroid carcinoma has rarely been identified (less than 1% of TDCs).

DERMOIDS. Dermoids are a form of teratoma that contain only ectoderm and mesoderm. These cysts are lined with stratified squamous epithelium and contain hair follicles and sweat and sebaceous glands. Dermoids are relatively rare in the neck but may occur in the midline submental region. As noted, they are a major differential diagnosis in all surgical procedures performed in this area. They do not move on tongue protrusion. The treatment of choice is surgical removal.

NEOPLASTIC LESIONS. Lipomas may be found in the midline in the submental space. Once they have been differentiated from lymphoma, they either can be removed or treated by observation.

Submandibular Region

DERMOIDS. Dermoids also can be found in the submandibular region.

SUBMANDIBULAR SIALADENITIS. This process occurs secondary to obstruction of Wharton's duct, usually by a stone, with secondary infection of the gland. During an acute episode, the patient should be treated with antibiotics and a sialagogue. If the stone is distal, an attempt can be made to dilate the duct and remove the stone. A plane radiograph will demonstrate the calculus in most instances. Little diagnostic information is obtained by sialography, and this procedure has the potential to cause infection. If the nature of the tumefaction in the submandibular gland is in doubt, a needle aspiration biopsy should be performed or a CT scan obtained. Surgery is generally not performed for the first occurrence, but it is appropriate for cases of recurrent sialadenitis.

NEOPLASTIC LESIONS. Submandibular tumors are rare in adolescents. When they do occur, they are more likely to be malignant than parotid gland tumors.

Upper Jugular Region

BRANCHIAL CLEFT CYSTS. Second branchial cleft anomalies are by far the most common of the branchial apparatus remnants. Nonetheless, they are three times less common than thyroglossal duct cysts. Roughly one third are cysts only, and two thirds are associated with fistulas or sinuses. Second branchial cleft cysts are more frequently identified in adolescents or young adults than in young children. This is postulated on the basis that time and perhaps recurrent infection is required to fill the cysts with secretions.

Second branchial cleft cysts present as soft cystic masses anterior and deep to the anterior border of the sternocleidomastoid muscle. Although bilaterality may occur, 90% to 95% are unilateral and two thirds present on the left side of the neck. They are frequently identified after an upper respiratory infection, and thus may present with erythema of the overlying skin and be tender to palpation. The anatomic relations are well defined. The cyst lies deep to the sternocleidomastoid muscle and lies just superficial to the bifurcation of the carotid artery. The associated sinus tract, when present, is superficial to the ninth cranial nerve and may extend up to and communicate with the palatine tonsil. Treatment consists of surgical removal.

LARYNGOCELE. Laryngoceles represent a herniation of the saccule of the laryngeal ventricle, which lies between the true and false vocal folds. They can be internal (presenting within the endolarynx) or external. Only external laryngoceles present as neck masses. They do so by passing through the thyrohyoid membrane and into the lateral neck in the upper jugular region. Causes include coughing, straining, and playing wind instruments. They can be bilateral. External laryngoceles are compressible and expand with a Valsalva maneuver. Treatment consists of surgical removal during which the existence of an endolaryngeal component can also be determined.

LYMPHADENITIS. The upper jugular region is the most common site in the neck for lymphadenitis in adolescents.

NEOPLASTIC LESIONS. Nodes in the upper jugular region represent a primary drainage site for nasopharyngeal carcinoma, as well as carcinomas of the tongue and floor of the mouth. Fine-needle (23-gauge) aspiration can be performed for diagnosis. There is virtually no danger that such aspiration will seed tumor.

Middle and Lower Jugular Regions

In general, inflammatory and neoplastic processes presenting in these regions may be related to the organs and regions that they drain (i.e., larynx, hypopharynx, thyroid, cervical esophagus).

Branchial cleft cysts may present in the midjugular region in combination with the upper jugular region. Lower jugular processes may be a manifestation of thyroid pathologic conditions.

CONGENITAL JUVENILE/PUBERTAL GOITERS. Goiters are quite common during the adolescent years, particularly when the individual resides in an area where there is low iodine intake. Goiters are typically characterized as hyperthyroidism (Graves' disease), euthyroidism (nontoxic nodular goiter), or hypothyroidism (autoimmune thyroiditis). Goiters can cause symptoms of dysphagia and dyspnea, as well as cosmetic deformity. They can fail medical therapy and increase in size, causing compressive symptoms. They can also increase in size if malignant degeneration takes place. Benign goiters have been associated with symptoms such as pain and hoarseness, but this is uncommon and should raise the suspicion of malignancy. The management of adolescent goiters is primarily pharmacologic with L-thyroxine hormone to suppress enlargement of the goiter. From 6 to 12 months of treatment may be required before any response is noticed. If suppression therapy with thyroid hormone does not work and the patient is symptomatic, surgical removal is indicated. (See Chapter 24, "Thyroid Disorders.")

Endemic goiters are no longer a health problem in the United States, but they remain a major health problem in mountainous, underdeveloped regions. Treatment usually involves the provision of adequate dietary iodide.

HASHIMOTO'S THYROIDITIS (CHRONIC LYMPHOCYTIC THYROIDITIS). Hashimoto's thyroiditis is the most common type of thyroiditis in young people, with a female preponderance. Frequently, other members of the patient's family have a history of thyroid disease. A genetic predisposition has been described with HLA-B8 and HLA-DR5 antigens in this clearly autoimmune process. The most common form is goitrous thyroiditis, associated with elevated levels of antithyroid antibodies. About 90% of patients are positive for antimicrosomal antibody. Hashimoto's is often associated with other autoimmune processes such as Graves' disease. Patients with Hashimoto's thyroiditis often present with a slowly progressive, firm, diffusely enlarged but irregular mass in the lower anterior neck with little or no tenderness. Histologically, lymphocytic infiltration with fibrosis and Hürthle cell change of the follicular cells is common. Up to 20% of adolescents with Hashimoto's thyroiditis also present with signs of hypothyroidism. After pharmacologic restoration of an euthyroid state, the gland should return to normal. If there is no regression of size while the patient is on suppression therapy, the presence of lymphoma or a neoplasm must be entertained, as both of these entities have been associated with Hashimoto's thyroiditis. Surgical treatment is reserved for cases in which the diagnosis is suspect, to relieve symptoms, or for cosmetic reasons.

CARCINOMA OF THE THYROID. The incidence of thyroid cancer is lower in children than in adults; however, the likelihood that a nodular thyroid in fact represents a malignancy is higher in young people than in adults. Previous radiation treatment to this area of the neck is a predisposing risk factor for such tumors, which are two to three times more common in girls. The usual histologic appearance is that of papillary carcinoma.

Evaluation includes an assessment of thyroid function and a thyroid scan, followed by a needle aspiration biopsy. CT can also help identify involved lymph nodes. As the incidence of malignancy is high in these nodular lesions, surgery is indicated for either proved malignancy or even suspicious test results on cytology. The incidence of positive nodes at the time of surgery is quite high, yet these tumors tend not to be highly malignant and long-term survival is commonplace. In fact, it is generally thought that the presence of positive lymph nodes has no effect upon survival.

The minimal management of the primary lesion is removal of the ipsilateral thyroid lobe and isthmus. The minimal management of palpable lymph nodes is a functional neck dissection in which all major structures are preserved. Many centers advocate total or near-total thyroidectomy to allow for more efficacious use of postoperative radioactive iodine.

It is also not uncommon for a young patient with thyroid cancer to present with a lymph node in the lower jugular chain or even in the posterior triangle, with no clinically obvious thyroid mass. Needle aspiration of the node is diagnostic under these circumstances. Special stains may be required to demonstrate the presence of thyroglobulin.

Posterior Triangle Region

Drainage to the posterior triangle is from the nasopharynx, posterior neck and scalp, thyroid gland, and cervical esophagus. Infectious processes of the posterior scalp can thereby cause adenopathy in this location. A mass in the posterior triangle may represent the initial manifestation of a nasopharyngeal primary tumor. Thus, all such lesions call for needle aspiration.

Supraclavicular Region

The supraclavicular region is an unusual drainage area of processes of head and neck origin. Masses are frequently a manifestation of disease processes in distant areas of the body. Lesions in the apex of the lung, the gastrointestinal tract, and the breast may cause nodes to develop in this area. Thus, any masses in the supraclavicular region require an extensive search for pathologic conditions beyond the head and neck.

Retropharyngeal (Rouviere) Region

The retropharyngeal space is significant in adolescents as an area of potential infection. Retropharyngeal nodal involvement and abscess can occur in a young person after an upper respiratory viral infection or a bacterial infection in the posterior nose, nasopharynx, or paranasal sinuses. Infected nodes that are left untreated may lead to abscess formation with the potential for respiratory embarrassment.

SUMMARY

The development of cervical adenopathy and other neck masses during adolescence is quite common. Most cases of such adenopathy represent acute self-limiting infectious processes that are frequently never brought to medical attention. However, patients with persistent cervical masses that may be secondary to an inflammatory process, a congenital anomaly, thyroid dysfunction, or malignancy sometimes present for medical attention. The evaluation of such masses relies on a directed history, laboratory assessment, and physical examination that pays particular attention to the anatomic location of the mass. On the basis of this assessment, surgical intervention for diagnosis or treatment may be indicated.

Suggested Readings

Androulakis M, Johnson JT, Wagner RL: Thyroglossal duct and second branchial cleft anomalies in adults, *Ear Nose Throat J* 69:318-322, 1990.

Batsakis JG: *Tumors of the head and neck,* ed 2, Baltimore, 1979, Williams & Wilkins.

Black RR, Maxon HR III: Benign diseases of the thyroid gland. In Paparella MM, Shumrick DA, Gluckman JL, Meyerhoff WL, editors: *Otolaryngology,* ed. 3, Philadelphia, 1991, WB Saunders; pp 2483-2497.

Bordley JE, Brookhouser PE, Tucker GF, editors: *Ear, nose and throat disorders in children,* New York, 1986, Raven Press; pp 383-404.

Boswell WC, Zoller M, Williams JS, Lord SA, Check W: Thyroglossal duct carcinoma, *Am Surg* 60:650-655, 1994.

Boyer KM, Cherry JD: Cat scratch disease. In Feigin RD, Cherry JD, editors: *Textbook of pediatric infectious diseases,* ed 2, Philadelphia, 1987, WB Saunders; pp 2165-2170.

Butler KM, Baker CJ: Cervical lymphadenopathy. In Feigin RD, Cherry JD, editors: *Textbook of pediatric infectious diseases,* ed 2, Philadelphia, 1987, WB Saunders; pp 250-260.

DiBartolomeo JR, Paparella MM, Meyerhoff WL: Cysts and tumors of the external ear. In Paparella MM, Shumrick DA, Gluckman JL, Meyerhoff WL, editors: *Otolaryngology,* ed 3, Philadelphia, 1991, WB Saunders; pp 1243-1258.

Favus MJ, Schneider AB, Stachura ME, Arnold JE, Yun R, Pinsky SM, Colman M, Arnold MJ, Frohman LA: Thyroid cancer occurring as a late consequence of head-and-neck irradiation: evaluation of 1056 patients, *N Engl J Med* 294:1019-1025, 1976.

Fernandez JF, Ordonez NG, Schultz PN, Samaan NA, Hickey RC: Thyroglossal duct carcinoma, *Surgery* 110:928-934, 1991.

Girard M, De Luca SA: Thyroglossal duct cyst, *Am Fam Physician* 42:665-668, 1990.

Guarisco JL: Congenital head and neck masses in infants and children, *Ear Nose Throat J* 70:40-47, 1991.

Handler SD: Evaluation of neck masses in children: benign, malignant, and congenital. In Healy GB, editor: *Common problems in pediatric otolaryngology,* Chicago, 1990, Mosby–Year Book; pp 329-339.

Handler SD, Raney RB Jr: Management of neoplasms of the head and neck in children. I. Benign tumors, *Head Neck Surg* 3:395, 1981.

Hayles AB, Johnson LM, Beahrs OH, Woolner LB: Carcinoma of the thyroid in children, *Am J Surg* 106:735-743, 1963.

Healy GB: Malignant tumors of the head and neck in children: diagnosis and treatment, *Otolaryngol Clin North Am* 13:483-488, 1980.

Huang RD, Pearlman S, Friedman WH, Loree T: Benign cystic vs. solid lesions of the parotid gland in HIV patients, *Head Neck* Nov/Dec: 522-527, 1991.

Jacobs JR, Negendank WG: Lymphomas of the head and neck. In Paparella MM, Shumrick DA, Gluckman JL, Meyerhoff WL, editors: *Otolaryngology,* ed 3, Philadelphia, 1991, WB Saunders; pp 2591-2598.

Jaffe BF, Jaffe N: Diagnosis and treatment: head and neck tumors in children, *Pediatrics* 51:731-740, 1973.

Karmody CS: Developmental anomalies of the neck. In Bluestone CD, Stool SE, Scheetz MD, editors: *Pediatric otolaryngology,* ed 2, vol 2, Philadelphia, 1990, WB Saunders; pp 1303-1316.

Kendig EL Jr: The clinical picture of sarcoidosis in children, *Pediatrics* 54:289-292, 1974.

Lack EE, Upton MP: Histopathologic review of salivary gland tumors in childhood, *Arch Otolaryngol Head Neck Surg* 114:898-906, 1988.

Lusk RP: Neck masses. In Bluestone CD, Stool SE, Scheetz MD, editors: *Pediatric otolaryngology,* ed 2, vol 2, Philadelphia, 1990, WB Saunders; pp 1294-1302.

Maziak D, Borowy ZJ, Deitel M, Jaksik T, Ralph-Edwards A: Management of papillary carcinoma arising in thyroglossal-duct anlage, *Can J Surg* 35:522-525, 1992.

Mounsey RA, Forte V, Friedberg J: First branchial cleft sinuses: an analysis of current management strategies and treatment outcomes, *J Otolaryngol* 22:457-461, 1993.

Myer CM: Congenital neck masses. In Paparella MM, Shumrick DA, Gluckman JL, Meyerhoff WL, editors: *Otolaryngology,* ed 3, Philadelphia, 1991, WB Saunders; pp 2535-2543.

Nyberg DA, Jeffrey RB, Brant-Zawadzki M, Federle M, Dillon W: Computed tomography of cervical infections, *J Comput Assist Tomogr* 9:288-296, 1985.

Pontell J, Rosenfeld RM, Kohn B: Kawasaki disease mimicking retropharyngeal abscess, *Otolaryngol Head Neck Surg* 110:428-430, 1994.

Radkowski D, Arnold J, Healy GB, McGill T, Treves ST, Paltiel H, Friedman EM: Thyroglossal duct remnants: preoperative evaluation and management, *Arch Otolaryngol Head Neck Surg* 117:1378-1381, 1991.

Samuel AM, Sharma SM: Differentiated thyroid carcinomas in children and adolescents, *Cancer* 67:2186-2190, 1991.

Schneider AB, Favus MJ, Stachura ME, Arnold MJ, Frohman LA: Salivary gland neoplasms as a late consequence of head and neck irradiation, *Ann Intern Med* 87:160-164, 1977.

Silverman JF, Gurley AM, Holbrook CT, Joshi VV: Pediatric fine-needle aspiration biopsy, *Am J Clin Pathol* 95:653-659, 1991.

Stanievich JF: Cervical adenopathy. In Bluestone CD, Stool SE, Scheetz MD, editors: *Pediatric otolaryngology,* ed 2, vol 2, Philadelphia, 1990, WB Saunders; pp 1317-1327.

Torsiglieri AJ, Tom LWC, Ross AJ III, Wetmore RF, Handler SD, Potsic WP: Pediatric neck masses: guidelines for evaluation, *Int J Pediatr Otorhinolaryngol* 16:199-210, 1988.

Yanagisawa K, Eisen RN, Sasaki CT: Squamous cell carcinoma arising in a thyroglossal duct cyst, *Arch Otolaryngol Head Neck Surg* 118:538-541, 1992.

CHAPTER 154

Pectus Excavatum

•

Sylvain Kleinhaus

Congenital chest deformities in children and adolescents have been described for hundreds of years, but only in the past 50 years have successful methods of treatment been achieved. The severity of the defects ranges from minor cosmetic problems, such as a bifid xiphoid, to severe, deforming conditions, such as Poland's syndrome in which there is an absence of ribs and overlying muscles. The most common chest wall deformity is pectus excavatum, which comprises over 75% of the correctable chest wall abnormalities.

As first described by Ravitch, the condition is actually composed of several malformations. These deformities include a sternum depressed most severely in its inferior segments (which explains the original theory of a shortened xiphoid tendon), sloped or rounded shoulders, a protuberant abdomen or potbelly, and slight to moderate kyphosis. When taking deep breaths, patients with pectus excavatum also exhibited a paradoxical motion of the sternum: instead of expanding with the rest of the ribcage, the sternum moves posteriorly toward the spine on inspiration.

Originally it was believed that a shortened subxiphoid tendon was responsible for tethering the sternum posteriorly and causing pectus excavatum or funnel chest deformity, and the first unsuccessful operations were attempts at releasing this "tendon."

In 1928 the German surgeon Sauerbruch reported the first series of children and adolescents in whom pectus excavatum was successfully corrected, and since then the surgical procedure has been improved and refined. In 1949 Ravitch described in detail the deformity and the operation for its surgical correction, which is now the most widely employed technique against which all other such procedures are measured. In terms of defining the etiology of pectus excavatum, Ochsner and DeBakey were among the first to advance the theory, which has since been accepted by most clinicians, that the sternum is pushed posteriorly by the longitudinal overgrowth of the costal cartilages.

INDICATIONS FOR OPERATION

The earliest observations of children with pectus excavatum seemed to indicate that these patients were minimally to moderately handicapped in their physical activities, especially when participating is strenuous sports in which large vital capacities and maximal cardiac outputs were required. When the earliest and most rudimentary physiologic tests were devised, however, they seemed to indicate that these children experienced little or no deficit. As a result, many physicians caring for these patients were reluctant to refer them for corrective surgery. The operative morbidity was considered too high and the risk of failure too great for what was considered a purely cosmetic operation. As the parameters for physiologic testing were expanded, as the tests became more sophisticated, and as the results became more reproducible and less invasive, it became increasingly clear that not only was there a cosmetic raison d'être, but there was also very sound functional physiologic indications for surgery. The original cardiac output tests were done with the patients at rest and supine, and the results demonstrated no real differences between controls and patients with pectus excavatum. The modern exercise stress tests now available have shown that young adults afflicted with pectus excavatum have some physiologic deficits in cardiac and respiratory dynamics as the degree of exertion increases. Although there is still some controversy over the significance and severity of these deficits, it is now more generally accepted that the indications for operative repair are not only cosmetic and psychologic but also physiologic and serve to improve the patients' functional capabilities. Only in the mildest cases should pectus excavatum not be surgically treated (Fig. 154-1).

Computed tomography (CT) has also contributed to the ability to measure the degree of deformity. In a normal individual the "pectus index," which is the widest transverse thoracic diameter divided by the shortest anteroposterior distance between the sternum and spine,

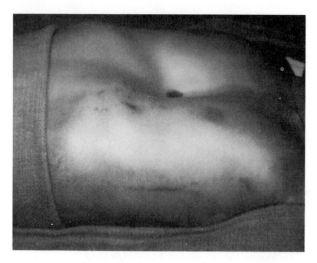

Fig. 154-1. Preoperative photograph of a 13-year-old boy with pectus excavatum. There is a small puddle of iodine solution at the bottom of the depression of the pectus.

should be below 3.25. CT scans allow the measurement of these dimensions.

OPERATIVE PROCEDURE

The operation performed by most surgeons is essentially as described by Ravitch in 1949. The original malformation is not always symmetric, but a complete bilateral operation should be performed except under the most unusual circumstances; only by performing a complete operation can the surgeon be sure of freeing the sternum and reducing the chances of recurrence. A transverse incision is made at the level of the fifth interspace and carried down to the periosteum of the sternum. In females, it is important to place the incision at or just below the inframammary fold in order to avoid future breast deformities. Flaps are then created to the sternal notch above and xiphoid below, and the costal cartilages are exposed. The third to sixth costal cartilages are removed bilaterally in a subperiosteal fashion. The seventh and rarely the eighth costal cartilage must sometimes be removed also if they are abnormal. An osteotomy of the anterior sternal cortex allows the inferior portion of the sternum to be straightened and brought back to its normal position. Some surgeons believe the results to be improved by the insertion of a strut beneath the sternum to maintain it in its corrected position; others believe this to be unnecessary.

Pneumothorax and wound hematomas are the most common early operative complications and are easily treated by appropriate aspiration and/or suction catheter drainage.

The optimal age for operation is between 6 and 10 years. By this time the deformity has stabilized and its extent can be properly assessed, but it is before the adolescent growth spurt and before the child must face potentially embarrassing situations in the gym locker room.

FOLLOW-UP

Long-term follow-up of these patients is important, because recurrences are often delayed. Recurrence may be due in part to the continued growth of any abnormal cartilaginous remnant and any added stress applied to the healing sternum and cartilages by the normal growth and expansion of the chest in adolescents. There is a postoperative recurrence rate of 5% to 10%, but many of these recurrences are minimal in severity and do not require reoperation.

The presternal area has a tendency to form hypertrophied or keloid scars, and because cosmesis is often a significant factor in the decision for surgery, the patients and family should be forewarned of this possibility.

Suggested Readings

Ghory MJ, James FW, Mays W: Cardiac performance in children with pectus excavatum, *J Pediatr Surg* 24:751, 1989.

Haller JA Jr, Kramer SS, Lietman SA: Use of CT scans in selection of patients for pectus excavatum surgery: a preliminary report, *J Pediatr Surg* 22:904, 1987.

Ravitch MM: The operative treatment of pectus excavatum, *Ann Surg* 129:429, 1949.

Shamberger RC, Welch KJ: Surgical repair of pectus excavatum, *J Pediatr Surg* 23:615, 1988.

CHAPTER 155

Breast Tumors

•

Richard G. Rosen

BENIGN TUMORS

Fibroadenomas

Fibroadenomas are the most frequent breast masses occurring in children and adolescents and are more common than all other breast masses combined. These tumors occur mainly in pubertal females but have on rare occasions been noted in children before menarche. They appear to be hormonally dependent in some way—not only are they found predominantly in the adolescent or young woman, but they rarely appear for the first time after menopause. Fibroadenomas are usually asymptomatic and are discovered accidentally by the patient or by a physician during a routine examination. They are firm, discrete, freely movable masses and are multiple or bilateral in up to 20% of patients. Although usually 1 to 3 cm in diameter at the time they are noticed, they may grow to great size. The term *fibroadenomatosis* has been used to describe the rare cases in which numerous tumors occur throughout both breasts. This condition would have to be differentiated from virginal hypertrophy in which similar histologic characteristics are found but in which the breast tissue is uniformly involved without encapsulated tumors.

The natural history of fibroadenomas is slow growth over a few years followed by a period during which they may remain stationary in size. There is no long-term study of fibroadenomas that were not excised, but one study interpreted the variation in histologic appearance of fibroadenomas excised at different ages to indicate that regression may occur after many years. A minor percentage of fibroadenomas remain small for 3 to 5 years and then grow rapidly to a very large size. These giant fibroadenomas can be differentiated histologically from

unilateral virginal hypertrophy and from cystosarcoma phyllodes, although all three can produce massive enlargement and distortion of one breast. Prominent dilated veins, adherence, and ulceration of the overlying skin can occur with these very large tumors, whose average weight in one study was 7.6 pounds.

The necessity for excising fibroadenomas of the breast has been questioned by some nonsurgeons since these are benign tumors and appear to be easily identified. Excision remains mandatory for three reasons: (1) an absolute diagnosis cannot be made by physical examination (one such lesion in our experience turned out to be a histologically malignant cystosarcoma phyllodes arising from a preexisting fibroadenoma); (2) small fibroadenomas may undergo sudden rapid growth, causing permanent alterations in breast contour; and (3) phychologic studies of girls with breast tumors that were not excised reveal that the girls suffer significant continuing anxiety.

Excision of most fibroadenomas can be performed through a circumareolar incision and undermining of the skin. Enucleation of the tumor without removing any normal breast tissue is all that is required and is associated with few recurrences.

Cystosarcoma Phyllodes

This impressive tumor is much less common than the fibroadenoma, from which it is sometimes derived, and represents only 2% to 3% of the fibroepithelial tumors. They are usually clinically indistinguishable from fibroadenomas, but their large size and sometimes rapid growth can suggest the diagnosis. The diagnosis of cystosarcoma is based on the presence of stromal overgrowth and hypercellularity in association with intracystic stromal projections on histologic section. The disease is more common in patients over the age of 40, but numerous reports of cystosarcoma in adolescents have appeared. These tumors can even occur before menarche.

Although listed here with the benign tumors, a minority of these tumors have the microscopic features of

Modified from Rosen RG: Disorders of the Breast. In Boley SJ, Cohen MI, editors: *Surgery of the adolescent,* Orlando FL, 1986, Grune & Stratton; pp 10-14. Copyright WB Saunders.

malignancy, and some of them metastasize and cause death. The metastasizing malignant form has been reported in adolescents and, in one case, in a prepubertal girl. Treatment consists of wide local excision, including a margin of normal breast tissue. Recurrences of the benign form are not uncommon, and malignant transformations upon recurrence have occurred. If the malignant variety is diagnosed and the original excision was inadequate (e.g., when the excision was performed for a presumed fibroadenoma), immediate reexcision is indicated. Mastectomy is reserved for cases of recurrence or when the tumor involves the entire breast.

Intraductal Papillomas

Solitary intraductal papillomas usually present with serous or serosanguineous nipple discharge. A palpable mass is unusual. This lesion is not common in the young: only two of 173 cases reported by Haagensen occurred in women under 20—both were 18 years old. This lesion consists of a grossly visible papillary tumor arising in, and often filling, a lactiferous duct and sometimes extending up the duct a few centimeters. It can even grow into an adjacent cyst. The involved duct or ducts can almost always be identified preoperatively by careful, stepwise, circumferential palpation. Treatment of this benign lesion consists of excision of the involved ductal system through a circumareolar incision. The duct containing the papilloma can be identified and defined at operation by gross examination and meticulous dissection. Cosmetic and functional postoperative results are excellent.

Multiple papillomatosis is a different disease. Aside from the obvious difference of multiplicity, the lesion is much rarer but much more likely than solitary papillomas to occur in the adolescent. It is also a more serious lesion, as it either is premalignant itself or occurs in patients who frequently develop cancer of the breast later in life. Only wide local excision is advised, but careful follow-up is indicated for many years, if not for life.

Other Benign Tumors

Benign tumors of the skin and soft tissues occur in and around the breast and generally behave as they do elsewhere. Lipomas, keratomas, papillomas, lymphangiomas, and hemangiomas are not uncommon, with hemangiomas often presenting at birth and growing rapidly during the first 2 years of life. Hemangiomas rarely should be excised, since in most instances they spontaneously regress. Resection may also injure or remove part of the undeveloped breast. Other benign tumors should be removed, while resection of the breast itself should be avoided.

MALIGNANT TUMORS

Breast cancer is rare in patients under the age of 25 but not unknown. In a 1977 review of the literature through 1972, Ashikari et al were able to find reports of 74 cancers in patients under the age of 20; seven patients were male. There have been enough additional reports since then to bring the total close to 100 cases. All the patients presented with a firm or hard mass, usually subareolar in location. Obvious metastases at the time of diagnosis were unusual.

For most adolescent patients, treatment should be similar to that in adults. A modified radical mastectomy (total mastectomy and axillary dissection) is the currently preferred operation if there is no fixation of the tumor to the muscle. For tumors in prepubertal children, wide excision may be adequate. There is currently a strong trend in the treatment of early breast cancer to perform less radical surgery and only with combination therapy. Wide excision of the primary tumor, axillary sampling, and postoperative radiotherapy is probably as adequate as modified radical mastectomy for most breast cancers and has the advantage of preserving the patient's original breast. The radical radiotherapy required, however, may not be advisable in a teenager and carries complications of its own. A lumpectomy alone can be done, but this is still unproved therapy. In view of the remarkable improvements in the technique and results of breast reconstruction during the past decade, a total mastectomy, axillary dissection, and either immediate or delayed reconstruction is our choice.

Most malignant breast tumors in adolescents are typical adenocarcinomas as seen in adults. However, about one third of young patients with breast cancer have a variant characterized by (1) less intense staining of cytoplasm with eosin, simulating the clear cell appearance of some renal tumors; and (2) the presence of eosinophilic secretory material in the cytoplasm of tumor cells and in rudimentary ductlike spaces formed by the tumor. Tumors with this pattern, described initially by McDivitt and Steward as "juvenile adenocarcinomas," have been renamed "secretory carcinomas" by Tavassoli and Norris, since not all appear in juveniles. They appear to have a better prognosis than the usual intraductal carcinomas. Modified radical mastectomy is probably the safest treatment for secretory carcinomas, although their more favorable prognosis has prompted some researchers to recommend only wide excision.

Angiosarcoma and other soft tissue sarcomas have been described in the breast of the adolescent but are extremely rare. Treatment is based on the principles appropriate for the specific type of sarcoma rather than on the location. Surgical excision, radiotherapy, and chemotherapy are all part of the therapeutic regimen.

Suggested Readings

Ashikari H, Jun MY, Farrow JH, et al: Breast carcinomas in children and adolescents, *Clin Bull* 7:55, 1977.

Haagensen CD: *Diseases of the breast,* ed 3, Philadelphia, 1986, WB Saunders; p 138.

Hoover HC, Trestioreann A, Ketcham AS: Metastatic cystosarcoma phyllodes in an adolescent girl. An unusually malignant tumor, *Ann Surg* 181:279, 1975.

McDivitt RW, Steward FW: Breast carcinoma in children, *JAMA* 195:388, 1966.

Rosenthal TM, Weiss E: Precocious puberty and sexual immaturity. In Gold JJ, Josimovich JB, editors: *Gynocologic endocrinology,* ed 3, New York, 1980, Harper & Row; pp 625-641.

Tavassoli FA, Norris HJ: Secretory carcinoma of the breast, *Cancer* 45:2404, 1980.

CHAPTER 156

Management of Solid Tumors

•

Ronald Nathaniel Kaleya

The role of the surgical oncologist in the treatment of solid malignancies in the pediatric and adolescent population extends from the diagnosis to the planning of definitive treatment and requires integration with the pediatric oncologist, radiotherapist, and pediatrician or internist. (See also Chapter 51 for a discussion of solid tumors.)

Although malignant diseases are uncommon in youth, cancer accounts for approximately 11% of all deaths in patients under 15 years of age. Sixty percent of the malignancies in this age group are solid tumors (Box 156-1). If lymphomas are included in this consideration, the surgeon has a significant role in the treatment of 75% of all pediatric and adolescent cancers.

DIAGNOSIS

The initial therapy for a solid mass is determined by its histology. The biopsy technique is extremely important in the planning of definitive surgery. Several biopsy techniques are presently available; however, each type has specific indications, applications, and limitations.

Fine-Needle Aspiration Biopsy

Cells are aspirated with a 21-gauge needle, smeared onto glass slides, and fixed in 95% alcohol. In general, this type of biopsy is useful in the evaluation of thyroid nodules and metastases once the histologic diagnosis of the primary tumor is known. It is not helpful in most of the intraabdominal tumors found in the pediatric and adolescent age group, nor is it useful in the diagnosis of lymphoma.

Core-Needle Biopsy

This biopsy method provides a $2 \times 2 \times 10$ mm core of tissue that can be evaluated by routine histologic techniques. However, this method is inadequate when special stains are required, as in the case with lymphomas and soft tissue sarcomas.

Incisional or Excisional Biopsy

An open biopsy technique is required in all cases in which a large amount of tissue is required for histologic diagnosis, immunophenotyping, and immunohistochemical analysis. Although small (<2 cm) tumors can be excised, large or deep tumors are best assessed through a generous incisional biopsy. The site and orientation of an incisional biopsy must be chosen so that the performance of future definitive surgery will not be compromised. Therefore, biopsies on the trunk should be performed along the skin lines, and biopsies on the extremities should be oriented along the axis of the limb.

BOX 156-1
BOX 156-1
Solid Tumors of Adolescents

Lymphoma
Neuroblastoma (rare)
Soft tissue sarcomas
Wilms' tumor (uncommon)
Bone tumors

LYMPHOMA

Lymphoma is the second most common solid malignancy in children. There are two distinct forms: Hodgkin's and non-Hodgkin's lymphomas. The incidence of non-Hodgkin's lymphoma is about 1.5 times that of Hodgkin's lymphomas in the adolescent and preadolescent age groups. Up to the age of 10 years, there is a significant male predominance, which decreases rapidly after puberty.

The surgeon's role in these diseases is limited to biopsy and treatment planning. A patient presenting with painless adenopathy should undergo an excisional biopsy of an enlarged lymph node. The node should be excised in its entirety and delivered to the pathologist without formalin fixation. It should also be sent for immunophenotyping, which can be performed only on a fresh specimen.

Hodgkin's Disease

Surgical staging remains a controversial issue in the treatment of Hodgkin's disease in the adolescent. Despite optimal preoperative evaluation with chest computed tomography (CT) scans, abdominal CT scans, and lymphangiography, surgical staging of the pediatric Hodgkin's patient will alter therapy in approximately 30% of patients. There is minimal operative morbidity associated with such staging. The procedures performed during the staging laparotomy include splenectomy, multiple liver biopsies, and node sampling, and their performance is directed by both clinical examination and the presence of abnormalities on the preoperative lymphangiogram.

Current treatment programs vary among institutions, and therefore surgical staging should be used only in those centers in which primary radiation therapy is considered an appropriate therapeutic alternative for early-stage disease. Staging laparotomy is not indicated in those instances in which the patient will be treated by chemotherapy irrespective of the finding at laparotomy. These include involvement of more than one third of the diameter of the chest, B-type symptoms (fevers, weight loss, sweats), and bone marrow involvement. There are

some periods in a child's life when there is an increased risk of growth retardation and deformity as a result of primary radiation therapy, and the decision as to whether radiation therapy is appropriate for an individual patient should be decided before a staging laparotomy is performed.

Non-Hodgkin's Lymphomas

This group of lymphomas generally presents with stage III or IV disease, making staging laparotomy unwarranted in these patients. The surgeon's role is limited to diagnosis. On occasion, after the completion of therapy, the surgeon may have a role in the evaluation of a residual intraabdominal mass detected through an imaging modality. The mainstay therapy for non-Hodgkin's lymphomas is chemotherapy.

NEUROBLASTOMA

Neuroblastoma is the most common intraabdominal malignancy in the child, with approximately 500 new cases diagnosed each year in the United States. More than half of the cases are manifested within the first year of life, with a peak incidence at 2 years of age. It is relatively rare during adolescence.

This disease is considered a congenital neoplasm of the fetal neural crest tissues. It can arise anywhere along the sympathetic nervous system, including the adrenal medulla and the paravertebral ganglia from the cervical to the lumbar regions. Approximately 65% of these tumors are in the abdomen.

Presenting symptoms are usually nonspecific and include irritability, weight loss, anemia, fatigue, and bone pain; less frequently, oculogyric crisis, cerebellar ataxia, and diarrhea occur. Although most neuroblastomas are metabolically functional, with secretion of vasoactive amines in more than 90% of cases, hypertension in this patient population remains uncommon.[1]

Preoperative evaluation should include an abdominal or chest CT scan. Magnetic resonance imaging (MRI) has proved to be as accurate as CT in the diagnosis of neuroblastoma. The adrenal lesions are frequently shown to displace the kidney inferiorly and outwardly as the adrenal mass enlarges. About half of the lesions are calcified. An intravenous pyelogram is not essential; when performed, it will show no involvement of the renal parenchyma. The possibility of metastases to the lungs and bones should be evaluated with a chest radiograph and bone scintigraphy. Meta-iodobenzylguanidine, a norepinephrine analog concentrated by the neuroblastoma cells, can be tagged to a radioisotope and used for more precise localization of primary and metastatic tumor deposits.[2]

Laboratory aids in the evaluation of a suspected neuroblastoma include liver function tests and determination of lactate dehydrogenase levels and levels of vanillylmandelic acid (VMA) and homovanillic acid (HVA) in the urine. Liver function tests are useful to screen for hepatic metastases. In up to 80% of patients with neuroblastoma, the VMA and HVA urinary levels are found to be elevated. The level tests are fairly good markers of response to therapy. However, in some cases the levels of these by-products of catecholamine metabolism remain elevated for years after a clinical complete response to therapy.

Although there are several staging systems for this disease (Box 156-2), the Pediatric Oncology Group staging system, the St. Jude's Children Research Hospital staging system, and the Evans' staging system are used most frequently. Retrospective analysis of survival has shown that large tumor size, tumor extension beyond the anatomic midline, nonresectability, and older age are poor prognostic variables. Other prognostic variables, including thoracic versus abdominal site; degree of regional lymph node involvement; and elevated serum levels of GD_2 ganglioside antigen, serum ferritin, and neuron-specific enolase, have been associated with a decreased survival rate in some studies.[3]

The treatment of neuroblastoma in the pediatric and adolescent populations is determined by both the stage of the disease and the age of the patient. Patients with Evans' stage I or II disease may need no further therapy after complete tumor excision, depending on other prognostic factors such as favorable histology or markers. At the time of surgery, it is essential to evaluate the status of the regional lymph nodes, because in some studies discontinuous involvement of the lymph nodes has had grave prognostic implications. The addition of chemotherapy or radiation therapy to the treatment of young children with neuroblastoma is not advised, because there is excellent long-term survival (>90%) with surgery alone and the salvage therapy is reasonably good. For children with extensive disease that is found to be unresectable at the time of exploratory laparotomy, only a biopsy is indicated. The patient is treated for 4 to 6 months with chemotherapy, which is followed by "second look" laparotomy. At the time of the second laparotomy, unresectable disease should be debulked in preparation for further therapy. In the older child and adolescent, radiation therapy may be added to the treatment regimen.

An exception to this treatment protocol is stage IVS neuroblastoma, which is disease that would otherwise be considered stage I or II but with remote disease confined to the liver, bone marrow, or skin. Patients with stage IVS disease who are untreated or who receive chemotherapy do surprisingly well (50% to 80% 5-year survival). The chemotherapy group experiences more rapid regression of the enormous tumor burden. Surgery in patients with

---

BOX 156-2
Staging of Neuroblastoma

Stage I   Tumor confined to a single organ or structure amenable to complete resection.

Stage II   Tumor extends beyond organ of origin but does not cross midline. Ipsilateral lymph nodes may be positive.

Stage III   Tumors that cross midline. Bilateral nodes may be positive.

Stage IV   Distant metastases to bone, other organs, and distant lymph nodes.

Stage IVS   Stage I or II disease with metastases confined to liver, skin, or bone marrow

---

stage IVS disease is often limited to biopsy or excision of the primary tumor. Children in whom the disease is asymptomatic should receive no further therapy. Therapy is reserved for palliation of feeding problems or other total local effects of the tumor mass.

Surgery has almost no role in the primary treatment of diffusely metastatic neuroblastoma other than to palliate symptoms and provide access for chemotherapy. Infants treated with one of several aggressive multimodality regimens have up to 80% survival, whereas only 3% of children over the age of 1 year are disease free at 2 years.[4] Traditional cytoreductive surgery (debulking) prior to initial therapy with chemotherapy has not been shown to improve survival in this group of patients. However, surgical restaging after induction chemotherapy may improve survival. Cyclophosphamide, vincristine, dacarbazine (DTIC), doxorubicin, teniposide, and cisplatin are the most active chemotherapeutic agents for this disease. Currently, the PACE regimen[5] (cyclophosphamide, etoposide, cisplatin, and doxorubicin) is the most commonly used combination. Bone marrow transplantation is being evaluated for the treatment of patients with disseminated disease or those children in whom standard therapies fail.

WILMS' TUMOR

Wilms' tumor is the most common, although not the only, malignancy of the renal parenchyma in children and adolescents. It occurs in familial and sporadic forms. The familial form has been associated with several congenital syndromes and chromosomal abnormalities. Bilateral disease is encountered in up to 25% of cases of the congenital form compared with only 5% to 10% of the sporadic cases.[6]

These patients usually present with a painless flank mass that is noted by them or the caregiver. Approximately one third of patients present with abdominal pain with or without fever. Anemia and hypertension are rare, but when present they usually indicate hemorrhage into the tumor.

The preoperative evaluation of the patient with suspected Wilms' tumor includes abdominal and chest radiography, sonography of the abdomen, intravenous pyelography, and CT of the abdomen. Angiography is rarely helpful in these cases. However, when a tumor thrombus in the renal vein or inferior vena cava is suspected on the sonogram, a contrast inferior vena-cavogram may be useful. MRI is gaining favor in the diagnosis of malignancies in adolescents because it does not expose the patient to unnecessary radiation.

Staging in this disease is determined surgically except in advanced cases. The staging system proposed by the National Wilms' Tumor Study Group is currently used (Box 156-3). Stage I disease is confined to the kidney, stage II disease extends beyond the kidney but is completely excised, stage III disease is unresectable without distant metastases, stage IV disease has systemic metastases, and stage V disease includes all cases with bilateral involvement irrespective of the extent of each primary tumor.

Surgical therapy is directed toward complete excision at the initial laparotomy. Because the tumor frequently invades the renal vein or vena cava, it has been recommended that the renal pedicle be clamped as early as possible to prevent tumor emboli. When the tumor is adherent to the vena cava, a partial excision of the vena cava wall may be necessary. If the tumor thrombus has extended into the superior vena cava or right atrium, cardiopulmonary bypass may be necessary to perform complete excision. More recently, surgeons are inducing deep hyperthermia and cardiac arrest in patients with more extensive tumors involving the right atrium in order to perform optimal excision.

Generally, these tumors are approached through a transverse abdominal incision so that both kidneys can be evaluated easily for bilateral disease. Gerota's fascia of

---

BOX 156-3
Staging of Wilms' Tumor

Stage I — Tumor limited to kidney and completely excised with spillage. No invasion of capsule.

Stage II — Extends beyond kidney but is totally excised. Local spillage or local vascular invasion may be present.

Stage III — Residual local disease, massive tumor spillage, or lymph node involvement.

Stage IV — Distant metastases.

Stage V — Bilateral disease.

---

the contralateral kidney must be opened for complete evaluation. Because Wilms' tumors tend to be friable, the plane of resection is outside Gerota's fascia to avoid causing spillage. The regional lymph nodes should be removed at the time of initial surgical therapy.

All areas of residual disease are marked with titanium clips for subsequent radiation therapy. Biopsy alone is indicated for patients with locally extensive disease and is followed by chemotherapy and/or radiation therapy. After induction therapy in cases of advanced disease, "second look" laparotomy is performed with attempted resection of residual disease.

Patients with stage I disease are treated immediately with chemotherapy and have an approximately 90% relapse-free survival. Adjuvant radiation therapy is of minimal benefit and is not advised for stage I disease. In more advanced disease, chemotherapy has proved beneficial. The agents currently used to treat Wilms' tumor include actinomycin D, vincristine, cyclophosphamide, and doxorubicin with or without radiation therapy. The length of treatment is 15 months. For stage I lesions, patients receive only 10 weeks of therapy.[7]

RHABDOMYOSARCOMA

Rhabdomyosarcoma is the most common soft tissue tumor of the pediatric age group. It is of mesenchymal origin and therefore can occur wherever there is skeletal muscle. The most common sites include the head and neck, genitourinary tract, extremities, and trunk. The incidence of rhabdomyosarcoma is bimodal in the pediatric and adolescent age groups. Infants (2 to 4 years) tend to develop bladder, prostate, or head and neck disease; adolescents (12 to 16 years) develop truncal, paratesticular, or abdominal disease. The disease usually becomes apparent as a painless mass or as a result of impingement on a vital structure (e.g., proptosis or diplopia with rhabdomysarcoma of the orbit).

This disease has a propensity to metastasize to the lungs, liver, lymph nodes, bones, bone marrow, and brain; the preoperative evaluation should include examination of these areas. Lesions of the head and neck are evaluated best with a CT or MRI. MRI may produce a somewhat better image with less bony artifact and also has the ability to recreate multiple planes, which allows improved operative or radiation treatment planning.

Diagnosis is made by excisional biopsy or (more frequently) incisional biopsy. In cases in which complete excision cannot be accomplished, cytoreduction can change the stage classification, thereby decreasing the intensity and duration of chemotherapy and radiation therapy. Cytoreductive surgery should not be performed if a major functional or cosmetic disability will be inflicted by the surgery.

Primary tumors of the genitourinary system should be

excised only if the vagina, uterus, bladder, or prostate can be preserved. Alternatively, the patient can undergo biopsy followed by chemotherapy. If residual disease is present after chemotherapy, radiation therapy is recommended. Persistent disease after radiation therapy necessitates an anterior pelvic exenteration. Paratesticular rhabdomyosarcoma, however, is treated primarily by radical inguinal orchiectomy and retroperitoneal lymph node dissection followed by chemotherapy. A transscrotal biopsy should never be undertaken in this or any other malignant disease involving the testicle.

Head and neck rhabdomyosarcomas are rarely amenable to surgical extirpation and therefore are treated primarily with chemotherapy. In cases of extremity rhabdomyosarcoma, wide local excision with elective lymph node dissection for staging purposes is recommended. Amputations are no longer considered appropriate therapy except in extraordinary situations.

Adjuvant radiation therapy is of benefit in reducing local and regional recurrences only in patients with the unfavorable alveolar and pleomorphic subtypes of the disease. In general, radiation therapy is used as primary treatment with or without chemotherapy to treat unresectable disease, or to avoid mutilating or function-compromising surgery (i.e., amputation of an extremity).

Chemotherapy with a combination of vincristine, actinomycin D, and cyclophosphamide (VAC regimen) is used as an adjuvant therapy for stage I patients. Stage II patients are treated with radiation therapy to the tumor bed as well as with vincristine and actinomycin D (VA regimen) or the VAC regimen. Stages III and IV patients currently receive the VA regimen with or without doxorubicin followed by radiation therapy. These approaches have yielded survivals of 80%, 70%, 70%, and 30% for stages I, II, III, and IV, respectively.[8]

SOFT TISSUE SARCOMAS

Soft tissue sarcomas are a nonhomogeneous group of more than 50 different malignancies. They arise in mesoderm-derived tissue and therefore are found most frequently in the extremities, retroperitoneum, and trunk. Treatment is based on grade, size, site, and depth of the tumor mass.

Initially, an open biopsy is performed as described earlier so as not to compromise subsequent excision. Once the diagnosis is made, the patient should undergo a work-up consisting of either MRI or CT of the involved area and the lung, because the lung is the most common site of metastasis in this group of patients.

Patients without synchronous lung metastases should be treated by wide local excision. Depending on the location of the sarcoma, significant functional impairments resulting from the excision of the sarcoma may occur. There is no improvement in disease-free survival

or overall survival with amputation; therefore amputation should be avoided. Patients with high-grade tumors and those with close but uninvolved margins should be treated with external radiation or brachytherapy. The adjuvant use of radiation decreases the incidence of local recurrences but has no effect on overall patient survival. The routine use of adjuvant chemotherapy, except in the case of osteosarcoma, is associated with a small improvement in disease-free interval. However, since no clear improvement in survival is demonstrated after chemotherapy, chemotherapy is generally not recommended.

Patients with synchronous metastases to the lung should undergo resection of the primary tumor if it is believed that all the lung metastases are resectable and if the primary tumor can be excised completely. Patients are followed up with serial chest radiographs every 3 months in the postoperative period to screen for pulmonary recurrences. Most recurrences become evident within 18 months of initial therapy. Resection of bilateral pulmonary metastases is performed through a median sternotomy, whereas unilateral metastases are approached through a lateral thoracotomy. Survival after resection of pulmonary metastases is related to the number of metastases and the disease-free interval. Approximately 30% to 40% of the patients survive for 5 years after metastasectomy of soft tissue sarcomas.

CONCLUSION

Although surgery remains an integral part of therapy for most pediatric and adolescent malignancies, it is likely that further advances in survival rates will result from a better integration and sequencing of the different oncologic disciplines.

References

1. Laug WE, Siegel SE, Shaw K, et al: Initial urinary catecholamine metabolite concentrations and prognosis in neuroblastoma, *Pediatrics* 62:77-84, 1978.
2. Muller-Gartner HW, Erttmann R, Helmke K: Meta-iodobenzylguanidine scintigraphy in neuroblastoma. a comparison with conventional x-ray and ultrasound, *Pediatr Hematol Oncol* 3:97-109, 1986.
3. Zelter PM, Marangos PJ, Evans AE: Serum neuron specific enolase in children with neuroblastoma, *Cancer* 57:1230-1234, 1986.
4. Evans AE, D'Angio GJ, Propert K, et al: Prognostic factors in neuroblastoma, *Cancer* 59:1853-1859, 1987.
5. Hartmann O, Pinkerton CR, Phillip T, et al: Very high dose cisplatin and etoposide in children with untreated advanced neuroblastoma, *J Clin Oncol* 6:44-50, 1988.
6. Coppes MJ, DeKraker J, Van Dijken PJ, et al: Bilateral Wilms's tumors: longterm survival and some epidemiological features, *J Clin Oncol* 7:310-315, 1989.
7. D'Angio GJ, Breslow N, Beckwith JB, et al: Treatment of Wilms' tumor: results of the third national Wilms' tumor study, *Cancer* 64:349-360, 1989.
8. Maurer HM, Beltangady M, Gehan EA, et al: The intergroup rhabdomyosarcoma, study I, *Cancer* 61:209-220, 1988.

CHAPTER 157

Appendicitis

•

Robert Sammartano, Mary Beth Gregor, and Sylvain Kleinhaus

The incidence of acute appendicitis is highest in adolescence and early adulthood and is the most common indication for abdominal surgery in this age group. Appreciation of the early signs and symptoms of appendicitis is of the utmost importance in diagnosing and treating the patient in an expedient manner, thus avoiding the complications associated with appendiceal perforation and peritonitis. Although the exact etiology of acute appendicitis is not always evident, obstruction of the appendiceal lumen is believed to be the cause in most cases. After obstruction, the mucosa distal to the obstruction continues to secrete mucus, and intestinal content continues to ferment in a closed system. The appendiceal lumen distends as the pressure increases, compressing the submucosal vessels and resulting in ischemia of the appendiceal wall. If this ischemia is not corrected, gangrene and necrosis will ensue, with resultant perforation, peritoneal contamination, and peritonitis. Obstruction is most commonly caused by a fecalith, which may or may not be radiopaque. Other causes such as foreign bodies, tumors, and parasitic infestation, although less frequent, are not unusual. The terminal ileum and pericecal area are rich in lymphatics (Peyer's patches), especially in this age group, and lymphoid hypertrophy, which sometimes occurs during an acute viral illness, may also compress the appendiceal lumen, resulting in appendicitis.

DIAGNOSIS

Classically, the pain associated with appendicitis first presents periumbilically; this is because the appendix originates from the same dermatome as the umbilical region. Gradually, as the appendiceal inflammation and periappendiceal reaction develop, the pain shifts to the right lower quadrant. The exact location of the pain depends on the anatomic position of the appendix. If the appendix lies in the pelvis, the primary symptom may be dysuria; if it is in the cul-de-sac, tenesmus may be the most prominent sign; if the appendix lies in the right paracolic gutter, the pain may mimic cholecystitis or renal colic; if it points medially, the periumbilical pain may not shift to the right lower quadrant but remain in the midabdomen. Retrocecal appendicitis is often very difficult to diagnose, since the overlying cecum can mask the evolving pathologic condition in the appendix.

The earliest symptoms are usually anorexia, nausea, and/or vomiting, which may precede or follow the onset of pain. The patient initially may be afebrile, but a low-grade fever soon develops. The patient's temperature rises as the inflammatory response to the appendicitis progresses. By the time gangrene sets in and the patient's appendix perforates, the patient's temperature has usually risen to 39°C (102°F) unless antipyretic agents have been administered.

The physical examination is the most important factor in diagnosing appendicitis. Palpation of the abdomen should be preceded by auscultation for the presence or absence of bowel sounds. In acute appendicitis the bowel sounds are usually diminished or absent, a direct result of localized or generalized peritonitis. If a perforation has occurred, intestinal motility is reduced so that the patient avoids painful stretching of the peritoneum as much as possible and therefore reduces the amount of spillage of intestinal contents. The presence of hyperactive bowel sounds should call into question the diagnosis of acute appendicitis.

The most tender area on palpation of the abdomen is usually in the right lower quadrant overlying McBurney's point, which is at the junction of the lateral third and medial two thirds of a line joining the umbilicus and anterosuperior iliac spine. As mentioned, the point of maximal tenderness also depends on the location of the appendix. As the degree of inflammation increases, so does the ability of the patient to localize the pain to one small specific area.

If the diagnosis is not made and the process is allowed to progress, perforation will eventually occur. If the perforation is localized and contained by the omentum, small bowel, cecum, and adnexa, or any combination of contiguous structures, the pain will remain localized to the right lower quadrant. If there is a free perforation, generalized peritonitis will ensue with its typical signs and symptoms. Abdominal guarding will be more generalized with rebound tenderness throughout, the abdomen will be silent, the patient will attempt to remain motionless, and paradoxically the pain will be subjectively less for a short time.

The rectal examination is most likely to be positive if the tip of the appendix lies in the posterior cul-de-sac. However, a normal rectal examination does not preclude appendicitis. The digital examination may not elicit any pain if the appendix is retrocecal or in the right pericolic gutter. If the appendix has already perforated, a pelvic abscess will often be palpable through the anterior rectal wall.

Laboratory results may also be helpful in confirming the diagnosis. Leukocytosis, which is almost always present from the onset, will progressively increase to the 12,000 to 18,000 range, with a progressive left shift as the process continues. The urinalysis may be positive, especially if the appendix overlies the ureter and/or dome of the bladder. If only the ureter is involved, a small number of white or red blood cells may be seen; if the inflammation involves the bladder wall, the cell count per high-power field may be higher. On occasion, urinary tract symptoms are so prominent in the early stages of the disease that it may even be mistaken for cystitis.

Adolescent females present greater difficulties in diagnosis. Pelvic inflammatory disease and ovarian cysts are the entities most commonly confused with appendicitis. Although pelvic inflammatory disease is associated with a history of previous sexual activity, it must be suspected even if no such history is obtained. Mittelschmerz also varies from patient to patient and from one menstrual cycle to another. Patients with pelvic inflammatory disease are most likely to present with acute abdominal pain in the immediate postmenstrual period, whereas the pain accompanying a ruptured follicular cyst occurs in midcycle. If a patient has pelvic inflammatory disease, the pelvic examination will frequently disclose a pelvic infection, and a Gram's stain of any discharge may reveal intracellular diplococci. Of course, the presence of one entity does not preclude concomitant appendicitis.

Radiographs of the chest and abdomen are helpful in diagnosing acute appendicitis. Lower lobar pneumonia, especially on the right side, may be confused with appendicitis, and recognition of a lower lobar infiltrate on a chest film can prevent the performance of an unnecessary appendectomy. On the other hand, several findings on abdominal flat films may reinforce the clinical impression of appendicitis. A localized right lower quadrant ileus and/or a mass effect in the area of the cecum are often seen in appendicitis (Fig. 157-1). The presence of a fecalith is considered an absolute indication for appendectomy. Not only is obstruction of the appendiceal lumen more likely in the presence of an appendicolith, but data indicate that perforation occurs more frequently and earlier in the course of the disease in patients with calcified fecaliths than in patients without fecaliths. For this reason, we recommend elective appendectomy in the absence of symptoms in any patient with an appendicolith evident on an abdominal film (Fig. 157-2). Some radiologists have recommended barium enema studies for the diagnosis of appendicitis; a nonfilling appendix and cecal edema are the criteria for diagnosis (Fig. 157-3).

Ultrasonography has become an important diagnostic tool in cases in which the diagnosis of appendicitis is unclear. With ultrasonography, the pelvic organs can be visualized well in most cases in females, and the presence of an unsuspected pregnancy can be excluded. Ovarian cysts and/or fluid in the cul-de-sac can be demonstrated, as well as adnexal abnormalities such as torsion, inflammation, and extrauterine gestation. In some cases the appendix itself can be visualized, and in some studies

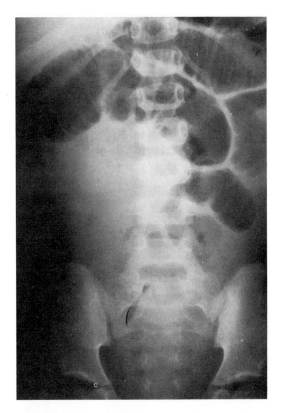

Fig. 157-1. Flat plate of the abdomen showing distended loops of small bowel surrounding a relatively air-free right lower quadrant. An appendicolith and several small air bubbles can be seen in the center of the right lower quadrant, which is consistent with acute appendicitis with periappendiceal abscess. (Courtesy of H. Pritzker, MD, Bronx, NY.)

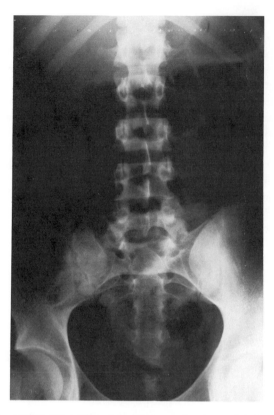

Fig. 157-2. Flat plate of the abdomen showing a right lower quadrant fecalith. (Courtesy of H. Pritzker, MD, Bronx, NY.)

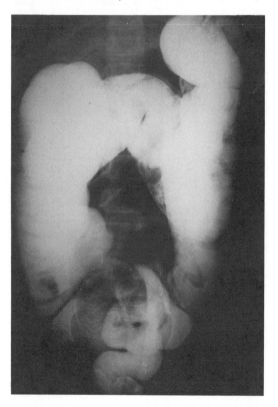

Fig. 157-3. Barium enema showing concentric edematous folds in the cecum characteristic of acute appendicitis. (Courtesy of H. Pritzker, MD, Bronx, NY.)

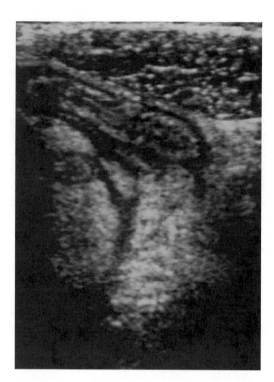

Fig. 157-4. Ultrasound appearance of acute appendicitis showing debris in the lumen, a thickened appendiceal wall, and a sonolucent border representing edema fluid.

this finding has been used to make a presumptive radiologic diagnosis of appendicitis (Fig. 157-4).

TREATMENT

The definitive treatment of appendicitis is appendectomy. Once the diagnosis is made, appendectomy should be performed as expeditiously as possible to prevent perforation. Even if there is a high degree of suspicion without clinical certainty, it is considered safer to perform an appendectomy than to delay treatment for observation. These patients are usually mildly dehydrated and require fluid resuscitation before induction of anesthesia. Serum electrolyte levels, as determined by serial serum analysis, are corrected and adequate urinary output is ensured. If there is peritonitis, the fluid requirements may be impressive. In addition, intravenous antibiotics are administered in the pre- and postoperative periods. A nasogastric tube is placed in most patients, especially those in whom an ileus has been demonstrated. Intraoperatively, the operative site should be irrigated profusely with a 0.1% kanamycin solution before closing the peritoneum, and the same solution is used to vigorously irrigate the muscle, fascia, and subcutaneous layers. In grossly contaminated cases the skin is closed over a subcutaneous Penrose drain brought out through the lateral end of the incision.

There is still a difference of opinion over surgical treatment of the perforated appendix with a periappendiceal mass or abscess. Some surgeons prefer to operate immediately, drain the abscess, and remove the appendix after proper rehydration and fluid resuscitation. Others believe that it is safer to delay the appendectomy until the patient is no longer toxic and the abdominal signs and symptoms have abated. An elective appendectomy can then be performed, usually several weeks later, without the risk of opening the contained perforation and spreading the contamination to the remainder of the peritoneal cavity. However, it is not uncommon for the patient to redevelop acute appendicitis while awaiting interval appendectomy. If the patient does not respond to nonoperative therapy, including appropriate antibiotic administration, fluid resuscitation, and nasogastric suction, the operation should be performed immediately despite the associated risks.

Laparoscopic Appendectomy

The increasing availability and variety of laparoscopic surgical instrumentation, and the large number of surgeons trained in laparoscopic operative technique for cholecystectomy, have made laparoscopic appendectomy possible at most institutions. Since laparoscopic appendectomy for acute appendicitis was first reported by Semm in 1983, numerous authors have reported both randomized and nonrandomized prospective experiences comparing laparoscopic and open appendectomy.

The surgical indications in patients presenting with acute, noncomplicated appendicitis are the same for laparoscopic appendectomy and open appendectomy. For the patient whose clinical presentation suggests an intraabdominal process that is not clearly appendicitis, laparoscopic evaluation of the abdomen is a valuable tool. This is especially so for the adolescent female patient who has reached menarche; who presents with right-sided, lower abdominal pain; and in whom the clinical investigation is equivocal for an acute abdomen. Laparoscopy allows direct visualization of the intraabdominal and pelvic viscera and permits the surgeon to delineate the extensive differential diagnoses for the patient's symptoms. If no pelvic or abdominal pathology is found at laparoscopy, an appendectomy is performed so that if the patient presents with similar abdominal pain at a later date, a diagnosis of acute appendicitis is eliminated, sparing the patient a possible right lower quadrant laparotomy.

If the appendix is perforated, laparoscopic appendectomy affords a complete view of the abdominal viscera, as well as the ability to assess the extent of the spillage of intestinal contents into the peritoneal cavity. It also enables the surgeon to irrigate effectively those areas that are not readily accessible through a small classic open incision.

The results of treatment of acute appendicitis using an open or laparoscopic approach have been compared by various authors. Bonanni et al reported 300 consecutive open as compared with 66 laparoscopic appendectomies, finding essentially no differences in operative complications, postoperative morbidity, pain medication requirements, or time to resumption of a regular diet. In their experience, for complicated appendicitis, laparoscopic appendectomy carried a higher postoperative rate of abscess formation. Other authors have reported an opposite experience with complicated appendicitis treated by laparoscopy or by an open operation.

Varlet et al, in a retrospective study, reported that of 403 appendectomies (200 laparoscopic and 203 open) there were definite advantages in laparoscopic appendectomy. These were noted as ease of treatment for ectopic appendix, less operative trauma, efficient peritoneal lavage, less frequent postoperative complications, and better postoperative comfort.

As for any abdominal surgery, there is an occurrence of symptomatic postoperative adhesions after open and laparoscopic appendectomy. These adhesions can present as partial or complete bowel obstruction, adnexal torsion, and also recurrent intermittent abdominal pain. Laparoscopic exploration with adhesiolysis has been used effectively to treat patients presenting with postappendectomy abdominal pain.

Overall, the benefits of laparoscopic appendectomy for noncomplicated acute appendicitis are seen in reduced length of hospital stay, decreased use of postoperative pain medications, and faster return to a normal active life style. The added expense because of the use of disposable laparoscopic instrumentation noted by some authors is easily offset by the decreased length of hospital stay and the increased availability of reusable instruments. In the hands of a trained surgical staff, laparoscopic appendectomy is becoming a safe, efficient alternative to conventional open appendectomy.

COMPLICATIONS

The complications of acute appendicitis are many despite optimal therapy. The most common is infection. Superficial wound infections occur in 6% to 15% of patients with nonsuppurative acute appendicitis, with or without perioperative antibiotic therapy. In cases in which appendicitis is more advanced at the time of operation, the rate of infection is even higher.

The second most common infectious complication is a pelvic abscess, which develops 4 to 7 days after appendectomy. The patient develops a spiking fever and lower abdominal pain; a rectal examination demonstrates a tender anterior rectal wall that bulges into the lumen. Sonography confirms the presence and extent of the abscess, as well as any other coexistent intraabdominal collections. Many of these abscesses respond to intravenous antibiotic and symptomatic treatment without drainage. Some pelvic collections drain spontaneously through the rectum, as manifested by a transanal gush of foul-smelling mucopurulent material. Some cases require surgical drainage in the operating room; when possible, this is done transanally. In the more complicated cases, ultrasonographic guidance is used to place a catheter within the abscess cavity.

Before the availability of antibiotics, one of the most feared complications of appendicitis was pylephlebitis: infectious thrombosis of the portal vein. Fortunately, this occurrence is now rare. Inflammatory involvement of the right uterine adnexa often produces adhesions that incorporate the fimbria and may result in occlusion of the fallopian tube.

CONCLUSION

Acute appendicitis is a common disease in the adolescent. The treatment goal is to diagnose the condition as early as possible in the disease course so that complications can be minimized. This requires appropriate pre- and postoperative care and frequent sequential examinations by the same practitioner in cases in which the diagnosis is unclear.

Suggested Readings

Attwood SEA, Hill ADK, et al: A prospective randomized trial of laparoscopic versus open appendectomy, *Surgery* 112:497-501, 1992.

Bagi P, Dueholm S, et al: Percutaneous drainage of appendiceal abscess: an alternative to conventional treatment, *Dis Colon Rectum* 30:532-535, 1987.

Bonnani F, Reed J III, Hartzell G, et al: Laparoscopic versus conventional appendectomy, *J Am Coll Surg* 179:273-278, 1994.

Gaensler EHL, Jeffery RB, et al: Sonography in patients with suspected acute appendicitis: value in establishing alternative diagnoses, *AJR* 152:49-51, 1989.

Gilchrist BF, Lobe TE, et al: Is there a role for laparoscopic appendectomy in pediatric surgery?, *J Pediatr Surg* 127:209-214, 1992.

Heinzelmann M, Simmen HP, et al: Is laparoscopic appendectomy the new "gold standard"?, *Arch Surg* 130:782-785, 1995.

Jeffery RB Jr, Laing FC, et al: Acute appendicitis: sonographic criteria based on 250 cases, *Radiology* 167:327-329, 1988.

Jeffery RB Jr, Laing FC, et al: Acute appendicitis: high resolution real-time US findings, *Radiology* 163:11-14, 1987.

Kleinhaus S: Laparoscopic lysis of adhesions for postappendectomy pain, *Endoscopy* 30:304-305, 1985.

Pulaert JBCM, Rutgers PH, et al: A prospective study of ultrasonography in the diagnosis of appendicitis, *N Engl J Med* 317:666-669, 1987.

Rabau MY, Dreznik Z, et al: Indications for interval appendectomy in the management of appendicular abscess, *J Abdom Surg* 22:73-74, 1980.

Rajagopalan AE, Mason JH, et al: The value of the barium enema in the diagnosis of acute appendicitis, *Arch Surg* 112:531-533, 1977.

Reiertsen O, Trondsen E, et al: Prospective non-randomized study of conventional versus laparoscopic appendectomy, *World J Surg* 18:411-416, 1994.

Samuelson SL, Reyes HM: Management of perforated appendicitis in children—revisited, *Arch Surg* 112:531-533, 1977.

Schirmer BD, Schmieg RE, et al: Laparoscopic versus traditional appendectomy for suspected appendicitis, *Am J Surg* 165:670-675, 1993.

Seal A: Appendicitis: an historical review, *Can J Surg* 24:427-433, 1981.

Semm K: Endoscopic appendectomy, *Endoscopy* 15:59-64, 1983.

Varlet F, Tardieu D, et al: Laparoscopic versus open appendectomy in 403 children—comparative study, *Eur J Surg* 4:333-337, 1994.

Williams MD, Miller D, et al: Laparoscopic appendectomy, is it worth it?, *South Med J* 87:592-598, 1994.

CHAPTER 158

Surgical Aspects of Inflammatory Bowel Disease

•

Sylvain Kleinhaus

The two most common types of inflammatory bowel disease (IBD) experienced by adolescents are ulcerative colitis and Crohn's disease (CD). Surgery for IBD is essentially surgery for the complications of IBD. In many cases the distinctions between ulcerative colitis (UC) and CD are unclear and the indications overlap, so the physician must take care to distinguish between the two entities.

CROHN'S DISEASE

CD can involve the entire gastrointestinal tract from the mouth to the anus but not necessarily all areas at once. In a study from St. Justine's Hospital in Montreal involving 230 children and adolescents, three (1%) had disease limited to the upper gastrointestinal tract; 37 (16%) to the small bowel alone; 169 (74%) to the small and large bowel; and 21 (9%) to the colon and/or rectum alone. This distribution is representative of the results of many other surveys, and complications requiring surgical intervention in these anatomic areas occur in similar proportion. Thus, surgery of the oropharynx, esophagus, stomach, and/or duodenum is rarely indicated. The presenting features of the most common form of CD, which afflicts the stomach and duodenum, are similar to those of peptic ulcer disease—pain, bleeding, or stricture—and are treated accordingly.

The surgical treatment of small bowel disease, the classic "regional enteritis," has undergone considerable evolution. Originally, it was considered essential to resect the entire bowel involved with the disease, and it was routine to perform frozen section analysis of the margins of resection to avoid anastomosing involved bowel. Rather, a clinical judgment is made based on the gross appearance of the bowel, and a "healthy" area is chosen for anastomosis. Indications for surgery are failure of medical treatment as manifested by intestinal obstruction, intractable pain, fistula formation with or without abscess (which may be intramesenteric or intraperitoneal), and

perforation. Situations that involve fistula formation and/or perforation are generally the most complicated and life threatening. Of these indications, obstruction is the most common, and resection is usually performed. Since most of these cases involve the ileocecal area, the most common procedure performed is an ileocecectomy. As much of the ascending colon is saved as possible and only the most diseased ileum is removed. The presence of creeping fat does not preclude the use of a bowel segment as long as the bowel wall itself is salvageable. Since there are often "skip" areas (obviously diseased areas alternating with less involved segments), it is important to examine the entire small bowel and institute treatment as is appropriate.

Multiple strictures are not uncommon, and more and more often stricturoplasties are performed in situations in which the strictures are short and relatively widely separated. If there are several strictures close to one another, it is sometimes safer to resect them and perform one anastomosis than to create several suture lines, even though the suture line in a stricturoplasty may not be completely circumferential. Bypass surgery is generally contraindicated except in the most complicated cases and under special circumstances, since the unresected diseased bowel is a source of continued inflammation and secondary complications such as fistulas and cancers.

Fistulas can develop between loops of adjacent bowel and are often multiple. They are frequently ileoileal and relatively asymptomatic. However, ileocolic fistulas can be more serious because they form a spontaneous bypass and significantly alter the patient's nutritional capabilities. Some fistulas respond to nonsurgical treatment, such as elemental diet or long-term hyperalimentation, but eventually most patients with fistulas require surgery. Ileocolic fistulas usually require resection of the involved small bowel with an anastomosis. It is often possible to close the colonic end of the fistula without resection. If the colonic disease is too extensive, colonic resection is also required. Depending on the extent and location of the disease and the technical difficulty of the anastomoses, a proximal diverting loop ileostomy or jejunostomy may be advisable.

Fistulas may also develop between the bowel and the genitourinary system. Enterovesical fistulas occur in 5% to 10% of patients with complicated CD, as manifested by pyuria, pneumaturia, and fecaluria. This type of fistula is almost always an indication for early surgery, with resection of the involved bowel, multilayered closure of the bladder, and Foley catheter drainage until healing occurs. Female patients may also have fistulas to the fallopian tubes, uterus, and vagina. These fistulas are often difficult to repair surgically and may also require proximal diversion.

Enterocutaneous fistulas may develop spontaneously, but they usually follow surgical intervention and are the result of an anastomotic leak or an unrecognized perforation. Small fistulas may heal with the aid of hyperalimentation, but in most cases they require reintervention with re-resection and anastomosis once the acute inflammatory reaction has subsided. If the fistula is "high output," with most of the fecal stream diverted through the fistula, reoperation is usually indicated. Late enterocutaneous fistulas through an incisional or ileostomy site indicate recurrent disease.

Perianal disease is unfortunately quite common and, though not frequently life threatening, both debilitating and psychologically disheartening. Sometimes the first indication of IBD is a nonhealing perianal fistula. Although treated by the conventional surgical approaches, these fistulas are frequently slow to heal and often persist for months or years without resolution. They may exist in the absence of any recognizable evidence of proximal disease. On occasion, rectal and perirectal disease may be so extensive that a proximal ostomy, and sometimes even proctectomy in the extreme case, is required.

Free perforation into the peritoneal cavity is very rare because the inflammatory reaction around the involved bowel usually causes the omentum and/or adjacent bowel to adhere and wall off the perforation. When free perforation occurs, emergency surgery is indicated, and the procedure selected depends on the condition of the patient and the anatomic considerations at the time of laparotomy. The minimal procedure would be proximal diversion and drainage. In selected cases a primary anastomosis may be performed.

Intraabdominal abscesses are almost always the result of a contained perforation. If the patient is toxic, only drainage of the abscess may be indicated, with subsequent enterocutaneous fistula formation. Once the patient has been stabilized and diagnostic studies have been obtained, surgery is almost always indicated for resection of the involved bowel.

Ileostomy complications are also not infrequent, and revisions of the ileostomy for local fistulas and/or repositioning of the ileostomy because of recurrent disease at or near the stoma are unfortunately commonplace.

In adolescents, there is an additional unique indication for surgery: sexual maturation and growth. It is well known that any chronic debilitating disease can retard the adolescent growth spurt and concomitant sexual development. This situation can be further aggravated by corticosteroid therapy administered in high and prolonged dosage. In these young teenagers, extirpation of the most inflamed bowel, followed by gradual reduction and subsequent cessation of steroid therapy, frequently results in a rapid catch-up growth spurt and normal sexual maturation. For these reasons, young teenagers require a more aggressive surgical approach than older adolescents who have already passed growth and sexual maturation milestones.

ULCERATIVE COLITIS

All the complications of CD are also associated with UC, which complicates and sometimes prevents unequivocal identification of and distinction between the two diseases. The upper gastrointestinal manifestations, however, are essentially limited to CD. The two complications essentially limited to UC and rarely seen in CD are toxic megacolon and fulminant colitis with hemorrhage.

Toxic megacolon is associated with very high morbidity and mortality; the key to treatment is prevention. All efforts must be made to prevent perforation of the toxic megacolon, which has a mortality rate approaching 50%. Medical treatment includes nasogastric suction, steroid therapy, and antibiotic administration. If these actions do not result in improvement in 48 to 72 hours and/or if the patient's condition deteriorates, surgery is indicated. The procedure of choice is subtotal colectomy and mucous fistula with the construction of an ileostomy. At a later date, once the patient has recovered, restoration of intestinal continuity can be considered. Ileoproctostomy and endorectal pull-through procedures with or without a pouch are restorative options to consider; the condition of the rectal mucosa influences the final operative decision.

Acute colitis without dilation may also occur and is frequently accompanied by life-threatening hemorrhage. Emergency surgery is indicated if medical measures fail. Elective resection in the quiescent phase can be performed as described above.

POSTOPERATIVE COMPLICATIONS

Postoperative complications after surgical treatment of both CD and UC are frequent. The most common complication is wound infection, especially after emergency procedures when patients are most toxic and adequate bowel preparation is impossible. Less common but more serious are intraabdominal abscesses, which often are the result of or lead to intestinal fistulas. These complications may occur despite the most meticulous regard to surgical technique and peritoneal and wound antisepsis.

Recurrence in CD is not uncommon and may be early or late. Surgical intervention at the time of a recurrence should be considered only when medical management has failed. The removal of involved intestine is not curative of the underlying disease, and introduces problems with postoperative healing and the potential loss of significant lengths of bowel. Retained colon in ulcerative colitis is well known to be the site of malignancy, and monitoring for the emergence of cancerous lesions and consideration for colectomy must be a part of the ongoing management.

CONCLUSION

In summary, surgery in UC and CD is part of the management of these diseases, not the cure. IBD is difficult to manage, and surgery is indicated only for those complications that cannot otherwise be treated. Morbidity and mortality are considerable, and until a cure is found the goal is to minimize the incidence and severity of complications as much as possible.

Suggested Readings

Fry RD, Shemesh EI, Kodner IJ, Timmcke A: Techniques and results in the management of anal and perianal Crohn's disease, *Surg Gynecol Obstet* 168:42-48, 1989.

Glotzer DJ: Surgical therapy for Crohn's disease, *Gastroenterol Clin North Am* 24:577-596, 1995.

Kahng KU, Roslyn JJ: Surgical treatment of inflammatory bowel disease, *Med Clin North Am* 78:1427-1441, 1994.

Lenaerts C, Roy CC, Vaillancourt M, Weber AM, Morin CL, Seidman E: High incidence of upper gastrointestinal tract involvement in children with Crohn's disease, *Pediatrics* 83:777-781, 1989.

Longo WE, Oakley JR, Laveny IC, Church JM, Fazio VW: Outcome of ileorectal anastomosis for Crohn's colitis, *Dis Colon Rectum* 35:1066-1071, 1992.

Palder SB, Shandling B, Bilik R, Griffiths AM, Sherman P: Perianal complications of Pediatric Crohn's disease, *J Pediatr Surg* 26:513-515, 1991.

Sharif H, Alexander-Williams J: Stricturoplasty for ileo-colic anastomotic strictures in Crohn's disease, *Int J Colorect Dis* 6:214-216, 1991.

CHAPTER 159

Cholelithiasis

•

Gerard Weinberg

INCIDENCE

The incidence of cholelithiasis in children and adolescents compared with that in adults is quite low. A study of 1570 healthy adults in Italy using standard ultrasound techniques showed an overall prevalence of 0.13% (two females, no males).[1] Other studies, especially those of older adolescents up to age 21, have reported a somewhat higher prevalence of cholelithiasis, ranging up to 1%; this incidence is, however, still much below that of older populations.[2]

There are several groups of children and adolescents who are at greater risk of developing biliary stones.[3,4]

Group I includes children who produce higher than normal levels of bilirubin, usually secondary to chronic hemolysis: for example, children with sickle cell disease or congenital spherocytosis. Group II includes children who have an abnormal or impaired enterohepatic circulation, such as those who have undergone ileal resection, those with inflammatory bowel disease, and those who have experienced severe dehydration or sepsis. Group III includes children with a genetic or familial predisposition to secrete bile containing a higher than normal concentration of cholesterol, such as the Pima Indians of

Arizona. Group IV includes adolescent females, especially those who have been or are pregnant. The ratio of adolescent females to adolescent males with cholelithiasis is 19:1. A study has shown that 65% of 14- to 18-year-old girls with gallstones were or had been pregnant.[5] It has been postulated that the higher estrogen levels produced during pregnancy reduce the concentration of bile acids in the bile but do not affect the concentration of cholesterol, thus increasing the lithogenicity of the bile. Another factor that may also contribute to the higher incidence of cholelithiasis in these girls is decreased gallbladder motility, which can result in bile stasis. Stasis may also explain the higher incidence of stones in obese patients, since these patients are also known to have a higher incidence of gallbladder stasis.

PATHOLOGY

Most of the stones found in adolescents are in the gallbladder, but several large series of adolescents have reported stones in the common duct. These patients present with the classic signs of biliary tract obstruction: jaundice, fever, and cholangitis. Most of the stones in adolescents are composed of pigment, calcium, and cholesterol. Calcium bilirubinate stones are usually found in children who have hemolytic disorders, whereas older adolescents without hemolytic disorders usually have cholesterol gallstones.

PRESENTATION

The signs and symptoms of cholelithiasis in adolescents are very similar to those demonstrated in other age groups. These symptoms include colicky, epigastric, and right upper quadrant pain; a history of fatty food intolerance; nausea; and vomiting. A small number of patients may have had transient jaundice or hyperamylasemia. Unless the patient currently has acute cholecystitis, the physical examination and laboratory study results are normal. Only about 10% of gallstones are radiopaque, and therefore most are not visible on plain abdominal films. Diagnosis is usually made on the basis of a suggestive history coupled with the results of real-time ultrasonography. With ultrasonography, the stones as well as the anatomy of biliary tree are defined. Ultrasonography is also helpful in defining the size of the gallbladder and diameter of the common duct, and it shows possible common duct stones and/or signs of pancreatitis. The oral cholecystogram is used less often than in the past, since most stones are now identified with ultrasonography.

MANAGEMENT

Unless there is a medical contraindication, a cholecystectomy should be performed in adolescents who have cholelithiasis, since in most cases complications from the stones will eventually develop. An elective cholecystectomy carries no mortality and very little morbidity. The traditional cholecystectomy has been an open cholecystectomy, necessitating a hospital stay of 3 to 5 days. There are now several alternatives to open cholecystectomy that may be offered to the adolescent. The most widely accepted innovation is the endoscopic or laparoscopic cholecystectomy performed via a laparoscope with the patient under general anesthesia. Unlike open cholecystectomy, there is no large incision and the postoperative recovery period is much shorter. Patients often can be discharged from the hospital the day of the surgery and can resume normal activities 1 week later.

There are other alternatives to cholecystectomy. Biliary stones can be dissolved by administration of high doses of oral bile salts such as ursodeoxycholic acid. This therapy has been used in Europe in adults and achieves stone dissolution in over 10% of patients. The drug, however, has not been approved for use in children. Since many of these stones recur once therapy is discontinued, drug dissolution of stones will probably be rarely indicated for use in children and adolescents.

Another option is extracorporeal shock wave lithotripsy. Most of the experience with this modality has also been in adults. Some reports have shown dissolution of gallstones in over 90% of patients in 12 to 18 months. A number of complications have been associated with lithotripsy, including pancreatitis and hematuria. Given the success rate and increasingly wide acceptance of endoscopic cholecystectomy, lithotripsy will probably not play a significant role in the management of biliary stones in adolescents and is being performed less often in adults also.

Adolescents with sickle cell disease and symptomatic cholelithiasis present a special problem in management.[6] These patients are more likely to develop serious complications of cholelithiasis, including sickle cell crisis, necrosis of the gallbladder wall due to intramural sickling, and sepsis from ascending cholangitis should stones become impacted in the common duct. Therefore, in these patients, cholecystectomy should be performed as soon as possible. To minimize the risk of a sickle cell crisis in the perioperative period, patients with sickle cell disease should have repeat transfusions several weeks before the scheduled cholecystectomy to decrease the hemoglobin S concentration to less than 30% and to increase the hemoglobin to at least 11 g/dl. Patients should be well hydrated before and during surgery and should be well oxygenated. When these precautions are taken, patients with sickle cell disease who undergo a cholecystectomy have no mortality and a highly acceptable morbidity rate. Most physicians caring for children with sickle celll disease do not recommend cholecystectomy if the stones are truly asymptomatic. The difficulty with this approach is that it can sometimes be difficult to detect whether a child with sickle cell disease who presents with right upper quadrant symptoms is suffering from biliary colic or is having a sickle cell crisis.

ACUTE CHOLECYSTITIS

Acute cholecystitis is an inflammation of the gallbladder that usually results from a stone impacted in the cystic duct or gallbladder neck. These patients present with severe pain in the right upper quadrant or epigastrium that radiates to the right shoulder or the back. Nausea and vomiting occur frequently and may be accompanied by fever. Patients may be mildly jaundiced even though there is no stone in the common duct. Physical examination reveals peritoneal signs in the right upper quadrant characterized by abdominal muscle guarding and rebound. Often a tender mass can be palpated below the right costal margin. Laboratory studies show leukocytosis with a shift to the left. Bilirubin, alkaline phosphatase, and amylase levels may also be elevated.

Patients with acute cholecystitis should be admitted to the hospital and treated with bed rest, nasogastric suction, and intravenous antibiotic administration. Diagnosis is confirmed by a sonogram and a cholescintigram using one of the technetium-99m—labeled hepatic-iminodiacetic acid (HIDA) agents. The radionuclide is absorbed by the liver, is excreted into the biliary tree, and enters the small bowel in rapid sequence. If the cystic duct is blocked because of an impacted stone or inflammation, the gallbladder will not be visualized, thus confirming the diagnosis of acute cholecystitis.

Most surgeons opt for cholecystectomy as soon as the diagnosis of cholecystitis is established, because they believe that such a treatment plan shortens hospitalization and makes the operation technically easier to perform. Other surgeons treat these patients nonoperatively: they allow the cholecystitis to subside, discharge the patient, and schedule elective cholecystectomy 6 weeks later.[7] The first option is preferable since it results in an earlier return to normal activities. Cholecystectomy, when performed early in the course of acute cholecystitis, is safe and carries very little morbidity and no mortality.

A number of patients have choledocholithiasis and may present with jaundice, fever, and chills. Any patient who has an elevation in bilirubin or amylase levels should undergo an intraoperative cholangiogram at the time of cholecystectomy. If the cholangiogram shows stones in the common duct, a common duct exploration with removal of the stones should be performed.

CONCLUSION

Cholecystitis and cholelithiasis in the adolescent are not uncommon. They are more common in patients with hemolytic diseases and in females who have been pregnant. These entities are best treated by surgery, and at the present time laparoscopic cholecystectomy is the method of choice.

References

1. Palasciano G, Portincasa P, Vinciguerra V, Velard A, Tardi S, et al: Gallstone prevalence and gallbladder volume in children and adolescents, *Am J Gastroenterol* 84:1378, 1989.
2. Robertson JRF, Carachi CR, Sweet EM, et al: Cholelithiasis in childhood, *J Pediatr Surg* 23:246, 1988.
3. Holcomb GW Jr, Holcomb GW III: Cholelithiasis in infants, children and adolescents, *Pediatr Rev* 11:268, 1990
4. Bailey PV, Connors RH, Tracy TF Jr, Sotel-Auila C, Lewis JE, Weber TR: Changing spectrum of cholelithiasis and cholecystitis in infants and children, *Am J Surg* 158:585, 1989.
5. Bujumsohn A, Albo E, Grest PH, Subbarao MJ: Cholelithiasis and teenage mothers, *J Adolesc Health Care* 11:339, 1990.
6. Ware R, Filston HC, Schultz WH, et al: Elective cholecystectomy in children with sickle hemoglobinopathies, *Ann Surg* 208:1722, 1988.
7. Weinberg G: Diseases of the biliary tract. In Boley SJ, Cohen MI, editors: *Surgery of the adolescent,* Orlando, 1986, Grune & Stratton; p 33.

CHAPTER 160

Pilonidal Disease

•

Sylvain Kleinhaus

Pilonidal disease consists of cysts and sinuses originating in the intergluteal fold overlying the posterior aspect of the lower sacrum and coccyx. These cysts and sinuses become infected and painful, causing the patient to seek medical attention. Although they occur at all ages, the incidence of pilonidal infections is highest in the second and third decades of life, and the disease frequently first becomes symptomatic in the middle to late teens. Both sexes are affected, but pilonidal disease is more common in men.

ETIOLOGY

The etiology of pilonidal disease is no longer controversial. When it was originally described as a separate clinical entity, its origins were ascribed to the presence of a congenital malformation, possibly related to notochordal remnants. However, the theory has gradually become accepted that pilonidal cysts and sinuses are an acquired disease resulting most certainly from infected hair follicles and ingrown hair. Several observations have led to this conclusion: (1) infants and young children are rarely if ever affected, (2) there is a significant incidence of recurrent cysts even though the entire primary cyst and area has been excised, and (3) there is an absence of hair follicles from most of the sinus tracts. Additional evidence pointing to their acquired origin is the prevalence of the disease in hirsute patients with deep intergluteal folds. Within these deep folds, hairs from one side constantly irritate the opposite epiderm, inciting an inflammatory reaction. Any break in the skin caused by trauma or irritation allows the hair to grow into the defect, resulting in further inflammation until finally an infected sinus develops. There is also some evidence that these same factors can lead to edema and inflammation of the hair follicles themselves, with temporary obstruction leading to dilation of the follicular sac, infection, and subsequent abscess formation. This entity is most prevalent in obese sedentary individuals with a history of local trauma. The classic example is the high incidence of

pilonidal disease among jeep and truck drivers during World War II. It is not uncommon for several family members to have similar symptoms if they are hirsute.

CLINICAL COURSE

Most patients present for the first time to the emergency room with a painful pilonidal abscess that prevents them from sitting or walking without discomfort. On further questioning, the patient usually discloses a history of several days of increasing intergluteal pain, and perhaps describes a similar previous episode that resulted in the discharge of a foul-smelling exudate and temporary relief. It is frequently difficult to examine these patients without sedation because any attempt to spread the buttocks produces intense pain. Surrounding the abscess there is usually an area of erythema and edema, which may be symmetric or extend to one side. There may be one visible sinus tract or several, with or without hair, and scarring from previous spontaneous drainage or surgical incision may be present. Absence of perianal induration on rectal examination will differentiate this entity from a perianal or perirectal abscess. In addition, closer inspection will reveal that the inflammatory process is centered in the sarcococcygeal region and not in the perianal area.

TREATMENT

In the acute phase, which is when most patients present for the first time, major surgical procedures should be avoided. If the area surrounding a pilonidal sinus is swollen, indurated, and erythematous but there is no fluctuant area, four to six warm sitz baths a day and administration of oral analgesics and antibiotics should be prescribed. If the patient is toxic, he or she is admitted to the hospital and intravenous antibiotics are administered. Broad-spectrum antibiotics are administered for both coliform organisms and *Staphylococcus aureus,* which are the most common offenders. In most cases a fluctuant area will form in the ensuing hours or days. If the abscess does not drain spontaneously, it should be incised and the collection of pus drained. Depending on the circumstances and the patient, this procedure may be done safely and adequately with the patient under general anesthesia, sedation and local anesthesia, or sometimes even without anesthesia if the patient presents when the abscess is about to rupture spontaneously. Sitz baths and antibiotic administration are continued until the acute phase is over. Antibiotic therapy is then discontinued and the patient scheduled for elective surgery.

It is most important to stress to the patient and the family that regardless of what type of operation is to be performed, the patient will be required to keep the intergluteal area scrupulously clean forever. In most patients, this means sitz baths, in addition to the daily shower or bath, and the use of a depilatory on a weekly basis. This attendance to personal hygiene cannot be overemphasized. As most of these patients are hirsute and have a relatively deep intergluteal cleft, there is a tendency for these abscesses to recur, sometimes even if the patient does follow the prescribed regimen.

If the involved area is small, the sinuses appear superficial, and the residual induration is minimal, the pilonidal sinus and indurated area should be excised and a primary closure performed. This surgical approach can be performed in only a small percentage of patients, but it is the simplest and quickest way to heal the involved site. If the primary closure is performed under excess tension, it will separate in the early postoperative period and then heal by secondary intention. This process is disappointing, painful, and long.

In most cases the preferred method of treatment is marsupialization. The central involved area is excised and the sinus tracts are then opened. The old granulation tissue is removed with curettage, and the skin is sewn down to the base of the tracts and presacral fascia. This procedure results in a stellate wound, which heals relatively quickly and is surprisingly pain free or only minimally painful to the patient, who usually can return to school or work within a few days.

In the most difficult cases in which there have been recurrences despite proper treatment and care, it is sometimes necessary to rotate gluteal flaps in an attempt to obliterate the intergluteal crease entirely. This procedure is more formidable and fortunately is rarely indicated.

CONCLUSION

The most important element in the treatment of pilonidal disease is meticulous cleanliness and fastidious care of the intergluteal region. Patients must learn to perform this hygienic regimen to avoid recurrences, for no matter how well conceived or optimally performed the surgery for pilonidal disease may be, its ultimate success depends on the local care provided by the patient.

Suggested Readings

Alver O, Kayabasi B, Ozcan M, Tortum O: The complete rhombic excision of pilonidal sinus with primary closure by the use of fasciocutaneous Limberg flap, *Contemp Surg* 33:54-56, 1988.

Bascom J: Pilonidal disease: origin from follicles of hairs and results of follicle removal as treatment, *Surgery* 87:567-572, 1980.

Lamke LA, Larsson J, Nylen B: Results of different types of operation for pilonidal sinus, *Acta Chir Scand* 140:321-324, 1974.

CHAPTER 161

Plastic Surgery

•

Bruce Greenstein, Craig D. Hall, and Berish Strauch

ADOLESCENT PSYCHOLOGY AND PLASTIC SURGERY

Adolescence is a period of awakening, a transition from childhood to adulthood. This transition may be a period of instability for adolescents, since it is during this time that they establish a self-identity. This establishment of self requires a separation from a familial dependence and an incorporation into a vast social network. During this period of transition, insecurities and feelings of inadequacy may develop. Because of adolescents' magnified focus and emphasis on self-image, they may blame perceived or real physical deficits for their inadequate sense of self, and thus seek plastic surgery for correction of the defect and achievement of a secure and positive self-identity. The primary goal of the plastic surgeon when dealing with an adolescent patient is to interact with the adolescent, family, and pediatrician and determine whether a surgical correction is warranted on the basis of functional or psychosocial indications.

Functional indications such as nasal airway problems or dental malocclusion are usually clear-cut and therefore readily identified. Psychosocial indications are much more difficult to determine; however, failure to address them may lead to long-term consequences as severe and damaging as any mechanical problem. An illustrative example is a port-wine stain of the cheek. Functionally, it is of no clinical significance except in terms of its possible correlation with other birth defects. Skin with a port-wine stain does not have a greater incidence of infection, malignancy, or ulceration than surrounding uninvolved skin. However, a port-wine stain is clinically relevant in its psychologic importance. It is a "birthmark," an abnormality, something that makes the individual feel different and thus separate from others. Such patients may feel stigmatized to the point that they believe they can never feel attractive or accepted. They may attempt to compensate for having the birthmark or they

may avoid interpersonal contact. These reactions represent alterations in behavior caused by a skin hematoma, the functional significance of which is simply that it exists.

The example of a port-wine stain is simple to comprehend because it is visibly obvious. The psychosocial import of prominent ears, an ethnic nose, or small breasts is just as significant, although the perceived "deformity" may be less obvious, if not at all apparent, to the observer. The psychosocial issue is adolescents' internalization of externally derived expectations, which, when they measure themselves according to these standards and find themselves lacking, leads to a loss of self-esteem. Issues of self-esteem for adolescents are foremost as they strive to establish themselves as social entities apart from their family units. The adolescent's self-perception is in a state of flux. This inherent instability can produce profound self-doubt, but it also allows adolescents to adapt to changes in their physical appearance rapidly—a plasticity of self-perception that works in the plastic surgeon's behalf.

BREAST SURGERY

Breasts have always been symbols of femininity and fertility. Given this perspective, it is of little wonder that women in general, and adolescent girls in particular, frequently base a great deal of their sexual identity and self-esteem on the appearance of their breasts. An individual's sexual identity and self-esteem can suffer in a society in which "perfect" breasts are amply displayed in the media.

The idealized breast is societally defined most often by the fashions of the times. During the 1960s, relative hypomastia was the vogue, whereas more recent fashions have flattered fuller breasts. Given these generalizations, how may breast form be dealt with clinically?

Hypomastia

Micromastia refers to an arrest of breast development in which the lobule architecture develops but the size and shape of the breast remain juvenile. Hypomastia is the condition in which the breasts are judged by the patient and the clinician to be small relative to the body build of the patient. These two conditions represent the most common developmental breast complaints. Small breasts, by engendering feelings of inadequacy, may lead to shy, withdrawn social behavior.

Infrequently, hypoplastic breast development may be asymmetric. Tuberous breasts have an elongated shape, with most of the breast tissue located beneath the nipple-areola complex and a constricted base. In Poland's syndrome there is a partial or complete lack of growth of one breast, and there may be upper limb abnormalities on the same side and complete or partial absence of the pectoral muscle on the same side.

Surgery is generally considered after full physical maturation of the patient and stabilization of any further breast growth. The surgical correction of hypomastia requires making the breast mound larger. Breast augmentation is usually accomplished with synthetic implants. Only in cases of Poland's syndrome, in which there is a congenital absence of the pectoralis major muscle, does the surgeon consider using autogenous tissue. The latissimus dorsi muscle may be used in addition to an implant to reconstruct the breast.

The use of implants for reconstruction or augmentation of the breast carries its own attendant problems. Since the implant is not of the patient's own tissue, the body develops a reaction to wall off the implant and creates a capsule surrounding the implant. Recently, textured surfaces have been applied to the implants to attempt to disturb the laminar nature of the capsule formation and thus prevent capsular contracture. Secondary procedures may be necessary if contracture becomes painful or otherwise symptomatic.

Saline-filled implants are in common use at present. These are likely to require replacement as a result of deflation during the course of a lifetime when placed in a young patient.

Breast implant augmentation has not been found to correlate with an increased incidence of human breast carcinoma. It does place greater technical demand on mammography technicians, since the breast mound is less compressible after augmentation. Postaugmentation mammography requires multiview examinations so that as much of the breast as possible can be seen. Sonography and magnetic resonance imaging are becoming useful adjuncts to study the status and integrity of implants.

Breast augmentation is usually performed on an ambulatory basis with the patient under local anesthesia and also receiving intravenous sedation medication. The breast implant may be placed either beneath the breast tissue above the pectoralis or beneath the pectoralis major muscle. Subpectoral implants are recommended in patients with profound hypomastia because the implant is placed beneath a greater volume of soft tissue.

Three types of incisions may be used for placement of the implant: periareolar, axillary, and inframammary. The periareolar incision is made at the junction of the inferior pole of the areola and the adjacent breast skin. It is well camouflaged by the textured glandular nature of the areola but is limited in its application by the size of the areola itself: the areola must be at least 4 cm in diameter. Axillary incisions are placed transversely in an axillary fold and are extremely well concealed. The limitations of the axillary approach arise from an inability to develop the inferior pole of the implant pocket adequately at the level of the inframammary crease. The use of the endoscope has facilitated this approach. Placement by means of an intraumbilical incision has been described. Many technical compromises are necessitated by this approach, which therefore has not become a generally accepted mode of placement. Exposure and operative visualization are minimal, making this approach difficult. The inframammary approach provides direct access to the implant pocket, the scar being hidden in the inframammary crease or the undersurface of the breast.

Macromastia

Macromastia is defined as a condition in which breasts are disproportionately large compared with the body build of the patient. Two clear clinical entities are virginal hypertrophic macromastia and symptomatic macromastia, the former usually blending into the latter.

In some patients, owing to involutional changes, the breast becomes severely ptotic. In these cases, correction will involve a procedure similar to that used for macromastia or use of a prosthesis alone, with revision of the nipple-areola site (Fig. 161-1).

In virginal hypertrophic macromastia, the breast parenchymal development induced by pubertal hormones is profound. The breasts are firm and large, tending toward gigantomastia. Patients complain of self-consciousness about their excessive breast development and an inability to find clothes that adequately accommodate their breasts. They frequently report that their social interactions are constrained by inappropriate attention to their breasts. Surgery is generally considered when no further growth of the patient's breasts has occurred for a period of 1 year. However, intervention may become necessary if there is no cessation of breast growth and if the breasts are extremely large. Secondary procedures may be necessary should the breast continue to be large after a successful operation.

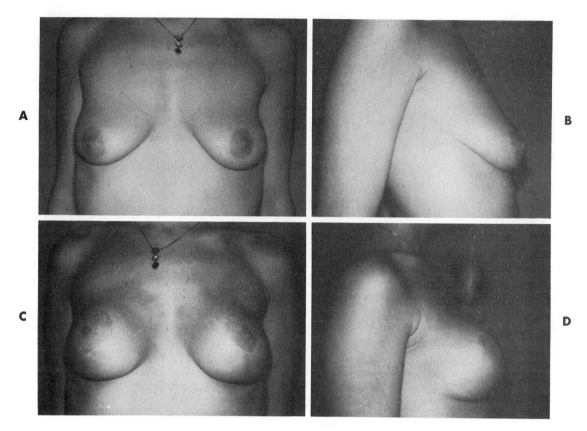

Fig. 161-1. Ptosis. **A** and **B,** Preoperative views. **C** and **D,** Postoperative views after mastopexy and augmentation.

Symptomatic macromastia arises from long-term postural compensation for excessive breast development. The patient's shoulders and upper back round, failing in their support of upper body weight. Secondary complaints of chronic back pain, bra-strap grooving, and even symptoms of ulnar nerve compression may arise from postural compensations. The patient may also suffer from intertrigo of the inframammary crease secondary to macromastia. Patients with fully grown breasts, stable in size and causative of symptoms, are considered for reduction mammaplasty.

Reduction mammaplasty operations are based on preservation of the circulation to the nipple-areola complex where feasible. Circulation can be maintained by basing the pedicle on superior, lateral, or inferior circulation. The choice of specific technique is based on patient attributes and physician preference (Fig. 161-2).

Complications, although infrequent, may include hematoma, nipple loss, skin slough, infection, and scar hypertrophy.

Breast sensitivity is generally retained after a reduction. However, it may be reduced in a few patients, and totally absent in the rare patient. Depending on the extent of the retention of the glandular duct system to the nipple,

some patients may be able to lactate; however, the volume of milk may be significantly reduced.

Gynecomastia

Gynecomastia, the excessive development of male mammary glands, occurs during puberty in 95% of cases. Breast hypertrophy may be unilateral or bilateral. Most instances are related to increasing testosterone levels and to a large extent involute over the course of several years. Gynecomastia has also been associated with hypothyroidism and hyperthyroidism, pituitary adenomas, acromegaly, juvenile cirrhosis, marijuana use (as well as certain therapeutic medication use), male pseudohermaphroditism, obesity, Klinefelter's syndrome, and testicular tumors, especially seminomas. Steroid use by weight lifters may result in gynecomastia.

Gynecomastia tends to be devastating to the psyche of the affected adolescent male and, if left untreated, can result in significant psychologic problems. The patient is embarrassed to undress in front of his peers in the locker room and to engage in sports.

Preoperatively, the breasts and testes are carefully examined and a thorough history and review of systems

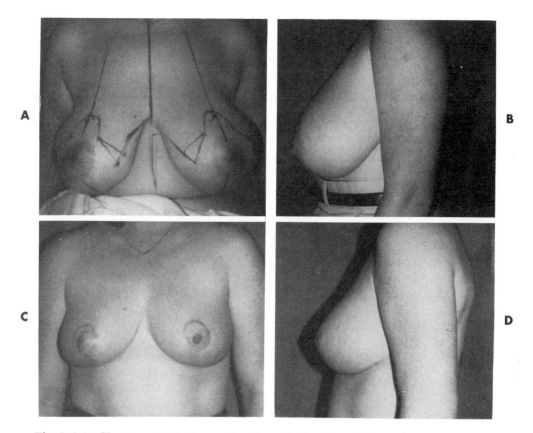

Fig. 161-2. Gigantomastia. **A,** Preoperative view with planned surgical markings. **B,** Preoperative view. **C** and **D,** Postoperative views after reduction mammaplasty.

obtained; any evidence of endocrinopathy is sought. Endocrinologic consultation is often sought to rule out systemic abnormalities.

Once it is decided to proceed with surgical correction, the nature of the scarring is discussed with the patient. For mild to moderate cases of gynecomastia, a periareolar incision is used and excess breast tissue removed. Liposuction has become a mainstay in cases of mild to moderate hypertrophy and is often an adjunct procedure in which direct excision is required. The resulting scar is well hidden in the junction of the pigmented nipple, areolar skin, and chest skin. Suction lipectomy of excess fat, but not breast tissue, may be used as an adjunct to the procedure. The concentric circle technique resects skin circumferentially around the nipple, areola, and breast tissue, while nipple viability is maintained on a superior dermal pedicle. A circumferential scar around the areola results. Cases of significant skin excess necessitate horizontal and perhaps vertical chest scars, which will be visible even after complete healing has been achieved. The nipple may also be elevated with this technique, using a minor variation. On occasion, drains may be needed postoperatively. A compressive dressing is usually maintained over the chest for several days to minimize bleeding.

Complications, although infrequent, are similar to those of reduction mammaplasty in the female (e.g., hematoma, nipple loss, skin slough, infection, scar hypertrophy).

SUCTION LIPECTOMY

Suction lipectomy is a relatively new technique for body contouring. The adolescent patient who is a candidate for this technique may reap its maximal benefits. Youthful skin is more supple and better able to recontour after removal of localized areas of unsightly fat padding. However, suction lipectomy is not a method for generalized weight loss. Its major indication is for local areas of excess fat distribution around the knee, trochanteric area, thighs, and abdomen; less frequently, the neck, ankle, and buttocks are amenable to surgical correction. The adolescent's need to "look good" in fashionable, tight-fitting clothing can sometimes be met by removal of discrete collections of adipose tissue.

The procedure may be performed on an outpatient basis under either local or general anesthesia.

The liposuction cannulas are introduced through small incisions near the area to be treated. Negative pressures just under 1 atm are generated. The cannulas are passed back and forth through the preoperatively marked areas, suctioning adipose tissue, and the edges of the suctioned areas are feathered. Septa containing neurovascular structures are left intact, maintaining major nerves and vessels. Most liposuctions are performed using a "tumescent" or "wet" technique. High volumes of very dilute local anesthetic and epinephrine solutions are infiltrated to allow for ease of fat removal and reduction of bleeding. Postoperatively, the patient wears compression garments for several weeks. Autotransfusion is occasionally required when large volumes of fat are removed. Untoward sequelae have been infrequent, consisting of hypesthesia, seroma, edema formation, and (to a lesser degree) hematomas, infections, and skin slough. There have been rare reports of pulmonary emboli. Secondary procedures can be performed.

LASER TREATMENT OF CUTANEOUS VASCULAR LESIONS

Benign vascular lesions such as telangiectasias, port-wine stains, and hemangiomas, especially when they involve the face and other exposed areas of the body, are of major concern to both patients and parents. The treatment of these lesions has been markedly improved by the use of tunable pulsed dye lasers. Selective photothermocoagulation of blood vessels occurs at a wavelength of 585 nm with the production of yellow light. Hemoglobin selectively absorbs yellow light, and thus the vessels differentially absorb the thermal energy. Little scarring results from laser treatment because of the minimal absorption of thermal energy at the dermal-epidermal junction.

With cooperative patients, the procedure may be performed with little discomfort; it often requires no anesthesia and can be carried out on an outpatient basis. Further advances in laser technology may broaden its application to the treatment of other cutaneous lesions. Superficial pigmented legions may be treated with the carbon dioxide laser as well as certain acne scars. Future improvements in this technology may be expected.

RHINOPLASTY

Rhinoplasty remains the most common aesthetic plastic surgery procedure in adolescents. Enormous psychologic, emotional, and social significance is attributed to the nose because it constitutes the central element of the face. During adolescence, maturation of the face includes growth of the nose. A cute childhood button nose gives way, under the influence of pubertal hormones, to reflections of ethnic and genetic heritage. Adolescents whose self-image is externally derived may be unable to incorporate a prominent nose or a large bump on the nose into a healthy self-perception.

A successful rhinoplasty can greatly enhance self-image; the change is clear both to the patient and to other people, whose favorable response contributes to the adolescent's enhanced self-image. Rhinoplasties can be performed in adolescents as young as 13 years of age who are demonstrating no unusual growth of the nose and who already have a large nose with a projecting tip.

Rhinoplasties, as well as all surgical corrections in adolescents, are best deferred until completion of growth and maturation. This delay eliminates the possibility of persistent growth and development attenuating the postoperative outcome. Female nasal development is 90% complete by 13 to 16 years of age; male nasal development is similarly complete by 15 to 18 years of age. These timetables refer to completion of the cartilaginous and bony architecture of the nose; changes in the integument continue throughout life.

Preoperatively, attentive listening to the patient remains the most important aspect of the examination. Complaints in excess of physical findings may indicate psychologic disturbances. In such cases, counseling is recommended. Similarly, different ethnic groups have different aesthetic values, and surgeons who ignore the desires of the patient and create a nose with their own personal stamp may produce an outcome that is unacceptable to the patient. It is critically important to ask patients to describe specifically the change they would like in the nasal appearance. Any airway obstruction should be evaluated preoperatively, and concomitant septal surgery can be performed, if necessary.

The current standard of beauty is a nose that is almost completely straight on the side view. Many consider the scooped-out, "ski-jump" type of nasal profile to be a deformity. The appearance of the nostrils must also be taken into consideration; the patient may feel that wide, flaring nostrils require surgical correction.

Almost all adolescent rhinoplasties are performed with the patient under local anesthesia, combined with pre- and intraoperative use of sedation medication. Rhinoplasties are performed through intranasal incisions. A recent modification in technique involves making a small incision at the base of the columella so that an "open" rhinoplasty can be done. This technique allows for better visualization and sculpting of the nasal cartilages. If areas of the nose such as the dorsum or the tip require augmentation, cartilage from the septum and, should it prove necessary, from the ear may be harvested. Major dorsal profile augmentations may require the use of tissues from other donor sites or autologous grafts such as irradiated rib cartilage grafts. Bone or cartilage grafts can be harvested from the calvarium, ribs, iliac crest, or ears.

All internal incisions are sutured with absorbable materials that do not require removal. The nose is then packed to prevent adhesions from forming between the intranasal incisions. This packing is removed after 24 to 48 hours, unless septal surgery has been performed, in which case packing remains in place for longer periods. An external splint is then worn for 1 week to maintain the nasal bones in position. The patient is placed on a diet that requires minimal mastication and is discharged 24 hours after the procedure.

The most common postoperative complication is epistaxis. Bleeding may occur either immediately postoperatively or after an interval of 10 to 14 days. Most bleeding can be treated with repeat packing.

Infection after rhinoplasty is rare. Swelling of the nose after surgery, especially at the tip, is not unusual and may last for several weeks to months.

After technically successful rhinoplasty, most properly selected adolescent patients express satisfaction with the postoperative results as they receive positive reinforcement from their own favorable assessment and from the response of their peers to the change in their appearance (Fig. 161-3).

CRANIOFACIAL SURGERY

The philosophy of craniofacial surgery involves the notion that the correction of any facial deformity requires that the facial skeleton be made anatomically normal. This simple concept has opened new vistas in the

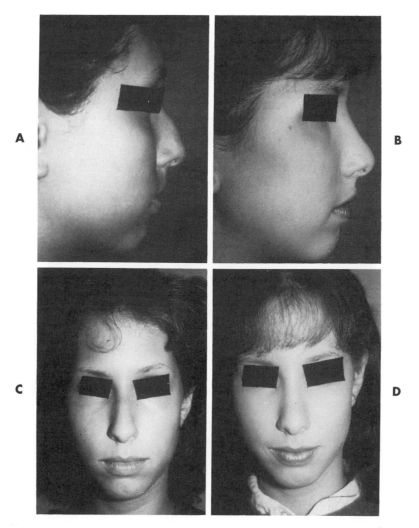

Fig. 161-3. A, Preoperative lateral view. **B,** Postoperative lateral view after rhinoplasty. **C,** Preoperative front view. **D,** Postoperative front view after rhinoplasty.

correction of congenital craniofacial disorders. Before Tessier's work, most congenital craniofacial disorders were treated by camouflage procedures in which bone grafts were onlayed to the facial skeleton in hopes of augmenting the bony deficits and filling in bony defects. The challenge to the craniofacial surgeon is to restructure the abnormal facial skeleton, bringing the bones into a normal anatomic relationship through the use of carefully placed osteotomies within the facial skeleton.

The original craniofacial procedures were performed on adolescents and young adults in the belief that their ability to tolerate both the length and magnitude of the operative procedure made them the best candidates for this surgery. As the constructs and techniques of craniofacial surgery have been refined, the age at which this surgery can be performed has become progressively younger. Psychosocial considerations often dictate the timing of current craniofacial reconstructions. However, the adolescent and young adult period of life remain the ideal time for reconstructions of the orbit and midface. During late adolescence, the facial skeleton undergoes its final maturation. The surgeon can approach the patient at this age confident that the surgical reconstruction will not destroy areas of active growth nor be altered by unarrested growth processes.

The operations performed by the craniofacial surgeon may be considered in three distinct categories: orbitotomy, midfacial advancement, and mandibulotomy. Orbitotomy is a procedure in which the orbital skeleton is separated from the cranium and maxilla to correct orbital dystopia and ocular hypertelorism (Fig. 161-4).

In the surgical correction of orbital dystopia, a C-osteotomy that includes the lateral portion of the superior orbital brow, lateral orbital wall, and inferior orbital rim is performed, and these structures are moved as a unit.

This unit may be moved superiorly, laterally, or inferiorly to bring the bony orbital wall of one orbit into alignment with the anatomic position of the orbit on the contralateral side.

In the surgical correction of ocular hypertelorism, both orbits are operated on simultaneously. Osteotomies of the superior orbital wall, superior orbital rim, medial orbital walls, inferior orbital floors, and lateral orbital walls are performed so that each orbit constitutes a bony rectangle. The nasal ethmoid region is then resected, allowing these bony rectangles to be moved closer to the midline, thereby eliminating the increased intercanthal space.

Midfacial advancement is indicated when the patient has a clinical class III malocclusion in which the maxillary arch lies posterior to the mandibular arch and in which the position of the mandible is normal relative to the cranial base. Midfacial advancements can be performed at various levels. LeFort I advancement brings the alveolar segment of the maxilla with its dentition forward, affecting only the tip and base of the nose. LeFort I midfacial advancement is frequently used for correction of mandibular maxillary dental disharmony. The LeFort II operation advances the nasal root and the central pyramid of the maxilla, leaving the inferior orbital rims and zygomas of the face unaffected. The LeFort III midfacial advancement advances the entire maxilla, zygomas, and inferior orbital floors relative to the mandible and the cranial base. The LeFort II procedure is frequently performed for correction of posttraumatic facial deformities; the LeFort III midfacial advancement is most often employed for correction of congenital midfacial deficiencies, such as those demonstrated in Crouzon's, Apert's, and Pfeiffer's syndromes.

Mandibulotomies are surgical osteotomies within the bony arch of the mandible. In craniofacial surgery, man-

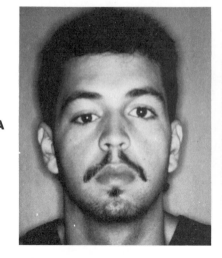
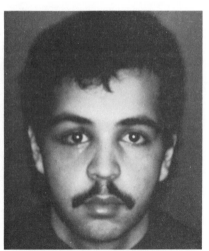

Fig. 161-4. A 20-year-old man with congenital orbital dystopia. **A,** Preoperative view. **B,** postoperative view after 6 weeks.

dibular osteotomies are frequently limited to genioplasties in which a horizontal mandibular osteotomy is used to advance or reduce the prominence of the chin.

Craniofacial surgery is a dynamic subarea of plastic surgery that can create a striking semblance of normal facial appearance in even the most severe congenital deformities. The surgery places great demands on the patient and the physician, but at its best it can provide patients with an improved facial appearance and give them the confidence to become integrated members of society.

MENTOPLASTY

The optimal results of a rhinoplasty can be obtained only if the chin position is in harmony with the rest of the face. The aesthetic balance between the forehead, nose, and chin is of major importance. Major chin deformities are usually associated with dental occlusive abnormalities and require mandibular and perhaps maxillary surgery for correction.

Most patients with chin deformities are unaware of their abnormal profile beyond attributing their dissatisfaction with their appearance to the nose. In this situation, the surgeon must examine the chin position carefully. The chin should project beyond the line drawn through the glabella and upper lip. Prognathism, or the prominence of the jaw in both full-face and profile views, may also require treatment. Rarely, the chin alone may be excessively large, with a normal occlusive relationship, and this condition is considered true macrogenia. Preoperatively, cephalometric radiograph studies, which are the standard for measuring dental and facial proportions, may be helpful in determining how much correction a patient requires.

For a retruded or small chin, two procedures are possible. In the more common approach, a Silastic or Proplast implant is placed through either an intraoral or a submental incision while the patient is under local anesthesia. The implant is then supported for several weeks with external taping to avoid displacement.

The alternative procedure is a sliding genioplasty, which is a repositioning of the chin by the performance of a horizontal osteotomy within the mandible. The chin can be advanced by sliding the segment forward, reduced by lowering the height of the segment, or retruded by sliding the segment backward. Internal wires or plates are used to maintain the corrected chin position. Immediately postoperatively, the patient is placed on a liquid diet, which is followed by a diet requiring minimal mastication.

Potential complications include hypesthesia secondary to injury of the inferior alveolar nerve. This problem rarely occurs with implants and, although more common

with osteotomies, permanent severe alterations in sensibility remain rare. Hematoma is also a rare postoperative problem. Infections are unusual; however, they may necessitate removal of the implant and/or wires placed for the genioplasty. Extrusion of the implants, if Silastic, can occur. Secondary correction may then be required.

Suggested Readings

General Considerations

Gifford S: Cosmetic surgery and personality change: a review and some clinical observations. In Goldwyn RM, editor: *The unfavorable results in plastic surgery,* Boston, 1972, Little, Brown.

Goin JM, Goin MK: *Changing the body: psychological effects of plastic surgery,* Baltimore, 1986, Williams & Wilkins.

Hill G, Silver AG: Psychodynamic and esthetic motivations for plastic surgery, *Psychosom Med* 12:345, 1950.

Jacobsen WE, Edgerton MT, Meyer E, et al: Psychiatric evaluation of male patients seeking cosmetic surgery, *Plast Reconstr Surg* 26:356, 1960.

Kalick SM: Aesthetic surgery: how it affects the way patients are perceived by others, *Ann Plast Surg* 2:128, 1979.

Knorr NJ, Hoopes JE, Edgerton MT: Psychiatric-surgical approach to adolescent disturbance in self-image, *Plast Reconstr Surg* 41:249, 1968.

Kolin IS, Baber JL, Bartlett ES: Psychosexual aspects of mammary augmentation, *Med Aspects Hum Sex* 12:88, 1974.

Lerner RM, Karabenick SA: Physical attractiveness, body attitudes, and self concept in late adolescents, *J Youth Adolesc* 23:307, 1974.

Macgregor FC, Schaffner B: Screening patients for nasal plastic operations: some sociologic and psychiatric considerations, *Psychosom Med* 12:277, 1950.

Breast Augmentation

De Cholnoky T: Augmentation mammaplasty: survey of complications of 10,941 patients by 265 surgeons, *Plast Reconstr Surg* 45:573, 1970.

de la Fuente A, Martin del Yerro JL: Periareolar mastopexy with mammary implants, *Aesthetic Plast Surg* 16:337, 1992.

Dempsey WC, Latham WD: Subpectoral implants in augmentation mammaplasty, *Plast Reconstr Surg* 42:515, 1968.

Fredericks S: Management of mammary hypoplasia. In Goldwyn RM, editor: *Plastic and reconstructive surgery of the breast,* Boston, 1976, Little, Brown; p 387.

Gifford S: Emotional attitudes toward cosmetic breast surgery: loss and restitution of the ideal self. In Goldwyn RM, editor: *Plastic and reconstructive surgery of the breast,* Boston, 1976, Little, Brown; p 103.

Harris HI: Survey of breast implants from the point of view of carcinogenesis, *Plast Reconstr Surg* 28:81, 1961.

Rose NR: Nonimmunogenicity of Silastic (letter). In Additional Comments from Plastic Surgery to the FDA, prepared by members of the Silicone Implant Research Committee of the Plastic Surgery Educational Foundation, February 1991.

Silver HL: Treating the complications of augmentation mammaplasty, *Plast Reconstr Surg* 49:637, 1972.

Vinnick CA: Spherical contracture of fibrous capsules around breast implants: prevention and treatment, *Plast Reconstr Surg* 58:555, 1976.

Williams JE: Augmentation mammaplasty inframammary approach. In Georgiade N, editor: *Reconstructive breast surgery,* St. Louis: 1976, Mosby–Year Book; p 50.

Williams JE: Experience with a large series of Silastic breast implants, *Plast Reconstr Surg* 49:253, 1972.

Breast Reduction

Born G: The "L" reduction mammoplasty, *Ann Plast Surg* 32:383, 1994.

Courtiss EH, Goldwyn RM: Breast sensation before and after plastic surgery, *Plast Reconstr Surg* 58:1, 1976.

Goin MK, Goin JM, Gianini MH: The psychic consequences of a reduction mammaplasty, *Plast Reconstr Surg* 59:530, 1977.

Juma A, Miller JG, Laitung JK: Pedicle deepithelialization in breast reduction and mastopexy using the electric dermatome (letter), *Plast Reconstr Surg* 95:216, 1995.

Lejour M: Vertical mammaplasty and liposuction of the breast, *Plast Reconstr Surg* 94:100, 1994.

McKissock PK: Correction of macromastia by the bipedicle vertical dermal flap. In Goldwyn RM, editor: *Plastic and reconstructive surgery of the breast,* Boston, 1976, Little, Brown.

Owsley JQ, Peterson RA, editors: *Symposium on aesthetic surgery of the breast,* vol 18, St. Louis, 1978, Mosby–Year Book.

Regnault P: Breast ptosis: definition and treatment, *Clin Plast Surg* 3:193, 1976.

Robbins LB, Hoffman DK: The superior dermoglandular pedicle approach to breast reduction, *Ann Plast Surg* 29:211, 1992.

Strombeck JO: Reduction mammaplasty, *Surg Clin North Am* 51:453, 1971.

Wise RJ: Breast reduction with nipple transplantation. In Goldwyn RM, editor: *Plastic and reconstructive surgery of the breast,* Boston, 1976, Little, Brown.

Mastopexy

Brink RR: Management of true ptosis of the breast, *Plast Reconstr Surg* 91:657, 1993.

de la Fuente A, Martin del Yerro JL: Periareolar mastopexy with mammary implants, *Aesthetic Plast Surg* 16:337, 1992.

Juma A, Miller JG, Laitung JK: Pedicle deepithelialization in breast reduction and mastopexy using the electric dermatome (letter), *Plast Reconstr Surg* 95:216, 1995.

Sandsmark M, Amland PF, Samdal F, et al: Clinical results in 87 patients treated for asymmetrical breasts: a follow-up study, *Scand J Plast Reconstr Surg Hand Surg* 26:321, 1992.

Gynecomastia

Davidson B: Concentric circle operation for massive gynecomastia to excise the redundant skin, *Plast Reconstr Surg* 63:350, 1979.

Huang TT, Hidalgo JE, Lewis SR: A circumareolar approach in surgical management of gynecomastia, *Plast Reconstr Surg* 69:35, 1982.

Nuttall FQ: Gynecomastia as a physical finding in normal men, *J Clin Endocrinol Metab* 48:338, 1979.

Suction Lipectomy

Courtiss EH: A retrospective analysis of 100 patients, *Plast Reconstr Surg* 73:780, 1984.

Illouz YG: Body contouring by lipolysis: a five-year experience with over 3000 cases, *Plast Reconstr Surg* 72:591, 1983.

Kesselring VK: Regional fat aspiration for body contouring, *Plast Reconstr Surg* 72:610, 1983.

Pitman GH, Temourian B: Suction lipectomy: complications and results by survey, *Plast Reconstr Surg* 76:65, 1985.

Temourian B, Adham MD, Gulin S, Shapiro C: Suction lipectomy: a review of 200 patients over a six-year period and a study of the technique in cadavers, *Ann Plast Surg* 11:93, 1983.

Laser Treatment of Cutaneous Vascular Lesions

Achauer BM, Vandenkam VM: Capillary hemangioma of infancy: comparison of argon and Nd:YAG laser treatment, *Plast Reconstr Surg* 84:60, 1989.

Anderson RR, Parrish JA: Selective photothermolysis: precise microsurgery by selective absorption of pulsed radiation, *Science* 220:524, 1983.

Dixon JA: *Surgical application of lasers,* Chicago, 1987, Mosby–Year Book.

Mulliken JB, Young AE: *Vascular birthmarks, hemangiomas and malformations,* Philadelphia, 1988, WB Saunders.

Tan OT, Sherwood R, Gilchrest BA: Treatment of children with port wine stains using the flashlamp pulsed tunable dye laser, *N Engl J Med* 320:416, 1989.

Thomson HG: Cutaneous hemangiomas and lymphangiomas, *Clin Plast Surg* 14:341, 1987.

Thomson HG: Common benign pediatric cutaneous tumors: timing and treatment, *Clin Plast Surg* 17:55, 1990.

Rhinoplasty

Converse JM, Wood-Smith D, Waring MKH, et al: Deformities of the nose. In Converse JM, editor: *Plastic and reconstructive surgery,* Philadelphia, 1964, WB Saunders; p 869.

Diamond H: Rhinoplasty techniques, *Surg Clin North Am* 51:317, 1971.

Goin MK, Goin JM: Psychoanalytic perspectives of rhinoplasty. Presented at the American Society of Plastic and Reconstructive Surgeons, Toronto, Canada, October 1979.

Gordon HL, Baker TJ: Primary cosmetic rhinoplasty, *Clin Plast Surg* 4:9, 1977.

Hull HF, Mann JM, Sands CJ, et al: Toxic shock syndrome related to nasal packing, *Arch Otolaryngol* 109:624, 1983.

Jacobson W, Edgerton M, Meyer E, et al: Psychiatric evaluation of male patients seeking cosmetic surgery, *Plast Reconstr Surg* 26:356, 1966.

Meyer R, Kesselring VK: Sculpturing and reconstructive procedures in aesthetic and functional rhinoplasty, *Clin Plast Surg* 4:15, 1977.

Millard DR: *Symposium on corrective rhinoplasty,* vol 13, St. Louis, 1976, Mosby–Year Book.

Rees TD: *Aesthetic plastic surgery,* vol 1, Philadelphia, 1980, WB Saunders.

Rogers BO: Rhinoplasty. In Goldwyn RM, editor: *The unfavorable result in plastic surgery,* Boston, 1972, Little, Brown.

Sheen JH: *Aesthetic rhinoplasty,* St. Louis, 1978, Mosby–Year Book.

Toback J, Fayerman JW: Toxic shock syndrome following septo-rhinoplasty: implications for the head and neck surgeon, *Arch Oto-laryngol* 109:627, 1983.

Craniofacial Surgery

Caronni EP: *Craniofacial surgery,* Boston, 1985, Little, Brown.

Goodrich JT, Poast KD, Argamaso RV: *Plastic techniques in neuro-surgery,* New York, 1991, Thieme.

Jackson IT, Munro IR, Salyer KE, Whitaker LA: *Atlas of craniomax-illofacial surgery,* St. Louis, 1982, Mosby–Year Book.

Whitaker LA: Aesthetic surgery of the facial skeleton, *Clin Plast Surg* 18:153, 1991.

Wolfe AN, Berkowitz S: *Plastic surgery of the facial skeleton,* Boston, 1989, Little, Brown.

Zins JE, Whitaker LA: Membranous versus endochondral bone: implications for craniofacial reconstruction, *Plast Reconstr Surg* 72:778, 1983.

Mentoplasty

Flowers RS: Alloplastic augmentation of the anterior mandible, *Clin Plast Surg* 18:107, 1991.

Gonzalez-Uloa M, Stevens E: Role of chin correction in profile plasty, *Plast Reconstr Surg* 41:477, 1968.

Hinds EC, Kent JN: Genioplasty: the versatility of the horizontal os-teotomy, *Oral Surg* 27:690, 1969.

Jobe R, Iverson R, Vistnes L: Bone deformation beneath alloplastic implants, *Plast Reconstr Surg* 51:169, 1973.

McCarthy JG, Ruff GL, Zide BM: A surgical system for the correction of bony chin deformity, *Clin Plast Surg* 18:139, 1991.

Millard R: Augmentation mentoplasty, *Surg Clin North Am* 61:333, 1971.

Pitanguy I: Augmentation mentoplasty, *Plast Reconstr Surg* 42:5, 1968.

Rish BB: Profile-plasty: report on plastic chin implants, *Laryngo-scope* 74:144, 1964.

Stambaugh KI: Chin augmentation: an important adjunctive procedure to rhinoplasty, *Arch Otolaryngol Head Neck Surg* 118:682, 1992.

Wolfe SA: Chin advancement as an aid in correction of deformities of the mental and submental regions, *Plast Reconstr Surg* 67:624, 1981.

Wolfe SA, Berkowitz S: The chin. In Wolfe SA, Berkowitz S, editors: *Plastic surgery of the facial skeleton,* Boston, 1989, Little, Brown; p 111.

INDEX